INFLAMMATION

4TH EDITION: THE COLORFUL AND DEFINITIVE GUIDE TOWARD HEALTH AND VITALITY AND AWAY FROM THE BOREDOM, RISKS, COSTS, AND INEFFICACY OF ENDLESS ANALGESIA, IMMUNOSUPPRESSION, AND POLYPHARMACY

A Three-Part Learning System of Text, Images, and Video

ALEX VASQUEZ D.C. N.D. D.O. F.A.C.N.

- Doctor of Osteopathic Medicine, graduate of University of North Texas Health Science Center, Texas College of Osteopathic Medicine (2010)
- Doctor of Naturopathic Medicine, graduate of Bastyr University (1999)
- Doctor of Chiropractic, graduate of University of Western States (1996)
- Fellow of the American College of Nutrition (2013-present)
- Former Overseas Fellow of the Royal Society of Medicine
- Editor, *International Journal of Human Nutrition and Functional Medicine* IntJHumNutrFunctMed.org. Former Editor, *Naturopathy Digest*; Former/Recent Reviewer for *Journal of Naturopathic Medicine, Alternative Therapies in Health and Medicine, Autoimmune Diseases, International Journal of Clinical Medicine,* and *PLOS One*
- Private practice of integrative and functional medicine in Seattle, Washington (2000-2001), Houston, Texas (2001-2006), Portland, Oregon (2011-2013), consulting practice (present)
- Consultant Researcher and Lecturer (2004-present), Biotics Research Corporation
- Teaching and Academics:
  - Director of Programs, International College/Conference on Human Nutrition and Functional Medicine ICHNFM.org
  - Founder and Former Program Director of the world's first accredited university-affiliated graduate-level program in Functional Medicine
  - Adjunct Professor, Integrative and Functional Nutrition in Immune Health, Doctor of Clinical Nutrition program
  - Former Adjunct Professor (2009-2013) of Laboratory Medicine, Master of Science in Advanced Clinical Practice
  - Former Faculty (2004-2005, 2010-2013) and Forum Consultant (2003-2007), The Institute for Functional Medicine
  - Former Adjunct Professor (2011-2013) of Pharmacology, Evidence-Based Nutrition, Immune and Inflammatory Imbalances, Principles of Functional Medicine, Psychology of Wellness
  - Former Adjunct Professor of Orthopedics (2000), Radiographic Interpretation (2000), and Rheumatology (2001), Naturopathic Medicine Program, Bastyr University
- Author of more than 100 articles and letters published in *JAMA—Journal of the American Medical Association, BMJ—British Medical Journal,* TheLancet.com, *JAOA—Journal of the American Osteopathic Association, Annals of Pharmacotherapy, Journal of Clinical Endocrinology and Metabolism, Alternative Therapies in Health and Medicine, Nutritional Perspectives, Journal of Manipulative and Physiological Therapeutics, Integrative Medicine, Current Allergy and Asthma Reports, Nutritional Wellness, Evidence-based Complementary and Alternative Medicine, Nature Reviews Rheumatology* and *Arthritis & Rheumatism*: Official Journal of the American College of Rheumatology

INTERNATIONAL COLLEGE OF HUMAN NUTRITION & FUNCTIONAL MEDICINE

ICHNFM.ORG

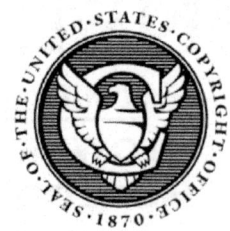
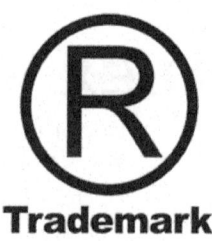

Dedications: I dedicate this book to the following people in appreciation for their works, their direct and indirect support of this work, and for their contributions to the advancement of true healthcare.

- **To the students and practitioners of naturopathic/functional medicine**, those who continue to learn so that they can provide the best possible care to their patients
- **To the researchers** whose works are cited in this text
- **To Dr Alan Gaby and Dr Jeffrey Bland,** my most memorable and influential *personal* professors and mentors
  - Dr Gaby's diligent scholarship of the medical nutrition literature laid the evidence-based foundation for nearly all of us; his *Nutritional Medicine* is an excellent companion text to compliment this volume
  - Dr Bland deserves credit for being the primary developer of the American rendition of "functional medicine", a conceptual framework and clinical model used and discussed in this text. While development and continuous maturation of the functional medicine model has depended upon numerous researchers and clinicians, Dr Bland was clearly the pioneer for this concept circa 1993 and the nucleus around which many of us have worked (at least initially) in this regard.
- **To Henry Rollins**, in particular for his prose book *One from None*, which completely changed my life in 1991
- **To Dr Linus Pauling**, for modeling the combination of scientific scholarship (Nobel Prize in Chemistry 1954) and social engagement (Nobel Peace Prize 1962)
- **To Dr Friedrich Nietzsche and Dr Noam Chomsky,** my most memorable and influential *virtual* professors and mentors, both of whom exemplify profound scholarship and intellectual independence in favor of developing the highest possible human culture on earth
- **To Dr Robert Richard**, my clinical mentor in general outpatient medicine—a truly exemplary clinician
- **To Dr Bruce Ames**[1] **and Dr Roger J Williams**[2], for proving the importance of biochemical individuality
- **To Dr Chester Wilk**[3,4] **and important others**[5,6,7] for documenting and resisting the organized oppression of natural, non-pharmaceutical, non-surgical healthcare
- **To Jorge Strunz and Ardeshir Farah,** for daily artistic inspiration since my first listen of *Primal Magic* in 1992

Acknowledgments for Peer and Editorial Review of Earlier Versions of This Work: Most of the sections that comprise the current work have been previously reviewed/published/presented; peer/editorial reviews are acknowledged below. Acknowledgement here does not imply that the reviewer fully agrees with or endorses the material in this text but rather that they were willing to review specific sections of the book for clinical applicability and clarity and to make suggestions to their own level of satisfaction.

- 2016 Edition of *Inflammation Mastery* and the excerpt *Pain Revolution for Migraine and Fibromyalgia*: Sabrina Piper BSc (2016 ND candidate), John Bartemus DC BCIM CFMP DACBN, Elizabeth Busetto DC ND, Kenneth Cintron MD
- 2015 Edition of *Human Microbiome and Dysbiosis in Clinical Disease*: Julie Jean BS BSN RN, Joseph Iaccino DC MSc
- 2014 Edition of *Antiviral Strategies and Immune Nutrition*: Annette D'Armata ND, Elizabeth Busetto DC ND
- 2014 Edition of *Naturopathic Rheumatology*: Annette D'Armata ND
- 2012 Edition of *Fibromyalgia in a Nutshell*: Lisa Scholl BA, Annette D'Armata ND
- 2012 Edition of *Migraine Headaches, Hypothyroidism, and Fibromyalgia*: Holly Furlong DC
- 2011 Edition of *Integrative Chiropractic Management of High Blood Pressure and Chronic Hypertension*: Barry Morgan MD, Holly Furlong DC, Kris Young DC, Erika Mennerick DC, and J William Beakey DOM
- 2011 Edition of *Integrative Medicine and Functional Medicine for Chronic Hypertension*: Erika Mennerick DC, JoAnn Fawcett DC, Ileana Bourland MSOM LAc, James Bogash DC, J William Beakey DOM
- 2010 Edition of *Chiropractic Management of Chronic Hypertension*: Joseph Paun MS DC, David Candelario OMS4 (TCOM c/o 2010), James Bogash DC, Bill Beakey DOM, Robert Richard DO
- 2009 Edition of *Chiropractic and Naturopathic Mastery of Common Clinical Disorders*: Heather Kahn MD, Robert Richard DO, James Leiber DO, David Candelario (UNT-HSC TCOM OMS4)
- 2007 Edition of *Integrative Orthopedics*: Barry Morgan MD, Dennis Harris DC, Richard Brown DC (DACBI candidate), Ron Mariotti ND, Patrick Makarewich MBA, Reena Singh (SCNM ND4), Zachary Watkins DC, Charles Novak MS DC, Marnie Loomis ND, James Bogash DC, Sara Croteau DC, Kris Young DC, Joshua Levitt ND, Jack Powell III MD, Chad Kessler MD, Amy Neuzil ND
- 2006 Edition of *Integrative Rheumatology*: Amy Neuzil ND, Cathryn Harbor MD, Julian Vickers DC, Tamara Sachs MD, Bob Sager BSc MD DABFM (Clinical Instructor in the Department of Family Medicine, University of Kansas), Ron

---

[1] Ames BN, et al. High-dose vitamin therapy stimulates variant enzymes with decreased coenzyme binding affinity (increased K(m). *Am J Clin Nutr.* 2002 Apr;75:616-58
[2] Williams RJ. *Biochemical Individuality: The Basis for the Genetotrophic Concept.* Austin and London: University of Texas Press; 1956
[3] Wilk CA. *Medicine, Monopolies, and Malice: How the Medical Establishment Tried to Destroy Chiropractic.* Garden City Park: Avery, 1996
[4] Getzendanner S. Permanent injunction order against AMA. *JAMA.* 1988 Jan 1;259(1):81-2
[5] Carter JP. *Racketeering in Medicine: The Suppression of Alternatives.* Norfolk: Hampton Roads Pub; 1993
[6] Morley J, Rosner AL, Redwood D. A case study of misrepresentation of the scientific literature: recent reviews of chiropractic. *J Altern Complement Med.* 2001;7:65-78
[7] Terrett AG. Misuse of the literature by medical authors in discussing spinal manipulative therapy injury. *J Manipulative Physiol Ther.* 1995 May;18(4):203-10

Mariotti ND, Titus Chiu (DC4), Zachary Watkins (DC4), Gilbert Manso MD, Bruce Milliman ND, William Groskopp DC, Robert Silverman DC, Matthew Breske (DC4), Dean Neary ND, Thomas Walton DC, Fraser Smith ND, Ladd Carlston DC, David Jones MD, Joshua Levitt ND

- 2004 Edition of *Integrative Orthopedics*: Peter Knight ND, Kent Littleton ND MS, Barry Morgan MD, Ron Hobbs ND, Joshua Levitt ND, John Neustadt (Bastyr ND4), Allison Gandre BS (Bastyr ND4), Peter Kimble ND, Jack Powell III MD, Chad Kessler MD, Mike Gruber MD, Deirdre O'Neill ND, Mary Webb ND, Leslie Charles ND, Amy Neuzil ND

Format and Layout: The format/layout of this book is designed to efficiently take the reader through the clinically relevant spectrum of considerations for each condition that is detailed. Important topics are given their own section within each chapter, while other less important or less common conditions are only described briefly in terms of the four "clinical essentials" of 1) definition/pathophysiology, 2) clinical presentation, 3) assessment/diagnosis, and 4) treatment/management. Each of the expanded sections that details the more important/common conditions maintains a consistent format, taking the reader through the spectrum of primary clinical considerations: definition/pathophysiology, clinical presentations, differential diagnoses, assessments (physical examination, laboratory, imaging), complications, management, and treatment. As my books have progressed, I am increasingly using an article-by-article review format (especially in the sections on management and treatment) so that readers have more direct access to the information so as to understand and *incorporate* more deeply what the research actually states; the goal and general approach here is to use a *representative sampling* of the research literature.

References and Citations: Citations to articles, abstracts, texts, and personal communications are footnoted throughout the text to provide supporting information and to provide interested readers the resources to find additional information. Many of the cited articles are available on-line for free, and often I have included the website addresses so that readers can easily access the complete article.

Peer-review and Quality Control: Peer-review is essential to help ensure accuracy and clinical applicability of health-related information. Consistent with the importance of these goals, I have employed several "checks and balances" to increase the accuracy and applicability of the information within my textbooks:
- Reliance upon authoritative references: Nearly all important statements are referenced to peer-reviewed biomedical journals or authoritative texts, examples of the latter include *The Merck Manual*, *Current Medical Diagnosis and Treatment*, and *5-Minute Clinical Consult*. Each citation is provided by a footnote at the bottom of each page so that readers will know quickly and easily exactly where the information was obtained.
- Extensive cross-referencing: Readers will notice the supranormal number of references and citations. Many important statements have several references. Many references (especially textbooks) are referenced several times even on the same page; the purpose of this extensive referencing is three-fold: 1) to guide you—the reader—to additional information, 2) to help me (as writer) stay organized, and 3) to help you and me (the practicing physicians) employ this information with confidence. In more recent updates/revisions, I have started shortening the number of listed authors by frequent use of *et al* with an interest in keeping each citation to one line of text on the page, likewise reducing mental and eye strain; quite obviously I respect each of the authors—even those whose names are not listed in the citation—and am implementing this solely for the sake of efficient book formatting (aiming for one citation per line) and information density (fewer lines dedicated to citations allows more space for text and images). Given hundreds of pages and thousands of citations, formatting considerations such as these are summatively significant.
- Periodic revision: Any significant errors that are discovered will be posted at InflammationMastery.com/volume1 (...volume2, etc); please check these folders periodically to ensure that you are working with the most accurate information of which I am aware.
- Peer-review: The peer-review process for my books takes several forms. First, colleagues and students are invited to review new and revised sections of the text before publication; every section of the book that you are holding has been independently reviewed by health science students and/or practicing clinicians from various backgrounds: allopathic, chiropractic, osteopathic, naturopathic. Second, you - the reader - are invited to provide feedback about the information in the book, typographical errors, syntax, case reports, new research, etc. If your ideas truly change the nature of the material, I will be glad to acknowledge you in the text (with your permission, of course). If your contribution is hugely significant, such as reviewing three or more chapters or helping in some important way, I will be glad to not only acknowledge you, but to also send you the next edition at a discount or courtesy when your ideas take effect. Third, I keep abreast of new literature by constantly perusing new research and advancements in the health sciences. Having been successful in three separate doctoral programs in the health sciences, I have learned not only to master large amounts of material but to also separate and integrate different viewpoints as appropriate. I also "field test" my protocols with patients in the various clinical arenas in which I work and also with professionals and

academicians via presentations and critical dialogue. By implementing these quality control steps, I hope to create a useful text and advance our professions and practices by improving the quality of care that we deliver to our patients.

How to Use This Book Most Effectively: Ideally, these books should be read cover-to-cover within a context of coursework that is supervised by a clinically experienced professor. For post-graduate professionals, they might consider forming a local or virtual "book club" and meeting for weekly or monthly discussions to check their understandings and share their clinical experiences to refine the application of clinical knowledge, perceptions, and skills. Virtual groups and internet forums—such as those hosted by International College of Human Nutrition and Functional Medicine at ICHNFM.ORG—can provide access to an assembly of international professional peers wherein sharing of clinical questions and experiences are synergistic. This book is not intended to extensively cover all aspects of clinical medicine, such as clinical pharmacology and prescribing (for which I recommend *Epocrates.com* and its associated app) and medical management (for which I recommend *5-Minute Clinical Consult* via book, website, and app).

Video access: Video access is provided via notices and footnotes appropriately placed and indicated throughout the book. Readers actually have to read the book to access the information and gain knowledge.
- Sample: vimeo.com/ichnfm/drv-functional-inflammology-intro2013
- Password: DrVprotocol

Notices: The intention and scope of this text are to provide health science students and doctorate-level clinicians with useful information and a familiarity with available research and resources pertinent to the management of patients in integrative primary care and specialty care settings. Specifically, the information in this book is intended to be used by licensed healthcare professionals who have received hands-on/residential clinical training and supervision at accredited health science colleges. Additionally, information in this book should be used in conjunction with other resources, texts, and in combination with the clinician's best judgment and intention to "*first, do no harm*" and second to provide effective healthcare. Information and treatments applicable to a specific *condition* may not be appropriate for or applicable to a specific *patient* in your office; this is especially true for patients with multiple

> ## Purpose, scope, recommended companion resources
>
> The purpose of this book is not to serve as a stand-alone "recipe book" for the complete management of all reviewed conditions; rather the focus of this book is the delivery of clinically important concepts and facts to enhance the management of various clinical disorders, in particular by documenting and explicating this author's naturopathic, allopathic, integrative and functional medicine approach. Readers and instructors using this book are encouraged to use whichever additional resources they choose, including but not limited to the supporting videos at Vimeo.com/DrVasquez and Vimeo.com/ICHNFM; in particular, *5-Minute Clinical Consult* and *Epocrates* are excellent and strongly advised companion guides for overall medical diagnosis/management and clinical pharmacology/prescribing, respectively. Clinicians need to have a good understanding of clinical medicine before applying many of the approaches described in this book; cross-referencing and double-checking management strategies and drug doses are essential components of quality care. Both *5-Minute Clinical Consult* and *Epocrates* are available as point-of-care references, and their use is advised.
>
> This work is best used with the relevant videos from DrV available online, some of which are linked and made password-accessible via this book; additional videos by Dr Vasquez are available online (occasionally with accompanying printed presentation slides); please see the following examples and locations:
> - vimeo.com/ichnfm
> - vimeo.com/drvasquez

comorbidities and those taking pharmaceutical medications with potential for multiple adverse effects and drug/nutrient/herb interactions. In my books and articles, I describe treatments—manual, dietary, nutritional, botanical, pharmacologic, and occasionally surgical—and their research support for the clinical condition being discussed; each practitioner must determine appropriateness of these treatments for his/her individual patient and with consideration of the doctor's scope of practice, education, training, skill, and—occasionally—the appropriateness of "off label" use of medications and treatments. This book has been carefully written and checked for accuracy by the author and professional colleagues. However, in view of the possibility of human error and new discoveries in the biomedical sciences, neither the author nor any party associated in any way with this text warrants that this text is perfect, accurate, or complete in every way, and we disclaim responsibility for harm or loss associated with the application of the material herein. With all conditions/treatments described herein, each physician must be sure to consider the balance between what is best for the patient and the physician's own level of ability, expertise, and experience. When in doubt, or if the physician is not a specialist in the treatment of a given severe condition, referral is appropriate. These notes are written with the routine "outpatient" in mind and are not tailored to severely injured patients or "playing field" or "emergency response" situations; consult your First Aid and Emergency Response texts and course materials for appropriate information. These notes represent the author's perspective based on academic education, experience, and post-graduate continuing education and are not inclusive of every fact that a clinician may need to know. This is not an "entry level" book except when used in an academic setting with a knowledgeable professor who can explain the concepts, tests, physical exam procedures, and treatments; this book requires a certain level of knowledge from the reader and familiarity with clinical concepts, laboratory assessments, and physical examination procedures. Suggested doses—if any—are for adults (not infants and children) unless otherwise specified in context; the responsibility for appropriate dosing is of course that of the prescribing clinician in view of the patient's age, weight, overall state, hepatic and renal function, comorbidities, polypharmacy, etc.

Updates, Corrections, and Newsletter: When and if omissions, errata, and the need for important updates become clear, I will post these at the website InflammationMastery.com. A reader might access this page periodically to ensure staying informed of any corrections that might have clinical relevance. This book consists not only of the text in the printed pages you are holding, but also the footnotes and any updates at the website. If any clinically important corrections are made, they will be distributed by newsletter InflammationMastery.com/join_email.html and/or placed in the folder FunctionalInflammology.com/volume1/ (with analogous folders for subsequent volumes, e.g., volume2, etc) for constant availability. Be alerted to new integrative clinical research, updates to this textbook and other news/publications/conferences/videos by registering for the free newsletter at ICHNFM.ORG.

Language, Semantics, and Perspective: As a diligent student who previously aspired to be an English professor, I have written this text with great (though inevitably imperfect) attention to detail. Individual words were chosen with care. I confess to knowing, pushing, and creatively breaking several rules of grammar and punctuation. With regard to the he/she and him/her debacle of the English language, I've occasionally mixed singular and plural pronouns for the sake of being efficient and so that the images remain gender-neutral to the extent reasonable. In several previous publications, the subtitle *The art of creating wellness while effectively managing acute and chronic musculoskeletal/health disorders* was chosen to emphasize the intentional creation of wellness rather than a limited focus on disease treatment and symptom suppression; for the 2009 printing of *Chiropractic and Naturopathic Mastery of Common Clinical Disorders*, this subtitle was slightly modified from "creating" to "co-creating" to emphasize the team effort required between physician and patient. *Managing* was chosen to emphasize the importance of treating-monitoring-referring-reassessing, rather than merely *treating*. *Disorders* was chosen to reflect the fact that a distinguishing characteristic of *life* is the ability to regularly create *organized structure* and *higher order* from chaos and *disorder*. For example, plants organize the randomly moving molecules of air and water into the organized structure of biomolecules which eventually take shape as plant structure—fiber, leaves, flowers, petals. Similarly, the human body creates organized structure of increased complexity from consumed plants and other foods; molecules ingested and inhaled from the environment are organized into specific biochemicals and tissue structures with distinct characteristics and definite functions. Injury and disease *result in* or *result from* a lack of order, hence my use of the word "disorders" to characterize human illness and disease. For example, a motor vehicle accident that results in bodily injury, for example, is an example of an external chaotic force, which, when imparted upon human body tissues, results in a disruption (disorder) of the normal structure and organization that previously defined and characterized the now-damaged tissues of the body; likewise, an autoimmune disease process that results in tissue destruction is an *anti-evolutionary* process that takes molecules of higher complexity and reverts them to simpler, fragmented, and non-functional forms. From the perspective of "health" as *organized structure and meaningful function* and "disease" as *the reversion to chaos, destruction of structure, and the loss of function*, the task of healthcare providers is essentially to restore order, and to acutely reduce and proactively prevent/eliminate clinical-biochemical-biomechanical-emotional chaos insofar as it adversely affects the patient's life experience as an individual and our collective experience as an interdependent society. What is required of clinicians then is the ability *first* to create conceptual order from what appears to be chaotic phenomena, and then *second* to materialize—make real and practically applied for patients/people seeking improved health—that conceptual order into our physical world; this is our task, and no small task it is. Also under this heading of Semantics and Language, I will make readers aware of the following additional facts. First, I tend to write very long sentences, both in general and at times when I want to connect two or more complex ideas; rather than be dismayed or discouraged by this occurrence, readers are encouraged to read these longer sentences more than just once and to engage actively, perhaps by asking, *"Why is DrV making an effort to connect these ideas?"* **"What is the conceptual advantage to the binding of these ideas together?"** I am aware of most of the rules of grammar, and I am generally—but not always—compliant. Second, I create new words and phrases as needed; an index of some of these is provided toward the back of the book, whereas some of these new terms are self-explanatory, e.g., *hypoinsulinreception*—underreception or lack of receptor responsiveness to insulin. When possible, I strongly prefer to use single words when discussing concepts, rather than multiple disparate words for singular concepts. I have started to prefer using *italics* rather than "quotation marks" when introducing new terms or when using terms/phrases/words with emphasis; the main purpose of this is to reduce the number of punctuation marks and character spaces, both of which over the course of a multi-volume work of 2,000 pages and hundreds of thousands of words are numerically significant. Last for this section, the *colorization* process that I began in April 2014 for my (larger) books is intended to 1) bring out more detail in my increasingly complex diagrams, 2) bring emphasis and highlighting to areas of particular interest, 3) make the work more visually stimulating/pleasing over the previous black/white/grayscale versions, and—relatedly—4) to keep the work interesting as readers tread through a remarkable amount of complex and detailed information; I realize that some readers may at times find the colorization to be a small distraction, but I think this is better than the alternative of monotony induced by several hundred dense pages of grayscale.

Integrity and Creativity: I have endeavored to accurately represent the facts as they have been presented in texts and research, and to specifically resist any temptation to embellish or misrepresent data as others have done.[8,9] Conversely, I have not endeavored to make this book appeal to the "average" student or reader; my goal is to write and teach to the students at the top of the class, thereby affirming them and pulling the other students forward and upward. While I offer *explanations*, I intentionally resist *simplifications*, except when one simplification might facilitate the comprehension of a more complex phenomenon, or when such a simplification might facilitate the conveyance of information from clinician to patient. I have allowed this text to be unique in format, content, and style, so that the personality of this text can be contrasted with that of the instructor and reader, thus enabling the learner to at least benefit from an intentionally different – and intentionally honest – perspective and approach. Students using this text with the guidance of a qualified professor will benefit from the experience of "two teachers" rather than just one.

Linearity, Nonlinearity, Redundancy, Asynchronicity: Although the overall flow of the text is highly linear and sequential, occasionally I place a conclusion before its introduction for the sake of foreshadowing and therefore for preparing the reader for what is to come. The purpose of this is not simply one of preparation for the sake of allowing the reader to know what is already lying ahead on the path, but more to begin creating new "shelf space" in the reader's intellectual-neuronal "library" so that when the new—particularly if *neoparadigmatic*—information is encountered, a space will already exist for it; in other words: the intent is to make learning easier. Likewise, for the sake of *information retention*— or what is physiologically understood as synaptogenesis—important points are presented more than once, either identically or variantly. Given that *"No one ever reads the same book twice"*[10] (because the "person who starts" the reading of a meaningful book is changed into the "person who finishes" the reading of that book (assuming proper intentionality and application of one's "self"), the person reading these words might consider a second glace after the first. For the sake of efficient use of space I have tried to minimize redundancy; however, in a few locations, redundancy of text and images proved necessary as—for example—viewing the same diagram within two different conversations allows the reader to gain a more profound understanding of the concepts by viewing them from two different contexts.

Bon Voyage: All artists and scientists—regardless of genre—grapple with the divergent goals of *perfecting* their work and *presenting* their work; the former is impossible in the ultimate sense, while the latter is the only means by which the effort can create the desired effect in the world, whether that is pleasure, progress, or both. At some point, we must all agree that it is "good enough" and that it contains the essence of what needs to be communicated. While neither this nor any future edition of this book is likely to be "perfect", I am content with the literature reviewed, presented, and the new conclusions and implications which are described—many for the first time ever—in this text. Firstly in and progressively from my *Integrative Rheumatology* (2006), each chapter achieved/achieves a paradigm shift which distanced/distances us farther from the simplistic pathocentric and pharmacocentric model and toward one which authentically empowers both practitioners and patients. With time, I will make future editions more complete, consistently passionate, and either more or less polemical. I hope you are able to implement these conclusions and research findings *into your own life* and into the *treatment plans for your patients*. Hopefully this work's value and veracity will promote patients' vitality via the vigilant and virtuous clinicians viewing this volume; to the more attentive and thoroughgoing reader, more is revealed (for example, the last sentence is a reference to the descriptive and prophetic movie *V for Vendetta* (2006).

Thank you for engaging with this work, and I wish you and your patients the best of success and health.

Alex Vasquez, D.C., N.D., D.O., F.A.C.N.
March 14, 2016

---

[8] Vasquez A. Zinc treatment for reduction of hyperplasia of prostate. *Townsend Letter for Doctors and Patients* 1996; January: 100.
[9] Broad W, Wade N. *Betrayers of the Truth: Fraud and Deceit in the Halls of Science*. New York: Simon and Schuster; 1982
[10] Davies R. *Reading and Writing*. Salt Lake City: University of Utah Press; 1992, page 23

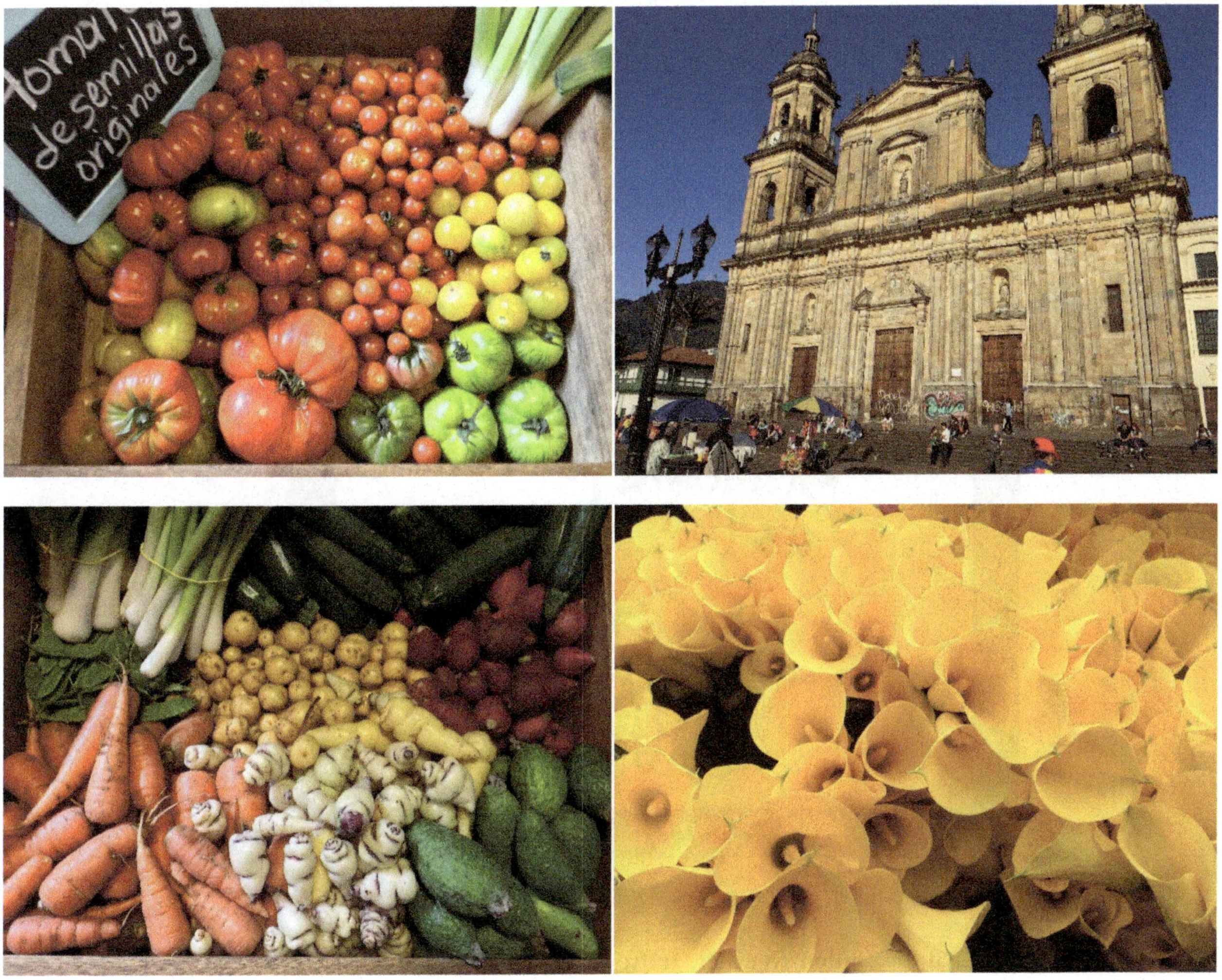

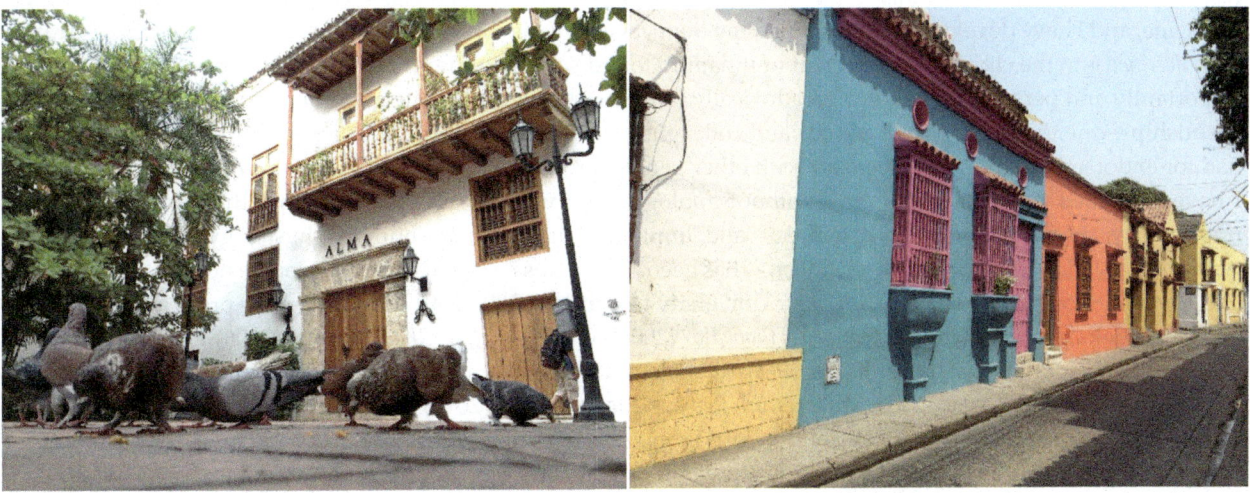

Living color, more vitality: The "colorization" process for the interior of this book began in April 2014 in Bogota (above) and Cartagena Colombia (below).

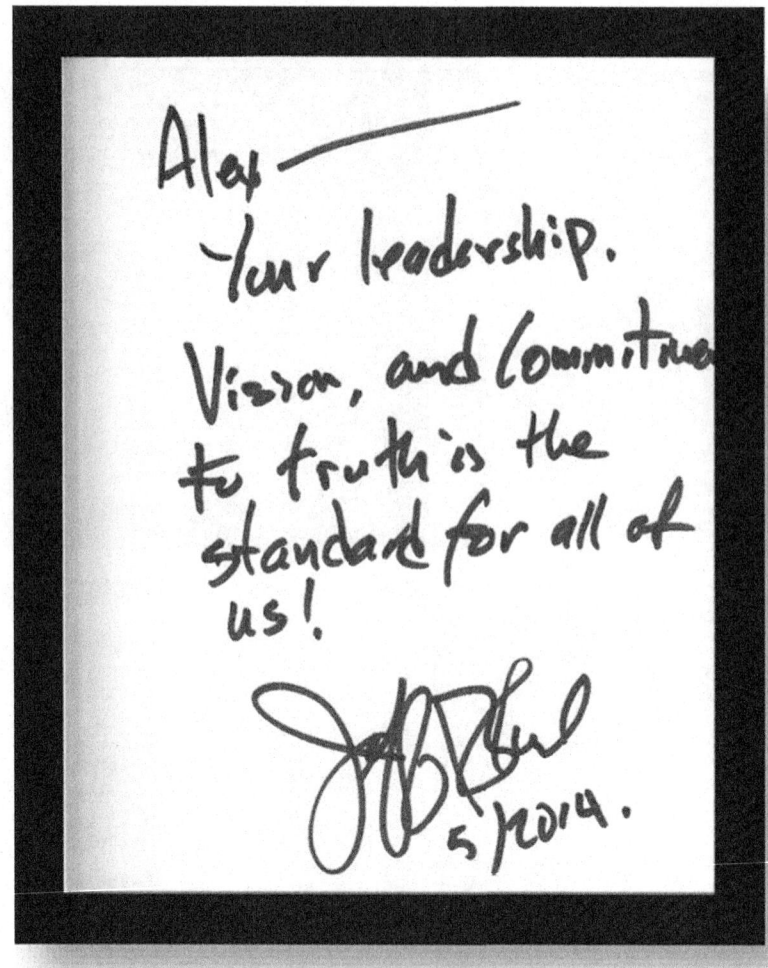

Pictured above—Personal inscription from Dr. Jeffrey Bland at a book signing event for his book *Disease Delusion*: My inclusion of Dr Bland's personal note above is not meant to imply that he is endorsing this book; he might very well reject any or all of it. Further, this inclusion does not imply that he carries those same sentiments beyond the day that he wrote them to me in May of 2014. Rather, my inclusion signifies our mutual respect as colleagues, and my personal respect for his thought and demeanor, and his influence on my life and work. I have respectfully honored him in this book as the founder of what most clinicians in America know as Functional Medicine, and I have developed and extended my own version of his concept—that disease states are *malleable* rather than *destined*—to the clinical management of inflammatory disorders under the name of Functional Inflammology. Importantly and personally—but not paradoxically if one understands the true goals of mentorship, affiliation, and friendship—due to the support of friends and colleagues, this book also represents a departure from concern that I had for endorsement from or agreement with other people, professions, universities, or organizations. In this book, I have presented the truth as I see it—without apology—and without any filtering other than as the limitations imposed by time, space, my own abilities, and limitations imposed by human physiology. This work—now published as *Inflammation Mastery, 4th Edition* —has been "in progress" since its origin as course notes for Orthopedics and Rheumatology which I taught at Bastyr University in Seattle in 2000-2001 and through its previous publications in many books starting with *Integrative Orthopedics* (2004) and *Integrative Rheumatology* (2006) and peer-reviewed publications in journals such as *Annals of Pharmacotherapy* (2005), *Alternative Therapies in Health and Medicine* (2004, 2014), *British Medical Journal* (2005), and *Nature Reviews Rheumatology* (2016). In addition to spanning more than 16 years, this work has also spanned various countries and cultures—including Houston, Fort Worth, Austin (Texas), Seattle (Washington), Portland (Oregon) in the United States, then to Bogota Colombia and Barcelona Spain. I consider this volume to be my highest presentation of truth, accuracy, clinical application and—most importantly for me: contextualization—that I could humanly muster while maintaining my own health, relationship, and other obligations. I will remain open to the correction and the updating of this work as the weight of evidence indicates. The goals of healthcare should be the optimization of physical health and psychosocial-intellectual freedom.

Reviews of previous and recent works:

- "Alex is the master of painful conditions and metabolic treatments." *Public comment by an award-winning neurosurgeon and functional medicine practitioner, 2016*

- "I love this course and your approach to the material. I am learning so much. Each article you assigned was strategically chosen and offered support and insight. I was pleasantly surprised by the exam and thought it was very fair. … Thank you for sharing your knowledge and experience with us!" *Doctorate Student under Dr Vasquez, 2016*

- "I appreciate the lecture yesterday and I am truly fascinated by your topic and your vast knowledge. ... I for one feel having people like you on our faculty can only strengthen the credibility of our school. ... I appreciate your education, knowledge and clearly you are the authority in your field. I have listened to all your lectures on YouTube - fantastic!" *University Faculty and Doctorate Student under Dr Vasquez, 2016*

- "Thank you most kindly for your incredible dedication and kindness in sharing your knowledge with us. I am due to start med school next semester and thanks to you and all those who have taught you, I'll be way ahead of the curve." *Premedical/Medical student 2015*

- "Dr Vasquez, I have followed your work extensively and admire your intellect and passion. Thank you for your passion for teaching with integrity!" *Chiropractic doctor 2015*

- "I just wanted to tell you how much I appreciate the information I have received from you. I am still digesting most of it. I feel I have learned quite a bit already yet also feel I have barely scratched the surface." *Doctor and Graduate student under Dr Vasquez, 2013*

- "Dr. Vasquez, Thank you for all you do. **Your conference was simply amazing**. No one wanted to leave the room. I met medical professionals and very interesting lay people who were stimulated and invigorated to change their lives and the lives of others. **I am in awe at your intellectual integrity and veracity.** Best of luck to you in all of your future endeavors." *Medical physician and ICHNFM 2013 Conference Attendee*

- **2014 review of Functional Inflammology, Volume 1:** "A truly comprehensive text on the vast subject of inflammation. I consider this book to be an essential addition to any health care practitioner who wishes to operate within the realm of Function Medicine. Please be aware that this book is dense in its content, and its 700 plus pages are full of deeply insightful information. I think Dr. Vasquez is one of the most prolific functional medicine contributors and books such as this should cement his reputation as such."

- "I attended the last ICHNFM conference in Portland (and am still basking in the amazing information received)." *Email from Clinical Oncology Dietitian, in late February 2014*

- "Thanks for a fantastic conference!" *ICHNFM 2013 Conference Attendee*

- "Your discourse today reflected not only your passion and commitment to the wellness of our planet but most importantly the clarity and sincerity of your spirit/ heart/ mind. Always good to be with you and look forward to seeing you soon. Hope we can spend more time then." *Medical physician attendee 2014*

- "I was so refreshed by the 'unfiltered excellence.' What humanness. Breaths of fresh air." *ICHNFM 2013 Attendee*

- "Keep in mind Alex, that humanity is a better place because of you. I know you can't undo it all, but think about how many people would be worse off if it wasn't for your wonderful knowledge being shared with all us docs. Things that I have learned from you have changed peoples' lives for the better." *Naturopathic physician, 2014*

- "Just got back to Guam. Great experience at the International Conference on Human Nutrition and Functional Medicine. Exciting concepts on functional medicine. Thanks Dr Alex Vasquez and team!" *ICHNFM 2013 Conference Attendee*

- "Already waiting in line to buy next year's ticket! **Dr. Vasquez you crushed it!** The future is looking fun already ☺" *ICHNFM 2013 Conference Attendee*

- "Had an incredible time at the 2013 International Conference on Human Nutrition and Functional Medicine. Got to meet some amazing people and hear from some of the top researchers/health professionals about human nutrition and functional medicine approaches. It was definitely worth every penny and can't wait to go back next year!" *ICHNFM 2013 Conference Attendee*

- "I miss you! Your confidence in a program you believed in. I miss your live classes where we would get off topic on a clinical pearl. I miss your way of teaching in a laid back atmosphere that made me feel comfortable, not intimidated. I just needed to let you know, this program is not the same, I am almost done, otherwise, I would have bailed out! I am grateful for the last 18 months I did have with you at the helm. ... You ignited in me my passion for learning again. You sparked the minds of all of us with your enthusiasm. Don't ever let anyone take that away. It has given birth to your new endeavor, and we will follow where you lead. Enjoy your new surroundings and celebrate your new beginnings. I know I look forward to what is ahead." *Doctor and Graduate student under Dr Vasquez, 2013*

- "Wonderful conference! Thanks so much." *ICHNFM 2013 Conference Attendee*

- "Really wonderful conference! Lots of material ready to implement Monday morning! **Congrats to Alex Vasquez on a herculean job very well done!**" *ICHNFM 2013 Conference Attendee*

- "Thanks for a great conference. I really enjoyed all of the speakers, but your lectures were by far the most useful for implementing ideas into my clinical practice. And the most entertaining." *ICHNFM 2013 Conference Attendee*

- "Thank you for your life-changing work." *Physician, 2011*
- "I want Dr. Vasquez to know that I have just received his book, *Chiropractic and Naturopathic Mastery of Common Clinical Disorders*. **It is a treasure. The best book in my library.** Thank you for the contribution that you are giving to the world of health care." *Clinician, 2010*
- "I appreciate the resources you offer the profession. I use your books and articles regularly." *Doctor, 2011*
- "Dr. Vasquez, I greatly appreciate your efforts. I am a student at ___, 8th trimester, and would like to express my gratitude for your research and works. After coming across your texts in the library, **I quickly found your insight and explanations of the current health care crisis, and in depth coverage and algorithms for inflammatory diseases as a profound inspiration and call to action. I appreciate your attention to detail, and have been taken back several times by the potency and meaning of your sentences. Thank you for your hard work, I will enjoy these books and will surely share with those that have the same drive for true and competent patient care.**" *Health Sciences Student, 2008*
- "I never told you this, but whenever I need to research a particular disease, **besides going on Pubmed and checking some classic Pathophysiology and Clinical Nutrition books, I use your books and I find them extremely well organized, concise, and up-to-date and with the functional/integrative medicine thinking I enjoy and believe it is the future of Health Care.**" *Nutrition Research Consultant and University Faculty in Europe, 2009*
- "Thanks so much. You are a great asset to our profession." *Doctor, 2010*
- "As a 7th trimester student quickly approaching 8th trimester and student clinic, I know I will be utilizing your books often. **Your "Chiropractic and Naturopathic Mastery of Common Clinical Disorders" book is referenced very frequently by many clinicians and faculty members at [our university]. Your work is highly regarded,** and I look forward to clinically utilizing the information I will obtain from your writings." *Health Sciences Student, 2011*
- "I am a chiropractic student at ___ Chiropractic College. I just wanted to drop a quick line thanking you for your thorough and accessible textbook Integrative Orthopedics. We are using it in our Differential Diagnosis class, and **it is the best book I've come across in Chiropractic College bar none. The writing is concise, informative and refreshingly eloquent. The material is super practical. I hope you continue putting out great resources.**" *Health Sciences Student, 2011*
- "I appreciate the resources you offer the profession. **I use your books and articles regularly.**" *Doctor, 2011*
- "**Your Integrated Orthopedics book is magnificent**. I wish all textbooks were structured and as thoughtful as that one." *Health Sciences Student, 2008*
- "By reading the introduction I realize that calling it an orthopedics book; does not do it justice. **It is far more than that. It looks to me that you have created, or are creating, the bible of Integrative Orthopedics and physical medicine.** *Physician, 2007*
- "First of all let me say how honored I am that you have allowed me to review this work. You have done an amazing job! In my opinion **every healthcare provider SHOULD have this on their bookshelf.**" *Physician, 2007*
- "Your work on Chapter 12: Hip and Thigh is very good. The chapter is inclusive of the typical pathologies seen in private practice and I particularly liked the separation of juvenile from adult pathologies. Your choice of tests to assess hip and thigh pathology on page 320 is very nice and inclusive. I appreciate your use of algorithms and find them very useful in teaching and in practice. In general, **I thought this chapter represents a quality, state of the art presentation!**" *Clinician and Professor in Clinical Sciences, 2007*
- "I saw your books in a colleague's office and was really impressed. Really appreciate the thoroughness you've put into them." *Doctor, 2010*
- "**It is with great interest and fascination that I have been reading your material both in your two books (Integrative Orthopedics and Integrative Rheumatology) and online. I consider myself very fortunate to have come across your work**, as many of the basic elements of health which you discuss I never learnt or even heard about while in chiropractic college." *Doctor, 2010*
- "I appreciate the resources you offer the profession. I use your books and articles regularly." *Doctor, 2011*
- "**I'm so pleased with your books and was inspired to let you know they have already been incredibly useful! Good index; well organized algorithms. Sometimes I buy educational material and it just sort of sits there... Your books now live on my main desk. Thanks.**" *Physician and Journal Editor, 2009*
- "I just wanted to let you know how much I am enjoying reading **your book Integrative Rheumatology. It is having an extremely positive impact in the way I view health and am having a tough time putting it down. It is very inspirational.** I have long felt that it is very important to set a good example for your patients and now try my best to be one for my future patients. I like how you stress this in your book. In order to be the best example for my patients I am going to need to address some problems with my own health. I look healthy from the outside but I have been suffering from fatigue for about 4 years. It has a very negative impact on my health. People say that doing the same thing and expecting different results is the definition of insanity so I think it is time that I attempt to make some

changes. ... **Thanks again for writing such a great book. I feel it is a must have for anyone in a musculoskeletal practice.**" *Health Sciences Student, 2010*

- "My name is [recent graduate], and I've been a fan of your books since I was in chiropractic college at [university] campus. Dr. [Author, Presenter] made your book, Integrative Rheumatology, required reading for his 9th quarter nutrition class. I never looked back, and have since purchased Chiropractic & Naturopathic Mastery of Common Clinical Disorders as well as Chiropractic Management of Chronic Hypertension." *Doctor, 2010*

- "I saw your books in a colleague's office and was really impressed. Really appreciate the thoroughness you've put into them." *Doctor, 2010*

- "Reading the new integrative management of high blood pressure book and I am thoroughly enjoying it; excellent job. **I am feeling so empowered I'm opening another office focusing on 'restoring the foundations of health' for the community** that I open it in. I am looking for a location and networking to find an internist and cardiologist that are forward thinking; I'm very excited!" *Doctor, 2011*

- "Thank you for the presentation at [the university] this past weekend. **My horizons about what can be done to help people were greatly expanded. I am now still studying the notes from the seminar and am looking forward to more study and learning on how to** *correctly* **manage diabetes and hypertension.**" *Doctor, 2011*

- "Thank you for exposing so many people to the results of our research on the treatment of hypertension. I hope you can pay us a visit during your next trip to our area so we can give you the tour of our new 50+ bed inpatient facility." *Dr Alan Goldhamer, Chief of Health Promoting Clinic, 2010*

- "**I always enjoy reading your work.** I personally gain a lot of knowledge through being a peer-reviewer for you and am better because of it!" *Doctor, Faculty Member, and Postgraduate Instructor, 2011*

- "**I attended your seminar at [University] in June and have been utilizing your hypertension protocols. In that short time, I have seen some marked progress with various patients.**" *Doctor, 2010*

- "I want to personally thank you for your expertise and books on...everything. I'm in my last year at SCNM (taking rheumatology right now) and I truly admire your research and ability to compile valuable information. Thank you." *Naturopathic Medical Student, 2014*

- "Doc, I really want to thank you for sharing some of the most important-relevant Facebook posts. **If we had more doctors, leaders and informed human beings (like yourself) our world would be a better place. Thank you for your commitment to truth and doing the right thing.**" *Doctorate Clinician, 2016*

- "I love your No BS approach to everything you do. I loved it in 2013 when you hosted the most informative conference I have ever had the opportunity to attend (because I could afford it at the time thank you). I wish there were more scientists/authors/academics/doctors like you! You are a breath of fresh air among the smell of BS and one can almost "smell" your intolerance to corruption. Please don't ever stop speaking your mind, disseminating information, and rebutting the "experts" because sadly, you're a rare breed." *Doctorate Clinician, 2016*

Work as love made tangible

"You work that you may keep pace with the earth and the soul of the earth.
For to be idle is to become a stranger unto the seasons, and to step out of life's
  procession. ...
Work is love made visible."

Kahlil Gibran (1883-1930). *The Prophet*, 1973

Begin at the beginning

"He who wishes one day to *fly*, must first learn *standing*
  and *walking*
    and *running*
      and *climbing*
        and *dancing*.
One does not *fly* into *flying*."

Friedrich Nietzsche (1845-1900). *Thus Spoke Zarathustra—A Book for All and None*, 1883-1885

CORRESPONDENCE

Neuroinflammation in fibromyalgia and CRPS is multifactorial

Alex Vasquez

In his Review article (Neurogenic neuro-inflammation in fibromyalgia and complex regional pain syndrome. *Nat. Rev. Rheumatol.* **11**, 639–648; 2015)[1], Geoffrey Littlejohn ascribes neuroinflammation to a "neurogenic" origin, presumably triggered by pain and stress. However, attribution of neuroinflammation and central sensitization to a primary neurogenic origin is premature without integrating the well-documented coexistence of small intestine bacterial overgrowth (SIBO, one type of gastrointestinal dysbiosis), vitamin D deficiency, and mitochondrial dysfunction.

Littlejohn[1] notes that chronic pain has been associated with lipopolysaccharide (LPS)–stimulated proinflammatory cytokines (particularly IFN-γ and TNF); however, he does not pursue this line of thought to connect it to relevant literature showing clear evidence of gastrointestinal dysbiosis and increased intestinal permeability in patients with fibromyalgia and complex regional pain syndrome (CRPS). The gastrointestinal tract is the most abundant source of LPS, systemic absorption of which is increased by SIBO and increased intestinal permeability. In 1999, Pimentel *et al.*[2] showed that oral administration of antibiotics led to alleviation of pain and other clinical measures of fibromyalgia. In 2004, Pimentel *et al.*[3] showed that among 42 fibromyalgia patients, all (100%) showed laboratory evidence of SIBO, severity of which correlated positively with severity of fibromalgia. In that same year, Wallace and Hallegua[4] showed that eradication of SIBO with antimicrobial therapy led to clinical improvements in fibromyalgia patients in direct proportion to antimicrobial efficacy. In 2008, Goebel *et al.*[5] documented that patients with fibromyalgia and CRPS have intestinal hyperpermeability; mucosal "leakiness" was highest in patients with CRPS, indicating a strong gastrointestinal component to the illness. In 2013, Reichenberger *et al.*[6] showed that CRPS patients have a distinct alteration in their gastrointestinal microbiome characterized by reduced diversity and significantly increased levels of Proteobacteria. LPS from Gram-negative bacteria is powerfully proinflammatory and is known to trigger microglial activation via Toll-like receptor 4; experimental studies have shown that LPS promotes muscle mitochondrial impairment, peripheral hyperalgesia, and central sensitization[7].

Vitamin D deficiency is prevalent in chronic pain and fibromyalgia patients and promotes pain sensitization, myalgia and bone pain (osteomalacia)[8]. Human clinical trials have shown that vitamin D supplementation can alleviate inflammation[9], intestinal hyperpermeability[10], fibromyalgia pain[11] and other neuromusculoskeletal pain. Vitamin D reduces experimental microglial activation[12], a component of neuroinflammation and central sensitization.

Mitochondrial dysfunction, noted in fibromyalgia[13] and CRPS[14], may be triggered by gastrointestinal dysbiosis via LPS, D-lactate, hydrogen sulfide, and inflammation; mitochondrial dysfunction exacerbates and perpetuates microglial activation and glutaminergic neurotransmission[15], thereby promoting pain sensitization centrally while also contributing to muscle pain peripherally[7]. Treatment of mitochondrial dysfunction with ubiquinone alleviates many biochemical and clinical manifestations of fibromyalgia[13].

Thus, neuroinflammation in fibromyalgia and CRPS has biological contributions including gastrointestinal dysbiosis, vitamin D deficiency, and mitochondrial dysfunction. These independent contributions commonly coexist, and each of these is additive/synergistic with the others in the promotion of peripheral and central hyperalgesia. The consistent pain-alleviating benefits of treatments for intestinal dysbiosis (antibiotics), vitamin D deficiency (supplementation) and mitochondrial dysfunction (ubiquinone) establish that these painful conditions are multifactorial and maintained by ongoing physiologic insults, each of which is treatable.

Alex Vasquez is at the International College of Human Nutrition and Functional Medicine, Calle Balmes 184, 3° 3ª, Barcelona, Spain 08006.
avasquez@ichnfm.org

doi:10.1038/nrrheum.2016.25
Published online 3 Mar 2016

1. Littlejohn, G. Neurogenic neuroinflammation in fibromyalgia and complex regional pain syndrome. *Nat. Rev. Rheumatol.* **11**, 639–648 (2015).
2. Pimentel, M. *et al.* Improvement of symptoms by eradication of small intestinal overgrowth in FMS: a double-blind study [abstract]. *Arthritis Rheum.* **42**, S343 (1999).
3. Pimentel, M. *et al.* A link between irritable bowel syndrome and fibromyalgia may be related to findings on lactulose breath testing. *Ann. Rheum. Dis.* **63**, 450–452 (2004).
4. Wallace, D. J. & Hallegua, D. S. Fibromyalgia: the gastrointestinal link. *Curr. Pain Headache Rep.* **8**, 364–368 (2004).
5. Goebel, A., Buhner, S., Schedel, R., Lochs, H. & Sprotte, G. Altered intestinal permeability in patients with primary fibromyalgia and in patients with complex regional pain syndrome. *Rheumatology* **47**, 1223–1227 (2008).
6. Reichenberger, E. R. *et al.* Establishing a relationship between bacteria in the human gut and complex regional pain syndrome. *Brain Behav. Immun.* **29**, 62–69 (2013).
7. Vasquez, A. *Human Microbiome and Dysbiosis in Clinical Disease 2015* (International College of Human Nutrition and Functional Medicine, 2015).
8. von Känel, R., Müller-Hartmannsgruber, V., Kokinogenis, G. & Egloff, N. Vitamin D and central hypersensitivity in patients with chronic pain. *Pain Med.* **15**, 1609–1618 (2014).
9. Timms, P. M. *et al.* Circulating MMP9, vitamin D and variation in the TIMP-1 response with VDR genotype: mechanisms for inflammatory damage in chronic disorders? *QJM* **95**, 787–796 (2002).
10. Raftery, T. *et al.* Effects of vitamin D supplementation on intestinal permeability, cathelicidin and disease markers in Crohn's disease: results from a randomised double-blind placebo-controlled study. *United European Gastroenterol. J.* **3**, 294–302 (2015).
11. Wepner, F. *et al.* Effects of vitamin D on patients with fibromyalgia syndrome: a randomized placebo-controlled trial. *Pain* **155**, 261–268 (2014).
12. Hur, J., Lee, P., Kim, M. J. & Cho, Y. W. Regulatory effect of 25-hydroxyvitamin D$_3$ on nitric oxide production in activated microglia. *Korean J. Physiol. Pharmacol.* **18**, 397–402 (2014).
13. Cordero, M. D. *et al.* Oxidative stress correlates with headache symptoms in fibromyalgia: coenzyme Q$_{10}$ effect on clinical improvement. *PLoS One* **7**, e35677 (2012).
14. Tan, E. C. *et al.* Mitochondrial dysfunction in muscle tissue of complex regional pain syndrome type I patients. *Eur. J. Pain* **15**, 708–715 (2011).
15. Nguyen, D. *et al.* A new vicious cycle involving glutamate excitotoxicity, oxidative stress and mitochondrial dynamics. *Cell Death Dis.* **8**, e240 (2011).

Competing interests statement
The author declares that he has worked as a consultant for Biotics Research Corporation (a nutraceutical company based in the USA), and that he has lectured and written for this company on various topics, including fibromyalgia.

2016 publication in *Nature Reviews Rheumatology* substantiating the model (at least partly, per the space limitations) of fibromyalgia described in this text: Provided here in printed format in accord with publisher's copyright agreement ("Authors retain the following nonexclusive rights to reproduce the contribution in whole or in part in any printed book of which they are the author"). The article needed to be added to this preface rather than deeper into the text in order to avoid the massive task of renumbering/indexing the entire book, and it serves as a validating foreshadowing of several of the concepts and clinical approaches contained herein. *Citation details*: Vasquez A. Neuroinflammation in fibromyalgia and CRPS is multifactorial. *Nat Rev Rheumatol*. 2016 Mar 3. doi: 10.1038/nrrheum.2016.25. PMID: 26935282. *Publisher site*: nature.com/nrrheum/journal/vaop/ncurrent/full/nrrheum.2016.25.html

Examples of commonly used abbreviations:

- **25-OH-D** = serum 25-hydroxy-vitamin D(3)
- **ACEi** = angiotensin-2 converting enzyme inhibitor
- **Alpha-blocker** = alpha-adrenergic antagonist
- **ANA** = antinuclear antibodies
- **ARB** = angiotensin-2 receptor blocker/antagonist
- **ARF** = acute renal failure
- **BB** = beta blocker or beta-adrenergic antagonist
- **bHB, BHB** = beta-hydroxy-butyrate
- **BMP** = basic metabolic panel, includes serum Na, K, Cl, CO2, BUN, creatinine, and glucose
- **BP** = blood pressure, relatedly **HBP** = high blood pressure
- **BUN** = blood urea nitrogen
- **C and S** = culture and sensitivity
- **CAD** = coronary artery disease
- **CBC** = complete blood count
- **CCB** = calcium channel blocker/antagonist
- **CE** = cardiac enzymes, including creatine kinase (CK), creatine kinase myocardial band (CKMB), and troponin-1, with the latter being the most specific serologic marker for acute myocardial injury; for the evaluation of acute MI, these are generally tested 2-3 times at 6-hour intervals with ECG performed at least as often.
- **CHF** = congestive heart failure
- **CHO, carb** = carbohydrate
- **CK** = creatine kinase, historically named creatine phosphokinase (CPK)
- **CKD** = chronic kidney disease, generally stratified into five stages based on GFR of roughly <90, 90-60, 60-30, 30-15, and >15, respectively
- **CMP** = comprehensive metabolic panel, also called a chemistry panel, includes the BMP along with markers of hepatic status albumin, protein, ALT, AST, may also include alkaline phosphatase and rarely GGT; panels vary per laboratory and hospital.
- **CNS** = central nervous system
- **COPD** = chronic obstructive pulmonary disease
- **CRF, CRI** = chronic renal failure/insufficiency
- **CRP** = c-reactive protein, hsCRP = high-sensitivity c-reactive protein

- **CT** = computed tomography
- **CVD** = cardiovascular disease
- **CXR** = chest X-ray
- **DM** = diabetes mellitus
- **DMARD** = disease-modifying antirheumatic drugs
- **ECG** or **EKG** = electrocardiograph
- **Echo** = echocardiography
- **ERS** = endoplasmic reticulum stress
- **GFR** = glomerular filtration rate
- **HDL** = high density lipoprotein cholesterol
- **HTN** = hypertension
- **Ig** = immune globulin = antibodies of the G, A, M, E, or D classes.
- **IHD** = ischemic heart disease
- **I+D** = incision and drainage
- **IM, IV** = intramuscular, intravenous
- **LPS** = bacterial lipopolysaccharide, endotoxin
- **MCV** = mean cell volume
- **MI** = myocardial infarction
- **Mito** = mitochondria(l)
- **MRI** = magnetic resonance imaging, **MRA** = magnetic resonance angiography
- **mTOR** = mechanistic or mammalian receptor of rapamycin; **TOR** is also reasonable
- **NFkB** = nuclear transcription factor kappa beta
- **PNS** = peripheral nervous system
- **PRN** = from the Latin "pro re nata" meaning "on occasion" or "when necessary"
- **PTH** = parathyroid hormone, iPTH = intact parathyroid hormone
- **PVD** = peripheral vascular disease
- **RA** = rheumatoid arthritis
- **RAD** = reactive airway disease, asthma
- **SIBO** = small intestine bacterial overgrowth
- **SLE** = systemic lupus erythematosus
- **TLR** = Toll-like receptor
- **TRIG(s)** = serum triglycerides
- **UA** = urinalysis
- **UPR** = unfolded protein response
- **US** = ultrasound

Dosing shorthand:

- **bid** = twice daily
- **cc** = with meals
- **hs** = at bedtime
- **ic** = between meals
- **po** = per os = by mouth
- **prn** = as needed (additional details above)

- **q** = each
- **qd** = each day, also /d or /day
- **qid** = four times per day
- **tid** = thrice daily
- **yo** = years old

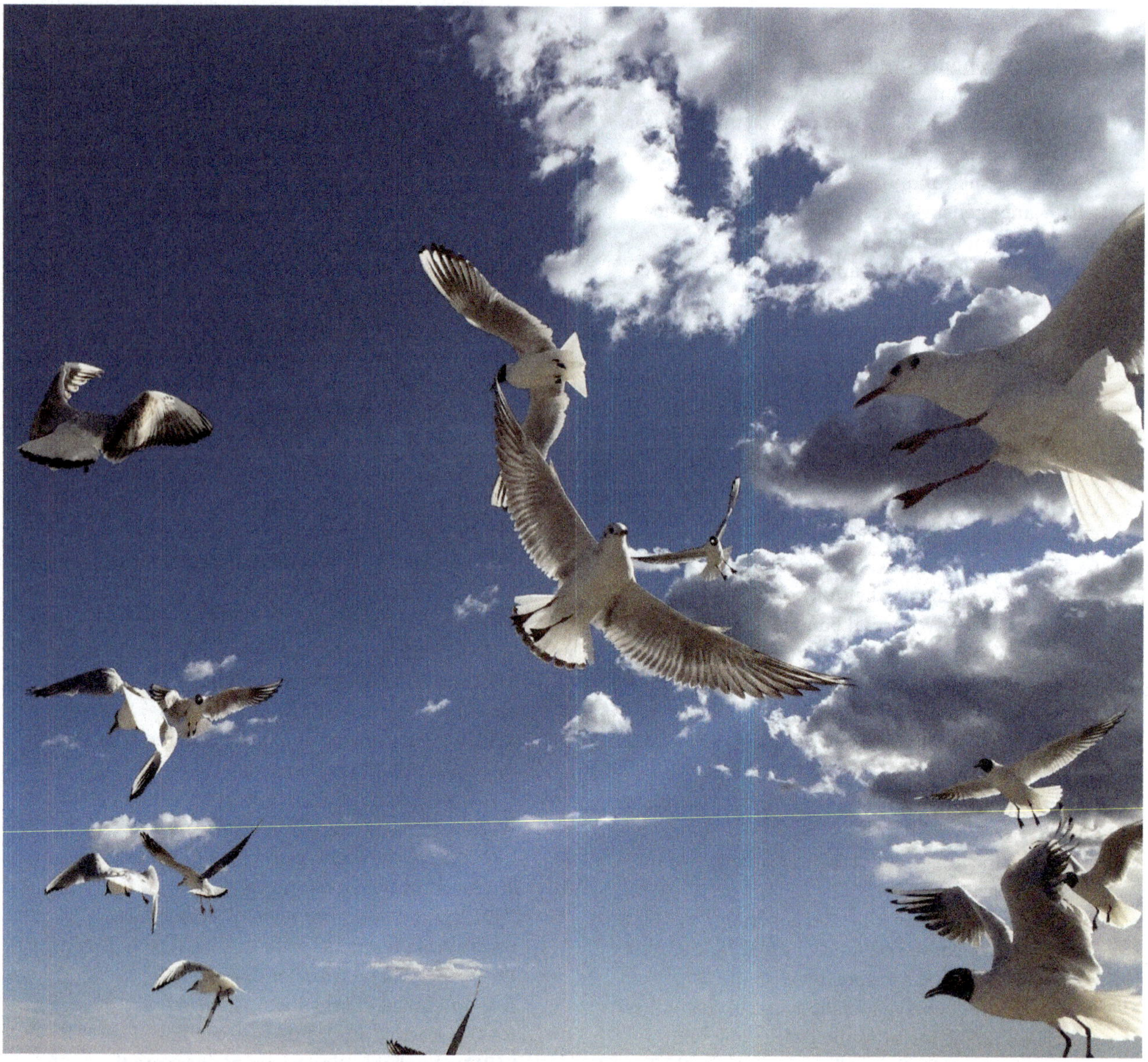

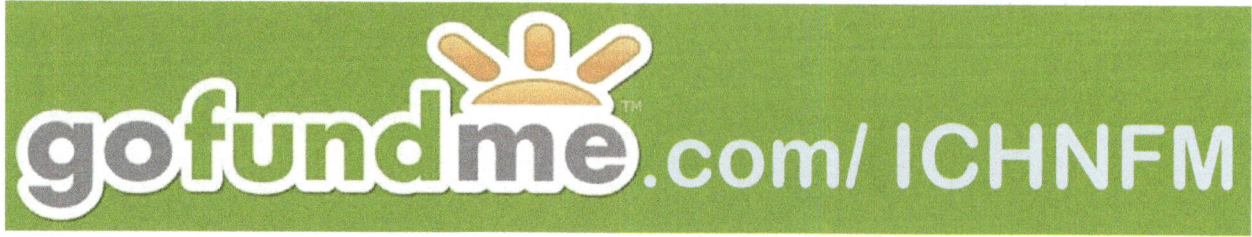

Seagulls in Sitges, Spain (2016 photo by DrV): "Most gulls don't bother to learn more than the simplest facts of flight — how to get from shore to food and back again." … "One school is finished, and the time has come for another to begin." … "We can lift ourselves out of ignorance, we can find ourselves as creatures of excellence and intelligence and skill." Richard Bach. *Jonathan Livingston Seagull*.1972

In 2016, ICHNFM initiated several new means by which students, clinicians, and benefactors can contribute to our ongoing efforts, ranging from supporting the Editorial and Review Staff of the *International Journal of Human Nutrition and Functional Medicine* (IntJHumNutrFunctMed.Org) to continue the free distribution of our publication and associated videos and interviews, to underwriting our ongoing certification efforts and joining as members to access the growing video archive and attend our webinars of case reports and research reviews. Support can also be sent directly via PayPal.com account admin@ichnfm.org; additionally, all of the ICHNFM print and ebook publications are available on Amazon.com listed under International College of Human Nutrition and Functional Medicine.

Chapter 1:
Initial Considerations in Patient Assessment and Management:
An Overview of Key Concepts and Facts in Patient History,
Physical Examination, Laboratory Interpretation,
Risk Management and Clinical Approach,
Common Clinical Considerations

Overview of this chapter

Reviewed herein are the three essential components of patient assessment:
1. History
2. Physical examination
3. Laboratory assessment

Additional concepts and perspectives are provided that will help facilitate risk management and promote and contextualize optimal patient care.

This chapter concludes with two new sections under the title of "Common Clinical Considerations", since these topics—hemochromatosis and hypothyroidism—are both commonly encountered in clinical practice and need to be considered in the routine evaluation of essentially all patients and especially those who present with disorders such as diabetes, depression, fatigue, and musculoskeletal pain. Previously, I had published these as separate chapters in various books, but—again—at this time I think these need to be integrated into basic/daily/routine clinical consideration.

Topics:

- **Moving past disease- and drug-centered medicine toward patient-centered health optimization: the goal is *wellness***
- **Acute Care and Musculoskeletal Care as Opportunities for Health Optimization**
- **Clinical Assessments**
  - History taking & physical examination
  - Orthopedic/musculoskeletal examination: Concepts and goals
  - Neurologic assessment: Review
  - Laboratory assessments: General considerations of commonly used tests
    - i. <u>Routine tests</u>: Chemistry/metabolic panel, lipid panel, CBC, 25(OH)-vitamin D, ferritin, thyroid stimulating hormone, CRP, ESR
    - ii. <u>Rheumatology/inflammation</u>: ANA (antinuclear antibodies), ANCA (antineutrophilic cytoplasmic antibodies), RF (rheumatoid factor), CCP (cyclic citrullinated protein antibodies), complement proteins, HLA-B27, additional tests for various immune/inflammatory disorders, tests for chronic infections/dysbiosis
    - iii. <u>Functional assessments</u>: Lactulose-mannitol assay, comprehensive stool analysis and comprehensive parasitology
- **High-Risk Pain Patients**
- **Clinical Concepts**
  - Not all injury-related problems are injury-related problems
  - Safe patient + safe treatment = safe outcome
  - Four clues to underlying problems
  - Special considerations in the evaluation of children
  - No errors allowed: Differences between primary healthcare and spectator sports
  - "Disease treatment" is different from "patient management"
  - Clinical practice involves much more than "diagnosis and treatment"
  - Clinical Management of Patients with Systemic Inflammatory/Autoimmune Diseases
  - Risk Management, Charting, and Avoiding Medical Errors: Useful Reminders and Acronyms
  - Risk Management: A note especially to students and recent licensees
- **Musculoskeletal Emergencies**
  - Acute compartment syndrome
  - Acute red eye, including acute iritis and scleritis
  - Atlantoaxial subluxation and instability
  - Cauda equina syndrome
  - Giant cell arteritis, temporal arteritis
  - Myelopathy, spinal cord compression
  - Neuropsychiatric lupus
  - Osteomyelitis
  - Septic arthritis, acute nontraumatic monoarthritis
- **Brief Overview of Integrative Healthcare Disciplines**
  - Naturopathic Medicine
  - Functional Medicine
  - Osteopathic Medicine
  - Chiropractic
- **Common Clinical Considerations**
  - Hemochromatosis and Iron Overload
  - Hypothyroidism, particularly Functional/Metabolic/Peripheral Hypothyroidism

Moving past diagnosis/disease/drug-centered medicine toward patient-centered health optimization: The goal is *wellness—optimal physical and psychosocial functioning*

Written for students and experienced clinicians, this chapter introduces and reviews many new and common terms, procedures, and concepts relevant to the management of patients with musculoskeletal disorders. Especially for students, the reading of this chapter is essential to understanding the extensive material in this book and will facilitate the clinical assessment and management of patients with various clinical presentations.

Healthcare is currently in a time of significant fluctuation and is ready for changes in the balance of power and the paradigms which direct our therapeutic interventions. For nearly a century, allopathic medicine has hailed itself as "the gold standard", and other professions have either submitted to or been crushed by their ongoing political/scientific manipulations and their continual proclamation of intellectual and therapeutic superiority[1,2,3,4,5,6,7,8,9,10,11,12,13] despite 180,000-220,000 iatrogenic *medically-induced* deaths per year (500-600 iatrogenic deaths per day)[14,15] and consistent documentation that most medical/allopathic physicians are unable to provide accurate musculoskeletal diagnoses due to pervasive inadequacies in medical training.[16,17,18,19] Increasing disenchantment with allopathic *heroic medicine* and its adverse outcomes of inefficacy, exorbitant expenses, and unnecessary death are

> **Medical iatrogenesis kills 493 Americans per day**
>
> "Recent estimates suggest that each year more than 1 million patients are injured while in the hospital and approximately 180,000 die because of these injuries. Furthermore, drug-related morbidity and mortality are common and are estimated to cost more than $136 billion a year."
>
> Holland, Degruy. *Am Fam Physician.* 1997 Nov

fostering change, such that allopathic medicine has been dethroned as the leading paradigm among American patients, who spend the majority of their discretionary healthcare dollars on consultations and treatments provided by "alternative" healthcare providers.[20,21] With the ever-increasing utilization of integrative medical services, we must see that our paradigms and interventions keep pace with the evolving research literature and our increasing professional responsibilities so that we can deliver the highest possible quality of care.

While we all readily acknowledge the importance of emergency care for emergency situations, those of us who advocate and practice a more complete approach to healthcare and life readily see the shortcomings of a limited and mechanical approach to healthcare, and we aspire to do more than simply fix problems. The implementation of *multidimensional* (i.e., *comprehensive* and *multifaceted*) treatment plans that address many aspects of pathophysiologic phenomena is a huge step forward in creating improved health and preventing future illness in the patients who seek our professional assistance. However, even complete multidimensional treatment plans still fall short of the goal of creating wellness, if for no other reasons than 1) they are still disease- and problem-

[1] Wilk CA. Medicine, Monopolies, and Malice: How the Medical Establishment Tried to Destroy Chiropractic. Garden City Park: Avery, 1996

[2] Getzendanner S. Permanent injunction order against AMA. *JAMA.* 1988 Jan 1;259(1):81-2

[3] Carter JP. Racketeering in Medicine: The Suppression of Alternatives. Norfolk: Hampton Roads Pub; 1993

[4] Morley J, Rosner AL, Redwood D. A case study of misrepresentation of the scientific literature: recent reviews of chiropractic. *J Altern Complement Med.* 2001 Feb;7:65-78

[5] Terrett AG. Misuse of the literature by medical authors in discussing spinal manipulative therapy injury. *J Manipulative Physiol Ther.* 1995;18(4):203-10

[6] National Alliance of Professional Psychology Providers. AMA Seeks To Control and Restrict Psychologist's Scope of Practice. nappp.org/scope.pdf Accessed Nov 2006

[7] "In an effort to marshal the medical community's resources against the growing threat of expanding scope of practice for allied health professionals, the AMA has formed a national partnership to confront such initiatives nationwide… The committee will use $25,000..." Daly R, American Psychiatric Association. AMA Forms Coalition to Thwart Non-M.D. Practice Expansion. *Psychiatric News* 2006 March; 41: 17 pn.psychiatryonline.org/cgi/content/full/41/5/17-a?eaf Accessed November 25, 2006

[8] Spivak JL. *The Medical Trust Unmasked.* Louis S. Siegfried Publishers; New York: 1961

[9] Trever W. *In the Public Interest.* Los Angeles; Scriptures Unlimited; 1972. This is probably the most authoritative documentation of the illegal actions of the AMA up to 1972; contains numerous photocopies of actual AMA documents and minutes of official meetings with overt intentionality of destroying Americans' healthcare options so that the AMA and related organizations would have a monopoly in national healthcare.

[10] Wenban AB. Inappropriate use of the title 'chiropractor' and term 'chiropractic manipulation' in the peer-reviewed biomedical literature. *Chiropr Osteopat.* 2006;14:16

[11] Orme-Johnson DW, Herron RE. An innovative approach to reducing medical care utilization and expenditures. *Am J Manag Care.* 1997 Jan;3:135-44

[12] van der Steen WJ, Ho VK. Drugs versus diets: disillusions with Dutch health care. *Acta Biotheor.* 2001;49(2):125-40

[13] Texas Medical Association. Physicians Ask Court to Protect Patients From Illegal Chiropractic Activities. texmed.org/Template.aspx?id=5259 Accessed Feb 2007

[14] Starfield B. Is US health really the best in the world? *JAMA.* 2000 Jul 26;284(4):483-5

[15] "Recent estimates suggest that each year more than 1 million patients are injured while in the hospital and approximately 180,000 die because of these injuries. Furthermore, drug-related morbidity and mortality are common and are estimated to cost more than $136 billion a year." Holland EG, Degruy FV. Drug-induced disorders. *Am Fam Physician.* 1997;56(7):1781-8, 1791-2

[16] Freedman KB, Bernstein J. The adequacy of medical school education in musculoskeletal medicine. *J Bone Joint Surg Am.* 1998;80(10):1421-7

[17] Freedman KB, Bernstein J. Educational deficiencies in musculoskeletal medicine. *J Bone Joint Surg Am.* 2002;84-A(4):604-8

[18] Matzkin E, Smith ME, Freccero CD, Richardson AB. Adequacy of education in musculoskeletal medicine. *J Bone Joint Surg Am.* 2005;87-A(2):310-4

[19] Schmale GA. More evidence of educational inadequacies in musculoskeletal medicine. *Clin Orthop Relat Res.* 2005 Aug;(437):251-9

[20] "…Americans made an estimated 425 million visits to providers of unconventional therapy. This number exceeds the number of visits to all U.S. primary care physicians (388 million)." Eisenberg DM, Kessler RC, et al. Unconventional medicine in the United States. Prevalence, costs, and patterns of use. *N Engl J Med.* 1993 Jan 28;328(4):246-52

[21] "Estimated expenditures for alternative medicine professional services increased 45.2% between 1990 and 1997 and were conservatively estimated at $21.2 billion in 1997, with at least $12.2 billion paid out-of-pocket. This exceeds the 1997 out-of-pocket expenditures for all US hospitalizations." Eisenberg DM, Davis RB, Ettner SL, Appel S, Wilkey S, Van Rompay M, Kessler RC. Trends in alternative medicine use in the United States, 1990-1997: results of a follow-up national survey. *JAMA* 1998 Nov 11;280(18):1569-75

oriented, rather than health-oriented, 2) they are prescribed from outside ("The doctor told me to do it.") rather than originating internally and spontaneously by the patient's own direction and affirmation ("I *do* this because I *am* this."), and, finally and most difficult to relay, 3) they are mechanistic rather than organic, they can do no better than the sum of their parts, they flow exclusively from the mind ("do") and not also from the body-soul ("am"). The art of creating wellness takes time to understand, longer to implement clinically, and even longer to apply to one's own life. Wellness is a state of being rather

than a checklist of activities in a "preventive health program." The subtle differences that distinguish "wellness" from any "program" or "prescription" are the differences between *leading* versus *following* and *flowing* versus *performing*. Wellness transcends mere health (e.g., vitality and absence of disease) and health (e.g., beyond physical, mental, and psychosocial wellbeing). **True and fully developed authentic wellness is the embodiment of multidimensional health; it is as-complete-as-possible (e.g., asymptotic) self-actualization, full integration of one's life—present, past, and future; it must ultimately be and manifest in physical, mental, emotional, spiritual, sociopolitical, transpersonal and multigenerational dimensions, inclusive of one's shadow[22], work[23], feelings, thoughts, and goals into a cohesive living whole – "a wheel rolling from its own center"[24] and beyond itself, beyond—ultimately—its own place and time.**

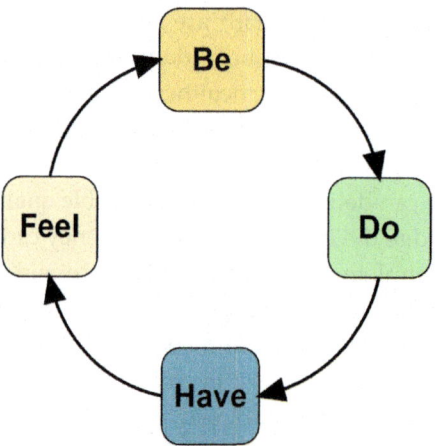

Self-reinforcing cycles of perception, manifestation, action, actualization, and reflection which reinforces (or changes) perception:
"Reciprocal causality" is the term popularized by psychologist Nathaniel Branden in his excellent works such as *Psychology of Self-Esteem*. Relatedly, "reciprocal determinism" is the psychosocial theory set forth by psychologist Albert Bandura that a person's behavior both influences and is influenced by personal factors and the social environment.

Authentic Selfhood, Internal Locus of Control, Creativity, Self-Direction
"Innocence is the child, and forgetfulness,
  a new beginning, a game,
   a self-rolling wheel,
   a first movement, a holy *Yea*.
Surely, for the game of creating, there is needed a holy *Yea* unto life."

Nietzsche FW. *Thus Spoke Zarathustra*. Part 1

---

[22] Robert Bly. *The Human Shadow*. Sound Horizons 1991 [audio cassette ISBN: 1879323001] and Bly R. *A Little Book on the Human Shadow*. ISBN: 0062548476
[23] Rick Jarow. *Creating the Work You Love: Courage, Commitment and Career*. Inner Traditions Intl Ltd; 1995. ISBN: 0892815426
[24] Friedrich Wilhelm Nietzsche. Walter Kaufmann (Translator). *Thus Spoke Zarathustra: A Book for None and All*. Penguin USA; 1978, page 27

Acute Care and Musculoskeletal Care: Opportunities for Health Optimization

Clinicians should appreciate that every patient encounter is an opportunity for comprehensive care, disease prevention, and health optimization. This is true whether the presenting complaint is acne, psoriasis, a respiratory infection, or musculoskeletal pain. Given the relatively high frequency of musculoskeletal complaints in clinical practice in general and chiropractic and osteopathic practices in particular, the following section will emphasize the clinical presentation of musculoskeletal complaints as an underappreciated opportunity for wellness care.

Since **approximately 1 of every 7 (14% of total) visits to a primary healthcare provider is for the treatment of musculoskeletal pain or dysfunction**[25], every healthcare provider needs to have 1) knowledge of important concepts related to musculoskeletal medicine, 2) the ability to recognize urgent and emergency conditions, 3) the ability to competently perform orthopedic examination procedures and interpret laboratory assessments, and 4) the knowledge and ability to design and implement effective treatment plans and to coordinate patient management.

In pharmacosurgical allopathic medicine, the goal of musculoskeletal treatment is to address the patient's injury or disorder by alleviating pain with the use of drugs, preventing further injury, and returning the patient to his/her previous status and activities. The most commonly employed interventions are 1) rest and "watchful waiting", 2) non-steroidal anti-inflammatory drugs (NSAIDS) and cyclooxygenase-2-inhibitors (COX-2 inhibitors, or "coxibs"), and 3) surgery. The more action-oriented approaches used by many chiropractic, naturopathic, and osteopathic physicians differs from the allopathic approach because, although avoidance of and "rest" from damaging activities is reasonable and valuable, too much rest without an emphasis on active preventive rehabilitation ❶ encourages patient passivity and ❷ the assumption of the sick role, and it ❸ fails to actively promote tissue healing and ❹ fails to address the underlying proprioceptive deficits that are common in patients with chronic musculoskeletal pain and recurrent injuries.[26,27,28] NSAIDs are considered "first line" therapy for musculoskeletal disorders by allopaths despite the data showing that "There is no evidence that widely used NSAIDs have any long-term benefit on osteoarthritis."[29] What is worse than this lack of efficacy is the evidence showing that NSAIDs *exacerbate* musculoskeletal disease (rather than *cure* it). NSAIDs are known to inhibit cartilage formation and to promote bone necrosis and joint degradation with long-term use[30,31,32,33] and NSAIDs are responsible for more than 16,000 gastrohemorrhagic deaths and 100,000 hospitalizations each year.[34] The "coxibs" were supposed to provide anti-inflammatory benefits with an enhanced safety profile, but the gastrocentric focus of the drug developers failed to appreciate that COX-2 is necessary for the formation of prostacyclin, a prostaglandin created from arachidonic acid via COX-2 that plays an important role in vasodilation and antithrombosis; not surprisingly therefore, use of COX-2-inhibiting drugs has consistently been associated with increased risk for adverse cardiovascular effects including myocardial infarction, unstable angina, cardiac thrombus,

> **Allopathic medicine has been described (ie, has described itself) as "scientific" since a time when this was clearly not the case**
>
> "...only about 15% of medical interventions are supported by solid scientific evidence..."
>
> Smith R. Where is the wisdom...? The poverty of medical evidence. *BMJ*. 1991 Oct

resuscitated cardiac arrest, sudden or unexplained death, ischemic stroke, and transient ischemic attacks.[35] Additionally, the use of a COX-2 inhibiting treatment in patients who overconsume arachidonic acid (i.e., most people in America and other industrialized nations[36]) would be expected to shunt bioavailable arachidonate into

[25] American College of Rheumatology Ad Hoc Committee on Clinical Guidelines. Guidelines for the initial evaluation of the adult patient with acute musculoskeletal symptoms. *Arthritis Rheum*. 1996 Jan; 39(1):1-8 See also: Vasquez A. Musculoskeletal disorders and iron overload disease. *Arthritis Rheum* 1996;39: 1767-8
[26] McPartland JM, Brodeur RR, Hallgren RC. Chronic neck pain, standing balance, and suboccipital muscle atrophy--a pilot study. *J Manipulative Physiol Ther*. 1997;20:24-9
[27] Bullock-Saxton et al. Reflex activation of gluteal muscles in walking. An approach to restoration of muscle function for patients with low-back pain. *Spine* 1993 May;18:704-8
[28] Sinaki M, Brey RH, Hughes CA, Larson DR, Kaufman KR. Significant reduction in risk of falls and back pain in osteoporotic-kyphotic women through a Spinal Proprioceptive Extension Exercise Dynamic (SPEED) program. *Mayo Clin Proc*. 2005 Jul;80(7):849-55
[29] Beers MH, Berkow R (Eds). *The Merck Manual. 17th Edition*. Whitehouse Station; Merck Research Laboratories 1999 page 451
[30] "At...concentrations comparable to those... in the synovial fluid of patients treated with the drug, several NSAIDs suppress proteoglycan synthesis... These NSAID-related effects on chondrocyte metabolism ... are much more profound in osteoarthritic cartilage than in normal cartilage, due to enhanced uptake of NSAIDs by the osteoarthritic cartilage." Brandt KD. Effects of nonsteroidal anti-inflammatory drugs on chondrocyte metabolism in vitro and in vivo. *Am J Med*. 1987 Nov 20; 83(5A): 29-34
[31] "The case of a young healthy man, who developed avascular necrosis of head of femur after prolonged administration of indomethacin, is reported here." Prathapkumar KR, Smith I, Attara GA. Indomethacin induced avascular necrosis of head of femur. *Postgrad Med J*. 2000 Sep; 76(899): 574-5
[32] "This highly significant association between NSAID use and acetabular destruction gives cause for concern, not least because of the difficulty in achieving satisfactory hip replacements in patients with severely damaged acetabula."Newman et al. Acetabular bone destruction related to non-steroidal anti-inflammatory drugs. *Lancet* 1985;2:11-4
[33] Vidal y Plana et al. Articular cartilage pharmacology: I. In vitro studies on glucosamine and non steroidal antiinflammatory drugs. *Pharmacol Res Commun*. 1978 Jun;10:557-69
[34] Singh G. Recent considerations in nonsteroidal anti-inflammatory drug gastropathy. *Am J Med*. 1998;105(1B):31S-38S
[35] Mukherjee D, Nissen SE, Topol EJ. Risk of cardiovascular events associated with selective COX-2 inhibitors. *JAMA*. 2001 Aug 22-29;286(8):954-9
[36] Seaman DR. The diet-induced proinflammatory state: a cause of chronic pain and other degenerative diseases? *J Manipulative Physiol Ther*. 2002;25(3):168-79

the formation of leukotrienes, a group of inflammatory mediators known to promote atherogenesis.[37] Thus, the outcome was entirely predictable: overuse of COX-2 inhibitors should have been expected to create a catastrophe of iatrogenic cardiovascular death, and this is exactly what was allowed to occur—clearly indicating independent but synergistic failures on the part of pharmaceutical companies, the FDA, and the medical profession.[38,39,40,41] According to statements by David J. Graham, MD, MPH, (Associate Director for Science, Office of Drug Safety, FDA) in 2005, an estimated 139,000 Americans who took Vioxx suffered serious complications including stroke or myocardial infarction; between 26,000 and 55,000 Americans died as a result of their doctors' prescribing Vioxx.[42] Additionally, the surgical procedures employed by allopaths for the treatment of musculoskeletal pain do not consistently show evidence of efficacy, safety, or cost-effectiveness. Arthroscopic surgery for osteoarthritis of the knee, for example, costs thousands of dollars to each individual and billions of dollars to the American healthcare system but is no more effective than placebo.[43,44,45] In a review which also noted that only 15% of medical procedures are supported by literature references and that only 1% of such references are deemed scientifically valid, Rosner[46] showed that the risks of serious injury (i.e., cauda equina syndrome or vertebral artery dissection) associated with spinal manipulation are *"400 times **lower** than the death rates observed from gastrointestinal bleeding due to the use of nonsteroidal anti-inflammatory drugs and 700 times **lower** than the overall mortality rate for spinal surgery."*

In integrative/functional medicine, the goal and means of musculoskeletal treatment is to address the patient's injury or disorder by simultaneously alleviating pain with the use of natural, noninvasive, low-cost, and low-risk interventions while improving the patient's overall health, preventing future health problems, and "upgrading" the patient's overall paradigm of health maintenance and disease prevention from one that is passive and reactive to one that is empowered and pro-active. Commonly employed therapeutics include spinal manipulation[47,48,49], exercise[50] and the use of nutritional supplements and botanical medicines[51,52] which have been demonstrated in peer-reviewed clinical trials to be safe and effective for the alleviation of musculoskeletal pain. In order to deliver competent drug-free pain management and to help patients who use nutritional supplements, today's clinicians need to be well-versed in the clinical utilization of such treatments as niacinamide[53], glucosamine and chondroitin sulfates[54], vitamin D[55], vitamin B-12[56], anti-inflammatory diets[57,58], balanced and complete fatty acid therapy[59], proteolytic/pancreatic enzymes[60], and botanical medicines such as *Boswellia*[61], *Harpagophytum*[62], *Uncaria*, and willow bark[63,64]—each of these interventions has been validated in peer-reviewed research for safety and effectiveness.[65] Furthermore, from the perspective of progressive/functional medicine, aiming for such a limited accomplishment as mere "returning the patient to previous status and activities" would be considered substandard, since the patient's overall health was neither addressed nor improved and since returning the patient to his/her previous status and activities would be a direct invitation for the problem to recur indefinitely. Astute physicians should appreciate that, especially regarding "~~chronic~~" (i.e., sustained) health problems, any treatment plan that

[37] Dwyer JH, et al. Arachidonate 5-lipoxygenase promoter genotype, dietary arachidonic acid, and atherosclerosis. *N Engl J Med*. 2004 Jan 1;350(1):29-37

[38] Topol EJ. Arthritis medicines and cardiovascular events--"house of coxibs". *JAMA*. 2005 Jan 19;293(3):366-8. Epub 2004 Dec 28

[39] Ray WA, Griffin MR, Stein CM. Cardiovascular toxicity of valdecoxib. *N Engl J Med*. 2004 Dec 23;351(26):2767. Epub 2004 Dec 17

[40] Topol EJ. Failing the public health--rofecoxib, Merck, and the FDA. *N Engl J Med*. 2004 Oct 21;351(17):1707-9

[41] Horton R. Vioxx, the implosion of Merck, and aftershocks at the FDA. *Lancet*. 2004 Dec 4-10;364(9450):1995-6

[42] David J. Graham, MD, MPH, (Associate Director for Science, Office of Drug Safety, USFDA) estimated that 139,000 Americans who took Vioxx suffered serious side effects; he estimated that the drug killed between 26,000 and 55,000 people. commondreams.org/views05/0223-35.htm and fda.gov/cder/drug/infopage/vioxx/vioxxgraham.pdf 2006 Nov

[43] Kolata G. A Knee Surgery for Arthritis Is Called Sham. *The New York Times*, July 11, 2002

[44] Moseley JB, et al. A controlled trial of arthroscopic surgery for osteoarthritis of the knee. *N Engl J Med*. 2002;347:81-8

[45] Bernstein J, Quach T. A perspective on the study of Moseley: questioning the value of arthroscopic knee surgery for osteoarthritis. *Cleve Clin J Med* 2003;70:401, 405-6, 408-10

[46] Rosner AL. Evidence-based clinical guidelines for the management of acute low-back pain: response. *J Manipulative Physiol Ther*. 2001;24(3):214-20

[47] Manga P, Angus D, Papadopoulos C, et al. *The Effectiveness and Cost-Effectiveness of Chiropractic Management of Low-Back Pain*. Richmond Hill, Ontario: Kenilworth; 1993

[48] Meade et al. Low-back pain of mechanical origin: randomised comparison of chiropractic and hospital outpatient treatment. *BMJ*. 1990;300(6737):1431-7

[49] Meade et al. Randomised comparison of chiropractic and hospital outpatient management for low-back pain: results from extended follow up. *BMJ*. 1995;311(7001):349-5

[50] Elrick H. Exercise is Medicine. *The Physician and Sportsmedicine*. 1996 Feb;24(2):72-6

[51] Vasquez A. Revisiting the Five-Part Nutritional Wellness Protocol: The Supplemented Paleo-Mediterranean Diet. *Nutritional Perspectives* 2011 Jan

[52] Vasquez A. Improving overall health while safely and effectively treating musculoskeletal pain. *Nutritional Perspectives* 2005; 28: 34-38, 40-42

[53] Kaufman W. Niacinamide therapy for joint mobility. Therapeutic reversal of a common clinical manifestation of the "normal" aging process. *Conn State Med J* 1953;17:584-591

[54] Reginster JY, et al. Long-term effects of glucosamine sulphate on osteoarthritis progression: a randomised, placebo-controlled clinical trial. *Lancet*. 2001;357(9252):251-6

[55] Vasquez A, Manso G, Cannell J. The clinical importance of vitamin D: a paradigm shift with implications for all healthcare providers. *Altern Ther Health Med* 2004;10:28-36

[56] Mauro et al. Vitamin B12 in low back pain: a randomised, double-blind, placebo-controlled study. *Eur Rev Med Pharmacol Sci*. 2000 May-Jun;4(3):53-8

[57] Seaman DR. The diet-induced proinflammatory state: a cause of chronic pain and other degenerative diseases? *J Manipulative Physiol Ther*. 2002 Mar-Apr;25(3):168-7

[58] Vasquez A. New Insights into Fatty Acid Biochemistry and the Influence of Diet. *Nutritional Perspectives* 2004; October: 5, 7-10, 12, 14

[59] Vasquez A. New Insights into Fatty Acid Supplementation and Its Effect on Eicosanoid Production and Genetic Expression. *Nutritional Perspectives* 2005; January: 5-16

[60] Trickett P. Proteolytic enzymes in treatment of athletic injuries. *Appl Ther*. 1964;30:647-52

[61] Kimmatkar et al. Efficacy and tolerability of Boswellia serrata extract in treatment of osteoarthritis of knee: controlled trial. *Phytomedicine*. 2003 Jan;10(1):3-7

[62] Chrubasik et al. Effectiveness of Harpagophytum extract WS 1531 in the treatment of exacerbation of low-back pain. *Eur J Anaesthesiol* 1999 Feb;16(2):118-29

[63] Chrubasik et al. Treatment of low-back pain exacerbations with willow bark extract: a randomized double-blind study. *Am J Med*. 2000;109:9-14

[64] Vasquez A, Muanza DN. Comment: Evaluation of Presence of Aspirin-Related Warnings with Willow Bark. *Ann Pharmacotherapy* 2005 Oct;39(10):1763

[65] Vasquez A. Improving overall health while safely and effectively treating musculoskeletal pain. *Nutritional Perspectives* 2005;28:34-42

allows the patient to resume his/her previous lifestyle is by definition doomed to fail because a return to the patient's previous lifestyle and activities that allowed the onset of the disease/disorder in the first place will most certainly result in the perpetuation and recurrence of the illness or disorder. **Stated more directly: for *healing* to truly be effective, the comprehensive treatment plan must generally result in a permanent and profound change in the patient's lifestyle and emotional climate, which are the primary modifiable determinants of either health or disease.**

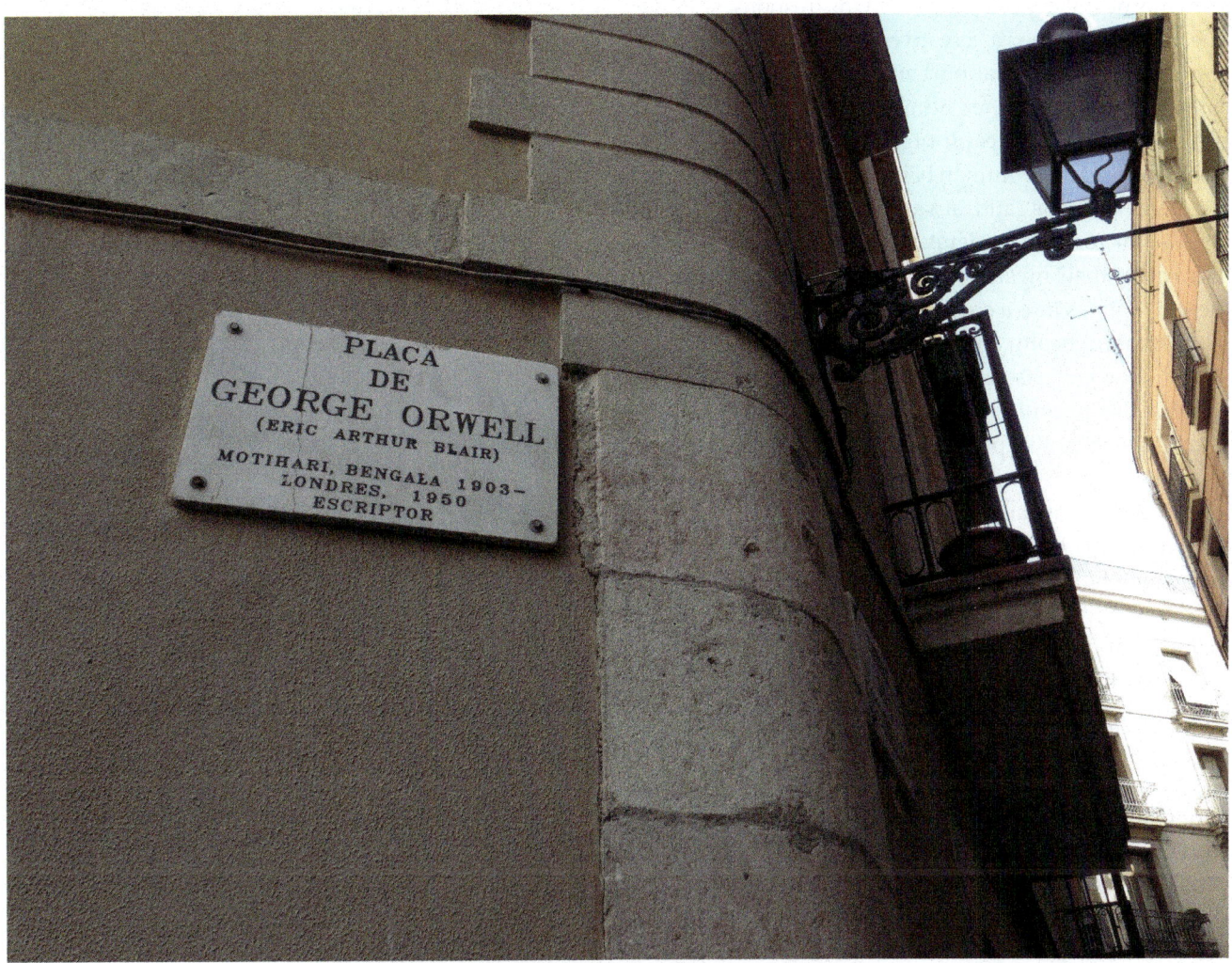

Barcelona's tradition of honoring intellectuals—Plaça de George Orwell: George Orwell is best known for his brilliant books *1984* and *Animal Farm* which creatively tell complex tales of herd mentality, politics, and various forms of social control and the manufacture of public consent and conformity. Less well-known is his *Homage to Catalonia*, in which he describes his experience as a volunteer in the Spanish Civil War (during which he was shot in the neck by a sniper) against the fascist regime of Francisco Franco, then supported by Hitler's Nazi Germany and Mussolini's Fascist Italy. His required-reading book *1984* has recently been summarized in a brilliant audio version[66] (and a short free video[67]) to increase its accessibility. In 2014, people protesting government surveillance and unjust imprisonments in Thailand were arrested for reading *1984*.[68]

---

[66] Moustaki N (Author), Podehl N (Narrator). *1984: CliffsNotes*. Audible. cliffsnotes.com/literature/n/1984/book-summary and amazon.com/1984-CliffsNotes/dp/B004S8NFZ2/
[67] Video SparkNotes: Orwell's 1984 Summary. https://youtube.com/watch?v=pTqIVvUPAjw
[68] Associated Press. 23 June, 2014. Protesting Thai reader of Orwell's *1984* dragged off by police in Bangkok. "Police in Thailand yesterday arrested eight people for demonstrating against the nation's increasingly repressive military junta, including a man dragged away by undercover officers for reading a copy of George Orwell's *Nineteen Eighty-Four*. The arrest was the first known case of anyone being detained for reading as a form of protest since the military seized power last month. ... A Thai reporter who witnessed the lone man reading Orwell's classic said he was taken away by half a dozen plainclothes police. The reporter said the man held the book up as officers approached. ... Another of the arrests was of a woman wearing a T-shirt with the words "Respect My Vote" on it." *South China Morning Post* scmp.com/news/asia/article/1538616/protesting-thai-reader-orwells-1984-dragged-police-bangkok. See also Campbell C. A Yellow Shirt Leader Says the Thai Coup Was Planned in 2010. *Time* 2014 Jun 23. time.com/2910484/thai-coup-planned-2010-suthep-thaugsuban/. "My friends told me when they read 1984 for the first time they could never imagine there would be a country like that, but it's happening now in Thailand," says Pimsiri. "People are really watching you, your computers are being monitored... and many people have been detained in undisclosed locations." *Christian Science Monitor* csmonitor.com/World/Asia-Pacific/2014/0530/Orwell-s-1984-suddenly-fashionable-on-Bangkok-streets

Clinical Assessments: Brief Review of Essential Concepts

The clinical assessments reviewed in the following sections are history-taking, orthopedic/musculoskeletal, and neurologic examinations, and commonly used laboratory tests. **History taking is the art of conducting an** *informative* **and** *collaborative* **patient interview.**

The role of the doctor during the interview process is not merely that of a data-collecting machine, spewing out questions and receiving responses. Patient interviews can be a creative, enjoyable, comforting opportunity to build rapport and to establish meaningful connection with another human being. Patients are not simply people with health problems – they are first and foremost our fellow human beings, not so dissimilar from ourselves perhaps, and always full of complexity. Our task is not to fully understand their complexity nor to solve all of their mysteries, but rather to help orchestrate these dynamics into a coordinated if not unified direction that promotes health and healing.

Beyond its diagnostic value, the interview process also provides a key opportunity to gain insight into the patient's psychoepistimology—the patient's operating system for interacting with data and the world and internalizing and metabolizing external inputs in such a way as to merge these with internal experiences (i.e., emotions, feelings, preferences, responses). Epistemology is the branch of philosophy concerned with the nature and scope of knowledge. Per Rand[69], psychoepistimology is a person's "method of awareness"; a person's psychoepistimology creates a "corollary view of existence" and in turn, "A man's method of using his consciousness determines his method of survival." By understanding how the patient views him/herself in the world, understanding his/her goals, and—in essence— what "drives" the patient and what "makes him/her tick", clinicians can shape the nuances of the conversation and the treatment plan to promote the desired cognitive-conceptual-behavioral changes in behavior that are prerequisite for the attainment of optimized health outcomes.

History & Assessment
History of the primary complaint: "D.O.P.P. Q.R.S.T." • Description/location • Onset • Provocation: exacerbates • Palliation: alleviates • Quality • Radiation of pain • Severity • Timing
Associated complaints • Additional manifestations • Concomitant diseases
Review of systems • Head-to-toe inventory of health status, associated health problems, and complications
Past health history • Surgeries • Hospitalizations • Traumas • Vaccinations and medications • Successful and failed treatments for the current complaint(s)
Family health history • Genotropic illnesses and predispositions • Lifestyle patterns • Emotional expectations
Social history • Hobbies, work, exposures • Relationships and emotional experiences • Interpersonal support • Malpractice litigation
Health Habits • Diet: appropriate intake of protein, fruits, vegetables, fats, sugars • Sleep • Stress management • Exercise / Sedentary Lifestyle • Spirituality / Centeredness • Caffeine and tobacco • Ethanol and recreational drugs
Medication and supplements • Reason, doses, duration, cost • Side-effects • Interactions
Responsibility and Compliance • Ability and willingness to comply with prescribed treatment plan and to incorporate the necessary diet-exercise-relationship-emotional-lifestyle modifications • *Internal* versus *external* locus of control

---

[69] Rand A. *For the New Intellectual*. New York; Signet:1961, page 16

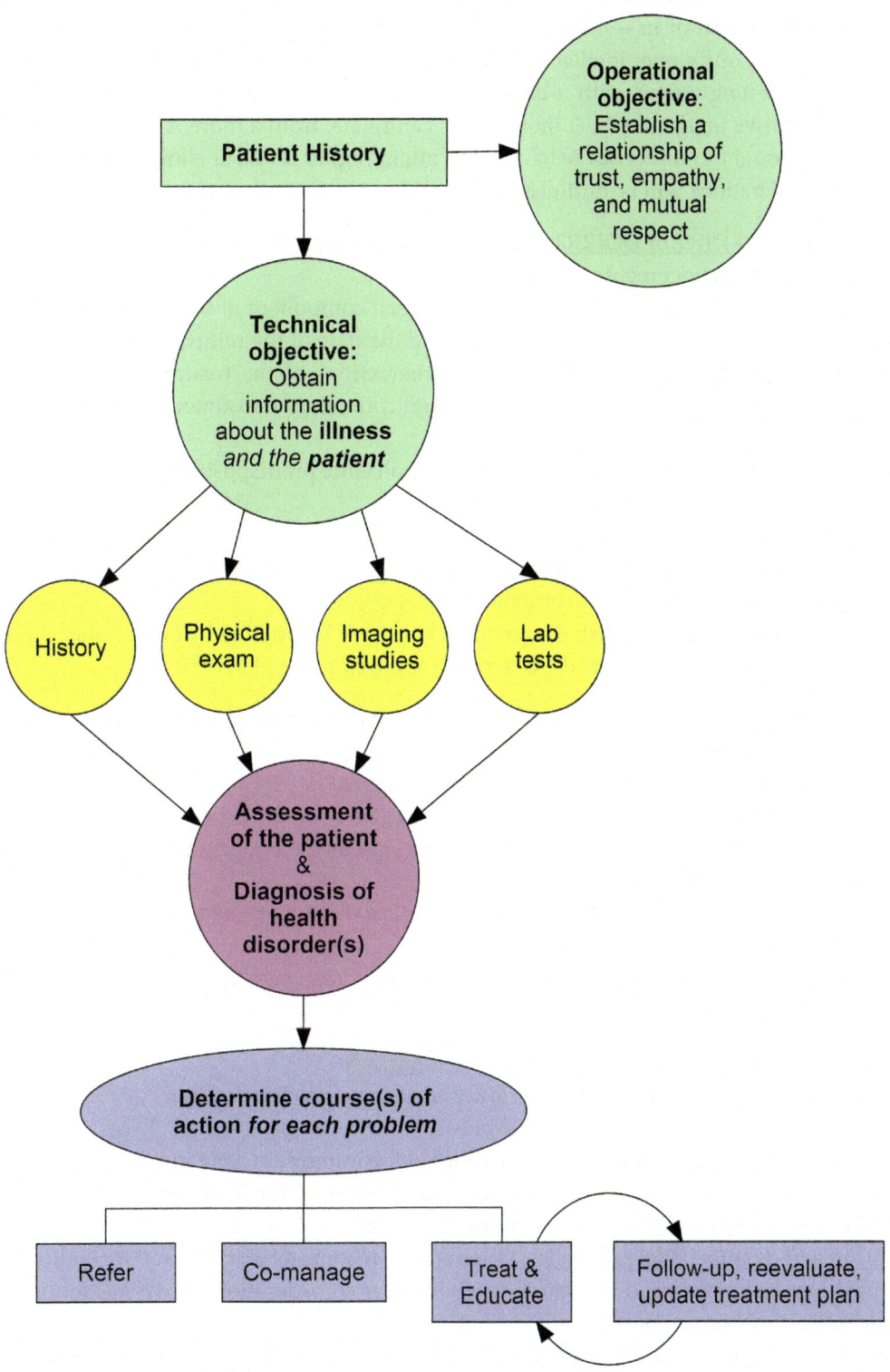

Key components of patient assessment and management: Patient assessment and management is an on-going process that begins with the initial history taken at the first clinical encounter and continues through the physical examination and laboratory assessments and thereafter by monitoring the patient's implementation of and response to the treatment plan. The plan is complete *not simply when it is designed and delivered*; the treatment plan is complete when the desired outcome of health optimization is achieved and sustained.

Clinical acronyms: Outlined here are some of my preferred and—in the case of D.I.R.T. and F.I.N.D.S.E.X.™—unique acronyms which help all of us—students and seasoned clinicians alike—to develop a system of thought which then frees us to apply our higher intellectual functions to the nuances of the clinical case/condition/situation we are considering. Interestingly (and with a bit of Dionysian humor), the sequential use of DIRT, SOAP, and FINDSEX creates an intuitive image to which most adults can relate; from a more Apollonian perspective, we can apply this structure of thought to direct our behavior and attain higher levels of clinical care with greater ease and consistency. These considerations will be outlined and developed in sections that follow.

Risk management acronym—==DIRT== or ==DDIRRT==: Start with the intention to practice defensively and effectively.
- Defensive mindset: Risk management must be pro-active,
- Duration of treatment: Define and limit the duration of each component of the treatment plan; define the next steps of care (e.g., continued care or laboratory tests) and the date of the return visit,
- Interactions—drugs and diseases: Double-check for interactions of the treatment plan with drugs and the patient's disease(s), especially renal insufficiency. Several commonly encountered clinical examples follow:
    o High-potassium diet ≠ renal insufficiency
    o Vitamin D ≠ hydrochlorothiazide or other hypercalcemic predisposition/state
    o Calcium and magnesium ≠ tetracycline antibiotics
    o Vitamin K ≠ warfarin
- Referral: Determine the need for additional consultation,
- Return visit: Specify and chart timeframe or date of next visit,
- Treatment plan, charted, dated, signed: Treatment plan must be archived in chart and should be given to patient; the clinician must sign and date the chart note and treatment plan.

Patient management acronym—==SOAP==: Competent care starts with an open-minded, compassionate, information-seeking excellence-aspiring clinician.
- Subjective: History of presenting complaints; patient's concerns,
- Objective: Physical exam, lab tests: always assess renal function and other basic biochemical parameters; more complex cases require evaluation of more sensitive markers of metabolic and immune imbalance, imaging, biopsy, procedures—as necessary,
- Assessment: Reach an assessment of the entire constellation of patient's situation; diagnosis and appropriate management of each true disease and concern,
- Plan: Informed consent (PARBQ): procedures, alternatives, risks, benefits, questions answered; treatments; follow-up, rescheduling, referral, co-management.

Functional medicine/inflammology treatment acronym—==FINDSEX==®
- Food: Diet and nutrition: input, metabolism, utilization, unique needs, excretion,
- Infections: Persistent microbial colonization, dysbiosis,
- Nutritional Immunomodulation: Integrative "shaping" of the immune system in favor of Treg at the expense of Th1/2/17. This clinical system has been organized and refined by Dr Vasquez since its first publication in *Functional Immunology and Nutritional Immunomodulation* (2012)
- Dysmetabolism and dysfunctional organelles: Originally in this protocol, dysfunctional mitochondrial was the focus; this has since been expanded to include much broader considerations of dysmetabolism in general and endoplasmic reticulum stress in particular.
- Special considerations, sleep, style of living: This section is intended to cover the basics of sleep, stress management, social considerations, special supplementation, surgery, somatic medicine and spinal manipulation, spirituality, etc.
- Endocrine: Hormonal imbalances must be assessed and corrected/optimized if metabolic and inflammatory balance are to be restored.
- Xenobiotics: Due mostly to the synergistic effects of failure of governmental regulatory agencies combined with careless and reckless corporate production of pollution and toxic chemicals, our world has become highly contaminated with chemicals that alter our hormonal, neurological, reproductive, and immune health. Because this phenomena is subtle, nonacute, and ubiquitous, it is easily overlooked despite its importance.

Components of a Complete Patient History: "D.O.P.P. Q.R.S.T."

Category	Patient history questions and implications
Description, Location: Always start with open-ended questions	• *What is it like for you?* • *What do you experience?* • *What are you feeling?* • *Where is the pain/sensation/problem?* • Ask about specifics: **Pain, numbness, weakness, tingling**, fatigue, recent or chronic infections, burning, aching, dull, sharp, cramping, stretching, pins and needles, weakness, changes in function (i.e., bowel and bladder continence, sexual function).
Onset	• *When did it begin? Have you ever had anything like this before?* • *Was there a specific event associated with the onset of the problem, such as an injury or an illness, or did the problem start gradually or insidiously?* • *How has it changed over time?* • *Prior injuries to site?* • *Why are you seeking care for this now (rather than last week or last month)?* • *What has changed? How is the pain/problem developing over time—getting worse or getting better?*
Palliation	• *How have you tried treating it? Does anything make it go away?* • *What makes it better? What relieves the pain?* • Ask about prior and current treatments, radiographs, medications, supplements (herbs, vitamins, minerals), injections, surgery, massage, manipulation, and counseling. • Knowing response/resistance to previous treatments can provide clinical insight.
Provocation	• *Are your symptoms constant, or does the problem come and go?* • *What makes it worse? What makes the pain worse?* • *When during the day/week/month/year are your symptoms the worst?*
Quality	• *Can you describe the pain to me?* • *What does it feel like?* • *What do you experience?* • Get a clear understanding of the type of sensation(s): stabbing, shooting pain, pins and needles, sharp pain, electric sensation, numbness, burning, aching, throbbing, weakness, tingling, gel phenomenon (stiffness worsened by inactivity), dizziness, confusion, fatigue, shortness of breath.
Radiation	• *Does the pain stay localized or does it move to your arm/leg/head/face?* • *Do you feel pain in other areas of your body?*
Severity	• *How bad is it? How would you rate it on a scale of one to ten if one were almost no pain and ten was the worst pain you could imagine?* Use the validated VAS—visual analog scale—to quantify the level of pain and impairment. • *Does this problem prevent you from engaging in your daily activities, such as work, exercise, or hobbies?* This is a very important question for determining functional impairment and internal consistency; if the patient is "too injured to work" yet is still able to fully participate in recreational activities that are physically challenging, then malingering is likely.
Timing	• *When do you notice this problem?* • *Is it constant, or does it come and go? Where are you when you notice it the most?* • *Is it worse in the morning, or worse in the evening?* • *Does anyone else in your [home/office/worksite] have this same problem?* • *What times of the day or what days of the week is it the worst?*

Category	Patient history questions and implications
Associated manifestations and constitutional symptoms	• *Have you noticed any other problems associated with this problem?* • ***Fatigue?*** • ***Fever?*** • ***Weight loss?*** *Weight gain?* • *Night **sweats?*** • ***Diarrhea? Constipation?*** • ***Weakness?*** • *Nausea?* • *Bowel or bladder difficulties or changes? Difficulty with sexual function?* These could be related to hormonal imbalances, drug side-effects, relationship problems, nutritional deficiencies, nerve compression, and/or depression. • *Change in sensation near your anus/genitals?* Cauda equina syndrome is an important consideration in patients with low-back pain. • *Loss of appetite?* • *Difficulty sleeping?* • *Skin rash or change in pigmentation?*
ROS: review of systems	• <u>**General constitution**</u>: fatigue, malaise, fever, chills, weight gain/loss… • *"Now we are going to conduct a head-to-toe inventory just to make sure that we have covered everything."* • <u>**Head**</u>: headaches, head pain, pressure inside head, difficulty concentrating, difficulty remembering, mental function • <u>**Ears:**</u> ringing in ears, dizziness, hearing loss, hypersensitivity to noise, ear pain, discharge from ear, pressure in ears • <u>**Eyes:**</u> eye pain, loss of vision or decreased vision or ability to focus, redness or irritation, seeing flashing lights or spots, double vision • <u>**Nose**</u>: sinus problems, chronically stuffy nose, difficulty smelling things, nose bleeds, change or decrease in sense of smell or taste • <u>**Mouth**</u>, teeth, TMJ, pain or sores in mouth, difficulty chewing, sensitive teeth, bleeding gums, pain in jaw joint, change or decrease in sense of taste • <u>**Neck:**</u> pain at the base of skull, pain in neck, stiffness • <u>**Throat:**</u> difficulty swallowing, pain in throat, feeling like things get stuck in throat, change in voice, difficulty getting air or food in or out • <u>**Chest and breasts**</u>: any chest pain, difficult breathing, wheezing, coughing, pain, lumps, or discharge from nipple • <u>**Shoulders:**</u> pain or aching in your shoulders, restricted motion or stiffness • <u>**Arms, elbows, hands:**</u> pain or problems with your arms, elbows, hands …in the joints or the muscles…, numbness, tingling, weakness, swelling, changes in fingernails, cold hands? • <u>**Stomach, abdomen, pelvis, genitals, urinary tract, rectum,**</u> **:** pain in stomach or abdomen, difficulty with digestion, gas, bloating, regurgitation, ulcer, any problems lower down in your abdomen—near your lower intestines? Pain, lumps, swelling, difficulty passing stool, pain or itching near your anus, genitalia; any genital pain, burning, discharge, redness, irritation, sexual dysfunction or impotence, loss of bowel or bladder control? Diarrhea or constipation? How often do you have a bowel movement? • <u>**Hips, legs, knees, ankles, feet:**</u> numbness, weakness, pain or tingling in the hips, knees, ankles, or feet; pain in calves with walking, swelling of ankles, cold feet • *Are you aware of anything else that you think I should know in order to help you?*

Components of a Complete Patient History: "D.O.P.P. Q.R.S.T."—*continued*

Category	Patient history questions and implications

Medical history	• *Are you taking any* **medications**? *What medications have you taken in the past few years?* Finding out that your new patient recently discontinued his 20-year regimen of valproic acid, lithium, and risperidone may significantly change your interpretation of the clinical interview. Likewise, a patient may not be taking immunosuppressive drugs on the day of your first clinical encounter—he or she may have discontinued such drugs against medical advice (AMA) the week prior to consulting with you.
	• *Have you been* **treated for any medical conditions** *or health problems?*
	• *Have you ever been* **hospitalized**?
	• *Have you ever had* **surgery**?
	• *Have you ever been* **diagnosed with any health problems** *such as high blood pressure or diabetes?*
	• Investigate for specific problems in the past health history that would be a major oversight to miss:
	   o Current or past diseases: cancer, diabetes, psychosis, infections, immune disorders
	   o Hypertension or high cholesterol
	   o Medications, especially corticosteroids
	   o Surgeries, hospitalizations, trauma or previous injuries

Social history	• **Work**—*What do you do for work? Are you exposed to chemicals or fumes at your workplace?* • **Hobbies**—*What do you do for recreation or hobbies? Are you exposed to chemicals or fumes at home or with your hobbies (e.g., painting, gardening)?* • **Eat**—*Tell me about your breakfast, lunch, dinner, snacks… Do you consume foods or drinks that contain aspartame* (linked to increased incidence of brain tumors[70]) *or carrageenan* (possibly linked to increased risk of breast cancer and inflammatory bowel disease[71,72])? • **Exercise**—*What do you do for exercise or physical activity?* • **Drink**—*Do you* **drink alcohol**? *Coffee/caffeine? Water?* • **Drugs**—*Do you use recreational* **drugs**? **Now or in the past?** • **Smoke**—*Do you* **smoke**? *Have you ever smoked on a regular basis?* • **Sex**—*Are you* **sexually active**? *If so, do you practice safer sex practices? For all women: Is there any chance you could be pregnant right now? A "yes" reply may contraindicate radiographic assessment and the use of certain nutrients, botanicals, and/or drugs.* • **Emotional support, family contact, relationships**: The typical American has no-one in whom to confide and has a social network of two people[73]; in all; Americans are the most medicated/drugged and most socially isolated society that has ever existed.
Family health history	• *Does anyone in your family have any health problems, especially your parents and siblings?* • *Do you have any children? Do they have any health problems?* • *Do any diseases "run in the family" such as cancer, diabetes, arthritis, heart disease?*
Additional questions	• *Do you have any other information for me? Is there anything that I did not ask?* • *What is your opinion as to why you are having this health problem?* • *Are you in litigation for your illness or injuries?*

---

[70] "In the past two decades brain tumor rates have risen in several industrialized countries, including the United States... Compared to other environmental factors putatively linked to brain tumors, the artificial sweetener aspartame is a promising candidate to explain the recent increase in incidence and degree of malignancy of brain tumors." Olney JW, Farber NB, Spitznagel E, Robins LN. Increasing brain tumor rates: is there a link to aspartame? *J Neuropathol Exp Neurol* 1996 Nov;55(11):1115-23

[71] Tobacman JK. Review of harmful gastrointestinal effects of carrageenan in animal experiments. *Environ Health Perspect.* 2001 Oct;109(10):983-94

[72] "However, the gum carrageenan which is comprised of linked, sulfated galactose residues has potent biological activity and undergoes acid hydrolysis to poligeenan, an acknowledged carcinogen." Tobacman JK, Wallace RB, Zimmerman MB. Consumption of carrageenan and other water-soluble polymers used as food additives and incidence of mammary carcinoma. *Med Hypotheses.* 2001 May;56(5):589-98

[73] "Discussion networks are smaller in 2004 than in 1985. The number of people saying there is no one with whom they discuss important matters nearly tripled. The mean network size decreases by about a third (one confidant), from 2.94 in 1985 to 2.08 in 2004. The modal respondent now reports having no confidant; the modal respondent in 1985 had three confidants." McPherson M, Smith-Lovin L, Brashears ME. Social Isolation in America. *American Sociological Review* June 2006 71: 353-375

Patients can be asked to <u>localize</u> and <u>describe</u> their pain/discomfort on drawings such as these. *Examples of descriptions:*

- Numb
- Hypersensitive
- Tingling

- Shooting pain
- Electrical pain
- Stabbing pain

- Burning pain
- Dull ache
- Muscle weakness

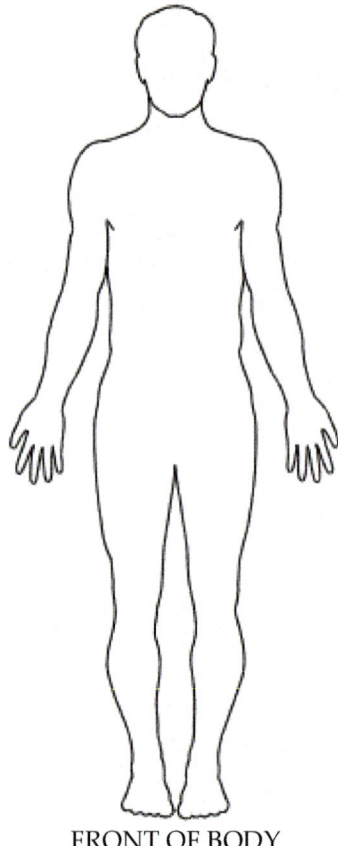

FRONT OF BODY

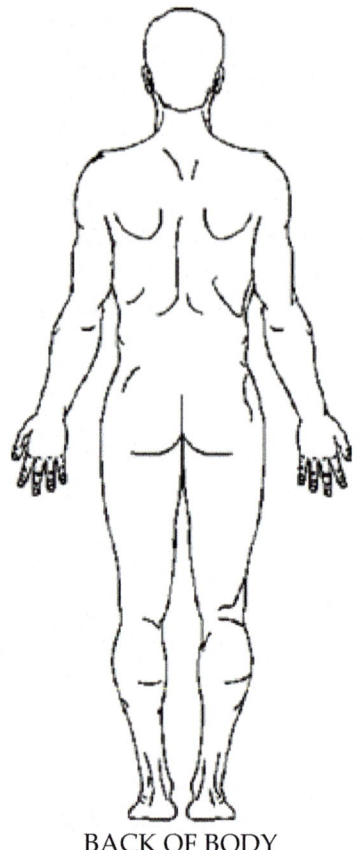

BACK OF BODY

On the lines below, indicate the location of pain/discomfort and then quantify it by placing an "X" on the line.

Location of pain:_____

No pain at all	Worst pain imaginable

Location of pain:_____

No pain at all	Worst pain imaginable

Location of pain:_____

No pain at all	Worst pain imaginable

Review of Systems—checklist: Patients/clients are asked to provide more information by the arrow "→", also at the bottom of each page, and/or whereever more detail is warranted. This form can be completed by the clinician and/or by the client.

GENERAL HEALTH	Very rare-None	Occasional-Mild	Intermittent-Moderate	Frequent-Severe
Fatigue, lack of energy, lack of stamina	❑ 0	❑ 1	❑ 2	❑ 3
Need to decrease or alter activities of daily living due to fatigue, pain, or illness	❑ 0	❑ 1	❑ 2	❑ 3
Insomnia, lack of sleep	❑ 0	❑ 1	❑ 2	❑ 3
Excessive tiredness and increased need for sleep	❑ 0	❑ 1	❑ 2	❑ 3
Tired and/or not hungry after waking	❑ 0	❑ 1	❑ 2	❑ 3
Pain at night, night sweats	❑ 0	❑ 1	❑ 2	❑ 3
Enlarged lymph nodes	❑ 0	❑ 1	❑ 2	❑ 3
Frequent infections	❑ 0	❑ 1	❑ 2	❑ 3
Undesired weight loss	❑ 0	❑ 1	❑ 2	❑ 3
Undesired weight gain, difficulty losing weight	❑ 0	❑ 1	❑ 2	❑ 3
Cold hands or feet	❑ 0	❑ 1	❑ 2	❑ 3
Compulsive/binge eating, increased appetite	❑ 0	❑ 1	❑ 2	❑ 3
Decreased appetite	❑ 0	❑ 1	❑ 2	❑ 3
Hypoglycemia, low blood sugar	❑ 0	❑ 1	❑ 2	❑ 3
Allergies to food or environment	❑ 0	❑ 1	❑ 2	❑ 3
Sensitivity to fumes, chemicals, odors, exhaust	❑ 0	❑ 1	❑ 2	❑ 3
Have you been tested for iron disorders?	❑ NO	❑ YES	❑ ?	
Past diagnosis of serious illness or chronic health condition such a systemic disease, cancer, HIV, mental condition, heart disease, infection, kidney problems, or other condition	❑ NO	❑ YES→		

MUSCLES and JOINTS	Very rare-None	Occasional-Mild	Intermittent-Moderate	Frequent-Severe
Pain, swelling, or limited motion in joint(s)	❑ 0	❑ 1	❑ 2	❑ 3
Pain, swelling, or weakness in muscle(s)	❑ 0	❑ 1	❑ 2	❑ 3
Cramps in muscles, grind teeth at night?	❑ 0	❑ 1	❑ 2	
Other problem, concerns, or questions in this area?	❑ NO	❑ YES→		

HEAD and MIND	Very rare-None	Occasional-Mild	Intermittent-Moderate	Frequent-Severe
Headaches	❑ 0	❑ 1	❑ 2	❑ 3
Feeling of pressure inside head	❑ 0	❑ 1	❑ 2	❑ 3
Faintness, loss of consciousness	❑ 0	❑ 1	❑ 2	❑ 3
Dizziness	❑ 0	❑ 1	❑ 2	❑ 3
Seizures, epilepsy	❑ 0	❑ 1	❑ 2	❑ 3
Difficulty thinking or processing information; confusion	❑ 0	❑ 1	❑ 2	❑ 3
Difficulty with concentrating or maintaining attention	❑ 0	❑ 1	❑ 2	❑ 3
Poor memory	❑ 0	❑ 1	❑ 2	❑ 3
Difficulty speaking or talking, slurred speech	❑ 0	❑ 1	❑ 2	❑ 3
Hyperactivity	❑ 0	❑ 1	❑ 2	❑ 3
Learning difficulties, dyslexia	❑ 0	❑ 1	❑ 2	❑ 3
Other problem, concern, or question in this area?	❑ NO	❑ YES→		

Additional notes or comments:

EMOTIONS and SOCIAL HEALTH	Very rare-None	Occasional-Mild	Intermittent-Moderate	Frequent-Severe
Depression, sadness	❑ 0	❑ 1	❑ 2	❑ 3
Anger, irritability, anxiety	❑ 0	❑ 1	❑ 2	❑ 3
Stressful situations	❑ 0	❑ 1	❑ 2	❑ 3
Apathy, lack of interest or concern	❑ 0	❑ 1	❑ 2	❑ 3
Use of alcohol, herbs, drugs, or medications to help manage emotions	❑ 0	❑ 1	❑ 2	❑ 3
Isolation, few friends, distant family	❑ 0	❑ 1	❑ 2	❑ 3
Problems with parents or family	❑ 0	❑ 1	❑ 2	❑ 3
Problems with employer(s) or coworker(s)	❑ 0	❑ 1	❑ 2	❑ 3
Sadness or recurrent problems from childhood or past events	❑ 0	❑ 1	❑ 2	❑ 3
Recent or current thoughts of suicide?	❑ **NO**	❑ **YES→**		
Diagnosed mental condition such as bipolar, schizophrenia, or other condition	❑ NO	❑ YES→		
Other problem, concern, or question in this area?	❑ NO	❑ YES→		
EYES	Very rare-None	Occasional-Mild	Intermittent-Moderate	Frequent-Severe
Watery, red, or itchy eyes	❑ 0	❑ 1	❑ 2	❑ 3
Dark circles under eyes	❑ 0	❑ 1	❑ 2	❑ 3
Decrease or loss of vision; cataracts, or glaucoma	❑ **0**	❑ **1**	❑ **2**	❑ **3**
Poor night vision, night blindness	❑ 0	❑ 1	❑ 2	❑ 3
Pain in eye(s)	❑ 0	❑ 1	❑ 2	❑ 3
Pain near or behind eye(s)	❑ 0	❑ 1	❑ 2	❑ 3
Other problem, concern, or question in this area?	❑ NO	❑ YES→		
EARS	Very rare-None	Occasional-Mild	Intermittent-Moderate	Frequent-Severe
Earaches, pain in ear(s)	❑ 0	❑ 1	❑ 2	❑ 3
Ringing in ear(s)	❑ 0	❑ 1	❑ 2	❑ 3
Ear infections	❑ 0	❑ 1	❑ 2	❑ 3
Decrease or loss of hearing	❑ 0	❑ 1	❑ 2	❑ 3
Other problem, concern, or question in this area?	❑ NO	❑ YES→		
MOUTH, NOSE, and THROAT	Very rare-None	Occasional-Mild	Intermittent-Moderate	Frequent-Severe
Swollen or tender tongue or gums	❑ 0	❑ 1	❑ 2	❑ 3
Decreased sense of taste or smell	❑ 0	❑ 1	❑ 2	❑ 3
Stuffy nose, nasal congestion	❑ 0	❑ 1	❑ 2	❑ 3
Sinus infections, sinus pain	❑ 0	❑ 1	❑ 2	❑ 3
Nasal polyps	❑ 0	❑ 1	❑ 2	❑ 3
Ulcers or sores in mouth or lips, oral herpes	❑ 0	❑ 1	❑ 2	❑ 3
Allergies/ sneezing/ runny nose	❑ 0	❑ 1	❑ 2	❑ 3
Excessive mucus formation	❑ 0	❑ 1	❑ 2	❑ 3
Drainage to back of throat	❑ 0	❑ 1	❑ 2	❑ 3
Sore throat	❑ 0	❑ 1	❑ 2	❑ 3
Cough or wheeze	❑ 0	❑ 1	❑ 2	❑ 3
Change in voice	❑ 0	❑ 1	❑ 2	❑ 3
Hoarseness, loss of voice	❑ 0	❑ 1	❑ 2	❑ 3
Other problem, concern, or question in this area?	❑ NO	❑ YES→		

LUNGS and HEART	Very rare-None	Occasional-Mild	Intermittent-Moderate	Frequent-Severe
Pain in left arm and/or left side of neck or face	❏ 0	❏ 1	❏ 2	❏ 3
Shortness of breath, difficulty breathing	❏ 0	❏ 1	❏ 2	❏ 3
Irregular heartbeat	❏ 0	❏ 1	❏ 2	❏ 3
Rapid or pounding heartbeat	❏ 0	❏ 1	❏ 2	❏ 3
Chest congestion, bronchitis	❏ 0	❏ 1	❏ 2	❏ 3
Asthma	❏ 0	❏ 1	❏ 2	❏ 3
Medications for lungs or heart	❏ 0	❏ 1	❏ 2	❏ 3
Current or past cigarette smoking or tobacco use	❏ 0	❏ 1	❏ 2	❏ 3
Pain in chest	❏ NO	❏ YES→		
High blood pressure, high cholesterol, or high triglycerides?	❏ NO	❏ YES→		
Other problem, concern, or question in this area?	❏ NO	❏ YES→		
SKIN, HAIR, and NAILS	Very rare-None	Occasional-Mild	Intermittent-Moderate	Frequent-Severe
Acne	❏ 0	❏ 1	❏ 2	❏ 3
Eczema	❏ 0	❏ 1	❏ 2	❏ 3
Psoriasis	❏ 0	❏ 1	❏ 2	❏ 3
Dry skin	❏ 0	❏ 1	❏ 2	❏ 3
Oily skin	❏ 0	❏ 1	❏ 2	❏ 3
Flushing, hot flashes	❏ 0	❏ 1	❏ 2	❏ 3
Itchy skin (with or without redness) or hives	❏ 0	❏ 1	❏ 2	❏ 3
Decrease in body or facial hair	❏ 0	❏ 1	❏ 2	❏ 3
Decrease in head hair (not male pattern baldness)	❏ 0	❏ 1	❏ 2	❏ 3
Increase in body or facial hair	❏ 0	❏ 1	❏ 2	❏ 3
Excessive sweating	❏ 0	❏ 1	❏ 2	❏ 3
Insufficient sweating when hot or active	❏ 0	❏ 1	❏ 2	❏ 3
Area(s) of numbness	❏ 0	❏ 1	❏ 2	❏ 3
Area(s) of tingling	❏ 0	❏ 1	❏ 2	❏ 3
Area(s) of pain	❏ 0	❏ 1	❏ 2	❏ 3
Weak or ridged fingernails	❏ NO	❏ YES		
Change in skin color or pigmentation, vitiligo	❏ NO	❏ YES		
Small rough bumps on back of upper arms	❏ NO	❏ YES		
Other problem, concerns, or questions in this area?	❏ NO	❏ YES→		
STOMACH and DIGESTIVE TRACT	Very rare-None	Occasional-Mild	Intermittent-Moderate	Frequent-Severe
Heartburn	❏ 0	❏ 1	❏ 2	❏ 3
Poor digestion	❏ 0	❏ 1	❏ 2	❏ 3
Nausea	❏ 0	❏ 1	❏ 2	❏ 3
Vomiting	❏ 0	❏ 1	❏ 2	❏ 3
Diarrhea	❏ 0	❏ 1	❏ 2	❏ 3
Constipation	❏ 0	❏ 1	❏ 2	❏ 3
Belching, intestinal bloating, gas or flatulence	❏ 0	❏ 1	❏ 2	❏ 3
Pain in stomach, intestines, colon	❏ 0	❏ 1	❏ 2	❏ 3
Rectal itching, pain, or bleeding	❏ 0	❏ 1	❏ 2	❏ 3
Hemorrhoids	❏ 0	❏ 1	❏ 2	❏ 3
Loss of bowel control, incontinence	❏ 0	❏ 1	❏ 2	❏ 3
Other problem, concern, or question in this area?	❏ NO	❏ YES→		

KIDNEYS and GENITALS	Very rare-None	Occasional-Mild	Intermittent-Moderate	Frequent-Severe
Kidney stones	❑ 0	❑ 1	❑ 2	❑ 3
Other kidney problems	❑ 0	❑ 1	❑ 2	❑ 3
Difficulty controlling urination, incontinence	❑ 0	❑ 1	❑ 2	❑ 3
Bladder problems (other than infections)	❑ 0	❑ 1	❑ 2	❑ 3
Frequent urination	❑ 0	❑ 1	❑ 2	❑ 3
Pain or burning with urination	❑ 0	❑ 1	❑ 2	❑ 3
Discharge or blood in urine	❑ 0	❑ 1	❑ 2	❑ 3
Urinary tract (kidney, bladder, urethra) infection(s)	❑ 0	❑ 1	❑ 2	❑ 3
Sexually transmitted disease(s)	❑ 0	❑ 1	❑ 2	❑ 3
Genital herpes	❑ 0	❑ 1	❑ 2	❑ 3
Low sex drive, low libido	❑ 0	❑ 1	❑ 2	❑ 3
Have you been tested for HIV?	❑ Negative	❑ Positive	❑ Not tested	
Other problem, concern, or question in this area?	❑ NO	❑ YES→		

For **WOMEN** only	Very rare-None	Occasional-Mild	Intermittent-Moderate	Frequent-Severe
Irregular menses	❑ 0	❑ 1	❑ 2	❑ 3
Painful menses	❑ 0	❑ 1	❑ 2	❑ 3
Pain between menses	❑ 0	❑ 1	❑ 2	❑ 3
Painful, swollen, or fibrocystic breasts	❑ 0	❑ 1	❑ 2	❑ 3
Water retention	❑ 0	❑ 1	❑ 2	❑ 3
Premenstrual syndrome	❑ 0	❑ 1	❑ 2	❑ 3
Excessive bleeding	❑ 0	❑ 1	❑ 2	❑ 3
Abnormal uterine/vaginal bleeding	❑ NO	❑ YES→		
Missed menses	❑ 0	❑ 1	❑ 2	❑ 3
Vaginal dryness, irritation, painful intercourse	❑ 0	❑ 1	❑ 2	❑ 3
Yeast infections	❑ 0	❑ 1	❑ 2	❑ 3
Uterine fibroids	❑ NO	❑ YES		
Menopausal symptoms or concerns	❑ NO	❑ YES→		
Infertility	❑ NO	❑ YES		
Annual Pap smear, breast examination, and health checkup?	❑ NO	❑ YES		
Family history of breast, uterine, or ovarian cancer	❑ NO	❑ YES→		
Other problem, injury, concern in this area?	❑ NO	❑ YES→		

For **MEN** only	Very rare-None	Occasional-Mild	Intermittent-Moderate	Frequent-Severe
Pain or difficulty obtaining or maintaining erection	❑ 0	❑ 1	❑ 2	❑ 3
Pain or difficulty with ejaculation	❑ 0	❑ 1	❑ 2	❑ 3
Pain or mass in testicles	❑ 0	❑ 1	❑ 2	❑ 3
Slow stream of urine or frequent urination	❑ 0	❑ 1	❑ 2	❑ 3
Undescended testis, testis in abdomen or pelvis	❑ NO	❑ YES		
Men over 50: annual PSA test and prostate exam?	❑ NO	❑ YES		
Family history of prostate cancer	❑ NO	❑ YES→		
Other problem, injury, concern in this area?	❑ NO	❑ YES→		

Additional notes or comments:

_____

_____

Physical Examination

Because these books are used in graduate/doctorate courses wherein students need to integrate—or at least have some exposure to—real-world clinical concepts, I have kept these sections from my teaching notes within the book. Experienced clinicians might appreciate the review, perhaps even learn something new.

<u>Goals and purpose of the orthopedic/musculoskeletal/neurologic examination</u>:
1. **To establish an** accurate diagnosis (or diagnoses),
2. To assess the patient's functional status and current condition,
   a. Range of motion,
   b. Muscle strength,
   c. Ability to perform activities/actions of daily living such as standing, walking, climbing stairs, reaching for overhead objects, etc.
3. To assess, quantify (amount), and qualify (type[s]) of pain—if present,
4. **To assess for** concomitant and/or underlying and preexisting problems,
5. To exclude ("rule out") emergency situations and occult-yet-impending disasters,
6. To contextualize/integrate all of the above into a cohesive multidimensional assessment and plan.
- *Example*: If your patient presents with low back and leg pain, and you determine that his fall off a horse resulted in ischial bursitis, have you also excluded a lumbar compression fracture? You can send the patient home with anti-inflammatory treatments and icepacks for the bursitis; but if you missed the spinal fracture, your patient could suffer neurologic injury resultant from your "failure to diagnose." Don't assume that the patient has only one problem until you have proven with your history and examination that other likely problems do not exist.

<u>Functional assessment</u>: When working with patients with acute injuries and systemic diseases, take a wider view of the patient than simply diagnosing the problem.
- Will she be able to return to work?
- Will he be able to drive home safely?
- Will she need help with activities of daily living?
- Is there an occult disease, infection, malignancy, or toxic exposure that is causing these problems?
- Is this an acute presentation of a new problem, or an acute exacerbation of a chronic problem?

<u>Neurologic examination</u>: One of the most important areas to assess when a patient presents with a musculoskeletal complaint is the neurologic system, especially if the complaint is related to a recent traumatic injury. Blood circulation is essential for life; but lack of circulation is only a major consideration in a small number of injuries, and it is usually readily apparent when severe because the problem will become acute quickly. Nerve injuries, however, can be subtle. All patients with spine (neck, thoracic, low back) pain must be questioned thoroughly for evidence of neurologic compromise. Neurologic insults—such as cauda equina syndrome and transverse myelitis—can be painless, can progress rapidly, and can lead to permanent functional disability from muscle weakness or paralysis. Every patient with pain, weakness, or recent trauma must be evaluated for neurologic deficits before the patient is treated and released from care. Neurologic examinations are briefly reviewed in the pages that follow; citations can be used for sources of additional information.

<u>Resources for students on neurologic assessment</u>:
- Goldberg S. *The Four-Minute Neurologic Exam*. Medmaster medmaster.net/
- neuroexam.com/neuroexam/ Information and free videos of a neurologic exam.
- Excellent interactive simulation of assessment of extraocular muscles in a neurologic examination: rad.usuhs.mil/rad/eye_simulator/eyesimulator.html
- Excellent review, noteworthy for its description of a "+5" level of reflex grading denoting sustained clonus: emedicine.medscape.com/article/1147993-overview

Orthopedic Musculoskeletal Examination: Concepts and Goals

Orthopedic tests are detailed or reviewed in each respective chapter of _Integrative Orthopedics_[74] (i.e., shoulder exams are in the chapter on shoulders, knee exams in the chapter on knees). This section reviews the concepts and goals that provide the rationale for performing these tests. Orthopedic tests are designed to place particular types of stress on specific body tissues. Types of stress include tension/distraction, compression/pressure, shear force, vibration, friction, and percussion. Each type of stress is applied to elicit specific information about the exact tissue or structure that is being tested. If you understand the reason for the type of stress that you are applying, and you are aware of the tissue/structure that you are testing, then you will find it much easier to perform the dozens of tests that are required in clinical practice. If you understand the "how" and the "why" then you won't be overwhelmed with named tests that otherwise appear illogical or superfluous.

The tests that are described in _Integrative Orthopedics_ meet at least one of the following two criteria: 1) it is a common test that all doctors know and which is needed for the sake of communication and for passing academic and licensing examinations, or 2) it is going to be a useful test in clinical practice.

Always remember that abnormalities found during the physical examination—particularly the neurologic examination—are often indicative of an underlying _nonmusculoskeletal_ problem that must be identified or—at the very least—considered and then excluded by additional testing. For example, a patient shoulder pain and neurologic deficits found during the neuromusculoskeletal portion of your examination could have a herniated cervical disc as the underlying cause; but the cause could also be syringomyelia, or an apical lung tumor that is invading local bone and destroying the nerves of the brachial plexus.[75]

As a clinician, the successful management and treatment of your patients depends in large part on the following: ❶ knowledge: your ability to conceptualize broadly and to consider many _functional_ and _pathologic_ causes of your patient's complaints, ❷ tact: the efficiency and accuracy with which you assess, accept, and exclude the various differential diagnoses into your final working diagnosis from which your treatment, management, referral, and co-management decisions are made, ❸ art: your ability to create the changes in your patient's outlook, lifestyle, biochemistry, biomechanics/anatomy, and physiology to effect the desired outcome.

Types of stress applied during the physical examination for specific purposes

- **Tension, traction**: To provoke pain from injured/compromised tissues: tendons, muscles, ligaments, and nerves
- **Compression, pressure**: To provoke pain from inflamed tissues; also used to assess for swelling and fluid accumulation in subcutaneous tissue, bursa, and joint spaces such as the knee
- **Shearing force**: To test the integrity of ligaments and intervertebral discs
- **Vibration (using ultrasound or 128 Hz tuning fork)**: To assess vibration sense (neurologic: peripheral nerves and dorsal columns) and screen for broken bones (orthopedic)
- **Friction, grinding**: To elicit pain from injured tissues (cross-fiber friction) and articular surfaces (grinding tests)
- **Percussion, over bone and discs**: To assess for bone fractures, bone infections, and acute disc injuries
- **Percussion, over peripheral nerves**: To assess hypesthesia/tingling suggesting reduced threshold for depolarization secondary to nerve irritation or compression, i.e., Tinel's sign
- **Fulcrum tests**: To assess for bone fractures: commonly the doctor's arm or a firm object is placed centrally under the bone in question and increasingly firm downward stress is applied to both ends of the bone to test for occult fracture
- **Torque, twisting**: To test joint integrity (restriction or laxity) or for occult bone fracture (particularly of the digits)

---

[74] Vasquez A. _Integrative Orthopedics_. InflammationMastery.com
[75] "Pancoast tumor has long been implicated as a cause of brachial plexopathy...The possibility of Pancoast lesion should be considered not only in the presence of brachial plexopathy, but also when C8 or T1 radiculopathy is found." Vargo et al. Pancoast tumor presenting as cervical radiculopathy. _Arch Phys Med Rehabil._ 1990 Jul;71(8):606-9

Neurologic Assessment

Clinical neurology is a complex yet very rewarding area of study. While most of us have the experience of extreme challenge when studying Neuroanatomy for the first time as medical/health science students, that initial confusion and apprehension eventually gives way to a relaxed understanding of the essential structures and pathways, allowing for facile clinical assessment and rapid localization of neurologic lesions. A reasonable strategy for managing the observance of abnormal findings on the neurologic exam is—just as with all other abnormal findings—to verify/qualify, assess, and manage.

1. **Presence**: Is this patient's presentation *neuropathologically* abnormal, a normal variant, or presentation of something otherwise explainable, such as an adverse drug effect or nutritional deficiency?

2. **Assessment**: If it is *neuropathologically* abnormal, does it indicate a specific disease or lesion? What is the appropriate assessment?

3. **Referral/management**: Does this condition require referral to a specialist or emergency care?

Reliable indicators of organic (real) neurologic disease:
These cannot be feigned and must be assumed to reveal organic neurologic illness that must be evaluated by a neurologist: • Significant asymmetry of pupillary light reflex,   • Ocular divergence,   • Papilledema,   • Marked nystagmus,   • Muscle atrophy and fasciculation,   • Muscle weakness with neurologic deficit; upper motor neuron lesions (UMNL) indicate a central nervous system (CNS) lesion and need to be fully evaluated by a specialist; the need for referral is less necessary in cases of peripheral neuropathy of known cause.

Every clinician needs thorough training in anatomy and clinical neurology to be competent in the management of patients, because even common problems such as "pain" and "fatigue" and "headache" may herald devastating neurologic illness that must be assessed accurately and managed skillfully. While a complete review of clinical neurology is beyond the scope of this text, the following section provides a basic review of the clinical essentials. The concise clinical reviews by Goldberg[76,77] are excellent.

The purpose of the neurologic examination is to qualify ("yes" or "no") the presence of a neurologic deficit, and—if present—to localize the lesion so that it can be further assessed with the proper laboratory, imaging, electrodiagnostic, or biopsy techniques. The following 9-point summary of localized lesions does not supplant independent studies of neurology and neuroanatomy but is useful for a quick clinically-relevant review:

1. **Cerebral cortex and internal capsule**: Neurologic deficit depends on location of lesion but is typically a combination of sensory/motor deficit and impaired higher neurologic function such as comprehension (superior temporal gyrus) or socially appropriate behavior (frontal lobe, ventral frontal gyri).

2. **Basal ganglia and striatal system**: Athetosis (lentiform nucleus: putamen and globus pallidus), (hemi)ballism (subthalamic nucleus), chorea (putamen), akinesia, bradykinesia, hypokinesia (lack of nigrostriatal dopamine).

3. **Cerebellum**: Ataxia, awkward clumsy execution of *intentional* motions; may have nystagmus, hypotonia.

4. **Brainstem**: Cranial nerve deficit(s) with contralateral distal sensory and/or UMN motor deficits.

5. **Spinal cord**: Cranial nerves and higher cortical functions are intact; lesion can be a combination of sensory and motor (UMN and LMN) deficits and the pattern distal to lesion may be a complete or incomplete pattern of sensory and motor deficits on one or both sides of body depending on area of spinal cord affected.

6. **Nerve root**: Segmental unilateral motor deficit; dermatomal distribution pain or sensory disturbance.

7. **Peripheral nerve**: Localized combination of sensory and motor deficits; may be bilateral or unilateral.

8. **Neuromuscular junction**: Painless weakness and "fatigable weakness": weakness that *worsens* with repeated testing; typically involves cranial nerves first in myasthenia gravis; also consider Lambert-Eaton Syndrome (LES: autoimmune neuromuscular junction disorder associated with occult malignancy; contrasts with myasthenia gravis in that in LES strength *increases* with repeated testing).

9. **Muscle disease**: Painless weakness, typically involving proximal hip/shoulder muscles first; test for elevated serum aldolase and (phospho)creatine kinase (aka, creatine phosphokinase, CK, CPK).

---

[76] Goldberg S. *Clinical Neuroanatomy Made Ridiculously Simple*. Miami, Medimaster, Inc, 1990. Now in a third edition with interactive CD.
[77] Goldberg S. *The Four-Minute Neurologic Exam*. Miami, Medimaster, Inc, 1992

Clinical assessments of neurologic function and structures

Cortex	Cerebellum
• <u>Orientation</u>: Person, place, time, situation • <u>Mood and cooperation</u>: E.g., calm vs agitated, cooperative vs noncooperative. • <u>Level of consciousness</u>: Alert, lethargic, stupor, coma (indirect assessment of reticular system in brainstem) • <u>Memory</u>: Remember objects or numbers; *recent* memory is most commonly affected by brain lesions: *What day of the month is it? How did you get here?* • <u>Mentation</u>: *Count backward from 100 by 7's.* • <u>Spelling</u>: *Spell the word "hand" backwards.* • <u>Stereognosis</u>: Identify by touch a familiar object such as a key or coin. • <u>Hoffman's reflex</u>: Doctor rapidly extends distal joint of patient's middle finger and watches for patient's hand to perform grasp reflex; this test is performed for motor tract lesions involving the cerebral cortex, cerebellum, and upper motor neurons of the spinal cord. • <u>Pronator drift</u>: Supinated hands and arms outstretched forward for 30 seconds; doctor taps on palms; falling of hands and arms into pronation suggests UMNL. • <u>Babinski reflex</u>: Scraping the bottom of the foot results in splaying and flexing of the toes and extension (dorsiflexion) of the big toe; normal in infants.	• <u>Gait</u> (lesion: ataxia) • <u>Heel-to-toe walk</u> • <u>Tandem gait</u> • <u>Hand flip</u>, <u>foot tap</u> (lesion: dysdiadochokinesia) • <u>Finger-to-nose</u>: Patient reaches out to doctor's finger, then patient touches patient nose, then back to new location of doctor's finger. • <u>Heel-to-shin</u>: Slide heel along shin. • <u>Walk in circle around chair</u> • <u>Move eyes in a rapid "figure 8"</u>: Technique for provoking latent nystagmus • <u>Rhomberg's test</u>: Patient stands with feet close together and eyes closed; tests proprioception (peripheral nerves, dorsal columns, spinocerebellar tracts); vision (eyes open tests optic righting reflex) and coordinated motor activity (cerebellum).

Several of the above '"cerebral" deficits may also result from intoxicative, nutritional, or metabolic disorders rather than an organic irreversible physical lesion. Likewise "cerebellar" deficits may also result from lesion of the brainstem tracts/nuclei and cerebellar peduncles, rather than the cerebellum itself.

Brainstem and Cranial Nerves	Spinal Cord, Roots, Nerves

1. Olfactory: **smell**
• Smell: Test with strong and common odors such as coffee; do not use ammonia or other irritants which are perceived via trigeminal nerve (cranial nerve 5)
• This is a worthwhile test in patients with recent head trauma (direct or indirect) such as from motor vehicle accidents (MVA); any violent motion of the head may result in injury to the olfactory fibers passing through the cribiform plate; patients may have associated anosmia or altered sense of flavor; frontal lobe disorders such as altered social behavior may be noted in lesioned patients
2. Ophthalmic: **reading, peripheral vision, fundoscopic**
• Snellen chart for far vision, Rosenbaum card for near vision
• Peripheral vision
• Fundoscopic examination
3. Oculomotor: **move eyes and constrict pupils**
• Eye motion in cardinal fields of gaze
• Pupil contraction to light
• Pupil contraction to accommodation
4. Trochlear: **motor to superior oblique**
• Look "down and in" toward nose
5. Trigeminal: **bite, sensory to face and eyes**
• Bite (motor to muscles of mastication)
• Feel (sensory to face, eyes, and tongue)
6. Abducens: **motor to lateral rectus**
• Looks laterally to the ear
7. Facial: **face muscles and taste to anterior tongue**
• Furrow forehead, close eyes forcefully, smile and frown
• Taste to anterior tongue
8. Vestibulocochlear: **hearing and balance**
• Hearing, Rinne-Weber tests[78]
• Balance: observe gait and Romberg test
9. Glossopharyngeal: **swallowing, and gag reflex**
• Swallow
• Gag reflex (sensory component)
10. Vagus: **motor to palate**
• Say "ahh" to raise uvula
• Gag reflex (motor component)
11. Spinal accessory: **motor to SCM and trapezius**
• Raise your shoulders (against resistance)
• Turn your head (against resistance)
12. Hypoglossal: **motor to tongue**
• Stick out tongue to front
	Motor and reflex
	• Strength: Specific muscles are tested and rated 0-5
	• Plantar (Babinski) reflex: Signifies UMNL
	• Abdominal reflexes: "Present" or "absent" (not rated 0-4); superficial reflexes are lost (rather than hyperactive) with UMNL
	    ○ Upper abdominal: T8-10
	    ○ Lower abdominal: T10-12
	• Anal reflex: Cauda equina and sacral nerve roots
	• Reflexes: Rate 0-4; asymmetric reflexes are more significant than finding absent or hyperactive (+3) reflexes; +4 reflex with sustained clonus is almost always pathologic and requires neurologist referral. Deep tendon reflexes with main spinal root levels are as follows:
	    ○ Biceps: C5
	    ○ Brachioradialis: C6
	    ○ Triceps: C7
	    ○ Patellar: L3-L4
	    ○ Hamstring: L5
	    ○ Achilles: S1
	Sensory
	• Light touch
	• Two-point discrimination
	• Vibration (use 128 Hz tuning fork)
	• Joint position sense and proprioception (eyes closed, locate position of joint)
	• Sharp and dull
	• Hot and cold
	• Sensory loss mapping (if deficits are found)
	• Romberg (peripheral nerves, dorsal columns, vestibular, cerebellar)
	• Nerve root tension tests such as straight leg raising
	• **Subjective pain and discomfort can be indicated on pain diagrams and VAS (visual analog scale) as shown on the following page**

---

[78] "The Rinne and Weber tuning fork tests are the most important tools in distinguishing between conductive and sensorineural hearing loss." Ruckenstein MJ. Hearing loss. A plan for individualized management. *Postgrad Med.* 1995 Oct;98(4):197-200, 203, 206

Deep tendon reflexes are summarized below and on the following page. Hyperreflexia is noted with upper motor neuron lesions (UMNL) in the cortex, subcortical nuclei, brainstem, or corticospinal tracts of the spinal cord, whereas hyporeflexia can result from lesions of lower motor neurons (LMNL) in spinal cord, peripheral nerves, as well as from sensory/afferent defects including diabetic neuropathy, vitamin B-12 deficiency, and Guillain-Barre disorder. Muscle strength should always be "five over five" to be considered normal, whereas in the testing of reflexes, symmetry/asymmetry is generally more important than the grade of response (except with sustained clonus). **Asymmetry of reflex or strength (especially when seen together) is never normal and requires clinical correlation and investigation.** Reflexes and strength are evaluated and graded per details in the following table.

Grading of deep tendon reflexes (DTR) and muscle strength

Deep tendon reflexes	Muscle strength
+5 <u>Hyperreflexia with sustained clonus</u>: Sustained clonus strongly suggests UMNL and requires investigation; most textbooks use a 0-4 scale, yet this 0-5 scale facilitates clear communication of observed lesions.[79]	5/5 <u>Normal: Full strength: able to withstand gravity and full resistance.</u>
+4 <u>Marked hyperreflexia</u>: Up to 4 beats of unsustained clonus may be normal[80]; suggests UMNL but may be caused by medications, electrolyte disturbances, etc.	4/5 <u>Partial strength</u>: Able to withstand gravity and partial resistance.
+3 <u>Hyperreflexia</u>: More than normal.	3/5 <u>Partial strength</u>: Only able to resist gravity.
+2 <u>Normal: Neither hyporeflexia nor hyperreflexia.</u>	2/5 <u>Partial strength</u>: Able to contract muscle but unable to resist gravity.
+1 <u>Hyporeflexia</u>: Less than normal	1/5 <u>Slight flicker of muscle contraction</u>: Does not result in joint movement.
0 <u>No reflex</u>: Requires clinical correlation for lesion of sensory receptors, peripheral nerve, spinal cord, anterior horn, or neuromuscular junction; this is a common finding in normal individuals.	0/5 <u>No clinically detectable contraction</u>: Correlate with lesion of peripheral nerve, cord, cerebrum, anterior horn, or neuromuscular junction.

---

[79] Oommen K, edited by Berman SA, et al. Neurological History and Physical Examination. Last Updated: October 4, 2006. *eMedicine* emedicine.com/neuro/topic632.htm
[80] "…three to four beats of clonus can be elicited at the ankles in some normal individuals." Waxman SG. *Clinical Neuroanatomy 25th Edition*. McGraw Hill, 2003, p 325

Laboratory Assessments: General Considerations of Commonly Used Tests

"The laboratory evaluation of patients with rheumatic disease is often informative but rarely definitive."[81]

Laboratory tests are immensely important in evaluating patients with musculoskeletal pain, as these tests allow the clinician to 1) assess for infection (e.g., subacute osteomyelitis), 2) quantify the degree of inflammation (i.e., with CRP or ESR), 3) assess or exclude other disease processes that may be the cause of pain or dysfunction, and 4) assess for concomitant diseases (e.g., septic arthritis complicating rheumatoid arthritis). Additionally, 5) these tests open the door to more complete patient care and holistic management of the whole person because they allow for a more comprehensive and complete understanding of the patient's underlying physiology. **The recommended routine is to use the following panel of tests when assessing patients with musculoskeletal pain: 1) CBC, 2) CRP, 3) chemistry/metabolic panel, and preferably also 4) ferritin, 5) 25(OH)-vitamin D, and 6) thyroid assessment, minimally including TSH** and optimally including free T4, total T3, reverse T3 and anti-thyroid antibodies. The use of a screening evaluation on a routine basis helps identify patients with occult diseases and also allows for more comprehensive management of the patient's overall health. Other tests are indicated in specific situations. *Orthopedics* relies heavily upon physical examination and imaging, whereas *Rheumatology* relies more heavily upon laboratory analysis. In Orthopedics, laboratory tests are used mainly for the purposes of discovering or excluding rheumatic and systemic diseases. In Rheumatology, lab tests are used to specifically identify the type of illness, quantify the severity of the condition, and to assess for concomitant illnesses and complications.

Essential Tests: These tests are *required* for *basic* patient assessment

Test	Purpose	Clinical application
CRP (or ESR)	Screening for infection, inflammation, and possibly cancer; if inflammation is present, then these tests allow for a generalized quantification of severity.	Useful in all new patients for helping to differentiate systemic/inflammatory disorders from those which are noninflammatory and mechanical. Also very helpful as a general "barometer" of health since higher values correlate with increased risk for diabetes mellitus and cardiovascular disease; thus this test helps bridge the gap between acute care and wellness promotion.
CBC	Screening for anemia, infection, certain cancers (namely leukemia).	Useful in any patient with nontraumatic musculoskeletal pain or systemic manifestations, especially fever or weight loss; occasionally detects occult B-12 and folate deficiencies.
Chemistry panel	Screening for diabetes, liver disease, kidney failure, bone lesions (alkaline phosphatase), electrolyte disturbances, adrenal insufficiency (hyponatremia with hyperkalemia), hypercalcemia, hyperparathyroidism, et al.	Use this panel in any patient with nontraumatic musculoskeletal pain or systemic manifestations; all patients with hypertension, diabetes, or who use medications that cause hepatotoxicity, nephrotoxicity, etc.
Thyroid assessments	Hypothyroidism is a common problem and is an often overlooked cause of musculoskeletal pain.[82]	This is a reasonable test panel (detailed later) for any patient with fatigue, cold extremities, depression, "arthritis", muscle pain, hypercholesterolemia, or other manifestations of hypothyroidism.
Serum ferritin	Determine iron status	Best test for iron overload and deficiency, both of which are of major importance—detailed in following sections

---

[81] Klippel JH (ed). *Primer on the Rheumatic Diseases. 11th Edition*. Atlanta: Arthritis Foundation. 1997 page 94
[82] "Hypothyroidism is frequently accompanied by musculoskeletal manifestations ranging from myalgias and arthralgias to true myopathy and arthritis." McLean RM, Podell DN. Bone and joint manifestations of hypothyroidism. *Semin Arthritis Rheum*. 1995 Feb;24(4):282-90

Overview of Important Tests: Additional Components of Routine Evaluation

Test	Purpose	Clinical Application
Ferritin— *recommended for all patients given the high prevalence and major significance of both iron overload and iron deficiency*	Important for assessing for iron overload (e.g., hemochromatoic polyarthropathy), and iron deficiency (e.g., low back pain due to colon cancer metastasis). Ferritin values less than 20 in adults (e.g., iron deficiency) or greater than 200 in women and 300 in men (e.g., iron overload) necessitate evaluation and effective treatment.	**Ferritin is the ideal test for both iron overload and iron deficiency.** All patients should be screened for hemochromatosis and other hereditary forms of iron overload regardless of age, gender, or ethnicity.[83] Iron deficiency—particularly in adults—may be the first clue to gastric/colon cancer and generally necessitates referral to gastroenterologist.
Serum 25-hydroxy-vitamin D, 25(OH)D	Vitamin D deficiency is a common cause of musculoskeletal pain and inflammation[84,85], and vitamin D deficiency is a significant risk factor for numerous serious health problems.[86,87,88]	Measurement of serum 25(OH) vitamin D (or empiric treatment with 2,000 – 4,000 IU vitamin D3 per day for adults) is indicated in patients with chronic musculoskeletal pain.[89,90] Optimal vitamin D status correlates with serum 25(OH)D levels of 50 – 100 ng/mL.[91]
Antinuclear antibodies (ANA)	Sensitive (but not specific) for the detection of several autoimmune diseases, especially systemic lupus erythematosus (SLE).	This test is particularly valuable for assessing patients with polyarthropathy, facial rash, and/or fatigue.
Rheumatoid factor (RF)	The primary value of this test is in supporting a diagnosis of rheumatoid arthritis; specificity is low.	RF may be positive in normal health, iron overload, chronic infections, hepatitis, sarcoidosis, and bacterial endocarditis.
Cyclic citrullinated protein (CCP) antibodies	Cyclic citrullinated protein (CCP) antibodies are currently the single best laboratory test for rheumatoid arthritis (RA) and have largely replaced RF.	Citrullinated protein antibodies are rapidly becoming *the test* for diagnosing and confirming RA; used with RF for highly specific "conjugate seropositivity."
Lactulose-mannitol assay	Assesses for malabsorption and excess intestinal permeability—"leaky gut."	Diagnostic test for intestinal damage; excellent nonspecific screening test for pathology or pathophysiology such as celiac and Crohn's disease.
Comprehensive parasitology, stool analysis	Identification and quantification of intestinal yeast, bacteria, and other microbes.	Extremely valuable test when working with patients with chronic fatigue syndromes, fibromyalgia, or autoimmunity.

[83] Vasquez A. Musculoskeletal disorders and iron overload disease: comment on the American College of Rheumatology guidelines for the initial evaluation of the adult patient with acute musculoskeletal symptoms. *Arthritis Rheum* 1996;39: 1767-8   InflammationMastery.com/reprints

[84] Masood et al. Persistent limb pain and raised serum alkaline phosphatase earliest markers subclinical hypovitaminosis D Kashmir. *Indian J Physiol Pharmacol* 1989;33:259-61

[85] Al Faraj S, Al Mutairi K. Vitamin D deficiency and chronic low back pain in Saudi Arabia. *Spine.* 2003 Jan 15;28(2):177-9

[86] Grant WB. An estimate of premature cancer mortality in the U.S. due to inadequate doses of solar ultraviolet-B radiation. *Cancer.* 2002;94(6):1867-75

[87] Zittermannn A. Vitamin D in preventive medicine: are we ignoring the evidence? *Br J Nutr.* 2003 May;89(5):552-72

[88] Holick MF. Vitamin D: importance in the prevention of cancers, type 1 diabetes, heart disease, and osteoporosis. *Am J Clin Nutr.* 2004;79(3):362-71

[89] Plotnikoff GA, Quigley JM. Prevalence of severe hypovitaminosis D in patients with persistent, nonspecific musculoskeletal pain. *Mayo Clin Proc.* 2003 Dec;78(12):1463-70

[90] Al Faraj S, Al Mutairi K. Vitamin D deficiency and chronic low back pain in Saudi Arabia. *Spine.* 2003 Jan 15;28(2):177-9

[91] Vasquez A, et al. The Clinical Importance of Vitamin D (Cholecalciferol). *Alternative Therapies in Health and Medicine* 2004;10:28-37 and *Integrative Medicine* 2004;3:44-54

Chemistry/metabolic panel	
Overview and interpretation:	<ul><li>Accurate interpretation requires knowledge and pattern-recognition by the doctor to translate numbers into differential diagnoses that are correlated with the clinical presentation, examination, and imaging findings to arrive at probable diagnoses.</li><li>Variation exists in the components and ranges offered by different laboratories.</li></ul>
Advantages:	<ul><li>Inexpensive and easy to perform—venipuncture + serum separator tube.</li><li>Provides a quick screen for diabetes, hepatitis, renal insufficiency, suggestions of alcohol abuse, hyperparathyroidism, electrolyte imbalances, etc.</li></ul>
Limitation and considerations:	<ul><li>Individual tests and the most common clinical considerations for low and high values are listed in the following section. These values and considerations are provided with the routine adult outpatient in mind and are not inclusive of every possible differential diagnosis and therapeutic consideration. Consult your laboratory texts and reference manuals as needed per patient.</li><li>Abnormal laboratory results are always due to one of four problems:<ol><li><u>Technical error</u>: Error with the laboratory analysis, improper patient identification correlating with the sample, alteration of the sample before delivery to the laboratory (e.g., too much time, too much heat, lysis of cells). Given the importance of laboratory accuracy and the life-and-death decisions that are based upon such reports, this type of error is inexcusable, however, it does occur, occasionally producing results that defy physiologic possibility or which contradict the clinical picture. Repeating the test is appropriate. *Example*: Hypercalcemia (elevated serum calcium) may be reported in error by the laboratory due to problems with the analyzing machinery.</li><li><u>Drug effect</u>: An otherwise healthy patient may develop a laboratory abnormality due to a drug effect. *Example*: Hypercalcemia can be secondary to the effect of a calcium-sparing diuretic, such as hydrochlorothiazide (HCTZ).</li><li><u>Pathology</u>: The patient has a diagnosable disease causing the laboratory abnormality. *Example*: Hypercalcemia can be secondary to a parathyroid adenoma which secretes abnormally high amounts of parathyroid hormone; hypercalcemia can also be a presentation of malignancy such as breast cancer or prostate cancer, or from a granulomatous disease such as sarcoidosis.</li><li><u>Physiologic abnormality</u>: The patient has a physiologic abnormality causing the laboratory abnormality. *Example*: Hypercalcemia can be secondary to excess intake of vitamin D. In practice, hypercalcemia from hypervitaminosis D is very rare because vitamin D has a wide safety margin; but for the sake of this discussion, vitamin D toxicity will be listed as a possible cause of hypercalcemia.</li></ol></li></ul>
Comments:	<ul><li>All abnormalities require follow-up—repeat test within 2-4 weeks as part of routine follow-up along with additional investigation and clinical re-assessment. Extraordinary abnormalities and those with life-threatening implications should of course be retested immediately; often, the laboratory will hold the blood sample for 7 days and the repeat analysis can be performed on the same blood sample to exclude technical error.</li><li>Many ill patients (such as those with chronic fatigue syndrome, fibromyalgia, etc) will have normal results with the metabolic panel and other basic routine laboratory assessments. Therefore, normal results do not ensure that the patient is healthy nor without life-threatening illness.</li><li>Generally, laboratory tests are performed in the morning under fasting conditions; such is the standard but is not necessarily required depending on the nature of the test, convenience, and the clinical situation.</li></ul>

Practical overview of common abnormalities on the chemistry/metabolic panel

Low values—considerations	Analyte: range[92]	High values—considerations
Technical error due to faulty processing of sample (i.e., hemolysis); insulinoma, exogenous insulin administration (test serum C-peptide), overdose of anti-hyperglycemic drugs, hypopituitarism and adrenal insufficiency.	**Glucose:** 65 - 99 mg/dL **Clinical pearl** Fasting glucose levels can fail to reveal the hyperglycemia of mild/moderate type-2 diabetes mellitus; a better test for long-term glucose status is hemoglobin A1c.	Postprandial sample, diabetes mellitus type-1 or type-2, Cushing disease or syndrome, acromegaly, pheochromocytoma, glucagonoma, hyperthyroidism. Fasting glucose >126 mg/dL on two or more occasions is consistent with the diagnosis of diabetes mellitus, as is the finding of nonfasting glucose >200 mg/dL on any one occasion. If glucose is >300 mg/dL and patient is unstable (e.g., tachypnic or stuporous), evaluate for diabetic ketoacidosis or hyperosmolar state. Optimal fasting serum glucose is in the range of 70-75 up to 85 mg/dL, since levels >85 mg/dL have been associated with increased mortality.
Hyponatremia[93,94] is potentially fatal and is also a cause of permanent neurologic injury (e.g., pontine myelinolysis). Clinicians should be particularly concerned when the sodium level drops below 125 mmol/L. Symptomatic hyponatremia is worthy of treatment in hospital setting; mild cases due to a recent event such as excess diaphoresis (e.g., prolonged sweating and exercise) or excess fluid intake (e.g., beer potomania [i.e., binge drinking], overhydration with unmineralized water) might be managed with sodium replacement and water restriction. Adrenal insufficiency classically presents with fatigue, hypotension, and hyponatremia with hyperkalemia; ACTH challenge test is the most sensitive and specific laboratory assessment. Older patients, patients with pulmonary disease, and patients taking certain drugs such as serotonin-reuptake inhibitors may develop a chronic and relatively benign mild hyponatremia associated with "reset osmostat syndrome." Sodium levels can be altered downward by conditions that introduce osmotically active substances into the serum, such as immunoglobulins (e.g., multiple myeloma), hyperglycemia, and hypertriglyceridemia; corrective equations are available for such situations.	**Sodium:** 136 - 144 mEq/L (mmol/L)	Hypernatremia in outpatients is rare; assess for drug effect and dehydration with hemoconcentration. Some clinicians will determine the free water deficit, while others will treat with oral or IV hydration with plain water or half-normal saline, respectively. Electrolyte abnormalities—particularly involving sodium—should generally be corrected slowly and with close supervision.

[92] The reference range for this table and some provisional information was derived from Medline Plus provided by the U.S. Department of Health and Human Services and National Institutes of Health. nlm.nih.gov/medlineplus/ency/article/003468.htm Accessed June 28, 2011. However, the majority of the information in this table comes from the author's (Dr Vasquez's) clinical training and experience. Editorial and peer reviews were provided by colleagues Barry Morgan MD, William J Beakey DOM, et al.
[93] Goh KP. Management of hyponatremia. *Am Fam Physician.* 2004;69:2387-94 aafp.org/afp/2004/0515/p2387.html Accessed June 2011.
[94] Decaux G, Musch W. Clinical laboratory evaluation of the syndrome of inappropriate secretion of antidiuretic hormone. *Clin J Am Soc Nephrol.* 2008 Jul;3(4):1175-84

Practical overview of common abnormalities on the chemistry/metabolic panel—*continued*

Low values—considerations	Analyte	High values—considerations
Hypokalemia can cause fatal cardiac arrhythmias and needs to be taken seriously. Replacement is generally via oral administration of potassium-rich foods, juices, or supplements such as potassium citrate (best option) or potassium chloride (KCl, inexpensive and therefore commonly used in medical settings even though KCl is clearly not optimal therapy due to the acidifying effect of the chloride anion). Recalcitrant hypokalemia is often a sign of magnesium depletion.[95] Causes of hypokalemia include diarrhea, vomiting, diuretics, Cushing disease/syndrome, dietary insufficiency, overhydration with mineral-free fluids, hyperaldosteronism and renal artery stenosis. Acute metabolic acidosis should cause relative or absolute elevations in serum K; the finding of normal or low serum K in a patient with acidosis (e.g., diabetic ketoacidosis) indicates (severe) potassium depletion.	<u>Potassium</u>: 3.6 - 5.2 mEq/L (mmol/L)	**Hyperkalemia is defined as a potassium level greater than 5.5 mmol/L. Severe hyperkalemia (>7 mmol/L) can be fatal and needs to be taken seriously.** In severe hyperkalemia, treatment and emergency management should be implemented before a complete evaluation and differential diagnosis are performed.[96] ❶ Ensure that blood sample was not hemolyzed. Repeat test if patient is stable and time allows. ❷ If hyperkalemia is severe or patient is symptomatic or has electrocardiographic changes, treat hyperkalemia with intravenous calcium, beta-adrenergic agonists (e.g., albuterol), bicarbonate, insulin and glucose; magnesium sulfate may also help alleviate arrhythmias; oral sodium polystyrene sulfonate (SPS, also known as Kayexalate) is a frequently used potassium-binding agent. ❸ DDX includes adrenal insufficiency, potassium-sparing diuretics, ACE-inhibitors and ARBs, NSAIDs, rhabdomyolysis, renal failure, and massive cell necrosis such as with tumor lysis syndrome.
Evaluate hypocalcemia clinically with Chvostek's sign (~30% sensitive) and Trousseau sign (~90% sensitive) which may also be present in hypomagnesemia; evaluate clinically for arrhythmia, muscle spasm/hypertonicity, and hyperreflexia. Measure serum albumin and perform equation for "corrected calcium" if albumin is low. DDX includes renal failure, hypoparathyroidism, malabsorption, and drug effect (e.g., rarely a loop diuretic such as furosemide). Chronic mild hypocalcemia is treated with oral vitamin D and calcium supplementation; subacute symptomatic hypocalcemia can be treated with intravenous calcium gluconate especially if cardiac arrhythmias are present.	<u>Calcium</u>: 8.6 - 10.2 mg/dL	Outpatient hypercalcemia is potentially serious and needs to be evaluated in a stepwise manner: ❶ repeat the test to rule out lab error unless you are confident in the performance of the laboratory and stability of the submitted sample, ❷ review drug list for adverse effect, such as from hydrochlorothiazide (HCTZ) or rarely from excess cholecalciferol intake, ❸ test intact parathyroid hormone (iPTH) to evaluate for hyperparathyroidism, ❹ evaluate for possible granulomatous disease such as sarcoidosis, tuberculosis, Crohn's disease, and possible leukemia or lymphoma, ❺ consider metabolic bone disease such as Paget disease of bone or metastatic bone disease, ❻ evaluate for cancer, ❼ test urine calcium for familial hypocalciuric hypercalcemia, ❽ refer to specialist such as internist or endocrinologist if hypercalcemia persists and answer is not forthcoming.

Corrected calcium (cCa) equations: Used when both serum calcium and albumin are low
<u>American units</u>: cCa (mg/dL) = serum Ca (mg/dL) + 0.8 (4.0 - serum albumin [g/dL])
<u>International units</u>: cCa (mmol/L) = measured total Ca (mmol/L) + 0.02 (40 - serum albumin [g/L])

---

[95] "Herein is reviewed literature suggesting that magnesium deficiency exacerbates potassium wasting by increasing distal potassium secretion." Huang CL, Kuo E. Mechanism of hypokalemia in magnesium deficiency. *J Am Soc Nephrol.* 2007;18:2649-52 jasn.asnjournals.org/content/18/10/2649

[96] "If the hyperkalemia is severe (potassium >7.0 mEq/L) or if the patient is symptomatic, begin treatment before diagnostic investigation of the underlying cause." Garth D. Hyperkalemia in emergency medicine treatment and management. *Medscape Reference* emedicine.medscape.com/article/766479-treatment#a1126 Accessed June 2011

Practical overview of common abnormalities on the chemistry/metabolic panel—*continued*

Low values—considerations	Analyte	High values—considerations
Clinically meaningful hypochloremia is rare among outpatients. Hypochloremic metabolic alkalosis is commonly seen after persistent vomiting. Consider syndrome of inappropriate diuretic hormone (SIADH) secretion, cardiopulmonary disease, and adrenal insufficiency.	**Chloride**: 97 - 111 mmol/L	Hyperchloremia in outpatients is rare; assess for drug effect and dehydration with hemoconcentration; assess for acid-base disturbance, especially acidosis.
Reduced CO2 correlates with hyperventilation; consider acid-base disturbance, salicylate overdose, asthma. Slight decrements in healthy outpatients are probably due to anxious hyperventilation at time of venipuncture.	**CO2 (carbon dioxide)**: 20 - 30 mmol/L	Elevated CO2 can suggest cardiopulmonary compromise and/or acid-base disturbance; assess clinically. Slight elevations in otherwise healthy outpatients are probably due to breath-holding at time of venipuncture.
Reduced total protein with normal albumin suggests hypogammaglobulinemia; evaluate for nephrotic syndrome, liver disease, protein deficiency and malabsorption/enteropathy, immunosuppressive syndromes and consider intravenous gammaglobulin therapy.	**Total protein (albumin + globulins)**: 6.3 - 8.0 g/dL	Elevated total protein with normal albumin suggests hypergammaglobulinemia, such as due to infection or plasma cell dyscrasia (e.g., multiple myeloma and Waldenstrom's disease). Evaluate within the clinical context; order serum protein electrophoresis if cause remains elusive, especially if patient has immune complex disease, neuropathy, or nephropathy.
Assess for liver disease, nephrotic syndrome, protein deficiency, malabsorption (consider celiac disease).	**Albumin**: 3.9 - 5.0 g/dL	Assess for dehydration/hemoconcentration.
Loss of hepatic mass due to cirrhosis, possible pyridoxine deficiency.	**ALT (alanine aminotransferase)**: 10 - 40 IU/L	Hepatocellular liver injury due to chemical toxicity, viral hepatitis, hemochromatosis, metastatic or infectious disease, muscle injury. ALT is preferentially elevated over AST in viral hepatitis.
Loss of hepatic mass due to cirrhosis, possible pyridoxine deficiency.	**AST (aspartate aminotransferase)**: 10 - 40 IU/L	Hepatocellular liver injury due to chemical toxicity, viral hepatitis, hemochromatosis, metastatic or infectious liver disease, myocardial infarct, muscle injury. AST is preferentially elevated over ALT in alcoholic hepatitis and rhabdomyolysis.
Consider zinc deficiency, malnutrition.	**Alkaline phosphatase (abbreviated as ALK PHOS or ALP)**: 44 - 147 IU/L	Metabolic bone disease, metastatic bone disease, vitamin D deficiency, congestive liver disease. Test isoenzymes to differentiate bone versus hepatic origin if cause of elevation remains unclear.

INFLAMMATION MASTERY & FUNCTIONAL INFLAMMOLOGY

Practical overview of common abnormalities on the chemistry/metabolic panel—*continued*

Low values—considerations	Analyte	High values—considerations
GGT levels are reduced in hypothyroidism, likely as a reflection of total reduction in protein synthesis. Oral contraceptive agents and clofibrate may also reduce levels. **GGT as a possible marker of oxidative stress and xenobiotic exposure** "It is possible that recently reported associations between serum GGT and various health outcomes may be explained by **increases in serum GGT due to the exposure to various environmental pollutants**." Lim et al. *Clin Chem* 2007 Jun	**GGT (Gamma-glutamyl transpeptidase)**: 0 - 51 IU/L *HgbA1c and serum insulin is discussed in the chapters and presentations on diabetes, hypertension, and metabolic syndrome.*	Because the GGT enzyme is highly represented in cells of the hepatobiliary tract, it is especially elevated in disorders of this region, especially obstructive jaundice, intrahepatic cholestasis, cholestasis of pregnancy, pancreatitis, liver metastases, alcohol/toxin/drug-induced liver disease, infectious mononucleosis, congestive heart failure, primary biliary cirrhosis, or biliary atresia. Clinicians should search for—when assessing a patient with possible/confirmed hepatobiliary obstruction—a triad of elevated GGT, ALP, and (conjugated) bilirubin. Combined elevations of GGT reflecting hepatic congestion and of MCV suggesting folate-cobalamin deficiency and/or bone marrow toxicity may suggest alcohol abuse. Milder elevations of GGT may be seen with systemic lupus erythematosus (SLE) or hyperthyroidism. GGT is considered the most sensitive laboratory marker for hepatobiliary obstruction; leucine aminopeptidase (LAP) or 5′ nucleotidase are additional/confirmatory tests. Unlike ALP which can be elevated in disorders of either liver or bone (thus possibly contributing to a diagnostic dilemma), GGT has no origin in bone. The correlation between elevated GGT and insulin resistance / diabetes mellitus type-2 / metabolic syndrome[97] may be mediated via increased activity of the glutathione and detoxification systems[98] appropriately upregulated in response to the increased body burden of persistent organic pollutants.[99]
Low values are rare but might be noted with severe chronic anemia.	**Total bilirubin**: 0.2 - 1.5 mg/dL Direct (conjugated) bilirubin: 0 - 0.3 mg/dL Indirect (unconjugated) bilirubin: Determined by subtracting the *direct* from the *total* bilirubin.	Indirect/unconjugated bilirubin is elevated with hemolysis (e.g., hemolytic anemia) and impaired enzymatic conjugation (e.g., Gilbert's syndrome) or both (e.g., neonates). Direct/conjugated bilirubin has been enzymatically conjugated with glucuronic acid but is blocked from hepatobiliary excretion; consider performing liver and gall bladder sonogram (or CT or MRI) to evaluate for causes of biliary obstruction in addition to a careful abdominal exam. In patients with advanced liver disease, perform the Model for End-Stage Liver Disease (MELD) score and/or the MELD-Na score to predict 3-month mortality.[100] Fluoridated water inhibits glucuronidation in some patients with Gilbert's syndrome; biochemical improvement follows avoidance of fluoridated water.[101]

---

[97] Grundy SM. Gamma-glutamyl transferase: another biomarker for metabolic syndrome and cardiovascular risk. *Arterioscler Thromb Vasc Biol.* 2007 Jan;27(1):4-7
[98] McLennan SV et al .Changes in hepatic glutathione metabolism in diabetes. *Diabetes.* 1991 Mar;40(3):344-8
[99] Lim et al. A strong interaction between serum gamma-glutamyltransferase and obesity on the risk of prevalent type 2 diabetes. *Clin Chem* 2007;53:1092-8
[100] MELD calculations are best performed electronically, such as with mayoclinic.org/meld/mayomodel8.html or other medical calculator.
[101] Lee J. Gilbert's disease and fluoride intake. *Fluoride* 1983; 16: 139-45

Practical overview of common abnormalities on the chemistry/metabolic panel—*continued*

Low values—considerations	Analyte	High values—considerations
Liver disease, nephrotic syndrome, protein deficiency and malabsorption.	**BUN (blood urea nitrogen)**: 7 - 20 mg/dL	Consider renal underperfusion (e.g., due to heart failure, GI bleeding, renal artery stenosis, and dehydration), intrinsic renal failure, and post-renal urinary tract obstruction. When renal disease is initially considered, order a urinalysis with microscopic analysis—see following section on urinalysis (UA).
BUN-to-creatinine ratio (normal = ~10) ≥10-20: Renal underperfusion, post-renal obstruction ≤10: Suggests intrinsic renal disease		
Sarcopenia (insufficient muscle mass), protein deficiency and malabsorption.	**Creatinine**: 0.8 - 1.3 mg/dL	Excess dietary protein, creatine supplementation, renal hypoperfusion; the most important consideration is intrinsic renal failure. Creatinine production (from arginine and creatine) is proportional to muscle mass. A rise in creatinine does not become evident until renal function (measured by glomerular filtration rate [GFR]) has fallen by approximately 50%. Creatinine levels indicative of impaired renal function to such an extent that modifications in diet, medications, and co-management become relevant are 1.4 mg/dL in women and 1.5 mg/dL in men. In the evaluation of renal function, the patient's age is a crucial determinant of how the serum creatinine is interpreted for the estimation of renal function (via GFR—see the Cockcroft-Gault equation). Cystatin C is more sensitive than are singular or conjugate interpretations of BUN and creatinine. If drug-induced nephritis is suspected, test urine eosinophils.
Laboratory assessment of renal function, creatinine clearance, glomerular filtration rate (GFR) 1. Routine urinalysis 2. Random urine albumin:creatinine ratio 3. Modification of Diet in Renal Disease (MDRD) equation*, 4. 24-hour urine creatinine measurement, 5. Serum cystatin-C measurement, 6. Cockcroft-Gault equation (below): $$GFR = \frac{(140 - age\ years) \times wt\ kg \times (0.85\ if\ female)}{72 \times serum\ creatinine\ in\ mg/dL}$$ Clinical pearls for managing the chronic kidney disease (CKD) patient with declining renal function: • When the GFR ≤ 60 (CKD stage 3): Modify dosages or withdraw certain drugs. Treat the causative problem and/or begin specialist co-management. • When the GFR ≤ 30 (CKD stage 4): The patient needs to consult a nephrologist. • When the GFR ≤ 15 (CKD stage 5): The patient needs a transplant or dialysis. *National Institute of Diabetes and Digestive and Kidney Diseases. GFR MDRD Calculator for Adults (Conventional units). Accessed June 2011 nkdep.nih.gov/professionals/gfr_calculators/idms_con.htm		

Cystatin C	

Overview and interpretation:	▪ Cystatin C is gaining acceptance as studies confirm and define its usefulness, especially as an early, sensitive marker for chronic kidney disease. Concentrations of cystatin C are not affected by gender, age, or race, and cystatin C is not affected by most drugs (prednisone increases; cyclosporine decreases), infections, diet, or inflammation.[102]
	▪ Produced at a constant rate by all nucleated cells.
	▪ Freely filtered by the glomerulus.
	▪ Elevated in: renal disorders.
	   ○ Cystatin C rises more rapidly than creatinine (Cr) in early renal impairment.
	   ○ Good predictor of the severity of ATN (acute tubular necrosis).
	   ○ The cystatin C concentration is an independent risk factor for heart failure, mortality, CVD and non-CVD outcomes in older adults and appears to provide a better measure of risk assessment than the serum Cr concentration.

Advantages:	▪ More accurate assessment of renal function than creatinine-based assessments. ▪ Can be used to accurately assess renal function when creatinine-based assessments suggest impending renal impairment inconsistent with clinical presentation.
Limitations:	▪ Cost is approximately US $80. ▪ False "non-renal" elevations may occur with cancer and/or rheumatic disease.

Clinical Case **40yo male presenting for follow-up on abnormal renal function assessment—use of cystatin C to confirm normal kidney function**: This apperantly healthy and athletic 40yo man displays consistently elevated creatinine and an estimated glomerular filtration rate (eGFR) that is close enough at 62 to warrant concern. Clinicians must appreciate that eGFR <60 is consistent with stage 3 chronic kidney disease (CKD) which warrants monitoring and which often necessitates changes in drug dosing (e.g., to avoid metformin-induced lactic acidosis) and diet (e.g., to avoid hyperkalemia).

Date and Time Collected	Date Entered	Date and Time Reported	Physician Name	NPI	Physician ID
12/07/11 11:10	12/08/11	12/13/11 04:07ET	VASQUEZ , A		

Tests Ordered
Comp. Metabolic Panel (14); FSH+TestT+LH+DHEA S+Prog+E2...; Chlamydia pneumoniae(IgG/M); Venipuncture

TESTS	RESULT	FLAG	UNITS	REFERENCE INTERVAL	LAB
Comp. Metabolic Panel (14)					
Glucose, Serum	89		mg/dL	65 – 99	01
BUN	18		mg/dL	6 – 24	01
Creatinine, Serum	**1.41**	**High**	mg/dL	0.76 – 1.27	01
eGFR If NonAfricn Am	62		mL/min/1.73	>59	
eGFR If Africn Am	72		mL/min/1.73	>59	
Note: A persistent eGFR <60 mL/min/1.73 m2 (3 months or more) may indicate chronic kidney disease. An eGFR >59 mL/min/1.73 m2 with an elevated urine protein also may indicate chronic kidney disease. Calculated using CKD-EPI formula.					
BUN/Creatinine Ratio	13			9 – 20	

In this situation, cystatin C was performed and confirmed normal renal function despite persistently elevated creatinine, which is probably attributable to this patient's athleticism and muscle mass.[103]

Date and Time Collected	Date Entered	Date and Time Reported	Physician Name	NPI	Physician ID
12/07/11 11:10	12/12/11	12/15/11 07:14ET	VASQUEZ , A		

Tests Ordered
Cystatin C; Written Authorization

TESTS	RESULT	FLAG	UNITS	REFERENCE INTERVAL	LAB
Cystatin C	0.71		mg/L	0.53 – 0.95	01

---

[102] labtestsonline.org/understanding/analytes/cystatin-c/tab/test Accessed April 2012
[103] Thank you, William J Beakey DOM of Professional Co-op Services, Inc. professionalco-op.com for provision of these laboratory services.

Clinical Case 69yo asymptomatic female presenting for routine visit found to have life-threatening hyperkalemia: Review the following labs and outline your treatment plan before reading the discussion below.

PATIENT NAME	PATIENT ID	ROOM NUMBER	AGE	SEX	PHYSICIAN
			69 Y 1941	F	Vasquez

REQUISITION NO	ACCESSION NO	ID.NO.	COLLECTION DATE & TIME	LOG-IN-DATE	REPORT DATE & TIME
			09/22/10 08:00 AM	09/22/10 06:37 PM	09/23/10 03:36AM

NOTES:
PT FASTING

TEST	RESULTS OUT OF RANGE	RESULTS WITHIN RANGE	UNITS	EXPECTED RANGE	LAB
BASIC METABOLIC PROFILE					
GLUCOSE		98	MG/DL	65-100	
BUN		19	MG/DL	8-25	
CREATININE		1.2	MG/DL	0.6-1.3	
EGFR AFRICAN AMER.	54		ML/MIN/1.73	>60	
EGFR NON-AFRICAN AMER.	45		ML/MIN/1.73	>60	
SODIUM		136	MEQ/L	133-146	
POTASSIUM	8.5		MEQ/L	3.5-5.3	

RESULTS RECHECKED AND VERIFIED
NOTE: NO VISIBLE HEMOLYSIS OBSERVED.

CHLORIDE		100	MEQ/L	97-110	
CARBON DIOXIDE		27	MEQ/L	18-30	
CALCIUM		10.0	MG/DL	8.5-10.5	
LIPID PANEL					
CHOLESTEROL		193	MG/DL	<200	
TRIGLYCERIDES		129	MG/DL	<150	
HDL CHOLESTEROL		52	MG/DL	>39	
CALCULATED LDL CHOL	115		MG/DL	<100	
RISK RATIO LDL/HDL		2.22	RATIO	<3.22	
HEMOGLOBIN A1C	7.0		%	4.0-5.6	

AMERICAN DIABETES ASSOCIATION GUIDELINES FOR HGB A1C:
GLYCEMIC GOAL IN DIABETES . . . . . . <7.0%
DIAGNOSIS OF DIABETES . . . . >/=6.5%
CONFIRMED ON REPEAT ANALYSIS OR
WITH APPROPRIATE SYMPTOMS.
INCREASED RISK FOR DIABETES 5.7-6.4%

TSH	10.6		UIU/ML	0.3-5.1	

PERFORMING LAB(S) LEGEND:

> **Chemistry/metabolic panels should be performed on all new patients prior to treatment and periodically on all established patients to monitor for disease emergence and response to treatment**
>
> Treating this diabetic patient with a potassium-rich diet emphasizing low-carbohydrate fruits and vegetables would exacerbate her already life-threatening hyperkalemia. Note also that her hypothyroidism would be expected to contribute to her obesity which is exacerbating her diabetes and that (somewhat theoretically since we don't have her vital signs here) hypothyroid bradycardia could also reduce renal perfusion and contribute to her low GFR and hyperkalemia.

Assessments and plan: ❶ Life-threatening hyperkalemia: The clinician must focus on the emergency issue(s). Many books quote a potassium of 6 mEq/L as a panic value; note that the laboratory already excluded technical error and checked for hemolysis, which are the two most common causes of spurious hyperkalemia. This patient should be called at home and advised to immediately seek transportation by a secondary driver (e.g., taxi, ambulance, friend, neighbor, or relative) to the nearest hospital. If the patient is demented or otherwise incompetent, the clinician should contact the patient's caretaker or call directly for an ambulance. Attention must be given to the reliability of the driver, the urgency of the situation, and the speed by which the driver can get the patient to the hospital; failure by the clinician to ensure proper patient care—which in this case and most situations is best ensured by enrolling the ambulance service—could easily result in medicolegal complications. Hospital treatment for hyperkalemia will include assessment for electrocardiographic changes and treatment of hyperkalemia with intravenous calcium to stabilize cardioelectroconductivity, beta-adrenergic agonists, bicarbonate, diuretics, insulin and glucose; magnesium may also help alleviate arrhythmias; oral sodium polystyrene sulfonate (Kayexalate) is a potassium-binding agent. ❷ Diabetes mellitus: Notice that this patient's fasting glucose level is "normal" and yet the patient is clearly diabetic per the hemoglobin A1c value >6.5%. This patient needs a comprehensive nutritional plan for diabetes management. Promoting dependence on drugs at this early point should be considered inappropriate. ❸ Hypothyroidism: The TSH >10 indicates primary hypothyroidism by any standard; in all probability, unless major contraindications exist (of which very few exist), this patient should be started on a thyroid hormone combination as discussed in the section on thyroid assessment. ❹ Renal insufficiency: This patient has stage-3 chronic kidney disease and should begin a renoprotective and renorestorative program—beyond the basics of hypertension and hyperglycemia control—as discussed in *Chiropractic and Naturopathic Mastery of Common Clinical Disorders*. Use of ACE-inhibitor or ARB is contraindicated due to hyperkalemia. ❺ Dyslipidemia: LDL cholesterol and triglycerides should both be below 100 mg/dL. Diet is key, followed by fatty acid therapy, niacin, and berberine.

Lipid panel

Overview and interpretation: **Understanding blood lipids** We now appreciate "blood lipids" in much greater detail, appreciating *subfractions* and *functionality* of these lipids; nonetheless, these considerations maintain some validity for general care	• "High cholesterol" was a buzz phrase many years ago indicating an unfavorable lipid profile causally associated with accelerated atherogenesis and the resultant CVD in its myriad forms. The next step was to identify low-density lipoprotein (LDL) cholesterol as the most obvious kingpin of vascular villains. Advances over the past decade include: 1. Appreciation that other non-lipid molecules such as homocysteine and c-reactive protein (CRP) are important contributors to the atherogenic process, 2. Renewed interest in the beneficial effects of high-density lipoprotein (HDL) cholesterol in mediating vasculoprotection, 3. "Non-standard" CVD risk factors such as very-low-density lipoprotein (VLDL), β-VLDL, intermediate-density lipoprotein (IDL) cholesterol, and lipoprotein-a (Lp-a) are also clinically important. For the sake of this introductory section on the basics of laboratory interpretation, the discussion will be limited to the components of the standard lipid panel; additional tests and details are provided in disease-specific chapters on metabolic/inflammatory disorders.

Lipids: Goals	**Clinical notes:**
Total cholesterol: < 200 mg/dL	• Higher cholesterol levels correlate with increased risk for CVD. Except in very rare cases of genotropic disease, the vast majority of humans should be able to achieve a total cholesterol <200 mg/dL via nutritional optimization, exercise, and proper endocrine (especially thyroid) status. The so-called "statin" drugs which block HMG-CoA reductase (3-hydroxy-3-methyl-glutaryl-CoA reductase, the rate-limiting enzyme for the endogenous production of cholesterol) would and should be *orphan drugs*. Reducing serum levels of insulin—the primary inducer of HMG-CoA reductase—is the most rational means by which to reduce total cholesterol levels. Thyroid hormone downregulates HMG-CoA reductase; this explains the well-established association of hypothyroidism with dyslipidemia and hypercholesterolemia.
LDL: <100 mg/dL	• O'Keefe and Cordain and colleagues[104] have noted that optimal LDL is 50-70 mg/dl and that lower is better and is physiologically normal for humans who eat appropriate diets and who are physically active.
HDL: >50-60 mg/dL	• Per the American Heart Association[105], "An HDL of 60 mg/dL and above is considered protective against heart disease." Of note, a recent report linked accumulation of persistent organic pollutants (POP) with elevated HDL levels.[106]
Triglycerides: <100 mg/dL	• Elevated serum triglycerides—except in rare cases of genotropic disease—are indicators of dietary carbohydrate excess and/or alcohol excess and/or insulin resistance. Hypertriglyceridemia is associated with increased CVD risk, higher body mass index (BMI), vitamin D deficiency, and increased risks of breast cancer and prostate cancer. Extreme hypertriglyceridemia (500 mg/dL or more) can cause pancreatitis; administration of omega-3 fatty acids from fish oil is protective.
Advantages	• Allows for the monitoring of established cardiovascular risk factors and a surrogate marker for dietary compliance and lifestyle optimization.
Limitations:	• Other non-lipid risk factors should also be monitored and optimized.
Comments:	• Important panel for overall patient management and disease prevention.

---

[104] O'Keefe JH Jr, Cordain L, et al. Optimal low-density lipoprotein is 50 to 70 mg/dl: lower is better and physiologically normal. *J Am Coll Cardiol*. 2004 Jun 2;43(11):2142-6
[105] American Heart Association. heart.org/HEARTORG/Conditions/What-Your-Cholesterol-Levels-Mean_UCM_305562_Article.jsp Accessed June 2011
[106] "However, unlike the findings with p,p'-DDE, after the initial decrease of HDL-cholesterol from the 1st to 2nd quartile, HDL-cholesterol increased from the 2nd to 4th quartile of these PCBs." Lee DH, Steffes MW, Sjödin A, Jones RS, Needham LL, Jacobs DR Jr. Low dose organochlorine pesticides and polychlorinated biphenyls predict obesity, dyslipidemia, and insulin resistance among people free of diabetes. *PLoS One*. 2011 Jan 26;6(1):e15977

Complete blood count: CBC	
Overview and interpretation:	This test measures numbers and indices of white and red blood cells and platelets. A routine "CBC with differential" is affordable, practical, and thus preferred for the vast majority of situations (step 1); the next step when the clinical picture remains unclear is—generally—to order a peripheral blood smear (step 2) before proceeding to a hematologist referral (step 3). Additional tests—more components of step 2—are listed below per topic. If all three blood cell populations are reduced (pancytopenia) consider nutritional anemia, hypersplenism (especially secondary to hepatic cirrhosis), autoimmunity (especially systemic lupus erythematosus), or bone marrow disorder such as myelofibrosis or aplastic anemia.

- WBC (white blood cells): The three most commonly encountered disorders that cause an abnormal WBC count are ❶ bone marrow suppression (causing low WBC count) and conditions associated with elevated WBC count including ❷ leukemia/lymphoma and ❸ response to infection. An elevated WBC count suggests the possibility of infection (especially bacterial infection) or leukemia/lymphoma and therefore requires the clinician's attention. However, relying on the WBC count for the assessment of serious infection is potentially misleading, particularly since, for example, it is elevated in less than 50% of patients with acute and chronic musculoskeletal infections; per Shaw et al[107] "Therefore, it [the WBC count] is helpful when it is high, but potentially misleading when it is normal." Clinicians can gain additional information by assessing percentage and quantitative indices of neutrophils, lymphocytes, and eosinophils, elevations of which may suggest bacterial infections, viral infections, or allergic or parasitic conditions, respectively. Primary care clinicians may also choose to perform lymphocyte immunophenotyping by flow cytometry in patients with unexplained lymphocytosis prior to hematologist consult.

  - Neutropenia: Severe suppression of WBC count resulting in neutropenia can occur in liver disease, viral infections (including but not limited to HIV), autoimmune disorders, bone marrow infiltration/failure, and toxin/alcohol exposure. For severe neutropenia, hospitalization, isolation precautions, prophylactic antibiotics, and marrow-stimulating agents are often indicated. Neutropenia is defined by an absolute neutrophil count (ANC) less than 1500 neutrophilic cells per mm3. Neutropenia is most commonly due to

    > **Absolute neutrophil count (ANC) = Total WBC x (% "Segs" + % "Bands")**
    > - Normal value: ≥ 1500 cells/mm3,
    > - Mild neutropenia: 1000-1500/mm3,
    > - Moderate neutropenia: 500-1000/mm3,
    > - Severe neutropenia: ≤ 500/mm3; hospitalization is generally advised

    use of anti-cancer cytotoxic agents; other drugs that can cause neutropenia include anticonvulsants (e.g., carbamazepine, valproic acid, diphenylhydantoin), thyroid inhibitors (carbimazole, methimazole, propylthiouracil), antibacterial drugs (penicillins, cephalosporins, sulfonamides, chloramphenicol, vancomycin, trimethoprim-sulfamethoxazole), antipsychotic drugs (clozapine), antiarrhythmics (procainamide), antirheumatic drugs (penicillamine, gold salts, hydroxychloroquine), and NSAIDs.[108] The ANC is calculated with "segs" (segmented neutrophils) and "bands" (band neutrophils) reported on CBC with differential: ANC = Total WBC x (% Segs + % Bands).

---

[107] Shaw BA, Gerardi JA, Hennrikus WL. How to avoid orthopedic pitfalls in children. *Patient Care* 1999; Feb 28: 95-116
[108] Tefferi A, Hanson CA, Inwards DJ. How to interpret and pursue an abnormal complete blood cell count in adults. *Mayo Clin Proc.* 2005 Jul;80(7):923-36 mayoclinicproceedings.com/content/80/7/923.long This article serves as the main review for this section on CBC interpretation.

Complete blood count: CBC—*continued*

Overview and interpretation —*continued:*	• **RBC (red blood cells and associated indices):** Since polycythemia is relatively rare, in most situations the clinician is looking for anemia, most often related to the categories in the subsections that follow this paragraph. The first step is to classify the anemia based on the mean corpuscular volume (MCV) as microcytic (MCV, <80 fL), normocytic (MCV, 80-95 fL), or macrocytic (MCV, >95 fL)—details on following page.

• Clinical notes on the most common anemias:

   o Nutritional deficiency of B-12 or folate: My approach is to critique the mean corpuscular volume (MCV) and to interpret MCV values greater than 90 with an increased suspicion for folate and/or B-12 deficiency. Clinical experience has shown that MCV values greater than 95 correlate with increased homocysteine levels, and a clinical response (improvement in mood, energy, and a reduction in MCV) is commonly seen following three months of nutritional supplementation. Deficiency of vitamin B-12 can easily be treated with oral administration of 2,000 mcg per day of vitamin B-12.[109] I generally use 5 mg (rarely up to 20 mg) per day of oral folate for the treatment of probable or documented folic acid deficiency; this is safe for most patients, excluding those on antiepileptic drugs.[110] Vitamin B-12 and folic acid *function together* and should be *administered together*. Cyanocobalamin should be avoided due to its cyanide; hydroxocobalamin, methylcobalamin, adenosylcobalamin are better.

   o Iron deficiency (confirmed with assessment of serum ferritin): While inadequate intake, malabsorption, or menstrual bleeding may cause iron deficiency, **adult patients with iron deficiency are at higher probability for gastrointestinal pathology and should therefore be evaluated with endoscopy or other comprehensive assessment** *beyond fecal occult-blood testing* **to rule out gastrointestinal disease.**[111,112] **The standard of care for all healthcare professionals is that adult patients with inexplicable iron deficiency are referred for gastroenteroscopic evaluation to assess for occult gastrointestinal pathology; the major concerns are gastric/colon carcinoma, but malabsorptive conditions and bleeding noncancerous polyps are also worthy of diagnosis.** Iron supplementation should be administered and can reasonably be withheld during acute viral and bacterial infections as it promotes bacterial and viral replication and pathogenicity.

   o The anemia of chronic disease: Generally associated with a corresponding disease history such as long-term RA or renal insufficiency and often associated with increased ESR, CRP, and ferritin. **Do not assume that an anemic patient has iron deficiency until proven with measurement of serum ferritin.** Anemia of chronic kidney disease (CKD) is associated with reduced renal production of erythropoietin, thereby resulting in understimulation of bone marrow.

   o Anemia caused by hemolysis or splenic sequestration: Autoimmune hemolytic anemia most commonly occurs in patients with systemic lupus erythematosus (SLE). Pancytopenia—reduced numbers of RBC, WBC, and platelets—is seen with chronic liver disease that has progressed to cirrhosis and has resulted in hemolysis and splenic sequestration of blood cells; such patients are at risk for esophageal varicies, encephalopathy, and ascites with spontaneous bacterial peritonitis and should be screened and treated appropriately.

---

[109] Kuzminski AM, et al. Effective treatment of cobalamin deficiency with oral cobalamin. *Blood* 1998 Aug 15;92(4):1191-8

[110] "PGA administered in doses up to 1,000 mg orally a day… The folate was well absorbed, as reflected by marked increases in the serum and erythrocyte folate concentrations… There was no evidence of clinical or laboratory toxicity at these high doses of folate." Boss GR, Ragsdale RA, Zettner A, Seegmiller JE. Failure of folic acid (pteroylglutamic acid) to affect hyperuricemia. *J Lab Clin Med* 1980 Nov;96(5):783-9

[111] Rockey DC, Cello JP. Evaluation of the gastrointestinal tract in patients with iron-deficiency anemia. *N Engl J Med.* 1993;329(23):1691-5

[112] "Endoscopy revealed a clinically important lesion in 23 (12%) of 186 patients. … CONCLUSIONS: Endoscopy yields important findings in premenopausal women with iron deficiency anemia, which should not be attributed solely to menstrual blood loss." Bini EJ, Micale PL, Weinshel EH. Evaluation of the gastrointestinal tract in premenopausal women with iron deficiency anemia. *Am J Med.* 1998 Oct;105(4):281-6

Anemia—the most common considerations in outpatient practice: Always assess patient for tachycardia, hypovolemia, orthostasis, and adequate perfusion; always test serum ferritin during the initial evaluation then perform peripheral blood smear (PBS) if diagnosis remains unclear

- Microcytic anemia:
  - Iron deficiency anemia (IDA): Test serum ferritin. The confirmation of iron deficiency in adults generally requires gastroenterologic consultation to assess for occult gastrointestinal blood loss; this is especially true for all men and post-menopausal women but also applies to premenopausal women.* Testing for celiac disease and hematuria is advised.**
  - Thalassemia: Check for polycythemia, test Hgb electrophoresis; because the diagnosis of the various thalassemias can be complex, consider consulting a hematologist,
  - Anemia of chronic disease (ACD): Assess patient, inflammatory markers, and renal function. The most common causes of ACD are temporal (giant cell) arteritis and polymyalgia rheumatica, rheumatoid arthritis, chronic infection, Hodgkin lymphoma, renal cell carcinoma, myelofibrosis, and Castleman disease (a noncancerous lymphoproliferative disorder).
- Normocytic anemia:
  - Nutritional anemia: Iron deficiency and vitamin B-12 deficiency can both cause normocytic anemia.
  - Bleeding: Assess patient for tachycardia, hypovolemia, and shock; consider transfusion and/or volume repletion as needed. Assess serum ferritin and the reticulocyte count.
  - Chronic renal failure (CRF): Anemia associated with elevated BUN and creatinine.
  - Hypersplenism: Assess for chronic hepatitis and cirrhosis. Cirrhotic patients are at increased risk for gastroesophageal hemorrhage and ascites with spontaneous bacterial peritonitis.
  - Hemolysis: Expect to see elevated reticulocytes (chronic) and lactate dehydrogenase (acute); expect high indirect bilirubin and low serum haptoglobin with intravascular hemolysis; assess for autoimmunity (ANA, direct Coombs test [direct antiglobulin test]), glucose-6-phosphate dehydrogenase (G6PD) deficiency, drug-induced hemolysis, and other causes as case warrants.
  - Bone marrow disorder: Correlate lab findings with patient presentation; consult hematologist if solution is not forthcoming.
- Macrocytosis:
  - Induced by toxins, drugs, alcohol: Assess per patient history and other findings; the most notorious offenders are hydroxyurea, zidovudine, and alcohol.
  - Vitamin B-12 and/or folate deficiency: Consider testing serum methylmalonate and homocysteine followed by empiric supplementation with B-12 at 2,000 or more micrograms per day and folate at 1-5 milligrams per day; determine cause of problem and strongly consider autoimmune gastritis, bacterial overgrowth, and celiac disease. Test serum ferritin because nutritional deficiencies commonly occur together. Administration of vitamin B-12 is advised in all patients suspected of having B-12 deficiency.*** Regarding the clinical presentation of vitamin B-12 deficiency, clinicians should remember the adage that one-third of patients will present with anemia, one-third with peripheral neuropathy, and one-third with central neurologic problems such as depression, psychosis, and/or other disturbances of mood, memory, or personality. Failure to diagnose and treat vitamin B-12 deficiency in a timely manner will result in permanent neurologic damage.
  - Hypothyroidism: Measure TSH and free T4 at a minimum; assess basal body temperature, and speed of Achilles reflex return.

* "A gastrointestinal source of chronic blood loss was identified in a substantial proportion of premenopausal women with iron deficiency anemia." Green BT, Rockey DC. Gastrointestinal endoscopic evaluation of premenopausal women with iron deficiency anemia. *J Clin Gastroenterol.* 2004 Feb

** Goddard et al on behalf of the British Society of Gastroenterology. Guidelines for the management of iron deficiency anaemia. *Gut.* 2011 Jun epocrates.com/dacc/1106/irondefbmj1106.pdf

*** "Thus, therapeutic trials of Cbl are warranted when clinical findings consistent with Cbl deficiency are present..." Solomon LR. Cobalamin-responsive disorders in the ambulatory care setting: unreliability of cobalamin, methylmalonic acid, and homocysteine testing. *Blood* 2005 Feb bloodjournal.hematologylibrary.org/content/105/3/978.full.pdf

CBC: complete blood count—*continued*	
Overview and interpretation—continued:	▪ <u>Platelets</u>: Elevated platelet count (thrombocytosis) can be due to malignant primary thrombocytosis, iron-deficiency anemia, hemolysis, asplenia, and reactive thrombocytosis due to cancer, infection, or chronic inflammation. Low platelet count (thrombocytopenia, fewer than 150,000 platelets per microliter) increases risk for spontaneous bleeding and can—rarely but importantly—be associated with serious and potentially life-threatening disorders such as thrombotic thrombocytopenic purpura/hemolytic uremic syndrome (TTP/HUS) and disseminated intravascular coagulation (DIC). In relatively asymptomatic and nonacute outpatients, the most common causes of thrombocytopenia are hypersplenism due to liver cirrhosis, idiopathic thrombocytopenic purpura (ITP), and drug reaction, most notoriously secondary to trimethoprim-sulfamethoxazole ("Bactrim"), cardiac medications (e.g., quinidine, procainamide, thiazide diuretics), antirheumatic drugs (gold salts [rarely used these days]), and heparin. Heparin-induced thrombocytopenia (HIT, type-2) is potentially fatal and requires immediate cessation of heparin administration. Patients with unexplained persistent thrombocytopenia should be tested for HIV, autoimmunity (ANA), and lymphoproliferative disorders (PBS, immunophenotyping, serum protein electrophoresis, and serum immunofixation). Isolated mild to moderate thrombocytopenia (75,000 – 150,000 platelets per microliter) during pregnancy generally is considered nonpathologic.
Advantages:	▪ The **CBC with differential** is inexpensive and easy to perform and is appropriate for asymptomatic patients. The "CBC with diff" is an appropriate first test for patients who are symptomatic (e.g., fatigue, fever) or have an ongoing history of health problems. In certain healthcare settings where cost containment is a major priority, CBC *without* differential is commonly ordered; however, in outpatient private practice, the additional expenditure of $2 for the CBC *with* differential is the preferred evaluation. It provides a quick screen for anemia, leukemia, infection, and for provisional evidence of B-12/folate and iron deficiencies. The CBC can also identify more complex conditions such as pancytopenia and thereby promote comprehensive patient management; for example, pancytopenia may unmask hepatic cirrhosis which may necessitate use of nadolol for prophylaxis against gastroesophageal variceal hemorrhage as well as use of prophylactic antibiotics against spontaneous bacterial peritonitis. ▪ The **peripheral blood smear (PBS)** is used to further evaluate leukocytosis, anemias, and other abnormalities. In the investigation of persistent leukocytosis, the PBS is of limited value and therefore, while the PBS should certainly be performed, it is generally followed by **immunophenotyping by flow cytometry** if not a direct referral to a hematologist. An excellent review by Tefferi et al[113] concluded, "In general, it is prudent to perform a PBS in most instances of abnormal CBC, along with basic tests that are dictated by the type of CBC abnormalities. The latter may include, for example, serum ferritin in patients with microcytic anemia or lymphocyte immunophenotyping by flow cytometry in patients with lymphocytosis..."
Limitations:	▪ WBC count may be normal even in patients with serious infections. ▪ RBC indices may be normal in people with severe iron deficiency. ○ **Dr Vasquez's experience**—*Many outpatients with no evidence of anemia on the CBC will be grossly iron deficient with ferritin values less than 6 mcg/L, clearly indicating iron deficiency. Nonanemic iron deficiency contributes to fatigue, depression, RLS, attention deficit.*
Comments:	▪ The **CBC** is a foundational part of the assessment for all new patients. Generally, "CBC *with* differential" should be ordered.

---

[113] Tefferi A, Hanson CA, Inwards DJ. How to interpret and pursue an abnormal complete blood cell count in adults. *Mayo Clin Proc* 2005;80(7):923-3

Clinical Case **Classic iron insufficiency in a healthy 32yo athletic female**: This limited laboratory report is from a 32yo athletic female whose primary complaint is that of "less endurance than expected" given her healthy lifestyle and frequent participation in physical exercise of various types such as running, biking, hiking, and kayaking. Her TSH is on the low end of normal consistent with her taking 17 mcg daily of liothyroinine (T3); note however that the total T3 level remains on the low end of the normal range, suggesting that she may benefit from additional T3 supplementation. The RBC parameters Hgb and Hct are on the low end of the normal range consistent with recent menstruation; the response of the bone marrow to recent blood loss is noted with the RDW being toward the high end of normal, refecting increased marrow production of reticulocytes. Ferritin is suboptimal at 25 ng/mL, given that the optimal range is approximately 40-70 ng/mL. Although various iron supplements are available on the market and high-iron foods such as beef and blackstrap molasis can be used, typical treatment is with iron 18 mg per day often provided as ferrous sulfate 90 mg; note that 5 mg ferrous sulfate = 1 mg elemental iron. Other forms of iron such as ferrous aspartate may be better tolerated. Daily iron supplementation for 2-3 months should elevate the ferritin level and improve the feeling of energy not simply by ❶ improving oxygen delivery to tissues but also by ❷ improving function of the electron transport chain where iron is a required cofactor, ❸ improving the conversion of thyroid hormone (T4) into the active form of T3, and by ❹ improving the production of dopamine and norepinephrine, since iron is a required cofactor for the enzyme tyrosine hydroxylase which converts the amino acid tyrosine into L-DOPA which is converted to dopamine and then partially to norepinephrine. Given that this patient menstruates monthly and has no significant medical history and—specifically—no gastrointestinal complaints; the probability is high that her state of iron insufficiency is due to physiologic blood loss; however, a case could be made for endoscopic evaluation[114], and in the event that the patient suffered from an diagnosed intestinal lesion such as colon cancer, the practitioner who did not refer for gastroenterologic evaluation would be challenged to produce effective medicolegal defense. Guidelines[115] published in 2011 support testing for celiac disease, *H. pylori* infection, and hematuria while reserving endoscopy in premenopausal women to those aged 50 years or older, or with symptoms of gastrointestinal disease, or those with a strong family history of colorectal cancer.

Reported: 07/07/2011 / 06:02 CDT

Test Name	In Range	Out Of Range	Reference Range
TSH, 3RD GENERATION	0.54		mIU/L

Reference Range

> or = 20 Years   0.40-4.50

Pregnancy Ranges
First trimester   0.20-4.70
Second trimester   0.30-4.10
Third trimester   0.40-2.70

Test Name	In Range	Reference Range
T3, TOTAL	97	76-181 ng/dL
CBC (INCLUDES DIFF/PLT)		
WHITE BLOOD CELL COUNT	7.1	3.8-10.8 Thousand/uL
RED BLOOD CELL COUNT	4.28	3.80-5.10 Million/uL
HEMOGLOBIN	12.1	11.7-15.5 g/dL
HEMATOCRIT	36.2	35.0-45.0 %
MCV	84.5	80.0-100.0 fL
MCH	28.4	27.0-33.0 pg
MCHC	33.6	32.0-36.0 g/dL
RDW	14.8	11.0-15.0 %
PLATELET COUNT	248	140-400 Thousand/uL
ABSOLUTE NEUTROPHILS	3586	1500-7800 cells/uL
ABSOLUTE LYMPHOCYTES	2854	850-3900 cells/uL
ABSOLUTE MONOCYTES	525	200-950 cells/uL
ABSOLUTE EOSINOPHILS	107	15-500 cells/uL
ABSOLUTE BASOPHILS	28	0-200 cells/uL
NEUTROPHILS	50.5	%
LYMPHOCYTES	40.2	%
MONOCYTES	7.4	%
EOSINOPHILS	1.5	%
BASOPHILS	0.4	%
FERRITIN	25	10-154 ng/mL

[114] "A gastrointestinal source of chronic blood loss was identified in a substantial proportion of premenopausal women with iron deficiency anemia." Green BT, Rockey DC. Gastrointestinal endoscopic evaluation of premenopausal women with iron deficiency anemia. *J Clin Gastroenterol*. 2004 Feb;38(2):104-9
[115] Goddard AF, James MW, McIntyre AS, Scott BB; on behalf of the British Society of Gastroenterology. Guidelines for the management of iron deficiency anaemia. *Gut*. 2011 Jun 6. [Epub ahead of print] epocrates.com/dacc/1106/irondefbmj1106.pdf

<mark>Clinical Case</mark> **Vitamin B-12 deficiency without hematologic abnormality—report and discussion**: This elderly patient shows no signs of anemia; note also that the MCV is perfectly normal. Given that the psychiatric literature supports a minimal serum vitamin B-12 level of 600 pg/ml, the advocation by medical reference laboratories of a lower "normal" limit of 200 pg/ml is scientifically absurd and ethically indefensible; this is yet another example of the importance of clinicians' knowledge of the literature overriding the laboratory's reference range. The consistent documentation of the rapid reversibility of severe neuropsychiatric illness with vitamin B-12 therapy as the only intervention[116,117] provides additional justification for empiric vitamin B-12 administration in patients with clinical symptoms consistent with vitamin B-12 deficiency regardless of hematologic and serologic findings.[118] Vitamin B-12 deficiency is very serious because it can lead to permanent brain damage, resulting in personality changes, memory impairment, and overt psychotic disorders, including catatonia; mechanisms of neurologic injury may include homocysteine toxicity, autoimmune neuronal demyelinization, and axonal degeneration and nerve-sheath demyelination especially in the median forebrain bundle.[119]

HEMATOLOGY

----- CBC - WBC STUDIES -----

Procedure:	WBC 10E3
Reference:	[4.50-11.00]
Units:	/CMM
07DEC06 0926 THU	7.32

----- CBC - RBC STUDIES -----

Procedure:	RBC 10E6	HEMOGLOBIN	HEMATOCRIT	MCV	MCH	MCHC	RDW-CV
Reference:	[4.50-5.90]	[13.5-17.5]	[41.0-53.0]	[80.0-94.0]	[27.0-31.0]	[32.0-36.0]	[11.0-16.0]
Units:	/CMM	G/DL	%	FL	PG	%	%
07DEC06 0926 THU	5.16	15.7	46.3	89.7	30.4	33.9	14.1

----- CBC - PLATELET STUDIES -----

Procedure:	PLATELET 10E3	MPV
Reference:	[150-500]	[9.0-13.0]
Units:	/CMM	FL
07DEC06 0926 THU	308	11.2

CHEMISTRY PROFILES

----- ROUTINE CHEMISTRY PROFILES -----

Procedure:	SODIUM	POTASSIUM	CHLORIDE	CO2	GLUCOSE	BUN	CREATININE	CALCIUM
Reference:	[133-145]	[3.5-5.3]	[100-110]	[22.0-29.0]	[70-110]	[5-25]	[0.5-1.4]	[8.3-10.3]
Units:	MMOL/L	MEQ/L	MMOL/L	MMOL/L	MG/DL	MG/DL	MG/DL	MG/DL
07DEC06 0926 THU	137	4.3	101	27.0	90	16	0.9	9.9

Procedure:	ANION GAP	OSMOLARITY	BUN/CREAT
Reference:	[6-14]	[272-305]	
Units:	MEQ/L	MOSM/K	MG/DL
07DEC06 0926 THU	13	275	17.8

SPECIAL CHEMISTRY

----- CHEMISTRY SPECIAL/MISCELLANEOUS -----

Procedure:	FOLATE	VITAMIN B-12
Reference:	[2.0-18.0]	[193-982]
Units:	NG/ML	PG/ML
07DEC06 0926 THU	14.7	182 L

[116] Berry N, Sagar R, Tripathi BM. Catatonia and other psychiatric symptoms with vitamin B12 deficiency. *Acta Psychiatr Scand.* 2003 ;108(2):156-9

[117] Newbold HL. Vitamin B-12: placebo or neglected therapeutic tool? *Med Hypotheses.* 1989 Mar;28(3):155-64

[118] Solomon LR. Cobalamin-responsive disorders in the ambulatory care setting. *Blood.* 2005;105:978-85. Very important article supporting empiric vitamin B12 supplementation.

[119] Catalano G, et al. Catatonia. Another neuropsychiatric presentation of vitamin B12 deficiency? *Psychosomatics.* 1998;39:456-60 psy.psychiatryonline.org/cgi/reprint/39/5/456

Nutritional deficiency, diet-responsive disorders, and the allopathic medical paradigm: Review and commentary with emphases on diabetes mellitus and vitamins D and B-12

Consequences of vitamin B-12 deficiency: Initially the manifestations are mild and reversible, but over time they become more severe and strongly refractory to treatment to the point that permanent damage (particularly in the CNS) is anticipated:

- "Bipolar disorder"—Vitamin B12 deficiency can result in a condition indistinguishable from a bipolar disorder,
- Organic brain syndrome, delirium, confusion, poor memory, impaired cognition,
- Dementia and erroneous diagnosis of "Alzheimer's disease",
- Mood disorders, depression, catatonia, paranoia, paranoid psychosis, violent behavior,
- Peripheral neuropathy, "combined degeneration" of anterior and posterior columns of the spinal cord,
- As a result of the above problems, patients who are mismanaged by doctors unknowledgeable about basic nutrition often suffer directly from these effects but also suffer from the medical management from these problems. Mood disorders and psychosis may result from B-12 deficiency, and the medical management of mood disorders and psychosis includes medicalization, electroconvulsive therapy (ECT), and institutionalization.

The medical profession's failure to train its students and doctors in nutrition is widely and consistently documented; given that such a profession-wide policy can do nothing other than result in patient harm and/or drug dependency under the guise of "healthcare", it is—borrowing a phrase from Nietzsche—"the highest of all conceivable corruptions."

- Nutritional deficiencies and the medical paradigm (*J Clin Endocrinol Metab* 2003 Nov): "But public health measures in the first half of the 20th century eradicated the most extreme of the vitamin deficiencies in the industrialized nations, and the physician's actual experience of [obvious] deficiency disease dropped to near zero. Perhaps as a result, the medical profession's approach to nutrition today is still dominated by the external agent paradigm, as witnessed in the national campaigns for cholesterol, saturated fat, and salt. Those who think more seriously in terms of the continuing importance of deficiency per se are often derogated or relegated to the quackery fringe. The result, at the very least, is inattention to the real deficiencies that may masquerade as other disorders, or that may simply be ignored altogether."
- Failure of surgical treatment for low-back pain caused by vitamin D deficiency (*J Am Board Fam Med* 2009 Jan): The author of this case series describes six cases of chronic debilitating back pain—three of which "required surgery"—which were greatly relieved or completely cured by correction of vitamin D deficiency. The author notes, "Chronic low back pain and failed back surgery may improve with repletion of vitamin D from a state of deficiency/insufficiency to sufficiency. Vitamin D insufficiency is common; repletion of vitamin D to normal levels in patients who have chronic low back pain or have had failed back surgery may improve quality of life or, in some cases, result in complete resolution of symptoms."

That nutritional deficiencies can cause mood disorders and mental disease is well-known; in contrast to what patients actually need, the general allopathic approach to these clinical presentations is founded upon the administration of drugs, followed by ECT, institutionalization, and psychosurgery and—lately, instead of scalpel-induced brain damage—radiofrequency heating (thermocapsulotomy) or gamma radiation (radiosurgery, gammacapsulotomy) for the destruction of brain structures, and the surgical implantation of brain electrostimulators. **Meanwhile, thousands of these psychiatrically-labeled patients simply need nutritional supplementation.** Minor exceptions noted, the medical profession as a whole chooses to remain blind to the value of nutrition so that the pharmacosurgical paradigm can remain dominant by continuing to *appear* omnipotent. The dual illusions that are maintained are "Drugs and surgery are the answers to all major health problems" and "If no drug exists for a condition, then it is idiopathic and no curative treatment is available."

Notable/additional publications relevant to this section:
1. Catalano G, Catalano MC, Rosenberg EI, Embi PJ, Embi CS. Catatonia. Another neuropsychiatric presentation of vitamin B12 deficiency? *Psychosomatics.* 1998 Sep-Oct;39(5):456-60
2. Newbold HL. Vitamin B-12: placebo or neglected therapeutic tool? *Med Hypotheses.* 1989 Mar;28(3):155-64
3. Solomon LR. Cobalamin-responsive disorders in the ambulatory care setting: unreliability of cobalamin, methylmalonic acid, and homocysteine testing. *Blood.* 2005 Feb 1;105(3):978-85
4. Christmas D, Eljamel MS, Butler S, et al. Long term outcome of thermal anterior capsulotomy for chronic, treatment refractory depression. *J Neurol Neurosurg Psychiatry.* 2011 Jun;82(6):594-600
5. Malone DA Jr. Use of deep brain stimulation in treatment-resistant depression. *Cleve Clin J Med.* 2010 Jul;77 Suppl 3:S77-80
6. Heaney RP. Vitamin D, nutritional deficiency, and the medical paradigm. *J Clin Endocrinol Metab.* 2003;88:5107-8
7. Schwalfenberg G. Improvement of chronic back pain or failed back surgery with vitamin D repletion: a case series. *J Am Board Fam Med.* 2009 Jan-Feb;22(1):69-74

Nutritional deficiency, diet-responsive disorders, and the allopathic medical paradigm: Review and commentary with emphases on diabetes mellitus and vitamins D and B-12—*continued*

The diabetes deception: Type-2 diabetes mellitus (T2DM) has burgeoned into an epidemic under the dominance of the allopathic disease model, and patients are told that the condition is genetic, progressive and incurable; a review published in the May 2011 issue of *Journal of the American Osteopathic Association* admonished physicians to (mis)educate their patients as follows, with Dr Vasquez's comments in brackets: "Be absolutely clear that T2DM is a lifelong disease [false statement] that will require lifelong treatment [false statement fostering dependency]. Success in controlling the disease and preventing future complications will depend on the patient and physician working together [creation of dependency under the guise of "working together"]. There is often a fatalistic attitude in patients with T2DM [perhaps because they have been lied to and disempowered], so it is important to establish a relationship that on one hand offers hope [creating the illusion of hope while enforcing drug dependency] and on the other does not suggest that the disease will be cured [although the diseases is generally curable with appropriate nutritional intervention]. Be up front with the patient from the first visit and make it clear that T2DM is a chronic illness [enforce drug dependency starting at the first visit]…" This babble was published in a peer-reviewed medical journal despite clear multi-decade evidence showing that T2DM is reversible with nutritional intervention.

T2DM is rapidly reversible with diet (*Diabetologia* 2011 Jun): "Normalization of both beta cell function and hepatic insulin sensitivity in type 2 diabetes was achieved by dietary energy restriction alone. This was associated with decreased pancreatic and liver triacylglycerol stores. **The abnormalities underlying type 2 diabetes are reversible by reducing dietary energy intake.**"
* Diet therapy effective, safe, and is at least as effective as injected insulin for reducing chronic hyperglycemia in T2DM (*Nutr Metab* 2009 May): "The number of patients on sulfonylureas decreased from 7 at baseline to 2 at 6 months. No patient required inpatient care or insulin therapy. In summary, the 30%-carbohydrate diet over 6 months led to a remarkable reduction in HbA1c levels, even among outpatients with severe type 2 diabetes, without any insulin therapy, hospital care or increase in sulfonylureas. **The effectiveness of the [low-carbohydrate] diet may be comparable to that of insulin therapy.**"

Ironically (or not), the first-line drug for T2DM—metformin—causes vitamin B-12 (cobalamin, Cbl) deficiency and exacerbation of the often debilitating peripheral neuropathy of T2DM which is often treated with the drugs gabapentin/Neurontin or pregabalin/Lyrica, which exacerbates obesity and T2DM, thereby promoting a vicious cycle.
* Pregabalin/Lyrica and gabapentin/Neurontin promote fat-weight gain, thereby exacerbating T2DM (*Prescrire Int* 2005 Dec): "Pregabalin, like gabapentin, can lead to weight gain and peripheral edema especially in elderly patients."
* Metformin causes vitamin B-12 deficiency and exacerbates diabetic peripheral neuropathy (*Diabetes Care* 2010 Jan): "Metformin-treated patients had depressed Cbl levels and elevated fasting MMA and Hcy levels. Clinical and electrophysiological measures identified more severe peripheral neuropathy in these patients; the cumulative metformin dose correlated strongly with these clinical and paraclinical group differences. CONCLUSIONS: Metformin exposure may be an iatrogenic cause for exacerbation of peripheral neuropathy in patients with type 2 diabetes."
* Vitamin B-12 deficiency secondary to metformin prescription (*Rev Assoc Med Bras* 2011 Jan): "The present findings suggest a high prevalence of vitamin B12 deficiency in metformin-treated diabetic patients [n=144]. Older patients, patients in long term treatment with metformin and low vitamin B12 intake are probably more prone to this deficiency."
* Metformin-induced vitamin B12 deficiency presenting as a peripheral neuropathy (*South Med J* 2010 Mar): "Chronic metformin use results in vitamin B12 deficiency in 30% of patients. … **Vitamin B12 deficiency, which may present without anemia and as a peripheral neuropathy, is often misdiagnosed as diabetic neuropathy, although the clinical findings are usually different. Failure to diagnose the cause of the neuropathy will result in progression of central and/or peripheral neuronal damage which can be arrested but not reversed with vitamin B12 replacement.**"
* Low vitamin B-12 status correlates with expedited brain atrophy (*Neurology* 2008 Sep): "The decrease in brain volume was greater among those with lower vitamin B(12) and holoTC levels and higher plasma tHcy and MMA levels at baseline. … Using the upper (for the vitamins) or lower tertile (for the metabolites) as reference in logistic regression analysis and adjusting for the above covariates, vitamin B(12) in the **bottom tertile (<308 pmol/L)** was associated with increased rate of brain volume loss (odds ratio 6.17)."

Notable/additional publications relevant to this section:
1. Gavin et al. Type 2 diabetes mellitus: practical approaches for primary care physicians. *J Am Osteopath Assoc* 2011;111(5s4):S3-S12
2. Lim EL, et al. Reversal of type 2 diabetes: normalisation of beta cell function. *Diabetologia*. 2011 Jun 9
3. Haimoto et al. Effects of a low-carbohydrate diet on glycemic control in outpatients with severe type 2 diabetes. *Nutr Metab* 2009;6;21
4. Gabapentin/Neurontin causes "Gains of up to 15 kg (33lbs) during 3 months of treatment." pacmedweightloss.com/docs/medications_that_cause_weight_gain.pdf Accessed July 2011.
5. Vogiatzoglou et al. Vitamin B12 status and rate of brain volume loss in community-dwelling elderly. *Neurology*. 2008;71(11):826-32
6. Wile DJ, Toth C. Association of metformin, elevated homocysteine, and methylmalonic acid levels and clinically worsened diabetic peripheral neuropathy. *Diabetes Care*. 2010 Jan;33(1):156-61
7. Nervo M, Lubini A, Raimundo FV, Faulhaber GA, Leite C, Fischer LM, Furlanetto TW. Vitamin B12 in metformin-treated diabetic patients: a cross-sectional study in Brazil. *Rev Assoc Med Bras*. 2011 Jan-Feb;57(1):46-9
8. Bell DS. Metformin-induced vitamin B12 deficiency presenting as a peripheral neuropathy. *South Med J*. 2010 Mar;103(3):265-7
9. [No authors listed] Pregabalin: new drug. Very similar to gabapentin. *Prescrire Int*. 2005 Dec;14(80):203-6

<u>Nutritional inertia: consequences for the clinician</u>: Given that the evidence in favor of early and empiric treatment for possible vitamin B-12 deficiency is stronger than evidence in favor of allowing vitamin B-12 deficiency or dependency to persist with potentially catastrophic outcomes, no scientific argument can be made in favor of failing to diagnose and treat vitamin B-12 deficiency/dependency. However, since, in general, the allopathic and osteopathic medical professions have failed to educate their students and doctors about nutrition, these professions have established ignorance as their defense and therefore no standard of care exists for the treatment or failure of treatment of chronic nutritional deficiencies. Ethically, the results are failure to achieve beneficence via failure to diagnose and treat, and the widespread implementation of malfeasance via diagnostic/therapeutic failure complicated by the unnecessary expenses and adverse effects of drugs/surgeries/interventions used in place of nutritional supplementation. **The enforcement of a standard of care is meaningless when nutritional incompetence is the standard.** Fortunately for patients, the biomedical literature uses increasingly strong language in favor of mandating standards for nutritional evaluation and treatment:

- <u>Nutritional deficiencies and the medical paradigm</u> (*J Clin Endocrinol Metab* 2003 Nov): "J. Cannell (submitted for publication) has written that measures such as this editorial will not change the situation, and that only tort litigation will work. One can only hope that he is wrong. Either way, something needs to change"
- <u>Physicians should routinely use vitamin supplementation as treatment for patients</u> (*JAMA* 2002 Jun): "Physicians should make specific efforts to ensure that patients are taking vitamins they should..."
- <u>Testing and treating for vitamin D deficiency among patients with chronic nonspecific musculoskeletal pain should be the standard of care</u> (*Mayo Clin Proc* 2003 Dec): "Because osteomalacia is a known cause of persistent, nonspecific musculoskeletal pain, screening all outpatients with such pain for hypovitaminosis D should be standard practice in clinical care."
- <u>Testing and treating for vitamin D deficiency among patients with chronic low-back pain should be the standard of care</u> (*Spine* 2003 Jan): "Screening for vitamin D deficiency and treatment with supplements should be mandatory in this setting."

<u>Notable/additional publications relevant to this section</u>:
1. Fletcher RH, Fairfield KM. Vitamins for chronic disease prevention in adults: clinical applications. *JAMA*. 2002;287:3127-9
2. Plotnikoff et al. Prevalence of severe hypovitaminosis D in patients persistent musculoskeletal pain. *Mayo Clin Proc*. 2003;78:1463-70
3. Al Faraj S, Al Mutairi K. Vitamin D deficiency and chronic low back pain in Saudi Arabia. *Spine* 2003 ;28:177-9

Urinalysis: UA	

Overview and interpretation:	▪ <u>Collection</u>: Unless catheterized, patients are advised to pass approximately one-third of their available urine into the toilet, then pass approximately the middle-third of their urine into the specimen container. Use of an antiseptic to clean the urethral meatus was once advocated to avoid/reduce specimen contamination, but this step is ineffective and therefore unnecessary because contamination rates remain similar at 32% and 29% whether or not, respectively, urethral meatus cleansing is performed.[120]
	
	▪ <u>Analysis</u>: Analysis should be performed on fresh urine, preferably within 1-2 hours; in outpatient clinical practice this two-hour timeframe is consistently possible only if the clinician performs in-office dipstick analysis (and perhaps microscopic visualization). Samples that cannot be analyzed within 1-2 hours or those which are destined for a reference laboratory should be refrigerated. Dipstick UA can be performed in office and is simple, inexpensive, and—when performed and interpreted with a modicum of competence—sufficiently accurate. Per Klatt[121], "The color change occurring on each segment of the strip is compared to a color chart to obtain results. However, a careless doctor, nurse, or assistant is entirely capable of misreading or misinterpreting the results." Urine samples can be sent to a reference laboratory for more accurate chemical analysis as well as microscopic analysis, culture and sensitivity. Whether infection is clinically suspected or not, clinicians might chose to order "UA with reflex to microscopy and culture" to ensure that urine samples are appropriately processed if the laboratory finds suspicion of UTI upon dipstick analysis.
	
	▪ <u>Scope of this review</u>: The purpose of this brief review is to concisely refresh clinicians' appreciation of the components of the routine urinalysis, one that is generally performed in-office with a dipstick reagent stick or that is performed by a reference laboratory. This is not an exhaustive review, and microscopic findings have not been detailed here because most clinicians do not perform microscopy in their offices; additional details on UA and microscopic assessment is available in articles such as the excellent review by Simerville, Maxted, and Pahira published in *American Family Physician* 2005 and available on-line at aafp.org/afp/2005/0315/p1153.html as of July 2011.
	
	▪ <u>Components of routine urinalysis</u>:
	  o <u>Visual inspection</u>: Urine should be clear with a color ranging from faint yellow (well hydrated, dilute urine) to bright yellow (especially with B-vitamin supplementation). An amber-brown hue might be due to dehydration or a pathologic process resulting in myoglobinuria (i.e., rhabdomyolysis) or the presence of bile pigments (i.e., biliary tract obstruction). A red color to urine suggests hematuria, recent beet consumption, or use of certain drugs or food dyes; the antibiotic rifampin/rifampicin is notorious for adding a red-orange color to the urine (and to a lesser extent to sweat and tears). The urine of patients with porphyria cutanea tarda will be red-brown in natural light and pink-red in fluorescent light.[122] Cloudy urine is due to pyruia (infection), proteinuria, or precipitated phosphate crystals in alkaline urine.
	  o <u>Strong odor</u>: Odiferous or malodorous urine suggests infection, recent ingestion of foods such as asparagus or nutritional supplements such as lipoic acid, certain medications, concentrated urine due to dehydration or underperfusion of the kidneys.
	  o <u>Specific gravity</u>: Specific gravity is a measure of solute concentration and thus is proportional to urine osmolality; as such it reflects renal perfusion, hydration, and the ability of the kidneys to perform their critical function of concentrating filtrate. Dilute urine has a specific gravity <1.010 and is seen with adequate/excessive hydration,

---

[120] Simerville JA, Maxted WC, Pahira JJ. Urinalysis: a comprehensive review. *Am Fam Physician.* 2005 Mar 15;71(6):1153-62 aafp.org/afp/2005/0315/p1153.html
[121] Klatt EC. WebPath. Savannah, Georgia, USA. library.med.utah.edu/WebPath/tutorial/urine/urine.html Accessed July 1, 2011
[122] Rich MW. Porphyria cutanea tarda. Don't forget to look at the urine. *Postgrad Med.* 1999 Apr;105(4):208-10, 213-4

diuretic use, diabetes insipidus, adrenal insufficiency, hyperaldosteronism, and impaired renal function (i.e., failure of the kidneys to concentrate urine). Concentrated urine has a specific gravity >1.020 and correlates with dehydration, renal artery stenosis, hypoperfusion/shock, glucosuria, and syndrome of inappropriate anti-diuretic hormone secretion (SIADH), which is often associated with hyponatremia.

o <u>pH</u>: Urine pH may range from 4.5 (very acidic) to as high as 8.5 (very alkaline). Urine pH correlates with serum pH except in patients with renal tubular acidosis (RTA type-1, a condition associated with chronically alkaline urine). Therefore, urine pH can be used to screen for various conditions of systemic alkalosis and acidosis. The Western diet—also called the standard American diet or S.A.D.—causes mild diet-induced metabolic acidosis[123] which promotes degenerative diseases; in contrast, a diet rich in fruits and vegetables such as the Paleo-Mediterranean diet[124] promotes mild systemic and urinary alkalinization.[125] From a wellness perspective, urine pH should be 7.5 up to 8.0 because urinary alkalinization facilitates xenobiotic excretion[126], promotes urinary retention of minerals such as potassium, magnesium, and calcium, and causes a reduction in serum cortisol.[127] Urine pH—like urine sodium:potassium ratio—can be used as a marker of compliance for intake of fruits, vegetables, and alkalinizing supplements such as potassium citrate. For some patients (mostly female), urine alkalinization may encourage urinary tract infection, especially if gastrointestinal dysbiosis[128] is present; in such situations, the often causative GI dysbiosis should be treated, and consistent or transient urinary acidification can be achieved with oral ascorbic acid. Urea-splitting bacteria can cause the urine to be alkaline, and such bacteria can also promote development of magnesium-ammonium phosphate crystals and so-called staghorn nephrolithiasis. Acidic urine promotes development of uric acid nephrolithiasis; therapeutic urinary alkalinization such as by use of supplemental potassium citrate or an alkalinizing diet is preventive and therapeutic. On this topic, Cicerello et al[129] wrote, "In conclusion urinary alkalization with maintaining continuously high urinary pH values, could be the treatment of choice for stone dissolution and prevention of uric acid stones."

o <u>Bilirubin in urine</u>: If present, bilirubin in urine is of the direct/conjugated fraction (rather than indirect/unconjugated, which is nonhydrosoluble) and indicates the need to evaluate for biliary tract obstruction.

o <u>Urobilinogen</u>: Urobilinogen is (direct) bilirubin that has been conjugated in the liver, passed through the biliary system into the intestine, partially metabolized by bacteria, then reabsorbed via the portal circulation and filtered by the kidney. Elevated urobilinogen is associated with liver disease and hemolytic diseases.

o <u>Glucose</u>: Glucose is found in the urine when the serum glucose exceeds approximately 190 mg/dL and overwhelms the reabsorptive/resorptive capacity of the proximal tubule. Glucose in the urine is presumptive evidence supporting the diagnosis of diabetes mellitus. Rare non-diabetic causes of glucosuria/glycosuria include liver disease, pancreatic disease, and Fanconi's syndrome (characterized by a failure of the proximal renal tubules to reabsorb glucose, amino acids, uric acid, phosphate and bicarbonate).

---

[123] "The modern Western-type diet is deficient in fruits and vegetables and contains excessive animal products, generating the accumulation of non-metabolizable anions and a lifespan state of overlooked metabolic acidosis, whose magnitude increases progressively with aging due to the physiological decline in kidney function." Adeva MM, Souto G. Diet-induced metabolic acidosis. *Clin Nutr.* 2011 Aug;30(4):416-21. Epub 2011 Apr 9.

[124] Vasquez A. Revisiting the Five-Part Nutritional Wellness Protocol: The Supplemented Paleo-Mediterranean Diet. *Nutritional Perspectives* 2011 Jan

[125] Cordain L, Eaton SB, Sebastian A, et al. Origins and evolution of the Western diet: health implications for the 21st century. *Am J Clin Nutr.* 2005 Feb;81(2):341-54

[126] Proudfoot AT, Krenzelok EP, Vale JA. Position Paper on urine alkalinization. *J Toxicol Clin Toxicol.* 2004;42(1):1-26

[127] Maurer et al. Neutralization of Western diet inhibitsbone resorption independently of K intake, reduces cortisol secretion in humans. *Am J Physiol Renal Physiol* 2003;:F32-40

[128] Vasquez A. Nutritional and Botanical Treatments Against "Silent Infections" and Gastrointestinal Dysbiosis, Commonly Overlooked Causes of Neuromusculoskeletal Inflammation and Chronic Health Problems. *Nutritional Perspectives* 2006; Jan

[129] Cicerello E, Merlo F, Maccatrozzo L. Urinary alkalization for the treatment of uric acid nephrolithiasis. *Arch Ital Urol Androl.* 2010 Sep;82(3):145-8

Urinalysis: UA

- o Ketones: Most UA dipsticks detect acetic acid; other products of fatty acid metabolism found in urine include acetone and beta-hydroxybutyric acid. Ketonuria indicates either metabolic disturbance such as diabetes mellitus or normal physiology in the fasting or lipolytic state. Many clinicians—particularly medical students and physicians[note 130]—have been taught to view ketonuria as synonymous with ketoacidosis; this is obviously inaccurate since lipolysis and the resulting ketonuria are normal *and quite desirable* physiologic states. Ketonuria can be measured with ketone-specific dipsticks as a marker of weight-loss efficacy and compliance with diet and exercise programs.

- o Protein: Urine should not contain measurable protein on routine urinalysis. Any finding of protein in the urine—even a "trace" amount—requires follow-up; specifically, the test should be repeated within 2-4 weeks and consistently positive results require more detailed testing including serum BUN and creatinine. Urine protein can also be measured in 24-hour urine collections and should not exceed 150 mg/day; greater than this amount is diagnostic of proteinuria, while ≥ 3.5 gm/day is consistent with nephrotic syndrome, mandating a much more comprehensive *and urgent* patient evaluation. Testing for "protein" with a routine urinalysis will not detect all forms of clinically relevant proteinuria; specifically and classically, routine UA is insensitive for the microalbuminuria of diabetes mellitus (detected with the urinary albumin:creatinine ratio) and also the Bence-Jones proteinuria seen with multiple myeloma.

Evaluation of persistent proteinuria

1. Comprehensive evaluation of patient history, physical exam, and overall clinical impression,
2. Measurement of serum BUN, creatinine, albumin, and lipids; consider measuring cystatin c,
3. Microscopic examination of urinary sediment,
4. Assessment for conditions that commonly cause proteinuria, especially hypertension (sphygmomanometry), diabetes (hemoglobin A1c), autoimmune conditions (screen with ANA);
5. Measurement of 24-hour urinary creatinine excretion (or spot urinary albumin-creatinine ratio),
6. Urinary protein electrophoresis,
7. If the above measures are pathoetiologically unfruitful, refer to an internist or nephrologist.

---

[130] One of the arguments most commonly leveled against the ketogenic diet—in particular the Atkins diet—is that the induction of ketosis, as measured by ketonuria, is a potentially problematic state that should be avoided. This is an example of selective medical ignorance since mild ketosis is physiologically normal is clinically advantageous for weight loss and seizure control. In our osteopathic medical school, one lecturer advised our student body of 170 that ketosis was evidence of the "danger from diet therapies." On the contrary, given that most of my medical school professors were obese, they should have more carefully considered the benefits of rational dietary therapy, including low-carbohydrate versions of the Paleo-Mediterranean diet (described in this text) which can produce mild ketosis en route to alleviating diabetes mellitus and hypertension. Examples of selective medical ignorance and bias against low-carbohydrate ketogenic diets abound from allopathic institutions. "One diet that has raised safety concerns among the scientific community is the low-carbohydrate, high-protein diet." Tapper-Gardzina Y, Cotugna N, Vickery CE. Should you recommend a low-carb, high-protein diet? *Nurse Pract.* 2002 Apr;27(4):52-3, 55-6, 58-9. "High Protein / Low Carb (Carbohydrate) Diets. Long term, these fad diets can be harmful. Many of the health claims about these diets are not based on scientific proof. Low carb diets are still just that – a diet. Most people find maintaining a low carb diet difficult if not impossible long term. Even if weight is lost, 90% of fad dieters gain all or most of the weight back in five years." Ohio State University. medicalcenter.osu.edu/PatientEd/Materials/PDFDocs/nut-diet/nut-other/high-pro.pdf 2011 Jul.

Overview and interpretation:	o <u>Nitrite</u>: Urinary nitrite is most often the result of bacterial action on excreted urinary nitrate; students and clinicians can remember this by recalling that nitrate is consumed in foods via the *a*limentary tract, while nitrite in the urine generally indicates urinary tract *i*nfection (UTI). A small amount of nitrate is naturally present in some foods, including tap water, beer, some cheese products, cured meats and bacon. Additional environmental sources of nitrate include the nitrates that are intentionally added to foods as preservatives, those which are contaminants from nitrate-containing fertilizers, and those which are present in our polluted environment from pesticides and the manufacture of rubber and latex. Not all bacteria can convert nitrate to nitrite; generally, this reaction indicates the presence of Gram-negative rods such as *Escherichia coli*, the causative agent in the vast majority of UTIs in both men and women. Much less commonly, Gram-positive bacteria may also cause nitrite-positive UTI. A negative urine nitrite does not exclude UTI as it may be due to either a low-nitrate diet, diuretic use, or infection with bacteria that are incapable of reducing nitrate to nitrite.
	
	       UTI management
	    Finding evidence of a UTI requires the clinician to determine the nature of that UTI—urethritis, prostatitis/vaginitis, cystitis, pyelonephritis—and to evaluate the severity of the infection in the context of the patient's age and comorbidities.
	
	o <u>Leukocyte esterase</u>: Leukocyte esterase—as its name suggests—is an enzyme produced by white blood cells and is therefore associated with urinary tract infection. Up to five minutes is required for the enzyme to fully react with the dipstick reagent. Obviously, a positive dipstick leukocyte esterase does not itself distinguish between benign infectious cystitis and life-threatening pyelonephritis.
	
	o <u>Red blood cells (RBC)</u>: On a dipstick urinalysis (in contrast to a legitimate microscopic exam), "RBC" are reported not because of the presence of cells but because of the peroxidase activity of erythrocytes, which is also noted with myoglobinuria or hemoglobinuria. Thus, a dipstick analysis "positive for RBC" could indicate legitimate hematuria, or the presence of hemoglobin or myoglobin such as from marked intravascular hemolysis or rhabdomyolysis, respectively. Red blood cells in urine are not "normal" per se, but are not necessarily pathologic. Microhematuria can be induced by many benign events, including sexual intercourse, exercise, and sample contamination from menstruation. Conversely, pathologic causes of hematuria include urinary tract infections, glomerulonephritis, IgA nephropathy, and nephrolithiasis; overt hematuria is often the first sign of renal or bladder carcinoma. Thus, when consistently present over 2-3 samples, overt or microscopic hematuria—just like any degree of proteinuria—always requires the clinician's attention.
	
	    Overt hematuria and cancer
	    "Up to 20 percent of patients with gross hematuria have urinary tract malignancy; a full work-up with cystoscopy and upper-tract imaging is indicated in patients with this condition."
	
	    Simerville et al. Urinalysis: a comprehensive review. *Am Fam Physician.* 2005 Mar

Advantages:	▪ Allows point-of-care testing and thereby facilitates assessment and treatment.
Limitations:	▪ Noted above, e.g., insensitivity to microalbuminuria and mild Bence-Jones proteinuria
Comments:	▪ For additional information, please see any of several excellent clinically-oriented reviews such as Simerville JA, Maxted WC, Pahira JJ. Urinalysis: a comprehensive review. *Am Fam Physician* 2005 Mar aafp.org/afp/2005/0315/p1153.html

Clinical Case **Routine lab evaluation in an asymptomatic elderly female—part 1**: Whereas a healthy young adult might be treated nonpharmacologically such as with fluid loading and cranberry juice for a routine UTI, clinicians should appreciate several nuances of this case that add to the complexity of appropriate management. This female patient presented for a routine annual examination. Note the patient's date of birth and the date of examination in the lower right-hand corner of the report. Because of the patient's advanced age, additional considerations are warranted. This patient was also noted to be vitamin D deficient and diabetic at the time of the exam—how does this change the overall management? Clinicians must appreciate that elderly patients are less likely to mount a symptomatic and febrile response to advanced urinary tract infections; therefore consideration to the possiblity of pyelonephritis (life-threatening) in contrast to a simple cystitis (benign) must be considered. If the patient has dementia or clinically significant forgetfulness (both of which are easily tested during the office visit), compliance with treatment is much less likely, particularly if the patient does not have access to home nursing and/or does not have a spouse, relative, friend or neighbor who can aid with the supervision of care. Urinary tract infections tend to be more aggressive in elderly patients, especially those who are diabetic, especially those with micronutrient deficiencies.

Questions:
1. What additional assessments are warranted?
2. Would fluid-loading and use of cranberry juice be appropriate treatment for this patient's UTI?
3. What follow-up is recommended?

```
URINALYSIS              01/06/10
                        11:21
U COLOR                  YELLOW
U CLARITY                CLOUDY**
U GLUCOSE              NEGATIVE
U BILE                 NEGATIVE
U KETONES             NEGATIVE
U SPEC GRAVITY           1.012
U BLOOD               NEGATIVE
U PH                       6.0
                        (NOTE06)
U PROTEIN QUAL            20**
U UROBILINOGEN           0.2
U NITRITE             NEGATIVE
U LEUK ESTERASE       MODERATE**
U WBC                     53*H
U WBCC                  RARE**
U RBC                      5*H
U SQUAM EPITH             13
U HYALINE CAST             2
U MUCOUS                 RARE
(NOTE06)
URINE SAMPLES SUBMITTED FOR TESTING MORE THAN 2 HOURS AFTER COLLECTION MAY
YIELD UNRELIABLE RESULTS WHICH INCLUDE INCREASED pH, INCREASED CRYSTAL
FORMATION AND BACTERIAL CONTENT, AND DEGRADATION OF CELLULAR ELEMENTS.
```

```
                          BDATE: 03/20/1926 SEX: F RACE:
                          13:59 01/29/10
```

Answers:
1. Assessments: Clinical examination must include cardiac auscultatory exam, careful pulmonary auscultation for basilar crackles, distal extremity examination for edema and peripheral vascular disease, assessment for tenderness of the flanks, abdomen, and back. Vital signs are assessed: ❶ temperature, ❷ pulse, ❸ blood pressure, ❹ respiratory rate, and ❺ pain. A chemistry panel, CBC with differential, and CRP or ESR should be performed. The urinalysis is sent for microbial culture and sensitivity. Review patient's current drug regimen. If WBC casts were noted on the microscopic exam, then suspected pyelonephritis would warrant hospitalization.
2. Treatments: Fluid-loading would not be appropriate in an elderly patient who might have cardiopulmonary failure, renal insufficiency, or plasma electrolyte imbalance. Cranberry juice is not universally effective and is generally used for UTIs in younger patients who have evidence of *E coli* infection as evidenced by positive urinary nitrite; because this patient's nitrite is negative, a more likely probability exists that the UTI is due to Gram-positive bacteria and thus cranberry juice is less likely to be effective. A clinician could reasonably label this a complicated UTI due to the patient's advanced age and diabetes; thus, either an extended course of Bactrim DS (po b.i.d. for 7-10 days), or Ciprofloxacin (250-500 mg po b.i.d. for 3 days), or Nitrofurantoin (50-100 mg po q6h x7 days or 100 mg ER po q12h x7 days; give w/ food) would be considered. Drug choice depends on patient's tolerance, recent exposure, renal status, drugs, and results of culture and sensitivity.
3. Follow-up: Review laboratory results as soon as possible; if this visit is occurring at the end of the week, the lab should be alerted to phone the clinician with results over the weekend because concomitant leukocytosis or severe acute phase response (suggesting possible pyelonephritis or urosepsis) would change the management on an urgent basis. Patient should return to the office within 24-48 hours for reassessment and repeat UA. Patient is advised to return to office or go to hospital if symptoms develop— especially fever, chills, dizziness, or persistent nausea.

Clinical Case—continued | Routine laboratory evaluation in an asymptomatic elderly female—part 2:

Readers should review the lab report in the left side of the page before reading the discussion on the right side of the page. *Write the appropriate interpretation and intervention before looking at the answers in the column on the right.* Normal ranges were not provided with the original report.

```
CBC                        01/06/10
                           11:21
WBC 10E3                   7.50
NRBC %                     0.0
NRBC 10E3                  0.00
RBC 10E6                   4.08*L
HGB                        11.7*L
HCT                        35.1*L
MCV                        86.0
MCH                        28.7
MCHC                       33.3
RDW-CV                     13.7
RDW-SD                     43.1
PLATELET 10E3              175
MPV                        12.3
-------------------------------------
CHEM PANEL                 01/06/10
                           11:21
SODIUM                     140
POTASSIUM                  4.2
CHLORIDE                   102
CO2 VENOUS                 27.0
GLUCOSE                    248*H
BUN                        22
SER CREATININE             1.2
CALCIUM                    9.5
GLOBULIN                   3.2
TOTAL PROTEIN              7.3
ALBUMIN TOT                4.1
BILI TOTAL                 0.5
ALKALINE PHOSPHA           63
SGOT (AST)                 15
CHOLESTEROL                186
                           (NOTE01)
TRIGLYCERIDES              122
SGPT (ALT)                 11
ANION GAP                  11
OSMOLRTY CALC              291
BUN/CREAT                  18.3
ALB/GLOB RATIO             1.30
HDL                        31
                           (NOTE02)
LDL CALC                   131*H
                           (NOTE03)
(NOTE01)
BORDERLINE HIGH RISK = 200-239
HIGH RISK = 240 AND ABOVE.
(NOTE02)
12-16 HR FASTING:
(NOTE03)
NORMAL = LESS THAN 130 MG/DL
130-159 BORDERLINE/HIGH RISK
>/= 160 HIGH RISK
-------------------------------------
CHEM SPECIAL               01/06/10
                           11:21
HEMOGLOBIN A1C             7.6*H
                           (NOTE04)
25-OHD TOTAL               29
-------------------------------------
BDATE: 03/20/1926 SEX: F
13:59 01/29/10 FROM E585
```

This patient is anemic. The anemia is not of a severity that would be expected to cause cardiopulmonary/perfusion deficits, but the patient should be assessed, particularly if he/she has history of heart failure or lung disease such as emphysema. The MCV is not elevated, nor is it low. This could be due to combined B-12/folate and iron deficiencies; the patient should be tested and treated appropriately. Assuming that the ferritin is low, what is the next mandatory step in the management of this patient? [Answer: Treat the iron deficiency with iron supplementation but be sure to refer the patient for gastrointestinal endoscopy because of the increased probability of intestinal lesion, especially colon cancer.]

This patient is diagnosed with diabetes mellitus because the glucose is above 200. Cardioprotective measures must be implemented, ophthalmologist eye exam initiated, and foot exam performed. An integrative anti-diabetes plan[131] should be implemented.

Clinicians must appreciate the importance of the MDRD equation in this case. The answer is provided below. Perform the Cockcroft-Gault equation on paper (with use of a calculator if necessary), then perform the MDRD equation. Does this change the management of this patient's UTI? Does this change the overall management of this patient? [Answer: This patient has renal insufficiency (GFR 48-55 if African-American and 42-45 if "other race") and therefore some drugs are now contraindicated. Patient is at increased risk of hyperkalemia, especially if taking ACEi or ARB medications. The wise clinician would consider referral to an internist or nephrologist in order to ensure that the patient receives proper monitoring; for example, if the diabetes and renal insufficiency progress, the patient may require dialysis and—possibly—renal transplant, although transplant is unlikely in a patient of this advanced age.][Note 132]

Triglycerides and LDL are higher than optimal. Diet therapy and combination fatty acid supplementation (described later in this text) is indicated. Berberine might be considered as an adjunct.

HgbA1c greater than 6.5% diagnoses diabetes mellitus.

The vitamin D level is low and should be supported with oral administration of 2,000 - 10,000 IU/d and retested at 2-6 months. Serum calcium should be tested after 2-4 weeks of therapy—sooner if the patient is taking a calcium-sparing drug such as hydrochlorothiazide—and again at about 6 and 12 months.

---

[131] Vasquez A. *Chiropractic and Naturopathic Mastery of Common Clinical Disorders, 2009.* See InflammationMastery.com for details and replacements starting in 2014.
[132] Review of this case by Dr Barry Morgan (MD, emergency medicine) is acknowledged and appreciated.

Clinical Case **45yo HLA-B27+ woman with recurrent UTIs and a 7-year history of ankylosing spondylitis treated with anti-TNF drugs**: Positive urine culture and positive stool culture demonstrating bacteria (*Escherichia coli* and *Klebsiella pneumoniae*) known to share molecular mimicry and cross-reactivity with HLA-B27: The Gram-negative bacterium *E. coli* produces a protein named "hypothetical protein 168" (Protein Identification Resource [PIR] data bank access code #jp0612) which shares the amino acid sequence **"RRYLE"** with HLA-B27, which contains the sequence "EWL**RRYLE**IGKETLQRVDP."[133] Per the same citation, *Klebsiella pneumoniae*'s protein (PIR s01840) nitrogenase (reductase) molybdenum-iron protein NifN contains the sequence "EWLRR." This amino acid homology confers validation to the phenomenon of molecular mimicry and thus that immune system components such as immunoglobulins and activated T-cells can cross-react between microbial peptides and human tissue antigens.[134] This patient was treated with the combination pharmaceutical antibiotic trimethoprim and sulfamethoxazole commonly referred to as "Bactrim DS" in addition to dietary optimization, hormonal optimization, and nutritional supplementation. Antimicrobial treatment with amoxicillin-clavulanate would have been reasonable, too, except for this patient's prior allergic reaction to the drug.

```
Urine Culture, Routine
Urine Culture, Routine        Final Report
Result 1
     Escherichia coli
     50,000-100,000 colony forming units per mL
Antimicrobial Susceptibility
     ***** S = Susceptible; I = Intermediate; R = Resistant *****
                 P = Positive; N = Negative
          MICS are expressed in micrograms per mL
```

Antibiotic	RSLT#1
Amoxicillin/Clavulanic Acid	S
Ampicillin	S
Cefazolin	S
Cefepime	S
Ceftriaxone	S
Cefuroxime	S
Cephalothin	I
Ciprofloxacin	R
ESBL	N
Ertapenem	S
Gentamicin	S
Imipenem	S
Levofloxacin	R
Nitrofurantoin	S
Piperacillin	S
Tetracycline	S
Tobramycin	S
Trimethoprim/Sulfa	S

Comprehensive Stool Analysis / Parasitology x3

BACTERIOLOGY CULTURE		
Expected/Beneficial flora	**Commensal (Imbalanced) flora**	**Dysbiotic flora**
4+ Bacteroides fragilis group	3+ Alpha hemolytic strep	3+ Klebsiella pneumoniae ssp pneumoniae
3+ Bifidobacterium spp.		
4+ Escherichia coli		
3+ Lactobacillus spp.		
NG Enterococcus spp.		
2+ Clostridium spp.		
NG = No Growth		

PRESCRIPTIVE AGENTS			
	Resistant	**Intermediate**	**Susceptible**
Amoxicillin-Clavulanic Acid			S
Ampicillin	R		
Cefazolin			S
Ceftazidime			S
Ciprofloxacin			S
Trimeth-sulfa			S

Susceptible results imply that an infection due to the bacteria may be appropriately treated when the recommended dosage of the tested antimicrobial agent is used.
Intermediate results imply that response rates may be lower than for susceptible bacteria when the tested antimicrobial agent is used.
Resistant results imply that the bacteria will not be inhibited by normal dosage levels of the tested antimicrobial agent.

---

[133] Scofield RH, Warren WL, Koelsch G, Harley JB. A hypothesis for the HLA-B27 immune dysregulation in spondyloarthropathy: contributions from enteric organisms, B27 structure, peptides bound by B27, and convergent evolution. *Proc Natl Acad Sci U S A.* 1993 Oct 15;90(20):9330-4
[134] Rashid T, Ebringer A. Ankylosing spondylitis is linked to Klebsiella—the evidence. *Clin Rheumatol.* 2007 Jun;26(6):858-64

C-reactive protein: CRP	

Overview and interpretation:	• CRP is a protein made by the liver in response to the immunologic activation characteristic of infectious and inflammatory conditions. Generally, any tissue injury or inflammatory process especially that involves the immune system's increased production of IL-6 will result in increased production of CRP.[135] High sensitivity CRP (hsCRP) is preferred over regular CRP due to its greater sensitivity and use in assessing cardiovascular risk.
	• Elevated values are seen with:
	   • <u>Infections</u>: Bacterial, fungal, parasitic, viral diseases; some patients with dysbiosis[136] will have mildly-moderately elevated CRP,
	   • <u>Inflammatory bowel disease</u>: Crohn's disease and ulcerative colitis (higher in CD than UC),
	   • <u>Autoimmune disease</u>: Rheumatoid arthritis, polymyalgia rheumatica, giant cell arteritis, polyarteritis nodosa, (not always SLE),
	   • <u>Acute myocardial infarction or other tissue ischemia</u>
	   • <u>Organ transplant rejection</u>: Renal, (not cardiac),
	   • <u>Trauma</u>: Burns, surgery,
	   • <u>Obesity</u>: Leads to modest elevations in CRP.

Advantages:	• This is an excellent screening test for differentiating "serious problems" (e.g., inflammatory and infectious arthropathy) from "benign problems" such as osteoarthritis. • Since higher values of CRP are a well-recognized risk factor for cardiovascular disease, screening "musculoskeletal patients" with hsCRP provides data for cardiovascular risk assessment and a more comprehensive and holistic treatment approach, thus bridging the gap between acute care and preventive care.
Limitations:	• Elevations in CRP are completely nonspecific, requiring clinical investigation to determine the underlying cause of the immune activation. • CRP may be normal in some patients with severe systemic diseases (such as lupus or cancer), and therefore a normal CRP does not entirely exclude the presence of significant illness.
Comments:	• Writing in *The New England Journal of Medicine*, authors Gabay and Kushner[137] note that measurements of plasma or serum **C-reactive protein can help differentiate inflammatory from non-inflammatory conditions and are useful in managing the patient's disease, since "the concentration often reflects the response to and the need for therapeutic intervention."** Additionally, they note, "Most normal subjects have plasma C-reactive protein concentrations of 2 mg per liter or less, but some have concentrations as high as 10 mg per liter." Deodhar[138] noted that **"Any clinical disease characterized by tissue injury and/or inflammation is accompanied by significant elevation of serum CRP…"** and that **CRP should replace ESR as a method of laboratory evaluation.** Deodhar also noted that **some patients with severe SLE will have normal CRP levels.**

[135] Deodhar SD. C-reactive protein: the best laboratory indicator available for monitoring disease activity. *Cleve Clin J Med* 1989 Mar-Apr;56(2):126-30
[136] See Chapter 4 of *Integrative Rheumatology* and Vasquez A. Nutritional and Botanical Treatments Against "Silent Infections" and Gastrointestinal Dysbiosis, Commonly Overlooked Causes of Neuromusculoskeletal Inflammation and Chronic Health Problems. *Nutr Perspect* 2006; Jan InflammationMastery.com/reprints
[137] Gabay C, Kushner I. Acute-phase proteins and other systemic responses to inflammation. *N Engl J Med*. 1999 Feb 11;340(6):448-54
[138] Deodhar SD. C-reactive protein: the best laboratory indicator available for monitoring disease activity. *Cleve Clin J Med* 1989 Mar-Apr;56(2):126-30

Clinical Case **Elevated hsCRP (high-sensitivity c-reactive protein) in a male patient with metabolic syndrome and rheumatoid arthritis—response to treatment protocol in *Integrative Rheumatology*:** This 52-year-old male patient presented with a 4-year history of rheumatoid arthritis which was unresponsive to prednisone and anti-TNF (tumor necrosis factor alpha) drugs, ie, "biologics." As expected, the prednisone exacerbated the patient's insulin resistance and hypertension; the drug failed to produce an anti-inflammatory benefit for this patient. At a cost of several thousand dollars per treatment, the anti-TNF "biologic" drugs failed to provide any benefit. At the intial visit in July 2005, the hsCRP level was 124 mg/L (normal range 0-3 mg/L), as shown in these lab results.

DATE OF SPECIMEN	TIME	DATE RECEIVED	DATE REPORTED	TIME		Houston		TX	77036-0000
7/08/2005	16:19	7/08/2005	7/11/2005	7:38	419	ACCOUNT NUMBER:	42407150		

TEST	RESULT	LIMITS	LAB
C-Reactive Protein, Cardiac			
> C-Reactive Protein, Cardiac	124.00H mg/L	0.00 - 3.00	HD
	Relative Risk for Future Cardiovascular Event		
	Low	<1.00	
	Average	1.00 - 3.00	
	High	>3.00	

The patient was treated with the protocol outlined in Chapter 4 of *Integrative Rheumatology*.[139] Stool testing showed *Citrobacter freundii* (renamed *Citrobacter rodentium*) which was addressed with botanical medicines; the insufficiency dysbiosis was also corrected per the five-part protocol. Slightly low testosterone and slightly elevated estradiol was optimized with a pharmaceutical aromatase inhibitor (Arimidex) given twice weekly. The five-part nutritional wellness protocol (supplemented Paleo-Mediterranean diet [SPMD]) was implemented.[140]

Comprehensive Parasitology, stool, x2

MICROBIOLOGY

Bacteriology Culture

Beneficial flora		Imbalances		Dysbiotic flora	
Bifidobacter	0+	Gamma strep	1+	Citrobacter freundii	1+
E. coli	2+	Enterobacter sp.	1+		
Lactobacillus	0+				

Mycology (Yeast) Culture

Normal flora	Dysbiotic flora
No yeast isolated	

PARASITOLOGY

	Sample 1		Sample 2
No	Ova or Parasites	No	Ova or Parasites

No anti-inflammatory drugs or botanicals were used. Within five weeks of treatment, the patient's hsCRP dropped from 124 mg/L to 7.58 mg/L—a reduction of approximately 95%—far superior to any previoius response to corticosteroid and biologic drugs. Patient experienced significant alleviation of pain and improved mobility.

8/17/2005	11:06	8/18/2005	8/18/2005	12:32	738	ACCOUNT NUMBER:	42407150		

TEST	RESULT	LIMITS	LAB
C-Reactive Protein, Cardiac			
C-Reactive Protein, Cardiac	7.58H mg/L	0.00 - 3.00	HD

---

[139] Vasquez A. *Integrative Rheumatology*. See InflammationMastery.com for newest edition, which in 2014 is *Naturopathic Rheumatology v3.5*.
[140] Vasquez A. Revisiting the Five-Part Nutritional Wellness Protocol. *Nutritional Perspectives* 2011 Jan   Reprinted and updated in Chapter 4.

Erythrocyte sedimentation rate: ESR	

Overview and interpretation:	▪ Values may be elevated even when no pathology is present because ESR increases with anemia and with age.
	
	▪ Much more sensitive than WBC count when screening for infection.[141]
	
	▪ May be normal in about 10% of patients who have pathology such as **giant cell arteritis** and **polymyalgia rheumatica** (conditions where it is generally the only lab abnormality, besides anemia); may also be normal in several other diseases.
	
	▪ **May be normal in patients with septic arthritis and patients with crystal-induced arthritis: joint aspiration for synovial fluid analysis is indicated if septic arthritis is suspected.**[142]
	
	▪ Increased with age, anemia, inflammation; higher in women than men. Age-adjusted normal ranges: any value over 25 is considered high in young people, or 40 in elderly women.
	
	▪ Age-related adjustments for men and women are as follows:
	    • Men: age divided by 2
	    • Women: (age + 10) divided by 2

Advantages:	▪ Inexpensive and easy to perform—use the same lavender-topped tube that you use for CBC. ▪ Provides a quick screen for infection, inflammation, and multiple myeloma—the most common primary bone tumor in adults. ▪ In patients with elevated levels, ESR can be used to monitor progression of disease and response to treatment.[143] However, a negative/normal test result does not exclude the presence of significant disease; some noteworthy examples include the following: 1) elderly—due to diminished ability to mount an inflammatory response, 2) patients taking anti-inflammatory drugs and immunosuppressants, 3) a significant proportion of patients with lupus will have normal ESR despite aggressive disease, and 4) some cancer patients with clinically significant tumor burden will not show signs of systemic inflammation. ▪ ESR may be more reliable than CRP for multiple myeloma.[144]
Limitations:	▪ ESR may be normal in a subset of patients with clinically significant infection or inflammation. ▪ Values are elevated in the elderly and patients with anemia and are thus not necessarily indicative of disease in these populations.
Comments:	▪ This test is generally considered *outdated* and has been replaced in most circumstances by CRP for the evaluation of inflammation and infection. ▪ The only time I use this test clinically is when I am highly suspicious of inflammation and the CRP is normal. Further, this test may be preferred when assessing for temporal arteritis and for multiple myeloma, two conditions which are classically associated with elevated ESR.

[141] Shaw BA, Gerardi JA, Hennrikus WL. How to avoid orthopedic pitfalls in children. *Patient Care* 1999; Feb 28: 95-116

[142] Klippel JH (ed). *Primer on the Rheumatic Diseases. 11th Edition*. Atlanta: Arthritis Foundation. 1997 page 94

[143] Shojania K. Rheumatology: 2. What laboratory tests are needed? *CMAJ*. 2000 Apr 18;162(8):1157-63 cmaj.ca/cgi/content/full/162/8/1157

[144] "ESR, a simple and easily performed marker, was found to be an independent prognostic factor for survival in patients with multiple myeloma." Alexandrakis et al. Clinical and prognostic significance of erythrocyte sedimentation rate (ESR), serum interleukin-6 (IL-6), acute phase protein levels in multiple myeloma. *Clin Lab Haematol*. 2003;25:41-6

Ferritin	
Overview and interpretation:	• Ferritin levels are directly proportional to body iron stores, except in patients with inflammation, infection, hepatitis, or cancer. Therefore, measuring ferritin allows assessment for iron deficiency (a cause of fatigue, or early manifestation of GI cancer) and allows for assessment of iron overload (as a cause of joint pain and arthropathy). This test should be performed in all African Americans[145,146], white men over age 30 years[147], diabetics[148], and patients with peripheral arthropathy[149], and exercise-associated joint pain[150,151] The research also justifies testing children[152], women[153], young adults[154] and the general asymptomatic public.[155] • Low ferritin = iron deficiency • High ferritin = iron overload, cancer, inflammation, infection, and/or hepatitis (viral, alcoholic, or toxic)
Advantages:	• Reliable screening test for iron overload when used in conjunction with patient assessment and evidence (e.g., normal CRP) of no infection or acute phase response. • This is the blood test of choice for iron deficiency *and* iron overload.
Limitations:	• Iron-deficient patients with an acute phase response may have a falsely normal level of ferritin since ferritin is an acute phase reactant and will be elevated *disproportionate to iron status* during inflammation. • Elevations of ferritin (i.e., >200 mcg/L in women and >300 mcg/L in men) need to be retested along with CRP (to rule out false elevation due to excessive inflammation) before making the presumptive diagnosis of iron overload. **In the absence of significant inflammation, ferritin values >200 mcg/L in women and >300 mcg/L in men indicate iron overload and the need for treatment regardless of the absence of symptoms or end-stage complications.**[156]
Comments:	• Note that since ferritin is an acute-phase reactant, a high level of serum ferritin by itself does not allow differentiation between iron overload, infection, and the inflammation associated with tissue injury or metastatic disease. Ferritin must be evaluated within the context of the patient's clinical condition and the assessment of at least one other marker for inflammation such as CRP. If the patient is not acutely ill or has not recently suffered tissue injury (e.g., myocardial infarction) and the CRP is normal, then an elevated ferritin value indicates iron overload until proven otherwise with diagnostic phlebotomy, which is safer and less expensive than liver biopsy or MRI. Transferrin saturation can also be measured when the interpretation of ferritin is unclear. By itself, serum iron is unreliable.

[145] Barton JC, Edwards CQ, Bertoli LF, Shroyer TW, Hudson SL. Iron overload in African Americans. *Am J Med.* 1995 Dec;99(6):616-23

[146] Wurapa RK, Gordeuk VR, Brittenham GM, et al. Primary iron overload in African Americans. *Am J Med.* 1996;101(1):9-18

[147] Baer DM, Simons JL, et al. Hemochromatosis screening in asymptomatic ambulatory men 30 years of age and older. *Am J Med.* 1995 May;98:464-8

[148] Phelps G, Chapman I, Hall P, Braund W, Mackinnon M. Prevalence of genetic haemochromatosis among diabetic patients. *Lancet* 1989; 2: 233-4

[149] Olynyk J, Hall P, Ahern M, KwiatekR, MackinnonM. Screening for hemochromatosis in a rheumatology clinic. *Aust NZ J Med* 1994; 24: 22-5

[150] McCurdie I, Perry JD. Haemochromatosis and exercise related joint pains. *BMJ.* 1999 Feb 13;318(7181):449-5

[151] "RESULTS: Our findings indicate a high prevalence of HFE gene mutations in this population (49.2%) compared with sedentary controls (33.5%). No association was detected in the athletes between mutations and blood iron markers. CONCLUSIONS: The findings support the need to assess regularly iron stores in elite endurance athletes." Chicharro JL, Hoyos J, Gomez-Gallego F, et al. Mutations in the hereditary haemochromatosis gene HFE in professional endurance athletes. *Br J Sports Med.* 2004 Aug;38(4):418-21. Erratum in: *Br J Sports Med.* 2004 Dec;38(6):793 bjsm.bmjjournals.com/cgi/content/full/38/4/418 Accessed September 12, 2005

[152] Kaikov Y, et al. Primary hemochromatosis in children: report of three newly diagnosed cases and review of the pediatric literature. *Pediatrics* 1992; 90: 37-42

[153] Edwards CQ, Kushner JP. Screening for hemochromatosis. *N Engl J Med* 1993; 328: 1616-20

[154] Gushusrt TP, Triest WE. Diagnosis and management of precirrhotic hemochromatosis. *W Virginia Med J* 1990; 86: 91-5

[155] Balan V, et al. Screening for hemochromatosis: a cost-effectiveness study based on 12, 258 patients. *Gastroenterology* 1994; 107: 453-9

[156] Barton JC, McDonnell SM, Adams PC, Brissot P, Powell LW, Edwards CQ, Cook JD, Kowdley KV. Management of hemochromatosis. Hemochromatosis Management Working Group. *Ann Intern Med.* 1998 Dec 1;129(11):932-9—one of the best papers ever written on this topic.

Ferritin—*Interpretation of serum levels*

Ferritin	Categorization and management
≥ 800 mcg/L	<u>Practically diagnostic of iron overload</u>[157]: Repeat tests; rule out inflammation or occult pathology. Initiate phlebotomy and consider liver biopsy or MRI.
≥ 300 mcg/L	<u>Probable iron overload</u>[158]: Repeat tests; rule out inflammation or occult pathology. In men, initiate phlebotomy and consider liver biopsy or MRI.[159]
≥ 200 mcg/L	<u>*In women*: Suggestive of iron overload</u>[160]: Repeat tests, rule out inflammation or occult pathology. In women, initiate phlebotomy and consider liver biopsy or MRI.[161] <u>*In men*: High-normal *unhealthy* iron status with increased risk of myocardial infarction</u>[162]: Rule out inflammation or occult pathology. No follow-up is mandated, yet blood donation and/or abstention from dietary iron are recommended preventative healthcare measures.
≥ 160 mcg/L	<u>*In women*: Abnormal iron status</u>[163]: Repeat tests, rule out inflammation or occult pathology. Consider phlebotomy and liver biopsy or MRI.
≥80-120 mcg/L	<u>High-normal unhealthy iron status</u>[164,165]: No follow-up is mandated; blood donation and abstention from dietary iron are suggested preventative healthcare measures. A subset of patients with restless leg syndrome (RLS, a condition also causally associated with intestinal bacterial overgrowth dysbiosis) have impaired transport of iron into the brain and therefore require slightly elevated ferritin/iron levels (up to 120) to enhance cerebral iron uptake.
40-70 mcg/L	**Optimal iron status for most people**[166,167]
< 20 mcg/L	<u>Iron deficiency</u>: Search for occult gastrointestinal blood loss with endoscopy or imaging assessments in adults; refer to gastroenterologist.[168,169]

Ferritin is an acute-phase reactant, which means that its production is increased during the acute phase of inflammatory and/or infectious disorders. Therefore the numeric value and hence its clinical meaning can be interpreted only within a context that also includes assessment of the patient's inflammatory status, which is best assessed with either ESR or CRP. If CRP/ESR is high, then the physician might assume that the ferritin value is "falsely elevated"—disproportionately elevated with respect to body iron stores. *Common clinical examples requiring use and skillful interpretation of ferritin*:

- **Elderly or arthritic patient with iron deficiency despite normal serum ferritin**: An elderly patient with normal ferritin and elevated CRP/ESR is probably iron deficient; retesting of ferritin and measurement of transferrin saturation and CBC should be performed promptly. If iron deficiency is confirmed or cannot be excluded, referral for endoscopic examination must be implemented. In a patient with known inflammatory arthropathy, the ferritin may appear normal even though the patient is iron deficient and in need of supplementation and endoscopy.
- **Non-anemic iron deficiency**: A middle-aged patient (commonly a premenopausal woman) presents with fatigue and during the course of evaluation is found to have a normal CBC. Do not let a normal CBC prevent you from assessing ferritin; many nonanemic patients are impressively iron deficient with ferritin values of 2-6 mcg/L and are in need of iron replacement as well as evaluation for conditions including celiac disease, *H. pylori* infection, hematuria, and gastrointestinal bleeding/lesions.

[157] Milman N, Albeck MJ. Distinction between homozygous and heterozygous subjects with hemochromatosis using iron status markers and receiver operating characteristic (ROC) analysis. *Eur J Clin Biochem* 1995; 33: 95-8. See also Milman N. Iron status markers in hereditary hemochromatosis. *Eur J Haematol* 1991;47:292-8

[158] Olynyk JK, Bacon BR. Hereditary hemochromatosis: detecting and correcting iron overload. *Postgrad Med* 1994;96: 151-65

[159] "Therapeutic phlebotomy is used to remove excess iron and maintain low normal body iron stores, …initiated in men with serum ferritin levels of 300 microg/L…and in women with serum ferritin levels of 200 microg/L…regardless of the presence or absence of symptoms." Barton et al. Management of hemochromatosis. *Ann Intern Med*. 1998;129:932-9

[160] Barton JC, Edwards CQ, Bertoli LF, Shroyer TW, Hudson SL. Iron overload in African Americans. *Am J Med* 1995; 99: 616-23

[161] Barton JC, McDonnell SM, Adams PC, et al. Management of hemochromatosis. *Ann Intern Med*. 1998 Dec 1;129(11):932-9

[162] Salonen JT, Nyyssonen K, Korpela H,et al. High stored iron levels are associated with excess risk of myocardial infarction in eastern Finnish men. *Circulation* 1992; 86: 803-11

[163] Nicoll D. Therapeutic drug monitoring and laboratory reference ranges. In: Tierney LM, McPhee SJ, Papadakis MA. *Current Medical Diagnosis and Treatment 1996 (35th Edition)*. Stamford: Appleton and Lange, 1996: 1442

[164] Lauffer, RB. *Iron and Your Heart*. New York: St. Martin's Press, 1991: 79-8, 83-88, 162

[165] Sullivan JL. Iron and the sex difference in heart disease risk. *Lancet*. 1981 Jun 13;1(8233):1293-4

[166] Lauffer, RB. *Iron and Your Heart*. New York: St. Martin's Press, 1991: 79-8, 83-88, 162

[167] Vasquez A. High body iron stores: causes, effects, diagnosis, and treatment. *Nutritional Perspectives* 1994; 17: 13, 15-7, 19, 21, 28 and Vasquez A. Men's Health: Iron in men: why men store this nutrient in their bodies and the harm that it does. *MEN Magazine* 1997; Jan:11,21-23 vix.com/menmag/alexiron.htm

[168] Rockey DC, Cello JP. Evaluation of the gastrointestinal tract in patients with iron-deficiency anemia. *N Engl J Med*. 1993;329(23):1691-5

[169] "Endoscopy revealed a clinically important lesion in 23 (12%) of 186 patients. … CONCLUSIONS: Endoscopy yields important findings in premenopausal women with iron deficiency anemia, which should not be attributed solely to menstrual blood loss." Bini EJ, Micale PL, Weinshel EH. Evaluation of the gastrointestinal tract in premenopausal women with iron deficiency anemia. *Am J Med*. 1998 Oct;105(4):281-6

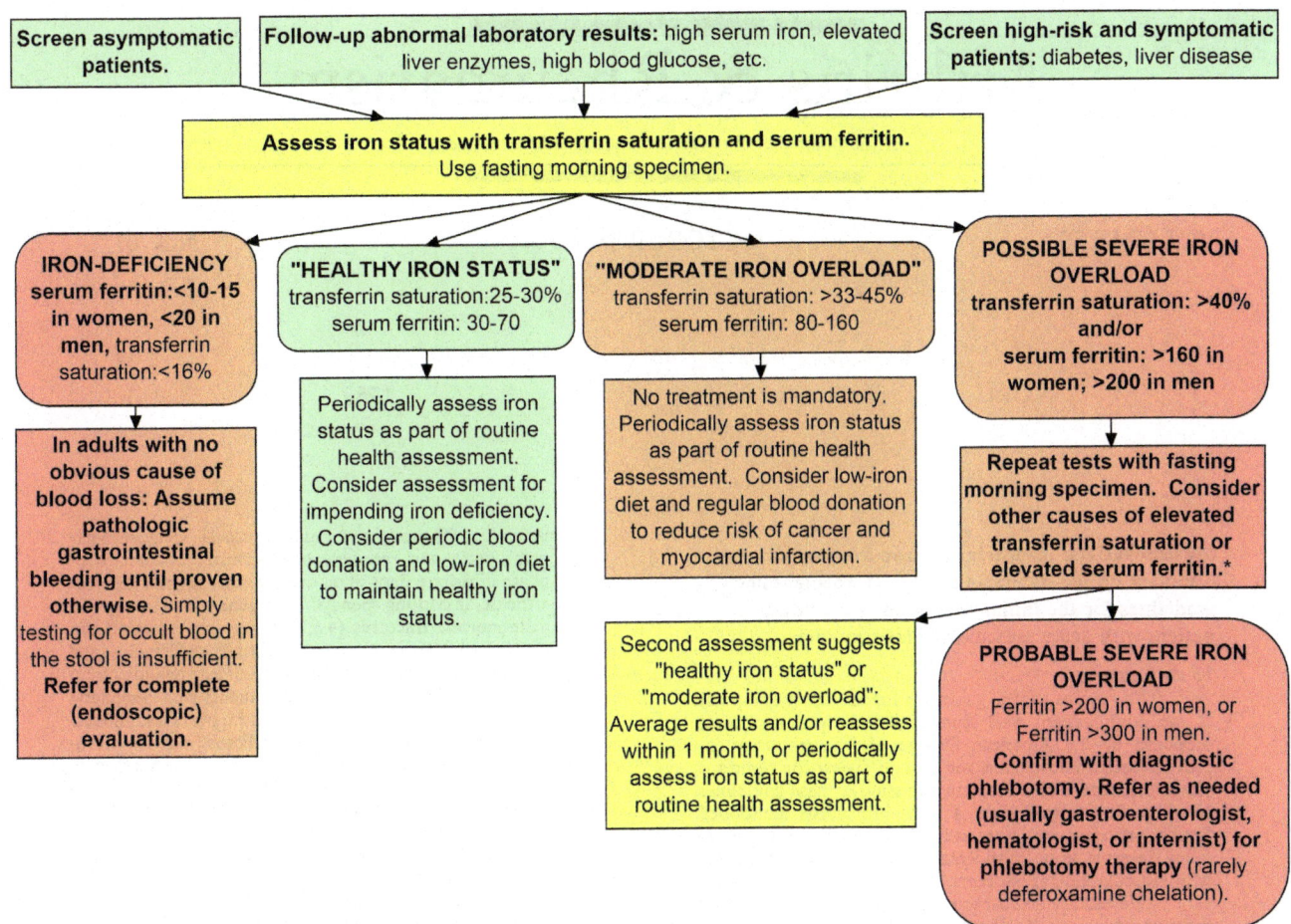

Algorithm for the comprehensive management of iron status based on the review and citations provided previously: The above flow-chart delineates patient management per iron status.

Basic treatments for severe iron overload:
- **Iron-removal therapy is mandatory:** Phlebotomy therapy is generally performed weekly or twice-weekly; deferoxamine chelation is reserved for patients who do not withstand phlebotomy (due to cardiomyopathy, severe anemia, or hypoproteinemia) or may be used concurrently with phlebotomy in some patients. Periodically assess hematologic and iron indexes. Continue with weekly iron removal therapy until patient reaches mild iron-deficiency anemia, then decrease frequency and continue phlebotomy as needed (e.g., 4 times per year).
- **Laboratory tests and physical examination:** Assess general physical condition and hepatic, cardiac, endocrine, and general health status.
- **Confirm diagnosis:** Liver biopsy ("gold standard") or diagnostic phlebotomy; perhaps MRI.
- **Assess liver status:** Liver biopsy or perhaps MRI. Cirrhosis indicates increased risk of hepatocellular carcinoma and reduced life expectancy. Consider liver ultrasound, serum liver enzyme measurement, and serum alpha-fetoprotein to screen for hepatocellular carcinoma every 6 months. Hepatoma surveillance is mandatory in cirrhotic patients.
- **Implement dietary modifications and nutritional therapies:** Avoid iron supplements, multivitamin supplements with iron, iron-fortified foods, liver, beef, pork, alcohol, and excess vitamin C. Ensure adequate protein intake to replace protein lost during phlebotomy. Diet modifications are not substitutes for iron removal therapy. Consider antioxidant therapy.
- **Screen all blood relatives of patients with primary iron overload**. *Mandatory!*
- **Monitor patient condition, and compliance** with lifelong phlebotomy therapy
- **Assess and address psychoemotional issues/concerns**

Arthritis & Rheumatism

Official Journal of the American College of Rheumatology

VOLUME 39   OCTOBER 1996   NO. 10

1767   1768

Musculoskeletal disorders and iron overload disease: comment on the American College of Rheumatology guidelines for the initial evaluation of the adult patient with acute musculoskeletal symptoms

To the Editor:

The recent clinical guidelines for the initial evaluation of the adult patient with acute musculoskeletal symptoms, proposed by the American College of Rheumatology (1), provide useful information and a good review for clinicians. However, there is one important omission in these guidelines. Nowhere in the guidelines is hemochromatosis mentioned. Such a prevalent and potentially life-threatening disease certainly deserves to be considered in the evaluation of patients with musculoskeletal disorders.

Hereditary hemochromatosis is now thought to be the most common genetic disorder in the white population (2). Approximately 1 in 250 persons is homozygous for this disorder and will develop the characteristic clinical manifestations such as diabetes, cardiomyopathy, liver disease, endocrine dysfunction, and, most notable for this discussion, arthropathy or other musculoskeletal disorders (2). Although hereditary iron overload disorders have traditionally been thought of as occurring exclusively in whites, recent research by Barton et al (3) indicates that approximately 1 in 67 African-Americans is affected by an etiologically distinct and severe form of iron overload. Hereditary iron overload disorders have been detected in persons of every ethnic background.

Arthropathy affects up to 80% of iron-overloaded patients and is often the only manifestation of this disease (4). Joint pain is a common and early symptom of iron overload, and "bone pain" has also been described as a common initial complaint (5). Clinically and radiographically, hemochromatoic arthropathy can resemble osteoarthritis, calcium pyrophosphate dihydrate deposition disease, pseudogout, rheumatoid arthritis, ankylosing spondylitis, or generalized osteopenia with osteoporotic fractures (4,6,7). Since iron overload can cause such a wide array of musculoskeletal manifestations and because definitive clinical differentiation of iron overload from other arthropathies is very difficult, patients with peripheral arthropathy should be screened for iron overload. Indeed, recent research by Olynyk et al (8) indicates that the prevalence of iron overload is 5 times higher in patients with peripheral arthropathy than in the general population. Therefore, screening of patients with peripheral arthropathy for the possible presence of iron overload is justified.

Thus, since iron overload affects such a large portion of the population and arthropathy is a common manifestation of this disorder, patients with musculoskeletal symptoms should be screened for iron overload (4,8). The current literature suggests that everyone should be screened for iron overload even if there are no symptoms (8–10).

Alex Vasquez, DC
Seattle, WA

1. American College of Rheumatology Ad Hoc Committee on Clinical Guidelines: Guidelines for the initial evaluation of the adult patient with acute musculoskeletal symptoms. Arthritis Rheum 39:1–8, 1996
2. Olynyk JK, Bacon BR: Hereditary hemochromatosis: detecting and correcting iron overload. Postgrad Med 96:151–165, 1994
3. Barton JC, Edwards CQ, Bertoli LF, Shroyer TW, Hudson SL: Iron overload in African Americans. Am J Med 99:616–623, 1995
4. Faraawi R, Harth M, Kertesz A, Bell D: Arthritis in hemochromatosis. J Rheumatol 20:448–452, 1993
5. Adams PC, Kertesz AE, Valberg LS: Clinical presentation of hemochromatosis: a changing scene. Am J Med 90:445–449, 1991
6. Bywaters EGL, Hamilton EBD, Williams R: The spine in idiopathic hemochromatosis. Ann Rheum Dis 30:453–465, 1971
7. Eyres KS, McCloskey EV, Fern ED, Rogers S, Beneton M, Aaron JE, Kanis JA: Osteoporotic fractures: an unusual presentation of hemochromatosis. Bone 13:431–433, 1992
8. Olynyk J, Hall P, Ahern M, Kwiatek R, Mackinnon M: Screening for hemochromatosis in a rheumatology clinic. Aust N Z J Med 24:22–25, 1994
9. Baer DM, Simmons JL, Staples RL, Runmore GJ, Morton CJ: Hemochromatosis screening in asymptomatic ambulatory men 30 years of age and older. Am J Med 98:464–468, 1995
10. Adams PC, Gregor JC, Kertesz AE, Valberg LS: Screening blood donors for hereditary hemochromatosis: decision analysis model based on a 30-year database. Gastroenterology 109:177–188, 1995

Vasquez A. Musculoskeletal disorders and iron overload disease: comment on the American College of Rheumatology guidelines for the initial evaluation of the adult patient with acute musculoskeletal symptoms. *Arthritis Rheum.* 1996 Oct;39(10):1767-8 ncbi.nlm.nih.gov/pubmed/8843875

25(OH)D: serum 25(OH) vitamin D	
Overview and interpretation:	▪ **Vitamin D deficiency is a common cause of musculoskeletal pain**[170,171,172], and vitamin D deficiency is a significant risk factor for cancer, autoimmunity, diabetes, mental illness, chronic pain and physical disability.[173,174,175] ▪ Measurement of serum 25(OH) vitamin D (or empiric treatment with 2,000 – 10,000 IU vitamin D3 per day for adults) is indicated in patients with chronic musculoskeletal pain, particularly low-back pain.[176] Optimal vitamin D status correlates with serum 25(OH)D levels of 50 – 100 ng/mL (125 - 250 nmol/L)—see our review article for more details[177]; levels greater than 100 ng/mL are unnecessary and increase the risk of hypercalcemia. **Excess vitamin D** > 100 ng/mL (250 nmol/L) with hypercalcemia **Optimal range** 50 - 100 ng/mL (125 - 250 nmol/L) **Insufficiency range** < 20- 40 ng/mL (50 - 100 nmol/L) **Deficiency** < 20 ng/mL (50 nmol/L) **Interpretation of serum 25(OH) vitamin D levels**. Modified from Vasquez et al, *Alternative Therapies in Health and Medicine* 2004 and Vasquez A. *Musculoskeletal Pain: Expanded Clinical Strategies* 2008.
Advantages:	▪ Accurate assessment of vitamin D status.
Limitations:	▪ Patients with certain granulomatous conditions such as sarcoidosis or Crohn's disease and patients taking certain drugs such as thiazide diuretics (hydrochlorothiazide) can develop hypercalcemia due to "vitamin D hypersensitivity" or drug side effects—these patients require frequent monitoring of serum calcium while taking vitamin D supplements.
Comments:	▪ **Routine measurement and/or empiric treatment with vitamin D3 needs to become a routine component of patient care.**[178] ▪ Periodic assessment of 25(OH)D and serum calcium are required to ensure effectiveness and safety of treatment, respectively. ▪ I'm increasingly convinced of the merit of measuring 1,25-dihydroxyvitamin D3, at least for the initial assessment of patients with inflammatory/autoimmune conditions.

[170] Masood et al. Persistent limb pain, raised serum alkaline phosphatase earliest markers of subclinical hypovitaminosis D Kashmir. *Indian J Physiol Pharmacol.* 1989;33:259-61

[171] Al Faraj S, Al Mutairi K. Vitamin D deficiency and chronic low back pain in Saudi Arabia. *Spine.* 2003 Jan 15;28(2):177-9

[172] Plotnikoff GA, Quigley JM. Prevalence of severe hypovitaminosis D in patients with persistent, nonspecific musculoskeletal pain. *Mayo Clin Proc.* 2003 Dec;78(12):1463-70

[173] Grant WB. An estimate of premature cancer mortality in the U.S. due to inadequate doses of solar ultraviolet-B radiation. *Cancer* 2002;94(6):1867-75

[174] Zittermannn A. Vitamin D in preventive medicine: are we ignoring the evidence? *Br J Nutr.* 2003 May;89(5):552-72

[175] Holick MF. Vitamin D: importance in the prevention of cancers, type 1 diabetes, heart disease, and osteoporosis. *Am J Clin Nutr.* 2004;79(3):362-71

[176] Al Faraj S, Al Mutairi K. Vitamin D deficiency and chronic low back pain in Saudi Arabia. *Spine.* 2003 Jan 15;28(2):177-9

[177] Vasquez A, et al. Clinical Importance of Vitamin D (Cholecalciferol): A Paradigm Shift with Implications for All Healthcare Providers. *AlternTherap Heal Med* 2004;10:28-37

[178] Heaney RP. Vitamin D, nutritional deficiency, and the medical paradigm. *J Clin Endocrinol Metab.* 2003;88:5107-8 jcem.endojournals.org/cgi/content/full/88/11/5107

Vitamin D, 1,25 + 25-Hydroxy

Test	Low	Normal	High	Reference Range	Units
Calcitriol(1,25 Di-Oh Vit D)			115.8	10.0-75.0	pg/mL
Vitamin D, 25-Hydroxy		53.1		30.0-100.0	ng/mL

Cmp14+Egfr

Test	Low	Normal	High	Reference Range	Units
Glucose, Serum		90		65-99	mg/dL
Bun		20		6-20	mg/dL
Creatinine, Serum		0.93		0.76-1.27	mg/dL
Egfr If Nonafricn Am		104		>59	mL/min/1.73
Egfr If Africn Am		120		>59	mL/min/1.73
Bun/Creatinine Ratio			22	8-19	1
Sodium, Serum		142		134-144	mmol/L
Potassium, Serum		4.8		3.5-5.2	mmol/L
Chloride, Serum		99		97-108	mmol/L
Carbon Dioxide, Total		26		18-29	mmol/L
Calcium, Serum		9.7		8.7-10.2	mg/dL

Cbc/Diff Ambiguous Default

Test	Low	Normal	High	Reference Range	Units
Wbc		5.8		3.4-10.8	x10E3/uL
Rbc		5.26		4.14-5.80	x10E6/uL

Ldh

Test	Low	Normal	High	Reference Range	Units
Ldh		123		121-224	IU/L

Homocyst(E)Ine, Plasma

Test	Low	Normal	High	Reference Range	Units
Homocyst(E)Ine, Plasma		10.7		0.0-15.0	umol/L

Laboratory results for a 39yoM with psoriasis and psoriatic arthritis: Abnormally increased conversion of 25-OH-cholecalciferol to 1,25-diOH-cholecalciferol is due expression of 25-hydroxyvitamin D3-1alpha-hydroxylase (1-OHase) in inflammatory tissue/cells. Note that serum calcium is normal, so no immediate threat is present (i.e., hypercalcemia) but of course the clinician has the responsibility to ❶ monitor periodically, ❷ inform the patient of symptoms of hypercalcemia such as headache and abdominal pain, and ❸ search for any predictive risk factors such as renal insufficiency or occult leukemia/lymphoma that could precipitate hypercalcemia. Assessment for hyperparathyroidism (e.g., iPTH) is reasonable but not completely necessary; likewise, cancer screening is not absolutely indicated, as it would be in the case of idiopathic hypercalcemia. Also noted is the elevated homocysteine, common in patients with psoriasis; increased cell turnover—dermal hyperproliferation—likely contributes to draining/catabolizing nutrients such as folate. Since this patient's 25-OH-D is plenty sufficient, I had the patient temporarily reduce/discontinue vitamin D supplementation to reduce risk of hypercalcemia given that he is clearly vitamin D sufficient.

INFLAMMATION MASTERY & FUNCTIONAL INFLAMMOLOGY

CME
CONTINUING MEDICAL EDUCATION

THE CLINICAL IMPORTANCE OF VITAMIN D (CHOLECALCIFEROL): A PARADIGM SHIFT WITH IMPLICATIONS FOR ALL HEALTHCARE PROVIDERS

Alex Vasquez, DC, ND, Gilbert Manso, MD, John Cannell, MD

Alex Vasquez, DC, ND is a licensed naturopathic physician in Washington and Oregon, and licensed chiropractic doctor in Texas, where he maintains a private practice and is a member of the Research Team at Biotics Research Corporation. He is a former Adjunct Professor of Orthopedics and Rheumatology for the Naturopathic Medicine Program at Bastyr University. **Gilbert Manso**, MD, is a medical doctor practicing integrative medicine in Houston, Texas. In practice for more than 35 years, he is Board Certified in Family Practice and is Associate Professor of Family Medicine at University of Texas Medical School in Houston. **John Cannell**, MD, is a medical physician practicing in Atascadero, California, and is president of the Vitamin D Council (Cholecalciferol-Council.com), a non-profit, tax-exempt organization working to promote awareness of the manifold adverse effects of vitamin D deficiency.

InnoVision Communications is accredited by the Accreditation Council for Continuing Medical Education to provide continuing medical education for physicians. The learner should study the article and its figures or tables, if any, then complete the self-evaluation at the end of the activity. The activity and self-evaluation are expected to take a maximum of 2 hours.

OBJECTIVES

Upon completion of this article, participants should be able to do the following:

1. Appreciate and identify the manifold clinical presentations and consequences of vitamin D deficiency
2. Identify patient groups that are predisposed to vitamin D hypersensitivity
3. Know how to implement vitamin D supplementation in proper doses and with appropriate laboratory monitoring

Reprint requests: InnoVision Communications, 169 Saxony Rd, Suite 103, Encinitas, CA 92024; phone, (760) 633-3910 or (866) 828-2962; fax, (760) 633-3918; e-mail, alternative.therapies@innerdoorway.com. Or visit our online CME Web site by going to http://www.alternative -therapies.com and selecting the Continuing Education option.

While we are all familiar with the important role of vitamin D in calcium absorption and bone metabolism, many doctors and patients are not aware of the recent research on vitamin D and the widening range of therapeutic applications available for cholecalciferol, which can be classified as both a vitamin and a pro-hormone. Additionally, we also now realize that the Food and Nutrition Board's previously defined Upper Limit (UL) for safe intake at 2,000 IU/day was set far too low and that the physiologic requirement for vitamin D in adults may be as high as 5,000 IU/day, which is less than half of the >10,000 IU that can be produced endogenously with full-body sun exposure.[1,2] With the discovery of vitamin D receptors in tissues other than the gut and bone—especially the brain, breast, prostate, and lymphocytes—and the recent research suggesting that higher vitamin D levels provide protection from diabetes mellitus, osteoporosis, osteoarthritis, hypertension, cardiovascular disease, metabolic syndrome, depression, several autoimmune diseases, and cancers of the breast, prostate, and colon, we can now utilize vitamin D for a wider range of preventive and therapeutic applications to maintain and improve our patients' health.[3] Based on the research reviewed in this article, the current authors believe that assessment of vitamin D status and treatment of vita-

CME: The Clinical Importance of Vitamin D

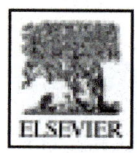

THE LANCET.com

May 6, 2005

Subphysiologic Doses of Vitamin D are Subtherapeutic: Comment on the Study by The Record Trial Group

Dear Editor,

Based on recently published research, it is clear that the study by The Record Trial Group [1] on vitamin D and calcium in the prevention of fractures suffered from at least four important shortcomings which negatively skewed their results.

First, and most important, the dose of vitamin D used in their study (800 IU/d) is subphysiologic and would therefore not be expected to produce a clinically meaningful effect. The physiologic requirement for vitamin D was determined scientifically in a recent study by Heaney and colleagues [2], who showed that healthy men utilize 3,000 to 5,000 IU of cholecalciferol per day, and several recent clinical trials have been published documenting the safety and effectiveness of administering vitamin D in physiologic doses of at least 4,000 IU per day.[3-5] In fact, studies have shown a dose-response relationship with vitamin D supplementation [6], and low doses (e.g., 600 IU) are clearly less effective than higher doses in the physiologic range (e.g., 4,000 IU).[5] It is important to note that the commonly used dose of vitamin D at 800 IU per day was not determined scientifically; rather this amount was determined arbitrarily before sufficient scientific methodology was available.[2,7] Given that the commonly recommended daily intake of vitamin D in the range of 200-800 IU is not sufficient for maintaining adequate serum levels of vitamin D [8], it is therefore incumbent upon modern researchers and clinicians to use doses of vitamin D that are consistent with the physiologic requirement as established in current research.

Second, the authors recognize that patient compliance in their study population was quite poor. This poor compliance obviously contributed to the purported lack of treatment efficacy.

Third, and consistent with recent data published elsewhere [8], virtually all of their patients were still vitamin D deficient at the end of one year of treatment, thereby affirming the inadequacy of the treatment dose. Vitamin D deficiency is common in industrialized nations, particularly those of northern latitudes [9-11], including the UK, where this study was performed. By modern criteria for serum vitamin D levels [12], virtually all of the patients in this study were vitamin D deficient at the beginning of the study, and the insufficient treatment dose of 800 IU/d failed to correct this deficiency even after 1 year of treatment. Given that vitamin D levels must be raised to approximately 40 ng/mL (100 nmol/L) in order to maximally reduce parathyroid hormone levels and bone resorption [13,14], supplementation that does not accomplish the goal of raising serum vitamin D levels into the optimal physiologic range cannot be considered adequate therapy.[12]

Fourth, and finally, there is reason to question the bioavailability of their vitamin D3 supplement, as the authors note that their dose-response was generally lower than that seen in other studies. Bioavailability is a prerequisite for treatment efficacy, and the elderly have higher likeliness of comorbid conditions that impair digestion and absorption of nutrients. Specifically, it is well documented that vitamin D absorption is decreased in elderly patients compared to younger controls [15,16], and this is complicated by an age-related reduction in renal calcitriol production [17,18] and intestinal vitamin D receptors [19], thereby further impairing vitamin D metabolism and calcium absorption. Since emulsification of fat soluble vitamins is required for their absorption [20], and since pre-emulsification of nutrients has been shown to increase absorption and dose-responsiveness of the fat-soluble nutrient coenzyme Q [21, 22], it seems apparent that attention to the form (not merely the dose) of nutrient supplementation is clinically important, particularly when working with elderly patients.

These shortcomings, when combined, could have led to an additive or synergistic reduction in treatment potency that skewed their results toward a conclusion of inefficacy. In order to produce more meaningful results in clinical trials, our group published guidelines [12] recommending that future studies 1) ensure patient compliance, 2) use physiologic doses of vitamin D (e.g., 4,000 IU per day), and 3) ensure that serum levels are raised to a minimum of 40 ng/mL (100 nmol/L), since levels below this threshold are associated with increased parathyroid hormone levels, increased bone resorption, and recalcitrance to bone-building interventions.[23,24]

Alex Vasquez

Competing Interests: Dr. Vasquez is a researcher at Biotics Research Corporation, an FDA-licensed drug manufacturing facility in the USA.

Citation: Vasquez A. Subphysiologic Doses of Vitamin D are Subtherapeutic: Comment on the Study by The Record Trial Group. *Lancet* 2005 published online May 6

Internet: Originally posted at thelancet.com/journals/lancet/article/PIIS0140673605630139/comments; for citations, see folder online: http://inflammationmastery.com/reprints/vasquez-2005-lancet-refined.pdf

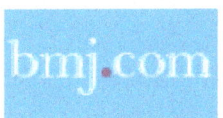

Calcium and vitamin D in preventing fractures

Data are not sufficient to show inefficacy

EDITOR—The study by Porthouse et al had two major design flaws.[1] Firstly, the dose of vitamin D (800 IU per day) is subphysiological and therefore subtherapeutic. Secondly, their use of "self report" as a measure of compliance is unreliable.

The dose of vitamin D at 800 IU daily was not determined scientifically but determined arbitrarily before sufficient scientific methodology was available.[2-4] Heaney et al determined the physiological requirement of vitamin D by showing that healthy men use 4000 IU cholecalciferol daily,[2] an amount that is safely attainable with supplementation[3] and often exceeded with exposure of the total body to equatorial sun.[4]

We provided six guidelines for interventional studies with vitamin D.[5] Dosages of vitamin D must reflect physiological requirements and natural endogenous production and should therefore be in the range of 3000-10 000 IU daily. Vitamin D supplementation must be continued for at least five to nine months. The form of vitamin D should be D_3 rather than D_2. Supplements should be assayed for potency. Effectiveness of supplementation must include measurement of serum 25-hydroxyvitamin D. Serum 25(OH)D concentrations must enter the optimal range, which is 40-65 ng/ml (100-160 nmol/l).

Since the study by Porthouse et al met only the second and third of these six criteria, their data cannot be viewed as reliable for documenting the inefficacy of vitamin D supplementation.

Alex Vasquez, *researcher*

Biotics Research Corporation, 6801 Biotics Research Drive, Rosenberg, TX 77471, USA avasquez@bioticsresearch.com

John Cannell, *president*

Vitamin D Council, 9100 San Gregorio Road, Atascadero, CA 93422, USA

Competing interests: AV is a researcher at Biotics Research Corporation, a drug manufacturing facility in the United States that has approval from the Food and Drug Administration.

References

1. Porthouse J, Cockayne S, King C, Saxon L, Steele E, Aspray T, et al. Randomised controlled trial of calcium and supplementation with cholecalciferol (vitamin D3) for prevention of fractures in primary care. *BMJ* 2005;330: 1003. (30 April.)[Abstract/Free Full Text]
2. Heaney RP, Davies KM, Chen TC, Holick MF, Barger-Lux MJ. Human serum 25-hydroxycholecalciferol response to extended oral dosing with cholecalciferol. *Am J Clin Nutr* 2003;77: 204-10.[Abstract/Free Full Text]
3. Vieth R, Chan PC, MacFarlane GD. Efficacy and safety of vitamin D3 intake exceeding the lowest observed adverse effect level. *Am J Clin Nutr* 2001;73: 288-94.[Abstract/Free Full Text]
4. Vieth R. Vitamin D supplementation, 25-hydroxyvitamin D concentrations, and safety. *Am J Clin Nutr* 1999;69: 842-56.[Abstract/Free Full Text]
5. Vasquez A, Manso G, Cannell J. The clinical importance of vitamin D (cholecalciferol): a paradigm shift with implications for all healthcare providers. *Altern Ther Health Med* 2004;10: 28-36.[ISI][Medline]

Related Article

Randomised controlled trial of calcium and supplementation with cholecalciferol (vitamin D₃) for prevention of fractures in primary care
Jill Porthouse, Sarah Cockayne, Christine King, Lucy Saxon, Elizabeth Steele, Terry Aspray, Mike Baverstock, Yvonne Birks, Jo Dumville, Roger Francis, Cynthia Iglesias, Suezann Puffer, Anne Sutcliffe, Ian Watt, and David J Torgerson
BMJ 2005 330: 1003. [Abstract] [Full Text]

Vasquez A, Cannell J. Calcium and vitamin D in preventing fractures: Data are not sufficient to show inefficacy. *BMJ*. 2005 Jul 9;331:108-9 ncbi.nlm.nih.gov/pubmed/16002891 InflammationMastery/reprints

Proof of the cause-and-effect relationship between vitamin D deficiency and chronic musculoskeletal pain comes from clinical trials among deficient patients showing that vitamin D monotherapy alleviates pain. The exemplary study by Al Faraj and Al Mutairi[35] showed that among patients with "idiopathic chronic low back pain," 83% (n = 299) were vitamin D deficient, and supplementation with 5000 to 10 000 IU/d of cholecalciferol for 3 months alleviated or cured the low back pain in more than 95% of patients. The authors concluded that, in the evaluation of chronic musculoskeletal pain among populations with a sufficiently high prevalence of vitamin D deficiency, "Screening for vitamin D deficiency and treatment with supplements should be mandatory in this setting."

Vitamin D has a wide range of safety according to an extensive review of the literature performed by Vieth.[228] Doses of 2000 IU/d of vitamin D3 have been given to children starting at 1 year of age and were not associated with toxicity but led to a reduction in the incidence of type 1 diabetes by 80%, consistent with the vitamin's anti-infective and immunomodulatory roles.[229] A 2004 review[36] on the clinical importance of vitamin D proposed that optimal vitamin D status is defined as 40 ng/mL to 65 ng/mL (100–160 nmol/L) and that "until proven otherwise, the balance of the research indicates that oral supplementation in the range of 1000 IU per day for infants, 2000 IU per day for children and 4000 IU per day for adults is safe and reasonable to meet physiological requirements, to promote optimal health, and to reduce the risk of several serious diseases. Safety and effectiveness of supplementation are assured by periodic monitoring of serum 25(OH)D and serum calcium." Current data and laboratory reference ranges support a higher top limit for serum 25(OH)D of approximately 100 ng/mL (250 nmol/L). Vitamin D hypersensitivity is seen with primary hyperparathyroidism, granulomatous diseases (such as sarcoidosis, Crohn's disease, and tuberculosis), adrenal insufficiency, hyperthyroidism, hypothyroidism, and various forms of cancer, as well as adverse drug effects, particularly with thiazide diuretics. Thiazide diuretics are known to potentiate hypercalcemia.

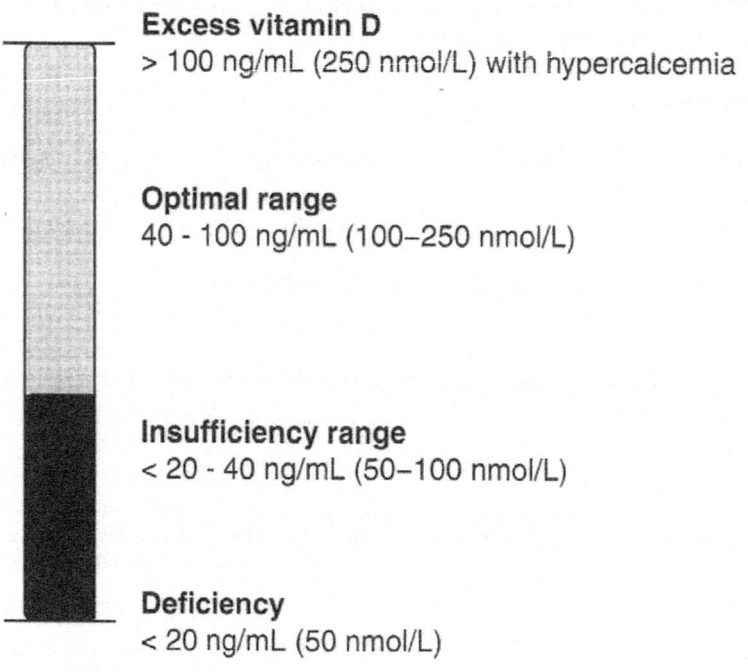

Excess vitamin D
> 100 ng/mL (250 nmol/L) with hypercalcemia

Optimal range
40 - 100 ng/mL (100–250 nmol/L)

Insufficiency range
< 20 - 40 ng/mL (50–100 nmol/L)

Deficiency
< 20 ng/mL (50 nmol/L)

Figure 2.1—Interpretation of Serum 25(OH)D Levels
Adapted from Vasquez A, Manso G, Cannell J. *Altern Ther Health Med.* 2004;10:28-37.36

35

Thyroid status — laboratory assessments	
Overview and interpretation:	▪ Context: Thyroid disorders are common in clinical practice and thus all clinicians need to have a clear understanding of the clinical presentations and laboratory assessments. Although various aspects of thyroid dysfunction, laboratory tests and clinical presentations will be reviewed here, the primary emphasis will be upon hypothyroidism, which is the most common and *unnecessarily* enigmatic of the thyroid disorders. ▪ Controversy: In the allopathic medical paradigm, much confusion exists regarding a common but "mysterious" and "enigmatic" condition known as hypothyroidism—low thyroid function. Its converse—**hyper**thyroidism and Graves disease—is well understood, easily diagnosed, and readily treated. Because the medical treatment for **hyper**thyroidism often leaves patients in a **hypo**thyroid state, affected patients thus transition from *clarity* (hyperthyroidism) wherein they feel ill due to the disease process into *"mystery"* (hypothyroidism) wherein they feel ill due to incomplete/inaccurate treatment. The basis for the confusion within the allopathic medical community about hypothyroidism is primarily two-fold: ❶ first, they rely on the wrong test (TSH) as the main basis for laboratory assessment, ❷ second, they use incomplete treatment (T4 without T3) which defies the known physiology of the thyroid gland, which makes at least two hormones rather than one. One might get the impression that perpetual confusion is at times the goal of the medical profession; we certainly see this with the management of hypertension, depression, diabetes mellitus, psoriasis and other inflammatory/autoimmune conditions. For people who seek clarity, it is available. ▪ Basic physiology: The hypothalamus produces thyrotropin-releasing hormone (TRH) which stimulates the anterior pituitary gland to make thyroid-stimulating hormone (TSH), which stimulates the thyroid gland to produce thyroxine (T4, approximately 85% of thyroid gland hormone production) and triiodothyronine (T3, approximately 15% of thyroid gland hormone production). In the periphery, the prohormone T4 is converted to active T3 by deiodinase enzymes. Stress, glucagon, and environmental toxins (halogenated phenolics, plastic monomers, flame retardants[179]) impair production of T3 and/or increase production of reverse T3, which is either inert or inhibitory to the action of T3. If the thyroid gland begins to fail, then TSH levels increase as the body attempts to stimulate production of thyroid hormones from a failing gland, which typically fails due to autoimmune attack (Hashimoto's thyroiditis); hence the association of elevated blood TSH levels with "primary hypothyroidism." Thyroid hormones have many different functions in the body, and one of the chief effects is contributing to maintenance of the basal metabolic rate, or the speed of reactions within and the temperature of the body. An insufficiency of thyroid hormone adversely effects numerous biochemical reactions and body/organ functions; hence the myriad of clinical presentations reflecting variations in biochemical and physiologic individuality. Conversely yet similarly, excess thyroid hormone (whether endogenously produced or exogenously administered) also affects numerous body systems. ▪ Clinical presentation of *hyper*thyroidism: The clinical pattern of thyroid excess is more narrowly-focused and thus more predictable and consistent than is the presentation of low thyroid function. The clinical manifestations of hyperthyroidism generally fall into three categories: hyper-adrenergic, hypermetabolic, and ophthalmologic/ocular. ❶ hyper-adrenergic: tachycardia, tremor, diaphoresis, insomnia and a feeling of nervousness and psychomotor agitation due to upregulation of adrenergic tone and generally some degree of relative or absolute hyperthermia; increased dopaminergic and noradrenergic tone in the brain accounts for the neuropsychiatric manifestations, such as mania, psychosis, and

---

[179] "All studied contaminants inhibited DI activity in a dose-response manner… This study suggests that some halogenated phenolics, including current use compounds such as plastic monomers, flame retardants and their metabolites, may disrupt thyroid hormone homeostasis through the inhibition of DI activity in vivo." Butt CM, Wang D, Stapleton HM. Halogenated Phenolic Contaminants Inhibit the In Vitro Activity of the Thyroid Regulating Deiodinases in Human Liver. *Toxicol Sci.* 2011 May 11. [Epub ahead of print]

hypersexuality, ❷ hyper-metabolic: fecal frequency often described as "diarrhea" due to expedited intestinal transit, elevated temperature, and weight loss due to increased overall metabolic rate, ❸ ophthalmologic/ocular: in chronic cases particularly of the autoimmune variety, exophthalmos develops secondary to retro-orbital connective tissue proliferation and autoimmunity directed toward the extraocular muscles; the histologic abnormalities are chiefly characterized by increased accumulation of collagen (behind the eye and within the extraocular muscles, leading to muscle weakness), accumulation of glycosaminoglycans (GAGs), and the attendant edema.

- Clinical presentation of **hypo**thyroidism: In his classic book _Biochemical Individuality_, Williams[180] noted that "a wide variation in thyroid activity exists among 'normal' human beings." Clearly, some patients do not make enough thyroid hormone to function optimally[181]; or, perhaps more precisely, they make enough thyroid hormone (T4) but do not efficiently convert it to the active form (T3) in the periphery. Further complicating the picture is that some patients make appropriate amounts of TSH, T4, and T3 but they make excess of inactive reverse T3 (rT3) which puts them into a physiologic state of hypothyroidism despite adequate glandular function. Patients may have one or more of the following: fatigue, depression, **cold hands and feet** (excluding Raynaud's syndrome, peripheral vascular disease), dry skin, menstrual irregularities, infertility, premenstrual syndrome (PMS), uterine fibroids, excess menstrual bleeding, **low basal body temperature**, weak fingernails, sleep apnea and increased need for sleep (hypersomnia), slow heart rate (relative or absolute **bradycardia**), easy weight gain and difficult weight loss (thus, predisposition to overweight and obesity), hypercholesterolemia, slow healing, decreased memory and concentration, frog-like husky voice, low libido, recurrent infections, hypertension especially diastolic hypertension, poor digestion (due to insufficient gastric production of hydrochloric acid), **delayed Achilles return** (due to delayed muscle relaxation), carotenodermia, vitamin A deficiency, and gastroesophageal acid reflux, constipation, and predisposition to small intestine bacterial overgrowth (SIBO) due to slow intestinal transit. Of these manifestations, cold hands and feet, low basal body temperature, bradycardia, and delayed Achilles return are the most specific; some very competent physicians will—following proper patient evaluation—treat with thyroid hormone based on the clinical presentation of the patient and _with proper consideration of_ and _without dependency upon_ laboratory findings.

- Overview of thyroid tests:
  - Thyrotropin-releasing hormone (TRH): The hypothalamus releases TRH to stimulate pituitary production of TSH. TRH is not routinely tested in clinical practice, although abnormalities of TRH secretion are noted in patients with mental "depression."
  - Thyroid-stimulating hormone (TSH: 0.4 - 5.0 mIU/L [milli-international units per liter]): TSH is the most commonly performed test for evaluating thyroid status; its frequent (over)use owes more to habit and inexpensiveness than to aspirations for clinical excellence. TSH values greater than 2 mIU/L represent a disturbance of the thyroid-pituitary axis and an increased risk for future thyroid problems[182], and the American Association of Clinical Endocrinologists states, "The target TSH level should be between 0.3 and 3.0 μIU/mL."[183] Clinical rationale is available to support implementation of a therapeutic trial of thyroid hormone treatment in patients who are clinically hypothyroid even if they are biochemically euthyroid (per TSH) provided that treatment is implemented cautiously, in appropriately selected

[180] Williams RJ. _Biochemical Individuality: The Basis for the Genetotrophic Concept_. Austin and London: University of Texas Press, 1956 page 82
[181] Broda Barnes MD, Lawrence Galton, _Hypothyroidism: The Unsuspected Illness_. Ty Crowell Co; 1976
[182] Weetman AP. Fortnightly review: Hypothyroidism: screening and subclinical disease. _BMJ: British Medical Journal_ 1997;314: 1175
[183] American Association of Clinical Endocrinologists. "The target TSH level should be between 0.3 and 3.0 μIU/mL." AACE Medical Guidelines for Clinical Practice for Evaluation and Treatment of Hyperthyroidism and Hypothyroidism. 2002, 2006 Amended Version. aace.com/sites/default/files/hypo_hyper.pdf Accessed Aug 2011

Thyroid status—laboratory assessments

patients, and patients are appropriately informed.[184,185] If the clinical world were as perfect as it is portrayed in basic physiology textbooks, then a clinician might fancifully rely on TSH to perform the diagnosis *prima facie*, with reduced TSH values correlating with glandular overperformance and negative feedback suppressing TSH secretion, whilst an underperforming gland would require greater stimulation with elevated TSH levels; however, TSH has never been thus vested with infallible reliability, which explains in part why doctors need brains of their own and why better clinicians have developed the capacity for independent thought.

o Free thyroxine (free T4: 4.5 - 11.2 mcg/dL): Unbound T4 is tested to provide evidence of glandular production of thyroid hormone(s). Because T4 is the major thyroid hormone produced by the thyroid gland it serves as an excellent marker for glandular productivity but it reveals nothing about peripheral conversion of T4 to the active thyroid hormone triiodothyronine (T3); in the practice of medicine, conversion of T4 to the active T3 is assumed to reliably occur unabated despite evidence to the contrary, especially among symptomatic patients.

o Triiodothyronine (T3: 100 - 200 ng/dL[186]): In textbook-perfect physiology, T4 is converted by deiodinase enzymes type-1 and type-2 to the active thyroid hormone T3; in reality, this is only part of the story. Because T3 is the active form of the hormone responsible for the physiologic functions of thyroid physiology, a clinician desiring to assess a patient's thyroid status might reasonably ask the proper question by performing the proper test. T3 is tested as "total T3" or "free T3" in large part based on the clinician's preference; the current author prefers total T3 because it can be compared to the total level of reverse T3 (rT3) in a ratio, the optimal range of which is generally considered to be 10-14 as originally presented by McDaniel[187] and reviewed in the following pages. Patients with psychiatric depression have lower levels of T3 than do healthy controls and have been described as having "low T3 syndrome"[188]; very obviously—whether cause or effect—the low T3 levels in these patients would serve to promote and perpetuate their state of mental depression. Although the focus of this review within the subject of laboratory evaluation is not to describe the implementation of thyroid hormone treatment, clinicians should be aware that T3 administration increases hepatic production of sex hormone binding globulin (SHBG) and that therefore T3 administration can reduce cellular bioavailability of protein-bound hormones. Many authoritative and clinically-experienced sources recommend using a time-released (e.g., sustained-release) form of T3 due to its shorter half-life compared with T4. However, obtaining time-released T3 via a compounding pharmacy can be cumbersome and expensive for the patient; clearly some patients respond to once daily dosing of *non*-time-released preparations with good effects and without adverse effects. Some patients can divide the immediate-release dose into two servings per day for enhanced effect and lessened physiologic fluctuations, if necessary. Per Drugs.com[189] in August 2011, "Since liothyronine sodium (T3) is not firmly bound to serum protein, it is readily available to body tissues. The onset of activity of liothyronine sodium is rapid, occurring within a few hours. Maximum pharmacologic response occurs within 2 or 3 days, providing early clinical response. The biological half-life is about 2.5 days." Very

[184] Skinner GR, et al. Thyroxine should be tried in clinically hypothyroid but biochemically euthyroid patients. *BMJ: British Medical Journal* 1997 Jun 14; 314(7096): 1764
[185] McLaren EH, Kelly CJ, Pollack MA. Trial of thyroxine treatment for biochemically euthyroid patients has been approved. *BMJ* 1997; 315: 1463
[186] U.S. National Library of Medicine (NLM) and National Institutes of Health (NIH) nlm.nih.gov/medlineplus/ency/article/003687.htm Accessed August 2011
[187] McDaniel AB. Thyroid Assessment: Controversies and Conundrums. Institute for Functional Medicine 14th International Symposium. Tucson, Arizona. May 23-26, 2007
[188] "Out of 250 subjects with major psychiatric depression, 6.4% exhibited low T3 syndrome (mean serum T3 concentration 0.94 nmol/l vs normal mean serum concentration of 1.77 nmol/l)." Premachandra BN, Kabir MA, Williams IK. Low T3 syndrome in psychiatric depression. *J Endocrinol Invest.* 2006 Jun;29(6):568-72
[189] drugs.com/pro/cytomel.html Accessed August 2011.

clearly, a significant portion of hypothyroid patients respond to T3 alone (either time-released, divided-dosing, or once-daily dosing) or a combination of T4 and T3 when other treatments have failed.[190,191]

- o Reverse triiodothyronine (rT3: 90 - 320 pg/mL[192]): T4 is converted by deiodinase enzymes type-1 and type-3 to the inactive thyroid hormone rT3; per a standard endocrinology textbook, "Approximately 70–80% of released T4 is converted by deiodinases to the biologically active T3, the remainder to reverse-T3 (rT3) which has no significant biological activity."[193] Clinicians must know that, "The prohormone T4 must be converted to T3 in the body before it can exert biological effects. **During periods of illness or stress, this conversion is often inhibited and can be diverted to the inactive reverse T3 (rT3) moiety.**"[194] Furthermore and very importantly, clinicians should appreciate that rT3 is not simply inactive but that it may actually impair production/utilization of normal T3; "T4-T3 and T4-rT3 conversion are provoked by different enzymes. **The elevation of rT3 might be a cause of the observed decrease in peripheral T3 generation** in old [elderly] subjects, acting via **inhibition of the T4-T3 conversion**."[195] During times of psychologic/physiologic stress and specific types of pharmacologic stress (e.g., propanolol[196] and corticosteroids), T4 metabolism is preferentially shunted away from T3 toward rT3; an anthropocentric explanation holds that by making less of the active T3 and more of the inactive rT3, the body is better able to conserve energy during times of stress by reducing overall metabolic rate, particularly resting energy expenditure and protein utilization. For example, caloric restriction and fasting result in a decrease in resting metabolic rate (RMR), and the reduced RMR persists for months after the fasting has ended and a normal diet is resumed.[197] This author (AV) terms this stress-induced impairment of thyroid hormone conversion "**metabolic hypothyroidism**" or "**functional hypothyroidism**" because the defect is in the metabolism (not the production) of thyroid hormone into its most active form; "**peripheral hypothyroidism**" might also be used to distinguish the fact that the defect is in the peripheral metabolism rather than located more centrally, within the thyroid gland itself. Because psychologic stress and certain pharmacologic exposures—as well as the thyro-metabolic stress of fasting and caloric restriction in which the counterregulatory hormone glucagon appears to trigger enhanced rT3 production—reduce T3 while simultaneously increasing rT3 levels, clinicians can appreciate that calculation of the T3/rT3 ratio will be more significantly altered (and thus a more sensitive indicator of metabolic disruption) than will be the isolated measurements of T3 or rT3 alone. Functional medicine clinicians[198] note the importance of the ratio of total T3 to reverse T3 (tT3:rT3 ratio) and consider the optimal range to be 10-14 with lower ratios indicating impaired formation or T3 and/or excess production of rT3.[199] Contrary to the previous view which held that rT3 was simply inactive, we now appreciate that rT3 actually impairs normal thyroid hormone metabolism thus functioning as an thyrometabolic monkeywrench or "brake" on normal metabolism.

[190] Bunevicius R, et al. Effects of thyroxine as compared with thyroxine plus triiodothyronine in patients with hypothyroidism. *N Engl J Med.* 1999 Feb 11;340(6):424-9

[191] Kelly T, Lieberman DZ. The use of triiodothyronine as an augmentation agent in treatment-resistant bipolar II and bipolar disorder NOS. *J Affect Disord.* 2009;116(3):222-6

[192] The reference range provided here for rT3 is a compilation from the laboratory reference ranges from the sample reports on the following pages, each of which is performed by either Quest Diagnostics or LabCorp, the two largest medical laboratories in the United States.

[193] Nussey S, Whitehead S. *Endocrinology: An Integrated Approach.* Oxford: BIOS Scientific Publishers, 2001. See also Box 3.29 Metabolism of thyroid hormones. ncbi.nlm.nih.gov/books/NBK28/box/A270/?report=objectonly Accessed July 2011

[194] *1998 Mosby's GenRX. Sixth Edition.* St. Louis Missouri; Mosby-Year Book, 1998

[195] Szabolcs I, Weber M, Kovács Z, et al. The possible reason for serum 3,3'5'-(reverse) triiodothyronine increase in old people. *Acta Med Acad Sci Hung.* 1982;39(1-2):11-7

[196] "Propranolol administration (40 mg t.i.d. for a week) caused a similar rT3 elevation in old persons (n = 18) as in 12 young ones." Szabolcs I, Weber M, Kovács Z, Irsy G, Góth M, Halász T, Szilágyi G. The possible reason for serum 3,3'5'-(reverse) triiodothyronine increase in old people. *Acta Med Acad Sci Hung.* 1982;39(1-2):11-7

[197] Elliot DL, Goldberg L, Kuehl KS, Bennett WM. Sustained depression of the resting metabolic rate after massive weight loss. *Am J Clin Nutr* 1989 Jan;49(1):93-96

[198] The conclusion of this paragraph is derived from Vasquez A. *Musculoskeletal Pain: Expanded Clinical Strategies.* Institute for Functional Medicine, 2008

[199] McDaniel AB. Thyroid Assessment: Controversies and Conundrums. Institute for Functional Medicine 14th International Symposium. Tucson, Arizona. May 23-26, 2007

Thyroid status—laboratory assessments	
	Elevated rT3 levels predict mortality among critically ill patients.[200] Aberrancies in thyroid hormone levels may reflect organic disease, psychoemotional stress, or nutritional deficiency[201], and therefore such serologic abnormalities warrant consideration of underlying problems and direct treatment when possible. If no underlying cause is apparent, then a trial of thyroid hormone/hormones is reasonable in appropriately selected patients. Beyond stress reduction, allergen/gluten avoidance, and nutritional supplementation with iodine, selenium, and zinc (as indicated per patient), correction of overt, subclinical, and functional hypothyroidism generally centers on the administration of natural or synthetic thyroid hormones in the form of T4 and T3. Correction of functional hypothyroidism (relatively reduced total T3 and increased rT3) is accomplished with either time-released or twice-daily dosing of T3 *without T4* to suppress endogenous T4 conversion to T3, thereby allowing rT3 levels to fall precipitously. T3 administration allows temporary downregulation of transforming enzymes so that rT3 production is reduced following withdrawal of T3 replacement; thus, short-term and/or periodic T3 administration helps normalize or "reset" peripheral thyroid metabolism so that, following withdrawal of T3 administration, T4 can be converted to T3 without excess production of rT3. The safety and effectiveness of this approach—using T3 administration (often twice daily or in a sustained-release compounded tablet or capsule) to recalibrate peripheral thyroid hormone metabolism—has documented safety and effectiveness.[202] Alleviation of symptoms, restoration of morning body temperature to 98.6° F (oral or axillary) and other clinical objective improvements achieved by the judicious and safe administration of T3 are the criteria of success; physiologic improvement following T3 administration retrospectively confirms the diagnosis.
	o <u>Antithyroid antibodies—antithyroglobulin (anti-TG) and anti-thyroid peroxidase (anti-TPO)</u>: Autoimmune thyroiditis (also called Hashimoto's disease or chronic lymphocytic thyroiditis) or is the most common cause of overt primary hypothyroidism. The diagnosis of autoimmune thyroiditis can be made clinically (i.e., without biopsy) upon detection of elevated blood levels of antibodies against thyroglobulin (anti-thyroglobulin antibodies) and anti-thyroid peroxidase (anti-TPO) antibodies. Autoimmune thyroiditis may present asymptomatically and with normal thyroid hormone levels; classically, patients may have a slightly hyperthyroid presentation as the inflamed gland releases extra thyroid hormone before becoming atrophic and hypofunctional.
Advantages:	▪ Thyroid disorders are quite common in general practice and are often undiagnosed, undertreated, or inappropriately treated. ▪ Consistent with the principle of beneficence, patients and doctors benefit when thyroid disorders are diagnosed and treated appropriately.
Limitations:	▪ A properly interpreted TSH may overlook problems of T4 production or conversion to active T3. Additionally, in some patients, all of these tests are normal but they may have thyroid autoimmunity (i.e., thyroid peroxidase antibodies, anti-TPO) and should receive

---

[200] Peeters RP, Wouters PJ, van Toor H, Kaptein E, Visser TJ, Van den Berghe G. Serum 3,3',5'-triiodothyronine (rT3) and 3,5,3'-triiodothyronine/rT3 are prognostic markers in critically ill patients and are associated with postmortem tissue deiodinase activities. *J Clin Endocrinol Metab*. 2005 Aug;90(8):4559-65

[201] Kelly GS. Peripheral metabolism of thyroid hormones: a review. *Altern Med Rev*. 2000 Aug;5(4):306-33

[202] Friedman M, et al. Supraphysiological cyclic dosing of sustained release T3 in order to reset low basal body temperature. *P R Health Sci J*. 2006 Mar;25(1):23-9

Thyroid status—laboratory assessments	
	treatment with thyroid hormone[203] or some other corrective treatment (e.g., selenium supplementation[204,205] and a gluten-free diet[206]) to normalize thyroid status.
Comments:	■ Comprehensive thyroid laboratory testing includes ❶ history, ❷ TSH, ❸ free T4, ❹ total T3, ❺ rT3, ❻ antithyroid antibodies, should be evaluated alongside the ❼ heart rate, ❽ cold extremities and basal body temperature, ❾ Achilles' return speed, and ❿ response to treatment.
	■ The combination of T3 and T4 (as in the prescription Liotrix/Thyrolar or Armour thyroid) appears to have similar safety to T4 alone (Levothyroxine, Synthroid) and may result in greater improvements in mood and neuropsychological function.[207]
	■ Glandular thyroid supplements and Armour thyroid generally should *not* be used in patients with thyroid autoimmunity (Hashimoto's thyroiditis) because the bovine/porcine antigens will exacerbate the anti-thyroid immune response as evidenced by increased anti-TPO antibodies.

Optimal thyroid status

<u>Concept by Dr Vasquez</u>: Optimal thyroid status is not defined by basic laboratory testing with TSH and free T4. It is defined *per patient* based on the levels and ratios of all major thyroid-related hormones and antibodies—in association with other hormonal, psychologic, dysbiotic, nutritional and environmental factors— that work best for that particular unique biochemically-individual patient. If a patient may benefit from a therapeutic trial of thyroid hormone (a substance produced naturally within the human body) and if no contraindications such as mania or cardiovascular disease are present, then a therapeutic trial of thyroid hormone is indeed quite likely reasonable and is arguably much more reasonable than the administration of foreign substances that do not correct or support normal physiologic functions.

<u>Laboratory interpretation by Dr McDaniel</u>: "Optimal hormone balance is debatable. My observations: A few "well" people and patients treated successfully with T4 and T3 seem best with:

- TSH around 0.7–0.9μIU/mL
- fT4 around 0.7–0.8ng/dL
- fT3 optimally 3.4–3.8pg/mL
- **Total T3-RT3 ratio 12 +/-2**"

McDaniel AB. Thyroid Assessment: Controversies and Conundrums. Institute for Functional Medicine Fourteenth International Symposium. Tucson, Arizona. May 23-26, 2007

---

[203] Beers MH, Berkow R (eds). *The Merck Manual. 17th Edition*. Whitehouse Station; Merck Research Laboratories 1999 page 96

[204] Duntas LH, Mantzou E, Koutras DA. Effects of a six month treatment with selenomethionine in patients with autoimmune thyroiditis. *Eur J Endocrinol*. 2003 Apr;148(4):389-93 eje-online.org/cgi/reprint/148/4/389

[205] Gartner R, Gasnier BC. Selenium in the treatment of autoimmune thyroiditis. *Biofactors*. 2003;19(3-4):165-70

[206] Sategna-Guidetti C, Volta U, Ciacci C, Usai P, Carlino A, De Franceschi L, Camera A, Pelli A, Brossa C. Prevalence of thyroid disorders in untreated adult celiac disease patients and effect of gluten withdrawal: an Italian multicenter study. *Am J Gastroenterol*. 2001 Mar;96(3):751-7

[207] "CONCLUSIONS: In patients with hypothyroidism, partial substitution of triiodothyronine for thyroxine may improve mood and neuropsychological function; this finding suggests a specific effect of the triiodothyronine normally secreted by the thyroid gland." Bunevicius R, Kazanavicius G, Zalinkevicius R, Prange AJ Jr. Effects of thyroxine as compared with thyroxine plus triiodothyronine in patients with hypothyroidism. *N Engl J Med*. 1999 Feb 11;340(6):424-9

Clinical Case 31yo female with fatigue, a recent history of extreme emotional stress, maternal history of Hashimotos thyroiditis—testing performed in 2010 by Quest Diagnostics: Outline plan before reading discussion.

Test Name	In Range	Out of Range	Reference Range
THYROGLOBULIN ANTIBODIES	<20		<20 IU/mL
THYROID PEROXIDASE ANTIBODIES		38 H	<35 IU/mL
T3, TOTAL	89		76-181 ng/dL
T3 UPTAKE		37 H	22-35 %
T4, FREE	1.6		0.8-1.8 ng/dL
T4 (THYROXINE), TOTAL			
T4 (THYROXINE), TOTAL	10.9		4.5-12.5 mcg/dL
FREE T4 INDEX (T7)		4.0 H	1.4-3.8
TSH, 3RD GENERATION	0.82		mIU/L

Reference Range

> or = 20 Years   0.40-4.50

Pregnancy Ranges
First trimester   0.20-4.70
Second trimester   0.30-4.10
Third trimester   0.40-2.70

Test Name	In Range	Out of Range	Reference Range
T3, FREE	318		230-420 pg/dL
T3, REVERSE		43 H	11-32 ng/dL

This test was performed using a kit that has not been approved or cleared by the FDA. The analytical performance characteristics of this test have been determined by Quest Diagnostics Nichols Institute, San Juan Capistrano. This test should not be used for diagnosis without confirmation by other medically established means.

Discussion: Note that the TSH is completely normal and thus would give the impression of normalcy and "health" if the clinician had not ordered the additional tests. Thyroid peroxidase antibodies are minimally elevated; this is consistent with thyroid autoimmunity but titers this low are of limited clinical importance. Note that the rT3 level is abnormally elevated. Note that because the units provided for total T3 (89 ng/dL) and rT3 (43 ng/dL) are identical, no unit conversion is required, thereby making the calculation of the ideal ratio (range: 10-14) very simple. In this patient's case, the ratio comes to 2.06 which is obviously significantly lower than the proposed optimal of 10-14; the patient responded well to liothyronine/Cytomel supplementation with 15 mcg/d. Patients with thyroid autoimmunity often benefit from a gluten-free diet[208] and supplementation with selenium 200 mcg/d.[209] Finally, note that the reference range for total T3 provided by this laboratory is 76-181 ng/dL which contrasts significantly from the range recommended by the US National Institutes of Health (NIH) 100 to 200 ng/dL[210]; using the NIH's reference range, this patient's T3 production is inadequate.

---

[208] "Hypothyroidism, diagnosed in 31 patients (12.9%) and nine controls (4.2%), was subclinical in 29 patients and of nonautoimmune origin in 21. ... In most patients who strictly followed a 1-yr gluten withdrawal (as confirmed by intestinal mucosa recovery), there was a normalization of subclinical hypothyroidism. The greater frequency of thyroid disease among celiac disease patients justifies a thyroid functional assessment. In distinct cases, gluten withdrawal may single-handedly reverse the abnormality." Sategna-Guidetti et al. Prevalence of thyroid disorders in untreated adult celiac disease patients and effect of gluten withdrawal: an Italian multicenter study. *Am J Gastroenterol.* 2001 Mar;96(3):751-7

[209] "Patients with HT assigned to Se supplementation for 3 months demonstrated significantly lower thyroid peroxidase autoantibodies (TPOab) titers (four studies, random effects weighted mean difference: −271.09, 95% confidence interval: −421.98 to −120.19, p< 10⁻⁴) and a significantly higher chance of reporting an improvement in well-being and/or mood (three studies, random effects risk ratio: 2.79, 95% confidence interval: 1.21-6.47, p= 0.016) when compared with controls. .. On the basis of the best available evidence, Se supplementation is associated with a significant decrease in TPOab titers at 3 months and with improvement in mood and/or general well-being."Toulis et al. Selenium supplementation in the treatment of Hashimoto's thyroiditis: a systematic review and a meta-analysis. *Thyroid.* 2010 Oct;20(10):1163-73

[210] U.S. National Library of Medicine and NIH nlm.nih.gov/medlineplus/ency/article/003687.htm Accessed Aug 2011

Toxic metal testing—emphasis on lead and mercury

Overview and application:	• **Introduction**: Per the US Department of Labor's Occupational Safety and Health Administration (OSHA)[211], toxic metals, including "heavy metals", are individual metals and metal compounds that negatively affect people's health. While lists of toxic metals can vary per source, OSHA names the following: arsenic, beryllium, cadmium, hexavalent chromium, lead, and mercury; of these, lead and mercury are the most commonly observed problematic toxic metals in outpatient practice. The three most important clinical concepts with regard to testing for "heavy metals" or "toxic metals" are as follows:

1. <u>Heavy metal toxicity/accumulation is not uncommon in clinical practice</u>: Toxic/heavy metal accumulation is clinically important due both to its frequency and its pathophysiologic consequences. An article published in *Journal of the American Medical Association (JAMA)*[212] showed that approximately 8% of [1,709 American] women had [blood mercury] concentrations higher than the US Environmental Protection Agency's recommended reference dose (5.8 µg/L), below which exposures are considered to be without adverse effects; stated more plainly, 8% of American women have (potentially) toxic levels of mercury *even when evaluated by the least sensitive of laboratory methods—blood mercury*, which represents only 5% of total body mercury. Another study, also published in *JAMA*[213], showed a positive relationship between blood lead levels and hypertension, even at blood lead levels considered within the normal range; the authors wrote, "At levels well below the current US occupational exposure limit guidelines (40 µg/dL), blood lead level is positively associated with both systolic and diastolic blood pressure and risks of both systolic and diastolic hypertension among women aged 40 to 59 years."

2. <u>The clinical presentation of heavy metal toxicity/accumulation is generally diverse and nonspecific</u>: Clinical presentations due to or associated with toxic metal accumulation can include dyscognition, fatigue, anemia, chronic pain from myalgia or neuropathy, hypertension, autism, and immune disorders including autoimmunity and allergy. In particular, autism[214,215,216] and hypertension[217,218] are noteworthy for their consistent associations with mercury and with mercury and lead, respectively.

3. <u>Therefore, clinicians should test for and treat toxic metal accumulation</u>: When problems are clinically significant and not extremely unlikely, clinicians have an obligation to test for and treat such problems for the benefit of the patient. Therefore, because toxic metal accumulation is common, clinically significant, and because it is a reversible cause of numerous symptoms, syndromes, and a contributing factor in the development/perpetuation of many other diagnosable conditions commonly labeled as "idiopathic" (e.g., hypertension, immune disorders, mood disorders), clinicians have an obligation to consider and test for toxic metals among their patients.

---

[211] osha.gov/SLTC/metalsheavy/index.html Accessed July 2011.

[212] Schober et al. Blood mercury levels in US children and women of childbearing age, 1999-2000. *JAMA* 2003;289:1667-74 jama.ama-assn.org/content/289/13/1667.long

[213] Nash D, Magder L, Lustberg M, Sherwin RW, Rubin RJ, Kaufmann RB, Silbergeld EK. Blood lead, blood pressure, and hypertension in perimenopausal and postmenopausal women. *JAMA*. 2003 Mar 26;289(12):1523-32. See also Muntner P, He J, Vupputuri S, Coresh J, Batuman V. Blood lead and chronic kidney disease in the general United States population: results from NHANES III. *Kidney Int*. 2003 Mar;63(3):1044-50 nature.com/ki/journal/v63/n3/pdf/4493526a.pdf

[214] Stamova B, Green PG, Tian Y, Hertz-Picciotto I, Pessah IN, Hansen R, Yang X, Teng J, Gregg JP, Ashwood P, Van de Water J, Sharp FR. Correlations between gene expression and mercury levels in blood of boys with and without autism. *Neurotox Res*. 2011;19:31-48. Epub 2009 Nov 24.

[215] "The results of the study indicated that the participants' overall ATEC scores and their scores on each of the ATEC subscales (Speech/Language, Sociability, Sensory/Cognitive Awareness, and Health/Physical/Behavior) were linearly related to urinary porphyrins associated with mercury toxicity. The results show an association between the apparent level of mercury toxicity as measured by recognized urinary porphyrin biomarkers of mercury toxicity and the magnitude of the specific hallmark features of autism as assessed by ATEC." Kern JK, Geier DA, Adams JB, Geier MR. A biomarker of mercury body-burden correlated with diagnostic domain specific clinical symptoms of autism spectrum disorder. *Biometals*. 2010 Dec;23(6):1043-51

[216] Kempuraj D, Asadi S, Zhang B, Manola A, Hogan J, Peterson E, Theoharides TC. Mercury induces inflammatory mediator release from human mast cells. *J Neuroinflammation*. 2010 Mar 11;7:20 jneuroinflammation.com/content/7/1/20

[217] Schober et al. Blood mercury levels in US children and women of childbearing age, 1999-2000. *JAMA* 2003;289:1667-74 jama.ama-assn.org/content/289/13/1667.long

[218] Nash D, et al. Blood lead, blood pressure, and hypertension in perimenopausal and postmenopausal women. *JAMA*. 2003 Mar 26;289(12):1523-32

Toxic metal testing—emphasis on lead and mercury

- **Additional details—mercury:** Mercury is an established neurotoxin, immunotoxin, and nephrotoxin. Because pathophysiologic effects are noted even with very small doses of exposure, one could reasonably argue that no safe amount exists and therefore that any detected mercury is an indication for therapeutic intervention to remove this toxicant. According to an article by Schober et al[219] published in *JAMA—Journal of the American Medical Association* in 2003, "Approximately 8% of [1,709 American] women had [blood mercury] concentrations higher than the US Environmental Protection Agency's recommended reference dose (5.8 μg/L), below which exposures are considered to be without adverse effects." Sources of exposure include dental amalgams, vaccinations, airborne pollution, deep-water fish such as tuna, some cosmetics[220], and selected herbicides, fungicides, and germicides; recently, high-fructose corn syrup was shown to contain mercury in clinically meaningful amounts.[221] Mercury impairs catecholamine degradation and can thereby cause a clinical syndrome that can include hypertension, tremor, tachycardia, diaphoresis, and neurocognitive changes.[222] Per Shih and Gartner[223], "Mercury combines with the sulfhydryl group of S-adenosylmethionine, which is a cofactor for catecholamine-O-methyltransferase (COMT), and this inhibition of COMT allows accumulation of norepinephrine, epinephrine, and dopamine." The clinical presentation of mercury toxicity can include any of the following: diffuse erythematosus rash, dermatitis (acrodynia), anorexia, malaise, fatigue, muscle pain, proximal and/or distal muscle weakness, tremor, weight loss, insomnia, night sweats, burning peripheral neuropathy (axonal neuropathy), renal insufficiency/failure, inattention, neurocognitive compromise, personality changes, depression, diaphoresis, tachycardia, and hypertension. Mercury poisoning/accumulation can occur in humans as a result of consumption of contaminated foods—especially seafood such as shark, swordfish, king mackerel, tilefish, and albacore ("white") tuna.[224] The immunologic effects of organic and/or inorganic mercury include immunosuppression, immunostimulation, formation of antinucleolar antibodies targeting fibrillarin, and formation and deposition of immune-complexes, resulting in a syndrome called "mercury-induced autoimmunity" which can be induced by exposure of susceptible animals to mercury.[225] Mercury/"silver" amalgam dental fillings rank highly among the most significant source of mercury exposure in humans, and implantation of mercury-silver dental amalgams in susceptible animals causes chronic stimulation of the immune system with induction of systemic autoimmunity.[226] Besides being a neurotoxin with no safe exposure limit[227], mercury is known to modify/antigenize/haptenize endogenous proteins to promote autoimmunity[228], and mercury may also promote autoimmunity by contributing to a pro-inflammatory environment that awakens quiescent autoreactive immunocytes via bystander activation.[229] For example,

[219] Schober SE, et al. Blood mercury levels in US children and women of childbearing age, 1999-2000. *JAMA*. 2003 Apr 2;289(13):1667-74
[220] "Most makeup manufacturers have phased out the use of mercury, but it's still added legally to some eye products as a preservative and germ-killer, said John Bailey, chief scientist with the Personal Care Products Council in Washington." Associated Press. Minnesota Bans Adding Mercury To Cosmetics. February 11, 2009. cbsnews.com/stories/2007/12/14/health/main3618048.shtml Accessed August 2011
[221] "Average daily consumption of high fructose corn syrup is about 50 grams per person in the United States. With respect to total mercury exposure, it may be necessary to account for this source of mercury in the diet of children and sensitive populations." Dufault R, LeBlanc B, Schnoll R, Cornett C, Schweitzer L, Wallinga D, Hightower J, Patrick L, Lukiw WJ. Mercury from chlor-alkali plants: measured concentrations in food product sugar. *Environ Health*. 2009 Jan 26;8:2. See also: "High fructose corn syrup has been shown to contain trace amounts of mercury as a result of some manufacturing processes, and its consumption can also lead to zinc loss." Dufault R, et al. Mercury exposure, nutritional deficiencies and metabolic disruptions may affect learning in children. *Behav Brain Funct*. 2009 Oct 27;5:44.
[222] Wössmann W, Kohl M, Grüning G, Bucsky P. Mercury intoxication presenting with hypertension and tachycardia. *Arch Dis Child*. 1999 Jun;80(6):556-7 ncbi.nlm.nih.gov/pmc/articles/PMC1717944/pdf/v080p00556.pdf
[223] Shih H, Gartner JC Jr. Weight loss, hypertension, weakness, and limb pain in an 11-year-old boy. *J Pediatr*. 2001 Apr;138(4):566-9
[224] See fda.gov/Food/FoodSafety/Product-SpecificInformation/Seafood/FoodbornePathogensContaminants/Methylmercury/ucm115662.htm for the white-washed version; see ewg.org/news/bamboozled-fish for a more accurate and complete perspective.
[225] Havarinasab S, Hultman P. Organic mercury compounds and autoimmunity. *Autoimmun Rev*. 2005;4(5):270-5 generationrescue.org/pdf/havarinasab.pdf Dec 2005
[226] "We hypothesize that under appropriate conditions of genetic susceptibility and adequate body burden, heavy metal exposure from dental amalgam may contribute to immunological aberrations, which could lead to overt autoimmunity." Hultman P, Johansson U, Turley SJ, Lindh U, Enestrom S, Pollard KM. Adverse immunological effects and autoimmunity induced by dental amalgam and alloy in mice. *FASEB J*. 1994 Nov;8(14):1183-90
[227] University of Calgary Faculty of Medicine. How Mercury Causes Brain Neuron Degeneration. commons.ucalgary.ca/mercury/ Current Aug 2011
[228] Havarinasab S, Hultman P. Organic mercury compounds and autoimmunity. *Autoimmun Rev*. 2005 Jun;4(5):270-5. generationrescue.org/pdf/havarinasab.pdf Dec 2005
[229] "It is therefore theoretically possible that compounds present in vaccines such as thiomersal or aluminium hydroxide can trigger autoimmune reactions through bystander effects." Fournie et al. Induction of autoimmunity through bystander effects. Lessons from immunological disorders induced by heavy metals. *J Autoimmun*. 2001 May;16:319-26

administration of mercury to "susceptible" mice induces autoimmunity via modification of the nucleolar protein *fibrillarin*[230]; noteworthy in this regard is the fact that antifibrillarin antibodies are characteristic of the human autoimmune disease scleroderma.[231] The mercury-based preservative thimerosol is a type-IV (delayed hypersensitivity) sensitizing agent[232], and recent research implicates mercury as a contributor to autism[233,234] and eczema.[235] A review and clinical report published by Bains et al[236], stated, "Eczematous eruptions may be produced through topical contact with mercury and by systemic absorption in mercury sensitive individuals. Mercury…may cause hypersensitivity leading to contact dermatitis or Coomb's Type IV hypersensitivity reactions. The typical manifestation is an urticarial or erythematous rash, and pruritus on the face and flexural aspects of limbs, followed by progression to dermatitis." Thus, this survey of the literature supports the notions that mercury toxicity—i.e., a level of mercury in human patients sufficient to cause adverse health effects—is ❶ common (e.g., 8% of American women), ❷ problematic via causation of or contribution to various health problems commonly encountered in clinical practice, ❸ diagnosable via laboratory testing followed by monitoring response to treatment, and ❹ treatable, most notably with DMSA but also to a lesser extent with potassium citrate, selenium, and phytochelatins.

- Additional details—lead: The International Agency for Research on Cancer (IARC, part of the World Health Organization [WHO]) classified lead as a "possible human carcinogen" in 1987. A 2003 review published in *British Medical Bulletin* by Järup[237] noted that lead exposure (which comes equally from air and food, particularly food served via lead-contaminated ceramics) should be avoided as much as possible because physiologic toxicity occurs with low-level exposure; "Blood levels in children should be reduced below the levels so far considered acceptable, recent data indicating that there may be neurotoxic effects of lead at lower levels of exposure than previously anticipated." Occupational exposure to lead occurs in mines, smelting plants, glass-manufacturing facilities, battery plants, and among workers who weld metals already painted with lead-containing paints; air emissions near such facilities and activities may also contaminate nonworkers. Air contamination frequently leads to water contamination, threatening wildlife and humans who are exposed to contaminated water. Children are particularly vulnerable to lead exposure due to very efficient (compared with adults) gastrointestinal absorption and a more permeable ("leaky") blood-brain barrier. Organic lead compounds such as tetramethyl-lead and tetraethyl lead easily penetrate skin and blood-brain barrier of children as well as adults. Classic, large-dose, acute and subacute lead poisoning manifests as anemia, renal tubular damage, and dark blue line of lead sulphide at the gingival margin; clinicians awaiting this classic presentation prior to considering lead toxicity should fortify their knowledge of and reconsider their perspective on this topic. Other symptoms of acute lead poisoning are headache, irritability, abdominal pain and various neurologic-psychiatric symptoms generally referred to as "lead encephalopathy" characterized by sleeplessness, restlessness, confusion/dyscognition, behavioral disturbances, particularly learning and concentration difficulties in children;

---

[230] Nielsen JB, Hultman P. Mercury-induced autoimmunity in mice. *Environ Health Perspect*. 2002 Oct;110 Suppl 5:877-81 ehp.niehs.nih.gov/docs/2002/suppl-5/877-881nielsen/abstract.html

[231] "Since anti-fibrillarin antibodies are specific markers of scleroderma, the present animal model may be valuable for studies of the immunological aberrations which are likely to induce this autoimmune response." Hultman P, Enestrom S, Pollard KM, Tan EM. Anti-fibrillarin autoantibodies in mercury-treated mice. *Clin Exp Immunol*. 1989;78(3):470-7

[232] "Thimerosal is an important preservative in vaccines and ophthalmologic preparations. The substance is known to be a type IV sensitizing agent. High sensitization rates were observed in contact-allergic patients and in health care workers who had been exposed to thimerosal-preserved vaccines." Westphal et al. Homozygous gene deletions of the glutathione S-transferases M1 and T1 are associated with thimerosal sensitization. *Int Arch Occup Environ Health*. 2000 Aug;73(6):384-8

[233] Vojdani A, Pangborn JB, Vojdani E, Cooper EL. Infections, toxic chemicals and dietary peptides binding to lymphocyte receptors and tissue enzymes are major instigators of autoimmunity in autism. *Int J Immunopathol Pharmacol*. 2003 Sep-Dec;16(3):189-99

[234] Geier DA, Geier MR. A comparative evaluation of the effects of MMR immunization and mercury doses from thimerosal-containing childhood vaccines on the population prevalence of autism. *Med Sci Monit*. 2004 Mar;10(3):PI33-9. medscimonit.com/pub/vol_10/no_3/3986.pdf

[235] Weidinger et al. Body burden of mercury is associated with acute atopic eczema and total IgE in children from southern Germany. *J Allergy Clin Immunol*. 2004;114(2):457-9

[236] Bains VK, Loomba K, Loomba A, Bains R. Mercury sensitisation: review, relevance and a clinical report. *Br Dent J*. 2008 Oct 11;205(7):373-8 intolsante.com/documents/publications/-mercury-sensitisation-review-relevance-and-clinical-report-22.pdf Accessed August 2011

[237] Järup L. Hazards of heavy metal contamination. *Br Med Bull*. 2003;68:167-82

Toxic metal testing—emphasis on lead and mercury	
	more extreme manifestations can include acute psychosis and stupor. Per the previously cited review by Järup, "Individuals [chronically exposed to lead] with average blood lead levels under 3 µmol/l may show signs of peripheral nerve symptoms with reduced nerve conduction velocity and reduced dermal sensibility."
Overview and application:	▪ No universally accepted consensus exists for the most accurate testing methodology. However, from the science-based perspectives that toxic metals have been proven to cause harm at levels previously believed to be "acceptable" and that—very importantly—toxic metals are exponentially more toxic when in combination than when present alone, reasonable clinicians can therefore conclude that the best test for clinical use is the one that is most sensitive, along with being reasonably convenient for the patient as well as affordable. For these reasons, the current author and many other clinicians chose DMSA-provoked urine toxic metal testing. Hair and nails can also be tested for chronic exposure, as can blood which is generally only useful for recent and relatively high-level exposure. Our clinical concern in general outpatient practice is not with recent and relatively high-level exposure, and therefore blood is not necessarily optimal. Our clinical concern in general outpatient practice is with chronic low-level exposure which leads to adverse cellular effects despite the failure to "spike" the serum level into the detectable toxic range. Arguments in favor of allowing symptomatic patients to persist untreated in a state of toxic metal accumulation would be difficult to justify scientifically and ethically.
Advantages:	▪ Toxic metal accumulation is ❶ sufficiently common to warrant testing in selected patients—such testing should be used frequently with a low threshold for implementation, ❷ problematic via causation of or contribution to various health problems commonly encountered in clinical practice, ❸ diagnosable via laboratory testing followed by monitoring response to treatment, and ❹ treatable. Therefore, clinicians should establish pathways for the assessment and treatment of metal toxicity.
Limitations:	▪ Patients with toxic metal accumulation frequently have accumulation of chemical xenobiotics as well; thus testing for and treating toxicity due to metals only relieves one type of toxicity.
Comments:	▪ Clinicians should establish pathways for the assessment and treatment of toxic metal accumulation.

Clinical Case **Widespread musculoskeletal pain resembling fibromyalgia secondary to lead and mercury accumulation**: This 54yo athletic female with healthy diet, lifestyle, and supportive relationship presented with chronic diffuse musculoskeletal pain. Health history was sigificant for decades of environmental illness/intolerance (EI) also known as multiple chemical sensitivity (MCS). Family history was positive for maternal temporal (giant cell) arteritis. Physical examination revealed numerous tender points consistent with fibromyalgia; yet the history and stool analysis with comprehensive bacteriology and parasitology were unsupportive of gastrointestinal dysbiosis, particularly of the subtype small intestine bacterial overgrowth, which is causal for fibromyalgia.[238] Laboratory investigations revealed normal results for hsCRP (high-sensitity c-reactive protein), CK (creatine kinase, a marker of muscle damage and myositis), ANA (anti-nuclear antibodies), vitamin D, calcium, phosphorus, and comprehensive thyroid evaluation. The patient was then (defensively) referred to an osteopathic internist who diagnosed fibromyalgia.

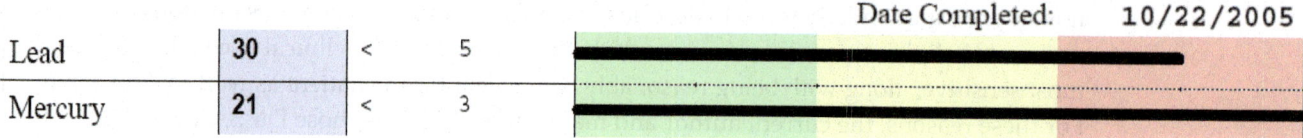

				Date Completed:	10/22/2005
Lead	30	<	5		
Mercury	21	<	3		

Discussion: The patient, unsatisfied with the diagnosis of fibromyalgia, returned to the current author, who then performed urine heavy metal testing provoked with 10 mg per kilogram of dimercaptosuccinic acid (DMSA). Results revealed the highest levels of lead and mercury encountered in the author's practice at that time. As shown above, lead levels were 6x above the reference range and mercury levels were 7x above the reference range. The patient was commenced on DMSA 10 mg/kg/d on alternating weeks to avoid toxicity in general and bone marrow toxicity (neutropenia) in particular, selenium 800 mcg/d to promote excretion of toxic metals and to support renal and antoxidant protection, vegetable juices to provide potassium and citrate for urinary alkalinization and enhanced excretion of xenobiotics[239], and a proprietary phytochelatin (metal-binding peptides from plants[240]) concetrate to bind toxic metals in the gut and thereby promote their fecal excretion by blocking enterohepatic recycling/recirculation. The use of DMSA for children and adults is supported by peer-reviewed literature.[241,242,243,244,245] DMSA chelation is approved by the US Food and Drug Administration (FDA) for the treatment of marked lead toxicity in children.[246] After approximately 8 months of treatment, the patient was completely free of pain, and the clinical improvement was associated with a reduction in both lead and mercury of approximately 50% as demonstrated by follow-up laboratory testing. Testing was performed by Doctors Data. This case was previously published in peer-reviewed literature for continuing education credits.[247]

				Date Completed:	6/30/2006
Lead	15	<	5		
Mercury	8.2	<	4		

[238] Vasquez A. *Integrative Orthopedics* and *Integrative Rheumatology* and *Fibromyalgia in a Nutshell* and newer versions in the Inflammation Mastery series.
[239] Crinnion WJ. Environmental medicine, part three: long-term effects of chronic low-dose mercury exposure. *Altern Med Rev.* 2000 Jun;5(3):209-23
[240] Cobbett CS. Phytochelatins and their roles in heavy metal detoxification. *Plant Physiol.* 2000;123:825-32 plantphysiol.org/content/123/3/825
[241] Bradstreet J, Geier DA, Kartzinel JJ, Adams JB, Geier MR. A case-control study of mercury burden in children with autistic spectrum disorders. *Journal of American Physicians and Surgeons* 2003; 8: 76-79 jpands.org/vol8no3/geier.pdf
[242] Crinnion WJ. Environmental medicine, part three: long-term effects of chronic low-dose mercury exposure. *Altern Med Rev.* 2000 Jun;5(3):209-23
[243] Forman J, Moline J, Cernichiari E, Sayegh S, Torres JC, Landrigan MM, Hudson J, Adel HN, Landrigan PJ. A cluster of pediatric metallic mercury exposure cases treated with meso-2,3-dimercaptosuccinic acid (DMSA). *Environ Health Perspect.* 2000 Jun;108(6):575-7 ehp.niehs.nih.gov/docs/2000/108p575-577forman/abstract.html
[244] Miller AL. Dimercaptosuccinic acid (DMSA), a non-toxic, water-soluble treatment for heavy metal toxicity. *Altern Med Rev.* 1998 Jun;3(3):199-207 thorne.com/altmedrev/.fulltext/3/3/199.pdf
[245] DMSA. *Altern Med Rev.* 2000 Jun;5(3):264-7 thorne.com/altmedrev/.fulltext/5/3/264.pdf
[246] "The Food and Drug Administration has recently licensed the drug DMSA (succimer) for reduction of blood lead levels >/= 45 micrograms/dl. This decision was based on the demonstrated ability of DMSA to reduce blood lead levels. An advantage of this drug is that it can be given orally." Goyer RA, Cherian MG, Jones MM, Reigart JR. Role of chelating agents for prevention, intervention, and treatment of exposures to toxic metals. *Environ Health Perspect.* 1995 Nov;103(11):1048-52 ehp.niehs.nih.gov/docs/1995/103-11/meetingreport.html
[247] Vasquez A. *Musculoskeletal Pain: Expanded Clinical Strategies*. Institute for Functional Medicine. 2008

Clinical Case **Chronic "idiopathic" hypertension associated with lead and mercury accumulation** (per DMSA-provoked urine testing): This 43yo male presents with recalcitrant stage-1 hypertension. His cardiologist prescribed drugs to "treat" (some would say "mask") his elevated blood pressure. Since hypertension always has an underlying cause, the ethical and appropriate course of action is to determine the cause of the problem rather than silencing the alarm that is alerting to an underlying dysfunction. While this case is currently in progress at the time of this writing (the patient's medical records arrived in July 2011), it does offer a model case for clinical decision-making. Clinicians should be aware that, per animal studies, the toxicity of lead and mercury are greatly enhanced when both toxins are present at the same time.

Date Collected: 6/3/2010

| Lead | 8.5 | < | 2 |
| Mercury | 17 | < | 3 |

Mercury and hypertension: Mercury is an established neurotoxin, immunotoxin, and nephrotoxin. Because pathophysiologic effects are noted even with very small doses of exposure, one could reasonably argue that no safe amount exists and therefore that any detected mercury is an indication for therapeutic intervention to remove this toxicant. Sources of exposure include dental amalgams, vaccinations, airborne pollution, and fish; recently, high-fructose corn syrup was shown to contain mercury.[248] Mercury impairs catecholamine degradation and can thereby cause a clinical syndrome that can include hypertension, tremor, tachycardia, diaphoresis, and neurocognitive changes.[249] Per Shih and Gartner[250], "Mercury combines with the sulfhydryl group of S-adenosylmethionine, which is a cofactor for catecholamine-O-methyltransferase (COMT), and this inhibition of COMT allows accumulation of norepinephrine, epinephrine, and dopamine."

Lead and hypertension: In the United States, a consistent correlation has been found between body burden of lead and HTN, even when blood lead levels are well below the current US occupational exposure limit guidelines (40 microg/dl).[251] Harlan et al[252] analyzed data from the second National Health and Nutrition Examination Survey (1976-1980) and thereby found a direct relationship between blood lead levels and systolic and diastolic pressures for men and women and for white and black persons aged 12 to 74 years; they concluded, "Blood lead levels were significantly higher in younger men and women (aged 21 to 55 years) with high blood pressure, but not in older men or women (aged 56 to 74 years)." Schwartz and Stewart[253] found that blood lead was the assessment that most strongly correlated with HTN; they concluded, "Systolic blood pressure was elevated by blood lead levels as low as 5 microg/dl." Thus, clinicians might first measure blood lead levels, which do not measure total body burden but rather the lead that is mobile or *in transit* within the body and which appears to have the best correlation with HTN; the finding of normal blood lead results could then be followed with the more sensitive DMSA-provoked heavy metal testing before concluding that heavy metals are noncontributory to that particular patient's HTN. For heavy metal testing in various clinical scenarios, this author's preference is to use DMSA-provoked measurement of urine toxic metals. After a minimal test dose of DMSA (e.g., in the range of 50-100 mg) to screen for hypersensitivity, patients take oral DMSA 10 mg/kg as a single oral dose in the morning on an empty stomach after emptying the bladder and send a sample from the next urination for laboratory analysis; follow laboratory protocol if different from these instructions. Use of DMSA for lead and mercury chelation/detoxification and for diagnostic purposes is generally safe and effective.[254,255,256]

---

[248] "Average daily consumption of high fructose corn syrup is about 50 grams per person in the United States. With respect to total mercury exposure, it may be necessary to account for this source of mercury in the diet of children and sensitive populations." Dufault R, LeBlanc B, Schnoll R, Cornett C, Schweitzer L, Wallinga D, Hightower J, Patrick L, Lukiw WJ. Mercury from chlor-alkali plants: measured concentrations in food product sugar. *Environ Health*. 2009 Jan 26;8:2. See also: "High fructose corn syrup has been shown to contain trace amounts of mercury as a result of some manufacturing processes, and its consumption can also lead to zinc loss." Dufault R, et al. Mercury exposure, nutritional deficiencies and metabolic disruptions may affect learning in children. *Behav Brain Funct*. 2009 Oct 27;5:44.

[249] Wössmann W, Kohl M, Grüning G, Bucsky P. Mercury intoxication presenting with hypertension and tachycardia. *Arch Dis Child*. 1999 Jun;80(6):556-7 ncbi.nlm.nih.gov/pmc/articles/PMC1717944/pdf/v080p00556.pdf

[250] Shih H, Gartner JC Jr. Weight loss, hypertension, weakness, and limb pain in an 11-year-old boy. *J Pediatr*. 2001 Apr;138(4):566-9

[251] Nash D, Magder L, Lustberg M, Sherwin RW, Rubin RJ, Kaufmann RB, Silbergeld EK. Blood lead, blood pressure, and hypertension in perimenopausal and postmenopausal women. *JAMA*. 2003 Mar 26;289(12):1523-32 jama.ama-assn.org/cgi/content/full/289/12/1523

[252] Harlan WR, et al. Blood lead and blood pressure. Relationship in the adolescent and adult US population. *JAMA*. 1985 Jan 25;253(4):530-4

[253] "Systolic blood pressure was elevated by blood lead levels as low as 5 microg/dl." Schwartz BS, Stewart WF. Different associations of blood lead, meso 2,3-dimercaptosuccinic acid (DMSA)-chelatable lead, and tibial lead levels with blood pressure in 543 former organolead manufacturing workers. *Arch Environ Health*. 2000 Mar-Apr;55(2):85-92

[254] Bradstreet J, Geier DA, Kartzinel JJ, Adams JB, Geier MR. A case-control study of mercury burden in children with autistic spectrum disorders. *Journal of American Physicians and Surgeons* 2003; 8: 76-79 jpands.org/vol8no3/geier.pdf

[255] Miller AL. Dimercaptosuccinic acid (DMSA), a non-toxic, water-soluble treatment for heavy metal toxicity. *Altern Med Rev*. 1998 Jun;3(3):199-207

[256] DMSA. *Altern Med Rev*. 2000 Jun;5(3):264-7

Antinuclear antibody: ANA	
Overview and interpretation:	▪ Good screening test for autoimmune conditions: SLE, Sjogren's syndrome, and various other "connective tissue" inflammatory/rheumatic/autoimmune diseases. ▪ Good and "highly sensitive" for initial assessment of SLE; positive in 95-98% of SLE patients; negative result strongly suggests against diagnosis of SLE.[257] Only 2% of patients with SLE have a negative ANA test—these patients may be identified by testing with anti-RO antibodies and CH50 (complement levels). ▪ This test measures for the presence of antibodies that react to nucleoproteins. Some labs report titers of 1:20 or 1:40 as "positive"; however, low levels of ANA are common (5-15%) in the general population. Thus, ANA is not specific for any one disease; may be positive in SLE, RA, scleroderma, Sjogren's, also seen with elderly, infected patients, cancer, and with certain medications. Titers less than 1:160 may not indicate the presence of *clinical* autoimmunity[258]; titers >=1:160 usually indicate the presence of active SLE, or other autoimmunity.[259] Titers greater than 1:320 are considered indicative of clinically significant autoimmunity. ▪ Methodologies (indirect immunofluorescence is most popular), subtypes, and patterns reported for ANA results may be irrelevant or clinically meaningful; the most common descriptors are provided in the table below. Clinicians should order quantitative ANA with reflex to FANA staining patterns

ANA patterns and descriptions[260,261]	Clinical correlation
Homogeneous, diffuse nuclear staining	SLE, lupus nephritis, and other autoimmunity
Speckled	SLE, scleroderma, Sjogren's, other autoimmunity
Rim or peripheral staining	Correlates with SLE and lupus nephritis
Anti-centromere: selective staining of the centromeres of nuclei in metaphase	Highly specific for the limited scleroderma subtype associated with **CREST** syndrome
Nucleolar	Correlated with diffuse scleroderma (systemic sclerosis), Sjogren's syndrome, SLE
FANA: fluorescent ANA	The standard ANA test in the US
Anti-Sm: anti-Smith[262]	**Highly specific for SLE**; insensitive: positive in 20-30% of SLE patients
Anti-dsDNA: anti-double stranded DNA	**Highly specific for SLE** and indicative of an increased likelihood of poor prognosis with major organ involvement[263] especially active renal disease
Anti-Ro (anti-SS-A)	Correlates with SLE, Sjögren's syndrome, and neonatal SLE
Anti-La (anti-SS-B)	Sjögren's syndrome or low risk of SLE nephritis
Anti-RNP	SLE and/or mixed connective tissue disease (MCTD)
Anti-Jo-1	Specific but not sensitive for polymyositis/dermatomyositis
Antihistone	SLE and especially drug-induced SLE
Antitopoisomerase (Scl-70)	**Correlates with diffuse scleroderma, especially with interstitial lung disease**

[257] Shojania K. Rheumatology: 2. What laboratory tests are needed? *CMAJ*. 2000 Apr 18;162(8):1157-63 cmaj.ca/cgi/content/full/162/8/1157
[258] Hardin JG, Waterman J, Labson LH. Rheumatic disease: Which diagnostic tests are useful? *Patient Care* 1999; March 15: 83-102
[259] Antinuclear Antibodies (ANA), Synonyms: FANA, Test Number: 164947, CPT Code: 86038. https://labcorp.com March 2013
[260] Shojania K. Rheumatology: 2. What laboratory tests are needed? *CMAJ*. 2000 Apr 18;162(8):1157-63 cmaj.ca/cgi/content/full/162/8/1157
[261] Ward MM. Laboratory testing for systemic rheumatic diseases. *Postgrad Med*. 1998 Feb;103(2):93-100.
[262] Lane SK, Gravel JW Jr. Clinical utility of common serum rheumatologic tests. *Am Fam Physician*. 2002;65:1073-80 aafp.org/afp/20020315/1073.html
[263] Shojania K. Rheumatology: 2. What laboratory tests are needed? *CMAJ*. 2000 Apr 18;162(8):1157-63 cmaj.ca/cgi/content/full/162/8/1157

Antinuclear antibody: ANA—*continued*	
Advantages:	▪ ANA has 98% sensitivity and 90% specificity for SLE in an unselected population. ▪ The negative predictive value in an unselected population is greater than 99%. ANA is therefore an excellent test for *excluding* the diagnosis of SLE.
Limitations:	▪ The positive predictive value in an unselected population is about 30%; only 30% of unselected people with a positive result will have SLE—this fact underscores the importance of patient selection and judicious interpretation of this test. ▪ Positive ANA is seen in patients with conditions other than SLE, including rheumatoid arthritis, Sjogren's syndrome, scleroderma, polymyositis, vasculitis, juvenile rheumatoid arthritis (JRA), and infectious diseases.
Comments:	▪ ANA is most often used to support the diagnosis of SLE in a patient with multisystemic illness and a clinical picture compatible with SLE. Nearly all patients with SLE will have positive ANA. **A positive ANA does not mean that the patient necessarily has SLE; be weary of paraneoplastic syndromes and viral hepatitis as underlying causative processes in patients with an unclear clinical picture.** ▪ I view any "positive ANA" as an indicator of poor health in general and immune dysfunction in particular. The goal, then, is to restore health. I have seen ANA show a trend toward normalization or completely normalize with effective health restoration as detailed in *Integrative Rheumatology* (Chapter 4). I realize that my experience in this regard contrasts sharply with the allopathic view that serial measurements of ANA are worthless because the result never normalizes once a patient is ANA-positive[264]; I consider this evidence of the effectiveness of my integrative-functional approach and the comparable failure of the allopathic approach.

Antineutrophilic cytoplasmic antibodies: ANCA	
Overview:	▪ ANCA are autoantibodies to the cytoplasmic constituents of granulocytes and are characteristically found in vasculitic syndromes and also in (Chinese) patients with inflammatory bowel disease[265] and nearly all patients with hepatic amebiasis due to *Entamoeba histolytica.*[266] Two types: ▪ Cytoplasmic ANCA (C-ANCA): classically seen in Wegener's granulomatosis; also seen in some types of glomerulonephritis and vasculitis; this test is highly sensitive and specific for these conditions. In fact, a positive C-ANCA result can replace biopsy in a patient with a clinical picture of Wegener's granulomatosis.[267] ▪ Perinuclear ANCA (P-ANCA): considered a nonspecific finding[268] that correlates with SLE, drug induced lupus, and some types of glomerulonephritis and vasculitis. Shojania[269] stated that this test must be confirmed with antimyeloperoxidase antibodies to evaluate for Churg–Strauss syndrome, crescentic glomerulonephritis, and microscopic polyarteritis.
Advantages, limitations, and comments	▪ Not to be used as a screening test, except in patients with idiopathic vasculitis or glomerulonephritis. ▪ The fact that hepatic amebiasis due to *Entamoeba histolytica* induces production of C-ANCA antibodies in nearly 100% of infected patients may support the hypothesis that autoimmunity can be induced or exacerbated by parasitic infections.

---

[264] Shojania K. Rheumatology: 2. What laboratory tests are needed? *CMAJ.* 2000 Apr 18;162(8):1157-63 cmaj.ca/cgi/content/full/162/8/1157
[265] "Fourteen patients (73.5%) were positive, of which six (31.5%) showed a perinuclear staining pattern and eight (42%) demonstrated a cytoplasmic pattern." Sung JY, Chan KL, Hsu R, Liew CT, Lawton JW. Ulcerative colitis and antineutrophil cytoplasmic antibodies in Hong Kong Chinese. *Am J Gastroenterol.* 1993 Jun;88(6):864-9
[266] "ANCA was detected in 97.4% of amoebic sera; the pattern of staining was cytoplasmic, homogeneous, without central accentuation (C-ANCA)." Pudifin DJ, Duursma J, Gathiram V, Jackson TF. Invasive amoebiasis is associated with the development of anti-neutrophil cytoplasmic antibody. *Clin Exp Immunol.* 1994 Jul;97(1):48-5
[267] Shojania K. Rheumatology: 2. What laboratory tests are needed? *CMAJ.* 2000 Apr 18;162(8):1157-63 cmaj.ca/cgi/content/full/162/8/1157
[268] Shojania K. Rheumatology: 2. What laboratory tests are needed? *CMAJ.* 2000 Apr 18;162(8):1157-63 cmaj.ca/cgi/content/full/162/8/1157
[269] Shojania K. Rheumatology: 2. What laboratory tests are needed? *CMAJ.* 2000 Apr 18;162(8):1157-63 cmaj.ca/cgi/content/full/162/8/1157

Overview and Application:	▪ Rheumatoid factor—"anti-IgG antibodies"—are antibodies directed to the Fc portion of the patient's own IgG. Rheumatoid factors are anti-immunoglobulin antibodies, classically anti-IgG IgM. RF are found in low levels in most patients, and despite the "rheumatoid" name, RF is not specific for rheumatoid arthritis.[270] Current tests (latex fixation or nephelometry) detect IgM anti-immunoglobulin antibodies; however IgA-RF appears to have clinical superiority over other forms of RF because it correlates more strongly with clinical status.[271]
	▪ This test is most commonly used to support the diagnosis of rheumatoid arthritis in a patient with a compelling clinical picture: peripheral polyarthritis lasting >6 weeks.[272] A negative result with a compelling clinical presentation of RA is termed "seronegative rheumatoid arthritis" by allopathic textbooks whereas a more appropriate term might be oligoarthritis, a condition described as "idiopathic" by allopathic text books despite the clear evidence that the majority of patients have one or more subsets of dysbiosis.[273]
	▪ Titers (latex fixation) of 1:160 are considered clinically significant, favoring the diagnosis of RA.[274] However the positive predictive value is low—only 20-34% of people in an unselected population with a positive test result actually have RA.[275,276]
Advantages:	▪ Supports the diagnosis of rheumatoid arthritis: about 60-85% positive/sensitive in patients with rheumatoid arthritis (RA).[277,278] Quantitative titers of RF correlate with prognosis: a very high RF value portends a poor prognosis.
Limitations:	▪ Positive findings are common in the following conditions: rheumatoid arthritis, viral hepatitis, Sjögren's syndrome, endocarditis, scleroderma, mycobacteria diseases, polymyositis and dermatomyositis, syphilis, systemic lupus erythematosus, old age, mixed connective tissue disease, sarcoidosis; positive results may also been noted in: cryoglobulinemia, parasitic infection, interstitial lung disease, asymptomatic relatives of people with autoimmune diseases.
	▪ Febrile patients with arthralgia are more likely to have endocarditis than RA.[279]
	▪ Patients with iron overload present with a similar clinical picture (i.e., polyarthropathy with systemic complaints) and may have a positive RF. Thus, patients with positive RF and polyarthropathy should be tested for iron overload; use serum ferritin.[280]
Comments:	▪ This test should only be used to confirm the diagnosis of rheumatoid arthritis in patients with a compelling clinical picture of the disease: inflammatory peripheral polyarthropathy with systemic complaints for > 6 weeks. A negative result does not mean that the patient *does not* have rheumatoid arthritis; a positive result does not mean that the patient *does* have rheumatoid arthritis.[281]
	▪ CCP (cyclic citrullinated protein) antibodies appear to be more specific and sensitive for RA and is becoming the test of choice for RA as described on the following page.

[270] Shojania K. Rheumatology: 2. What laboratory tests are needed? *CMAJ*. 2000 Apr 18;162(8):1157-63 cmaj.ca/cgi/content/full/162/8/1157
[271] Jonsson T, Valdimarsson H. What about IgA rheumatoid factor in rheumatoid arthritis? *Ann Rheum Dis*. 1998 Jan;57(1):63-4
[272] Shojania K. Rheumatology: 2. What laboratory tests are needed? *CMAJ*. 2000 Apr 18;162(8):1157-63 cmaj.ca/cgi/content/full/162/8/1157
[273] See Chapter 4 of *Integrative Rheumatology* and Vasquez A. Reducing Pain and Inflammation Naturally. Part 6: Nutritional and Botanical Treatments Against "Silent Infections" and Gastrointestinal Dysbiosis, Commonly Overlooked Causes of Neuromusculoskeletal Inflammation and Chronic Health Problems. *Nutr Perspect* 2006; Jan
[274] Beers MH, Berkow R (eds). *The Merck Manual. Seventeenth Edition*. Whitehouse Station; Merck Research Laboratories 1999 Page 417
[275] Ward MM. Laboratory testing for systemic rheumatic diseases. *Postgrad Med*. 1998 Feb;103(2):93-100.
[276] Shojania K. Rheumatology: 2. What laboratory tests are needed? *CMAJ*. 2000 Apr 18;162(8):1157-63 cmaj.ca/cgi/content/full/162/8/1157
[277] Tierney ML. McPhee SJ, Papadakis MA (eds). *Current Medical Diagnosis and Treatment 2002, 41st Edition*. New York: Lange Medical, 2002 p854
[278] Shojania K. Rheumatology: 2. What laboratory tests are needed? *CMAJ*. 2000 Apr 18;162(8):1157-63 cmaj.ca/cgi/content/full/162/8/1157
[279] Klippel JH (ed). *Primer on the Rheumatic Diseases. 11th Edition*. Atlanta: Arthritis Foundation. 1997 page 96
[280] Bensen WG, Laskin CA, Little HA, Fam AG. Hemochromatoic arthropathy mimicking rheumatoid arthritis. A case with subcutaneous nodules, tenosynovitis, and bursitis. *Arthritis Rheum* 1978; 21: 844-8
[281] Shojania K. Rheumatology: 2. What laboratory tests are needed? *CMAJ*. 2000 Apr 18;162(8):1157-63 cmaj.ca/cgi/content/full/162/8/1157

CCP: Cyclic citrullinated protein antibody; Citrullinated protein antibodies (CPA); anti-CCP antibodies	
Overview and use:	<ul><li>CCP—cyclic citrullinated protein antibodies; anticitrullinated protein antibodies: this is a relatively new auto-antibody marker that shows great promise and specificity for the early diagnosis of rheumatoid arthritis (RA). The test often becomes positive/present in asymptomatic patients years before the onset of clinical manifestations of RA.</li><li>As of the first inclusion of this information in my books in December 2006, the information on anti-CCP antibodies is so new that it is not even included in most 2006-edition medical and rheumatology reference textbooks; nonetheless, doctors nationwide are already starting to use this test for the early diagnosis of RA. This may be particularly important because some research has shown that *early* and *aggressive* treatment of RA has an important impact on long-term prognosis[282]; however, the importance of early intervention is debatable.[283]</li><li>Anti-CCP antibodies are directed toward several native proteins (e.g., filaggrin, fibrinogen, and vimentin) that have become posttranslationally modified by an uncharged citrulline in contrast to the normal positively charged arginine. This "citrullination" is catalyzed by a calcium-dependent enzyme, peptidylarginine deiminase (PAD). These changes in protein charge and sequence make the native protein a target of auto-antibody attack by IgG antibodies in RA.[284] However, this does not necessarily imply that citrullination of native proteins is "the cause" of RA because citrullination of native proteins can also occur *de novo* in inflamed joints, which are then further targeted for inflammatory destruction. Until more information is available, we should withhold final judgment as to the ultimate role and origin of anti-CCP antibodies and in the meanwhile view them as a very strong and sensitive association with RA that facilitates the early diagnosis of this disease.</li></ul>
Advantages:	<ul><li>Anti-CCP antibodies have 98% specificity for RA[285] and is likely to become the future laboratory standard in the diagnosis and prognosis of RA.[286] Anti-CCP antibodies with a positive rheumatoid factor (RF) is termed "composite seropositivity" and appears to be more specific than isolated anti-CCP antibodies or RF.[287]</li></ul>
Limitations:	<ul><li>The best current data indicates that anti-CCP antibodies are sensitive and specific for RA[288], and clinicians should use this test to diagnose and confirm RA.</li></ul>
Comments:	<ul><li>Healthy people do not generally have anti-CCP antibodies. Asymptomatic patients with anti-CCP antibodies are at increased risk for clinical RA and are probably *en route* to the manifestation of clinical autoimmunity—RA, Sjogren's disease, or SLE. *Holistically intervene.*</li><li>I hypothesize that PAD may become upregulated in synovial joints exposed to allergens, xenobiotics, bacterial debris/toxins/lipopolysaccharides and that the subsequent citrullination of joint proteins may lead to an autoimmune arthropathy that persists, perhaps despite removal of the inciting immunogen. More obviously (or perhaps more theoretically), given that PAD is calcium-dependent, it may be upregulated secondary to intracellular hypercalcinosis secondary to vitamin D deficiency, magnesium deficiency, or fatty acid imbalance.[289]</li></ul>

---

[282] "CONCLUSION: An initial 6-month cycle of intensive combination treatment that includes high-dose corticosteroids results in sustained suppression of the rate of radiologic progression in patients with early RA, independent of subsequent antirheumatic therapy." Landewe RB, et al. COBRA combination therapy in patients with early rheumatoid arthritis: long-term structural benefits of a brief intervention. *Arthritis Rheum*. 2002 Feb;46:347-56

[283] "By 5 years patients receiving early DMARDs had similar disease activity and comparable health assessment questionnaire scores to patients who received DMARDs later in their disease course." Scott DL. Evidence for early disease-modifying drugs in rheumatoid arthritis. *Arthritis Res Ther*. 2004;6(1):15-18 arthritis-research.com/content/6/1/15

[284] Hill J, Cairns E, Bell DA. The joy of citrulline. *J Rheumatol*. 2004 Aug;31(8):1471-3 jrheum.com/subscribers/04/08/1471.html

[285] Hill J, Cairns E, Bell DA. The joy of citrulline. *J Rheumatol*. 2004 Aug;31(8):1471-3

[286] "We conclude that, at present, the antibody response directed to citrullinated antigens has the most valuable diagnostic and prognostic potential for RA." van Boekel et al. Autoantibody systems in rheumatoid arthritis: specificity, sensitivity and diagnostic value. *Arthritis Res*. 2002;4(2):87-93 arthritis-research.com/content/4/2/87

[287] "…our findings suggest that a positive anti-CCP antibody result does not necessarily exclude SLE in African American patients presenting with inflammatory arthritis. In such patients, the additional assessment of IgA-RF or IgM-RF isotypes may be of added value since composite seropositivity appears to be nearly exclusive to patients with RA." Mikuls et al. Anti-cyclic citrullinated peptide antibody and rheumatoid factor isotypes in African Americans with early rheumatoid arthritis. *Arthritis Rheum*. 2006 Sep;54:3057-9

[288] "Serum antibodies reactive with citrullinated proteins/peptides are a very sensitive and specific marker for rheumatoid arthritis." Migliorini P, Pratesi F, Tommasi C, Anzilotti C. The immune response to citrullinated antigens in autoimmune diseases. *Autoimmun Rev*. 2005 Nov;4(8):561-4

[289] naturopathydigest.com/archives/2006/sep/vasquez.php

Exemplary case of clinical and laboratory evidence of reversal of "severe, aggressive, drug-resistant" rheumatoid arthritis in a 51yoWF following implementation of the Functional Inflammology Protocol: This summarizes the 13-month clinical outcome of the first patient treated with the updated functional inflammology protocol after its revision and expansion in March 2012.[290] After being diagnosed accurately by a rheumatologist—for this patient very clearly met diagnostic criteria—this patient presented for care following notably inefficacious treatment with the full medicopharmaceutical antirheumatic protocol comprised of NSAIDs, prednisone (she had only minimal response to prednisone >60mg/d), methotrexate, hydroxychloroquine, and "biologics" including etanercept/Enbrel; she was now being recommended to start newer "experimental" drugs. Following the failure of medical treatment, the patient was treated at the teaching clinic of a naturopathic college where her treatments included a clinician-supervised 26-day water-only fast, which resulted in the loss of 30 pounds (13.6 kilograms) but provided no clinical benefit for the rheumatoid arthritis. [Note: I/Dr Vasquez treat this patient at no charge. Dr William J Beakey of Professional Co-Op Services (Professionalco-op.com) generously donated these laboratory tests for collaborative/research purposes. Biotics Research Corporation (BioticsResearch.com) generously donates nutritional supplements for this patient.]

<u>March 2012—severe symptoms and CCP >250</u>: Patient reports suffering significantly with joint pain and lower extremity edema; foundational nutritional protocol[291] is implemented with antidysbiotic/antimicrobial intervention limited to emulsified oregano oil 600mg/d, mitochondrial support and the nutritional immunomodulation protocol. CCP level at this time is beyond laboratory testing limits, measured simply as "greater than" 250 units.

CCP Antibodies IgG/IgA	>250	High	units	0 – 19
			Negative	<20
			Weak positive	20 – 39
			Moderate positive	40 – 59
			Strong positive	>59

<u>January 2013—mild symptoms and CCP 195</u>: Few modifications are made for the first 9 months and patient feels progressively better, but wants to "move to the next level of improvement" because—despite feeling and functioning significantly better solely with dietary and nutritional interventions—patient still notes exacerbations of pain, particularly following extended manual farm labor. At this time, labs are drawn showing an impressive reduction in CCP levels from "greater than" 250 units to 195 units, correlating with a reduction of at least 22%. At this time, patient was commenced on additional treatments including cabergoline, oral vancomycin, and azithromycin.

CCP Antibodies IgG/IgA	195	High	units	0 – 19
			Negative	<20
			Weak positive	20 – 39
			Moderate positive	40 – 59
			Strong positive	>59

<u>April 2013—virtually normal, CCP 54</u>: Patient continues to improve clinically; her subjective and objective clinical improvements (including additional loss of 30 pounds [13.6 kilograms] and reduction in hand swelling necessitating resizing of wedding ring) correlate nicely with the reduction in CCP levels, which have reduced from >250 units to 54 units, for a reduction of more than 78%. Thus, by objective physical and laboratory criteria, this patient appears to be experiencing authentic reversal—cure—of her disease due to the functional inflammology protocol.

CCP Antibodies IgG/IgA	54	High	units	0 – 19
			Negative	<20
			Weak positive	20 – 39
			Moderate positive	40 – 59
			Strong positive	>59

---

[290] Vasquez A. Functional Immunology and Nutritional Immunomodulation. 2012 createspace.com/3899760 and updated as F.I.N.D. S.E.X® The Easily Remembered Acronym for the Functional Inflammology Protocol. 2013 createspace.com/4234627

[291] Vasquez A. Revisiting the Five-Part Nutritional Wellness Protocol: Supplemented Paleo-Mediterranean Diet. *Nutr Perspect* 2011 Jan ichnfm.org/faculty/vasquez/profile.html

HLA-B27: Human leukocyte antigen B-27	
Overview and interpretation:	▪ A common (5-10% of general population) genetic marker strongly associated with seronegative* spondyloarthropathy (all of which occur more commonly in men[292]): • Ankylosing spondylitis (90-95% of 'whites' and 50% of 'blacks')[293] • Reactive arthritis [formerly called Reiter's syndrome] (85%) • Enteropathic spondyloarthropathy • Psoriatic spondylitis (<60%) * Recall that "seronegative" in this context implies that the *rheumatoid factor is negative*, even though *the HLA-B27 may be positive.*
Advantages: *Limitations:* *Comments:*	▪ *From a diagnostic perspective*: The clinical application and significance of this test is of limited value. All of the above-listed conditions are better assessed with the combination of clinical assessment and radiographs. In a patient with early and mild disease, this test may add evidence either supporting or refuting the diagnosis; but the test itself is not diagnostic of anything other than a genetic/histologic marker associated with various types of infection-induced arthropathy and autoimmunity (dysbiotic arthropathy[294]). ▪ *From an integrative/functional medicine perspective*: This test can be of some value if the result is positive and the patient has evidence of a systemic inflammatory/autoimmune disorder since it therefore more strongly suggests that a dysbiotic locus is the cause of disease.[295] A consistent theme in the rheumatology literature is that of "molecular mimicry"—the phenomenon by which structural similarities between human and microbial structures lead to targeting of human tissues by immune responses aimed at microbial antigens. This topic is explored in considerable detail in the section on multifocal dysbiosis in *Integrative Rheumatology*. The important link between microbe-induced autoimmunity and HLA-B27 is that many dysbiotic bacteria produce an HLA-B27-like molecule that appears to trigger an immune response which then erroneously affects human tissues, leading to the clinical picture of autoimmune inflammation. Many of these HLA-B27-producing bacteria colonize the gastrointestinal and genitourinary tracts, promoting musculoskeletal inflammation via molecular mimicry and other mechanisms.[296,297] A strong and growing body of research shows that HLA-B27 is a risk factor for microbe-induced autoimmunity. "Autoimmune" patients positive for HLA-B27 are presumed to have an occult infection—especially gastrointestinal, genitourinary, or sinorespiratory—until proven otherwise. ▪ <u>Keep in mind that HLA-B27 itself is not a "disease"</u> and therefore a "positive" result merely means that the patient has this particular human leukocyte antigen; this test is not and will never be diagnostic of a specific disease—it simply correlates with increased propensity toward dysbiotic arthropathy and suggests the need for dysbiosis testing and the (re)establishment of eubiosis.[298]

[292] "The major diseases associated with HLA-B27 (Reiter's disease, ankylosing spondylitis, acute anterior uveitis, and psoriatic arthritis) all occur much more commonly in men." James WH. Sex ratios and hormones in HLA related rheumatic diseases. *Ann Rheum Dis*. 1991 Jun;50(6):401-4

[293] Shojania K. Rheumatology: 2. What laboratory tests are needed? *CMAJ*. 2000 Apr 18;162(8):1157-63 cmaj.ca/cgi/content/full/162/8/1157

[294] See Chapter 4 of *Integrative Rheumatology* and Vasquez A. Nutritional and Botanical Treatments Against "Silent Infections" and Gastrointestinal Dysbiosis, Commonly Overlooked Causes of Neuromusculoskeletal Inflammation and Chronic Health Problems. *Nutr Perspect* 2006; Jan InflammationMastery.com/reprints

[295] "The association between Klebsiella pneumoniae in AS and Proteus mirabilis in RA." Ebringer et al. HLA molecules, bacteria and autoimmunity. *J Med Microbiol*. 2000 Apr;49:305-11

[296] Inman RD. Antigens, the gastrointestinal tract, and arthritis. *Rheum Dis Clin North Am*. 1991 May;17(2):309-21

[297] Hunter JO. Food allergy--or enterometabolic disorder? *Lancet*. 1991 Aug 24;338(8765):495-6

[298] Dysbiotic arthropathy—joint inflammation and destruction as a result of a neuroimmune inflammatory response to microorganisms. Phrase coined by Alex Vasquez on December 15, 2005. No matching term on Medline or Google search.

Complement levels: CH50, C3, and C4	
Overview and interpretation:	• Complement proteins are consumed in the complement cascades (typically activated by immune complexes) and thus low levels of complement proteins provide indirect evidence of extensive consumption due to immune complex-mediated inflammation. *Low* levels of complement are seen with *increased* disease activity in immune complex disorders (such as SLE, vasculitis, mixed cryoglobulinemia, rheumatoid vasculitis, glomerulonephritis). As expected, low levels of complement are also seen with inherited complement deficiencies; 10%–15% of Caucasian patients with SLE have an inherited complement deficiency.[299] • "CH50" is a screening test for complement levels whereas "C3" and "C4" are more specific for the monitoring of disease activity in autoimmune diseases hallmarked by immune complex deposition, most typically systemic lupus erythematosus (SLE) but also chronic active hepatitis, some chronic infections, poststreptococcal and membranoproliferative glomerulonephritis, and others. Given the wide range of diseases that can cause alterations in complement levels, clinical correlation and differential diagnosis are essential.
Advantages:	• Low complement levels—if not due to genotropic deficiency—provide indirect evidence of immune complex-mediated inflammation. • Elevated levels of complement are seen in conditions of infection or inflammation.
Limitations:	• Some patients have a hereditary absence of complement proteins and thus their levels are always abnormally low; obviously the test cannot be used in these patients for monitoring inflammatory disease.

CIC: Circulating immune complexes	
Overview: 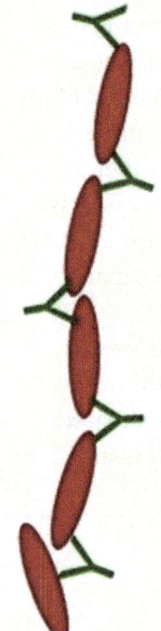	• Antibodies/immunoglobulins are produced in several different "classes": IgG, IgA, IgM, IgE, IgD. IgA antibodies are produced mostly in response to mucosal infections, such as from gastrointestinal dysbiosis or overt infections. When antibodies (in the shape of the letter "Y" with 2 antigen-binding sites on one end and the immuno-reactive site on the other) combine with the target antigen (depicted here in the shape of an oval, such as a bacteria or globular protein), "immune complexes" are formed which are chain-like links of antigens and antibodies. • Although formed in small amounts in healthy persons, in certain disease states, immune complexes may accumulate and initiate complement-dependent injury in various organs and tissues. This activation of complement may begin a series of potentially destructive events in the host, including anaphylatoxin production, cell lysis, leukocyte stimulation, and activation of macrophages and other cells. When immune complexes become fixed to vessel walls, destruction of normal tissue can occur, as in some types of glomerulonephritis and vasculitis. Predisposed to deposition in joints, vessels, and kidneys, immune complexes contribute directly to tissue injury in several autoimmune-inflammatory diseases.[300] **Immune Complexes, (Raji Cell), Quantitative** Reference Range: (Enzyme immunoassay [EIA]; cost $130) • Normal: ≤ 15.0 µg Eq/mL • Equivocal: 15.1-19.9 µg Eq/mL • **Positive: ≥20.0 µg Eq/mL**
Advantages:	• This test allows for direct quantification of immune-complex production.
Limitations:	• This test has only recently become available to practicing clinicians; however, it is very well supported by many publications in peer-reviewed research.[301]

[299] Shojania K. Rheumatology: 2. What laboratory tests are needed? *CMAJ*. 2000 Apr 18;162(8):1157-63 cmaj.ca/cgi/content/full/162/8/1157
[300] Jancar S, Sánchez Crespo M. Immune complex-mediated tissue injury: a multistep paradigm. *Trends Immunol*. 2005 Jan;26(1):48-55
[301] Davies KA,etal. Immune complex processing in patients with systemic lupus erythematosus. *J Clin Invest* 1992;90:2075-83 jci.org/articles/view/116090

Other tests for autoimmunity and immune dysfunction

Overview and interpretation:	▪ The table below is a quick reference guide to additional clinical disorders and *additional* laboratory tests; diagnostic criteria and lab tests change from time to time. Evaluation should always include history, physical exam, and basic labs such as CBC, UA, and chemistry panel.

Disease	Laboratory (or other) assessment
Autoimmune thyroid disease	• Anti(TPO) thyroid peroxidase antibodies: Hashimoto's thyroiditis • Antithyroglobulin antibodies: Hashimoto's thyroiditis • Thyroid stimulating immunoglobulins (TSI, 78%) and thyrotropin receptor antibodies (90%) are noted in Grave's disease
Latent autoimmune diabetes in adults (LADA), diabetes mellitus type 1.5	• Islet cell antibodies (ICA, also known as antipancreatic islet antibodies) and glutamic acid decarboxylase (GAD) antibodies • LADA/DM1.5 accounts for roughly 10 percent of cases of adult diabetes mellitus; has characteristics of type-1 (autoantibodies) and type-2 (insulin resistance); progresses to insulin-dependence within 6 years of diagnosis; assess beta-cell failure with C-peptide • Consider also tyrosine phosphatase (IA2) antibodies—positive in DM type-1 if this diagnosis is suspected
Autoimmune hepatitis	• Serum antinuclear antibodies (ANA) • Anti–smooth muscle antibodies (SMA) • Liver-kidney microsomal (type-1 [LKM-1]) antibodies • Anti–liver cytosol-1 (anti-LC1) antibodies • Consider also serum protein electrophoresis (SPEP) and quantitative immunoglobulin analysis; confirm with biopsy
Primary sclerosing cholangitis (PSC)	• ANA (53%), (p)ANCA (87%), anticardiolipin (66%) and anti-smooth muscle antibodies • Imaging of the bile duct, usually endoscopic retrograde cholangiopancreatography (ERCP)
Primary biliary cirrhosis (PBC)	• Anti-mitochondrial antibodies (AMA): 93% sensitivity, 98% specificity • ANA: positive in 20-50% of PBC patients • Imaging and biopsy; consider autoimmune cholangitis
Celiac disease	• IgA Anti-tissue Transglutaminase antibodies (anti-tTG) • IgG and IgA Anti-Gliadin antibodies (AGA) • IgA Deamidated Gliadin Peptide (DGP) antibodies • Quantitative immunoglobulin A (IgA)—performed to exclude selective sIgA deficiency, one of the most common immune deficiency disorders • > 95% of celiac patients have HLA-DQ2 or HLA-DQ8
Inflammatory bowel disease (IBD)	• IgA and IgG antibodies for *Saccharomyces cerevisiae*—nearly 80% of Crohn's disease patients are positive for either IgA or IgG. "In ulcerative colitis, <15% are positive for IgG, and <2% are positive for IgA. Fewer than 5% of healthy controls are positive for either IgG or IgA antibody, and no healthy controls had antibody for both."[302] • "Atypical ANCA"—positive in a significant percentage of patients with ulcerative colitis, primary sclerosing cholangitis, autoimmune hepatitis • P-ANCA antibodies—"found in 50-70% of ulcerative colitis (UC) patients, but in only 20% of Crohn disease (CD) patients"[303]
Antiphospholipid/ anticardiolipin/ Hughes syndrome	• IgA, IgG, IgM cardiolipin antibody and IgG, IgM (preferably with IgA) Beta-2 glycoprotein-I antibodies; lupus anticoagulant(s) • Clinical correlation is essential to determine significance

Advantages:	▪ Labs always provide additional data, some of which may be diagnostic.
Limitations:	▪ Laboratory data must be interpreted within a clinical context in order to properly inform clinical decision-making, diagnostic criteria, and therapeutic intervention.

[302] Inflammatory Bowel Disease (IBD) Profile. https://labcorp.com   March 2013
[303] Inflammatory Bowel Disease Differentiation Profile. aruplab.com/guides/ug/tests/0050567.jsp March 2013

Testing for Occult Infections and Dysbiosis—A Practical Introduction and Clinical Approach

Conceptual overview, advantages and limitations:	▪ With the publication of my *Integrative Rheumatology* textbook in 2006/2007, I was the first to promote the ideas that patients with systemic inflammation in general and autoimmunity in particular ***always*** have occult "infections" or microbial colonization—dysbiosis—and that this dysbiotic foci is general not singular, nor due to only one offending microbe; rather, inflammatory dysbiosis tends to be multifocal and polymicrobial—what I have termed "multifocal polydysbiosis." In the ensuing years, additional research has consistently proven this model to be correct. I have further defined dysbiosis as "a relationship of non-acute host-microorganism interaction that adversely affects the human host", and I have more recently subdivided the general effects of dysbiosis on the human host as either inflammatory/immunogenic ("inflammatory dysbiosis") or metabolic ("metabolic dysbiosis") although overlap clearly exists.

> **DrV's dysbiosis terminology**
>
> **Dysbiosis**: A relationship of non-acute non-infectious host-microorganism interaction that adversely affects the human host.
>
> Dysbiosis subtypes (based on location):
> 1. Orodental
> 2. Sinorespiratory
> 3. Gastrointestinal
> 4. Parenchymal, Tissue
> 5. Genitourinary
> 6. Cutaneous
> 7. Environmental
> 8. Microbial
>
> **Multifocal dysbiosis**: A clinical condition characterized by a patient's having more than one foci/location of dysbiosis; generally the adverse physiologic and clinical consequences are additive and synergistic.
>
> **Polydysbiosis**: Concurrent dysbiosis with several different microbes
>
> **Main treatment approaches for dysbiosis**: ❶ antimicrobial, ❷ immunorestorative, ❸ tolerogenic via nutritional immunomodulation

■ Microbial colonization is *necessary but not sufficient* for the existence of the host-microbe relationship that characterizes dysbiosis; the host must be susceptible to the effects of the microbes, and the hosts defense system must be sufficiently impaired to allow the microbial biomass to become qualitatively sufficient (and diverse) to surpass the host's threshold of immunologic and metabolic tolerance. Nevertheless, despite the tripartite requirements for the establishment of dysbiotic inflammation—microbes, immunoincompetence, and intolerance—the fact remains clear that dysbiosis requires microbes. Equally clear is the fact that microbes alone are insufficient for dysbiotic inflammation.

■ One of the first questions that arises for clinicians that of choosing methodology for the detection of the offending microbe(s). Briefly, the quest for the identification of the offending microbe(s) is simultaneously wise and sophomoric (soph-, "wise," and moros, "fool"). This approach is wise because the quest for identification and thereafter targeted eradication of the offending microbe is intellectually "clean", clinically efficient, and—most legitimately—allows for precise use of antimicrobial therapy; in reality, this approach is based on numerous erroneous presuppositions including:

   • Presumed physiologic reliability: A common error is that of using antibody assays for the detection of current "infections", especially of the dysbiotic type. Antigen detection is preferable to antibody measurement, given that antibodies may be present even when an infection is presently absent, and that infection/colonization may be present even when antibodies are absent.

   • Presumed equivalence of tests for acute infections and tests for chronic dysbiotic colonizations: Another common error is that of using testing methods developed for the detection of acute infections (e.g., the rapid strep test for acute [extracellular] streptococcal pharyngitis) when seeking to detect dysbiotic infections (e.g., chronic [intracellular] streptococcal pharyngeal colonization of psoriasis).

      • Concept: Microbial phenotype varies per type and chronicity of infection/colonization (*Clinical and Experimental Immunology* 2004 Jan[304]):

---

[304] Gudjonsson JE, Johnston A, Sigmundsdottir H, Valdimarsson H. Immunopathogenic mechanisms in psoriasis. *Clin Exp Immunol*. 2004 Jan;135(1):1-8

"Although streptococci have traditionally been viewed as *extracellular* pathogens, they are able to *invade several eukaryotic cell types* [i.e., manifest an intracellular phenotype] including squamous epithelium and macrophages, and this has been associated with persistent streptococcal carriage and recurrent infections."

- Presumed performance reliability: Culture-based methodology is notoriously insensitive for anaerobic bacteria, and it is impractical for the detection and identification of complex microbial quorums and biosystems. DNA-based tests exist as numerous methodologies—many of which are patented for research use and are therefore not commercially available; DNA-based testing is impractical for the detection and identification of complex microbial quorums and biosystems with thousands of different microbes.

- Presumed stability of identity of microbes: Microbes have historically been presumed to have stable identities and microbe-disease associations; what we now know is that microbes readily exchange genetic material and that microbial phenotype and metabolic and inflammatory/immunogenic properties can change for example in response to the host's diet or psychoemotional state (the latter described as the study of "microbial endocrinology"[305]).

  - Concept: The emerging irrelevance of microbial identification (*Autoimmune Reviews* 2009 Jul[306]): "These [human-colonizing] bacteria rapidly and frequently share their DNA with their fellow species – even distantly related species – through horizontal gene transfer. … Some argue that the number of microbes created through genetic recombination is so high that the concept of distinct bacterial species may become obsolete."

- Identification and eradication of a singular offending microbe is noted in the research literature and in clinical practice to occasionally produce brilliant and stunning clinical responses; more commonly—and even more powerfully supported by major trends in the research literature—what we find is a positive clinical response to the combination of ❶ nonspecific antimicrobial therapy (e.g., drugs or botanicals, often and preferably both synthetic and natural agents at the same time), ❷ immunorestorative interventions such as stress reduction and immunonutrition, and ❸ nutritional immunomodulation (detailed in my protocol) to induce immunotolerance. Therefore, the expense and pursuit of identifying the offending microbe(s) is not necessary for a therapeutic response; indeed, the expense and pursuit of identifying the offending microbe(s) may actually deter or delay implementation of effective therapy. However—and finally, the use of testing to determine the presence and persistence of dysbiotic microbial infections/colonizations is occasionally helpful to direct antimicrobial drug therapy especially when more dangerous antimicrobial agents are being employed and/or when previous empiric approaches have not been useful; clinicians can use these and other tests with consideration of the discussion provided above and the more extended discussion in Chapter 4 of *Integrative Rheumatology / Inflammation Mastery*. For the sake of organization, this author's more common test considerations will be listed here by location, with the appreciation that the concept of location is itself somewhat misleading, given that microbes may apparently affect/infect one location (e.g., herpes simplex virus infection of the oral mucosa and associated cranial nerve body) while occultly affecting/infecting a distant location (e.g., the hippocampus).[307]

[305] Freestone PP, Sandrini SM, Haigh RD, Lyte M. Microbial endocrinology: how stress influences susceptibility to infection. *Trends Microbiol*. 2008 Feb;16(2):55-64

[306] Proal AD, Albert PJ, Marshall T. Autoimmune disease in the era of the metagenome. *Autoimmun Rev*. 2009 Jul;8(8):677-81

[307] "HSV-1, for example, can infect oral and nasal mucosa and then travels through retrograde axonal transport to the trigeminal ganglion or the olfactory bulb, respectively, where it establishes a latent infection or may rapidly enter the CNS. … Periodic reactivations from latency are followed by axonal transport of newly produced HSV-1 virions either back to the site of primary infection, where they cause new skin vesicles or mucosal ulcers, or onward to the CNS, where they can cause a productive, but usually mild infection, which may later become latent, as described for rodents. In particular, newly produced virions may target the limbic system, which includes the hippocampus, thalamus and amygdala." De Chiara G, Marcocci ME, Sgarbanti R, et al. Infectious agents and neurodegeneration. *Mol Neurobiol*. 2012 Dec;46(3):614-38

Laboratory tests per location of dysbiotic microbial colonization:	▪ Per the above discussion and context, some of the more common and/or more useful laboratory tests are listed here; these are listed per location for organizational purposes only, with the full appreciation that the location itself is mostly irrelevant, with the possible exception of the gastrointestinal tract which harbors the greatest quantity and diversity of microbes and which harbors these microbes in intimate contact with the bulk of the human immune system—the gut-associated lymphoid tissue (GALT) possesses the largest mass of lymphoid tissue in the human body. In sum, testing for microbes provides either direct and specific evidence of microbes or indirect evidence (both with varying levels of sensitivity), or—at the opposite extreme—empiric evidence (i.e., monitoring response to antimicrobial or immunorestorative interventions) which is completely nonspecific yet much more clinically meaningful. ❶ Direct testing—culture/DNA/antigen: Swab for culture and sensitivity (C-S), DNA-based testing such as polymerase chain reaction (PCR), or antigen detection, ❷ Indirect testing—most commonly antibody assays: Various antibody tests against microbes are available and clinically meaningful, ❸ Empiric testing: Monitoring response to therapeutic-diagnostic intervention with antimicrobial therapy.
	
	Introduction to "dysbiosis by location"—essential for understanding and treating multifocal polydysbiosis as detailed in Chapter 4:
	
	▪ **Orodental dysbiosis/colonization—introduction to assessment**:
	   ❶ Direct testing—culture/DNA/antigen: Swabs of mucosa, gingiva, teeth, and dentures can be used for culture, DNA, and antigen testing.
	   ❷ Indirect testing—antibody assays: Antibody titers specific for oral/dental/periodontal microbes correlate with numerous inflammatory disorders, ranging from insulin resistance to rheumatoid arthritis (RA).
	   ❸ Empiric observation: Oral exam may reveal tooth and gum disease. *Example*—rheumatoid arthritis: "Control of periodontal infection and gingival inflammation by scaling/root planing and plaque control in subjects with periodontal disease may reduce the severity of RA."[308]
	▪ **Sinorespiratory dysbiosis/colonization—introduction to assessment**:
	   ❶ Direct testing—culture/DNA/antigen: Swabs of nasal and pharyngeal mucosa can be used for culture, DNA, and antigen testing. Sputum can be submitted for culture and direct microscopic analysis. *Example*—atopic dermatitis: In eczema, skin cultures yielded *Staphylococcus aureus* from lesional skin in 87.1% of patients and from the nares in 80.6% of patients.
	   ❷ Indirect testing—antibody assays: Antibody titers specific for respiratory microbes correlate with numerous inflammatory disorders, ranging from cardiovascular disease to oligoarthritis.
	   ❸ Empiric observation: *Example*—ANCA (previously Wegener's) granulomatosis/vasculitis: Treatment with trimethoprim-sulfamethoxazole (co-trimoxazole, a broad-spectrum antibiotic) reduces the incidence of relapses in patients with Wegener's granulomatosis in remission.[309,310]
	▪ **Gastrointestinal dysbiosis/colonization—introduction to assessment**:
	   ❶ Direct testing—culture/DNA/antigen: Jejunal aspiration is the gold standard for diagnosis of SIBO—small intestinal bacterial overgrowth; similarly, aspiration with or without biopsy followed by direct microscopy or culture is generally the gold standard for the identification of most infections. Stool tests are available using culture, DNA, and antigen-detecting methodology; routine pathogens such as *Salmonella, Shigella, Campylobacter*, and enterohemorrhagic *E coli* (EHEC) can be

---

308 Al-Katma MK, Bissada NF, Bordeaux JM, et al. Control of periodontal infection reduces the severity of active rheumatoid arthritis. *J Clin Rheumatol*. 2007 Jun;13(3):134-7
309 Zycinska K, et al. Co-trimoxazole and prevention of relapses of PR3-ANCA positive vasculitis with pulmonary involvement. *Eur J Med Res*. 2009 Dec 7;14 Suppl 4:265-7
310 Stegeman CA, et al. Trimethoprim-sulfamethoxazole (co-trimoxazole) for the prevention of relapses of Wegener's granulomatosis. *N Engl J Med*. 1996 Jul 4;335(1):16-20

detected by routine (i.e., standard, hospital-based) medical reference laboratories. When testing for dysbiotic-type colonizations, clinicians should utilize a specialty laboratory that presents the results within a context of additional markers for clinical decision-making as discussed in a following section on stool testing.

❷ Indirect testing—antibody assays, lactulose:mannitol assay, inflammatory markers, sIgA, breath hydrogen and methane: Antibody assays specific for gastrointestinal yeast, bacteria, and protozoans are available. In specific situations, very indirect testing such as the lactulose:mannitol assay can be used to determine increased intestinal permeability which can provide indirect evidence of intestinal dysbiosis; likewise, inflammatory markers such as calprotectin, lactoferrin, and lysozyme can also indicate intestinal inflammation which is commonly caused by intestinal microbial overgrowth/colonization. Secretory IgA is also measured in fecal samples and can be interpreted in clinical context; elevated levels suggest immunologic response to intraluminal antigens, the most offensive of which are microbial/dysbiotic. Exhaled hydrogen and methane can be measured following a carbohydrate challenge to assess for nonspecific SIBO. *Example*—fibromyalgia: "3/15 (20%) controls had an abnormal breath test compared with 93/111 (84%) subjects with IBS (p<0.01) and 42/42 (100%) with fibromyalgia (p<0.0001 v controls, p<0.05 v IBS). … The degree of somatic pain in fibromyalgia correlated significantly with the hydrogen level seen on the breath test. An abnormal lactulose breath test is more common in fibromyalgia than IBS. In contrast with IBS, the degree of abnormality on breath test is greater in subjects with fibromyalgia and correlates with somatic pain."[311]

❸ Empiric observation: Response to antimicrobial therapy confirms intestinal microbial overgrowth/dysbiosis/parasitosis; the retrospective diagnosis is made most clearly with observation of a positive clinical response following treatment with orally-administered nonabsorbed antimicrobial agents, such as oregano oil, berberine, nystatin, rifaximin, and vancomycin. *Example*—empiric diagnosis and treatment of small intestinal bacterial overgrowth: "For cases in which a firm diagnosis cannot be made, but clinical symptoms favor SIBO, empirical antibiotic use may be a more cautious approach to prevent delay of treatment and to prevent increases in symptom severity."[312]

- ==Genitourinary dysbiosis/colonization—introduction to assessment==:
  ❶ Direct testing—culture/DNA/antigen: Reactive/inflammatory arthritis secondary to genitourinary infection is well known, formerly called Reiter's syndrome; a similar association is established in chronic oligoarthritis. *Example*—reactive arthritis: "Urogenital swab cultures showed a microbial infection in 44% of the patients with oligoarthritis (15% *Chlamydia*, 14% *Mycoplasma*, 28% *Ureaplasma*), whereas in the control group only 26% had a positive result (4% *Chlamydia*, 7% *Mycoplasma*, 21% *Ureaplasma*) (P < 0.001). … Urogenital swab culture is the only useful diagnostic method for the detection of the arthritogenic infection in extra-articularly asymptomatic patients with undifferentiated oligoarthritis."[313]
  ❷ Indirect testing—antibody assays: Antibody assays specific for genitourinary microbes are available. *Example*—oligoarthritis: "A Chlamydia IgG-antibody titer > or = 1:256 was found in 22% of the patients in the oligoarthritis group and in 9% of

[311] Pimentel M, Wallace D, Hallegua D, Chow E, Kong Y, Park S, Lin HC. A link between irritable bowel syndrome and fibromyalgia may be related to findings on lactulose breath testing. *Ann Rheum Dis*. 2004 Apr;63(4):450-2

[312] Malik BA, Xie YY, Wine E, Huynh HQ. Diagnosis and pharmacological management of small intestinal bacterial overgrowth in childrenwith intestinal failure. *Can J Gastroenterol*. 2011 Jan;25(1):41-5. This is a very excellent article—highly recommended.

[313] Erlacher L, Wintersberger W, Menschik M, et al. Reactive arthritis: urogenital swab culture is the only useful diagnostic method for the detection of the arthritogenic infection in extra-articularly asymptomatic patients with undifferentiated oligoarthritis. *Br J Rheumatol*. 1995 Sep;34(9):838-42

the controls (P < 0.01). However, for only half of *Chlamydia* IgG-positive patients could a *Chlamydia* infection be confirmed by urogenital swab culture."[314]

❸ Empiric observation: Response to antimicrobial and immunorestorative interventions. *Example*—rheumatoid arthritis: "We propose that sub-clinical *Proteus* urinary tract infections are the main triggering factors and that the presence of molecular mimicry and cross-reactivity between these bacteria and RA-targeted tissue antigens assists in the perpetuation of the disease process through production of cytopathic auto-antibodies. Patients with RA especially during the early stages of the disease could benefit from *Proteus* anti-bacterial measures involving the use of antibiotics, vegetarian diets and high intake of water and fruit juices such as cranberry juice in addition to the currently employed treatments."[315]

- **Cutaneous dysbiosis/colonization—introduction to assessment**:
  ❶ Direct testing—culture/DNA/antigen: For bacterial infections/colonizations, culture and DNA methods can be used; for fungi, skin scraping followed by KOH wet-mount and microscopic examination is commonly used. *Example*—atopic dermatitis: In eczema, skin cultures yielded *Staphylococcus aureus* from lesional skin in 87.1% of patients and from the nares in 80.6% of patients.[316]
  ❷ Indirect testing—antibody assays: Antibodies to dermal microbes can be measured. *Example*—atopic dermatitis: Eczema patients commonly have serum IgE antibodies specific for *Malassezia sympodialis, Candida albicans*, and *Staphylococcus aureus*, and these antibody levels correlate with disease severity.[317]
  ❸ Empiric observation: *Example*—atopic dermatitis: "Patients with AD can have sudden exacerbations of AD attributable to overgrowth of *S aureus* that can be independent of true secondary bacterial infection, a notion supported by the clinical response of patients with severe AD to anti-staphylococcal antibiotics [*Dr Vasquez*: and other antimicrobial measures]."

- **Environmental dysbiosis/colonization—introduction to assessment**:
  ❶ Direct testing—culture/DNA/antigen: Home, work, and recreational environments can be surveyed for microbial contamination, particularly mold. Pier-and-beam homes should be inspected for mold and water in the crawlspace; likewise, attics should be inspected for occult leaks and mold. Mold plates, Petri dishes, and filter cartridges can be used to identify airborne microbes. *Fusarium, Trichoderma*, and *Stachybotrys* produce mycotoxins.[318]
  ❷ Indirect testing—antibody assays: Tests can be performed for evidence of microbial exposure and immune response (e.g., antibodies specific for microbes); correlative tests can also be performed to assess the clinical and immunological significance of the exposure (e.g., RF, ANA, CCP, and other autoantibodies). *Example*—inflammatory disease associated with working/living in moisture-damaged building: *Chlamydophila pneumoniae* antibodies may be elevated in correlation with clinical symptoms and environmental exposure to microbes.[319] *Example*—biochemical changes noted in persons exposed to microbial contamination: An article co-authored by Vojdani[320] noted, "biochemical abnormal concentrations in

[314] Erlacher L, Wintersberger W, Menschik M, et al. Reactive arthritis: urogenital swab culture is the only useful diagnostic method for the detection of the arthritogenic infection in extra-articularly asymptomatic patients with undifferentiated oligoarthritis. *Br J Rheumatol*. 1995 Sep;34(9):838-42

[315] Ebringer A, Rashid T. Rheumatoid arthritis is an autoimmune disease triggered by Proteus urinary tract infection. *Clin Dev Immunol*. 2006 Mar;13(1):41-8

[316] Huang JT, Abrams M, Tlougan B, Rademaker A, Paller AS. Treatment of Staphylococcus aureus colonization in atopic dermatitis decreases disease severity. *Pediatrics*. 2009 May;123(5):e808-14

[317] Sonesson A, Bartosik J, Christiansen J, et al. Sensitization to Skin-associated Microorganisms in Adult Patients with Atopic Dermatitis is of Importance for Disease Severity. *Acta Derm Venereol*. 2012 Oct 16. doi: 10.2340/00015555-1465. medicaljournals.se/acta/content/?doi=10.2340/00015555-1465

[318] Am Acad Pediatrics. Toxic effects of indoor molds. Committee on Environ Health. *Pediatrics* 1998;101(4 Pt1):712-4 aappolicy.aappublications.org/cgi/content/full/pediatrics;101/4/712

[319] Seuri M, Paldanius M, Leinonen M, Roponen M, Hirvonen MR, Saikku P. Chlamydophila pneumoniae antibodies in office workers with and without inflammatory rheumatic diseases in a moisture-damaged building. *Eur J Clin Microbiol Infect Dis*. 2005 Mar;24(3):236-7

[320] Anyanwu E, Campbell AW, Vojdani A, Ehiri JE, Akpan AI. Biochemical changes in the serum of patients with chronic toxigenic mold exposures: a risk factor for multiple renal dysfunctions. *ScientificWorldJournal*. 2003 Nov 3;3:1058-64

creatinine, uric acid, phosphorus, alkaline phosphatase, cholesterol, LDH [*Dr Vasquez*: LDH here is corrected from "HDH" per data in Table 1 of the full-text article], SGOT/AST, segmented neutrophils, lymphocytes, total T3, IgG and IgA immunoglobulins with significant differences between patients and controls."; the authors note an increased prevalence of renal disorders among such patients. *Example*—increased serum autoantibodies in patients exposed to environmental molds: "Abnormally high levels of ANA, ASM, and CNS myelin (immunoglobulins [Ig]G, IgM, IgA) and PNS myelin (IgG, IgM, IgA) were found; odds ratios for each were significant at 95% confidence intervals, showing an increased risk for autoimmunity."[321] *Example*—elevated mold counts, and elevations of non-IgE antibodies in mold-exposed persons: "Detection of high levels (colony-forming units per cubic meter) of molds—which, in this study, strongly suggested that there existed a reservoir of spores in the building at the time of sampling—along with a significant elevation in IgG, IgM, or IgA antibodies against molds and mycotoxins, could be used in future epidemiologic investigations of fungal exposure. In addition to IgE, measurements of IgG, IgM, and IgA antibodies should be considered in mold-exposed individuals."

❸ Empiric observation: Alleviation of clinical symptoms and signs following building evacuation or remediation substantiates the exposure-immunopathology link.

- <mark>Parenchymal dysbiosis/colonization—introduction to assessment</mark>: Many different "internal" infections/colonizations can contribute to chronic inflammatory disease and—at its most extreme—autoimmunity. Some of these situations are perhaps best described/characterized as true "infections" such as noted with hepatitis C infection contributing to immune-complex-mediated dermatitis and arthritis; infection in this context is noted to have the classic pathologic manifestations of histologic observability and tissue damage (e.g., viral hepatitis and cirrhosis). In other situations, the microbe is neither consistently observable in tissue nor does microbe-induced tissue damage characterize the clinical condition; these situations are perhaps better defined as "parenchymal dysbiosis"—a state of microbe-induced inflammation lacking the classic pathological findings of histologic observability and microbe-induced tissue damage. An example of the latter includes chronic systemic inflammation and—occasionally—inflammatory arthritis (but not septic arthritis) triggered by *Chlamydia/Chlamydophila pneumoniae*. See the following tables for microbe-specific assessments and disease associations.

  ❶ Direct testing—culture/DNA/antigen: *Example*—hepatitis C: Hepatitis C virus RNA detected by quantitative or qualitative PCR.

  ❷ Indirect testing—antibody assays: *Example*—chronic fatigue, chronic oligoarthritis: IgG antibodies specific for *Chlamydia/Chlamydophila pneumonia*.

  ❸ Empiric observation: *Example*—psoriasis: Beneficial response to empiric antimicrobial treatment with penicillin[322] or azithromycin[323] confirms the microbial basis of the disease.

[321] Gray MR, Thrasher JD, Crago R, Madison RA, Arnold L, Campbell AW, Vojdani A. Mixed mold mycotoxicosis: immunological changes in humans following exposure in water-damaged buildings. *Arch Environ Health*. 2003 Jul;58(7):410-20
[322] Saxena VN, Dogra J. Long-term use of penicillin for the treatment of chronic plaque psoriasis. *Eur J Dermatol*. 2005 Sep-Oct;15(5):359-62
[323] Saxena VN, Dogra J. Long-term oral azithromycin in chronic plaque psoriasis: a controlled trial. *Eur J Dermatol*. 2010 May-Jun;20(3):329-33

Parenchymal/internal/occult dysbiotic microbes and/or occult infections that can contribute to chronic inflammation, metabolic impairment, or autoimmunity

Viruses	Laboratory assessment	Disease association(s)
Cytomegalovirus (CMV)	IgM antibodies may not peak until 4-7 weeks after onset; IgG antibodies increase by 4x during acute infection; in immunosuppressed patients, PCR and antigen testing is preferred over antibody testing	Fatigue, mononucleosis-like illness, retinopathy in immunosuppressed
Epstein-Barr virus (EBV)	IgG and IgM antibodies to viral antigens are specific and include EBV-early antigen (EA) IgG, EBV-viral capsid antigen (VCA) IgG; EBV-VCA IgM; Epstein-Barr nuclear antigen antibodies (EBNA); IgG titers >1:640 appear to correlate with increased fatigue and clinical response to antiviral treatment in patients with chronic fatigue syndrome[324]	Fatigue, chronic fatigue syndrome, mononucleosis
Hepatitis B virus (HepB, HBV)	HepB surface antigen and DNA are most specific	Liver disease, immune complex (IC)-mediated vasculitis and arthritis
Hepatitis C virus (HepC, HCV)	HCV RNA becomes positive 1-3 weeks postexposure	Liver disease, immune complex (IC)-mediated vasculitis and arthritis
Human herpes virus type-6 (HHV-6)	IgG antibody titers >1:320 correlate with increased fatigue and clinical response to antiviral treatment in patients with chronic fatigue syndrome[325]; IgM and viral DNA levels are elevated in patients with multiple sclerosis[326]	Fatigue, chronic fatigue syndrome, multiple sclerosis
Human immunodeficiency virus (HIV)	Typical protocol is ELISA antibody testing (and/or Western blot) followed by PCR for viral load; for acute infection (prior to [antibody] seroconversion) and severe immunosuppression, DNA-based testing is preferred	Fatigue, peripheral neuropathy, opportunistic infections, severe acute psoriasis
Herpes simplex virus types 1 and 2 (HSV1, HSV2)	Measured by chemiluminescence (CI) or enzyme immunoassay (EIA), IgG antibody titers correlate with exposure/infection and level of viral replication (i.e., higher titers indicate higher viral replication); Western blot methodology is considered the epidemiologic gold standard[327] but IgG measurements by CI/EIA are clinically very reliable and are more widely available.	Fatigue, acute encephalitis, Alzheimer's disease, multiple sclerosis

---

[324] "Nine out of 12 (75%) patients experienced near resolution of their symptoms, allowing them all to return to the workforce or full time activities. In the nine patients with a symptomatic response to treatment, EBV VCA IgG titers dropped from 1:2560 to 1:640 (p = 0.008) and HHV-6 IgG titers dropped from a median value of 1:1280 to 1:320 (p = 0.271)." Kogelnik AM, Loomis K, Hoegh-Petersen M, et al. Use of valganciclovir in patients with elevated antibody titers against Human Herpesvirus-6 (HHV-6) and Epstein-Barr Virus (EBV) who were experiencing central nervous system dysfunction including long-standing fatigue. *J Clin Virol*. 2006 Dec;37 Suppl 1:S33-8

[325] "Nine out of 12 (75%) patients experienced near resolution of their symptoms, allowing them all to return to the workforce or full time activites. In the nine patients with a symptomatic response to treatment, EBV VCA IgG titers dropped from 1:2560 to 1:640 (p = 0.008) and HHV-6 IgG titers dropped from a median value of 1:1280 to 1:320 (p = 0.271)." Kogelnik AM, Loomis K, Hoegh-Petersen M, et al. Use of valganciclovir in patients with elevated antibody titers against Human Herpesvirus-6 (HHV-6) and Epstein-Barr Virus (EBV) who were experiencing central nervous system dysfunction including long-standing fatigue. *J Clin Virol*. 2006 Dec;37 Suppl 1:S33-8

[326] "Results demonstrate increased levels of anti-HHV6-IgG (78.2% versus 76.4% in controls; P = NS), and IgM (34.6% versus 6.5% in controls; P < 0.05) in MS patients. ... Moreover, load of cell-free viral DNA was higher in RRMS and SPMS patients and detected in 60.2% (47/78) of MS patients, compared with 14.6% (18/123) of healthy controls (P < 0.001)." Ramroodi N, Sanadgol N, Ganjali Z, Niazi AA, Sarabandi V, Moghtaderi A. Monitoring of active human herpes virus 6 infection in Iranian patients with different subtypes of multiple sclerosis. *J Pathog*. 2013;2013:194932

[327] Accessed in March 2013. "The Western Blot, the most accurate of these blood tests, is done at the University of Washington." depts.washington.edu/herpes/faq.php#faqCat-3. "The Western blot assay is the most validated method for identifying type-specific antibodies and is considered the gold standard. ... The Western blot assay is conducted exclusively at the University of Washington where clinical specimens can be sent and processed. Two type-specific glycoprotein G serological tests are commercially available in the United States. Sensitivity and specificity of these tests are comparable to the Western blot assay. These tests cost $10 to $40 (U.S. dollars)." uspreventiveservicestaskforce.org/uspstf05/herpes/herpesup.htm

Parenchymal/internal/occult dysbiotic microbes and/or occult infections that can contribute to chronic inflammation, metabolic impairment, or autoimmunity—*continued*

Viruses—continued	Laboratory assessment	Disease association(s)
Parvovirus B19	IgG and IgM antibodies are commonly used; however, "high-level viremia in acutely infected persons may cause virus-antibody complexes, which will result in a false-negative IgM test result. In this setting, polymerase chain reaction (PCR) may be a better diagnostic modality."[328]	Arthritis/arthralgia, which can mimic rheumatoid arthritis[329]

Bacteria, protozoa, etc.	Assessment	Disease association(s)
Infectious agents well-known to cause reactive/inflammatory arthritis: *Chlamydia trachomatis* and various species in the genera *Salmonella, Shigella, Campylobacter,* and *Yersinia*	Direct microscopy, culture, DNA-based testing; antibody testing is less commonly used for these acute and subacute infections; empiric antimicrobial treatment without laboratory testing is reasonable with a compelling clinical picture of infection and associated inflammopathy/arthropathy	Reactive arthritis, chronic arthritis, autoimmune thyroiditis (especially *Yersinia*, in which case anti-*Yersinia* antibodies are strongly correlated with thyroid disease[330])
Borrelia burgdorferi, Babesia species including *microti, divergens,* MO1, *duncani* (WA-1)	IgG and IgM antibodies, Western blot, PCR; many experienced clinicians prefer IGeneX testing; much controversy exists about the "best" testing method(s)	Fatigue, Lyme disease (erythema chronicum migrans, myocarditis, arthritis, meningitis, neuropathies)
Chlamydia/Chlamydophila pneumoniae	IgG titers > 1:64 correlate with chronic/persistent infection/colonization[331]; likewise, IgA titers > 1:20 correlate with chronic/persistent infection/colonization; IgA positivity and/or PCR positivity correlate with myocardial infarction[332]; as expected PCR is considered best evidence of current active infection, since antibody levels do not always correlate with active infection whereas nuclear material is rapidly degraded by human restriction endonucleases and therefore when present provides clear proof of current infection/colonization	Chronic fatigue, chronic inflammatory arthritis (responds to prolonged combination therapy with azithromycin and rifampin[333]), multiple sclerosis[334], myocardial infarction

---

[328] Cennimo DJ, Steele RW. Parvovirus B19 Infection Workup. emedicine.medscape.com/article/961063-workup Accessed March 2013

[329] Sabella C, Goldfarb J. Parvovirus B19 infections. *Am Fam Physician.* 1999 Oct 1;60(5):1455-60

[330] "In contrast to the low prevalence of antibodies in controls (less than 8%), 48 of 67 patients (75%) with a variety of thyroid disorders had titers greater than 1:8. Antibodies were found in 24 of 36 patients with Graves' disease, five of six with autonomous adenoma, seven of seven with Hashimoto's thyroiditis, three of five with idiopathic primary hypothyroidism, four of 11 with nontoxic nodular goiter, and one of two with thyroid carcinoma." Shenkman L, Bottone EJ. Antibodies to Yersinia enterocolitica in thyroid disease. *Ann Intern Med.* 1976 Dec;85(6):735-9

[331] "Because there is as yet no standardisation of serological criteria for persistent infection, we considered antibody titres of > 1/20 in the IgA fraction, together with IgG titres of 1/64 to 1/256, to be indicative of persistent infection." Ben-Yaakov M, Eshel G, Zaksonski L, Lazarovich Z, Boldur I. Prevalence of antibodies to Chlamydia pneumoniae in an Israeli population without clinical evidence of respiratory infection. *J Clin Pathol.* 2002 May;55(5):355-8

[332] Haider M, et al. Acute and chronic Chlamydia pneumoniae infection and inflammatory markers in coronary artery disease patients. *J Infect Dev Ctries.* 2011 Aug;5:580-6

[333] Carter JD, Espinoza LR, Inman RD, Sneed KB, Ricca LR, Vasey FB, Valeriano J, Stanich JA, Oszust C, Gerard HC, Hudson AP. Combination antibiotics as a treatment for chronic Chlamydia-induced reactive arthritis: a double-blind, placebo-controlled, prospective trial. *Arthritis Rheum.* 2010 May;62(5):1298-307

[334] "In clinically definite MS patients, the VUMC and USF detection rates were 72 and 61%, respectively, and in patients with monosymptomatic MS, the VUMC and USF detection rates were 41 and 54%, respectively. The PCR signal was positive for 7% of the OND controls at VUMC and for 16% at USF. These studies confirm our previous reports concerning the high prevalence of C. pneumoniae in the CSF of MS patients." Sriram S, Yao SY, Stratton C, et al. Comparative study of the presence of Chlamydia pneumoniae in cerebrospinal fluid of Patients with clinically definite and monosymptomatic multiple sclerosis. *Clin Diagn Lab Immunol.* 2002 Nov;9(6):1332-7.

Parenchymal/internal/occult dysbiotic microbes and/or occult infections that can contribute to chronic inflammation, metabolic impairment, or autoimmunity—*continued*

Bacteria, protozoa, etc.	Assessment	Disease association(s)
Helicobacter pylori	Serum IgA, IgM, IgG antibodies—IgG antibodies are the most useful *serologic* test (>90% sensitive and specific) for monitoring response to eradication therapy despite the fact that antibody titer may remain elevated for a long time after *H pylori* eradication; urea breath test (gives false-negative results with coccoid forms of *H pylori* that do not produce urease, use of antibiotics, bismuth, histamine-2 blockers, or proton pump inhibitors), stool antigen shows excellent specificity (98%) and sensitivity (94%) and is highly responsive to the presence or absence of the infection[335]	Chronic gastritis and gastroduodenal ulceration, hypochlorhydria and subsequent maldigestion and small intestine bacterial overgrowth (SIBO), Sjogren syndrome, GI lymphoma, migraine, reactive/chronic arthritis, Raynaud's phenomenon
Mycoplasma species including *pneumoniae, fermentans, hominis, penetrans, genitalium*	IgG and IgM antibodies to various subspecies; PCR showed positivity in patients with fatigue/fibromyalgia: *M. pneumoniae* (54/91), *M. fermentans* (44/91), *M. hominis* (28/91) and *M. penetrans* (18/91)[336]	Chronic fatigue syndrome and fibromyalgia, Gulf War Illness[337], autoimmunity
Pseudomonas aeruginosa, Acinetobacter spp	Culture of site (urine, stool, sputum, wounds, cerebrospinal fluid) as indicated, otherwise, use stool culture and urine culture if investigating neuronal autoimmunity; serum IgA and IgG antibodies against *Pseudomonas aeruginosa* and *Acinetobacter* spp antigens are elevated in patients with multiple sclerosis[338,339], however such testing is not widely commercially available for routine clinical use; the current author has found stool testing and culture for *Pseudomonas aeruginosa* to be valuable in the treatment of neuronal autoimmunity	Neuronal autoimmunity including peripheral neuropathy and multiple sclerosis
Streptococcal infections: *Streptococcus pyogenes,* streptococci hemolytic groups A, B, D, and G	Acute pharyngeal infections are generally diagnosed clinically, with or without the use of "rapid Strep tests" or throat culture and treated with short-term penicillin-based antibiotic. However, with chronic infections/colonizations, the microbiologic phenotype of the bacteria changes from the extracellular form prototypical of acute infections to that of an intracellular form; as a general guideline, acute/extracellular infections respond more rapidly to treatment than do chronic/intracellular infections. Standard laboratory testing includes culture, and serum measurements of antistreptolysin-O (ASO), antihyaluronidase, anti-DNase-B, and Streptozyme; diagnosis can also be supported by response to treatment.	Psoriasis, rheumatoid arthritis, polymyositis, dermatomyositis, rheumatic fever, and many other chronic inflammatory disorders

[335] Santacroce L, Katz J. Helicobacter Pylori Infection Workup. emedicine.medscape.com/article/176938-workup#a0719 Updated: Feb 15, 2013

[336] Nasralla M, Haier J, Nicolson GL. Multiple mycoplasmal infections detected in blood of patients with chronic fatigue syndrome and/or fibromyalgia syndrome. *Eur J Clin Microbiol Infect Dis.* 1999 Dec;18(12):859-65

[337] "In studies on hundreds of U.S. and British veterans with Gulf War Illness, approximately 40-50% of Gulf War Illness patients show evidence of mycoplasmal infections compared to 6-9% in non- deployed, healthy subjects." Nicolson GL, Nasralla MY, Nicolson NL, Haier J. High Prevalence of Mycoplasmal Infections in Symptomatic (Chronic Fatigue Syndrome) Family Members of Mycoplasma-Positive Gulf War Illness Patients. *J Chronic Fatigue Syndrome* 2003; 11(2): 21-36

[338] Hughes LE, Smith PA, Bonell S, et al. Cross-reactivity between related sequences found in Acinetobacter sp., Pseudomonas aeruginosa, myelin basic protein and myelin oligodendrocyte glycoprotein in multiple sclerosis. *J Neuroimmunol.* 2003 Nov;144(1-2):105-15

[339] Hughes LE, Bonell S, Natt RS, et al. Antibody responses to Acinetobacter spp. and Pseudomonas aeruginosa in multiple sclerosis: prospects for diagnosis using the myelin-acinetobacter-neurofilament antibody index. *Clin Diagn Lab Immunol.* 2001 Nov;8(6):1181-8

Clinical Case **Polymicrobial positivity in a patient diagnosed with systemic lupus erythematosus (SLE), mixed connective tissue disease (MCTD), Raynaud's syndrome, and secondary amyloidosis (inaccurately diagnosed as bilateral carpal tunnel syndrome and peripheral edema)**: Results show positivity toward *Mycoplasma*, *Chlamydia/Chlamydophila*, and parvovirus: Of these three results, the positivity against *Chlamydia/Chlamydophila pneumoniae* is the most actionable per published research; antibody titers against *Mycoplasma* and parvovirus are may indicate past "extinguished" or current "smouldering" infection/colonization—only a clinical trial with antibacterial and antiviral interventions (respectively) followed by monitoring 1) clinical response to treatment, 2) reduction in other markers of autoimmune disease activity, such as Sjogren's antibodies and anti-double-stranded DNA antibodies in this case, and 3) reduction in microbe-specific antibody titers would be able to prove or refute the microbe-autoimmunity links in this particular case. Negative results for anti-dsANA and CCP not shown.

DATE OF COLLECTION TIME		DATE RECEIVED	DATE REPORTED	TIME	
11/02/2012	13:15	11/03/2012	11/05/2012	14:11	

TEST	RESULT		LIMITS
Antiextractable Nuclear Ag			
> RNP Antibodies	5.6H	AI	0.0 - 0.9
> Smith Antibodies	1.8H	AI	0.0 - 0.9

Test	Result	Units	Flag	Reference Range
Sjorgren's Ant-SS-A	2.0	AI	H	0.0-0.9
Sjorgren's Ant-SS-B	<0.2			-

Account Number	Patient ID	Control Number	Date and Time Collected	Date Reported	Sex	Age(Y/M/D)	Date of Birth
		0	04/26/13 09:46	04/30/13	F	69	

TESTS	RESULT	FLAG	UNITS	REFERENCE INTERVAL	LAB
Mycoplasma pneu. IgG/IgM Abs					
M pneumoniae IgG Abs	203	High	U/mL	0 - 99	
			Negative:	<100	
			Indeterminate:	100 - 320	
			Positive:	>320	

The reference interval established is intended as a baseline only. Values >100 may indicate a recent infection with Mycoplasma pneumoniae and need to be confirmed either by a positive IgM result and/or an additional specimen drawn 2-4 weeks later showing a significant increase in antibody levels.

M pneumoniae IgM Abs	<770		U/mL	0 - 769	
			Negative	<770	

Clinically significant amount of M. pneumoniae antibody not detected.

Chl. pneumoniae (IgG/IgM/IgA)					
Chlamydia pneumoniae IgG	>1:256	High		Neg:<1:16	
Chlamydia pneumoniae IgM	<1:10			Neg:<1:10	
Chlamydia pneumoniae IgA	>1:256	High		Neg:<1:16	

Parvovirus, Antibody   Stage: **Final**   Resulted: 11/2/2012

Test	Result	Units	Flag	Reference Range
Parvo IgG 163303	5.7	index	H	0.0-0.8
Negative <0.9				
Equivocal 0.9 - 1.1				
Positive >1.1				
Parvo IgM 163303	0.1	index		0.0-0.8
Negative <0.9				
Equivocal 0.9 - 1.1				
Positive >1.1				

Results show positivity toward *Proteus* (most likely urogenital), inflammatory gastrointestinal dysbiosis (markedly elevated lysozyme and lactoferrin with no obviously dysbiotic microbes detected), and high-"normal" titers against ASO (most likely pharyngeal). Patient has three different autoimmune diseases, HTN, and severe obesity.

Date and Time Collected	Date Entered	Date and Time Reported	Physician Name	NPI	Physician ID
05/24/12 14:42	05/24/12	05/30/12 15:39ET	VASQUEZ , A		

Tests Ordered

Testosterone, F Eqlib+T LC/MS; Thyroid Antibodies; Hemoglobin A1c; Thyroxine (T4) Free, Direct, S; DHEA-Sulfate; TSH; Prolactin; Estradiol; Reverse T3, Serum; Vitamin D, 25-Hydroxy; t-Transglutaminase (tTG) IgA; Triiodothyronine (T3); Ferritin, Serum; Venipuncture

TESTS	RESULT	FLAG	UNITS	REFERENCE INTERVAL	LAB
Testosterone, F Eqlib+T LC/MS					
Testosterone, Total, LC/MS	**334.1**	**Low**	ng/dL	348.0 - 1197.0	
Testosterone, Free	7.85		ng/dL	5.00 - 21.00	
% Free Testosterone	2.35		%	1.50 - 4.20	
Thyroid Antibodies					
Thyroid Peroxidase (TPO) Ab	**235**	**High**	IU/mL	0 - 34	
		Please note reference interval change			
Antithyroglobulin Ab	<20		IU/mL	0 - 40	
Siemens (DPC) ICMA Methodology					
Hemoglobin A1c	5.4		%	4.8 - 5.6	

Increased risk for diabetes: 5.7 - 6.4
Diabetes: >6.4
Glycemic control for adults with diabetes: <7.0

TESTS	RESULT	FLAG	UNITS	REFERENCE INTERVAL	LAB
Thyroxine (T4) Free, Direct, S					
T4,Free(Direct)	1.12		ng/dL	0.82 - 1.77	
DHEA-Sulfate	267.7		ug/dL	160.0 - 449.0	
TSH	3.510		uIU/mL	0.450 - 4.500	
Prolactin	5.6		ng/mL	4.0 - 15.2	
Estradiol	28.4		pg/mL	7.6 - 42.6	
Roche ECLIA methodology					
Reverse T3, Serum	25.5		ng/dL	13.5 - 34.2	
Vitamin D, 25-Hydroxy	**19.4**	**Low**	ng/mL	30.0 - 100.0	

Date and Time Collected	Date Entered	Date and Time Reported	Physician Name	NPI	Physician ID
08/27/12 14:06	08/27/12	08/29/12 15:09ET	VASQUEZ , A		679

Tests Ordered

Anticardiolipin Ab, IgG/M, Qn; Immunoglobulin A, Qn, Serum; Antistreptolysin O Ab; Venipuncture

TESTS	RESULT	FLAG	UNITS	REFERENCE INTERVAL	LAB
Antistreptolysin O Ab	199.5		IU/mL	0.0 - 200.0	

PROTEUS OX - 19	**POSITIVO 1:80**	(This appears to be an antibody titer.)

ESTUDIO	RESULTADO		UNIDAD	REFERENCIA
Acs. ANTI PEPTIDO CICLICO CITRULINADO (Ac. CCP) IgG	**★200.0**		U/mL	0.00-5.00
Ac. ANTI-NUCLEARES	**NEGATIVOS**			NEGATIVOS
RHEUMATOID FACTOR	183 (H)			0 - 14 IU/mL
SED RATE WESTERGREN	28 (H)			0 - 15
C-REACTIVE PROTEIN	1.3 (H)			0 - 0.8 mg/dL
ANA TITER	1:80 (Abnl)			Negative
ANA PATTERN	Homogeneous (Abnl)			Negative
Result Narrative				
ANA TITER 2	1:160 (Abnl)			Negative
ANA PATTERN 2	Speckled (Abnl)			Negative

Clinical Case—continued **Multiple laboratory abnormalities and multifocal polydysbiosis in a patient diagnosed with RA, psoriasis, and Hashimoto's thyroiditis**: Inflammatory gastrointestinal dysbiosis, presumably due to low-level *Klebsiella* and nonculturable yeast

Comprehensive Stool Analysis / Parasitology x3

BACTERIOLOGY CULTURE		
Expected/Beneficial flora	**Commensal (Imbalanced) flora**	**Dysbiotic flora**
2+ Bacteroides fragilis group	1+ Klebsiella pneumoniae ssp pneumoniae	
3+ Bifidobacterium spp.		
4+ Escherichia coli		
3+ Lactobacillus spp.		
4+ Enterococcus spp.		
NG Clostridium spp.		
NG = No Growth		

BACTERIA INFORMATION
Expected /Beneficial bacteria make up a significant portion of the total microflora in a healthy & balanced GI tract. These beneficial bacteria have many health-protecting effects in the GI tract including manufacturing vitamins, fermenting fibers, digesting proteins and carbohydrates, and propagating anti-tumor and anti-inflammatory factors.
Clostridia are prevalent flora in a healthy intestine. Clostridium spp. should be considered in the context of balance with other expected/beneficial flora. Absence of clostridia or over abundance relative to other expected/beneficial flora indicates bacterial imbalance. If *C. difficile* associated disease is suspected, a Comprehensive Clostridium culture or toxigenic *C. difficile* DNA test is recommended.
Commensal (Imbalanced) bacteria are usually neither pathogenic nor beneficial to the host GI tract. Imbalances can occur when there are insufficient levels of beneficial bacteria and increased levels of commensal bacteria. Certain commensal bacteria are reported as dysbiotic at higher levels.
Dysbiotic bacteria consist of known pathogenic bacteria and those that have the potential to cause disease in the GI tract. They can be present due to a number of factors including: consumption of contaminated water or food, exposure to chemicals that are toxic to beneficial bacteria; the use of antibiotics, oral contraceptives or other medications; poor fiber intake and high stress levels.

YEAST CULTURE	
Normal flora	**Dysbiotic flora**
No yeast isolated	

MICROSCOPIC YEAST	
Result:	**Expected:**
Many	None - Rare

The microscopic finding of yeast in the stool is helpful in identifying whether there is proliferation of yeast. Rare yeast may be normal; however, yeast observed in higher amounts (few, moderate, or many) is abnormal.

YEAST INFORMATION

Yeast normally can be found in small quantities in the skin, mouth, intestine and mucocutaneous junctions. Overgrowth of yeast can infect virtually every organ system, leading to an extensive array of clinical manifestations. Fungal diarrhea is associated with broad-spectrum antibiotics or alterations of the patient's immune status. Symptoms may include abdominal pain, cramping and irritation. When investigating the presence of yeast, disparity may exist between culturing and microscopic examination. Yeast are not uniformly dispersed throughout the stool, this may lead to undetectable or low levels of yeast identified by microscopy, despite a cultured amount of yeast. Conversely, microscopic examination may reveal a significant amount of yeast present, but no yeast cultured. Yeast does not always survive transit through the intestines rendering it unvialble.

Despite lackluster results in the microbiologic section of this comprehensive stool/microbiology text, results show markedly elevated lysozyme and lactoferrin, most likely attributable to exaggerated "dysbiotic" immune response against *Klebsiella pneumoniae* and nonculturable yeast. This case exemplifies the importance of interpreting microbiologic tests in patient-specific context.

INFLAMMATION				
	Within	**Outside**	**Reference Range**	
→ Lysozyme*		1280	<= 600 ng/mL	
→ Lactoferrin		29.2	< 7.3 µg/mL	
White Blood Cells	None		None - Rare	
Mucus	Neg		Neg	

Lysozyme* is an enzyme secreted at the site of inflammation in the GI tract and elevated levels have been identified in IBD patients. **Lactoferrin** is a quantitative GI specific marker of inflammation used to diagnose and differentiate IBD from IBS and to monitor patient inflammation levels during active and remission phases of IBD. **White Blood Cells** (WBC): in the stool are an indication of an inflammatory process resulting in the infiltration of leukocytes within the intestinal lumen. WBCs are often accompanied by mucus and blood in the stool. **Mucus** in the stool may result from prolonged mucosal irritation or in a response to parasympathetic excitability such as spastic constipation or mucous colitis.

Clinical Case—continued Multiple laboratory abnormalities and multifocal polydysbiosis in a patient diagnosed with RA, psoriasis, and Hashimoto's thyroiditis: Urinalysis showing mild metabolic acidosis along with asymptomatic bacteruria/bacteriuria; urinary leukocytes (not normal) is noted.

FECHA   20/08/2011   # 200037

EXAMEN GENERAL DE ORINA

EDAD   33 AÑOS   **Sexo** M

PRUEBA	RESULTADO		REFERENCIA	
Densidad	+1.030		1.01 - 1.03	
pH	5.5		5.00 8.00	
Proteinas	0	mg/dl	0	mg/dl
Glucosa	0	mg/dl	0	mg/dl
Cetonas	0	mg/dl	0	mg/dl
Bilirrubinas	0		0	
Urobilinogeno	NORMAL		0.2	E.U./dl.
Hemoglobina	0		0	
Nitritos	NEGATIVO		Negativo	

Examen Microscopico 40x

Leucocitos:	0 A 1 POR 3 CAMPOS	Piocitos:	0
Eritrocitos:	0	Cilindros:	0
Cristales:	0	Bacterias:	MODERADAS
Filamento Moco:	MODERADO	Levaduras:	0

Clinical Case **Multiple laboratory abnormalities in a patient diagnosed with multiple sclerosis**: Elevated IgE corresponding with food allergies and immune dysfunction; oxidative stress indicated by low glutathione.

Test Name	In Range	Out Of Range	Reference Range
HOMOCYSTEINE, CARDIOVASCULAR	5.2		<10.4 umol/L
IMMUNOGLOBULIN E		862 H	<OR=114 kU/L
GLUTATHIONE		526 L	544-1228 umol

Immune reactivity suggesting chronic *Chlamydia/Chlamydophila pneumoniae* colonization; the particular relevance of this finding in this case is the correlation between *Chlamydophila pneumoniae* infection and multiple sclerosis.[340]

CHLAMYDIA/CHLAMYDOPHILA ANTIBODY PANEL 1 (IGG)			
C. TRACHOMATIS IGG	<1:64		
C. PNEUMONIAE IGG		1:256 H	
C. PSITTACI IGG	<1:64		
REFERENCE RANGE: <1:64			

Elevated IL-6 at 5.85 pg/ml (range 0.31-5.0) indicating immune activation; one might question the value of this test (ordered by another physician) except possibly for use in monitoring responsiveness to treatment.

INTERLEUKIN 6, HIGHLY SENSITIVE, ELISA		5.85 H	0.31-5.00 pg/mL

Low red blood cell magnesium at 3.9 mg/dl (range 4.0-6.4) correlates with 1) insufficient magnesium intake, 2) increased renal loss and metabolic acidosis, and 3) oxidative stress in general and gluathone depletion in particular.

MAGNESIUM, RBC		3.9 L	4.0-6.4 mg/dL

Clinical Case **Normalization of antibody titers against *Streptococcus* following antibiotic-immunorestorative treatment in a patient with difficult-to-treat rheumatoid arthritis**: Elevated anti-Streptococcal antibodies showing reduction/normalization following nutritional supplementation with immunorestorative vitamins, minerals and fatty acids and administration of azithromycin, emulsified oregano oil, and oral vancomycin. Patient also positive for *Chlamydia/Chlamydophila pneumoniae* at a titer of 1:256 (data not shown). Streptococcal bacteria can be involved in acute and chronic infections; typically the acute infection phenotype is extracellular while the chronic "dysbiotic" phenotype can be either/both extracellular and intracellular. Streptococcal bacteria are associated with numerous inflammatory and autoimmune diseases, particularly psoriasis, rheumatoid arthritis, and dermatomyositis. In brilliant research publshed by Svartz[341] rheumatoid arthritis was induced in animals by innoculating them with group B streptococci isolated from the nasopharynx of RA patients. Note also in the example below that in the intial testing, only 1 of the 3 tests was positive.

Account Number	Patient ID	Control Number	Date and Time Collected 12/22/12 09:22	Date Reported 12/26/12	Sex F	Age(Y/M/D)	Date of Birth

TESTS	RESULT	FLAG	UNITS	REFERENCE INTERVAL	LAB
Anti-DNase B Strep Antibodies					
	134	High	U/mL	0 - 120	
Streptozyme	Negative			Neg:<1:100	
Antistreptolysin O Ab	63.3		IU/mL	0.0 - 200.0	

Date and Time Collected 07/13/13 00:00	Date Entered 07/17/13	Date and Time Reported 07/22/13 04:05ET	Physician Name	NPI	Physician ID

Tests Ordered
Anti-DNase B Strep Antibodies; Written Authorization

TESTS	RESULT	FLAG	UNITS	REFERENCE INTERVAL	LAB
Anti-DNase B Strep Antibodies					
	99		U/mL	0 - 120	
Results verified by repeat testing					

---

[340] Sriram S, et al. Comparative study of the presence of Chlamydia pneumoniae in cerebrospinal fluid of Patients with clinically definite and monosymptomatic multiple sclerosis. *Clin Diagn Lab Immunol.* 2002 Nov;9(6):1332-7 cvi.asm.org/content/9/6/1332.long

[341] "In experimental arthritis, produced by streptococci group B (Svartz), there appears in rats the same type of joint disease as in human RA and, besides, a rheumatoid factor (RF)-like macroglobulin, which cannot be distinguished by available methods from human RF macroglobulin. ...The streptococci B used in our investigations were mostly isolated from the nasopharynx of RA patients. Svartz N. The origin of rheumatoid arthritis. *Rheumatology.* 1975;6:322-8

DrV's perspective on the relativity of microbial activity—herpes simplex virus (HSV) as an example: Too often, doctors and clinicians seem to misunderstand the complexity and relativity of human microbial colonization, which—in this conversation—very clearly includes occult viral activity, even and specifically that which is not clinically manifest, that which is nonacute, and/or which is commonplace. Distinctions will be presented in the following table with clinical examples of HSV infection to follow.

Common (mis)perceptions	More accurate perceptions
• Patients either have infections that are clinically apperant or they are unaffected by microbes.	• In the human metaorganism/superorganism, microbial cells outnumber human cells by a ratio of 10 to 1, meaning that for each human cell, the body harbors ~10 microbes, allowing the statement that "humans" are really 90% microbes/bacteria.[342] • "Each person is host to some 100 trillion microbes, predominantly bacteria."[343] Thus, the total microbial load (TML) and total antigenic immunostimulatory load (TAIL) is quite considerable, whether or not a patient has an obvious "infection".
• If a patient has had a common infection such as HSV-1 or *Chlamydophila/Chlamydia pneumoniae*, then —when the infection is not appearant even though it might be persistent— it is considered to be irrelevant.	• Just because an infection is common does not mean that it is benign; HSV-1 is an example of a common infection (seen in approximately 50% of people worldwide) which has been correlated with several chronic health problems ranging from multiple sclerosis to Alzheimer's disease. • Just because the infection is not clinically *appearant* does not mean that the infection is "cleared" or clinically *irrelevant*; many chronic and persistent infections/colonizations remain subclinically active despite — or perhaps because of— the absense of an obvious vigorous immunological response.
• Chronic infections are seen quantitatively (ie, "you either had/have it or you don't").	• Chronic infections are both quantitative (ie, present or absent) and qualitative with respect to the impact that they have on metabolic processes and immunological/inflammatory reponses. Thus, the degree of the microbal load and microbial activity/replication is important, not simply the presence or absense of the microbe(s).
• Chronic inflammatory disorders are idiopathic; they result from "a combination of genetic predisposition with unidentified environmental triggers."	• Total microbial load (TML) and total immunostimulatory load (TIL) contribute to activation of the innate immune response and the subsequent development of inflammatory diseases, the pattern of which will depend on other pro- and anti-inflammatory and immuno-regulatory and –dysregulatory balances.
• Microbial colonizations—like nutritional defiencies—are primarily singular.	• Microbial colonizations—like nutritional defiencies—are nearly always multiple—not singular. • The *patterns of inflammatory responses* are driven by the TML and TIL of the patient's genetic, nutritional, microbial, immunological, mitochondrial, psychosocial, hormonal and xenobiotic statuses.

Clinical Cases—HSV1 positivity with varying antibody levels correlating with clinical outbreaks **Lower antibody titers correlate with less viral activity**: Here we see evidence of HSV seropositivity with a relatively low titer in a patient who has never experienced a clinical herpetic outbreak.

```
HSV I/II, IgG/Rfx Type II IgG
   HSV I/II IgG                    21.6    High      index        0.0 - 0.8
```

Higher antibody titers correlate with more viral activity: Here we see evidence of HSV seropositivity with a relatively high titer in a patient who experiences frequent clinical (oral) herpetic outbreaks.

```
HSV I/II, IgG/Rfx Type II IgG
   HSV I/II IgG                    36.5    High      index        0.0 - 0.8
                                                     Negative        <0.9
                                                     Equivocal   0.9 - 1.0
                                                     Positive         >1.0
```

---

[342] Dizikes C. 'We are 90% bacteria,' says researcher for Hospital Microbiome Project. *Chicago Tribune* 2013, Jan 02 articles.chicagotribune.com/2013-01-02/news/ct-met-microbiome-20130102_1_human-microbiome-bacteria-human-life

[343] Betts KS. A study in balance: how microbiomes are changing the shape of environmental health. *Environ Health Perspect.* 2011 Aug;119(8):A340-6

Lactulose-mannitol assay: assessment for intestinal hyperpermeability and malabsorption	
Overview and interpretation:	▪ The lactulose-mannitol assay is a highly validated assessment for the accurate determination of small intestine permeability. This test is used to diagnose "leaky gut", which is a common problem and contributor to systemic inflammation in patients with inflammation and immune dysfunction—see Chapter 4 of *Integrative Rheumatology*. Intestinal hyperpermeability reflects inflammation of and damage to the small intestine mucosa and is seen in patients with parasite infections, food allergies, celiac disease, malnutrition, bacterial infections, systemic ischemia or inflammation, ankylosing spondylitis, Crohn's disease, eczema, psoriasis, and those who consume enterotoxins such as NSAIDs and excess ethanol.[344] ▪ Elevations of **lactulose** indicate increased **paracellular** permeability caused by intestinal damage and are diagnostic of "leaky gut." *Clinical pearl*: remember that the "L" in *lactulose* rhymes with *leaky*. Decrements in **mannitol** suggest impaired **transcellular** absorption and suggest malabsorption in general and villous atrophy in particular. *Clinical pearl*: remember that the "M" in *mannitol* rhymes with *malabsorption*. Classically, in patients with damaged intestinal mucosa, we see a combined *increase in paracellular* permeability (measured with lactulose) and a *reduction in transcellular* transport (measured with mannitol); these divergent effects result in an increased lactulose-to-mannitol ratio.
Advantages:	▪ This test is safe and affordable for the assessment of small intestine mucosal integrity. Abnormal results—"leaky gut" and/or malabsorption—generally indicate one or more of following, which can be recalled by the acronym M.E.D. F.I.T. [345] 1. <u>Malnutrition</u>: Such as due to poor intake, catabolism, or malabsorption; we might also consider in particular: zinc, glutamine, and vitamin D3. 2. <u>Enterotoxins</u>: Such as NSAIDs or ethanol. 3. <u>**Dysbiosis**</u>: **including yeast, bacteria, protozoa, amebas, worms, etc.**** 4. <u>**Food allergies**</u>: **Including celiac disease, but also with milder food allergies.**** 5. <u>Inflammatory bowel disease</u>: Crohn's disease, ulcerative colitis, or family history of IBD. 6. <u>Trauma or major injury/inflammation (sufficient to induce a catabolic response)</u>: Tissue hypoxia, trauma, recent surgery, etc. **Note that of these six items, all but two can be excluded by history and patient assessment; therefore, a clinician could very reasonably perform specialized stool testing to assess for dysbiosis since negative results in a patient with increased intestinal permeability would then point toward food allergy.
Limitations:	▪ Abnormalities and the identification of "leaky gut" are nonspecific and do not point to a specific or single diagnosis or treatment.
Comments:	▪ The value of this test is two-fold: 1) as a screening test for the above-mentioned disorders, and 2) as a method for determining the efficacy of treatment once the cause of the problem has been putatively identified and treated. ▪ This test can be used to promote compliance and to encourage the use of additional testing in patients who are otherwise prone to noncompliance or who resist other tests, such as stool testing. In other words, the clinician can gain an advantage by showing the patient an objective abnormality which then validates the need for treatment and additional testing. ▪ I only use this test on rare occasions because I more commonly either assume that a patient has leaky gut if he/she has one of the aforementioned conditions or we move directly to stool testing and comprehensive parasitology—clearly one of the most valuable tests in the management and treatment of systemic inflammation and immune dysfunction—otherwise known as "autoimmunity" and "allergy."

---

[344] Miller AL. The Pathogenesis, Clinical Implications, and Treatment of Intestinal Hyperpermeability. *Alt Med Rev 1997*:2(5):330-345
[345] Credit to Angelique Marquez for the MEDFIT acronym and proving that great teachers inspire genius in their students ☺

Clinical Case **Highly abnormal lactulose-mannitol ratio in a patient with idiopathic peripheral neuropathy prior to comprehensive stool analysis and parasitology showing intestinal dysbiosis**: This 40-yo man presented with a multiyear history of periodic febrile exacerbations of peripheral neuropathy that would cause severe paresthesias and motor deficits. Patient had been evaluated by several board-certified medical neurologists to no avail. Laboratory, imaging, electrodiagnostic studies, and cerebrospinal fluid (CSF) analysis revealed nonspecific abnormalities that did not lead to an established diagnosis. From an integrative naturopathic and functional medicine perspective, food allergy and intestinal dysbiosis are the most obvious probable etiologies; these clinical suspicions were confirmed with laboratory testing showing increased intestinal permeability and gastrointestinal dysbiosis.

Patient:	Order Number: 40220637	HOUSTON OPTIMAL HEALTH
	Completed: April 24, 2003	ALEX VASQUEZ DC ND
Age: 40	Received: April 22, 2003	
Sex: M	Collected: April 21, 2003	Houston, TX 77098
MRN:		

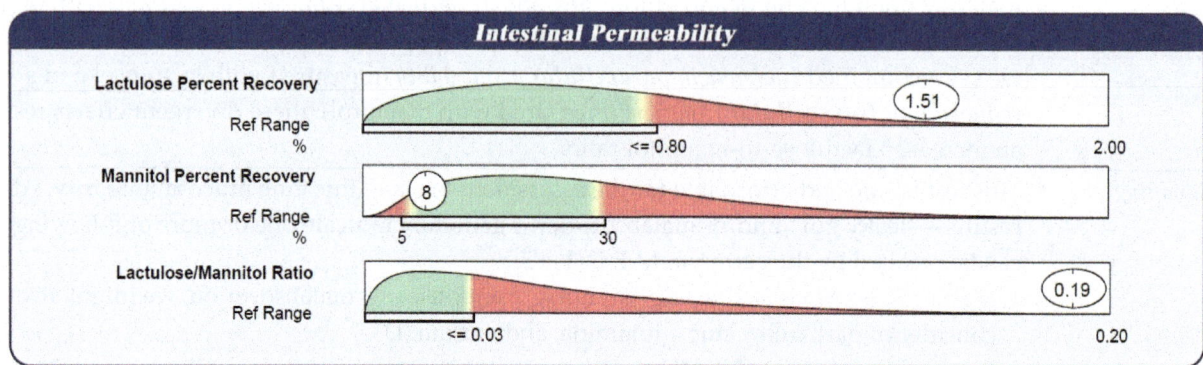

As expected, comprehensive parasitology showed intestinal dysbiosis, including insufficiency of *Lactobacillus* and presence of *Psuedomonas* and abnormal yeast species. Of particular note, *Psuedomonas aeruginosa* shows cross-reactivity with human neuronal tissues.[346,347] Eradication of the dysbiotic condition with a combination of dietary improvement, nutritional supplementation, hormonal optimization, and antimicrobial drugs and herbs lead to rapid and sustained remission of this "idiopathic peripheral neuropathy" which had defied standard medical diagnosis and treatment for many years.

Comprehensive Stool Analysis / Parasitology x3

MICROBIOLOGY

Bacteriology Culture					
Beneficial flora		**Imbalances**		**Dysbiotic flora**	
Bifidobacter	4+	Haemolytic E. coli	4+	Pseudomonas sp.	4+
E. coli	4+	Gamma strep	2+		
Lactobacillus	2+				

Mycology (Yeast) Culture			
Normal flora		**Dysbiotic flora**	
Candida glabrata	1+		
Rhodotorula sp.	1+		

[346] Hughes LE, Bonell S, Natt RS, et al. Antibody responses to Acinetobacter spp. and Pseudomonas aeruginosa in multiple sclerosis: prospects for diagnosis using the myelin-acinetobacter-neurofilament antibody index. *Clin Diagn Lab Immunol.* 2001 Nov;8(6):1181-8 cvi.asm.org/content/8/6/1181.full.pdf
[347] Hughes LE, Smith PA, Bonell S, Natt RS, Wilson C, Rashid T, Amor S, Thompson EJ, Croker J, Ebringer A. Cross-reactivity between related sequences found in Acinetobacter sp., Pseudomonas aeruginosa, myelin basic protein and myelin oligodendrocyte glycoprotein in multiple sclerosis. *J Neuroimmunol.* 2003 Nov;144(1-2):105-15

Comprehensive stool analysis and comprehensive parasitology

Overview and interpretation:	• **This is clearly one of the most valuable tests in clinical practice when working with patients with chronic fatigue, systemic inflammation, and autoimmunity. Second only to routine laboratory assessments such as CBC, chemistry panel, and CRP, the importance of stool testing and comprehensive parasitology assessments must be appreciated by progressive clinicians of all disciplines.**

- Stool testing must be performed by a specialty laboratory because the quality of testing provided by most standard "medical labs" and hospitals is completely inadequate. Initial samples should be collected on three separate occasions by the patient and each sample should be analyzed separately by the laboratory.

- Important qualitative and quantitative markers include the following:
  - **Beneficial bacteria ("probiotics")**: Microbiological testing should quantify and identify various beneficial bacteria, which should be present at "+4" levels on a 0-4 scale.
  - **Harmful and potentially harmful bacteria, protozoans, amebas, etc.**: Questionable or harmful microbes should be eradicated even if they are not identified as true pathogens in the Paleo-classic Pasteurian/Kochian sense.[348]
  - **Yeast and mycology**: At least two tests must be performed for a complete assessment: 1) yeast culture, and 2) microscopic examination for yeast elements. Both tests are necessary because some patients—perhaps those with the most severe symptomatology and the most favorable response to anti-yeast treatment—will have a negative yeast culture and positive findings on the microscopic examination. In other words, these patients have intestinal yeast that contributes to their disease/symptomatology but which does not grow on culture despite being clearly visible with microscopy; a similar pattern (using a swab of the rectal mucosa rather than microscopy) is referred to as "negative culture with positive smear."[349]
  - **Microbial sensitivity testing**: An important component to parasitology testing is the determination of which anti-microbial agents (natural and synthetic) the microbe is sensitive to. This helps to guide and enhance the effectiveness of anti-microbial therapy.
  - **Secretory IgA**: SIgA levels are elevated in patients who are having an immune response to either food or microbial antigens.[350] Thus, in a patient with minimal dysbiosis, say for example with *Candida albicans*, an elevated sIgA can indicate that the patient is having a hypersensitivity reaction to an otherwise benign microbe—in this case, eradication of the microbe is warranted and may result in a positive clinical response. Low sIgA suggests either primary or secondary immune defect such as selective sIgA deficiency[351] or malnutrition, stress, prednisone/corticosteroids, or possibly mycotoxicosis (immunosuppression due to fungal immunotoxins). In addition to addressing any systemic causative factors, a low sIgA may be addressed with the administration of bovine colostrum, glutamine, vitamin A, and *Saccharomyces boulardii*; the following doses may be considered for use in adults with proportionately smaller doses for children:
    - Bovine colostrum: 2.4 – 3.6 grams per day in divided doses for adults. No drug interactions are known. Side effects may include increased energy, insomnia, and stimulation. One study in particular used very large doses of 10 grams per

---

[348] Vasquez A. Reducing Pain and Inflammation Naturally. Part 6: Nutritional and Botanical Treatments Against "Silent Infections" and Gastrointestinal Dysbiosis, Commonly Overlooked Causes of Neuromusculoskeletal Inflammation and Chronic Health Problems. *Nutr Perspect* 2006; Jan

[349] "According to Galland, the best predictor of who will respond to anticandida medication is a negative stool culture combined with a positive smear of the rectal mucosa (for the identification of intracellular hyphal forms of the organism); however, even that test is not 100% reliable." Gaby AR. Before you order that lab test: part 2. *Townsend Letter for Doctors and Patients*. 2004; January findarticles.com/p/articles/mi_m0ISW/is_246/ai_112728028

[350] Quig DW, Higley M. Noninvasive assessment of intestinal inflammation: inflammatory bowel disease vs. irritable bowel syndrome. *Townsend Letter for Doctors and Patients* 2006;Jan:74-5

[351] "Selective IgA deficiency is the most common form of immunodeficiency. Certain select populations, including allergic individuals, patients with autoimmune and gastrointestinal tract disease and patients with recurrent upper respiratory tract illnesses, have an increased incidence of this disorder." Burks AW Jr, Steele RW. Selective IgA deficiency. *Ann Allergy*. 1986;57:3-13

day for four days in children and found no adverse effects[352]; another case report of a child involved the use of 50 grams per day for at least two weeks and showed no adverse effects.[353]

- ◆ Glutamine: 6 grams 3 times per day (18 grams per day) is a common dosage with significant literature support.
- ◆ Vitamin A: Correction of subclinical vitamin A deficiency improves mucosal integrity and increases sIgA production in humans.[354] Common doses used by integrative clinicians are in the range of 200,000 IU to 300,000 for a limited amount of time, generally 1-4 weeks; thereafter the dose is tapered. Patients are educated as to manifestations of toxicity (see the chapter on *Therapeutics* toward the end of this book) and the importance of limited duration of treatment.
- ◆ *Saccharomyces boulardii*: Common dose for adults is 250 mg thrice daily; ability of this treatment to increase sIgA levels and its anti-infective efficacy have been documented in human and animal studies.

- ▫ **Short-chain fatty acids**: These are produced by intestinal bacteria. Quantitative excess indicates bacterial overgrowth of the intestines, while insufficiency indicates a lack of probiotics or an insufficiency of dietary substrate, i.e., soluble fiber. Abnormal patterns of individual short-chain fatty acids indicate qualitative/quantitative abnormalities in gastrointestinal microflora, particularly anaerobic bacteria that cannot be identified with routine bacterial cultures.

- ▫ **Beta-glucuronidase**: This is an enzyme produced by several different intestinal bacteria. High levels of beta-glucuronidase in the intestinal lumen serve to nullify the benefits of detoxification (specifically glucuronidation) by cleaving the toxicant from its glucuronide conjugate. This can result in re-absorption of the toxicant through the intestinal mucosa which then re-exposes the patient to the toxin that was previously detoxified ("enterohepatic recirculation" or "enterohepatic recycling"[355]). This is an exemplary aspect of "auto-intoxication" that results in chronic fatigue and upregulation of Phase 1 detoxification systems (Chapter 4 of *Integrative Rheumatology*).

- ▫ **Lactoferrin**: The iron-binding glycoprotein lactoferrin is an inflammatory marker that helps distinguish functional disorders (i.e., IBS) from more serious diseases (i.e., IBD). Approximate values are as follows:
  - ◆ Healthy and IBS: 2 mcg/ml
  - ◆ Severe dysbiosis: up to 120 mcg/ml
  - ◆ Inactive IBD: 60-250 mcg/ml
  - ◆ Active IBD: > 400 mcg/ml.

- ▫ **Lysozyme**: Elevated in proportion to intestinal inflammation in dysbiosis and IBD.

- ▫ **Other markers**: Other markers of digestion, inflammation, and absorption are reported with the more comprehensive panels performed on stool samples. These tests are not always necessary, but such additional information is always helpful when working with complex patients. These markers are relatively self-explanatory and/or are described on the results of the test by the laboratory.

---

[352] "In this double blind placebo-controlled trial, 80 children with rotavirus diarrhea were randomly assigned to receive orally either 10 g of IIBC (containing 3.6 g of antirotavirus antibodies) daily for 4 days or the same amount of a placebo preparation." Sarker SA, Casswall TH, Mahalanabis D, Alam NH, Albert MJ, Brussow H, Fuchs GJ, Hammerstrom L. Successful treatment of rotavirus diarrhea in children with immunoglobulin from immunized bovine colostrum. *Pediatr Infect Dis J*. 1998 Dec;17(12):1149-54

[353] Lactobin-R is a commercial hyperimmune bovine colostrum with some specificity for cryptosporidiosis; administration to a 4 year old child with AIDS and severe diarrhea resulted in significant clinical improvement in the diarrhea and "permanent elimination of the parasite from the gut as assessed through serial jejunal biopsy and stool specimens." Shield et al. Bovine colostrum immunoglobulin concentrate for cryptosporidiosis in AIDS. *Arch Dis Child*. 1993 Oct;69(4):451-3

[354] "It can increase resistance to infection by increasing mucosal integrity, increasing surface immunoglobulin A (sIgA) and enhancing adequate neutrophil function. If infection occurs, vitamin A can act as an immune enhancer, increasing the adequacy of natural killer (NK) cells and increasing antibody production." Faisel H, Pittrof R. Vitamin A and causes of maternal mortality: association and biological plausibility. *Public Health Nutr*. 2000 Sep;3(3):321-7

[355] Parker RJ, Hirom PC, Millburn P.Enterohepatic recycling of phenolphthalein, morphine, lysergic acid diethylamide (LSD) and diphenylacetic acid in the rat. Hydrolysis of glucuronic acid conjugates in the gut lumen. *Xenobiotica*. 1980 Sep;10(9):689-70

Comprehensive stool analysis and comprehensive parasitology	
Advantages:	▪ **Stool analysis in general and parasitology assessments in particular provide supremely valuable information in the comprehensive assessment and treatment of patients with complex illnesses such as chronic fatigue, irritable bowel syndrome, fibromyalgia, and all of the autoimmune/rheumatic diseases.**
Limitations:	▪ Tests vary in price from $250-$400. ▪ Anaerobic bacteria are difficult to culture. ▪ Specialty examinations, such as for *Helicobacter pylori* antigen and enterohemorrhagic *E. coli* cytotoxin, must be requested specifically at additional cost.
Comments:	▪ I have found stool testing to be the single most powerful diagnostic tool for helping chronically ill patients to attain improved health. Insights from stool/parasitology testing can be used to implement powerfully effective treatments. The value of this test in the treatment of patients with rheumatic disease must be appreciated.

Concepts, facts, and tools to promote safe clinical practice

Concept: Not all "Apparent Injury-related Problems" are "Injury-related Problems"

In the case of most acute injuries, the underlying problem is often the injury itself. However, the physician must conduct a thorough history and examination to assess for possible underling pathologies that cause or contribute to the problem that "appears" to be injury-related. Congenital anomalies, underlying pathology, previous injury, occult infections, and psychoemotional disorders may have been present *before* the "injury."

> **"Pediatric infections and neoplasms are notorious for masquerading as sport injuries."**
>
> "...Take the relevant history directly from the patient, and keep tumors and infections high on your list of differential diagnoses... For example, about 15% of children with leukemia present with musculoskeletal complaints..."
>
> Shaw et al. How to avoid orthopedic pitfalls in children. *Patient Care* 1999 Feb

Just because the patient reports a problem such as pain following an injury does not mean that the injury is the *sole* cause of the pain. *Do not let a biased history lead you down the wrong path*. **In children and young adults, 5% of "sports-related" injuries are associated with preexisting infection, anomalies, or other conditions.** In adult women, "...between 9% and 20% of women with breast cancer attribute their symptoms to previous trauma to the breast. In these cases, the association of the breast mass with a traumatic event resulted in a delay in diagnosis ranging from four months to one year."[356]

A group of German physicians describe a man who presented with a soft-tissue pain following a soccer game; he was later diagnosed with a malignant tumor—synovial sarcoma.[357] Similarly, Wakeshima and Ellen[358] describe a young athletic woman who presented with chronic hip pain. The woman's history was significant for ulcerative colitis, but otherwise her radiographs were normal and her history and examination lead to a diagnosis of trochanteric bursitis. However, the patient's condition did not respond to routine treatment, and additional investigation over several months lead to a diagnosis of giant cell carcinoma. The authors concluded, "This case shows **the importance of repeat radiographic studies in patients whose joint pain does not respond or responds slowly to conservative therapy, despite initial normal findings."**

What you expect to find and hear when taking a trauma-related history is that **1) a healthy patient** with no previous health concerns was **2) exposed to a traumatic event**, the history and consequences of which perfectly coincide with the injury you are assessing in your office, and that **3) your physical examination findings are all consistent** and lead to a specific diagnosis, which then **4) responds to your treatment. If you find discrepancies between the history of the injury and your physical examination findings (e.g., fever after a "sports-related" injury), if the patient appears unhealthy in disproportion to the presenting complaint, or if the patient does not respond to your treatment, then you must consider the possibility of preexisting or concomitant disease.**

When treating children, be very careful to get an accurate history—this is difficult since your two sources of information are not very reliable: parents often think that they already have the problem figured out, and so their history will be biased toward convincing you of what they think is the problem and solution; children are often not good historians and can form illogical relationships between events that can be misleading.

Astute doctors search for and rule-out/exclude preexisting and underlying pathology before ascribing the problem to the "obvious cause." Always assess for consistency between the history, examination findings, and response to treatment—inconsistencies suggest the need for additional investigation.

---

[356] Seifert S. Medical Illness Simulating Trauma (MIST) syndrome: case reports and discussion of syndrome. *Fam Med* 1993 Apr;25(4):273-6
[357] Engel C, Kelm J, Olinger A. Blunt trauma in soccer. The initial manifestation of synovial sarcoma. [Article in German] *Zentralbl Chir* 2001 Jan;126(1):68-71
[358] Wakeshima Y, Ellen MI. Atypical hip pain origin in a young athletic woman: a case report of giant cell carcinoma. *Arch Phys Med Rehabil* 2001 Oct;82(10):1472-5

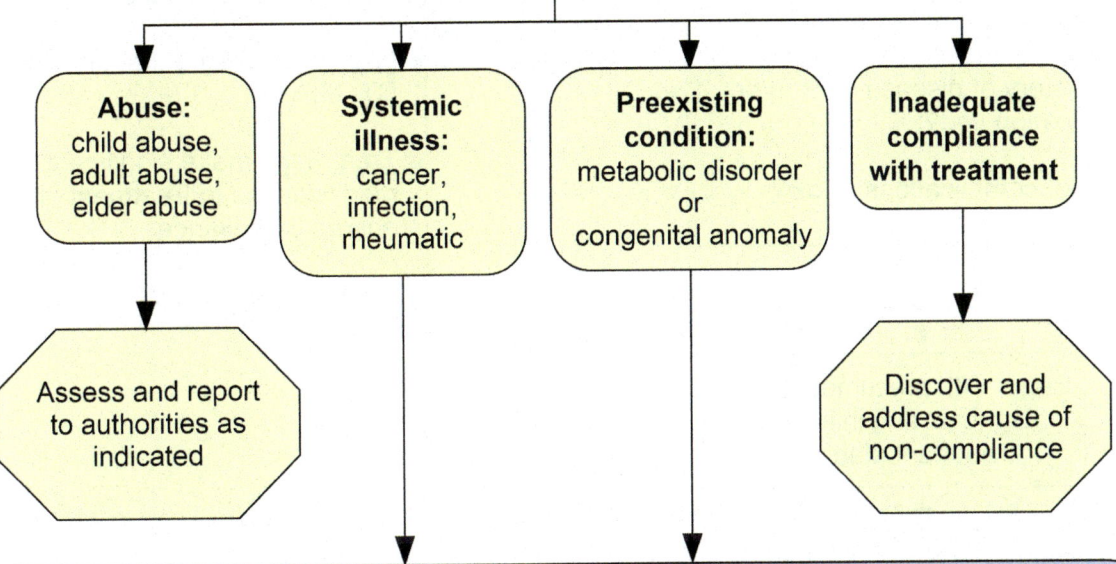

Previous health history
+
History of the present complaint
+
Clinical observations and physical examination findings
+
Response to treatment

If all 4 parts of the story do not add up perfectly, then you need to consider alternate diagnoses and take appropriate steps to ensure patient care.

Abuse:
child abuse,
adult abuse,
elder abuse

Systemic illness:
cancer,
infection,
rheumatic

Preexisting condition:
metabolic disorder
or
congenital anomaly

Inadequate compliance with treatment

Assess and report
to authorities as
indicated

Discover and
address cause of
non-compliance

If you have a specific condition in mind, then test specifically for it. If you suspect preexisting/concomitant illness but are unsure of exact nature of the condition, gather additional information by:

1) Taking a more detailed history,
2) Ordering lab tests: CBC, chemistry panel, ferritin, hsCRP, UA
3) Obtaining diagnostic imaging: radiographs, bone scan, MRI, CT, US
4) Reassessing patient within two weeks for progression of disease or crossing diagnostic threshold.
5) Referral or co-management: if the patient does not respond to your treatment and/or you suspect an underlying serious pathology, refer the patient to another physician at least for co-management. Put your referral in writing and chart appropriately. "When in doubt, refer it out."

<u>**Clinical management**</u>: Inconsistencies between the history, exams, and response to treatment indicate the need for additional investigation and additional diagnostic considerations.

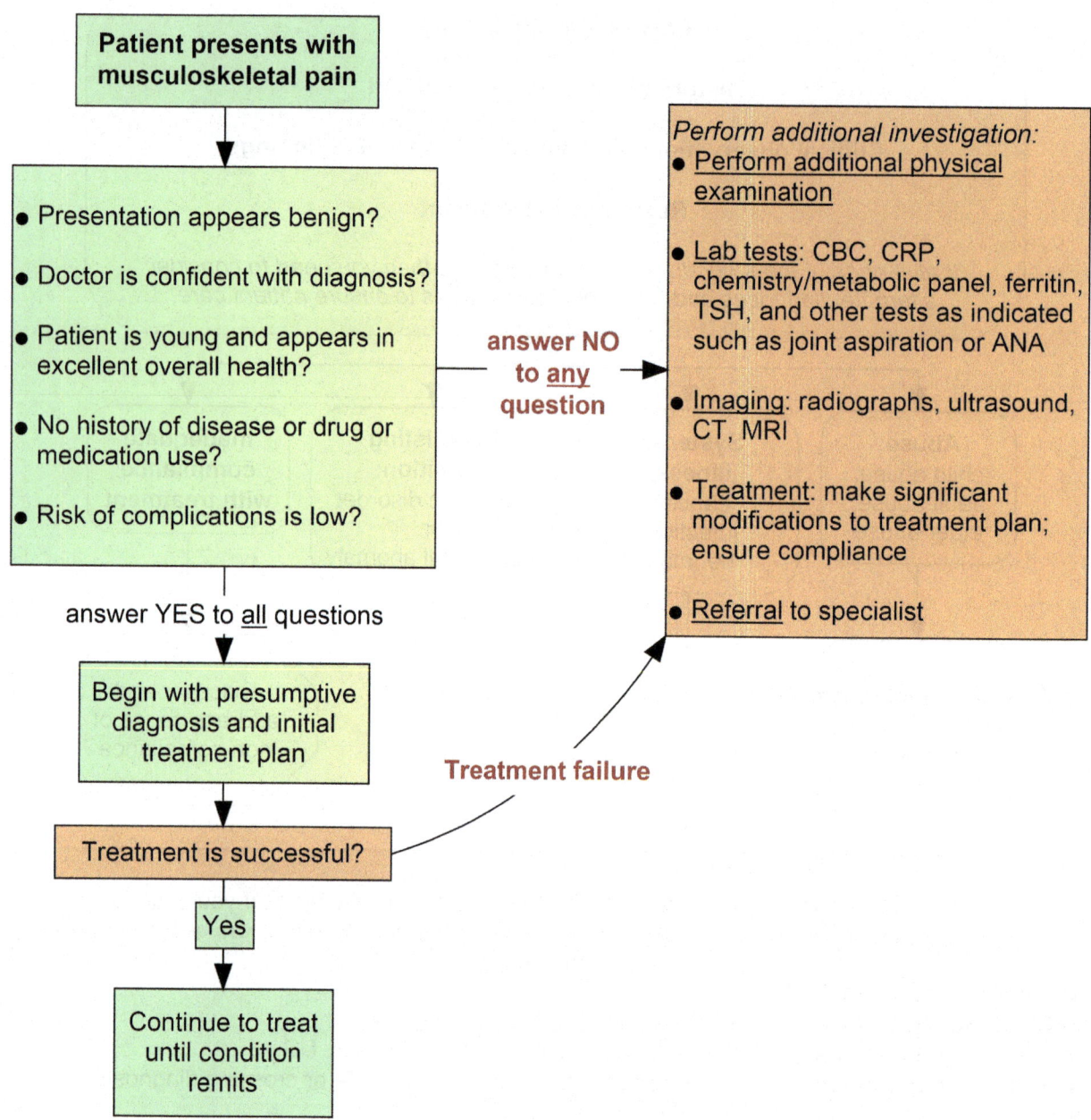

Patient presents with musculoskeletal pain

- Presentation appears benign?
- Doctor is confident with diagnosis?
- Patient is young and appears in excellent overall health?
- No history of disease or drug or medication use?
- Risk of complications is low?

answer NO to <u>any</u> question →

Perform additional investigation:
- <u>Perform additional physical examination</u>
- <u>Lab tests</u>: CBC, CRP, chemistry/metabolic panel, ferritin, TSH, and other tests as indicated such as joint aspiration or ANA
- <u>Imaging</u>: radiographs, ultrasound, CT, MRI
- <u>Treatment</u>: make significant modifications to treatment plan; ensure compliance
- <u>Referral</u> to specialist

answer YES to <u>all</u> questions

Begin with presumptive diagnosis and initial treatment plan

Treatment failure

Treatment is successful?

Yes

Continue to treat until condition remits

<u>**Clinical management**</u>: Inconsistencies between the history, exams, and response to treatment indicate the need for additional investigation and additional diagnostic considerations.

Concept: Identifying High-Risk Pain Patients

When a patient has musculoskeletal pain and any of the following characteristics, radiographs should be considered as an appropriate component of comprehensive evaluation. These considerations are particularly—though not exclusively—relevant for spine and low-back pain.[359]

1. More than 50 years of age
2. Physical trauma (accident, fall, etc.)
3. Pain at night
4. Back pain not relieved by lying supine
5. Neurologic deficits (motor or sensory)
6. Unexplained weight loss
7. Documentation or suspicion of inflammatory arthropathy[360] such as ankylosing spondylitis, SLE/lupus, RA/rheumatoid arthritis, JRA/juvenile rheumatoid arthritis, PsA/psoriatic arthritis
8. Drug or alcohol abuse (increased risk of infection, nutritional deficiencies, anesthesia)
9. History of cancer
10. Intravenous drug use
11. Immunosuppression, due to illness (e.g., HIV) or medications (e.g., steroids or cyclosporine)
12. History of corticosteroid use (causes osteoporosis and increased risk for infection)
13. Fever above 100° F or suspicion of septic arthritis or osteomyelitis
14. Diabetes (increased risk of infection, nutritional deficiencies, anesthesia)
15. Hypertension (abdominal aneurysm: low back pain, nausea, pulsatile abdominal mass)
16. Recent visit for same problem and not improved
17. Patient seeking compensation for pain/ injury (increased need for documentation)
18. Skin lesion (psoriasis, melanoma, dermatomyositis, the butterfly rash of lupus, scars from previous surgery, accident, etc....)
19. Deformity or immobility
20. Lymphadenopathy (suggests cancer or infection)
21. Elevated ESR/CRP (cancer, infection, inflammatory disorder)
22. Elevated WBC count
23. Elevated alkaline phosphatase (bone lesions, metabolic bone disease, hepatopathy, vitamin D deficiency)
24. Elevated acid phosphatase (occasionally used to monitor prostate cancer)
25. Positive rheumatoid factor and/or CCP—cyclic citrullinated protein antibodies
26. Positive HLA-B27 (propensity for inflammatory arthropathies)
27. Serum gammopathy (multiple myeloma is the most common primary bone tumor)
28. "High-risk for disease" *examples:*
    - Long-term heavy smoking of cigarettes
    - Long-term exposure to radiation
    - Obesity
29. Strong family history of inflammatory, musculoskeletal, or malignant disease
30. Others: _____

_____

_____

_____

_____

_____

---

[359] Remember that metastasis often travel first from the primary site to bone, therefore bone pain may be an early manifestation of occult cancer. Most of the above are from "Table 1: The high-risk patient: clinical indications for radiography in low back pain patients." J Taylor, DC, DACBR, D Resnick, MD. Imaging decisions in the management of low back pain. *Advances in Chiropractic*. Mosby Year Book. 1994; 1-28

[360] Radiographs are often essential for diagnosis or to rule out complications of the disease. For example, in patients with inflammatory arthropathies such as these, spontaneous rupture of the transverse ligament (at the odontoid process) has been reported; although rare, this complication could be life-threatening if mismanaged or undiagnosed.

Concept: Safe Patient + Safe Treatment = Safe Outcome

The purpose of performing the history and physical examination on a new *or established* patient is to determine their current health status—including their mental and emotional health and their physical health, particularly as this relates to important and life-threatening possibilities such as cancer, infections, fractures, systemic diseases, and neurologic compromise. The questions that lead this investigation are: **"What is this patient's current status?"** **"Does this patient have a serious disease, neurologic injury, or are they at high risk for developing a serious complication in the near future that can be prevented with appropriate care *now*?"**

Is your patient safe?

♦ The question to ask yourself is, "Is this patient's health problem or current complaint/exacerbation a manifestation of an underlying condition that could result in a negative outcome?

♦ If a patient comes to you with a headache, and you neglect to find that their blood pressure is 230/130, then you missed the opportunity to help them avoid the stroke that they could have after leaving your office.

♦ If a patient comes to you with a complaint of low back pain, and you neglect to perform a neurologic examination to find that *the patient already has a neurologic deficit even before you treated them*, then you have lost the opportunity to defend yourself in court when the patient later claims that *your* treatment and *your* management of their case is the reason that they now have a permanent neurologic deficit.

Is your treatment safe?: Have you been perfectly clear with the patient about the risks and benefits of your treatment plan? **Have you obtained informed consent?** Have you charted **"PAR-B"** to indicate that you have discussed the **P**rocedures, **A**lternatives, **R**isks, and **B**enefits of your treatment plan? Have you been clear about the duration of treatment and the need for appropriate follow-up? If you are prescribing nutrition or botanical medicines, have you informed the patient about the duration of treatment? **Have you looked for contraindications to your otherwise brilliant treatment plan?** What about the fact that this patient was on corticosteroids for the past

15 years and only discontinued prednisone 2 months before arriving at your office? *The patient may have steroid-induced osteoporosis even though he/she is no longer on prednisone.* When you recommend that your patient take 100,000 IU of vitamin A to treat her throat infection, what happens when she presents to your office 8 months later with signs of vitamin A toxicity because she continued her treatment plan indefinitely rather than using it only for 7 days as you had intended?

> **Check your work**
> Double-check to ensure that your patient is safe (no forthcoming complications or predictable emergencies) and that your treatment is safe (appropriate, effective, clearly communicated, and time-limited with instructions to return for office visit).

Be sure to put a time limit on your treatment plans. Every treatment plan should be 1) given to the patient in legible print and clear statements, 2) be copied for the chart, 3) include "what to do if things get worse" in the event of adverse treatment effect or exacerbation of problem, and 4) include patient's responsibility for returning to office/clinic for follow-up and reassessment.

Informed consent: From a legal standpoint, doctors can only treat a patient after the patient has given *consent to treatment*. Patients can only authoritatively consent to treatment after they have been educated about the treatment—thereafter, they can provide *informed consent*. Educating the patient requires discussion (and documentation) of each of the following:

• Procedures—what may take place, what is required; duration, costs, follow-up,
• Alternatives—what options are available,
• Risks—what risks are involved,
• Benefits—what benefits can be reasonably expected,
• Questions—allow for the patient to ask questions and receive answers.

This is commonly charted as **"PARB—no questions"** or **"PARB—questions answered"** once the patient gives consent to treatment; alternatively and more humorously, this may be charted as **"PAR-B-Q"**.

Concept: Four Clues to Discovering Underlying Problems

When I taught Orthopedics at Bastyr University I encouraged students to search for specific **sets of clues** when evaluating patients. These clues—often insignificant in isolation but meaningful in combination—were often the "red flags" that could help make the difference between an accurate diagnosis and a missed diagnosis. These four categories can be recalled with the acronym *"S.C.I.N."* or *"S.C.I.M."* These four areas of assessment/safety emphasis differ from the "vindicates" mnemonic which is used for differential diagnosis.

- **Systemic symptoms and signs**: Ask about systemic signs and symptoms such as fever, weight loss, lymphadenopathy, or skin rash in patients who present with pain because these "whole body" manifestations might indicate an underlying or concomitant disease that deserves attention, either independently from the musculoskeletal pain, or as a cause of the musculoskeletal pain. For example, "headache" may appear benign, whereas "headache with fever and skin rash" suggests meningitis—a medical emergency. "Low-back pain" is a common occurrence; yet "low-back pain with weight loss and fever" might suggest occult malignancy, osteomyelitis, or other systemic disease.

- **Complications**: We *ask about* and *look for* already existing complications, such as "numbness, weakness, tingling in the arms or hands, legs or feet" to rapidly screen for neurologic deficits and we follow this up with screening assessments such as "squat and rise", toe walk, heel walk, and reflexes for spinal cord and lower extremity neuromuscular integrity. Additionally, when dealing with patients with spine-related complaints or injuries, we also ask about changes or loss of function in bowel and bladder control and numbness near the anus or genitals, which may be the *only* clinical clues to cauda equina syndrome—a medical emergency. Ask about effects of the condition on ADL (activities of daily living) to attain a more comprehensive view of the condition and to ensure that the patient's story is consistent.

- **Indicators from the history**: We look for specific "red flags" and "yellow flags" such as trauma, risk factors (such as smoking, prednisone, alcohol), or a positive history of chronic infections or cancer. Nonmechanical musculoskeletal pain in a patient with a history of or high risk for cancer is highly suspicious and mandates thorough investigation.

- **Non-Mechanical pain**: Non-mechanical pain suggests a pathologic etiology rather than simple joint dysfunction. Pain at night, pain that occurs without an inciting injury, pain that is not strongly affected by motion and is not powerfully provoked by your physical examination assessments suggests the possibility of underlying disorder such as cancer, neuropathy, or infection. However, the ability to elicit an exacerbation of pain with "mechanical" maneuvers does not indicate that the pain is "mechanical" and therefore "non-pathologic." Mechanical pain can still be pathologic pain, such as the exquisite pain felt by patients with spinal fractures—they may be neurologically intact, they do have pain worse with motion, but they are not safe to manipulate, and they require appropriate treatment and referral on an urgent basis.

Vindicates: a popular mnemonic acronym for differential diagnosis	
V	Vascular / Visceral referral
I	Infectious / Inflammatory / Immunologic
N	Neurologic / Nutritional / New growth: neoplasia or pregnancy
D	Deficiency / Degenerative
I	Iatrogenic (drug related) / Intoxication / Idiosyncratic
C	Congenital / Cardiac or circulatory
A	Allergy / Autoimmune / Abuse: drugs, alcohol, physical
T	Trauma / Toxicity
E	Endocrine / Exposure
S	Subluxation / Somatic dysfunction / Structural / Stress / Secondary gain

Check your work
Keeping these four assessment categories in mind can serve as a useful "checkpoint" to ensure that your patient is safe, and that your treatment is appropriate and therefore safe, too.

"Pediatric infections and neoplasms are notorious for masquerading as sport injuries. … There is only one way to avoid this trap: Take the relevant history directly from the patient, and keep tumors and infections high on your list of differential diagnoses."[361]

- **Consider the possibility of child abuse when a child presents with an injury:** As a non-naïve physician, you always have to consider the possibility of child abuse when a child presents with an injury. Be detailed in your history taking, and be sure to search for discrepancies between 1) the child's version of the incident, 2) the adult's version of the incident, and 3) what is realistic (based on your practical life experience and clinical training). As a primary care physician, you are obligated to report your *suspicion* of child abuse to law enforcement agencies and/or child protective services.
- **Children heal quickly:** This rapid healing is good as long as tissues are approximated. But if a fractured bone is displaced and not correctly replaced, then problematic malunion deformities may result *within days*.
- **Children are more susceptible to rapidly progressing infections than are adults:** Soft tissue, joint, and bone infections need to be diagnosed expeditiously and treated aggressively.
- **Children are radiographically different from adults:** Make sure that your radiographs are interpreted by a competent radiologist with experience in the interpretation of *pediatric radiographs*. Radiographic considerations specific to children include:

  - Epiphyseal growth plates
  - Secondary ossification centers
  - Variants in trabecular patterns and bone densities
  - Specific conditions that happen only in children, such as slipped capital femoral epiphysis
  - Congenital anomalies
  - Difficulty following directions with positioning (applies to some adults, too!)
  - Bone scans can be difficult to interpret in children: Bone scans derive their value from the demonstration of a focal increase

  in uptake of radioactive isotopes, which demonstrates and localizes an area of increased metabolic activity. In adults, this increased and localized activity generally indicates pathology, especially malignant disease in bone (primary or metastatic) and recent fracture. In children, however, since their bones are already highly metabolically active due to the normal growth process, bone scans are difficult to interpret and are not highly reliable for the demonstration of focal lesions.

> **Playground injury or child abuse? Infection or cancer? Undiagnosed developmental disorder, congenital anomaly, or metabolic illness?**
>
> Always consider the possibility of abuse, cancer, infection, or congenital anomaly as a cause of musculoskeletal pain in children, even if the injury appears to be related to injury or trauma. Strongly consider lab tests, as well as radiographs (interpreted by a pediatric radiologist). When in doubt, refer for second opinion. If you suspect abuse, you have a legal and ethical obligation to report your _suspicion_.

> **Don't be naïve**
>
> While your compassion for human suffering and your love of nutrition and exercise may have directed you into healthcare, your professional success and survival will depend in large part on your ability to manage the technical and defensive aspects of clinical practice.
>
> Neuromusculoskeletal disorders and autoimmune diseases are "big league" clinical problems, and they need to be taken seriously.

---

[361] Shaw BA, Gerardi JA, Hennrikus WL. How to avoid orthopedic pitfalls in children. *Patient Care* 1999; Feb 28: 95-116

Concept: Differences between Primary Healthcare and Spectator Sports

This following mini-section was originally written for *Integrative Orthopedics* in 2004. In 2016, I reviewed this section, which occurred to me as possibly pedantic, added this first paragraph, and decided to let the original version stand as it was originally written (below) primarily for the following reason: In early 2016, I had a conversation with an academic administrator who nonchalantly proclaimed that not all health professionals manage life and death problems—"we refer to physicians for that." While she claimed that doctorate-level nutritionists had no need to understand or be aware of hyperkalemia despite routinely recommending high-potassium diets to patients with renal insufficiency (see video: vimeo.com/152296851), I offered a correction to the attempt to circumnavigate responsibilities by stating "the fact that you are training people for a *healthcare* profession at the *doctorate* level indicates that they will have responsibility for—and therefore need to know and appreciate—the risks of treatment and the possible complications that might exist prior to that treatment." The sports metaphor used below originated from a conversation I had with a hospital vice president in 2001 when we were discussing one of my SLE/lupus patients; his remark to me at that early time in my clinical career—"lupus is a big league disease"—obviously made an impression upon me, reminding me that these diseases are serious and need to be taken seriously by the practitioner. Too often, clinicians do not appreciate the gravity of the situations in their clinical practices; better to be overcautious than to face a clinical complication and medicolegal engagement.

In baseball, "errors" have been defined as "a defensive mistake that allows a batter to stay at the plate or reach first base, or that advances a base runner."[362] In baseball, a few errors can make the difference between winning and losing a particular game or season. However, a few errors in a game are to be expected, and ultimately the team can start over at the next game or season and try to do better.

Healthcare, however, is not a game, and even relatively minor errors such as the doctor's forgetting to ask a particular question or perform a specific test can result in a patient's catastrophic injury or death. In healthcare, when we are dealing with serious injuries and illnesses, even a single "error" is not allowed. "Failure to diagnose" is one of the biggest reasons for malpractice claims against doctors; such judgments often result in loss of licensure and awards of hundreds of thousands of dollars. "Failure to treat" results when the patient is injured because the doctor failed to effectively treat the patient or when the doctor failed to provide the appropriate referral to a specialist in a timely manner. Such failures are not only capable of destroying a physician's career and forcing the liquidation of his/her possessions, but such cases can also greatly damage the integrity of whole professions, especially the naturopathic and chiropractic professions which are generally *guilty until proven innocent* due to the double standards imposed by those adherent to the "always right" dogma of the medical paradigm.[363] Stated differently, **if the doctor does not ask the right questions and perform the right tests, then the doctor may miss an emergency diagnosis. Missing an emergency diagnosis can result in patient death. Patient death may result in litigation, loss of license for the doctor, and irreparable harm to the profession.** The upcoming section on **Musculoskeletal Emergencies** represents *core competencies* that every clinician must keep present in his/her mind during each interaction with a patient with musculoskeletal complaints, especially patients who are elderly, on medications such as prednisone, and those with known autoimmune or immunosuppressive disorders.

Concept: "Disease Treatment" is Different from "Patient Management"

> "The key to successful intervention for orthopedic problems in a primary care practice is to know what conditions to refer and when and to whom to refer the refractory patient."[364]

Treating a problem is one thing, managing a patient is something different. "Problems" such as "low back pain" are abstract concepts, and we automatically form mental lists of treatments for problems that are irrespective of the patient who has the condition. However this list may be of only very limited applicability to the individual patient with whom you are working. Management of patients includes ❶ assessing and reassessing the differential diagnoses, ❷ monitoring compliance with treatments, including the treatments of other healthcare providers, ❸ co-treating with other healthcare providers, ❹ assessing for contraindications, ❺ monitoring patient status and

---

[362] nocryinginbaseball.com/glossary/glossary.html Accessed November 11, 2006
[363] Micozzi MS. Double standards and double jeopardy for CAM research. *J Altern Complement Med.* 2001 Feb;7(1):13-4
[364] Brier S. *Primary Care Orthopedics*. St. Louis: Mosby, 1999 page ix

effectiveness of treatments, and also ❻ the office-related tasks of charting, documentation, billing, and correspondence. The management of emergency conditions often involves transport to the nearest hospital. In some situations, the patient will be able to drive himself/herself without difficulty. In other situations, the patient should be driven by friend, family, or taxi. In the most extreme, the patient should be transported by ambulance. When in doubt about the mode of transport, do not hesitate to call 911 for an ambulance. If the taxi driver gets lost on the way to the hospital, or your patient goes into shock while being driven by a friend, the liability will come back to haunt the *doctor*, not the *friend* or the *taxi driver*.

Concept: Clinical Practice Involves Much More than "Diagnosis and Treatment"

Emergency room and hospital-based physicians are appropriately able to focus solely on diagnosis and treatment as their primary spheres of activity and interaction with patients. However, those of us in private practice learn that *healthcare* involves much more than simply being a "good doctor." From an integrative perspective we have to go beyond diagnosis and treatment *for each health disorder* with each patient. Beyond *diagnosis* and *treatment* are *understanding* and *integration*. Orchestrating all of this into a treatment plan that the patient can actually implement requires creativity, resourcefulness, and the ability to enroll patients in the process of *redesigning*—often *rebuilding*— their lives.

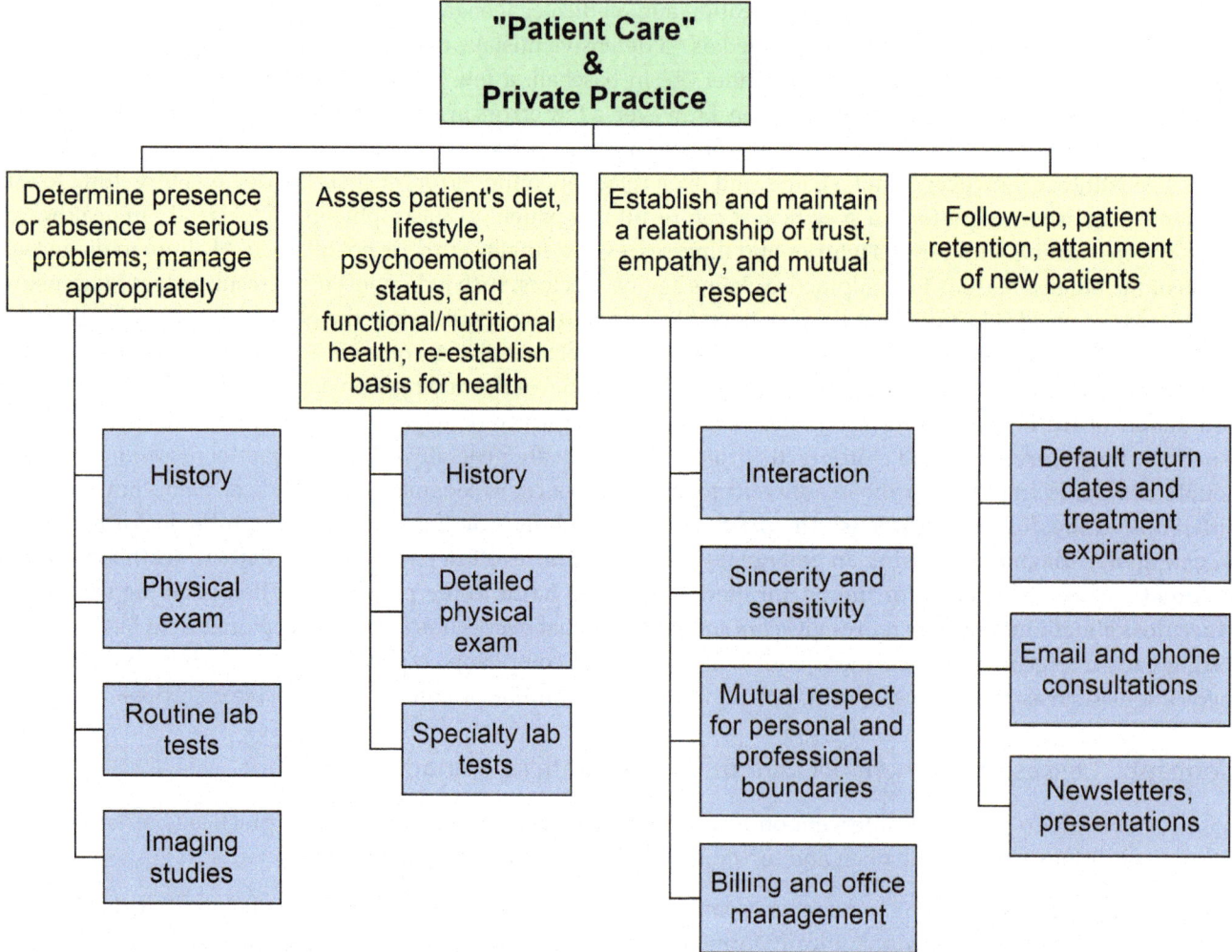

Components of Patient Care and Practice Management: Recall that **28% of malpractice claims involve mistakes made by medical office staff**; this includes unreturned phone calls which can culminate in malpractice by way of "patient abandonment." Similarly, inability to get a timely consultation may result in sufficient "sense of harm" that a patient may decide to sue; this is a factor in 10% of malpractice cases.[365]

---

[365] James R. Hall, Ph.D., L.Psych., FABMP, FGICPP. Departments of Internal Medicine and Psychology, UNT Health Science Center at Fort Worth. "Communication and Medico-Legal Issues." October 19, 2006

Clinical Management of Patients with Systemic Inflammatory/Autoimmune Diseases

In *Integrative Rheumatology* (2006, 2007, 2014), other peer-reviewed publications[366,367,368], and later the *Inflammation Mastery* multivolume series starting in 2014, I provide—what is to the best of my knowledge—an original conceptualization of rheumatic diseases:

1) Autoimmunity is a manifestation of immune dysfunction.

2) "Different" autoimmune diseases have much in common despite the different labels applied and manifestations observed. The commonalities in their etiologies and pathogenesis provides the rationale for the similarities in their treatments and a focus on identifying and ameliorating the underlying causes of autoimmunity as detailed: 1) food allergies/incompatibilities, 2) multifocal dysbiosis, 3) hormonal imbalances, 4) xenobiotic immunotoxicity, and 5) a pro-inflammatory diet and lifestyle. The new additions to this list starting in 2012[369] and 2013[370] are 6) mitochondrial dysfunction—in 2014 endoplasmic reticulum stress was added, and 7) nutritional immunomodulation.

3) Autoimmunity can be *ameliorated* (not always eliminated) MD the majority of patients with combined and coordinated effort on the part of the physician and the patient to address the most common causes of immune dysfunction, which rarely operate in isolation and are generally found in synergistic combination.

4) Since the etiopathogenesis is generally complex and multifaceted, treatment must be assertive and likewise multifaceted. Only rarely will a simple "silver bullet" cure be effective and sustainable.

Of the four major healthcare paradigms in Western medicine—i.e., osteopathic, chiropractic, naturopathic, and allopathic—the naturopathic paradigm is uniquely—and perhaps *solitarily*—well-suited for the successful assessment of and intervention for most autoimmune diseases. For it is only in naturopathic medicine that we find the specific admonishment to *Treat the Cause*, and this is a critical differentiation from the allopathic model which codifies and compels the use of symptom-suppressing and immune-suppressing medications. The original chiropractic model acknowledges the multifaceted nature of health and disease but is too vague in this context to direct assessment and treatment. The original osteopathic model did not include an appreciation of biochemical/nutritional considerations and environmental contributions which are essential for the treatment of autoimmunity. Obvious to any student of rheumatology is that the allopathic paradigm turns to symptom-suppressing drugs as "first line treatment" for rheumatic disease; this is—in the long-term—an abysmal failure except for suppression of acute inflammation and that it reduces symptomatology. Drug-only management of autoimmunity protracts the disease while imposing an impressive array of medication side-effects and nearly unbearable financial burdens. The failure of the modern allopathic medical paradigm is evidenced in the increased utilization of high-dose chemotherapy and stem-cell transplantation for the treatment of autoimmune diseases[371], an action which seems to confess, "Since we were unsuccessful with our first use of a hammer, instead of trying a different approach, we will just use a bigger hammer." The data is quite clear that even with "optimal drug therapy" and subspecialist management, the majority of patients with rheumatoid arthritis are "poorly controlled" with regard to disease activity—in other and more direct terms: medical management fails.[372]

> **Failure of long-term drug management of rheumatic disease**
>
> - < 50% of subjects remained in remission 1 year later.
> - Other studies have described sustained remission in daily practice as uncommon, being reached by only 17% to 36% of RA patients for up to 6 months. These studies did not evaluate time in remission beyond 6 months. A recent study...also concluded that long-term remission is rare, considering that the probability of a remission lasting 2 years was 6% to 14%.
> - Conclusions: This study shows that in clinical practice, a minority of RA patients are in sustained remission.
>
> Prince et al. Sustained rheumatoid arthritis remission is uncommon in clinical practice. *Arthritis Res Ther* 2012 Mar arthritis-research.com/content/14/2/R68

---

366 Vasquez A. "Inflammation and Autoimmunity: A Functional Medicine Approach." David S. Jones, MD (Editor-in-Chief). *Textbook of Functional Medicine*. Gig Harbor, WA; Institute for Functional Medicine: 2006, pages 409-417

367 Vasquez A. Web-like Interconnections of Physiological Factors. *Integrative Medicine: A Clinician's Journal* 2006, April/May, 32-37

368 Vasquez A. Reducing Pain and Inflammation Naturally. Part 6: Nutritional and Botanical Treatments Against "Silent Infections" and Gastrointestinal Dysbiosis, Commonly Overlooked Causes of Neuromusculoskeletal Inflammation and Chronic Health Problems. *Nutritional Perspectives* 2006; January

369 Vasquez A. *Functional Immunology and Nutritional Immunomodulation*. 2012

370 Vasquez A. *Integrative Rheumatology*, *Nutritional Immunomodulation*, and *Functional Inflammology*. 2013

371 "Hematopoietic stem cell transplantation is an increasingly used therapy for treatment of autoimmune diseases and severe immune-mediated disorders." Burt RK, Verda L, Statkute L, Quigley K, Yaung K, Brush M, Oyama Y. Stem cell transplantation for autoimmune diseases. *Clin Adv Hematol Oncol*. 2004 May;2(5):313-9

372 Prince et al. Sustained rheumatoid arthritis remission is uncommon in clinical practice. *Arthritis Res Ther* 2012 Mar arthritis-research.com/content/14/2/R68

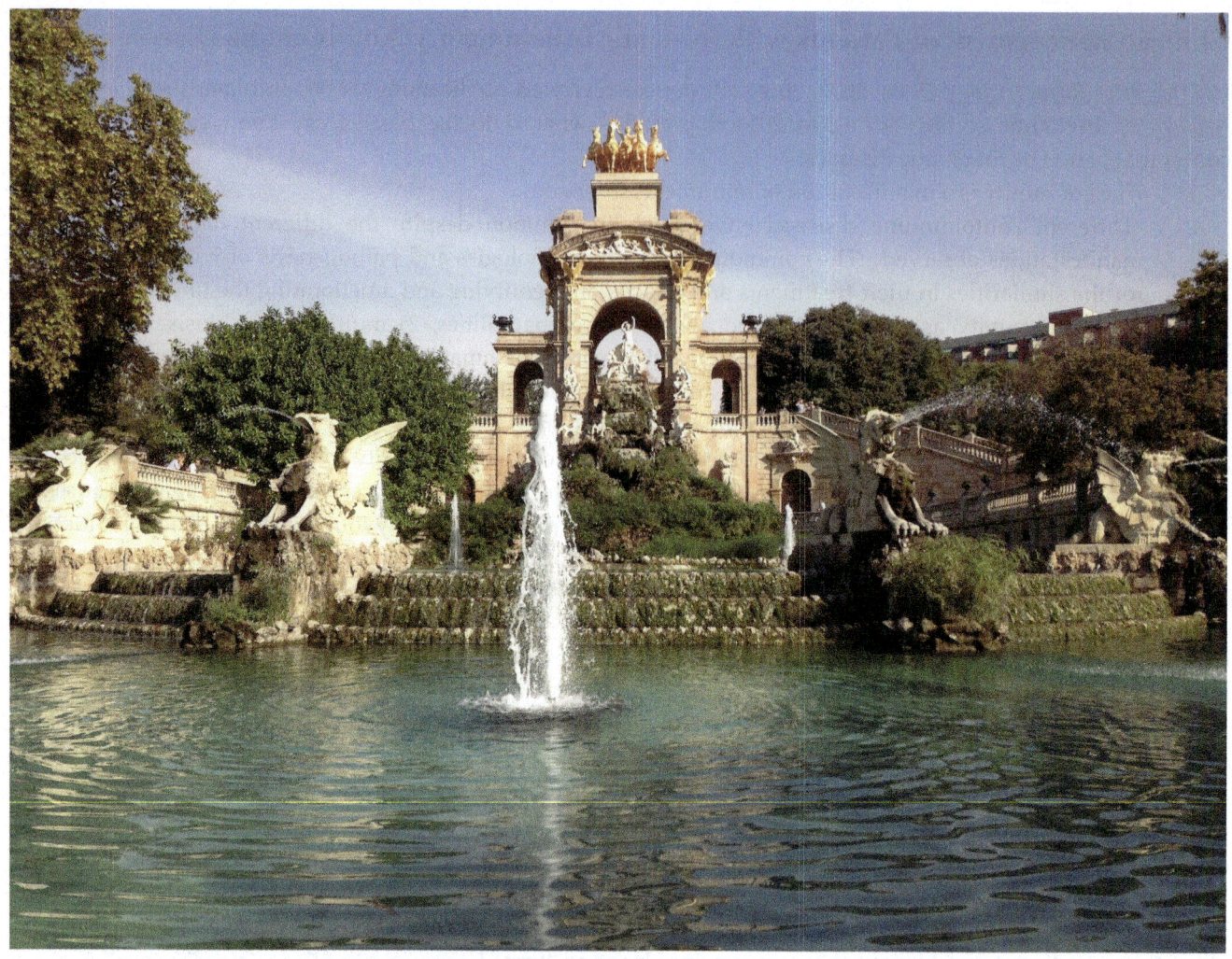

Parc de la Ciutadella, Venus, and Quadriga de l'Aurora: Grandeur of this scale reflects and reinforces true culture—a society's aspiration toward higher ideals, and a progressively better life. Societal aspirations are virtually nonexistent in modern times, wherein indifference, inertia, and ignorance are more apparent than are concern, progress, and knowledge. *What would be the characteristics of a modern aspirational culture?* An aspirational human culture seeks to develop the positive potentialities of life in general and human life in particular. As such, it provides for the maximal development of human intellectual, creative, and social potential, thus allowing people to achieve the optimal development of those qualities that are generally considered to be "most truly human." Consistent with these goals, systems of education, work, production, transportation are orchestrated to maximize learning, participation, efficient implementation, and sustainability (etc). Democratic and meritocratic ideas and ideals pervade educational, occupational, and political systems. From an

> **Culture: humanity with a goal**
> "There is lacking the one goal. As yet humanity has not a goal. But pray tell me, my brethren, if the goal of humanity be still lacking, is there not also still lacking *humanity itself?*"
>
> Nietzsche FW. *Thus Spoke Zarathustra*, *The Thousand and One Goals*

early age, students are taught intellectual skills, history, health/physicality, practical life skills, at least two languages, and effective communication and conflict resolution skills. I would consider these essentials to be a reasonable point from which we might start[373], and I trust that we could collectively improve upon and practically implement such a foundation for humanity. World leaders have grossly failed to orchestrate humanity toward basic unfying goals that transcend superficial differences and which promote the optimization of human experience and survival.

---

[373] This is not an exhaustive treatise on the possible positive future of humanity; I wrote it on my phone to assuage boredom while waiting on air cargo to be released in Spain. Have you ever waited on a government process in Spain that requires more than 1 person and more than one piece of paper? It's like standing still in slow motion, like sleeping in frozen oatmeal, like moving at glacial speed. Actually, with the government-facilitated melting of the ice caps, glacial speed these days is becoming a metaphor for speed. ... For a more developed discussion of this topic, see Largent C, Breton D. *The Paradigm Conspiracy: Why Our Social Systems Violate Human Potential—And How We Can Change Them Paperback*. Hazelden Publishing: 1998

Risk Management, Charting, and Avoiding Medical Errors: Useful Reminders & Acronyms

This page conveniently summarizes the most important acronyms for risk management, documentation, treatment, and patient education.

Acronym	Components	Exegesis
D.I.R.T.	Defensive mindset	Start with the conscious intention to practice defensively and effectively
	Duration of treatment	Define and limit the duration of each component of the treatment plan; define the next steps of care (e.g., continued care or laboratory tests) and the date of the return visit
	Interactions with disease and drugs	Double-check for interactions of the treatment plan with drugs and the patient's disease(s), especially renal insufficiency
	Referral	Determine the need for additional consultation
	Treatment plan, charted, dated, signed	Treatment plan must be archived in chart and should be given to patient; the clinician must sign and date the chart note and treatment plan
S.O.A.P.	Subjective	Patient's concerns, goals, changes in status
	Objective	Clinician's findings, including physical examination, reports from laboratory, imaging, biopsy, and consultations
	Assessments	Global assessments, firm diagnoses
	Plan	Treatments—definitions, durations for each concern, goal, assessment, diagnosis
F.I.N.D. S.E.X.® [374]	Food and nutrition	5-part nutritional wellness protocol—supplemented Paleo-Mediterranean diet: low-carbohydrate Paleo diet, multivitamin/mineral, physiologic doses of cholecalciferol, combination fatty acid therapy (CFAT), probiotics, allergy elimination-challenge, avoid genetically modified pseudofoods
	Infections and dysbiosis	Assess or treat empirically; components of treatment include antimicrobial, immunomodulation, immunorestoration
	Nutritional immunomodulation	See *Integrative Rheumatology, Inflammation Mastery* (2014 and beyond) for the latest update to the protocol—component #10 added in 2014 Jan.
	Dysfunctional mitochondria	Optimize mitochondrial function via mitophagy, resuscitation, and interventional disinhibition
	Stress, sleep, spinal health, sociology, sweat/exercise	Stress management and lifestyle/psychosocial optimization, sleep, spinal manipulation as indicated, sweat via daily exercise
	Endocrine/hormonal optimization	Especially assess and correct thyroid, prolactin, estradiol, insulin, DHEA, testosterone, and cortisol
	Xenobiotics and toxins	Toxicity is pandemic, therefore daily detoxification is mandatory and should target metals and organic/carbon-based toxins
P.A.R.B.Q.	Procedures	Explain the components of the treatment plan
	Alternatives	Explain what options and modifications exist
	Risks	Explain the risks of treatment, consider the aforementioned components of drug-interactions, disease-interactions, referral, and duration of treatment
	Benefits	Explain the anticipated benefits in realistic terms; never guarantee efficacy since "Each patient is different and each patient's response to treatment is unique."
	Questions answered	Document that questions—if any—were answered

---

[374] The FINDSEX acronym is a registered trademarkby Dr Vasquez associated with Functional Immunology and Nutritional Immunomodulation (2012), "F.I.N.D. S.E.X®" The Easily Remembered Acronym for the Functional Inflammology Protocol (2013), and updated books in the Inflammation Mastery series from InflammationMastery.com

Even if you are a board-certified rheumatologist and an assertive and astute clinician with years of experience, the consideration of these guidelines may help protect **you** from malpractice liability and **your patient** from harm. Practicing "good medicine" is inherently defensive and in the best interests of the patient and the doctor.

1. **Document the specifics of your treatment plan and the rationale behind it.**
2. **Do not tell your patient to discontinue their anti-rheumatic drugs unless these drugs are in your scope of practice _and_ discontinuing such drugs is therapeutically appropriate.**
3. **Give your patient written instructions, and specifically delineate time parameters for the next visit to monitor for therapeutic effectiveness, adverse effects, and disease progression/regression.**
4. **Always have an internist or rheumatologist (or appropriate specialist) on-board as part of the clinical team in case the patient experiences an exacerbation and needs to be hospitalized or acutely immunosuppressed.**
5. **When working with patients that have potentially serious diseases such as most of the autoimmune diseases, you should have a back-up plan integrated into your treatment plan from day one.** You might consider having patients sign a consent form that includes language consistent with the following:

   ▪ _"Due to the uniqueness of each disease and each individual, including his or her willingness and ability to implement the treatment plan, no guarantees of successful treatment can be offered."_

   _"Dr.___ is not available on a 24-hour basis at all times. If you have a serious health problem that requires immediate attention, you should call your other doctors(s), call 911, or have someone take you to the nearest hospital emergency room. If you notice an adverse effect from one of the components of your health plan, you should discontinue it then call Dr.___ and inform him/her of what occurred."_

   ▪ _"Treatments with other physicians or healthcare providers are not necessarily to be discontinued. Please let Dr.___ know if you are being treated by other healthcare providers (physicians, counselors, therapists, etc.). Consult your prescribing doctor before discontinuing medications."_

6. **Test responsibly.**
7. **Treat responsibly.**
8. **Re-test to document effectiveness of your intervention.**
9. **When in doubt, refer the patient for co-management.** If you are working with a serious life-threatening disease, and _your plan_ or _the patient's implementation of it_ is unable to produce **documentable results**, then you should refer the patient for allopathic/osteopathic/specialist co-management for the sake of protecting the patient from harm and for protecting yourself from undue liability.
10. **Practice defensively.** You will thereby safeguard your patient and your livelihood.

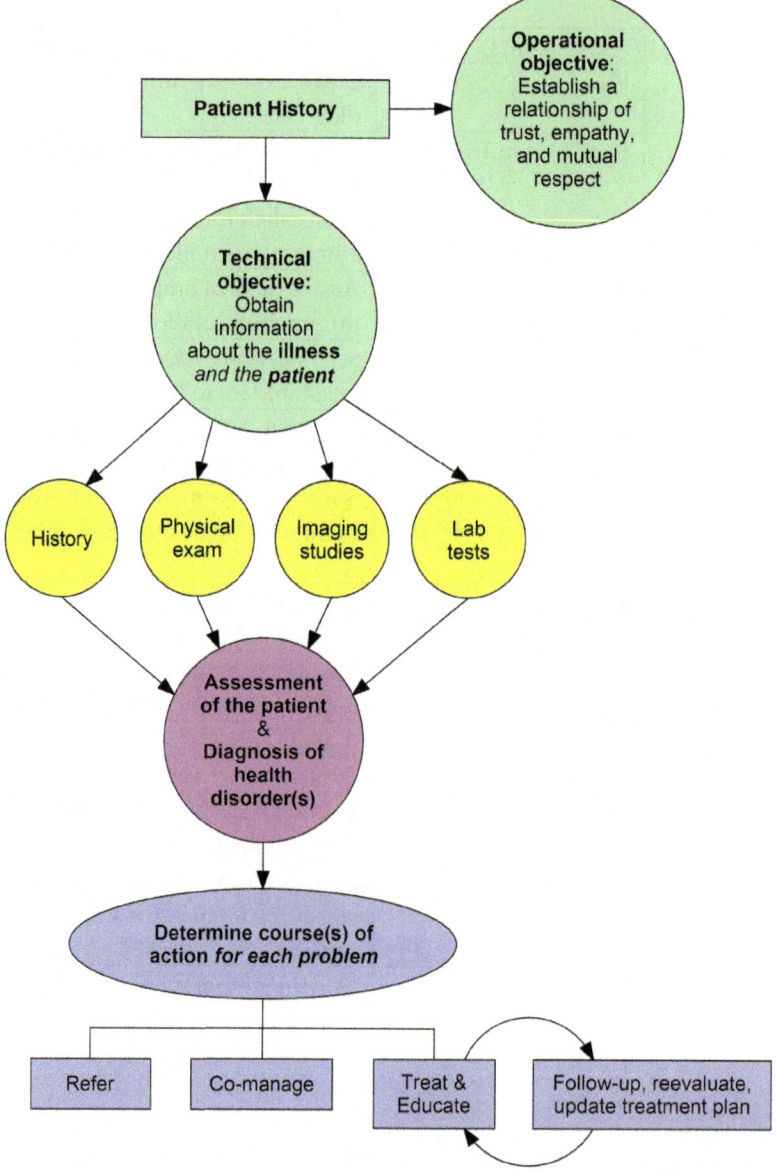

Musculoskeletal Emergencies

These are some of the "core competencies" that clinicians can never afford to miss, and these are pertinent to patients with musculoskeletal disorders, whether structural/orthopedic or metabolic/rheumatic. With these conditions, clinicians are wise to err on the side of caution— *"When in doubt, refer out"*—and implement the appropriate referral on an expedient (either urgent or emergency) basis. These are organized in a categorical/regional manner rather than listed alphabetically.

Neurovascular Disorders

Problem	Presentation	Assessment	Management
Neuropsychiatric lupus	<ul><li>Psychosis</li><li>Seizures</li><li>Transient ischemic attacks</li><li>Severe depression</li><li>Delirium, confusion</li></ul>	<ul><li>Neuropsychiatric manifestations with history of lupus</li></ul>	<ul><li>Emergency or prompt referral as indicated</li></ul>
Giant cell arteritis, Temporal arteritis: Considered a medical emergency since it may rapidly progress to blindness due to associated involvement of the ophthalmic artery: *"Loss of vision is the most feared manifestation and occurs quite commonly."*[375]	Presentation typically includes the following: <ul><li>Headache, scalp tenderness</li><li>Jaw claudication</li><li>Changes in vision</li><li>Systemic manifestations of rheumatic disease: fever, weight loss, muscle aches</li></ul>	<ul><li>Palpation of the temporal artery may reveal a "cord-like" artery</li><li>Elevated ESR</li><li>CBC may show anemia</li><li>Temporal artery biopsy is diagnostic</li></ul>	<ul><li>Standard medical treatment is with immediate prednisone</li><li>Implement treatment that is immediately effective or refer patient for medical treatment</li></ul>
Acute red eye: General term including acute iritis and scleritis; despite the name of this condition, redness may actually be rather minimal, and it is typically accompanied by cloudy changes in region of the iris and lens	<ul><li>Eye pain and redness</li><li>May have facial pain</li><li>May be the presenting manifestation of rheumatic disease</li></ul>	<ul><li>Red eye</li><li>Photophobia</li><li>Reduced vision</li><li>May have fixed pupil</li><li>Differential diagnosis includes acute glaucoma, bacterial/amebic/viral conjunctivitis or keratitis, allergy, and irritation due to contact lens</li></ul>	<ul><li>"The **acute** onset of a **painful**, **red** eye, even in the absence of visual upset, should be regarded primarily as an ophthalmological emergency."[376]</li><li>**Granulomatous uveitis** occurs in 15% of patients with sarcoidosis and can result in bilateral blindness—this must be managed as a medically urgent condition</li></ul>

---

[375] Tierney ML. McPhee SJ, Papadakis MA (eds). *Current Medical Diagnosis and Treatment, 41st Edition*. New York: Lange Medical; 2002. P999-1005
[376] McInnes I, Sturrock R. Rheumatological emergencies. *Practitioner*. 1994 Mar;238(1536):220-4

Neural canal compression

Problem	Presentation	Assessment	Management
Atlantoaxial instability: Excess mobility between the atlas and axis (commonly due to lesion of the dens or transverse ligament) makes the spinal cord vulnerable to compressive injury when the atlas translates anteriorly on the axis especially during cervical flexion; may progress to neurologic compromise including respiratory and somatic paralysis	▪ Post-traumatic neck injury ▪ Down's syndrome ▪ May present spontaneously (without trauma) in patients with inflammatory rheumatic disease, especially rheumatoid arthritis and ankylosing spondylitis ▪ May have gradual or sudden onset of myelopathy: upper motor neuron lesion (UMNL) signs (e.g., spastic weakness), changes in bowel-bladder function, numbness	▪ Clinical suspicion is followed by lateral cervical and APOM (anteroposterior open mouth) radiographs to assess ADI (atlantodental interval) and dens ▪ MRI should be performed in patients with suspected myelopathy ▪ Neurologic examination of the upper and lower extremities ▪ Do not force neck flexion; do not perform the Soto Hall test	▪ **Urgent neurosurgical consultation is recommended; stabilizing surgery is the best option for the prevention of neurologic catastrophes**[377] ▪ Onset of myelopathy mandates referral to ER and/or neurosurgeon; immobilize with spine board or hard cervical collar and transport appropriately ▪ Asymptomatic and mild increases in ADI (< 5mm) might be managed conservatively with activity restriction, exercises, and bracing/collars) ▪ PAR discussion and referral for surgical consultation is necessary for informed consent and safe management
Myelopathy, spinal cord compression or lesion: May occur due to infection, edema, tumor, spinal fracture, stenosis, or inflammatory disease	▪ **Spastic weakness** ▪ Bowel-bladder dysfunction ▪ Numbness ▪ Problems are distal to cord lesion	▪ Hyperreflexia ▪ Rigidity ▪ Muscle weakness ▪ MRI (with and without contrast) should be performed in patients with suspected myelopathy; CT may also be indicated	▪ Obtain MRI to confirm diagnosis ▪ Immobilize spine and transport if necessary ▪ Acute myelopathy is a medical emergency that can result in rapid-onset paralysis
Cauda equina syndrome: Compression of the sacral nerve roots due to lumbar disc herniation **Cauda equina syndrome is a surgical emergency.**	▪ History of sciatic low back pain ▪ Urinary retention, perineal numbness, and fecal incontinence are common ▪ May have lower extremity weakness	▪ Assess for bladder distention ▪ Assess anal sphincter strength with rectal exam ▪ Lower extremity neurologic examination	▪ Urgent referral for CT/MRI to confirm diagnosis ▪ If diagnosis is confirmed or strongly suspected clinically, urgent referral for surgical decompression is mandatory

---

[377] "When atlantoaxial stability is lost...it is thought that surgical stabilisation of the atlantoaxial joint is more reasonable and beneficial than conservative management. Minimal trauma of an unstable atlantoaxial joint can lead to serious neurological injury." Moon MS, Choi WT, Moon YW, Moon JL, Kim SS. Brooks' posterior stabilization surgery for atlantoaxial instability: review of 54 cases. *J Orthop Surg* (Hong Kong). 2002 Dec;10(2):160-4. josonline.org/PDF/v10i2p160.pdf

Acute peripheral nerve compression

Problem	Presentation	Assessment	Management
Acute compartment syndrome: acute onset of *potentially irreversible* muscle and/or nerve compression injury due to inflammation, swelling, or bleeding within a fascial compartment **Acute compartment syndrome is a surgical emergency.**	▪ Most commonly occurs in the anterior leg; may also occur in the posterior leg as well as forearm—these are the areas most notable anatomically for the investment of muscle in tight and resilient fascial sheaths ▪ Onset generally follows strenuous exercise that leads to reactive hyperemia and secondary edema ▪ May occur following trauma or fracture	Assess for: ▪ Pulselessness ▪ Palor ▪ Painful passive stretch ▪ Weakness ▪ **Numbness** ▪ Assessment and treatment should be performed on an emergency basis since irreversible nerve damage begins within 6 hours of intracompartmental hypertension	▪ Decompressive fasciotomy is the standard treatment for acute compartment syndrome that could result in permanent muscle necrosis and/or permanent nerve death ▪ Acute compartment syndrome can be fatal if rhabdomyolysis precipitates renal failure[378]

Musculoskeletal infections

Problem	Presentation	Assessment	Management
Septic arthritis: intraarticular bacterial infection; complications of septic arthritis are 1) articular destruction and 2) **death in 5-10% of patients**[379] **Septic arthritis is a medical emergency**	▪ **Febrile** patient has **acute/subacute mono/oligo-arthritis** ▪ Some patients may not have fever ▪ Other possible findings: Immuno-suppression due to medications, concomitant disease (RA, DM), elderly ▪ In some patients with concomitant disease or medications, the clinical picture can be blurred.	▪ **Warm, swollen, tender joint** ▪ Clinical assessment with **immediate referral for joint aspiration**, which reveals manifestations of infection such as WBC's and bacteria ▪ Differential diagnosis includes trauma, gout, CPPD, hemochromatosis	▪ **Immediate referral for joint aspiration** ▪ **An aggressive and prolonged course of IV and oral antimicrobials** ▪ "Immune support" such as vitamin A and glutamine and general measures to improve health and prevent recurrence
Osteomyelitis, infectious discitis: considered a medical emergency[380] **Osteomyelitis—especially vertebral osteomyelitis—is a medical emergency**	▪ Febrile patient with bone pain ▪ Assess for constitutional manifestations such as weight loss, night sweats, and malaise	▪ Exacerbation of bone pain when stress/percussion is applied to the bone ▪ Lab: CRP & WBC may be elevated ▪ MRI is more sensitive than CT, bone scan, or radiography[381]	▪ Emergency referral for vertebral osteomyelitis, since **up to 15% of patients will develop nerve lesions or cord compression**[382] ▪ Urgent referral for other types of osteomyelitis

[378] Paula R. Compartment Syndrome, Extremity. *eMedicine* June 22, 2006 emedicine.com/emerg/topic739.htm Accessed November 26, 2006
[379] Tierney ML. McPhee SJ, Papadakis MA. *Current Medical Diagnosis and Treatment. 35th edition*. Stamford: Appleton & Lange, 1996 page 759
[380] American College of Rheumatology Ad Hoc Committee on Clinical Guidelines. Guidelines for the initial evaluation of the adult patient with acute musculoskeletal symptoms. *Arthritis Rheum*. 1996;39(1):1-8. Also note my accompanying reply in *Arthritis Rheum*. 1996 Oct;39(10):1767-8
[381] Tierney ML. McPhee SJ, Papadakis MA (eds). *Current Medical Diagnosis and Treatment 2002, 41st Edition*. New York: Lange Medical; 2002. p 883
[382] King RW, Johnson D. Osteomyelitis. Updated July 13, 2006. *eMedicine* emedicine.com/emerg/topic349.htm Accessed Dec 24, 2006

Acute Nontraumatic Monoarthritis and Septic Arthritis

General Approach:

- "Acute monoarthritis is a potential medical emergency that must be investigated and treated promptly."[383]
- "Monoarthropathies should initially be investigated to exclude sepsis. ... Diagnostic joint aspiration ... should be carried out immediately."[384]
- "In acute monoarthritis, it is essential that infection of a joint be diagnosed or excluded, and this can only be done by joint aspiration and synovial fluid culture."[385]
- "Acute monoarthritis should be considered infectious until proven otherwise."[386]

Clinical presentations:

- Patient presents with acute joint pain in one joint (occasionally more than one joint may be involved).
- May or may not have fever and other systemic manifestations of infection.

> **Clinical Pearl**
>
> The primary goal of this section is to solidify your awareness of septic arthritis, its differential diagnoses, and the method and importance of assertive diagnosis and management.
>
> Septic arthritis is a medical emergency, and some authoritative textbooks report a mortality rate of 5-10%.
>
> Septic arthritis must be diagnosed urgently with joint aspiration, and it must be treated with antibiotics in order to preserve the joint and prevent spread of the infection.

Major Differential Diagnoses for Nontraumatic Monoarthritis

Problem	Presentation	Assessment & Management
Septic arthritis: intraarticular bacterial infection; complications of septic arthritis are 1) articular destruction and 2) **death in 5-10% of patients**[387]	• **Febrile** patient has **acute/subacute mono/oligo-arthritis** • **Onset over hours or days** Other possible findings: • Immuno-suppression due to medications, concomitant disease (RA, DM), elderly • Some patients may not have fever • In some patients with a previous or concomitant disease process, the clinical picture can be blurred	• **Warm, swollen, red, painful joint** • Clinical assessment with **immediate referral for joint aspiration**, which reveals characteristic manifestations of infection such as WBCs and bacteria • **Immediate joint aspiration** • An aggressive and prolonged course of IV and oral antimicrobials • "Immune support" and general measures to improve health and prevent recurrence

> **Septic arthritis is life-threatening**
>
> "Septic arthritis is still a life-threatening disease with a mortality of 2–5% and high morbidity."
>
> Zacher J, Gursche A. Regional musculoskeletal conditions: 'hip' pain. *Best Practice & Research Clinical Rheumatology*. 2003 Feb;17:71-85

---

[383] Cibere J. Rheumatology: 4. Acute monoarthritis. *CMAJ (Canadian Medical Association Journal)*. 2000;162(11):1577-83 cmaj.ca/cgi/content/full/162/11/1577 Jan 2004
[384] McInnes I, Sturrock R. Rheumatological emergencies. Practitioner. 1994 Mar;238(1536):220-4
[385] American College of Rheumatology Ad Hoc Committee on Clinical Guidelines. Guidelines for the initial evaluation of the adult patient with acute musculoskeletal symptoms. *Arthritis Rheum*. 1996 Jan;39(1):1-8
[386] Cibere J. Rheumatology: 4. Acute monoarthritis. CMAJ (*Canadian Medical Association Journal*). 2000;162(11):1577-83 cmaj.ca/cgi/content/full/162/11/1577 Jan 2004
[387] Tierney ML. McPhee SJ, Papadakis MA. *Current Medical Diagnosis and Treatment. 35th edition*. Stamford: Appleton and Lange, 1996 page 759

Major differential diagnoses for non-traumatic monoarthritis—*continued*

Problem	Presentation	Assessment & Management
Osteochondritis dissecans: A disorder of unclear etiology (trauma and/or avascular necrosis) which results in the death and subsequent fragmentation of subchondral bone[388]	▪ Primarily affects ages 10-30 years ▪ **Most common in the knees and elbows** ▪ Locking and crepitus due to intraarticular loose bodies ("joint mice") ▪ Some patients are almost asymptomatic, while others have acute pain ▪ Swelling of the affected joint	▪ Radiographs—consider to assess both knees as the condition is bilateral in 30% ▪ MRI is used to assess severity and need for surgical intervention ▪ Stable and nondisplaced lesions may be managed nonsurgically; larger and displaced fragments require surgical repair to reduce long-term complications[389]
Transient synovitis, irritable hip: Non-specific short-term inflammation and effusion of the hip joint	▪ Acute onset of painful hip and limp ▪ Decreased pain with hip in flexion and abduction ▪ Considered the most common cause of hip pain in children[390] ▪ More common in boys, age 3-6 years and generally younger than 10 years ▪ May have recent history of viral infection, and some children (1.5-10%) eventually manifest RA or AVN[391]	▪ May have slight elevation of ESR ▪ Normal WBC ▪ <u>No</u> fever; the child appears <u>healthy</u> ▪ "…radiography is indicated to exclude osseous pathological conditions…"[392] ▪ **Joint aspiration is indicated if septic arthritis is suspected**[393] ▪ Conservative treatment, restricted exertion and weight-bearing for several weeks
Legg-Calve-Perthe's disease: Idiopathic ischemic necrosis of the femoral head occurring in children **Avascular necrosis (AVN) of the femoral head, osteonecrosis**: Ischemic necrosis of the femoral head	Perthe's disease: ▪ 80% occur in children generally between ages of 4-9 years; more common in boys; may present with hip pain or knee pain AVN: ▪ Ages 20-40 years ▪ Unilateral hip pain ▪ May have knee pain ▪ History of trauma is common AVN associations: ▪ Steroid use, prednisone ▪ Hyperlipidemia ▪ Alcoholism ▪ Pancreatitis ▪ Hemoglobinopathies ▪ Smoking ▪ Fatty liver disease: "fat globules from the liver"[394]	▪ Limited ROM ▪ **Radiographs**; if normal and clinical suspicion is high order MRI or bone scan ▪ **Crutches** ▪ **Orthopedic referral is recommended** although not all patients will require surgery and some may be managed conservatively[395]

[388] Tatum R. Osteochondritis dissecans of the knee: a radiology case report. *J Manipulative Physiol Ther* 2000 Jun;23(5):347-51

[389] Browne RF, Murphy SM, Torreggiani WC, Munk PL, Marchinkow LO. Radiology for the surgeon: musculoskeletal case 30. Osteochondritis dissecans of the medial femoral condyle. *Can J Surg*. 2003;46(5):361-3 cma.ca/multimedia/staticContent/HTML/N0/l2/cjs/vol-46/issue-5/pdf/pg361.pdf

[390] Maroo S. Diagnosis of hip pain in children. *Hosp Med* 1999 Nov;60(11):788-93

[391] Souza TA. *Differential Diagnosis for the Chiropractor: Protocols and Algorithms*. Gaithersberg, Maryland: Aspen Publications. 1997 page 265

[392] Maroo S. Diagnosis of hip pain in children. *Hosp Med* 1999 Nov;60(11):788-93

[393] Maroo S. Diagnosis of hip pain in children. *Hosp Med* 1999 Nov;60(11):788-93

[394] Skinner HB, Scherger JE. Identifying structural hip and knee problems. *Postgrad Med* 1999;106(7):51-2, 55-6, 61-4

[395] Souza TA. *Differential Diagnosis for the Chiropractor: Protocols and Algorithms*. Gaithersberg, Maryland: Aspen Publications. 1997 page 263

Major differential diagnoses for non-traumatic monoarthritis—*continued*

Problem	Presentation	Assessment & Management
<u>Gout</u>	• **Febrile** patient has **acute/subacute mono/oligo-arthritis** • **Onset over hours or days** • "A history of discreet attacks, usually affecting one joint, that precede the onset of fixed symmetric arthritis is the major clue."[396] • May have fever, chills, tachycardia, leukocytosis—just like septic arthritis	• Clinical presentation may be sufficient for DX; however septic arthritis should be excluded • Serum uric acid is generally meaningless for the diagnosis of gout since many gout patients will have normal serum uric acid • Medical treatment is rest, NSAID's, and allopurinol • Fluid loading: >3 liters per day; monitor for electrolyte imbalances and hyponatremia as needed • Integrative assessment and treatment for insulin resistance, hormonal imbalances, and nutritional deficiencies
<u>CPPD</u>: Calcium pyrophosphate dihydrate deposition disease	• Idiopathic • May be caused by iron overload in some patients • Presentation may be acute or subacute	• Medical diagnosis is by synovial biopsy • Radiographs reveal chondrocalcinosis • Allopathic treatment is NSAIDs; phytonutritional anti-inflammatory treatments may also be used (see Chapter 3 of *Integrative Orthopedics/Rheumatology*) • Oral colchicine 0.5 to 1.5 mg per day prevents attacks[397]
<u>Hemarthrosis</u>: Generally associated with trauma, anticoagulation (i.e., coumadin), leukemia, hemophilia	• Monoarthralgia with limited motion • May follow direct trauma • Nontraumatic hemarthrosis may be due to anticoagulation, leukemia, hemophilia	• Synovial fluid analysis reveals blood • Treatment of underlying disorder; refer as indicated
<u>Slipped capital femoral epiphysis (SCFE)</u>: The most common cause of hip pain in adolescents[398]	• Seen in adolescents generally 8-17 years of age • Classic presentation is a tall overweight boy with **hip pain**, knee pain, and/or a painful limp: *"Slipped femoral capital epiphysis is a developmental injury that must be considered in any adolescent who presents with hip pain."*[399]	• **Radiographs** of both hips (bilateral SCFE in 40%): "AP and frog lateral views are recommended in all children over age of 9 years with hip pain."[400] • Orthopedic referral—"…the patient should be referred immediately to an orthopedist for surgical stabilization."[401]

[396] Hardin JG, Waterman J, Labson LH. Rheumatic disease: Which diagnostic tests are useful? *Patient Care* 1999; March 15: 83-102
[397] Beers MH, Berkow R (eds). *The Merck Manual. Seventeenth Edition*. Whitehouse Station; Merck Research Laboratories 1999 Page
[398] Maroo S. Diagnosis of hip pain in children. *Hosp Med* 1999 Nov;60(11):788-93
[399] O'Kane JW. Anterior hip pain. *Am Fam Physician* 1999 Oct 15;60(6):1687-96
[400] Maroo S. Diagnosis of hip pain in children. *Hosp Med* 1999 Nov;60(11):788-93
[401] O'Kane JW. Anterior hip pain. *Am Fam Physician* 1999 Oct 15;60(6):1687-96

Clinical assessment of non-traumatic monoarthritis:
- History and orthopedic assessment of the joint
- Laboratory assessments and joint aspiration should be performed with suspicion of infection

History/subjective:
- Acute or subacute joint pain with or without systemic manifestations and fever.
- History or may not be significant; other than the obvious risk factor of immunosuppression, septic arthritis can occur with impressive spontaneity and randomness

Differential physical examination and objective findings:
- **Septic arthritis**: pain and limitation of motion, swelling, redness; patient may have systemic symptoms of fever and malaise
- **Gout**: pain and limitation of motion, swelling, redness; patient may have systemic symptoms of fever and malaise
- **Pseudogout and calcium pyrophosphate dihydrate deposition disease (CPDD/CPPD)**: pain and limitation of motion, swelling, redness; patient may have systemic symptoms of fever and malaise
- **Ischemic necrosis**: pain and limitation of motion; swelling, redness and systemic symptoms are less likely.
- **Hemarthrosis**: pain and limitation of motion; often associated with trauma, use of anticoagulant medications[402], or hemophilia and other hematologic abnormalities[403]
- **Tumor**: assess with history, imaging, and biopsy if possible
- **Injury**: Meniscal injury, fracture, ligament injury; physical examination procedures are described in the chapters that follow

Imaging and laboratory assessments:
- **Septic arthritis**: joint aspiration; STAT CBC (for WBC count) and CRP
- **Gout**: joint aspiration; CBC (for WBC count) and CRP
- **Pseudogout and PPDD**: rule out septic arthritis with joint aspiration, CBC, and CRP; radiographs often show chondrocalcinosis
- **Ischemic necrosis**: radiographs are diagnostic
- **Hemarthrosis**: joint aspiration and assessment for underlying disease or medication, especially if the condition was not trauma-induced
- **Tumor**: assess with radiographs
- **Injury**: rule out infection; consider imaging with radiography or MRI.

Establishing the diagnosis:
- The aforementioned examinations and lab assessments should establish the exact diagnosis. **The priorities are 1) first exclude life-threatening illness (i.e., septic arthritis), then 2) to exclude serious injury or illness,** and finally 3) to help manage the exact problem.

Complications:
- **Septic arthritis can result in death in 5-10% of patients. "Five to 10 percent of patients with an infected joint die, chiefly from respiratory complications of sepsis. The mortality rate is 30% for patients with polyarticular sepsis. Bony ankylosis and articular destruction commonly also occur if the treatment is delayed or inadequate."[404]** Complications vary per location, infecting organism, severity, and patient.

---

[402] Riley SA, Spencer GE. Destructive monarticular arthritis secondary to anticoagulant therapy. *Clin Orthop*. 1987 Oct;(223):247-51

[403] Jean-Baptiste G, De Ceulaer K. Osteoarticular disorders of haematological origin. *Baillieres Best Pract Res Clin Rheumatol*. 2000 Jun;14(2):307-23

[404] Tierney ML. McPhee SJ, Papadakis MA. *Current Medical Diagnosis and Treatment. 35th edition*. Stamford: Appleton & Lange, 1996 page 759

Clinical management of non-traumatic monoarthritis:

- **Suspected septic arthritis requires referral for joint aspiration and antimicrobial drugs.**
- Referral if clinical outcome is unsatisfactory or if serious complications are evident.
- Treatment of other conditions that cause acute monoarthritis (such as gout and calcium pyrophosphate dihydrate deposition disease) is based on the problem and individual patient.

Treatments:

- **Septic arthritis requires IV/oral antimicrobial drugs:** Intravenous antibiotics are generally started before culture results are available. After results and culture from synovial fluid analysis have been considered, the dose, combination, and administration of antibiotics can be fine-tuned. Frequently, antibiotics are administered intravenously for at least 3-4 weeks. Surgical/endoscopic drainage/debridement and immobilization during the acute phase may also be implemented.[405]
- **Immunonutrition considerations:** Immunonutritional considerations are listed below; doses listed are for adults. Although studies have not been performed specifically in patients with bone/joint infections, general benefits derived from the use of immunonutrition are reductions in severity/frequency/duration of major infections, abbreviated hospitalization (i.e., early discharge due to expedited healing and recovery), reductions in the need for medications, significant improvements in survival, and hospital savings.[406,407,408,409,410,411,412]
  - Paleo-Mediterranean diet: as detailed later in this text and elsewhere[413,414]
  - Vitamin and mineral supplementation: anti-infective benefits shown in elderly diabetics[415]
  - High-dose vitamin A: Vitamin A shows potent immunosupportive benefits, and vitamin A stores are depleted by the stress of infection and injury. Consider 200,000-300,000 IU per day of retinol palmitate for 1-4 weeks, then taper; reduce dose or discontinue with onset of toxicity symptoms such as skin problems (dry skin, flaking skin, chapped or split lips, red skin rash, hair loss), joint pain, bone pain, headaches, anorexia (loss of appetite), edema (water retention, weight gain, swollen ankles, difficulty breathing), fatigue, and/or liver damage.
  - Arginine: Dose for adults is in the range of 5-10 grams daily
  - Fatty acid supplementation: In contrast to the higher doses used to provide an anti-inflammatory effect in patients with autoimmune/inflammatory disorders, doses used for immunosupportive treatments should be kept rather modest to avoid the *relative* immunosuppression that has been controversially

---

[405] Brusch JL. Septic Arthritis (Last Updated: October 18, 2005). *eMedicine*. emedicine.com/med/topic3394.htm Accessed Nov 25, 2006

[406] "To evaluate the metabolic and immune effects of dietary arginine, glutamine and omega-3 fatty acids (fish oil) supplementation, we performed a prospective study... CONCLUSIONS: The feeding of Neomune in critically injured patients was well tolerated as Traumacal and significant improvement was observed in serum protein. Shorten ICU stay and wean-off respirator day may benefit from using the immunonutrient formula." Chuntrasakul C, Siltham S, Sarasombath S, Sittapairochana C, Leowattana W, Chockvivatananvanit S, Bunnak A. Comparison of a immunonutrition formula enriched arginine, glutamine and omega-3 fatty acid, with a currently high-enriched enteral nutrition for trauma patients. *J Med Assoc Thai*. 2003 Jun;86(6):552-6

[407] "CONCLUSIONS: In conclusion, arginine-enhanced formula improves fistula rates in postoperative head and neck cancer patients and decreases length of stay." de Luis DA, Izaola O, Cuellar L, Terroba MC, Aller R. Randomized clinical trial with an enteral arginine-enhanced formula in early postsurgical head and neck cancer patients. *Eur J Clin Nutr*. 2004;58(11):1505-8

[408] "In this prospective, randomised, double-blind, placebo-controlled study, we randomly assigned 50 patients who were scheduled to undergo coronary artery bypass to receive either an oral immune-enhancing nutritional supplement containing L-arginine, omega3 polyunsaturated fatty acids, and yeast RNA (n=25), or a control (n=25) for a minimum of 5 days... Intake of an oral immune-enhancing nutritional supplement for a minimum of 5 days before surgery can improve outlook in high-risk patients who are undergoing elective cardiac surgery." Tepaske R, et al. Effect of preoperative oral immune-enhancing nutritional supplement on patients at high risk of infection after cardiac surgery: a randomised placebo-controlled trial. *Lancet*. 2001 Sep 1;358(9283):696-701

[409] "The feeding of IMMUNE FORMULA was well tolerated and significant improvement was observed in nutritional and immunologic parameters as in other immunoenhancing diets. Further clinical trials of prospective double-blind randomized design are necessary to address the so that the necessity of using immunonutrition in critically ill patients will be clarified." Chuntrasakul C, et al. Metabolic and immune effects of dietary arginine, glutamine and omega-3 fatty acids supplementation in immunocompromised patients. *J Med Assoc Thai*. 1998 May;81(5):334-43

[410] "enteral diet supplemented with arginine, dietary nucleotides, and omega-3 fatty acids (IMPACT, Sandoz Nutrition, Bern, Switzerland) " Senkal M, et al. Early postoperative enteral immunonutrition: clinical outcome and cost-comparison analysis in surgical patients. *Crit Care Med* 1997;25(9):1489-96

[411] "supplemented diet with glutamine, arginine and omega-3-fatty acids... It was clearly established in this trial that early postoperative enteral feeding is safe in patients who have undergone major operations for gastrointestinal cancer. Supplementation of enteral nutrition with glutamine, arginine, and omega-3-fatty acids positively modulated postsurgical immunosuppressive and inflammatory responses." Wu GH, Zhang YW, Wu ZH. Modulation of postoperative immune and inflammatory response by immune-enhancing enteral diet in gastrointestinal cancer patients. *World J Gastroenterol*. 2001 Jun;7(3):357-62 wjgnet.com/1007-9327/7/357.pdf

[412] "using a formula supplemented with arginine, mRNA, and omega-3 fatty acids from fish oil (Impact)... CONCLUSIONS: Immune-enhancing enteral nutrition resulted in a significant reduction in the mortality rate and infection rate in septic patients admitted to the ICU. These reductions were greater for patients with less severe illness." Galban C, Montejo JC, Mesejo A, Marco P, Celaya S, Sanchez-Segura JM, Farre M, Bryg DJ. An immune-enhancing enteral diet reduces mortality rate and episodes of bacteremia in septic intensive care unit patients. *Crit Care Med*. 2000 Mar;28(3):643-8

[413] Vasquez A. A Five-Part Nutritional Protocol that Produces Consistently Positive Results. *Nutritional Wellness* 2005 Sep. Reprinted and updated in Chapter 4.

[414] Vasquez A. Implementing the Five-Part Nutritional Wellness Protocol for the Treatment of Various Health Problems. *Nutritional Wellness* 2005 November. Reprinted and updated in Chapter 4.

[415] "CONCLUSIONS: A multivitamin and mineral supplement reduced the incidence of participant-reported infection and related absenteeism in a sample of participants with type 2 diabetes mellitus and a high prevalence of subclinical micronutrient deficiency." Barringer TA, Kirk JK, Santaniello AC, Foley KL, Michielutte R. Effect of a multivitamin and mineral supplement on infection and quality of life. A randomized, double-blind, placebo-controlled trial. *Ann Intern Med*. 2003 Mar;138:365-71 annals.org/cgi/reprint/138/5/365

reported in patients treated with EPA and DHA. Reasonable doses are in the following ranges for adults: EPA+DHA: 500-1,500, and GLA: 300-500 mg.

o Glutamine: Glutamine enhances bacterial killing by neutrophils[416], and administration of 18 grams per day in divided doses to patients in intensive care units was shown to improve survival, expedite hospital discharge, and reduce total healthcare costs.[417] Another study using glutamine 12-18 grams per day showed no benefit in overall mortality but significant benefits in terms of reduced healthcare costs (-30%) and significantly reduced need for medical interventions.[418] After administering glutamine 26 grams/d to severely burned patients, Garrel et al[419] concluded that glutamine reduced the risk of infection by 3-fold and that oral glutamine "may be a life-saving intervention" in patients with severe burns. A dose of 30 grams/d was used in a recent clinical trial showing hemodynamic benefit in patients with sickle cell anemia.[420] The highest glutamine dose that the current author is aware of is the study by Scheltinga et al[421] who used 0.57 gm/kg/day in cancer patients following chemotherapy administration; for a 220-lb-pt, this would be approximately 57 grams of glutamine per day.

o Melatonin: 20-40 mg hs (*hora somni*—Latin: sleep time). Immunostimulatory anti-infective action of melatonin was demonstrated in a small clinical trial wherein septic newborns administered 20 mg melatonin showed significantly increased survival over nontreated controls.[422]

---

[416] Furukawa et al. Glutamine-enhanced bacterial killing by neutrophils from postoperative patients. *Nutrition* 1997;13(10):863-9. *In vitro* study.

[417] Griffiths RD, Jones C, Palmer TE. Six-month outcome of critically ill patients given glutamine-supplemented parenteral nutrition. *Nutrition* 1997;13(4):295-302

[418] "There was no mortality difference between those patients receiving glutamine-containing enteral feed and the controls. However, there was a significant reduction in the median postintervention ICU and hospital patient costs in the glutamine recipients $23 000 versus $30 900 in the control patients." Jones C, Palmer TE, Griffiths RD. Randomized clinical outcome study of critically ill patients given glutamine-supplemented enteral nutrition. *Nutrition*. 1999 Feb;15(2):108-15

[419] The glutamine dose in this study was "a total of 26 g/day" administered in four divided doses. CONCLUSION: "The results of this prospective randomized clinical trial show that enteral G reduces blood culture positivity, particularly with P. aeruginosa, in adults with severe burns and may be a life-saving intervention." Garrel D, Patenaude J, Nedelec B, et al. Decreased mortality and infectious morbidity in adult burn patients given enteral glutamine supplements. *Crit Care Med*. 2003 Oct;31(10):2444-9

[420] Niihara Y, Matsui NM, Shen YM, et al. L-glutamine therapy reduces endothelial adhesion of sickle red blood cells to human umbilical vein endothelial cells. *BMC Blood Disord*. 2005 Jul 25;5:4 biomedcentral.com/1471-2326/5/4

[421] "Subjects with hematologic malignancies in remission underwent a standard treatment of high-dose chemotherapy and total body irradiation before bone marrow transplantation. After completion of this regimen, they were randomized to receive either standard parenteral nutrition (STD, n = 10) or an isocaloric, isonitrogenous nutrient solution enriched with crystalline L-glutamine (0.57 g/kg/day, GLN, n = 10)." Scheltinga MR, Young LS, Benfell K, Bye RL, Ziegler TR, Santos AA, Antin JH, Schloerb PR, Wilmore DW. Glutamine-enriched intravenous feedings attenuate extracellular fluid expansion after a standard stress. *Ann Surg*. 1991 Oct;214(4):385-93; discussion 393-5 pubmedcentral.nih.gov/articlerender.fcgi?tool=pubmed&pubmedid=1953094 For additional review, see Ziegler TR. Glutamine supplementation in cancer patients receiving bone marrow transplantation and high dose chemotherapy. J Nutr. 2001 Sep;131(9 Suppl):2578S-84S jn.nutrition.org/cgi/content/full/131/9/2578S

[422] Gitto E, et al. Effects of melatonin treatment in septic newborns. *Pediatr Res*. 2001;50:756-60 pedresearch.org/cgi/content/full/50/6/756

Naturopathic Medicine, Functional Medicine, Osteopathic Medicine, Chiropractic

Introduction

In these following sections, I provide some review and insights about each of the main integrative healthcare disciplines; these are distinguished by their relatively greater eclecticism contrasted to the narrow range of allopathic medicine, which relies almost exclusively on drugs and surgery and—again in contrast—requires greater passivity on the part of the clinician and the patient.

All institutions and professions have their shadow—that part that is disowned, denied, repressed; to appreciate the whole and maintain honesty and integrity, the totality should be appreciated, lest our apprehension and vision become and remain selective. This closing paragraph for each section will be further developed over the next few years. I might hope that readers were first familiarized with the concept of shadow during previous courses in Psychology, since the concept is well popularized after having originated from the work of the famous psychologist Carl Jung PhD who founded analytical psychology and introduced concepts such as *synchronicity*, *individuation*, *extraversion/extroversion*, *introversion*, *archetypes*, *collective unconscious*, and *shadow* into the psychological and social sciences and eventually common conversation. "In Jungian psychology, the shadow or "shadow aspect" may refer to 1) an unconscious aspect of the personality which the conscious ego does not identify in itself. Because one tends to reject or remain ignorant of the least desirable aspects of one's personality, the shadow is largely negative, or 2) the entirety of the unconscious, i.e., everything of which a person is not fully conscious. … "Everyone carries a shadow," Jung wrote, "and the less it is embodied in the individual's conscious life, the blacker and denser it is."[423]

---

[423] wikipedia.org/wiki/Shadow_(psychology) 2014

Naturopathic Medicine

"The work of the naturopathic physician is to elicit healing by helping patients to create or recreate conditions for health to exist within them. Health will occur where the conditions for health exist. Disease is the product of conditions which allow for it." Jared Zeff, ND[424]

The diagram on this page is derived from the review by Zeff published in 1997 in *Journal of Naturopathic Medicine* entitled "The process of healing: a unifying theory of naturopathic medicine." By my interpretation, the diagram is important for at least three reasons.

First, whereas the allopathic profession describes the genesis of most diseases as *idiopathic* and therefore [somehow] exclusively serviceable by drugs and surgery, the naturopathic profession describes disease processes as *multifactorial* and *logical* and therefore treatable by the skilled discovery and treatment of the underlying causes. Such underlying causes, which nearly always occur as a plurality, may vary mildly or significantly even within a group of patients with the same diagnosis.

Second, the diagram shows that the development of disease and the restoration of health are both *processes*. The restoration and retention of health requires *intentionality* and *tenacity* in lieu of the simplistic *miracle medicines* and *passive treatments* proffered by the pharmaceutical industry. Generally, disease does not arrive from outside; it is the result of one or more internal imbalances. Chronic illness is generally the result of manifold internal imbalances that culminate in numerous physiologic insults which compromise essential functions to the point that one or more organ systems begin to fail; we as patients and doctors generally label this as some specific "disease" or other, and the general—often erroneous—assumption has been that each *specific disease* (i.e., label, …abstraction, …conceptual entity) requires a *specific treatment* rather than a generalized health-restorative approach. Health is restored through a progressive and stepwise program that addresses as many facets of the illness as possible while vigorously supporting optimal physiologic function.

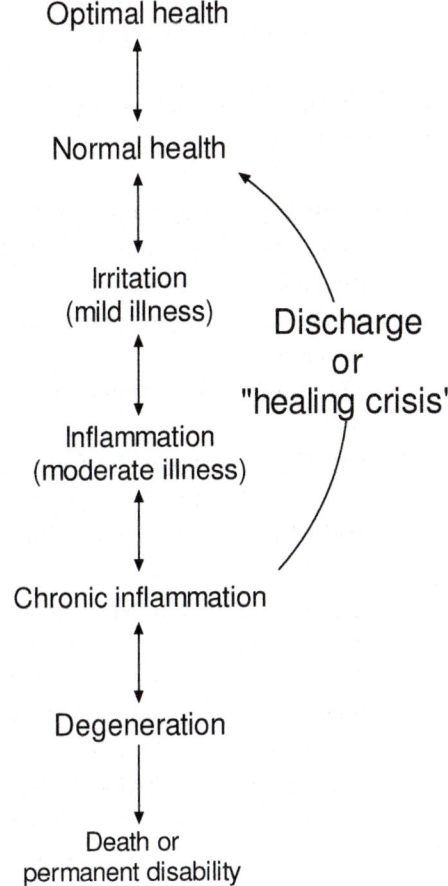

Third, the fact that Zeff considered the discharge or "healing crisis" so important that it merited inclusion in this diagram shows, indirectly, the naturopathic emphasis on detoxification and the eradication of dysbiosis. Both in the treatment of toxic metal/chemical exposure and in the treatment of chronic infections, patients often go through an acute or subacute phase of feeling ill before experiencing a dramatic alleviation of symptoms; the fact that symptoms may temporarily "get worse before getting better" has been referred to as the "healing crisis." This can occur for at least three reasons. First, in the elimination of chemicals and metals from the body, they must first be released from the tissues; the transition from tissues to blood is similar to a subacute re-exposure which triggers symptoms of toxicity until the toxin is excreted via sweat, urine, bile, or breath. Similarly, improvement in nutritional status—a cornerstone of all naturopathic interventions—expedites/facilitates/restores physiologic processes that have been relatively dormant due to lack of enzymatic cofactors such as vitamins and minerals[425]; optimization of nutritional status provides an opportunity for these pathways (such as detoxification of stored xenobiotics) to function again at which time they must "catch up" on work that has not been performed during the time of nutritional deficiency. The activation of these pathways is an essential step toward health restoration but results in an initial upregulation of hepatic phase-1/oxidative biotransformation which often results in the formation of reactive intermediates that temporarily impair physiologic processes and cause an initial exacerbation of symptoms. Third, whether through immunorestoration or the use of botanical/pharmacologic antimicrobial

---

[424] Zeff JL. The process of healing: a unifying theory of naturopathic medicine. *Journal of Naturopathic Medicine* 1997; 7: 122-5
[425] Ames BN. The metabolic tune-up: metabolic harmony and disease prevention. *J Nutr*. 2003 May;133(5 Suppl 1):1544S-8S

agents, the symptom-exacerbating "die off" reaction—classically called the Jarisch-Herxheimer reaction in the context of treating syphilis—is a result of increased (endo)toxin production/release by bacteria/microbes in response effective antimicrobial processes, whether physiologic or pharmacologic.

Modern naturopathic medicine has grown from deeply rooted European healing traditions reaching back several centuries. Naturopathic physicians have unwaveringly demonstrated respect, love, and appreciation for the healing powers of nature and the process of life itself.[426] Following their coursework in the basic biomedical sciences, naturopathic physicians are trained in urology, oncology, neurology, pediatrics, obstetrics and gynecology, urology, manual physical manipulation (including spinal manipulation), minor surgery, medical procedures, professional ethics, therapeutic diets, clinical and interventional nutrition, botanical medicines, psychological counseling, environmental medicine, and other modalities. Licensed naturopathic physicians commonly practice as generalists and family doctors.[427,428,429,430]

Naturopathic Principles, Concepts, & the *Vis Medicatrix Naturae*

> **Vis Medicatrix Naturae:
> the healing power of nature**
>
> "The healing power of nature is the inherent self-organizing and healing process of living systems… It is the naturopathic physician's role to support, facilitate and augment this process by identifying and removing obstacles to health and recovery, and by supporting the creation of a healthy internal and external environment."[431]

1. **First, Do No Harm (*Primum Non Nocere*)**: Naturopathic physicians use good judgment and compassion to ensure that the treatment does not cause harm to the patient. This contrasts with the effects of allopathic treatment, which collectively kill more than 180,000-220,000 patients per year, at least 493 American patients per day.[432]

2. **Identify and Treat the Causes (*Tolle Causam*)**: "*Illness does not occur without cause.*" Naturopathic physicians focus on identifying and addressing the underlying deficiency, toxicity, impairment, or imbalance that is the cause of the health problem or disease.

3. **Treat the Whole Person**: "*The multifactorial nature of health and disease requires a personalized and comprehensive approach to diagnosis and treatment.*" On some occasions the illness does take precedence over the person who has it—such in emergency situations like septic arthritis, acute ischemia, and pulmonary edema. In these cases, the situation must be managed appropriately, and these situations are not immediately amenable to long-term lifestyle changes—they require immediate treatment. However, the vast majority of cases in routine outpatient clinical practice will require detailed and bipartite attention to the facets of both **the disease process** and **the person who has the illness**. Our focus as naturopathic physicians on the individual patient is what sets our healing profession apart from others that focus exclusively on the disease and do not consider the manifold intricacies of the individual patient.

4. **The Healing Power of Nature: *Vis Medicatrix Naturae***: Naturopathic medicine recognizes an inherent self-healing process in the person that is ordered and intelligent. The body has many highly efficient mechanisms for sustaining and regaining health. These mechanisms have their specific and necessary components (e.g., nutrients) and means by which they can be impaired (e.g., xenobiotic immunosuppression). Poor health and disease can result from impairment of these self-healing processes and biologic mechanisms, and thus the body's inherent, natural, self-healing mechanisms—the "healing power of nature"—can be diminished to the state of ineffectiveness or harm (e.g., autoimmunity). Recognizing that the body has this inherent goal of and movement toward self-healing, naturopathic physicians start by identifying and removing "obstacles to cure" rather than ignoring these factors and masking the manifestations of dysfunction with symptom-suppressing drugs.

[426] Kirchfeld F, Boyle W. *Nature Doctors: Pioneers in Naturopathic Medicine*. Portland, Oregon; Medicina Biologica (Buckeye Naturopathic Press, East Palestine, Ohio), 1994

[427] Boon HS, et al. Practice patterns of naturopathic physicians: results from a random survey of licensed practitioners in two US States. *BMC Complement Altern Med*. 2004;4:14

[428] Smith MJ, Logan AC. Naturopathy. *Med Clin North Am*. 2002 Jan;86(1):173-84

[429] Cherkin DC, et al. Characteristics of visits to licensed acupuncturists, chiropractors, massage therapists, and naturopathic physicians. *J Am Board Fam Pract*. 2002;15:463-72

[430] Cherkin DC, et al. Characteristics of licensed acupuncturists, chiropractors, massage therapists, and naturopathic physicians. *J Am Board Fam Pract*. 2002 Sep-Oct;15:378-90

[431] Quoted from the American Association of Naturopathic Physicians website aanp.net/Basics/h.naturo.philo.html on February 4, 2001. Other italicized quotes in this section are from the same source. This website has since been replaced by naturopathic.org/

[432] "Recent estimates suggest that each year more than 1 million patients are injured while in the hospital and approximately 180,000 die because of these injuries. Furthermore, drug-related morbidity and mortality are common and are estimated to cost more than $136 billion a year." Holland EG, Degruy FV. Drug-induced disorders. *Am Fam Physician*. 1997;56(7):1781-8, 1791-2

5. **Prevention**: Healthy lifestyle, proper nutrition, and emotional hygiene go a long way toward preventing (and treating) most conditions. Specific conditions have specific risk factors and causes that have to be considered per patient and condition.

> **Physician, heal thyself.**
> _____
> "Physician, heal thyself; thus you help your patient, too.
> Let this be his best medicine
> that he beholds with his eyes:
> the doctor who heals himself."
>
> Nietzsche FW. *Thus Spoke Zarathustra* (1892). [Kaufmann W, translator]. Viking Penguin: 1954, page 77

6. **Doctor as Teacher (*Docere*)**: Naturopathic physicians explain the situation and the proposed solution to the patient so that the patient is empowered with understanding and with the comfort of knowing what has happened, what is happening, and the proposed course of upcoming events. Naturopathic physicians strive to let their own lives serve as a models for our patients. This does not mean that naturopathic doctors have to feign perfection; the task is to live the best and most conscious life that we can, to be present with our emotions, qualities, and faults and to treat ourselves with respect and acceptance. We can exemplify health (rather than perfection) to our patients by being who we authentically are and by so doing we can facilitate their own acceptance of their current health situation, which is a prerequisite to self-initiated change.

7. **Re-Establish the Foundation for Health**: An overview of this important naturopathic concept is provided throughout this chapter.

8. **Removing "obstacles to cure"**: *examples*

Obstacle to the optimization of health	Example of possible intervention
Toxic exposures, medication side-effects	Reduce drug use and dependency
Toxic relationships, emotional obstacles, past events, unfulfilling occupation,	Improve self-esteem, develop conflict resolution skills, determine life goals and values and a plan for their pursuit
Social isolation: the typical American has only two friends no-one in whom to confide[433]	Encourage social interaction
Diet with excess fat, arachidonate, sugar, additives, colorants, and insufficiency of protein, fiber, phytonutrients, and health-promoting fatty acids: ALA, GLA, EPA, DHA, and oleic acid	Diet improvement and nutritional supplementation
Sedentary lifestyle, lack of exercise	Encourage exercise
Weight gain/loss as necessary for weight optimization	Encourage self-valuing
Epidemic exposure to mercury, lead, and xenobiotics	Support detoxification process as a lifestyle; what we see these days is an increasing number of conditions complicated/caused by mitochondrial dysfunction induced by xenobiotics

Hierarchy of Therapeutics: This naturopathic concept articulates the importance of addressing *the underlying cause* rather than simply focusing on *the presenting problem*, which is the *symptom of the cause*. Further, interventions are **prioritized**, *for example*:

- Patient-implemented *before* doctor-implemented.
- Removal of harming agent *before* addition of a therapeutic agent: e.g., stop smoking *before* investing in respiratory therapy; implement healthy diet and exercise before higher-risk and higher-cost drugs for hypertension and hypercholesterolemia.
- Low-force interventions *before* high-force interventions.
- Generally: Diet *before* nutritional supplements; nutrients *before* botanicals; botanicals *before* drugs; modulatory drugs *before* suppressive/inhibitory drugs; integrative care *before* surgery.
- *See examples below.*

---

[433] McPherson M, Smith-Lovin L, Brashears ME. Social Isolation in America: Changes in Core Discussion Networks over Two Decades. *American Sociological Review* 2006; 71: 353-75 asanet.org/galleries/default-file/June06ASRFeature.pdf

Hierarchy of Therapeutics (specifically sequential)	Example of possible intervention
1. Reestablishing the foundation for health	• Mental/emotional/spiritual health • Meditation, freeze-frame, "time out", relaxation • Positive visualization, positive expectation, affirmation • Counseling, social contact, group work • Family contact and resolution • Dietary intake and nutritional health which addresses the patient's biochemical individuality[434] and correction of deficiencies or excesses • Identification and elimination of food allergies/sensitivities • Reduce toxin exposure, promote detoxification • Identification and elimination of exposure to xenobiotics • Remove or reduce specific "obstacles to cure"
2. Stimulation of the "healing power of nature" and the "vital force"	• Constitutional hydrotherapy • Homeopathy, Botanical adaptogens • Tai Chi, Qigong: "energy-cultivation" • Acupuncture, Spinal manipulation • Meditation, rest
3. Tonification of weakened systems	• Botanical medicines and nutritional supplementation to help restore normal cellular/tissue function • Spinal manipulation to address the primary somatovisceral dysfunction and/or secondary musculoskeletal disorders • Hormonal supplementation, exercise, hydrotherapy
4. Correction of structural integrity	• Spinal manipulation, deep tissue massage, visceral manipulation, lymphatic pump to promote immune surveillance[435], stretching, balancing, muscle strengthening, and proprioceptive retraining • Surgery, as a last resort

The shadow of the naturopathic profession: I would say that the weakness of the naturopathic profession is simply that—its lack of power *internally* to translate to power *externally*. Naturopathic physicians are few in number, and their incomes do not rival those of allopathic/osteopathic physicians (and thus cannot collectively afford powerful state organizations and paid lobbyists as can allopathic-pharmaceutical groups); they do not have the cultural authority of allopathic physicians, and they do not have the *carte blanche* backing of the pharmaceutical industry, whose financial power and thus political influence are both massive in the United States.[436] Naturopathic physicians have faced in the past and continue to face in recent/current times opposition/oppression by groups such as the AMA whose deep pockets and political contacts are used for legal/legislative initiatives such as marshalling "the medical community's resources against the growing threat of expanding scope of practice for allied health professionals."[437] The

> **Physician-philosophers of the future**
>
> "*Where must we reach with our hopes*? We have no option: we must reach for new philosophers, for those spirits strong and original enough to provide the stimuli for an opposing way of estimating current values [seeing things anew] and to initiate a revaluation and [if necessary] reversal of 'eternal values'."
>
> Nietzsche FW. *Beyond Good and Evil: Prelude to a Philosophy of the Future* (1886). Essay #203. Cambridge Texts in the History of Philosophy, page 91

---

[434] Williams RJ. *Biochemical Individuality: The Basis for the Genetotrophic Concept*. Austin and London: University of Texas Press, 1956

[435] "Lymph flow in the thoracic duct increased from 1.57±0.20 mL·min-1 to a peak TDF of 4.80±1.73 mL·min-1 during abdominal pump, and from 1.20±0.41 mL·min-1 to 3.45±1.61 mL·min-1 during thoracic pump." Knott EM, Tune JD, Stoll ST, Downey HF. Increased lymphatic flow in the thoracic duct during manipulative intervention. *J Am Osteopath Assoc*. 2005 Oct;105(10):447-56 jaoa.org/cgi/content/full/105/10/447

[436] This is only one of many documented examples. "The legislation was the cornerstone of Republican's domestic agenda and would extend limited prescription drugs coverage under Medicare to 41 million Americans, including 13 million who had never been covered before. At an estimated cost of just under $400 billion over 10 years, it was the largest entitlement program in more than 40 years, and the debate broke down along party lines." Under the Influence: Steve Kroft Reports On Drug Lobbyists' Role in Passing Bill That Keeps Drug Prices High cbsnews.com/news/under-the-influence/ Originally broadcast on April 1, 2007, updated on July 23, 2007. 2014 Jun

[437] "In an effort to marshal the medical community's resources against the growing threat of expanding scope of practice for allied health professionals, the AMA has formed a national partnership to confront such initiatives nationwide... The committee will use $25,000..." Daly R, American Psychiatric Association. AMA Forms Coalition to Thwart Non-M.D. Practice Expansion. Psychiatric News 2006 March; 41: 17 pn.psychiatryonline.org/cgi/content/full/41/5/17-a?eaf Accessed November 25, 2006

nutritional supplement and whole foods industries have failed to provide adequate support for the naturopathic profession in proportion to the increase in nutrition supplement sales and the public's increasing appreciation for *and purchase of* whole and organic foods, both of which have been supported by the naturopathic profession. Naturopathic schools are not without some occasional administrative incompetence and political pettiness; notable events during 2013 within two schools caused the unnecessary loss of intellectual power and internationally-respected irreplaceable academic/clinical/intellectual leadership from the profession in ways that clearly violate the profession's social, humanitarian, and intellectual values, despite administrative declarations to the opposite. Overall, the naturopathic profession continues to make positive albeit slow progress. Because the naturopathic profession's philosophy of healthcare stems from and extends back to life itself, naturopathic medicine is, at present and without any legitimate question, the only philosophy and model of primary healthcare (contrasted to allopathic and osteopathic) capable of salvaging, reforming, and optimizing healthcare outcomes in particular and human life in general.

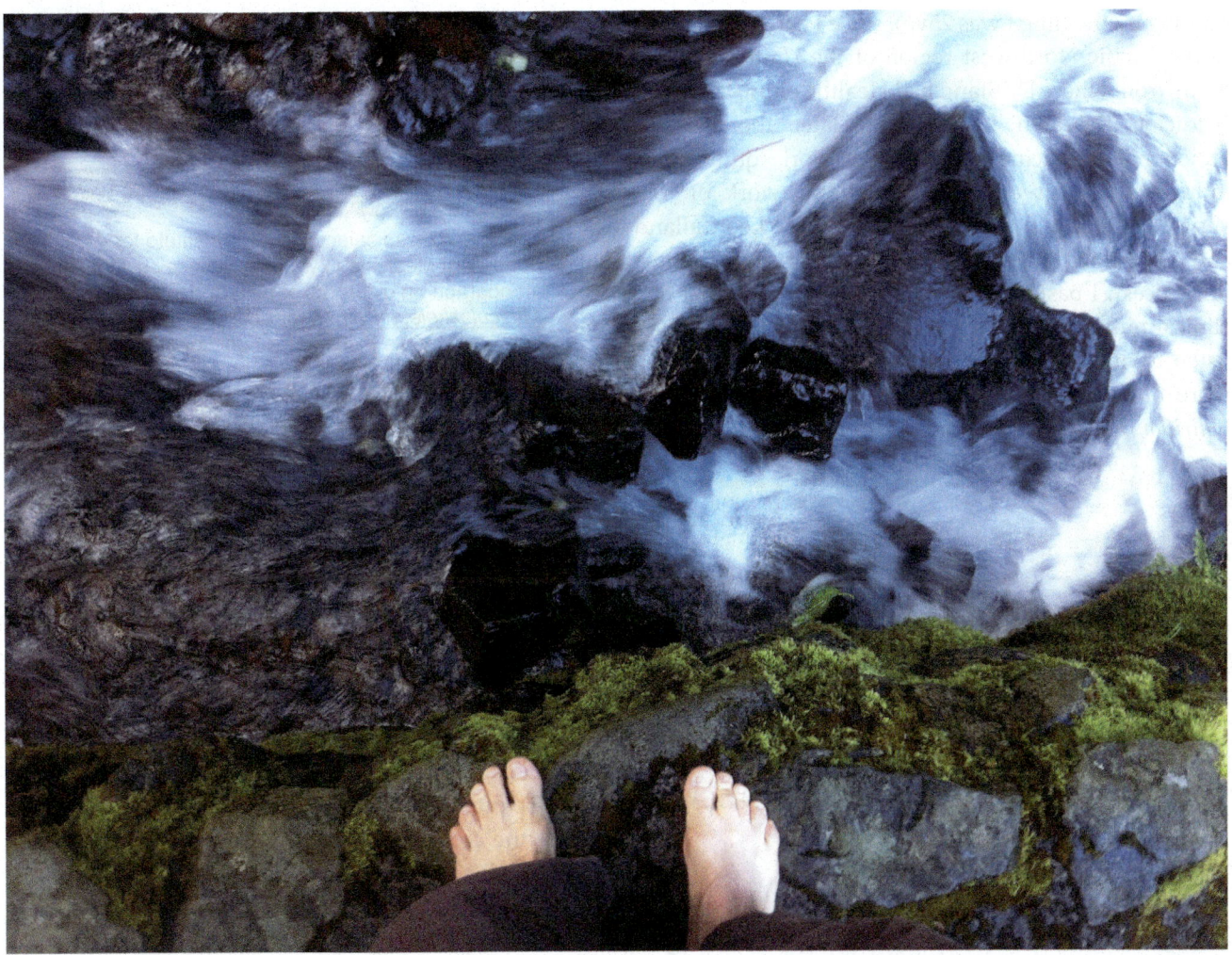

Barefoot physician (Wahkeena Falls, Oregon): "Let us spend one day as deliberately as Nature, and not be thrown off the track by every nutshell and mosquito's wing that falls on the rails [train tracks]. Let us rise early and fast, or let us break the fast gently and without perturbation; let company come and let company go, let the bells ring and the children cry—determined to make a day of it. Why should we knock under and go with the stream? ... Let us settle ourselves, and work and wedge our feet downward through the mud and slush of opinion, and prejudice, and tradition, and delusion, and appearance, that alluvion which covers the globe, through Paris and London, through New York and Boston and Concord, through Church and State, through poetry and philosophy and religion, until we come to a hard bottom and rocks in place, which we can call *reality*." Thoreau HD. *Walden*. 1854

Functional Medicine

Introduction and personal experiences/perspectives: "Functional Medicine" as most of us know and appreciate it was developed from initial concepts that spawned from the genius of Dr Jeffrey Bland, a PhD biochemist drawn into the world of nutrition by a project of one of his graduate students, and who later made many paradigm-shifting contributions to the fields of clinical biochemistry and clinical practice of physicians world-wide. I (DrV) consider myself to have been a student and apprentice of Dr Bland starting in 1994, when I started attending his *Nutritional Biochemistry* presentations (vicariously, via audio cassettes) and every post-graduate conference and symposium I could attend, which was a considerable number (more than 300 hours of post-graduate training by the time I was 25yo), since I had by then relocated to the Pacific Northwest region of the United States, a few hours from where Dr Bland had HealthComm, the Functional Medicine Research Center, and later the Institute for Functional Medicine. Dr Bland's work quite obviously influenced me greatly, along with the work of Jonathan Wright MD (also in the Pacific Northwest), Leo Galland MD, and especially Alan Gaby MD; under their "nutritional influences", I basically "grew up" in an intellectual house of clinical nutrition and functional medicine. I would basically listen to audios of their lectures constantly, until the tapes wore out. Dr Bland's presentation *Advancement in Clinical Nutrition* in 1994 (cherished audio cassette pictured below)

A Functional Medicine Monograph

MUSCULOSKELETAL PAIN:
Expanded Clinical Strategies

Alex Vasquez, DC, ND

THE INSTITUTE FOR FUNCTIONAL MEDICINE

Dr Vasquez was selected by the Institute for Functional Medicine to write its peer-reviewed CME monograph on disorders of pain and inflammation: *Musculoskeletal Pain: Expanded Clinical Strategies*, published by the Institute for Functional Medicine in 2008. Parts of this section were originally derived from the pre-edited draft of the introduction to that book, and any variations are used here with permission. Modifications were made to this section during revisions in 2011 and again in 2014. *Musculoskeletal Pain* contained an introduction to functional medicine and a review of assessments and therapeutics, followed by the clinical topics: migraine headaches, fibromyalgia, back pain, and rheumatoid arthritis. As would be expected, all of these topics have been discussed to a higher level of detail in more recent editions of *Integrative Orthopedics* (3rd Edition and later), *Integrative Rheumatology* (3rd Edition and later), *Fibromyalgia in a Nutshell* (2012), and the *Inflammation Mastery* series starting in 2014.

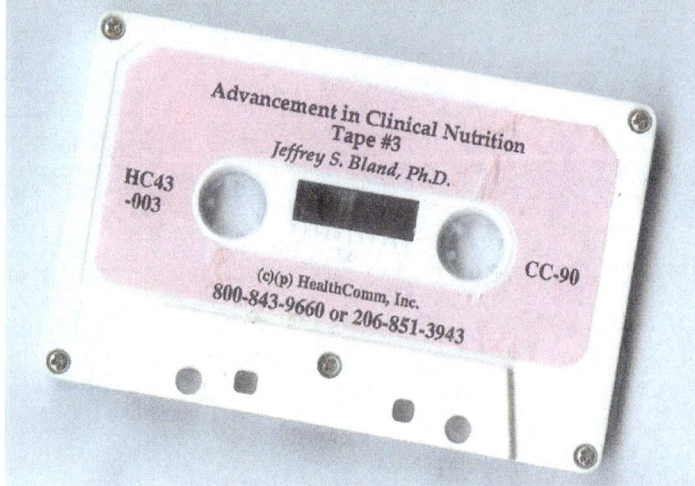

struck me with particular profundity; I listened to it so often that I had parts of it memorized because of the combination of verbal eloquence for which Dr Bland is famous and for the intellectual independence and lucidity with which Dr Bland articulated a new vision for medicine: that of moving beyond the *static* pathology-based models of disease toward appreciating illnesses as disorders of impaired *function*. Most people familiar with my work know that nutritional biochemistry and functional medicine are best described as my second interests following psychology and philosophy; indeed, I spent most of any "free time" during my 20s while completing two consecutive doctorates engaged with athletics, philosophy/psychology, and functional nutrition/medicine. The combination(s) of studying Gaby, Wright, Bland, Galland simultaneously with Rollins, Nietzsche, Bradshaw, Bly, Hillman, Lee, Meade, Kipnis, Moore, Miller, Deida, Branden, professionals and various personal groups gave me a unique view of health(care) and human potential; what appeared clear and obvious from these eclectic viewpoints was unknown or unspeakable among the majority of professors and students in the classes and clinics where I studied and learned.

Dr Bland's declaration that health and disease are *dynamic states of function* and *not static states of determinism* is powerful because Dr Bland uniquely had the ability to communicate his model with articulate clarity and the scientific knowledge to support every component. His model of *health as a dynamic entity* clearly opposed the static Pathology-based view of disease upon which allopathic medicine is founded: generally that disease states are constant and require life-long drug treatment (or surgery). The idea that clinicians should focus on improving *dynamic* function (mostly via nutrition and lifestyle) rather than treating *static* disease (always with drugs and surgery) was about as radical in Western medicine as analogous scientific landmarks such as the earth is round (Aristotle, et al), that the sun is the center of our planetary system (Aristarchus, Copernicus, Galileo), the evolution and interconnection of species (Darwin), and the denial of metaphysics and affirmation of earthly life (Nietzsche).

Evolution of medicine, from metaphysical determinism to dynamic molecular biology: Historically, prevailing views of disorders of pain and inflammation were conceptually similar to those of most other diseases and premodern accounts of life in general. Our clinical predecessors did the best they could to understand, describe, and treat the health problems with which their patients presented, and the paradigms from which these clinical entities were viewed and addressed were shaped by the social, religious, and scientific views and limitations of their time. Lacking a molecular and physiologic understanding of disease origination, and restrained by metaphysical and simplistic models of "cause and effect", premodern clinicians devised models for the understanding and treatment of disease that generally appear unsatisfactory today in light of the advances in our understanding in disparate yet interrelated fields such as psychoneuroimmunology, molecular biology, nutrigenomics, environmental medicine and toxicology. Despite these advances, we as a human society and as healthcare providers still carry many of these previous conceptualizations and misconceptualizations with us as we move forward toward a future wherein our views and interventions will be much more precise and "objective" in contrast to the generalized and phenomenalistic approaches that typified premodern medicine and which still permeate certain aspects of clinical care today. For example, we still use the term "stroke" to describe acute cerebrovascular insufficiency, although the term originated from the view that affected patients had been "struck" by the gods or fates perhaps as a form of punishment for some ethical or religious transgression. Even today, patients and clinicians commonly interpret disease as some form of punishment or as an extension of spiritual or intrapersonal shortcoming. Advancing science allows us to disassemble complex events that were previously experienced as *phenomena*, that is, as undecipherable and enigmatic events that overwhelmed comprehension. Dr Bland's functional medicine concept and the clinical tools that were developed from it began the process of helping clinicians grasp a science-based and systems-based multidimensional and decipherable view of diseases and corresponding treatments; as such, it has facilitated the achievement of higher clinical efficacy, improved patient outcomes, and more favorable safety and cost-effectiveness profiles.

Whereas the advancement of our scientific knowledge often leads us to discard previous models and interventions, occasionally modern science helps us to understand and revisit previous interventions that may have been prematurely or unduly discarded. For example, Hippocrates' admonition to "Let thy food be thy medicine, and thy medicine be thy food" experienced decades of devaluation when dietary, nutritional, and other natural interventions were misbranded as "quackery." On the contrary to these premature and unsubstantiated condemnations, simple natural interventions such as therapeutic fasting and augmentation of vitamin D3 status (via nutritional supplementation or exposure to ultraviolet-B radiation) have shown remarkable safety and efficacy in the mitigation of chronic hypertension, musculoskeletal pain, and autoimmunity.[438,439,440,441,442,443,444,445,446] Relatedly, newer research has also shown that the appropriate use of vitamin supplementation helps prevent

[438] Goldhamer A, et al. Medically supervised water-only fasting in the treatment of hypertension. *J Manipulative Physiol Ther* 2001 Jun;24(5):335-9
[439] Goldhamer AC, et al. Medically supervised water-only fasting in the treatment of borderline hypertension. *J Altern Complement Med*. 2002 Oct;8(5):643-50
[440] Goldhamer AC. Initial cost of care results in medically supervised water-only fasting for treating high blood pressure and diabetes. *J Altern Complement Med* 2002 Dec;8:696-7
[441] Krause R, Bühring M, Hopfenmüller W, Holick MF, Sharma AM. Ultraviolet B and blood pressure. *Lancet*. 1998 Aug 29;352(9129):709-10
[442] Pfeifer et al. Effects of a short-term vitamin D(3) and calcium supplementation on blood pressure and parathyroid hormone. *J Clin Endocrinol Metab*. 2001 Apr;86(4):1633-7
[443] McCarty MF. Preliminary fast may potentiate response to a subsequent low-salt, low-fat vegan diet in management of hypertension. *Med Hypotheses*. 2003 May;60(5):624-33
[444] Hyppönen E, Läärä E, Reunanen A, Järvelin MR, Virtanen SM. Intake of vitamin D and risk of type 1 diabetes: a birth-cohort study. *Lancet*. 2001 Nov 3;358(9292):1500-3
[445] Fuhrman J, et al. Brief case reports of medically supervised, water-only fasting associated with remission of autoimmune disease. *Altern Ther Health Med*. 2002;8:112,110-1
[446] Holick MF. Vitamin D deficiency: what a pain it is. *Mayo Clin Proc*. 2003 Dec;78(12):1457-9

chronic disease by numerous mechanisms including modulation of gene transcription, enhancement of DNA repair and stability, and enhancement of metabolic efficiency.[447,448,449]

While all clinicians can appreciate the importance of protocols and clinical practice guidelines, we must also perpetually ratify the preeminence of patient individuality and therefore the importance of tailoring treatment to the patient's unique combination of biochemical individuality, comorbid conditions, drug use, personal goals, and willingness to participate in a health-promoting lifestyle. Standardized protocols and practice guidelines are founded on the fallacy of disease homogeneity and the irrelevance of physiologic, psychosocial, and biochemical individuality.

A clinician who is unaware of the political forces that shape healthcare policy and research is analogous to a captain of an oceangoing ship not knowing how to use a compass, sextant, or coastline map. Medical science and healthcare policy are influenced by a myriad of powerful private interests which are motivated by their own goals, at times different from the stated goals of medicine, which purports to hold paramount the patient's welfare. Scientific objectivity and the guiding ethical principles of informed consent, beneficence, autonomy, and non-malfeasance are subject to different interpretations depending upon the lens through which a dilemma is viewed. When this "dilemma" is the whole of healthcare, what first appears as order and structure now appears as the disarrayed tug-of-war between factions and private interests, with paradigmatic victory often being awarded to those with the best marketing campaigns and political influence with less importance given to safety, efficacy, and the economic burden to consumers.[Compilation footnote 450] To be ignorant of such considerations is to be blind to the nature of research, policy, and our own biased inclinations for and against particular paradigms, assessments, and interventions. Research articles and sources of authority must be approached with an artist's delicacy, and with a

---

[447] Fletcher RH, Fairfield KM. Vitamins for chronic disease prevention in adults: clinical applications. *JAMA*. 2002 Jun 19;287(23):3127-9

[448] Heaney RP. Long-latency deficiency disease: insights from calcium and vitamin D. *Am J Clin Nutr*. 2003 Nov;78(5):912-9

[449] Ames BN. The metabolic tune-up: metabolic harmony and disease prevention. *J Nutr*. 2003 May;133(5 Suppl 1):1544S-8S

[450] Supporting citations include all of the following: Editorial. Drug-company influence on medical education in USA. *Lancet*. 2000 Sep 2;356(9232):781

1. Horton R. Lotronex and the FDA: a fatal erosion of integrity. *Lancet*. 2001 May 19;357(9268):1544-5
2. Editorial. Politics trumps science at the FDA. *Lancet*. 2005 Nov 26;366(9500):1827
3. Topol EJ. Failing the public health—rofecoxib, Merck, and the FDA. *N Engl J Med*. 2004 Oct 21;351(17):1707-9
4. Wolinsky H, Brune T. The Serpent on the Staff: The Unhealthy Politics of the American Medical Association. GP Putnam and Sons, New York, 1994
5. Wilk CA. Medicine, Monopolies, and Malice: How the Medical Establishment Tried to Destroy Chiropractic. Garden City Park: Avery, 1996
6. Carter JP. Racketeering in Medicine: The Suppression of Alternatives. Norfolk: Hampton Roads Pub; 1993
7. National Alliance of Professional Psychology Providers. AMA Seeks To Control and Restrict Psychologist's Scope of Practice. nappp.org/scope.pdf 2006 Nov
8. Daly R, American Psychiatric Association. AMA Forms Coalition to Thwart Non-M.D. Practice Expansion. *Psychiatric News* 2006 March; 41: 17
9. Angell M. The Truth About the Drug Companies: How They Deceive Us and What to Do About it. Random House; August 2004
10. Terrett AG. Misuse of the literature by medical authors in discussing spinal manipulative therapy injury. *J Manipulative Physiol Ther*. 1995 May;18(4):203-10
11. Morley et al. A case study of misrepresentation of the scientific literature: recent reviews of chiropractic. *J Altern Complement Med*. 2001 Feb;7(1):65-78
12. Wenban AB. Inappropriate use of title 'chiropractor' and term 'chiropractic manipulation' in peer-reviewed biomedical literature. *Chiropr Osteopat*. 2006 Aug;14:16
13. Spivak JL. *The Medical Trust Unmasked*. Louis S. Siegfried Publishers; New York: 1961
14. Trever W. *In the Public Interest*. Los Angeles; Scriptures Unlimited; 1972. This is probably the most authoritative documentation of the illegal actions of the AMA up to 1972; contains numerous photocopies of actual AMA documents and minutes of official meetings with overt intentionality of destroying Americans' healthcare options so that the AMA and related organizations would have a monopoly in healthcare.
15. Getzendanner S. Permanent injunction order against AMA. *JAMA*. 1988 Jan 1;259(1):81-2
16. "A national study released today reports 20 million American families — or one in seven families — faced hardships paying medical bills last year, which forced many to choose between getting medical attention or paying rent or buying food…" Freeman, Liz. 'Working poor' struggle to afford health care. *Naples Daily News*. naplesnews.com/npdn/news/article/0,2071,NPDN_14940_3000546,00.html
17. "The USA's 5.8 million small companies… Health care costs are rising about 15% this year for those with fewer than 200 workers vs. 13.5% for those with 500 or more… But many small employers cite increases of 20% or more. That's made insurance the No. 1 small business problem…" Jim Hopkins. Health care tops taxes as small business cost drain. *USA TODAY*. usatoday.com/news/health/2003-04-20-small-business-costs_x.htm.
18. "Though the U.S. has slightly fewer doctors per capita than the typical developed nation, we have almost twice as many MRI machines and perform vastly more angioplasties. …at least 31 percent of all the incremental income we'll earn between 1999 and 2010 will go to health care." Regnier P. Healthcare myth: We spend too much. *Money Magazine* October 13, 2003: 11:29 AM EDT money.cnn.com/2003/10/08/pf/health_myths_1/
19. "Although they spend more on health care than patients in any other industrialized nation, Americans receive the right treatment less than 60 percent of the time, resulting in unnecessary pain, expense and even death…" Ceci Connolly. U.S. Patients Spend More but Don't Get More, Study Finds: Even in Advantaged Areas, Americans Often Receive Inadequate Health Care. *Washington Post*, May 5, 2004; Page A15washingtonpost.com/ac2/wp-dyn/A1875-2004May4
20. McGlynn et al. The quality of health care delivered to adults in the United States. *N Engl J Med*. 2003 Jun 26;348(26):2635-45
21. Brennan et al. Incidence of adverse events and negligence in hospitalized patients. *Qual Saf Health Care*. 2004 Apr;13(2):145-51
22. "Basically, you die earlier and spend more time disabled if you're an American rather than a member of most other advanced countries." Christopher Murray MD PhD, Director of World Health Organization's Global Program on Evidence for Health Policy who.int/inf-pr-2000/en/pr2000-life.html Accessed July 12, 2004
23. Shi L. Health care spending, delivery, and outcome in developed countries: a cross-national comparison. *Am J Med Qual* 1997;12(2):83-93
24. Holland EG, Degruy FV. Drug-induced disorders. *Am Fam Physician*. 1997 Nov 1;56(7):1781-8, 1791-2
25. Brennan et al. Incidence of adverse events and negligence in hospitalized patients. *Qual Saf Health Care*. 2004 Apr;13(2):145-51
26. Whitaker R. The case against antipsychotic drugs: a 50-year record of doing more harm than good. *Med Hypotheses*. 2004;62(1):5-13
27. Use of horse estrogens in humans as "hormone replacement therapy" exemplified the application of a strong carcinogen to millions of unsuspecting women: Zhang et al. Major metabolite of equilin, 4-hydroxyequilin, autoxidizes to an o-quinone which isomerizes to potent cytotoxin 4-hydroxyequilenin-o-quinone. *Chem Res Toxicol*. 1999 Feb;12(2):204-13; Pisha et al. Evidence that a metabolite of equine estrogens, 4-hydroxyequilenin, induces cellular transformation in vitro. *Chem Res Toxicol*. 2001;14:82-90; Zhang et al. Equine estrogen metabolite 4-hydroxyequilenin induces DNA damage in rat mammary tissues. *Chem Res Toxicol*. 2001 Dec;14:1654-9
28. Newman NM, Ling RS. Acetabular bone destruction related to non-steroidal anti-inflammatory drugs. *Lancet*. 1985 Jul 6; 2(8445): 11-4
29. "In 1983, 2876 people died from medication errors. ... By 1993, this number had risen to 7,391 - a 2.57-fold increase." Phillips DP, Christenfeld N, Glynn LM. Increase in US medication-error deaths between 1983 and 1993. *Lancet*. 1998 Feb 28;351(9103):643-4
30. Smith R. Medical journals are an extension of the marketing arm of pharmaceutical companies. *PLoS Med*. 2005 May;2(5):e138
31. van der Steen WJ, Ho VK. Drugs versus diets: disillusions with Dutch health care. *Acta Biotheor*. 2001;49(2):125-40

willingness to receive new information as worthy of preeminence over deeply rooted and well ensconced institutionalized fallacies.

Understanding How Interconnected Systems Participate in Health and Disease: When viewed as a diagram, the web of major influences reveals the interconnected nature of causes, effects, and body systems and how imbalance or disruption in one area can lead to problems in another. Once homeostatic reserves and compensatory mechanisms are depleted, the patient experiences progressively worsening health (which may be asymptomatic) and the eventual manifestation of clinical disease.

Although newer versions of this diagram have been developed over the past few years, replacing the previous version provided below, the original diagram—interconnected by Vasquez in 2003—is the most efficient and practical for demonstrating the body systems and external inputs most important to the maintenance of health and genesis of disease. These systems and inputs described in following pages with particular consideration given to pain and inflammation, both of which are leading causes of disability and illness among patients seen in general practice and specialty and subspecialty care on a daily basis.

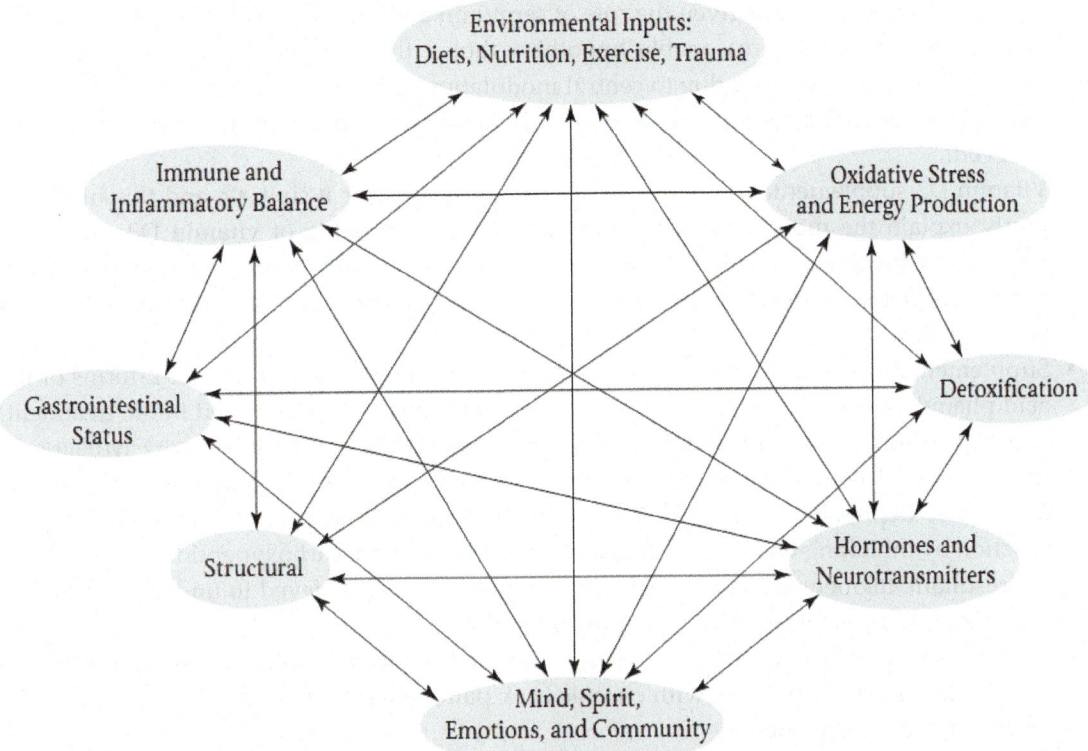

Interconnected Physiologic Web illustrated by Alex Vasquez (circa 2003): This version of "the Functional Medicine Matrix" interconnected by Alex Vasquez provides an illustration of the interdependency of physiologic factors and organ systems; this version was published in Vasquez A. Web-like Interconnections of Physiological Factors. *Integrative Medicine* 2006 Apr/May. "The Matrix" is owned and has since been completely changed by the Institute for Functional Medicine. A reprint of this article is available at InflammationMastery.com/reprints/vasquez-2006-weblike-connections.pdf

Exploring the Different Aspects of the Interconnected Physiologic Web

1. Hormonal and neurotransmitter imbalances: While most clinicians are aware that neurotransmitters can either transmit pain signals or dampen their reception, many clinicians are not aware that neurotransmitter status is somewhat malleable and can be modulated with nutritional supplementation and botanical medicines. The examples that will be considered here are the tryptophan-serotonin-melatonin and the phenylalanine-tyrosine-dopamine-norepinephrine-epinephrine and enkephalin pathways.

- Tryptophan and 5-hydroxytryptophan (5HTP) are prescription and nonprescription nutritional supplements that are the amino acid precursors for the formation of the neurotransmitter serotonin and the pineal hormone melatonin. Biochemically, these conversions are linear as follows: tryptophan → 5HTP → serotonin → melatonin. Tryptophan depletion and low levels of serotonin are consistently associated with depression, anxiety, exacerbation of eating disorders, and increased sensitivity to acute and chronic pain. Serotonergic pathways are impaired by chronic stress due to increased utilization of serotonin (e.g., serotonin-dependent cortisol release) and increased hepatic degradation of tryptophan by cortisol-stimulated tryptophan pyrrolase.[451] Therapeutically, supplementation with 5HTP augments serotonin and melatonin synthesis and has specific applicability in the alleviation of depression and pain syndromes such as fibromyalgia and headache, including migraine, tension headaches, and juvenile headaches.[452,453] Certainly part of the benefit from 5HTP supplementation is derived from the increased formation of melatonin, as the biological effects of melatonin extend beyond its sleep-promoting role to include powerful antioxidation, anti-infective immunostimulation[454], and preservation of mitochondrial function, a benefit which is of particular relevance to the treatment of fibromyalgia.[455]

- The conditionally essential fatty acids found in fish oil modulate serotonergic and adrenergic activity in the human brain[456], and given the role of serotonin and norepinephrine in the central processing of pain perception[457], a reasonable hypothesis holds that the pain-relieving activity of fish oil supplementation[458] is partly due to central modulation of pain perception and is not wholly due to modulation of eicosanoid production and inflammatory mediator transcription as previously believed.

- Vitamin D3 supplementation may also augment serotonergic activity[459], and this mechanism may partly explain the mood-enhancing and pain-relieving benefits of vitamin D3 supplementation. Attentive readers will note that this brief discussion has already begun to bridge the gaps between nutritional status, neurotransmitter synthesis, pain sensitivity, immune function, and mitochondrial bioenergetics.

- Supplementation with DL-phenylalanine (DLPA; racemic mixture of D- and L-forms of the amino acid phenylalanine derived from synthetic production) has long been used in the treatment of pain and depression.[460] The nutritional L-isomer is converted from phenylalanine → tyrosine → L-dopa → dopamine → norepinephrine → epinephrine. Augmentation of this pathway promotes resistance to fatigue, depression, and pain. The synthetic D-isomer augments pain-relieving enkephalin function by inhibiting enkephalin degradation by the enzyme carboxypeptidase A (enkephalinase); the resultant augmentation of enkephalin levels is generally believed to underlie the analgesic and mood-enhancing benefits of DLPA supplementation.

- Therapeutic massage is yet another means to modulate neurotransmitter synthesis for the alleviation of pain. In a study of patients with chronic back pain, massage increased serotonin and dopamine levels (measured in urine).[461]

Hormonal imbalances are particularly relevant to the discussion of chronic pain caused by inflammation characteristic of autoimmune diseases such as rheumatoid arthritis (RA). Often clinically subtle but nonetheless of extreme importance, these hormonal influences on painful inflammation are worthy of their own detailed discussion and thus will be reviewed later in this textbook. Generally speaking and with a few noted exceptions, the research literature points to a specific pattern of hormonal imbalances among patients with autoimmunity, and this pattern is consistent with the pro-inflammatory and immunodysregulatory effects of estrogens and prolactin and the anti-inflammatory and

[451] Sandyk R. Tryptophan availability and the susceptibility to stress in multiple sclerosis: a hypothesis. *Int J Neurosci.* 1996 Jul;86(1-2):47-53
[452] Turner EH, Loftis JM, Blackwell AD. Serotonin a la carte: supplementation with the serotonin precursor 5-hydroxytryptophan. *Pharmacol Ther.* 2006 Mar;109(3):325-38
[453] Birdsall TC. 5-Hydroxytryptophan: a clinically-effective serotonin precursor. *Altern Med Rev.* 1998 Aug;3(4):271-80
[454] Gitto E, et al. Effects of melatonin treatment in septic newborns. *Pediatr Res.* 2001 Dec;50(6):756-60
[455] Acuna-Castroviejo D, Escames G, Reiter RJ. Melatonin therapy in fibromyalgia. *J Pineal Res.* 2006 Jan;40(1):98-9
[456] Hibbeln et al. Omega-3 fatty acid deficiencies in neurodevelopment, aggression and autonomic dysregulation: opportunities for intervention. *Int Rev Psychiatry* 2006;18:107-18
[457] Wise TN, Fishbain DA, Holder-Perkins V.Painful physical symptoms in depression: a clinical challenge. *Pain Med.* 2007 Sep;8 Suppl 2:S75-82
[458] Goldberg RJ, Katz J. A meta-analysis of the analgesic effects of omega-3 polyunsaturated fatty acid supplementation for inflammatory joint pain. *Pain.* 2007;129(1-2):210-23
[459] Lansdowne AT, Provost SC. Vitamin D3 enhances mood in healthy subjects during winter. *Psychopharmacology* (Berl). 1998 Feb;135(4):319-23
[460] Russell AL, McCarty MF. DL-phenylalanine markedly potentiates opiate analgesia. *Med Hypotheses.* 2000 Oct;55(4):283-8
[461] Hernandez-Reif M, Field T, Krasnegor J, Theakston H. Lower back pain is reduced and range of motion increased after massage therapy. *Int J Neurosci* 2001;106(3-4):131-45

immunomodulatory effects of cortisol, dehydroepiandrosterone (DHEA), and testosterone. Patients with autoimmune neuromusculoskeletal inflammation generally display a complete or partial pattern of hormonal disturbances typified by elevated estrogen and prolactin and lowered testosterone, DHEA, and cortisol; appropriate therapeutic correction of these imbalances can safely result in disease amelioration. Rectification of endocrinologic imbalances ("orthoendocrinology") is detailed later in this book.

2. <u>Oxidation-reduction imbalances and mitochondriopathy</u>: Oxidative stress results from the chronic systemic inflammation seen in painful inflammatory disorders such as RA, and oxidative stress contributes to the perpetuation and exacerbation of inflammatory diseases via expedited tissue destruction and alterations in gene transcription and resultant enhancement of inflammatory mediator production.[462] Immune activation increases production of reactive oxygen species (ROS; "free radicals"), and oxidant stress increases activation of pro-inflammatory transcription factors (such as nuclear factor KappaB, NFkB) and also increases spontaneous oxidative modification of endogenous proteins such as cartilage matrix which then undergoes expedited degradation or immunologic attack; thus a vicious cycle of oxidation and inflammation exacerbates and perpetuates various inflammation-associated diseases, resulting in therapeutic recalcitrance and autonomous disease progression.[463,464] A rational clinical approach to breaking this vicious pathogenic cycle can include simultaneous antioxidation and immunomodulation, the former with diet optimization and nutritional supplementation and the latter with allergen avoidance, hormonal correction, xenobiotic detoxification, and specific phytonutritional modulation of pro-inflammatory pathways. Severe and acute inflammation can and often should be suppressed pharmacologically, but sole reliance on pharmacologic immunosuppression leaves the patient vulnerable to iatrogenic immunosuppression and the well-known increased risk for cardiovascular disease, osteoporosis, infection, and clinical malignancy while failing to address the underlying biochemical and immunologic imbalances which generate and maintain all chronic inflammatory and autoimmune diseases. The contribution of mitochondrial dysfunction to chronic recurrent or persistent pain is most plainly demonstrated in migraine and fibromyalgia. An important characteristic of migraine is mitochondrial dysfunction, the severity of which correlates positively with the severity of the headache syndrome.[465] In fibromyalgia, numerous abnormalities in cellular bioenergetics are noted, which correlate clinically with the lowered lactate threshold, persistent muscle pain, reduced functional capacity, and the subjective fatigue that characterize the disorder.[466] Nutritional preservation and enhancement of mitochondrial function was termed "mitochondrial resuscitation" by Jeffrey Bland PhD in the 1990s, and clinical implementation of such an approach generally includes, in addition to diet and lifestyle modification, supplementation with coenzyme Q-10, niacin, riboflavin, thiamin, lipoic acid, magnesium, and other nutrients and botanical medicines which enhance production of adenosine triphosphate (ATP).[467]

3. <u>Detoxification and biotransformational imbalances</u>: As our environment becomes increasingly polluted and as researchers and clinicians expand their appreciation and knowledge of the adverse effects of xenobiotics (toxic metals and chemicals), healthcare providers will need to attend to their patients' detoxification capacity and xenobiotic load as a component of the prevention and treatment of disease. By now, senior students and practicing clinicians should be aware of the association of xenobiotics in prototypic diseases such as Parkinson's disease[468,469], adult-onset diabetes mellitus[470,471,472,473], and attention-

[462] Hitchon CA, El-Gabalawy HS. Oxidation in rheumatoid arthritis. *Arthritis Res Ther*. 2004;6(6):265-78

[463] Tak PP, et al. Rheumatoid arthritis and p53: how oxidative stress might alter the course of inflammatory diseases. *Immunol Today*. 2000 Feb;21(2):78-82

[464] Kurien BT, Hensley K, Bachmann M, Scofield RH. Oxidatively modified autoantigens in autoimmune diseases. *Free Radic Biol Med*. 2006 Aug 15;41(4):549-56

[465] Lodi R, et al. Quantitative analysis of skeletal muscle bioenergetics and proton efflux in migraine and cluster headache. *J Neurol Sci*. 1997 Feb 27;146(1):73-80

[466] Park et al. Use of P-31 magnetic resonance spectroscopy to detect metabolic abnormalities in muscles of patients with fibromyalgia. *Arthritis Rheum*. 1998 Mar;41(3):406-13

[467] Pieczenik SR, Neustadt J. Mitochondrial dysfunction and molecular pathways of disease. *Exp Mol Pathol*. 2007 Aug;83(1):84-92

[468] Corrigan FM, et al. Organochlorine insecticides in substantia nigra in Parkinson's disease. *J Toxicol Environ Health A*. 2000 Feb 25;59(4):229-34

[469] Fleming L, Mann JB, Bean J, Briggle T, Sanchez-Ramos JR. Parkinson's disease and brain levels of organochlorine pesticides. *Ann Neurol*. 1994 Jul;36(1):100-3

[470] Fujiyoshi et al. Molecular epidemiologic evidence for diabetogenic effects of dioxin exposure in U.S. Air force veterans of the Vietnam War. *Environ Health Perspect*, 2006 Nov;114(11):1677-83

[471] Lee DH, Lee IK, Song K, Steffes M, Toscano W, Baker BA, Jacobs DR Jr. A strong dose-response relation between serum concentrations of persistent organic pollutants and diabetes: results from the National Health and Examination Survey 1999-2002. *Diabetes Care* 2006 Jul;29(7):1638-44

[472] Lee DH, Lee IK, Jin SH, Steffes M, Jacobs DR Jr. Association between serum concentrations of persistent organic pollutants and insulin resistance among nondiabetic adults: results from the National Health and Nutrition Examination Survey 1999-2002. *Diabetes Care*, 2007 Mar;30(3):622-8

[473] Remillard RB, Bunce NJ. Linking dioxins to diabetes: epidemiology and biologic plausibility. *Environ Health Perspect*, 2002 Sep;110(9):853-8

deficit hyperactivity disorder.[474,475,476] The role of xenobiotic exposure and impaired detoxification in neuromusculoskeletal pain and inflammatory disorders is more subtle and is generally mediated through the resultant immunotoxicity that manifests as autoimmunity. Occasionally, clinicians will encounter patients with musculoskeletal symptomatology that defies standard diagnosis and treatment but which responds remarkably and permanently to empiric clinical detoxification treatment. The numerous roles of xenobiotic exposure in the genesis and perpetuation of chronic health problems and the role of clinical detoxification in the treatment of such problems has been detailed elsewhere by Crinnion[477,478,479,480,481], Rea[482], Bland[483,484], Vasquez[485,486], and others.[487,488]

4. <u>Immune imbalances</u>: Immune imbalances have an obvious role in musculoskeletal inflammation when discussed in the context of autoimmune diseases such as rheumatoid arthritis, ankylosing spondylitis, and systemic lupus erythematosus. While the standard medical approach to this pathophysiology has focused almost exclusively on the pharmacologic suppression of resultant inflammation and tissue destruction, other disciplines such as naturopathic medicine and functional medicine have emphasized the importance of determining and addressing the underlying causes of such immune imbalance. While clinicians of all disciplines must appreciate the important role of pharmacologic immunosuppression in the treatment of inflammatory exacerbations as seen with giant cell arteritis or neuropsychiatric lupus, they should also appreciate that sole reliance on immunosuppression for long-term management of inflammatory disorders is destined to therapeutic failure insofar as it does not correct the underlying cause of the disease and creates dependency upon perpetual immunosuppression with its attendant costs (not uncommonly in the range of $20,000 - 50,000 per year) and adverse effects including infection and increased risk for cancer. Rather than presuming that immune dysfunction and the resultant inflammation and autoimmunity are results of spontaneous generation, astute clinicians seek to identify and correct the causes of these immune imbalances. By identifying and correcting the underlying causes of immune imbalance (when possible), clinicians can lessen or obviate the need for chronic polypharmaceutical treatment with anti-inflammatory and immunosuppressive agents. Vasquez[489] proposed that secondary immune imbalances (distinguished from primary congenital disorders) generally arise from one or more of five main problems: ❶ habitual consumption of a pro-inflammatory diet, ❷ food allergies and intolerances, ❸ microbial dysbiosis, including multifocal polydysbiosis, ❹ hormonal imbalances, and ❺ xenobiotic exposure and accumulation resulting in immunotoxicity via bystander activation and enhanced processing of autoantigens as well as haptenization and neoantigen formation. These influences may act singularly or when combined may be additive and synergistic.

5. <u>Inflammatory imbalances</u>: Inflammatory imbalances may be distinguished from immune imbalances insofar as inflammatory imbalances connote disorders of inflammatory mediator production in the absence of the immunodysfunction that typifies allergy, autoimmunity, or immunosuppression. Here again, long-term consumption of a pro-inflammatory diet[490] is a primary consideration because such a diet typically oversupplies inflammatory precursors such as arachidonate and undersupplies anti-inflammatory phytonutrients such as vitamin D, zinc, selenium, and the numerous phytochemicals that reduce activation

---

[474] Rauh VA, et al. Impact of prenatal chlorpyrifos exposure on neurodevelopment in the first 3 years of life among inner-city children. *Pediatrics*. 2006 Dec;118(6):e1845-59

[475] Cheuk DK, Wong V. Attention-deficit hyperactivity disorder and blood mercury level: a case-control study in Chinese children. *Neuropediatrics*. 2006 Aug;37(4):234-40

[476] Nigg et al. Low blood lead levels with clinically diagnosed attention-deficit/hyperactivity disorder and mediated by weak cognitive control. *Biol Psychiatry*. 2008;63:325-31

[477] Crinnion W. Results of a Decade of Naturopathic Treatment for Environmental Illnesses: A Review of Clinical Records. *J Naturopathic Medicine* vol. 7; 2, 21-27

[478] Crinnion WJ. Environmental medicine, part 1: the human burden of environmental toxins and their common health effects. *Altern Med Rev*. 2000 Feb;5(1):52-63

[479] Crinnion WJ. Environmental medicine, part 2: health effects of and protection from ubiquitous airborne solvent exposure. *Altern Med Rev*. 2000 Apr;5(2):133-43

[480] Crinnion WJ. Environmental medicine, part 3: long-term effects of chronic low-dose mercury exposure. *Altern Med Rev*. 2000 Jun;5(3):209-23

[481] Crinnion WJ. Environmental medicine, part 4: pesticides - biologically persistent and ubiquitous toxins. *Altern Med Rev*. 2000 Oct;5(5):432-47

[482] Rea WJ, Pan Y, Johnson AR. Clearing of toxic volatile hydrocarbons from humans. *Bol Asoc Med P R*. 1991 Jul;83(7):321-4

[483] Bland JS, et al. A Medical Food-Supplemented Detoxification Program in the Management of Chronic Health Problems. *Altern Ther Health Med*. 1995 Nov 1;1(5):62-71

[484] Minich DM, Bland JS. Acid-alkaline balance: role in chronic disease and detoxification. *Altern Ther Health Med*. 2007 Jul-Aug;13(4):62-5

[485] Vasquez A. *Integrative Rheumatology: Second Edition*. Fort Worth, Texas; Integrative and Biological Medicine Research and Consulting, 2007

[486] Vasquez A. Diabetes: Are Toxins to Blame? *Naturopathy Digest* 2007; April

[487] Kilburn et al. Neurobehavioral dysfunction in firemen exposed to polycholorinated biphenyls (PCBs): improvement after detoxification. *Arch Environ Health* 1989;44:345-50

[488] Cecchini M, LoPresti V. Drug residues store in the body following cessation of use: impacts on neuroendocrine balance and behavior--use of the Hubbard sauna regimen to remove toxins and restore health. *Med Hypotheses*. 2007;68(4):868-79

[489] Vasquez A. *Integrative Rheumatology: Second Edition*. Fort Worth, Texas; Integrative and Biological Medicine Research and Consulting, 2007

[490] Seaman DR. The diet-induced proinflammatory state: a cause of chronic pain and other degenerative diseases? *J Manipulative Physiol Ther*. 2002 Mar-Apr;25(3):168-79

of inflammatory pathways.[491,492,493,494] Three of the best examples of correctable inflammatory imbalances are those due to vitamin D deficiency, fatty acid imbalances, and overconsumption of simple sugars and saturated fats. Vitamin D deficiency is a widespread and serious health problem that spans nearly all geographic regions and socioeconomic strata with several important adverse effects. Vitamin D deficiency results in systemic inflammation[495] and chronic musculoskeletal pain[496] which both resolve quickly upon correction of the nutritional deficiency. Similarly and consistent with the Western/American pattern of dietary intake, overconsumption of alpha-linoleic acid and arachidonate along with underconsumption of alpha-linolenic acid (ALA), gamma-linolenic acid (GLA), eicosapentaenoic acid (EPA), docosahexaenoic acid (DHA), and oleic acid subtly yet powerfully shift nutrigenomic tendency and precursor availability in favor of enhanced systemic inflammation. Correction of this imbalance such as with reduced consumption of arachidonate and increased consumption of EPA and DHA has consistently proven to be of significant clinical value in the management of chronic inflammatory disorders.[497,498] Measurable increases in systemic inflammation and oxidative stress follow glucose challenge[499], consumption of saturated fatty acids as found in cream[500], and consumption of a "fast food" breakfast, which triggers the prototypic inflammatory activator NF-kappaB for enhanced production of inflammatory mediators.[501] This triad (vitamin D deficiency, fatty acid imbalance, and overconsumption of sugars and saturated fats) is typical of the Western/American pattern of dietary intake, and the molecular means and clinical consequences of such dietary choices is quite clear, evidenced by burgeoning epidemics of metabolic and inflammatory diseases.

6. Digestive, absorptive, and microbiological imbalances: The grouping of digestive and absorptive considerations suggests that the alimentary tract and its accessory organs of the liver, gall bladder and pancreas will be the focus of these core clinical imbalances, and the addition of microbiological imbalances should remind current clinicians that gastrointestinal dysbiosis is an important and frequent clinical consideration. Impaired digestion begins neither in the stomach nor in the mouth, but it stems rather from any socioeconomic milieu which deprives people of the means to prepare wholesome health-promoting meals and the time to consume those meals in a relaxed parasympathetic-dominant mode, preferably among good company, stimulating conversation, and appropriate ambiance. Poor dentition, xerostomia, hypochlorhydria, cholestasis or cholecystectomy, pancreatic insufficiency, mucosal atrophy, altered gut motility, and bacterial overgrowth of the small bowel are important and common contributors to impaired digestion and absorption; clinicians should consider these frequently and implement treatment with a low threshold for intervention. The relevance of these problems to pain and the musculoskeletal system is generally that of malnutrition and its macro- and micronutrient consequences. Sunlight-deprived individuals must rely on dietary sources of vitamin D, which are hardly adequate for the prevention of overt deficiency; any impairment in digestion, emulsification, or absorption of this fat-soluble vitamin can readily lead to hypovitaminosis D and its resultant musculoskeletal consequences of osteomalacia and unremitting pain.[502] Consumption of foods to which the individual is sensitized ("food allergies") can trigger migraine and other chronic headaches[503,504] as well as generalized musculoskeletal pain and arthritis.[505,506,507] Avoidance of the offending foods often results in amelioration or complete remission of the painful syndrome at low cost and high efficacy without reliance on expensive or potentially harmful or addictive pain-relieving drugs. Occasionally, gluten enteropathy (celiac disease) presents with arthritic pain

[491] Vasquez A. New Insights into Fatty Acid Biochemistry and the Influence of Diet. *Nutr Perspectives* 2004; Oct: 5,7-10,12,14
[492] Vasquez A. New Insights into Fatty Acid Supplementation and Its Effect on Eicosanoid Production and Genetic Expression. *Nutritional Perspectives* 2005; January: 5-16
[493] Vasquez A. Improving overall health while safely and effectively treating musculoskeletal pain. *Nutritional Perspectives* 2005; 28: 34-38, 40-42
[494] Vasquez A. Nutritional and Botanical Inhibition of NF-kappaB, the Major Intracellular Amplifier of the Inflammatory Cascade. *Nutritional Perspectives* 2005;July: 5-12
[495] Timms PM, et al. Circulating MMP9, vitamin D and variation in the TIMP-1 response with VDR genotype. *QJM*. 2002 Dec;95(12):787-96
[496] Al Faraj S, Al Mutairi K. Vitamin D deficiency and chronic low back pain in Saudi Arabia. *Spine*. 2003 Jan 15;28(2):177-9
[497] James MJ, Gibson RA, Cleland LG. Dietary polyunsaturated fatty acids and inflammatory mediator production. *Am J Clin Nutr*. 2000 Jan;71(1 Suppl):343S-8S
[498] James et al. Dietary n-3 fats as adjunctive therapy in a prototypic inflammatory disease. Prostaglandins *Leukot Essent Fatty Acids*. 2003 Jun;68(6):399-405
[499] Mohanty P, et al. Glucose challenge stimulates reactive oxygen species (ROS) generation by leucocytes. *J Clin Endocrinol Metab*. 2000 Aug;85(8):2970-3
[500] Mohanty et al. Both lipid and protein intakes stimulate increased generation of reactive oxygen species. *Am J Clin Nutr*. 2002 Apr;75(4):767-72
[501] Aljada et al. Increase in intranuclear nuclear factor kappaB and decrease in inhibitor kappaB in mononuclear cells after a mixed meal. *Am J Clin Nutr*. 2004 Apr;79(4):682-90
[502] Basha B, Rao DS, Han ZH, Parfitt AM. Osteomalacia due to vitamin D depletion: a neglected consequence of intestinal malabsorption. *Am J Med*. 2000 Mar;108(4):296-300
[503] Grant EC. Food allergies and migraine. *Lancet*. 1979 May 5;1(8123):966-9
[504] Millichap JG, Yee MM. The diet factor in pediatric and adolescent migraine. *Pediatr Neurol*. 2003 Jan;28(1):9-15
[505] van de Laar MA, Aalbers M, Bruins FG, et al. Food intolerance in rheumatoid arthritis. II. Clinical and histological aspects. *Ann Rheum Dis*. 1992 ;51(3):303-6
[506] Golding DN. Is there an allergic synovitis? *J R Soc Med*. 1990 May;83(5):312-4
[507] Hvatum M, Kanerud L, Hällgren R, Brandtzaeg P. The gut-joint axis: cross reactive food antibodies in rheumatoid arthritis. *Gut*. 2006 Sep;55:1240-7

and chronic synovitis; the pain and inflammation remit on a gluten-free diet.[508] Alterations in intestinal microbial balance or an individual's unique response to endogenous bacteria (i.e., dysbiosis) can lead to systemic inflammation, arthritis, vasculitis, and musculoskeletal pain; clinical nuances and molecular mechanisms of gastrointestinal dysbiosis will be surveyed later in this monograph based on a previous review by Vasquez.[509] Clinicians should appreciate that dysbiosis can occur at sites other than the gastrointestinal tract, most importantly the nasopharynx and genitourinary tracts. Eradication of the occult infection or mucosal colonization often results in marked reductions in systemic inflammation and its clinical complications. Interested readers are directed to the excellent review by Noah[510] on the relevance of dysbiosis and its treatment relative to psoriasis; additional citations and clinical applications will be discussed later in this book.

7. <u>Structural imbalances from cellular membrane function to the musculoskeletal system</u>: Molecular structural imbalances lie at the heart of the concept of "biochemical individuality" originated by Roger J. Williams[511] in 1956, and this concept was soon thereafter expanded into the theory and practice of "orthomolecular medicine" pioneered by Linus Pauling and colleagues.[512,513] Pauling is considered by many authorities to be the original source of the concept of molecular medicine because he coined the phrase "molecular disease" after his team's discovery in 1949 that sickle cell anemia resulted from a single amino acid substitution that caused physical deformation of the hemoglobin molecule in hypoxic conditions.[514] One of

2013 INTERNATIONAL CONFERENCE ON HUMAN NUTRITION AND FUNCTIONAL MEDICINE

PORTLAND OREGON CONVENTION CENTER • SEPTEMBER 25-29, 2013

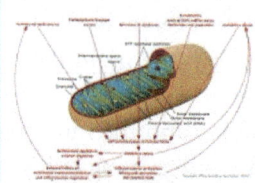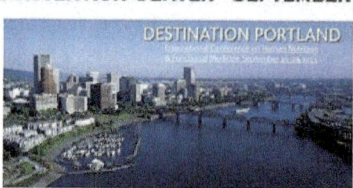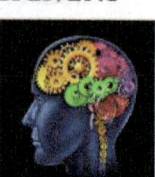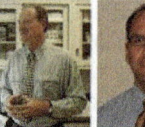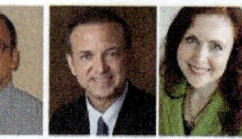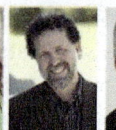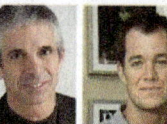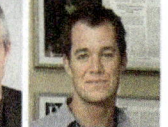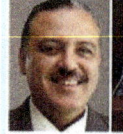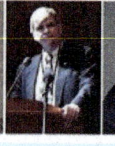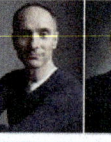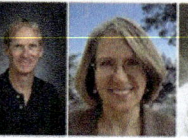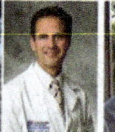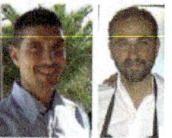

For additional and more current video discussions of functional medicine, please see videos and new CME events from International College of Human Nutrition and Functional Medicine: ICHNFM.ORG
- NutritionAndFunctionalMedicine.org—courses for professionals.
- Vimeo.com/ICHNFM—videos
- Facebook.com/ICHNFM—news updates
- IntJHumNutrFunctMed.org—peer-reviewed journal

Pauling's students, Jeffery Bland, continued this legacy with the organization of "functional medicine.[515] Single nucleotide polymorphisms (SNP; pronounced "snip") are DNA sequence variations that can result in amino acid substitutions that render the final protein (e.g., structural protein or enzyme) abnormal in structure and therefore function. This aberrancy may or may not cause clinical disease (depending on the severity and importance of the variation), and consequences of the dysfunction may be occult, subtle, or obvious. One of the most powerful and effective means for treating diseases resultant from SNPs that result in enzyme defects is the use of high-dose vitamin supplementation, and this forms the scientific basis for "mega-vitamin therapy" as elegantly and authoritatively reviewed by Bruce Ames, et al.[516] SNP-induced alterations in enzyme structure reduce affinity for vitamin-derived coenzyme binding; this reduced affinity can be "overpowered" by administration of high doses of the required vitamin cofactor to increase tissue concentrations of the nutrient to promote binding of the enzyme with its ligand for the performance of

[508] Bourne JT, Kumar P, Huskisson EC, Mageed R, Unsworth DJ, Wojtulewski JA. Arthritis and coeliac disease. *Ann Rheum Dis.* 1985 Sep;44(9):592-8

[509] Vasquez A. Nutritional and Botanical Treatments against "Silent Infections" and Gastrointestinal Dysbiosis. *Nutr Perspect* 2006; Jan: 5-21

[510] Noah PW. The role of microorganisms in psoriasis. *Semin Dermatol.* 1990 Dec;9(4):269-76

[511] Williams RJ. *Biochemical Individuality: The Basis for the Genetotrophic Concept.* Austin and London: University of Texas Press, 1956. Page x

[512] Pauling L. On the Orthomolecular Environment of the Mind. In: Williams RJ, Kalita DK. *Physician's Handbook on Orthomolecular Medicine.* Keats Publishing: 1977. p 76

[513] Pauling L, Robinson AB, Teranishi R, Cary P. Quantitative analysis of urine vapor and breath by gas-liquid partition chromatography. *Proc Natl Acad Sci* 1971 Oct;68:2374-6

[514] Pauling L, Itano HA, Singer SJ, Wells IC. Sickle cell anemia, a molecular disease. *Science.* 1949 Nov 25;110(2865):543-8

[515] Bland JS. Jeffrey S. Bland, PhD, FACN, CNS: functional medicine pioneer. *Altern Ther Health Med.* 2004 Sep-Oct;10(5):74-81

[516] Ames BN, et al. High-dose vitamin therapy stimulates variant enzymes with decreased coenzyme binding affinity (increased K(m)). *Am J Clin Nutr.* 2002 Apr;75(4):616-58

enzymatic function. Thus, the scientific rationale for nutritional therapy is derived in part from the recognition that altered enzymatic function due to altered enzyme structure can often be corrected by administration of supradietary doses of nutrients. Relatedly, the structure and function of cell membranes is determined by their composition, which is influenced by dietary intake of fatty acids, and which influences production prostaglandins and leukotrienes. This is an important aspect of the scientific rationale for the use of specific fatty acid supplements in the prevention and treatment of painful inflammatory musculoskeletal disease. Cell membrane structure and function can also be altered by systemic oxidative stress; the concomitant alterations in intracellular ions (e.g., calcium) and receptor function along with activation of transcription factors such as NF-kappaB contribute to widespread physiologic impairment which creates a vicious cycle of inflammation, metabolic disturbance, and additional free radical generation.[517,518] Somatic dysfunction, musculoskeletal disorders, and inefficient biomechanics contribute to pain, increased production of inflammatory mediators, and the expedited degeneration of tissues such as collagen and cartilage matrix. Physicians trained in clinical biomechanics and physical medicine appreciate the subtle nuances of musculoskeletal structure-function relationships and address these problems directly with physical and manual means rather than ignoring the physical problem and only treating its biochemical sequelae. While biomechanics, palpatory diagnosis, and manual therapeutics takes years of diligent study for the achievement of proficiency, some of these concepts will be reviewed later in this book, particularly in the section on integrative pain management.

8. Psychological and Spiritual Equilibrium: The connections between physical pain and psychoemotional status and events is worthy of thorough discussion and not merely for the sake of improving upon outdated clinical practices which have typically marginalized these ethereal considerations or considered them only long enough to substantiate psychopharmaceutical intervention. A survey of the literature makes clear the interconnected nature of pain, inflammation, psychoemotional stress, depression, social isolation, and nutritional status; due to space and time limitations, a brief overview must necessarily suffice for the exemplification of representative concepts. Stressful and depressive life events promote the development, persistence, and exacerbation of disorders of pain and inflammation through nutritional, hormonal, immunologic, oxidative, and microbiologic mechanisms. Stated most simply, the perception of stressful events and the resultant neurohormonal cascade results in expedited metabolic utilization and increased urinary excretion of nutrients (e.g., tryptophan , and zinc, magnesium, retinol, respectively) which sum to effect nutritional imbalances and depletion, particularly when the stress response is severe and prolonged.[519,520,521] Specific to the consideration of pain, the depletion of tryptophan (and thus serotonin and melatonin) leaves the patient vulnerable to increased pain from lack of antinociceptive serotonin and to increased inflammation due to impaired endogenous production of anti-inflammatory cortisol, the adrenal release of which requires serotonin-dependent stimulation.[522] Severe stress, inflammation, and drugs used to suppress immune-mediated tissue damage (e.g., cyclosporine) increase urinary excretion of magnesium[523], and the eventual magnesium depletion renders the patient more vulnerable to hyperalgesia, depression, and other central nervous system and psychiatric disorders.[524,525] Furthermore, experimental and clinical data have shown that magnesium deficiency leads to a systemic pro-inflammatory state associated with oxidative stress and increased levels of the nociceptive and proinflammatory neurotransmitter substance P.[526] Stress increases secretion of prolactin, a hormone which plays an important pathogenic role in chronic inflammation and autoimmunity.[527,528] An abundance of experimental and clinical research supports the model that chronic psychoemotional stress reduces mucosal immunity,

[517] Evans JL, Maddux BA, Goldfine ID. The molecular basis for oxidative stress-induced insulin resistance. *Antioxid Redox Signal*. 2005 Jul-Aug;7(7-8):1040-52

[518] Joseph et al. Membrane and receptor modifications of oxidative stress vulnerability in aging. Nutritional considerations. *Ann N Y Acad Sci*. 1998 Nov 20;854:268-76

[519] Stephensen CB, Alvarez JO, et al. Vitamin A is excreted in the urine during acute infection. *Am J Clin Nutr*. 1994 Sep;60(3):388-92

[520] Ingenbleek Y, Bernstein L. The stressful condition as a nutritionally dependent adaptive dichotomy. *Nutrition*. 1999 Apr;15(4):305-20

[521] Henrotte et al. Blood and urinary magnesium, zinc, calcium, free fatty acids, and catecholamines in type A and type B subjects. *J Am Coll Nutr*. 1985;4(2):165-72

[522] Sandyk R. Tryptophan availability and the susceptibility to stress in multiple sclerosis: a hypothesis. *Int J Neurosci*. 1996 Jul;86(1-2):47-53

[523] DiPalma JR. Magnesium replacement therapy. *Am Fam Physician*. 1990 Jul;42(1):173-6

[524] Murck H. Magnesium and affective disorders. *Nutr Neurosci*. 2002 Dec;5(6):375-89

[525] Hashizume N, Mori M. An analysis of hypermagnesemia and hypomagnesemia. *Jpn J Med*. 1990 Jul-Aug;29(4):368-72

[526] Weglicki W, et al. Potassium, magnesium, and electrolyte imbalance and complications in disease management. *Clin Exp Hypertens*. 2005 Jan;27(1):95-112

[527] Imrich R. The role of neuroendocrine system in the pathogenesis of rheumatic diseases (minireview). *Endocr Regul*. 2002 Jun;36(2):95-106

[528] Orbach H, Shoenfeld Y. Hyperprolactinemia and autoimmune diseases. Autoimmun Rev. 2007 Sep;6(8):537-42

increases intestinal permeability, and allows for increased intestinal colonization by microbes that then stimulate immune responses that cross-react with musculoskeletal tissues and result in the clinical manifestation of autoimmunity and painful rheumatic syndromes which appear clinically as variants of acute and chronic reactive arthritis[529,530,531,532,533,534,535,536], formerly Reiter' syndrome.[537] Very interestingly, certain intestinal bacteria can sense when their human host is stressed, and they take advantage of the situation by becoming more virulent whereas previously these same bacteria may have been incapable of causing disease.[538,539] Psychoemotional stress also reduces mucosal immunity and increases colonization in locations other than the gastrointestinal tract. Microbial colonization of the genitourinary tract ("genitourinary dysbiosis") appears highly relevant in the genesis and perpetuation of rheumatoid arthritis.[540,541,542,543] Stressful life events also lower testosterone in men and the resultant lack of hormonal immunomodulation can increase the frequency and severity of exacerbations of rheumatoid arthritis[544]; resultant inflammation further suppresses testosterone production and bioavailability[545] leading to a self-perpetuating cycle of hypogonadism and inflammation. Thus, by numerous routes and mechanisms, psychoemotional stress increases the prevalence, persistence, and severity of musculoskeletal inflammation and pain.

Psychiatric codiagnoses are common among patients with painful neuromusculoskeletal disorders, and when the prevailing medical logic cannot solve the musculoskeletal riddle, the disorder is often ascribed to its accompanying mental disorder. The "appropriate" treatment from this perspective is the prescription of psychoactive drugs, generally of the "antidepressant" class. Science-based explanations are needed to expand clinicians' consideration of new possibilities which may someday prevail over commonplace suppositions that leave both clinician and patient trapped within a paradigm of futilely cyclical reasoning and its resultant simplistic symptom-targeting interventions. The following subsections provide alternatives to the "idiopathic pain is caused by its associated depression and both should be treated with antidepressant drugs" hypothesis.

a. <u>Pain, inflammation, and mental depression are final common pathways for nutritional deficiencies and imbalances</u>: As a scientific community we now know that the epidemic problem of vitamin D deficiency leads to both musculoskeletal pain[546] as well as depression[547], and that supplementation with physiologic doses of vitamin D results in an enhanced sense of well-being[548] and high-efficacy alleviation of musculoskeletal pain and depression while providing other major collateral benefits.[549] Since the existence of vitamin D deficiency is more probable than that of antidepressant deficiency, the appropriate intervention for the former is more scientific and rational than that of the latter. Relatedly, research in various fields has shown that Western/American lifestyle and diet patterns diverge radically from human physiologic expectations and human nutritional

[529] Tlaskalová-Hogenová et al. Commensal bacteria (normal microflora), mucosal immunity and chronic inflammatory and autoimmune diseases. *Immunol Lett.* 2004 May 15;93(2-3):97-108

[530] Collins SM. Stress and the Gastrointestinal Tract IV. Modulation of intestinal inflammation by stress. *Am J Physiol Gastrointest Liver Physiol.* 2001 Mar;280(3):G315-8

[531] Hart A, Kamm MA. Review article: mechanisms of initiation and perpetuation of gut inflammation by stress. *Aliment Pharmacol Ther.* 2002 Dec;16(12):2017-28

[532] Farhadi A, Fields JZ, Keshavarzian A. Mucosal mast cells are pivotal elements in inflammatory bowel disease that connect the dots: stress, intestinal hyperpermeability and inflammation. *World J Gastroenterol.* 2007 Jun 14;13(22):3027-30

[533] Yang PC, et al. Chronic psychological stress in rats induces intestinal sensitization to luminal antigens. *Am J Pathol.* 2006 Jan;168(1):104-14

[534] Rashid T, Ebringer A. Ankylosing spondylitis is linked to Klebsiella--the evidence. *Clin Rheumatol.* 2007 Jun;26(6):858-64

[535] Vasquez A. *Integrative Rheumatology*. Fort Worth, Texas; Integrative and Biological Medicine Research and Consulting, 2007 InflammationMastery.com

[536] Samarkos M, Vaiopoulos G. The role of infections in the pathogenesis of autoimmune diseases. *Curr Drug Targets Inflamm Allergy.* 2005 Feb;4(1):99-103

[537] Panush RS, Wallace DJ, Dorff RE, Engleman EP. Retraction of the suggestion to use the term "Reiter's syndrome" sixty-five years later: the legacy of Reiter, a war criminal, should not be eponymic honor but rather condemnation. *Arthritis Rheum.* 2007 Feb;56(2):693-4

[538] Alverdy J, Holbrook C, Rocha F, Seiden L, Wu RL, Musch M, Chang E, Ohman D, Suh S. Gut-derived sepsis occurs when the right pathogen with the right virulence genes meets the right host: evidence for in vivo virulence expression in Pseudomonas aeruginosa. *Ann Surg.* 2000 Oct;232(4):480-9

[539] Wu L, Holbrook C, Zaborina O, Ploplys E, Rocha F, Pelham D, Chang E, Musch M, Alverdy J. Pseudomonas aeruginosa expresses a lethal virulence determinant, the PA-I lectin/adhesin, in the intestinal tract of a stressed host: the role of epithelia cell contact and molecules of the Quorum Sensing Signaling System. *Ann Surg.* 2003;238(5):754-64

[540] Ebringer A, Rashid T. Rheumatoid arthritis is an autoimmune disease triggered by Proteus urinary tract infection. *Clin Dev Immunol.* 2006 Mar;13(1):41-8

[541] Erlacher L, Wintersberger W, Menschik M, et al. Reactive arthritis: urogenital swab culture is the only useful diagnostic method for the detection of the arthritogenic infection in extra-articularly asymptomatic patients with undifferentiated oligoarthritis. *Br J Rheumatol.* 1995 Sep;34(9):838-42

[542] Rashid T, Ebringer A. Rheumatoid arthritis is linked to Proteus--the evidence. *Clin Rheumatol.* 2007 Jul;26(7):1036-43

[543] Ebringer A, Rashid T, Wilson C. Rheumatoid arthritis: proposal for the use of anti-microbial therapy in early cases. *Scand J Rheumatol.* 2003;32:2-11

[544] James WH. Further evidence that low androgen values are a cause of rheumatoid arthritis: the response to seriously stressful life events. *Ann Rheum Dis* 1997;56:566

[545] Karagiannis A, Harsoulis F. Gonadal dysfunction in systemic diseases. *Eur J Endocrinol.* 2005 Apr;152(4):501-13

[546] Plotnikoff GA, Quigley JM. Prevalence of severe hypovitaminosis D in patients with persistent, nonspecific musculoskeletal pain. *Mayo Clin Proc.* 2003 Dec;78(12):1463-70

[547] Wilkins et al. Vitamin D deficiency is associated with low mood and worse cognitive performance in older adults. *Am J Geriatr Psychiatry.* 2006 Dec;14(12):1032-40

[548] Vieth R, Kimball S, Hu A, Walfish PG. Randomized comparison of the effects of the vitamin D3 adequate intake versus 100 mcg (4000 IU) per day on biochemical responses and the wellbeing of patients. *Nutr J.* 2004 Jul 19;3:8

[549] Vasquez et al. The clinical importance of vitamin D (cholecalciferol): a paradigm shift with implications for all healthcare providers. *Altern Ther Health Med.* 2004;10:28-36

requirements.[550] With regard to fatty acid intake and the resultant effects on inflammation and neurotransmission, modernized diets are a "set-up" for musculoskeletal pain and mental depression, which frequently occur concomitantly and which are both alleviated by corrective fatty acid intervention such as fish oil supplementation as a source of EPA and DHA.[551,552] Correction of fatty acid imbalance is therefore more rational in the comanagement of pain and depression than is sole reliance on antidepressant and anti-inflammatory drugs; the latter have their place in treatment but neither addresses the primary cause of the problem and both drug classes have important adverse effects and significant costs in contrast to the safety, affordability, and collateral benefits derived from fatty acid supplementation. Also relevant to this discussion of chronic pain triggered and perpetuated by nutritional imbalances are the pro-inflammatory nature of the Western/American diet[553] and the pain-sensitizing effects of epidemic magnesium deficiency.[554] Therefore, correction of nutritional deficiencies and optimization of nutritional status should generally logically supersede the prescription of drugs in patients with concomitant depression and pain. See review of microglial activation and altered neurotransmission detailed in Chapter 5

b. Pain, inflammation, and depression are final common pathways of physical inactivity: Exercising muscle elaborates cytokines ("myokines") with anti-inflammatory activity; a sedentary lifestyle fails to stimulate this endogenous anti-inflammation and is therefore relatively pro-inflammatory.[555] Further, exercise has antidepressant benefits mediated by positive influences on neurotransmission, growth factor elaboration, endocrinologic function, self-image, skill-building, and social contact.[556] Patients with musculoskeletal pain should be encouraged to exercise to the extent possible given the individual's capacity and type of injury and/or degree of disability. Thus, a prescription for exercise might supersede the prescription of drugs in patients with concomitant depression and pain. Exercise prescriptions must consider frequency, duration, intensity, variety, safety, enjoyment, accountability and objective measures of compliance and progress, as well as appropriate combinations of components which emphasize aerobic fitness, strengthening, flexibility, muscle balancing, coordination, skill-building and functional/practical applications.

c. Pain and depression are final common pathways of inflammation: Several pro-inflammatory cytokines are psychoactive and cause depression, social withdrawal, impaired cognition, and sickness behavior.[557] As an alternative to the use of antidepressant drugs, correction of the underlying inflammatory disorder by natural, pharmacologic, or integrative means may subsequently promote restoration of normal affect and cognitive function. (See Chapter 5.)

d. Pain, inflammation, and mental depression are final common pathways for hormonal deficiencies and imbalances: Deficiencies of thyroid hormones, testosterone, cortisol, and DHEA, and/or insufficiency or excess of estrogen can cause depression and impaired neuroemotional status. Hormonal aberrations are common in patients with chronic musculoskeletal pain, particularly of the inflammatory and autoimmune types. Clinical trials have shown that administration of thyroid hormones, testosterone, DHEA, cortisol and suppression prolactin can each provide anti-inflammatory, analgesic, and antidepressant benefits among appropriately selected patients. Thus, identification and correction of hormonal imbalances might supersede the prescription of antidepressant drugs in patients with concomitant depression, inflammation, and pain.

Our cultural and scientific advancements in the knowledge of how the brain and mind function have been paradoxically paralleled by social trends showing increasing depression and social isolation; the typical American has only two friends and no one in whom to confide.[558] In the United States, violent injuries are epidemic, and the level of firearm morbidity and mortality in the US is far higher than anywhere else in the

[550] O'Keefe JH Jr, Cordain L. Cardiovascular disease resulting from a diet and lifestyle at odds with our Paleolithic genome. *Mayo Clin Proc*. 2004 Jan;79(1):101-8

[551] Kiecolt-Glaser JK, et al. Depressive symptoms, omega-6:omega-3 fatty acids, and inflammation in older adults. *Psychosom Med*. 2007 Apr;69(3):217-24

[552] Simopoulos AP. Omega-3 fatty acids in inflammation and autoimmune diseases. *J Am Coll Nutr*. 2002 Dec;21(6):495-505

[553] Aljada et al. Increase in intranuclear nuclear factor kappaB and decrease in inhibitor kappaB in mononuclear cells after a mixed meal. *Am J Clin Nutr*. 2004 Apr;79(4):682-90

[554] Park JH, Niermann KJ, Olsen N. Evidence for metabolic abnormalities in the muscles of patients with fibromyalgia. *Curr Rheumatol Rep*. 2000 Apr;2(2):131-40

[555] Petersen AM, Pedersen BK. The anti-inflammatory effect of exercise. *J Appl Physiol*. 2005 Apr;98(4):1154-62

[556] Cotman CW, Berchtold NC, Christie LA. Exercise builds brain health: key roles of growth factor cascades and inflammation. *Trends Neurosci*. 2007 Sep;30(9):464-72

[557] Wilson CJ, Finch CE, Cohen HJ. Cytokines and cognition--the case for a head-to-toe inflammatory paradigm. *J Am Geriatr Soc*. 2002 Dec;50(12):2041-56

[558] McPherson M, Smith-Lovin L, Brashears ME. Social Isolation in America: Changes in Core Discussion Networks over Two Decades. *Am Sociological Rev* 2006; 71: 353-75

industrialized world.[559] This does to some extent beg the question of the value of "scientific knowledge" of the brain and mind within a social structure that is increasingly violent and fragmented. ==Further, the mental depression resultant from pandemic social isolation would be better served by physicians' admonition for increased social contact than by the continued overuse of drugs which inhibit neurotransmitter reuptake.==

<u>Conclusion</u>: The clinical employment of the functional medicine approach to chronic disease management and health promotion rests upon a foundation of competent patient management and then extends to consider the well-documented contributions of the causative *internal and external imbalances* that have allowed the genesis and perpetuation of the problem(s) under consideration. ==The attainment of wellness, the success of preventive medicine, and the optimization of socioemotional health cannot be attained by pharmacological suppression of the manifestations of dysfunction that result from nutritional and neuroendocrine imbalances, xenobiotic accumulation, sedentary lifestyles, social isolation, and mucosal microbial colonization.== Rather, these problems are addressed directly, and these and other causative considerations must remain foremost in the mind of the physician committed to the successful, ethical, and cost-effective long-term prevention and management of chronic health disturbances, particularly those characterized by inflammation and pain.

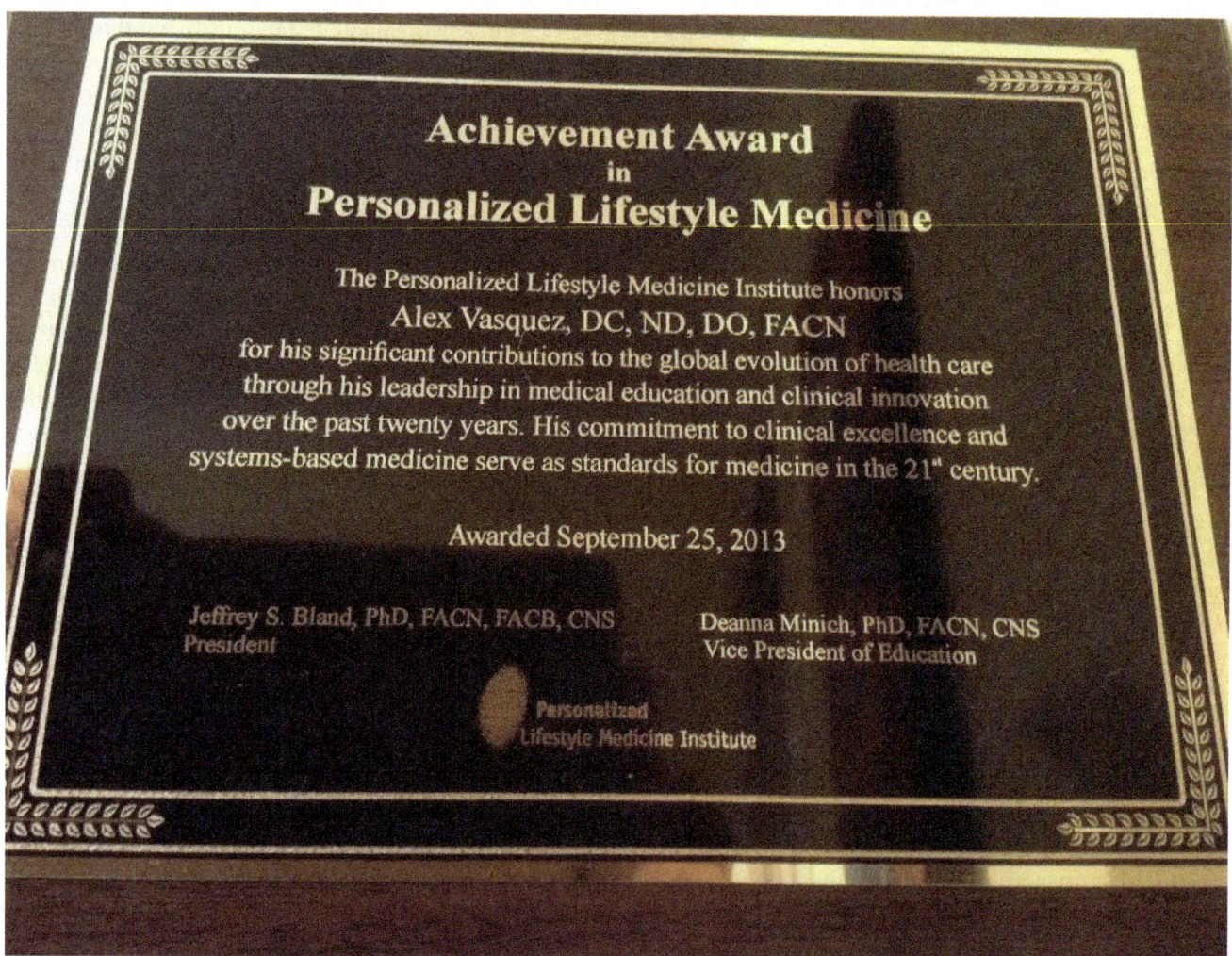

Achievement award: Sincere appreciation was shared at our 2013 International Conference on Human Nutrition and Functional Medicine, wherein Dr Vasquez and Dr Bland received awards for their contributions to the fields of nutrition and functional medicine. vimeo.com/ichnfm/2013keynote or vimeo.com/100562693 Password: Keynote

---

[559] Preventing firearm violence: a public health imperative. American College of Physicians. *Ann Intern Med.* 1995 Feb 15;122(4):311-3

The shadows of functional medicine: The single biggest shadow of functional medicine is pretty obvious to those of us who have been involved with what has now been described/degraded by some as a "movement" as if it were a social fad or cult rather than the culmination of biomedicine's potential: it is the *gross profiteering* off of the intellectual foundation provided by Dr Jeffrey Bland and of functional medicine's image as *a more sophisticated alternative to alternative medicine*. Some "authorities" within functional medicine grossly overcharge their clinical patients (real-world example $15,000 for initial patient consultation), and some prominent organizations beg for donations (including occasional crying on stage) under the pretense of working as a "nonprofit organization" while the internal mechanics of the organization overpay a select few administrators and undermine speaking careers and profitability of teaching faculty. Functional medicine as a discipline should not profess *health* and *holism* on the stage and then behave differently behind closed doors; functional medicine should manifest the same integrity, authenticity, and cohesiveness *in practice* that it promotes *for healthcare*.

Examples of dysfunction in functional medicine:

- Overpaying a select few: Using nonprofit status to grossly overpay part-time employees, e.g., more than $164,000 in a single year for part-time work or less.[560] Among the consequences of this are the demoralization of expert teaching faculty who are underpaid for their talent and hard work. The other obvious issue is that of integrity, or—more accurately—lack thereof. Personally, I think using "nonprofit status" to pay luxurious salaries to people who work (far) less than part-time is disingenuous and misleading; probably, donors would be less enthusiastic about their donations if they knew the "nonprofit" money was being used to overpay a small group of employees. Other *constantly elevating* salaries of $140,000 and $144,000 are far out of range for their corresponding US national average pay of $54,000-64,000 with a top 10% of $110,000.[561] From experience, I've learned to be wary when I see accountants of organizations being overpaid. At one particular so-called "non-profit" physician-education institution, we note that the accountant's salary exceeds the annual salary of many doctorate-level clinicians and certainly exceeds the salary of most college, university, and medical school professors (including full professors with hard-earned tenure); this is even more noteworthy during a time of major economic recession which particularly impacts the cash-only practices of many functional medicine clinicians. Larger payments by nonprofit groups are available via obligatory public disclosures: GuideStar.org

- Forcing members/attendees to pay *more* to receive *less*: Diluting educational quality for the intentional purpose of enlarging the quantity so that members/attendees will have to pay for additional courses to receive what would have otherwise been more/better information for less cost. Entrapping people in a "certification" process of diluted material makes them pay *more* while the organization works *less*.

- Exploitation of experts: Exploiting expert's knowledge by video-recording their presentations and then selling those presentations to third parties without informing or paying the expert, thus forcing the experts to essentially *compete with themselves* as lecturers. For me as a lecturer, I find it wholly unacceptable that an organization would pay me once for a presentation, and then record and sell my presentation to other audiences without compensating me; in this instance, the organization would be profiting far more from my own work—simply for pushing the "record" button—than would I after decades and long hours of work.

- Laboratory profiteering: A "functional medicine laboratory" used worthless laboratory methods[562] to profiteer millions of dollars from functional medicine clinicians and patients. Likely, the doctors and customers deserve a refund or compensation for this falsity, which likely lead to instances of misdiagnosis, delayed diagnosis, and erroneous treatment. Given the high cost of laboratory assessments in functional medicine—wherein a single panel of tests can cost $500-700 easily—the use of bogus laboratory methods cost patients and any unwitting insurance companies (tens of) millions of dollars in aggregate.

- Overzealous infatuation with technology and testing: Despite having a great model for disease genesis and treatment, functional medicine has factions that are intoxicated by laboratory testing and new technology, despite the high costs, dubious value, and the fact that treatment of phenotype (ie, the hologram) is generally more effective and cost-effective than is extensive and expensive laboratory testing, even if under the guise/auspice of "personalized treatment", which as a concept is unassailable. The overuse of lab testing gives the appearance of objectivity, despite the huge profiting/profiteering by companies and boutique practices.

---

[560] guidestar.org/ "Trusted nonprofit information. Search GuideStar for the most complete, up-to-date nonprofit data available." 2013 Jun and rechecked in 2014 Jul

[561] "According to the BLS, the median annual salary for an accountant was $63,550 in 2012, or $30.55 per hour. The best-paid 10 percent earned roughly $111,510," money.usnews.com/careers/best-jobs/accountant/salary

[562] Gingras BA, Duncan SB, Scheuller NJ, Schreckenberber PC. Assessment of diagnostic accuracy of recently introduced DNA stool screening test. *International Journal of Human Nutrition and Functional Medicine* 2014: 2(1);1 intjhumnutrfunctmed.org

- Serving "trends" and the healthcare needs of the financial elite; ignoring population-wide needs; silence on major issues: Functional medicine has a tendency to ignore the strength of its own model by jumping on popular trends; infatuation with testing and technology by definition means that functional medicine is preferentially serving the needs and interests of the financial upper class, thereby contributing to the very same social inequality that fuels health discrepancies. Major nonprofit groups in functional medicine and nutrition, despite claiming "independence" from commercial interests, clearly serve major commercial interests by advocating expensive tests and treatments, and by remaining silent on major issues such as the overuse of pesticides and the resultant contamination of the entire nation's/world's food, air, and water. Further, the lack of social diversity among functional medicine administrators and presenters is brightly obvious.

- Standing on the shoulders of giants does not make one a giant: Self-evident but frequently forgotten, this "esteem via association" has caused some people—indeed entire organizations—to consider themselves genius simply because they have (peripherally) associated with a genius. The fallacy is pretty clear from outside the organizational bubble.

- Misguided truths: Misusing the name(s) of intellectual giants such as Bland and Pauling and allowing low performers to undermine standards of excellence; bestowing grand namesake awards to people based on financial return and petty friendships rather scientific contribution, intellectual development, or exemplification of a better way of life.

- Verbal abuse and internet bullying: I observed an email discussion (2014 Jul) among many prominent "functional medicine experts" wherein one participant assumed the right to character assassinate another person merely for asking questions that were beyond the "bully's" intellectual ability to process and respond. This became a classic demonstration of the well-known Karpman drama triangle, wherein the bully/aggressor was clearly the offender— including using profanity and the insinuation of physical threat—yet he claimed to be the rescuer/defender of some of the more feeble participants and—as is classic and common—the victim. That such a conversation would occur among the highest members of the functional medicine community is an embarrassment to the very idea of functional medicine and how it should manifest in the real world.

- Arrogance, elitism, and profiteering—recent clinical experience: A patient of mine was charged $15,000 by a prominent functional medicine clinician for an initial evaluation of a previous diagnosis of rheumatoid arthritis; most of this profiteering was secured via overcharging for laboratory tests, the vast majority of which were unnecessary, as they simply lead to the assessment of inflammation (which we already knew) and need for nutritional supplementation (which we already knew). Originally, functional medicine was based in part on the idea that we could help patients become healthier in a less costly and more efficient manner by treating the causes of their problems; in this clinician's case, he chose to exploit the patient's illness, desire for healing, and the fame of functional medicine by cashing-in on her desperation—$15,000 for a one-time consultation and lab tests is pure exploitation, made even worse by the clinician's inefficacy.

- Unfair and unreasonable contracts for faculty: Contract clauses that force employees to resign their intelligence and self-respect by agreeing that the organization has no accountability whatsoever, even if it violates its own self-same contract. "Faculty agrees to indemnify, defend, and hold harmless from any and all actions, causes of action, claims, demands, costs, liabilities, expenses, and damages (including attorney's fees) arising out of or in connection with any breach of this Agreement."

- "We care (but we really don't)": Having a touchy-feely appearance and then refusing to accept feedback from paid members and faulty, alienating membership and faculty.

- Firing faculty members who have worked hard for the organization for more than 10 years and not even having the courage to let them know they have been replaced, e.g., faculty members who find out on Facebook that they are no longer employed despite 10 years of either no/low payment (ie, volunteer work) for high loyalty and valuable material/monetary contributions.

- Telling people how lucky they are to be in attendance: Modeling arrogance while talking humility, e.g., traditions of self-congratulatory behavior: telling audience members how lucky they are to be in attendance, after these same audience members have paid thousands of dollars to travel, attend, lodge, and take time away from clinical practice and family in order to attend educational events. In one example, a lecturer gave 15 self-congratulatory comments in the first 17 minutes of her presentation.

- Submit to my entitlement: In accord with the gross differential between image and reality, I know one notable presenter within the functional medicine movement who lectures on the importance of *the healing/therapeutic power of relationships* and then demanded (from me) free admission to my presentations and teaching materials because he said I had an obligation to "honor" our "relationship." Any relationship that includes **haughty demands for submission** and **arrogant assumptions of entitlement** is *not* a healing relationship and *not* one that should be modeled by someone well-positioned in the leadership of a major functional medicine institution.

Osteopathic Medicine

Osteopathy was founded by Andrew Taylor Still, a medical doctor who sought to reform what was then called the "Heroic" paradigm of medicine, which embraced bloodletting and the administration of leeches, purgatives, emetics, and poisons such as mercury as means for "rebalancing" what were perceived to be internal causes of disease, namely the "four humours" of the body which were thought to be blood, phlegm, black bile, and yellow bile. In part because of his training within and identification with the medical profession, Still sought to *reform* rather than *directly oppose* the "mainstream medicine" of his day; in contrast, chiropractic's founder Daniel David Palmer was more strongly opposed to the horrific medicine of his time and thus was more *revolutionary* than *evolutionary* in his approach to forging a new paradigm of health and healthcare. Still's willingness to align with the medical profession and the increasingly powerful and influential pharmaceutical industry unquestionably helped his fledgling profession survive the extinction that otherwise would have been swift at the hands of allopathic groups such as the American Medical Association (AMA), which labeled osteopathic physicians as "cultists" and systematically restricted inclusion of the osteopathic profession into mainstream healthcare by proclamation in 1953 that "…all voluntary associations with osteopaths are unethical." When osteopathic resistance mounted, the AMA and its co-conspirators, who were later found guilty of violating the nation's antitrust laws by illegally suppressing competition and attempting to build a medical monopoly[563], acquiesced and accepted osteopaths into its ranks—a strategy which the medical profession believed would eventually destroy the osteopathic profession by forcing it to resign its ideals and identity. In his review of osteopathic history, Gevitz[564] writes, "…the M.D.'s gradually came to believe that the only way to destroy osteopathy was through the absorption of D.O.'s, much as the homeopaths and eclectics [naturopaths] had been swallowed up early in the century." Even recently, the AMA has listed osteopathic medicine under "alternative medicine"[565] although several osteopathic medical colleges have consistently provided training that is superior to most "conventional" allopathic medical schools.[566] Today, osteopathic physicians practice in most ways similarly to allopaths—i.e., with unlimited scope of practice in all 50 states, full access to the use of drugs and surgery, and with a very pharmacosurgical paradigm of disease and healthcare. Osteopathic medicine is one of the fastest growing healthcare professions in America.

Osteopathic Manipulative Medicine: Osteopathic manipulative medicine (OMM) is similar to and yet distinct from chiropractic manipulation; the naturopathic profession—true to its eclectic roots—incorporates techniques from all professions. In contrast to chiropractic, OMM terminology and therapeutics focus much more on soft tissues, and the osteopathic lesion—"somatic dysfunction"—is clearly originated from soft tissues in contrast to the chiropractic lesion—the "vertebral subluxation"—which obviously originates from spinal articulations. Whereas the chiropractic intent of correcting or "adjusting" the "subluxation" was historically to improve function of the nervous system, the osteopathic lesion is addressed to more fully improve not only function of the nervous system but also of the vascular, lymphatic, and myofascial systems, too.[567] With regard to the latter, the osteopathic profession has always emphasized the importance of fascia in the genesis of "somatic dysfunction." Indeed, fascia appears to play an important and dynamic (not passive) role in neuromusculoskeletal health, particularly as it is a major contributor to proprioception and may also have a more direct effect through the recently described ability of fascia to actively contract in a smooth-muscle-like manner.[568]

From this author's perspective, two of the most widely used osteopathic texts—*Osteopathic Principles in Practice* (1994) by Kuchera and Kuchera[569], and *Outline of Osteopathic Manipulative Procedures* (2006) by Kimberly[570]—both leave very much to be desired with respect to their clarity, terminology, clinical applicability, and referencing to the scientific literature. *Manipulation of the Spine, Thorax and Pelvis: An Osteopathic Perspective* (2006) by Gibbons

---

[563] Getzendanner S. Permanent injunction order against AMA. *JAMA*. 1988 Jan 1;259(1):81-2

[564] Gevitz N. *The D.O.'s: Osteopathic Medicine in America*. Johns Hopkins University Press; 1991; pages 100-103

[565] American Medical Association. Report 12 of the Council on Scientific Affairs (A-97) Full Text ama-assn.org/ama/pub/category/13638.html November 23, 2006

[566] Special report. America's best graduate schools. Schools of Medicine. The top schools: primary care. *US News World Rep*. 2004 Apr 12;136(12):74

[567] Williams N. Managing back pain in general practice--is osteopathy the new paradigm? *Br J Gen Pract*. 1997 Oct;47(423):653-5

[568] "…the existence of an active fascial contractility could have interesting implications for the understanding of musculoskeletal pathologies with an increased or decreased myofascial tonus. It may also offer new insights and a deeper understanding of treatments directed at fascia, such as manual myofascial release therapies or acupuncture." Schleip et al. Active fascial contractility: Fascia may be able to contract in a smooth muscle-like manner and thereby influence musculoskeletal dynamics. *Med Hypotheses*. 2005;65:273-7

[569] Kuchera WA, Kuchera ML. *Osteopathic Principles in Practice, revised second edition*. Kirksville, MO, KCOM Press; 1994

[570] Kimberly PE. *Outline of Osteopathic Manipulative Procedures.The Kimberly Manual 2006*. Kirksville College Osteopathic Medicine. Walsworth Publish. Co., Marceline, Mo

and Tehan[571] is much more accessible and clinically applicable; however the text focuses exclusively on high-velocity low-amplitude (HVLA) techniques and therefore does not provide sufficient background and training for students in the very techniques that distinguish osteopathic from chiropractic techniques, namely heightened attention to the myofascial dysfunction that (appropriately) underlies the osteopathic lesion.

Ironically, the very growth and "allopathicization" of the profession that has threatened the profession's adherence to its holistic tenets has caused a reflexive re-affirmation of these tenets, and the profession has responded with a well-funded and intentional directive to scientifically investigate the mechanisms and efficacy of osteopathic manipulative medicine.[572,573] Recent findings include improved function and reduced pain in patients treated with a comprehensive manipulative technique for the shoulder[574], as well as the significant efficacy of ankle manipulation for patients with recent ankle injuries.[575] Further, OMM treatment of patients medicated for depression was found to triple the effectiveness of drug monotherapy.[576] Other studies have shown benefit of OMM in the treatment of geriatric pneumonia[577], pediatric asthma[578], pediatric dysfunctional voiding[579], carpal tunnel syndrome[580], low-back pain[581], and recovery from cardiac bypass surgery.[582] Replication and validation of these studies—many of which are small or of nonrigorous design (e.g., open clinical trials with no control group)—is important to further define and establish the value of osteopathic manipulation in clinical care.

The shadow of osteopathic medicine: Most insiders will agree that—with all due respect for the tremendous progress made by the osteopathic profession, having gone from *medical oppression* to *medical acceptance* to now *medical parity* and some would argue *medical superiority* due to the equivalent *quality* of education and (with the discipline of osteopathic manipulative medicine) greater *quantity* of medical education compared with allopaths—the challenge for the profession now is that of identity, or—more accurately—integrity. Can and will the osteopathic profession maintain and champion its holistic perspective on health and all that such a perspective entails, or will it continue to genuflect to the pathocentric and pharmacodependent model of allopathic medicine? These are obviously important questions with implications for the educational process, clinical practice, and professional differentiation and post-graduate education. In our osteopathic college at University of North Texas Health Science Center Texas College of Osteopathic Medicine, we obviously proved ourselves to be a top medical school in Primary Care Medicine (*U.S. News & World*

Osteopathic Interventions need to be Consistent with Osteopathic Philosophy

"In contrast to the description of the osteopathic medical profession by the American Osteopathic Association, namely, "doctors of osteopathic medicine, or D.O.s, apply the philosophy of treating the whole person to the prevention, diagnosis and treatment of illness, disease and injury," [the authors of the article in question] essentially reviewed only pharmacologic treatment. ...It is hoped that future reviews in this journal can include a more balanced survey of the literature, inclusive of non-pharmacologic and "holistic" interventions that are consistent with osteopathic philosophy."

Vasquez A. Interventions need to be Consistent with Osteopathic Philosophy. [Letter] *JAOA: Journal of the American Osteopathic Association* 2006 Sep jaoa.org/cgi/content/full/106/9/528

---

[571] Gibbons P, Tehan P. Manipulation of the Spine, Thorax and Pelvis: An Osteopathic Perspective. Churchill Livingstone; 2006. Isbn: 044310039X

[572] Wisnioski SW 3rd. "Circle Turns Round" to "Allopathic Osteopathy." *J Am Osteopath Assoc* 2006; 106: 423-4 jaoa.org/cgi/content/full/106/7/423

[573] Teitelbaum HS, et al. Osteopathic medical education: renaissance or rhetoric? *J Am Osteopath Assoc.* 2003 Oct;103(10):489-90 jaoa.org/cgi/reprint/103/10/489

[574] Knebl JA, Shores JH, Gamber RG, Gray WT, Herron KM. Improving functional ability in the elderly via the Spencer technique, an osteopathic manipulative treatment: a randomized, controlled trial. *J Am Osteopath Assoc.* 2002 Jul;102(7):387-96 jaoa.org/cgi/reprint/102/7/387

[575] This study shows the rapid onset and benefit of manipulative medicine for the treatment of acute ankle sprains: Eisenhart AW, Gaeta TJ, Yens DP. Osteopathic manipulative treatment in the emergency department for patients with acute ankle injuries. *J Am Osteopath Assoc.* 2003 Sep;103(9):417-21 jaoa.org/cgi/reprint/103/9/417

[576] This study impressively showed that musculoskeletal manipulation improved treatment effectiveness for depression from 33% to 100%. "After 8 weeks, 100% of the OMT treatment group and 33% of the control group tested normal by psychometric evaluation. ... The findings of this pilot study indicate that OMT may be a useful adjunctive treatment for alleviating depression in women." Plotkin et al. Adjunctive osteopathic manipulative treatment in women with depression. *J Am Osteopath Assoc.* 2001 Sep;101(9):517-23

[577] This study showed improved clinical outcomes and reduced antibiotic use in elderly patients with pneumonia when treated with manipulative medicine: "The treatment group had a significantly shorter duration of intravenous antibiotic treatment and a shorter hospital stay." Noll DR, Shores JH, Gamber RG, Herron KM, Swift J Jr. Benefits of osteopathic manipulative treatment for hospitalized elderly patients with pneumonia. *J Am Osteopath Assoc.* 2000 Dec;100(12):776-82 jaoa.org/cgi/reprint/100/12/776

[578] Osteopathic manipulation improved pulmonary function in pediatric patients with asthma: "With a confidence level of 95%, results for the OMT group showed a statistically significant improvement of 7 L per minute to 9 L per minute for peak expiratory flow rates. These results suggest that OMT has a therapeutic effect among this patient population." Guiney PA, Chou R, Vianna A, Lovenheim J. Effects of osteopathic manipulative treatment on pediatric patients with asthma: a randomized controlled trial. *J Am Osteopath Assoc.* 2005 Jan;105(1):7-12 jaoa.org/cgi/content/full/105/1/7

[579] Nemett et al. Randomized controlled trial of effectiveness of osteopathy-based manual physical therapy treating pediatric dysfunctional voiding. *J Pediatr Urol* 2008 Apr:100-6

[580] Sucher BM, Hinrichs RN, Welcher RL, Quiroz LD, St Laurent BF, Morrison BJ. Manipulative treatment of carpal tunnel syndrome: biomechanical and osteopathic intervention to increase the length of the transverse carpal ligament: part 2. Effect of sex differences and manipulative "priming". *J Am Osteopath Assoc.* 2005 May;105(5):238 jaoa.org/cgi/content/full/105/3/135

[581] "CONCLUSION: OMT significantly reduces low back pain. The level of pain reduction is greater than expected from placebo effects alone and persists for at least three months." Licciardone JC, Brimhall AK, King LN. Osteopathic manipulative treatment for low back pain: a systematic review and meta-analysis of randomized controlled trials. *BMC Musculoskelet Disord.* 2005 Aug 4;6;43 biomedcentral.com/1471-2474/6/43

[582] This study showed benefit from osteopathic manipulation administered immediately after coronary artery bypass graft surgery: "The observed changes in cardiac function and perfusion indicated that OMT had a beneficial effect on the recovery of patients after CABG surgery. The authors conclude that OMT has immediate, beneficial hemodynamic effects after CABG surgery when administered while the patient is sedated and pharmacologically paralyzed." O-Yurvati et al. Hemodynamic effects of osteopathic manipulative treatment immediately after coronary artery bypass graft surgery. *J Am Osteopath Assoc.* 2005 Oct;105(10):475-81 jaoa.org/cgi/content/full/105/10/475

Report, 2002 through present), Top 15 Specialty Ranking in Rural Medicine, Geriatrics (2013), Top 20 Specialty Ranking in Family Medicine (2013), and our students in particular attained top performance on US Medical Licensing Examination (USMLE) and Comprehensive Osteopathic Medical Licensing Examination (COMLEX) wherein I personally scored in the top 1% and 5% nationally for each of the medical licensing exams I took; but at times we seemed to have nearly paid for our education with our souls: I have never worked so hard in my life as I did in osteopathic medical school, and while I wished some less brutal methods might have been used, I am authentically grateful for the transformative experience. However, when I look at the profession as a reader of the *Journal of American Osteopathic Association* (JAOA), I often get the impression I am looking at a profession that has sold itself for too low a price to the pharmaceutical paradigm; reading the *JAOA* often leaves me with the impression that I just read some very noncomplex articles, many of which seem/are directly authored promotional material from the pharmaceutical industry. I continue to hope that "future reviews in this journal [and perspectives from the profession it represents] can include a more balanced survey of the literature, inclusive of non-pharmacologic and "holistic" interventions that are consistent with osteopathic philosophy."[583]

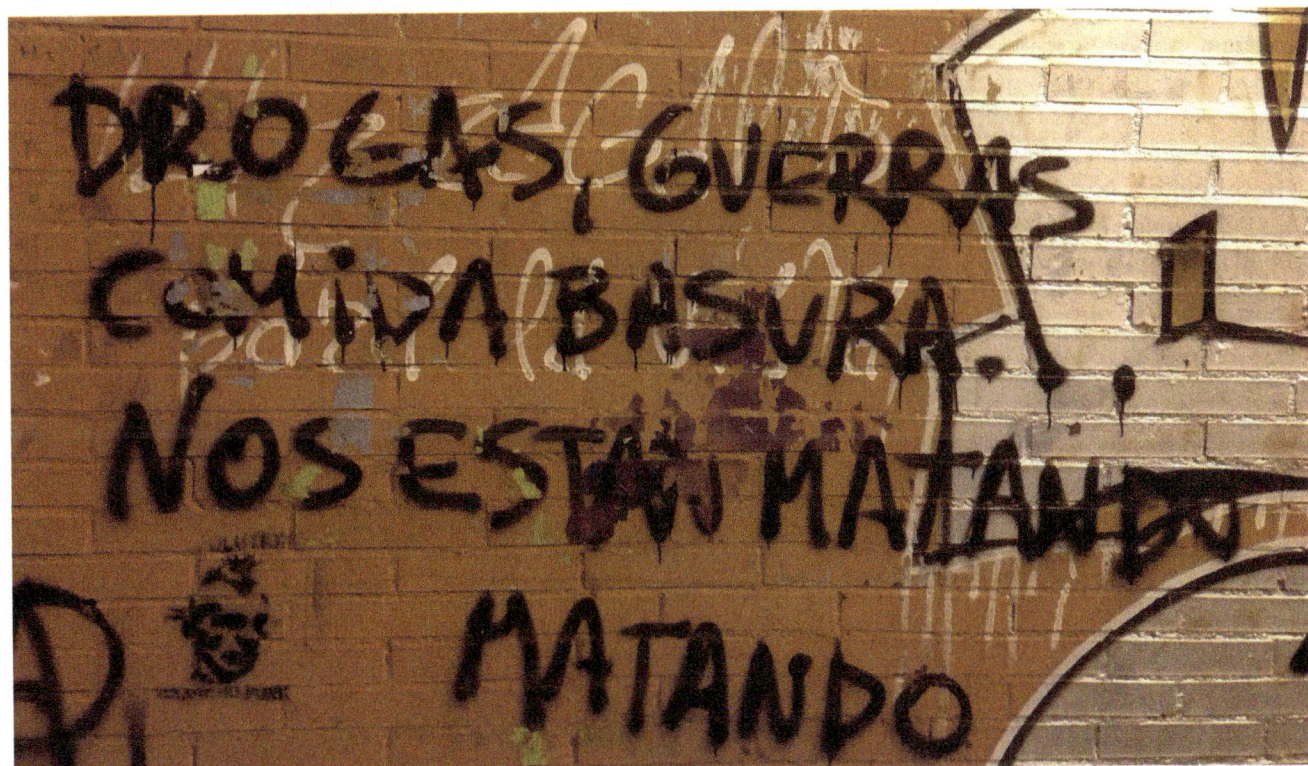

The population is increasingly aware of the hazards of medicines, junk foods (made cheap and convenient by government subsidies) and paradigms of endless war—Photo of graffiti in Merida Spain 2013 by DrV: Translates from Spanish to English as "Drugs, wars, and junk [garbage] food are killing us." One might wonder if "drogas/drugs" is meant to imply recreational drugs or prescriptions drugs, the latter of which—in the form of "adverse drug effects" and other iatrogenesis—kill 3,500 patients per week in the United States alone; per the excellent clinical review published in *American Family Physician* (1997 Nov): "Recent estimates suggest that each year more than 1 million patients are injured while in the hospital and approximately 180,000 die because of these injuries. Furthermore, drug-related morbidity and mortality are common and are estimated to cost more than $136 billion a year."

---

[583] Vasquez A. Interventions need to be Consistent with Osteopathic Philosophy. [Letter] *JAOA: Journal of the American Osteopathic Association* 2006 Sep jaoa.org/cgi/content/full/106/9/528

"The human body represents the actions of three laws—spiritual, mechanical, and chemical— united as one triune. As long as there is perfect union of these three, there is health." Daniel David Palmer—the founder of chiropractic

The basic philosophical model which is taught in many chiropractic colleges is to envision health, disease, and patient care from a conceptual model named the "triad of health" which gives its attention to the three fundamental foundations for well-being: namely, the physical/structural, mental/emotional, and biochemical/nutritional aspects of health. Revolutionary at the time of its inception in the early 1900's, this model now forms the foundation for the increasingly dominant and very popular paradigm of "holistic medicine." It remains a powerful contrast and an attractive alternative to the reductionistic allopathic approach, which generally approaches the human body as if it were simply a conglomerate of independent organ systems that have little or no functional relationship to each other.[584]

Using the state of the sciences before the year 1910, chiropractic was founded with a profound appreciation of the integrated nature of health, and the therapeutic focus was on spinal manipulation. In describing the chiropractic model of health, DD Palmer[585] wrote, "The human body represents the actions of three laws—spiritual, mechanical, and chemical—united as one triune. As long as there is perfect union of these three, there is health." While the therapeutic focus of the profession has been spinal manipulation, from its inception the chiropractic profession has emphasized a holistic, integrative model of therapeutic intervention, health, and disease, and chiropractic was the first healthcare profession in America to specifically claim that the optimization of health requires attention to spiritual-emotional-psychological, mechanical-physical-structural, and biochemical-nutritional-hormonal-chemical considerations.

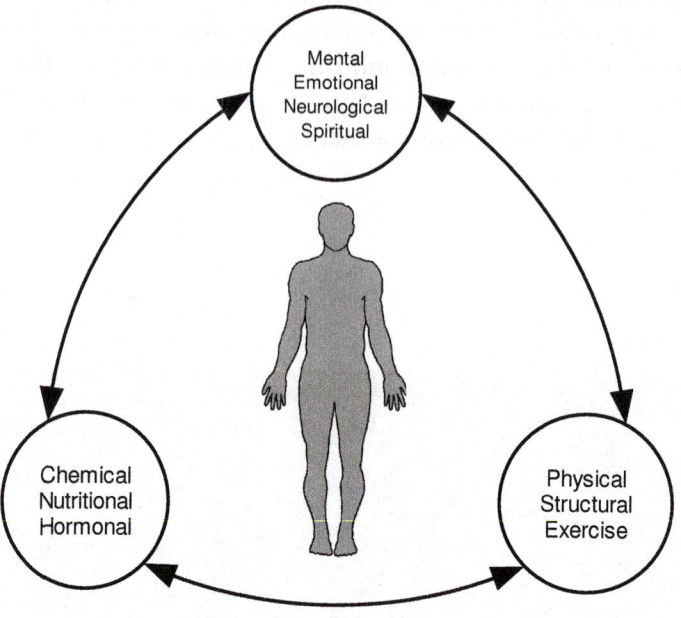

The chiropractic "triad of health"

From its inception, chiropractic has been a philosophy of healing that considered the entire health of the patient by addressing the interconnected aspects of our chemical-spiritual-physical being. Later, intraprofessional factions polarized between holistic and vitalistic paradigms; the latter has been presumed to be the philosophy of the entire profession by organizations such as the American Medical Association[586] that have sought to contain and eliminate chiropractic and other forms of natural healthcare[587] by falsifying research[588,589], intentionally misleading the public and manipulating politicians[590,591,592], arriving at illogical conclusions which support the medical paradigm and refute the value of manual therapies[593], and exploiting weaknesses within the profession for its own financial profitability and political advantage.[594] Intentional misrepresentation and defamation of chiropractic continues to occur to recent times, as documented by the 2006 review by Wenban.[595]

[584] Beckman JF, Fernandez CE, Coulter ID. A systems model of health care: a proposal. *J Manipulative Physiol Ther.* 1996 Mar-Apr; 19(3): 208-15

[585] Palmer DD. *The Science, Art, and Phiosophy, of Chiropractic.* Portland, OR; Portland Printing House Company, 1910: 107

[586] American Medical Association. Report 12 of the Council on Scientific Affairs (A-97) Full Text. ama-assn.org/ama/pub/category/13638.html Accessed Sep 10, 2005

[587] Getzendanner S. Permanent injunction order against AMA. *JAMA.* 1988 Jan 1;259(1):81-2

[588] Terrett AG. Misuse of the literature by medical authors in discussing spinal manipulative therapy injury. *J Manipulative Physiol Ther.* 1995 May;18(4):203-10

[589] Morley J, Rosner AL, Redwood D. A case study of misrepresentation of the scientific literature: recent reviews of chiropractic. *J Altern Complement Med.* 2001 Feb;7(1):65-78

[590] Spivak JL. *The Medical Trust Unmasked.* Louis S. Siegfried Publishers; New York: 1961

[591] Trever W. *In the Public Interest.* Los Angeles; Scriptures Unlimited; 1972. This is probably the most authoritative documentation of the illegal actions of the AMA up to 1972; contains numerous photocopies of actual AMA documents and minutes of official meetings with overt intentionality of destroying Americans' healthcare options so that the AMA and related organizations would have a monopoly in healthcare.

[592] Wolinsky H, Brune T. The Serpent on the Staff: The Unhealthy Politics of the American Medical Association. GP Putnam and Sons, New York, 1994

[593] Mein EA, et al. Manual medicine diversity: research pitfalls and the emerging medical paradigm. *J Am Osteopath Assoc.* 2001 Aug;101(8):441-4

[594] Wilk CA. Medicine, Monopolies, and Malice: How the Medical Establishment Tried to Destroy Chiropractic. Garden City Park: Avery, 1996

[595] Wenban AB. Inappropriate use of the title 'chiropractor' and term 'chiropractic manipulation' in the peer-reviewed biomedical literature. *Chiropr Osteopat.* 2006;14:16

In accord with the comprehensive chiropractic training in musculoskeletal management, numerous sources of evidence demonstrate that chiropractic management of the most common spinal pain syndromes is safer and less expensive than allopathic medical treatment, particularly for the treatment of low-back pain. In their extensive review of the literature, Manga et al[596] published in 1993 that chiropractic management of low-back pain is superior to allopathic medical management in terms of greater safety, greater effectiveness, and reduced cost; they concluded, "There is an overwhelming body of evidence indicating that chiropractic management of low-back pain is more cost-effective than medical management" and "There would be highly significant cost savings if more management of LBP [low-back pain] was transferred from medical physicians to chiropractors." In a randomized trial involving 741 patients, Meade et al[597] showed, "Chiropractic treatment was more effective than hospital outpatient management, mainly for patients with chronic or severe back pain... The benefit of chiropractic treatment became more evident throughout the follow up period. Secondary outcome measures also showed that chiropractic was more beneficial." A 3-year follow-up study by these same authors[598] in 1995 showed, "At three years the results confirm the findings of an earlier report that when chiropractic or hospital therapists treat patients with low-back pain as they would in day to day practice, those treated by chiropractic derive more benefit and long term satisfaction than those treated by hospitals." In 2004 Legorreta et al[599] reported that the availability of chiropractic care was associated with significant cost savings among 700,000 patients with chiropractic coverage compared to 1 million patients whose insurance coverage was limited to allopathic medical treatments; whether the cost savings associated with chiropractic availability are due to 1) improved overall health and reduced need for pharmacosurgical intervention, 2) greater safety and lower cost of chiropractic treatment versus pharmacosurgical treatment, and/or 3) self-selection by wellness-oriented, perhaps healthier, and higher-income patients, remains to be determined. A literature review by Dabbs and Lauretti[600] showed that spinal manipulation is safer than the use of NSAIDs in the treatment of neck pain; of note beyond NSAIDs is the finding that Coxibs have injured and killed tens of thousands of patients. [601] Contrasting the rates of manipulation-associated cerebrovascular accidents to the dangers of medical and surgical treatments for spinal disorders, Rosner[602] noted, "These rates are 400 times lower than the death rates observed from gastrointestinal bleeding due to the use of nonsteroidal anti-inflammatory drugs and 700 times lower than the overall mortality rate for spinal surgery." Similarly, in his review of the literature comparing the safety of chiropractic manipulation in patients with low-back pain associated with lumbar disc herniation, Oliphant[603] showed that, "The apparent safety of spinal manipulation, especially when compared with other [medically] accepted treatments for [lumbar disk herniation], should stimulate its use in the conservative treatment plan of [lumbar disk herniation]."

Osteopathic medicine, discussed in a previous section, shares a few features in common with chiropractic. Osteopathic medicine and chiropractic are American-born healthcare professions and paradigms that started at nearly the same time in history and from many of the same foundational principles. Both professions were started in the late 1800's and early 1900's and were founded upon the philosophical premise that the body functioned as a whole and that therefore healthcare and therapeutic interventions needed to be comprehensive in scope and multifaceted in their application. Further, both professions emphasized the importance of structural integrity as a foundational component of health and thus embraced manual manipulative therapy and spinal manipulation. From their common origins, subtle differences and chance historic events shaped and further separated these professions from each other.

[596] Manga P, et al. The Effectiveness and Cost-Effectiveness of Chiropractic Management of Low-Back Pain. Richmond Hill, Ontario: Kenilworth Publishing; 1993

[597] Meade TW, et al. Low-back pain of mechanical origin: randomised comparison of chiropractic and hospital outpatient treatment. *BMJ*. 1990;300(6737):1431-7

[598] Meade TW, et al. Randomised comparison of chiropractic and hospital outpatient management for low-back pain: results from extended follow up. *BMJ*. 1995;311(7001):349-5

[599] Legorreta et al. Comparative analysis of individuals with and without chiropractic coverage: patient characteristics, utilization, and costs. *Arch Intern Med*. 2004;164:1985-92

[600] Dabbs V, Lauretti WJ. A risk assessment of cervical manipulation vs. NSAIDs for the treatment of neck pain. *J Manipulative Physiol Ther*. 1995;18:530-6

[601] Topol EJ. Failing the public health--rofecoxib, Merck, and the FDA. *N Engl J Med*. 2004 Oct 21;351(17):1707-9

[602] Rosner AL. Evidence-based clinical guidelines for the management of acute low-back pain: response to the guidelines prepared for the Australian Medical Health and Research Council. *J Manipulative Physiol Ther*. 2001;24(3):214-20

[603] Oliphant D. Safety of spinal manipulation in the treatment of lumbar disk herniations: a systematic review and risk assessment. *J Manipulative Physiol Ther*. 2004;27:197-210

The shadow(s) of the chiropractic profession: Coming face-to-face with the shadow(s) of the chiropractic profession has easily been one of the biggest disappointments in my life. Like many young athletic students who are attracted to the profession, I fell in love with the profession's *image* and its *potential*—before I knew about the *realities* within the schools and the larger profession. That I have/had been a major cheerleader for the chiropractic profession—advocating for the profession's scope expansion, for high professional standards, and for greater integrative chiropractic care—is well documented in my many publications for the chiropractic profession starting in 1994[604], including my being the first (to my knowledge) chiropractic doctor published in the American College of Rheumatology's journal *Arthritis & Rheumatism*[605], my writing of the profession's first clinical textbook on the management of hypertension and differential diagnosis of high blood pressure[606], and my numerous other *pro-chiropractic* books, articles, and editorials.[607] However, after working

The price of our commitment to truth

"We have had to pay dearly for every atom of truth. We have had to pay for it with almost everything that our hearts, our love, our trust cling to. This requires greatness of soul. The service of truth is the hardest service."

Nietzsche FW. *Cambridge University Texts in the History of Philosophy*; 2005, p. 49

Truth can—and often does—hurt

"Your pain is the breaking of the shell that encloses your understanding. It is the bitter potion by which the physician within you heals your sick self; so therefore, trust the physician and drink his remedy in silence and tranquility."

Kahlil Gibran. *The Prophet*; 1923

---

[604] Vasquez A. High body iron stores: causes, effects, diagnosis, and treatment. *Nutritional Perspectives* 1994
[605] Vasquez A. Musculoskeletal disorders and iron overload disease. [Letter] *Arthritis & Rheumatism* 1996; 39:1767-8
[606] Vasquez A. Chiropractic Management of Chronic Hypertension 2010, Integrative Chiropractic Management of High Blood Pressure: Updated & Expanded 2nd Edition 2011
[607] A sample listing of additional pro-chiropractic, chiropractic-specific, and chiropractic-friendly books, articles, and editorials by Dr Vasquez:

1. Vasquez A. *Integrative Orthopedics*: 2004, 2007, 2012
2. Vasquez A. *Integrative Rheumatology*: 2006, 2007, 2014
3. Vasquez A. *Musculoskeletal Pain: Expanded Clinical Strategies*: Printed monograph approved for ACCME PRA-1 Continuing Medical Education. 2008 May
4. Vasquez A. Chiropractic and Naturopathic Mastery of Common Clinial Disorders: 2009
5. Vasquez A. Selected Topics in NeuroMusculoskeletal Medicine: 2013
6. Vasquez A. Chiropractors Managing Chronic Hypertension An Idea Who's Time Has Arrived. *Dynamic Chiropractic* 2010 Jun
7. Vasquez A. Affirmation and Rebirth of the Chiropractic Profession, Part 1. Setting New Standards in Office-Based Musculoskeletal Care and Health Promotion. *Dynamic Chiropractic* 2007 Apr
8. Vasquez A. Affirmation and Rebirth of the Chiropractic Profession, Part 2. *Dynamic Chiropractic* 2007 Apr
9. Vasquez A. Chiropractic Musculoskeletal Competence: Is Being "Best" Good Enough? *Dynamic Chiropractic* 2007 Mar
10. Vasquez A. Implementing the Five-Part Nutritional Wellness Protocol for the Treatment of Various Health Problems. *Nutritional Wellness*—a chiropractic nutrition magazine 2005 Nov
11. Vasquez A. The Importance of Integrative Chiropractic Health Care in Treating Musculoskeletal Pain and Reducing the Nationwide Burden of Medical Expenses and Iatrogenic Injury and Death: A Concise Review of Current Research and Implications for Clinical Practice and Healthcare Policy. *The Original Internist*—a chiropractic magazine/journal 2005; 12(4): 159-182
12. Vasquez A. Revisiting the Five-Part Nutritional Wellness Protocol: The Supplemented Paleo-Mediterranean Diet. *Nutritional Perspectives*—published by the American Chiropractic Association's Council on Nutrition 2011 January
13. Vasquez A. Five-Part Nutritional Wellness Protocol That Produces Consistently Positive Results. *Nutritional Wellness*—chiropractic nutrition magazine 2005 Sep
14. Vasquez A. The Science of Chiropractic and Spinal Manipulation, Part 2 mercola.com/2005/mar/12/chiropractic_spine.htm 2005, March 12
15. Vasquez A. The Science of Chiropractic and Spinal Manipulation, Part 1 mercola.com/2005/mar/9/chiropractic_spine.htm 2005, March 9
16. Vasquez A. Vitamin D Supplementation in the Treatment of Musculoskeletal Pain. *The Original Internist*—a chiropractic magazine/journal 2004; 11: 7-9
17. Vasquez A, John Cannell, MD. Better Bones and Beyond: Vitamin D Plays Role in Inflammatory and Metabolic Disease. *Holistic Primary Care* 2004; (Fall) 5: 3,6,7
18. Vasquez A. Integrative Orthopedics and Vitamin D: Testing, Administration, and New Relevance in the Treatment of Musculoskeletal Pain. *Townsend Letter for Doctors and Patients* 2004; October, 75-77
19. John Cannell, MD and Vasquez A. Measuring Your Vitamin D Levels: Your Most Important Blood Test? mercola.com/2004/jul/3/vitamin_d_levels.htm 2004, July 3
20. Vasquez A. Interventions Need to Be Consistent with Osteopathic Philosophy. *JAOA: Journal of the American Osteopathic Association* 2006 Sep
21. Vasquez A. Web-like Interconnections of Physiological Factors. *Integrative Medicine: A Clinician's Journal* 2006 Apr/May
22. Vasquez A. Reducing pain and inflammation naturally - Part 6: Nutritional and Botanical Treatments against "Silent Infections" and Gastrointestinal Dysbiosis, Commonly Overlooked Causes of Neuromusculoskeletal Inflammation and Chronic Health Problems. *Nutritional Perspectives*—by ACA Council on Nutr 2006 Jan
23. Vasquez A. "Chapter 10: Organ System Function and Underlying Mechanisms: The Interconnected Web." In Jones DS (Editor-in-Chief). *Textbook of Functional Medicine*. Institute for Functional Medicine. 2005
24. Vasquez A. "Chapter 25: Structural Imbalances." In Jones DS (Editor-in-Chief). *Textbook of Functional Medicine*. Institute for Functional Medicine. 2005
25. Vasquez A. "Chapter 27: Inflammation and Autoimmunity: A Functional Medicine Approach." In Jones DS (Editor-in-Chief). *Textbook of Functional Medicine*. Institute for Functional Medicine. 2005
26. Vasquez A, Murray MT. Chapter 188 "Inflammatory Bowel Diseases: Ulcerative Colitis and Crohn's Disease" in Pizzorno JE, Murray MT (Eds). *Textbook of Natural Medicine: Third Edition*. Churchill Livingstone. 2005 Nov
27. Vasquez A. Reducing pain and inflammation naturally - Part 5: Improving neuromusculoskeletal health by optimizing immune function and reducing allergic reactions: a review of 16 treatments and a 3-step clinical approach. *Nutritional Perspectives*—published by the ACA's Council on Nutrition 2005 Oct
28. Vasquez A, Muanza DN. Comment: evaluation of presence of aspirin-related warnings with willow bark.[letter] *Annals of Pharmacotherapy* 2005 Oct
29. Vasquez A, Cannell J. Calcium and vitamin D in preventing fractures: data are not sufficient to show inefficacy.[letter] *BMJ: British Medical Journal* 2005 May
30. Vasquez A. Reducing pain and inflammation naturally - Part 4: Nutritional and Botanical Inhibition of NFkappaB, the Major Intracellular Amplifier of the Inflammatory Cascade. A Practical Clinical Strategy Exemplifying Anti-Inflammatory Nutrigenomics. *Nutritional Perspectives*—published by the American Chiropractic Association's Council on Nutrition 2005 July
31. Vasquez A. Subphysiologic Doses of Vitamin D are Subtherapeutic: Comment on the Study by The Record Trial Group. *TheLancet.com* 2005 May online
32. Vasquez A. Reducing pain and inflammation naturally - Part 3: Improving overall health while safely and effectively treating musculoskeletal pain. *Nutritional Perspectives*—published by the American Chiropractic Association's Council on Nutrition 2005; 28: 34-38, 40-42
33. Vasquez A. Healthcare for our bones: Practical nutritional approach to preventing osteoporosis. [Letter]. *JManipulative and Physiological Therapeutics* 2005;28:213
34. Vasquez A. Reducing Pain and Inflammation Naturally. Part 2: New Insights into Fatty Acid Supplementation and Its Effect on Eicosanoid Production and Genetic Expression. *Nutritional Perspectives*—published by the American Chiropractic Association's Council on Nutrition 2005; January: 5-16
35. Muanza DN, Vasquez A, et al. Isoflavones and Postmenopausal Women. [Letter] *JAMA: Journal of the American Medical Association* 2004; 292: 2337
36. Vasquez A. Reducing Pain and Inflammation Naturally. Part 1: New Insights into Fatty Acid Biochemistry and the Influence of Diet. *Nutritional Perspectives*—published by the American Chiropractic Association's Council on Nutrition 2004 Oct
37. Vasquez A, Gilbert Manso, M.D., John Cannell, M.D. The Clinical Importance of Vitamin D (Cholecalciferol). *Alternative Therapies in Health and Medicine* 2004
38. Vasquez A. A brief review of two potential adverse effects of zinc supplementation. *Nutritional Perspectives*—published by the ACA's Council on Nutrition 1995

within the profession in the post-graduate arena and — very especially— within several chiropractic colleges, I learned more than a few distasteful lessons by direct observation and experience; being the diligent researcher that I am, I've ensured that all of these experiences have been corroborated by other staff and professionals within the school(s) and/or documented with archived emails, internal documents, and meeting transcripts.

The degree of administrative incompetence that I have witnessed within chiropractic academics, and which I have seen other professors abused by, and which has been independently documented in *The Chronicle of Higher Education*[608,609,610] is simply stunning and bewildering; **for those who love academics and education and who hold / have held a high vision for the chiropractic profession, these experiences are particularly painful.** My observations, experiences, and those of others include but are not limited to the following: petty politics carried to the extreme, and repeated and sequential *constructive dismissals* (illegal); lowering of academic standards to lessen the burden on administrators and to increase enrollment; familial and nonfamilial nepotism (e.g., hiring and overpaying unqualified family members and "friends"); misleading the Board of Directors/Trustees by misrepresenting facts about critical institutional issues such as finances, and usurping money from one program to compensate for another program's failings so that the Board would not know the truth; using school money to pay-off fired administrators with *nondisclosure agreements* so that administrative corruption/incompetence remains hidden, and using school attorneys and thus school money to threaten professors who disagree with administrative recklessness; implementing sweeping changes within the faculty, staff, and Board of Directors/Trustees (i.e., administrative *scorched earth policy*) in such a way that institutional accountability becomes a practical impossibility because the "people who know" are excised from the campus and are replaced by newbies just trying to learn the ropes and keep their jobs; allowing email and phone privacy to be breached (e.g., eavesdropping, selective deletion of sensitive emails); lying to students and other faculty about the inappropriate political genesis of administrative changes; intentionally false advertising to attract students; blocking professor's school email during final exam week thus prohibiting communication with students and support staff and then accusing professor of "failing to honor contract obligations and teaching duties"; accepting huge sums of money from corporate interests and misdirecting the educational course –e.g., allowing the insertion of corporate-produced "educational material" into the official doctorate-level clinical curriculum and allowing corporate-friendly "administrators" to replace established expert teachers and clinicians; maintaining appearances (such as with glossy catalogs and visitor gifts) rather than supporting quality education and faculty needs (e.g., radiology departments without basic modern radiology equipment); failing to support basic science and clinical faculty[611]; falsifying

---

Pitfalls and misadventures in chiropractic academics

All-to-common themes in chiropractic academics:
- Administrative mistreatment of teaching faculty
- Gross overpayment of upper administrators: drains monies from academics, demoralizes teaching faculty
- Exclusion of teaching faculty from Board meetings, so that a very "selective truth" can be presented
- Selection of admin-friendly Board members who overlook and remain voluntarily blind to school problems and administrative misbehavior
- Inappropriate firing and constructive dismissal of qualified and performing middle admin and professors for political purposes

Chronicle of Higher Education 2012 Apr15
chronicle.com/article/Chiropractic-Colleges-Ruling/131539/

Some of the biggest problems and challenges for the chiropractic profession—e.g., quality of education, issues of professionalism and ethics, retention of quality faculty and clinicians, maintaining and educating for the desired scope of practice—stem from chiropractic colleges and "university" administrators themselves

"But concerns about management are central to the issues surrounding chiropractic colleges, and overcoming them may be key to the institutions' efforts to build their reputations in mainstream higher education, draw more students, and ultimately, survive."

Fuller A. Chiropractic Colleges Seek Legitimacy Amid Financial Woes. *Chronicle of Higher Education* 2012

The opportunity to make things better is in the hands of chiropractic clinicians, students, teachers, alumni

Chiropractic clinicians, students, teachers, and alumni have the option to run and hide from these problems, or to acknowledge them and then use the information to demand accountability and authentic professionalism from upper administrators and the weak Boards that have allowed chaos to reign.

---

608 Fuller A. Chiropractic Colleges Seek Legitimacy Amid Financial Woes. *Chronicle of Higher Education*. 2012 Apr 15.
609 Stripling J. Presidential Couple at Chiropractic College Draws Fire Over Wife's Role. *Chronicle of Higher Education*. 2012 Apr15.
610 Stripling J. Dogged by Nepotism Charges, Chiropractic College Reveals Earnings of Chief's Family. *Chronicle of Higher Education*. 2012 Oct 17
611 Comic video with a lot of painful accuracy about chiropractic academics: "So you're thinking of going to chiropractic college? youtube.com/watch?v=TqpAvaSUnkY

meeting minutes and/or the data presented within those meetings; lying to students about the safety/application of carcinogenic chemicals to the school's landscape; exorbitant and extended presidential vacations abroad during times of institutional initiatives and crises; bypassing criteria for advancement for a select few administrators and thereby undermining the legitimacy of academic titles and effort by honest faculty; ultimately but not exclusively, these result in the repulsion of quality students and faculty from the chiropractic profession, diminution of educational quality, impairment of clinical performance, and retardation of the profession *from within* from delivering the highest quality of care and achieving greater professional success for its members. Any true proponent of the chiropractic profession will acknowledge that these problems need to be addressed *at their sources within chiropractic academics* if the profession is to move forward toward greater authenticity, cultural authority, and professional success; the shame of chiropractic's self-sabotage—and how this blocks the profession *from within* from moving forward—is well reflected in the African proverb, "If there is no enemy within, the enemy outside can do us no harm." Chiropractic clinicians, students, teachers, and alumni have the option to run and hide from these problems, or to acknowledge them and then use the information to demand accountability and authentic professionalism from upper administrators. Smaller minds will get angry at the revelation and realization of inconvenient truths, but the only way to help the situation get better is to address these problems in chiropractic schools—not continue to deny and cover them. These problems are not isolated in one particular chiropractic school or another but are disappointingly common and chronic across several chiropractic schools; greater oversight by regional accreditors is also needed since unfortunately the administrators are often not accountable and the Boards of these schools impose no accountability either, via ignorance, neglect, or the common combination of the two: intentional ignorance. The problem is compounded exponentially when school administrators have positions within the offices of the regional accreditors; this gross conflict of interest creates a situation where *the fox is guarding the henhouse*, and "accountability" is just a joke at the expense of students, professors, and the public who deserve it.

Examples of these problems have been documented in articles published in *The Chronicle of Higher Education* and while this documentation is important, that two of the articles cited refer to a single chiropractic college thereby might contribute to a false impression that similar events are not occurring in other colleges, which is *very* clearly not the situation. Other noteworthy problems are the profession's persistent lack of use of laboratory testing[612] and additional evidence proving that the profession *as a whole* is not engaged in primary care[613], the overuse of radiography[614], and the error in logic that suppression of the profession by medical groups indicates parity with those medical groups. Despite all of this, chiropractic-specific musculoskeletal manipulation—"the adjustment"—remains an impressively potent therapeutic tool: alleviating pain and musculoskeletal dysfunction for many and delivering the occasional "chiropractic miracle" for few. Similarly, some chiropractors with additional post-graduate training and certification deliver clinically brilliant and highly competent primary and specialist care.

A common experience in chiropractic academics: micromanagement for short-term gain at the expense of the future of the profession and quality of education

"The administration does not care about quality control: they consistently undermine the efforts of the basic science professors and clinical faculty. It is dangerous and irresponsible on the part of the administration of the schools. You will find that the administrations of chiropractic colleges are hell-bent on destroying their own profession in exchange for short-term monetary gains."

To be sure, this is a social rather than scientifically-referenced quote, but it is largely consistent with what I and many other students and faculty in chiropractic colleges have experienced. youtube.com/watch?v=TqpAvaSUnkY

Wilk vs American Medical Association: The successful antitrust case against medical monopolization

The following 2 pages provide the transcript of the 1987 judgment that was intended to end AMA's attempt to eliminate chiropractic.

---

[612] National Board of Chiropractic Examiners. *Practice Analysis of Chiropractic 2010*. Chapter 9. "Draw blood, collect urine and/or perform other laboratory tests in your office = 0.3/range 0-5 = Virtually Never." "Order blood, urine, or other laboratory tests from an outside facility = 0.8 = Yearly." "Perform a focused cardiopulmonary examination = 0.9 = Yearly" "Review laboratory studies and interpret the results = 1.6 = Monthly." nbce.org/wp-content/uploads/analysis_chapter_09.pdf

[613] National Board of Chiropractic Examiners. *Practice Analysis of Chiropractic 2010*. Chapter 8, Patient Conditions. nbce.org/wp-content/uploads/analysis_chapter_08.pdf

[614] Some sample citations are provided at ncahf.org/pp/chirop.html#hazardous; note "In addition, across all five vignettes, 25% of chiropractors would take, or order, a full spine plain x-ray. ... There is no evidence that full spine x-rays are warranted in these vignettes and this finding is troubling considering the radiation dose that the patient would receive." Walker et al. Management of people with acute low-back pain. *Chiropr Man Therap*. 2011 Dec 15;19(1):29 While the overuse of radiography within the chiropractic profession has abated in recent years, no reasonable person within the profession will deny that the profession as a whole has overused radiography to assess *functional* rather than *pathologic* problems of the spine and that most of these same functional problems could have been diagnosed *without radiography* and treated successfully *without radiography*. As a gross example, virtually our entire freshman class in chiropractic school received full-spine radiographs and a full set of regional radiographs during our introduction to clinical services in the first year of chiropractic college; generally this means that hundreds and thousands of chiropractic students have been exposed unnecessarily to a significant amount of ionizing radiation, pseudo-justified by minimal or facticious criteria and for the need to give graduating students the radiography credits needed per school accreditation.

Special Communication

IN THE UNITED STATES DISTRICT COURT
FOR THE NORTHERN DISTRICT OF ILLINOIS
EASTERN DIVISION

```
CHESTER A. WILK, et al.,         )
                                 )
                  Plaintiffs,    )
                                 )
        v.                       )   No. 76 C
                                 )     3777
AMERICAN MEDICAL ASSOCIATION,    )
et al.,                          )
                                 )
                  Defendants.    )
```

PERMANENT INJUNCTION ORDER AGAINST AMA

Susan Getzendanner, District Judge

The court conducted a lengthy trial of this case in May and June of 1987 and on August 27, 1987, issued a 101 page opinion finding that the American Medical Association ("AMA") and its members participated in a conspiracy against chiropractors in violation of the nation's antitrust laws. Thereafter an opinion dated September 25, 1987 was substituted for the August 27, 1987 opinion. The question now before the court is the form of injunctive relief that the court will order.

See also p 83.

As part of the injunctive relief to be ordered by the court against the AMA, the AMA shall be required to send a copy of this Permanent Injunction Order to each of its current members. The members of the AMA are bound by the terms of the Permanent Injunction Order if they act in concert with the AMA to violate the terms of the order. Accordingly, it is important that the AMA members understand the order and the reasons why the order has been entered.

The AMA's Boycott and Conspiracy

In the early 1960s, the AMA decided to contain and eliminate chiropractic as a profession. In 1963 the AMA's Committee on Quackery was formed. The committee worked aggressively—both overtly and covertly—to eliminate chiropractic. One of the principal means used by the AMA to achieve its goal was to make it unethical for medical physicians to professionally associate with chiropractors. Under Principle 3 of the AMA's Principles of Medical Ethics, it was unethical for a physician to associate with an "unscientific practitioner," and in 1966 the AMA's House of Delegates passed a resolution calling chiropractic an unscientific cult. To complete the circle, in 1967 the AMA's Judicial Council issued an opinion under Principle 3 holding that it was unethical for a physician to associate professionally with chiropractors.

The AMA's purpose was to prevent medical physicians from referring patients to chiropractors and accepting referrals of patients from chiropractors, to prevent chiropractors from obtaining access to hospital diagnostic services and membership on hospital medical staffs, to prevent medical physicians from teaching at chiropractic colleges or engaging in any joint research, and to prevent any cooperation between the two groups in the delivery of health care services.

Published by order of Susan Getzendanner, US District Judge, Sept 25, 1987.

The AMA believed that the boycott worked—that chiropractic would have achieved greater gains in the absence of the boycott. Since no medical physician would want to be considered unethical by his peers, the success of the boycott is not surprising. However, chiropractic achieved licensing in all 50 states during the existence of the Committee on Quackery.

The Committee on Quackery was disbanded in 1975 and some of the committee's activities became publicly known. . Several lawsuits were filed by or on behalf of chiropractors and this case was filed in 1976.

Change in AMA's Position on Chiropractic

In 1977, the AMA began to change its position on chiropractic. The AMA's Judicial Council adopted new opinions under which medical physicians could refer patients to chiropractors, but there was still the proviso that the medical physician should be confident that the services to be provided on referral would be performed in accordance with accepted scientific standards. In 1979, the AMA's House of Delegates adopted Report UU which said that not everything that a chiropractor may do is without therapeutic value, but it stopped short of saying that such things were based on scientific standards. It was not until 1980 that the AMA revised its Principles of Medical Ethics to eliminate Principle 3. Until Principle 3 was formally eliminated, there was considerable ambiguity about the AMA's position. The ethics code adopted in 1980 provided that a medical physician "shall be free to choose whom to serve, with whom to associate, and the environment in which to provide medical services."

The AMA settled three chiropractic lawsuits by stipulating and agreeing that under the current opinions of the Judicial Council a physician may, without fear of discipline or sanction by the AMA, refer a patient to a duly licensed chiropractor when he believes that referral may benefit the patient. The AMA confirmed that a physician may also choose to accept or to decline patients sent to him by a duly licensed chiropractor. Finally, the AMA confirmed that a physician may teach at a chiropractic college or seminar. These settlements were entered into in 1978, 1980, and 1986.

The AMA's present position on chiropractic, as stated to the court, is that it is ethical for a medical physician to professionally associate with chiropractors provided the physician believes that such association is in the best interests of his patient. This position has not previously been communicated by the AMA to its members.

Antitrust Laws

Under the Sherman Act, every combination or conspiracy in restraint of trade is illegal. The court has held that the conduct of the AMA and its members constituted a conspiracy in restraint of trade based on the following facts: the purpose of the boycott was to eliminate chiropractic; chiropractors are in competition with some medical physicians; the boycott had substantial anti-competitive effects; there were no pro-competitive effects of the boycott; and the plaintiffs were injured as a result of the conduct. These facts add up to a violation of the Sherman Act.

In this case, however, the court allowed the defendants the opportunity to establish a "patient care defense" which has the following elements:

(1) that they genuinely entertained a concern for what they perceive as scientific method in the care of each person with whom they have entered into a doctor-patient relationship; (2) that this concern is objectively reasonable; (3) that this concern has been the dominant motivating factor in defendants' promulgation of Principle 3 and in the

conduct intended to implement it; and (4) that this concern for scientific method in patient care could not have been adequately satisfied in a manner less restrictive of competition.

The court concluded that the AMA had a genuine concern for scientific methods in patient care, and that this concern was the dominant factor in motivating the AMA's conduct. However, the AMA failed to establish that throughout the entire period of the boycott, from 1966 to 1980, this concern was objectively reasonable. The court reached that conclusion on the basis of extensive testimony from both witnesses for the plaintiffs and the AMA that some forms of chiropractic treatment are effective and the fact that the AMA recognized that chiropractic began to change in the early 1970s. Since the boycott was not formally over until Principle 3 was eliminated in 1980, the court found that the AMA was unable to establish that during the entire period of the conspiracy its position was objectively reasonable. Finally, the court ruled that the AMA's concern for scientific method in patient care could have been adequately satisfied in a manner less restrictive of competition and that a nationwide conspiracy to eliminate a licensed profession was not justified by the concern for scientific method. On the basis of these findings, the court concluded that the AMA had failed to establish the patient care defense.

None of the court's findings constituted a judicial endorsement of chiropractic. All of the parties to the case, including the plaintiffs and the AMA, agreed that chiropractic treatment of diseases such as diabetes, high blood pressure, cancer, heart disease and infectious disease is not proper, and that the historic theory of chiropractic, that there is a single cause and cure of disease is wrong. There was disagreement between the parties as to whether chiropractors should engage in diagnosis. There was evidence that the chiropractic theory of subluxations was unscientific, and evidence that some chiropractors engaged in unscientific practices. The court did not reach the question of whether chiropractic theory was in fact scientific. However, the evidence in the case was that some forms of chiropractic manipulation of the spine and joints was therapeutic. AMA witnesses, including the present Chairman of the Board of Trustees of the AMA, testified that some forms of treatment by chiropractors, including manipulation, can be therapeutic in the treatment of conditions such as back pain syndrome.

Need for Injunctive Relief

Although the conspiracy ended in 1980, there are lingering effects of the illegal boycott and conspiracy which require an injunction. Some medical physicians' individual decisions on whether or not to professionally associate with chiropractors are still affected by the boycott. The injury to chiropractors' reputations which resulted from the boycott has not been repaired. Chiropractors suffer current economic injury as a result of the boycott. The AMA has never affirmatively acknowledged that there are and should be no collective impediments to professional association and cooperation between chiropractors and medical physicians, except as provided by law. Instead, the AMA has consistently argued that its conduct has not violated the antitrust laws.

Most importantly, the court believes that it is important that the AMA members be made aware of the present AMA position that it is ethical for a medical physician to professionally associate with a chiropractor if the physician believes it is in the best interests of his patient, so that the lingering effects of the illegal group boycott against chiropractors finally can be dissipated.

Under the law, every medical physician, institution, and hospital has the right to make an individual decision as to whether or not that physician, institution, or hospital shall associate professionally with chiropractors. Individual choice by a medical physician voluntarily to associate professionally with chiropractors should be governed only by restrictions under state law, if any, and by the individual medical physician's personal judgment as to what is in the best interest of a patient or patients. Professional association includes referrals, consultations, group practice in partnerships, Health Maintenance Organizations, Preferred Provider Organizations, and other alternative health care delivery systems; the provision of treatment privileges and diagnostic services (including radiological and other laboratory facilities) in or through hospital facilities; association and cooperation in educational programs for students in chiropractic colleges; and cooperation in research, health care seminars, and continuing education programs.

An injunction is necessary to assure that the AMA does not interfere with the right of a physician, hospital, or other institution to make an individual decision on the question of professional association.

Form of Injunction

1. The AMA, its officers, agents and employees, and all persons who act in active concert with any of them and who receive actual notice of this order are hereby permanently enjoined from restricting, regulating or impeding, or aiding and abetting others from restricting, regulating or impeding, the freedom of any AMA member or any institution or hospital to make an individual decision as to whether or not that AMA member, institution, or hospital shall professionally associate with chiropractors, chiropractic students, or chiropractic institutions.

2. This Permanent Injunction does not and shall not be construed to restrict or otherwise interfere with the AMA's right to take positions on any issue, including chiropractic, and to express or publicize those positions, either alone or in conjunction with others. Nor does this Permanent Injunction restrict or otherwise interfere with the AMA's right to petition or testify before any public body on any legislative or regulatory measure or to join or cooperate with any other entity in so petitioning or testifying. The AMA's membership in a recognized accrediting association or society shall not constitute a violation of this Permanent Injunction.

3. The AMA is directed to send a copy of this order to each AMA member and employee, first class mail, postage prepaid, within thirty days of the entry of this order. In the alternative, the AMA shall provide the Clerk of the Court with mailing labels so that the court may send this order to AMA members and employees.

4. The AMA shall cause the publication of this order in JAMA and the indexing of the order under "Chiropractic" so that persons desiring to find the order in the future will be able to do so.

5. The AMA shall prepare a statement of the AMA's present position on chiropractic for inclusion in the current reports and opinions of the Judicial Council with an appropriate heading that refers to professional association between medical physicians and chiropractors, and indexed in the same manner that other reports and opinions are indexed. The court imposes no restrictions on the AMA's statement but only requires that it be consistent with the AMA's statements of its present position to the court.

6. The AMA shall file a report with the court evidencing compliance with this order on or before January 10, 1988.

It is so ordered.

Susan Getzendanner
United States District Judge

Common Clinical Considerations: Hemochromatosis and Hypothyroidism

Iron Overload and Genetic Hemochromatosis:
Identification and Management

Introduction to Iron Overload

In its "classic" form, homozygous genetic hemochromatosis is noted in about 1 per 200-250 Caucasian persons, with a similar incidence among Hispanics. The incidence among persons of African descent is notably higher, reported as high as 1 per 80 among hospitalized African Americans. The heterozygous form of iron overload which is phenotypically milder occurs in as many as 1 per 7 (14% of total) persons; any disorder that is common in the general population will be even more common in a clinical population of symptomatic care-seeking patients, especially those with musculoskeletal disorders and complaints.[615]

Testing serum ferritin on a routine basis in clinical practice allows for the detection of iron deficiency (very common, even among non-anemic patients) and iron overload (quite common, especially among patients with joint pain, diabetes, heart failure, and liver disease as well as many other clinical manifestations—most common of which is asymptomaticity.

Description/pathophysiology:

- Hereditary iron overload disorders are now recognized as being among the most common genetic diseases in the human population.[616,617,618,619,620,621,622]

- Iron overload is a phenotypic state to which a patient arrives by either genetic or environmental/iatrogenic routes. The severity of iron overload can range from moderate to severe.

- Excess iron catalyzes oxidative stress which damages body tissues and structures in which the iron is stored. In patients with genetic hemochromatosis, two problems exist simultaneously: 1) a disproportionately large amount of iron is absorbed from the gastrointestinal tract (i.e., these patients' iron absorption is "too efficient"), and 2) iron is preferentially deposited in parenchymal tissues such as the heart, liver, pancreas, pituitary gland, and joints rather than being stored safely within the reticuloendothelial system. The deposition of excess iron in parenchymal tissues promotes destruction of these organs/tissues via oxidative mechanisms and subsequent tissue necrosis and fibrosis, leading to the protean manifestations of the disease dependent upon which organs are most affected in the individual patient: heart failure, hepatic fibrosis, hypoinsulinemic diabetes, hypopituarism, and hemochromatoic arthropathy.

- Iron overload can be defined as a state of "iron toxicity" similar to mercury toxicity or poisoning with any other heavy metal or toxin, except that the mechanism is more related to the *quantity* of the iron rather than the unique characteristics or *quality* of iron itself. In other words, whereas the toxicity of mercury can be seen even when only small amounts of the metal are present, the toxicity of iron is directly related to the amount of the excess iron (ie, dose-response relationship of free-radical generation).

> **Iron overload disorders are common in all ethnic/racial populations**
>
> Genetic hemochromatosis is considered one of the most common hereditary disorders in the Caucasian population with a homozygote frequency of 1 per 200-250 (approx 0.5%) and a heterozygote frequency of about 1 in 7 (approx 14%); the condition is at least as common in other ethnic groups except that this predisposition toward iron overload is more common in Africans (as high as 1 in 20) and African-Americans (as high as about 1 in 80 in some series among hospitalized patients). Of course, the expected frequency would be even higher among symptomatic patients than among the general population. **Thus, for a clinician in full-time practice, the only reason for not appreciating this condition among one's patient population several times per year is because one is simply not sufficiently looking and testing for this condition.**

---

[615] Vasquez A. Musculoskeletal disorders and iron overload disease: comment on the American College of Rheumatology guidelines for the initial evaluation of the adult patient with acute musculoskeletal symptoms. *Arthritis & Rheumatism*: Official Journal of the American College of Rheumatology 1996; 39:1767-8

[616] Olynyk JK, Bacon BR. Hereditary hemochromatosis: detecting and correcting iron overload. *Postgrad Med* 1994; 96: 151-65

[617] Phatak PD, Cappuccio JD. Management of hereditary hemochromatosis. *Blood Rev* 1994; 8: 193-8

[618] Rouault TA. Hereditary hemochromatosis. *JAMA* 1993; 269: 3152-4

[619] Crosby WH. Hemochromatosis: current concepts and management. Hosp Pract 1987; 22:173-92

[620] Bloom PD, Gordeuk VR, MacPhail AP. HLA-linked hemochromatosis and other forms of iron overload. *Dermatol Clin* 1995; 13: 57-63

[621] Barton JC, Bertoli LF. Hemochromatosis: the genetic disorder of the twenty-first century. *Nat Med* 1996; 2: 394-5

[622] Lauffer, RB. *Iron and Your Heart*. New York: St. Martin's Press, 1991

Clinical presentations:

- **Many patients are asymptomatic.**
- **Most patients eventually present with a problem that is attributed to another disorder:**
  - <u>Diabetes</u>: Patients may present with diabetes, which is erroneously attributed to metabolic syndrome or type-2 diabetes.[623]
  - <u>Musculoskeletal pain</u>: Patients may present with joint pain that is erroneously attributed to osteoarthritis[624], rheumatoid arthritis[625], or some other musculoskeletal syndrome.[626]
  - <u>Cardiomyopathy</u>: Patients may present with heart failure that is written off as "idiopathic cardiomyopathy."[627]
  - <u>Liver disease</u>: Hemochromatosis liver disease resembles and exacerbates viral hepatitis, alcoholic hepatitis, and porphyria.
- <u>Fatigue, lethargy, weakness</u>
- <u>Chronic abdominal pain</u>
- <u>Liver damage</u>: Hepatomegaly, elevated serum levels of liver enzymes and alkaline phosphatase, fibrosis and cirrhosis, hepatocellular carcinoma, or other findings such as hematemesis and melena, ascites, hyperbilirubenemia and jaundice, hypoalbuminemia, hepatic encephalopathy, clotting dysfunction, anemia, liver abscess, increased incidence of esophageal carcinoma.
- <u>Abnormal glucose metabolism or diabetes mellitus</u>: Elevated glucose levels. Usually asymptomatic, yet can cause weight loss, polyuria, polyphagia, polydypsia.
- <u>Musculoskeletal disorders</u>: Arthritis and arthralgia, generalized osteoporosis, bone pain, myalgia. Especially arthropathy of the hands and wrists, hips, and knees.
- <u>Cardiac dysfunction</u>: Cardiomyopathy, arrhythmia, fibrillation, congestive heart failure; shortness of breath or dyspnea on exertion, fatigue.
- <u>Cutaneous manifestations</u>: Slate-gray or ashen coloration, increased pigmentation ('tan') of the skin, atrophy of the skin, ichthyosis, koilonychia, loss of body hair, increased incidence of malignant melanoma.
- <u>Endocrine disorders</u>: Hypogonadotrophic hypogonadism, (autoimmune) hypothyroidism, hyperthyroidism; manifest as decreased libido, impotence, testicular atrophy, or sterility in males, amenorrhea or difficulty conceiving in females, loss of body hair.
- <u>Susceptibility to increased frequency and severity of infections</u>: Especially infections due to *Yersinia enterocolitica*, *Vibrio vulnificus*, HIV, and *Mycobacterium tuberculosis*.
- <u>Neurologic symptoms</u>: Blurred vision, sensorineural hearing loss, hyperactivity, dementia, attention deficit disorder, ataxia, lightheadedness, dizziness, anxiety, depression, tinnitus, confusion, lethargy, memory loss, disorientation, headaches and migraine headaches, personality changes, hallucinations, paranoia, chronic treatment-resistant psychiatric illness such as schizophrenia, compulsive disorders, bipolar affective disorder.
- <u>'Alcoholism'</u>: Alcoholism can cause elevated liver enzymes and liver damage, and many iron overload patients are erroneously diagnosed as alcoholics despite their abstinence from alcohol when the clinician fails to consider iron overload as the cause for the hepatopathy.
- <u>Any race, nationality, or ethnic background</u>: Hereditary iron overload conditions have been identified in people of all ethnic backgrounds and nationalities. Secondary iron overload conditions can occur irrespective of genetic predisposition.
- <u>Either gender</u>: Iron overload conditions occur in both men and women

---

Rationale for screening all patients

1. Hereditary iron-accumulation disorders occur in a large percentage of the population.
2. Persons with the disease usually have no symptoms.
3. Clinical manifestations are often indicative of irreversible organ damage or organ failure.
4. Iron overload can cause death if not treated early.
5. Early treatment ensures normal life expectancy.
6. **Therefore, early detection (before the onset of symptoms and organ damage) requires screening asymptomatic patients.**

Test of choice: Serum ferritin, shows the best correlation with body iron stores and thus prognosis and need for treatment.

---

[623] "Most of the patients (95%) had one or more of the following conditions; obesity, hyperlipidaemia, abnormal glucose metabolism, or hypertension. INTERPRETATION: We have found a new non-HLA-linked iron-overload syndrome which suggests a link between iron excess and metabolic disorders." Moirand R, Mortaji AM, Loreal O, Paillard F, Brissot P, Deugnier Y. A new syndrome of liver iron overload with normal transferrin saturation. *Lancet.* 1997 Jan 11;349(9045):95-7

[624] Axford JS, Bomford A, Revell P, et al. Hip arthropathy in genetic hemochromatosis: radiographic and histologic features. *Arthritis Rheum* 1991; 34: 357-61

[625] Bensen et al. Hemochromatoic arthropathy mimicking rheumatoid arthritis. A case with subcutaneous nodules, tenosynovitis, and bursitis. *Arthritis Rheum* 1978; 21: 844-8

[626] Olynyk J, Hall P, et al. Screening for genetic hemochromatosis in a rheumatology clinic. *Australian and New Zealand Journal of Medicine* 1994; 24: 22-25

[627] [No authors listed] Case records of the Massachusetts General Hospital. Weekly clinicopathological exercises. Case 31-1994. A 25-year-old man with the recent onset of diabetes mellitus and congestive heart failure. *N Engl J Med.* 1994 Aug 18;331(7):460-6

- A family history of, or suggestive of, a hereditary iron overload condition: Family history of iron overload, hereditary anemia or iron-loading anemia, cardiac disorders or "heart disease", arthritis, diabetes, neurologic disorders, liver disease, impotence, amenorrhea, sterility.

Differential diagnoses:
- Diabetes mellitus: Remember that the classic presentation of hemochromatosis is "bronze diabetes with cirrhosis." **All patients with diabetes should be tested for iron overload.**[628,629]
- Cardiomyopathy:
- Hepatopathy: **Iron overload is one of the most important rule-outs in patients with liver disease.**[630] Liver biopsy is often indicated to assess condition and disease co-existence.
- Musculoskeletal disorders: **Patients with polyarthropathy should be tested for iron overload.**[631]
  - Degenerative arthritis or osteoarthritis
  - Pseudogout, calcium pyrophosphate dihydrate deposition disease
  - Rheumatoid arthritis[632]
  - Ankylosing spondylitis: The resemblance here is only superficial, related primarily to calcification of the intervertebral discs and ligaments.[633]
- Hyperthyroidism and hypothyroidism[634,635]
- Hypogonadotrophic hypogonadism: Erectile dysfunction in men, subfertility in women[636]
- Porphyria cutanea tarda: "Virtually all patients have increased iron stores; serum iron, iron saturation, and ferritin values."[637] **All patients with porphyria cutanea tarda must be tested for iron overload.**

Conditions associated with iron overload
Primary/genetic disorders
1. Homozygous genetic hemochromatosis
2. Heterozygous genetic hemochromatosis
3. African iron overload
4. African-American hemochromatosis (African-American iron overload)
5. Non-HLA-linked hemochromatosis
6. Juvenile hemochromatosis
7. Neonatal hemochromatosis
Secondary and metabolic disorders
8. Dietary excess of iron
9. Parenteral administration of iron in the form of iron injections and blood transfusions
10. Porphyria cutanea tarda
11. Portacaval shunt
12. Hepatic cirrhosis, portal hypertension, and splenomegaly
13. AIDS
14. Sudden infant death syndrome
15. Alcoholism
16. Metabolic syndrome
Inherited red blood cell abnormalities ("iron-loading anemias", hemoglobinopathies)
17. Alpha-thalassemia
18. Beta-thalassemia
19. Thalassemia intermedia
20. Sideroblastic anemia
21. Aplastic anemia
22. Anemia associated with pyruvate kinase deficiency
23. AC hemoglobinopathy
24. AS hemoglobinopathy
25. X-linked hypochromic anemia
26. Pyridoxine-responsive anemia
27. Atransferrinemia

Clinical assessment:
- **History/subjective:**
  - The manifestations of the condition are so protean that history is generally non-sensitive and non-specific for the disorder. Rarely, a patient will mention that a relative was diagnosed with iron overload or that a relative had an unusual heart or liver disease, and this clue may lead to a diagnosis of iron overload in unsuspecting family members.
- **Physical examination/objective:**
  - The classic presentation of the fully developed disease is "bronze diabetes with arthritis and cirrhosis."
  - Physical examination should be specific for the patient's complaint(s) of arthritis, cardiomyopathy, diabetes, etc.

[628] Czink E, Tamas G. Screening for idiopathic hemochromatosis among diabetic patients. *Diabetes Care* 1991; 14: 929-30
[629] Phelps G, Chapman I, Hall P, Braund W, Mackinnon M. Prevalence of genetic haemochromatosis among diabetic patients. *Lancet* 1989; 2: 233-4
[630] Herrera JL. Abnormal liver enzyme levels: clinical evaluation in asymptomatic patients. *Postgrad Med* 1993; 93: 119-32
[631] M'Seffar AM, Fornasier VL, Fox IH. Arthropathy as the major clinical indicator of occult iron storage disease. *JAMA* 1977; 238: 1825-8
[632] Bensen WG, Laskin CA, Little HA, Fam AG. Hemochromatoic arthropathy mimicking rheumatoid arthritis. *Arthritis Rheum* 1978; 21: 844-8
[633] Bywaters EGL, Hamilton EBD, Williams R. The spine in idiopathic hemochromatosis. *Ann Rheum Dis* 1971; 30: 453-65
[634] Edwards CQ, Kelly TM, Ellwein G, Kushner JP. Thyroid disease in hemochromatosis. Increased incidence in homozygous men. *Arch Intern Med* 1983 Oct;143(10):1890-3
[635] Phillips G Jr, Becker B, Keller VA, Hartman J 4th. Hypothyroidism in adults with sickle cell anemia. *Am J Med* 1992 May;92(5):567-70
[636] Tweed MJ, Roland JM. Haemochromatosis as an endocrine cause of subfertility. *BMJ*. 1998 Mar 21;316(7135):915-6 bmj.bmjjournals.com/cgi/content/full/316/7135/915
[637] "Virtually all patients have increased iron stores; serum iron, iron saturation, and ferritin values." Rich MW. Porphyria cutanea tarda. *Postgrad Med*. 1999;105: 208-10, 213-4

- **Imaging & laboratory assessments:**
  - **Routine screening with serum ferritin for iron overload among all patients should be the standard of care in clinical practice.**
    - "In view of the high prevalence of hereditary hemochromatosis, its dire consequences when untreated, and its treatability, screening for the disorder should be performed routinely."[638]
    - "Screening for hemochromatosis is both feasible and cost-effective, and we recommend its use in patients seeking medical care."[639]
    - "The high gene frequency in the general population warrants routine screening tests in asymptomatic healthy young adults."[640]
    - "Primary iron overload occurs in African Americans... Clinicians should look for this condition."[641]
  - <u>Imaging</u>: The radiographic findings are nearly identical to those of osteoarthritis, except more joints are typically involved and that the distribution is typically symmetric (both due to the systemic/metabolic nature of the disease). Hook-like osteophytes at the metacarpal heads—with the "hooks" pointing proximally (rather than distally, as in rheumatoid arthritis) may be the only finding that could be called pathognomonic. Flattened or "squared-off" metacarpal heads are also seen. See previous table labeled *Musculoskeletal manifestations of iron overload* for more details.
  - <u>Laboratory evaluation</u>: Serum ferritin is the test of choice when looking for primary iron overload, secondary iron overload, and/or iron deficiency and should be a component of each new patient's evaluation, just as are CBC and the chemistry/metabolic panel. Transferrin saturation is a common test used for the detection of genetic hemochromatosis in research studies because it measures both iron levels but also disordered iron handling; this is why this test is best used in research screening of large populations. For clinicians, serum ferritin is very obviously the superior lab test for iron overload and deficiency.
    - <u>Transferrin saturation</u>: Good test for detecting genetic hemochromatosis before iron overload has occurred; values greater than 40% should be repeated *in conjunction with a measurement of serum ferritin*. Guidelines for screening for genetic hemochromatosis advocate the transferrin saturation test because it is a more sensitive assessment (compared to serum ferritin) for the hemochromatosis genotype which manifests phenotypically not simply as increased iron absorption and accumulation but also as an abnormality in iron handling which preferentially alters the transferrin saturation value, which is the ratio of serum iron to serum transferrin; the former rises due to increased iron absorption while the latter declines due to impaired hepatic synthetic function secondary to the preferential intraparenchymal deposition of iron in genetic hemochromatosis. Thus, genetic hemochromatosis is not simply a disorder characterized by increased iron absorption; it is also a disorder of iron handling/metabolism wherein iron is stored intracellularly in tissue parenchyma rather than (as in non-GH persons) in the reticuloendothelial system.

Musculoskeletal manifestations of iron overload
Clinical findings may include
• **Joint pain**
• **Bone pain**
• Joint swelling
• Loss of motion
• Bursitis
• Tendonitis
• Tenosynovitis
• Subcutaneous nodules
Sites of involvement
• **Metacarpophalangeal joints**
• **Wrist**
• **Hip**
• **Knee**
• Shoulder
• Ankle
• Metatarsophalangeal joints
• Elbow
• Spine
• Symphysis pubis
• Achilles tendon
• Plantar fascia
Radiographic findings
• **Joint space narrowing**
• **Sclerosis**
• Cysts
• Pseudocysts
• Osteophytes
• **Hook-like osteophytes at the metacarpal heads (high specificity)**
• Flattened or "squared-off" metacarpal heads
• Generalized osteopenia
• Generalized osteoporosis
• Chondrocalcinosis
• Subchondral cysts
• Carpal erosions
• Calcific tendonitis

[638] Fairbanks VF. Laboratory testing for iron status. *Hosp Pract* (Off Ed) 1991 Suppl 3:17-24
[639] Balan V, Baldus W, Fairbanks V, et al. Screening for hemochromatosis: a cost-effectiveness study based on 12, 258 patients. *Gastroenterology* 1994; 107: 453-9
[640] Gushusrt TP, Triest WE. Diagnosis and management of precirrhotic hemochromatosis. *W Virginia Med J* 1990; 86: 91-5
[641] Wurapa RK, Gordeuk VR, Brittenham GM, Khiyami A, Schechter GP, Edwards CQ. Primary iron overload in African Americans. *Am J Med.* 1996 Jul;101(1):9-18

- **Ferritin**: Routine use of serum ferritin is the most reasonable and cost-effective means for diagnosing this condition in symptomatic and asymptomatic patients. Elevations of ferritin (i.e., >200 mcg/L in women and >300 mcg/L in men) need to be retested along with CRP (to rule out false elevation due to excessive inflammation) before making the presumptive diagnosis of iron overload. **In the absence of significant inflammation, ferritin values >200 mcg/L in women and >300 mcg/L in men indicate iron overload and the need for treatment/phlebotomy regardless of the absence of symptoms or end-stage complications.**[642] Another benefit to the use of serum ferritin is the frequent detection of iron deficiency

Interpretation of iron status based on serum ferritin (in descending order)

Ferritin	Categorization and management
≥ 800 mcg/L	<u>Practically diagnostic of severe iron overload</u>[643]: Repeat tests; rule out inflammation or occult pathology. Initiate phlebotomy and consider liver biopsy or MRI.
≥ 300 mcg/L	<u>Probable iron overload; clear predisposition to iron accumulation</u>[644]: Repeat tests; rule out inflammation or occult pathology. In men, initiate phlebotomy and consider liver biopsy or MRI.[645]
≥ 200 mcg/L	*In women*: <u>Probable iron overload; clear predisposition to iron accumulation</u>[646]: Repeat tests, rule out inflammation or occult pathology. In women, initiate phlebotomy and consider liver biopsy or MRI.[647] *In men*: <u>High-normal *unhealthy* iron status with increased risk of myocardial infarction</u>[648]: Rule out inflammation or occult pathology. No follow-up is mandated, yet blood donation and/or abstention from dietary iron are recommended preventative healthcare measures.
≥ 160 mcg/L	*In women*: <u>Abnormal iron status</u>[649]: Repeat tests, rule out inflammation or occult pathology. Consider phlebotomy and liver biopsy or MRI.
≥80-120 mcg/L	<u>High-normal unhealthy iron status</u>[650,651]: No follow-up is mandated; blood donation and abstention from dietary iron are suggested preventative healthcare measures. A subset of patients with restless leg syndrome (RLS, a condition also causally associated with intestinal bacterial overgrowth dysbiosis) have impaired transport of iron into the brain and therefore require slightly elevated ferritin/iron levels (up to 120) to enhance cerebral iron uptake.
40-70 mcg/L	**Optimal iron status for most people**[652,653]
< 20 mcg/L	<u>Iron deficiency</u>: Search for occult gastrointestinal blood loss with endoscopy or imaging assessments in adults; refer to gastroenterologist.[654,655]

---

[642] Barton JC, McDonnell SM, Adams PC, Brissot P, Powell LW, Edwards CQ, Cook JD, Kowdley KV. Management of hemochromatosis. Hemochromatosis Management Working Group. *Ann Intern Med*. 1998 Dec 1;129(11):932-9

[643] Milman N, Albeck MJ. Distinction between homozygous and heterozygous subjects with hemochromatosis using iron status markers and receiver operating characteristic (ROC) analysis. *Eur J Clin Biochem* 1995; 33: 95-8. See also Milman N. Iron status markers in hereditary hemochromatosis: distinction between individuals being homozygous and heterozygous for the hemochromatosis allele. *Eur J Haematol* 1991;47:292-8

[644] Olynyk JK, Bacon BR. Hereditary hemochromatosis: detecting and correcting iron overload. *Postgrad Med* 1994;96: 151-65

[645] "Therapeutic phlebotomy is used to remove excess iron and maintain low normal body iron stores, ... initiated in men with serum ferritin levels of 300 microg/L or more and in women with serum ferritin levels of 200 microg/L or more, regardless of the presence or absence of symptoms." Barton JC, McDonnell SM, Adams PC, Brissot P, Powell LW, Edwards CQ, Cook JD, Kowdley KV. Management of hemochromatosis. Hemochromatosis Management Working Group. *Ann Intern Med*. 1998 Dec 1;129(11):932-9

[646] Barton JC, Edwards CQ, Bertoli LF, Shroyer TW, Hudson SL. Iron overload in African Americans. *Am J Med* 1995; 99: 616-23

[647] Barton JC, McDonnell SM, Adams PC, et al. Management of hemochromatosis. *Ann Intern Med*. 1998 Dec 1;129(11):932-9

[648] Salonen JT, Nyyssonen K, Korpela H,et al. High stored iron levels are associated with excess risk of myocardial infarction in eastern Finnish men. *Circulation* 1992; 86: 803-11

[649] Nicoll D. Therapeutic drug monitoring and laboratory reference ranges. In: Tierney LM, et al. *Current Medical Diagnosis and Treatment.* Appleton and Lange, 1996: 1442

[650] Lauffer, RB. *Iron and Your Heart*. New York: St. Martin's Press, 1991: 79-8, 83-88, 162

[651] Sullivan JL. Iron and the sex difference in heart disease risk. *Lancet*. 1981 Jun 13;1(8233):1293-4

[652] Lauffer, RB. *Iron and Your Heart*. New York: St. Martin's Press, 1991: 79-8, 83-88, 162

[653] Vasquez A. High body iron stores: causes, effects, diagnosis, and treatment. *Nutritional Perspectives* 1994; 17: 13, 15-7, 19, 21, 28 and Vasquez A. Men's Health: Iron in men: why men store this nutrient in their bodies and the harm that it does. *MEN Magazine* 1997; Jan:11,21-23 vix.com/menmag/alexiron.htm

[654] Rockey DC, Cello JP. Evaluation of the gastrointestinal tract in patients with iron-deficiency anemia. *N Engl J Med*. 1993;329(23):1691-5

[655] "Endoscopy revealed a clinically important lesion in 23 (12%) of 186 patients. ... CONCLUSIONS: Endoscopy yields important findings in premenopausal women with iron deficiency anemia, which should not be attributed solely to menstrual blood loss." Bini EJ, Micale PL, Weinshel EH. Evaluation of the gastrointestinal tract in premenopausal women with iron deficiency anemia. *Am J Med*. 1998 Oct;105(4):281-6

- CRP: Should be relatively normal as iron overload is not inflammatory, per se. If the ferritin is elevated and the CRP is markedly elevated, then inflammatory and hepatic diseases must be considered, namely advanced cancer, viral hepatitis or other hepatopathy, and alcoholic liver disease. If the ferritin is elevated and the CRP is normal, then the most likely diagnosis is iron overload, which should be confirmed either with liver biopsy or diagnostic/therapeutic phlebotomy.
- CBC: may show anemia, but the findings here are nonspecific
- Chemistry panel: may show evidence of diabetes and hepatopathy
- Thyroid assessment: may show hyperthyroidism or hypothyroidism, both of which are more common in patients with iron overload.
- Bone marrow biopsy: unnecessary and archaic in this setting, now that serum ferritin is widely available.
- Liver biopsy: traditionally considered the "gold standard" for diagnosing iron overload but is now clearly unnecessary for the diagnosis, which can be established by monitoring the response to therapeutic phlebotomy, which is the treatment of choice.[656] **Life-saving diagnostic and therapeutic phlebotomy should never be denied or delayed for lack of liver biopsy in patients with laboratory indicators of iron overload.**[657]
- Genetic testing, such as for the HFE mutation: This is a waste of time and money in most clinical situations; these tests should be reserved for research purposes and for evaluation of affected relatives—especially children—of index cases. The only value these tests may have in clinical practice is that of supporting a diagnosis in a patient with elevated serum ferritin who refuses biopsy, liver MRI, or phlebotomy; however, a negative result is meaningless if the ferritin is high and the clinical picture is compatible with iron overload. If the diagnosis is established, genetic relatives must be tested.

Establishing the diagnosis: Any *one* of the following three is sufficient:
- Diagnostic liver biopsy shows heavy iron deposits.
- Characteristic laboratory findings (ferritin >200 in women or >300 in men) *and* the ability to resist intractable anemia with serial/weekly phlebotomies.
- Characteristic MRI of liver *and* the ability to tolerate serial/weekly phlebotomies.

Complications:
- Patients diagnosed *and effectively treated* before the onset of signs and symptoms have normal life expectancy.
- The most common causes of premature mortality in undiagnosed and untreated patients are related to heart failure, liver failure, infections and/or complications of diabetes.

Clinical management:
- Treatment for severe iron overload is iron-removal therapy. Since blood is high in iron, the removal of blood—therapeutic phlebotomy—is the treatment of choice. Deferoxamine chelation can be administered to patients who refuse or cannot withstand phlebotomy (i.e., patients with cardiomyopathy, severe anemia, hypoproteinemia) but is much less effective, much more expensive, and with side effects such as neurotoxicity. Adjunctive nutritional and lifestyle modifications are no substitute for iron-removal therapy, and weekly phlebotomy is the treatment of choice.
- When a hereditary iron overload disorder is diagnosed, all (first-degree) blood relatives must be screened for iron overload.

> **Initiation of therapeutic phlebotomy is based on serum ferritin and does not require liver biopsy**
>
> "Therapeutic phlebotomy is used to remove excess iron and maintain low normal body iron stores, and it should be initiated in men with serum ferritin levels of 300 microg/L or more and in women with serum ferritin levels of 200 microg/L or more, regardless of the presence or absence of symptoms."
>
> Barton et al. Management of hemochromatosis.
> *Ann Intern Med.* 1998 Dec

---

[656] "Therapeutic phlebotomy is used to remove excess iron and maintain low normal body iron stores, and it should be initiated in men with serum ferritin levels of 300 microg/L or more and in women with serum ferritin levels of 200 microg/L or more, regardless of the presence or absence of symptoms." Barton JC, McDonnell SM, Adams PC, Brissot P, Powell LW, Edwards CQ, Cook JD, Kowdley KV. Management of hemochromatosis. Hemochromatosis Management Working Group. *Ann Intern Med.* 1998 Dec 1;129:932-9
[657] Sullivan JL, as quoted in Crawford R, ed. "The debate." In: *Ironic Blood: information on iron overload.* West Palm Beach: Iron Overload Diseases Association. 1996; 16 (2)

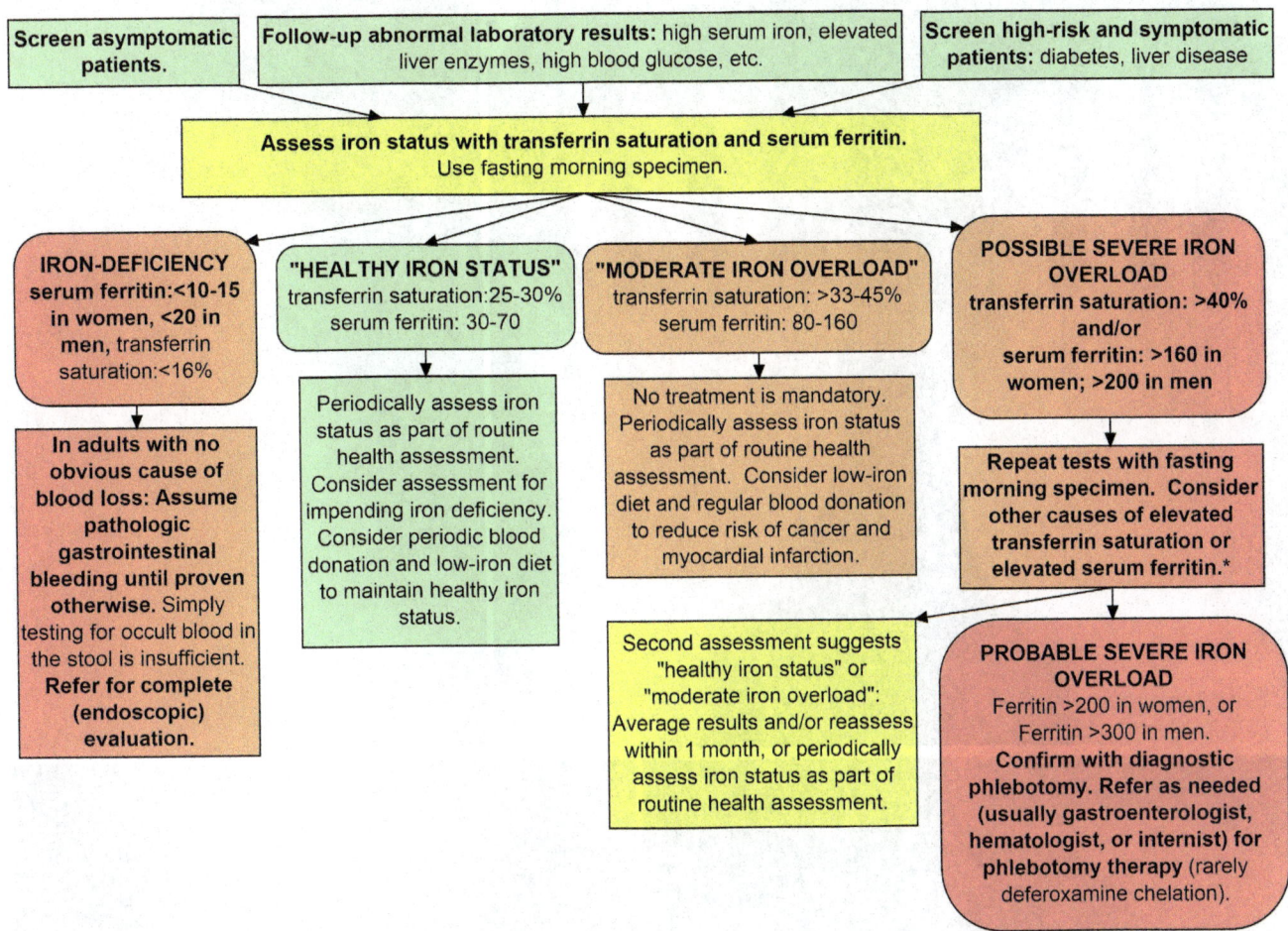

Guide to Patient Management Based on Iron Status:

- Deficiency: Adult patients with iron deficiency must generally be presumed to have occult gastrointestinal blood loss and should therefore be referred for gastrointestinal endoscopy; this is consistent with the standard of care in medicine.

- Optimal: Ferritin levels between 40-70 mcg/L are generally optimal for most men and women; up to 120 mcg/L is reasonable for subsets of patients with restless leg syndrome, perhaps also those with recalcitrant depression and/or Parkinsonian features to allow sufficient iron entry into the brain for maximal dopamine production.

- Excess: Levels greater than 200 mcg/L in a woman or 300 mcg/L in a man are suggestive of iron overload and/or tendency toward accumulation and are physiologically unnecessary and medically unjustifiable, particularly as increased iron stores correlate with increased cancer mortality, increased cardiovascular mortality, and increased all-cause mortality.

- Overload: Diagnosis and treatment for iron overload can occur simultaneously with diagnostic/therapeutic phlebotomy. Genetic testing and liver biopsy are generally inefficient expenditures of financial and medial resources; genetic testing is largely irrelevant in the presence of the hemochromatosis phenotype (i.e., otherwise inexplicable iron accumulation) while liver biopsy exposes the patient to unnecessary treatment delays, risk, and expenses. Identification of idiopathic or genotropic iron overload requires testing of genetic relatives.

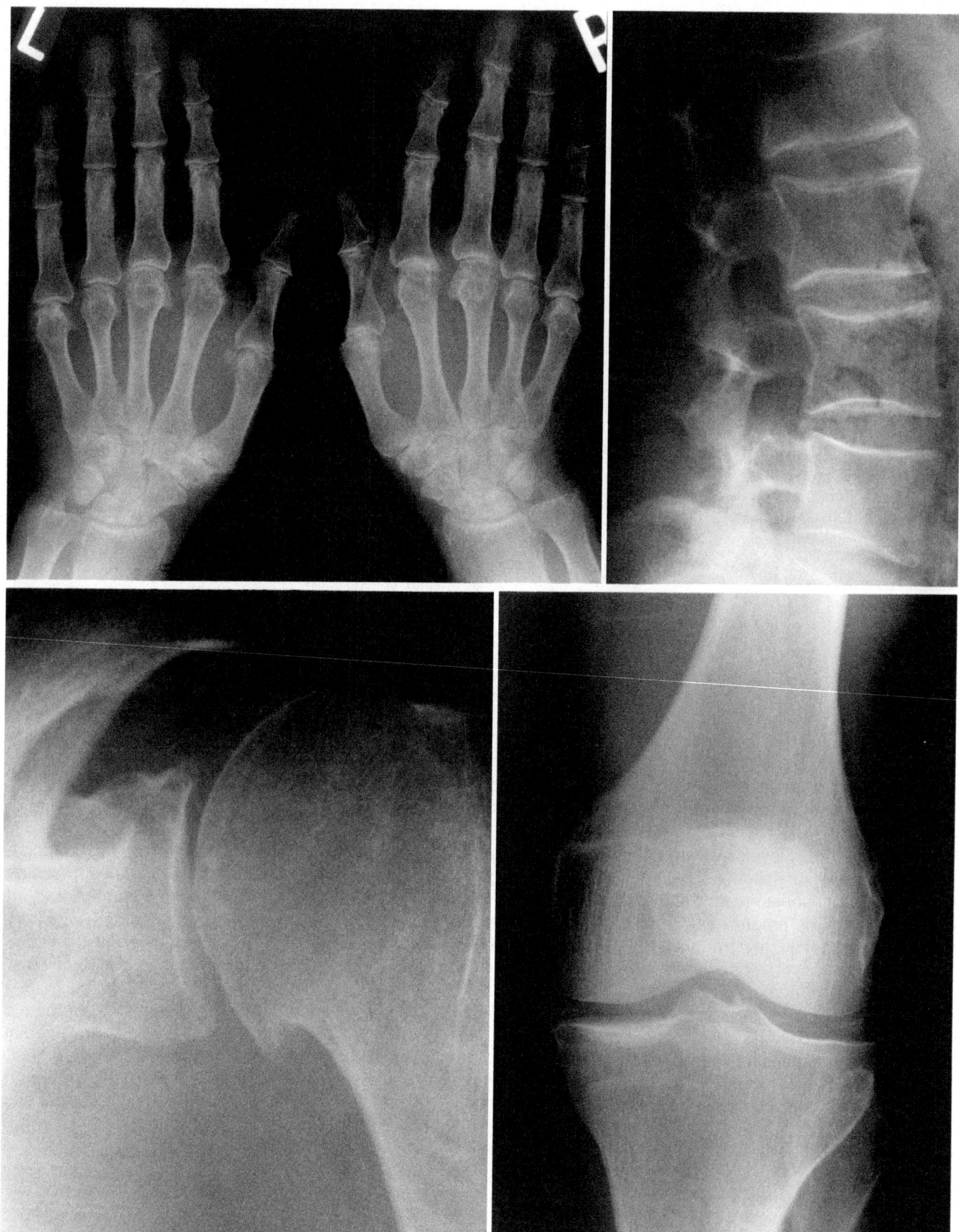

Musculoskeletal findings in genetic hemochromatosis: The only specific finding is the retrograde hook-like osteophytes at the metacarpal heads; other findings of intervertebral disc calcification, osteophytosis of the humeral head, and meniscal chondrocalcinosis are nonspecific and therefore easily nondiagnosed or misdiagnosed. Images here are respectfully used with kind permissions of Dr Manfred Harth and *Journal of Rheumatology* (hands and knee) and Dr JD Macfarlane and *Journal of Bone and Joint Surgery* (spine and shoulder) per personal correspondence, written permission, and provision of radiographs.

Treatments:

- <u>Medical standard</u>: <mark>Iron-removal is accomplished by weekly phlebotomy of 1-2 units (250-500 mL of blood, each of which removes 250 mg of iron)</mark>, and deferoxamine chelation is used in patients who cannot tolerate phlebotomy. Complications of the disease, such as arthritis, heart failure, hypogonadism, and diabetes are treated appropriately. Cirrhotic patients must be monitored for hepatoma with twice-yearly liver ultrasound and measurement of serum alpha-fetoprotein. Always, when a hereditary iron overload disorder is diagnosed, all (first-degree) blood relatives must be screened for iron overload.

- <u>Diet modifications</u>: These are no substitute for iron-removal therapy with phlebotomy and are weak in their effectiveness by comparison.
  - Decrease consumption of foods and nutritional supplements which are significant sources of iron: Iron supplements, iron-fortified foods and supplements, liver, beef, pork, lamb.
  - Increase consumption of foods that will decrease intestinal absorption of iron from ingested food: tannins in tea, phytates (in whole-grain products, bran, legumes, nuts, and seeds), soy protein, egg, calcium supplements.
  - Ensure adequate protein intake to replace protein lost during phlebotomy.
  - Decrease consumption of excess ascorbic acid (vitamin C); high-dose vitamin C supplementation is clearly contraindicated.[658]
  - Alcohol consumption should be avoided because ethanol exacerbates liver damage and increases iron absorption from the gut.

- <u>Silymarin</u>: Milk thistle has proved benefit in an animal model of iron overload[659] and is probably suitable for use in patients with iron overload, particularly given its ability to reverse cirrhosis.[660] More recently, silybin has been shown to chelate iron in the gastrointestinal tract and reduce its absorption; the more important finding here is that silybin is safe for patients with hemochromatosis.
  - <u>Iron-chelating potential of silybin in patients with hereditary hemochromatosis</u> (*Eur J Clin Nutr* 2010 Oct[661]): "Milk thistle contains silybin, which is a potential iron chelator. ... In this crossover study, on three separate occasions, 10 patients who were homozygous for the C282Y mutation in the HFE gene (and fully treated) consumed a vegetarian meal containing 13.9 mg iron with: 200 ml water; 200 ml water and 140 mg silybin (Legalon Forte); or 200 ml tea. Blood was drawn once before, then 0.5, 1, 2, 3 and 4 h after the meal. Consumption of silybin with a meal resulted in a reduction in the postprandial increase in serum iron (AUC±s.e.) compared with water (silybin 1726.6±346.8 versus water 2988.8±167; P<0.05) and tea (silybin 1726.6±346.8 versus tea 2099.3±223.3; P<0.05). In conclusion, silybin has the potential to reduce iron absorption, and this deserves further investigation, as silybin could be an adjunct in the treatment of hemochromatosis."

- <u>Antioxidant supplementation (excluding high-dose ascorbate)</u>: Oxidative stress is increased and antioxidant reserves are decreased in patients with iron overload.

- <u>Coenzyme Q10</u>: CoQ-10 probably has a role in the treatment of hemochromatoic cardiomyopathy given its safety and efficacy in other cardiomyopathies.[662,663,664,665,666,667,668,669]

Musculoskeletal disorders and iron overload disease—reminder to review the previous article on page 57

"Approximately one and a 250 persons is homozygous for this disorder and will develop the characteristic clinical manifestations such as diabetes, cardiomyopathy, liver disease, endocrine dysfunction, and, most notable for this discussion, arthropathy or other musculoskeletal disorders. ... The current literature suggests that everyone should be screened for iron overload, regardless of the presence or absence of symptoms."

Vasquez A. *Arthritis Rheum.* 1996 Oct

---

[658] Mclarlan et al. Congestive cardiomyopathy and hemochromatosis: rapid progression possibly accelerated by excessive ingestion of ascorbic acid. *Aust NZ J Med* 1982;12:187-8

[659] "CONCLUSIONS: Oral administration of silybin protects against iron-induced hepatic toxicity in vivo. This effect seems to be caused by the prominent antioxidant activity of this compound." Pietrangelo A, et al. Antioxidant activity of silybin in vivo during long-term iron overload in rats. *Gastroenterology.* 1995 Dec;109(6):1941-9

[660] Salmi et al. Effect of silymarin and chemical, functional, and morphological alterations of the liver. A double-blind controlled study. *Scand J Gastroenterol* 1982;17:517-21

[661] Hutchinson et al. The iron-chelating potential of silybin in patients with hereditary haemochromatosis. *Eur J Clin Nutr.* 2010 Oct;64(10):1239-41

[662] Greenberg S, Frishman WH. Co-enzyme Q-10: a new drug for cardiovascular disease. *J Clin Pharmacol* 1990; 30: 596-608

[663] Langsjoen PH, Langsjoen PH, Folkers K. Long-term efficacy and safety of coenzyme Q-10 therapy for idiopathic dilated cardiomyopathy. *Am J Cardiol* 1990; 65: 521-3

[664] Manzoli U, Rossi E, Littarru GP, et al. Coenzyme Q-10 in dilated cardiomyopathy. *Int J Tiss Reac* 1990; 12: 173-8

[665] Langsjoen et al. Pronounced increase of survival of patients with cardiomyopathy when treated with coenzyme Q-10 and conventional therapy. *Int J Tiss Reac* 1990;12:163-8

[666] Folkers K. Heart failure is a dominant deficiency of coenzyme Q-10 and challenges for future clinical research on CoQ-10. *Clin Investig* 1993; 71: s51-s54

[667] Folkers K, et al. Therapy with coenzyme Q-10 of patients in heart failure who are eligible or ineligible for a transplant. *Biochem Biophys Res Commun* 1992;182:247-53

[668] Mortensen SA, et al. Coenzyme Q-10: clinical benefits with biochemical correlates suggesting a scientific breakthrough.... *Int J Tiss Reac* 1990;12:155-62

[669] Langsjoen PH, Langsjoen PH, Folkers K. A six-year clinical study of therapy of cardiomyopathy with coenzyme Q-10. *Int J Tiss Reac* 1990; 12: 169-71

Hypothyroidism:
Clinical, Functional, and Practical Considerations

Introduction:
Due mostly to the allopathic medical profession's limited view of hypothyroidism—ie, as the presence or absence of gland failure without proper consideration of peripheral metabolism— the condition has remained enigmatic, and both doctors and patients have been rendered ineffective in their ability to understand and treat this common clinical condition. In the following few pages, the illusion of complexity and incomprehensibility will be deflated. This chapter details the most important considerations in the assessment and treatment of various types of low thyroid function. As with the other chapters of the book, information will be presented in an outlined format.

Description/pathophysiology:

- **Anatomy and normal physiology of thyroid hormone production and function**: The base of the brain contains a region called the hypothalamus, which coordinates many body functions and secretes thyrotropin releasing hormone (TRH) which stimulates the nearby pituitary gland to produce thyroid stimulating hormone (TSH). The TSH produced from the pituitary gland on the underside of the brain provides the stimulating signal to the thyroid gland, located at the front of the neck, for it to produce its hormones. The main hormones secreted by the thyroid gland are thyroxine (also called "T4" because it is the thyroid hormone made from the amino acid tyrosine [T] that has four [4] molecules of iodine) and triiodothyronine, also called "T3" because it has three molecules of iodine. Most of the hormone produced by the thyroid gland is in the form of T4, which is much less biologically active than T3. T4 is converted into T3 in the liver and in the peripheral tissues of the body, with the notable exception of the brain. Although the thyroid gland's production of T3 is quantitatively less than that of T4, because T3 is the active form of the hormone, the direct production of T3 from the thyroid gland itself is important for peripheral tissues such as the brain which are unable to sufficiently convert T4 into T3.

Illustration of thyroid hormone production, stimulation, and peripheral metabolism: Although most doctors have been taught to focus only on thyroid production, updated clinicians realize the importance of considering thyroid production in conjunction with peripheral thyroid metabolism and the differential conversion from the inactive T4 to the reciprocally produced active T3 and reverse T3, the latter of which is either biologically inert or—

Hypothalamus produces thyrotropin releasing hormone (TRH)

↓

TRH stimulates the pituitary gland to produce thyroid stimulating hormone (TSH)

↓

TSH stimulates the thyroid gland to produce mostly T4 with some T3 (and other hormones)

↓

T4 is released into the blood and must be converted to the active T3 form to be biologically active

↓

T4

Generally speaking and during states of health, T4 is converted to T3, which is the most active form of the hormone

↓

Normal health and normal hormone levels

During times of stress, the body produces more of the inactive reverse T3 (rT3) which actually blocks the function of normal T3, causing the manifestations of hypothyroidism even when other aspects of thyroid hormone production are normal

↓

Impaired health despite normal levels of TSH and T4; T3 may be low, and rT3 is elevated

more likely—counteractive to normal T3 utilization. Conversion of T4 to active T3 is achieved by type-1 and type-2 deiodinase (5' [five prime] iodinase) while conversion of T4 to reverse T3 is achieved by types-2 deiodinase (5-iodinase).[670] Impaired glandular production of thyroid hormones is appropriately termed central or glandular hypothyroidism, while impaired peripheral conversion or utilization of thyroid hormone is appropriately termed metabolic or peripheral or functional hypothyroidism.

---

[670] Kansagra et al. The Challenges and Complexities of Thyroid Hormone Replacement. *Lab Med.* 2010;41(6):229-348 medscape.com/viewarticle/722086_8

- **Hormones and feedback mechanisms**: When thyroid hormone production is insufficient, receptors in the hypothalamus and pituitary sense the hormone deficiency and respond by increasing the production of TSH to stimulate hormone production from the thyroid gland; when thyroid hormone production increases, feedback to the hypothalamus and pituitary reduces TSH production to lower thyroid hormone production. In these ways, as with many other body systems and physiological processes, the body is able to maintain a steady state of thyroid hormone production; most people have heard of this phenomenon of self-regulation referred to as *homeostasis*, even though a more accurate term is *homeodynamics*, because it is an active (not static) process in constant fluctuation and regulation. If a patient is given too much thyroid hormone by prescription, then the TSH level will be reduced; if a patient has hypothyroidism and is undertreated with an insufficient amount of thyroid hormone, then the TSH will remain elevated. Lab tests and optimal hormone levels will be discussed later in this chapter.
- **Problems that may arise in thyroid hormone production and metabolism**: In this section, details will be provided about common problems that can arise in thyroid hormone production and metabolism:
  - Problems of the hypothalamus: Damage to the hypothalamus from an injury such as head trauma, cancer, or infection can result in an inability to produce TRH; these problems are very rare. Doctors do not generally test for TRH production; however, some abnormalities in TRH production have been noted in patients with chronic depression. "Hypothalamic hypothyroidism" is hypothyroidism resulting from a problem in the hypothalamus; this is also called *tertiary hypothyroidism*, because it is two "steps" away from the primary location of thyroid hormone production—the thyroid gland itself.
  - Problems of the pituitary gland: Rarely, the pituitary gland might overproduce TSH and function autonomously from TRH stimulation; this will result in excess thyroid hormone production. More commonly but still rare, damage to the pituitary gland—for example if a nearby tumor compresses the gland, or if the gland is damaged by a disease like iron overload (e.g., hemochromatosis) or by a stroke (e.g., Sheenan's syndrome)—can cause a reduction in TSH production. Problems localized to the pituitary gland resulting in either excess or deficient production of TSH are very rare and are not responsible for the majority of thyroid disorders. Hypothyroidism caused by problems in the pituitary gland is called *secondary hypothyroidism* because it is *secondary* to (i.e., caused by) problems *outside* of the thyroid gland.
  - Problems of the thyroid gland: Several problems can affect the thyroid gland and its ability to produce the proper amount of thyroid hormone. Some of the more relevant disorders are discussed in the following subsections:
    - Graves' disease—autoimmune *hyper*thyroidism: Graves' disease is a fairly common autoimmune disease wherein the body's immune system creates antibodies to the TSH receptor. These antibodies stimulate the TSH receptor just as would the normal TSH hormone, and thus the result is an increased production of thyroid hormones from the gland, causing excess thyroid gland function and the clinical manifestations of hyperthyroidism. Common manifestations of the disease are weight loss, excess body heat, diarrhea due to more rapid gastrointestinal transit, and tremor (shakiness) and tachycardia (fast heart rate) due to increased stimulation of the sympathetic nervous system. Another common trademark manifestation of Graves' disease is exophthalmos—"bulging of the eyes"—because excess fibrous tissue is deposited behind the eyes and because the muscles surrounding the outside of the eyes are weakened by immune (antibody) damage. Graves' disease is most commonly treated with drugs that block the metabolism of thyroid hormones, or with other drugs such as radioactive iodine which cause destruction of the thyroid gland, resulting in hypothyroidism which is then treated with prescription thyroid hormone. Graves' disease can be considered a form of *primary* hyperthyroidism because it is hyperthyroidism resulting from abnormal function of the gland *itself*, even though the cause of the problem is the antibodies that are interacting with the gland receptors. With Graves' disease or any other cause of primary hyperthyroidism, lab tests will show that TSH is low and T4 is high. Occasionally noted clinically is a mixed hyper-/hypo- picture, Graves' with Hashimoto's.
      - Nonpharmacologic treatment options for Graves's disease: The best nonpharmacologic treatment for hyperthyroidism is the amino acid L-carnitine 1-4 grams/d orally; carnitine blocks entry of thyroid hormone into the nucleus of the cell, thereby blocking most of the effects of excess thyroid

hormone.[671] Very interestingly, when researchers or we as clinicians use carnitine in patients with normal thyroid status, we do not see adverse effects consistent with "carnitine-induced hypothyroidism", which is to say that carnitine appears to block *excess* thyroid hormone reception but appears to not have a blocking effect on *normal* thyroid function/reception. Since Graves' disease is an autoimmune disorder, attention should be given to normalizing immune function (nutritional immunomodulation) and removing triggers of autoimmunity such as allergenic/immunogenic foods, dysbiotic microbial infections, and xenobiotics—all of these are discussed in Chapter 4 of this book. Finally, patients with the iron-accumulating disease hemochromatosis have an increased risk for developing Graves disease; thus, patients with Graves disease—especially males—should be tested and treated for iron overload, specifically using the blood test serum ferritin, as detailed in Chapter 1.

- **Viral infection, acute viral thyroiditis**: The thyroid gland can be infected by a viral infection, perhaps as a consequence of an upper respiratory infection; this is called "viral thyroiditis." (Keep in mind that the suffix "-itis" simply means inflammation, so "thyroiditis" just means inflammation of the thyroid gland, whether from infection, trauma [rare], or autoimmune disease [most common].) Classically, the patient has had a recent viral infection—such as a common cold—and the thyroid gland, located at the anterior lower neck just barely above the rib cage, is tender and slightly swollen. In these situations, infection of the gland causes release of thyroid hormone from the gland, temporarily resulting in hyperthyroidism. If the gland is damaged by the infection, then the period of transient *hyper*thyroidism may be followed by *hypo*thyroidism due to failure of the gland to produce sufficient thyroid hormone. This resulting hypothyroidism may be mild or severe, temporary or permanent.

- **Hashimoto's disease, autoimmune thyroiditis, autoimmune *hypo*thyroidism**: The most common cause of *primary hypothyroidism*—hypothyroidism resulting from failure of the thyroid gland—is autoimmune destruction of the thyroid gland, also called Hashimoto's thyroiditis in recognition of the Japanese medical scientist Hashimoto Hakaru who first described the condition in 1912. The condition is also called lymphocytic thyroiditis because biopsy of the thyroid gland will show infiltration of immune cells called lymphocytes, which cause damage to the glandular tissue. In this condition, the body's own immune system—specifically the T-cells and the antibodies/immunoglobulins made by the B-cells or plasma cells—causes injury to and eventual destruction of the thyroid gland. Autoimmune destruction of the thyroid gland can occur as a solitary phenomenon, or it may occur as part of another autoimmune disorder, such as rheumatoid arthritis (RA), systemic lupus erythematosus (SLE, lupus), or Sjögren's syndrome. If the thyroid gland itself is failing to produce sufficient amounts of thyroid hormone, then feedback mechanisms will cause TSH to increase; thus, what most doctors look for when screening for hypothyroidism is simply an elevated TSH. For many doctors, if they fail to find an elevated TSH, then they will exclude hypothyroidism as a diagnosis and will not treat the patient with thyroid hormone even if the patient is *clinically hypothyroid*, that is, showing all the clinical manifestations expected with

---

If autoimmune hypothyroidism is the problem, then what is the cause of the problem?

Given that an autoimmune disease process (involving auto-antibodies and auto-reactive T-cells) can lead to inflammatory destruction of the thyroid gland, a reasonable question becomes "What triggers the immune system to attack the thyroid gland?" The top six answers to this question are:

❶ Exposure to the dietary protein gluten, found in grains such as wheat, rye, barley,
❷ Nutritional deficiency of selenium, and possibly vitamins D and A,
❸ Localized viral infection, noted to result commonly in self-limited thyroid disease,
❹ Infection with specific bacteria—such as *Yersinia enterocolitica*—anywhere in the body but especially the gastrointestinal tract,
❺ Xenobiotic exposure,
❻ Iron overload—patients and especially men with hemochromatosis have a higher risk of developing autoimmune thyroid disease especially Graves disease.

A genetic predisposition atop any of these other six triggers will increase the probability of developing autoimmune thyroiditis but is by itself insufficient.

---

[671] "In conclusion, L-carnitine is effective in both reversing and preventing symptoms of hyperthyroidism and has a beneficial effect on bone mineralization. Because hyperthyroidism depletes the body deposits of carnitine and since carnitine has no toxicity, teratogenicity, contraindications and interactions with drugs, carnitine can be of clinical use." Benvenga et al. Usefulness of L-carnitine, a naturally occurring peripheral antagonist of thyroid hormone action, in iatrogenic hyperthyroidism: a randomized, double-blind, placebo-controlled clinical trial. *J Clin Endocrinol Metab.* 2001 Aug;86(8):3579-94. "Taken together, all these experiments indicate that L-carnitine decreases the access of thyroid hormone to thyroid hormone receptors by decreasing the amount of hormone having access to cell nuclei, and not by inhibiting thyroid hormone interaction with the nuclear receptors." Benvenga et al. Effects of carnitine on thyroid hormone action. *Ann N Y Acad Sci* 2004 Nov;1033:158-67

hypothyroidism. Blood levels of T4 may be normal due to compensatory stimulation by extra TSH; T4 levels might also be reduced. Most often, laboratory tests will also reveal elevated levels of antibodies which specifically target components of the thyroid gland. The two most common antibodies seen in Hashimoto/autoimmune thyroiditis are directed toward thyroglobulin, which is a protein found in the thyroid gland, and against the enzyme peroxidase; these are called anti-thyroglobulin antibodies and anti-thyroid peroxidase (anti-TPO) antibodies, respectively.

- o <u>Problems of peripheral metabolism</u>: As reviewed above in the section on normal thyroid metabolism, the thyroid gland's production of thyroid hormone—mostly T4—is followed by conversion of T4 into the active form of thyroid hormone, which is T3. During times of stress, the body's ability to produce and utilize T3 is impaired because the enzymes that catalyze this conversion change in a way that produces a different hormone called "reverse T3" (rT3), which is certainly less active than normal T3 and which appears to actually block the function of the normal T3 that is produced. In these situations, TSH and T4 levels are generally normal, and since most doctors do not test the levels of T3 and rT3, the problem is almost never discovered. Reliable test for T3 and rT3 have been available for many years; the reason that most doctors do not use these tests is that they were not taught to do so in medical school and because most textbooks have not yet incorporated this relatively new information. A well-known paradox is that medical education and clinical training are very slow to change certain ideas despite the clarity of science (such as the importance of optimal nutrition—see extensive reviews in Chapters 2,3,4), and yet are very fast to accept unscientific changes that support drug over-prescribing and nutritional ignorance, such the widespread overuse of unproven drugs (such as rofecoxib/Vioxx, which was a new anti-inflammatory drug that was not very effective for pain but which caused tens of thousands of deaths before its withdrawal[672]) and the American Medical Association's discouragement of GMO labeling—keeping the public ignorant about the food they eat—despite clear scientific evidence of adverse effects.[673]

- **Definitions and descriptions of hypothyroidism**: The American Thyroid Association has described hypothyroidism as follows in a 2003 publication—ATA Hypothyroidism Booklet[674]—available on their website in December 2011: "Hypothyroidism is an underactive thyroid gland ("hypo-"means *under* or below *normal*). Hypothyroidism means that the thyroid gland cannot make enough thyroid hormone to keep the body running normally. People are hypothyroid if they have too little thyroid hormone in their blood." Patients and clinicians should appreciate that while this definition is accurate, it is incomplete because hypothyroidism involves more than the state of insufficient hormone production from the gland; in some situations we see that patients make sufficient thyroid hormone from their thyroid gland, but that the peripheral metabolism of their thyroid hormone is impaired, thereby creating the paradox of hypothyroid manifestations despite normalcy of commonly performed lab tests. Hypothyroidism should therefore be at least partially defined as a clinical syndrome of health problems which are fully or partly reversible with proper replacement of thyroid hormones.

- <u>A new practical definition of hypothyroidism</u>: Rather than defining hypothyroidism by "hormone levels in the blood", a wiser and more accurate definition of hypothyroidism holds that the condition should be defined as "an adverse physiological state caused by insufficient function of thyroid hormone at the *cellular* (not *serum*) level, resulting in clinical manifestations consistent with hypothyroidism and which respond wholly or partly to appropriately dosed and formulated thyroid replacement therapy, notably with T4 and T3 in combination, or T3 alone, but generally not T4—the inactive hormone—alone." This definition of hypothyroidism is based on physiology, i.e., the fact that the purpose of thyroid hormone is to effect action and changes at the cellular level to support optimal health and vitality; defining the presence or absence of hypothyroidism on the clinician's measurement of TSH is myopic and doctorcentric/anthropocentric, if not misanthropic. The purpose of the

---

[672]Topol EJ. Failing the public health--rofecoxib, Merck, and the FDA. *N Engl J Med.* 2004 Oct 21;351(17):1707-9 nejm.org/doi/pdf/10.1056/NEJMp048286

[673] "...there is no scientific justification for special labeling of bioengineered foods, as a class, and that voluntary labeling is without value unless it is accompanied by focused consumer education." Nestle M. The AMA's Strange Position on GM Foods. *THE ATLANTIC* 2012 Jun theatlantic.com/health/archive/2012/06/the-amas-strange-position-on-gm-foods-test-but-dont-label/258968/ Finamore et al. Intestinal and peripheral immune response to MON810 maize ingestion in weaning and old mice. *J Agric Food Chem.* 2008 Dec 10;56(23):11533-9 pubs.acs.org/doi/abs/10.1021/jf802059w Krüger et al. Detection of Glyphosate Residues in Animals and Humans. *Environmental & Analytical Toxicology* 2014 Jan:4;2 omicsonline.org/open-access/detection-of-glyphosate-residues-in-animals-and-humans-2161-0525.1000210.pdf Gammon C. Weed-whacking herbicide proves deadly to human cells. *Scientific American* 2009 Jun scientificamerican.com/article/weed-whacking-herbicide-p/

[674] American Thyroid Association. ATA Hypothyroidism Booklet. 2003 Available at thyroid.org/patients/brochures/Hypothyroidism%20_web_booklet.pdf on December 2011. "This booklet was prepared by the American Thyroid Association (ATA), a professional society of physicians and researchers specializing in the thyroid gland. Founded in 1923, the ATA fosters excellence and innovation in patient care, research, education, and public advocacy. The recommendations given here are those of the ATA."

thyroid gland is to make sufficient thyroid hormone to effect normal healthy physiology; the purpose of the thyroid gland is not to produce a level of thyroid hormone that fits within a laboratory reference range defined by a small group of laboratories, researchers, and clinicians based on small numbers of patients, many of whom were likely not optimally healthy. Therefore, any accurate definition of hypothyroidism must be based on physiology rather than on blood tests; again, the purpose of the hormonal system is to create certain physiologic effects consistent with health and vitality, not to produce an amount of hormone considered "normal."

- <u>**One way to explain this to patients**</u>: The way that I have often explained this to patients—verbally or as below from my written patient education materials—is so say something to the effect that, "Thyroid hormones have many different functions in the body, and their chief effect is contributing to the control of the basal metabolic rate, or the *speed of biochemical reactions and physiologic processes* and the *temperature of the body.* For reasons that are not entirely clear, some people do not make enough thyroid hormone to function optimally.[675] Other people make enough to be considered "normal" but they do not feel well, and they often feel better when taking additional thyroid hormone as prescribed by their doctor.[676,677] Indeed, a famous physiology researcher at the University of Texas at Austin—Dr. Roger J Williams—noted in his classic book *Biochemical Individuality*, "a wide variation in thyroid activity exists among 'normal' human beings."[678]

<u>Clinical presentations</u>:

- **Prevalence**: Hypothyroidism is common, affecting about 10% of the population. It is more commonly diagnosed in women than in men; this may be because autoimmune disorders (such as autoimmune thyroiditis) are generally more common in women—some of these reasons (and solutions) are discussed in Chapter 4.
  - o <u>Fatigue</u>: Fatigue and "not enough energy" are among the most common complaints of patients with hypothyroidism. Fatigue and low energy are nonspecific subjective complaints that correlate with innumerable health conditions, including depression, existential crisis, anemia, hypothyroidism, infection, cancer, autoimmune diseases, cardiopulmonary disease, nutritional deficiency, and many others.
  - o <u>Depression, lack of energy, lack of appetitive drives</u>: Depression is common among patients with hypothyroidism. The most direct explanations for this are ❶ reduced function of the adrenergic nervous system, specifically the reception of neurotransmitters norepinephrine and dopamine, which support energy/attention/vigilance and drive/direction/pleasure, respectively, ❷ reduced metabolic function overall due to lower body temperature (most enzymes function most efficiently within a narrow range of temperatures), ❸ nutritional deficiencies due to reduced stomach acid production (noted in patients with hypothyroidism) and/or bacterial overgrowth of the small bowel (SIBO) secondary to slow intestinal transit, which is well noted in patients with hypothyroidism. Additionally, patients with hypothyroidism often have weight gain, difficult weight loss, reduced appetite and sex drive, various health problems such as hypertension and headaches, and also the experience of being underdiagnosed/undertreated and feeling misunderstood by their doctors and perhaps by friends, family, and intimate/romantic partners as well; these can all contribute to the psychological and social aspects of depression and feelings of sadness, despair, and isolation. Notice from above the combination of reduced food appetite/intake with weight gain and difficult weight loss; this paradox has very few explanations and is therefore a clue in the patient's history suggesting hypothyroidism. Many patients diagnosed with "depression" actually have "depression secondary to hypothyroidism"; rather than being treated with potentially dangerous so-called "anti-depressant drugs" these patients would be better treated for improved mood and enhanced overall health by receiving treatment to optimize thyroid function, namely thyroid hormone.
  - o <u>Low body temperature, cold hands and feet</u>: Because T3 increases energy expenditure and therefore increases body heat, patients with an insufficiency of thyroid hormone commonly notice feeling cold and also not tolerating cold weather—a phenomenon referred to as cold intolerance. This can be assessed simply by touching the skin and hands of a person with hypothyroidism; often the initial handshake at the start of the patient's office visit is the first clue to hypothyroidism. Many of these patients have low oral temperatures that never reach the normal temperature of 98.6° Fahrenheit (F) or 37° Celsius (C); often they

---

[675] Broda Barnes MD, Lawrence Galton, <u>*Hypothyroidism: The Unsuspected Illness*</u>. Ty Crowell Co; 1976

[676] Skinner GR, et al. Thyroxine should be tried in clinically hypothyroid but biochemically euthyroid patients. *BMJ: British Medical Journal* 1997 Jun 14; 314(7096): 1764

[677] McLaren EH, Kelly CJ, Pollack MA. Trial of thyroxine treatment for biochemically euthyroid patients has been approved. *BMJ* 1997; 315: 1463

[678] Williams RJ. <u>*Biochemical Individuality: The Basis for the Genetotrophic Concept*</u>. Austin and London: University of Texas Press, 1956 page 82

report that the only time their oral temperature reaches the normal temperature is when they have a "fever" due to an infection. Very few conditions cause low body temperature; therefore, the finding of a consistently low body temperature is a clinical finding that is objective and significant and which warrants evaluation. Low body temperature is most consistent with hypothyroidism; to a lesser extent it is consistent with high estrogen levels, low testosterone levels and—in women and on a menstrual/periodic basis—low progesterone levels. Poor peripheral circulation to the extremities can also produce the feeling of localized coldness; the main conditions to consider in this regard are peripheral arterial disease (PAD, generally seen in elderly patients with other manifestations of cardiovascular disease) and Raynaud's phenomenon (periodic vasoconstriction secondary to vasomotor instability, commonly noted with other autoimmune diseases such as scleroderma and lupus and/or bacterial infections such as with the common bacteria *Helicobacter pylori*, detailed in Chapters 4 (and 5 of DrV's *Naturopathic Rheumatology*).

o <u>Dry skin</u>: Dry skin is commonly noted in patients with hypothyroidism. This may be due to a combination of impaired nutrient absorption and also impaired function of the oil-producing glands of the skin.

o <u>Constipation, poor digestion, acid reflux</u>: Because hypothyroidism leads to a generalized slowing of the body's functions, it commonly leads to slower intestinal transit, which manifests as constipation. Impaired gastrointestinal motility can also promote acid reflux. Approximately 30% of patients with Hashimoto's/autoimmune thyroiditis also make antibodies to the acid-producing cells in the stomach (parietal cells), and this can eventually lead to damage to the stomach lining and reduced stomach acid production, thereby impairing protein digestion. The lack of stomach acid and/or the slowing of intestinal transit promotes excessive growth of bacteria in the intestines because they are not being killed by stomach acid and/or "moved along" by normal peristaltic motions; this small intestinal bacterial overgrowth (SIBO) can lead to other problems such as fatigue, fibromyalgia, chemical sensitivity, and inflammatory arthritis.

o <u>Menstrual irregularities, premenstrual syndrome (PMS), uterine fibroids, excess menstrual bleeding, polycystic ovarian syndrome (PCOS)</u>: Women with hypothyroidism commonly have one or more menstrual or reproductive disorders[679]; these are generally reversible or at least partially treatable with normalization of thyroid hormone status and optimization of other health factors. Women with polycystic ovary syndrome have higher-than-normal rates of goiter and autoimmune hypothyroid disease.[680]

o <u>Infertility and the feeling and experience of not having enough sex hormones</u>: Proper thyroid status is needed for the complexities of gonadal function and reproductive success. Men and women with hypothyroidism may have problems with regard to sexual function, desire, and reproduction; infertility and subfertility are common among this patient population. Thyroid hormone is directly necessary for sex hormone production and for the successful maintenance of pregnancy. Primary hypothyroidism associated with elevated TSH levels commonly leads to elevated levels of a pituitary hormone called prolactin, which causes infertility either by direct mechanisms or by secondary mechanisms, such as increasing the liver's production of a protein called sex-hormone-binding globulin (SHBG) which binds to sex hormones (estrogen and testosterone) so tightly that they are unavailable to cells to complete their functions, such as supporting sex drive, sexual function, and

> **Hypothyroidism is a cause of sexual dysfunction and reproductive disorders in men and women**
>
> "Via its interaction in several pathways, normal thyroid function is important to maintain normal reproduction. ... Male reproduction is adversely affected by both thyrotoxicosis [hyperthyroidism] and hypothyroidism. Erectile abnormalities have been reported. ... In females, thyrotoxicosis and hypothyroidism can cause menstrual disturbances. Thyrotoxicosis is associated mainly with hypomenorrhea and polymenorrhea, whereas hypothyroidism is associated mainly with oligomenorrhea [reduced frequency of menstruation]. Thyroid dysfunction has also been linked to reduced fertility. ... Autoimmune thyroid disease is present in 5-20% of unselected pregnant women. ... Overt hypothyroidism has been associated with increased rates of spontaneous abortion, premature delivery and/or low birth weight, fetal distress in labor, and perhaps gestation-induced hypertension and placental abruption."
>
> Krassas et al. Thyroid function and human reproductive health. *Endocr Rev* 2010 Oct

---

[679] Weeks AD. Menorrhagia and hypothyroidism. Evidence supports association between hypothyroidism and menorrhagia. *BMJ*. 2000 Mar 4;320(7235):649

[680] "In this case-control study, anti-thyroid antibodies and goiter prevalence were significantly higher in PCOS patients. These data suggest that thyroid exam and evaluation of thyroid function and autoimmunity should be considered in such patients." Kachuei M, Jafari F, Kachuei A, Keshteli AH. Prevalence of autoimmune thyroiditis in patients with polycystic ovary syndrome. *Arch Gynecol Obstet*. 2012 Mar;285(3):853-6

reproductive capability.[681] As a cause of low libido, hypothyroidism impairs neurotransmitters such as norepinephrine and dopamine which promote sex drive in men and women. Hypothyroidism also impairs internal production of testosterone, which is a necessary hormone for sex drive and sexual performance.

o **Weak fingernails, hair loss:** The weak fingernails seen in hypothyroidism are almost certainly due to impaired protein digestion and amino acid and mineral absorption, as well as metabolic impairment of the cells in the nail matrix which produces the toenails and fingernails. Via similar mechanisms, hypothyroidism also causes loss of head hair, which is particularly notable in women. The finding of weak fingernails is a relatively specific finding for a limited number of considerations; generally these are protein deficiency (due to insufficient intake, impaired digestion or absorption, or increased metabolic consumption or increased renal excretion), deficiency of minerals such as zinc, and hypothyroidism. Severe cases of skin diseases such as psoriasis can also affect the nails, but generally these conditions are evident upon observation of the patient; the clinical findings are also different from those seen in hypothyroidism (i.e., flaking of the nails in hypothyroidism versus pitting of the nails with psoriasis).

o **Increased need for sleep:** An increased need for sleep—termed either hypersomnia or hypersomnolence—is sometimes noted among hypothyroid patients, who might have the experience of needing extra sleep (e.g., > 9 hours per night) and yet not feeling refreshed after a good night's sleep. Other causes of increased need for and/or reduced quality of sleep are heart failure and sleep apnea; these can generally be distinguished from hypothyroidism based on history, physical exam, laboratory tests, and—more accurately but not generally needed—special tests such as echocardiography and sleep tests (polysomnography).

o **Overweight, gain weight easily, difficulty losing weight:** Thyroid hormone is an important factor energy utilization and thus caloric expenditure and therefore calorie intake-expenditure balance. Any low thyroid condition will promote weight gain and reduced weight loss because the overall metabolic rate is lowered in states of low thyroid status. The caveat to this situation is that patients with hypothyroidism often have reduced appetite, and therefore food intake may be reduced and thereby mask reduced caloric expenditure because body weight may not change much. When present, the paradox of "weight gain despite reduced food intake" strongly suggests hypothyroidism.

o **High cholesterol, dyslipidemia, cardiovascular risk:** Patients with hypothyroidism commonly have elevated blood cholesterol levels (as well as triglycerides and lipoprotein-a levels), and ridiculously and unfortunately, many patients who need thyroid treatment are forced to take cholesterol-lowering "statin" drugs instead of receiving the proper treatment for hypothyroidism, which is generally thyroid hormone. We now know that the cause of the elevation of cholesterol is not due to an effect on the cholesterol producing enzyme HMG-CoA reductase, but rather the elevated cholesterol levels noted in hypothyroidism are due to reduced uptake/reception and subsequent breakdown/catabolism of LDL cholesterol in the liver, while elevated triglyceride levels are due to reduced activity of the enzyme lipoprotein lipase.[682] Hypothyroidism is also well-known to cause (reversible) hyperhomocysteinaemia. Many patients noted to have high cholesterol levels are prescribed a lifetime of cholesterol-lowering drugs; this is unfortunate because what these patients often need is thyroid hormone.

o **Slow heart rate, heart abnormalities (asymmetric septal hypertrophy, similar to and often confused with idiopathic hypertrophic subaortic stenosis):** The average adult heart rate of the "textbook-normal" adult is approximately 72 beats per minute (b/m); abnormally slow heart rate (bradycardia) is defined as less than 60 b/m and excessively fast heart rate is greater than 100 b/m. In certain situations, a fast or slow heart rate might be normal for the situation at hand; for example, well-trained athletes may have a "normal" heart rate in the 50s, and an individual who is anxious, severely anemic, sick with an infection, or over-caffeinated might have an elevated heart rate that does not indicate a serious/real disease. If I see a patient with a heart rate <65 b/m and the patient is not athletic and does not have a heart condition or is not taking a medication that slows the heart rate, then I become suspicious of hypothyroidism and will look for other historical, physical, or laboratory evidence of hypothyroidism. Hypothyroidism can also cause a rare heart disorder called asymmetric septal hypertrophy (ASH), which is very similar to and often confused with

---

[681] Hardy KJ, Seckl JR. Endocrine assessment of impotence—pitfalls of measuring serum testosterone without sex-hormone-binding globulin. *Postgrad Med J* 1994 Nov;70:836-7
[682] "Decreased activity of LDL-receptors' resulting in decreased receptor-mediated catabolism of LDL and IDL is the main cause of the hypercholesterolemia observed in hypothyroidism." Liberopoulos EN, Elisaf MS. Dyslipidemia in patients with thyroid disorders. *Hormones* (Athens). 2002 Oct-Dec;1(4):218-23

idiopathic hypertrophic subaortic stenosis (IHSS); treatment with thyroid hormone generally cures this heart problem.[683]

o **High blood pressure, diastolic hypertension**: Hypothyroidism is a well-known cause of high blood pressure, specifically a type of high blood pressure called diastolic hypertension; treatment with thyroid hormone generally cures this problem.

o **Slow healing**: Reduced overall metabolic rate and impaired protein digestion and utilization—both of which are noted in patients with hypothyroidism—leads to impaired healing of wounds and injuries.

o **Decreased memory and concentration**: Reduced overall metabolic rate and impaired protein digestion and utilization—both of which are noted in patients with hypothyroidism—leads to impaired memory and cognition. Protein is the source of amino acids, which are used by the body to make neurotransmitters such as serotonin, dopamine, and norepinephrine. Low thyroid state also impairs the function of the nervous system, specifically the adrenergic aspect of the nervous system which uses dopamine and norepinephrine to promote attention, mood, and pleasure.

o **Muscle weakness**: In more severe cases, hypothyroidism can cause a muscle disease (hypothyroid myopathy); this can lead to muscle weakness.

o **Sleep apnea**: Hypothyroidism contributes to sleep apnea (impaired breathing during sleep).

o **Frog-like husky voice**: Changes in voice is commonly noted among patients with reduced thyroid function.

o **Recurrent infections**: Hypothyroidism impairs immune function, resulting in more severe and more frequent infections.

o **Many other manifestations**: Because thyroid hormone is necessary for every body system, its lack or insufficiency thereby also affects all body systems. Thus, *many* adverse health effects and symptoms may result from an insufficiency of thyroid hormone.

Major differential diagnoses for hypothyroidism:

- Because hypothyroidism can result in so many different health problems and subjective symptoms, the list of diagnostic considerations that share similarities with hypothyroidism is virtually endless. Each of the symptoms above has its own list of possible different diagnostic considerations. However, despite the confusion and similarity shared with other diseases, careful study of hypothyroidism from my experience with patients and with the fruits of reflection have revealed a pattern of symptoms in hypothyroidism that is indeed unique:

  ❶ The symptom cluster of "fatigue, depression, cold hands and feet, dry skin, constipation…"

  ❷ Weight gain despite reduced appetite and reduced food intake

  ❸ Persistently low body temperature—described in adjacent text box

  ❹ Slow or relatively slow heart rate—what I call "relative bradycardia"

  ❺ Delayed Achilles reflex return (discussed below).

How to measure first-morning axillary temperature
1. Shake down mercury thermometer before going to bed; leave thermometer near bedside (but obviously not in the bed where it could be warmed or broken),
2. Immediately upon wakening, before any other activity, place thermometer deep in axilla (armpit) and measure temperature for 7-10 minutes,
3. Normal is 97.8-98.2°F; less than this temperature warrants consideration of hypothyroidism.

Clinical assessment:

- **History/subjective**: Historical findings and clinical presentations are listed above. The symptom cluster of "fatigue, depression, cold hands and feet, dry skin, constipation" is classic and may be present in whole (rare) or in part (common).

- **Physical examination/objective**: The most relevant clinical findings are discussed here:

  o **Low body temperature**: Very few conditions result in persistently low body temperature; clearly the most common and important of these conditions is hypothyroidism. Patients who are persistently uncomfortable with cold hands and feet and persistent cold intolerance are worthy of assessment and treatment. Objectively, the physician will note that upon the welcoming handshake, the patient's hands feel cold; this

---

[683] "In 10 patients who returned to euthyroid state with L-thyroxine therapy, these abnormalities resolved. We conclude that long-standing hypothyroidism leads to a reversible cardiomyopathy, manifested by asymmetric septal hypertrophy with or without other echocardiographic features of a hypertrophic obstructive cardiomyopathy." Santos et al. Echocardiographic characterization of the reversible cardiomyopathy of hypothyroidism. *Am J Med*. 1980 May;68(5):675-82

assessment will be invalidated if the patient recently washed hands in hot or cold water, is wearing gloves, or if the physician also has hypothyroidism and is therefore equally cold. A persistently low first-morning *oral* temperature below 98.6° F warrants consideration for hypothyroidism. A persistently low first-morning *axillary* (underarm) temperature below 97.8-98.2° F warrants consideration of hypothyroidism.

- o Delayed Achillies reflex return: The deep tendon reflexes assessed by doctors during most clinical encounters contain two components: the contraction phase and the relaxation phase. Most of the time, we as doctors are primarily concerned with the contraction phase, which tells us about the integrity of the neuromuscular system. However, when we are looking for hypothyroidism, we are more concerned with the relaxation phase of the reflex; patients with hypothyroidism have reduced speed of muscular relaxation, and therefore the relaxation phase of the reflex cycle is prolonged. This finding is highly specific for hypothyroidism; some earlier medical diagnosis textbooks stated that a delayed Achilles reflex return "indicates" hypothyroidism, which is to say it is practically a diagnostic finding.

- o Slow heart rate—bradycardia: A heart rate less than 65 b/m suggests the possibility of hypothyroidism unless the patient is a well-conditioned athlete, has heart conduction problems, or is taking a medication such as a beta-blocking drug which will slow the rate of heart contractions.

- **Imaging & laboratory assessments**:
  - o Imaging: Imaging is not routinely relevant in the assessment and monitoring of hypothyroidism. Ultrasound scans and radionucleotide scans can be used to assess for more serious thyroid diseases, such as thyroid cancer.

  - o Laboratory evaluation: Laboratory evaluation of the patient with clinical manifestations of low thyroid function should be tertiary in importance to 1) the physician's assessment, judgment, and experience and 2) the patient's need for effective treatment for his/her complaints. As is stated with regard to the treatment of hypertension: *the physician's judgment remains paramount*.

    - ▪ Thyrotropin-releasing hormone—TRH: TRH is not routinely tested in clinical practice, although abnormalities of TRH secretion are noted in patients with mental "depression."

    - ▪ Thyroid-stimulating hormone—TSH (reference range 0.4 - 5.0 mIU/L [milli-international units per liter]): TSH is the most commonly performed test for evaluating thyroid status; its frequent (over)use owes more to habit and

> ### Optimal thyroid status
>
> <u>Concept by Dr Vasquez</u>: Optimal thyroid status is not defined by basic laboratory testing with TSH and free T4. It is defined *per patient* based on the levels and ratios of all major thyroid-related hormones and antibodies—in association with other hormonal, psychologic, dysbiotic, nutritional and environmental factors—that work best for that *biochemically unique* patient.
>
> <u>Laboratory interpretation by Dr McDaniel</u>: "Optimal hormone balance is debatable. My observations: A few "well" people and patients treated successfully with T4 and T3 seem best with:
> - TSH around 0.7–0.9 µIU/mL
> - fT4 around 0.7–0.8 ng/dL
> - fT3 optimally 3.4–3.8 pg/mL
> - **Total T3-RT3 ratio 12 +/-2**"
>
> McDaniel AB. Thyroid Assessment: Controversies and Conundrums. Institute for Functional Medicine Fourteenth International Symposium. Tucson, Arizona. May 23-26, 2007

inexpensiveness than to aspirations for clinical excellence. TSH values greater than 2 mIU/L represent a disturbance of the thyroid-pituitary axis and an increased risk for future thyroid problems[684], and the American Association of Clinical Endocrinologists stated initially in 2006 (and again in 2011), "The target TSH level should be between 0.3 and 3.0 µIU/mL."[685] Clinical rationale is available to support implementation of a therapeutic trial of thyroid hormone treatment in patients who are *clinically hypothyroid* even if they are *biochemically euthyroid* (per TSH) provided that treatment is implemented cautiously, in appropriately selected patients, and patients are appropriately informed.[686,687] If the clinical world were as perfect as it is portrayed in basic physiology textbooks, then a clinician might fancifully rely on TSH to perform the diagnosis *prima facie*, with reduced TSH values correlating with glandular overperformance and negative feedback suppressing TSH secretion, whilst an underperforming gland would require greater stimulation with elevated TSH levels; however, TSH

---

[684] Weetman AP. Fortnightly review: Hypothyroidism: screening and subclinical disease. *BMJ: British Medical Journal* 1997;314: 1175

[685] American Association of Clinical Endocrinologists. "The target TSH level should be between 0.3 and 3.0 µIU/mL." AACE Medical Guidelines for Clinical Practice for Evaluation and Treatment of Hyperthyroidism and Hypothyroidism. 2002, 2006 Amended Version. https://aace.com/sites/default/files/hypo_hyper.pdf Accessed Aug 2011

[686] Skinner GR, et al. Thyroxine should be tried in clinically hypothyroid but biochemically euthyroid patients. *BMJ: British Medical Journal* 1997 Jun 14; 314(7096): 1764

[687] McLaren EH, Kelly CJ, Pollack MA. Trial of thyroxine treatment for biochemically euthyroid patients has been approved. *BMJ* 1997; 315: 1463

has never been thus vested with infallible reliability, which explains in part why doctors need brains of their own and why better clinicians have developed the capacity for independent thought.

- Free thyroxine—free T4 (reference range 4.5 - 11.2 mcg/dL): Unbound T4 is tested to provide evidence of glandular production of thyroid hormone(s). Because T4 is the major thyroid hormone produced by the thyroid gland, it serves as an excellent marker for glandular productivity but it reveals nothing about peripheral conversion of T4 to the active thyroid hormone triiodothyronine (T3); in the practice of medicine, conversion of T4 to the active T3 is assumed to reliably occur unabated despite evidence to the contrary, especially among symptomatic and ill patients, the exact patients to whom we are providing care.

- Triiodothyronine—free T3 or total T3, the active form of thyroid hormone (reference range: 100 - 200 ng/dL[688]): Yes, contrary to what I was taught in medical school, I actually perform and advocate testing for the active form of the thyroid hormone when assessing patients for low thyroid function; some (non)experts/thinkers might consider this heretical or a waste of money, but I consider it to be a manifestation of common sense in the interest of providing efficient and cost-effective care. In textbook-perfect physiology, T4 is converted by the selenium-dependent deiodinase enzymes to the active thyroid hormone T3; in reality, this is only part of the story. Because T3 is the active form of the hormone responsible for the physiologic functions of thyroid physiology, a clinician desiring to assess a patient's thyroid status might reasonably ask the proper question by performing the proper test. T3 is tested as "total T3" or "free T3" in large part based on the clinician's preference; the current author prefers total T3 because it can be compared to the total level of reverse T3 (rT3) in a ratio, the optimal range of which is generally considered to be 10-14 as originally presented by McDaniel[689] and reviewed in the following pages. Patients with psychiatric depression have lower levels of T3 than do healthy controls and have been described as having "low T3 syndrome"[690]; very obviously, the low T3 levels in these patients would serve to promote and perpetuate their state of mental depression. Clinicians should be aware that T3, like estrogens, increases hepatic production of sex hormone binding globulin (SHBG) and that therefore T3 (and estrogen) administration can reduce cellular bioavailability of protein-bound hormones such as testosterone. Many authoritative and clinically-experienced sources recommend using a time-released (e.g., sustained-release) form of T3 due to its shorter half-life compared with T4. However, obtaining time-released T3 via a compounding pharmacy can be cumbersome and expensive for the patient; clearly many patients respond to once daily dosing of *non*-time-released T3 preparations—Cytomel or its generic equivalent—with good effects and without adverse effects. Some patients can divide the immediate-release dose into two servings per day for enhanced effect and lessened physiologic fluctuations, if necessary. Per Drugs.com[691] in August 2011, "Since liothyronine sodium (T3) is not firmly bound to serum protein, it is readily available to body tissues. The onset of activity of liothyronine sodium is rapid, occurring within a few hours. Maximum pharmacologic response occurs within 2 or 3 days, providing early clinical response. The biological half-life is about 2.5 days." Very clearly, a significant portion of hypothyroid patients respond to T3 alone (either time-released, divided-dosing, or once-daily dosing) or a combination of T4 and T3 when other treatments have failed.[692,693]

- Reverse triiodothyronine—rT3 (reference range: 90 - 320 pg/mL[694]): In addition to its conversion into the active T3 hormone, T4 can also be converted by deiodinase enzymes into the inactive thyroid hormone rT3; per a standard endocrinology textbook, "Approximately 70–80% of released T4 is converted by deiodinases to the biologically active T3, the remainder to reverse-T3 (rT3) which has no

[688] U.S. National Library of Medicine (NLM) and National Institutes of Health (NIH) nlm.nih.gov/medlineplus/ency/article/003687.htm Accessed August 2011
[689] McDaniel AB. Thyroid Assessment: Controversies and Conundrums. Institute for Functional Medicine Fourteenth International Symposium. Tucson, Az. May 23-26, 2007
[690] "Out of 250 subjects with major psychiatric depression, 6.4% exhibited low T3 syndrome (mean serum T3 concentration 0.94 nmol/l vs normal mean serum concentration of 1.77 nmol/l)." Premachandra BN, Kabir MA, Williams IK. Low T3 syndrome in psychiatric depression. *J Endocrinol Invest*. 2006 Jun;29(6):568-72
[691] drugs.com/pro/cytomel.html August 2011.
[692] Bunevicius R, et al. Effects of thyroxine as compared with thyroxine plus triiodothyronine in patients with hypothyroidism. *N Engl J Med*. 1999 Feb 11;340(6):424-9
[693] Kelly T, Lieberman DZ. The use of triiodothyronine as an augmentation agent in treatment-resistant bipolar II and bipolar disorder NOS. *J Affect Disord*. 2009;116(3):222-6
[694] The reference range provided here for rT3 is a compilation from the laboratory reference ranges from the sample reports on the following pages, each of which is performed by either Quest Diagnostics or LabCorp, the two largest medical laboratories in the United States.

significant biological activity."[695] Clinicians must know that, "The prohormone T4 must be converted to T3 in the body before it can exert biological effects. **During periods of illness or stress, this conversion is often inhibited and can be diverted to the inactive reverse T3 (rT3) moiety.**"[696] Furthermore and very importantly, clinicians should appreciate that rT3 is not simply inactive but that it may actually impair production/utilization of normal T3; "T4-T3 and T4-rT3 conversion are provoked by different enzymes. **The elevation of rT3 might be a cause of the observed decrease in peripheral T3 generation** in old [elderly] subjects, acting by an **inhibition of the T4-T3 conversion**."[697] During times of psychologic/physiologic stress and specific types of pharmacologic stress (e.g., propanolol[698] and corticosteroids), T4 metabolism is preferentially shunted away from T3 toward rT3; an anthropocentric explanation holds that by making less of the active T3 and more of the inactive rT3, the body is better able to conserve energy during times of stress by reducing overall metabolic rate, particularly resting energy expenditure and protein utilization. For example, caloric restriction and fasting result in a decrease in resting metabolic rate (RMR), and the reduced RMR persists for months after the fasting has ended and a normal diet is resumed.[699] This author (AV) terms this stress-induced impairment of thyroid hormone conversion "**metabolic hypothyroidism**" or "**functional hypothyroidism**" because the defect is in the metabolism (not the production) of thyroid hormone into its most active form; "**peripheral hypothyroidism**" might also be used to distinguish the fact that the defect is in the peripheral metabolism rather than located more centrally, within the thyroid gland itself. Because psychologic stress and certain pharmacologic exposures—as well as the thyro-metabolic stress of fasting and caloric restriction in which the counterregulatory hormone glucagon appears to trigger enhanced rT3 production—*reduce* active T3 while simultaneously *increasing* rT3 levels, clinicians can appreciate that calculation of the T3/rT3 ratio will be more significantly altered (and thus a more sensitive indicator of metabolic disruption) than will be the isolated measurements of T3 or rT3 alone. Functional medicine clinicians[700] note the importance of the ratio of total T3 to reverse T3 (tT3:rT3 ratio) and consider the optimal range to be 10-14 with lower ratios indicating impaired formation or T3 and/or excess production of rT3.[701] Contrary to the previous view which held that rT3 was simply inactive, we now appreciate that rT3 actually impairs normal thyroid hormone metabolism thus functioning as an thyrometabolic monkeywrench or "brake" on normal metabolism. Even if rT3 were only *inactive* and not *counteractive*, measuring its levels and the T3:rT3 ratio would still be appropriate. Elevated rT3 levels predict mortality among critically ill patients.[702] Aberrancies in thyroid hormone levels may reflect organic disease, psychoemotional stress, or nutritional deficiency[703], and therefore such serologic abnormalities warrant consideration of underlying problems and direct treatment when possible. If no underlying cause is apparent, then a trial of thyroid hormone/hormones is reasonable in appropriately selected patients. Beyond stress reduction, allergen/gluten avoidance, and nutritional supplementation with iodine, selenium, and zinc (as indicated per patient), correction of overt, subclinical, and functional hypothyroidism generally centers on the administration of natural or synthetic thyroid hormones in the form of T4 and T3. Correction of functional hypothyroidism (relatively reduced total T3 and increased rT3) is accomplished with either time-released or twice-daily dosing of T3 *without T4* to suppress endogenous T4 conversion to T3, thereby allowing rT3 levels to fall precipitously. T3 administration allows temporary downregulation of transforming enzymes so that rT3 production is reduced following withdrawal of T3 replacement; thus, short-term and/or periodic T3 administration helps normalize or "reset" peripheral thyroid metabolism so that, following withdrawal of T3 administration, T4 can be converted to T3 without excess production of rT3. The

[695] Nussey S, Whitehead S. *Endocrinology: An Integrated Approach*. Oxford: BIOS Scientific Publishers; 2001. See also Box 3.29 Metabolism of thyroid hormones. ncbi.nlm.nih.gov/books/NBK28/box/A270/?report=objectonly Accessed July 2011

[696] *1998 Mosby's GenRX. Sixth Edition*. St. Louis Missouri; Mosby-Year Book, Inc., 1998

[697] Szabolcs I, et al. The possible reason for serum 3,3'5'-(reverse) triiodothyronine increase in old people. *Acta Med Acad Sci Hung*. 1982;39(1-2):11-7

[698] "Propranolol administration (40 mg t.i.d. for a week) caused a similar rT3 elevation in old persons (n = 18) as in 12 young ones." Szabolcs I, et al. The possible reason for serum 3,3'5'-(reverse) triiodothyronine increase in old people. *Acta Med Acad Sci Hung*. 1982;39(1-2):11-7

[699] Elliot DL, et al. Sustained depression of the resting metabolic rate after massive weight loss. *Am J Clin Nutr* 1989 Jan;49(1):93-96

[700] The conclusion of this paragraph is derived from Vasquez A. *Musculoskeletal Pain: Expanded Clinical Strategies*. Published 2008 by The Institute for Functional Medicine.

[701] McDaniel AB. Thyroid Assessment: Controversies and Conundrums. Institute for Functional Medicine Fourteenth International Symposium. Tucson, Az. May 23-26, 2007

[702] Peeters RP, et al. Serum 3,3',5'-triiodothyronine (rT3) and 3,5,3'-triiodothyronine/rT3 are prognostic markers in critically ill patients and are associated with postmortem tissue deiodinase activities. *J Clin Endocrinol Metab*. 2005 Aug;90(8):4559-65

[703] Kelly GS. Peripheral metabolism of thyroid hormones: a review. *Altern Med Rev*. 2000 Aug;5(4):306-33

safety and effectiveness of this approach—using T3 administration (often twice daily or in a sustained-release compounded tablet or capsule) to recalibrate peripheral thyroid hormone metabolism—has documented safety and effectiveness.[704] Alleviation of symptoms, restoration of morning body temperature to 98.6° F (oral or axillary) and other clinical objective improvements achieved by the judicious and safe administration of T3 are the criteria of success; physiologic improvement following T3 administration retrospectively confirms the diagnosis of either hypothyroidism generally or functional hypothyroidism in particular.

- Antithyroid antibodies—antithyroglobulin (anti-TG) and anti-thyroid peroxidase (anti-TPO): Autoimmune thyroiditis (also called Hashimoto's disease or chronic lymphocytic thyroiditis) or is the most common cause of overt primary hypothyroidism. The diagnosis of autoimmune thyroiditis can be made clinically (i.e., without biopsy) upon detection of elevated blood levels of antibodies against thyroglobulin (anti-thyroglobulin antibodies) and anti-thyroid peroxidase (anti-TPO) antibodies. Autoimmune thyroiditis may present asymptomatically and with normal thyroid hormone levels; classically, patients may have a slightly hyperthyroid presentation as the inflamed gland releases extra thyroid hormone before becoming atrophic and hypofunctional.

Establishing the diagnosis:

- Hypothyroidism: The diagnosis of hypothyroidism is supported by the constellation of ❶ the patient's history and subjective complaints, ❷ physical examination findings, ❸ laboratory findings, and ❹ response to a clinical trial of thyroid hormone, preferably T3 alone or the combination of T4 and T3 which are consistent with the physiologic production of thyroid hormones from the thyroid gland. Treatment with T4 alone cannot be considered optimal therapy, if for no other reason than *the supremely important reason* that the brain cannot adequately convert T4 to T3; given the importance of the brain for our subjective feelings and perceptions as well as objective homeodynamic regulation, common sense argues against giving the hypothyroid brain a hormone that it cannot use.

- Autoimmune thyroiditis: The diagnosis of Hashimoto's/autoimmune thyroiditis is strongly suggested by the finding of elevated antibody levels against thyroglobulin and/or TPO.

DrV's perspective on the complexity and frequent lack of success in treating autoimmune hypothyroidism

The treatment of hypothyroidism has been a clinical conundrum for doctors for many years; it is the topic of many journal articles, debate and confusion, and well-ensconced views and opinions. Here, I will deconstruct the conundrum:

- Errors in testing and treating: From my perspective, the obvious reason for this confusion is that doctors—as medical students and as post-graduate readers of textbooks and journal articles that have inaccurate information—are trying to do the right thing (help patients) with the wrong information about testing (i.e., that TSH is the best [and almost exclusive] test for evaluating thyroid function) and treating (that the inactive T4 hormone should be used). Both of these promulgations are absurdly wrong. The reason that this topic is so confusing and contentious is that doctors have been misled to use the wrong test (TSH only) and the wrong treatment (T4 only); this explains why hypothyroid patients rarely receive any helpful treatment and are even more rarely treated to fully satisfactory result.

- Failure to consider, appreciate, and test for the important peripheral metabolism of thyroid hormones: Most doctors do not test for T3 levels; this erudite and unintellectual considering that if they are considering "hypothyroidism" as a diagnosis they should use testing that includes assessment of the active hormone in question. Fewer clinicians test for reverse T3, and fewer still appreciate the importance—conceptual more than mathematical—of the reciprocal T3:rT3 ratio. Given that T3 is the active hormone, doctors should test for and treat with T3—alone or in combination with T4—when working with hypothyroid patients. In my experience, proof that rT3 is *antagonistic* and not merely *inactive* is shown by the tolerance "high rT3 patients" have to treatment with high doses of T3 which should otherwise be and later are excessive, but which are tolerated during initial treatment when rT3 levels are still elevated.

- Not knowing how to treat autoimmunity, naively believing that giving thyroid hormone will be sufficient to resolve the immune imbalance that is manifesting as thyroid autoimmunity: If patients have thyroid autoimmunity as the cause of their hypothyroidism, simply giving thyroid hormone appears to me to be a rather ridiculous idea because it leaves the primary disease—the autoimmunity—untreated and therefore persistent. Many integrative doctors have used nonspecific health-improvement measures such as dietary improvement, general nutritional supplementation, and avoidance of common dietary allergens/immunogens to provide better care and alleviate immune dysfunction, but these general measures pale in comparison to what can be achieved with the more contemporary and comprehensive applications of functional inflammology and nutritional immunomodulation (Chapter 4). Thus, the autoimmunity needs to be treated directly, independently from and yet in conjunction with the hypothyroidism.

---

[704] Friedman M, et al. Supraphysiological cyclic dosing of sustained release T3 in order to reset low basal body temperature. *P R Health Sci J.* 2006 Mar;25(1):23-9

Complications:

- **Complications of hypothyroidism**: The complications of hypothyroidism are mainly continuations of the health problems previously mentioned in the sections on clinical presentations and clinical assessments. The most common and "important" problems from a clinical/medical perspective are depression, cardiovascular/hypertensive/hypercholesterolemic/hyperhomocysteinemic risks, reproductive/sexual problems, and increased susceptibility to infection. From a more personal perspective for the patients with *undiagnosed*, *untreated* or *insufficiently treated* hypothyroidism, the impaired quality of life, the chronic tiredness and fatigue, the lack of mental clarity and chronic low-grade depression, plus the feeling that "something is wrong with me" and the lack of understanding from doctors, friends, family, and intimate partners can be very distressing.

Clinical management:

- **Implementation of effective treatment**: Patients with laboratory evidence of hypothyroidism and/or a compelling clinical picture of hypothyroid deserve treatment with thyroid hormone—T3 alone, or T3 and T4 in combination—if no important conditions contraindicate its use. Conditions such as mania, seizure disorder, cardiac arrhythmia, coronary artery disease, and adrenal insufficiency are the main—but not absolute—contraindications.
- **Consideration of other immune disorders**: Patients with autoimmune thyroiditis have higher-than-normal rates of celiac disease (gluten intolerance) and other autoimmune disorders; these should be assessed and treated per the applied functional inflammology protocol with disease-specific considerations.[705]
- **Periodic monitoring**: Patients should be monitored for safety with clinical assessment and laboratory tests at the initiation of treatment and at approximately 3-6 months after the initiation of treatment and then yearly thereafter.

Treatments:

- **Overall considerations**: Treatment of low thyroid function generally centers on the administration of thyroid hormone(s), although some patients are able to restore normal thyroid function with specific dietary modification (e.g., avoidance of allergens and gluten-containing grains) and nutritional supplementation (e.g., selenium). A few people are able to take thyroid hormone treatment for a few months or years, and then discontinue the medication and yet maintain normal function; these are likely cases of transient thyroiditis and/or peripheral/functional hypothyroidism that either self-resolved or resolved with supportive thyroid treatment. Many people take the hormones for life. As implied previously, my position on this is that hypothyroidism and autoimmunity are separate issues and each needs to be addressed directly and effectively for optimal outcome.
- **Thyroid hormone replacement—physiologically appropriate—with T4 and T3**: Patients with insufficient function of thyroid hormone generally need *more* thyroid hormone to overcome their *hypo*thyroidism expeditiously, which is generally delivered in the form of biologically identical synthetic thyroid hormones, T4 and/or T3. Unfortunately, most (allopathic) doctors have been trained to use T4 without T3; this is nonphysiologic and therefore neither intellectually nor scientifically nor physiologically valid. When patients are hypothyroid, they generally need T4 and T3 together because the thyroid gland makes both of these hormones, and they are both required for optimal and normal thyroid status. Studies that have used T4 alone without T3 may have found "lack of effectiveness" not because the patients did not stand to benefit from thyroid hormone(s) but because the patients were given *inactive* T4 when they needed *active* T3, or a combination of T4 with T3. The three most common types of thyroid hormone replacement are described as follows.

> **Patients often feel better with combination T4 and T3 rather than T4 alone**
>
> "Twelve patients preferred combination treatment, 6 patients preferred the add-on combination treatment, 2 patients preferred standard treatment, and 6 patients had no preference."
>
> Escobar-Morreale et al. Thyroid hormone replacement therapy in primary hypothyroidism. *Ann Intern Med.* 2005 Mar

  - **Synthetic T4: L-thyroxine, Levothyroxine**: L-thyroxine is synthetic T4; it is chemically the same as the hormone produced in the body. Because it is synthetic and not derived from animal tissue, it does not contain antigens that can provoke an immune response. Levothyroxine/T4 must be converted in the body

---

[705] See various and upcoming books on rheumatology, most recent of which in 2014 is Vasquez A. *Naturopathic Rheumatology and Integrative Inflammology—v3.5*. ISBN-13: 978-0990620426. An update to this work is anticipated in 2015/2016 and will be noted at the website InflammationMastery.com

to liothyronine/T3 in order to be active; therefore, T4 administration is more safe and "stable" than is the administration of T3 but it is also generally less effective, especially for neuropsychiatric symptoms of depression, anhedonia, and fatigue. The standard allopathic medical approach is to use T4 *without T3*[706,707] and the presumed—not examined—"logic" of using an inactive hormone when these patients need and benefit from the active form continues to elude ascriptions of logic.

> **Combination T4 and T3 (not T4 alone) provides a mood-elevating antidepressant effect**
>
> "Fourteen of 17 patients showed improvement. … **This case series shows that T3 may be successfully employed as a long term treatment augmentation of major depression if over time dosage levels are increased beyond the traditional 50 mcg.**"
>
> Kelly TF, Lieberman DZ. Long term augmentation with T3 in refractory major depression. *J Affect Disord.* 2009 May

- **Available dose forms (amount per tablet)**: 25, 50, 75, 88, 100, 112, 125, 137, 150, 175, 200, 300 mcg.
- **Conversion equivalents of various forms of thyroid hormone**: levothyroxine 100 mcg = liothyronine 25 mcg = Liotrix 1 grain = thyroid (porcine) 1 grain.
- **Dose for adults**: 50-200 to a max of 300 mcg PO (by mouth) qd (daily) with a starting dose of 12.5-50 mcg PO qd; doses are smaller for children. Levothyroxine appears to be slightly more effective if taken at night rather than in the morning.[708]
- **Info**: Give on empty stomach between meals; specifically avoid soy products within 2 hours of thyroid hormone administration because constituents of soy bind thyroid hormone in the gastrointestinal tract.
- **Contraindications and cautions**: Allergy to the preparation, recent heart attack, adrenal insufficiency; caution with cardiovascular disease, cardiac arrhythmia, diabetes mellitus, and elderly patients.
- **Drug/botanical/nutrient interactions**: L-carnitine 1-4 grams/d can clearly block the hyperthyroid state via blocking thyroid hormone entry into the nucleus[709]; this treatment is effective for Graves disease, iatrogenic hyperthyroidism (thyroid hormone overdose), and thyroid storm. The botanical medicine lemon balm (*Melissa officinalis*) is claimed to block TSH binding to the thyroid gland receptor, but scientific data—let alone a quality clinical trial in humans—is lacking to support this contention.
- **Adverse effects—generally not noted with proper dosing**: Unmasking of cardiac arrhythmias, angina if cardiovascular disease and arterial stenosis is present. Excessive dosing or overdose can cause palpitations, tachycardia, nervousness, tremor, weight loss (long-term), diaphoresis/sweating, diarrhea/loose stools, abdominal cramps, anxiety.
- **Safety/Monitoring**: *Pregnancy*: A, *Lactation*: Safe
- **Half-life**: 6-7 days

o **Synthetic T3—Liothyronine, Cytomel**: T3 is the active form of thyroid hormone and it is therefore rapidly utilized and thus has a shorter half-life than does T4. T3 is the preferred form of thyroid hormone administration for the treatment of the previously described peripheral/metabolic hypothyroidism, treatment of which must be accomplished via suppressing endogenous T4 production to reduce the amount of rT3 being produced by stress-induced physiologic/enzymatic adaptations.[710]

- **Available dose forms (amount per tablet)**: 5, 25, 50 mcg
- **Conversion equivalents of various forms of thyroid hormone**: levothyroxine 100 mcg = liothyronine 25 mcg = Liotrix 1 grain = thyroid (porcine) 1 grain.
- **Dose for adults**: 25-75 mcg PO qd; for severe hypothyroidism start with a low dose of 5-10 mcg PO qd.
- **Info**: Give on empty stomach between meals; specifically avoid soy products within 2 hours of thyroid hormone administration because constituents of soy bind thyroid hormone in the gastrointestinal tract.

---

[706] Escobar-Morreale HF, et al. Treatment of hypothyroidism with combinations of levothyroxine plus liothyronine. *J Clin Endocrinol Metab.* 2005 Aug;90(8):4946-54

[707] Joffe RT, et al. Treatment of clinical hypothyroidism with thyroxine and triiodothyronine: a literature review and metaanalysis. *Psychosomatics.* 2007 Sep-Oct;48(5):379-84

[708] "Levothyroxine taken at bedtime significantly improved thyroid hormone levels. Quality-of-life variables and plasma lipid levels showed no significant changes with bedtime vs morning intake. Clinicians should consider prescribing levothyroxine intake at bedtime." Bolk N, Visser TJ, Nijman J, Jongste IJ, Tijssen JG, Berghout A. Effects of evening vs morning levothyroxine intake: a randomized double-blind crossover trial. *Arch Intern Med.* 2010 Dec 13;170(22):1996-2003

[709] "In conclusion, L-carnitine is effective in both reversing and preventing symptoms of hyperthyroidism and has a beneficial effect on bone mineralization. Because hyperthyroidism depletes the body deposits of carnitine and since carnitine has no toxicity, teratogenicity, contraindications and interactions with drugs, carnitine can be of clinical use." Benvenga et al. Usefulness of L-carnitine, a naturally occurring peripheral antagonist of thyroid hormone action, in iatrogenic hyperthyroidism: a randomized, double-blind, placebo-controlled clinical trial. *J Clin Endocrinol Metab.* 2001 Aug;86(8):3579-94. "Taken together, all these experiments indicate that L-carnitine decreases the access of thyroid hormone to thyroid hormone receptors by decreasing the amount of hormone having access to cell nuclei, and not by inhibiting thyroid hormone interaction with the nuclear receptors." Benvenga et al. Effects of carnitine on thyroid hormone action. *Ann N Y Acad Sci* 2004 Nov;1033:158-67

[710] Friedman M, et al. Supraphysiological cyclic dosing of sustained release T3 in order to reset low basal body temperature. *P R Health Sci J.* 2006 Mar;25(1):23-9

- Contraindications and cautions: Allergy to the preparation, recent heart attack, adrenal insufficiency; caution with cardiovascular disease, cardiac arrhythmia, diabetes mellitus, and elderly patients.

Contraindications to T3, liothyronine
Absolute contraindications:
• Anaphylaxis or severe hypersensitivity,
• Acute (current) myocardial infarction,
• Hyperthyroidism,
• Untreated adrenal insufficiency.
Relative contraindications and cautions:
• CAD, angina pectoris, or cardiac arrhythmia,
• Elderly patients, severe hypothyroidism—start with low dose and titrate as tolerated.

- Adverse effects—generally not noted with proper dosing: Unmasking of cardiac arrhythmias, angina if cardiovascular disease and arterial stenosis is present. Excessive dosing or overdose can cause palpitations, tachycardia, nervousness, tremor, weight loss, diaphoresis/sweating, diarrhea, abdominal cramps, anxiety.

- Safety/Monitoring: *Pregnancy*: A, *Lactation*: Safe

- Half-life: 1 day; I think this is perfect, since if the dose is not correct—let's say for example, that the dose is too high initially—the patient can skip the dose on the following day and then resume with a lower dose on the following day.

- Noteworthy proof of safety and remarkable efficacy of T3—triiodothyronine as an augmentation agent in treatment-resistant bipolar II and bipolar disorder NOS (*J Affect Disord* 2009 Aug[711]): "The charts of 125 patients with bipolar II disorder and 34 patients with bipolar disorder NOS were reviewed. Patients had been unsuccessfully treated with an average of 14 other medications before starting T3. At an average dose of 90.4 mcg (range 13 mcg-188 mcg) the medication was well tolerated. None of the patients experienced a switch into hypomania, and only 16 discontinued due to side effects. Improvement was experienced by 84%, and 33% experienced full remission. ... Augmentation with supraphysiologic doses of T3 should be considered in cases of treatment resistant bipolar depression."

o Synthetic T4 with synthetic T3—Liotrix, Thyrolar: This is a convenient yet more expensive way to obtain synthetic T4 along with synthetic T3 in an attempt to most closely mimic normal thyroid hormone production. It is dosed orally between meals in strengths of "1", "2", and "3". This product can be very difficult to obtain. Some but not all studies show clinical improvement in patients who use combination T4 and T3 rather than T4 alone.

o Animal-derived glandular products with either T4 and T3, or T3 alone: Glandular products derived from the thyroid glands of cows and pigs contain T4 and T3; these preparations of desiccated/dried thyroid gland are available by prescription such as Armour Thyroid generic desiccated thyroid. T3 derived from desiccated thyroid is also available without prescription. Patients who show greater benefit with these products than they did with synthetic T4 alone are probably responding to the T3, but the possibility exists that other nutritive factors or hormones in the whole gland are providing benefit. My preference is to avoid the use of glandular products in patients with thyroid autoimmunity due to the possible/documented exacerbation of the (auto)immune response, which can be monitored by measurement of blood levels of anti-TPO and anti-thyroglobulin antibodies. Furthermore, in these modern times, in America wherein most of the corn and soy fed to cows and pigs is genetically manipulated and overtreated with herbicides like glyphosate, my educated opinion is that the food supply in general and commercially/corporate-raised non-organic animal products are contaminated with GMO toxins (see Chapter 4), some of which are mitochondrial toxins and others of which have been shown to promote pro-inflammatory immune responses in animal experiments. Likewise, I advocate that all patients with inflammatory/autoimmune conditions consume an organic diet, as discussed in Chapter 4.

- **Nonpharmacologic and nonhormonal treatments, including nutritional and botanical supplementation:**
  o Zinc—15-50 mg per day: Zinc is necessary for the proper metabolism of thyroid hormones. Many patients—especially the elderly—are deficient in zinc. Zinc supplementation is quite safe and the pill(s) should be taken with food in order to avoid stomach upset. Long-term high-dose zinc supplementation can cause deficiency of copper. I always recommend use of a high-potency multivitamin-multimineral supplement to patients as part of the foundational treatment plan—see my review[712] which is also reprinted and updated/amended in Chapter 4.

---

[711] Kelly et al. The use of triiodothyronine as an augmentation agent in treatment-resistant bipolar II and bipolar disorder NOS. *J Affect Disord.* 2009 Aug;116(3):222-6
[712] Vasquez A. Five-Part Nutritional Wellness Protocol: The Supplemented Paleo-Mediterranean Diet. *Nutritional Perspectives* 2011 Jan InflammationMastery.com/reprints

- o <u>Selenium—200-800 mcg per day</u>: Selenium, zinc, and iron are all necessary for the biochemical pathways necessary for the peripheral metabolism of thyroid hormones, specifically the conversion of T4 to T3; deficiency of these nutrients can induce a "metabolic hypothyroidism" or "nutritional hypothyroidism" due to impairment of thyroid hormone metabolism and utilization. Further, zinc and selenium support antioxidant defenses; whereas iron is an antioxidant a low doses and a potent pro-oxidant in when present in higher amounts. Several studies have shown that nutritional supplementation with selenium 200 micrograms (mcg) per day for adults lowers the levels of anti-thyroid antibodies within three months and to an even greater extent by the end of nine months[713]; although this simple treatment is not always effective, it is clearly benign, and higher doses of selenium 400-800 mcg/d—especially in combination with the other components of the nutritional immunomodulation protocol detailed in Chapter 4—would very clearly be expected to produce better results.

- o <u>Iron—only for patients with iron deficiency documented by the lab test serum ferritin</u>: Iron is necessary for the proper metabolism of thyroid hormones. Iron status is assessed with a lab test called serum ferritin, and the optimal range is 40-70 ng/mL for most people; for patients with restless leg syndrome their ferritin can be up to 120 ng/mL to overcome defects in blood-brain transport. Iron deficiency in adults can be a sign of gastrointestinal blood loss such as from a stomach ulcer or colon cancer and must therefore always be evaluated appropriately.

- o <u>Food allergen avoidance, especially gluten</u>: Among food "allergy" disorders (discussed in Chapter 4) associated with thyroid autoimmunity, allergy to the protein gluten found in grains such as wheat, rye, and barley is clearly preeminent. A specific "gluten related disorder"—celiac disease—is associated with autoimmunity in general and thyroid autoimmunity in particular. Approximately 15% of patients with celiac disease have thyroid autoimmunity (i.e., Hashimoto's thyroiditis), and this is reversible in a large percentage of patients following the adoption of a gluten-free diet; however, this simple treatment is not always effective. Furthermore, food allergic reactions in general and celiac disease in particular can cause damage to the absorptive gastrointestinal mucosa, and the resulting malabsorption can reduce uptake of thyroid hormone administration; treatment options include allergen avoidance such as a gluten-free diet (GFD) or—less optimally—use of higher doses of thyroid hormone to overcome the malabsorption.[714]

  - ▪ <u>Positive study—Prevalence of thyroid disorders in untreated adult celiac disease patients and effect of gluten withdrawal</u> (*Am J Gastroenterol* 2001 Mar[715]): "241 consecutive untreated patients and 212 controls were enrolled. ... In most patients who strictly followed a 1-yr gluten withdrawal (as confirmed by intestinal mucosa recovery), there was a normalization of subclinical hypothyroidism. ... The greater frequency of thyroid disease among celiac disease patients justifies a thyroid functional assessment. In distinct cases, gluten withdrawal may single-handedly reverse the abnormality."

  - ▪ <u>Negative study—Gluten-free diet and autoimmune thyroiditis in patients with celiac disease</u> (*Scand J Gastroenterol.* 2012 Jan[716]): "During the follow-up, the thyroid volume decreased significantly in the patients with celiac disease compared with the controls, indicating the progression of thyroid gland atrophy despite the gluten-free diet. CONCLUSIONS: Celiac patients had an increased risk of thyroid autoimmune disorders. A gluten-free diet seemed not to prevent the progression of autoimmune process during a follow-up of 1 year."

- o *Coleus forskolii*: *Coleus forskolii* is a useful botanical medicine that is often stated to enhance thyroid function; but the research supporting this effect is weak at best. One recent study showed that the extract forskolin

---

[713] "We prospectively studied 80 women with HT, median age 37 (range 24-52) years, for 1 year. All patients received 200 microg Se in the form of l-selenomethionine orally for 6 months. ... An overall reduction of 21% (p < 0.0001) compared with the basal values was noted in Group A. ... Our study showed that in HT patients 6 months of Se treatment caused a significant decrease in serum anti-TPO levels, which was more profound in the second trimester. The extension of Se supplementation for 6 more months resulted in an additional 8% decrease, while the cessation caused a 4.8% increase, in the anti-TPO concentrations." Mazokopakis et al. Effects of 12 months treatment with L-selenomethionine on serum anti-TPO Levels in Patients with Hashimoto's thyroiditis. *Thyroid*. 2007 Jul;17(7):609-12 "L-selenomethionine substitution suppresses serum concentrations of TPOAb in patients with AIT, but suppression requires doses higher than 100 microg/day which is sufficient to maximize glutathione peroxidase activities. The suppression rate decreases with time." Turker et al. Selenium treatment in autoimmune thyroiditis: 9-month follow-up with variable doses. *J Endocrinol*. 2006 Jul;190(1):151-6 "We demonstrate that Se administration in our AIT patient's cohort does not induce significant immunological changes, either in terms of cytokine production patterns of peripheral T lymphocytes or of TPOAb levels. Our data suggest that AIT patients with moderate disease activity (in terms of TPOAb and cytokine production patterns) may not (equally) benefit as patients with high disease activity." Karanikas et al. No immunological benefit of selenium in consecutive patients with autoimmune thyroiditis. *Thyroid*. 2008 Jan;18(1):7-12

[714] "Atypical CD increases need for T4. The effect was reversed by GFD or by increasing T4 dose. Malabsorption of T4 may provide opportunity to detect CD that was overlooked until the patients were put under T4 therapy." Virili et al. Atypical celiac disease as cause of increased need for thyroxine. *J Clin Endocrinol Metab*. 2012 Mar;97:E419-22

[715] Sategna-Guidetti et al. Prevalence of thyroid disorders in untreated adult celiac disease patients and effect of gluten withdrawal. *Am J Gastroenterol*. 2001 Mar;96(3):751-7

[716] Metso et al. Gluten-free diet and autoimmune thyroiditis in patients with celiac disease. A prospective controlled study. *Scand J Gastroenterol*. 2012 Jan;47(1):43-8

promoted weight loss and muscle gain in overweight and obese men, but these benefits were not attributed to improved thyroid function.

- o <u>7-keto-DHEA, also called 7-oxo-DHEA</u>: 7-keto-DHEA is a metabolite of the hormone DHEA (dehydroepiandrosterone) which is a weak androgen (i.e. similar to but less potent than testosterone); 7-keto-DHEA metabolite does not have hormonal effects per se. One small study showed that administration of 7-keto-DHEA resulted in an increase in T3 levels.

- o <u>Detoxification and avoidance of chemicals/xenobiotics</u>: Xenobiotic exposure is ubiquitous due to chemical contamination of our food, air, water and surroundings, and thyroid autoimmunity and impaired thyroid function occur early following chemical exposure and bioaccumulation.[717] The common-sense solutions are 1) avoidance of exposure to the extent possible—this obviously includes mandating tighter government-corporate regulations on pollution production, and 2) promotion of optimal detoxification. Detoxification is introduced in Chapter 1 and given more detail in Chapter 4 and the accompanying video presentations.

- **<u>Specific treatment for the autoimmunity—implementation of the functional immunology protocol, especially the nutritional immunomodulation component</u>**: As stated above, my position is that the greatest success is achieved in the treatment of autoimmune hypothyroid thyroiditis by treating the hypothyroidism separately from the autoimmunity. My opinion is that treatment of hypothyroidism has been unnecessarily obfuscated when in reality the treatment options are few, the worst option (generally, although it might be useful for some patients)—T4—is overused, and the best options—T3 alone or combinations of T3 and T4—have been underused. Furthermore, most doctors have not until recently had an effective and comprehensive plan for reversing autoimmunity; I have provided such a plan in my Functional Inflammology Protocol (Chapter 4) and with clinical applications for specific autoimmune disorders in my updated *Rheumatology* textbooks.

Clinical Case **38yo male under extreme psychological stress with constantly cold extremities**—testing performed by LabCorp (2010): Clinicians should appreciate the stunning suppression of T3 combined with the marked elevation of rT3; note that the T4 level is normal and that if this had been the only test performed then the patient's underlying and obvious functional/metabolic/peripheral hypothyroidism would have been missed.

TESTS	RESULT	FLAG	UNITS	REFERENCE INTERV
Triiodothyronine (T3)				
Triiodothyronine (T3)	57	Low	ng/dL	71-180
Reverse T3				
Reverse T3	312		pg/mL	90-350
Triiodothyronine,Free,Serum				
Triiodothyronine,Free,Serum	2.5		pg/mL	2.0-4.4

Step-by-step conversion from ng/dL to pg/mL—end result is multiply by 10 (i.e., 10x)

Original units	Convert ng to pg[718]	Convert dL to mL	Simplify the fraction
1 ng / 1 dL	1,000 pg/ 1 dL	1,000 pg/ 100 mL	10 pg/ 1 ml
57 ng/ 1 dL	57,000 pg / 1 dL	57,000 pg / 100 mL	570 pg / 1 mL

Discussion: In this case, because the T3 level is low, *prima facie* justification for administration of T3 is provided, assuming that the clinical picture is compatible and that no contraindications to treatment are present. To calculate the total T3/rT3 ratio, equilibrate the units (multiply total T3 in ng/dL x 10 to convert to pg/mL; 1 pg = 0.001 ng [1 ng = 1,000 pg]; 1 dl = 100 ml). The total T3/rT3 ratio should be >10-14 (per McDaniel, op cit), but in this patient's case 570/312 = 1.8. Remember, more T3 than rT3 is better; hence, the higher ratio is better. On-line calculators for this conversion have been developed and surely more will be available in the future. This athletic and otherwise healthy 220-lb (100 kg) patient responded very well to T3 (liothyronine/Cytomel) with a starting dose of 150 mcg which was eventually tapered to 25 mcg and then to 12.5 mcg; in this patient's case, the initial high dose of T3 was well-tolerated because of the initially low level of T3, the elevated rT3 which appears to block T3 function, and the

---

[717] Schmidt MA, Bland JS. Thyroid gland as sentinel: interface between internal and external environment. *Altern Ther Health Med*. 1997 Jan;3(1):78-81 "However, there is now reasonably firm evidence that PCBs have thyroid-disrupting effects, and there is emerging evidence that also phthalates, bisphenol A, brominated flame retardants and perfluorinated chemicals may have thyroid disrupting properties." Boas et al. Thyroid effects of endocrine disrupting chemicals. *Mol Cell Endocrinol*. 2012 May 22;355(2):240-8 "Thyroid autoimmune disease, a multifactorial organ-specific autoimmune disorder, is marking a constant increase worldwide. It is thought to be caused by multiple environmental factors triggering autoimmune response in genetically susceptible individuals, though the exact mechanisms linking environmental factors to thyroid autoimmunity are not as yet well understood. Nevertheless, there is increasing evidence that mainly nutritive factors and environmental pollution by metals and chemicals (e.g. organochlorines, pesticides) are the main factors in the present-day spread of this disease." Duntas LH. Environmental factors and thyroid autoimmunity. *Ann Endocrinol* (Paris). 2011 Apr;72(2):108-13 Zoeller TR. Environmental chemicals targeting thyroid. Hormones (Athens). 2010 Jan-Mar;9(1):28-40

[718] Double-checked with unitconversion.org/weight/nanograms-to-picograms-conversion.html July 2011

patient's overall excellent cardiovascular fitness. A reasonable dosage range for liothyronine/Cytomel supplementation is 12.5-50 mcg for most patients tapered to the constellation of patient tolerance, patient preference, heart rate, basal body temperature optimization to 98.6° F, suppression of TSH and T4, resolution of symptoms and objective markers, and clinician's impression and experience.

Clinical Case **A 42yo male with fatigue**—testing performed by Quest Diagnostics (2010): Review the labs and outline your treatment plan before reading the discussion below. Note that the "optimal ratio" provided by the laboratory in this example was performed using free T3 rather than total T3 and without converting to equal units; regardless of the mathematics, clinicians should think conceptually and physiologically since doing so makes appropriate treatment very obvious and intuitive.

```
FREE T3/REVERSE T3 RATIO
    FREE T3/REVERSE T3 RATIO                          0.93 L          1.05-1.91**
    FREE T3                              325                           230-420 pg/dL
    REVERSE T3                                         350 H           100-340*** pg/mL

            **Ratio= Free T3 in pg/dL : reverse T3 in pg/mL. Ratio for reference
            range is calculated by dividing the lower and upper end of free T3
            with the mean of reverse T3 (220 pg/mL).

            ***Observed reference range is reported for reverse T3 per client
            request.
```

Step-by-step conversion from pg/dL to pg/mL—end result is divide by 100 (i.e., 0.01x): Provided for the sake of completeness even though the conversion is not necessary per the laboratory interpretation provided above.

Original units	Convert dL to mL	Simplify the fraction
1 pg / 1 dL	1 pg/ 100 mL	0.01 pg / 1 mL
325 pg/ 1 dL	325 pg / 100 mL	3.25 pg / 1 mL

Discussion: Note that if the T3 had been tested without rT3 the results would have been reported as "normal" and that a "depressed" patient so assessed would have likely been given an "antidepressant" medication and a diagnosis of depression rather than the proper treatment with T3 and a diagnosis of functional hypothyroidism. Luckily for this patient, his clinician tested rT3 and upon finding it impressively elevated treated with patient with T3 to suppress rT3 production by temporarily suppressing T4 production. The ratio calculation is provided and interpreted by the laboratory; notice that the "ideal ratio" for **total** T3/rT3 (>10) differs from that of **free** T3/rT3 (>1.05) *and that per the ratio provided by the labotatory does not equilibriate the measurement units*. This method is acceptable but is not the preferred method for determining functional thyroid status. The preferred method is the one presented by McDaniel (op cit) who advocated using total T3 (not free T3) in comparison with rT3 interpreted by an optimal ratio of 10-14.

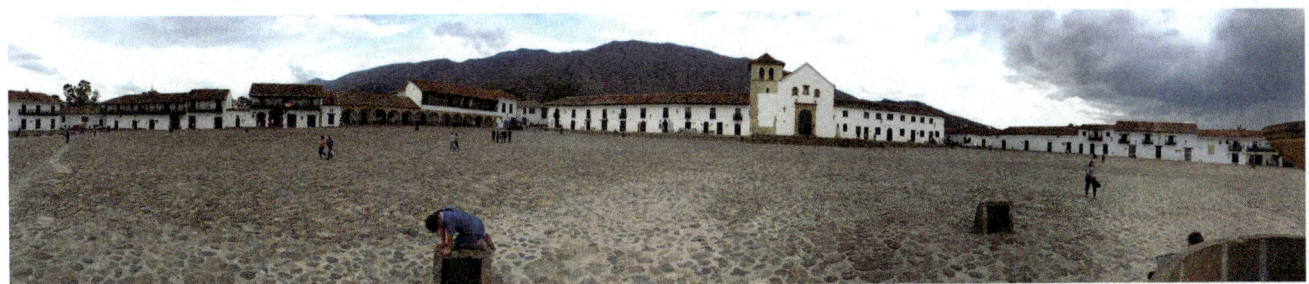

Plaza Mayor (Main Square) of Villa de Leyva, Colombia: Several formatting changes and updates to *Edition 3.5* were made in Villa de Leyva, Colombia in 2014 Sep. Panoramic photo above by DrV.

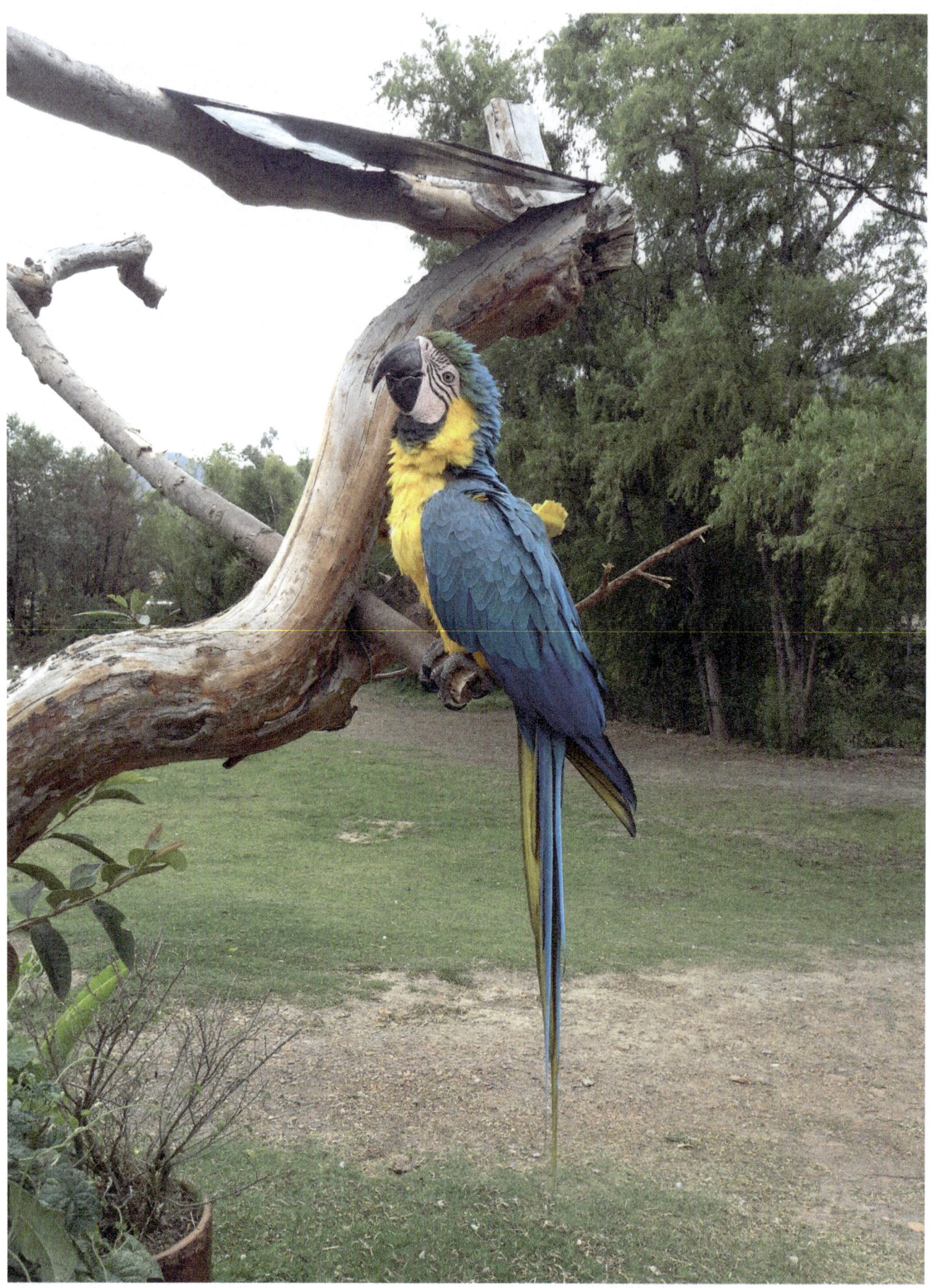

Blue and gold/yellow macaw, *Ara ararauna*, outside the short-term "editorial office" in Villa de Leyva: Photo by DrV.

Chapter 2:
Wellness Promotion
&
(Re)Establishing the Foundation for Health

Introduction to Lifestyle Optimization, Wellness Promotion, and Disease Prevention

This section details the lifestyle modifications that support a wellness-promoting whole-health program.

Among the four major primary healthcare professions in the United States and most other countries—chiropractic, osteopathy, naturopathy, and allopathy—the naturopathic profession stands preeminent in its emphasis upon wellness promotion and lifestyle optimization. This chapter reviews wellness promotion from the current author's perspective and experience—both personal and professional—which is consistent with but not officially representative of the naturopathic profession's concepts "re-establish the foundation of health" and "hierarchy of therapeutics."

This chapter originated many years ago as a handout for patients wherein it explained and described basic concepts that are foundational to health restoration, preservation, and optimization. Over the years that this handout has evolved into a chapter for my books, it has become more detailed and more relevant for clinicians treating patients. In essence, this chapter is a blueprint for the construction of a healthy lifestyle. While it may not cover every consideration, it covers the basics in sufficient detail so as to allow patients to change tracks from the downward descent of the disease-promoting lifestyle to the upward ascent of the health-promoting lifestyle.

Replacing the passive and disempowering drug-surgery paradigm with an active and empowering integrative/functional model of healthcare is one goal of this section.

This section can be thought of as a collection of essays. The review and consideration of a wide range of topics—which might otherwise appear random and nontopical to a reader accustomed to a more limited scope of discussion—is necessary due to the multifaceted nature of human experience and the widely ranging influences on health and disease outcomes.

Topics:

- **Re-establishing the Foundation for Health**
  - **Healthcare, Health, and Wellness**
  - **Daily living**
    - Lifestyle habits
    - Motivation: background and clinical applications
    - Exceptional living: the key to exceptional results
    - Recognize and affirm individual uniqueness
    - Individuation & conscious living: alternatives to common paradigms
    - Quality and quantity of sleep: concepts and clinical applications
    - Exercise, obesity, BMI, and proinflammatory activity of adipose tissue
  - **Diet is a powerful tool for the prevention and treatment of disease**
    - Make "whole foods" the foundation of the diet
    - Increase consumption of fruits and vegetables
    - Phytochemicals: food-derived anti-inflammatory nutrients
    - Eat the right amount of protein
    - Reducing consumption of sugars: exceptions for supercompensation
    - Avoiding artificial sweeteners, colors, and other additives, reducing caffeine
    - To the extent possible, eat "organic" foods
    - Recognize the importance of avoiding food allergens
    - Supplement your healthy diet with vitamins, minerals, and fatty acids
    - General guidelines for the safe use of nutritional supplements
  - **Advanced concepts in nutrition**
    - "Biochemical Individuality" and "Orthomolecular Medicine"
    - Nutrigenomics: Nutritional genomics
    - Putting it all together: *the supplemented Paleo-Mediterranean diet*
  - **Emotional, mental, and social health**
    - Stress management and authentic living
    - Stress always has a biochemical/physiologic component
    - The body functions as a whole
    - Healing past experiences
    - Autonomization, intradependence, emotional literacy, corrective experience
  - **Environmental health**
    - Environmental exposures and the importance of detoxification
    - Avoid unnecessary chemical medications and medical procedures
    - Intestinal health, bowel function, and introduction to dysbiosis
- **Natural holistic healthcare contrasted to standard medical treatment**
- **Opposite influences of health promotion vs. disease promotion**

Introduction to Wellness Promotion: Re-Establishing the Foundation for Health

"The work of the naturopathic physician is to elicit healing by helping patients to create or recreate conditions for health to exist within them.
Health will occur where the conditions for health exist.
Disease is the product of conditions which allow for it." *Jared Zeff, N.D.*[1]

One of the most important concepts within the philosophy and practice of naturopathic medicine is that of "re-establishing the foundation for health." This means that instead of first looking to a specific treatment or "magic bullet" to solve a health problem, we first look at the environment in which the problem arose to determine if the patient's environment has initiated or perpetuated the problem. The term *environment* as used here means much more than the patient's immediate surroundings at home and work; it includes all modifiable factors that may have an effect on the patient's health, such as lifestyle, diet, exercise, supplementation, chronic and situational stress, medications with positive and negative effects, exposure to toxicants and microbes, nutritionally-modifiable genetic factors[2], emotions, feelings, and unconscious assumptions[3], and many other considerations. Although the genes that we and our patients have inherited cannot be changed, we can very often modulate the expression of those genes (e.g., via nutrigenomics, described later) by modifying the biochemical, microbial, toxicologic, and neurohormonal milieu that bathes our cells and thus our genes; this concept was expressed in a statement by the US Centers for Disease Control and Prevention in its "Gene-Environment Interaction Fact Sheet" available on-line.[4]

"Optimal health" does not and never will come in a pill or tonic—the human body and the interactions that we each have between our genes, outlooks, environments, and lifestyles are far too complex to ever be addressed wholly and completely by a simplistic paradigm or single treatment. Even a superficial observation of the complexity of human physiology and the complexity of our environments (including noise, toxins such as benzene and mercury, chemicals such as formaldehyde from building materials, work stress and multitasking, ionizing and electromagnetic radiation exposure, microwaves, etc) shows that **our modern lifestyles subject the human body to many more "stressors" than ever before in the history of human existence.** Each of these stressors depletes our psychic and physiologic reserves, such that daily replenishment and protection are necessary.

> **Environment—lifestyle, diet, stresses, microbes, toxins—influences genetic expression and the manifestation of health or disease**
>
> "Virtually all human diseases result from the interaction of genetic susceptibility factors and modifiable environmental factors, broadly defined to include infectious, chemical, physical, nutritional, and behavioral factors. ...
>
> "Even so-called single-gene disorders actually develop from the interaction of both genetic and environmental factors. ...
>
> "We do not inherit a disease state per se. Instead, we inherit a set of a susceptibility factors to certain effects of environmental factors and therefore inherit a higher risk for certain diseases."
>
> Gene-Environment Interaction Fact Sheet by the Centers for Disease Control and Prevention, August 2000

Research in nutrition and physiology is revealing the mechanisms by which "simple" lifestyle practices and dietary interventions exert their powerful benefits. For example, whole foods such as fruits and vegetables contain over 8,000 phytochemicals with different physiologic effects[5], and simple practices such as meditation and massage can significantly alter hormone and neurotransmitter levels.[6,7] On the surface, a simple practice such as consumption of fruits and vegetables and a multivitamin/multimineral supplement may seem to be a way to provide merely "good nutrition"; however the clinical effects can include antidepressant[8] and anti-inflammatory

---

[1] Zeff JL. The process of healing: a unifying theory of naturopathic medicine. *Journal of Naturopathic Medicine* 1997; 7: 122-5
[2] Kaput J, Rodriguez LR. Nutritional genomics: the next frontier in the postgenomic era. *Physiol Genomics* 16:166–177 physiolgenomics.physiology.org/cgi/content/full/16/2/166
[3] Miller A. *The truth will set you free: overcoming emotional blindness and finding your true adult self.* New York: Basic Books; 2001
[4] Gene-Environment Interaction Fact Sheet by the US CDC, 2000 ashg.org/pdf/CDC%20Gene-Environment%20Interaction%20Fact%20Sheet.pdf Reviewed 2014 Jun
[5] "We propose that the additive and synergistic effects of phytochemicals in fruit and vegetables are responsible for their potent antioxidant and anticancer activities, and that the benefit of a diet rich in fruit and vegetables is attributed to the complex mixture of phytochemicals present in whole foods." Liu RH. Health benefits of fruit and vegetables are from additive and synergistic combinations of phytochemicals. *Am J Clin Nutr.* 2003 Sep;78(3 Suppl):517S-520S
[6] "The significant decrease of the catecholamine metabolite VMA (vanillic-mandelic acid) in meditators, that is associated with a reciprocal increase of 5-HIAA supports as a feedback necessity the "rest and fulfillment response" versus "fight and flight"." Bujatti M, Riederer P. Serotonin, noradrenaline, dopamine metabolites in transcendental meditation-technique. *J Neural Transm.* 1976;39(3):257-67
[7] "By the end of the study, the massage therapy group, as compared to the relaxation group, reported experiencing less pain, depression, anxiety and improved sleep. They also showed improved trunk and pain flexion performance, and their serotonin and dopamine levels were higher." Hernandez-Reif et al. Lower back pain is reduced and range of motion increased after massage therapy. *Int J Neurosci* 2001;106(3-4):131-45
[8] Benton D, Haller J, Fordy J. Vitamin supplementation for 1 year improves mood. *Neuropsychobiology.* 1995;32(2):98-105

benefits[9] by enhancing the efficiency of biochemical reactions[10] and by reducing excess activity of NF-kappaB[11], respectively. The power of interventional nutrition utilizing high-doses and/or synergistic formulations of nutraceuticals and phytonutraceuticals becomes much more clinically apparent when patients first (re)establish a healthy foundation of diet and lifestyle practices upon which these treatments can be added; **I estimate that the effectiveness of treatments for complex illness such as inflammatory diseases and cancer is** *at least* **doubled when patients implement these lifestyle changes in addition to specific treatments rather than relying on specific treatments alone without a healthy supportive lifestyle.** In other words, *"foundation for health* + specific treatments" is much more effective than *"unhealthy lifestyle* + specific treatments." This explains, in part, the discrepancy between the relatively lackluster response seen in *single-intervention* clinical trials* compared to the better results that we attain clinically when using a holistic approach characterized by *multicomponent* treatment plans. The biochemical and "scientific" reasons for this positive/negative synergism will become more clear during the course of this chapter and textbook.

Single-intervention clinical trials (i.e., clinical trials that utilize only one treatment) are the "gold standard" in allopathic drug-based research because in that setting the goal is to quantify and qualify the nature of positive and negative responses to a single intervention, generally a drug. However, this approach loses much of its luster and relevance in clinical settings where neither patients nor their environments and treatment plans can be standardized due to the unique constitution, lifestyle, history, and other nuances of each patient. Single intervention clinical trials have a place in the researching of all treatments, including natural interventions. However, clinicians—especially recent graduates—must pry themselves away from this research tool when it comes to treating individual patients in clinical practice, where **single interventions are the antithesis of holistic treatment**.

Daily Living: Life occurs on a moment-to-moment and daily basis. Choices that we make in relationships, occupations, exercise, and diet have profound and powerful influence over the course of our lives—particularly our health and happiness. Despite the previous and current obfuscation of health information by allopathic groups[12,13,14,15,16] and the pharmaceutical industry[17,18], enough valid information and common sense is available to doctors and the public such that **ignorance is no longer a viable excuse for deferring responsibility for lifestyle-induced disease and misery.**[19] Eating too much sugar and fat while not eating enough fruits and vegetables is making a choice to have an increased probability of developing diabetes, cancer, heart disease, arthritis, and obesity. Exercising regularly, eating a healthy diet, and supplementing the diet with high-quality nutrients and botanicals is making the choice to greatly reduce one's risk of health problems[20,21] and to nurture one's life and one's body so that one can make the most of one's life experience and enjoy life, hobbies, life purpose(s), travel, creativity, community involvement, and time with friends and family.

When we were children, we looked to other people to provide for us and to "take care of us." **As adults, we have to assume responsibility for the course of our own lives, to make decisions based on long-term considerations rather than instant gratification and selective ignorance.** Of course, this does not mean that we have to abandon enjoyment; but it does mean that we can make decisions based on priorities, and if health is a priority then we should take steps to attain and maintain it. For people who have chosen to make their health a priority, sugar- and fat-laden food begins to lose its appeal, and exploring new health-building experiences such as

[9] Church TS, Earnest CP, Wood KA, Kampert JB. Reduction of C-reactive protein levels through use of a multivitamin. *Am J Med.* 2003;115(9):702-7

[10] Ames BN, Elson-Schwab I, Silver EA. High-dose vitamin therapy stimulates variant enzymes with decreased coenzyme binding affinity (increased K(m)): relevance to genetic disease and polymorphisms. *Am J Clin Nutr.* 2002 Apr;75(4):616-58 ajcn.org/cgi/content/full/75/4/616

[11] Vasquez A. Reducing pain and inflammation naturally - part 4: nutritional and botanical inhibition of NF-kappaB, the major intracellular amplifier of the inflammatory cascade. A practical clinical strategy exemplifying anti-inflammatory nutrigenomics. *Nutritional Perspectives*, July 2005:5-12

[12] Wolinsky H, Brune T. *The Serpent on the Staff: The Unhealthy Politics of the American Medical Association*. GP Putnam and Sons, New York, 1994

[13] Wilk CA. *Medicine, Monopolies, and Malice: How the Medical Establishment Tried to Destroy Chiropractic*. Garden City Park: Avery, 1996

[14] Carter JP. *Racketeering in Medicine: The Suppression of Alternatives*. Norfolk: Hampton Roads Pub; 1993

[15] National Alliance of Professional Psychology Providers. AMA Seeks To Control and Restrict Psychologist's Scope of Practice. nappp.org/scope.pdf 2006 Nov

[16] "In an effort to marshal the medical community's resources against the growing threat of expanding scope of practice for allied health professionals, the AMA has formed a national partnership to confront such initiatives nationwide… The committee will use $25,000…" Daly R, American Psychiatric Association. AMA Forms Coalition to Thwart Non-M.D. Practice Expansion. *Psychiatric News* 2006 March; 41: 17 pn.psychiatryonline.org/cgi/content/full/41/5/17-a?eaf Accessed November 25, 2006

[17] Angell M. *The Truth About the Drug Companies: How They Deceive Us and What to Do About It*. Random House; August 2004

[18] "It begins on the first day of medical school… It starts slowly and insidiously, like an addiction, and can end up influencing the very nature of medical decision-making and practice… Attempts to influence the judgment of doctors by commercial interests serving the medical industrial complex are nothing if not thorough." Editorial. Drug-company influence on medical education in USA. *Lancet.* 2000 Sep 2;356(9232):781

[19] "Error is not blindness, error is cowardice. Every acquisition, every step forward in knowledge is the result of courage, of severity towards oneself, of cleanliness with respect to oneself." Nietzsche FW. *Ecce Homo: How One Becomes What One Is*. [Translator: Hollingdale RJ] Penguin Books:1979,34

[20] Orme-Johnson DW, Herron RE. An innovative approach to reducing medical care utilization and expenditures. *Am J Manag Care.* 1997;3(1):135-44

[21] Vasquez A. Five-Part Nutritional Protocol that Produces Consistently Positive Results.*Nutr Wellness* 2005Sep

healthy cooking, outdoor activities, and community involvement can become an empowering lifestyle that can be transformed into an art—one that is particularly amenable to building relationships and connections with other people. **The improved sense of well-being and improved physical and intellectual performance obtained from consumption of a health-promoting Paleo-Mediterranean diet (described later) supersedes any short-term gratification from the disease-promoting diet commonly referred to as the Standard American Diet (SAD).** When people want to be healthy,

> **Health living: lifestyle as living art**
>
> "What one should learn from artists: How can we make things beautiful, attractive, and desirable for us when they are not?—and I rather think that in themselves they never are! ... This we should learn from artists, while being wiser than they are in other matters. For with them this subtle power usually comes to an end where art ends and life begins; but we want to be the poets of our lives—first of all in the smallest, most everyday matters."
>
> Nietzsche FW. *Joyful Knowledge*, 1882. Essay #299

exercising and spending enjoyable time outdoors becomes more fun than the inactivity and passivity of watching television. When we consider that the average American watches at least 3-4 hours of television per day then we should not be surprised that, with physical inactivity as such a major component of the day, Americans show progressively higher rates of obesity, cancer, heart disease, and diabetes. Such an inactive lifestyle also affects our children: on average, each American child watches more than 23 hours of television per week[22]—a national habit that unquestionably contributes to the high levels of obesity and (social) illiteracy demonstrated by America's youth. Adults who watch average amounts of television are exposed to—some might say "...indoctrinated by...") more than 30 hours of drug advertisements per year—far exceeding their exposure to other, potentially more authentic, health-promoting health information.[23] Not only does television siphon time and energy that could be used more productively, more socially, or more enjoyably, but at a cost of $50-100 per month ($600 to $1,200 per year) **cable television subtracts from the available resources (i.e., time, money, and attention) that could be directed toward health-promoting choices.** Cable television—because of its financial cost and time commitment—is only one of many examples of how everyday lifestyle choices can have an impact on long-term health/disease outcomes. **Clinicians should encourage patients to become mindful of their choices and the impact these choices have on long-term health and vitality.**

<u>Lifestyle habits</u>: Without the conscious decision that **health is a priority** and the realization that **optimal health has to be earned rather than taken for granted,** patients and doctors alike can fall into the belief that healthcare and health maintenance are *burdens* and *inconveniences* rather than opportunities for fulfillment and self-care. Taking an **empowered** and **pro-active** role in one's healthcare may include a coordinated program of diet changes (i.e., eating certain foods, avoiding other foods, modulating total intake), regular exercise, nutritional supplementation, stress reduction, and relationship improvement. Unhealthy habits such as eating junk foods, using tobacco, and watching too much television rob people of the time, energy, motivation, and financial resources that could otherwise be used to improve health and prevent unnecessary illness. As described later in this chapter, the choices that are made on a daily basis from this point forward are the most powerful predictors of future health and are generally more powerful than past habits or genetic inheritance. We can all greatly increase our probability of enjoying a future of high-energy health rather than painful illness by consistently choosing health-promoting options instead of foods, behaviors, and emotional states that promote illness.

---

[22] "American children view over 23 hours of television per week. * Teenagers view an average of 21 to 22 hours of television per week. * By the time today's children reach age 70, they will have spent 7 to 10 years of their lives watching television." American Academy of Pediatrics aapca1.org/aapca1/tv.html accessed September 30, 2003

[23] "...many ads may be targeted specifically at women and older viewers. Our findings suggest that Americans who watch average amounts of television may be exposed to more than 30 hours of direct-to-consumer drug advertisements each year, far surpassing their exposure to other forms of health communication." Brownfield et al. Direct-to-consumer drug advertisements on network television: an exploration of quantity, frequency, and placement. *J Health Commun.* 2004 Nov-Dec;9(6):491-7

One hour of time per day and/or about $2 - $8 per day:

Active self-care lifestyle	*Distraction & inactive lifestyle*
1. Meditation	1. Cable television
2. Yoga, stretching	2. 1 pack of cigarettes per day
3. Walking, jogging, biking, no-cost calisthenics	3. Designer coffee such as Grande Café Latte
4. Martial arts, Tai Chi	
5. Hot bath	
6. Cooking new healthy meals	
7. Herbal teas (especially green tea) provide anti-inflammatory, anticancer, and antioxidant benefits	
8. Basic nutritional supplementation (less than $2 per day): 1) High-potency multivitamin and multimineral supplement, 2) Complete balanced, fatty acid supplementation, 3) 2,000 – 4,000 IU vitamin D per day for adults, 4) probiotics and/or symbiotic.	
Benefits	**Results**
1. Increased flexibility and joint mobility	1. Cable television: Cost $2 - $4 per day = average $1,095 per year)
2. Reduction in blood pressure	2. 1 pack of cigarettes per day ($3 per day = $1,095 per year)
3. Reduced risk of cancer	3. Grande Café Latte ($4 per day = average $1,460 per year)
4. Increased strength	
5. Improved cognitive function	
6. New and enjoyable meals	
7. Relaxation	
8. New life skills	
9. Improved heart health	
10. The opportunity to develop social skills and more friends and a better social support network	
11. Reduced risk for Alzheimer's and Parkinson's diseases	
Cost: At $2 per day for meditation, stretching, calisthenics, (etc.) and basic supplementation, the total comes to $730 per year.	**Cost:** For cable television, cafe coffee, and cigarettes, the total comes to approximately $3,600 per year.

Motivation: We all have a combination of reasons, feelings, inclinations, and unconscious influences that support and perpetuate our health behaviors.[24,25,26] Getting in touch with those motivations can help us to better understand the healthy/functional (health-promoting) and unhealthy/dysfunctional (illness-promoting) aspects of our psyches. Uncovering and "upgrading" these motivations can help us and our patients to develop more authentic lives and improved health. Self-defeating behaviors, such as 1) a willingness to remain ignorant of factors which influence health, 2) a willingness to frequently consume disease-promoting processed convenience foods, and 3) submission to confinement within the boundaries of one's insurance coverage (which often confines one to drugs and surgery as the only treatment options), reflect—*at best*—the willingness to settle for mediocrity and—*at worst*—an unconscious movement in the direction of illness and early death—masochism and suicide by lifestyle. Conversely, an unencumbered drive toward health will create the greatest opportunity for wellness. Since **actions originate from beliefs and goals**, we can surmise much about undisclosed beliefs and goals in others and ourselves simply by observing outward behavior. Effectively changing actions (such as diet and lifestyle choices) therefore must include not only behavior modification but also careful examination and reconsideration of largely unconscious goals and beliefs that motivate and underlie those behaviors. **When a fully empowered motivation toward health is matched with accurate informational insight, we have the** *potential* **for health-promoting change—***potential* **which only becomes** *manifest* **after the habitual application of appropriate** *action*. Patients and doctors alike can benefit from considering the factors that incline them *toward* or *away* from behaviors that promote health or disease.

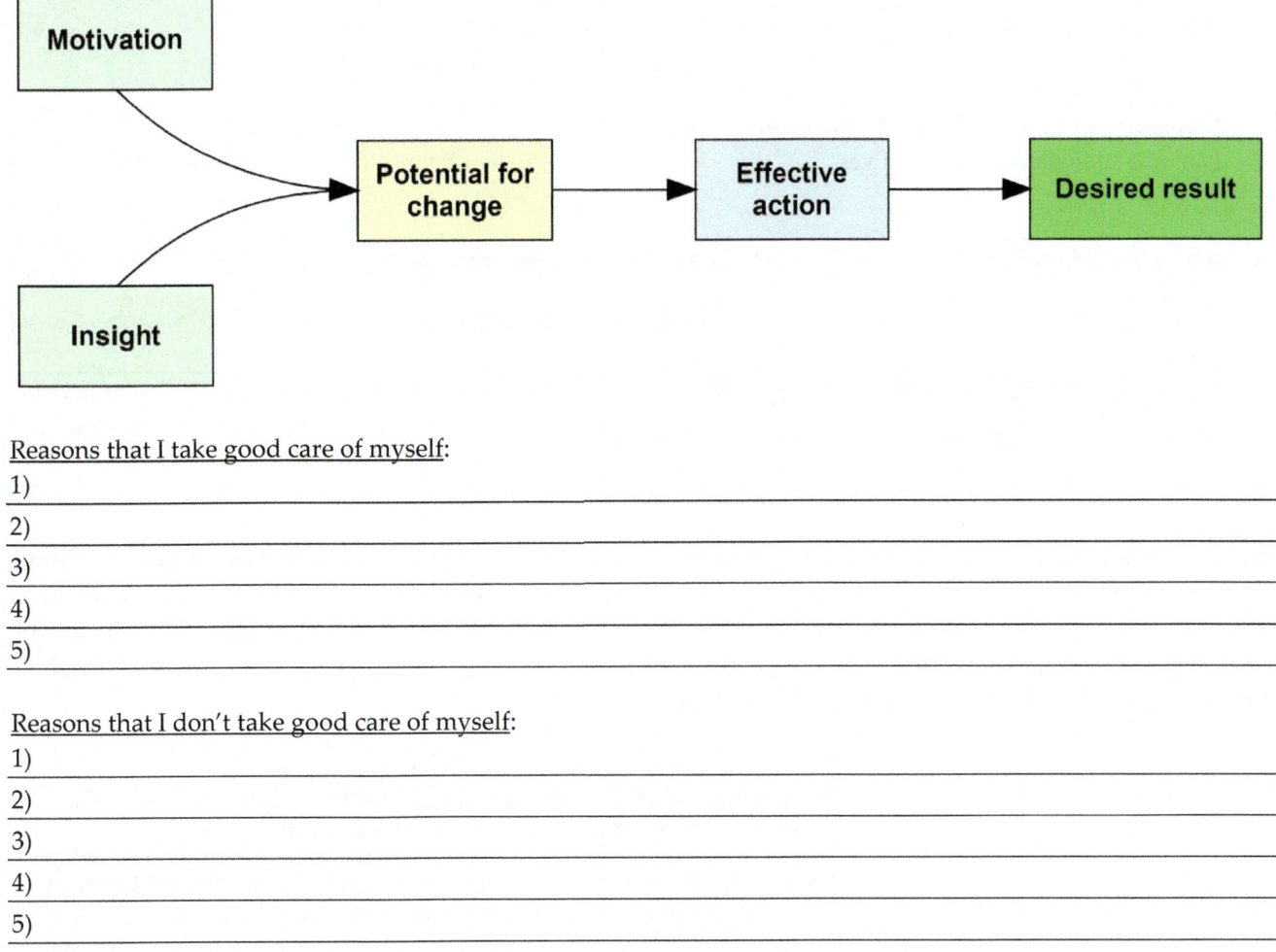

Reasons that I take good care of myself:

1) _____

2) _____

3) _____

4) _____

5) _____

Reasons that I don't take good care of myself:

1) _____

2) _____

3) _____

4) _____

5) _____

[24] Bradshaw J. *Healing the Shame that Binds You* [Audio Cassette (April 1990) Health Communications Audio; ISBN: 1558740430]
[25] Miller A. *The Drama of the Gifted Child: The Search for the True Self.* Basic Books: 1981. The book is brilliant, brave, and classic; the audiocassette version is also wonderful.
[26] Prochaska, JO, Norcross, JC, and DiClemente, CC (1994). *Changing for Good.* NY, William Morrow and Company; 1994

Motivation: moving from theory to practice: Many recently-graduated doctors start with the erroneous assumption that all patients actually want to become healthier, and furthermore, that all that the doctor has to do is "enlighten" them to the error of their ways and the patient will be dutifully compliant unto the attainment of his or her health-related goals. In reality, many people are surprisingly indifferent about their health. Many people do not care if they are 30 lbs overweight or have hypertension or will die early as a result of their lifestyle; they often have to be encouraged to begin to *consider* making positive changes.

Dr. James Prochaska[27] has elucidated the different stages of patient preparedness, and we note that each of these five levels of thought and action produces specific results and requires different types of support from the doctor. I have summarized and modified Dr. Prochaska's lecture in the following table; for additional discussion and details, see his book *Changing for Good*.[28]

Level of preparedness and readiness for change

Stage: representative statement	Doctor's interventions and social support
1. **Pre-contemplation**: "I am not seriously thinking about making a change to be healthier."	<ul><li>Outreach</li><li>Retainment</li></ul>
2. **Contemplation**: "I am thinking about making a change, but I am not ready for action."	<ul><li>Resolve resistance</li><li>Emphasize benefits</li><li>Address ambivalence</li></ul>
3. **Preparation**: "I am getting ready to make a change, but I am not taking effective action yet."	<ul><li>Ensure adequate preparation</li><li>Prevent relapse following initial action</li></ul>
4. **Action**: "I am beginning to make changes to become healthier."	<ul><li>Support (group support is best)</li><li>Encouragement</li><li>Reward system</li></ul>
5. **Maintenance**: "I take action every day and on a consistent basis to reach my goals."	<ul><li>Continued provision for continuation of health changes: facilities, supplements, social support, affirmation</li></ul>

Recognizing the different levels of patient preparedness and addressing individual patients with a customized approach not only for their *disease* but also for their *level of preparedness* for action can help doctors deliver more effective healthcare. Also, patients may have different levels of preparedness for different aspects of their treatment plans. He/she may be ready for **action** with regard to exercise, in **preparation** for dietary change, but in **precontemplation** for the use of supplements and botanicals.

---

[27] Prochaska JO. *Changing for good: motivating diabetic patients*. The Coming Storm: Reversing the Rising Pandemic of Diabetes and Metabolic Syndrome. The Eleventh International Symposium on Functional Medicine. May 13-15, 2004 in Vancouver, British Columbia, Canada. Pages 173-180. Institute for Functional Medicine
[28] Prochaska, JO, Norcross, JC, and DiClemente, CC (1994). *Changing for Good*. NY, William Morrow and Company; 1994

<u>**The secret to being exceptionally healthy:**</u> *One has to live in an exceptional (unique, personalized) way*. We cannot expect to achieve the goal of being vibrantly healthy or exceptionally happy if we live in the same way as everyone else, particularly when our fellow citizens are likely to be overweight, depressed, socially isolated[29], requiring multiple pharmaceutical medications[30], and experiencing a state of progressively declining health.[31] *Healthy lifestyle* not only includes the basics of adequate sleep, healthy whole-foods diet, supportive relationships, and regular exercise, but it also includes preventive medicine and pro-active healthcare. **Despite the fact that we in the United States (US) spend more on medical treatments than does any other country in the world, Americans have the worst health outcomes of all the major industrialized countries.**[32,33,34] This is largely because *American medicine* is centered on a *disease-oriented model of medicine* which means that instead of having a healthcare system and social structure that proactively promotes health and prevents disease before it happens, our systems are *reactive*—treating disease *after* it occurs rather than emphasizing the prevention of disease *before* it occurs. The dominant allopathic model in the US is also reductionistic: focusing on the small problem (micromanagement) rather than the big picture (macromanagement).

> **Americans have poor health outcomes compared to citizens of other industrialized nations**
>
> "Basically, you die earlier and spend more time disabled if you're an American rather than a member of most other advanced countries."
>
> Christopher Murray MD PhD, Director of World Health Organization's Global Program on Evidence for Health Policy. Jun 4, 2000 who.int/inf-pr-2000/en/pr2000-life.html

> **Approximately 493 Americans are killed daily by hospital injuries and drug-prescribing errors**
>
> "Recent estimates suggest that each year more than 1 million patients are injured while in the hospital and approximately 180,000 die because of these injuries. Furthermore, drug-related morbidity and mortality are common and are estimated to cost more than $136 billion a year."
>
> Holland EG, Degruy FV. Drug-induced disorders. *Am Fam Physician*. 1997

Clearly, the most effective method for avoiding expensive and potentially dangerous medical procedures and drug treatments is for us as a nation and as individuals to shift our thinking from a *disease treatment* model of healthcare to a more logical program of aggressive *disease prevention* and *wellness promotion* via the use of safe natural treatments rather than heroic interventions.[35,36] Of course, this means that our concept and view of health and healthcare will have to change. As noted by Shi[37], **"Redesigning the system of health care delivery in the United States may be the only viable option to improve the quality of health care."** In the meantime, while we work for change on a national level, we are wise to change our personal habits and healthcare choices in favor of natural and preventive healthcare.

> **Medical drug (in)efficacy**
>
> "The vast majority of drugs —more than 90 percent— only work in 30 or 50 percent of the people."
>
> Allen Roses, M.D., worldwide vice-president of genetics at GlaxoSmithKline. Published Dec 8, 2003 ttp://commondreams.org/headlines03/1208-02.htm

<u>**Healthy lifestyle and** *biochemical individuality* **credo: Recognize and affirm that you are a unique individual with unique needs**</u>: For each of us, our "personality" extends far beyond and far deeper than our sense of humor and our choice of clothing; we are very unique on a physiologic and biochemical level as well. So-called *normal* and *apparently healthy* individuals vary greatly in their biochemical efficiency and nutritional needs. This is the concept of "biochemical individuality" which was first detailed in 1956 by the renowned scientist Roger J Williams from the University of Texas. In his historic work *Biochemical Individuality: The Basis for the Genetotrophic Concept*, Dr.

[29] McPherson M, et al. Social Isolation in America: Changes in Core Discussion Networks over Two Decades. *American Sociological Review* 2006; 71: 353-75

[30] "According to the latest available data, total health care costs reached $1.3 trillion in 2000. This represents a per capita health care expenditure of $4,637. The total prescription drug expenditure in 2000 was $121.8 billion, or approximately $430 per person." Presentation to the U.S. Senate Commerce Committee April 23, 2002 "Drug Pricing & Consumer Costs" Kathleen D. Jaeger, R.Ph., J.D. commerce.senate.gov/hearings/042302jaegar.pdf

[31] Zack MM, Moriarty DG, Stroup DF, Ford ES, Mokdad AH. Worsening trends in adult health-related quality of life and self-rated health-United States, 1993-2001. *Public Health Rep*. 2004 Sep-Oct;119(5):493-505 pubmedcentral.nih.gov/articlerender.fcgi?tool=pubmed&pubmedid=15313113

[32] "[America] also has the fewest hospital days per capita, the highest hospital expenditures per day, and substantially higher physician incomes than the other OECD countries. On the available outcome measures, the United States is generally in the bottom half, and its relative ranking has been declining since 1960." Anderson GF, Poullier JP. Health spending, access, and outcomes: trends in industrialized countries. *Health Aff* (Millwood) 1999 May-Jun;18(3):178-92 content.healthaffairs.org/cgi/reprint/18/3/178.pdf

[33] "However, on outcomes indicators such as life expectancy and infant mortality, the United States is frequently in the bottom quartile among the twenty-nine industrialized countries, and its relative ranking has been declining since 1960." Anderson GF. In search of value: an international comparison of cost, access, and outcomes. *Health Aff* 1997 Nov-Dec;16(6):163-71

[34] "Basically, you die earlier and spend more time disabled if you're an American rather than a member of most other advanced countries," says Christopher Murray, MD, PhD, Director of WHO's Global Program on Evidence for Health Policy. who.int/inf-pr-2000/en/pr2000-life.html

[35] "Systematic access to managed chiropractic care not only may prove to be clinically beneficial but also may reduce overall health care costs." Legorreta A, et al N. Comparative Analysis of Individuals With and Without Chiropractic Coverage. *Archives of Internal Medicine* 2004; 164: 1985-1992

[36] Orme-Johnson DW, Herron RE. An innovative approach to reducing medical care utilization and expenditures. *Am J Manag Care*. 1997;3(1):135-44

[37] Shi L. Health care spending, delivery, and outcome in developed countries: a cross-national comparison. *Am J Med Qual* 1997;12(2):83-93

Williams[38] reviews research that conclusively proves that among *apparently healthy* individuals, we can objectively determine great differences in physiology, organ efficiency, enzyme function, and nutritional needs. For example, variables that promote health include increased enzyme efficiency and efficient digestion and assimilation of nutrients, while internal factors that reduce health can include inadequate digestion, inefficient absorption, increased excretion of nutrients, impaired detoxification, poor enzyme function and "partial genetic blocks"—a term now understood to imply single nucleotide polymorphisms[39] and related enzyme defects, which result in **supradietary requirements for specific vitamins and minerals** for the prevention of disease and maintenance of health.[40] What this means for us as doctors and for our patients in practical terms is that in order for us to become as healthy as possible, we will almost certainly have to give attention to each person's unique biochemical abilities/disabilities in order to maximize the function of the various body systems, enzymes, and to optimize genetic expression.[41] This means that what works for one's neighbor, spouse, or best friend in terms of exercise, diet and nutrition may not work for one's unique physiology. We must all muster the courage to affirm that, in order to attain the goal of stable or progressively better health, we will each have to learn about how our unique bodies work—what conditions of health must be created. We will have to learn to make changes in lifestyle and daily routine which reflect and honor our bodies' ways of working. This may mean modifying work, sleep, and exercise schedules, avoiding some foods and eating others, and customizing nutrient intake to meet the body's needs as they are *in the present*—the health program that appears to have worked last year may not be appropriate at the present time. The process of learning how a person's body works requires time, patience, and the process of trial and error—from patient and doctor—but achieving the goal of improved health and increased energy are well worth the effort.

Individuation and the practice of conscious living: Our visions of reality are influenced by religious institutions, large corporations, advertising networks[42], corporate-owned mass media[43], and what Professors Stevens and Glatstein called "the medical-industrial complex."[44] Some of the paradigms that are advocated are both *unhistorical* (having no historical precedent) and *antihistorical* (contrary to the available historical precedent, which includes sustainability). Some of these companies and organizations offer us a view of reality and vision of our individual potentials that is fashioned in such a way as to promote the financial and political interests of the company or organization. Conversely, the actualization of our true physical, emotional, intellectual, and spiritual potentials may require that we separate from or at least attain a conscious appreciation of the (pseudo)reality that we have been advised to follow.[45,46] Critiques of and reasonable alternatives to our current paradigms of school[47], work[48,49], and money[50] have been

> **The importance of living consciously**
>
> "Consciousness is our basic tool for successful adaptation to reality. The more conscious we are in any situation, the more possibilities we tend to perceive, the more options we have, the more powerful we are — perhaps even the longer we will live.
>   Living consciously means **seeking to be aware of everything** that bears on our actions, purposes, values, and goals — and **behaving in accordance** with that which we see and know."
>
> Branden N. *The Art of Living Consciously*.

discussed elsewhere and are worthy of consideration. Becoming mindful of the paradigms and assumptions under which we live is the first step in true individuation, characterized by choosing (*creating* the best option: freedom) rather than deciding (*selecting* one of the offered options: the illusion of freedom). Various conscious thoughts and unconscious assumptions create our "working reality" which represents the way that we see things and the paradigm by which we *act in* and *interact with* the larger world. These layers come from our own families, schools,

[38] Williams RJ. *Biochemical Individuality: The Basis for the Genetotrophic Concept*. Austin and London: University of Texas Press, 1956

[39] Ames BN. Cancer prevention and diet: help from single nucleotide polymorphisms. *Proc Natl Acad Sci U S A*. 1999 Oct 26;96(22):12216-8

[40] Ames BN, Elson-Schwab I, Silver EA. High-dose vitamin therapy stimulates variant enzymes with decreased coenzyme binding affinity (increased K(m)): relevance to genetic disease and polymorphisms. *Am J Clin Nutr*. 2002 Apr;75(4):616-58 ajcn.org/cgi/content/full/75/4/616

[41] "The combination of biochemical individuality and known functional utilities of allelic variants should converge to create a situation in which nutritional optima can be specified as part of comprehensive lifestyle prescriptions tailored to the needs of each person." Eckhardt RB. Genetic research and nutritional individuality. *J Nutr* 2001;131(2):336S-9S

[42] "Patients' requests for medicines are a powerful driver of prescribing decisions. In most cases physicians prescribed requested medicines but were often ambivalent about the choice of treatment. If physicians prescribe requested drugs despite personal reservations, sales may increase but appropriateness of prescribing may suffer." Mintzes et al. Influence of direct to consumer pharmaceutical advertising and patients' requests on prescribing decisions: two site cross sectional survey. *BMJ*. 2002 Feb 2; 324(7332): 278-9

[43] *Manufacturing Consent: Noam Chomsky and the Media*. Movie directed by Achbar M and Wintonick P. 1992. See also zeitgeistmovie.com/

Stevens CW, Glatstein E. Beware the Medical-Industrial Complex. *Oncologist* 1996;1(4):IV-V theoncologist.alphamedpress.org/cgi/reprint/1/4/190-iv.pdf

[45] Breton D, Largent C. *The Paradigm Conspiracy*. Center City; Hazelden: 1996

[46] Pearce JC. *Exploring the Crack in the Cosmic Egg: Split Minds and Meta-Realities*. New York: Washington Square Press; 1974

[47] Gatto JT. *Dumbing us down: the hidden curriculum of compulsory education*. Gabriola Island, Canada; New Society Publishers: 2005

[48] "No one should ever work. In order to stop suffering, we have to stop working. That doesn't mean we have to stop doing things. It does mean creating a new way of life based on play..." Black B. *The abolition of work and other essays*. Port Townsend: Loompanics Unlimited; 1985, pages 17-33

[49] Jarow R. *Creating the Work You Love: Courage, Commitment and Career*; Inner Traditions Intl Ltd; 1995 [ISBN: 0892815426]

[50] Dominguez JR. *Transforming Your Relationship with Money*. Sounds True; Book and Cassette edition: 2001 Audio tape.

teachers, churches, companies, friends, parents, and ourselves—our previous interpretations and misinterpretations of ourselves and events; in sum, our responses to outer events combined with our internal experiences meld into our perception of ourselves (known as "the genesis of personal identity") and how we as individuals relate to our inner ourselves and [our perception of] the outer world. Becoming conscious of these realities and illusions allows us the opportunity to discard those views that are inaccurate, dysfunctional, and harmful and to accept a truer reality based on what we experience, feel, and know to be real—in the present, as adults. Once we are freed from *unreality*, we can live true to ourselves in a way that is authentically responsible to our own needs *and* the needs of our communities so that we can simultaneously sustain our obligations to society[51,52] while being free to be unique individuals.[53,54]

Examples of commonly accepted paradigms and their reasonable alternatives

Commonly accepted paradigms ↳ Implication and effect	Alternate paradigm ↳ Implication and effect
It is OK to be irresponsible in daily choices and then blame health problems on bad luck, bad genes, or both. ↳ Many people fail to take responsibility for their lives and thereby become victims of circumstances—negative circumstances that they themselves helped to create.	**Lifestyle, especially diet and nutrition, is the most powerful influence on health outcomes. Therefore, an educated patient is empowered to direct his/her health destiny.** ↳ Optimal health *per individual* is attained when people take responsibility for their lives, seek health information, and then incorporate this information into their daily routine in the form of healthy living: health-promoting lifestyle, eating, exercise, supplementation, relationships, and occupational and social activities, including socio-political involvement to protect the environment and resist the privatization of life and the spoliation of the environment in which we live and upon which our lives and health depend.[55,56]
In general, chemical medications are the answer to nearly all health problems. ↳ The belief in medications as the primary treatment of disease creates a patient population that is apathetic, disempowered, and dependent upon the medical-pharmaceutical industry, which grows richer and more powerful despite so-called 'earnest' attempts at cost containment.[57]	**Many acute and chronic problems can be more effectively managed in terms of prevention, safety, efficacy, and cost-effectiveness when phytonutritional interventions are either used as primary therapy or, when necessary, used in conjunction with medications.** ↳ A reduction in disease prevalence via health-promoting diet and lifestyle along with integrative treatments offers the best opportunity for benefit to patients, doctors, and third-party payers.[58]

[51] Bly R. *The Sibling Society*. Vintage Books USA; Reprint edition (June 1, 1997) ISBN: 0679781285 (Abridged audio edition (May 1, 1996)

[52] Bly R. *Where have all the parents gone? A talk on the Sibling Society*. New York: Sound Horizons, 1996 Highly recommended.

[53] Bradshaw J. *Healing the Shame that Binds You* [Audio Cassette (April 1990) Health Communications Audio; ISBN: 1558740430]

[54] Miller A. *The truth will set you free: overcoming emotional blindness and finding your true adult self*. New York: Basic Books; 2001

[55] "Your lack of interest in the past, your lack of involvement, your unwillingness to develop coherent strategies, your unwillingness to challenge authority - these have created a vacuum in decision-making, that has been filled by professional groups with close relationships with the chemical industries..." Samuel Epstein MD, 1993. Professor of Occupational and Environmental Medicine at the School of Public Health, University of Illinois Medical Center Chicago. converge.org.nz/pirm/pestican.htm

[56] Kristin S. Schafer, Margaret Reeves, Skip Spitzer, Susan E. Kegley. Chemical Trespass: Pesticides in Our Bodies and Corporate Accountability. Pesticide Action Network North America. May 2004 Available at panna.org/campaigns/docsTrespass/chemicalTrespass2004.dv.html on August 1, 2004

[57] "In this paper I offer four hypotheses to help explain why use of pharmaceuticals has continued to grow even as managed care and other cost containment efforts have flourished." Berndt ER. The U.S. pharmaceutical industry: why major growth in times of cost containment? *Health Aff* (Millwood). 2001 Mar-Apr;20(2):100-14

[58] "Hospital admission rates in the control group were 11.4 times higher than those in the MVAH group for cardiovascular disease, 3.3 times higher for cancer, and 6.7 times higher for mental health and substance abuse. ...MVAH patients older than age 45...had 88% fewer total patients days compared with control patients." Orme-Johnson DW, Herron RE. An innovative approach to reducing medical care utilization and expenditures. *Am J Manag Care*. 1997 Jan;3(1):135-44

Examples of commonly accepted paradigms and their reasonable alternatives—*continued*

Commonly accepted paradigms ↳ Implication and effect	Alternate paradigm ↳ Implication and effect
Work ethic: a belief that "hard work" has moral value and makes a person "better." ↳ Belief in the principle of "work ethic" encourages people to mindlessly engage in work for the sake of engaging in work without considering the implications of their actions or other alternatives that might produce a more beneficial outcome.[59]	**Work is the means rather than an end unto itself (except when the "work" is enjoyable, in which case it is no longer "work").** ↳ Occupations and professions can be designed for the enhancement of life (health, pleasure, relationships, the environment, care of the poor) rather than as an end to themselves at the expense of the individual, society, and the environment.
Adults should give 10.5-12 hours per day 5 days per week to work. ↳ In most corporate environments, employee's work at least 8.5 hours per day, with 1 additional hour spent in commuting[60] and another hour spent in preparation, transportation, and maintenance of work-related clothing, preparing work-related meals, maintaining the auto that is used for work-related tasks. With 10.5 hours given directly to work, 0.5-1 additional hours are needed for recuperation from work-related stress ("daily decompression"); thus the average amount of time given to work-related activities is much larger than commonly believed.[61] Because of the time and energies devoted to "work" the vast majority of people feel that they do not have sufficient time for themselves, their families and friends, their creativity, learning about the world, political involvement, and other more important aspects of life. "Not enough time" is the most common reason given by patients for not exercising.	**A paradigm of a 4-day workweek is just as valid and perhaps more valid than one that advocates a 5-day workweek. A paradigm of a 6-hour workday is at least as valid as one of an 8-10 hour workday.** ↳ Many people in our culture are chronically overworked, undernourished, tired and suffer from an insufficiency of time to simply be in community, to rest, to be creative. Living with such limitations and pressures should be expected to produce a population that is reactively hedonistic, impulsive, and prone to addiction. Behaviors that are addictive (e.g., drugs, alcohol) and destructive (e.g., over-eating, alcohol, sugar, fat) are simply frustrated and maladaptive coping strategies to combat the stress caused by a damaging, unnatural paradigm from which most people cannot escape.[62] Redesigning our societal structures and expectations in ways that conform to our natural humanity and biologic, nutritional, and emotional needs is more rational than forcing *en masse* all of humanity to contort and conform to an artificial posture and cadence of performance, productivity, "professionalism", and other unnatural expectations. Less time dedicated to work and all that it entails leaves more time for 1) healthy cooking, 2) relaxed, conscious, and enjoyable eating, 3) exercise, 4) creativity and hobbies, 5) keeping informed of and involved with political change, and 6) participation in social relationships.[63] ↳ Readers of my books know that I advocated the 4-day workweek since the publication of my *Integrative Orthopedics* in 2004 and *Integrative Rheumatology* in 2006; finally, in 2014 this idea has made headlines: "One of Britain's leading doctors has called for the country to switch to a four-day week to help combat high levels of work-related stress, let people spend more time with their families or exercising, and reduce unemployment. Bringing the standard working week down from five to four days would also help address medical conditions, such as high blood pressure and the mental ill-health associated with overwork or lack of work, Prof John Ashton said."[64]

---

[59] "Conventional wisdom is the habitual, the unexamined life, absorbed into the culture and the fashion of the time, lost in the mad rush of accumulation, lulled to sleep by the easy lies of political hacks and newspaper scribblers, or by priests who wouldn't know a god if they met one." Nisker W. *Crazy Wisdom*. Berkeley; Ten Speed Press: 1990, p 7

[60] Sep 8, 2003: Average daily one-way commute to work in the United States takes just over 26 minutes, according to the Bureau of Transportation Statistics' Omnibus Household Survey. Omnibus Household Survey Shows Americans' Average Commuting Time is Over 26 Minutes. bts.gov/press_releases/2003/bts020_03/html/bts020_03.html

[61] Dominguez JR. *Transforming Your Relationship with Money*. Sounds True; Book and Cassette edition: 2001

[62] Breton D, Largent C. *The Paradigm Conspiracy: Why Our Social Systems Violate Human Potential-And How We Can Change Them*. Hazelden: 1998

[63] "Take back your time" is a major U.S./Canadian initiative to challenge the epidemic of overwork, over-scheduling and time famine that now threatens our health, our families and relationships, our communities and our environment. simpleliving.net/timeday/ on August 3, 2004

[64] Campbell D. UK needs four-day week to combat stress, says top doctor. *The Guardian* 2014 theguardian.com/society/2014/jul/01/uk-four-day-week-combat-stress-top-doctor

Quality and quantity of sleep: A sleep duration of less than 8 hours of deep solid sleep each night is physiologically insufficient for most of people; many people feel best with 9 hours of sleep, yet some people appear to function well on about 6 hours of sleep per night. Not only is it important to get a sufficient *quantity* of sleep, but we need to ensure that the *quality* of the sleep receives appropriate attention, as well. Sleep should be mostly continuous, not "broken" or interrupted. Some experts

> **The Importance of Sleep**
> Regulation of sleep-wake cycles and the regular satisfaction of sleep needs are important for preservation of immune function, intellectual performance, emotional stability, and the internal regulation of the body's inflammatory tendency.

believe that people should be able to recall their dreams at night, as this may be a sign of proper neurotransmitter status, especially with regard to serotonin, which is affected by pyridoxine[65] as well as other factors. Going to bed at a regular hour (not later than 10 or 11 at night) helps to synchronize the daily schedule with the body's inherent hormonal rhythms and "physiological clock" which expects one to be in deep sleep by midnight and to be waking at approximately 8 o'clock in the morning. Recent research has shown that **sleep deprivation causes a systemic inflammatory response manifested objectively by increases in high-sensitivity C-reactive protein (hsCRP)**.[66] Correspondingly, sleep apnea, a condition associated with repetitive sleep disturbances, is also associated with an elevation of CRP[67], and effective treatment of sleep apnea results in a normalization of CRP levels.[68] We could therefore conclude that **sleep deprivation creates a proinflammatory condition**. Furthermore, **sleep deprivation has been proven to impair intellectual functioning, emotional state, and immune function**, with abnormalities in immune status already evident the morning after sleep deprivation.[69] Wakefulness and exposure to light at night result in a suppression of melatonin production and may therefore contribute to cancer development since melatonin has anticancer actions that would be abrogated by its reduced endogenous production.[70,71] Limited evidence also suggests that melatonin production is altered in patients with the inflammatory conditions eczema[72] and psoriasis[73] and that this sleep-related hormone has anti-inflammatory/anti-autoimmune benefits that may be relevant for the suppression of diseases such as multiple sclerosis[74] and sarcoidosis.[75]

- Sleep disturbance, immune dysregulation, and disturbed inflammatory regulation (*Am J Geriatr Psychiatry.* 2012 Sep[76]): "Poor sleep diminishes mental and physical health. ... Participants categorized as poor sleepers on the basis of Pittsburgh Sleep Quality Index scores had significantly larger IL-6 responses to the cognitive stressors than good sleepers. The association between poor sleep and heightened IL-6 response to acute stress was not explained by other psychosocial factors previously linked to immune dysregulation, including depressive symptoms, perceived stress, and loneliness. CONCLUSIONS: Findings add to the growing evidence for poor sleep as an independent risk factor for poor mental and physical health. Older adults may be particularly vulnerable to effects of sleep disturbance due to significant age-related changes in both sleep and inflammatory regulation."

---

[65] " ...a significant difference in dream-salience scores (this is a composite score containing measures on vividness, bizarreness, emotionality, and color) between the 250-mg condition and placebo over the first three days of each treatment... An hypothesis is presented involving the role of B-6 in the conversion of tryptophan to serotonin." Ebben M, Lequerica A, Spielman A. Effects of pyridoxine on dreaming: a preliminary study. *Percept Mot Skills* 2002 Feb;94(1):135-40

[66] "CONCLUSIONS: Both acute total and short-term partial sleep deprivation resulted in elevated high-sensitivity CRP concentrations... We propose that sleep loss may be one of the ways that inflammatory processes are activated and contribute to the association of sleep complaints, short sleep duration, and cardiovascular morbidity observed in epidemiologic surveys." Meier-Ewert et al. Effect of sleep loss on C-reactive protein, an inflammatory marker of cardiovascular risk. *J Am Coll Cardiol.* 2004 Feb 18;43:678-83

[67] "OSA is associated with elevated levels of CRP, a marker of inflammation and of cardiovascular risk. The severity of OSA is proportional to the CRP level." Shamsuzzaman et al. Elevated C-reactive protein in patients with obstructive sleep apnea. *Circulation.* 2002 May 28;105(21):2462-4

[68] "CONCLUSIONS: Levels of CRP and IL-6 and spontaneous production of IL-6 by monocytes are elevated in patients with OSAS but are decreased by nCPAP." Yokoe T, Minoguchi K, Matsuo H, Oda N, Minoguchi H, Yoshino G, Hirano T, Adachi M. Elevated levels of C-reactive protein and interleukin-6 in patients with obstructive sleep apnea syndrome are decreased by nasal continuous positive airway pressure. *Circulation.* 2003 Mar 4;107(8):1129-34 circ.ahajournals.org/cgi/reprint/107/8/1129.pdf

[69] "Taken together, SD induced a deterioration of both mood and ability to work, which was most prominent in the evening after SD, while the maximal alterations of the host defence system could be found twelve hours earlier, i.e., already in the morning following SD." Heiser P, et al. Alterations of host defense system after sleep deprivation are followed by impaired mood and psychosocial functioning. *World J Biol Psychiatry* 2001 Apr;2(2):89-94

[70] "Observational studies support an association between night work and cancer risk. We hypothesise that the potential primary culprit for this observed association is the lack of melatonin, a cancer-protective agent whose production is severely diminished in people exposed to light at night." Schernhammer ES, Schulmeister K. Melatonin and cancer risk: does light at night compromise physiologic cancer protection by lowering serum melatonin levels? *Br J Cancer.* 2004 Mar 8;90(5):941-3

[71] "This is the first biological evidence for a potential link between constant light exposure and increased human breast oncogenesis involving MLT suppression and stimulation of tumor LA metabolism." Blask DE, Dauchy RT, Sauer LA, Krause JA, Brainard GC. Growth and fatty acid metabolism of human breast cancer (MCF-7) xenografts in nude rats: impact of constant light-induced nocturnal melatonin suppression. *Breast Cancer Res Treat.* 2003 Jun;79(3):313-20

[72] "In 6 patients exhibiting low serum levels of melatonin, the circadian melatonin rhythm was found to be abolished. In 8 patients a diminished nocturnal melatonin increase was observed compared with the controls (n = 40)." Schwarz W, et al. Alterations of melatonin secretion in atopic eczema. *Acta Derm Venereol.* 1988;68(3):224-9

[73] "Our results show that psoriatic patients had lost the nocturnal peak and usual circadian rhythm of melatonin secretion." Mozzanica N, Tadini G, Radaelli A, et al. Plasma melatonin levels in psoriasis. *Acta Derm Venereol.* 1988;68(4):312-6

[74] "This hypothesis is supported by the observation that administration of melatonin (3 mg, orally) at 2:00 p.m., when the patient experienced severe blurring of vision, resulted within 15 minutes in a dramatic improvement in visual acuity and in normalization of the visual evoked potential latency after stimulation of the left eye." Sandyk R. Diurnal variations in vision and relations to circadian melatonin secretion in multiple sclerosis. *Int J Neurosci.* 1995 Nov;83(1-2):1-6

[75] Cagnoni ML, Lombardi A, Cerinic MC, Dedola GL, Pignone A. Melatonin for treatment of chronic refractory sarcoidosis. *Lancet.* 1995;346:1229-30

[76] Heffner et al. Sleep disturbance and older adults' inflammatory responses to acute stress. *Am J Geriatr Psychiatry.* 2012 Sep;20(9):744-52

Helping patients improve quality and quantity of sleep

- Schedule sufficient time for sleep; generally this is 9 hours to allow time for "winding down" and "daily decompression" so that a full 8 hours of sleep can ensue.
- Reduce intake of stimulants such as caffeine, tobacco, and aspartame. Some patients will need to reduce intake only in the evening, while others will need to reduce intake even in the morning in order to have improved quality and quantity of sleep later at night.
- Exercise early in the day (morning or early afternoon) to promote restful sleep at night.[77]
- Avoid aggressive or arousing physical activity in the evening to avoid increases in norepinephrine, epinephrine, and cortisol, which can discourage sleep.
- Dim lights at night to promote melatonin production. Beginning one to two hours before bedtime, turn off bright lights and use only dim lighting. Bright lights reduce melatonin secretion and stimulate neocortical activity and thereby inhibit sleep.
- Have an evening ritual/pattern that helps the psyche recognize that the time for sleep has arrived. Such practices can include relaxing warm tea, meditation, prayer, and daily reflection.
- For patients with a pattern of falling asleep and then waking approximately 4-6 hours later with feelings of hunger or anxiety (nocturnal hypoglycemia), they should eat a small meal or snack of complex carbohydrates, protein, and fat before going to bed. For example, the combination of nuts (or nut butter) with whole fruit such as apples provides protein, fat, and complex carbohydrate with a low glycemic index to provide sustenance throughout the night. Protein powders and other sources of "predigested" amino acids should generally be avoided late at night because an excess consumption of high protein foods can reduce tryptophan entry into the brain and thus reduce serotonin and melatonin synthesis. Most amino acid-derived neurotransmitters such as dopamine, glutamate, and norepinephrine are excitatory/stimulatory in nature.
- Vitamin and mineral supplementation is commonly beneficial, particularly with thiamine[78], methylcobalamin (weak evidence[79]), and magnesium (particularly sleep disturbance associated with restless leg syndrome[80]). Vitamins should be taken earlier in the day (with breakfast and lunch; not before bed); however calcium and magnesium can be taken before bed.
- Earplugs, window covers, and a quiet, snore-free environment are generally conducive to better sleep.
- For patients with difficulty falling asleep, consider 5-hydroxytryptophan consumed with simple carbohydrate (50-200 mg for adults, up to 2 mg/kg[81] for children), melatonin (0.5-10 mg), valerian-hops tea or capsules[82] 60-90 minutes before bedtime.

---

[77] "This is the first report to demonstrate that low intensity activity in an elderly population can increase deep sleep and improve memory functioning." Naylor E, et al. Daily social and physical activity increases slow-wave sleep and daytime neuropsychological performance in the elderly. *Sleep.* 2000 Feb 1;23(1):87-95

[78] Wilkinson TJ, Hanger HC, Elmslie J, George PM, Sainsbury R. The response to treatment of subclinical thiamine deficiency in the elderly. *Am J Clin Nutr.* 1997;66(4):925-8

[79] "However, because the percentage of improvement was low and significant improvement was inconsistent, Met-12 might be considered to have a low therapeutic potency and possible use as a booster for other treatment methods of the disorders." Takahashi K, et al. Double-blind test on the efficacy of methylcobalamin on sleep-wake rhythm disorders. *Psychiatry Clin Neurosci.* 1999 Apr;53(2):211-3

[80] "Our study indicates that magnesium treatment may be a useful alternative therapy in patients with mild or moderate RLS-or PLMS-related insomnia." Hornyak M, Voderholzer U, et al. Magnesium therapy for periodic leg movements-related insomnia and restless legs syndrome: an open pilot study. *Sleep.* 1998 Aug 1;21(5):501-5

[81] Bruni O, Ferri R, Miano S, Verrillo E. l-5-Hydroxytryptophan treatment of sleep terrors in children. *Eur J Pediatr.* 2004 May 14

[82] "Sleep improvements with a valerian-hops combination are associated with improved quality of life. Both treatments appear safe and did not produce rebound insomnia upon discontinuation during this study. Overall, these findings indicate that a valerian-hops combination and diphenhydramine might be useful adjuncts in the treatment of mild insomnia." Morin et al. Valerian-hops combination and diphenhydramine for treating insomnia: a randomized placebo-controlled clinical trial. *Sleep.* 2005 Nov 1;28:1465-71

Exercise: Human existence has changed radically over the past few millennia, centuries, and decades, and one of the most profound changes has been in our relationship to physical activity. Paleologists and historical scientists agree that physical activity among humans is at its all-time historical low, and that levels of exertion that we now call "vigorous and frequent exercise" would have been *completely normal* in the daily lives of our ancestors, who engaged in at least four times more physical activity than their modern-day progeny.[83] At one time—a time in which vigorous physical activity was a normal part of daily life—probably no word existed for what modern people describe and often resist as "exercise."

Our current mode of compulsory primary and secondary education prioritizes "being still" over physical exertion/expression for the vast majority of students' time. Thus having been separated from their inherent tendency to be physically active and emotionally expressive, many children grow into adults who have to be *retaught to inhabit their bodies* and to engage in physical activity on a daily basis. Basic science has proven that this is true: when animals are restrained, they show less activity when freed and no longer tied down.

Daily exercise is health-promoting and restorative
"The health rewards of exercise extend far beyond its benefits for specific diseases."   1. Exercise reduces blood clotting,   2. ...lowers blood pressure,   3. ...lowers cholesterol,   4. ...improves glucose tolerance and insulin sensitivity,   5. ...enhances self-image, elevates mood,   6. ...reduces stress,   7. ...creates a feeling of well-being,   8. ...reinforces other positive life-style changes,   9. ...stimulates creative thinking,   10. ...increases muscle mass,   11. ...increases basal metabolic rate,   12. ...promotes improved sleep,   13. ...stimulates healthy intestinal function,   14. ...promotes weight loss, and   15. ...enhances appearance.   "Furthermore, **the ability of exercise to restore function to organs, muscles, joints, and bones is not shared by drugs or surgery.**"
Harold Elrick, MD. Exercise is medicine. *Physician and Sportsmedicine*. 1996 Feb

Conversely, when animals are rigorously exercised, they show higher levels of *spontaneous physical activity* when left to their own discretion. A probable sociological parallel is at work in human cultures where, under the guise of *office work* (sitting still), driving in cars (sitting still), and *spectator entertainment* (sitting still), people are corralled into lifestyles of physical inactivity in a wide range of apparently divergent activities. Watching television, driving a car, seeing a movie, doing computer/desk work at the office, attending a sports event or educational lecture, seeing the opera—all of these are simply different forms of ***sitting***, of physical inactivity. Changing our social structure in a way that prioritizes *life* over *work*, such as moving toward a 4-day work week and/or a 6-hour work day, would allow people more time to live their lives, to pursue healthy diets and relationships, to be creative, and to engage in more physical activity; thus, "escape entertainment" such as fiction books and movies and processed "fast foods"—the latter of which are inherently unhealthy[84]—would become less necessary and less attractive.

Daily exercise is the body's physiological expectation
"Although modern technology has made physical exertion optional, it is still important to exercise as though our survival depended on it, and in a different way it still does.   **We are genetically adapted to live an extremely physically active lifestyle.**"
O'Keefe JH Jr, Cordain L. Cardiovascular disease resulting from a diet and lifestyle at odds with our Paleolithic genome. *Mayo Clin Proc*. 2004 Jan

---

[83] Eaton SB, Cordain L, Eaton SB. An evolutionary foundation for health promotion. *World Rev Nutr Diet* 2001; 90:5-12
[84] For an additional social-experimental perspective see movie directed by Morgan Spurlock. *Super Size Me*. supersizeme.com released in 2004

Exploring the spectrum of physical activity from inactivity to athleticism

Inactivity	Minimally active	Active	Healthy	Athletic
• Bed-ridden • Chair-ridden • Minimal activity, such as walking to car or bathroom or to buy groceries • Activity in this category is equivalent to or barely above that which is necessary to sustain life	• Periodic performance of more activity than the minimal needed to sustain life, such as walking around the block after dinner, or taking a brief stroll at a park or at the beach	• Regular performance of low/moderate levels of activity at work or leisure, at least 30-60 minutes of physical activity per day	• 60-120 minutes of activity such as running, swimming, cycling, or other physical training 4-7 days per week	• More than 2 hours devoted to conditioning, strengthening, and skill-building 4-7 days per week

At least 30-45 minutes of exercise four days per week is the *absolute minimum*. Ideally, patients who have been sedentary and are over age 45 years would have a pre-exercise physical exam that might also include electrocardiography before embarking on a program of vigorous exercise. Patients who have been sedentary for many years can start slowly with their new exercise program, gradually increasing the duration and

> **Industrialized Westernized societies' disregard/disdain for connection with the body**
>
> "That I deemed it an imposition to have to make use of my perfectly adequate coordination, or resented—from unexamined principle—**the use of time to fill a need**, was an **arbitrary assignment of values** that [this other culture] did not share."
>
> Liedloff J. *The Continuum Concept*, 1977, page 15

intensity. With the simple addition of regular exercise to their routine, patients will have significantly reduced risk for problems such as depression, chronic pain, cancer, coronary artery disease, stroke, hypertension, diabetes, arthritis, osteoporosis, dyslipidemia, obesity, chronic obstructive pulmonary disease, constipation, and other problems.[85] Furthermore, successful prevention and treatment of health problems with exercise and lifestyle modifications reduces dependency on pharmaceutical drugs, thereby further saving lives. O'Keefe and Cordain[86] report that **during the hunter-gatherer period, humans averaged 5-10 miles of daily running and walking.** Additionally, **other physical activities such as heavy lifting, digging, and climbing would have been considered "normal" aspects of daily life rather than "exercise"—an achievement for which modern/industrialized people seek recognition.** Thus, when sedentary patients achieve the first-step goal of walking around the block after dinner, we can commend them for making a significant stride forward in ultimately attaining better health, but we cannot stop there nor delude them into believing that this is adequate.

- Physical activity can prevent physical and cognitive decline in postmenopausal women (*Maturitas* 2014 Jun[87]): Results of this systematic review of the literature showed that all previous studies found that physical activity was associated with lower rates of cognitive and physical decline and a significant reduction in all-cause mortality; exercise interventions (or lifestyle activities) that improved cardiorespiratory exercise capacity showed the most positive impact on physical health. The authors encouraged the embedding of physical activity programs into public health initiatives, developing home-based exercise programs that require few resources, and creating interventions that can incorporate physical activity within a healthy lifestyle. The review also suggests that clinicians should consider prescribing exercise that it is of a high enough intensity to obtain the positive sustained effects of exercise.

> **The philosophy of physicality**
>
> "There is more wisdom in your body than in your deepest philosophy."
>
> Nietzsche FW, *Thus Spoke Zarathustra*

---

[85] Harold Elrick, MD. Exercise is Medicine. *The Physician and Sportsmedicine* 1996 Feb

[86] O'Keefe JH Jr, Cordain L. Cardiovascular disease resulting from a diet and lifestyle at odds with our Paleolithic genome. *Mayo Clin Proc*. 2004 Jan;79(1):101-8

[87] Anderson et al. Can physical activity prevent physical and cognitive decline in postmenopausal women? A systematic review. *Maturitas*. 2014 Jun. pii: S0378-5122(14)00206-0

Common physical activities: a buffet of options from which to choose
☑ **"Boot camp"-style aerobics classes**: excellent variety and fast-pace maintains oxygen debt for the entire session (generally 60 minutes) even among reasonably well trained "healthy" people
☑ **Aerobic machines such as elliptical runners and stair-climbing machines**: easy on joints; accessible during inclement weather; easy to integrate with weight-lifting which is commonly available at the same facility
☑ **Baseball**: requires some skill in throwing and batting, but otherwise this is a very inactive sport
☑ **Football**: much of the game is spent in inactivity; most of the fitness comes from preparation for the game, not the game itself; high impact activity wherein injuries are expected
☑ **Hiking**: virtually free of expense; allows for conversation, exploration, and time in nature; mountains required
☑ **Indoor aerobics**: excellent for cardiovascular fitness and weight loss, requires and thus promotes coordination and timing
☑ **Indoor cycling**: excellent for cardiovascular fitness and weight loss, easy on the joints; accessible during inclement weather
☑ **Jogging and running**: easy, accessible, virtually free; allows for conversation and exploration; increases endorphin production and promotes a sense of well-being; detoxification via sweating
☑ **Kayaking and canoeing**: excellent combination of relaxation and exertion; develops upper body strength and balance
☑ **Martial arts**: requires more balance, coordination, timing, strategy, endurance; injuries are to be expected, as is enhanced sense of security and confidence
☑ **Outdoor cycling (mountain and trail)**: same as above; requires more balance and coordination
☑ **Outdoor cycling (road)**: same as above with added bonus of being outdoors; promotes independence from automobiles and petroleum products – thereby reducing pollution and sustaining the environment
☑ **Rock-climbing (indoor and outdoor)**: requires upper body and grip strength; promotes agility, resourcefulness, courage, and trust; good for building stronger relationships assuming that your partner does not drop the rope or get distracted; carries some inherent risk
☑ **Skiing, snowboarding, cross-country skiing**: Require balance and coordination, costly equipment, and appropriate season and climate; risk of traumatic injury due to speed in skiing and snowboarding. Cross-country skiing is generally safe from trauma and provides excellent cardiovascular exertion, in addition to exposure to nature
☑ **Soccer**: excellent for lower-body conditioning, teamwork, and coordination, the rapid stops and turns can be hard on joints
☑ **Surfing**: paddling requires upper body endurance and strength; some leg strength is required but is not strongly developed during the riding portion of surfing, which is mostly technique and "style"; excellent proprioceptive training
☑ **Swimming**: requires access to a pool or suitable body of water; excellent for promoting fitness in a way that is generally easy on joints and muscles and is without impact; requires and thus promotes coordination and timing
☑ **Tennis and racket sports**: requires more balance, coordination, timing, strategy, endurance; the rapid stops, starts, and turns can be hard on joints; upper body exertion is asymmetric and can promote muscle imbalance
☑ **Volleyball**: good team activity; not highly exertional in terms of either aerobic fitness nor strength acquisition
☑ **Walking**: easy, accessible, virtually free; allows for conversation and exploration; allows for time outdoors
☑ **Weight lifting, bodybuilding, and powerlifting**: excellent for increasing lean body mass – one of the primary determinants of basal metabolic rate; promotes bone strengthening
☑ **Yoga, Calisthenics**: inexpensive, can be done alone or in groups; does not require much/any equipment, therefore costs are low and access is near universal

Obesity: Obesity is a major risk factor for cardiovascular disease, cancer, diabetes mellitus, depression, joint degeneration and pain. Obese people also commonly report difficulties with performing daily activities, and they also report higher rates of depression and social isolation than do people of normal weight. "Body Mass Index" is a clinically valuable measure of height-weight proportionality and therefore adiposity, since an excess of height-proportionate weight is more commonly due to excess adipose than to excess muscle. To calculate BMI simply chart height and weight in the table below. Numbers greater than 25 correlate with being "overweight" while numbers greater than 30 meet the criteria for "obesity." BMI determinations may not be reflective of disease risk for people who are pregnant, highly muscular, or for young children or the frail elderly. BMI is interpreted as follows:

- Severely underweight: < 16.5
- Underweight: 16.5 - 18.4
- **Normal: 18.5 - 24.9**
- Overweight: 25 - 29.9
- Obese Class 1: 30 - 34.9
- Obese Class 2 (severe obesity): 35 - 39.9
- Obese Class 3 (morbid obesity): 40 - 47.9
- Obese Class 4 (supermorbid obesity): ≥ 48

Weight in kilograms (*derived from pounds and inches from original table below; BMI is approximate)

Height: (cm*)	45	50	55	59	63	68	73	77	82	86	90	95	100	104	109	114
152	20	21	23	25	27	29	31	33	35	37	39	41	43	45	47	49
155	19	21	23	25	26	28	30	32	34	36	38	40	42	43	45	47
157	18	20	22	24	26	27	29	31	33	35	37	38	40	42	44	46
160	18	19	21	23	25	27	28	30	32	34	35	37	39	41	43	44
162	17	19	21	22	24	26	27	29	31	33	34	36	38	39	41	43
165	17	18	20	22	23	25	27	28	30	32	33	35	37	38	40	42
167	16	18	19	21	23	24	26	27	29	31	32	34	36	37	39	40
170	16	17	19	20	22	23	25	27	28	30	31	33	34	36	38	39
173	15	17	18	20	21	23	24	26	27	29	30	32	33	35	36	38
175	15	16	18	19	21	22	24	25	27	28	30	31	32	34	35	37
177	14	16	17	19	20	22	23	24	26	27	29	30	32	33	34	36
180	14	15	17	18	20	21	22	24	25	26	27	28	30	32	33	35
182	14	15	16	18	19	20	22	23	24	26	27	28	30	31	33	34
185	13	15	16	17	18	20	21	22	24	25	26	28	29	30	32	33
188	13	14	15	17	18	19	21	22	23	24	26	27	28	30	31	32
190	12	14	15	16	17	19	20	21	22	24	25	26	27	29	30	31
193	12	13	15	16	17	18	19	21	22	23	24	26	27	28	29	30

Weight in pounds

Height: (Ft'inch")	100	110	120	130	140	150	160	170	180	190	200	210	220	230	240	250
5'0"	20	21	23	25	27	29	31	33	35	37	39	41	43	45	47	49
5'1"	19	21	23	25	26	28	30	32	34	36	38	40	42	43	45	47
5'2"	18	20	22	24	26	27	29	31	33	35	37	38	40	42	44	46
5'3"	18	19	21	23	25	27	28	30	32	34	35	37	39	41	43	44
5'4"	17	19	21	22	24	26	27	29	31	33	34	36	38	39	41	43
5'5"	17	18	20	22	23	25	27	28	30	32	33	35	37	38	40	42
5'6"	16	18	19	21	23	24	26	27	29	31	32	34	36	37	39	40
5'7"	16	17	19	20	22	23	25	27	28	30	31	33	34	36	38	39
5'8"	15	17	18	20	21	23	24	26	27	29	30	32	33	35	36	38
5'9"	15	16	18	19	21	22	24	25	27	28	30	31	32	34	35	37
5'10"	14	16	17	19	20	22	23	24	26	27	29	30	32	33	34	36
5'11"	14	15	17	18	20	21	22	24	25	26	27	28	30	32	33	35
6'0"	14	15	16	18	19	20	22	23	24	26	27	28	30	31	33	34
6'1"	13	15	16	17	18	20	21	22	24	25	26	28	29	30	32	33
6'2"	13	14	15	17	18	19	21	22	23	24	26	27	28	30	31	32
6'3"	12	14	15	16	17	19	20	21	22	24	25	26	27	29	30	31
6'4"	12	13	15	16	17	18	19	21	22	23	24	26	27	28	29	30

Adipose tissue is biologically active, promoting systemic inflammation and "estrogen dominance", thereby promoting the development of inflammatory and malignant diseases such as psoriasis and cancers of the breast, prostate, and colon. The previous view that fat (adipose) tissue was merely serving as an inert and inactive depot for lipid/energy storage is now replaced with the view that adipose tissue is biologically-active, influencing overall health via complex mechanisms that are biochemical-inflammatory-endocrinologic and not merely mechanical (i.e., excess weight, excess mass).[88] **Excess fat tissue—especially visceral/abdominal adipose—creates a systemic proinflammatory state** evidenced most readily by the elevations in hsCRP commonly seen in patients with obesity and the metabolic syndrome.[89] Adipokines are cytokines secreted by adipose tissue and include tumor necrosis factor-alpha, interleukin-6, and leptin—a cytokine derived from fat cells that promotes inflammation and immune activation; levels are higher in obese patients and decrease after weight loss. Obese patients also appear to have "leptin resistance" with regard to the suppression of appetite by leptin. **Adipose creates excess estrogens;** concomitant hyperglycemia increases androgen production[90], and these androgens are subsequently converted to estrogens by aromatase in the adipose tissue. For example, the adrenal gland makes androstenedione, which can be converted by aromatase in adipose tissue into estrone.[91] These proinflammatory and hormonal perturbations manifest clinically as an increased risk for breast, prostate, endometrial, colon and gallbladder cancers, insulin resistance and cardiovascular disease. The combination of inflammation, reduced testosterone, and elevated estrogen is also predisposes toward the development of autoimmune/inflammatory diseases.

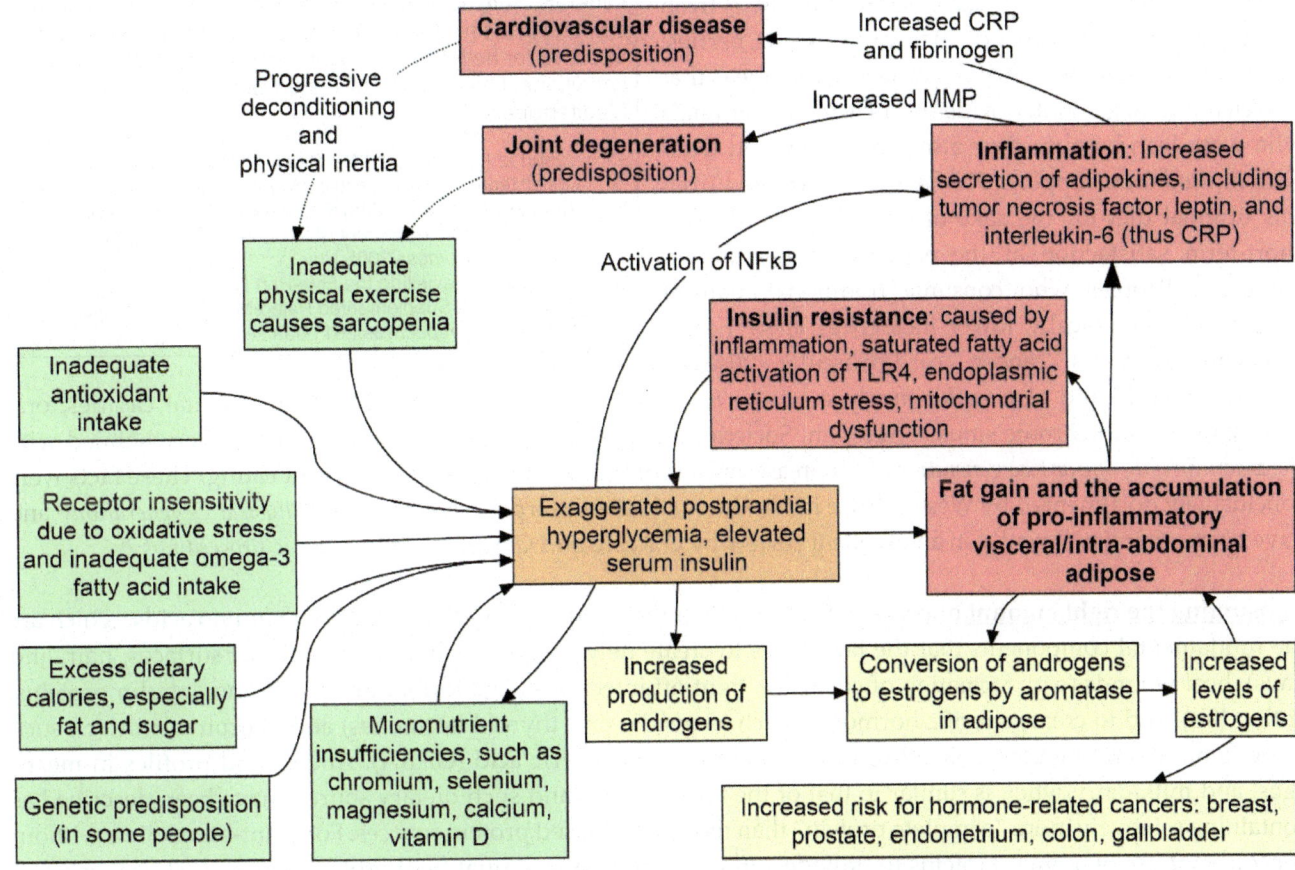

Overview of the proinflammatory and endocrinologic activity of adipose tissue: Adipose promotes systemic inflammation via adipokines and expedites the production of estrogens at the expense of androgens via aromatase.

---

88 "The fat cell is a true endocrine cell that secretes a variety of factors, including metabolites such as lactate, fatty acids, prostaglandin derivatives and a variety of peptides, including cytokines (leptin, tumor necrosis factor, interleukin-1 and -6, adiponectin), angiotensinogen, complement D (adipsin), plasminogen activator inhibitor-1 and undoubtedly many others." Bray GA. The underlying basis for obesity: relationship to cancer. *J Nutr.* 2002 Nov;132(11 Suppl):3451S-3455S

89 "Our results indicate a strong relationship between adipocytokines and inflammatory markers, and suggest that cytokines secreted by adipose tissue could play a role in increased inflammatory proteins secretion by the liver." Maachi M, et al. Systemic low-grade inflammation is related to both circulating and adipose tissue TNFalpha, leptin and IL-6 levels in obese women. *Int J Obes Relat Metab Disord.* 2004;28:993-7

90 Christensen et al. Elevated levels of sex hormones and sex hormone binding globulin in male patients with insulin dependent diabetes mellitus. *Dan Med Bull.* 1997;44:547-50

91 "Conversion of androstenedione secreted by adrenal gland into estrone by aromatase in adipose tissue stroma provides an important source of estrogen for the postmenopausal woman. This estrogen may play an important role in development of endometrial and breast cancer." Bray GA. Underlying basis for obesity. *J Nutr* 2002;3451S-3455S

The Daily Diet—Powerful Intervention for the Prevention and Treatment of Disease: "Whole foods" should form the foundation and majority of the diet. As doctors and patients, we should emphasize whole fruits, vegetables, nuts, seeds, berries, and lean sources of protein. "Whole foods" are foods that are found in nature, and they should be eaten as closely as possible to their natural state—preferably *unprocessed* and *raw*. Creating a diet based on whole, natural foods by emphasizing the consumption of fruits, vegetables, and lean meats and excluding high-fat factory meats, high-sugar foods like white potatoes, and milled grains like wheat and corn is essential for our efforts of promoting health by matching the human *diet* with the human *genome*.[92] Our genetic make-up was co-created over a period of more than 2.6 million years by interaction with the environment as it exists in its natural state. This environment mandated daily physical activity and a diet that was exclusively composed of 1) fresh fruits, 2) fresh vegetables (mostly uncooked), 3) raw nuts, seeds, berries, roots, and 4) generous portions of lean game meat that was rich in omega-3 fatty acids from free-living animals who were lean because they also ran, fasted, and dealt with limited food supplies. Humans have deviated from this original diet for the sake of ease, conformity, and short-term satisfaction at the expense of health and longevity. Peoples who consume traditional, natural diets have dramatically lower incidences *major* health problems such as cancer, cardiovascular disease,

> ### The Supplemented Paleo-Mediterranean Diet
>
> My conclusion after reading several hundred articles on epidemiology, nutritional biochemistry, and dietary intervention studies is that the Paleo-Mediterranean diet—particularly its pesco-vegetarian version—is the single most healthy dietary regimen for the broadest range of patients and for the prevention of the widest range of diseases including cancer, hypertension, diabetes, dermatitis, depression, obesity, arthritis and all inflammatory and autoimmune diseases. By definition, this is a diet that helps patients increase their intake of fruits and vegetables (fiber, antioxidants, phytonutrients), increases their intake of fish (for the anti-inflammatory omega-3 fats EPA and DHA) while reducing intake of the pro-cancer and pro-inflammatory omega-6 fats linoleic acid and arachidonic acid), and it is naturally low in sugars and cholesterol (for alleviating hyperglycemia and dyslipidemia). This dietary pattern helps patients avoid grains, particularly wheat (a common allergen), and it reduces the intake of the high-fermentation carbohydrates in breads, pasta, pastries, potatoes, and sucrose which promote overgrowth of bacteria and yeast in the intestines. Supplementing this pesco-vegetarian diet with vitamins, minerals, fatty acids such as fish oil and GLA (from borage oil), and protein from soy and whey makes this diet effective for both the treatment and prevention of many conditions; I have called this "the Supplemented Paleo-Mediterranean Diet."
>
> 1. Vasquez A. A Five-Part Nutritional Protocol that Produces Consistently Positive Results. *Nutritional Wellness* 2005 Sep
> 2. Vasquez A. Implementing the Five-Part Nutritional Wellness Protocol for the Treatment of Various Health Problems. *Nutritional Wellness* 2005 Nov
> 3. Vasquez A. Revisiting the Five-Part Nutritional Wellness Protocol: The Supplemented Paleo-Mediterranean Diet. *Nutritional Perspectives* 2011 Jan

diabetes, obesity and also suffer much less from *milder* problems such as acne, psoriasis, dental cavities, oral malocclusion, and chronic sinus congestion. Societies that are free of these disorders become overwhelmed with them *within only one or two generations* as soon as they adopt the American/Western style of eating. These facts were conclusively documented by Weston Price in his famous 1945 masterpiece *Nutrition and Physical Degeneration*[93] and have been reiterated recently in an excellent review by O'Keefe and Cordain in *Mayo Clinic Proceedings*.[94]

Consuming the right amount of protein: Dietary protein is eaten to provide the body with amino acids, which are the fundamental components that the body uses to create new tissues (such as skin, mucosal surfaces, hair, and nails), heal wounds (e.g., formation of collagen), fight off infections (e.g., formation of immunoglobulin proteins, antibodies), and to create specific hormones (such as insulin and thyroid hormones) and neurotransmitters, such as dopamine, serotonin, norepinephrine, and gamma-aminobutyric acid (GABA). Amino acid profiles in meats, eggs, and milk/dairy/whey is similar to that of the human body and such dietary sources have been described as containing relatively more "complete protein" than most plant-based protein sources. For plant-based diets without concomitant use of animal proteins to provide sufficient quantity and quality of protein, foods must be combined with respect to one another's amino acid profiles; beyond learned attention to *quality*, additional attention is needed to ensure sufficient *quantitative* intake, especially for vegetarian athletes, particularly those engaged in resistance training.

For most people (without kidney or liver problems) the goal for daily protein intake should be 0.50-0.75 grams of protein per pound of lean body weight, depending on activity level and other health needs (see table). Sufficient dietary protein is essential for patients with musculoskeletal injuries because tissue healing relies on the

---

[92] O'Keefe JH Jr, Cordain L. Cardiovascular disease resulting from a diet and lifestyle at odds with our Paleolithic genome. *Mayo Clin Proc.* 2004 Jan;79(1):101-8
[93] Price WA. *Nutrition and Physical Degeneration*. Santa Monica; Price-Pottinger Nutrition Foundation: 1945
[94] O'Keefe JH Jr, Cordain L. Cardiovascular disease resulting from a diet and lifestyle at odds with our Paleolithic genome. *Mayo Clin Proc.* 2004 Jan;79(1):101-8

constant availability of amino acids and micronutrients[95], which should be supplied by a healthy, balanced, whole-foods diet that may be supplemented with specific vitamins, minerals, and phytonutrients. Low-protein diets suppress immune function, reduce muscle mass, and impair healing[96,97] whereas intakes of higher amounts of protein safely facilitate healing and the maintenance of muscle mass. Increased protein intake does not adversely affect bone health as long as dietary calcium intake is adequate.[98] According to the 1998 review by Lemon[99], "Those involved in strength training might need to consume as much as …1.7 g protein x kg(-1) x day(-1)…while those undergoing endurance training might need about 1.2 to 1.6 g x kg(-1) x day(-1)… **…there is no evidence that protein intakes in the range suggested will have adverse effects in healthy individuals."**

Recommended <u>Grams of Protein</u> per <u>Patient Profile</u> and <u>Body Weight</u> Per Day		
Patient Profile	*Per* **pound** of weight[100]	*Per* **kilogram** of weight
Infants and children ages 1-6 years[101]	0.45-0.68	0.99-1.4
RDA for sedentary adult and children ages 6-18 years[102]	0.4	0.88
Adult recreational exerciser—average for adults	**0.5-0.75**	**1.1-1.65**
Adult competitive athlete	0.6-0.9	1.32-1.98
Adult building muscle mass	0.7-0.9	1.54-1.98
Dieting athlete	0.7-1.0	1.54-2.2
Growing teenage athlete	0.9-1.0	1.98-2.2
Pregnant women need additional protein	Add 15-30 grams/d[103]	Same

For patients who are completely sedentary, multiply body weight in pounds by 0.4 and this will give the number of grams of protein that should be eaten each day.[104] For patients who are very active (frequent weight lifting, or competitive athlete), multiply body weight in pounds by 0.7-0.9 and this will give the number of grams of protein that should be eaten each day.

Again, compared with sedentary people, *sick people, injured people,* and *athletes* need more protein to maintain weight, fight infections, repair injuries, and build and maintain muscle. Not only can insufficient protein intake cause muscle weakness and loss of weight, but recent articles have also suggested that low-protein diets can cause suppression of the immune system[105] and impairment of healing after injury or surgery.[106]

For example, in most instances and according to the data presented in and reviewed for this section, a person weighing 120 pounds should aim for at least 60 grams of protein per day, or 90 grams of protein per day if he/she is more physically active, ill, or injured. A can of tuna has 30 grams of protein; one egg has 6 grams of protein. If she is going to eat eggs as a source of protein for a meal, she might have to eat as many as five eggs to reach a target of 30 grams of protein per meal. When eating meat, visualize the amount of meat in a can of tuna to estimate the amount of protein being eaten—for example, if the portion of meat at a given meal is about the size of a half can of tuna, then we can estimate that the serving contains 15-20 grams of high-quality protein. By knowing the "target intake" for the day, and by estimating the amount of protein eaten with each meal, patients will be able to modify their protein intake to ensure that they reach their protein intake goal.

Protein supplements—most common of which are based on concentrates of or isolated components of egg, soy, or cow's milk— can be used *in conjunction with a healthy diet.* Patients using a protein supplement should eat a healthy diet and then add protein supplements between regular meals. If they substitute a protein supplement for

[95] "Supplementation with protein and vitamins, specifically arginine and vitamins A, B, and C, provides optimum nutrient support of the healing wound." Meyer NA, Muller MJ, Herndon DN. Nutrient support of the healing wound. *New Horiz* 1994 May;2(2):202-14
[96] Castaneda et al. Elderly women accommodate to a low-protein diet with losses of body cell mass, muscle function, and immune response. *Am J Clin Nutr* 1995 Jul;62(1):30-9
[97] [No author listed]. Vegetarians and healing. *JAMA* 1995; 273: 910
[98] Heaney RP. Excess dietary protein may not adversely affect bone. *J Nutr* 1998 Jun;128(6):1054-7
[99] Lemon PW. Effects of exercise on dietary protein requirements. *Int J Sport Nutr* 1998 Dec;8(4):426-47
[100] Slightly modified from Nancy Clark, MS, RD. Protein Power. *The Physician and Sportsmedicine* 1996, volume 24, number 4
[101] 1.5-1 g/kg/d (0.68-0.45 grams per pound of body weight. Younger people need proportionately more protein.) Brown ML (ed). *Present Knowledge in Nutrition. Sixth Edition.* Washington DC: International Life Sciences Institute Nutrition Foundation; 1990 page 68
[102] 0.83 g.kg-1.d-1 (equivalent to 0.37 grams per pound of body weight) Pellet PL. Protein requirements in humans. *Am J Clin Nutr* 1990 May;51:723-37
[103] Weinsier RL, Morgan SL (eds). *Fundamentals of Clinical Nutrition.* St. Louis: Mosby, 1993 page 50
[104] Pellet PL. Protein requirements in humans. *Am J Clin Nutr* 1990 May;51(5):723-37
[105] Castaneda et al. Elderly women accommodate to a low-protein diet with losses of body cell mass, muscle function, and immune response. *Am J Clin Nutr* 1995 Jul;62:30-9
[106] Vegetarians and healing. *Journal of the American Medical Association* 1995; 273: 910

a regular meal, then they may not actually increase protein intake. Whole *real* foods should form the foundation for the diet—patients should not rely too heavily on *protein supplements* when patients can get better results *and improved overall health* with *whole foods*. Whey, casein, and lactalbumin are proteins from milk and dairy products, and may therefore be allergenic in people allergic to cow's milk; however, I (DrV) generally enjoy and endorse the use of whey protein isolate given its high-quality protein, convenience, low cost, antioxidant benefits via glutathione precursors, satiating effect via tryptophan provision, gut-

Proteins, fruits, vegetables—not grains

"Historical and archaeological evidence shows hunter-gatherers generally to be lean, fit, and largely free from signs and symptoms of chronic diseases. When hunter-gatherer societies transitioned to an agricultural grain-based diet, their general health deteriorated. ... When former hunter-gatherers adopt Western lifestyles, obesity, type-2 diabetes, atherosclerosis, and other diseases of civilization become commonplace."

O'Keefe JH Jr, Cordain L. Cardiovascular disease resulting from a diet and lifestyle at odds with our Paleolithic genome. *Mayo Clin Proc.* 2004;79:101-8

healing effects and immune-supporting and anti-dysbiotic immunoglobulins. Soy protein is safe and a source of high-quality protein for adults[107], and research shows that consumption of soy protein can help reduce the risk of cancer and heart disease[108]; however, I do not recommend the use of large quantities of supplemental soy protein for pregnant women, or for children due to the potential for disrupting endocrine function. Patients may have to experiment with different products until they find one that is suitable in regard to taste, texture, digestibility, hypoallergenicity, nutritional effects, ease of preparation, and affordability.

Recall again that the goal is *improved health*, not simply *adequate protein intake*. If we focus solely on "grams of protein" then we might overlook adverse effects that are associated with certain protein sources. Cow's milk is a high quality protein, but it is commonly allergenic and can exacerbate joint pain in sensitive individuals.[109] Beef, liver, pork and other land animal meats are excellent sources of protein, but they are also generally rich sources of arachidonic acid[110] (if not grass-fed) and iron[111], both of which have been shown to exacerbate joint pain and inflammation. Fish is an excellent source of protein, but fish are often poisoned with mercury and other toxicants, which can be ingested by humans to produce negative health effects.[112,113]

Most patients (and doctors) need to increase consumption of fruits and vegetables: Encourage consumption of collard greens, broccoli, kale, spinach, chard, lettuce, onions, red peppers, green beans, carrots, apples, oranges, nuts, blueberries and other fruits and vegetables. Patients can find or make a good low-carbohydrate dressing (such as lemon-garlic tahini[114]) to make these vegetables taste great. Fresh fruits and vegetables are best; but frozen fruits and vegetables are acceptable. Patients can buy a package of (organic) frozen vegetables; then when they are ready for a healthy-and-fast meal, simply thaw the vegetables or warm/steam them on the stovetop. In just a few minutes and with only minimal effort, by regularly eating vegetables, they will have significantly reduced their risk for heart disease, diabetes, cancer, hemorrhoids, constipation, and many other chronic health problems. Using frozen vegetables and eating vegetables only twice per day is not *optimal*—it is *minimal*. For many patients, consuming two servings of vegetables per day is a major lifestyle change. Ultimately, the goal is for fresh fruits and vegetables to form a major portion of the diet, to be the main course rather than simply a side dish. A diet based on fruits and vegetables is a powerful nutritional strategy for reducing the risk for cancer, heart disease, and autoimmune and inflammatory disorders.[115]

Phytochemicals—important antioxidant and anti-inflammatory nutrients from fruits, vegetables, nuts, seeds, berries, and many herbs and spices: While we have all commonly thought of the benefits of fruits and vegetables as being derived from the vitamins, minerals, and fiber, we are learning from new research that many if not most

---

[107] "These results indicate that for healthy adults, the isolated soy protein is of high nutritional quality, comparable to that of animal protein sources, and that the methionine content is not limiting for adult protein maintenance." Young et al. Evaluation of the protein quality of an isolated soy protein in young men: relative nitrogen requirements and effect of methionine supplementation. *Am J Clin Nutr.* 1984 Jan;39(1):16-24

[108] Lissin LW, Cooke JP. Phytoestrogens and cardiovascular health. *J Am Coll Cardiol.* 2000 May;35(6):1403-10

[109] Golding DN. Is there an allergic synovitis? *J R Soc Med* 1990 May;83(5):312-4

[110] Adam O, et al. Anti-inflammatory effects of a low arachidonic acid diet and fish oil in patients with rheumatoid arthritis. *Rheumatol Int* 2003 Jan;23(1):27-36

[111] Dabbagh AJ, Trenam CW, Morris CJ, Blake DR. Iron in joint inflammation. *Ann Rheum Dis* 1993; 52:67-73

[112] "These fish often harbor high levels of methylmercury, a potent human neurotoxin." Evans EC. The FDA recommendations on fish intake during pregnancy. *J Obstet Gynecol Neonatal Nurs* 2002 Nov-Dec;31(6):715-20

[113] "Geometric mean mercury levels were almost 4-fold higher among women who ate 3 or more servings of fish in the past 30 days compared with women who ate no fish in that period.." Schober SE, et al. Blood mercury levels in US children and women of childbearing age, 1999-2000. *JAMA* 2003 Apr 2;289(13):1667-74

[114] Mollie Katzen. *The New Moosewood Cookbook*, Ten Speed Press; page 103

[115] "...one of the most consistent research findings is that those who consume higher amounts of fruits and vegetables have lower rates of heart disease and stroke as well as cancer..." Seaman DR. The diet-induced proinflammatory state: a cause of chronic pain and other degenerative diseases? *J Manipulative Physiol Ther.* 2002;25(3):168-79

of the health-promoting benefits of fruit and vegetable consumption comes from the unique plant-based chemicals—phytochemicals—contained therein. For example, while in the past we might have thought of the benefits of eating apples as being derived from the vitamin C content, we now know that vitamin C only provides 0.4% of the antioxidant action contained within a whole apple—obviously the other components of the apple, namely the phenolic compounds are responsible for most of an apple's antioxidant activity.[116] Recent research has shown that cranberries, apples, red grapes, and strawberries have the most antioxidant power of the fruits[117], while red peppers, broccoli, carrots, and spinach are the best antioxidant vegetables[118]; see the tables that follow. This is a very important concept to appreciate and remember: **the benefits derived from fruits and vegetables are _not_ derived principally from the vitamins and therefore can never be obtained from the use of multivitamin pills as a substitute for whole foods. Multivitamin and multimineral supplements are valuable and worthwhile _supplements_ to a whole-foods diet but should not be used as _substitutes_ for a whole-foods diet. Fruits and vegetables contain more than 8,000 phytochemicals, most of which have anti-inflammatory, anti-proliferative, and anti-cancer benefits**[119]—**the best and only way to benefit from these chemicals is to change the diet in favor of relying principally on fruits and vegetables as the major component of the diet**, and the easiest way to do this is to eliminate carbohydrate-rich antioxidant-poor foods such as bread, pasta, rice, sweets, crackers, chips and "junk foods."

Phenolic content and antioxidant capacity of common vegetables and fruits[120,121]

Vegetables				Fruits			
Phenolic content		**Antioxidant capacity**		**Phenolic content**		**Antioxidant capacity**	
1.	**Broccoli**	1.	**Red pepper**	1.	**Cranberry**	1.	**Cranberry**
2.	**Spinach**	2.	**Broccoli**	2.	**Apple**	2.	**Apple**
3.	**Yellow onion**	3.	**Carrot**	3.	**Red grape**	3.	**Red grape**
4.	**Red pepper**	4.	**Spinach**	4.	**Strawberry**	4.	**Strawberry**
5.	Carrot	5.	Cabbage	5.	Pineapple	5.	Peach
6.	Cabbage	6.	Yellow onion	6.	Banana	6.	Lemon
7.	Potato	7.	Celery	7.	Peach	7.	Pear
8.	Lettuce	8.	Potato	8.	Lemon	8.	Banana
9.	Celery	9.	Lettuce	9.	Orange	9.	Orange
10.	Cucumber	10.	Cucumber	10.	Pear	10.	Grapefruit
				11.	Grapefruit	11.	Pineapple

Different fruits and vegetables contain different types, quantities, and ratios of vitamins, minerals, and phytochemicals; therefore, *dietary diversity* **will therefore help patients obtain a broad spectrum of and maximum benefit from these different nutrients**. Taking appropriate action with the data that a fruit/vegetable-based diet has powerful health-promoting benefits means that we as doctors and patients have to change our lifestyles with regard to how we plan our meals, what we buy, what we prepare, and what we eat. Behavior modification is a tremendous challenge for people, especially those who lack sufficient motivation or insight. This text is providing the *insight*—the data, references, and concepts. But without *motivation*—from doctors to help their patients attain the highest levels of health, and from patients to change their lifestyles to become as healthy as possible—the research itself does little to promote health.

Many people (most Americans especially) need to increase potassium intake: The physiologic effect of potassium is influenced by the potassium:sodium ratio (sodium reduces effectiveness and retention of potassium),

---

[116] "We propose that the additive and synergistic effects of phytochemicals in fruit and vegetables are responsible for their potent antioxidant and anticancer activities, and that the benefit of a diet rich in fruit and vegetables is attributed to the complex mixture of phytochemicals present in whole foods." Liu RH. Health benefits of fruit and vegetables are from additive and synergistic combinations of phytochemicals. *Am J Clin Nutr*. 2003 Sep;78(3 Suppl):517S-520S

[117] "Cranberry had the highest total antioxidant activity (177.0 +/- 4.3 micromol of vitamin C equiv/g of fruit), followed by apple, red grape, strawberry, peach, lemon, pear, banana, orange, grapefruit, and pineapple." Sun et al. Antioxidant and antiproliferative activities of common fruits. *J Agric Food Chem*. 2002 Dec 4;50(25):7449-54

[118] "Red pepper had the highest total antioxidant activity, followed by broccoli, carrot, spinach, cabbage, yellow onion, celery, potato, lettuce, and cucumber." Chu YF, Sun J, Wu X, Liu RH. Antioxidant and antiproliferative activities of common vegetables. *J Agric Food Chem*. 2002 Nov 6;50(23):6910-6

[119] Liu RH. Health benefits of fruit and vegetables are from additive and synergistic combinations of phytochemicals. *Am J Clin Nutr*. 2003 Sep;78(3 Suppl):517S-520S

[120] Chu YF, Sun J, Wu X, Liu RH. Antioxidant and antiproliferative activities of common vegetables. *J Agric Food Chem*. 2002;50:6910-6

[121] Sun J, Chu YF, Wu X, Liu RH. Antioxidant and antiproliferative activities of common fruits. *J Agric Food Chem*. 2002;50:7449-54

potassium:chloride ratio (chloride reduces effectiveness and retention of potassium), and the overall pH/acid-base balance of the human host (i.e., metabolic acidosis reduces effectiveness and retention of potassium, while an alkaline state improves retention and effectiveness of potassium). Importantly, magnesium status is an important positive-direct determinant of potassium status, particularly in patients with recalcitrant hypokalemia and/or hyperaldosteronism.[122] Respective amounts of potassium per serving of food or juice (1 cup = 8 fluid ounces =240 milliliters) are provided in the table below; renal insufficiency and potassium-sparing drugs/diuretics promote hyperkalemia, generally contraindicate high intake of potassium, and mandate periodic assessment of serum potassium.

Potassium content of common foods

Food serving	Potassium in mg (Na as available)	
One papaya	780	
One cup of mixed vegetable juice	740 (35-630 mg Na)	**The importance of potassium**
One cup of prune juice	700	"Adults should consume at least 4.7 grams of potassium per day to lower blood pressure, blunt the effects of salt, and reduce the risk of kidney stones and bone loss. However, most American women 31 to 50 years old consume no more than half of the recommended amount of potassium, and men's intake is only moderately higher."
One cup of carrot juice	520 (160 mg Na)	
One cup plain low-fat yogurt	510 (150 mg Na)	
One cup of cantaloupe	490	
One cup of orange juice	470	
One small banana	465	
One cup of honeydew melon	460	
One-third cup of raisins	365	Food and Nutrition Board of the Institute of Medicine of the National Academies. "Dietary Reference Intakes: Water, Potassium, Sodium, Chloride, and Sulfate." Released: February 11, 2004 iom.edu/Reports/2004/Dietary-Reference-Intakes-Water-Potassium-Sodium-Chloride-and-Sulfate.aspx
One cup of carrot-orange juice	360 (35 mg Na)	
One medium mango	320	
One medium kiwi	250	
One small orange	240	
One medium pear	210	

Antihypertensive mechanisms of potassium include vasodilator activity, diuretic and naturietic effects, and suppression of renin, angiotensin, and adrenergic tone.[123] In February 2004, the Institute of Medicine (IOM) set the Adequate Intake of potassium for adults at 4.7 grams a day—more than double previous recommendations; more than 90% of American adults do not meet these recommendations. If 90% of the population is not meeting recommended intakes of potassium, and these recommendations from the IOM come after an extensive review of the scientific literature, then potassium assessment and supplementation should be routine components of patient care; furthermore, this shows to the inadequacy of current laboratory assessments for evaluating potassium status and potassium balance.

- Randomized trial with 1-year follow-up and a title that says it all: Increasing the dietary potassium intake reduces the need for antihypertensive medication (*Annals of Internal Med* 1991 Nov): Forty-seven patients with medication-controlled hypertension completed one year of dietary treatment (or control nonintervention); dietary intervention focused on potassium-rich foods, with compliance monitored by 3-day food records and 24-hour urinary potassium excretion. Results showed: "After 1 year, the average drug consumption (number of pills per day) relative to that at baseline was 24% in group 1 (potassium-rich diet) and 60% in group 2 (control diet). By the end of the study, blood pressure could be controlled using less than 50% of the initial [drug] therapy in 81% of the patients in group 1 compared with 29% of the patients in group 2. ... CONCLUSION: Increasing the dietary potassium intake from natural foods is a feasible and effective measure to reduce antihypertensive drug treatment."

---

[122] "Magnesium deficiency is frequently associated with hypokalemia. Concomitant magnesium deficiency aggravates hypokalemia and renders it refractory to treatment by potassium. Herein is reviewed literature suggesting that magnesium deficiency exacerbates potassium wasting by increasing distal potassium secretion. A decrease in intracellular magnesium, caused by magnesium deficiency, releases the magnesium-mediated inhibition of ROMK channels and increases potassium secretion. Magnesium deficiency alone, however, does not necessarily cause hypokalemia. An increase in distal sodium delivery or elevated aldosterone levels may be required for exacerbating potassium wasting in magnesium deficiency." Huang CL, Kuo E. Mechanism of hypokalemia in magnesium deficiency. *J Am Soc Nephrol.* 2007 Oct;18(10):2649-52
[123] Patki et al. Efficacy of potassium and magnesium in essential hypertension: a double-blind, placebo controlled, crossover study. *BMJ.* 1990 Sep 15;301(6751):521-3

<u>**Eat "complex carbohydrates"—emphasizing whole foods and avoiding grains and sugars—to stabilize blood sugar, mood, and energy**</u>: Choose items with a "low glycemic index"[124] to stabilize blood sugar and—for many people—to lower triglycerides and cholesterol levels. Foods with a low Glycemic Index (GI < 55)[125] include yogurt, apple (36), whole orange (43), peach (28), legumes, lentils (28), and soybeans (18), cherries, dried apricots, nuts, most meats, and most vegetables. Foods that have both a low *glycemic index* as well as a low *glycemic load* include: apples, carrots, chick peas, grapes, green peas, kidney beans, oranges, peaches, peanuts, pears, pinto beans, red lentils, and strawberries.[126]

<u>**Reduce or eliminate simple sugars from the diet (as necessary)**</u>: Nearly everyone should minimize intake of table sugar (sucrose), fructose and high-fructose corn syrup, and all artificial sweeteners. Of important and recent note, high-fructose corn syrup has been shown to be contaminated by mercury due to the manufacturing process[127], and fructose has been shown to induce hypertension and the metabolic syndrome in humans.[128] Chronic overconsumption of refined carbohydrates promotes disease by 1) increasing urinary excretion of magnesium and calcium, 2) inducing oxidative stress, 3) promoting fat deposition and obesity, which then generally leads to insulin resistance and hyperinsulinemia with an increase in production of cholesterol, triglycerides, and proinflammatory adipokines[129], and 4) reducing function of leukocytes.[130] Among sweeteners, honey is the best choice since it is the only natural sweetener available with a wide range of health-promoting benefits including anti-inflammatory, antibacterial, antioxidant and anti-allergy effects.[131] Also consider the herb stevia as a non-caloric and nutritive sweetener. Occasional intake of sweets is likely to be of little consequence for people who are generally healthy and who are willing to sustain relatively short-term endothelial dysfunction[132], oxidative stress[133], increased LDL oxidation[134], and activation of NF-kappaB[135] as a result of their self-induced hyperglycemia. Postexertional hyperglycemia can be used to enhance athletic performance by sustaining and inducing glycogen storage following and during exercise (i.e., carbohydrate loading for glycogen "supercompensation"[136,137]). Similarly, consumption of "simple" carbohydrate without protein can be used to promote entry of tryptophan across the blood-brain barrier and into the brain to promote serotonin synthesis.[138] In summary, *habitual overconsumption* of simple carbohydrates promotes disease by numerous oxidative and pro-inflammatory mechanisms, while conversely *periodic consumption* of simple carbohydrates can be used to promote athletic performance and to increase brain tryptophan uptake and thus serotonin synthesis for the promotion of enhanced mood and cognitive performance and for the regulation of food intake.

---

[124] For more information on glycemic index, consult a nutrition book or website such as stanford.edu/~dep/gilists.htm

[125] Janette Brand-Miller, Kaye Foster-Powell. Diets with a low glycemic index. *Nutr Today* 1999 Mar findarticles.com/cf_dls/m0841/2_34/54654508/p1/article.jhtml

[126] Mendosa D. Glycemic Values of Common American Foods mendosa.com/common_foods.htm Accessed on August 4, 2004

[127] "Average daily consumption of high fructose corn syrup is about 50 grams per person in the United States. With respect to total mercury exposure, it may be necessary to account for this source of mercury in the diet of children and sensitive populations." Dufault et al. Mercury from chlor-alkali plants. *Environ Health*. 2009 Jan 26;8:2. See also: "High fructose corn syrup has been shown to contain trace amounts of mercury as a result of some manufacturing processes, and its consumption can also lead to zinc loss." Dufault et al. Mercury exposure, nutritional deficiencies and metabolic disruptions may affect learning in children. *Behav Brain Funct*. 2009 Oct 27;5:44.

[128] News release from American Heart Association's 63rd High Blood Pressure Research Conference. High-sugar diet increases men's blood pressure; gout drug protective. Abstract P127. Sept. 23, 2009. americanheart.mediaroom.com/index.php?s=43&item=829 Accessed December 19, 2009

[129] "Because visceral and subcutaneous adipose tissues are the major sources of cytokines (adipokines), increased adipose tissue mass is associated with alteration in adipokine production (eg, overexpression of tumor necrosis factor-a, interleukin-6, plasminogen activator inhibitor-1, and underexpression of adiponectin in adipose tissue)." Aldahhi W, Hamdy O. Adipokines, inflammation, and the endothelium in diabetes. *Curr Diab Rep*. 2003 Aug;3(4):293-8

[130] Sanchez A, et al. Role of sugars in human neutrophilic phagocytosis. *Am J Clin Nutr*. 1973 Nov;26(11):1180-4

[131] Al-Waili NS. Effects of daily consumption of honey solution on hematological indices and blood levels of minerals and enzymes. *J Med Food*. 2003 Summer;6(2):135-4

[132] "Modest hyperinsulinemia, mimicking fasting hyperinsulinemia of insulin-resistant states, abrogates endothelium-dependent vasodilation in large conduit arteries, probably by increasing oxidant stress. These data may provide a novel pathophysiological basis to the epidemiological link between hyperinsulinemia/insulin-resistance and atherosclerosis in humans." Arcaro G, et al. Insulin causes endothelial dysfunction in humans: sites and mechanisms. *Circulation*. 2002 Feb 5;105(5):576-82

[133] "Hyperglycemia increased plasma MDA concentrations, but the activities of GSH-Px and SOD were significantly higher after a larger dose of glucose only. Plasma catecholamines were unchanged. These results indicate that the transient increase of plasma catecholamine and insulin concentrations did not induce oxidative damage, while glucose already in the low dose was an important triggering factor for oxidative stress." Koska J, Blazicek P, Marko M, Grna JD, Kvetnansky R, Vigas M. Insulin, catecholamines, glucose and antioxidant enzymes in oxidative damage during different loads in healthy humans. *Physiol Res*. 2000;49 Suppl 1:S95-100

[134] "In conclusion, insulin at physiological doses is associated with increased LDL peroxidation independent of the presence of hyperglycemia." Quinones-Galvan et al. Evidence that acute insulin administration enhances LDL cholesterol susceptibility to oxidation in healthy humans. *Arterioscler Thromb Vasc Biol*. 1999 Dec;19(12):2928-32

[135] "These data show that the intake of a mixed meal results in significant inflammatory changes characterized by a decrease in IkappaBalpha and an increase in NF-kappaB binding, plasma CRP, and the expression of IKKalpha, IKKbeta, and p47(phox) subunit." Aljada A, Mohanty P, Ghanim H, Abdo T, Tripathy D, Chaudhuri A, Dandona P. Increase in intranuclear nuclear factor kappaB and decrease in inhibitor kappaB in mononuclear cells after a mixed meal. *Am J Clin Nutr*. 2004 Apr;79(4):682-90

[136] "A significant glycogen sparing, as well as supercompensation within 24 h of recovery, was observed after [carbohydrate] supplementation." Brouns F, Saris WH, Beckers E, Adlercreutz H, et al. Metabolic changes induced by sustained exhaustive cycling and diet manipulation. *Int J Sports Med*. 1989 May;10 Suppl 1:S49-62

[137] "The accepted method of increasing muscle glycogen stores is by "glycogen loading," which classically involves depletion of muscle glycogen, usually by exercise, followed by consumption of a high-CHO diet for several days (e.g., 3, 39). ...increase muscle glycogen concentrations ([glycogen]) to between 150 and 200% of normal resting levels." Robinson et al. Role of submaximal exercise in promoting creatine and glycogen accumulation in human skeletal muscle. *J Appl Physiol*. 1999 Aug;87(2):598-604

[138] "Our results suggest that high-carbohydrate meals have an influence on serotonin synthesis. We predict that carbohydrates with a high glycemic index would have a greater serotoninergic effect than carbohydrates with a low glycemic index." Lyons PM, Truswell AS. Serotonin precursor influenced by type of carbohydrate meal in healthy adults. *Am J Clin Nutr*. 1988 Mar;47(3):433-9

Avoid artificial sweeteners, colors and other additives: Absolutely never use **aspartame**—this is a synthetic chemical that is easily converted to the toxin formaldehyde.[139] Aspartame causes cancer in animals and is strongly linked to brain tumors in humans.[140,141] **Sodium benzoate** is a food preservative that can cause asthma[142] and skin rashes[143] in sensitive individuals. **Tartrazine (yellow dye #5)** is a food/drug coloring agent that can cause asthma and skin rashes in sensitive individuals.[144] **Carrageenan** is a naturally-occurring carbohydrate extracted from red seaweed. Common sources of carrageenan are certain brands of "rice milk" and "soy milk." In addition to suppressing immune function[145], carrageenan causes intestinal ulcers and inflammatory bowel disease in animals[146] and some research indicates that carrageenan consumption is associated with an increased risk for cancer in humans.[147,148]

Consume sufficient daily water in the form of water and health-promoting teas and juices: Daily "water" intake should be approximately 30 ml/kg; thus, for a 150-lb (70-kg) person, fluid intake should be at least 2.1 liters, and for a person who weighs 220 lbs (100 kg) the daily intake should be approximately 3 liters. More fluids may be used during times of exercise, heat exposure, illness, or detoxification, while fluid restriction can be indicated in patients with heart failure, renal failure, anasarca (generalized edema), and hyponatremia.

Consider reducing or eliminating caffeine: This is especially important for people with reactive hypoglycemia, insomnia, anxiety, hypertension, low-back pain, and for women with fibrocystic breast disease. Caffeine ingestion also leads to the activation of brain noradrenergic receptors; activation of noradrenergic receptors can cause inhibition of dopaminergic neurotransmission.[149] For people who are in good health, 1-3 servings of caffeine per day are not harmful. Herbal teas in general and green tea in particular have significant health-promoting effects due to their phytonutrient components and antioxidant, anti-inflammatory, and anticancer properties.

To the extent possible, eat "organic" foods rather than industrially-produced foods: Organic foods (i.e., foods which are *naturally grown* rather than being treated with insect poisons, synthetic fertilizers, and chemicals to enhance shelf-life) tend to cost more than chemically-produced foods; but the increased phytonutrient content justifies the cost. Organic foods contain more nutrients than do chemically-produced foods.[150] More importantly, recent research has also indicated that organic foods are better able to prevent the genetic damage that can lead to cancer than are foods that have been grown in an environment of artificial fertilizers and pesticides.[151]

- Reduction in urinary organophosphate pesticide metabolites in adults after a week-long organic diet. (*Environ Res* 2014 Jul[152]): Industrial/corporate food production commonly uses organophosphate (OP) pesticides; this prospective, randomised, crossover study was conducted to determine if an organic food diet reduces organophosphate exposure in adults. "Thirteen participants were randomly allocated to consume a diet of at least 80% organic or conventional food for 7 days and then crossed over to the opposite diet. Urinary levels of six dialkylphosphate (DAP) metabolites were analysed in first-morning voids collected on day 8 of each phase using GC-MS/MS with detection limits of 0.11-0.51μg/L. RESULTS: The mean total DAP results in the organic phase were 89% lower than in the conventional phase. For total

---

[139] Trocho C, et al. Formaldehyde derived from dietary aspartame binds to tissue components in vivo. *Life Sci.* 1998;63(5):337-4949

[140] Compared to other environmental factors putatively linked to brain tumors, the artificial sweetener aspartame is a promising candidate to explain the recent increase in incidence and degree of malignancy of brain tumors. ...exceedingly high incidence of brain tumors in aspartame-fed rats compared to no brain tumors in concurrent controls..." Olney JW, Farber NB, Spitznagel E, Robins LN. Increasing brain tumor rates: is there a link to aspartame? *J Neuropathol Exp Neurol* 1996;55(11):1115-23

[141] Russell Blaylock MD. *Excitotoxins*. Health Press; December 1996 [ISBN: 0929173252] Pages 211-214

[142] "Adverse reactions to benzoate in this patient required avoidance of some drugs, some of those classically prescribed under the form of syrups in asthma." Petrus M, Bonaz S, Causse E, Rhabbour M, Moulie N, Netter JC, Bildstein G. [Asthma and intolerance to benzoates] [Article in French] *Arch Pediatr.* 1996;3(10):984-7

[143] Munoz FJ, et al. Perioral contact urticaria from sodium benzoate in a toothpaste. *Contact Dermatitis.* 1996 Jul;35(1):51

[144] "Tartrazine sensitivity is most frequently manifested by urticaria and asthma... Vasculitis, purpura and contact dermatitis infrequently occur as manifestations of tartrazine sensitivity." Dipalma JR. Tartrazine sensitivity. *Am Fam Physician.* 1990 Nov;42(5):1347-50

[145] "Impairment of complement activity and humoral responses to T-dependent antigens, depression of cell-mediated immunity, prolongation of graft survival and potentiation of tumour growth by carrageenans have been reported." Thomson AW, Fowler EF. Carrageenan: a review of its effects on the immune system. *Agents Actions.* 1981;11:265-73

[146] Watt J, Marcus R. Experimental ulcerative disease of the colon. *Methods Achiev Exp Pathol.* 1975;7:56-71

[147] Tobacman JK. Review of harmful gastrointestinal effects of carrageenan in animal experiments. *Environ Health Perspect.* 2001 Oct;109(10):983-94

[148] "However, the gum carrageenan which is comprised of linked, sulfated galactose residues has potent biological activity and undergoes acid hydrolysis to poligeenan, an acknowledged carcinogen." Tobacman JK, Wallace RB, Zimmerman MB. Consumption of carrageenan and other water-soluble polymers used as food additives and incidence of mammary carcinoma. *Med Hypotheses.* 2001 May;56(5):589-98

[149] "The results suggest that noradrenergic innervation of dopamine cells can directly inhibit the activity of dopamine cells." Paladini CA, Williams JT. Noradrenergic inhibition of midbrain dopamine neurons. *J Neurosci.* 2004 May 12;24(19):4568-75

[150] Smith B. Organic Foods versus Supermarket Foods: element levels. *Journal of Applied Nutrition* 1993; 45(1), p35-9

[151] "Against BaP, three species of OC vegetables showed 30-57% antimutagenecity, while GC ones did only 5-30%." Ren H, Endo H, Hayashi T. The superiority of organically cultivated vegetables to general ones regarding antimutagenic activities. *Mutat Res.* 2001 Sep 20;496(1-2):83-8

[152] Oates L, Cohen M, Braun L, et al. Reduction in urinary organophosphate pesticide metabolites in adults after a week-long organic diet. *Environ Res.* 2014 Jul;132:105-11

dimethyl DAPs there was a 96% reduction. Mean total diethyl DAP levels in the organic phase were half [-50% reduction] those of the conventional phase, yet the wide variability and small sample size meant the difference was not statistically significant. CONCLUSIONS: The consumption of an organic diet for one week significantly reduced organophosphate pesticide exposure in adults. Larger scale studies in different populations are required to confirm these findings and investigate their clinical relevance."

Recognize the importance of avoiding food allergens: Biomedical research has established that adverse food reactions, regardless of the underlying mechanisms or classification of allergy, intolerance, or sensitivity, can exacerbate a wide range of human illnesses, including thyroid disease[153], mental depression[154,155], asthma, rhinitis,[156] recurrent otitis media[157], migraine[158,159,160], attention deficit and hyperactivity disorders[161], epilepsy[162,163,164], gastrointestinal inflammation[165], hypertension[166], joint pain and inflammation[167,168,169,170,171,172,173,174] and a wide range of other health problems. Any program of health promotion and health maintenance must include consideration of food allergies, food intolerances, and food sensitivities. The elimination-and-challenge technique is the most cost-effective and it also teaches patients how to identify their own food allergies and intolerances, which may change for the better or worse over time; when the patient is empowered with this technique, he/she can take an active and on-going role in his/her own healthcare. Patients may be allergic to foods that are generally considered healthy, including whole organic foods. The more common food allergens—exemplified here by a list of offending foods identified in a study of patients with migraine[175]—are wheat (78%), orange (65%), eggs (45%), tea and coffee (40% each), chocolate and milk (37% each), beef (35%), and corn, cane sugar, and yeast (33% each).

Avoid microwave heating/cooking: Microwave ovens have been noted to exude electromagnetic radiation and may also structurally change native amino acids, forming racemic derivatives that might have no nutritional value (e.g., when converted from the natural L isomer to the abnormal R isomer) and/or toxic effects. In his extensive and clinically-experienced review of the nutrition literature, Gaby[176] writes, "Microwaving of infant formulas caused racemization of some amino acids that did not occur with conventional heating. One of these racemized amino acids, D-proline, has been shown to be neurotoxic, nephrotoxic, and hepatotoxic."

Supplement the health-promoting whole-foods diet with specific vitamins, minerals, fatty acids, and probiotics: Despite the fact that America is one of the richest nations on earth, and that we produce more than enough food to feed ourselves and many other nations with a healthy diet, Americans tend to have poor dietary habits and

[153] Sategna-Guidetti et al. Prevalence of thyroid disorders in untreated adult celiac disease patients and effect of gluten withdrawal. *Am J Gastroenterol.* 2001 Mar;96(3):751-7

[154] "The detection and treatment of psychological dysfunction related to food intolerance with particular reference to the problem of objective evaluation is discussed… Long-term follow-up revealed maintenance of marked improvements in psychological and physical functioning." Mills N. Depression and food intolerance: a single case study. *Hum Nutr Appl Nutr.* 1986 Apr;40(2):141-5

[155] "OBJECTIVE: To describe a patient with food intolerance probably contributing to depressive symptoms, intolerance to psychotropic medication and treatment resistance… RESULTS: The patient's course improved considerably with an elimination diet." Parker G, Watkins T. Treatment-resistant depression: when antidepressant drug intolerance may indicate food intolerance. *Aust N Z J Psychiatry.* 2002 Apr;36(2):263-5

[156] Speer F. The allergic child. *Am Fam Physician.* 1975 Feb;11(2):88-94

[157] Juntti H, Tikkanen S, Kokkonen J, Alho OP, Niinimaki A. Cow's milk allergy is associated with recurrent otitis media during childhood. *Acta Otolaryngol.* 1999;119:867-73

[158] "Foods which provoked migraine in 9 patients with severe migraine refractory to drug therapy were identified… These observations confirm that a food-allergic reaction is the cause of migraine in this group of patients." Monro J, Carini C, Brostoff J. Migraine is a food-allergic disease. *Lancet.* 1984 Sep 29;2(8405):719-21

[159] Egger J, Carter CM, Wilson J, et al. Is migraine food allergy? A double-blind controlled trial of oligoantigenic diet treatment. *Lancet.* 1983 Oct 15;2(8355):865-9

[160] Monro J, Brostoff J, Carini C, Zilkha K. Food allergy in migraine. Study of dietary exclusion and RAST. *Lancet.* 1980 Jul 5;2(8184):1-4

[161] Boris M, Mandel FS. Foods and additives are common causes of the attention deficit hyperactive disorder in children. *Ann Allergy.* 1994 May;72(5):462-8

[162] Egger J, Carter CM, Soothill JF, Wilson J. Oligoantigenic diet treatment of children with epilepsy and migraine. *J Pediatr.* 1989;114(1):51-8

[163] Pelliccia et al. Partial cryptogenetic epilepsy and food allergy/intolerance. Reflections on three clinical cases. *Minerva Pediatr.* 1999 May;51(5):153-7

[164] Frediani T, Lucarelli S, Pelliccia A, Vagnucci B, et al. Allergy and childhood epilepsy: a close relationship? *Acta Neurol Scand.* 2001;104(6):349-52

[165] Marr HY, Chen WC, Lin LH. Food protein-induced enterocolitis syndrome: report of one case. *Acta Paediatr Taiwan.* 2001;42(1):49-52

[166] Grant EC. Food allergies and migraine. *Lancet.* 1979 May 5;1(8123):966-9

[167] "Food allergy appeared to be responsible for the joint symptoms in three patients and in one it was possible to precipitate swelling of a knee due to synovitis with effusion by drinking milk a few hours beforehand, the synovial fluid having mildly inflammatory features and a relatively high eosinophil count." Golding DN. Is there an allergic synovitis? *J R Soc Med.* 1990 May;83(5):312-4

[168] Panush RS. Food induced ("allergic") arthritis: clinical and serologic studies. *J Rheumatol.* 1990 Mar;17(3):291-4

[169] Pacor ML, Lunardi C, Di Lorenzo G, Biasi D, Corrocher R. Food allergy and seronegative arthritis: report of two cases. *Clin Rheumatol.* 2001;20(4):279-81

[170] Schrander JJ, Marcelis C, de Vries MP, van Santen-Hoeufft HM. Does food intolerance play a role in juvenile chronic arthritis? *Br J Rheumatol.* 1997 Aug;36(8):905-8

[171] van de Laar MA, van der Korst JK. Food intolerance in rheumatoid arthritis. I. A double blind, controlled trial of the clinical effects of elimination of milk allergens and azo dyes. *Ann Rheum Dis.* 1992 Mar;51(3):298-302

[172] Haugen MA, Kjeldsen-Kragh J, Forre O. A pilot study of the effect of an elemental diet in the management of rheumatoid arthritis. *Clin Exp Rheumatol.* 1994;12(3):275-9

[173] van de Laar MA, Aalbers M, Bruins FG, et al. Food intolerance in rheumatoid arthritis. II. Clinical and histological aspects. *Ann Rheum Dis.* 1992;51(3):303-6

[174] Panush RS, Stroud RM, Webster EM. Food-induced (allergic) arthritis. Inflammatory arthritis exacerbated by milk. *Arthritis Rheum* 1986; 29(2): 220-6

[175] Grant EC. Food allergies and migraine. *Lancet.* 1979 May 5;1(8123):966-9

[176] Gaby AR. *Nutritional Medicine.* 2011

inadequate levels of nutritional intake that do not meet the minimal standards, such as the Recommended Daily Allowance (RDA, now Daily Reference Intake (DRI)).[177] Many people are under the misperception that if they appear healthy or are even overweight then they could not possibly have nutritional deficiencies. The truths of this matter are that 1) gross/obvious nutritional deficiencies are common among "apparently healthy" individuals, 2) common situations like stress, poor diets, and use of medications predispose people to nutritional deficiencies, 3) hereditary/genetic disorders affect a large portion of the population and lead to an increased need for nutritional intake which can generally only be met with supplementation in addition to a healthy whole-foods diet. Taking a "one-a-day" multivitamin is insufficient for people who truly desire significant benefit from supplementation. These one-a-day preparations generally only provide the minimum daily allowance—this dose is not large enough to provide truly preventive medicine results; also, such one-a-day products tend to contain low-quality nutrients, such as ergocalciferol rather than cholecalciferol[178], cyanocobalamin rather than the hydroxyl-, methyl-, or adenosyl- forms[179], and DL-tocopherol or exclusively L-alpha-tocopherol rather than a mix of tocopherols with a high concentration (generally approximately 40%) of gamma tocopherol.[180] Additional rationale for the routine and case-specific use of nutritional supplements is provided in later sections of this book and in the clinical protocols published in following volumes; the points below serve to introduce a few basic concepts:

- Many people think that eating a "healthy diet" will supply them with the nutrients that they need and that they do not need to take a vitamin supplement. This may have been true 2000 years ago, but today's industrially produced "foods" are generally stripped of much of their nutritional value long before they leave the factory. Industrially-produced fruits and vegetables contain lower quantities of nutrients than does naturally raised "organic" produce.[181]

- The reason that people can be of normal weight or can even be overweight and obese and still have nutrient deficiencies is that the body lowers the metabolic rate when the intake of vitamins and minerals is low. This is referred to as the "physiologic adaptation to marginal malnutrition." Even though people may eat enough calories and protein, they can still suffer from growth retardation and behavioral problems as a result of micronutrient malnutrition, even though they *appear* nourished.[182]

- Most nutrition-oriented doctors will agree that magnesium is one of the most important *supplemental* nutrients, especially for helping prevent heart attack and stroke. **Magnesium deficiency is an epidemic in so-called "developed" nations, with 20-40% of different populations showing objective laboratory evidence of magnesium deficiency.**[183,184,185,186]

- Add to the above that every day we are confronted with more chronic emotional stress and toxic chemicals than has ever before existed on the planet, and it becomes easy to see that basic nutritional support and an organic whole foods diet is just the start of attaining improved health.

General Guidelines for the Safe Use of Nutritional Supplements:
Supplementation with vitamins and minerals is generally safe, especially if the following guidelines are followed:

- <u>Vitamins and minerals should generally be taken with food in order to eliminate the possibility of nausea and to increase absorption</u>: Most vitamins and other supplements should be taken with food so that nausea is avoided.

---

[177] "Most people do not consume an optimal amount of all vitamins by diet alone. Pending strong evidence of effectiveness from randomized trials, it appears prudent for all adults to take vitamin supplements." Fletcher RH, Fairfield KM. Vitamins for chronic disease prevention in adults: clinical applications. *JAMA* 2002 Jun 19;287(23):3127-9

[178] "Vitamin D(2) potency is less than one third that of vitamin D(3). Physicians resorting to use of vitamin D(2) should be aware of its markedly lower potency and shorter duration of action relative to vitamin D(3)." Armas et al. Vitamin D2 is much less effective than vitamin D3 in humans. *J Clin Endocrinol Metab*. 2004 Nov;89(11):5387-91

[179] Freeman AG. Cyanocobalamin--a case for withdrawal: discussion paper. *J R Soc Med*. 1992 Nov;85(11):686–687

[180] "gamma-tocopherol is the major form of vitamin E in many plant seeds and in the US diet, but has drawn little attention compared with alpha-tocopherol, the predominant form of vitamin E in tissues and the primary form in supplements. However, recent studies indicate that gamma-tocopherol may be important to human health and that it possesses unique features that distinguish it from alpha-tocopherol." Jiang Q, Christen S, Shigenaga MK, Ames BN. gamma-tocopherol, the major form of vitamin E in the US diet, deserves more attention. *Am J Clin Nutr*. 2001 Dec;74(6):714-22 ajcn.org/content/74/6/714.full.pdf

[181] Smith B. Organic Foods versus Supermarket Foods: element levels. *Journal of Applied Nutrition* 1993; 45(1), p35-9

[182] Allen LH. The nutrition CRSP: what is marginal malnutrition, and does it affect human function? *Nutr Rev* 1993 Sep;51(9):255-67

[183] "The American diet is low in magnesium, and with modern water systems, very little is ingested in the drinking water." Innerarity S. Hypomagnesemia in acute and chronic illness. *Crit Care Nurs Q*. 2000 Aug;23(2):1-19

[184] "Altogether 43% of 113 trauma patients had low magnesium levels compared to 30% of noninjured cohorts." Frankel et al. Hypomagnesemia in trauma patients. *World J Surg*. 1999 Sep;23(9):966-9

[185] "There was a 20% overall prevalence of hypomagnesemia among this predominantly female, African American population." Fox et al. An investigation of hypomagnesemia among ambulatory urban African Americans. *J Fam Pract*. 1999 Aug;48(8):636-9

[186] "Suboptimal levels were detected in 33.7 per cent of the population under study. These data clearly demonstrate that the Mg supply of the German population needs increased attention." Schimatschek HF, Rempis R. Prevalence of hypomagnesemia in an unselected German population of 16,000 individuals. *Magnes Res*. 2001 Dec;14(4):283-90

- <u>Iron is potentially harmful</u>: Iron promotes the formation of reactive oxygen species ("free radicals") and is thus implicated in several diseases, such as infections, cancer, liver disease, diabetes, and cardiovascular disease. Iron supplements should not be consumed except by people who have been definitively diagnosed with iron deficiency by measurement of serum ferritin. Iron supplementation without documentation of iron deficiency by measurement of serum ferritin is inappropriate. [187]

- <u>Vitamin A is one of the only vitamins with the potential for serious toxicity even at low doses</u>: Attention should be given to vitamin A intake so that toxicity is avoided. Total intake of vitamin A must account for all sources—foods, fish oils, and vitamin supplements. Manifestations of vitamin A toxicity include: skin problems (dry skin, flaking skin, chapped or split lips, red skin rash, hair loss), joint pain, bone pain, headaches, anorexia (loss of appetite), edema (water retention, weight gain, swollen ankles, difficulty breathing), fatigue, and/or liver damage. Whenever vitamin A is used in high doses, it must be used for a defined period of time in order to avoid the toxicity that will result from high-dose long-term vitamin A supplementation.

  o <u>Adults</u>: Women who are pregnant or might become pregnant and who are planning to carry the baby to full term delivery should not ingest more than 10,000 IU of vitamin A per day. Vitamin A toxicity is seen with chronic ingestion of therapeutic doses (for example: 25,000 IU per day for 6 years, or 100,000 IU per day for 2.5 years[188]). Most patients should not consume more than 25,000 IU of vitamin A per day for more than 2 months without express supervision by a healthcare provider. Vitamin A is present in some multivitamins, in animal liver and products such as fish liver oil, and in other supplements—read labels to ensure that the total daily intake is not greater than 25,000 IU per day.

  o <u>Infants and Children</u>: Different studies have used either daily or monthly schedules of vitamin A supplementation. In a study with extremely low-birth weight infants, 5,000 IU of vitamin A per day for 28 days was safely used.[189] In another study conducted in sick children, those aged less than 12 months received 100,000 IU on two consecutive days, while children between ages 12-60 months received a larger dose of 200,000 IU on two consecutive days.[190]

- <u>Preexisting kidney problems (such as renal insufficiency) increase the risks associated with nutritional supplementation</u>: Supplementation with vitamins and minerals does not cause kidney damage. However, if a patient already has kidney problems, then nutritional supplementation may become hazardous; this is particularly true with magnesium and potassium and perhaps also with vitamin C. Assessment of renal function with serum or urine tests is encouraged before beginning an aggressive plan of supplementation. Conditions which cause kidney damage include use of specific drugs (e.g., acetaminophen, aspirin, contrast and chemotherapy agents, cocaine), acute or chronic high blood pressure, diabetes mellitus and other diseases such as lupus (SLE), polycystic kidney disease, and scleroderma.

- <u>Pre-existing medical conditions may make supplementation unsafe</u>: A few rare medical conditions may cause nutritional supplementation to be unsafe, including severe liver disease, renal failure, electrolyte imbalances, hyperparathyroidism and other vitamin D hypersensitivity syndromes.

- <u>Several drugs/medications may adversely interact with vitamin/mineral supplements and with botanical medicines</u>: Vitamins/minerals may reduce the effectiveness of some prescription medications. For example, taking certain antibiotics such as ciprofloxacin or tetracycline with calcium reduces absorption of the drugs, therefore rendering the drugs much less effective. Taking botanical medicines with medications may make the drugs dangerously less effective (such as when St. John's Wort is combined with protease inhibitor drugs[191]) or may make the drug dangerously more effective (such when Kava is combined with the anti-

[187] Hollán S, Johansen KS. Adequate iron stores and the 'Nil nocere' principle.*Haematologia* (Budap). 1993;25(2):69-84

[188] "The smallest continuous daily consumption leading to cirrhosis was 25,000 IU during 6 years, whereas higher daily doses (greater than or equal to 100,000 IU) taken during 2 1/2 years resulted in similar histological lesions. ... The data also indicate that prolonged and continuous consumption of doses in the low "therapeutic" range can result in life-threatening liver damage." Geubel et al. Liver damage caused by therapeutic vitamin A administration: estimate dose-related toxicity in 41 cases. *Gastroenterol* 1991 Jun:1701-9

[189] "Infants with birth weight < 1000 g were randomised at birth to receive oral vitamin A supplementation (5000 IU/day) or placebo for 28 days." Wardle SP, Hughes A, Chen S, Shaw NJ. Randomised controlled trial of oral vitamin A supplementation in preterm infants to prevent chronic lung disease. *Arch Dis Child Fetal Neonatal Ed.* 2001 Jan;84(1):F9-F13 Available on-line at adc.bmjjournals.com/cgi/content/full/fetalneonatal%3b84/1/F9

[190] "Children were assigned to oral doses of 200 000 IU vitamin A (half that dose if <12 months) or placebo on the day of admission, a second dose on the following day, and third and fourth doses at 4 and 8 months after discharge from the hospital, respectively." Villamor E, Mbise R, Spiegelman D, Hertzmark E, Fataki M, Peterson KE, Ndossi G, Fawzi WW. Vitamin A supplements ameliorate the adverse effect of HIV-1, malaria, and diarrheal infections on child growth. *Pediatrics.* 2002 Jan;109(1):E6

[191] Piscitelli SC, Burstein AH, Chaitt D, Alfaro RM, Falloon J. Indinavir concentrations and St John's wort. *Lancet.* 2000 Feb 12;355(9203):547-8

anxiety drug alprazolam[192]). If vitamin D is used in doses greater than 1,000 IU/d in patients taking hydrochlorothiazide or other calcium-retaining drugs, serum calcium should be monitored at least monthly until safety (i.e., lack of hypercalcemia) has been established per patient.[193] Patients should not combine nutritional or botanical medicines with chemical/synthetic drugs without specific advice from a knowledgeable doctor. Do not increase vitamin K consumption from supplements or dietary improvements in patients taking coumadin/warfarin. A reasonable recommendation is that nutritional supplements be taken 2 hours away from pharmaceutical medications to avoid complications such as intraintestinal drug-nutrient binding.

Advanced concepts in nutrition—an introduction

<u>**Biochemical Individuality and Orthomolecular Medicine**</u>: "Biochemical individuality" was the term coined by biochemist Dr. Roger Williams of the University of Texas[194] to describe the genetic and physiologic variations in human beings that produced different nutritional needs among individuals. Some enzymes essential for proper cellular function are adversely affected by defects in their construction (i.e., amino acid sequence) that reduce their efficiency. Dr. Linus Pauling, who discovered the molecular basis for the hemoglobinopathy of sickle cell anemia, noted that single amino acid substitutions could produce dramatic alterations in protein function.[195] Pauling discovered that sickle cell disease was caused by a single amino acid substitution in the hemoglobin molecule, and for this discovery he won the Nobel Prize in Chemistry in 1954.[196] With recognition of the importance of individual molecules in determining health or disease, Pauling coined the phrase "orthomolecular medicine" based on his thesis that many diseases could be effectively prevented and treated if we used the "right molecules" to correct abnormal physiologic function. Pauling contrasted the clinical use of nutrients for the improvement of physiologic function (orthomolecular medicine) with the use of chemical drugs, which generally work by interfering with normal physiology (toximolecular medicine). Since nutrients are the fundamental elements of the human body from which all enzymes, chemicals, and cellular structures are formed, Pauling advocated that the use of customized nutrition and nutritional

> ### Orthomolecular precepts
> - The functions of the body are dependent upon thousands of enzymes. Because of genetic defects that are common in the general population, some of these enzymes are commonly defective – even if only slightly – in large portions of the human population.
> - Enzyme defects reduce the function and efficiency of important chemical reactions. Because enzymes are so important for normal function and the prevention of disease, defects in enzyme function can result in disruptions in physiology and the creation of what later manifests as "disease."
> - Rather than treating these diseases with synthetic chemical drugs, it is commonly possible to prevent and treat disease with high-doses of vitamins, minerals, and other nutrients to compensate for or bypass metabolic dysfunctions, thus allowing for the promotion of optimal health by promoting optimal physiologic function.
>
> Ames et al. High-dose vitamin therapy stimulates variant enzymes with decreased coenzyme binding affinity (increased K(m)). *Am J Clin Nutr*. 2002 Apr

supplements could promote optimal health by optimizing cellular function and efficiency. More recently, Dr. Bruce Ames has thoroughly documented the science of the orthomolecular precepts[197] and has advocated optimal diets along with nutritional supplementation as a highly efficient and cost-effective method for preventing disease and optimizing health.[198,199] In sum, we see that 1) the foundational diet must be formed from whole foods such as fruits, nuts, seeds, vegetables, and lean meats, 2) processed and artificial foods should be avoided, and 3) the use of nutritional supplements is necessary to provide sufficiently high levels of nutrition to overcome defects in enzymatic activity.

---

[192] Almeida JC, Grimsley EW. Coma from the health food store: interaction between kava and alprazolam. *Ann Intern Med*. 1996 Dec 1;125(11):940-1

[193] Vasquez A, Manso G, Cannell J. The clinical importance of vitamin D (cholecalciferol): a paradigm shift. *Altern Ther Health Med*. 2004 Sep-Oct;10(5):28-36

[194] "Every individual organism that has a distinctive genetic background has distinctive nutritional needs which must be met for optimal well-being. …[N]utrition applied with due concern for individual genetic variations…offers the solution to many baffling health problems." Williams RJ. *Biochemical Individuality*. University of Texas, 1956. Page x

[195] "…the concentration of coenzyme [vitamins and minerals] needed to produce the amount of active enzyme required for optimum health may well be somewhat different for different individuals. …many individuals may require a considerably higher concentration of one or more coenzymes than other people do for optimum health…" Pauling L. On the Orthomolecular Environment of the Mind: Orthomolecular Theory. In: Williams RJ, Kalita DK. *A Physician's Handbook on Orthomolecular Medicine*. Keats Publ: 1977, p76

[196] nobel.se/chemistry/laureates/1954/pauling-bio.html on April 4, 2004

[197] "About 50 human genetic dis-eases due to defective enzymes can be remedied or ameliorated by the administration of high doses of the vitamin component of the corresponding coenzyme, which at least partially restores enzymatic activity." Ames BN, Elson-Schwab I, Silver EA. High-dose vitamin therapy stimulates variant enzymes with decreased coenzyme binding affinity (increased K(m)): relevance to genetic disease and polymorphisms. *Am J Clin Nutr*. 2002 Apr;75(4):616-58

[198] "An optimum intake of micronutrients and metabolites, which varies with age and genetic constitution, would tune up metabolism and give a marked increase in health, particularly for the poor and elderly, at little cost." Ames BN. The metabolic tune-up: metabolic harmony and disease prevention. *J Nutr*. 2003 May;133(5 Suppl 1):1544S-8S

[199] "Optimizing micronutrient intake [through better diets, fortification of foods, or multivitamin-mineral pills] can have a major impact on public health at low cost." Ames BN. Cancer prevention and diet: help from single nucleotide polymorphisms. *Proc Natl Acad Sci* U S A. 1999 Oct 26;96(22):12216-8

Molecular rationale for high-dose nutrient supplementation

"As many as **one-third of mutations** in a gene result in the corresponding enzyme having an increased Michaelis constant, or Km, (decreased binding affinity) for a coenzyme, resulting in a lower rate of reaction. **About 50 human genetic diseases due to defective enzymes can be remedied or ameliorated by the administration of high doses of the vitamin component of the corresponding coenzyme**, which at least partially restores enzymatic activity."

"**High doses of vitamins are used to treat many inheritable human diseases**. The molecular basis of disease arising from as many as one-third of the mutations in a gene is an increased Michaelis constant, or Km, (decreased binding affinity) of an enzyme for the vitamin-derived coenzyme or substrate, which in turn lowers the rate of the reaction."

Ames BN, et al. High-dose vitamin therapy stimulates variant enzymes. *Am J Clin Nutr.* 2002 Apr;75:616-58

Nutrigenomics—Nutritional Genomics: "Genome" refers to all of the genetic material in an organism, and "genomics" is the field of study of this information. The field of nutritional genomics—nutrigenomics—refers to the clinical synthesis of 1) research on the human genome, and 2) the advancing science of clinical nutrition, including research on nutraceuticals (nutritional medicines) and phytomedicinals (botanical medicines). Nutrigenomics represents a major advance in our understanding of the underlying biochemical and physiologic mechanisms of the effects of nutrition.

Nutrition is far more than "fuel" for our biophysiologic machine; we know now that nutrition—the consumption of specific proteins, amino acids, vitamins, minerals, fatty acids, and phytochemicals—can alter genetic expression and can thus either promote health or disease at the very fundamental level of genetic expression. The commonly employed excuse that many patients use—"I just have bad genes"—now takes on a whole new meaning; it may be that these patients suffer from the expression of "bad genes" *because of the food that they eat.*

The concept and phenomenon of nutrigenomics can be described by saying that each of us has the genes for health, as well as the genes for disease; what largely determines our level of health is how we treat our genes with environmental inputs, especially nutrition. We appear able, to a large extent, to "turn on" disease-promoting genes with poor nutrition and a pro-inflammatory lifestyle[200,201], while, to a lesser extent, we are able to activate or "turn on" health-promoting genes with a healthy diet[202] and with proper nutritional supplementation.[203]

Putting it all together with "the supplemented Paleo-Mediterranean diet": The health-promoting diet of choice for the majority of people is a diet based on abundant consumption of fruits, vegetables, seeds, nuts, omega-3 and monounsaturated fatty acids, and lean sources of protein such as lean meats, fatty cold-water fish, soy and whey proteins. This diet prohibits and obviates overconsumption of chemical preservatives, artificial sweeteners, and carbohydrate-dominant foods such as candies, pastries, breads, potatoes, grains, and other foods with a high glycemic load and high glycemic index. This "Paleo-Mediterranean Diet" is a combination of the "Paleolithic" or "Paleo diet" and the well-known "Mediterranean diet", both of which are well described in peer-reviewed journals and the lay press. The Mediterranean diet is characterized by increased proportions of legumes, nuts, seeds, whole grain products, fruits, vegetables (including potatoes), fish and lean meats, and monounsaturated and n-3 fatty acids.[204] Consumption of the Mediterranean diet is associated with improvements in insulin sensitivity and reductions in cardiovascular disease, diabetes, cancer, and all-cause mortality when contrasted to the effects of *ad libitum* eating, particularly in the standard American diet (SAD) eating pattern.[205] The Paleolithic diet detailed by collaborators Eaton[206], O'Keefe[207], and Cordain[208] is similar to the Mediterranean diet except for stronger emphasis on fruits and vegetables (preferably raw or minimally cooked), omega-3-rich lean meats, and reduced consumption of starchy foods such as potatoes and grains, the latter of which were not staples in the human diet until the last few thousand years. Emphasizing the olive oil and red wine of the Mediterranean diet and the absence of grains and potatoes per the Paleo diet appears to be the way to get the best of both dietary worlds; the remaining diet is characterized by fresh whole fruits, vegetables, nuts (especially almonds), seeds, berries, olive oil, lean meats rich

---

[200] Rusyn et al. Corn oil rapidly activates nuclear factor-kappaB in hepatic Kupffer cells by oxidant-dependent mechanisms. *Carcinogenesis.* 1999 Nov;20(11):2095-100

[201] Aljada et al. Increase in intranuclear nuclear factor kappaB and decrease in inhibitor kappaB in mononuclear cells after a mixed meal. *Am J Clin Nutr.* 2004 Apr;79(4):682-90

[202] OKeefe JH Jr,Cordain L.Cardiovascular disease resulting from a diet and lifestyle at odds with our Paleolithic genome.*Mayo Clin Proc.*2004;79:101-8

[203] Kaput J, Rodriguez LR. Nutritional genomics: the next frontier in the postgenomic era. *Physiol Genomics* 16: 166–177

[204] Curtis BM, O'Keefe JH Jr. Understanding the Mediterranean diet. Could this be the new "gold standard" for heart disease prevention? *Postgrad Med.* 2002;112:35-8,41-5

[205] Knoops KT, et al. Mediterranean diet, lifestyle factors, and 10-year mortality in elderly European men and women: the HALE project. *JAMA.* 2004 Sep 22;292(12):1433-9

[206] Eaton SB, Shostak M, Konner M. *The Paleolithic Prescription: A program of diet & exercise and a design for living*, New York: Harper & Row, 1988

[207] O'Keefe JH Jr, Cordain L. Cardiovascular disease resulting from a diet and lifestyle at odds with our Paleolithic genome. *Mayo Clin Proc.* 2004 Jan;79(1):101-8

[208] Cordain L. *The Paleo Diet.* Indianapolis; John Wiley and Sons, 2002

in n-3 fatty acids, and red wine in moderation. In sum, this dietary plan along with the inclusion of garlic and dark chocolate (a rich source of cardioprotective, antioxidative, antihypertensive, and anti-inflammatory polyphenolic flavonoids[209,210]) is expected to reduce adverse cardiovascular events by more than 76%.[211] Biochemical justification for this type of diet is ample and is well supported by numerous long-term studies in humans wherein both Mediterranean and Paleolithic diets result in statistically significant and clinically meaningful reductions in disease-specific and all-cause mortality.[212,213,214,215] Diets rich in fruits and vegetables are sources of more than 8,000 phytochemicals, many of which have antioxidant, anti-inflammatory, and anti-cancer properties.[216] Oleic acid, squalene, and phenolics in olive oil and phenolics and resveratrol in red wine have antioxidant, anti-inflammatory, and anti-cancer properties and also protect against cardiovascular disease.[217] N-3 fatty acids have numerous health benefits via multiple mechanisms as described in the sections that follow. Increased intake of dietary fiber from fruits and vegetable favorably modifies gut flora, promotes xenobiotic elimination (via flora modification, laxation, and overall reductions in enterohepatic recirculation), and is associated with reductions in morbidity and mortality. Such a "Paleolithic diet" can also lead to urinary alkalinization (average urine pH of ≥ 7.5 according to Sebastian et al[218]) which increases renal *retention of minerals* for improved musculoskeletal health[219,220,221] and which increases *urinary elimination of many toxicants and xenobiotics* for a tremendous reduction in serum levels and thus adverse effects from chemical exposure or drug overdose.[222] Furthermore, therapeutic alkalinization was recently shown in an open trial with 82 patients to reduce symptoms and disability associated with low-back pain and to increase intracellular magnesium concentrations by 11%.[223] **Ample intake of amino acids via dietary proteins supports phase-2 detoxification** (amino acid and sulfate conjugation) for proper xenobiotic elimination[224,225], **provides amino acid precursors for neurotransmitter synthesis** and maintenance of mood, memory, and cognitive performance[226,227,228,229], **and prevents the immunosuppression and decrements in musculoskeletal status caused by low-protein diets.**[230] Described originally by this author[231], the "supplemented Paleo-Mediterranean diet" provides patients the best of current knowledge in nutrition by relying on a foundational diet plan of fresh fruits, vegetables, nuts, seeds, berries, fish, and lean meats which is adorned with olive oil for its squalene, phenolic antioxidant/anti-inflammatory and monounsaturated fatty acid content. Inclusive of medical foods such as red wine, garlic, and dark chocolate which may synergize to effect at least a 76% reduction in cardiovascular disease[232], this diet also reduces the risk for cancer[233] and can be an integral component of a health-promoting lifestyle.[234] Competitive athletes are allowed increased carbohydrate consumption before and after training and competition to promote glycogen storage supercompensation.[235,236]

---

[209] Schramm et al. Chocolate procyanidins decrease the leukotriene-prostacyclin ratio in humans and human aortic endothelial cells. *Am J Clin Nutr*. 2001;73(1):36-40

[210] Engler et al. Flavonoid-rich dark chocolate improves endothelial function and increases plasma epicatechin concentrations in healthy adults. *J Am Coll Nutr* 2004;23:197-204

[211] Franco et al. The Polymeal: a more natural, safer, and probably tastier (than the Polypill) strategy to reduce cardiovascular disease by more than 75%. *BMJ*. 2004:1447-50

[212] de Lorgeril M, et al. Mediterranean dietary pattern in a randomized trial: prolonged survival and possible reduced cancer rate. *Arch Intern Med*. 1998 Jun 8;158(11):1181-7

[213] Knoops KT, et al. Mediterranean diet, lifestyle factors, and 10-year mortality in elderly European men and women: the HALE project. *JAMA*. 2004 Sep 22;292(12):1433-9

[214] Lindeberg S, Cordain L, and Eaton SB. Biological and clinical potential of a Paleolithic diet. *J Nutri Environ Med* 2003; 13:149-160

[215] O'Keefe JH Jr, Cordain L, et al. Optimal low-density lipoprotein is 50 to 70 mg/dl: lower is better and physiologically normal. *J Am Coll Cardiol*. 2004 Jun 2;43(11):2142-6

[216] Liu RH. Health benefits of fruit and vegetables are from additive and synergistic combinations of phytochemicals. *Am J Clin Nutr*. 2003;78(3 Sup):517S-520S

[217] Alarcon de la Lastra C, Barranco MD, Motilva V, Herrerias JM. Mediterranean diet and health: biological importance of olive oil. *Curr Pharm Des*. 2001;7:933-50

[218] Sebastian, Frassetto et al. Estimation of the net acid load of the diet of ancestral preagricultural Homo sapiens and their hominid ancestors. *Am J Clin Nutr* 2002;76:1308-16

[219] Sebastian A, et al. Improved mineral balance and skeletal metabolism in postmenopausal women treated with potassium bicarbonate. *N Engl J Med*. 1994;330(25):1776-81

[220] Tucker et al. Potassium, magnesium, fruit and vegetable intakes are associated with greater bone mineral density in elderly men and women. *Am J Clin Nutr*. 1999;69:727-36

[221] Whiting et al. Dietary protein, phosphorus, potassium are beneficial to bone mineral density in men consuming adequate dietary calcium. *J Am Coll Nutr*. 2002;21:402-9

[222] Proudfoot AT, Krenzelok EP, Vale JA. Position Paper on urine alkalinization. *J Toxicol Clin Toxicol*. 2004;42(1):1-26

[223] "The results show that a disturbed acid-base balance may contribute to the symptoms of low back pain. The simple and safe addition of an alkaline multimineral preparate was able to reduce the pain symptoms in these patients with chronic low back pain." Vormann J, et al. Supplementation with alkaline minerals reduces symptoms in patients with chronic low back pain. *J Trace Elem Med Biol*. 2001;15:179-83

[224] Liska DJ. The detoxification enzyme systems. *Altern Med Rev*. 1998;3:187-9

[225] Anderson KE, Kappas A. Dietary regulation of cytochrome P450. *Annu Rev Nutr*. 1991;11:141-67

[226] Rogers et al. Tryptophan depletion alters the decision-making of healthy volunteers through altered processing of reward cues. *Neuropsychopharmacology*. 2003;28:153-62

[227] Arnulf I, et al. Mid-morning tryptophan depletion delays REM sleep onset in healthy subjects. *Neuropsychopharmacology*. 2002;27(5):843-51

[228] Thomas JR, Lockwood PA, Singh A, Deuster PA. Tyrosine improves working memory in a multitasking environment. *Pharmacol Biochem Behav*. 1999;64:495-500

[229] Markus CR, et al. The bovine protein alpha-lactalbumin increases the plasma ratio of tryptophan to the other large neutral amino acids, and in vulnerable subjects raises brain serotonin activity, reduces cortisol concentration, and improves mood under stress. *Am J Clin Nutr*. 2000;71:1536-44

[230] Castaneda C, et al. Elderly women accommodate to a low-protein diet with losses of body cell mass, muscle function, and immune response. *Am J Clin Nutr*. 1995;62:30-9

[231] Vasquez A. Five-Part Nutritional Protocol that Produces Consistently Positive Results. *Nutr Wellness* 2005 Sept. InflammationMastery.com/reprints and updated in Chapter 4.

[232] Franco et al. The Polymeal: a more natural, safer, and probably tastier (than the Polypill) strategy to reduce cardiovascular disease by more than 75%. *BMJ* 2004;329:1447-50

[233] "The combination of 4 low risk factors lowered the all-cause mortality rate to 0.35 (95% CI, 0.28-0.44). In total, lack of adherence to this low-risk pattern was associated with a population attributable risk of 60% of all deaths, 64% of deaths from coronary heart disease, 61% from cardiovascular diseases, and 60% from cancer." Knoops KT, de Groot LC, Kromhout D, et al. Mediterranean diet, lifestyle factors, and 10-year mortality in elderly European men and women: the HALE project. *JAMA*. 2004 Sep 22;292(12):1433-9

[234] Orme-Johnson DW, Herron RE. An innovative approach to reducing medical care utilization and expenditures. *Am J Manag Care*. 1997;3(1):135-44

[235] "A significant glycogen sparing, as well as supercompensation within 24 h of recovery, was observed after [carbohydrate] supplementation." Brouns F, Saris WH, Beckers E, Adlercreutz H, et al. Metabolic changes induced by sustained exhaustive cycling and diet manipulation. *Int J Sports Med*. 1989 May;10 Suppl 1:S49-62

[236] "The accepted method of increasing muscle glycogen stores is by "glycogen loading," which classically involves depletion of muscle glycogen, usually by exercise, followed by consumption of a high-CHO diet for several days (e.g., 3, 39). ...increase muscle glycogen concentrations ([glycogen]) to between 150 and 200% of normal resting levels." Robinson TM, et al. Role of submaximal exercise in promoting creatine and glycogen accumulation in human skeletal muscle. *J Appl Physiol*. 1999 Aug;87(2):598-604

Profile of the Supplemented Paleo-Mediterranean Diet (Vasquez 2005, 2011)[237]

Foods to consume:	Foods to avoid:
☺ **Everything organic**: to enhance nutrition, avoid pesticides/herbicides, and to avoid GMO as much as possible (detailed and cited later)	☒ **Avoid as much as possible fat-laden arachidonate-rich meats like beef, liver, pork, and lamb, as well as high-fat cream and other dairy products with emulsified, readily absorbed saturated fats and arachidonic acid**
☺ **Lean sources of protein**	☒ **High-sugar pseudofoods**:
• Fish (avoiding tuna which is commonly loaded with mercury)	• Corn syrup
• Chicken and turkey	• Cola and soda
• Lean cuts of free-range grass-fed meats: beef, buffalo, lamb are occasionally acceptable	• Donuts, candy, etc...."junk food"
• Soy protein[238] and whey protein isolate[239,240]	☒ **Grains such as wheat, rye, barley**: These have only existed in the human diet for less than 10,000 years and are consistently associated with increased prevalence of degenerative diseases due to the allergic response they invoke and because of their high glycemic load and high glycemic index.
☺ **Fruits and fruit juices**	
☺ **Vegetables and vegetable juices**	
☺ **Nuts, seeds, berries**	☒ **Potatoes and rice**: High in sugar, low in phytonutrients
☺ **Generous use of olive oil**: On sautéed vegetables and fresh salads	☒ **Avoid allergens**: Determined per individual
☺ **Daily vitamin/mineral supplementation**: With a high-potency broad-spectrum multivitamin and multimineral supplement[241]	☒ **Chemicals to avoid**:
	• Pesticides, Herbicides, Fungicides
☺ **Sun exposure or vitamin D3 supplementation**: To ensure provision of 2,000-5,000 IU of vitamin D3 per day for adults[242]	• Carcinogenic sweeteners: aspartame[244]
	• Artificial flavors
	• Artificial colors: tartrazine
☺ **Balanced broad-spectrum fatty acid supplementation**: With ALA, GLA, EPA, and DHA[243]	• Preservatives: benzoate
	• Flavor enhancers: carrageenan and monosodium glutamate
☺ **Water, tea, home-made fruit/vegetable juices**: Commercial vegetable juices are commonly loaded with sodium chloride; choose appropriately. Fruit juices can be loaded with natural and superfluous sugars. Herbal teas can be selected based on the medicinal properties of the plant that is used.	• GMO: avoid genetically manipulated corporate products and do not contribute to unethical profiteering businesses; rather support local and sustainable farmers as much as possible for a wide range of ethical, nutritional, and environmental reasons

---

[237] Vasquez A. Five-Part Nutritional Protocol. *Nutritional Wellness* 2005 Sept. and Vasquez A. The Supplemented Paleo-Mediterranean Diet. *Nutritional Perspectives* 2011 Jan

[238] "These results indicate that for healthy adults, the isolated soy protein is of high nutritional quality, comparable to that of animal protein sources, and that the methionine content is not limiting for adult protein maintenance." Young et al. Evaluation of the protein quality of an isolated soy protein in young men. *Am J Clin Nutr.* 1984 Jan;39:16-24

[239] Bounous G. Whey protein concentrate (WPC) and glutathione modulation in cancer treatment. *Anticancer Res.* 2000 Nov-Dec;20(6C):4785-92

[240] Markus CR, et al. The bovine protein alpha-lactalbumin increases the plasma ratio of tryptophan to the other large neutral amino acids, and in vulnerable subjects raises brain serotonin activity, reduces cortisol concentration, and improves mood under stress. *Am J Clin Nutr.* 2000 Jun;71(6):1536-44

[241] "Most people do not consume an optimal amount of all vitamins by diet alone. ...it appears prudent for all adults to take vitamin supplements." Fletcher RH, Fairfield KM. Vitamins for chronic disease prevention in adults: clinical applications. *JAMA.* 2002;287:3127-9

[242] Vasquez A, et al.The clinical importance of vitamin D (cholecalciferol). *Altern Ther Health Med.* 2004Sep10:28-36

[243] Vasquez A. New Insights into Fatty Acid Supplementation and Its Effect on Eicosanoid Production and Genetic Expression. *Nutr Perspectives* 2005; Jan: 5-16

[244] "In the past two decades brain tumor rates have risen in several industrialized countries, including the United States... Compared to other environmental factors putatively linked to brain tumors, the artificial sweetener aspartame is a promising candidate to explain the recent increase in incidence and degree of malignancy of brain tumors." Olney JW, Farber NB, Spitznagel E, Robins LN. Increasing brain tumor rates: is there a link to aspartame? *J Neuropathol Exp Neurol* 1996 Nov;55(11):1115-23

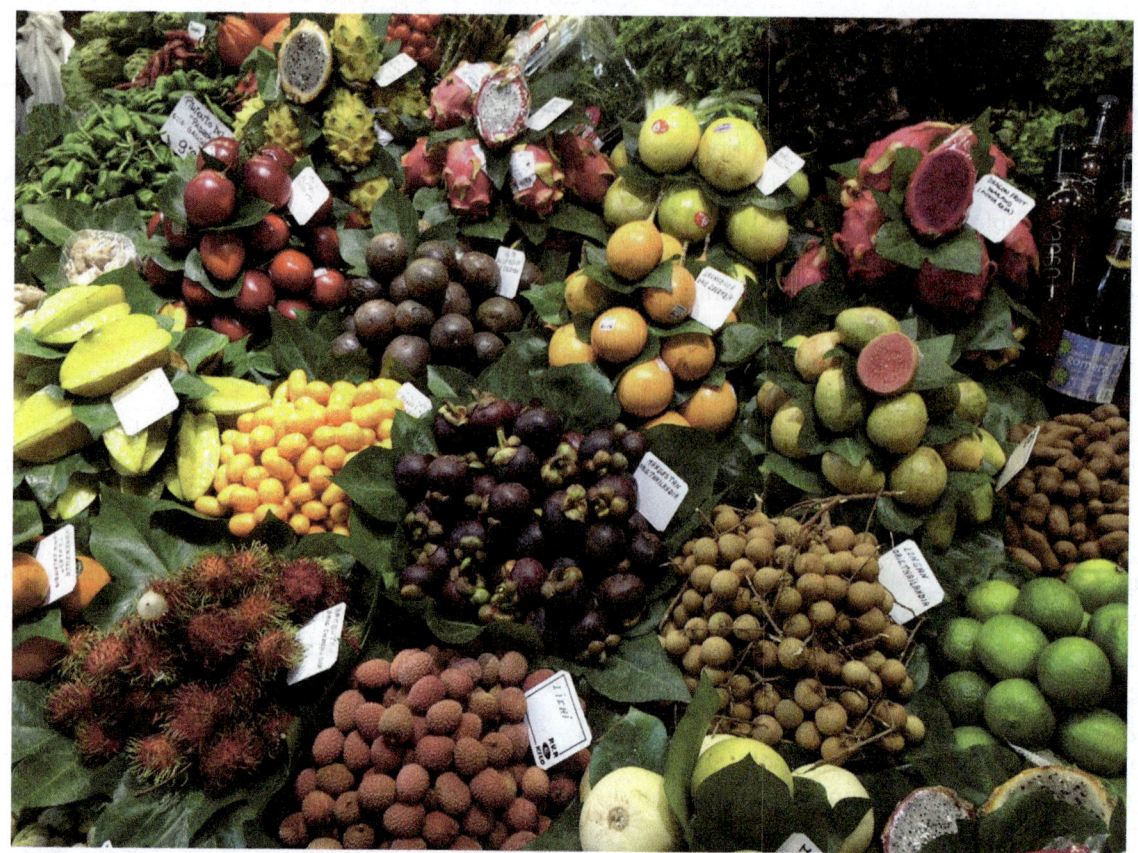

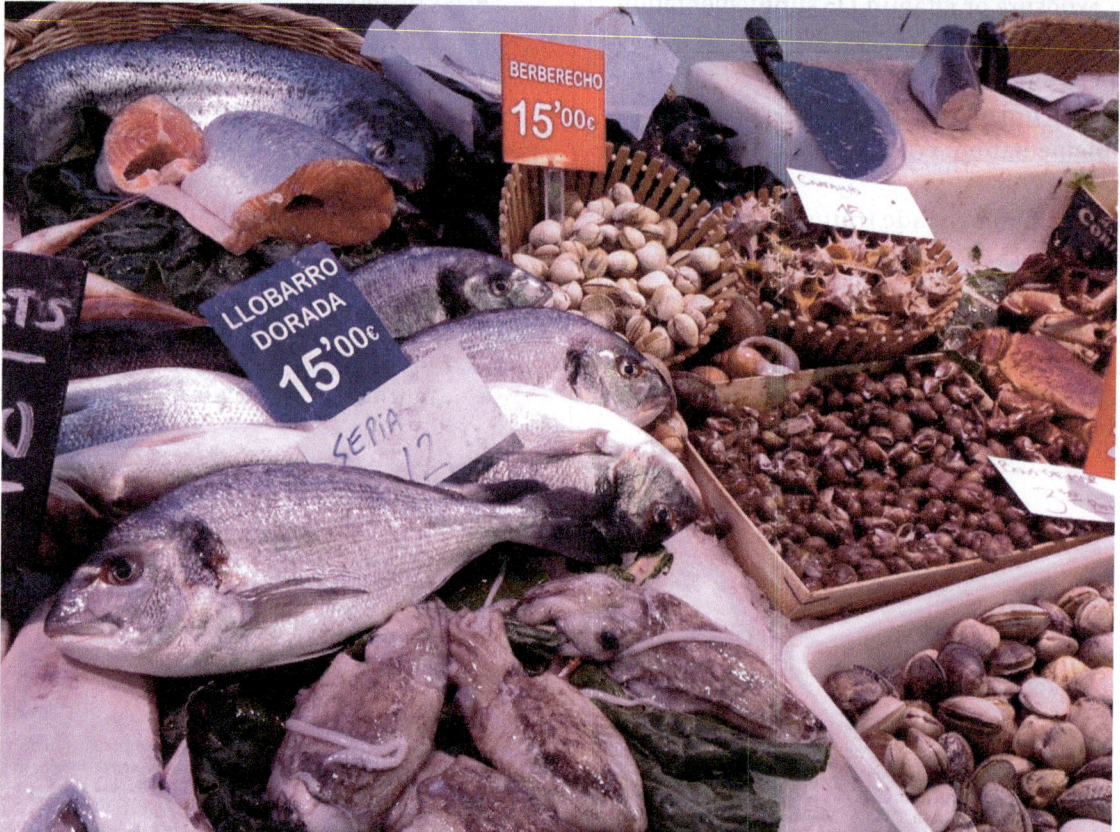

Local Mediterranean market fare: Plants provide fiber, antioxidants, numerous functional phytochemicals with anti-inflammatory properties, and prebiotic and antimicrobial constituents that favorably modulate human gastrointestinal flora to provide anti-inflammatory immunomodulation; seafood generally provides low-fat high-quality protein with favorable fatty acid profiles. Supporting local farmers, fishers, and personal store owners helps promote environmental and community sustainability.

Emotional, Mental, and Social Health

Stress management and authentic living: Mental, emotional, and physical "stress" describes any unpleasant living condition which can lead to negative effects on health, such as increased blood pressure, depression, apathy, increased muscle tension, and, according to some research, increased risk of serious health problems such as early death from cardiovascular disease and cancer. Many people find that their modern lives are characterized by excess amounts of multitasking, job responsibilities, family responsibilities, commuter traffic, financial pressures in combination with an insufficient amount of relaxation, sleep, community support, exercise, time in nature, healthy nutrition, and time to simply *be* rather than *do*. Stress comes in many different forms and includes malnutrition, trauma, insufficient exercise (epidemic), excess exercise (rare), sleep deprivation, emotional turmoil, and exposure to chemicals and radiation. When most people talk about "stress" they are referring to either chronic anxiety (such as with high-pressure work situations or dysfunctional interpersonal relationships) or the acute stress reaction that is typical of unpredictable rapid-onset events such as an injury, accident, or other physically threatening situation. These **"different types of stress" are not separate from each other; rather, they are interconnected:**

- Emotional stress causes nutritional depletion, particularly of vitamin A[245], magnesium, tryptophan, and vitamin C—most mammals (other than those that lost L-gulonolactone oxidase function such as humans/primates, guinea pigs, most bats, some birds and fish[246]) can internally produce ascorbate and greatly increase endogenous production during times of stress,
- Sleep deprivation alters immune response and mental functioning,[247]
- Emotional stress triggers increased microbial virulence, growth, and mucosal adhesion; the sensing of the neuroendocrine stress response by microorganisms, many of which have receptors for catecholamines, is termed "microbial endocrinology",[248]
- Chemical exposure can disrupt endocrine function.[249]

Therefore, **any type of [emotional] stress can cause other types of [physiologic] stress**. Avoiding stressful situations is, of course, an effective way to avoid being bothered or harmed by them. If work-related stress is the problem, then finding a new position or occupation is certainly an option worth considering and implementing. High-stress jobs are often high-paying jobs; but if in the process of making money, a person ruins her health and loses years from her life, then no one would ever say, "It was worth it." **Money, success, and freedom only have value for the person alive and healthy to enjoy them.** Toxic relationships, whether at home or work, are relationships that cause more harm than good by re-injuring old emotional wounds and by creating new emotional injuries. We can all benefit from affirming our right to a happy and healthy life by minimizing/eliminating contact with people who cause emotional harm to us—this requires conscious effort.[250] Engel[251] provides a clear articulation and description of abusive relationships, along with checklists for their recognition and exercises for their remediation. Healthy relationships are difficult to create and maintain these days, and probably a few basic components contribute to this phenomenon. ❶ With the society-wide disintegration of the extended family, most people in our society have never even seen a healthy family unit and therefore have no model and no available mentors to help them recreate a lasting family structure. ❷ Due specifically to the structure of our educational systems and (pseudo)culture of entertainment, most people have very short attention spans and are accustomed to inattention, distraction, and externally derived entertainment and gratification. ❸ Modern schools and fragmented families both fail to teach conflict resolution and relationship skills. ❹ Poor nutritional status—very common in the general population—promotes impulsivity, irritability, depression, and mood instability.

> **How to test relationship quality at home/work**
>
> "Good relationships make you feel loved, wanted, and cared for."
>
> Malcolm. *Health Style*. 2001,133

[245] Ingenbleek Y, Bernstein L. The stressful condition as a nutritionally dependent adaptive dichotomy. *Nutrition* 1999 Apr;15(4):305-20

[246] Drouin et al. The genetics of vitamin C loss in vertebrates. *Curr Genomics*. 2011 Aug;12(5):371-8 and "...bats lost the ability to biosynthesize vitamin C recently by exhibiting stepwise mutation patterns during GULO evolution..." Cui et al. Recent Loss of Vitamin C Biosynthesis Ability in Bats. *PLoS ONE* 2011;6(11):e27114

[247] Heiser P, e. Alterations of host defense system after sleep deprivation are followed by impaired mood and psychosocial functioning. *World J Biol Psychiatry* 2001 Apr;2:89-94

[248] Freestone et al. Microbial endocrinology: how stress influences susceptibility to infection. *Trends Microbiol.* 2008 Feb;16(2):55-64

[249] "Evidence suggests that environmental exposure to some anthropogenic chemicals may result in disruption of endocrine systems in human and wildlife populations." epa.gov/endocrine on March 7, 2004

[250] Collins BC. *How to Recognize Emotional Unavailability and Make Healthier Relationship Choices*. [Mjf Books; ISBN: 1567313442]

[251] Engel B. *The Emotionally Abusive Relationship: How to Stop Being Abused and How to Stop Abusing*. Wiley Publishers: 2003

<table>
<tr><td>

Stress affects the whole body.

Therefore, a complete stress management program must address the whole body:

Physical Structural

Biochemical Hormonal Nutritional

Mental Emotional Spiritual

</td><td>

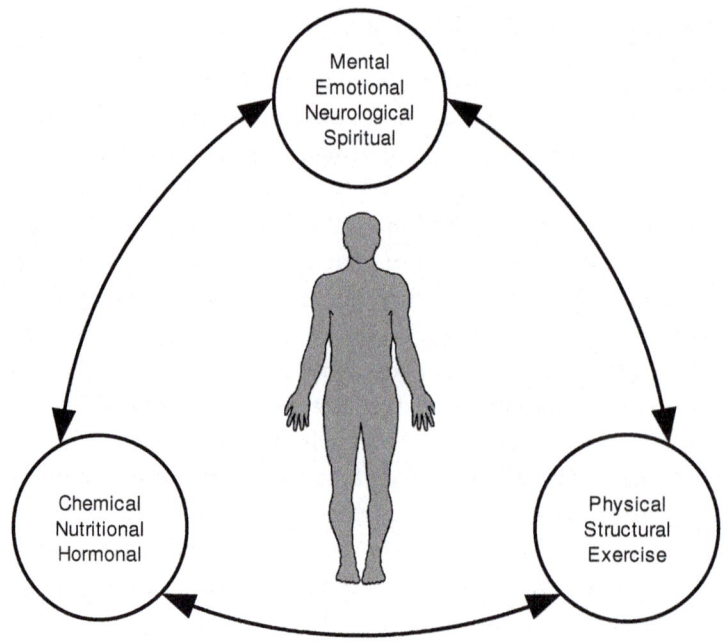

</td></tr>
</table>

An important concept is that ==**psychoemotional stress is a "whole body" phenomenon**==: affecting the mind, the brain, emotional state, the physical body (including musculoskeletal, immune, and cardiovascular systems), as well as the nutritional status of the individual. The adverse effects of stress can be reduced with an integrated combination of therapeutics that addresses each of the major body systems affected by stress, which are 1) mental/emotional, 2) physical, and 3) nutritional/biochemical.

Approaching stress management from a tripartite perspective

	Mental/emotional	**Physical**	**Nutritional/biochemical**
Therapeutic considerations	<ul><li>Social support</li><li>Re-parenting</li><li>Conversational style[252]</li><li>Meditation, prayer</li><li>Healthy boundaries</li><li>Books, tapes, groups</li><li>REST—reduced environmental stimulation therapy[253]</li><li>Expressive writing[254]</li><li>Time to simply rest and relax</li></ul>	<ul><li>Yoga</li><li>Massage</li><li>Exercise</li><li>Stretching</li><li>Swimming</li><li>Resting</li><li>Biking</li><li>Hiking</li><li>Physical touch and affection</li></ul>	<ul><li>Vitamins, especially vitamin C[255]</li><li>Fish oil[256]</li><li>Hormones, cytokines, neurotransmitters, and eicosanoids</li><li>Tryptophan, pyridoxine, whey protein</li><li>Botanical medicines such as *kava*[257], *Ashwaganda,* and *Eleutherococcus*</li></ul>

[252] Rick Brinkman ND and Rick Kirschner ND. *How to Deal With Difficult People* [Audio Cassette. Career Track, 1995]

[253] For more information on REST and its use in weight loss and alcohol consumption: Borrie et al. Restricted environmental stimulation therapy in a weight reduction program. *J Behav Med*. 1980 Jun;3(2):147-61. Cooper et al. Reduced Environmental Stimulation Therapy (REST) and reduced alcohol consumption. *J Subst Abuse Treat*. 1988;5(2):61-8

[254] Smyth et al. Effects of writing about stressful experiences on symptom reduction in patients with asthma or rheumatoid arthritis. *JAMA*. 1999 Apr 14;281(14):1304-9

[255] Brody S, Preut R, Schommer K, Schurmeyer TH. A randomized controlled trial of high dose ascorbic acid for reduction of blood pressure, cortisol, and subjective responses to psychological stress. *Psychopharmacology* (Berl). 2002 Jan;159(3):319-24

[256] Hamazaki T, Itomura M, Sawazaki S, Nagao Y. Anti-stress effects of DHA. *Biofactors*. 2000;13(1-4):41-5

[257] Cagnacci A, et al. Kava-Kava administration reduces anxiety in perimenopausal women. *Maturitas*. 2003 Feb 25;44(2):103-9

The body functions as a whole—not as independent, autonomous organ systems: Problems with one aspect of health create problems in other aspects of health. **Treatment of disease and promotion of wellness must therefore improve overall health and functioning while simultaneously addressing the disease or presenting complaint.**

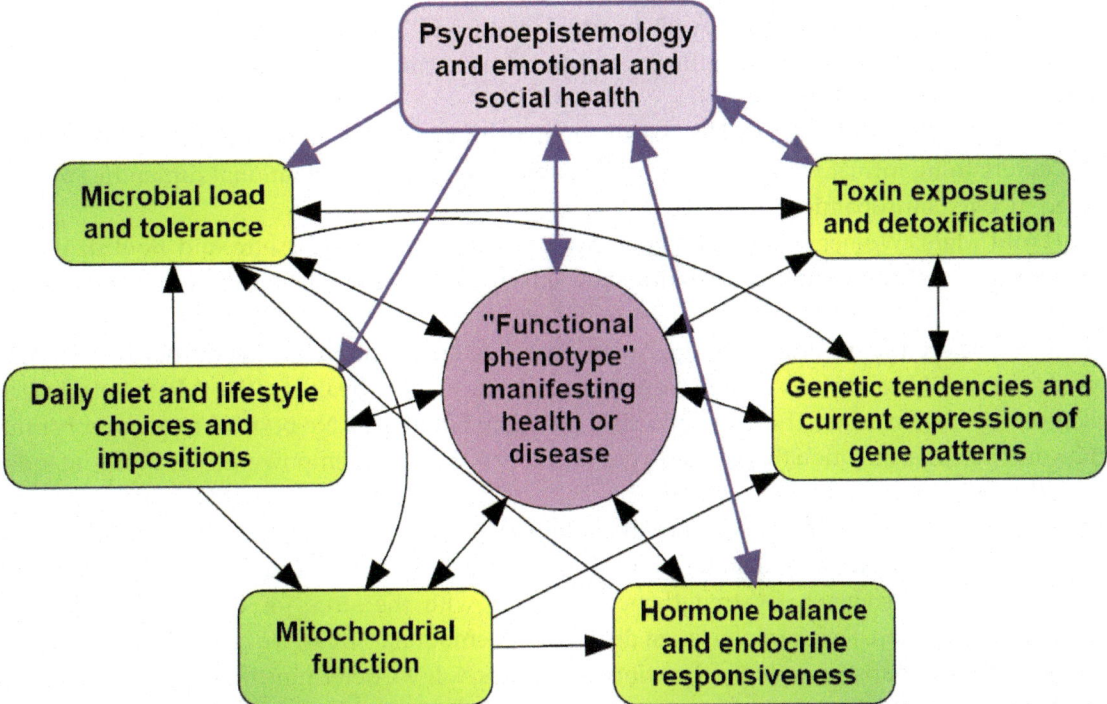

The influences on "functional phenotype" can originate from psychosocial health or dysfunction or "toxic" emotional exposures and the resulting physiologic and microbial responses: The model presented here is a simple one, but it serves to demonstrate how psychological health status can affect the entirety of all body systems, either directly or indirectly. Due to the interconnected nature of each component/system, problems can become synergistic and reinforced and thus self-perpetuating. For example, psychological stress increases microbial virulence (e.g., microbial endocrinology) and total microbial load while reducing mucosal immunity (e.g., reduced secretory IgA) and immunomodulating hormones (e.g., DHEA and testosterone are reduced with severe stress); complicating these are the facts that people tend to make poor dietary choices when they are stressed (e.g., "stress eaters") and that xenobiotic accumulation can only follow xenobiotic exposure and that most xenobiotic exposure results from corporate irresponsibility, government complicity, and population-wide sociopolitical ineffectiveness.

Stress always has a biochemical/physiologic component: Regardless of its origins, stress invariably takes a toll on the body—*the whole body*. Well-documented effects of stress include:

1. Increased levels of cortisol—higher levels are associated with osteoporosis, memory loss, slow healing, and insulin resistance.
2. Reduced function of thyroid hormones[258] (i.e., induction of peripheral/metabolic hypothyroidism)
3. Reduced levels of testosterone (in men)
4. Increased intestinal permeability and "leaky gut"[259]
5. Increased excretion of minerals in the urine
6. Increased need for vitamins, minerals, and amino acids
7. Suppression of immune function and of natural killer cells that fight viral infections and tumors
8. Decreased production of sIgA—main defense of the lungs, gastrointestinal tract, and genitourinary tract
9. Increased populations of harmful bacteria in the intestines and an associated increased rate of lung and upper respiratory tract infections
10. Increased incidence of food allergies[260]
11. Sleep disturbance

[258] Ingenbleek Y, Bernstein L. The stressful condition as a nutritionally dependent adaptive dichotomy. *Nutrition* 1999 Apr;15(4):305-20
[259] Hart A, Kamm MA. Review article: mechanisms of initiation and perpetuation of gut inflammation by stress. *Aliment Pharmacol Ther* 2002;16(12):2017-28
[260] Anderzen et al. Stress and sensitization: controlled prospective psychophysiological study of children exposed to international relocation. *J Psychosom Res* 1997;43:259-69

Sometimes a stressful situation can be modified into one that is less stressful or dysfunctional, so that the benefits are retained, yet the negative aspects are reduced. Of course, the best example of this is interpersonal relationships, which easily lend themselves to improvement with the application of conscious effort. Many audiotapes, books, and seminars are available for people interested in having improved interpersonal relationships. Selected resources are listed here:

- Men and Women: Talking Together by Deborah Tannen and Robert Bly [Sound Horizons, 1992. ISBN: 1879323095] A lively discussion of the different communication and relationship styles of men and women by two respected experts in their fields.
- How to Deal with Difficult People by Drs. Rick Brinkman and Rick Kirschner. [Audio Cassette. Career Track, 1995] An entertaining format with solutions to common workplace and situational difficulties. Authored and performed by two naturopathic physicians.
- Men are From Mars, Women are From Venus by John Gray. [Audio Cassette and Books]. Phenomenally popular concepts in understanding, accepting, and effectively integrating the differences between men and women.
- The ManKind Project (ManKindProject.org). An international organization hosting events for men and women. The men's events, formats, and groups are authentic, clear, and healthy. The ManKind Project has an organization for women called The WomanWithin (WomanWithin.org). No book or tape can substitute for the dynamics and personal attention that can be experienced by a conscious, empowered, and well-intended group.

When "the problem" cannot be avoided, and the interaction/relationship with the problem cannot be improved, a remaining option is to supplement the internal environment so that it is somewhat "strengthened" to deal with the stress of the bothersome event or situation. For example, when dealing with emotional stress, we can use counseling, support groups, or various relaxation techniques.[261] If we determine that the emotional stress has a biochemical component, then we can use specific botanical and nutritional supplementation to safely and naturally support and restore normal function. Moving deeper into the issue of "stress management" requires that we ask why a person is in a stressful situation to begin with. Of course, with *random acts of chaos* like car accidents, we cannot always ascribe the problem to the person, unless the accident resulted from their own negligence. But **when people are chronically stressed and unhappy about their jobs and/or relationships, then we need to employ more than stress reduction techniques**, and as clinicians we need to offer more than the latest adaptogen. **We have to ask why a person would subject himself/herself to such a situation, and what fears or limitations (self-imposed and/or externally applied) keep him/her from breaking free into a life that works**.[262,263,264,265,266,267]

> **Six fundamental components of Self-esteem**
> 1. Living consciously
> 2. Self-acceptance
> 3. Self-responsibility
> 4. Self-assertiveness
> 5. Living purposefully
> 6. Personal integrity
>
> Branden N. *Six Pillars of Self-Esteem*. Bantam: 1995

Autonomization, intradependence, emotional literacy, corrective experience:

> "None of us are completely developed people when we reach adulthood.
> We are each incomplete in our own way." *Merle Fossum*[268]

Consciousness-raising is a keystone gift that holistic physicians can impart to their patients and one which may be necessary for true healing to be manifested and maintained. Healthcare providers are quick to enlighten their patients to the details of diet, exercise, nutrition, medications, surgeries, and other *biomechanical* and *biochemical* aspects of health, but are routinely negligent when it comes to sharing with patients the emotional tools that may be necessary to repair or construct the "self" which is supposed to implement the treatment plan that the doctor has designed. Passivity and ignorance are not hindrances to the success of the *medical paradigm*, which requires that

[261] Martha Davis PhD, Matthew McKay MSW, Elizabeth Robbins Eshelman PhD. *The Relaxation & Stress Reduction Workbook 5th edition*. New Harbinger Publishers; 2000
[262] Rick Jarow. *Creating the Work You Love: Courage, Commitment and Career*; Inner Traditions Intl Ltd; 1995 [ISBN: 0892815426]
[263] Breton D, Largent C. *The Paradigm Conspiracy: Why Our Social Systems Violate Human Potential-And How We Can Change Them*. Hazelden: 1998
[264] Dominguez JR. *Transforming Your Relationship with Money*. Sounds True; Book and Cassette edition: 2001 Audio tape.
[265] Miller A. *The truth will set you free: overcoming emotional blindness and finding your true adult self*. New York: Basic Books; 2001
[266] Bradshaw J. *Healing the Shame that Binds You* [Audio Cassette (April 1990) Health Communications Audio; ISBN: 1558740430]
[267] Miller A. *The Drama of the Gifted Child: The Search for the True Self*. Basic Books: 1981
[268] Fossum M. *Catching Fire: Men Coming Alive in Recovery*. New York; Harper/Hazelden: 1989, 4-7

patients are "compliant" rather than self-directed; however, for *authentic, holistic healthcare* to be successful, it must empower the patient sufficiently such that he/she attains/regains appropriate *autonomy*—an "internal locus of control"—sufficient for lifelong internally-driven health maintenance. Health implications of autonomy (or its absence) are obvious and intuitive. Patients with an underdeveloped internal locus of control appear to experience greater degrees of social stress which can lead to hypercortisolemia and hippocampal atrophy.[269] A developed internal locus of control correlates strongly with the success of weight-loss programs, and for nonautonomous patients it is necessary to encourage the development of autonomous self-care behavior in addition to the provision of information about diet and exercise.[270]

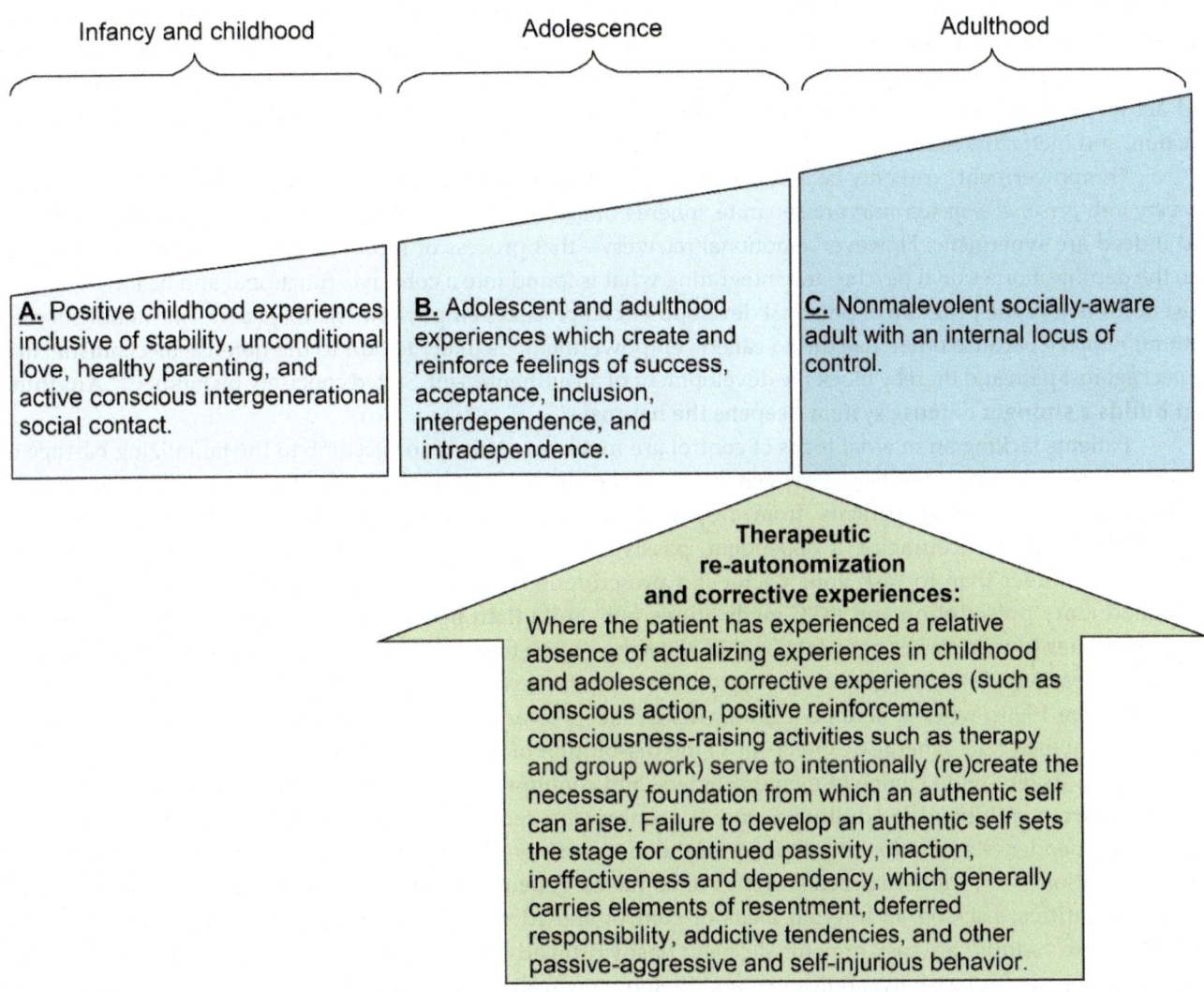

Primary, secondary, and tertiary means for developing an autonomous, authentic self: Ideally, positive childhood experiences (A) merge into adolescent and adult experiences of confidence and maturity (B) for the development of a true adult (C). If A or B is lacking or insufficient, the result is an incomplete self often incapable of *effective* and *appropriate* action. Corrective experiences must then be pursued to re-establish the foundation from which an authentic self can arise.

Completely formed internal identities are the natural result of the *continuum* of positive childhood experiences (inclusive of stability, "unconditional love", healthy parenting, and active, conscious intergenerational social contact) which are ideally merged into adolescent and adulthood experiences of success, acceptance, inclusion, independence, interdependence, and intradependence with the end result being a socially-conscious adult with an

---

[269] "Cumulative exposure to high levels of cortisol over the lifetime is known to be related to hippocampal atrophy... Self-esteem and internal locus of control were significantly correlated with hippocampal volume in both young and elderly subjects." Pruessner JC, Baldwin MW, Dedovic K, Renwick R, Mahani NK, Lord C, Meaney M, Lupien S. Self-esteem, locus of control, hippocampal volume, and cortisol regulation in young and old adulthood. *Neuroimage.* 2005 Dec;28(4):815-26

[270] "Their weight loss was significant and associated with an internal locus of control orientation (P < 0.05)... Participants with an internal orientation could be offered a standard weight reduction programme. Others, with a more external locus of control orientation, could be offered an adapted programme, which also focused on and encouraged the participants' internal orientation." Adolfsson B, Andersson I, Elofsson S, Rossner S, Unden AL. Locus of control and weight reduction. *Patient Educ Couns.* 2005 Jan;56:55-61

internal locus of control. Where the patient has experienced a relative absence of these natural and expected prerequisites, a truncated—wounded, reactive, shame-based, dissatisfied—self is likely to result. The failure to develop self-esteem and an internal locus of control largely explains why so many adult patients feign that they are incapable of action, "can't exercise", and "can't leave" their abusive jobs and relationships, and "can't resist" the dietary habits which daily contribute to their physical and psychoemotional decline. Thus, for more than a few patients, a therapeutic path must be explored which helps to re-create the foundation from which an autonomous adult and authentic self can grow—it is a *process* (not an event) of **emotional recovery**.[271] To this extent, interventional or therapeutic *autonomization* resembles a *recovery program* that can include various forms of conscious action, including goal-setting, positive reinforcement, developing emotional literacy[272] and emotional intelligence[273], and consciousness-raising experiences such as therapy and group work—all of which serve to intentionally (re)create and maintain the necessary climate for authentic selfhood. Therewith, the patient can accept challenges to further develop an *empowered self* by participating in exercises in which the ability to decide, choose, and act responsibly and appropriately are reinforced to eventually become second nature, replacing passivity, inaction, and ineffectiveness.[274]

"Empowerment" can only be authentic if it is built on the foundation of a developed self. While *emotional recovery* and *personal empowerment* are separate spheres of activity and attention, they are not mutually exclusive and indeed are synergistic. However, emotional recovery—that process of recounting one's own history, delving into the depths of one's own psyche, and integrating what is found into a cohesive, functional and healthy whole— must occur before the program of personal development emphasizes empowerment. *Empowerment* cannot succeed without *recovery* because otherwise the so-called "empowerment" is likely to add to the defense mechanisms that protect against pain and thereby block the development of an authentic self. Stated concisely by Janov[275], "**Anything that builds a stronger defense system deepens the neurosis.**"

Patients lacking an internal locus of control are much more likely to succumb to the tantalizing barrage of direct-to-consumer drug advertising[276] which infantilizes patients by 1) oversimplifying diseases, their causes, and treatments, 2) exonerating patients from responsibility and reinforcing the illusion of victimization and helplessness, and 3) encouraging a dependent, passively receptive role by telling patients that they have no proactive role other than to "ask your doctor if a prescription is right for you." **Americans have traditionally consumed more prescription and OTC medications per capita than people in any other country**[277,278]**, and this trend continues to worsen per new data in 2013 showing** "More than 4 billion prescriptions were written in 2011. That is the most ever. Everything from sleeping pills to drugs for anxiety and depression—you name it." "Something changed in the 1990s, when it became legal for drug makers to advertise. ... Demand for drugs skyrocketed."[279] With the combined and synergistic effects of 1) the dissolution of first the extended family and now the nuclear family[280], 2) a society-wide famine of mentors, elders, and community[281,282,283], 3) a dearth of autonomous, genuine exploration from childhood to adulthood, and 4) primary and secondary "educational" institutions designed to squelch independence and autonomy in favor of the more efficient, predictable, and controllable conformity and "standardization"[284,285], **industrialized societies have raised generations of people who lack completely formed internal identities**. Lacking an internal locus of control and identity from which to think independently and critically, these "adults" are easy prey for slick and flashy drug advertisements that promise the illusion of perfect health in exchange for passivity, abdication, and lifelong medicalization. That the typical American watches four hours of television per day[286] is bad enough, what makes this worse is that "Americans who watch average amounts

[271] Bradshaw J. *Healing the Shame that Binds You* [Audio Cassette (April 1990) Health Communications Audio; ISBN: 1558740430]
[272] Dayton T. *Trauma and Addiction: Ending the Cycle of Pain through Emotional Literacy*. Deerfield Beach; Health Communications, 2000
[273] Goleman D. *Emotional Intelligence*. New York; Bantam Books: 1995. Although the book as a whole was considered pioneering for its time, and the book continues to make a valuable contribution, a few of the concepts and author's personal stories are embarrassingly simplistic.
[274] Gatto JT. *A Schooling Is Not An Education: interview by Barbara Dunlop*. johntaylorgatto.com/bookstore/index.htm
[275] Janov A. *The Primal Scream*. New York; GP Putnam's Sons: 1970, page 20
[276] Aronson E. *The Social Animal*. San Fransisco; WH Freeman and company: 1972: 21-22, 53
[277] America the medicated. cbsnews.com/stories/2005/04/21/health/printable689997.shtml, msnbc.msn.com/id/7503122/, usgovinfo.about.com/od/healthcare/a/usmedicated.htm.
[278] Kivel P. *You Call This a Democracy*? Apex Press (August, 2004). ISBN: 1891843265 paulkivel.com/
[279] Costello T. *Pill Nation: are we too reliant on prescription meds*? 2013 Apr today.com/video/today/51490407/#51490407
[280] Bly R. *Iron John*. Reading, Mass.: Addison Wesley, 1990
[281] Bly R. *The Sibling Society*. Vintage Books USA; Reprint edition (June 1, 1997) ISBN: 0679781285 (Abridged audio edition (May 1, 1996), ASIN: 0679451609)
[282] Bly R. *Where have all the parents gone? A talk on the Sibling Society*. New York: Sound Horizons, 1996 Highly recommended.
[283] Bly R, Hillman J, Meade M. *Men and the Life of Desire*. Oral Tradition Archives. ISBN: 1880155001. Audio Cassette
[284] Gatto JT. *Dumbing Us Down: the Hidden Curriculum of Compulsory Education*. Gabriola Island, Canada; New Society Publishers: 2005
[285] Gatto JT. *The Paradox of Extended Childhood*. [From a presentation in Cambridge, Mass. October 2000] johntaylorgatto.com/bookstore/index.htm
[286] "American children view over 23 hours of television per week. Teenagers view an average of 21 to 22 hours of television per week. By the time today's children reach age 70, they will have spent 7 to 10 years of their lives watching television." Am. Acad.Pediatrics aapca1.org/aapca1/tv.html

of television may be exposed to more than 30 hours of direct-to-consumer drug advertisements each year, far surpassing their exposure to other forms of health communication."[287] If we are to wean our suckling culture from undue dependence on the pharmaceutical industry, we have to address our patient population directly and transform them from *passive, nonautonomous, and ignorant about health and disease* to pro-active, autonomous, and well-informed about health and the means required to obtain and sustain it.

> **Health ⇔ Healing**
> "The object of healing is...
> to move closer to wholeness."
> Kreinheder A. *Body and Soul*, 1991,p 38

Insight into a patient's internal dynamic can provide the clinician with an understanding that explains the phenomena of *non-compliance* and *disease identification*. Rather than seeing non-compliance as "weakness of will", non-compliance as a form of "disobedience" may be a reflection of the patient's unconscious need to wrestle with and resolve parental introjects. For example, if a patient had a rejecting, nonaffirming parent, he/she may need to find another rejecting authority figure in order to continue playing the role of the child; by assuming this role and "setting the stage", the patient is unconsciously attempting to create a situation wherein the primary relationship can be healed.[288] Complicating this is *disease identification*—in which patients use their disease as a source of identity and secondary gain for martyrdom, social support, group participation, acceptance, admiration, purpose, excitement, and—perhaps and at times—the drama of victimization, usually by the universe/life/world, thus confirming one's importance in that sense. Maxwell Maltz MD provided an alternate approach in his classic *PsychoCybernetics*, 1960 (page 121): "Stop dramatizing yourself as an object of pity and injustice."

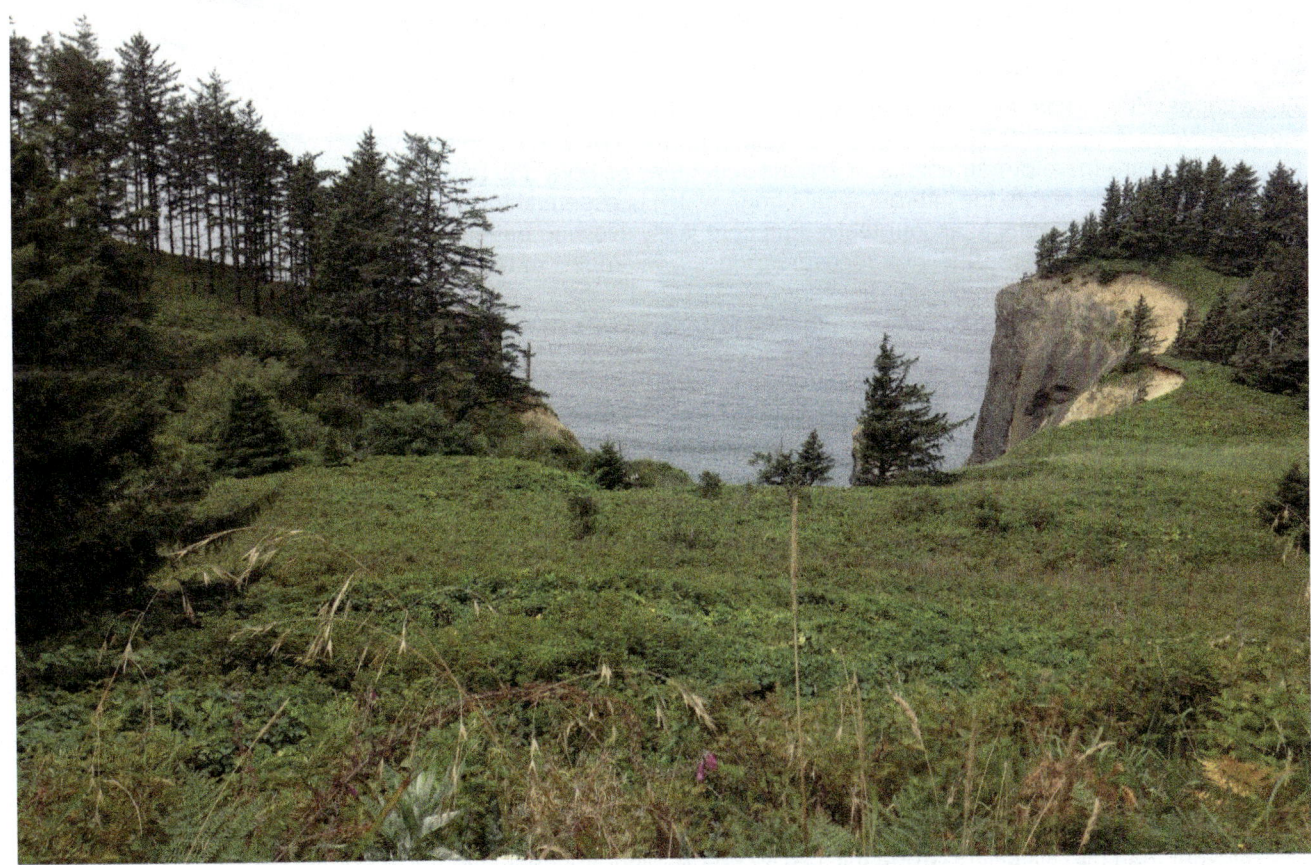

Spiritual strength: "How much truth can a spirit bear, how much truth can a spirit dare? ... That became for me more and more the real measure of value." "For a tree to become great, it seeks to twine hard roots around hard rocks." Nietzsche FW. *Ecce homo*, Introduction, sect. #3, and *Thus spoke Zarathustra*, Diminishing virtue, sect. #3; photo by DrV, Oregon coast near Astoria 2013 Aug.

---

[287] Brownfield ED, et al. Direct-to-consumer drug advertisements on network television. *J Health Commun*. 2004 Nov-Dec;9(6):491-7
[288] Miller A. *The Drama of the Gifted Child: The Search for the True Self*. Basic Books: 1981, page 88

Helping patients create and maintain authentic selves

An absent or underdeveloped locus of control is the key problem that underlies many anxiety disorders, addictive behavioral traits such as overeating, overworking, codependency, as well as chronic ineffectiveness in the pursuit of one's goals. The solutions to this problem are logical, practical, and accessible to everyone; the major costs associated with each are open-mindedness, attentiveness, discipline and persistence. There is scant mention of this concept and its intervention in the biomedical literature; however, it is well described in the psychological literature, particularly that which focuses on various types of "recovery" such as that from addiction, co-dependence, and low self-esteem, the latter two of which are virtually synonymous with an insufficient internal locus of control.

There is no single path here. There are many paths. The goal is not to choose the right path; rather the goal is to travel several paths to the degree necessary, implement what has been learned, travel other paths, and return to the same path again to retrace one's steps in new ways. The process is similar to that of *ceremonial initiation*, the purpose of which is to formally mark the *beginning* of a process that is *ongoing* and *infinite*.[1] Each path and each process has its gifts, significance, and limitations. However, the ultimate goal of each must be a tangible and positive change in the ways which the patient feels and/or behaves in and interacts with the world on a day-to-day basis.

In no particular order (since the proper sequence will have to be customized to the situation and willingness of the patient), the following are some of the more commonly cited exercises, processes, and sources of additional information:

Apprenticeship and Mentoring: books, tapes, and lectures: Children and non-autonomous adults are pulled into authentic adulthood by mentors, elders, and true adults. The therapeutic encounters thus provided— whether interpersonal or vicarious in the form of lectures, books, or audiotapes— serve as sources of information from which new possibilities can be gleaned, and these therefore serve as infinitely valuable resources for expanding the narrow horizons that characterize an underdeveloped internal locus of control. In essence, books, tapes, and lectures allow the patient to become a student and to choose a vicarious mentor. *Advantages*: Books and tapes allow access to many of the best minds in psychology; books and tapes are inexpensive; allow patients to explore and benefit from many different perspectives; books and tapes are always available and are therefore amenable to various schedules of work and responsibility. *Disadvantages*: Books and tapes do not re-create the interpersonal bridge which is essential for authentic recovery; do not provide a direct and objective means of accountably, thus potentially allowing patients to delude themselves about the effectiveness (or lack thereof) of their recovery process. Examples of better-known books, tapes and recorded lectures on the *process* of emotional recovery:

- *The Six Pillars of Self-Esteem* by Nathaniel Branden PhD. This is a very accessible yet very structured work in which Dr Branden brilliantly elucidates key concepts in psychology relevant to self-efficacy and self-esteem; also available as an audiobook excellently narrated by Dr Branden.
- *Healing the Shame that Binds You* by John Bradshaw [Audio Cassette (April 1990) Health Communications Audio; ISBN: 1558740430] Available as book and cassette with identical titles and different content.
- *A Little Book on the Human Shadow* by Robert Bly. Certainly among the most concise, accessible, and complete books ever written on the processes involved in losing and recovering the self; also available as an audio presentation.
- *The Drama of the Gifted Child* by Alice Miller. This internationally acclaimed book is considered a true classic among therapists and patients alike. Available as book and a brilliantly performed audio cassette.
- *You Can Heal Your Life* by Louise Hay. Another standard for recovery; very "new age."
- *Codependent No More: How to Stop Controlling Others and Start Caring for Yourself* by Melody Beattie. Pioneering for its time.
- *The Artist's Date Book* by Julia Cameron. Each page has a new creative idea for creative expression and "creative recovery."
- *The Psychology of Self-Esteem* by Nathaniel Branden PhD. More advanced and perhaps less widely relevant than his "six pillars" work, this is also an excellent encapsulation of important concepts in personal psychology.

Helping patients create and maintain authentic selves—*continued*

Therapy: *"Therapy is a conversation that matters."* Therapy in this context specifically means face-to-face, active interaction, either one-on-one or in a group setting, with the specific intention to give and/or provide support for personal growth. Whether 12-step groups such as Codependents Anonymous qualify as a form of therapy depends entirely upon the level of engagement of the participant; sitting in a room while *other people* do *their* work provides slow or no benefit for the passive observer. **Recovery is an *active* process, which is why it is antithetical to depression, which is a *passive* state of being.** Patients should go in knowing that this is a *process* and to not expect to be "fixed" after the first hour or even the first month. **Advantages**: Therapists can provide crucial support and insight while the client wrestles with undecipherable and convoluted emotional and psychic data. Therapists can help the client set goals ("stretches" and "homework") by which the client reaches beyond his/her comfort zone to attain the next expansion in being and experience. Therapists must create a safe space or "container" in which ideas and feelings can be brought forth to intermingle and be consciously appreciated. **Disadvantages**: Requires a flexible and disciplined schedule; costs money; bad therapists can do more harm than good if they misdirect their clients away from volatile and core issues and authentic expression. Therapy can be disempowering if the patient continues to project his/her locus of control onto the therapist.

Some of the more commonly used tools of the psychotherapeutic trade include:
- **Active listening**
- **Insight, explanation of events**: their origins, reasons, and significance
- **Reminders** of previous conclusions and stories
- **Challenge old ideas and habits**: Therapy that generally or completely lacks confrontation and accountability is ineffective.
- **Encourage exploration and new modes of being and interacting**
- **Creating a safe container wherein the client can review the details, significance, and feelings associated with past events**
- **Modeling the expression of feeling**
- **Defining goals and helping the client focus on what is significant**
- **Correcting distortions of reality**
- **Asking patients to get in touch with and then express their feelings**
- **Support and encourage clients to take calculated risks for the sake of self-expansion**
- **Pointing out errors in logic**
- **Coaching patients in the proper and responsible use of emotional language**
- **Discouraging evasiveness; requiring accountability**[1]

Creativity: All types of self-expression reinforce and validate the patient's sense of self. Creative self-expression, such as writing about thoughts and feelings about significant experiences, can reduce symptomatology in patients with rheumatoid arthritis and asthma.[1]

Experiential: Corrective experiences can be obtained in therapy, with friends and family, in integration groups, and during "experiential" retreats. **Advantages**: Experiential events orchestrated by therapists and various groups such as ManKind Project (mkp.org) and WomanWithin.org can rapidly facilitate personal growth while also providing an ongoing container and support system that encourages self-development rather than the ego-inflation that accompanies short-term events. **Disadvantages**: "Adventures" like driving across the nation or climbing a mountain are unconscious and largely impotent attempts at self-initiation; authentic initiation has always been supervised by community elders. However, once a well-founded initiation has taken place, preferably with an on-going community that facilitates continued refinement and self-exploration, then "adventures" can be undertaken consciously to maintain and reinforce the experience of autonomy and competent selfhood. Eventually, transformative and sustentative experiences can be integrated and created in the daily life experience so that dramatic adventures become unnecessary for the continued renewal and "recharging" of the self.

Creating and Re-Creating the Self: An on-going process that involves various types of "therapy" such as healthy formal/informal interpersonal and group relationships, creative expression and exploration, the periodic infusion of new ideas from teachers and mentors, attendance in workshops and seminars (and other forms of on-going consciousness-raising), reflection, and the integration of transformative and sustentative significance into everyday life, in such a way that daily life itself becomes *therapeutic* and *affirmative*.

Become your own source of transformation

"However you may be, be your own source of experience! Throw off your discontent about your nature; forgive yourself *your own self*, for you have in your life experience a ladder with a hundred rungs, on which you can climb to knowledge. ... You have it in your power to merge everything you have lived through—attempts, false starts, errors, delusions, passions, your love and your hope—into your future self and goal, with nothing left over."

Nietzsche FW. *Human, All Too Human: A Book for Free Spirits*. Essay #292

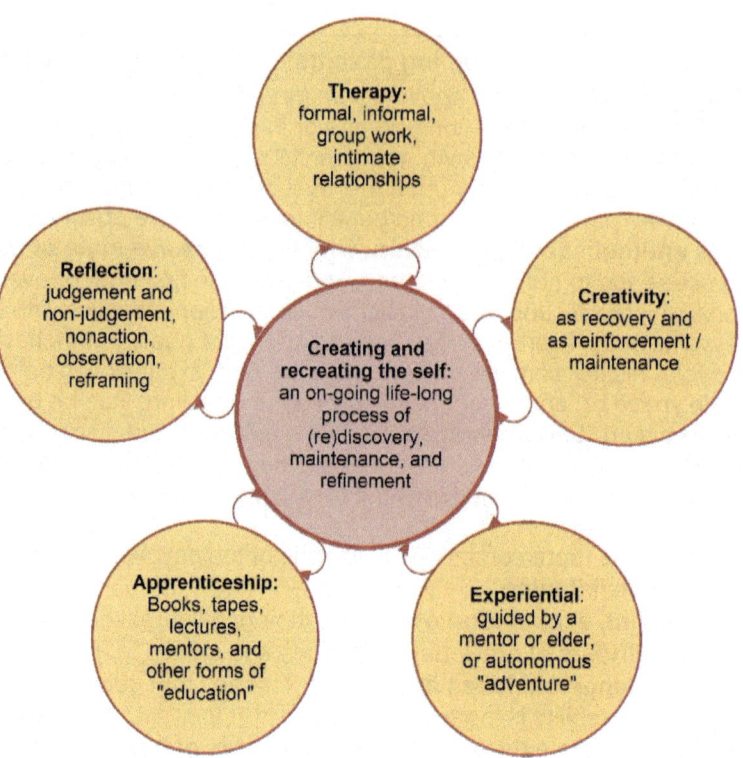

One possible sequence of events for effective, lasting, and authentic autonomization: The caterpillar does not blossom into a butterfly without spending time in its cocoon. The airborne seed descends into the earth for its nourishment before it sprouts and searches for the sun. Similarly, gratification of our ascentionist and impatient ego must be deferred for the sake of allowing the time and descent that provide "grounding" and developing of a solid foundation from which authentic growth can arise. The Western view of "personal development" idealizes a life course of constant ascension that is generally inconsistent with living in a real world fraught with imperfections; two of the major complications arising from such a perfectionistic paradigm are 1) that it causes people to feel anxious and ashamed when confronted with otherwise normal delays and failures, and 2) that it biases people into believing that improvement comes only from advancement rather than also from the return and short-term regression that are characteristic of most historically-proven societal traditions. With modification of the stepwise model proposed by Bradshaw[289], here I propose the following sequence:

1. **Short-term behavior modification**: For people whose behavior is acutely dysfunctional or harmful to themselves or others, they must stop the "acting out" that is the symptom of the underlying emotional injury or schism. Accepting abuse—at work or home—is a form of **acting out** that perpetuates old wounds and saps the strength required for recovery. Enacting addictive behavior is injurious to the psyche because self-injurious behavior reinforces the image of oneself as an object of contempt while also reinforcing the image of psychological dependency and emotional helplessness.

2. **Emotional recovery**: Complete healing is only possible when consciously pursued, and conscious healing can only be pursued after one has become conscious of the wounds, injuries, absences, dynamics, and events that lead to the current state. This process of recovery is referred to mythologically as the "descent" or the time of "eating ashes" that is a recurrent theme in various fairy tales ("Cinderella" literally means "ash girl") and cultural-religious histories (such as Jesus' *descent* into the tomb).[290] The biggest blockades to this process are 1) the ego, which prefers to ascend and to deny intrapersonal "negativity"[291], and 2) the challenge in finding elders and mentors in a society that constantly perpetuates and encourages immaturity, materialism, and superficiality.[292] In the words of famed psychologist Carl Jung, "One does not become enlightened by imagining figures of light, but by making the darkness *conscious*. The latter procedure, however, is disagreeable, and

289 Bradshaw J. *Healing the Shame that Binds You* [Audio Cassette (April 1990) Health Communications Audio; ISBN: 1558740430]
290 Bly R, Hillman J, Meade M. *Men and the Life of Desire*. Oral Tradition Archives. ISBN: 1880155001
291 Robert Bly. *The Human Shadow*. Sound Horizons, New York 1991 [ISBN: 1879323001] and Bly R. *A Little Book on the Human Shadow*.[ISBN: 0062548476]
292 Bly R. *Where have all the parents gone? A talk on the Sibling Society*. New York: Sound Horizons, 1996

therefore unpopular." People often have tremendous resistances to the process of self-exploration and internal learning; as Jeffrey Kottler[293] wrote of his own experience in *The Compleat Therapist*, "...like most prospective consumers of therapy, I made up a bunch of excuses for why I could handle this on my own... I was smiling like an idiot..."

3. <u>**Long-term behavior modification and integration**</u>: Insight allows for an illumination of the internal mental-emotional landscape, and effective insight must then be manifested externally by changes/modifications in behavior, habits, and interaction in the world. **Externalized behaviors simultaneously reflect and reinforce thoughts and feelings.** According to Grieneeks[294], patients (and their healthcare providers) can "*think* their way into new ways of *acting*" and "*act* their way into new ways of *thinking*." Eventually, a consciously designed life can be created so that actions, interactions, thoughts, and feelings are melded together in such ways that everyday life itself becomes simultaneously *therapeutic, affirmative, sustentative,* and *empowering*. In this way, the person and his/her life are unified in such ways as to become self-perpetuating and self-sustaining cycles of ascents and descents, thought-feeling and action, reflection and courage, independence and interdependence—in sum: "a wheel rolling from its own center."[295] At this point the self is established, though it must be maintained and developed with the continuous application of consciousness, reflection, and action.

4. <u>**Metapersonal involvement in community, religion, spirituality, and the world**</u>: Many people are tempted to move from a state of woundedness, relative incompleteness and the feelings of shame and disempowerment to a state of illusory *perfection, enlightenment* and *omnipotence* without doing the requisite hard work that makes authentic personal growth possible. People with unhealed emotional wounds often seek to camouflage those deficiencies by becoming pious and projecting an image of completeness and of "having it all figured out" and "having it all together"; religion and the acquisition of power are often misused for this purpose. Many people are successful in wearing this mask for many years; but its crumbling—often manifested as the "midlife crisis"—heralds an opportunity for personal growth if not medicated with anti-depressants, vacations, affairs, gambling, new cars and other distractions common in the American "midlife crisis." The temptation to bypass Stages 2 [emotional recovery] and 3 [integration] and leapfrog from Stage 1 [woundedness] to Stage 4 [spirituality] should be resisted because the religion or spirituality is then used as a shield *against authenticity* and as a tool for illusory control. Religion can be misused in this way by providing an "identity" and sense of redemption for people with incompletely formed identities and for those with incompletely reconciled shadows and unresolved childhood-parental introjects.[296,297,298] Nietzsche's[299] response to this problem was to encourage self-knowledge and self-reconciliation as prerequisites to religious devotion, hence his admonition, "By all means love your neighbor as yourself – but *first* be such that you love yourself." Historical and recent events remind us of how religion can be misused for misanthropic ends.[300] What is commonly referred to as "spiritual development"—a level of resolution, reconciliation, and autonomy that allows for compassionate interdependence with people, the planet and the larger "world"—is synergistic with and can be supported by religion; but the latter is not a substitute for the former.[301,302] Religion and other forms of metapersonal involvement (e.g., community participation and social generosity) are *important* and *necessary* extensions of self-development. In order for personal development to blossom from the germ of necessary narcissism into its flower of functional completeness, it must eventually manifest in the larger community and the world.

[293] Kottler JA. *The Compleat Therapist*. San Francisco; Jossey-Bass publishers; 1991, pages 2-3
[294] Keith Grieneeks PhD. "Psychological Assessment" taught in 1998 at Bastyr University.
[295] Friedrich Wilhelm Nietzsche, Walter Kaufmann (Translator). *Thus Spoke Zarathustra*. Penguin USA; 1978, page 27
[296] Bradshaw J. *Healing the Shame that Binds You* [Audio Cassette (April 1990) Health Communications Audio; ISBN: 1558740430]
[297] Miller A. *The Drama of the Gifted Child: The Search for the True Self*. Basic Books: 1981
[298] Miller A. *The truth will set you free: overcoming emotional blindness and finding your true adult self*. New York: Basic Books; 2001
[299] Nietzsche N. *Thus spoke Zarathustra*. Read by Jon Cartwright and Alex Jennings and published by Naxos AudioBooks. I think this is among the more brilliant achievements in human history. naxosaudiobooks.com/nabusa/pages/432512.htm
[300] *Bonhoeffer*, movie documentary by director/writer Martin Doblmeier described online bonhoeffer.com
[301] Lozoff B. *It's a Meaningful Life: It Just Takes Practice*. March 1, 2001. ISBN: 0140196242
[302] Bradshaw J. *Healing the Shame that Binds You* [Audio Cassette Version (April 1990) Health Communications Audio; ISBN: 1558740430]

5. _Acceptance of mortality and death_: No individual person or any system of thought, whether scientific or religious, can feign completeness without accounting for the end of life and incorporating this account into its overarching paradigm. The event is too significant, and the fear and concerns it provokes are too weighty to not be addressed directly and held in consciousness on a periodic—if not frequent—basis. This topic is of practical importance, too, not only in our own lives and those of our friends and family, but also to the national healthcare system, which currently spends the bulk of its money and resources vainly attempting to preserve life in the last few years and months after which disease or age call unrelentingly for the end of life. Perhaps if we as individuals and as participants in the healthcare system could accept and deal with our own deaths, then we would not have to panic and participate in such superfluous expenditures of time, energy, emotion, and money when death seeks to arrive, either for our patients, our friends and family, or ourselves. Proximal to the panic and aversion that characterizes the West's relationship to death is the "subclinical" panic and aversion that infiltrate the lives, practices, and policies that we experience every day. Surely, many unconscious events and subconscious influences contribute to the "lives of quiet desperation"[303] and "universal anxiety"[304] that subtly yet

> **Failure to accept aging and death can only create a fragmented and neurotic society**
>
> "**The event of death is not a tragedy**—to rabbit, fox or man. But **the _concept_ of death _is_ a tragedy,** for man, and _indirectly_ for poor fox, rabbit, bush, bird, just anything and everything in man's path."
>
> Pearce JC, _Exploring the Crack in the Cosmic Egg_. Washington Square Press; 1974, page 59

powerfully afflict most people; surely, lack of reconciliation with death is a major contributor. Especially in western cultures, death is commonly seen as some type of failure or shortcoming, either on behalf of the patient or his/her doctors, and the most common questions asked on the topic of death are _"how can this be avoided?"_ before the event and _"who is to blame?"_ after the event. Other cultures accept death as a natural part of life, and indeed, people are seen to have an obligation to die so that the next generations can have their turn in the cycle of life. Alternatives to western hysteria are founded on acceptance of death, and the prerequisites for the acceptance of death are 1) the dedication of sufficient time for its consideration (most people would rather watch a bad movie or attend spectator sports), 2) reframing the event in terms of its being a natural part of our lives, certainly nothing to be ashamed of (discussed below), 3) making necessary logistical preparations (e.g., writing of wills, providing for dependents, and other obvious technicalities), and 4) living as completely, consciously, compassionately, effectively, and authentically as possible so that remorse can be minimized, perhaps completely mitigated. Reframing the event of death begins with its description in general terms so that its enigma, from which its power over the hearts and minds of humanity is derived, can be deciphered and thus deflated. The main characteristics of death which precipitate its fear are 1) the unpredictability of its arrival, 2) the duration of the dying process, and 3) the quality of that process, for example whether it is painful or associated with or precipitated by severe illness or injury. The first characteristic of _timeliness_—the unpredictability of its arrival—stresses people because of their inadequate preparation and the feeling that they have only recently begun to live or have not quite yet begun to live their authentic lives. These concerns are allayed by preparation, both logistical and intrapersonal. Each of us has the responsibility to "become authentically whole" so that we do not inflict our incompleteness onto others, either directly through various forms of transference or deprivation or indirectly though the more subtle means of politics and cultural mores.[305,306] If a person can live with vitality, authenticity,

> **Failure to accept aging and death can only create a fragmented and neurotic society**
>
> "Once accepted, death is an integral component of every event, as the left hand to the right. The cultural death concept could only be instilled in a mind split from its own life flow."
>
> Pearce JC, _Exploring the Crack in the Cosmic Egg_.1974, p59

compassion and effectiveness then little is left to want, and fears of death and its untimely arrival are diminished. The remaining variables are both controllable and uncontrollable; they are uncontrollable to the extent that we are all subject to chaos and accidents, whether in cars, planes, or bathtubs. _Duration_ and _quality_

[303] Throeau HD, (Thomas O, ed). _Walden and Civil Disobedience_. New York: WW Norton and Company; 1966, page 5
[304] Becker E. _The Denial of Death_. New York: Free Press; 1973, pages 11 and 21
[305] Miller A. _The Drama of the Gifted Child: The Search for the True Self_. Basic Books: 1981
[306] Robert Bly. _The Human Shadow_. Sound Horizons, New York 1991 [ISBN: 1879323001] and Bly R. _A Little Book on the Human Shadow_.[ISBN: 0062548476

are both controllable on an inpatient setting to the extent that palliative care and autonomous decision-making is made available.[307,308]

Life can only be authentically and completely experienced after one has created an authentic self and has thereafter accepted life *as it is*. Since death is part of life, the full engagement of life requires *acceptance of* and *reconciliation with* death. Acceptance of death does not necessarily entail that life becomes permeated with nihilistic resignation; on the contrary, it infuses daily events with significance and makes all experiences unique and worthy of appreciation.

Growth, integration, and acceptance: Starting at the top, the progression of personal growth, emotional recovery, integration and daily practice is followed by the more advanced integration of one's chosen purpose, mission, and life work with one's chosen spiritual/religious practice, family and community involvement, and acceptance of and preparation for the end of life and the continuity of society and the environment.

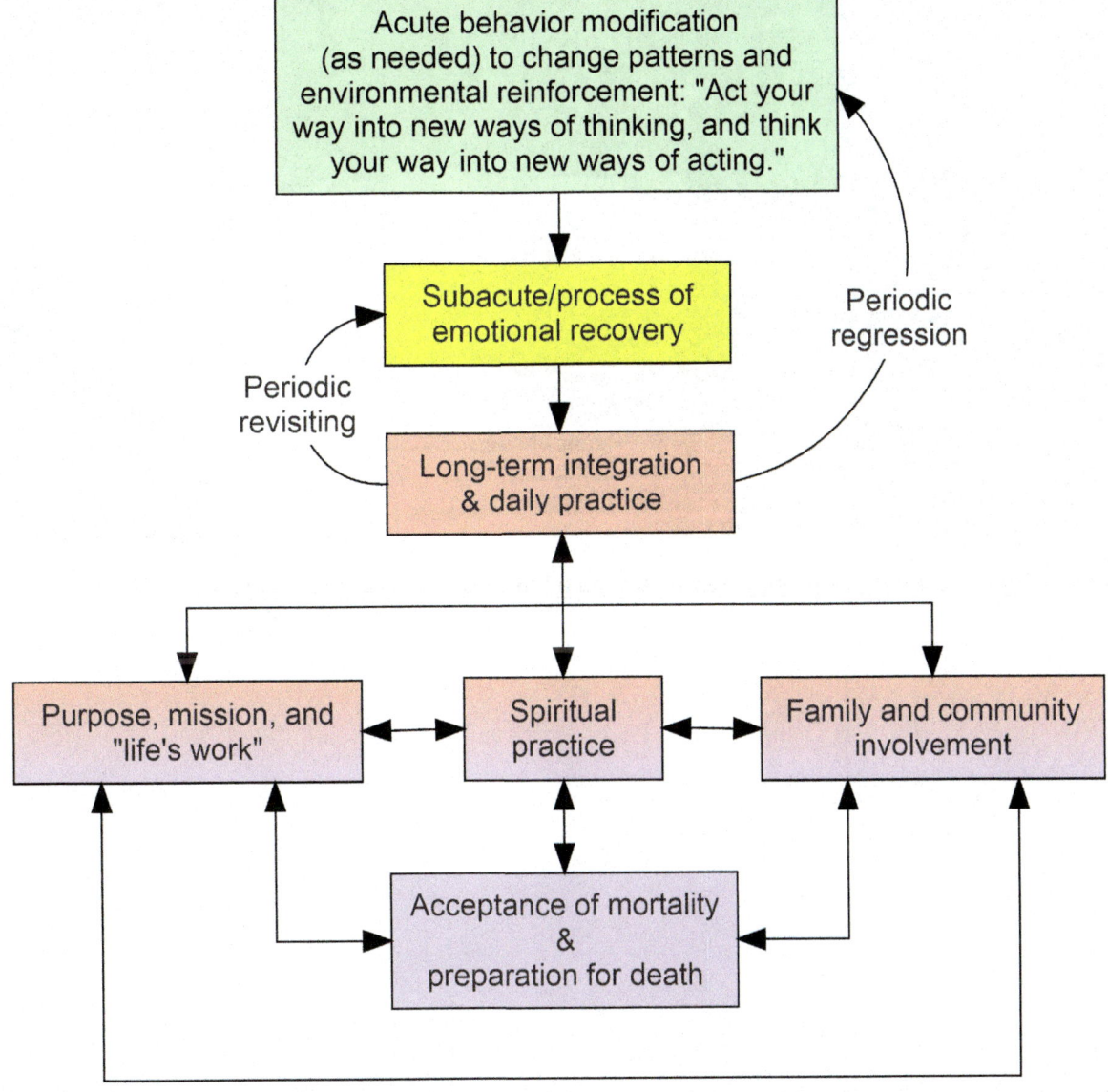

"They say there's no future for us. They're right, which is fine with us."

Rumi[309]

---

[307] Steinbrook R. Medical marijuana, physician-assisted suicide, and the Controlled Substances Act. *N Engl J Med*. 2004 Sep 30;351(14):1380-3

[308] "Failure to give an effective therapy to seriously ill patients, either adults or children, violates the core principles of both medicine and ethics… Therefore, in the patient's best interest, patients and parents/surrogates, have the right to request medical marijuana under certain circumstances and physicians have the duty to disclose medical marijuana as an option and prescribe it when appropriate." Clark PA. Medical marijuana: should minors have the same rights as adults? *Med Sci Monit*.2003;9:ET1-9

[309] Rumi in Barks C (translator). *The Essential Rumi*. HarperSanFransisco: 1995, page 2

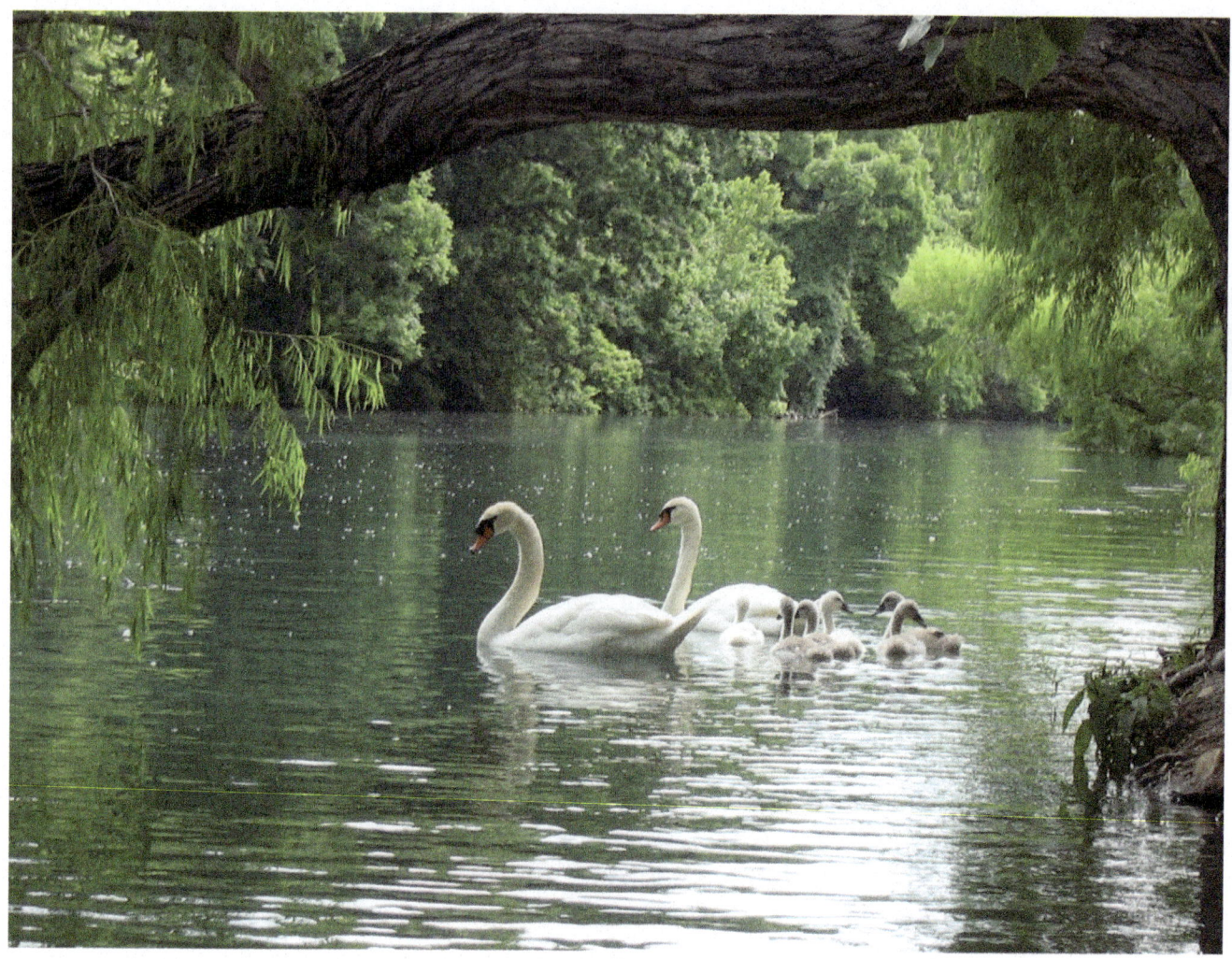

Town Lake (Colorado River) in Austin, Texas just as a light rain began, circa 2004: Photo by Dr V

Environmental Health, Toxicity, and Detoxification

"Man's attitude toward nature is today critically important simply because we have now acquired a fateful power to alter and destroy nature. But man is a part of nature, and his war against nature is inevitably a war against himself." *Rachel Carson*[310]

Environmental exposures to chemicals and toxic substances: Studies using blood tests and tissue samples from Americans across the nation have consistently shown that all Americans have toxic chemical accumulation whether or not they work in chemical factories or are obviously exposed at home or work.[311,312] **The recent report from the CDC found toxic chemicals such as pesticides in all Americans, especially minorities, women, and children.**[313] Nearly all of these chemicals are known to contribute to health problems in humans—problems such as cancer, fatigue, poor memory, endocrinopathy, subfertility/infertility, Parkinson's disease, autoimmune diseases like lupus, and many other serious conditions. Therefore, *detoxification programs are a necessity—not a luxury*.

Examples of toxicants commonly found in Americans

Environmental pollutant (population frequency)	Biologic effects as quoted from HSDB: Hazardous Substances Data Bank. National Library of Medicine, NIH[314] or other reference as noted
DDE (found in 99% of Americans): DDE is the main metabolite of DDT, a pesticide that was presumably banned in the US in 1972	• DDT is known to be immunosuppressive in animals. • A study published in 2004 showed that increasing levels of DDE in African-American male farmers in North Carolina correlated with a higher prevalence of antinuclear antibodies and up to 50% reductions in serum IgG.[315] • Other studies in humans have shown an estrogenic or anti-androgenic effect.[316] • Virtually all US women have evidence of DDT/DDE accumulation. Women with higher levels of DDT and/or its metabolites show pregnancy and childbirth complications and have higher rates of infant mortality.[317]
Glyphosate: The main active ingredient in Monsanto's Roundup ® herbicide	• Percentage of exposed population is essentially 100% because the US FDA has failed to regulate or even measure glyphosate residues in food • Now that massive percentages of American and international food is sprayed with glyphosate, either as a part of the genetic manipulation of foods debacle or as systemic overuse for example desiccation of grains for easier processing, glyphosate permeates the international environment • Thanks to independently funded research to compensate for the lack of government supervision, glyphosate has been detected in all types of food products including beer, wine baby food, cereals and food animals • Glyphosate and the Roundup formula have been shown to cause DNA damage, endocrine disruption, and mitochondrial dysfunction in various in vitro and in vivo studies, including human studies

---

[310] Rachel Carson. *Silent Spring*. Boston, Houghton Mifflin Company (2002). ISBN: 0395683297. See also Rachel Carson Dies of Cancer; 'Silent Spring' Author Was 56. New York Times 1956. rachelcarson.org/ on August 1, 2004

[311] "The average concentration of 2,3,7,8-tetrachlorodibenzo-p-dioxin in the adipose tissue of the US population was 5.38 pg/g, increasing from 1.98 pg/g in children under 14 years of age to 9.40 pg/g in adults over 45." Orban JE, Stanley JS, Schwemberger JG, Remmers JC. Dioxins and dibenzofurans in adipose tissue of the general US population and selected subpopulations. *Am J Public Health* 1994 Mar;84(3):439-45

[312] "Although the use of HCB as a fungicide has virtually been eliminated, detectable levels of HCB are still found in nearly all people in the USA." Robinson PE, Leczynski BA, Kutz FW, Remmers JC. An evaluation of hexachlorobenzene body-burden levels in the general population of the USA. *IARC Sci Publ* 1986;77:183-92

[313] "Many of the pesticides found in the test subjects have been linked to serious short- and long-term health effects including infertility, birth defects and childhood and adult cancers." panna.org/campaigns/docsTrespass/chemicalTrespass2004.dv.html July 25, 2004

[314] Primary source for this data is the Hazardous Substances Data Bank. National Library of Medicine, National Institutes of Health: toxnet.nlm.nih.gov/cgi-bin/sis/htmlgen?HSDB accessed on August 1, 2004

[315] Cooper GS, Martin SA, Longnecker MP, Sandler DP, Germolec DR. Associations between plasma DDE levels and immunologic measures in African-American farmers in North Carolina. *Environ Health Perspect*. 2004 Jul;112(10):1080-4

[316] Dalvie MA, Myers JE, Lou Thompson M, Dyer S, Robins TG, Omar S, Riebow J, Molekwa J, Kruger P, Millar R. The hormonal effects of long-term DDT exposure on malaria vector-control workers in Limpopo Province, South Africa. *Environ Res*. 2004 Sep;96(1):9-19

[317] "The findings strongly suggest that DDT use increases preterm births, which is a major contributor to infant mortality. If this association is causal, it should be included in any assessment of the costs and benefits of vector control with DDT." Longnecker MP, Klebanoff MA, Zhou H, Brock JW. Association between maternal serum concentration of the DDT metabolite DDE and preterm and small-for-gestational-age babies at birth. *Lancet*. 2001 Jul 14;358(9276):110-4

Environmental pollutant (population frequency)	Biologic effects as quoted from HSDB: Hazardous Substances Data Bank. National Library of Medicine, NIH[318] or other reference
2,5-dichlorophenol (88% nationally and up to 96% in select children populations): Dichlorophenols can occur in tap water as a result of standard chlorination treatment. General population may be exposed to 2,5-dichlorophenol through oral consumption or dermal contact with chlorinated tap water. 2,5-Dichlorophenol was identified in 96% of the urine samples of children residing in Arkansas near an herbicide plant at concentrations of 4-1,200 ppb. The sole manufacturer for herbicide use is Sandoz (Clariant Corporation).	• Human Toxicity Excerpts: 1. Burning pain in mouth and throat. White necrotic lesions in mouth, esophagus, and stomach. Abdominal pain, vomiting ... and bloody diarrhea. 2. Pallor, sweating, weakness, headache, dizziness, tinnitus. 3. Shock: Weak irregular pulse, hypotension, shallow respirations, cyanosis, pallor, and a profound fall in body temperature. 4. Possibly fleeting excitement and confusion, followed by unconsciousness. ... 5. Stentorous breathing, mucous rales, rhonchi, frothing at nose and mouth and other signs of pulmonary edema are sometimes seen. Characteristic odor of phenol on the breath. 6. Scanty, dark-colored ... urine ... moderately severe renal insufficiency may appear. 7. Methemoglobinemia, Heinz body hemolytic anemia and hyperbilirubinemia have been reported. ... 8. Death from respiratory, circulatory or cardiac failure. 9. If spilled on skin, pain is followed promptly by numbness. The skin becomes blanched, and a dry opaque eschar forms over the burn. When the eschar sloughs off, a brown stain remains.
Chlorpyrifos (found in 93% of Americans): Insecticide used on corn and cotton and for termite control. Conservative estimates hold that 80% of the chlorpyrifos in the US was produced directly or indirectly by Dow Chemical Corporation.[319] **This pesticide is routinely used in schools and is thus found in blood and tissue samples of nearly all American children.**	• Toxic if inhaled, in contact with skin, and if swallowed. • All the organophosphorus insecticides have a cumulative effect by progressive inhibition of cholinesterase. • The symptoms of chronic poisoning due to organophosphorus pesticides include headache, weakness, feeling of heaviness in head, decline of memory, quick onset of **fatigue, disturbed sleep**, loss of appetite, and loss of orientation. Other manifestations of accumulation include **tension, anxiety, restlessness, insomnia, headache, emotional instability, fatigue...** • Chlorpyrifos is a suspected endocrine disruptor.[320] • **Higher chlorpyrifos levels in children correlate with higher incidences attention problems, attention-deficit/hyperactivity disorder, and pervasive developmental disorder.[321]**

[318] Primary source for this data is the Hazardous Substances Data Bank, National Institutes of Health: toxnet.nlm.nih.gov/cgi-bin/sis/htmlgen?HSDB accessed on August 1, 2004

[319] Kristin S. Schafer, Margaret Reeves, Skip Spitzer, Susan E. Kegley. Chemical Trespass: Pesticides in Our Bodies and Corporate Accountability. Pesticide Action Network North America. May 2004 Available at panna.org/campaigns/docsTrespass/chemicalTrespass2004.dv.html on August 1, 2004

[320] panna.org/resources/documents/factsChlorpyrifos.dv.html accessed August 1, 2004

[321] "Highly exposed children (chlorpyrifos levels of >6.17 pg/g plasma) scored, on average, 6.5 points lower on the Bayley Psychomotor Development Index and 3.3 points lower on the Bayley Mental Development Index at 3 years of age compared with those with lower levels of exposure. Children exposed to higher, compared with lower, chlorpyrifos levels were also significantly more likely to experience Psychomotor Development Index and Mental Development Index delays, attention problems, attention-deficit/hyperactivity disorder problems, and pervasive developmental disorder problems at 3 years of age." Rauh VA, Garfinkel R, Perera FP, Andrews HF, Hoepner L, Barr DB, Whitehead R, Tang D, Whyatt RW. Impact of prenatal chlorpyrifos exposure on neurodevelopment in the first 3 years of life among inner-city children. *Pediatrics*. 2006 Dec;118(6):e1845-59

Examples of toxicants commonly found in Americans—*continued*

Environmental pollutant (population frequency)	Biologic effects as quoted from HSDB: Hazardous Substances Data Bank. National Library of Medicine, NIH[322] or other reference as noted
Mercury (8% of American women of reproductive age have mercury levels high enough to cause adverse health effects)	▪ Mercury is a well-known neurotoxin, immunotoxin, and nephrotoxin. Mercury toxicity is also a known cause of hypertension in humans. ▪ A recent study published in *JAMA—Journal of the American Medical Association*[323] noted that "Humans are exposed to methylmercury, a well-established neurotoxin, through fish consumption. The fetus is most sensitive to the adverse effects of exposure. … **approximately 8% of women had concentrations higher than the US EPA's recommended reference dose (5.8 microg/L),** below which exposures are considered to be without adverse effects." **The most obvious interpretation of this data published in *JAMA* is that 8% of American women have chronic mercury poisoning—poisoning in this case refers specifically to elevated blood levels of a known toxicant that consistently demonstrates adverse effects on human health.** Logical deduction holds that such a high prevalence of human poisoning should be unacceptable and should lead directly to legislative restrictions on corporate emissions to protect and salvage the health of the public.
2,4-dichlorophenol (found in 87% of Americans): Pesticide	▪ Human Toxicity Excerpts: same as for 2,5-dichlorophenol ▪ In males, significant increases in relative risk ratios for lung cancer, rectal cancer, and soft tissue sarcomas were reported; in females, there were increases in the relative risk of cervical cancer.

Toxicity and detoxification—basics: The physiologic processes by which toxins—whether chemicals or metals—are referred to generally as "detoxification." Clinically, doctors can implement treatment interventions to promote and facilitate the removal of chemical and metal toxins; this, too, is generally referred to as detoxification or clinical/therapeutic detoxification programs. Detoxification programs are popular with patients and some doctors and are most often misused and misapplied. The recent findings that mercury poisoning can result from once-weekly consumption of tuna[324] and that the average American has 13 pesticides in his/her body[325] should be seen as an indication of how dangerously toxic our environment has become, largely due to irresponsible corporate and government policies that value profitability over sustainability.

Detoxification procedures: Though a detailed clinical explanation of detoxification procedures will not be included here (see Chapter 4 of *Integrative Rheumatology*[326]), the general concepts for detoxification are as follows:
1. **Avoidance**: reduced exposure = reduced problem
    a. If there were less chemical pollution, then our environment would be less toxic and therefore we would not have such problems with environmental poisoning.
    b. Limit or eliminate exposure to paint fumes, car exhaust, new carpet, solvents, adhesives, artificial foods, synthetic chemical drugs, copier fumes, pesticides, herbicides, chemical fertilizers, etc.
2. **Depuration**: "The act or process of freeing from foreign or impure matter"[327]
    a. Exercise and sauna
    b. Bowel cleansing, fiber, probiotics, antibiotics, laxatives

---

[322] Primary source for this data is the Hazardous Substances Data Bank, National Institutes of Health: toxnet.nlm.nih.gov/cgi-bin/sis/htmlgen?HSDB Accessed Aug 1, 2004
[323] Schober SE, Sinks TH, Jones RL, Bolger PM, McDowell M, Osterloh J, Garrett ES, Canady RA, Dillon CF, Sun Y, Joseph CB, Mahaffey KR. Blood mercury levels in US children and women of childbearing age, 1999-2000. *JAMA.* 2003 Apr 2;289(13):1667-74
[324] "The neurobehavioral performance of subjects who consumed tuna fish regularly was significantly worse on color word reaction time, digit symbol reaction time and finger tapping speed (FT)." Carta P, Flore C, Alinovi R, Ibba A, Tocco MG, Aru G, Carta R, Girei E, Mutti A, Lucchini R, Randaccio FS. Sub-clinical neurobehavioral abnormalities associated with low level of mercury exposure through fish consumption. *Neurotoxicology.* 2003 Aug;24(4-5):617-23
[325] "A comprehensive survey of more than 1,300 Americans has found traces of weed- and bug-killers in the bodies of everyone tested, …. The survey, conducted by the U.S. Centers for Disease Control and Prevention, found that the body of the average American contained 13 of these chemicals." Martin Mittelstaedt. 13 pesticides in body of average American. *The Globe and Mail.* Friday, May 21, 2004 - Page A17 theglobeandmail.com/servlet/ArticleNews/TPStory/LAC/20040521/HPEST21/TPEnvironment/ 2004 Aug
[326] Vasquez A. *Integrative Rheumatology.* InflammationMastery.com
[327] Webster's 1913 Dictionary

    c. Liver and bile stimulators

    d. Cofactors for phase 1 oxidation and phase 2 conjugation

    e. Chelation for heavy metals

    f. Urine alkalinization

3. **Damage control**: managing the consequences of chemical and heavy metal toxicity

    a. Hormone replacement

    b. Antioxidant therapy

    c. Occupational and rehabilitative training

    d. Management of resultant diseases, particularly autoimmune diseases

4. **Political and social action**: Due in large part to corporate influence and government deregulation, environmental contamination with pesticides from American corporations has increased to such an extent over the past few decades that now all Americans show evidence of pesticide accumulation in their bodies. Failure to hold corporations to tight regulatory standards has jeopardized the future of humanity. Voter passivity combined with collusion between multinational corporations and government officials is the underlying problem. Political action is the solution. The past and recent history on this topic is clear and well documented for those who wish to access the facts.[328,329,330,331,332,333,334,335,336]

The most obvious problem in functional medicine and integrative/naturopathic healthcare with regard to population-wide xenobiotic exposure is the failure of political engagement to actually help solve the cause of the problem—failure or complete lack of government regulations at the corporate source of chemical production. The obviously problem with reliance on "detoxification programs" of various types is that these are generally accessible only by the more educated and wealthy sections of society, and are completely unavailable among poorer populations, which clearly bear the brunt of corporate irresponsibility and chemical trespass/assault. By failing to address the political root of the problem, healthcare groups allow the problem to fester, affecting the entire population, and then profiting either from those with xenobiotic-induced illness (all strata) or from the richer/educated strata of patients who seek "therapeutic detoxification programs"; basically what is happening is population-wide poisoning with occasional and selective salvation of a few people (generally wealthy/educated) who seek treatment for chemical exposure and accumulation.

> **"The only thing necessary for the triumph of evil is for good men to do nothing."** Edmond Burke (1729 – 1797)
>
> "Your lack of interest in the past, your lack of involvement, your unwillingness to develop coherent strategies, your unwillingness to challenge authority - these have created a vacuum in decision-making, that has been filled by professional groups with close relationships with the chemical industries…"
>
> Samuel Epstein, M.D.[337]

---

[328] Van den Bosch R. *The pesticide conspiracy*. Garden City, NY: Doubleday, 1978. ISBN: 0385133847

[329] "Monsanto Corporation is widely known for its production of the herbicide Roundup and genetically engineered Roundup-ready crops… altered to survive a dousing of the toxic herbicide. …glyphosate, is known to cause eye soreness, headaches, diarrhea, and other flu-like symptoms, and has been linked to non-Hodgkin's lymphoma." Bush Names Former Monsanto Executive as EPA Deputy Administrator. Daily News Archive From March 29, 2001 beyondpesticides.org/NEWS/daily_news_archive/2001/03_29_01.htm accessed on August 1, 2004

[330] "They pointed to budgets cuts for research and enforcement, to steep declines in the number of cases filed against polluters, to efforts to relax portions of the Clean Air Act, to an acceleration of federal approvals for the spraying of restricted pesticides and more." Patricia Sullivan. Anne Gorsuch Burford, 62, Dies; Reagan EPA Director. *Washington Post*. Thursday, July 22, 2004; Page B06 washingtonpost.com/wp-dyn/articles/A3418-2004Jul21.html on August 2, 2004

[331] "In fact, amongst the crimes of Reagan and Bush which will go down in history are their emasculation of Federal regulatory apparatus… But in 1988, under the Bush administration, the EPA - illegally, in our view - revoked the Dellaney Law…" Samuel Epstein MD, 1993. Professor of Occupational and Environmental Medicine at the School of Public Health, University of Illinois Medical Center Chicago. converge.org.nz/pirm/pestican.htm accessed August 1, 2004

[332] "The Environmental Protection Agency will be free to approve pesticides without consulting wildlife agencies to determine if the chemical might harm plants and animals protected by the Endangered Species Act, according to new Bush administration rules…. It also is intended to head off future lawsuits, the officials said." Associated Press. Bush Eases Pesticide Laws cbsnews.com/stories/2004/07/29/tech/main633009.shtml accessed August 1, 2004

[333] "The new policy also could bolster pesticide makers' contention that federal labeling insulates them from suits alleging that their products cause illness or environmental damage, Olson says. 'It . . . could really be disastrous for public health.'" Bush Exempts Pesticide Companies from Lawsuits. Law on Pesticides Reinterpreted: Government Alters Policy in Effort to Protect Manufacturers. Peter Eisler. *USA TODAY*. October 6, 2003 organicconsumers.org/foodsafety/bushpesticides100703.cfm Accessed Aug 2004

[334] "The Environmental Protection Agency will be free to approve pesticides without consulting wildlife agencies to determine if the chemical might harm plants and animals protected by the Endangered Species Act, according to new Bush administration rules." Bush eases pesticide reviews for endangered species. usatoday.com/news/washington/2004-07-29-epa-pesticides_x.htm?csp=34 Accessed August 2004

[335] "It is simply intolerable that the EPA, instead of providing an example for open scientific discussion, has continuously violated key environmental legislation, stifling legitimate dissent. The failure of EPA to properly encourage and protect whistleblowing has undermined the ability of the EPA and state environmental agencies to enforce environmental laws." Letter to Carol Browner, Administrator U.S. Environmental Protection Agency from Stephen Kohn, Chair National Whistleblower Center Board of Directors dated March 23, 1999. Availble at whistleblowers.org/statements.htm on October 10, 2004

[336] "The Bush administration has imposed a gag order on the U.S. Environmental Protection Agency from publicly discussing perchlorate pollution, even as two new studies reveal high levels of the rocket-fuel component may be contaminating the nation's lettuce supply." Peter Waldman. Rocket Fuel Residues Found in Lettuce: Bush administration issues gag order on EPA discussions of possible rocket fuel tainted lettuce. *THE WALL STREET JOURNAL*. See organicconsumers.org/toxic/lettuce042903.cfm rhinoed.com/epa's_gag_order.htm peer.org/press/508.html yubanet.com/artman/publish/article_13637.shtml

[337] Excerpted from lecture by Samuel Epstein MD, 1993. Professor of Occupational and Environmental Medicine at the School of Public Health, University of Illinois Medical Center Chicago. converge.org.nz/pirm/pestican.htm Accessed 2004 Sep and reviewed again 2014 Jun

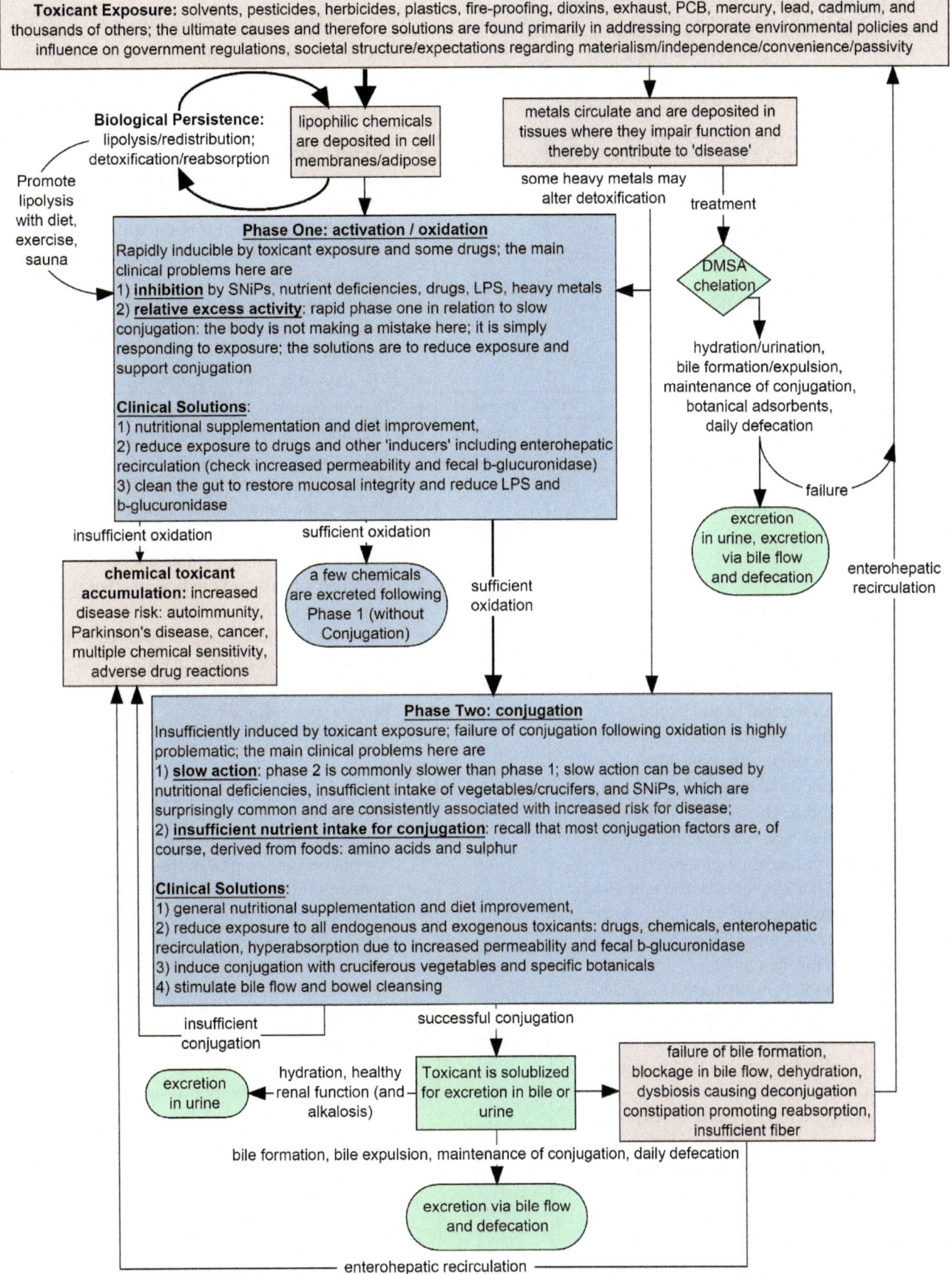

Toxicant Exposure: solvents, pesticides, herbicides, plastics, fire-proofing, dioxins, exhaust, PCB, mercury, lead, cadmium, and thousands of others; the ultimate causes and therefore solutions are found primarily in addressing corporate environmental policies and influence on government regulations, societal structure/expectations regarding materialism/independence/convenience/passivity

Biological Persistence: lipolysis/redistribution; detoxification/reabsorption

lipophilic chemicals are deposited in cell membranes/adipose

metals circulate and are deposited in tissues where they impair function and thereby contribute to 'disease'

Promote lipolysis with diet, exercise, sauna

some heavy metals may alter detoxification

treatment

Phase One: activation / oxidation
Rapidly inducible by toxicant exposure and some drugs; the main clinical problems here are
1) **inhibition** by SNiPs, nutrient deficiencies, drugs, LPS, heavy metals
2) **relative excess activity**: rapid phase one in relation to slow conjugation: the body is not making a mistake here; it is simply responding to exposure; the solutions are to reduce exposure and support conjugation

Clinical Solutions:
1) nutritional supplementation and diet improvement,
2) reduce exposure to drugs and other 'inducers' including enterohepatic recirculation (check increased permeability and fecal b-glucuronidase)
3) clean the gut to restore mucosal integrity and reduce LPS and b-glucuronidase

DMSA chelation

hydration/urination, bile formation/expulsion, maintenance of conjugation, botanical adsorbents, daily defecation

failure

excretion in urine, excretion via bile flow and defecation

enterohepatic recirculation

insufficient oxidation

sufficient oxidation

chemical toxicant accumulation: increased disease risk: autoimmunity, Parkinson's disease, cancer, multiple chemical sensitivity, adverse drug reactions

a few chemicals are excreted following Phase 1 (without Conjugation)

sufficient oxidation

Phase Two: conjugation
Insufficiently induced by toxicant exposure; failure of conjugation following oxidation is highly problematic; the main clinical problems here are
1) **slow action**: phase 2 is commonly slower than phase 1; slow action can be caused by nutritional deficiencies, insufficient intake of vegetables/crucifers, and SNiPs, which are surprisingly common and are consistently associated with increased risk for disease;
2) **insufficient nutrient intake for conjugation**: recall that most conjugation factors are, of course, derived from foods: amino acids and sulphur

Clinical Solutions:
1) general nutritional supplementation and diet improvement,
2) reduce exposure to all endogenous and exogenous toxicants: drugs, chemicals, enterohepatic recirculation, hyperabsorption due to increased permeability and fecal b-glucuronidase
3) induce conjugation with cruciferous vegetables and specific botanicals
4) stimulate bile flow and bowel cleansing

insufficient conjugation

successful conjugation

excretion in urine

hydration, healthy renal function (and alkalosis)

Toxicant is solublized for excretion in bile or urine

failure of bile formation, blockage in bile flow, dehydration, dysbiosis causing deconjugation constipation promoting reabsorption, insufficient fiber

bile formation, bile expulsion, maintenance of conjugation, daily defecation

excretion via bile flow and defecation

enterohepatic recirculation

Overview of toxicant exposure and detoxification/depuration: Details are discussed later in this text.

Integrative/functional/naturopathic healthcare empowers patients with the ability to understand and effectively participate in the course of their life and health

Drug/surgery-based medicine	Paradigm	Holistic natural healthcare
• Doctor as "savior" and indifferent "objective" observer	*Role of the doctor*	• Doctor as "teacher" and active caring partner and co-participant in the process
• Helpless victim, disempowered, dependent	*Role of the patient*	• Active participant, empowered, responsible
• <mark>Idiopathic</mark>: Illness is impossibly complex, and treating this with natural means is generally impossible • Treatment is simple: you have this disease, and you need to take one or more drugs for every problem • Diet and lifestyle modifications are generally viewed as secondary to drugs • The disease is more important than the patient	*Nature of illness*	• <mark>Multifactorial</mark>: involving many different aspects of lifestyle, diet, exercise, genetic inheritance, psychology, and environment • Many causes allows for many different treatment approaches and different ways of attaining health • Illness can be modified via selective dietary and lifestyle changes and a custom-tailored treatment plan • The patient is more important than the disease
• Disease-centered, drug-centered	*Viewpoint*	• Patient-centered, wellness-centered
• Drugs, including chemotherapy • Surgery • Radiation • Electroconvulsive treatment • Vaccinations	*Treatment and options*	• Diet and lifestyle improvement • Relationship/emotional work • Botanical and nutritional medicines • Physical medicine, chiropractic, exercise • Acupuncture • *Selective* rather than *first-line* use of pharmaceuticals and medical procedures
• Symptom suppression • Drug side-effects are a significant cause of death in the US • Only *treats disease*, does not *promote health*; cannot reach optimal health by only reactively treating established problems • Enormous expense, often subsidized by private or public "insurance"	*Long-term outcome*	• Improved health • Potential for successful prevention, treatment or eradication of chronic disease • Potential to become optimally healthy • Proven cost-reduction
• Heightened risk, since drugs are foreign chemicals that have action in the body by interfering with normal processes • Every drug has side-effects, some of which can be life-threatening • Surgery causes irreparable changes to the body, often for the worse. • Radiation and chemotherapy can cause a secondary cancer to develop	*Risks*	• Reduced risk, since most of the botanical treatments and all of the nutritional medicines have been a major part of the human diet for centuries/millennia and have proven safety • Delayed onset of action: most treatments are not fast-acting enough to be of value in traumatic or acutely life-threatening situations • Patients must be willing to adopt healthier lifestyles
• Allows a doctor to see many patients within a short amount of time, thus increasing profitability • Since drugs do not cure problems, patients must return for lifelong prescription renewals, thereby ensuring return visits • Therapeutic passivity: minimal action or effort required by patient and doctor • The doctor holds all the power, and the patient is completely dependent on the doctor for treatment	*Benefits*	• Improved short-term and long-term health • Empowerment • Understanding of body processes as well as healthcare directions and goals • Options

Health-promoting:

- Frequent exercise and physical activity
- Plenty of sleep
- Maintaining ideal body weight
- Avoiding exposure to chemicals, drugs, pollution, exhaust, tobacco smoke
- Daily consumption of fruits and vegetables
- Ideal protein intake for body size, physical activity, and health status
- Diet high in fiber and complex carbohydrates
- Use of health-promoting beverages such as green tea, fruit/vegetable juices, water, and light consumption of beer or red wine
- Increased intake of ALA, EPA, DHA, GLA, and oleic acid
- Multi-vitamin and multi-mineral supplementation
- Optimal vitamin D and iron status
- Beneficial gastrointestinal flora
- Natural and phytonutraceutical interventions to promote optimal health
- Pro-active healthcare
- Healthy and supportive relationships that foster responsibility, independence, interdependence, health and feelings of being wanted and cared for
- Work environments that promote collaboration and creativity and which appreciate personal time and allow for schedule flexibility

Disease-promoting:

- Physical inactivity and sedentary lifestyle
- Insufficient sleep
- Obesity
- Frequent exposure to chemicals, drugs, pollution, exhaust, tobacco smoke
- Daily consumption of processed and artificial foods
- Insufficient (common) or excessive (rare) protein
- Diet high in simple carbohydrates and sugars
- Use of disease-promoting beverages such as cola, artificially colored/flavored/sweetened drinks, and hard liquor
- Increased intake of linoleic acid (vegetable oils) and arachidonic acid (beef, liver, pork, lamb and most farm-raised land animals)
- Low intake of vitamins and minerals
- Excess iron and insufficient vitamin D
- Dysbiosis: intestinal overgrowth of yeast, parasites, and harmful bacteria
- Use of synthetic chemical drugs to suppress symptoms of poor health
- Reactive healthcare that only responds to problems after they have developed
- Dysfunctional relationships that enable and foster illness, dependency and isolation
- Work environments that promote isolation, pressure, perfectionism and which disapprove of creativity, personal time, and flexibility

Maximize factors that promote health ☯ Minimize factors that promote disease

Opposite influences of health promotion vs. disease promotion: Lifestyle concept: Improved clinical outcomes will be attained when doctors and patients attend to both **prescription of health-promoting activities** and **proscription of disease-promoting activities**. Indeed, attention needs to be given to the **ratio** of these disparate and opposing forces, which ultimately influence genetic expression and physiologic function of many organ systems.

Optimize the influences on the health-disease continuum
"The work of the naturopathic physician is to elicit healing by helping patients to create or recreate conditions for health to exist within them. Health will occur where the conditions for health exist. Disease is the product of conditions which allow for it." Jared Zeff, N.D. *Journal of Naturopathic Medicine* 1997

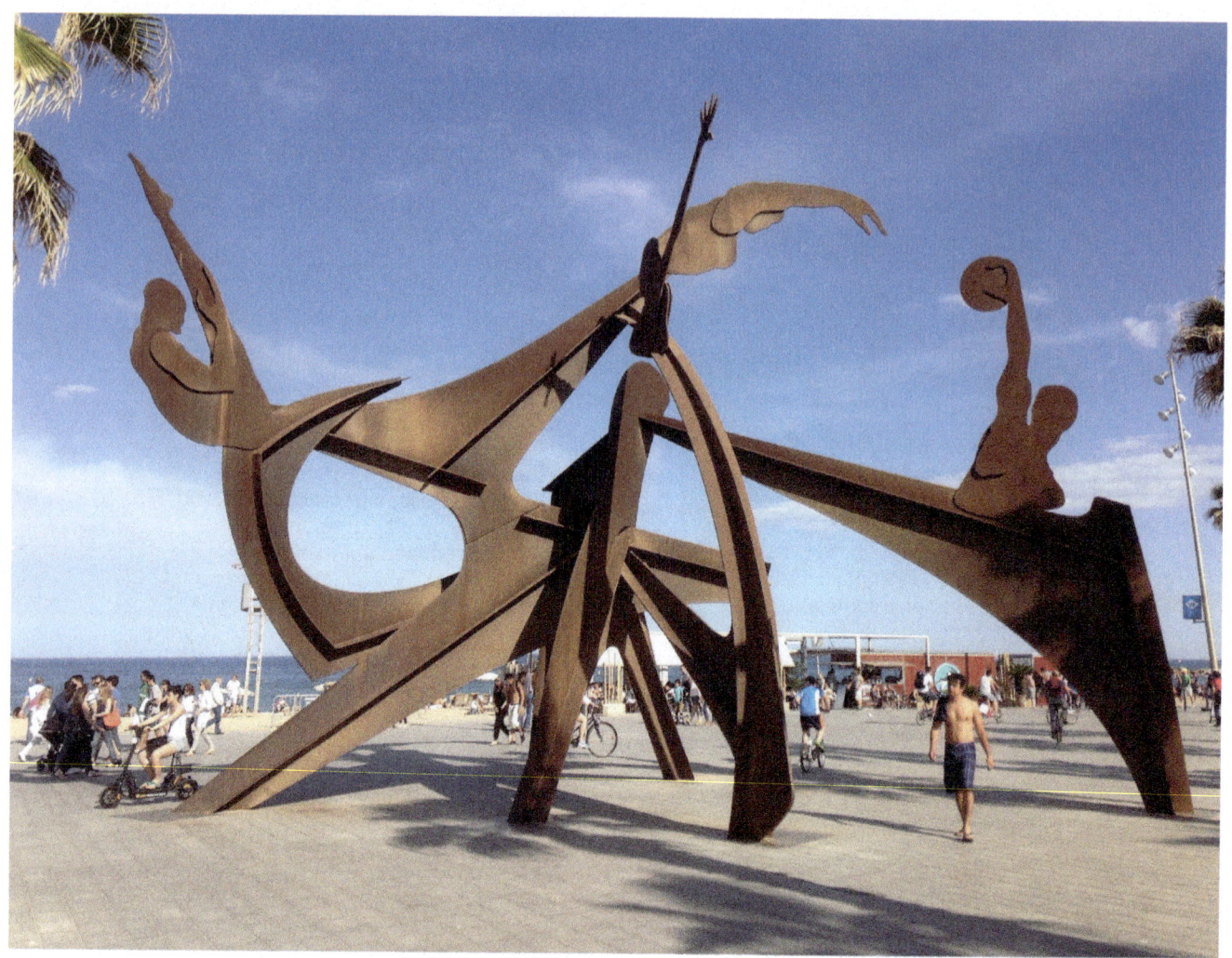

The experience and celebration of health and physicality: Playa Barceloneta 2013, photo by Dr Vasquez.

Chapter 3:
Basic Concepts and Therapeutics in (Nondrug) Musculoskeletal Care and Integrative Pain Management

Introduction

Nonpharmacologic management of musculoskeletal problems is preferred over pharmacologic (e.g., NSAID, Coxib, steroid, opioid) management because of the collateral benefits, safety, and cost-effectiveness associated with manual, dietary, botanical, and physiologic/physiotherapeutic treatments. A brief discussion of **the current "crisis in musculoskeletal medicine"** is provided for contextualization and emphasis of the importance of expanding clinicians' knowledge of effective nondrug treatments; the image below graphically demonstrates the *b.e.n.d. s.t.e.m.s.* acronym for treatments for pain and inflammation outlined later in this chapter.

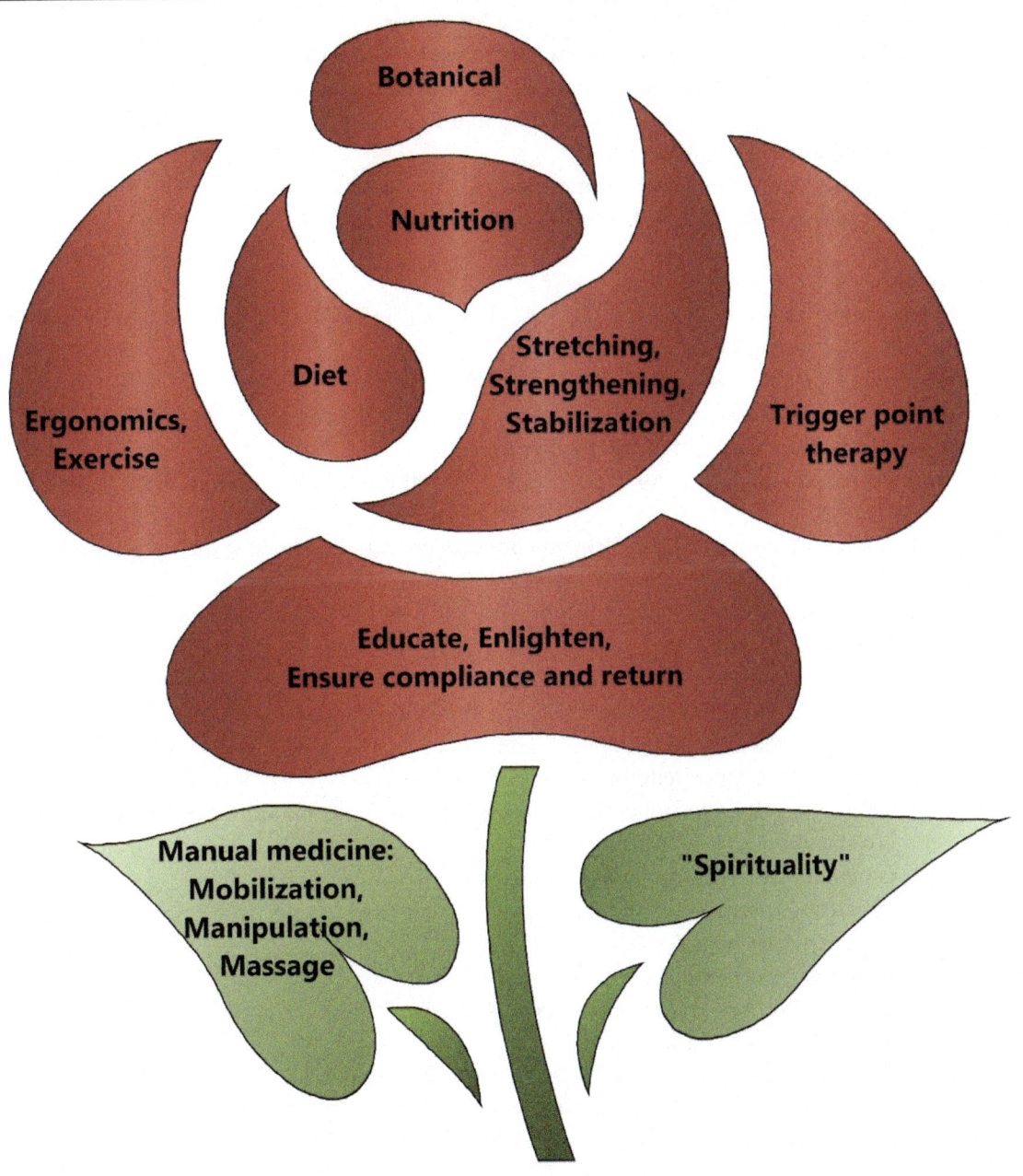

- **Introduction**
- **Pervasive and persistent inadequacies in musculoskeletal education and training among physicians**
- **Adverse effects of nonsteroidal anti-inflammatory drugs (NSAIDs) and COX-2 inhibitors (coxibs)**
- **Nonpharmacologic Musculoskeletal Care & Integrative Pain Management**
  - Protect, prevent re-injury
  - Relative rest
  - Ice/heat, individualize treatment
  - Compression
  - Elevation, establish treatment program
  - Anti-inflammatory & analgesic treatments
  - Treat with physical/manual medicine
  - Uncover the underlying problem
  - Re-educate, rehabilitate, resourcefulness, return to active life, refer to specialist
  - Nutrition, diet, and supplements
- **Myofascial trigger points (MFTP): diagnosis and treatment**
- **Musculoskeletal Manipulation and Manual Medicine: Brief Introduction and Sample Techniques**
  - Carpal Tunnel Syndrome as an example of a neuromusculoskeletal problem that responds very well to the combination of nutritional and manual manipulative interventions
- **Proprioceptive retraining/rehabilitation**
- **Introduction to Injection Therapies: Trigger Points, Anesthetics, Viscous Agents, Prolotherapy**
- **Additional clinical tool: the B.E.N.D.S.T.E.M.S. treatment acronym**

Core Competencies:

- Provide one example from each letter of the *p.r.i.c.e. a. t.u.r.n.* and/or *b.e.n.d. s.t.e.m.s.* mnemonic acronyms for integrative care for musculoskeletal injuries.
- List at least 6 of the 10 mechanisms of action of spinal manipulative therapy.
- List the two most common clinical findings associated with myofascial trigger points and describe appropriate physical/manual and nutritional treatments.
- Describe plans for low-back and ankle proprioceptive retraining/rehabilitation for a patient who has no exercise equipment.
- Describe the effects of stereotypic NSAIDs on chondrocyte metabolism and the long-term effects on joint structure.
- Name four biochemical/physiologic mechanisms by which COX-2 inhibiting drugs predispose to cardiovascular death.
- Demonstrate the proper clinical use of the following non-drug therapeutics for pain:
  - Fish oil: Eicosapentaenoic acid (EPA), Docosahexaenoic acid (DHA)
  - Gamma-linolenic acid (GLA)
  - Vitamin D3: Cholecalciferol
  - Vitamin E: Alpha-tocopherol, beta-tocopherol, delta-tocopherol, gamma-tocopherol
  - Niacinamide
  - Glucosamine sulfate and Chondroitin Sulfate
  - Pancreatin, bromelain, papain, trypsin and alpha-chymotrypsin: "proteolytic enzymes" and "pancreatic enzymes"
  - *Zingiber officinale*, Ginger
  - *Uncaria tomentosa, Uncaria guianensis*, "Cat's claw", "una de gato"
  - *Salix alba*, Willow Bark
  - *Capsicum annuum, Capsicum frutescens*, Cayenne pepper, hot chili pepper
  - *Boswellia serrata*, Frankincense, Salai guggal
  - *Harpagophytum procumbens*, Devil's claw

Introduction to Basic Musculoskeletal Care and Integrative Nonpharmacologic Pain Management: Whether dealing with a *recent and acutely painful injury* or an *exacerbation of a chronic injury or musculoskeletal disease*, all integrative clinicians are wise to have at their disposal a comprehensive protocol for the management of acute and subacute pain and exacerbations of joint inflammation. Undertraining and incompetence in musculoskeletal medicine are very common among healthcare providers[1,2,3,4,5], leaving doctors to overuse simplistic and dangerous treatments (i.e., pharmaceutical drugs) because they are unaware of better options.[6] Failure to understand how to arrive at an accurate diagnosis and subsequent failure to know how to manage musculoskeletal pain leaves doctors *and thus their patients* with "no other option" than the overuse of so-called anti-inflammatory drugs such as non-steroidal anti-inflammatory drugs (NSAIDs, such as aspirin), which kill at least 17,000 patients per year[7], and the cyclooxygenase-2 inhibiting drugs (COX-2 inhibitors, coxibs, such as Vioxx and Celebrex) which have killed tens of thousands of patients.[8,9,10,11]

- Opioid epidemic in the United States (*Pain Physician.* 2012 Jul[12]): "Over the past two decades, as the prevalence of chronic pain and health care costs have exploded, an opioid epidemic with adverse consequences has escalated. …dramatic increases in opioid use… …aggressive marketing by the pharmaceutical industry. These positions are based on unsound science and blatant misinformation, and accompanied by the dangerous assumptions that opioids are highly effective and safe, and devoid of adverse events when prescribed by physicians. … The escalating use of therapeutic opioids shows hydrocodone topping all prescriptions with 136.7 million prescriptions in 2011, with all narcotic analgesics exceeding 238 million prescriptions. It has also been illustrated that opioid analgesics are now responsible for more deaths than the number of deaths from both suicide and motor vehicle crashes, or deaths from cocaine and heroin combined. … The majority of [opioid-induced] deaths (60%) occur in patients when they are given prescriptions based on prescribing guidelines by medical boards, with 20% of deaths in low dose opioid therapy of 100 mg of morphine equivalent dose or less per day and 40% in those receiving morphine of over 100 mg per day. In comparison, 40% of deaths occur in individuals abusing the drugs obtained through multiple prescriptions, doctor shopping, and drug diversion. … The obstacles that must be surmounted are primarily inappropriate prescribing patterns, which are largely based on a lack of knowledge, perceived safety, and inaccurate belief of undertreatment of pain."

- Influence of profiteering public and private interests in drug regulation (*The Nation* 2014 July[13]): "Prescription opioids…are the most dangerous drugs abused in America, with more than 16,000 deaths annually linked to opioid addiction and overdose. The Centers for Disease Control and Prevention report that more Americans now die from painkillers than from heroin and cocaine combined. … People in the United States, a country in which painkillers are routinely overprescribed, now consume more than 84 percent of the entire worldwide supply of oxycodone and almost 100 percent of hydrocodone opioids. In Kentucky, to take just one example, about one in fourteen people is misusing prescription painkillers…."

The crisis in pain medicine and rheumatology: The epidemic of opioid overuse, the paucity of musculoskeletal training among medical physicians, the spike in analgesic and anti-inflammatory drug-related deaths, and the heightened costs of treating musculoskeletal conditions compared with other conditions[14] are summatively

---

[1] Joy EA, Hala SV. Musculoskeletal Curricula in Medical Education: Filling In the Missing Pieces. *The Physician and Sportsmedicine*. 2004; 32: 42-45

[2] Freedman KB, Bernstein J. The adequacy of medical school education in musculoskeletal medicine. *J Bone Joint Surg Am*. 1998;80(10):1421-7

[3] Freedman KB, Bernstein J. Educational deficiencies in musculoskeletal medicine. *J Bone Joint Surg Am*. 2002;84-A(4):604-8

[4] Matzkin E, Smith ME, Freccero CD, Richardson AB. Adequacy of education in musculoskeletal medicine. *J Bone Joint Surg Am*. 2005 Feb;87-A(2):310-4

[5] Schmale GA. More evidence of educational inadequacies in musculoskeletal medicine. *Clin Orthop Relat Res*. 2005 Aug;(437):251-9

[6] See Vasquez A. *Integrative Orthopedics, Third Edition* (2012), *Fibromyalgia in a Nutshell* (2012), *Inflammation Mastery and Integrative Rheumatology, Third Edition* (2014)

[7] Singh G. Recent considerations in nonsteroidal anti-inflammatory drug gastrophathy. *Am J Med*. 1998;105(1B):31S-38S

[8] "The results from VIGOR showed that the relative risk of developing a confirmed adjudicated thrombotic cardiovascular event (myocardial infarction, unstable angina, cardiac thrombus, resuscitated cardiac arrest, sudden or unexplained death, ischemic stroke, and transient ischemic attacks) with rofecoxib treatment compared with naproxen was 2.38." Mukherjee D, Nissen SE, Topol EJ. Risk of cardiovascular events associated with selective COX-2 inhibitors. *JAMA*. 2001 Aug 22-29;286(8):954-9

[9] Topol EJ. Failing the public health--rofecoxib, Merck, and the FDA. *N Engl J Med*. 2004 Oct 21;351(17):1707-9

[10] Ray WA, Griffin MR, Stein CM. Cardiovascular toxicity of valdecoxib. *N Engl J Med*. 2004;351(26):2767

[11] "Patients in the clinical trial taking 400 mg. of Celebrex twice daily had a 3.4 times greater risk of CV events compared to placebo. For patients in the trial taking 200 mg. of Celebrex twice daily, the risk was 2.5 times greater. The average duration of treatment in the trial was 33 months." FDA Statement on the Halting of a Clinical Trial of the cox-2 Inhibitor Celebrex. fda.gov/bbs/topics/news/2004/NEW01144.html Available on January 4, 2005

[12] Manchikanti L, Helm S 2nd, Fellows B, Janata JW, Pampati V, Grider JS, Boswell MV. Opioid epidemic in the United States. *Pain Physician*. 2012 Jul;15(3 Suppl):ES9-38

[13] Fang L. The Real Reason Pot Is Still Illegal. *The Nation* 2014 July 21-28 thenation.com/article/180493/anti-pot-lobbys-big-bankroll. For additional social context see JF. What civil-asset forfeiture means. *The Economist* 2014 Apr 14 economist.com/blogs/economist-explains/2014/04/economist-explains-7

[14] European League Against Rheumatism. Higher health care cost burden of musculoskeletal conditions. eurekalert.org/pub_releases/2014-06/elar-hhc061114.php. 2014 Jun

contributing to what is now called a **crisis in pain medicine**[15] and **rheumatology**[16]. For these reasons—and the humanitarian need to alleviate human suffering—this chapter provides an important review of nondrug treatments for musculoskeletal pain.

Previously, any medical treatment that was non-surgical was commonly described as "conservative" simply because it was *non-invasive/non-surgical*. However, many so-called "conservative" drug treatments are dangerously lethal and expensive, as the coxibs (cyclooxygenase-2 inhibitors), with their lethality and high costs, have demonstrated. Further, "conservative" has become such a confusing term in modern politics that even people who identify themselves as such are often at a loss for an accurate definition of the term. This updated version of this chapter will provide an expedient review of clinically relevant considerations in the management of pain and should be used in conjunction with the information in other chapters and volumes of this work.

The audience for this book—health science students and healthcare providers—should already be familiar with the components of basic care for injuries and the popular—yet overly simplistic—*r.i.c.e.* acronym, which stands for *rest, ice, compression, elevation* and is an easy and convenient approach to managing minor injuries, such as occurs during sports/athletics, e.g., the classic sprained ankle. When I taught Orthopedics at Bastyr University in 2000, I expanded this list to include protect, prevent re-injury, relative rest, ice, individualize treatment, compression, elevation, establish treatment program, anti-inflammatory and analgesic treatments, treat with physical/manual medicine,

Higher cost burden of musculoskeletal conditions compared to other diseases— Press Release from European League against Rheumatism (EULAR) 2014

In a new study released at the European League Against Rheumatism Annual Congress (EULAR 2014), **health care costs associated with musculoskeletal conditions were noted to be almost 50% higher for people with a musculoskeletal condition compared to any other singly occurring condition**.

- Musculoskeletal conditions have a larger impact on healthcare costs than any other disease category, whether occurring alone or as co-morbidity.
- "It is clear that the cost of delivering care to those patients with musculoskeletal conditions is considerably higher than those with other diseases."
- More than 150 conditions affect the muscles, bones, and joints, and these are collectively described as musculoskeletal conditions, and their prevalence increases considerably with age making them **the main cause of disability among the elderly**.
- Healthcare costs increase steeply as the number of diseases in an individual increased, but the presence of musculoskeletal conditions has a larger impact on the total cost than any other condition.

European League Against Rheumatism (EULAR), 2014 Jun eurekalert.org/pub_releases/2014-06/elar-hhc061114.php

uncover the underlying problem, re-educate, rehabilitate, retrain, resourcefulness, return to active life, and nutrition including diet and nutritional and botanical supplements. The mnemonic acronym spells *p.r.i.c.e. a. t.u.r.n.* which is cumbersome but perhaps easy to remember and therefore useful; the major point is to think outside of the *r.i.c.e.* box. As integrative doctorate and multidoctorate clinicians, we certainly have much more to offer our patients than rest, ice, compression, and elevation; this chapter reviews some of these options using an outline based on the previous *p.r.i.c.e. a. t.u.r.n.* acronym and then concludes with the more pleasant *b.e.n.d. s.t.e.m.s.* acronym which was graphically demonstrated on the first page of this chapter.

Whereas the allopathic/drug-based approach stops with minimal pain/injury treatment and provides essentially nothing in terms of prevention or comprehensive patient management—let alone promotion of optimal health—the holistic and integrative approach is centered on the *patient* and seeks to help him/her attain optimal health while being treated for the musculoskeletal disorder. We can and must help our patients attain optimal health while effectively managing their acute and chronic musculoskeletal problems.[17,18,19] **Indeed, since for many patients their only interaction with the healthcare system is when they are injured or in pain, we must seize upon this opportunity to enroll patients in preventive and pro-active healthcare**; the alternative to *proactive* healthcare (maintaining/optimizing health and addressing health problems *before* they start or are still small) is *reactive* healthcare (managing problems *after* they have fully developed), which is now proven to be a colossal failure in terms of finances, health outcomes, resource utilization and other ethical considerations.

---

[15] "The main causes of this crisis are: 1) the high prevalence of chronic pain, reaching levels of 17% in the adult population;2) the lack of appropriate training of primary care physicians in the field of chronic pain management; and 3) the paucity of consultation services in the field of chronic pain." Minerbi et al. Pain Medicine in Crisis—A Possible Model toward a Solution: Empowering Community Medicine to Treat Chronic Pain. Rambam Maimonides Med J. Oct 2013; 4(4): e0027

[16] Morris AJ. The approaching crisis in rheumatologic care. *J Rheumatol* 2003; 30: 1890

[17] Vasquez A. New Insights into Fatty Acid Supplementation and Its Effect on Eicosanoid Production and Genetic Expression. *Nutritional Perspectives* 2005; January: 5-16

[18] Vasquez A. Improving overall health while safely and effectively treating musculoskeletal pain. *Nutritional Perspectives* 2005; 28: 34-38, 40-42

[19] Vasquez A. The Importance of Integrative Chiropractic Health Care in Treating Musculoskeletal Pain and Reducing the Nationwide Burden of Medical Expenses and Iatrogenic Injury and Death: A Concise Review of Current Research and Implications for Clinical Practice and Healthcare Policy. *The Original Internist* 2005; 12(4): 159-182

Persistent inadequacies in musculoskeletal education/training among physicians: The need to advance clinicians' knowledge in musculoskeletal care, pain management, and nutrition

Question: What would be the expected clinical/financial outcome of physicians' being inadequately trained in musculoskeletal medicine and then given prescriptive rights for potent NSAIDs, coxibs, steroids, DMARDs, etc and placed in a position of ethical and professional responsibility for managing patients' pain?

Answer: We would reasonably expect the profession to misdiagnose various conditions, overuse drugs, overuse expensive (and with regard to computed tomography, dangerous) imaging technology to compensate for poor diagnostic skills, and to overuse procedures/surgery in an attempt to provide (the appearance of) competence in the clinical management of musculoskeletal problems. These are exactly the outcomes that we see in clinical practice: inaccurate diagnoses followed by inefficacious treatments, overuse of imaging, drugs, and surgery.

- Medical student musculoskeletal education (*J Bone Joint Surg Am* 2012 Oct[20]): "The survey contained a validated orthopedic examination of musculoskeletal competency (passing grade, 70% ... The mean score was 51.1%; only sixty-seven (19.3%) of the students passed. Fourth-year students scored significantly higher (59.0% [which is still an average grade of failure]) compared with first-year students (37.3%), but 65% of students in both groups failed. Only 34.2% of the graduating students had completed a musculoskeletal elective. Students who participated in elective musculoskeletal education had a higher pass rate (67.5%) than those who did not (43.9%)."

- Musculoskeletal education in US medical schools (*Curr Rev Musculoskelet Med* 2011 Sep[21]): "Despite the prevalence of musculoskeletal disorders in the United States, physicians have received inadequate training during medical school on how to examine, diagnose, and manage these conditions."

- Assessment of the musculoskeletal medicine attitudes and knowledge of medical students at Harvard Medical School (*Acad Med* 2007 May[22]): "Participants were asked to fill out a 30-question survey and a nationally validated basic competency exam in musculoskeletal medicine. ... Medical students rated musculoskeletal education to be of major importance (3.8/5) but rated the amount of curriculum time spent on musculoskeletal medicine as poor (2.1/5). Third-year students felt a low to adequate level of confidence in performing a musculoskeletal physical examination (2.7/5) and failed to demonstrate cognitive mastery in musculoskeletal medicine (passing rate on competency exam: 7%), whereas fourth-year students reported a similar level of confidence (2.7/5) and exhibited a higher passing rate (26%). ... These findings, which are consistent with those from other schools, suggest that medical students do not feel adequately prepared in musculoskeletal medicine and lack both clinical confidence and cognitive mastery in the field."

- Musculoskeletal cognitive competency in chiropractic interns (*J Manipulative Physiol Ther* 2007 Jan[23]): 123 fourth-year chiropractic students at a single school (Canadian Memorial Chiropractic College) were given a standardized musculoskeletal examination (basic competency examination [BCE], originally developed by Freedman and Bernstein, cited below, 1998 and 2002); very tellingly, these chiropractic researchers decided that twenty percent (5 questions) of the standardized musculoskeletal examination were not relevant to or were outside of the scope of chiropractic practice, i.e., that chiropractic practice scope is narrower than that of primary care and medical training. "Interns achieved a 51.2% passing rate (mean score, 73.2%) for the 25-item BCE,... For the modified 20-item BCE [narrowed for chiropractic education and practice scope], the interns' mean score was 80.8%..." This study is interesting in that, while chiropractic students performed better (51.5% for >73% passing grade; 64.7% for >70% passing grade) than their allopathic counterparts as would be expected for a four-year training program that focuses with near exclusively on musculoskeletal diagnosis and management, nearly half of them failed the exam if 73% accuracy is the standard; further, the researchers' modification of the exam appears to be an admission that chiropractic education/training scope is not on par with that of medical students and clinicians as they noted that 20% of questions "fell outside the scope of chiropractic practice." *What were the topics of these questions that were excluded?*: Congenital hip dislocation, knee dislocation following motor vehicle accident,

[20] Skelley NW, Tanaka MJ, Skelley LM, LaPorte DM. Medical student musculoskeletal education: an institutional survey. *J Bone Joint Surg Am.* 2012 Oct 3;94(19):e146(1-7)

[21] Monrad SU, et al. Musculoskeletal education in US medical schools: lessons from the past and suggestions for the future. *Curr Rev Musculoskelet Med.* 2011 Sep;4(3):91-8

[22] Day CS, et al. Musculoskeletal medicine: an assessment of the attitudes and knowledge of medical students at Harvard Medical School. *Acad Med.* 2007 May;82(5):452-7

[23] Humphreys et al. An examination of musculoskeletal cognitive competency in chiropractic interns. *J Manipulative Physiol Ther.* 2007 Jan;30(1):44-9

skin laceration and metacarpal fracture of the hand following minor trauma, appropriate indications for radiographs in patients with low-back pain, and simple clinical anatomy of the femoral neck and head. Thus, the admission by these researchers/clinicians that chiropractic students/clinicians are not prepared to deal with these issues is also a clear statement from them that they perceive that the profession is not prepared to deal with routine musculoskeletal issues at the primary care level.

- Insufficient musculoskeletal knowledge among academic primary care physicians (*J Bone Joint Surg Am* 2006 Jul[24]): "RESULTS: ... Fifty-nine (64%) of the ninety-two physicians scored < 70% [on an examination of basic musculoskeletal knowledge]. Higher examination scores were associated with male gender (p = 0.01) and participation in a musculoskeletal course (p = 0.009). Practitioners who took elective courses demonstrated higher scores compared with those who took required courses (p = 0.014). Greater musculoskeletal confidence was associated with the number of years in clinical practice (p = 0.045), male gender (p = 0.01), residency training in family practice (p < 0.00001), and prior participation in a musculoskeletal course (p = 0.0004). ... CONCLUSIONS: Although a large proportion of primary care visits are for musculoskeletal symptoms, the majority of primary care providers tested at a large, regional, academic primary care institution failed to demonstrate adequate musculoskeletal knowledge...."

- More evidence of educational inadequacies in musculoskeletal medicine (*Clin Orthop Relat Res* 2005 Aug[25]): "In their study, Freedman and Bernstein suggested that 80% of a group of graduates from many of the best medical schools in the United States were deficient in their knowledge of basic facts and concepts in musculoskeletal medicine. ... Despite generally improved levels of competency with each year at medical school, less than 50% of fourth-year students showed competency."

- Educational deficiencies in musculoskeletal medicine (*J Bone Joint Surg Am* 2002 Apr[26]): "Two hundred and forty (58%) of the 417 program directors of internal medicine residency departments responded. They suggested a mean passing score (and standard deviation) of 70.0% +/- 9.9%. As reported previously, the mean test score of the eighty-five examinees was 59.6%. Sixty-six (78%) of them failed to demonstrate basic competency on the examination according to the criterion set by the internal medicine program directors. ... According to the standard suggested by the program directors of internal medicine residency departments, a large majority of the examinees once again failed to demonstrate basic competency in musculoskeletal medicine on the examination. It is therefore reasonable to conclude that medical school preparation in musculoskeletal medicine is inadequate."

- Inadequacy of medical school education in musculoskeletal medicine (*J Bone Joint Surg Am* 1998 Oct[27]): "Seventy (82 per cent) of the eighty-five residents failed to demonstrate basic competency on the examination according to the chairpersons' criterion. In summary, seventy (82 per cent) of eighty-five medical school graduates failed a valid musculoskeletal competency examination. We therefore believe that medical school preparation in musculoskeletal medicine is inadequate."

- Training and clinical competency in musculoskeletal medicine (*Sports Med* 1993 May[28]): "Injuries and diseases of the musculoskeletal system account for more than 20% of patient visits to primary care and emergency medical practitioners. However, less than 3% of the pre-clinical medical school curriculum is devoted to teaching all aspects of musculoskeletal disease... Available elective training in musculoskeletal injuries and diseases is commonly taught by hospital-affiliated physicians and surgeons, with the result that this teaching case load is typically skewed towards serious and/or surgical problems."

In sum: The data and conclusions consistently report the fact that health professional education and training are both inadequate to ensure competence among (American) physicians in the understanding, diagnosis, and management of musculoskeletal disorders based on a verified and standardized *yet very basic* examination of musculoskeletal competence. The anticipated implications and consequences—inadequate care with overuse of invasive, expensive, and dangerous drugs, procedures, and surgeries—is well borne-out.

> **What purpose education?**
>
> "Education is a system of imposed ignorance."
>
> Chomsky N. *Manufacturing Consent*, 1992 documentary film

[24] Lynch et al. Important demographic variables impact musculoskeletal knowledge and confidence of academic primary care physicians. *J Bone Joint Surg Am* 2006;88:1589-95
[25] Schmale GA. More evidence of educational inadequacies in musculoskeletal medicine. *Clin Orthop Relat Res.* 2005 Aug;(437):251-9
[26] Freedman KB, Bernstein J. Educational deficiencies in musculoskeletal medicine. *J Bone Joint Surg Am.* 2002 Apr;84-A(4):604-8
[27] Freedman KB, Bernstein J. The adequacy of medical school education in musculoskeletal medicine. *J Bone Joint Surg Am.* 1998 Oct;80(10):1421-7
[28] Craton N, Matheson GO. Training and clinical competency in musculoskeletal medicine. Identifying the problem. *Sports Med.* 1993 May;15(5):328-37

Persistent inadequacies in nutrition education/training among physicians

Introduction: Despite the acknowledged importance of diet in the prevention of obesity, diabetes, hypertension and other components of cardiometabolic syndrome/disease, physicians are consistently and systematically untrained in nutrition. A few exemplary citations are summarized per the following:

- What do resident physicians know about nutrition? (*J Am Coll Nutr* 2008 Apr[29]): "OBJECTIVE: Despite the increased emphasis on obesity and diet-related diseases, nutrition education remains lacking in many internal medicine training programs. We evaluated the attitudes, self-perceived proficiency, and knowledge related to clinical nutrition among a cohort of internal medicine interns. METHODS: Nutrition attitudes and self-perceived proficiency were measured using previously validated questionnaires. Knowledge was assessed with a multiple-choice quiz. ... RESULTS: Of the 114 participants, 61 (54%) completed the survey. Although 77% agreed that nutrition assessment should be included in routine primary care visits, and 94% agreed that it was their obligation to discuss nutrition with patients, only 14% felt physicians were adequately trained to provide nutrition counseling. ... CONCLUSIONS: Internal medicine interns' perceive nutrition counseling as a priority, but lack the confidence and knowledge to effectively provide adequate nutrition education." These are impressive results showing that internal medicine doctors—specialists who commonly deal with diabetes, hypertension, obesity, and metabolic syndrome—do not have competence in nutrition, even by weak and basic standards.

- Relevance of clinical nutrition education and role models to the practice of medicine (*Eur J Clin Nutr*. 1999 May[30]): "Yet, despite the prevalence of nutritional disorders in clinical medicine and increasing scientific evidence on the significance of dietary modification to disease prevention, present day practitioners of medicine are typically untrained in the relationship of diet to health and disease."

- How much do gastroenterology fellows know about nutrition? (*J Clin Gastroenterol*. 2009 Jul[31]): "The mean total test score was 50.04%. ...CONCLUSIONS: Gastroenterology fellows think their knowledge of nutrition is suboptimal; objective evaluation of nutrition knowledge in this cohort confirmed this belief. A formal component of nutrition education could be developed in the context of GI fellowship education and continuing medical education as necessary."

In sum: The data consistently demonstrate that healthcare providers at the doctorate level are untrained in nutrition when assessed by rather simple standards; their knowledge of functional nutrition at the level of clinical intervention in the treatment of serious disease would reasonably be expected to be approximately zero. Thus, given that doctors are trained neither in musculoskeletal management (despite the fact that all patients have musculoskeletal systems and that related disorders represent no less than 20% of general practice) nor nutrition (despite the fact that all patients eat food and that such dietary habits (and/or the use of nutritional interventions) impact nearly all known diseases in the known universe), one might wonder as to the cause and perpetuation of this *systematically imposed ignorance* on such topics of major importance. Consistent faults in medical education are not accidental.

> **Dumbing Us Down: The Hidden Curriculum of Educational Systems**
>
> "Look again at the seven lessons of school teaching: confusion, class position, indifference, emotional and intellectual dependency, conditional self-esteem, and surveillance. All of these lessons are prime training for permanent underclasses, people deprived forever of finding the center of their own special genius."
>
> Such a curriculum produces physical, moral, and intellectual paralysis, and no curriculum of content will be sufficient to reverse its hideous effects. ... Schools teach exactly what they are intended to teach and they do it well."
>
> Gatto JT. *Dumbing Us Down: The Hidden Curriculum of Compulsory Schooling*, p. 16

Adverse effects of nonsteroidal anti-inflammatory drugs (NSAIDs), COX-2 inhibitors (coxibs)

Introduction: Nonsteroidal anti-inflammatory drugs (NSAIDs) have many common and serious adverse effects, including the promotion of joint destruction. Paradoxically, these drugs *cause* or *exacerbate* the very symptoms and disease they are supposed to treat: joint pain and destruction. In a tragic exemplification of Orwellian newspeak[32],

---

[29] Vetter et al. What do resident physicians know about nutrition? An evaluation of attitudes, self-perceived proficiency and knowledge. *J Am Coll Nutr*. 2008 Apr;27(2):287-98
[30] Halsted CH. The relevance of clinical nutrition education and role models to the practice of medicine. *Eur J Clin Nutr*. 1999 May;53 Suppl 2:S29-34
[31] Raman M, Violato C, Coderre S. How much do gastroenterology fellows know about nutrition? *J Clin Gastroenterol*. 2009 Jul;43(6):559-64
[32] Orwell G. *1984*. Harcourt Brace Jovanovich: 1949. "Newspeak" is defined by the Merriam-Webster Dictionary (m-w.com) as "propagandistic language marked by euphemism, circumlocution, and the inversion of customary meanings" and as "a language designed to diminish the range of thought," in the novel *1984* (1949) by George Orwell.

the habitual utilization and long-term prescription of NSAIDs for joint pain and inflammation as advocated by the pharmaceutical industry[33] and medical textbooks[34] is not described as *malpractice*; rather it is described as the *"standard of care"* and *"first-line therapy."* Adverse effects include:

- Promotion of bone necrosis and cartilage destruction: Several NSAIDs cause osteonecrosis[35] and many of these drugs interfere with chondrocyte function and cartilage formation and thus promote the destruction of joints.[36] As noted by Newman and Ling[37], **"...femoral head collapse and acceleration of osteoarthritis have been well documented in association with the NSAIDs..."** The subchondral osteonecrosis induced by many NSAIDs may both necessitate and complicate arthroplasty (joint replacement with prosthesis) because of extensive joint damage and because the underlying bone that must hold the new implant is too weak to provide a stable foundation.[38] *In vivo* studies have shown that salicylate, acetylsalicylic acid, fenoprofen, isoxicam, tolmetin, and ibuprofen reduce glycosaminoglycan synthesis.[39] COX-2 inhibition impairs anabolic bone activity that is necessary for the preservation of bone strength.[40,41]

- Gastric ulceration and gastrointestinal bleeding: Nearly all NSAIDs promote gastric ulceration and gastrointestinal bleeding. Among patients who chronically use NSAIDs 65% will develop intestinal inflammation[42] and up to 30% will develop gastroduodenal ulceration.[43] Drugs differ greatly in their propensity to damage the gastrointestinal mucosa and cause bleeding, and aspirin appears to be the most problematic.[44] NSAIDs can also promote and exacerbate colitis and inflammation of the large intestine.[45]

- Increased intestinal permeability: NSAIDs damage the mucosa of the small intestine and promote macromolecular absorption and paracellular permeability—"leaky gut." As described in greater detail later in this text, increased intestinal permeability most certainly contributes to the exacerbation and perpetuation of many rheumatic and musculoskeletal disorders by inducing inflammation via immune activation and by promoting the formation of immune complexes that are then deposited into synovial tissues for the induction of a local inflammatory response inside the joint.[46]

- Promotion of hepatic and renal injury and failure: Chronic use of NSAIDs is an important risk factor for the development of renal failure.[47] Hepatic injury is less common than NSAID-induced renal failure but can be achieved with higher drug doses (especially with the non-NSAID analgesic acetaminophen), coadministration of drugs, and concomitant consumption of alcohol.

- Death: NSAIDs have been an impressively significant cause of death in countries wherein they are used and overused. According to the 1998 review by Singh in *American Journal of Medicine*[48], **"Conservative calculations estimate that approximately 107,000 patients are hospitalized annually for nonsteroidal anti-inflammatory drug (NSAID)-related gastrointestinal (GI) complications and at least 16,500 NSAID-related deaths occur each year among arthritis patients alone. The figures for all NSAID users would be overwhelming, yet the scope of this problem is generally under-appreciated."** The profile of NSAID-

[33] "Congratulations: you've joined the 20 million people who have taken CELEBREX, the #1 doctor-prescribed brand of arthritis medication." celebrex.com 2004 Jan

[34] "The first drug to treat rheumatoid arthritis is an NSAID." Tierney et al (eds). *Current Medical Diagnosis and Treatment 2002, 41st Edition*. Lange Medical; 2002. Page 856

[35] "The case of a young healthy man, who developed avascular necrosis of head of femur after prolonged administration of indomethacin, is reported here." Prathapkumar KR, Smith I, Attara GA. Indomethacin induced avascular necrosis of head of femur. *Postgrad Med J*. 2000 Sep; 76(899): 574-5

[36] "At...concentrations comparable to those... in the synovial fluid of patients treated with the drug, several NSAIDs suppress proteoglycan synthesis... These NSAID-related effects on chondrocyte metabolism ... are much more profound in osteoarthritic cartilage than in normal cartilage, due to enhanced uptake of NSAIDs by the osteoarthritic cartilage." Brandt KD. Effects of nonsteroidal anti-inflammatory drugs on chondrocyte metabolism in vitro and in vivo. *Am J Med*. 1987 Nov 20; 83(5A): 29-34

[37] Newman NM, Ling RS. Acetabular bone destruction related to non-steroidal anti-inflammatory drugs. *Lancet*. 1985 Jul 6; 2(8445): 11-4

[38] "This highly significant association between NSAID use and acetabular destruction gives cause for concern, not least because of the difficulty in achieving satisfactory hip replacements in patients with severely damaged acetabula." Newman et al. Acetabular bone destruction related to non-steroidal anti-inflammatory drugs. *Lancet*. 1985; 2: 11-4

[39] Brandt KD. Effects of nonsteroidal anti-inflammatory drugs on chondrocyte metabolism in vitro and in vivo. *Am J Med*. 1987 Nov 20; 83(5A): 29-34

[40] "Histological observations suggest that cox-2 is required for normal endochondral ossification during fracture healing. Because mice lacking Cox2 form normal skeletons, our observations indicate that fetal bone development and fracture healing are different and that cox-2 function is specifically essential for fracture healing." Simon AM, Manigrasso MB, O'Connor JP. Cyclo-oxygenase 2 function is essential for bone fracture healing. *J Bone Miner Res*. 2002 Jun;17(6):963-76

[41] "The results indicate that cox-2 and constitutive NOS are important signaling molecules in the anabolic responses of neonatal tibial bone to the micromechanical load in vitro." Kunnel JG, Igarashi K, Gilbert JL, Stern PH. Bone anabolic responses to mechanical load in vitro involve cox-2 and constitutive NOS. *Connect Tissue Res*. 2004;45(1):40-9

[42] "NSAIDs cause small intestinal inflammation in 65% of patients receiving the drugs long-term." Bjarnason I, Macpherson AJ. Intestinal toxicity of non-steroidal anti-inflammatory drugs. *Pharmacol Ther*. 1994 Apr-May;62(1-2):145-57

[43] "Endoscopic studies indicate that up to 30% of chronic NSAID users will develop gastroduodenal ulceration." Blower AL. Considerations for nonsteroidal anti-inflammatory drug therapy: safety. *Scand J Rheumatol Suppl*. 1996;105:13-24

[44] "ASA (1,500 mg/day for 5 days) caused about a 6-fold increase in blood loss. Four days after withdrawal of ASA, faecal blood was still about twice as high as in faeces of subjects given ibuprofen and indoprofen." Porro GB, et al. Gastro-intestinal blood loss during administration of indoprofen, aspirin and ibuprofen. *J Int Med Res* 1977;5(3):155-60

[45] "Non-steroidal anti-inflammatory drugs (NSAIDs) may adversely affect the colon, either by causing a non-specific colitis or by exacerbating a preexisting colonic disease. ... Local and/or systemic effects of NSAIDs on mucosal cells might lead to an increased intestinal permeability, which is a prerequisite for colitis." Faucheron JL, Parc R. Non-steroidal anti-inflammatory drug-induced colitis. *Int J Colorectal Dis*. 1996;11(2):99-101

[46] Inman RD. Antigens, the gastrointestinal tract, and arthritis. *Rheum Dis Clin North Am*. 1991 May; 17(2): 309-21

[47] "Patients with chronic arthritis who consume excessive amount of NSAIDs are at risk of developing renal papillary necrosis and chronic renal impairment." Segasothy M, Chin GL, Sia KK, Zulfiqar A, Samad SA. Chronic nephrotoxicity of anti-inflammatory drugs used in the treatment of arthritis. *Br J Rheumatol*. 1995 Feb; 34(2): 162-5

[48] Singh G. Recent considerations in nonsteroidal anti-inflammatory drug gastropathy. *Am J Med*. 1998 Jul 27; 105(1B): 31S-38S

induced death is likely very different from country to country, and would be expected to change over time as new drugs are introduced; however, one should—ultimately—look at the aggregate of, in this example, not only NSAIDs but also their modern replacements, particularly the Coxibs, which cause *fewer gastrohemorrhagic deaths* but *more cardiovascular deaths*.

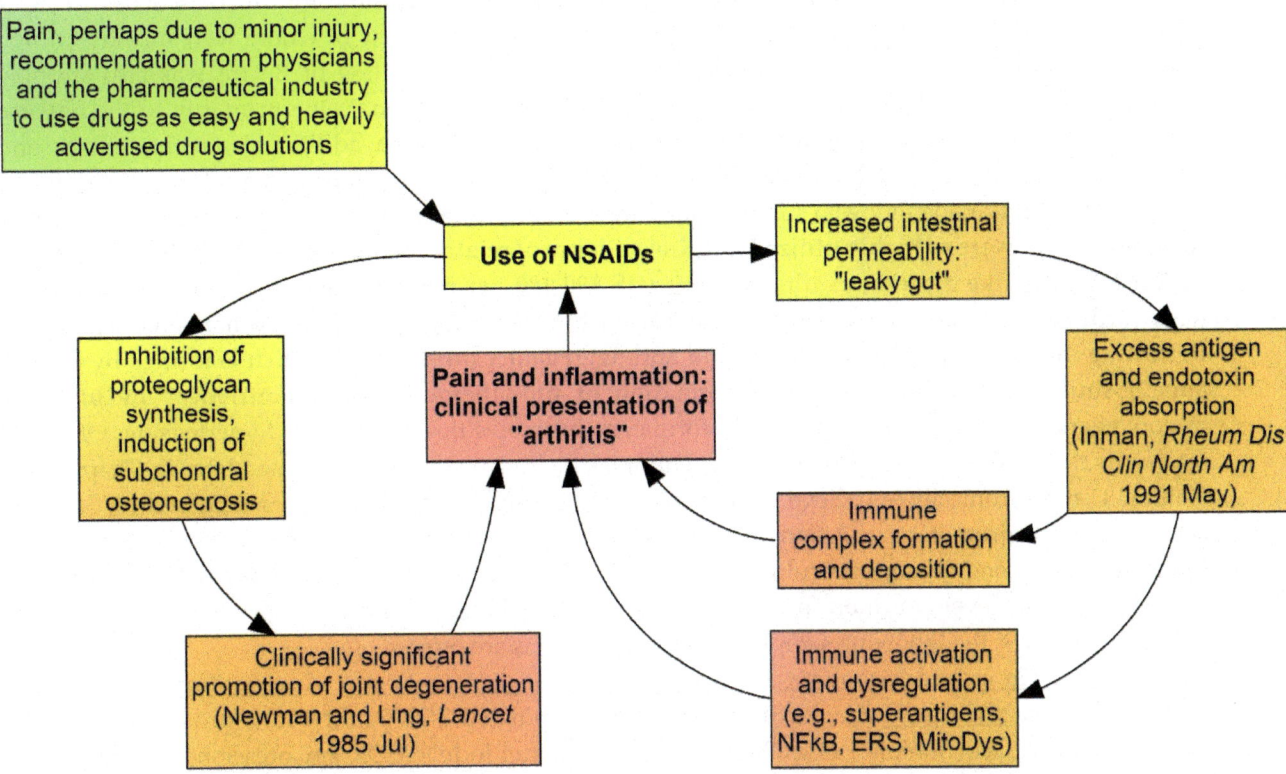

The vicious cycle of NSAID use: Pain prompts use of NSAIDS, which promote joint destruction and increased intestinal permeability, promoting systemic inflammation which then contribute(s) to the perpetuation of joint pain.

- Adverse effects specific to Coxibs: Drugs specifically designed to inhibit the isoform of cyclooxygenase known as cyclooxygenase-2 (coxibs) carry their own list of adverse effects, namely membranous glomerulopathy and acute interstitial nephritis[49], acute cholestatic hepatitis[50], toxic epidermal necrolysis[51,52], and—perhaps most importantly—increased risk for cardiovascular disease (e.g., stroke, hypertension, myocardial infarction) and cardiovascular death. Immediately following the withdrawal of the arthritis drug rofecoxib (Vioxx) in late September 2004, Topol[53] extrapolated that as many as 160,000 adverse cardiovascular events (including stroke, myocardial infarction, and death) may have resulted from the overuse of Vioxx/rofecoxib due to the collusion of Merck's intentional failure to withdraw what was known for years to be a dangerous drug, the FDA's failure to enforce regulatory standards to protect the public, and the overutilization of Vioxx by the medical profession, which was well informed of the lethality of Vioxx for several years[54] before Merck's confessionary and belated withdrawal of the drug. Soon thereafter, several other so-called "anti-inflammatory drugs" such as valdecoxib (Bextra)[55], celecoxib (Celebrex)[56], and naproxen (Aleve)[57] were likewise associated with excess cardiovascular injury and death. Although the

[49] Markowitz GS, et al. Membranous glomerulopathy and acute interstitial nephritis following treatment with celecoxib. *Clin Nephrol.* 2003;59(2):137-42

[50] Grieco A, Miele L, Giorgi A, Civello IM, Gasbarrini G. Acute cholestatic hepatitis associated with celecoxib. *Ann Pharmacother.* 2002;36(12):1887-9

[51] Berger P, Dwyer D, Corallo CE. Toxic epidermal necrolysis after celecoxib therapy. *Pharmacotherapy.* 2002 Sep;22(9):1193-5.

[52] Friedman B, Orlet HK, Still JM, Law E. Toxic epidermal necrolysis due to administration of celecoxib (Celebrex). *South Med J.* 2002;95(10):1213-4

[53] Topol EJ. Failing the public health--rofecoxib, Merck, and the FDA. *N Engl J Med.* 2004 Oct 21;351(17):1707-9

[54] Mukherjee D, Nissen SE, Topol EJ. Risk of cardiovascular events associated with selective cox-2 inhibitors. *JAMA* 2001; 286(8):954-9

[55] Ray WA, Griffin MR, Stein CM. Cardiovascular toxicity of valdecoxib. *N Engl J Med.* 2004;351(26):2767

[56] "Patients in the clinical trial taking 400 mg. of Celebrex twice daily had a 3.4 times greater risk of CV events compared to placebo. For patients in the trial taking 200 mg. of Celebrex twice daily, the risk was 2.5 times greater. The average duration of treatment in the trial was 33 months." FDA Statement on the Halting of a Clinical Trial of the cox-2 Inhibitor Celebrex. fda.gov/bbs/topics/news/2004/NEW01144.html Available on January 4, 2005

[57] "Preliminary information from the study showed some evidence of increased risk of cardiovascular events, when compared to placebo, to patients taking naproxen." FDA Statement on Naproxen. fda.gov/bbs/topics/news/2004/NEW01148.html Available on January 4, 2005

advertising-induced feeding frenzy on Celebrex made it the most "successful" drug launch in US history with more than 7.4 million prescriptions written within its first 6 months[58], major adverse effects due to the drug were noted within 2 years of its release onto the medical market[59]; current guidelines hold that patients must be informed of the excess cardiovascular risk associated with this drug and that its use should be limited to the lowest dose for the shortest time possible (weeks).[60] When compared with placebo in cardiac surgery patients, Bextra/valdecoxib is associated with a 3-fold to 4-fold increased risk of heart attack, stroke, and death[61], and recently 7 million arthritis patients, many of whom were already at high risk for cardiovascular disease, were being treated with this drug.[62] Use of Bextra was also strongly associated with toxic epidermal necrolysis, a potentially fatal condition.[63] Due primarily to the adverse cardiovascular effects[64], in the interest of protecting the public from additional adverse effects and unnecessary deaths, in April 2005 the FDA ordered that Bextra/valdecoxib be taken off the market in the US[65], and Health Canada followed suit by removing the drug from Canadian markets.[66] **It is inexcusable that these drugs were so highly utilized despite evidence of relative analgesic inefficacy (not better than earlier NSAIDs like aspirin), exorbitant costs (US $90-180 per month[67]) and clear evidence of danger (e.g., cardiovascular death) by two well-identified biochemical/physiologic mechanisms, namely: 1) inhibiting the formation of vasodilating and anti-aggregatory prostacyclin, which is formed by COX-2, and 2) shunting arachidonate toward formation of pro-atherosclerotic leukotrienes[68] by blocking cyclooxygenase.** Inhibition of prostacyclin formation promotes thrombosis and hypertension. Of recent interest is the finding that celecoxib induces endoplasmic reticulum stress (detailed later in Chapter 4 of Volume 1) and—ironically—cox2 expression; thus, per the research cited below presented in 2013, this drug actually induces/promotes expression of the same enzyme it is designed to inhibit. In order to foreshadow the discussion on endoplasmic reticulum stress (ERS) and the unfolded protein response (UPR) and to help readers begin to develop a more profound understanding of the subtle *pro-inflammatory effects of anti-inflammatory drugs*, the following sample quotes and citations are offered:

- Celecoxib induces apoptosis, ER stress, and cyclooxygenase-2 expression on lung cancer cells (*J Immunol* 2013 May[69]): "Paradoxically, celecoxib stimulated COX-2 mRNA and protein on A549, but indomethacin, inhibitor of COX-1 and COX-2 did not induce COX-2 expression. Taken together, we suggest that celecoxib induces apoptosis and ER stress on lung cancer cell line."
- Drug-induced perturbation of ER stress and the unfolded protein response (*Toxicol Pathol* 2013 Feb[70]): "Marketed pharmaceuticals developed for various diseases can also cause ER stress by either on- or off-target mechanisms for which they were developed including bortezomib, nelfinavir, atazanavir, ritonavir, lopinavir, sorafenib, indomethacin, and celecoxib."

Perspective: If we summarize that at least 17,000 people die each year from NSAIDs, that other "medication errors" kill over 7,000 people in America[71] and that an additional 180,000 Americans die due to hospital errors[72], then we have a situation where at least 200,000 Americans die each year due to drug effects and hospital/physician errors. Furthermore, according to estimates by David Graham, MD, MPH, (Associate Director for Science, Office of Drug

---

[58] Monsanto, Pfizer celebrate Celebrex. *St. Louis Business Journal*. July 20, 1999 bizjournals.com/stlouis/stories/1999/07/19/daily5.html Accessed on January 5, 2005

[59] Mukherjee D, Nissen SE, Topol EJ. Risk of cardiovascular events associated with selective cox-2 inhibitors. *JAMA*. 2001 Aug 22-29;286(8):954-9

[60] "Celecoxib should be used in the lowest effective doses for short periods (weeks) only. A risk–benefit discussion is necessary for those requiring the drug for a longer period." Cotter J, Wooltorton E. New restrictions on celecoxib (Celebrex) use and the withdrawal of valdecoxib (Bextra). *CMAJ*. 2005 May 10;172(10):1299

[61] Lenzer J. Pfizer criticised over delay in admitting drug's problems. *BMJ*. 2004;329(7472):935

[62] Ray WA, Griffin MR, Stein CM. Cardiovascular toxicity of valdecoxib. *N Engl J Med*. 2004;351(26):2767

[63] "There is a strong association between Stevens-Johnson syndrome/toxic epidermal necrolysis and the use of the sulfonamide cox-2 inhibitors, particularly valdecoxib." La Grenade et al. Comparison of Reporting of Stevens-Johnson Syndrome and Toxic Epidermal Necrolysis in Association with Selective cox-2 Inhibitors. *Drug Saf*. 2005;28:917-24

[64] Nussmeier NA, et al. Complications of the cox-2 inhibitors parecoxib and valdecoxib after cardiac surgery. *N Engl J Med*. 2005 Mar 17;352(11):1081-91

[65] "On April 7, the Food and Drug Administration requested that Pfizer suspend sales of BEXTRA in the United States. As a result, BEXTRA will no longer be available to patients in the United States... In light of the FDA's position that there is an increased cardiovascular risk for all prescription non-steroidal anti-inflammatory medicines, as well as the increased rate of rare, serious skin reactions with BEXTRA, the FDA has requested that sales of BEXTRA be suspended." bextra.com/ September 28, 2005

[66] Sibbald B. Pfizer withdraw valdecoxib (Bextra) at Health Canada's request. *CMAJ*. 2005 May 10;172(10):e1298. Epub 2005 Apr 7 cmaj.ca/cgi/reprint/172/10/e1298

[67] walgreens.com/library/finddrug/druginfo1.jsp?particularDrug=Celebrex&id=15102 Accessed September 29, 2005

[68] "CONCLUSIONS: Variant 5-lipoxygenase genotypes identify a subpopulation with increased atherosclerosis. The observed diet-gene interactions further suggest that dietary n-6 polyunsaturated fatty acids promote, whereas marine n-3 fatty acids inhibit, leukotriene-mediated inflammation that leads to atherosclerosis in this subpopulation." Dwyer JH, et al. Arachidonate 5-lipoxygenase promoter genotype, dietary arachidonic acid, and atherosclerosis. *N Engl J Med*. 2004 Jan 1;350(1):29-37

[69] Kim et al. Celecoxib induces apoptosis, ER stress, and cyclooxygenase-2 expression on lung cancer cells (P2090). *J Immunol* 2013 May; 190 (Meeting Abstract) 132.35

[70] Lafleur MA et al. Xenobiotic perturbation of ER stress and the unfolded protein response. *Toxicol Pathol*. 2013 Feb;41(2):235-6

[71] "In 1983, 2876 people died from medication errors. ... By 1993, this number had risen to 7,391 - a 2.57-fold increase." Phillips DP, Christenfeld N, Glynn LM. Increase in US medication-error deaths between 1983 and 1993. *Lancet*. 1998 Feb 28;351(9103):643-4

[72] "Recent estimates suggest that each year more than 1 million patients are injured while in the hospital and approximately 180,000 die because of these injuries. Furthermore, drug-related morbidity and mortality are common and are estimated to cost more than $136 billion a year." Holland EG, Degruy FV. Drug-induced disorders. *Am Fam Physician*. 1997;56(7):1781-8, 1791-2

Safety, US FDA), more than 139,000 Americans who took Vioxx suffered serious side effects and between 26,000 and 55,000 people died from using the drug.[73] This aggregate is significantly greater than the annual deaths due to diabetes (71,000), suicide (30,000), homicide (20,000) [74], and—as a most dramatic example—the September 11, 2001 American terrorist attack (up to 3,000) *combined*.[75] Data suggests that nondrug treatments such as spinal manipulation[76], glucosamine sulfate[77], *Harpagophytum*[78] and capsicum are safer and/or more effective than pharmaceutical drugs for the relief of many types of pain. The increased utilization of these and other nonpharmacologic treatments would result in reductions in morbidity, mortality, and overall healthcare expenses when compared to our current overutilization of NSAIDs and other medical/allopathic pharmacosurgical treatments.[79]

> **In the US, 493 patients die each day —3,452 deaths per week— due to adverse events in hospitals**
>
> "Recent estimates suggest that each year more than 1 million patients are injured while in the hospital and approximately 180,000 die because of these injuries. Furthermore, drug-related morbidity and mortality are common and are estimated to cost more than $136 billion a year."
>
> Holland, Degruy. *Am Fam Physician*, 1997

Basic Concepts and Commonly Employed Therapeutics in Integrative Pain Management

The following pages summarize the basic therapeutics most commonly employed by integrative physicians in the treatment of acute and chronic musculoskeletal conditions. Knowledge of some of the clinical skills relied upon in orthopedics[80] is necessary when treating rheumatic musculoskeletal problems[81] because an acutely inflamed joint associated with a *chronic* and *systemic* disorder may need to be treated as if it were a *recent* and *focal* injury. Although *rheumatology* is generally concerned with the treatment of *non-traumatic* disorders of an inflammatory or autoimmune nature, knowledge of orthopedics is necessary during the course of evaluating and treating patients with autoimmunity because differential diagnosis, qualification/quantification, and comanagement of joint disorders *within the same patient* are commonly necessary. For example, a patient with rheumatoid arthritis (long-term autoimmune disease) affecting the knees and hips may also develop carpal tunnel syndrome (orthopedic problem) and later present with neck pain and leg spasticity secondary to atlantoaxial instability (neuro-orthopedic emergency).

Orthopedics generally centers on the clinical management of 1) **acute injuries** (e.g., whiplash), 2) **chronic repetitive strain injuries** (tendonitis and myofasciitis/myofascitis), and 3) **congenital/developmental anomalies**, (odontoid hypoplasia and scoliosis). For most clinicians, management of congenital anomalies centers on accurate diagnosis and then either observation or appropriate referral. For the treatment of common acute and chronic injuries encountered in general practice, integrative clinical care can include the facets described in the following section, modified for the clinical situation and individual patient.

Generally, different types and locations of injuries can be treated from a common framework of interventions that are then customized for the three following primary considerations:

1) Location: The specific location and associated functional considerations, e.g., lower extremity injuries may require crutches while upper extremity injuries may benefit from a brace or sling; ergonomic modifications,
2) Tissue: The type of tissue that is injured—i.e., muscle, cartilage, tendons, or ligaments—may respond to a customized nutritional and rehabilitative protocol,
3) Patient: The specific goals, needs, comorbidities, medications, occupation, recreational activities, age, and other characteristics of the individual patient. Also included here is consideration/correction of the patient's *internal inflammatory tendency* and *inflammatory balance/imbalance*, e.g. pro-inflammatory diet, acid-base balance, mitochondrial function, AGE and allergen consumption, etc.

---

[73] commondreams.org/views05/0223-35.htm and fda.gov/cder/drug/infopage/vioxx/vioxxgraham.pdf Accessed July 26, 2006
[74] Centers for Disease Control and Prevention (CDC), National Center for Health Statistics. Deaths: Final Data for 2001. 116 pp. (PHS) 2003-1120. Available at cdc.gov/nchs/releases/03facts/mortalitytrends.htm on January 18, 2004
[75] "On September 11, 2001, four U.S. planes hijacked by terrorists crashed into the World Trade Center, the Pentagon and a field in Pennsylvania killing nearly 3,000 people in a matter of hours." From cnn.com/SPECIALS/2001/memorial/ on January 26, 2004
[76] "CONCLUSION: The best evidence indicates that cervical manipulation for neck pain is much safer than the use of NSAIDs, by as much as a factor of several hundred times. There is no evidence that indicates NSAID use is any more effective than cervical manipulation for neck pain." Dabbs V, Lauretti WJ. A risk assessment of cervical manipulation vs. NSAIDs for the treatment of neck pain. *J Manipulative Physiol Ther*. 1995 Oct;18(8):530-6
[77] Muller-Fassbender H, et al. Glucosamine sulfate compared to ibuprofen in osteoarthritis of the knee. *Osteoarthritis Cartilage*. 1994 Mar;2(1):61-9
[78] Chrubasik S, et al. A randomized double-blind pilot study comparing Doloteffin and Vioxx in the treatment of low back pain. *Rheumatology* (Oxford). 2003 Jan;42(1):141-8
[79] Orme-Johnson DW, Herron RE. An innovative approach to reducing medical care utilization and expenditures. *Am J Manag Care*. 1997 Jan;3:135-44
[80] Vasquez A. *Integrative Orthopedics*. Third Edition (2012) or later. InflammationMastery.com
[81] Vasquez A. *Integrative Rheumatology*. Third Edition (2014) or later. InflammationMastery.com

<u>**Protect & prevent re-injury**</u>:
- **Avoid motions and activities that cause significant pain, as pain indicates that damaged/inflamed tissues are being stressed.** The goals are 1) to allow healing of injured tissues, and 2) to promote maximal physical restoration and functional ability. An excess of rest promotes functional disability, muscle atrophy, and psychological dysfunction (e.g., iatrogenic neurosis, inaccurate perception of patient being permanently damaged or defective, loss of confidence, loss of social contact [especially for children, and adults for whom physical activity is important]). Returning to activities and work too quickly may not allow time for sufficient healing and may thus promote re-injury, temporary exacerbation, progression from mild to severe injury, and/or progression to repetitive strain injury.
- **Use bracing, taping, bandages, wrapping, canes, crutches, and walkers as needed.**[82,83]

<u>**Relative rest**</u>:
- **"Relative rest" simply means to take time away from the activities that either promote additional injury or that unnecessarily drain energies which could otherwise be used for healing and recuperation.** For some patients, this means avoiding certain exercises during a workout, while for other patients this may mean using a crutch or taking days off from work.
- "Bed rest" is generally to be avoided since it promotes muscle atrophy, intraarticular adhesions, loss of neuromuscular coordination, constipation, and patients' assumption of the sick role.[84]

<u>**Ice/heat**</u>:
- <u>**First 48-72 hours after injury:**</u> **Apply ice or cold pack for 10 minutes each 30-60 minutes for reduction in pain and inflammation.** The best protocol appears to be interrupted application of ice to maximize deep cooling of tissues while minimizing cold-induced damage to the skin.[85] Ice massage is more effective than stationary application of ice or an ice bag.[86] Intraarticular temperatures can be lowered with topical application of ice[87], and immersion into ice water appears to be the best method for reducing intraarticular temperature according to an animal study.[88] Greater skin thickness due to subcutaneous adipose increases the amount of time needed to achieve clinically significant cooling of deep tissues.[89] Avoid frostbite and cold injuries to skin and superficial nerves. Use caution in patients with decreased skin sensitivity, circulatory insufficiency, and/or suboptimal ability to follow directions and employ good judgment.
- <u>**After 48-72 hours post-injury:**</u> **Apply gentle heat as needed for the relief of pain and reduction in muscle spasm and to promote healing by increasing circulation.** Avoid heat injuries to skin. Use caution in patients with decreased skin sensitivity (e.g., diabetics and the elderly) or suboptimal ability to follow directions and employ good judgment.

<u>**Individualize treatment**</u>:
- **The cornerstone of effective holistic and integrative treatment is to design treatment plans that simultaneously 1) address "the problem" while also 2) improving the patient's overall health.** Often, serious and so-called "untreatable" diseases can be ameliorated or eradicated simply with general, non-specific, overall health improvement even when these conditions repeatedly fail to respond to specific "disease-targeting" medical treatments.

<u>**Compression**</u>:
- Snug bandages/wraps may help to reduce swelling and can provide support for injured tissues and weakened joints. Care must be utilized to avoid arterial, venous, or lymphatic obstruction. Overuse of

---

82 Van Hook FW, Demonbreun D, Weiss BD. Ambulatory devices for chronic gait disorders in the elderly. *Am Fam Physician*. 2003 Apr 15;67(8):1717-24
83 Joyce BM, Kirby RL. Canes, crutches and walkers. *Am Fam Physician*. 1991 Feb;43(2):535-42
84 "Glucose intolerance, anorexia, constipation, and pressure sores might develop. Central nervous system changes could affect balance and coordination and lead to increasing dependence on caregivers." Teasell R, Dittmer DK. Complications of immobilization and bed rest. Part 2: Other complications. *Can Fam Physician*. 1993 Jun;39:1440-2, 1445-6
85 "… melting iced water applied through a wet towel for repeated periods of 10 minutes is most effective." MacAuley DC. Ice therapy. *Int J Sports Med*. 2001 Jul;22(5):379-84
86 Zemke JE, et al. Intramuscular temperature responses in the human leg to two forms of cryotherapy: ice massage and ice bag. *J Orthop Sports Phys Ther*. 1998 Apr;27(4):301-7
87 Martin SS, et al. Cryotherapy: an effective modality for decreasing intraarticular temperature after knee arthroscopy. *Am J Sports Med*. 2001 May-Jun;29(3):288-91
88 Bocobo C, Fast A, Kingery W, Kaplan M. The effect of ice on intra-articular temperature in the knee of the dog. *Am J Phys Med Rehabil*. 1991 Aug;70(4):181-5
89 Otte JW, et al. Subcutaneous adipose tissue thickness alters cooling time during cryotherapy. *Arch Phys Med Rehabil*. 2002 Nov;83(11):1501-5

bandages/wraps/braces limits motion and thereby promotes neuromuscular discoordination, which can promote local instability and re-injury.

Educate, establish treatment program, elevation:

- Educate patient about the injury. Educate patient about the need for appropriate follow-up office visits for reexamination, reassessment, and treatment.
- Estimate the amount of time during which most recovery will take place. Estimate the extent of return to previous status.
- Elevate the injured part to minimize swelling and edema.

Anti-inflammatory & analgesic treatments:

- <u>Avoidance of pro-inflammatory foods</u>: **Arachidonic acid** (high in cow's milk, beef, liver, pork, and lamb) is the direct precursor to pro-inflammatory prostaglandins and leukotrienes[90] and pain-promoting isoprostanes.[91] **Saturated fats** promote inflammation by activating/enabling pro-inflammatory Toll-like receptors, which are otherwise "specific" for inducing pro-inflammatory responses to microorganisms.[92] Consumption of saturated fat in the form of **cream** creates marked oxidative stress and lipid peroxidation that lasts for at least 3 hours postprandially.[93] **Corn oil** rapidly activates NFkB (in hepatic Kupffer cells) for a pro-inflammatory effect[94]; similarly, consumption of **linoleic acid** promotes intracellular antioxidant depletion and may thus promote oxidation-mediated inflammation via activation of NFkB. **Linoleic acid** causes intracellular oxidative stress and calcium influx and results in increased NFkB-stimulated transcription of pro-inflammatory genes.[95] **High glycemic foods** cause oxidative stress[96,97] and inflammation via activation of NFkB and other mechanisms—e.g., *white bread causes inflammation*[98] as **does a high-fat high-carbohydrate fast-food breakfast.**[99] **High glycemic foods** suppress immune function[100,101] and thus promote the development of infection/dysbiosis.[102] Delivery of a **high carbohydrate load** to the gastrointestinal lumen promotes bacterial overgrowth[103,104], which is inherently pro-inflammatory[105,106] and which appears to be myalgenic in humans[107] at least in part due to the ability of endotoxin to impair muscle function.[108] Overconsumption of high-carbohydrate low-phytonutrient **grains, potatoes, and manufactured foods** displaces phytonutrient-dense foods such as fruits, vegetables, nuts, seeds, and berries which contain more than 8,000 phytonutrients, many of which have antioxidant and thus anti-inflammatory actions.[109,110]

- <u>Anti-inflammation versus hemostasis</u>: Anti-inflammatory/analgesic medications that impair coagulation (e.g., aspirin) are contraindicated in patients with possible internal bleeding such as severe hematoma,

[90] Vasquez A. New Insights into Fatty Acid Supplementation and Its Effect on Eicosanoid Production and Genetic Expression. *Nutritional Perspectives* 2005; January: 5-16

[91] Evans AR, et al. Isoprostanes, novel eicosanoids that produce nociception and sensitize rat sensory neurons. *J Pharmacol Exp Ther*. 2000 Jun;293(3):912-20

[92] Lee et al. Saturated fatty acids but not unsaturated fatty acids induce expression of cyclooxygenase-2 mediated through Toll-like receptor 4. *J Biol Chem* 2001 May;276:16683-9

[93] "CONCLUSIONS: Both fat and protein intakes stimulate ROS generation. The increase in ROS generation lasted 3 h after cream intake and 1 h after protein intake. Cream intake also caused a significant and prolonged increase in lipid peroxidation." Mohanty P, Ghanim H, Hamouda W, Aljada A, Garg R, Dandona P. Both lipid and protein intakes stimulate increased generation of reactive oxygen species by polymorphonuclear leukocytes and mononuclear cells. *Am J Clin Nutr*. 2002 Apr;75(4):767-72

[94] Rusyn I, et al. Corn oil rapidly activates nuclear factor-kappaB in hepatic Kupffer cells by oxidant-dependent mechanisms. *Carcinogenesis*. 1999 Nov;20(11):2095-100

[95] "Exposing endothelial cells to 90 micromol linoleic acid/L for 6 h resulted in a significant increase in lipid hydroperoxides that coincided wih an increase in intracellular calcium concentrations." Hennig B, Toborek M, Joshi-Barve S, Barger SW, Barve S, Mattson MP, McClain CJ. Linoleic acid activates nuclear transcription factor-kappa B (NF-kappa B) and induces NF-kappa B-dependent transcription in cultured endothelial cells. *Am J Clin Nutr*. 1996 Mar;63(3):322-8 ajcn.org/cgi/reprint/63/3/322

[96] Mohanty et al. Glucose challenge stimulates reactive oxygen species (ROS) generation by leucocytes. *J Clin Endocrinol Metab*. 2000 Aug;85(8):2970-3

[97] Koska J, et al. Insulin, catecholamines, glucose and antioxidant enzymes in oxidative damage during different loads in healthy humans. *Physiol Res*. 2000;49 Suppl 1:S95-100

[98] "Conclusion - The present study shows that high GI carbohydrate, but not low GI carbohydrate, mediates an acute proinflammatory process as measured by NF-kappaB activity." Dickinson S, et al. High glycemic index carbohydrate mediates acute proinflammatory process measured by NF-kappaB activation. *Asia Pac J Clin Nutr*. 2005;14:S120

[99] Aljada A, et al. Increase in intranuclear nuclear factor kappaB and decrease in inhibitor kappaB in mononuclear cells after a mixed meal. *Am J Clin Nutr*. 2004 Apr;79(4):682-90

[100] Sanchez A, Reeser JL, Lau HS, et al. Role of sugars in human neutrophilic phagocytosis. *Am J Clin Nutr*. 1973 Nov;26(11):1180-4

[101] "Postoperative infusion of carbohydrate solution leads to moderate fall in the serum concentration of inorganic phosphate. ... The hypophosphatemia was associated with significant reduction of neutrophil phagocytosis, intracellular killing, consumption of oxygen and generation of superoxide during phagocytosis." Rasmussen A, Segel E, Hessov I, Borregaard N. Reduced function of neutrophils during routine postoperative glucose infusion. *Acta Chir Scand*. 1988 Jul-Aug;154(7-8):429-33

[102] Vasquez A. Part 6: Nutritional and Botanical Treatments against "Silent Infections" and Gastrointestinal Dysbiosis. *Nutritional Perspectives* 2006; January

[103] Ramakrishnan et al. Beneficial effects of fasting and low carbohydrate diet in D-lactic acidosis with short-bowel syndrome. *JPEN J Parenter Enteral Nutr* 1985;9:361-3

[104] Gottschall E. *Breaking the Vicious Cycle: Intestinal Health through Diet*. Kirkton Press; Rev edition (August 1, 1994)

[105] Lin HC. Small intestinal bacterial overgrowth: a framework for understanding irritable bowel syndrome. *JAMA*. 2004 Aug 18;292(7):852-8

[106] Lichtman SN, et al. Reactivation of arthritis induced by small bowel bacterial overgrowth in rats. *Infect Immun*. 1995 Jun;63(6):2295-301

[107] Pimentel M, et al. A link between irritable bowel syndrome and fibromyalgia may be related to findings on lactulose breath testing. *Ann Rheum Dis*. 2004 Apr;63(4):450-2

[108] Bundgaard H, et al. Endotoxemia stimulates skeletal muscle Na+-K+-ATPase and raises blood lactate. *Am J Physiol Heart Circ Physiol*. 2003 Mar;284(3):H1028-34

[109] "We propose that the additive and synergistic effects of phytochemicals in fruit and vegetables are responsible for their potent antioxidant and anticancer activities, and that the benefit of a diet rich in fruit and vegetables is attributed to the complex mixture of phytochemicals present in whole foods." Liu RH. Health benefits of fruit and vegetables are from additive and synergistic combinations of phytochemicals. *Am J Clin Nutr*. 2003 Sep;78(3 Suppl):517S-520S

[110] Seaman DR. The diet-induced proinflammatory state: a cause of chronic pain and other degenerative diseases? *J Manipulative Physiol Ther*. 2002;25(3):168-79

hemarthrosis, spleen injury, intracranial hemorrhage (i.e., subdural hematoma following a whiplash injury) and in patients about to undergo surgery. Theoretically, some caution might also be used with nutritional/botanical supplements that have anti-coagulant effects, such as *Ginkgo biloba*[111] and garlic.[112]

- <u>Anti-inflammatory diet, the "supplemented Paleo-Mediterranean diet"</u>: The health-promoting diet of choice for the majority of people is a diet based on **abundant consumption of fruits, vegetables, nuts, seeds, berries, omega-3 and monounsaturated fatty acids, and lean sources of protein such as lean (e.g., grass-fed or game) meats, fatty cold-water fish, soy and whey protein isolate.** This diet obviates overconsumption of chemical preservatives, artificial sweeteners, and carbohydrate-dominant foods such as candies, pastries, breads, potatoes, grains, and other foods with a high glycemic load and high glycemic index. This "Paleo-Mediterranean Diet" is a combination of the "Paleolithic" or "Paleo diet" and the well-known "Mediterranean diet", both of which are well described in peer-reviewed journals and the lay press, particularly by Eaton[113], O'Keefe[114], and Cordain[115]—see Chapter 2 and my other reviews[116,117,118] (included in Chapter 4 of *Inflammation Mastery: Volume 1* series starting in 2014) for details. This diet is the most nutrient-dense diet available, and its benefits are further enhanced by supplementation with vitamins, minerals, probiotics, and the health-promoting polyunsaturated fatty acids: ALA, GLA, EPA, and DHA.

- <u>Anti-inflammatory nutrients and botanicals</u>: Nutritional and botanical therapeutics are prescribed *per patient* and *per condition*. Doses listed are for adults and can be reduced when numerous interventions are simultaneously applied.

  o <u>Fish oil: EPA with DHA</u>: Three grams per day (3,000 mg/d) of combined EPA and DHA is a reasonable therapeutic dose[119] and is generally supplied in one tablespoon of liquid fish oil. Encapsulated fish oil supplements vary tremendously in their concentration of EPA and DHA and may require consumption of as few as five and as many as 21 capsules per day to achieve the same dosage and of EPA+DHA found in one tablespoon of liquid fish oil; encapsulated fish oil supplements also generally cost significantly more than do liquid fish oil supplements. The routine use of eicosapentaenoic acid (EPA) and docosahexaenoic acid (DHA) supplements is justified based on the following data: ❶ Most modern diets are profoundly deficient in omega-3 fatty acids[120], ❷ Dietary/supplemental intake of omega-3 fatty acids is a necessary prerequisite to reducing the pro-inflammatory effects of omega-6 fatty acids[121], ❸ Supplementation with

> **Importance of removing/counteracting the common pro-inflammatory diet**
>
> "RESULTS: The typical American diet is deficient in fruits and vegetables and contains excessive amounts of meat, refined grain products, and dessert foods. **Such a diet can have numerous adverse biochemical effects, all of which create a proinflammatory state and predispose the body to degenerative diseases.** It appears that an inadequate intake of fruits and vegetables can result in a suboptimal intake of antioxidants and phytochemicals and an imbalanced intake of essential fatty acids. Through different mechanisms, **each nutritional alteration can promote inflammation and disease.** CONCLUSION: We can no longer view different diseases as distinct biochemical entities. Nearly all degenerative diseases have the same underlying biochemical etiology, that is, a **diet-induced proinflammatory state.** Although specific diseases may require specific treatments, such as adjustments for hypomobile joints, beta-blockers for hypertension, and chemotherapy for cancer, **the treatment program must also include nutritional protocols to reduce the proinflammatory state.**"
>
> Seaman DR. The diet-induced proinflammatory state. *J Manipulative Physiol Ther* 2002 Mar

---

[111] "A structured assessment of published case reports suggests a possible causal association between using ginkgo and bleeding events... Patients using ginkgo, particularly those with known bleeding risks, should be counseled about a possible increase in bleeding risk." Bent S, Goldberg H, Padula A, Avins AL. Spontaneous bleeding associated with ginkgo biloba: a case report and systematic review of the literature: a case report and systematic review of the literature. *J Gen Intern Med.* 2005 Jul;20(7):657-61

[112] "The authors report a case of spontaneous spinal epidural hematoma causing paraplegia secondary to a qualitative platelet disorder from excessive garlic ingestion." Rose KD, et al. Spontaneous spinal epidural hematoma with associated platelet dysfunction from excessive garlic ingestion: a case report. *Neurosurgery.* 1990 May;26(5):880-2

[113] Eaton SB, Shostak M, Konner M. *The Paleolithic Prescription*, New York: Harper & Row, 1988

[114] O'Keefe JH Jr, Cordain L. Cardiovascular disease resulting from a diet and lifestyle at odds with our Paleolithic genome. *Mayo Clin Proc.* 2004 Jan;79(1):101-8

[115] Cordain L. *The Paleo Diet*. Indianapolis; John Wiley and Sons, 2002

[116] Vasquez A. A Five-Part Nutritional Protocol that Produces Consistently Positive Results. *Nutritional Wellness* 2005 Sep

[117] Vasquez A. Implementing the Five-Part Nutritional Wellness Protocol for the Treatment of Various Health Problems. *Nutritional Wellness* 2005 Nov

[118] Vasquez A. Revisiting the five-part nutritional wellness protocol: the supplemented Paleo-Mediterranean diet. *Nutritional Perspectives* 2011 Jan

[119] "...clinical benefits of the n-3 fatty acids were not apparent until they were consumed for > or =12 wk. It appears that a minimum daily dose of 3 g eicosapentaenoic and docosahexaenoic acids is necessary to derive the expected benefits [in patients with rheumatoid arthritis]." Kremer JM. n-3 fatty acid supplements in rheumatoid arthritis.*Am J Clin Nutr.*2000;71(1Suppl):349S-51S

[120] Simopoulos AP. Essential fatty acids in health and chronic disease. *Am J Clin Nutr.* 1999 Sep;70(3 Suppl):560S-569S

[121] Rubin D, Laposata M. Cellular interactions between n-6 and n-3 fatty acids: a mass analysis of fatty acid elongation/desaturation, distribution among complex lipids, and conversion to eicosanoids. *J Lipid Res.* 1992 Oct;33(10):1431-40.

EPA+DHA is safe and reduces all-cause mortality[122], ❹ Supplementation with EPA+DHA consistently provides clinically significant benefits in the treatment of a wide range of painful/inflammatory conditions.[123,124]

Clinical review of fatty acid metabolism

Chapter 4 (2014 and later) includes an update of previous reviews published on clinical applications of CFAT—combination fatty acid therapy.

- **Clinical trial—Omega-3 fatty acids (fish oil) as an anti-inflammatory alternative to NSAIDs for discogenic back pain (*Surg Neurol* 2006 Apr[125]):** The authors note that the use of NSAID medications is a well-established effective therapy for both acute and chronic nonspecific neck and back pain and yet can carry "extreme complications, including gastric ulcers, bleeding, myocardial infarction, and even deaths." 250 patients who had been seen by a neurosurgeon and were found to have nonsurgical neck or back pain were asked to take a total of 1200 mg per day of omega-3 EFAs (eicosapentaenoic acid and docosahexaenoic acid) found in fish oil supplements. ... Seventy-eight percent were taking 1200 mg and 22% were taking 2400 mg of EFAs. Fifty-nine percent discontinued to take their prescription NSAID medications for pain. Sixty percent stated that their overall pain was improved, and 60% stated that their joint pain had improved. Eighty percent stated they were satisfied with their improvement, and 88% stated they would continue to take the fish oil. There were no significant side effects reported. ... omega-3 EFA fish oil supplements appear to be a safer alternative to NSAIDs for treatment of nonsurgical neck or back pain in this selective group."

- **GLA, Gamma-linolenic acid:** Approximately 500 mg per day is the common anti-inflammatory dose[126] although higher doses of 2.8 grams per day have been safely used in patients with rheumatoid arthritis.[127] Except in the rarest circumstances (perhaps including temporal lobe epilepsy[128]), **GLA (most concentrated in borage oil) should always be co-administered with EPA and DHA (from fish oil) in order to obtain maximal benefit and avoid the increased formation of arachidonic acid that occurs when GLA is administered alone and the reduction in GLA/DGLA that occurs when fish oil is administered alone.**

  - **Clinical trial—Alpha-lipoic acid (ALA), gamma linolenic acid (GLA) and rehabilitation in the treatment of back pain (*Int J Immunopathol Pharmacol* 2009 Jul-Sep[129]):** This is a very interesting study which applied a partial nutritional protocol for the treatment of neuropathy as adjunct to usual rehabilitation in the treatment of neuropathic pain associated with disc herniation/degeneration and associated nerve root compression. The treatment group (n=101) received oral alpha-lipoic acid (ALA) 600 mg/d and gamma-linolenic acid (GLA) 360 mg/d and a physical rehabilitation program for six weeks, the second (n = 102) treated with only rehabilitation program. The authors noted and concluded, "Significant improvements was noted in the ALA and GLA group for paresthesia, stabbing and burning pain, as showed by VAS (Visual Analogue Scale), Oswestry Low Back Pain Disability Questionnaire, Aberdeen Low Back Pain Scale; also, improvements of quality of life has been noted, in the same group, as showed by SF-36, LDQ (Revised Leeds Disability Questionnaire), Roland and Morris disability

[122] "The recent GISSI (Gruppo Italiano per lo Studio della Sopravvivenza nell'Infarto miocardico)-Prevention study of 11,324 patients showed a 45% decrease in risk of sudden cardiac death and a 20% reduction in all-cause mortality in the group taking 850 mg/d of omega-3 fatty acids. These fatty acids have potent anti-inflammatory effects and may also be antiatherogenic." O'Keefe JH Jr, Harris WS. From Inuit to implementation: omega-3 fatty acids come of age. *Mayo Clin Proc.* 2000 Jun;75(6):607-14

[123] "Many of the placebo-controlled trials of fish oil in chronic inflammatory diseases reveal significant benefit, including decreased disease activity and a lowered use of anti-inflammatory drugs." Simopoulos AP. Omega-3 fatty acids in inflammation and autoimmune diseases. *J Am Coll Nutr.* 2002 Dec;21(6):495-505

[124] Vasquez A. New Insights into Fatty Acid Supplementation and Its Effect on Eicosanoid Production and Genetic Expression. *Nutritional Perspectives* 2005; January: 5-16

[125] Maroon et al. Omega-3 fatty acids (fish oil) as an anti-inflammatory: alternative to nonsteroidal anti-inflammatory drugs for discogenic pain. *Surg Neurol.* 2006 Apr;65:326-31

[126] "Forty patients with rheumatoid arthritis and upper gastrointestinal lesions due to non-steroidal anti-inflammatory drugs entered a prospective 6-month double-blind placebo controlled study of dietary supplementation with gamma-linolenic acid 540 mg/day…" Brzeski M, Madhok R, Capell HA. Evening primrose oil in patients with rheumatoid arthritis and side-effects of non-steroidal anti-inflammatory drugs. *Br J Rheumatol.* 1991 Oct;30(5):370-2

[127] Zurier RB, Rossetti RG, Jacobson EW, DeMarco DM, Liu NY, Temming JE, White BM, Laposata M. gamma-Linolenic acid treatment of rheumatoid arthritis. A randomized, placebo-controlled trial. *Arthritis Rheum.* 1996 Nov;39(11):1808-17

[128] "Three long-stay, hospitalised schizophrenics who had failed to respond adequately to conventional drug therapy were treated with gamma-linolenic acid and linoleic acid in the form of evening primrose oil. They became substantially worse and electroencephalographic features of temporal lobe epilepsy became apparent." Vaddadi KS. The use of gamma-linolenic acid and linoleic acid to differentiate between temporal lobe epilepsy and schizophrenia. *Prostaglandins Med.* 1981 Apr;6(4):375-9

[129] Ranieri et al. Use of alpha-lipoic acid (ALA), gamma linolenic acid (GLA) and rehabilitation in treatment of back pain. *Int J Immunopathol Pharmacol.* 2009 Jul-Sep;22:45-50

questionnaire. All these outcome measure showed statistically significant decreases. Oral treatment with alpha-lipoic acid (ALA) and gamma-linolenic acid (GLA) for six weeks in synergy with rehabilitation therapy improved neuropathic symptoms and deficits in patients with radicular neuropathy."

- o *Zingiber officinale* (Ginger): Ginger is a well-known spice and food with a long history of use as an anti-inflammatory, anti-nausea, and gastroprotective agent[130], and components of ginger have been shown to reduce production of the leukotriene LTB4 by inhibiting 5-lipoxygenase and to reduce production of the prostaglandin PGE2 by inhibiting cyclooxygenase.[131,132] With its dual reduction in the formation of pro-inflammatory prostaglandins and leukotrienes, ginger has been shown to safely reduce nonspecific musculoskeletal pain[133,134] and to provide relief from osteoarthritis of the knees[135] and migraine headaches.[136] Ginger can be consumed liberally as a supplement or as whole food, and it is safe for use in pregnancy up to one gram per day.[137]

- o Willow bark *(Salix* spp): In a double-blind placebo-controlled clinical trial in 210 patients with moderate/severe low-back pain (20% of patients had positive straight-leg raising test), willow bark extract showed a dose-dependent analgesic effect with benefits beginning in the first week of treatment.[138] In a head-to-head study of 228 patients comparing willow bark (standardized for 240 mg salicin) with Vioxx (rofecoxib), treatments were equally effective yet willow bark was safer and 40% less expensive.[139] Because willow bark's salicylates were the original source for the chemical manufacture of acetylsalicylic acid (aspirin), researchers and clinicians have erroneously mistaken willow bark to be synonymous with aspirin; this is certainly inaccurate and therefore clarification of willow's mechanism of action will be provided here. Aspirin has two primary effects via three primary mechanisms of action: 1) anticoagulant effects mediated by the acetylation and permanent inactivation of thromboxane-A synthase, which is the enzyme that makes the powerfully proaggregatory thromboxane-A2; 2) antiprostaglandin action via acetylation of both isoforms of cyclooxygenase (COX-1 inhibition 25-166x more than COX-2) with widespread inhibition of prostaglandin formation, and 3) antiprostaglandin formation via retroconversion of acetylsalicylate into salicylic acid which then inhibits cyclooxygenase-2 gene transcription.[140] Notice that the acetylation reactions are specific to aspirin and thus actions #1 and #2 are not seen with willow bark; whereas #3—inhibition of COX-2 transcription by salicylates—appears to be the major mechanism of action of willow bark extract. Proof of this principle is supported by the lack of adverse effects associated with willow bark in the research literature. If willow bark were pharmacodynamically synonymous with aspirin, then we would expect case reports of gastric ulceration, hemorrhage, and Reye's syndrome to permeate the research literature; this is not the case and therefore—**with the exception of possible allergic reactions in patients previously allergic/anaphylactic to aspirin and salicylates—extensive "warnings" on willow bark products**[141] **are unnecessary.**[142] Salicylates are widely present in fruits, vegetables, herbs and spices and are partly responsible for the anti-cancer, anti-inflammatory, and health-promoting benefits of fruit and vegetable consumption.[143,144] With willow bark products, the daily dose should not exceed 240 mg of salicin, and products should include other components of the whole plant. **Except for rare allergy in patients previously sensitized to aspirin or salicylates, no adverse effects are**

[130] Langner E, Greifenberg S, Gruenwald J. Ginger: history and use. *Adv Ther* 1998 Jan-Feb;15(1):25-44

[131] Kiuchi F, et al. Inhibition of prostaglandin and leukotriene biosynthesis by gingerols and diarylheptanoids. *Chem Pharm Bull* (Tokyo) 1992 Feb;40(2):387-91

[132] Tjendraputra E, et al. Effect of ginger constituents and synthetic analogues on cyclooxygenase-2 enzyme in intact cells. *Bioorg Chem* 2001 Jun;29(3):156-63

[133] Srivastava KC, Mustafa T. Ginger (Zingiber officinale) in rheumatism and musculoskeletal disorders. *Med Hypotheses*. 1992 Dec;39(4):342-8

[134] Srivastava KC, Mustafa T. Ginger (Zingiber officinale) and rheumatic disorders. *Med Hypotheses*. 1989 May;29(1):25-8

[135] Altman RD, Marcussen KC. Effects of a ginger extract on knee pain in patients with osteoarthritis. *Arthritis Rheum.* 2001 Nov;44(11):2531-8

[136] Mustafa T, Srivastava KC. Ginger (Zingiber officinale) in migraine headache. *J Ethnopharmacol.* 1990 Jul;29(3):267-73

[137] "...oral ginger 1 g per day... No adverse effect of ginger on pregnancy outcome was detected." Vutyavanich T, Kraisarin T, Ruangsri R. Ginger for nausea and vomiting in pregnancy: randomized, double-masked, placebo-controlled trial. *Obstet Gynecol* 2001 Apr;97(4):577-82.

[138] Chrubasik S, et al. Treatment of low-back pain exacerbations with willow bark extract: a randomized double-blind study. *Am J Med.* 2000;109:9-14

[139] Chrubasik S, et al. Treatment of low-back pain with a herbal or synthetic anti-rheumatic: a randomized controlled study. *Rheumatology* (Oxford). 2001;40:1388-93

[140] Hare LG, Woodside JV, Young IS. Dietary salicylates. *J Clin Pathol* 2003 Sep;56(9):649-50 jcp.bmj.com/cgi/content/full/56/9/649

[141] Clauson KA, et al. Evaluation of Presence of Aspirin-Related Warnings with Willow Bark (July/August). *Ann Pharmacother.* 2005 Jul-Aug;39(7-8):1234-7 The article by Clauson et al contained/s numerous inaccuracies and should either be withdrawn or read only in conjunction with my refutation: Vasquez A, Muanza D. Evaluation of Presence of Aspirin-Related Warnings with Willow Bark: Comment on the Article by Clauson et al. *Ann Pharmacotherapy* 2005 Oct;39(10):1763

[142] Vasquez et al. Evaluation of Presence of Aspirin-Related Warnings with Willow Bark: Comment on the Article by Clauson et al. *Ann Pharmacotherapy* 2005 Oct;39(10):1763

[143] Lawrence JR, et al. Urinary excretion of salicyluric and salicylic acids by non-vegetarians, vegetarians, and patients taking low dose aspirin. *J Clin Pathol.* 2003 Sep;56:651-3

[144] Paterson JR, Lawrence JR. Salicylic acid: a link between aspirin, diet and the prevention of colorectal cancer. *QJM.* 2001 Aug;94(8):445-8

known; to be on the medicolegal safe side, use is discouraged during pregnancy, before surgery, or when anti-coagulant medications are being used.

- o *Uncaria guianensis* and *Uncaria tomentosa* ("cat's claw", "una de gato"): A double-blind placebo-controlled study using 100 mg daily of highly-concentrated freeze-dried aqueous extract of *Uncaria tomentosa* found significant pain relief (reduction by 36%) and minimal adverse effects after 4 weeks of treatment in 30 male patients with osteoarthritis of the knees, a benefit mediated via antioxidant activities and inhibition of NF-kappaB, TNFα, COX-2, and PGE-2 production.[145] Inhibition of NFkB and iNOS are of primary importance in the treatment of inflammatory conditions.[146] A year-long study of patients with active rheumatoid arthritis (RA) treated with sulfasalazine or hydroxychloroquine showed "relative safety and modest benefit" of coadministration of *Uncaria tomentosa*.[147] Other studies with *Uncaria tomentosa* have shown enhancement of post-vaccination immunity[148] and enhancement of DNA repair in humans.[149] Traditional uses have included the use of the herb as a contraceptive and as treatment for gastrointestinal ulcers.

- o *Boswellia serrata*: *Boswellia* inhibits 5-lipoxygenase[150] with no apparent effect on cyclooxygenase[151] and has been shown effective in the treatment of osteoarthritis of the knees[152] as well as asthma[153] and ulcerative colitis.[154] When used as monotherapy, the target dose is approximately 150 mg of boswellic acids TID.

- o *Harpagophytum procumbens* (Devil's claw): The safety and effectiveness of *Harpagophytum* has been established in patients with hip pain, low-back pain, and knee pain.[155,156,157] The mechanisms of action include weak anti-inflammatory effects and a stronger analgesic effect.[158,159] Research suggests that *Harpagophytum* is an effective analgesic for low back pain[160], including low back pain with radiculitis and radiculopathy.[161] The common dose is 60 mg harpagoside per day.[162]

- o Topical application of *Capsicum annuum, Capsicum frutescens* (Cayenne pepper, hot chili pepper): Capsaicin reduces pain perception by depleting sensory fibers of substance P—blocking transport as well as de-novo synthesis of substance P. Topical capsaicin alleviates diabetic neuropathy[163], low back pain[164], chronic neck pain[165], osteoarthritis[166], rheumatoid arthritis[167], notalgia paresthetica[168],

[145] Piscoya J, et al. Efficacy and safety of freeze-dried cat's claw in osteoarthritis of the knee. *Inflamm Res*. 2001 Sep;50(9):442-8

[146] Sandoval-Chacon M, et al. Antiinflammatory actions of cat's claw: the role of NF-kappaB. *Aliment Pharmacol Ther*. 1998 Dec;12(12):1279-89

[147] "This small preliminary study demonstrates relative safety and modest benefit to the tender joint count of a highly purified extract from the pentacyclic chemotype of UT in patients with active RA taking sulfasalazine or hydroxychloroquine." Mur E, Hartig F, Eibl G, Schirmer M. Randomized double blind trial of an extract from the pentacyclic alkaloid-chemotype of uncaria tomentosa for the treatment of rheumatoid arthritis. *J Rheumatol*. 2002 Apr;29(4):678-81

[148] "…Uncaria tomentosa or Cat's Claw which is known to possess immune enhancing and antiinflammatory properties in animals. There were no toxic side effects observed as judged by medical examination, clinical chemistry and blood cell analysis. However, statistically significant immune enhancement for the individuals on C-Med-100 supplement was observed..." Lamm S, Sheng Y, Pero RW. Persistent response to pneumococcal vaccine in individuals supplemented with a novel water soluble extract of Uncaria tomentosa, C-Med-100. *Phytomedicine*. 2001;8(4):267-74

[149] Sheng Y, Li L, Holmgren K, Pero RW. DNA repair enhancement of aqueous extracts of Uncaria tomentosa in a human volunteer study. *Phytomedicine*. 2001 Jul;8(4):275-82

[150] Wildfeuer A, Neu IS, Safayhi H, Metzger G, Wehrmann M, Vogel U, Ammon HP. Effects of boswellic acids extracted from a herbal medicine on the biosynthesis of leukotrienes and the course of experimental autoimmune encephalomyelitis. *Arzneimittelforschung* 1998 Jun;48(6):668-74

[151] Safayhi H, et al. Boswellic acids: novel, specific, nonredox inhibitors of 5-lipoxygenase. *J Pharmacol Exp Ther* 1992 Jun;261(3):1143-6

[152] Kimmatkar N, et al. Efficacy and tolerability of Boswellia serrata extract in treatment of osteoarthritis of knee. *Phytomedicine*. 2003 Jan;10(1):3-7

[153] Gupta I, et al. Effects of Boswellia serrata gum resin in patients with bronchial asthma. *Eur J Med Res*. 1998 Nov 17;3(11):511-4

[154] Gupta I, et al. Effects of Boswellia serrata gum resin in patients with ulcerative colitis. *Eur J Med Res*. 1997 Jan;2(1):37-43

[155] Chrubasik S, et al. Comparison of outcome measures during treatment with the proprietary Harpagophytum extract doloteffin in patients with pain in the lower back, knee or hip. *Phytomedicine* 2002 Apr;9(3):181-94

[156] Chantre P, et al. Efficacy and tolerance of Harpagophytum procumbens versus diacerhein in treatment of osteoarthritis. *Phytomedicine* 2000 Jun;7(3):177-83

[157] Leblan D, Chantre P, Fournie B. Harpagophytum procumbens in the treatment of knee and hip osteoarthritis.. *Joint Bone Spine* 2000;67(5):462-7

[158] Whitehouse et al. Devil's Claw (Harpagophytum procumbens): no evidence for anti-inflammatory activity in treatment of arthritic disease. *Can Med Assoc J* 1983;129:249-51

[159] Moussard C, Alber D, Toubin MM, Thevenon N, Henry JC. A drug used in traditional medicine, harpagophytum procumbens: no evidence for NSAID-like effect on whole blood eicosanoid production in human. *Prostaglandins Leukot Essent Fatty Acids* 1992 Aug;46(4):283-6

[160] Chrubasik S, et al. A randomized double-blind pilot study comparing Doloteffin and Vioxx in the treatment of low back pain. *Rheumatology* (Oxford). 2003 Jan;42(1):141-8

[161] "The majority of responders' were patients who had suffered less than 42 days of pain, and subgroup analyses suggested that the effect was confined to patients with more severe and radiating pain accompanied by neurological deficit... There was no evidence for Harpagophytum-related side-effects, except possibly for mild and infrequent gastrointestinal symptoms." Chrubasik S, Junck H, Breitschwerdt H, Conradt C, Zappe H. Effectiveness of Harpagophytum extract WS 1531 in the treatment of exacerbation of low back pain: a randomized, placebo-controlled, double-blind study. *Eur J Anaesthesiol* 1999 Feb;16(2):118-29

[162] "They took an 8-week course of Doloteffin at a dose providing 60 mg harpagoside per day... Doloteffin is well worth considering for osteoarthritic knee and hip pain and nonspecific low back pain." Chrubasik S, Thanner J, Kunzel O, Conradt C, Black A, Pollak S. Comparison of outcome measures during treatment with the proprietary Harpagophytum extract doloteffin in patients with pain in the lower back, knee or hip. *Phytomedicine* 2002 Apr;9(3):181-94

[163] "Study results suggest that topical capsaicin cream is safe and effective in treating painful diabetic neuropathy. "[No authors listed] Treatment of painful diabetic neuropathy with topical capsaicin. A multicenter, double-blind, vehicle-controlled study. The Capsaicin Study Group. *Arch Intern Med*. 1991 Nov;151(11):2225-9

[164] Keitel W, et al. Capsicum pain plaster in chronic non-specific low back pain. *Arzneimittelforschung*. 2001 Nov;51(11):896-903

[165] Mathias BJ, Dillingham TR, Zeigler DN, Chang AS, Belandres PV. Topical capsaicin for chronic neck pain. A pilot study. *Am J Phys Med Rehabil* 1995 Jan-Feb;74(1):39-44

[166] McCarthy GM, McCarty DJ. Effect of topical capsaicin in the therapy of painful osteoarthritis of the hands. *J Rheumatol*. 1992;19(4):604-7

[167] Deal CL, et al. Treatment of arthritis with topical capsaicin: a double-blind trial. *Clin Ther*. 1991 May-Jun;13(3):383-95

[168] Leibsohn E. Treatment of notalgia paresthetica with capsaicin. *Cutis* 1992 May;49(5):335-6

reflex sympathetic dystrophy[169], and cluster headache (intranasal application).[170,171,172] Notable with capsaicin are the absence of adverse effects (other than local burning sensation, which abates), high efficacy, and lower cost—all of which are often superior to prescription drug analgesics; an outline of notable studies is provided below:

- **Topical capsaicin versus oral amitriptyline for diabetic neuropathy**: An 8-week, double-blind, multicenter parallel study compared the safety and efficacy of topical capsaicin and oral amitriptyline in 235 patients with painful diabetic neuropathy involving the feet; pain relief and reduction in disability were comparable, but topical capsaicin was much safer and avoided the costs and adverse effects of amitriptyline (somnolence [46%], neuromuscular [23%] and cardiovascular [9%] effects). The authors concluded, "Topically applied capsaicin is an equally effective but considerably safer alternative to amitriptyline for relief of the pain of diabetic neuropathy."[173]
- **High-potency topical capsaicin 5-10% for severe intractable pain**: A very assertive intervention study by Robbins et al[174] used high-concentration (5%–10%) capsaicin administered with regional anesthesia in patients with intractable pain, complex regional pain syndromes and neuropathic pain; the effectiveness of this approach lead the authors to conclude, "The intermittent application of large-dose topical capsaicin may provide significant pain relief, decrease chronic analgesic dependence, and decrease aggregate health care expenditures."
- **Topical capsaicin for pediatric hernia repair analgesia**: A double-blind, placebo-controlled study among 108 children undergoing pediatric hernia repair showed that acupoint capsaicin application provided pain relief and allowed for reduced dependence on meperidine (opioid analgesic).[175]
- **Topical capsaicin for hysterectomy analgesia**: A double-blind, placebo-controlled study among 90 women undergoing abdominal hysterectomy showed that topical capsaicin reduced the need for morphine and postoperative antiemetics.[176]
- **Topical capsaicin for low-back pain**: A double-blind, randomized, placebo-controlled, multicenter parallel study with 320 patients with chronic low back pain used topical capsicum to safely obtain clinically relevant reductions in pain and disability.[177]
- **Intranasal capsaicin for cluster headache**: Treatment of active cluster headache with intranasal capsaicin (compared with placebo) reduced severity after 7 days of treatment.[178]
- **Intranasal capsaicin for migraine headache**: In a small controlled trial, patients stated that intranasal application of capsaicin alleviated migraine suffering by 50% to 80%.[179]

Capsaicin is applied externally and therefore has no internal adverse effects; delivery is typically via inexpensive OTC cream or patch with strengths ranging from 0.025, 0.075, 0.1%; more potent and expensive physician-authorized and physician-applied patches are also available. Capsaicin products are applied topically per product instructions and patient tolerance; the medically benign burning sensation abates with continued use. Doctors should experiment on themselves with this treatment before administering to patients in order to gain understanding by experience; care must always be used to avoid contact with eyes or genitals, especially at the same time, because that would

---

[169] "Capsaicin is effective for psoriasis, pruritus, and cluster headache; it is often helpful for itching and pain of postmastectomy pain syndrome, oral mucositis, cutaneous allergy, loin pain/hematuria syndrome, neck pain, amputation stump pain, and skin tumor; and it may be beneficial for neural dysfunction (detrusor hyperreflexia, reflex sympathetic dystrophy, and rhinopathy)." Hautkappe et al. Review of effectiveness of capsaicin for painful cutaneous disorders and neural dysfunction. *Clin J Pain* 1998;14:97-106

[170] "Capsaicin application to human nasal mucosa was found to induce painful sensation, sneezing, and nasal secretion. All of these factors exhibit desensitization upon repeated applications." Sicuteri F, et al. Beneficial effect of capsaicin application to the nasal mucosa in cluster headache. *Clin J Pain*. 1989;5(1):49-53

[171] "The efficacy of repeated nasal applications of capsaicin in cluster headache is congruent with previous reports on the therapeutic effect of capsaicin in other pain syndromes (post-herpetic neuralgia, diabetic neuropathy, trigeminal neuralgia) and supports the use of the drug to produce a selective analgesia." Fusco BM, Marabini S, Maggi CA, Fiore G, Geppetti P. Preventative effect of repeated nasal applications of capsaicin in cluster headache. *Pain*. 1994 Dec;59(3):321-5

[172] "These results indicate that intranasal capsaicin may provide a new therapeutic option for the treatment of this disease." Marks DR, Rapoport A, Padla D, Weeks R, Rosum R, Sheftell F, Arrowsmith F. A double-blind placebo-controlled trial of intranasal capsaicin for cluster headache. *Cephalalgia*. 1993 Apr;13(2):114-6

[173] Biesbroeck et al. A double-blind comparison of topical capsaicin and oral amitriptyline in painful diabetic neuropathy. *Adv Ther*. 1995 Mar-Apr;12(2):111-20

[174] Robbins WR, et al. Treatment of intractable pain with topical large-dose capsaicin: preliminary report. *Anesth Analg*. 1998 Mar;86(3):579-83

[175] Kim KS, Kim DW, Yu YK. The effect of capsicum plaster in pain after inguinal hernia repair in children. *Paediatr Anaesth*. 2006 Oct;16(10):1036-41

[176] Kim KS, Nam YM. The analgesic effects of capsicum plaster at the Zusanli point after abdominal hysterectomy. *Anesth Analg*. 2006;103(3):709-13

[177] Frerick H, Keitel W, Kuhn U, Schmidt S, Bredehorst A, Kuhlmann M. Topical treatment of chronic low back pain with a capsicum plaster. *Pain*. 2003 Nov;106(1-2):59-64

[178] Marks et al. A double-blind placebo-controlled trial of intranasal capsaicin for cluster headache. *Cephalalgia*. 1993 Apr;13(2):114-6

[179] Fusco BM, Barzoi G, Agrò F. Repeated intranasal capsaicin applications to treat chronic migraine. *Br J Anaesth*. 2003 Jun;90(6):812

really hurt, and would be socially awkward (contorted body posturing, facial grimacing, futile cries for help, etc—especially at a medical conference with colleagues or fine dining events with friends and family), and would make washing/rinsing difficult for technical (reduced vision due to excess lacrimation) and psychoepistimological (how to prioritize?) reasons.

o   *Cannabis sativa* and related variants (Cannabis): Cannabis is an inexpensive and impressively safe botanical providing therapeutic efficacy against a wide range of debilitating medical disorders (notably chronic pain), and it is readily cultivable by individual citizens/patients and increasingly available through decriminalized commercial channels. Clinicians and "premedical healers" have used Cannabis for its medicinal benefits for more than five thousand years; the world's oldest surviving medical text, the Chinese *Shen-nung Pen-tshao Ching* (*Divine Farmer's Materia Medica*), recommends Cannabis to reduce the pain of rheumatism and to address digestive disorders.[180] The plant has

> **The Responsibility of Intellectuals**
>
> "It is the responsibility of intellectuals to speak the truth and to expose lies."
>
> Chomsky N. *New York Review of Books* 1967 nybooks.com

been used medically for thousands of years with an objectively favorable risk:benefit ratio with the added benefit of low cost and notably easy cultivation. The plant was later made illegal for purposes of social divisiveness/targeting (e.g., independent thinkers, and because of its low cost and numerous medical uses, it was preferentially used by poor sections of the population, particularly minorities) and for market protection (i.e., because the medical and social uses of the drug dissuaded people from using patentable high-profit pharmaceutical drugs, taxable high-profit corporate-produced alcoholic beverages and tobacco products); currently, the criminalization of Cannabis is financially supported by police unions, privatized prison corporations in America, alcoholic beverage companies, prescription drug companies, and prison guard unions; see compilation footnote for citations.

The criminalization of Cannabis use has no legitimate medical or social basis especially when contrasted against costlier, riskier, less effective, and readily available ethanol/alcohol, tobacco, and innumerable government-approved pharmaceutical drugs, particularly analgesic, opioid, antispasmodic, antidepressant and antianxiety drugs. Recently and only after spending trillions of dollars and wasting innumerable *tens-hundreds of thousands* of human lives, laws regarding Cannabis are being relaxed internationally. Oral consumption of Cannabis products obviates concern regarding adverse effects from inhalation of smoked (and therefore chemically altered) plant material. See compilation footnote for citations/information.[181]

> **Private interests supporting criminalization of Cannabis and therefore penalization/incarceration of citizens**
>
> 1. Prescription drug makers: **Purdue Pharma** makes OxyContin, **Abbott Laboratories** makes Vicodin, **Alkermes** makes Zohydrol ("reportedly ten times stronger than OxyContin"), **Janssen Pharmaceutical** is a **Johnson & Johnson** subsidiary that makes Nucynta, and **Pfizer** makes several opioid drugs
> 2. Alcohol and beer companies
> 3. Privatized prison corporations
> 4. Police unions and (privatized) prison guard unions: recipients of federal funding; police departments, as authorized by the Reagan administration, gained the ability to financially profit via the seizure and sale of personal property ("asset forfeiture") called "policing for profit"
> 5. Community nonprofit groups: recipients of federal funding connected to the "War on Drugs"
> 6. Drug rehabilitation centers: benefit from court-ordered rehabilitation sentences
> 7. Partnership for Drug-Free Kids, formerly Partnership for a Drug-Free America: paid by opioid manufacturers and other pharmaceutical companies.
>
> Fang L, *Nation* 2014 Jul and JF, *The Economist* 2014 Apr. See compilation footnote.

- Pharmacologic and clinical effects of medical cannabis (*Pharmacotherapy* 2013 Feb[182]): "Pain and muscle spasms are the most common reasons that medical cannabis is being recommended. Studies of medical cannabis show significant improvement in various types of pain and muscle spasticity. Reported adverse effects are typically not serious, with the most common being dizziness."

- Cannabis as an adjunct to or substitute for opiates in the treatment of chronic pain (*J Psychoactive Drugs* 2012 Apr[183]): "There is a growing body of evidence to support the use of medical cannabis as an adjunct to or substitute for prescription opiates in the treatment of chronic pain. When used in conjunction with opiates, cannabinoids lead to a greater cumulative relief of pain, resulting in a reduction in

---

[180] Thomas J. The Past, Present, and Future of Medical Marijuana in the United States. *Psychiatric Times* 2010 Jan psychiatrictimes.com/articles/
[181] Compilation footnote: Brecher EM. *Licit and Illicit Drugs: The Consumers Union Report on Narcotics, Stimulants, Depressants, Inhalants, Hallucinogens, and Marijuana.* 1972. Fang L. The Real Reason Pot Is Still Illegal. *The Nation* 2014 July 21-28. JF. What civil-asset forfeiture means. *Economist* 2014 Apr
[182] Borgelt et al. The pharmacologic and clinical effects of medical cannabis. *Pharmacotherapy.* 2013 Feb;33(2):195-209
[183] Lucas P. Cannabis as an adjunct to or substitute for opiates in the treatment of chronic pain. *J Psychoactive Drugs.* 2012 Apr-Jun;44(2):125-33

the use of opiates (and associated side-effects) by patients in a clinical setting. Additionally, cannabinoids can prevent the development of tolerance to and withdrawal from opiates, and can even rekindle opiate analgesia after a prior dosage has become ineffective."

- Medical uses of Cannabis (*J Am Board Family Med* 2011 Jul[184]): Accepted applications of Cannabis per Canadian regulations: "end-of-life care; seizures from epilepsy; severe pain and/or persistent muscle spasms caused by multiple sclerosis, spinal cord diseases, or spinal cord injury; severe pain; cachexia; anorexia; weight loss and/or severe nausea from cancer or HIV/AIDS infection."

- Modulation of amygdala-cortical connectivity contributes to the dissociative effect of cannabis on pain perception (*Pain* 2013 Jan[185]): Functional magnetic resonance imaging was used to investigate the effects of delta-9-tetrahydrocannabinol (THC), a naturally occurring cannabinoid, on brain activity related to cutaneous ongoing pain and hyperalgesia that were temporarily induced by capsaicin in healthy volunteers. THC reduced reported unpleasantness but not intensity of ongoing pain and hyperalgesia. ... THC significantly reduced primary sensorimotor functional connectivity between the right amygdala and the primary sensorimotor cortex during the ongoing pain state."

- Low-dose vaporized cannabis significantly improves neuropathic pain (*J Pain* 2013 Feb[186]): "The analgesia obtained from a low dose of delta-9-tetrahydrocannabinol (1.29%) in patients, most of whom were experiencing neuropathic pain despite conventional treatments, is a clinically significant outcome. ...As a result, one might not anticipate a significant impact on daily functioning."

- **Medical cannabis reduces opioid analgesic overdose mortality (*JAMA Intern Med* 2014 Aug[187]): "States with medical cannabis laws had a 24.8% lower mean annual opioid overdose mortality rate (95% CI, -37.5% to -9.5%; P = .003) compared with states without medical cannabis laws. ... Medical cannabis laws are associated with significantly lower state-level opioid overdose mortality rates."**

- Pharmacological Basis of Cannabis Therapy for Epilepsy (*J Pharmacol Exp Ther* 2016 Apr[188]): "The two chief cannabinoids are delta-9-tetrahyrdrocannabinol [THC], the major psychoactive component of marijuana, and cannabidiol (CBD), the major nonpsychoactive component of marijuana. ... CBD is anticonvulsant..."

- Cannabidiol: a drug with wide spectrum of action (*Rev Bras Psiquiatr* 2008 Sep): "The last five years have shown a remarkable increase in publications on cannabidiol mainly stimulated by the discovery of its anti-inflammatory, anti-oxidative and neuroprotective effects. These studies have suggested a wide range of possible therapeutic effects of cannabidiol on several conditions, including Parkinson's disease, Alzheimer's disease, cerebral ischemia, diabetes, rheumatoid arthritis, other inflammatory diseases, nausea and cancer."

Cannabis' medical uses
"Various well-designed, randomized, placebo-controlled trials have shown that smoked cannabis can relieve peripheral, posttraumatic, and HIV-induced neuropathic pain." Evidence from Clinical Studies: • Tourette syndrome • Glaucoma • Post-operative pain • Refractory neuropathic pain • Nausea due to many causes • HIV anorexia, weight loss • Multiple sclerosis spasticity, central pain, bladder dysfunction • Opioid synergism Safety: "much less dangerous than opiates, amphetamines, and barbiturates and also less dangerous than alcohol." Leung, *Journal of the American Board Family Medicine* 2011 Jul

---

SUMMARY: *Cannabis* provides psychoemotional relaxation via THC and profound anti-inflammation via CBD
Cannabis was blacklisted by governments as a means of (excuse for) social control and to maintain social desperation and pharmaceutical dependency; no legitimate medical nor social reason exists for its criminalization. The so-called "criminal justice" system was co-opted to meet the government's political goal of selective suppression of social factions (e.g., anti-war groups, intellectuals, minorities), to protect and thereby promote sales of pharmaceutical drugs, and—later—to profit America's for-profit police and prison systems. An efficient and effective means to target intellectuals and free/independent thinkers is to criminalize reasonable and rational behavior; the illogical criminalization of *Cannabis* has been a perfect example of such. By extension, the medical profession allowed itself—via its perpetual and self-serving acquiescence on this subject—to aid and abet both social and medical injustice by allowing the unnecessary incarceration of millions of otherwise innocent people and by denying safe/effective/natural/affordable treatment to millions of patients who suffer from *Cannabis*-responsive conditions such as chronic pain, epilepsy, nausea and anorexia.

---

[184] Leung L. Cannabis and its derivatives: review of medical use. *J Am Board Fam Med*. 2011 Jul-Aug;24(4):452-62
[185] Lee et al. Amygdala activity contributes to the dissociative effect of cannabis on pain perception. *Pain*. 2013 Jan;154(1):124-34
[186] Wilsey et al. Low-dose vaporized cannabis significantly improves neuropathic pain. *J Pain*. 2013 Feb;14(2):136-48
[187] Bachhuber et al. Medical Cannabis Laws and Opioid Analgesic Overdose Mortality in the United States, 1999-2010. *JAMA Intern Med*. 2014 Aug;174(10):1668-1673
[188] Reddy DS, Golub VM. Pharmacological Basis of Cannabis Therapy for Epilepsy. *J Pharmacol Exp Ther*. 2016 Apr;357(1):45-55

Treat with physical/manual medicine:

- Massage: Gentle massage provides comfort, increases circulation, reduces edema, and promotes healing. After the acute phase, deeper massage may help restore range of motion by breaking adhesions and reducing the feeling of vulnerability that may occur after injury. Research indicates that massage can reduce adolescent aggression[189], improve outcome in preterm infants[190], alleviate premenstrual syndrome[191], improve flexibility, reduce pain, increase serotonin and dopamine in patients with low back pain[192], and improve function and alleviate depression in patients with Parkinson's disease (Alexander technique).[193]

- Joint mobilization and manipulation: Applied as appropriate (after contraindications have been excluded) and to the level of patient comfort. Mechanisms of action and sample techniques are listed later in this section.

- Treatment of associated muscle spasm and myofascial trigger points (MFTP): Such treatment can increase range of motion and decrease pain. See notes on the diagnosis and treatment of MFTP in the following section in this chapter.

Uncover the underlying problem:

- In the case of most acute injuries, the underlying problem is often the injury itself. However, the physician must not be overly naïve and must conduct a thorough history and examination to assess for possible underlying pathologies that cause or contribute to the problem that "appears" to be injury related. Congenital anomalies, underlying pathology, previous injury, and psychoemotional disorders may have been present before the "injury."
  - In children and young adults, 5% of "sports-related" injuries are associated with preexisting infection, anomalies, or other conditions.
  - In adult women: "In three cases of carcinoma, the breast mass was not noticed until after the [auto accident] and was initially thought by the patient to have been caused by the trauma. Indeed between 9% and 20% of women with breast cancer attribute their symptoms to previous trauma to the breast."[194]

- Look for leg length inequalities and biomechanical faults such as hyperpronation and pelvic torque.

- Assess and correct poor posture, poor ergonomics, lack of flexibility, muscle strength imbalances, and proprioceptive/coordination deficits.

- Patients may experience a reduction in pain—particularly low-back pain and osteoarthritis pain—when they eliminate coffee/caffeine, food allergens, and/or specific foods to which they are sensitive, most notably the *Solanaceae*/nightshade family—eggplant, tobacco, tomatoes, potatoes, and bell peppers. Foods in the *Solanaceae* family contain anti-acetylcholinesterases[195] that may effect increased synaptic transmission of afferent pain sensations.

- Correction of **diet-induced chronic metabolic acidosis**[196] with the use of alkalinizing diets/supplements can alleviate musculoskeletal pain, at least in part by raising/normalizing intracellular magnesium levels and by reducing intracellular calcium levels. Additional benefits of alkalinization include increased mineral retention, reduced bone resorption[197] and enhanced clearance of toxic xenobiotics and toxins (per the excellent internationally endorsed position paper by Proudfoot et al[198]). Generally speaking and after renal

---

[189] Diego MA, et al. Aggressive adolescents benefit from massage therapy. *Adolescence* 2002 Fall;37(147):597-607

[190] Mainous RO. Infant massage as a component of developmental care: past, present, and future. *Holist Nurs Pract* 2002 Oct;16(5):1-7

[191] Hernandez-Reif M, et al. Premenstrual symptoms are relieved by massage therapy. *J Psychosom Obstet Gynaecol* 2000 Mar;21(1):9-15

[192] "RESULTS: By the end of the study, the massage therapy group, as compared to the relaxation group, reported experiencing less pain, depression, anxiety and improved sleep. They also showed improved trunk and pain flexion performance, and their serotonin and dopamine levels were higher." Hernandez-Reif M, Field T, Krasnegor J, Theakston H. Lower back pain is reduced and range of motion increased after massage therapy. *Int J Neurosci* 2001;106(3-4):131-45

[193] Stallibrass C, Sissons P, Chalmers C. Randomized controlled trial of the Alexander technique for idiopathic Parkinson's disease. *Clin Rehabil* 2002 Nov;16(7):695-708

[194] Seifert S. Medical Illness Simulating Trauma (MIST) syndrome: case reports and discussion of syndrome. *Fam Med* 1993 Apr;25(4):273-6

[195] Krasowski MD, McGehee DS, Moss J. Natural inhibitors of cholinesterases: implications for adverse drug reactions. *Can J Anaesth.* 1997 May;44(5 Pt 1):525-34

[196] "Results of recent observational studies confirm an association between insulin resistance and metabolic acidosis markers, including low serum bicarbonate, high serum anion gap, hypocitraturia, and low urine pH." Adeva MM, Souto G. Diet-induced metabolic acidosis. *Clin Nutr.* 2011 Aug;30(4):416-21

[197] "In postmenopausal women, the oral administration of potassium bicarbonate at a dose sufficient to neutralize endogenous acid improves calcium and phosphorus balance, reduces bone resorption, and increases the rate of bone formation." Sebastian A, Harris ST, Ottaway JH, Todd KM, Morris RC Jr. Improved mineral balance and skeletal metabolism in postmenopausal women treated with potassium bicarbonate. *N Engl J Med.* 1994 Jun 23;330(25):1776-81 content.nejm.org/cgi/content/abstract/330/25/1776

[198] "Urine alkalinization is a treatment regimen that increases poison elimination by the administration of intravenous sodium bicarbonate to produce urine with a pH > or = 7.5." Proudfoot AT, et al. Position Paper on urine alkalinization. *J Toxicol Clin Toxicol.* 2004;42:1-26 eapcct.org/publicfile.php?folder=congress&file=PS_UrineAlkalinization.pdf

and electrolyte disorders have been excluded, the goal is to achieve and maintain a urine pH of 7.5 or slightly higher.

- o Clinical trial—Alkaline mineral supplementation decreases pain in rheumatoid arthritis patients (*Open Nutrition Journal* 2008[199]): Thirty-seven patients with active RA of at least two years duration receiving drug treatment participated in this 12-week study. "All patients were randomly allocated to a supplemented group (30g of an alkaline mineral supplement daily) or to an unsupplemented group. … DAS 28 and VAS decreased in the supplemented group, whereas there was no change in these parameters during the trial in the control group. The functions (HAQ) of the supplemented patients improved. The immunoreactive ==endorphin levels increased== in both groups but to a higher degree in the supplemented group. During the trial, ==medication (NSAIDs and steroids) could be reduced== in the supplemented group only. Conclusion: This study suggests that an alkaline supplement may improve function and pain in rheumatoid arthritis and may represent an easy and safe addition to the usual treatment of RA patients."

- o Clinical trial—Supplementation with alkaline minerals alleviates low back pain (*J Trace Elem Med Biol* 2001[200]): "The results show that a disturbed acid-base balance may contribute to the symptoms of low back pain. The simple and safe addition of an ==alkaline multimineral preparate was able to reduce the pain symptoms in these patients with chronic low back pain.=="

> **Correcting the common diet-induced metabolic acidosis: the importance of maintaining urinary alkalinization**
>
> Benefits of alkalinization correlating with urine pH 7.5 – 8, reasonably up to 8.5:
> - **Elevated endorphins** improves mood and alleviates pain (thereby alleviating depression, addiction, and need for analgesic/anti-inflammatory drugs)
> - **Reduced cortisol** (thereby lessening insulin resistance and hippocampal atrophy)
> - **Enhanced retention of minerals** (improved nutritional status)
> - **Enhanced excretion of poisons** (reduced xenobiotic load)
>
> For patients who do not achieve alkalinization with diet alone, oral administration of potassium/magnesium citrate/bicarbonate should be used.
>
> Proudfoot et al. *J Toxicol Clin Toxicol*. 2004
> Vormann et al. *J Trace Elem Med Biol*. 2001
> Maurer et al. *Am J Physiol Renal Physiol*. 2003

Re-educate, rehabilitate, resourcefulness, return to active life, reassure, referral:

- Educate patient on ways to avoid re-injury and to decrease likelihood of recurrence.
- Pre-rehabilitation assessment has three main goals: 1) identification of the type of injury, 2) quantification of the severity of the injury, and 3) determining the appropriate interventions.[201] Rehabilitative exercises **emphasizing strength, coordination, proprioception, range of motion, and functional utility** (appropriate per occupation and hobbies) should be employed.
- **Isometric exercises** can be used to maintain/increase muscle strength in patients for whom range-of-motion exercises are painful or contraindicated.
- **Work hardening** has been defined by the American Physical Therapy Association as "a highly structured goal-oriented, individualized treatment program designed to return a person to work. Work Hardening programs…use real or simulated work activities designed to restore physical, behavioral, and vocational functions."[202] Teperman[203] defined the specific goals of work hardening as:
  1. Improved lifting strength (loading and unloading) to/from different heights, including overhead,
  2. Improved carrying capacity (various objects, different distances, unilateral and bilateral),
  3. Improved functional tolerance (coordination and manipulation) at different levels,
  4. Improved cardiovascular endurance,
  5. Improved dexterity tasks (counting, weighing, sorting, packaging/unpacking),
  6. Improved biomechanics in any setting (work/leisure).
- **Work conditioning** has been defined as "a work-related, intensive, and goal-oriented treatment program specifically designed to restore an individual's systemic, neuromuscular (strength, endurance, flexibility,

---

[199] Cseuz et al. Alkaline mineral supplementation decreases pain in rheumatoid arthritis patients: a pilot study. *Open Nutrition Journal* 2008:10;2

[200] Vormann J, et al. Supplementation with alkaline minerals reduces symptoms in patients with chronic low back pain. *J Trace Elem Med Biol*. 2001;15(2-3):179-83

[201] Geffen SJ. 3: Rehabilitation principles for treating chronic musculoskeletal injuries. *Med J Aust*. 2003 Mar 3;178(5):238-42

[202] American Physical Therapy Association, "Guidelines for Programs for Injured Workers" 1995. Quoted by Washington State Department of Labor and Industries. lni.wa.gov/Main/MostAskedQuestions/ClaimsIns/WorkHardFaq.asp. Accessed July 23, 2006

[203] Teperman LJ. Active functional restoration and work hardening program returns patient with 2½-year-old elbow fracture-dislocation to work after 6 months: a case report. *J Can Chiropr Assoc* 2002; 46(1): 22-30 jcca-online.org/client/cca/JCCA.nsf/objects/Active+functional+restoration+elbow+fracture-dislocation/$file/5-Teperman.pdf

etc.) and cardiopulmonary function."[204] While overlaps exist between work hardening and work conditioning, and both are generally designed to "return the patient to work", work hardening is focused more on the performance of work-related tasks (task-oriented) while work conditioning tends to focus more on the cardiopulmonary and neuromuscular fitness of the patient (fitness-oriented).

- **Rehabilitation can become more than *restorative*; if the plan is comprehensive and it effects long-term improvements in overall health, then such a program can become *transformative*.** For example, while the oversimplified medical model as commonly practiced in HMO and PPO systems might describe a patient's problem as "low-back pain, refer for physiotherapy and begin Vioxx 25 mg b.i.d.", a more comprehensive assessment and treatment of the same patient's problem might be described as "low-back pain secondary to sedentary lifestyle, obesity, mild systemic inflammation, hypovitaminosis D, and proprioceptive deficits. Begin program of daily general exercise along with specific exercises for low-back region, low-carbohydrate diet to promote weight loss, balance training twice daily, begin supplementation with cholecalciferol 4,000 IU/d and fish oil 3 g/d." Notice that the typical allopathic plan *requires* and *thus ensures* patient passivity and does nothing to promote overall health, whereas the comprehensive natural/integrative plan is more in accord with current biomedical literature, requires active patient participation, offers the probability of improved overall health, and will reduce the severity and risk of present and future diseases, respectively.

- Patients should be supported in the tolerance of minor discomfort to avoid overuse of analgesics, to avoid an excessive reduction in activities, and to avoid playing the "sick role." While validating the patient's concerns, physicians should not encourage dysfunctional behavior or contribute to "iatrogenic neurosis."

- **Symptomatic treatment that provides no lasting benefit can foster psychological dependency and therapeutic passivity.** "Therapeutic dependency" describes the situation wherein the patient becomes dependent on treatment sessions for secondary gain of attention, physical contact, and time off from work (etc.) rather than focusing on the goal of getting as healthy as possible as quickly as possible. Therapeutic dependency is fostered by doctors who fail to educate patients to take an active role in their own care and by doctors who take on the role of "savior" rather than empowering patients to take effective action in improving their health. **Therapeutic passivity** is related to **therapeutic dependency** since patients who fail to take responsible action tend to become dependent on healthcare providers to "cure me", "fix me" and "rescue me."

- Modify home and occupational workstations to minimize strain and stress on injured tissues. Educate patients to use tools, machines, props, and stepstools to work efficiently and to reduce unnecessary lifting and straining motions.

- Physical activities can be fully resumed when symptoms have decreased and when physical examination findings (e.g., reflexes, strength, range of motion, spinal segmental function, and trigger points) are within normal limits. Note that in many situations returning the patient to their previous duration, frequency, and intensity of activity may predispose to re-injury since the patient is re-entering the situation wherein the original injury occurred; therefore at least one of these lifestyle/occupational/recreational variables must change in order to reduce the likeliness of re-injury.

- Books, websites, and national/local support groups and organizations may be available for emotional, physical, psychological-emotional, and legal assistance.

- While detailed individual descriptions of therapeutic exercise and rehabilitative programs are not the subject of this book, we can readily appreciate the many options that are available to us for the rehabilitation of injuries:
  - <u>Weight optimization</u>: For the majority of patients living in our society where obesity is pandemic, weight reduction is important not only to improve overall health and to reduce mechanical stresses on joints, but perhaps even more importantly to reduce the production of proinflammatory chemicals made in adipose tissue (adipokines) which promote an overall internal climate of pain and inflammation. Some patients may need to gain muscle strength to promote healing and avoid

---

[204] Howar JM. Keys to Effective Work Hardening and Limited Duty Programs. eh.doe.gov/feosh/contacts/LimitedDutyPrograms.pdf Accessed July 23, 2006. Ironically, even though the third page of this presentation clearly shows the use of spinal manipulation, chiropractic doctors are notably absent from the list of "Industrial Rehab Specialists."

re-injury; this can generally be achieved with resistance training and increased protein consumption.

- o Therapeutic exercise: Includes strength training, stretching, improving endurance, and functional training specific to the patient's occupational or athletic activities. These can be tailored to great detail to the patient's condition and goals.[205]

- o Proprioceptive retraining/rehabilitation: As discussed later in this chapter, restoration and optimization of proprioceptive function and balance control is especially important for the long-term functional improvement of patients with proprioceptive deficits, commonly seen in patients with chronic low-back pain[206], neck pain[207], knee arthritis[208], and ankle instability.[209]

- o Treatment of myofascial trigger points: Since joint injuries and chronic pain—*especially in the neck, back and shoulder*—are commonly associated with trigger points[210], addressing this secondary and occult cause of pain is important to maximize pain relief and functional restoration.

- o Analgesic and anti-inflammatory botanicals and nutraceuticals: Safe and effective natural means for achieving a timely reduction in pain include topical capsaicin, *Harpagophytum*, *Uncaria*, acupuncture, willow, and spinal manipulation. Fish oil, GLA, vitamin E, *Boswellia*, willow bark, *Harpagophytum*, and *Zingiber* are just a few of the effective natural anti-inflammatory treatments available.

- o Manipulation, mobilization, and massage: Joint manipulation has numerous physiologic and anatomic effects, most of which are relevant for the alleviation of pain and improvement of joint function. These mechanisms include:
  1. Releasing entrapped intraarticular menisci and synovial folds,
  2. Acutely reducing intradiscal pressure, thus promoting replacement of decentralized disc material,
  3. Stretching of deep periarticular muscles to break the cycle of chronic autonomous muscle contraction by lengthening the muscles and thereby releasing excessive actin-myosin binding,
  4. Promoting restoration of proper kinesthesia and proprioception,
  5. Promoting relaxation of paraspinal muscles by stretching facet joint capsules,
  6. Promoting relaxation of paraspinal muscles via "postactivation depression", which is the temporary depletion of contractile neurotransmitters,
  7. Temporarily elevating plasma beta-endorphin,
  8. Temporarily enhancing phagocytic ability of neutrophils and monocytes,
  9. Activating the diffuse descending pain inhibitory system located in the periaqueductal gray matter—this is an important aspect of nociceptive inhibition by intense sensory/mechanoreceptor stimulation, and
  10. Improving neurotransmitter balance and reducing pain (soft-tissue manipulation).[211]

Additional details are provided in numerous published reviews and primary research[212,213,214,215,216,217,218] and by Leach[219], whose extensive description of the mechanisms of action of spinal manipulative therapy is unsurpassed. Given such a wide base of experimental and clinical support published in peer-reviewed journals and widely-available textbooks, denigrations

[205] Basmajian JV (ed). *Therapeutic Exercise. Fourth Edition*. Baltimore: Williams and Wilkins. 1984

[206] Newcomer KL, et al. Muscle activation patterns in subjects with and without low back pain. *Arch Phys Med Rehabil*. 2002;83(6):816-21

[207] McPartland JM, et al. Chronic neck pain, standing balance, and suboccipital muscle atrophy--a pilot study. *J Manipulative Physiol Ther*. 1997 Jan;20(1):24-9

[208] Callaghan MJ, et al. The Effects of Patellar Taping on Knee Joint Proprioception. *J Athl Train*. 2002 Mar;37(1):19-24

[209] Olmsted LC, et al. Efficacy of the Star Excursion Balance Tests in Detecting Reach Deficits in Subjects With Chronic Ankle Instability. *J Athl Train*. 2002 Dec;37(4):501-506

[210] "The mean number of TrPs present on each neck pain patient was 4.3, of which 2.5 were latent and 1.8 were active TrPs. Control subjects also exhibited TrPs (mean: 2; SD: 0.8). All were latent TrPs." Fernandez-de-Las-Penas C, et al. Myofascial trigger points in subjects presenting with mechanical neck pain. *Man Ther*. 2006 Jun 10

[211] "RESULTS: By the end of the study, the massage therapy group, as compared to the relaxation group, reported experiencing less pain, depression, anxiety and improved sleep. They also showed improved trunk and pain flexion performance, and their serotonin and dopamine levels were higher." Hernandez-Reif M, Field T, Krasnegor J, Theakston H. Lower back pain is reduced and range of motion increased after massage therapy. *Int J Neurosci* 2001;106(3-4):131-45

[212] Maigne JY, Vautravers P. Mechanism of action of spinal manipulative therapy. *Joint Bone Spine*. 2003;70(5):336-41

[213] Brennan PC, et al. Enhanced neutrophil respiratory burst as a biological marker for manipulation forces. *J Manipulative Physiol Ther*. 1992 Feb;15(2):83-9

[214] Brennan PC, et al. Enhanced phagocytic cell respiratory burst induced by spinal manipulation: potential role of substance P. *J Manipulative Physiol Ther*. 1991;14(7):399-408

[215] Heikkila et al. Effects of acupuncture, cervical manipulation, NSAID therapy on dizziness and impaired head repositioning of suspected cervical origin. *Man Ther* 2000;5:151-7

[216] Rogers RG. The effects of spinal manipulation on cervical kinesthesia in patients with chronic neck pain: a pilot study. *J Manipulative Physiol Ther*. 1997;20(2):80-5

[217] Bergman, Peterson, Lawrence. *Chiropractic Technique*. New York: Churchill Livingstone 1993. An updated edition is now availabe published by Mosby.

[218] Herzog WH. Mechanical and physiological responses to spinal manipulative treatments. *JNMS: J Neuromusculoskeltal System* 1995; 3: 1-9

[219] Leach RA. (ed). *The Chiropractic Theories: A Textbook of Scientific Research, Fourth Edition*. Baltimore: Lippincott, Williams & Wilkins, 2004

directed toward spinal manipulation on the grounds that it is "unscientific" or "unsupported by research" are unfounded and are indicative of selective ignorance.[220]

- **Eicosanoid modulation**: Historically, the balance of omega-3 to omega-6 fatty acids in the human diet has been approximately 1:1 or 1:2.[221] Since omega-3 fatty acids are generally *anti-inflammatory* while omega-6 fatty acids are generally proinflammatory (with the exception of GLA/DGLA), the former *quantitative* dietary balance translated to a *qualitative* balance with regard to the body's inherent inflammatory tendency. Modern diets today, however, provide a ratio of 1:30, with anti-inflammatory omega-3 fatty acids greatly outnumbered by the proinflammatory omega-6 fatty acids. Thus, human physiology has been altered by the widespread consumption of a *pro-inflammatory acidogenic diet*.[222,223] **Correction of these problems at the level of dietary intake rather than by the use of** *and dependence upon by both doctors and patients* **anti-inflammatory medications is essential for the attainment of health and the long-term relief of pain and inflammation.**[224,225]

- **Reassurance**: Education, explanation, reassurance, and support help to address the mental and emotional aspects of injury.

- **Alkalinization**: The American/Western style of eating results in subclinical diet-induced pathogenic chronic metabolic acidosis[226] which can be corrected with a Paleo-Mediterranean diet[227] or alkalinizing supplements[228] (including potassium citrate and magnesium bicarbonate) for the alleviation of musculoskeletal pain in general and low-back pain in particular.[229]

- **Referral: Patients with severe pain, serious conditions/complications, or documented noncompliance are excellent candidates for co-management or unidirectional referral.**

Nutrition:

- **Supplementation with a high-potency broad-spectrum multivitamin and multimineral product**: This will help correct common nutritional deficiencies and support optimal healing. Certain nutrients such as vitamin C, zinc, and copper are commonly considered "specific" for promoting optimal repair of connective tissue.

- **Dietary protein for tissue repair**: In otherwise healthy patients with no liver, renal, or other metabolic disorders, ensure adequate intake of 0.5-0.9 gram of protein per pound of body weight.[230] Vegetarians may heal more slowly after injury than do omnivores; vegetarians and lacto-vegetarians undergoing cosmetic surgery reportedly have more complications and slower healing than do people eating a diet containing meat.[231] Additionally, low-protein diets have shown to reduce muscle mass and suppress immune function.[232] See the table below for protein intake recommendations:

---

[220] Vasquez A. The Science of Chiropractic and Spinal Manipulation, Part 2. mercola.com/2005/mar/12/chiropractic_spine.htm

[221] Simopoulos AP. Essential fatty acids in health and chronic disease. *Am J Clin Nutr*. 1999 Sep;70(3 Suppl):560S-569S

[222] Seaman DR. The diet-induced proinflammatory state: a cause of chronic pain and other degenerative diseases? *J Manipulative Physiol Ther*. 2002;25(3):168-79

[223] Adeva MM1, Souto G. Diet-induced metabolic acidosis. *Clin Nutr*. 2011 Aug;30(4):416-21

[224] Vasquez A. A Five-Part Nutritional Protocol that Produces Consistently Positive Results. *Nutritional Wellness* 2005 September

[225] Vasquez A. Dietary, Nutritional and Botanical Interventions to Reduce Pain and Inflammation. *Naturopathy Digest* 2006, March *Nutritional Wellness* 2006, March

[226] "As a result, healthy adults consuming the standard US diet sustain a chronic, low-grade pathogenic metabolic acidosis that worsens with age as kidney function declines." Cordain L, Eaton SB, Sebastian A, Mann N, Lindeberg S, Watkins BA, O'Keefe JH, Brand-Miller J. Origins and evolution of the Western diet: health implications for the 21st century. *Am J Clin Nutr*. 2005 Feb;81(2):341-54 ajcn.org/cgi/content/full/81/2/341

[227] Cordain L. *The Paleo Diet*. John Wiley and Sons, 2002

[228] "An acidogenic Western diet results in mild metabolic acidosis in association with a state of cortisol excess, altered divalent ion metabolism, and increased bone resorptive indices." Maurer et al. Neutralization of Western diet inhibits bone resorption independently of K intake and reduces cortisol secretion in humans. *Am J Physiol Renal Physiol*. 2003 Jan;284(1):F32-40

[229] "The results show that a disturbed acid-base balance may contribute to the symptoms of low back pain. The simple and safe addition of an alkaline multimineral preparate was able to reduce the pain symptoms in these patients with chronic low back pain." Vormann J, Worlitschek M, Goedecke T, Silver B. Supplementation with alkaline minerals reduces symptoms in patients with chronic low back pain. *J Trace Elem Med Biol*. 2001;15(2-3):179-83

[230] Nancy Clark, MS, RD. The Power of Protein. *The Physician and Sportsmedicine* 1996, volume 24, number 4. physsportsmed.com/issues/1996/04_96/protein.htm

[231] Vegetarians and healing. *JAMA* 1995; 273: 910

[232] Castaneda C, et al. Elderly women accommodate to a low-protein diet with losses of body cell mass, muscle function, and immune response. *Am J Clin Nutr* 1995 Jul;62:30-9

Recommended Grams of Protein per Patient Profile and Body Weight Per Day		
Patient Profile	Per pound of weight[233]	Per kilogram of weight
RDA for sedentary adult and children ages 6-18 years[234]	0.4	0.88
Adult recreational exerciser—average for adults	0.5-0.75	1.1-1.65
Adult competitive athlete	0.6-0.9	1.32-1.98
Adult building muscle mass	0.7-0.9	1.54-1.98
Dieting athlete	0.7-1.0	1.54-2.2
Growing teenage athlete	0.9-1.0	1.98-2.2

- **Vegetables, fruit, and fiber**: Whole foods provide micronutrients, natural anti-inflammatory components, and immune modulators; the fiber/phytonutrient content provides positive effects on gut flora while maintaining proper waste elimination and reducing straining (e.g., reduced need for the Valsalva maneuver).

- **Carbohydrates**: Carbohydrate intake should be adequate to supply energy-expenditure needs and to support healing but should not be excessive such as to unfavorably increase body weight during times of decreased physical activity. Preferred sources of carbohydrates are fruits and vegetables.

- **Water**: Adequate intake of water is important to flush out wastes, toxins, and to prevent constipation. Eight glasses per day is the classic recommendation; however increased fluid intake is appropriate during exercise, heat exposure, stress, and to promote clearance of nitrogenous wastes and xenobiotics. Fluid restriction may be appropriate for persons with adrenal insufficiency to avoid hyponatremia and those with cardiovascular failure, fluid overload, or edema.

- **Identification and elimination of adverse food reactions**: Adverse food reactions—regardless of the underlying mechanism(s) or classification of allergy, intolerance, or sensitivity—can precipitate joint pain and inflammation[235,236,237,238,239,240,241] and a wide range of other health problems.

- **Vitamin D3**: The data is very clear that 1) vitamin D deficiency causes pain—both axial and peripheral, 2) the pain of vitamin D deficiency is difficult-to-treat or unresponsive to NSAIDs and opioids, thus forcing pharmacocentric physicians to use higher and thus more dangerous doses of drugs, 3) replacement with vitamin D3 quickly and effectively alleviates the pain of vitamin D deficiency, 4) all "pain patients" should have their vitamin D levels tested and optimized per the data in this book. For adults without existing or predisposition toward hypercalcemia, the appropriate dose of vitamin D3 is typically 4,000-10,000 IU/d; serum calcium is periodically monitored for safety while serum 25-hydroxy-vitamin D is optimize per the graphic that follows.[242] Given the quantity and consistency of the data substantiating the causative connection between vitamin D3 deficiency and pain, the high frequency of this problem in clinical practice, the consequences of nontreatment, and the dependable success of treatment, failure to assess and treat vitamin D deficiency in patients with persistent major pain is not consistent with quality contemporary clinical care.

  - **Exemplary case report—A woman who left her wheelchair** (*Lancet* 1999 Mar[243]): 32yo patient with progressive muscular weakness of her legs and diffuse skeletal pain and required used of crutches or wheelchair. She had waddling gait, proximal hip-muscle weakness and hypotonia, and from the age of 21 she had been treated with steroids for ileal Crohn's disease, for which she had one small-bowel resection. She was given parenteral 1,25-dihydroxyvitaminD3 (1 microg/d) and

[233] Slightly modified from Nancy Clark, MS, RD. Protein Power. *The Physician and Sportsmedicine* 1996, volume 24, number 4
[234] 0.83 g.kg-1.d-1 (equivalent to 0.37 grams per pound of body weight) Pellet PL. Protein requirements in humans. *Am J Clin Nutr* 1990 May;51:723-37
[235] Golding DN. Is there an allergic synovitis? *J R Soc Med*. 1990 May;83(5):312-4
[236] Panush RS. Food induced ("allergic") arthritis: clinical and serologic studies. *J Rheumatol*. 1990 Mar;17(3):291-4
[237] Pacor ML, Lunardi C, Di Lorenzo G, Biasi D, Corrocher R. Food allergy and seronegative arthritis: report of two cases. *Clin Rheumatol*. 2001;20(4):279-81
[238] Schrander JJ, Marcelis C, de Vries MP, van Santen-Hoeufft HM. Does food intolerance play a role in juvenile chronic arthritis? *Br J Rheumatol*. 1997 Aug;36(8):905-8
[239] van de Laar et al. Food intolerance in rheumatoid arthritis. *Ann Rheum Dis*. 1992;51:298-302
[240] Haugen et al. A pilot study of the effect of an elemental diet in the management of rheumatoid arthritis. *Clin Exp Rheumatol*. 1994 May-Jun;12(3):275-9
[241] van de Laar et al. Food intolerance in rheumatoid arthritis. II. *Ann Rheum Dis*. 1992 Mar;51(3):303-6
[242] Vasquez A, Manso G, Cannell J. The clinical importance of vitamin D (cholecalciferol): a paradigm shift with implications for all healthcare providers. *Altern Ther Health Med*. 2004 Sep-Oct;10(5):28-36 Full-text available at ICHNFM.org/pdf
[243] Mingrone G et al. A woman who left her wheelchair. *Lancet*. 1999 Mar 6;353(9155):806

enhanced oral intake of calcium and phosphate-rich food (meat, fish, liver, and root vegetables), and "after 3 weeks she could walk again, and her muscle weakness and bone pain disappeared."

o Severe hypovitaminosis D in patients with persistent, nonspecific musculoskeletal pain (*Mayo Clin Proc* 2003 Dec[244]): "All patients with persistent, nonspecific musculoskeletal pain are at high risk for the consequences of unrecognized and untreated severe hypovitaminosis D. ... Because osteomalacia is a known cause of persistent, nonspecific musculoskeletal pain, screening all outpatients with such pain for hypovitaminosis D should be standard practice in clinical care."

o Clinical trial—Vitamin D deficiency and chronic low back pain (*Spine* 2003 Jan[245]): "Findings showed that 83% of the study patients (n = 299) had an abnormally low level of vitamin D before treatment with vitamin D supplements. After treatment, clinical improvement in symptoms was seen in all the groups that had a low level of vitamin D, and in 95% of all the patients (n = 341). Vitamin D deficiency is a major contributor to chronic low back pain in areas where vitamin D deficiency is endemic. Screening for vitamin D deficiency and treatment with supplements should be mandatory in this setting."

o Clinical trial—Vitamin D supplementation for diffuse musculoskeletal pain (*Eur J Gen Pract* 2014 Mar[246]): Patients 18-50yo with pain or unexplained asthenia/fatigue with hypovitaminosis D (average 25[OH]D level 23.7 nmol/l). After vitamin D supplementation, the adjusted mean serum 25ohD level increased to 118.8 nmol/l, the quality of life score increased and the pain evaluation score decreased. In this study, vitamin D supplementation decreased pain scores in adult patients with diffuse musculoskeletal pain and vitamin D deficiency.

o Review of 450 cases—Low vitamin D as a risk factor for the development of myalgia in patients taking high-dose simvastatin (*Clin Ther* 2014 May[247]): "This was a retrospective medical record review of 450 patients who were prescribed simvastatin 80 mg at the Veterans Affairs Western New York Healthcare System between August 1, 2006, and July 31, 2011. ... The mean vitamin D level in patients experiencing myalgia was 26.2 versus 36.3 ng/mL. The 25-hydroxyvitamin D level in those who reported myalgia was approximately 10 ng/mL lower compared with those who tolerated simvastatin 80 mg. Vitamin D insufficiency appears to be a risk factor for the development of [statin-induced] myalgia." *Comment by DrV*: Several studies have documented the correlation between statin-induced myalgia and vitamin D deficiency; sadly, both the vitamin D deficiency and the overuse of statin drugs would be avoided if clinicians and physicians had a better knowledge of nutrition.

o Case series—Improvement of chronic back pain or failed back surgery with vitamin D repletion (*J Am Board Fam Med* 2009 Jan-Feb[248]): "Chronic low back pain and failed back surgery may improve with repletion of vitamin D from a state of deficiency/insufficiency to sufficiency. Vitamin D insufficiency is common; repletion of vitamin D to normal levels in patients who have chronic low back pain or have had failed back surgery may improve quality of life or, in some cases, result in complete resolution of symptoms."

o Severity of vitamin D deficiency correlates with opioid drug need (dose and duration) for pain control (*Pain Med* 2008 Nov[249]): Among 267 chronic pain patients, the prevalence of vitamin D inadequacy was 26%. "Among patients using opioids, the mean morphine equivalent dose for the inadequate vitamin D group was 133.5 mg/day compared with 70.0 mg/day for the adequate group. The mean duration of opioid use for the inadequate and adequate groups were 71.1 months and 43.8 months, respectively. Opioid users with inadequate [vitamin D] levels reported worse physical functioning and health perception than opioid users with adequate levels."

[244] Plotnikoff GA, Quigley JM. Prevalence of severe hypovitaminosis D in patients with persistent, nonspecific musculoskeletal pain. *Mayo Clin Proc.* 2003 Dec;78(12):1463-70
[245] Al Faraj S, Al Mutairi K. Vitamin D deficiency and chronic low back pain in Saudi Arabia. *Spine* 2003 Jan 15;28(2):177-9
[246] Le Goaziou MF et al. Vitamin D supplementation for diffuse musculoskeletal pain: results of a before-and-after study. *Eur J Gen Pract.* 2014 Mar;20(1):3-9
[247] Mergenhagen K et al. Low vitamin d as a risk factor for the development of myalgia in patients taking high-dose simvastatin. *Clin Ther.* 2014 May 1;36(5):770-7
[248] Schwalfenberg G. Improvement of chronic back pain or failed back surgery with vitamin D repletion: a case series. *J Am Board Fam Med.* 2009 Jan-Feb;22(1):69-74
[249] Turner et al. Prevalence and clinical correlates of vitamin D inadequacy among patients with chronic pain. *Pain Med.* 2008 Nov;9(8):979-84

Excess vitamin D
> 100 ng/mL (250 nmol/L) with hypercalcemia

Optimal range
50 - 100 ng/mL (125 - 250 nmol/L)

Insufficiency range
< 20- 40 ng/mL (50 - 100 nmol/L)

Deficiency
< 20 ng/mL (50 nmol/L)

Serum 25(OH) vitamin D levels: Modified from earlier peer-reviewed versions published in Vasquez et al, *Alternative Therapies in Health and Medicine* 2004

- **Other specific supplements/botanicals:** Supplementation is tailored to the type of tissue that has been injured, such as calcium, magnesium, and vitamins D and K for bone fractures, glucosamine sulfate and niacinamide for cartilage injuries, and proteolytic enzymes for muscle strains.
  - Niacinamide: The niacinamide form of vitamin B3 was proven effective against osteoarthritis by Kaufman more than 50 years ago.[250] Furthermore, Kaufman's documentation of an "anti-aging" effect of vitamin supplementation in general and niacinamide therapy in particular[251] is consistent with recent experimental data demonstrating rapid reversion of aging phenotypes by niacinamide through modulation of histone acetylation.[252] A recent double-blind placebo-controlled repeat study found that niacinamide therapy improved joint mobility, reduced objective inflammation as assessed by ESR, reduced the impact of the arthritis on the activities of daily living, and allowed a reduction in analgesic/anti-inflammatory medication use.[253] While the mechanism of action is probably multifaceted, inhibition of joint-destroying nitric oxide appears to be an important benefit.[254] The standard dose of 500 mg given orally 6 times per day is more effective than 1,000 mg 3 times per day. Hepatic dysfunction is rare when daily doses are kept below 3,000 mg per day, yet Gaby[255] suggests measurement of liver enzymes after 3 months of treatment and yearly thereafter. Antirheumatic benefit is generally significant following 2-6 weeks of treatment, and patients may also notice an anxiolytic benefit, possibly mediated by the binding of niacinamide to GABA/benzodiazepine receptors.[256]
  - Glucosamine sulfate and chondroitin sulfate: Glucosamine and chondroitin are the "building blocks" from which cartilage is built and oral supplementation is intended to enhance cartilage anabolism and to thus counteract the enhanced cartilage catabolism seen in destructive arthritic processes.[257] Clinical trials with glucosamine and chondroitin sulfates have shown consistently positive results in clinical trials involving patients with osteoarthritis of the hands, hips, knees,

[250] Kaufman W. Niacinamide therapy for joint mobility. Therapeutic reversal of a common clinical manifestation of the normal aging process. *Conn State Med J* 1953;17:584-591
[251] Kaufman W. The use of vitamin therapy to reverse certain concomitants of aging. *J Am Geriatr Soc* 1955;3:927-936
[252] Matuoka K, et al. Rapid reversion of aging phenotypes by nicotinamide through possible modulation of histone acetylation. *Cell Mol Life Sci.* 2001;58(14):2108-16
[253] Jonas WB, Rapoza CP, Blair WF. The effect of niacinamide on osteoarthritis: a pilot study. *Inflamm Res* 1996 Jul;45(7):330-4
[254] McCarty et al. Niacinamide therapy for osteoarthritis--does it inhibit nitric oxide synthase induction by interleukin 1 in chondrocytes? *Med Hypotheses.* 1999;53(4):350-60
[255] Gaby AR. Literature review and commentary: Niacinamide for osteoarthritis. *Townsend Letter for Doctors and Patients.* 2002: May; 32
[256] Mohler H, Polc P, Cumin R, Pieri L, Kettler R. Nicotinamide is a brain constituent with benzodiazepine-like actions. *Nature.* 1979; 278(5704): 563-5
[257] Vidal y Plana et al. Articular cartilage pharmacology: I. In vitro studies on glucosamine and non steroidal antiinflammatory drugs. *Pharmacol Res Commun* 1978;10:557-69

temporomandibular joint, and low-back.[258,259,260,261,262,263,264] For example, glucosamine sulfate was superior to placebo for pain reduction and preservation of joint space in a 3-year clinical trial in patients with knee osteoarthritis.[265] Arguments against the use of glucosamine due to inflated concern about inefficacy or exacerbation of diabetes[266] are without scientific merit[267,268] as evidenced by a 90-day trial of diabetic patients consuming 1500 mg of glucosamine hydrochloride with 1200 mg of chondroitin sulfate which showed no significant alterations in serum glucose or hemoglobin A1c[269] and by the previously cited 3-year study which found significant clinical benefit and no adverse effects on glucose homeostasis.[270] The adult dose of glucosamine sulfate is generally 1500-2000 mg per day in divided doses, and the dose of chondroitin sulfate is approximately 1000 mg daily; these treatments can be used singly, in combination, and with other treatments. Both treatments are safe for multiyear use, and rare adverse effects include allergy and nonpathologic gastrointestinal upset. Clinical benefit is generally significant following 4-6 weeks of treatment and is maintained for the duration of treatment. In contrast to coxib and other mislabeled "anti-inflammatory" drugs that consistently elevate the incidence of cardiovascular disease, death, and other adverse effects[271,272,273,274,275], supplementation with chondroitin sulfate appears to safely reduce the pain and disability associated with osteoarthritis while simultaneously reducing incidence of cardiovascular morbidity and mortality.[276,277] In a study with animals that spontaneously develop atherosclerosis[278], administration of chondroitin sulfate induced regression of existing atherosclerosis. In a six-year study with 120 patients with established cardiovascular disease, 60 chondroitin-treated patients suffered 6 coronary events and 4 deaths compared to 42 events and 14 deaths in a comparable group of 60 patients receiving "conventional" therapy; chondroitin-treated patients reported enhancement of well-being while no adverse clinical or laboratory effects were noted during the 6 years of treatment.[279] Glucosamine sulfate is strongly preferred over glucosamine hydrochloride due to higher efficacy of the former. The negative study by Clegg et al[280] in *New England Journal of Medicine* 2006 was not a scientific study, but rather it was a pseudostudy designed with the intention to make "glucosamine and chondroitin sulfate" appear inefficacious so that drug sales of coxibs would remain high—this study is so ridiculously corrupt that 1) it should have never been published, 2) it should be withdrawn, and 3) it exemplifies the extent to which the *New England Journal of Medicine* panders to the pharmaceutical industry at the expense of quality patient care and good science.

[258] "...patients taking GS had a significantly greater decrease in TMJ pain with function, effect of pain, and acetaminophen used between Day 90 and 120 compared with patients taking ibuprofen." Thie et al. Evaluation of glucosamine sulfate compared to ibuprofen for the treatment of temporomandibular joint osteoarthritis. *J Rheumatol* 2001;28:1347-55

[259] Braham R, Dawson B, Goodman C. The effect of glucosamine supplementation on people experiencing regular knee pain. *Br J Sports Med*. 2003;37(1):45-9

[260] "...oral glucosamine therapy achieved a significantly greater improvement in articular pain score than ibuprofen, and the investigators rated treatment efficacy as 'good' in a significantly greater proportion of glucosamine than ibuprofen recipients. In comparison with piroxicam, glucosamine significantly improved arthritic symptoms after 12 weeks of therapy..." Matheson AJ, Perry CM. Glucosamine: a review of its use in the management of osteoarthritis. *Drugs Aging*. 2003; 20(14): 1041-60

[261] Uebelhart D, Malaise M, Marcolongo R, DeVathaire F, Piperno M, Mailleux E, Fioravanti A, Matoso L, Vignon E. Intermittent treatment of knee osteoarthritis with oral chondroitin sulfate: a one-year, randomized, double-blind, multicenter study versus placebo. *Osteoarthritis Cartilage*. 2004;12:269-76

[262] van Blitterswijk WJ, et al. Glucosamine and chondroitin sulfate supplementation to treat symptomatic disc degeneration. *BMC Complement Altern Med*. 2003;3(1):2

[263] Morreale P, et al. Comparison of the antiinflammatory efficacy of chondroitin sulfate and diclofenac sodium in patients with knee osteoarthritis. *J Rheumatol*. 1996;23:1385-91

[264] Mazieres B, et al. Chondroitin sulfate in osteoarthritis of the knee: a prospective, double blind, placebo controlled multicenter clinical study. *J Rheumatol*. 2001;28(1):173-81

[265] Reginster JY et al. Long-term effects of glucosamine sulphate on osteoarthritis progression: a randomised, placebo-controlled clinical trial. *Lancet*. 2001;357(9252):251-6

[266] Adams ME. Hype about glucosamine. *Lancet*. 1999;354(9176):353-4

[267] Cumming A. Glucosamine in osteoarthritis. *Lancet*. 1999;354(9190):1640-1

[268] Rovati LC, Annefeld M, Giacovelli G, Schmid K, Setnikar I. *Glucosamine in osteoarthritis*. Lancet. 1999;354(9190):1640

[269] Scroggie et al. Effect of glucosamine-chondroitin supplementation on glycosylated hemoglobin in patients with type 2 diabetes mellitus. *Arch Intern Med* 2003;163:1587-9

[270] Reginster JY, et al. Long-term effects of glucosamine sulphate on osteoarthritis progression: a randomised, placebo-controlled clinical trial. *Lancet*. 2001;357(9252):251-6

[271] Topol EJ. Failing the public health--rofecoxib, Merck, and the FDA. *N Engl J Med*. 2004 Oct 21;351(17):1707-9

[272] Mukherjee D, Nissen SE, Topol EJ. Risk of cardiovascular events associated with selective cox-2 inhibitors. *JAMA* 2001; 286(8):954-9

[273] Ray WA, Griffin MR, Stein CM. Cardiovascular toxicity of valdecoxib. *N Engl J Med*. 2004;351(26):2767

[274] "Patients in the clinical trial taking 400 mg. of Celebrex twice daily had a 3.4 times greater risk of CV events compared to placebo. For patients in the trial taking 200 mg. of Celebrex twice daily, the risk was 2.5 times greater. The average duration of treatment in the trial was 33 months." FDA Statement on the Halting of a Clinical Trial of the cox-2 Inhibitor Celebrex. fda.gov/bbs/topics/news/2004/NEW01144.html Available on January 4, 2005

[275] "Preliminary information from the study showed some evidence of increased risk of cardiovascular events, when compared to placebo, to patients taking naproxen." FDA Statement on Naproxen. fda.gov/bbs/topics/news/2004/NEW01148.html Available on January 4, 2005

[276] Morrison LM. Treatment of coronary arteriosclerotic heart disease with chondroitin sulfate-A: preliminary report. *J Am Geriatr Soc*. 1968;16(7):779-85

[277] Morrison LM, et al. The prevention of coronary arteriosclerotic heart disease with chondroitin sulfate A: preliminary report. *Exp Med Surg*. 1969;27(3):278-89

[278] Morrison et al. Absence of naturally occurring coronary atherosclerosis in squirrel monkeys (Saimiri sciurea) treated with chondroitin sulfate A. *Experientia* 1972 ;28:1410-1

[279] Morrison LM, Enrick N. Coronary heart disease: reduction of death rate by chondroitin sulfate A. *Angiology*. 1973 May;24(5):269-87

[280] Clegg DO, Reda DJ, Harris CL, et al. Glucosamine, chondroitin sulfate, and the two in combination for painful knee osteoarthritis. *N Engl J Med*. 2006;354:795-808

<table>
<tr><td colspan="2">Characteristics of the (pseudo)study by Clegg et al published and widely cited from New England J Med 2006</td></tr>
</table>

- <u>Misleading title</u>: The term "glucosamine and chondroitin sulfate" gives the impression that—if a distinction is being made—glucosamine sulfate is being used in the study, rather than glucosamine hydrochloride. Given that glucosamine sulfate is more popular among consumers and more clinically efficacious, one would reasonably assume that this is the form being used; in fact, the opposite is true: the authors used glucosamine hydrochloride, which is notably less effective than glucosamine sulfate (GS). This suggests that the authors were either ignorant or intentionally designing the study to produce negative results.
- <u>Misleading title</u>: The title makes no mention of the use of Celebrex/celecoxib in the study, while in fact the study was designed as a competition between these two interventions.
- <u>Unequal study design—duration</u>: GS typically takes several months to be effective, with optimal results not appreciated until treatment has been continued up to 3 years. In contrast, celecoxib is known to be much faster acting. By using a shorter term trial duration, the researchers gave the advantage to celecoxib.
- <u>Unequal study design—dose</u>: The dosing of celecoxib was more assertive than the dosing of GS and chondroitin.
- <u>Misleading conclusions published versus the authors' data</u>: According to Figure 2 of the article, glucosamine and chondroitin—alone or in combination—was equal to or generally better than placebo in every measure. Yet, the published conclusion and popular headlines in the lay press conclude that the nondrug treatments were inefficacious; this study has also been cited in otherwise reputable medical textbooks, such as <u>Cecil's Essentials of Medicine</u>, a medical textbook widely read by medical students and allopathic clinicians.
- <u>Several of the authors had received payment from Pfizer</u>, the drug company that makes Celebrex/celecoxib: Drs. Brandt, Moskowit z, Schnitzer, and Schumacher report having received consulting fees or having served on advisory boards for Pfizer. Dr. Brandt reports having equity interests in Pfizer. Drs. Moskowitz and Weisman report having received lecture fees from Pfizer. Drs. Bingham, Clegg, Hooper, Jackson, Molitor, Sawitzke, and Schnitzer, grant support from Pfizer. Dr. Moskowitz reports having served as an expert consultant for Pfizer.

Clegg DO, Reda DJ, Harris CL, Klein MA, O'Dell JR, Hooper MM, Bradley JD, Bingham CO 3rd, Weisman MH, Jackson CG, Lane NE, Cush JJ, Moreland LW, Schumacher HR Jr, Oddis CV, Wolfe F, Molitor JA, Yocum DE, Schnitzer TJ, Furst DE, Sawitzke AD, Shi H, Brandt KD, Moskowitz RW, Williams HJ. Glucosamine, chondroitin sulfate, and the two in combination for painful knee osteoarthritis. *N Engl J Med.* 2006;354:795-808. This article is an embarrassment to science; note the long list of agreeable authors.

- Vitamin E, with an emphasis on gamma-tocopherol: The *gamma* form of tocopherol inhibits cyclooxygenase and has anti-inflammatory activity.[281] Clinical trials and case reports have demonstrated benefit of vitamin E supplementation in patients with rheumatoid arthritis[282,283], spondylosis[284] and osteoarthritis[285], and autoimmune diseases including scleroderma, discoid lupus erythematosus, porphyria cutanea tarda, vasculitis, and polymyositis.[286,287,288] In 2013, we as clinicians gained valuable insight into the mechanism of action of vitamin E thanks to the work of Salinthone et al[289] who showed that, rather than functioning simply/solely as an antioxidant, vitamin E significantly raises cyclic adenosine monophosphate (cAMP) levels and thereby has an anti-inflammatory effect; they showed that "vitamin E resulted in a greater than 2-fold increase in cAMP level (29.19 pmol/mg protein) compared to baseline. Lipoic acid was used as a positive control, which generated 45.49 pmol/mg protein of cAMP." Elevation of cAMP—such as by alpha-tocopherol and lipoic acid—results in a dose-dependent inhibition of inflammatory IL-2 and IL-17 cytokine generation and by this mechanism—additive/synergistic with the antioxidant and mitochondrial-supportive effects—reduces inflammation. Generally, cAMP-elevating agents

---

[281] Jiang Q, Christen S, Shigenaga MK, Ames BN. gamma-tocopherol, the major form of vitamin E in the US diet, deserves more attention. *Am J Clin Nutr* 2001 Dec;74(6):714-22

[282] Helmy M, Shohayeb M, Helmy MH, el-Bassiouni EA. Antioxidants as adjuvant therapy in rheumatoid disease. A preliminary study. *Arzneimittelforschung.* 2001;51(4):293-8

[283] Edmonds SE, et al. Putative analgesic activity of repeated oral doses of vitamin E in the treatment of rheumatoid arthritis. *Ann Rheum Dis.* 1997 Nov;56(11):649-55

[284] "Vitamin E administration at a dose of 100 mg daily for three weeks resulted in a significant increase in serum vitamin E level accompanied by complete relief of pain... The results therefore strongly indicate that vitamin E is effective in curing spondylosis and most probably due to its antioxidant activity." Mahmud Z, Ali SM. Role of vitamin A and E in spondylosis. *Bangladesh Med Res Counc Bull.* 1992 Apr;18(1):47-59. See also "The results of this double-blind controlled clinical trial showed that vitamin E was superior to placebo with respect to the relief of pain (pain at rest, pain during movement, pressure-induced pain) and the necessity of additional analgetic treatment. Improvement of mobility was better in the group treated with vitamin E." Blankenhorn G. [Clinical effectiveness of Spondyvit (vitamin E) in activated arthroses. A multicenter placebo-controlled double-blind study] [Article in German—information from abstract] *Z Orthop Ihre Grenzgeb* 1986;124:340-3. See also This is a very interesting study because the clinical response to vitamin E was proportional to the increase in plasma levels of vitamin E, thus confirming the dose-response relationship that implies causality as well as indicating that the failure of such treatment in some patients may be due to malabsorption or unquenchable systemic oxidative stress rather than the inefficacy of vitamin E supplementation. "There were no significant differences in the efficacy of the two drugs, although one patient of the V-group refused further treatment after 8 days because of inefficacy. V reduced or abolished the pain at rest in 77% (D in 85%), the pain on pressure in 67% (D in 50%), and the pain on movement in 62% (D in 63%). Both treatments appeared to be equally effective in reducing the circumference of the knee joints (p = 0.001) and the walking time (p less than 0.001) and in increasing the joint mobility (p less than 0.002)." Scherak O, et al. [High dosage vitamin E therapy in patients with activated arthrosis] [Article in German—information from abstract] *Z Rheumatol.* 1990 Nov-Dec;49(6):369-73

[285] Machtey I, Ouaknine L. Tocopherol in Osteoarthritis: a controlled pilot study. *J Am Geriatr Soc.* 1978 Jul;26(7):328-30

[286] Killeen RN, Ayres S Jr, Mihan R. Polymyositis: response to vitamin E. *South Med J.* 1976 Oct;69(10):1372-4

[287] Ayres S Jr, Mihan R. Lupus erythematosus and vitamin E: an effective and nontoxic therapy. *Cutis.* 1979 Jan;23(1):49-52, 54

[288] Ayres S Jr, Mihan R. Is vitamin E involved in the autoimmune mechanism? *Cutis.* 1978 Mar;21(3):321-5

[289] Salinthone et al. α-Tocopherol stimulates cyclic AMP production in human peripheral mononuclear cells and alters immune function. *Mol Immunol.* 2013 Mar;53(3):173-8

demonstrate anti-inflammatory actions by increasing production of anti-inflammatory IL-10 and reducing production of pro-inflammatory TNF-alpha.[290]

o <u>Vitamin C</u>: Doses of 1-2 grams per day have been suggested to reduce pain and the need for surgery in patients with low-back pain by improving disc integrity.[291] Vitamin C reduces production of isoprostanes, which promote inflammation and pain. Ascorbate is also necessary for the production of the anti-inflammatory prostaglandin E-1. Supplemental vitamin C may also reduce the severity and progression of osteoarthritis.[292]

o <u>Pancreatic/proteolytic enzymes</u>: Orally-administered pancreatic and proteolytic enzymes are absorbed from the gastrointestinal tract into the systemic circulation[293,294] to exert analgesic, anti-inflammatory, anti-edematous benefits with therapeutic relevance for acute and chronic musculoskeletal disorders.[295,296,297,298]

---

[290] Eigler et al. Anti-inflammatory activities of cAMP-elevating agents: enhancement of IL-10 synthesis and suppression of TNF production. *J Leukoc Biol*. 1998 Jan;63(1):101-7

[291] Greenwood J. Optimum vitamin C intake as a factor in the preservation of disc integrity. *Med Ann Dist Columbia*. 1964 Jun;33:274-6

[292] "A 3-fold reduction in risk of OA progression was found for both the middle tertile and highest tertile of vitamin C intake. This related predominantly to a reduced risk of cartilage loss. Those with high vitamin C intake also had a reduced risk of developing knee pain." McAlindon TE, et al. Do antioxidant micronutrients protect against the development and progression of knee osteoarthritis? *Arthritis Rheum*. 1996 Apr;39(4):648-56

[293] Gotze H, Rothman SS. Enteropancreatic circulation of digestive enzymes as a conservative mechanism. *Nature* 1975; 257(5527): 607-609

[294] Liebow C, Rothman SS. Enteropancreatic Circulation of Digestive Enzymes. *Science* 1975; 189(4201): 472-474

[295] Trickett P. Proteolytic enzymes in treatment of athletic injuries. *Appl Ther*. 1964;30:647-52

[296] Walker JA, Cerny FJ, Cotter JR, Burton HW. Attenuation of contraction-induced skeletal muscle injury by bromelain. *Med Sci Sports Exerc*. 1992 Jan;24(1):20-5

[297] Walker et al. Bromelain reduces mild acute knee pain and improves well-being in a dose-dependent fashion in an open study of healthy adults. *Phytomedicine*. 2002;9:681-6

[298] Brien S, et al. Bromelain as a Treatment for Osteoarthritis: a Review of Clinical Studies. *Evidence-based Complementary and Alternative Medicine*. 2004;1(3)251–257

Myofascial trigger points (MFTP)

<u>Description/pathophysiology</u>:

- Many patients suffer from chronic pain that originates from myofascial trigger points—localized areas within muscle tissue that produce chronic pain, promote muscle contraction and tightness, and which mediate autonomous autonomic responses. Physicians who take the time to locate and treat MFTP and educate patients about effective home care can often rapidly and permanently reduce their patients' pain in a safe and highly cost-effective manner.
- MFTP have been defined as "a highly localized and hyperirritable spot in a palpable taut band of skeletal muscle fibers"[299] characterized by the following:
  1. <u>Referred pain with compression</u>: Digital compression of the MFTP causes local pain and most often causes referred pain in a distribution similar or identical to the patient's presenting complaint. The distribution of pain may appear radicular and may thus be described as "pseudoradicular."
  2. <u>Twitch response</u>: When digital pressure is applied perpendicularly to the direction of muscle fibers at the location of the MFTP and the muscle is "plucked" or allowed to "snap" as if one were plucking a taut rubber band or the string of a guitar, the muscle being assessed undergoes a rapid contraction.
  3. <u>Muscle tightness</u>: The muscle involved is tighter than usual, and it is resistant to stretch.
  4. <u>Associated autonomic phenomena</u>: Regions of the body near a localized MFTP may display associated autonomic dysregulation such as vasoconstriction, sweating, pilomotor response, and the patient may experience nausea, dizziness, light-headedness[300] or atrial fibrillation.[301]
  5. <u>MFTP may be "active" or "latent"</u>: Active MFTP are those which cause spontaneous pain with joint motion or muscle contraction, whereas latent MFTP cause pain only when provoked by an examiner's deep palpation and physical compression.[302]
  6. <u>Normal muscle strength</u>: Muscle weakness and atrophy are not associated with MFTP unless the weakness or atrophy is secondary to pain.
- The initiation and perpetuation of MFTP is complex and commonly associated with previous injury or chronic static posturing (such as sitting in front of a computer for 8-14 hours per day) and also with emotional stress. Since **intrafusal fibers of muscle spindles receive direct sympathetic innervation**, and since adrenaline/epinephrine directly increases the contractile tone and tension of muscles, it is reasonable to conclude that attention to emotional stress and stress management techniques should be part of the comprehensive treatment plan for MFTP. A significant reduction in emotional tension and work-related repetitive strain injuries may follow a comprehensive and "body-based" approach to healthy living and appropriate career choices.[303]
- The pathogenesis and physiology-based treatment of MFTP follow this route are as follows:

  <u>Pathogenesis</u>[304]
  1. Excess calcium is released from the sarcoplasmic reticulum, leading to local muscle fiber contraction.
  2. Intense and chronic muscle contractions cause relative local ischemia.
  3. The reduction in local blood supply limits energy replacement and leads to the depletion of adenosine triphosphate (ATP).
  4. The muscle cell now has insufficient ATP for the active return of calcium from the contractile elements to the sarcoplasmic reticulum, thus maintaining the muscle fibers in a contracted state.

  <u>Physiology-based treatment</u>:
  5. Stretching the muscle fibers reduces the overlap between actin and myosin, which then leads to a reduction in energy demand of the cell and thus helps to "break the cycle" of **contraction** *leading to* **energy depletion** *leading to* **contraction** *leading to* **energy depletion...**

---

[299] Hong CZ, Simons DG. Pathophysiologic and electrophysiologic mechanisms of myofascial trigger points. *Arch Phys Med Rehabil*. 1998;79(7):863-72

[300] Hubbard DR, Berkoff GM. Myofascial trigger points show spontaneous needle EMG activity. *Spine*. 1993 Oct 1;18(13):1803-7

[301] Simons DG. Cardiology and myofascial trigger points: Janet G. Travell's contribution. *Tex Heart Inst J*. 2003;30(1):3-7

[302] Hubbard DR, Berkoff GM. Myofascial trigger points show spontaneous needle EMG activity. *Spine*. 1993 Oct 1;18(13):1803-7

[303] Jarrow R. *Creating the Work You Love: Courage, Commitment and Career*. Inner Traditions Intl Ltd; December 1995) [ISBN: 0892815426]

[304] Simons DG. Cardiology and myofascial trigger points: Janet G. Travell's contribution. *Tex Heart Inst J*. 2003;30(1):3-7

6. Application of ice (or other benign, intense afferent stimuli such as capsaicin or spinal manipulation) floods the dorsal horn and thus blocks transmission of nociceptive stimuli via the hypothesized "gate control" mechanism of pain reception.

7. Magnesium supplementation is appropriate for many patients with MFTP since many patients do not consume sufficient dietary magnesium and since magnesium inhibits calcium release from the sarcoplasmic reticulum[305] and thereby has a muscle relaxing effect. **Magnesium deficiency is an epidemic** in so-called "developed" nations, with 20-40% of different populations showing objective serologic/cytologic evidence of magnesium deficiency.[306,307,308,309]

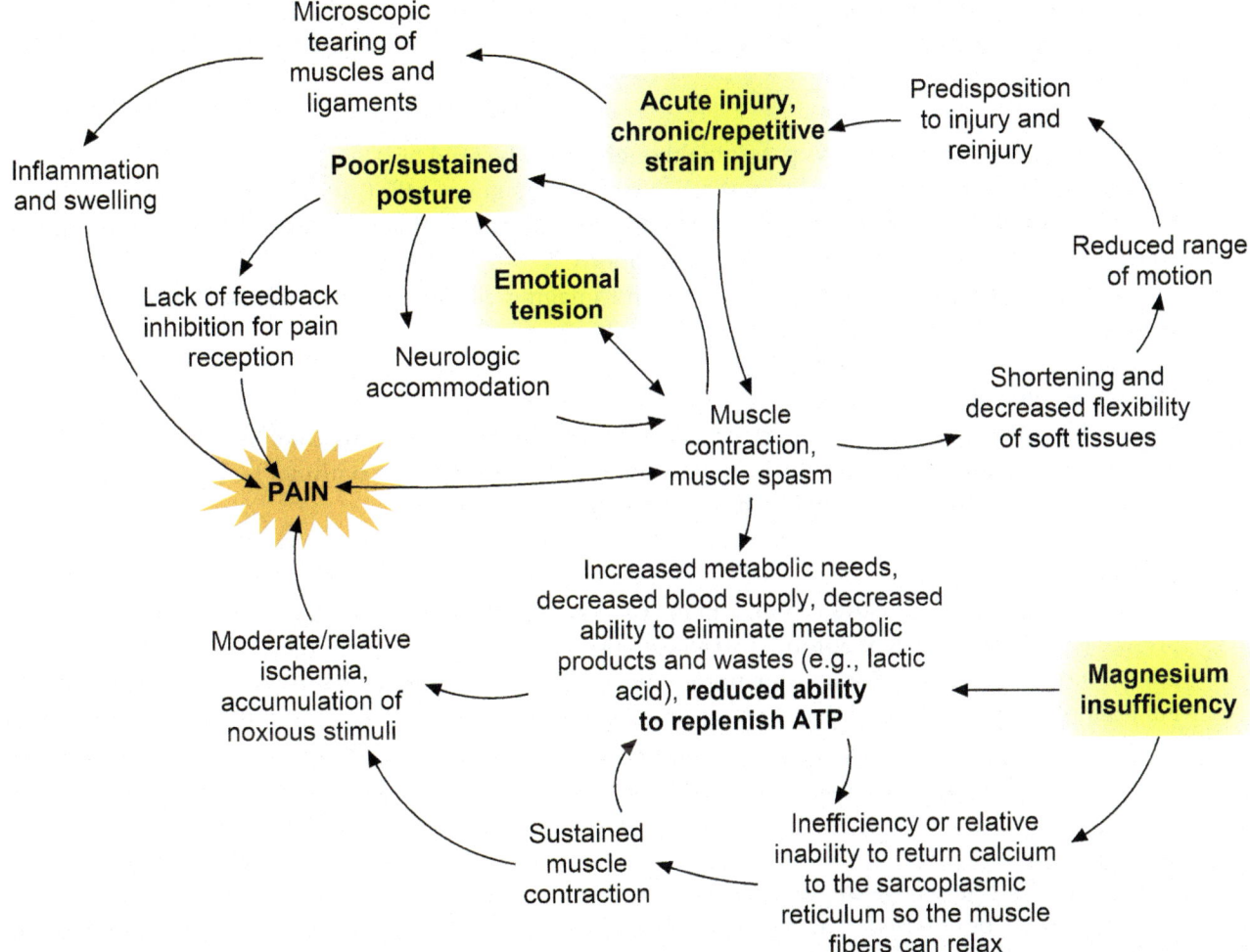

Reasonable and simple model for the initiation and promotion of myofascial trigger points with self-perpetuating cycles: Emotional tension, sustained posturing, and magnesium deficiency are a few of the "entry points" to neuromuscular pain.

Clinical presentations:

- The pain pattern from MFTP is varied and is dependent on the muscle(s) involved. Each muscle has a unique pattern of pain referral; e.g., a MFTP in the deltoid or supraspinatus may cause shoulder pain and arm pain that can mimic cervical radiculitis. MFTP in the sternocleidomastoid commonly causes

---

305 "Mg2+ inhibits Ca2+ release from the sarcoplasmic reticulum." Mathew R, Altura BM. The role of magnesium in lung diseases: asthma, allergy and pulmonary hypertension. *Magnes Trace Elem*. 1991-92;10(2-4):220-8

306 "The American diet is low in magnesium, and with modern water systems, very little is ingested in the drinking water." Innerarity S. Hypomagnesemia in acute and chronic illness. *Crit Care Nurs Q*. 2000 Aug;23(2):1-19

307 "43% of 113 trauma patients had low magnesium levels compared to 30% of noninjured cohorts." Frankel etal.Hypomagnesemia in trauma patients.*World J Surg* 1999;23:966-9

308 "There was a 20% overall prevalence of hypomagnesemia among this predominantly female, African American population." Fox CH, Ramsoomair D, Mahoney MC, Carter C, Young B, Graham R. An investigation of hypomagnesemia among ambulatory urban African Americans. *J Fam Pract*. 1999 Aug;48(8):636-9

309 "Suboptimal levels were detected in 33.7 per cent of the population under study. These data clearly demonstrate that the Mg supply of the German population needs increased attention." Schimatschek HF, Rempis R. Prevalence of hypomagnesemia in an unselected German population of 16,000 individuals. *Magnes Res*. 2001 Dec;14(4):283-90

"headache" and pain over the side of the face and TMJ; MFTP in the psoas can cause low back and leg pain. Patients may also report subjective numbness or tingling in addition to pain. Differentiation of MFTP pain from radiculitis and radiculopathy should be pursued clinically and documented in the patient chart.

Major differential diagnoses:
- Arthropathy and arthritis: Passive joint provocation tests are negative with MFTP; no laboratory abnormalities (such as elevated CRP) are seen with MFTP.
- Acute muscle injury, strain: History of *recent* injury is often negative; history of *chronic* strain and *previous* injury are common with MFTP
- Radiculitis: The pain associated with MFTP is not dermatomal and is reproduced with local muscle compression, whereas the pain of radiculitis is dermatomal and reproduced with nerve tension tests.
- Radiculopathy: Radiculopathy is associated with muscle weakness, which is not a characteristic of MFTP.

Clinical assessments:
- History/subjective: Pain is always present (although it may be mild or latent).
- Physical examination/objective: The most reliable physical signs of MFTP are **1) spot tenderness within a taut band of muscle, 2) reproduction of pain and referred pain with palpation and provocation**, and 3) local twitch response with palpation and provocation.
- Imaging & laboratory assessments: Lab tests and imaging assessments are normal. Myofascial trigger points show spontaneous electromyographic activity.[310]

Establishing the diagnosis:
- Reasonable clinical exclusion of acute strain, radiculopathy and radiculitis combined with characteristic clinical findings mentioned above, including at least **1) spot tenderness within a taut band of muscle, 2) reproduction of pain and referred pain with palpation/provocation**.

Complications:
- Many patients with MFTP suffer from pain for years before being properly diagnosed. Many patients are prescribed hazardous and inappropriate medications to treat the pain and symptoms of MFTP, and surgical interventions are periodically used inappropriately in patents who have not been accurately diagnosed. For example when a patient with low back pain due to MFTP is found to have an incidental disc herniation, the patient may undergo surgery on the intervertebral disc only to have pain continue postoperatively until it is treated with simple techniques directed at the MFTP.[311]

Clinical management:
- Simple nutritional and physical treatments as described below.
- Patients should be advised that deep massage of the area is often necessary and that pain may be temporarily exacerbated.

Treatments:
- Post-isometric stretching: Lewit and Simons described this simple and highly effective treatment succinctly in a highly recommended article[312], "The post-isometric relaxation technique begins by placing the muscle in a stretched position. Then an isometric contraction is exerted against minimal resistance. Relaxation and then gentle stretch follow as the muscle releases." In a large study involving 244 patients, post-isometric stretching "produced **immediate pain relief in 94%, lasting pain relief in 63%**, as well as lasting relief of point tenderness in 23% of the sites treated. Patients who practiced autotherapy on a home program were more likely to realize lasting relief." Clinically the technique is simultaneously performed, explained, and taught by the clinician: 1) stretch the target muscle, 2) weakly contract the target muscle against resistance for 10 seconds, 3) stretch the target muscle to a greater length than before for at least 20 seconds, 4) repeat

---

[310] Hubbard DR, Berkoff GM. Myofascial trigger points show spontaneous needle EMG activity. *Spine*. 1993 Oct 1;18(13):1803-7
[311] Rubin D. Myofascial trigger point syndromes: an approach to management. *Arch Phys Med Rehabil*. 1981 Mar;62(3):107-10
[312] Lewit K, Simons DG. Myofascial pain: relief by post-isometric relaxation. *Arch Phys Med Rehabil*. 1984 Aug;65(8):452-6

this procedure 2-3 times. Pretreatment heating or exercising of the target muscles along with post-treatment application of ice helps to increase treatment efficacy and minimize post-treatment soreness, respectively.

- <u>Cold and stretch</u>: The application of cold and the simultaneous stretching of the muscle is an effective treatment for MFTP.[313] Cold can be applied with ice. The previously popular "spray and stretch" technique that used a vapocoolant spray such as Fluori-Methane is unnecessary and is environmentally irresponsible.

- <u>Dry needling or injection of local anesthetic or saline</u>: While local injection of anesthetic or saline may appear more complex and therefore more effective, dry needling (rapid insertion and withdrawal of a needle) directly into the MFTP is just as effective, safer, and is less complicated than using anesthetic or saline solution. Increased efficacy of this technique is associated with the elicitation of a local twitch response immediately upon insertion and withdrawal of the needle. The accuracy of the needle insertion directly into the "sensitive locus" of the MFTP is essential for the effectiveness of this approach. Common locations for MFTP correlate with commonly used acupuncture points, and the technique of acupuncture is analogous to the dry needling technique except that dry needling is performed more quickly and with highly localized precision into the MFTP sensitive locus. [314]

- <u>Topical application</u>: Capsaicin helps to relieve neuromuscular pain, too, and may help break the cycle of pain and spasm by 1) providing afferent stimuli to block nociceptive stimuli, and 2) by depleting local tissues of substance P, which not only serves as a transmitter of pain sensations, but may also perpetuate muscle contraction and spasm. Another mechanism by which capsaicin can alleviate trigger points is by desensitizing the vanilloid receptor (VR-1) to ultimately decrease local neurotransmitter release.[315]

- <u>Adjunctive nutritional support</u>: Supplementation with **magnesium** (600 mg per day or to bowel tolerance[316]) and **calcium** are often helpful, particularly when used with an **alkalinizing Paleo-Mediterranean diet** (as discussed in Chapter 2), which—at the very least—promotes renal retention of calcium and magnesium to thus facilitate mineral retention. Other treatments to reduce intracellular calcium levels (intracellular hypercalcinosis[317]) include supplementation with **physiologic doses of vitamin D3** and **fish oil for EPA**[318] along with avoidance/reduction of factors which promote renal loss of calcium and magnesium such as caffeine, sugar, alcohol/ethanol, and psychoemotional stress.

---

[313] Rubin D. Myofascial trigger point syndromes: an approach to management. *Arch Phys Med Rehabil*. 1981 Mar;62(3):107-10

[314] Hong CZ, Simons DG. Pathophysiologic and electrophysiologic mechanisms of myofascial trigger points. *Arch Phys Med Rehabil*. 1998 Jul;79(7):863-72

[315] "Massage with capsaicin cream (0.075%, available over the counter) is useful for treating TrPs located in surgical scars,36 which are particularly refractory to treatment." McPartland JM. Travell trigger points—molecular and osteopathic perspectives. *J Am Osteopath Assoc*. 2004 Jun;104(6):244-9 jaoa.org/cgi/content/full/104/6/244

[316] "When the practitioner has been convinced to start Mg on the basis of his diagnosis or through insistence of the patient, the often recommended dose of 300 mg per day is insufficient. Experience of successful therapy indicates that no less than 600 mg per day is required." Liebscher DH, Liebscher DE. About the misdiagnosis of magnesium deficiency. *J Am Coll Nutr*. 2004 Dec;23(6):730S-1S coldcure.com/html/misdiagnosis-magnesium-deficiency.pdf

[317] naturopathydigest.com/archives/2006/sep/vasquez.php for additional discussion

[318] "This is a consequence of the ability of EPA to release Ca2+ from intracellular stores while inhibiting their refilling via capacitative Ca2+ influx that results in partial emptying of intracellular Ca2+ stores and thereby activation of protein kinase R." Palakurthi SS, Fluckiger R, Aktas H, Changolkar AK, Shahsafaei A, Harneit S, Kilic E, Halperin JA. Inhibition of translation initiation mediates the anticancer effect of the n-3 polyunsaturated fatty acid eicosapentaenoic acid. *Cancer Res*. 2000 Jun 1;60(11):2919-25

Musculoskeletal Manipulation and Manual Medicine: Introduction and Sample Techniques

Manual medicine in general and spinal manipulation in particular are mentioned in nearly every section of **_Integrative Orthopedics_**, and select techniques are described with accompanying text and photographs. Manipulative techniques are included in this textbook to remind practitioners of a few of the more useful and commonly applied maneuvers and to provide descriptions and citations for refinement of their application. However, the level of detail provided here is insufficient unless the reader has received hands-on professionally-supervised training in an accredited institution wherein other important concepts have been taught and implemented under experienced guidance. Competence and proficiency in the art and skill of manipulation cannot be learned from a textbook; these can only be approached with personal mentoring and in-person coursework amply provided in colleges and post-graduate trainings specializing in manipulative technique. **Manipulative medicine** is a _time-space_ objective-subjective-intuitive **kinesthetic phenomenon** which might be described as occurring in four dimensions—_anteroposterior, transverse/horizontal, vertical_, and _chronological_ due to variations in speed and power; all the while, the doctor is monitoring subjective and objective responses of the what might be considered the fifth dimension—the doctor's dynamic _perception of, influence upon_, and _interaction with_ the patient's affect, posture, muscle tension, dynamic joint positioning, tissue response, and compressive tension. As the doctor assesses and provides force, the patient's response changes the target, and so the doctor must adapt to a constantly moving target—the lesion being treated.

The intention with the following descriptions and examples is to remind clinicians of manipulation in general and these specific techniques in particular; only a few _subjectively chosen_ techniques are included from the several hundred vertebral, myofascial, visceral, and extravertebral/extremity maneuvers that are available.

General Layout and Description of Manipulative Techniques	
Patient position:	• Patient position may be prone, supine, lateral recumbent or "side-posture", standing, or seated
Doctor position:	• Usually standing, either _upright, forward flexed_, or using an oblique _fencer's stance_; knees are almost always bent in order to bring doctor's torso near treatment area to increase mechanical force from the upper limbs
Assessment:	• <u>Subjective</u>: Patient's experience, sensations, and effect on daily living • <u>Motion palpation</u>: Intersegmental motion analysis generally used for assessing the presence of vertebral motion restrictions or aberrant motion. The patient is relaxed and passive while the doctor takes the joint that is being assessed through its normal range of motion in various directions while palpating near adjacent joint surfaces for nuance of pattern and end-feel. Motion lesions are generally described as **restrictions** and/or **hypermobility** • <u>Static palpation</u>: Boney and other landmarks are compared symmetrically and to the practitioner's experience for the detection of abnormality consistent with subjective, motion, and soft tissue findings; static palpations are usually described in terms of prominence or relative superiority/inferiority when compared symmetrically • <u>Soft tissue palpation</u>: Subcutaneous tissues, tendons, ligaments, muscles, and joint spaces can be palpated to assess myofascial status and function. Soft tissue findings commonly include edema, joint swelling, bogginess, "ropiness" of muscles, tenderness, restricted motion of soft tissues, hypertonicity, spasm, and adhesions
Treatment contact, directive hand:	• Generally the doctor provides therapeutic contact with one of the contact surfaces of the hands—digital, hypothenar, pisiform, index, thumb, thenar, or "calcaneal" when using the heel of the hand[319]; other contacts such as the elbow or chest might be used for deep myofascial or compressive manipulative procedures, respectively. The _treatment contact_ is provided by the _directive hand_—the hand that is delivering the therapeutic _thrust_ or _direction_; the treatment contact of the directive hand works in cooperation with the _supporting contact_ of the _supporting hand_

---

[319] Kirk CR, et al. _States Manual of Spinal, Pelvic, and Extravertebral Technics. Second Edition_. Lombard, Il: National College of Chiropractic; 1985, page 20

Supporting contact:	This generally refers to the supportive hand, the one that is either holding or stabilizing the patient in contrast to the hand that is delivering the manipulative force. The indirect hand can provide at least three different types of support • <u>Neutral/stabilizing support</u>: The supportive hand plays a relatively neutral role with regard to the manipulative force • <u>Synergistic/cooperative/assistive support</u>: In this situation, the supportive hand moves with the therapeutic force in the same direction. An example of this would be the head-holding hand moving in the same direction as the directive/treatment hand when performing manipulation of the upper cervical spine • <u>Counterthrust/resistive support</u>: In this situation, the supportive hand moves counter/against the direction of the directive force. A common example is the force applied to the upper torso when performing a side-posture manipulation of the lumbar spine or pelvis. Another important example is the counterthrust by the supportive hand when performing a more forceful manipulation of the cervical spine; in this case the supportive hand is serving to limit the motion that would otherwise be imposed by forceful motion by the directive hand; more forceful manipulations such as used to increase afferent input to joint proprioceptors should *not* result in more motion; rather the increased speed and force of the directive hand is countered rather than assisted by the supportive hand
Pretreatment positioning:	• Joints are generally—but not always—taken to the end range of motion before the manipulative thrust is applied because the general purpose of high-velocity low-amplitude manipulation is to break myofascial restrictions and/or forcefully activate joint proprioceptors. In chiropractic terms, this is described as taking the joint into the **paraphysiologic space** because the physiologic range of motion is temporarily though safely exceeded[320]; in osteopathic terms, this part of the range of motion is described as being within the range of **passive motion** but still within the **anatomic barrier**[321]
Therapeutic action:	• For joint manipulation, this is usually the **chiropractic adjustment** or the **osteopathic HVLA** (high-velocity low-amplitude thrust); <u>thrust vectors</u> can be *straight, curvilinear,* or *rotary* into <u>**segmental directions**</u> of *rotation, extension, flexion, side-bending, traction,* and combinations of those directions • Other common manual techniques include stretching, post-isometric stretching, massage, compression, percussion, joint springing, mobilization, articulation, traction
Image:	• Photographs will be provided when relevant and available
Resources:	Textbook and article citations for additional information will be provided in this last row when relevant and available; the most commonly cited works include: • *States Manual, Second Edition*[322] by Constance Kirk DC, Dana Lawrence DC, Nila Valvo DC • *Kimberly Manual, 2006 Edition*[323] by Paul Kimberly DO • *Chiropractic Technique*[324] by Thomas Bergmann DC, David Peterson DC, Dana Lawrence DC • *Chiropractic Management of Spine-Related Disorders*[325] edited by Meridel Gatterman DC

Examples of manipulative medicine techniques

The following samples are an obvious underrepresentation of the diversity of manipulative techniques available, which easily numbers into the hundreds. Various techniques are—of course—described with greater range and depth in textbooks wholly dedicated to the topic of manipulation, which by itself is not the subject of this text. Rather, **use these samples as reminders to include or at least consider manipulative therapy** when composing your treatment plan; oftentimes, the manipulative therapy is the fastest and shortest route between *pain* and *relief from pain*.

[320] Leach RA. (ed). *The Chiropractic Theories: A Textbook of Scientific Research, Fourth Edition*. Baltimore: Lippincott, Williams & Wilkins, 2004, page 32-33
[321] Kimberly PE. *Outline of Osteopathic Manipulative Procedures. The Kimberly Manual 2006*. Kirksville College of Osteopathic Medicine. Walsworth Publishing, page 7
[322] Kirk CR, et al. *States Manual of Spinal, Pelvic, and Extravertebral Technics. Second Edition*. Lombard, Illinois: National College of Chiropractic; 1985
[323] Kimberly PE. *Outline of Osteopathic Manipulative Procedures. The Kimberly Manual 2006*. Kirksville College of Osteopathic Medicine. Walsworth Publishing
[324] Bergmann TF, Peterson DH, Lawrence DJ. *Chiropractic Technique*. New York; Churchill Livingstone: 1993
[325] Gatterman MI. *Chiropractic Management of Spine Related Disorders*. Baltimore; Williams and Wilkins: 1990

Cervical Spine: Rotation Emphasis

Patient position:	• Supine, neck slightly flexed
Doctor position:	• At 45° angle from head of table; may also be in a more lateral position aside the patient's head and neck; while it is acceptable to assess and set-up with straight legs, at the time of impulse, doctor's legs should be bent to provide the doctor with greater power, stability, and biomechanical safety
Assessment:	• <u>Subjective</u>: neck pain, headaches
	• <u>Motion palpation</u>: rotation restriction; primary or compensatory hypermobile segments may be detected above or below the restricted segment
	• <u>Static palpation</u>: vertebra may feel relatively posterior on the side opposite the rotational restriction, e.g., a right rotational restriction may present with a relative left rotational malposition that brings the vertebral lamina and articular pillars posterior on the left
	• <u>Soft tissue</u>: tenderness, may also have muscle spasm
Treatment contact:	• Doctor uses either an index or proximal phalange contact on the posterior aspect of the transverse process and/or articular pillar
	• The doctor's vector and hence the positioning of the forearm of the contact hand must change depending on the level of the cervical spine that is being treated
	• Notice in this photograph that the thumb of the doctor's contact hand is placed on the angle of the mandible, this is more to help anchor the contact and stabilize the doctor's wrist than to assist with the manipulation; very little pressure and zero thrust are applied to the mandible
Supporting contact:	• Head is held into rotation and slight flexion; as with all techniques, nuanced adjustments in flexion-extension, rotation, and side-bending are made until the premanipulative tension is localized to the specific direction/tissue of restriction
Pretreatment positioning:	• Slight flexion and extension may be used below and above the treatment contact to create motion restriction at the adjacent motion segments; this helps to focus the motion and therapeutic force at the specific; importantly the support hand is largely responsible for proper positioning with the correct amount of nuanced flexion-extension and side-bending so that the rotational force is accurately delivered
Thrust:	• Rotational thrust with contact hand; support hand keeps head off table allowing rotation
Image:	

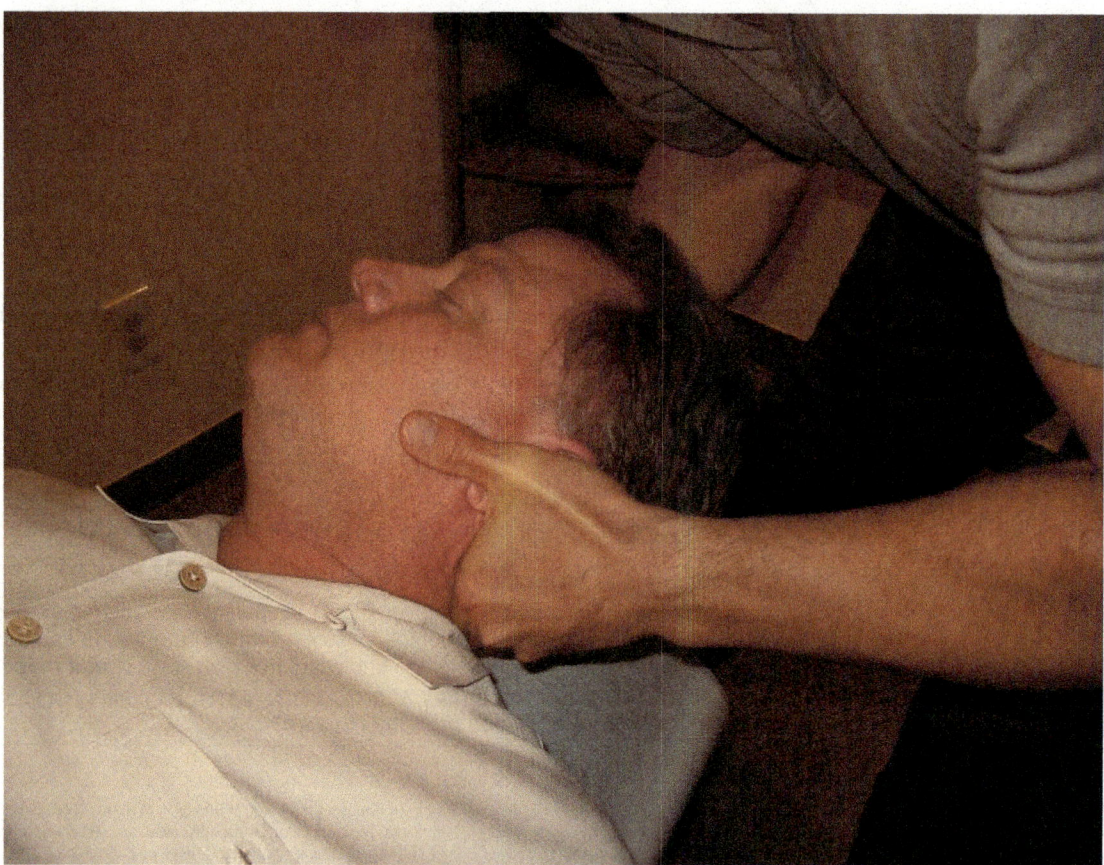

Cervical Spine: Lateral Flexion (Side-Bending) Emphasis; Treatment of Lateral Malposition

Patient position:	• Supine, head is neutrally placed—neither flexed nor extended; slight flexion is allowed; this technique can also be adapted for use in a seated position
Doctor position:	• At 45° angle from head of table; may also be in a more lateral position aside the patient's head and neck
Assessment:	• <u>Subjective</u>: neck pain, headaches
	• <u>Motion palpation</u>: lateral flexion restriction
	• <u>Static palpation</u>: vertebra may feel laterally displaced
	• <u>Soft tissue</u>: tenderness, may also have muscle spasm
Treatment contact:	• Using an index (metacarpal-phalangeal) contact at the tip of the transverse process or slightly posterior to the transverse process; an index phalangeal contact can also be used on the articular pillars as long as doctor is careful not to thrust in a rotational direction; notice in this picture how Dr Harris has the forearm of his contact hand perfectly aligned in the treatment vector, which is almost purely in the patient's transverse/horizontal plane; notice also that Dr Harris has his knees bent and is forward flexed to bring his torso closer to his contact and thereby minimize stress and strain on his own shoulders; with slight modifications in vector direction, this technique can be applied throughout the cervical spine from C0-C7
Supporting contact:	• Lateral aspect of head, opposite contact; generally the supporting hand is neutral, however it can supply some traction and can help induce lateral flexion at impulse; with more aggressive adjustments, the supporting hand can supply a counterforce to minimize motion following the application of a faster and more powerful thrust
Pretreatment positioning:	• Lateral flexion at the targeted segment; the slightest amount of contralateral rotation is applied
Therapeutic action:	• Establish minimal premanipulative tension once the end range of motion has been reached, then use quick and very shallow trust to induce lateral flexion
Image:	

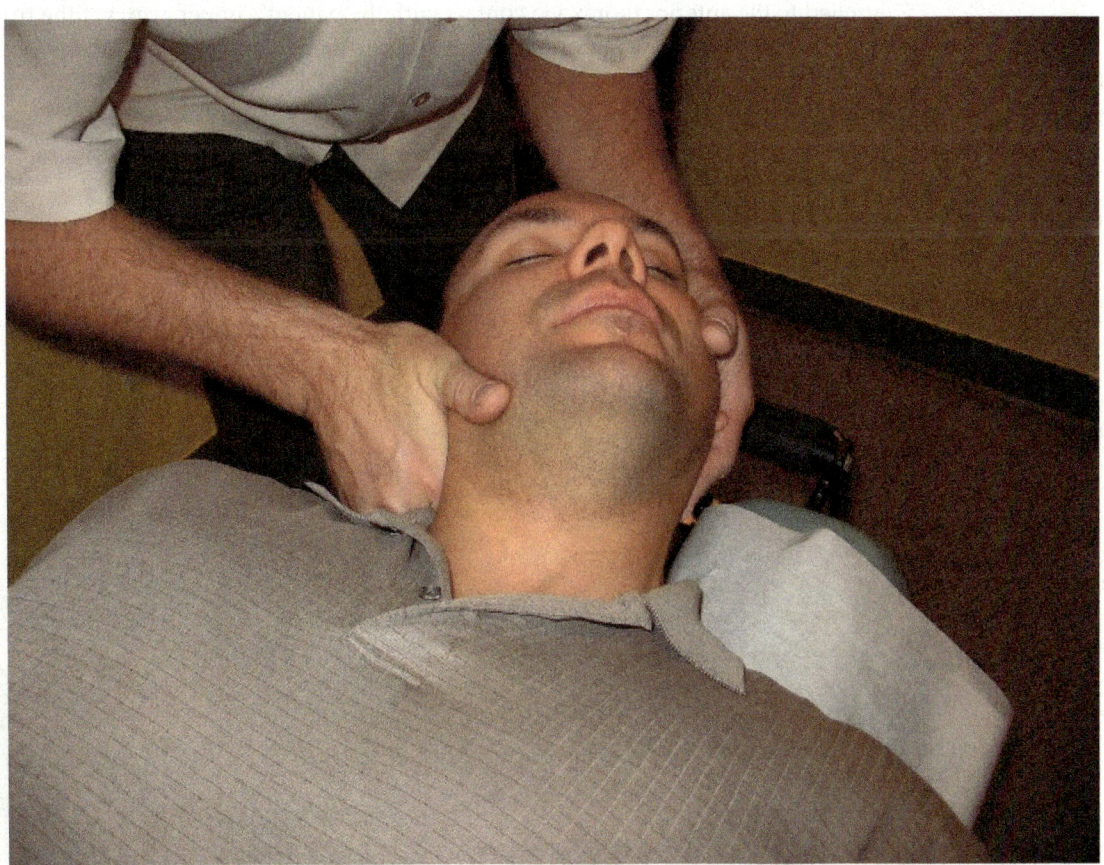

Posterior Ribs: Manipulation of the Costovertebral Junction

Patient position:	• Supine on table; to facilitate positioning, patient's leg opposite doctor may be flexed at hip and knee with foot flat on table. Patient's arms are crossed over the front of their body; my preference is that the arm closest to the doctor (the arm opposite to the side of the thorax being treated) is atop.
Doctor position:	• Modified fencer's stance facing cephalad
Assessment:	• <u>Subjective</u>: mechanical paraspinal pain; often discomfort with inhalation.
	• <u>Motion palpation</u>: stiffness at the affected costotransverse junction.
	• <u>Static palpation</u>: prominence in the posterior direction of the rib near the costotransverse junction.
	• <u>Soft tissue</u>: local tenderness to palpation is very common
Treatment contact:	• Contact on the specific rib immediately lateral to the costotransverse junction is made with the doctor's thenar eminence with the doctor's hand in a firm, pursed position. Initial contact is made superior and medial to the final location of manipulative contact in order to attain proper premanipulative tissue tension; pulling the contact hand inferiorly and laterally after some pressure has been applied helps ensure properly placed contact with premanipulative tension
Supporting contact:	• The doctor's supporting (noncontact) hand along with the doctor's torso deliver the manipulative thrust through the patient's arm atop the patient's thorax
Pretreatment positioning:	• Patient is supine; after positioning the contact hand posteriorly, the doctor grasps the patient's upper arm, then pulls downward and then applies progressive compressive force (body weight, not muscular force) while raising the supporting contact and rolling the patient over atop the contact hand
Thrust:	• Body-drop thrust generally superiorly and laterally in the direction of the patient's opposite shoulder; the angle of the thrust changes depending on the spinal-costal level being treated, with more superior segments requiring a more superiorly directed thrust, while lower segments require a progressively laterally-yet-sagittally directed thrust. Notably, the manipulative thrust is applied to the anterior thorax via contact with the patient's upper arm, yet the true manipulative force is from posterior to anterior via the doctor's thenar eminence positioned posteriorly.
Image:	

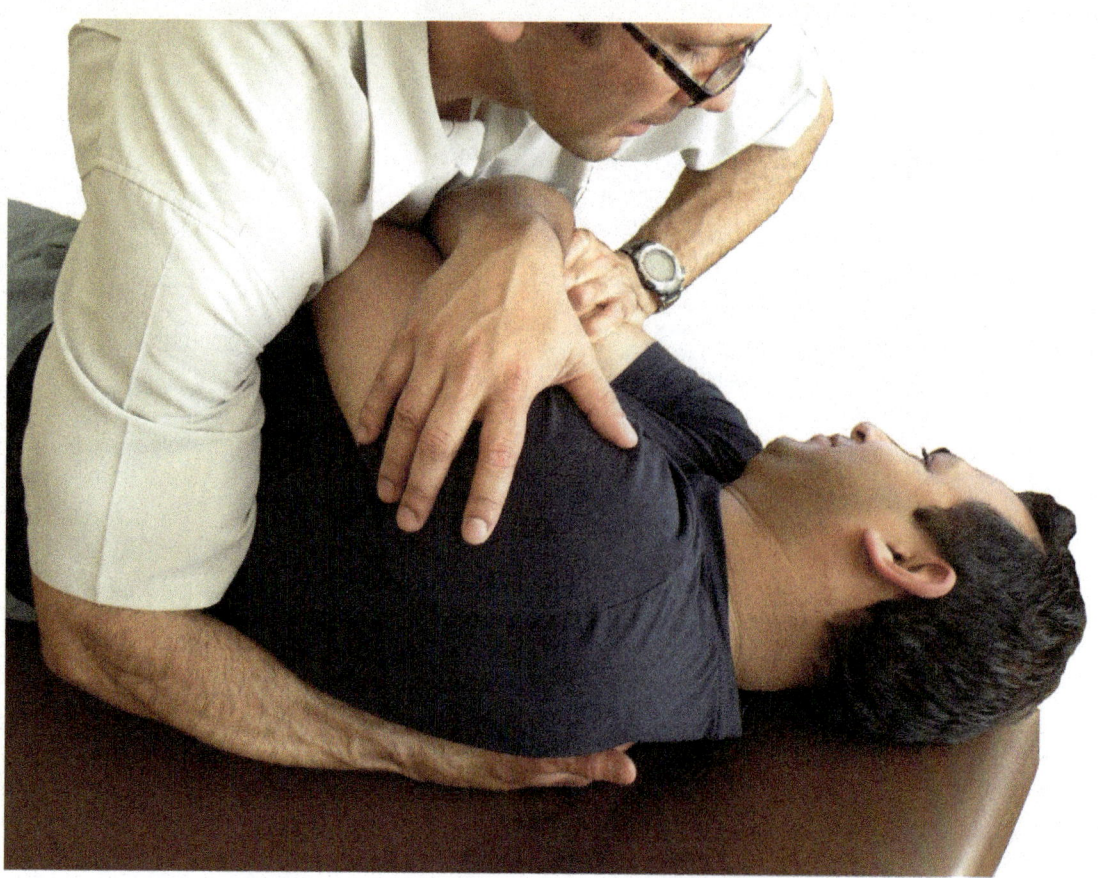

Thoracic Spine: Supine Thoracic Flexion, "Anterior Thoracic"

Patient position:	• Supine on table; to facilitate positioning, patient's leg opposite doctor may be flexed at hip and knee with foot flat on table
	• Patient is instructed to place right hand on right trapezius and left hand on left trapezius; the patient is instructed, "Do not place your hands behind your neck and do not interlace your fingers."
Doctor position:	• Facing table at 45° angle in fencer stance with feet apart and knees bent
	• Doctor must be midline and balanced at time of impulse in order to provide symmetric force
Assessment:	• <u>Subjective</u>: mechanical midback pain
	• <u>Motion palpation</u>: flexion restriction
	• <u>Static palpation</u>: extension malposition; focal loss of thoracic kyphosis; focal approximation of spinous processes consistent with extension malposition; vertebra may feel anteriorly displaced
	• <u>Soft tissue</u>: local paravertebral myohypertonicity is common; local paresthesia is very common, and patients are often exquisitely sensitive to the lightest touch
Treatment contact:	• Closed fist contact with spinous processes between doctor's distal interphalangeal joints and thenar eminence; the trust is delivered from the doctor's chest through the patient's arms which compress the patient's chest; Dr Harris (pictured as patient) prefers to use a forearm contact to reduce wear-and-tear on his hands and wrists
Supporting contact:	• The supporting contact is the hand-arm that supports the patient's upper torso; the supporting contact pulls toward the doctor and superiorly at time of impulse
Pretreatment positioning:	• Patient lifts head from table; doctor uses supporting hand and arm to lift patient off table to allow placement of contact hand and to facilitate spinal flexion
Therapeutic action:	• Doctor uses **body drop thrust** technique at 45° toward ground and toward the head of the table; the trust should simultaneously generate compression and long-axis traction; the contact hand remains tense to provide solid leverage *inferior* to the targeted motion segment; the supporting hand and arm pull toward doctor at time of impulse to accentuate traction and spinal flexion; patient is instructed to breathe deeply then relax and exhale; upon exhalation, the doctor establishes and maintains premanipulative tension to achieve joint flexion, then applies HVLA thrust; the thrust must be fast and shallow; slow and deep impulses can sprain the interspinous ligaments

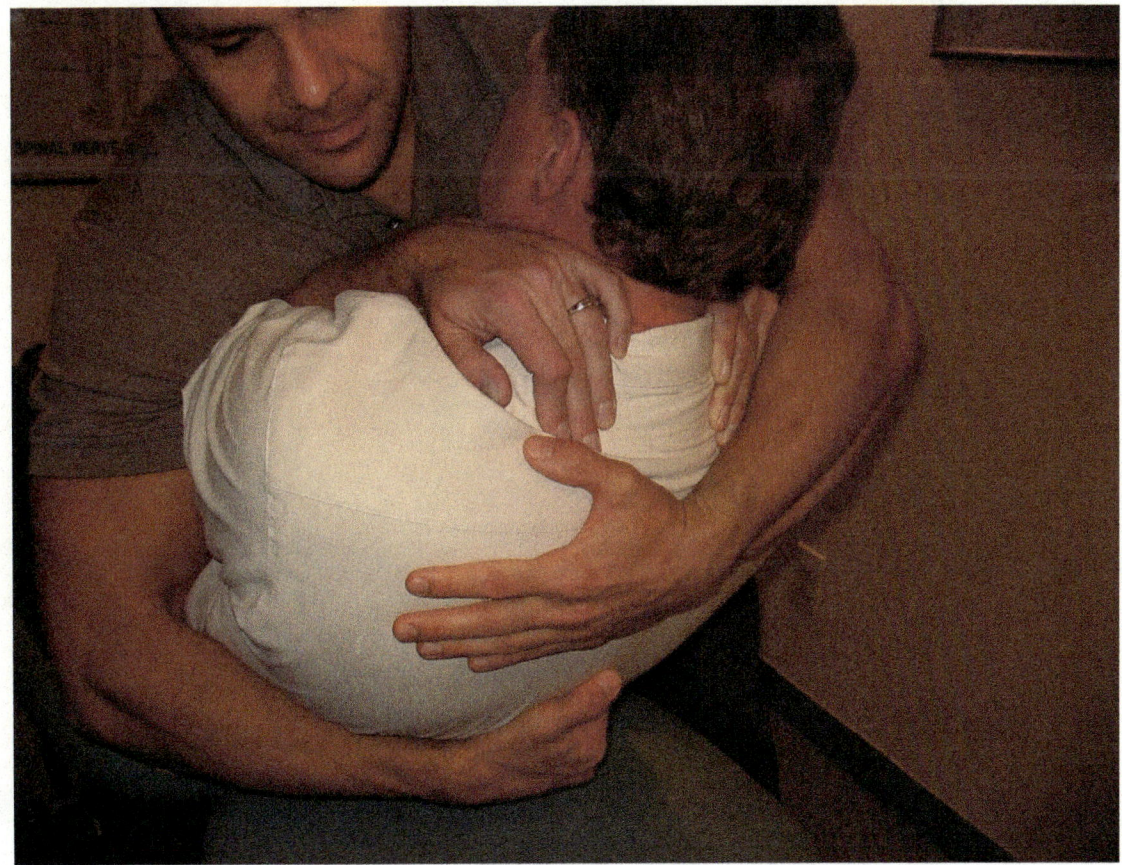

Lumbar Side-Posture Rotational Manipulation/Mobilization, "Lumbar Roll"

Patient position:	• Side-posture, lateral recumbent; lower leg is straight; upper leg is flexed at hip and knee with foot behind calf of the leg that is straight on the table
Doctor position:	• Facing table at 45° angle in fencer stance with feet apart and knees bent
	• Notice in the photograph how Dr Harris approximates his center of gravity and biomechanical leverage directly over his therapeutic contact
Assessment:	• <u>Subjective</u>: asymptomatic or with lumbar pain; lumbar disc herniation[326], use a cautious and gentle technique if the patient has radicular symptoms, and as a rule of thumb the patient should be positioned with the symptomatic leg down on the table (e.g., "good leg *up*, bad leg *down*")
	• <u>Motion palpation</u>: focal restrictions with focal pain are perhaps better treated with a lesion-specific technique such as the "push-pull" maneuver; this is an excellent technique if the patient has general discomfort without localization, or has pain and will benefit from rotational manipulation for its muscle stretching and afferent-stimulating analgesic benefits
	• <u>Static palpation</u>: minor displacements and malpositions may be noted; if specific biomechanical lesions are found, use a more specific technique such as the "push-pull" maneuver
	• <u>Soft tissue</u>: palpate for hypertonicity/spasm with or without relative muscle atrophy; patients with chronic low-back pain tend to have weaker extensor muscles than the general population; however, during an acutely painful episode, their otherwise weakened muscles will be hypertonic thus leading to a paradoxical **atrophic hypertonicity**
Treatment contact:	• Doctor uses a palmar/calcaneal ("heel of the hand") contact over the lumbar facet joints
	• Rotation and traction are provided at the time of impulse with the doctor's thigh which is compressed and providing long-axis traction against the patient's upper leg, which is flexed at the hip and knee
Support:	• Doctor's cephalad hand applies rotational resistance to patient's shoulder as shown
Pretreatment positioning:	• Premanipulative tension is attained and maintained prior to **body drop impulse**
	• The premanipulative tension and the therapeutic impulse are established and delivered through the contact hand and the doctor's caudad leg which has compressive contact with the patient's flexed leg
Therapeutic action:	• Body drop thrust impulse with rotational emphasis; notice how the forearm of his contact hand perpendicular to the patient's coronal plane to direct his impulse in a posterior-to-anterior direction

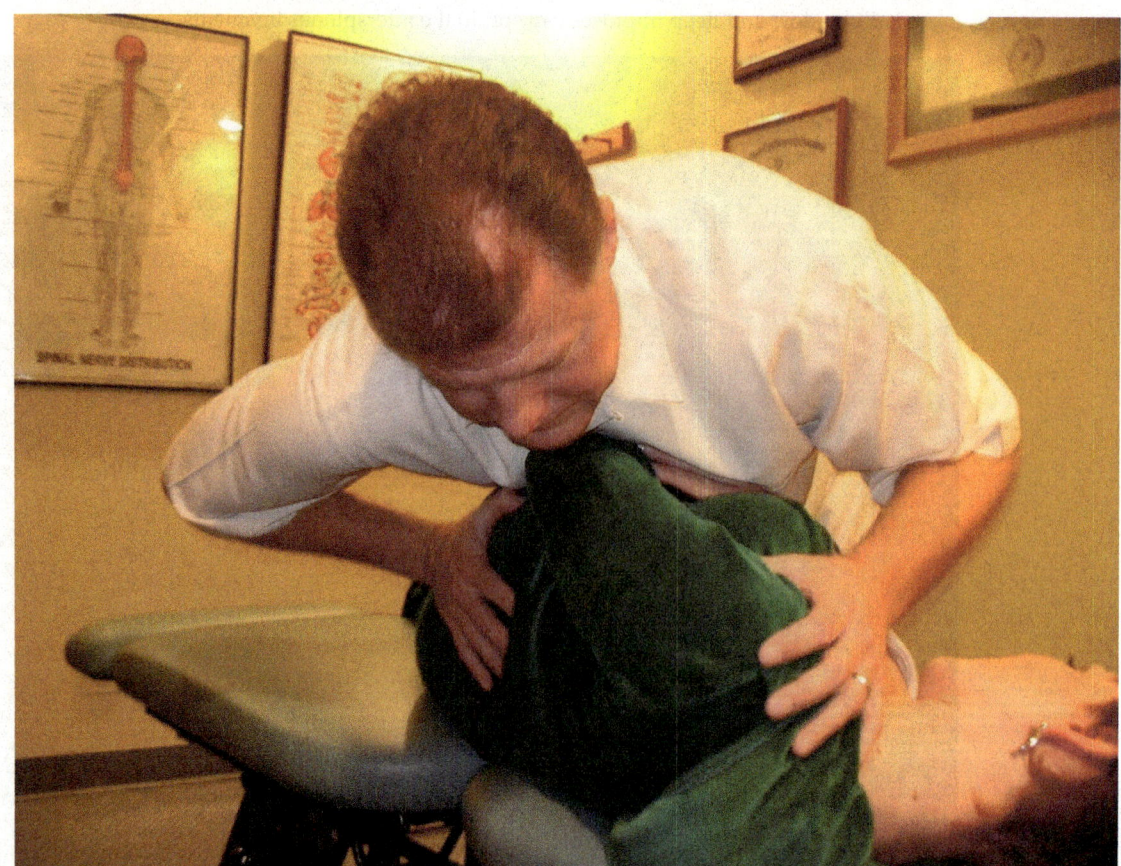

---

[326] Quon JA, et al. Lumbar intervertebral disc herniation: treatment by rotational manipulation. *J Manipulative Physiol Ther.* 1989 Jun;12(3):220-7

Lumbar Spine: Side-Posture Segmental Rotation (Lumbar "Push-Pull")

Patient position:	• Lateral recumbent (side-posture) with no/minimal lateral flexion and minimal thoracic rotation; upper leg is flexed at hip and knee, with foot placed/locked behind the calf that is on the table; the patient grasps his/her own forearms and maintains modest tension to provide anchoring for the doctor's caudad arm, which is placed under the patient's superior arm; the patient's lower leg is straight
Doctor position:	• Doctor is facing the table standing on the cephalad leg while the caudad leg is flexed at the hip and knee and placed atop the patient's flexed upper leg to provide additional leverage at the time of manipulative thrust. Regarding the doctor's cephalad arm, the humerus is directed toward the patient's shoulder, and the elbow is bent allowing the forearm to push into the sulcus formed by the pectoralis major and deltoid; doctors forearm emerges under patient's elbow, so that fingertips are on the superior/lateral aspect of the lumbar spinous process of the superior vertebra of the targeted motion segment. Regarding the doctor's caudad arm, the elbow is flexed and the forearm is placed along the posterior aspect of the patient's superior ilium; fingers hook the inferior/lateral aspect of the lumbar spinous process of the inferior vertebra of the targeted motion segment
Assessment:	• <u>Subjective</u>: asymptomatic or lumbar pain, which may not be at the affected segment • <u>Motion palpation</u>: rotational restriction • <u>Static palpation</u>: may have rotational malposition • <u>Soft tissue</u>: may have muscle spasm at nearby area of hypermobility
Treatment contact:	• The doctor's cephalad contacts are at the patient's deltopectoral sulcus and directly on the superior/lateral aspect of the lumbar spinous process of the superior vertebra of the targeted motion segment. This maneuver has three caudad contacts: 1) doctor's fingertips pull directly on the inferior/lateral aspect of the lumbar spinous process of the inferior vertebra of the targeted motion segment; 2) doctor's forearm on patient's ilium; 3) doctors caudad lower leg is atop patient's flexed leg
Support:	• All contacts are active
Pretreatment positioning:	• Rotational tension is applied and focused at the lumbar spinal segment being treated • Thoracic rotation and lateral flexion are minimized to the extent possible • Modest lumbar lateral flexion toward the table helps to gap the inferior articular process of the superior segment from the superior articular process of the inferior segment
Therapeutic action:	• 1) Doctor's cephalad elbow thrusts toward patient's shoulder to create simultaneous rotation and long-axis traction; 2) cephalad fingertips push toward the ground while atop the superior/lateral aspect of the lumbar spinous process of the superior vertebra of the targeted motion segment; 3) doctor's caudad fingertips hook and pull the inferior vertebra; 4) forearm pushes patient's ilium into rotation; 5) extension "kick" of doctor's knee quickly creates rotational force. All five actions occur simultaneously
Image:	

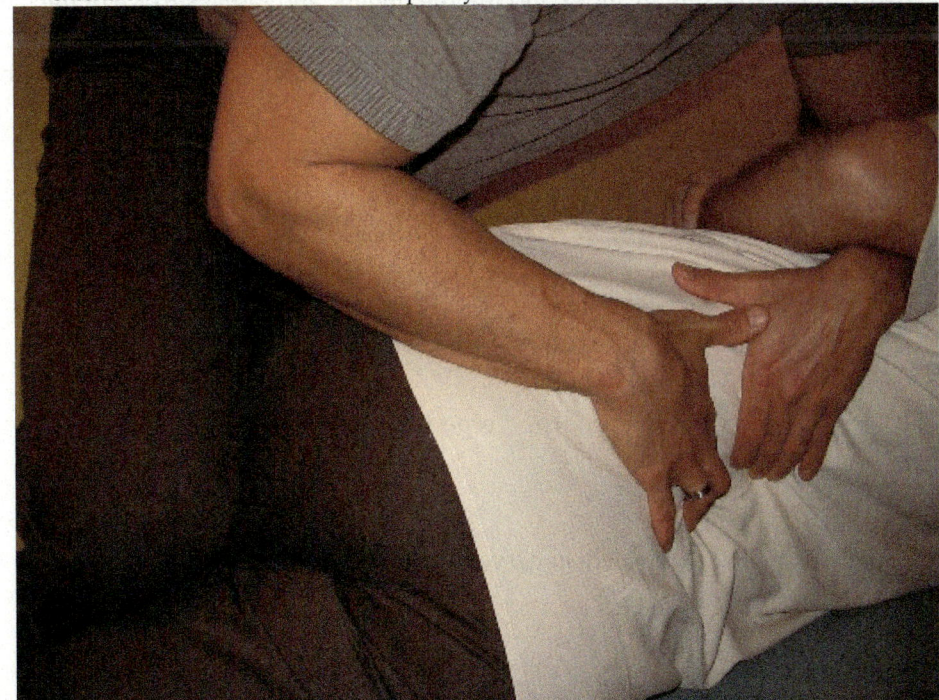

Carpal tunnel syndrome, CTS

Description/pathophysiology:
- Symptoms resultant from compression of the median nerve in the osteofibrous tunnel bordered by the carpal bones and the transverse carpal ligament. This compression may be due to:
  - Inflammatory edema of the finger flexor tendons and their associated synovial sheaths as they traverse the carpal tunnel; inflammation/edema may be due to overuse, injury, systemic edema (e.g., secondary to estrogen excess, pregnancy), hypothyroidism, or inflammatory process such as RA
  - May be exacerbated by external compression due to poor ergonomics, posture, or habits, such as sleeping prone on wrists, working with wrist on edge of desk/table, working with wrists in extreme flexion or extension
  - Rarely caused by congenital stenosis of the carpal tunnel
  - Specific nutritional deficiencies responsive to nutritional supplementation in many patients[327]
  - The median nerve can be compressed anywhere from its origin at the nerve roots all the way to the carpal tunnel. The concept of the "double crush" holds that two or more areas of minor compression to a nerve can result in a functional lesion similar to what would be expected with a single major compression; these compressive locations and their clinical assessment will be reviewed later in this section on CTS.

Complications:
- Loss of strength, muscle atrophy (intrinsic thenar muscles), and compromise of function of the hand; in severe cases, patients lose function of one or both hands and may be largely unable to work and function in their daily lives.
- Pain, paresthesia in the distribution of the median nerve

Clinical presentations:
- Pain-numbness-tingling in the thumb, index and middle fingers, and radial surface of the palm
- Symptoms are often worse at night
- May also have weakness of grip strength and loss of coordination of fine motor skills of the hand

Major differential diagnoses and contributing conditions:
- Double crush syndrome[328]
- Hypothyroidism
- Diabetes mellitus
- Acromegaly
- Amyloidosis
- Estrogen excess
- Pregnancy
- Nutritional deficiency or nutritional dependency, especially pyridoxine and riboflavin

Clinical assessments:
- History:
  - Pain, numbness, tingling in the median nerve distribution
  - Symptoms are worse at night.
  - May also have weakness of grip strength

---

[327] Folkers K, et al. Enzymology of the response of carpal tunnel syndrome to riboflavin and to combined riboflavin and pyridoxine. *Proc Natl Acad Sci* 1984 Nov;81(22):7076-8
[328] "Results supported the DCS hypothesis. DCS evaluation requires both structural and functional diagnosis of peripheral neurones ...." Flak et al. Double crush syndrome evaluation in the median nerve in clinical, radiological and electrophysiological examination. *Stud Health Technol Inform.* 2006;123:435-41

- Physical examination:
  - Intrinsic thumb muscles may be weak
  - Assess for atrophy of the thenar eminence by observation and bilateral comparison
  - Positive neuro-orthopedic assessment:
    - Phalen's test
    - Reverse Phalen's test
    - Tinel's test
    - Direct pressure at the carpal tunnel reproduces symptoms, i.e., numbness or tingling of the thenar palm
  - Assessment for compression of the median nerve and its contributory nerve roots:

Location	Screening assessments	Therapeutic considerations
Intervertebral disc of any level from C5-T1	<ul><li>Cervical compression tests</li><li>MRI if clinically warranted</li></ul>	<ul><li>Consider traction for disc decompression</li></ul>
Intervertebral foramina on the affected side	<ul><li>Provocative positioning to exacerbate hand paresthesia: combinations of ipsilateral side-bending and extension to exacerbate foraminal compression of nerve root</li><li>Cervical oblique radiographs to assess IVFs</li></ul>	<ul><li>Osseous and soft-tissue manipulation as indicated per patient to cervical and shoulder region</li><li>Improve spinal health and posture</li><li>Ergonomic and workstation improvements</li></ul>
Compression of brachial plexus due to thoracic outlet compression at anterior-middle scalenes, costoclavicular space, or secondary to tight pectoralis major	<ul><li>Tests for TOS (see Chapter on shoulder)</li></ul>	<ul><li>Stretch scalenes and pectoralis minor to relieve chronic compression of neurovascular bundle</li><li>Improve posture</li><li>Ergonomic and workstation improvements</li></ul>
Compression of median nerve at pronator teres	<ul><li>Palpation and provocation at dual origin of pronator teres: proximal medial ulna and medial epicondyle</li></ul>	<ul><li>Osseous and soft-tissue manipulation as indicated per patient to elbow region and pronator teres</li></ul>

Imaging & laboratory assessments:

- Assessment for hypothyroidism with TSH, free T4, free T3, and anti-TPO antibodies: **Hypothyroidism is relatively common among patients with CTS.**[329] **Musculoskeletal complaints are common in patients with thyroid problems, particularly hypothyroidism.**[330] With a suggestive or compelling clinical presentation, treatment of overt or subclinical hypothyroidism with thyroid hormone replacement is justified unless specifically contraindicated when the TSH value is greater than 2 μIU/mL[331], greater than 3 μIU/mL[332], or when antithyroid antibodies are present.[333] For most patients, treatment of hypothyroidism is best accomplished with a natural glandular source of thyroid hormone (such as a "nutritional" glandular product

[329] Palumbo CF, et al. The effects of hypothyroidism and thyroid replacement on the development of carpal tunnel syndrome. *J Hand Surg* [Am]. 2000 Jul;25(4):734-9

[330] Cakir M, Samanci N, Balci N, Balci MK. Musculoskeletal manifestations in patients with thyroid disease. *Clin Endocrinol* (Oxf). 2003 Aug;59(2):162-7

[331] Weetman AP. Hypothyroidism: screening and subclinical disease. *BMJ*. 1997 Apr 19;314(7088):1175-8 bmj.com/cgi/content/full/314/7088/1175

[332] "Now American Association of Clinical Endocrinologists encourages doctors to consider treatment for patients who test outside the boundaries of a narrower margin based on a target TSH level of 0.3 to 3.04. AACE believes the new range will result in proper diagnosis for millions of Americans who suffer from a mild thyroid disorder, but have gone untreated until now." aace.com/pub/tam2003/press.php 2004 Jan

[333] Beers MH, Berkow R (eds). *The Merck Manual of Diagnosis and Therapy, 17th Edition*. Whitehouse Station; Merck Research Laboratories 1999 page 96

or Armour thyroid) or a hypoallergenic synthetic bioidentical combination of both T3 and T4[334] (such as Liotrix/Thyrolar) and should also be accompanied by general nutritional supplementation with a high-potency broad-spectrum multivitamin/multimineral supplement that contains 200-600 mcg of selenium[335,336] and 15-25 mg of zinc.[337] Zinc, selenium, and iron are required for peripheral conversion and function of thyroid hormones; corresponding mineral deficiencies can precipitate a mild functional hypothyroidism.

- **Basic routine laboratory assessment with CBC, CRP, CCP, and chemistry/metabolic panel**: This approach is sufficient to screen for diabetes and rheumatoid arthritis, both of which are more common in patients with CTS.[338,339]
- **Assessment of vitamin levels and functional enzyme status**: This is generally not necessary; consider assessment of vitamin B6 status with erythrocyte glutamic oxaloacetic transaminase (EGOT) and/or serum P5P levels.
- **Electromyography**: EMG can be used to objectively quantify impaired nerve conduction
- **Serum ferritin**: Assess for iron overload or iron deficiency.

Clinical management: Referral if clinical outcome is unsatisfactory.

Treatments:

- **Pyridoxine (vitamin B-6; concomitant administration with magnesium)**: Many patients with CTS have serum and biochemical evidence of pyridoxine deficiency[340] which remit along with the CTS following supplementation with pyridoxine, thus helping to obviate the need for surgery.[341,342,343,344,345,346] *The Merck Manual of Diagnosis and Therapy, 17th Edition* advocates a trial of 50 mg twice daily[347] while others have recommended a dose of 200 mg per day.[348] A recent clinical trial[349] showed that enzyme saturation proceeds from 83% with 30 mg of pyridoxine to 93% with 200 mg of pyridoxine, thus proving again that dose-responsiveness is not maximized until higher *supranutritional* doses are used; this precept was previously reviewed in a brilliant *required reading* article by Bruce Ames et al.[350] In my practice I commonly use at least 250 mg daily with breakfast for a *loading dose* trial period of 2-12 weeks before tapering down to a maintenance dose of 50 mg/day. Long-term ultrahigh-dose administration of pyridoxine HCL can be neurotoxic, producing a peripheral neuropathy that is not unlike the presentation of carpal tunnel syndrome. One of the problems with supplementation with vitamin B-6 in the form of pyridoxine HCL is that this particular synthetic form of vitamin B-6 appears to be mildly neurotoxic and must be converted to the active form(s) of the vitamin before becoming harmless and physiologically functional. The phosphorylation of pyridoxine HCL into its active phosphorylated forms (e.g., pyridoxal-5-phosphate, P5P) requires the presence of magnesium. Many people are deficient in magnesium and therefore may not respond to supplementation with pyridoxine HCL because of deficiency-induced biochemical inability to convert the vitamin to its active form in sufficient quantities to achieve a therapeutic effect. Obviously, either using an activated form of pyridoxine such as the commercially available pyridoxal-5-phosphate would obviate this problem; gastrointestinal absorption of P5P appears to be limited. Coadministration of magnesium is advised with the

[334] Bunevicius R, et al. Effects of thyroxine as compared with thyroxine plus triiodothyronine in patients with hypothyroidism. *N Engl J Med.* 1999 Feb 11;340(6):424-9

[335] Duntas LH, et al. Effects of a six month treatment with selenomethionine in patients with autoimmune thyroiditis. *Eur J Endocrinol.* 2003 Apr;148(4):389-93

[336] Olivieri et al. Selenium, zinc, and thyroid hormones in healthy subjects: low T3/T4 ratio in elderly is related to impaired selenium status. *Biol Trace Elem Res* 1996;51:31-41

[337] Nishiyama S, et al. Zinc supplementation alters thyroid hormone metabolism in disabled patients with zinc deficiency. *J Am Coll Nutr.* 1994 Feb;13(1):62-7

[338] Van Dijk MA, et al. Indications for requesting laboratory tests for concurrent diseases in patients with carpal tunnel syndrome:. *Clin Chem.* 2003 Sep;49(9):1437-44

[339] Solomon DH, Katz JN, Bohn R, Mogun H, Avorn J. Nonoccupational risk factors for carpal tunnel syndrome. *J Gen Intern Med.* 1999 May;14(5):310-4

[340] Fuhr JE, Farrow A, Nelson HS Jr. Vitamin B6 levels in patients with carpal tunnel syndrome. *Arch Surg.* 1989 Nov;124(11):1329-30

[341] Ellis et al, Folkers K. Vitamin B6 deficiency in patients with clinical syndrome including the carpal tunnel defect. *Res Commun Chem Pathol Pharmacol* 1976 Apr;13:743-57

[342] Ellis J, Folkers K, et al. Clinical results of a cross-over treatment with pyridoxine and placebo of the carpal tunnel syndrome. *Am J Clin Nutr.* 1979 Oct;32(10):2040-6

[343] Ellis J, Folkers K, Levy M, Takemura K, Shizukuishi S, Ulrich R, Harrison P. Therapy with vitamin B6 with and without surgery for treatment of patients having the idiopathic carpal tunnel syndrome. *Res Commun Chem Pathol Pharmacol.* 1981 Aug;33(2):331-44

[344] Ellis JM, Folkers K, et al. Response of vitamin B-6 deficiency and the carpal tunnel syndrome to pyridoxine. *Proc Natl Acad Sci* U S A. 1982 Dec;79(23):7494-8

[345] Kasdan ML, Janes C. Carpal tunnel syndrome and vitamin B6. *Plast Reconstr Surg.* 1987 Mar;79(3):456-62

[346] Ellis JM. Treatment of carpal tunnel syndrome with vitamin B6. *South Med J.* 1987 Jul;80(7):882-4

[347] Beers MH, Berkow R (eds). *The Merck Manual of Diagnosis and Therapy, 17th Edition*. Whitehouse Station; Merck Research Laboratories 1999 Page 492

[348] "Current treatment for carpal tunnel syndrome should include NSAIDs, nighttime splinting, ergonomic workstation review, and vitamin B6 200 mg per day." Holm G, Moody LE. Carpal tunnel syndrome: current theory, treatment, and the use of B6. *J Am Acad Nurse Pract.* 2003 Jan;15(1):18-22

[349] "The in vivo study showed increasing aspartate aminotransferase saturation with increasing pyridoxine doses. 83% saturation was reached with 30 mg daily, 88% with 100 mg, and 93% with 200 mg after 20 days of oral supplementation." Oshiro M, Nonoyama K, Oliveira RA, Barretto OC. Red cell aspartate aminotransferase saturation with oral pyridoxine intake. *Sao Paulo Med J.* 2005 Mar 2;123(2):54-7 scielo.br/scielo.php?script=sci_arttext&pid=S1516-31802005000200004&tlng=es&lng=en&nrm=iso

[350] Ames BN, Elson-Schwab I, Silver EA. High-dose vitamin therapy stimulates variant enzymes with decreased coenzyme binding affinity (increased K(m)): relevance to genetic disease and polymorphisms. *Am J Clin Nutr.* 2002 Apr;75(4):616-58 ajcn.org/cgi/content/full/75/4/616

use of pyridoxine HCL, and generally long-term high-dose (i.e., bowel tolerance) supplementation is necessary to replenish body magnesium levels. If necessary, assessment of magnesium status is performed by measuring either RBC or WBC intracellular magnesium levels; serum levels of magnesium are generally meaningless from a nutritional standpoint. Furthermore, magnesium supplementation should occur along with concomitant urinary alkalinization so that supplemented magnesium will be retained. Failure to alkalinize the urine with either diet[351] or alkalinization therapy such as sodium bicarbonate and/or potassium citrate[352], or alkaline minerals[353] allows for facilitated excretion of magnesium and subsequent "failure" of pyridoxine therapy due to insufficient magnesium-dependent phosphorylation and activation of the vitamin. Vitamin B6 probably exerts its beneficial effects in the treatment of CTS via several mechanisms, including:

- o Facilitating biosynthesis of pain-relieving serotonin
- o Reducing excitatory glutamate levels
- o Diuretic effect: perhaps via inhibition of anti-diuretic hormone (ADH) secretion
- o Diuretic effect via estrogen-lowering[354]: probably effected via upregulation of hepatic transaminases but possibly also via a direct pituitary effect[355]

Likewise, magnesium supplementation appears to provide some analgesic benefit which is at least partially due to its role in inhibiting activation of NMDA receptors and reducing/normalizing neuronal transmission. Magnesium is a required co-factor for tissue alkaline phosphatase, the enzyme required for pyridoxine dephosphorylation prior to tissue uptake of pyridoxal-5-phosphate; thus, magnesium deficiency appears to cause tissue/cellular deficiency of vitamin B6 by reducing cellular uptake of the vitamin.[356]

- o **Drug-nutrient interactions**: High doses of **vitamin B6** can reduce blood levels and effectiveness of **barbiturate drugs** such as pentobarbital [Nembutal], phenobarbital [Phenobarbitone], secobarbital [Seconal], and thiopental [Pentothal]
- o **Drug-nutrient interactions**: High doses of **magnesium** may decrease the absorption or effectiveness of several drugs, including: Azithromycin (Zithromax), Cimetidine (Tagamet), Ciprofloxacin (Ciloxan, Cipro), Doxycycline (Atridox, Doryx, Doxy, Monodox, Periostat, Vibramycin), Famotidine (Mylanta-AR, Pepcid, Pepcid AC), Hydroxychloroquine (Plaquenil), Levofloxacin (Levaquin), Nitrofurantoin (Furadantin, Macrobid, Macrodantin), Nizatidine (Axid, Axid AR), Ofloxacin (Floxin, Ocuflox), Tetracycline (Achromycin, Sumycin, Helidac), Warfarin (Coumadin). Misoprostol (Cytotec, Arthrotec) with magnesium may result in diarrhea. Spironolactone (Aldactone, Aldactazide) or Amiloride (Midamor, Moduretic) may cause dangerously high levels of magnesium

Before moving on to the next section readers should have crystalline clarity with regard to the following:

- o Most patients consuming an American/Western-style diet have subtle chronic metabolic acidosis, which results in many adverse effects, one of which is increased urinary excretion of magnesium and reduced tissue/intracellular levels of magnesium.
- o This acidotic predisposition toward magnesium deficiency is exacerbated by low dietary intake of magnesium, as well as other factors such as overconsumption of caffeine, sugar, and also by chronic mental/emotional stress.
- o The resultant magnesium deficiency thus impairs activation/phosphorylation of pyridoxine HCL into the active form pyridoxal-5-phosphate via magnesium-dependent pyridoxal kinase; this results in a simultaneous diminution of effectiveness and enhancement of pyridoxine HCL-mediated neurotoxicity. Cofactors for various tissue-specific isoforms of pyridoxal kinase include magnesium, zinc, cobalt, and manganese; of these, zinc appears most important, particularly in the liver and brain.

[351] Cordain L. *The Paleo Diet*. Indianapolis; John Wiley and Sons, 2002
[352] Maurer et al.Neutralization of Western diet inhibitsbone resorption independently of K intake, reduces cortisol secretion in humans.*Am J PhysiolRenalPhysiol* 2003;284:F32-40
[353] Vormann J, et al. Supplementation with alkaline minerals reduces symptoms in patients with chronic low back pain. *J Trace Elem Med Biol*. 2001;15(2-3):179-83
[354] "Administration of vitamin B6 at doses of 200-800 mg/day reduces blood estrogen, increases progesterone and results in improved symptoms under double-blind conditions." Abraham GE. Nutritional factors in the etiology of the premenstrual tension syndromes. *J Reprod Med*. 1983 Jul;28(7):446-64
[355] "These results indicate that pharmacological doses of PLP inhibit pituitary cell proliferation and hormone secretion, in part mediated through PLP-induced cell-cycle arrest and apoptosis. Pyridoxine may therefore be appropriate for testing as a relatively safe drug for adjuvant treatment of hormone-secreting pituitary adenomas." Ren SG, Melmed S. Pyridoxal phosphate inhibits pituitary cell proliferation and hormone secretion. *Endocrinology*. 2006 Aug;147(8):3936-42
[356] "Mg deficiency impairs vitamin B6 status by depleting intracellular Mg and thus inhibits the activity of alkaline phosphatase, a metalloenzyme required for the uptake of pyridoxal phosphate by tissues." Planells E, et al. Effect of magnesium deficiency on vitamin B2 and B6 status in the rat. *J Am Coll Nutr*. 1997 Aug;16(4):352-6

The final production of active P5P requires a (ribo)flavin-dependent oxidase; thus, *B2 quantitative insufficiency* precipitates *B6 functional insufficiency*.[357]

- o Furthermore, magnesium deficiency impairs alkaline phosphatase, the enzyme required for cellular uptake of pyridoxal-5-phosphate; in this way, magnesium deficiency causes tissue insufficiency of pyridoxine.

- o Additionally, chronic metabolic acidosis further impairs intracellular accumulation of magnesium, apparently because the elevated intracellular concentration of hydrogen ions creates an electrochemically repulsive force, given that both hydrogen and magnesium are positively-charged cations.

- o In this situation, if a patient is supplemented with pyridoxine HCL *without magnesium* and *without systemic alkalinization*, we should not expect that optimal clinical responsiveness will be observed even if the patient is functionally vitamin B6 deficient and if the condition is pyridoxine responsive. Thus, the *correct treatment* in the *correct patient* **fails** not because of failure of the treatment *per se*, but rather due failure to create an internal milieu wherein vitamin B6 can function optimally.

  - ▪ Readers should now understand the inherent bias of the medical studies that have "proved" the "ineffectiveness" of vitamin B6 supplementation. Why did so many of these studies fail to show positive benefit? *The supplementation failed because the doctors had no training in nutrition and thus implemented a treatment that had little hope for optimal success because the researchers failed to* ❶ *improve the diet,* ❷ *correct the diet-induced metabolic acidosis, and* ❸ *provide co-factors necessary for B6 function.*

  - ▪ Readers should now understand how to reduce B6 toxicity while increasing its effectiveness. *Alkalinization followed by supplementation with zinc, magnesium, and riboflavin.*

  - ▪ Readers should now understand why an alkalinizing Paleo-Mediterranean diet is *primarily* essential for creating an internal environment wherein the *secondary* addition of high-dose nutritional supplements can function.

- Riboflavin (vitamin B2): ==Patients with CTS may respond to riboflavin therapy alone, and the combination of riboflavin 50 mg with pyridoxine 500 mg appears more efficacious than the use of either B2 or B6 alone.==[358] Per data that migraine headaches are alleviated with riboflavin 400 mg/d[359], in patients with CTS we may safely proceed with riboflavin 400 mg, preferably administered with breakfast.

- Yoga: Yoga postures and relaxation showed superior results compared to use of a night splint in the treatment of CTS.[360] In contrast to surgical lesion of the transverse carpal ligament, yoga is fun, feels good, and can improve aspects of overall health[361] and socioemotional wellbeing.

- Mobilization and manipulation of the carpal bones, myofascial release: Symptoms of CTS may be effectively reduced simply by a mobilization technique of squeezing the metacarpal heads together and also stretching the third and fourth digits into extension.[362] Osteopathic-type manipulation (similar to chiropractic manipulation) of the wrist has shown clinical, electromyographic, and MRI evidence of efficacy[363,364], and the technique is intuitive and commonly known among clinicians with training in manipulation. Additional effectiveness can be obtained when patients are taught to regularly perform stretching maneuvers with the forearm in supination, wrist in forced extension, and the thumb brought firmly back toward the body with the use of the contralateral hand.

- Trial of anti-inflammatory botanicals: Particularly bromelain and proteolytic enzymes.

- Reduce intake of dietary salt: Excess sodium ingestion promotes water retention and magnesium excretion (among many other adverse effects).

---

[357] Holman P. Pyridoxine - Vitamin B6. *Journal of the Australasian College of Nutritional & Environmental Medicine*, Vol. 14, No. 1, July 1995, pages 5-16 acnem.org/journal/14-1_july_1995/pyridoxine-vitamin_b6.htm Congratulations to Mr. Holman for his excellent summation of pyridoxine metabolism.

[358] Folkers et al. Enzymology of the response of the carpal tunnel syndrome to riboflavin and to combined riboflavin and pyridoxine. *Proc Natl Acad Sci* 1984 Nov;81(22):7076-8

[359] Schoenen J, Jacquy J, Lenaerts M. Effectiveness of high-dose riboflavin in migraine prophylaxis. A randomized controlled trial. *Neurology* 1998 Feb;50(2):466-70

[360] Garfinkel MS, Singhal A, Katz WA, et al. Yoga-based intervention for carpal tunnel syndrome: a randomized trial. *JAMA*. 1998 Nov 11;280:1601-3

[361] "It is likely that the yoga practices of controlling body, mind, and spirit combine to provide useful psychophysiological effects for healthy people and for people compromised by musculoskeletal and cardiopulmonary disease." Raub JA. Psychophysiologic effects of Hatha Yoga on musculoskeletal and cardiopulmonary function: a literature review. *J Altern Complement Med.* 2002 Dec;8(6):797-812

[362] Manente G, Torrieri F, Pineto F, Uncini A. A relief maneuver in carpal tunnel syndrome. *Muscle Nerve*. 1999 Nov;22(11):1587-9

[363] "All participants who were treated improved clinically, with decrease in both symptoms and palpatory restriction." Sucher BM. Palpatory diagnosis and manipulative management of carpal tunnel syndrome. *J Am Osteopath Assoc.* 1994 Aug;94(8):647-63

[364] Sucher BM. Myofascial manipulative release of carpal tunnel syndrome: documentation with magnetic resonance imaging. *J Am Osteopath Assoc.* 1993 Dec;93(12):1273-8

- <u>Deep tissue massage to the muscles of the forearm</u>: The median nerve can be compressed proximal to the carpal tunnel at its relationships to the flexor digitorum superficialis, pronator teres[365], and/or the lacertus fibrosus extension from the biceps tendon.[366] Soft-tissue manipulative treatments should be used as part of the comprehensive treatment plan for CTS before any patient is considered a surgical candidate.
- <u>Behavioral and occupational ergonomic modifications</u>: Improve work station functionality, avoid overuse of the hands and wrists, and particularly avoid direct compression of the wrist while working.
- <u>Treatment of endocrine abnormalities and concomitant disease</u>: Diabetes mellitus, thyroid disease, rheumatoid arthritis, in women: assess for high estrogen/ low progesterone, or the use of estrogen supplementation.[367]
- <u>Weight loss</u>: If the patient is overweight, the patient should lose weight.
- <u>Use of a wrist splint at night</u>: A commonly advocated treatment in allopathic textbooks.
- <u>Surgery</u>: For non-responsive cases only as a last resort after nutrition, diet, weight loss, ergonomics, and competent manipulation, mobilization, and massage have been utilized *in combination* along with assessment for and treatment of endocrinologic contributions.

---

[365] Olehnik WK, Manske PR, Szerzinski J. Median nerve compression in the proximal forearm. *J Hand Surg* [Am]. 1994 Jan;19(1):121-6

[366] Wertsch JJ, Melvin J. Median nerve anatomy and entrapment syndromes: a review. *Arch Phys Med Rehabil.* 1982 Dec;63(12):623-7

[367] "Recent weight gain and use of estrogen replacement therapy were identified as possible risk factors; this provides some support for the theory that fluid retention in the soft tissues of the carpal tunnel is etiologically involved, although these results are preliminary and further research must be carried out to refute or support these findings." Dieck GS, Kelsey JL. An epidemiologic study of the carpal tunnel syndrome in an adult female population. *Prev Med.* 1985 Jan;14(1):63-9

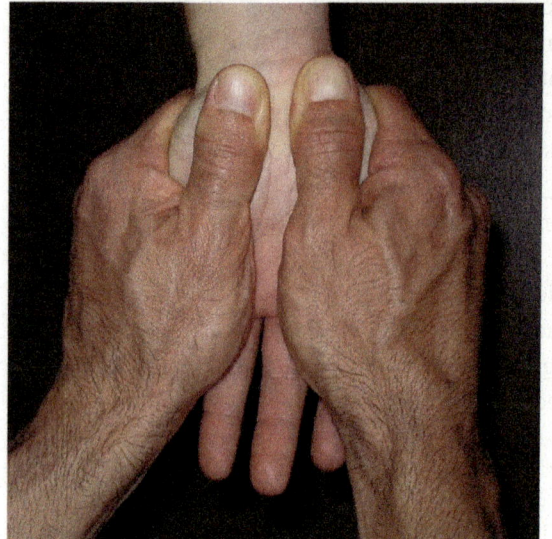

In this demonstration, the doctor is working on the patient's right wrist. In the doctor's right hand, the patient's pisiform, triquetral, and hamate bones are grasped and rolled externally, in a clockwise direction. In the doctor's left hand, the patient's scaphoid and trapezium bones are grasped and rolled externally from midline, in a counterclockwise direction. The combination of these two motions generates strong tension in the transverse carpal ligament (flexor retinaculum) that eventually leads to relaxation of the ligament and allows for increased cross-sectional area within the carpal tunnel, thus relieving pressure on its contents, particularly the median nerve. This maneuver is generally referred to as the *opponens roll*, and the following techniques are variations of same.

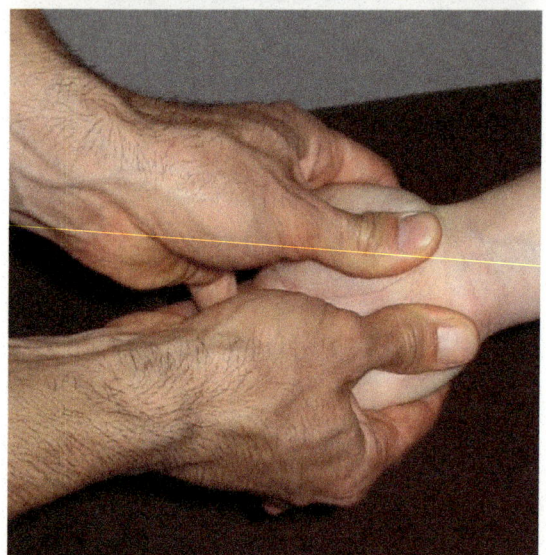

In this maneuver, the doctor's contacts and motions are the same as above, except that in this case the doctor's fingers are interposed between those of the patient. This positioning provides for greater control of the patient's distal palm, allowing the doctor to force the patient's wrist into extension while applying tension to the transverse carpal ligament. The addition of wrist extension appears to increase the clinical efficacy of the maneuver.

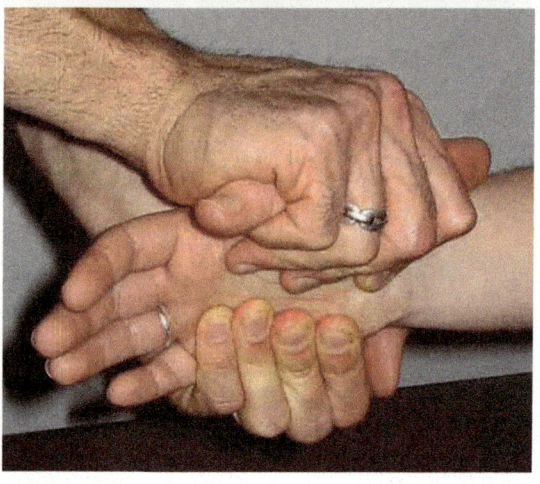

In this positioning, the actions are the same as above, but the doctor is using his fingers rather than thumbs to apply the mobilizing force. In the doctor's right hand, the patient's scaphoid and trapezium bones are grasped and rolled externally from the palmar surface, in a counterclockwise direction. In the doctor's left hand, the patient's pisiform, triquetral, and hamate bones are grasped and rolled externally from the palmar surface, in a clockwise direction. The action and concept are to "open" the carpal tunnel by tractioning the transverse carpal ligament.

[368] Sucher BM. Palpatory diagnosis and manipulative management of carpal tunnel syndrome. *J Am Osteopath Assoc.* 1994 Aug;94(8):647-63
[369] Sucher BM. Myofascial manipulative release of carpal tunnel syndrome: documentation with magnetic resonance imaging. *J Am Osteopath Assoc.* 1993 Dec;93(12):1273-8
[370] Sucher BM, et al. Manipulative treatment of carpal tunnel syndrome: biomechanical and osteopathic intervention to increase the length of the transverse carpal ligament: part 2. Effect of sex differences and manipulative "priming". *J Am Osteopath Assoc.* 2005 Mar;105(3):135-43 jaoa.org/cgi/content/full/105/3/135

Proprioceptive Rehabilitation: Essential for Treatment of Chronic/Back/Knee/Ankle Pain/Injuries

The central nervous system plays a silent and often underappreciated role in the maintenance of joint integrity and the prevention of joint injuries. Finely coordinated, minute alterations in muscle tension and joint position are essential for proper musculoskeletal biomechanics. Impaired coordination of this delicate neuromuscular system—either by injury or more commonly by disuse—predisposes to subtle and gross injuries and the perpetuation of chronic pain. **Muscle spasm, myofascial trigger points, and neuromuscular uncoupling must be viewed within a context that appreciates how the Western diet and lifestyle contribute to the genesis and perpetuation of painful musculoskeletal problems.**

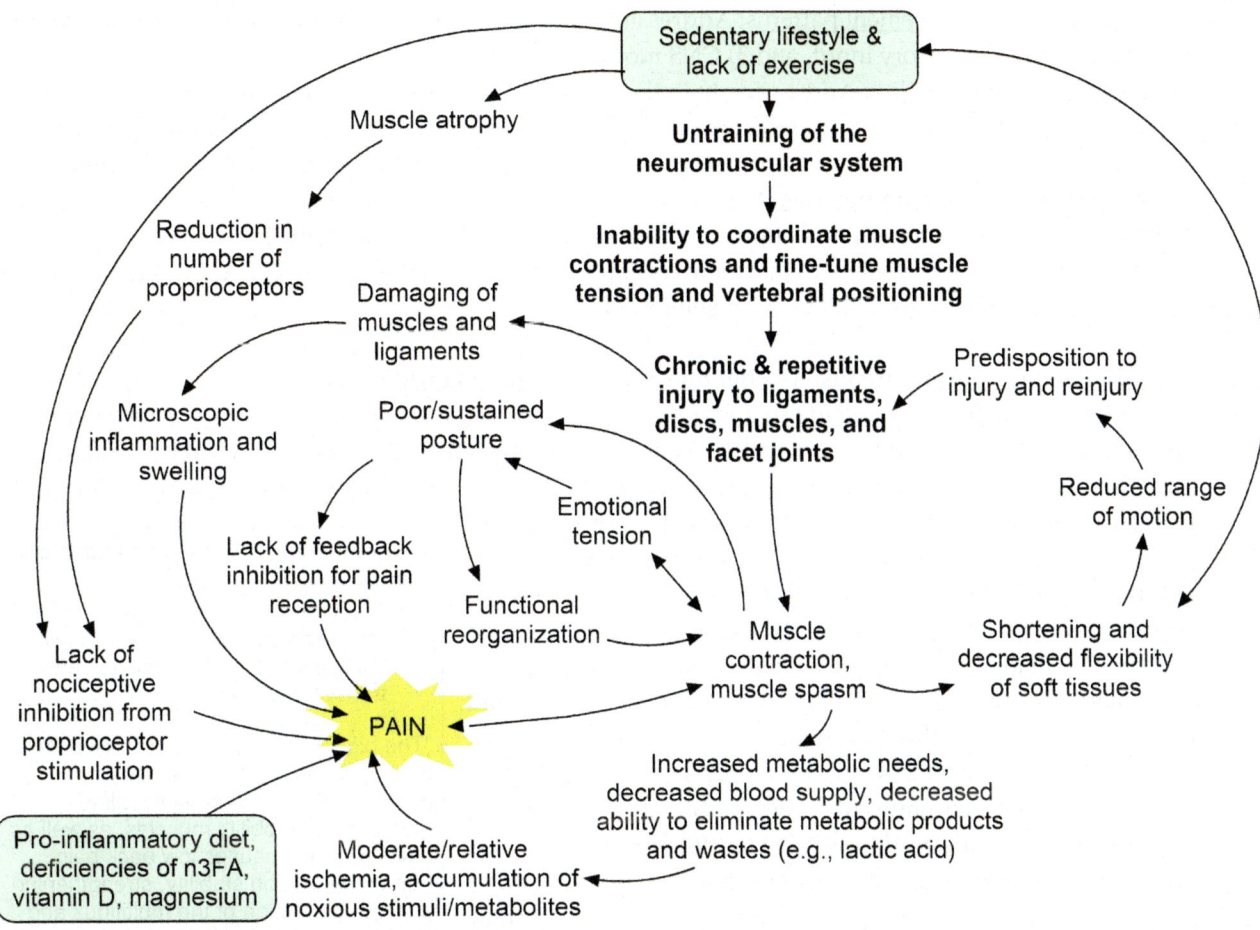

<u>Processed pro-inflammatory nutrient-poor diet and sedentary lifestyle contribute to the genesis and perpetuation of painful musculoskeletal problems</u>: Many people have undernourished (nutritional deficiencies promote pain) overfed (carbohydrates promote inflammation) bodies with weak muscles (lack of exercise) and an untrained (lack of coordination due to sitting nearly motionless most of the day) nervous system.

Proprioceptive deficits are common in patients with chronic low-back pain[371], neck pain[372], knee pain and arthritis[373], and ankle instability.[374] Not only does poor proprioception leave joints vulnerable to recurrent microtrauma, but also lack of proprioceptive inhibition of nociceptors negates the proposed "gate-control" mechanism of pain inhibition and thus opens the door to the perception of chronic pain.[375] Thus, **proprioceptive deficits both increase**

---

[371] Newcomer KL, et al. Muscle activation patterns in subjects with and without low back pain. *Arch Phys Med Rehabil*. 2002;83(6):816-21

[372] McPartland JM, Brodeur RR, Hallgren RC. Chronic neck pain, standing balance, and suboccipital muscle atrophy. *J Manipulative Physiol Ther*. 1997 Jan;20(1):24-9

[373] Callaghan MJ, Selfe J, Bagley PJ, Oldham JA. The Effects of Patellar Taping on Knee Joint Proprioception. *J Athl Train*. 2002 Mar;37(1):19-24

[374] Olmsted LC, et al. Efficacy of the Star Excursion Balance Tests in Detecting Reach Deficits in Subjects with Chronic Ankle Instability. *J Athl Train*. 2002 Dec;37(4):501-506

[375] "The lack of proprioceptive inhibition of nociceptors at the dorsal horn of the spinal cord would result in chronic pain and a loss of standing balance." McPartland JM, Brodeur RR, Hallgren RC. Chronic neck pain, standing balance, and suboccipital muscle atrophy--a pilot study. *J Manipulative Physiol Ther*. 1997 Jan;20(1):24-9

joint injury and increase pain perception. Chronic pain may lead to functional reorganization in the central nervous system and self-perpetuate pain as "pain memories"[376] — rewiring of the nervous system to maintain pain.

An important component to injury rehabilitation and prevention is proprioceptive retraining.[377] Proprioceptive retraining programs have been shown to reduce the severity of pain and the occurrence and recurrence of injuries. With the simple investment of a few minutes per day, patients and athletes can retrain their nervous systems to respond more quickly and to increase the accuracy of proprioception. Muscle-strengthening rehabilitative programs that fail to address proprioceptive retraining do not result in improved neuromuscular coordination as evaluated by electromyography.[378] Furthermore, muscle-strengthening programs may actually lead to a reduction in postural stability when compared to balance training.[379] The **physical medicine portion** of musculoskeletal rehabilitative programs should generally include:

- <u>Correction of faulty movement patterns</u>: Addressing each of the three major components: 1) initial posture, 2) quality of somatosensory input, and 3) CNS motor programs,
- <u>Promotion of spinal stability</u>: Addressing both the *active* and the *passive* components,
- <u>Proprioceptive/sensorimotor training</u>: Target the neck, torso, lumbar spine, pelvis, and lower extremity,
- <u>Strengthening exercises</u>: Strengthen the neck, shoulders, back, legs, and abdominal and oblique muscles,
- <u>Myofascial and spinal manipulative therapy</u>: Use manual medicine to alleviate pain, facilitate and effect proprioceptive/sensorimotor restoration, and promote optimal joint biomechanics.

A very comprehensive and dense review of this topic was published by Murphy[380] in 2000, and this article is highly recommended for practitioners specializing in rehabilitation.

Clinical techniques for proprioceptive/sensorimotor retraining and rehabilitation:

- <u>Wobble board, balance shoes, standing foam, exercise ball, or other labile support surface</u>: At the very least, patients should be advised to use a wobble board, balance board, balance shoes or exercise sandals for *at least* 5 minutes 2 times per day every day of the week. Exercise sandals appear to be highly efficient for increasing muscular activity in the lower leg and ankle.[381] Sedentary patients can easily integrate proprioceptive training into their lives — they can use the wobble board or balance shoes while they are watching television. This easy treatment has been shown to facilitate rapid subconscious neuromuscular coordination of the gluteal muscles, thus enhancing pelvic and low-back stability.[382] Other techniques include standing on thick foam or walking in thick sand, which are labile surfaces that require increased neuromuscular control. Standing on one leg and performing gentle motions while blindfolded or with closed eyes further challenges *and therefore improves* the coordination of proprioceptive input with neuromuscular responsiveness.[383,384,385]

  - o <u>Reflex activation of gluteal muscles in walking (*Spine* 1993 May[386])</u>: In this very important and notably brief report, the authors note that gluteal activation and pelvic stability often are decreased in chronic low-back pain

> **Neuromuscular faults in low back pain**
> ❶ Weak spinal extensors,
> ❷ Weak abdominal muscles,
> ❸ Delayed activation of deep stability muscles especially multifidus and transversus abdominis
>
> "The biggest problem of low back pain is lumbar instability. Unbalanced mobilization order among stability muscles and mobility muscles, as well as muscle length, causes low back pain. ... For lumbar region stability, strengthening and co-contraction of the multifidus and transversus abdominis (TA), which are deep stability muscles, and the erector spinae (ES) and abdominal muscles, which are superficial stabilizer muscles, is required."
>
> Lee et al. *J Phys Ther Sci.* 2014 Jan

---

[376] "Functional reorganisation in both the somatosensory and motor system... In patients with chronic low back pain and fibromyalgia... reorganisational change increases with chronicity; ...cortical reorganisation is correlated with the amount of pain... central alterations may be viewed as pain memories ... influence the processing of both painful and nonpainful input..." Flor H. Cortical reorganisation and chronic pain: implications for rehabilitation. *J Rehabil Med.* 2003 May;(41 Suppl):66-72

[377] Murphy DR. Chiropractic rehabilitation of the cervical spine. *J Manipulative Physiol Ther.* 2000 Jul-Aug; 23(6): 404-8

[378] "Unbalanced electromyographic patterns found in patients with LBP given symmetrical tasks were not affected by rehabilitation treatment." Lu WW, et al. Back muscle contraction patterns of patients with low back pain before and after rehabilitation treatment: an electromyographic evaluation. *J Spinal Disord.* 2001 Aug;14(4):277-82

[379] "RESULTS: After 1 month, back extensor strengthening led to decreased postural stability on hard surface... Balance skill training, however, increased postural stability as indicated by a decreased low-frequency component." Kollmitzer J, Ebenbichler GR, Sabo A, Kerschan K, Bochdansky T. Effects of back extensor strength training versus balance training on postural control. *Med Sci Sports Exerc.* 2000 Oct;32(10):1770-6

[380] Murphy DR. Chiropractic rehabilitation of the cervical spine. *J Manipulative Physiol Ther.* 2000 Jul-Aug;23(6):404-8

[381] Troy Blackburn J, et al. Exercise Sandals Increase Lower Extremity Electromyographic Activity during Functional Activities. *J Athl Train.* 2003 Sep;38(3):198-203

[382] Bullock-Saxton JE, Janda V, Bullock MI. Reflex activation of gluteal muscles in walking. *Spine* 1993 May;18(6):704-8

[383] Olmsted LC, et al. Efficacy of the Star Excursion Balance Tests in Detecting Reach Deficits in Subjects with Chronic Ankle Instability. *J Athl Train.* 2002 Dec;37(4):501-506

[384] Troy Blackburn et al. Exercise Sandals Increase Lower Extremity Electromyographic Activity during Functional Activities. *J Athl Train.* 2003 Sep;38(3):198-203

[385] Willems T, et al. Proprioception and Muscle Strength in Subjects with a History of Ankle Sprains and Chronic Instability. *J Athl Train.* 2002 Dec;37(4):487-493

[386] Bullock-Saxton JE, Janda V, Bullock MI. Reflex activation of gluteal muscles in walking. *Spine* 1993 May;18(6):704-8

sufferers. "Labile support, through wearing "balance shoes," offered facilitation of cerebellovestibular circuits." With ==one week of treatment== the authors note "Significant increases in ==gluteal activity== and significant decreases in time to 75% maximum contraction, demonstrated the value of sensorimotor elicitation of subconscious and automatic responses in muscles often weakened in back pain sufferers."

○ <u>Combination patterns of proprioceptive neuromuscular facilitation and ball exercise on pain and muscle activity of chronic low back pain patients</u> (*J Phys Ther Sci* 2014 Jan[387]): This study shows that pain measured by the validated visual analog scale (VAS) and muscle electromyographic activity (EMG) were both improved to a greater extent in patients using proprioceptive neuromuscular facilitation (PNF). ==The alleviation of low back pain with proprioceptive training proves the causative relationship between proprioceptive loss and low back pain and—perhaps even more importantly—the therapeutic value of proprioceptive rehabilitation for alleviation of back pain.== "VAS and EMG activity were significantly reduced in the PNF combination pattern group and the ball exercise group. A comparison of the groups showed significant differences. In VAS and EMG activity; in particular, the combination pattern group using PNF increased EMG activity more than the ball exercise group did after six weeks of intervention.

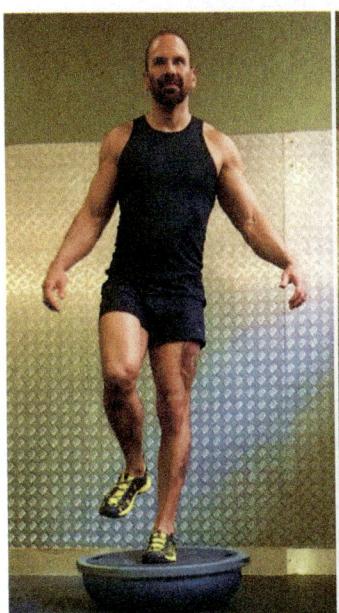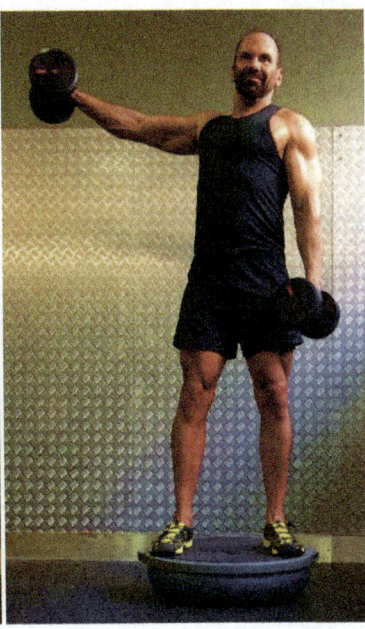

Wobble board (and other labile surface) variations
<u>Foot variations:</u> • Two feet wide, two feet narrow • One foot centered, other leg for balance **pictured** • One food centered, other leg moving in controlled pattern in all directions, e.g., star pattern • One foot centered, other leg moving somewhat randomly, i.e., dancing to music <u>Arm variations:</u> • Arms for balance • Arms moving in symmetry • Arms moving differently, randomly, e.g., dance • Arms lifting weights: biceps curl, lateral raises for deltoids and shoulders (single-sided **pictured** and double-sided) <u>Eye variations:</u> • Open or closed; closed eyes forces greater/exclusive reliance on proprioceptive input <u>Posture:</u> • As perfect as possible while retraining the nervous system to improved posture **not pictured**

<u>Proprioceptive rehabilitation—demonstration of use of wobble-board for single-leg empty-arm exercise and double-leg weight-lifting (single-side lateral raises for deltoids and shoulders)</u>: These pictured examples show the simple implementation of proprioceptive retraining, which is generally the simple implementation of proprioceptive/cerebellar challenge to enhance neuromuscular coordination. The effect (enhanced neuromuscular coordination) is rapid (occurring within 3 sessions of 5 minutes each) and the results (alleviation of pain) are clinically significant. For most purposes, wobble boards and other labile surfaces can be made from items purchased locally or found in-house. The brief original video is available online: vimeo.com/drvasquez/proprioceptive1

- <u>Spinal manipulation</u>: Spinal manipulation appears to improve proprioceptive function.[388]
- <u>Barefoot exercise</u>: Barefoot exercise increases proprioceptive input and helps alleviate back pain.[389]
- <u>Vigorous full-body exercise of any and all types</u>, especially those that are relatively fast and require high-frequency complex neuromuscular responses, such as:

---

[387] Lee CW et al. The effects of combination patterns of proprioceptive neuromuscular facilitation and ball exercise on pain and muscle activity of chronic low back pain patients. *J Phys Ther Sci.* 2014 Jan;26(1):93-6

[388] "RESULTS: Subjects receiving manipulation demonstrated a mean reduction in visual analogue scores of 44%, along with a 41% improvement in mean scores for the head repositioning skill." Rogers RG. The effects of spinal manipulation on cervical kinesthesia in patients with chronic neck pain. *J Manipulative Physiol Ther* 1997 Feb;20(2):80-5

[389] Bullock-Saxton JE, Janda V, Bullock MI. Reflex activation of gluteal muscles in walking. *Spine* 1993 May;18(6):704-8

- o <u>Swimming</u>: Excellent for promoting fitness in a way that is generally easy on joints and muscles and is without impact; requires and thus promotes coordination and timing
- o <u>Indoor aerobics</u>: Excellent for cardiovascular fitness and weight loss, requires and thus promotes coordination and timing
- o <u>Outdoor cycling (road)</u>: Excellent for cardiovascular fitness and weight loss, easy on the joints; requires and promotes coordination and balance.
- o <u>Outdoor cycling (mountain and trail)</u>: Same as above; requires more balance and coordination than road cycling due to unpredictability of surface; rough surfaces provide flood of afferent stimuli through feet and hands.
- o <u>Hiking</u>: Excellent combination of lower extremity strengthening and aerobics; random and uneven trails provide proprioceptive challenge; helps people get in touch with nature.
- o <u>Yoga, Pilates, Calisthenics</u>: Yoga and calisthenics are ways convenient, can be done alone or with others, do not require expensive equipment, and can be tailored for low-back rehabilitation.[390,391,392]

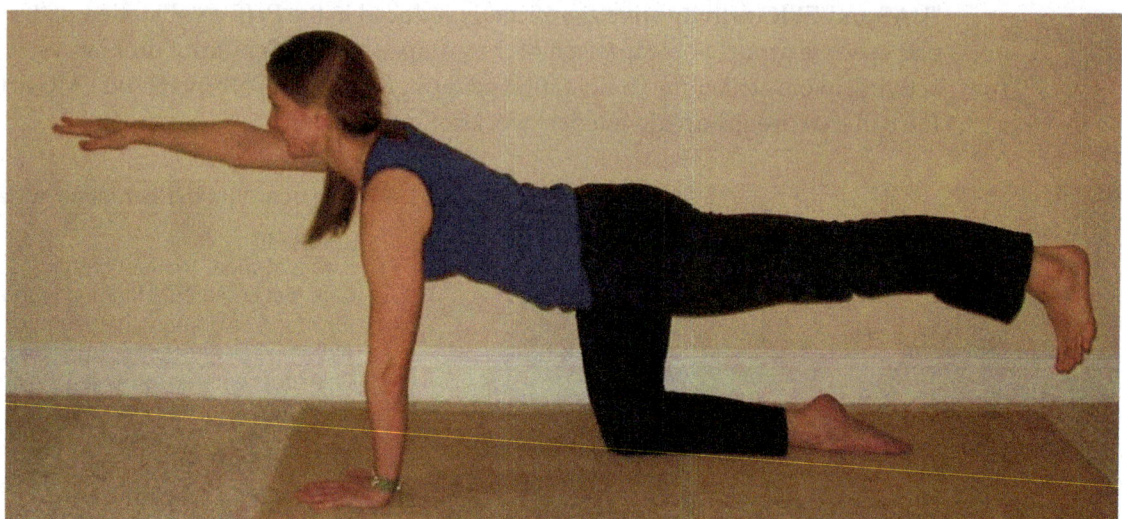

Relaxing, convenient, yoga/calisthenics for improved strength and neuromuscular control: The yoga/calisthenics exercise demonstrated above promotes strengthening of gluteal muscles and spinal extensors; the crossed pattern of (right) arm and (left) leg raising requires much more neuromuscular control than would be required if both hands were being used for stabilization. Repetitions should be repeated until muscular failure is achieved.

> **Correction of vitamin D deficiency improves muscle strength and neuromuscular coordination**
>
> "Vitamin D supplementation, in fallers with vitamin D insufficiency, has a **significant beneficial effect on functional performance, reaction time and balance**... This suggests that **vitamin D supplementation improves neuromuscular or neuroprotective function**, which may in part explain the mechanism whereby vitamin D reduces falls and fractures."
>
> Dhesi et al. *Age Ageing.* 2004 Nov

- <u>Skin taping to increase afferent stimuli</u>: Applying tape to the skin can increase sensory input from cutaneous mechanoreceptors and can improve sensorimotor coordination.[393,394,395,396]
- <u>Vitamin D3</u>: Identification and correction of vitamin D deficiency has been shown to improve muscular strength, alleviate pain, improve neuromuscular coordination, and—in several studies—reduce the incidence of falling and osteoporotic fractures. The increasingly

390 Shiple B. Relieving Low-Back Pain with Exercise. *Physician and Sportsmedicine* 1997; 25: physsportsmed.com/issues/1997/08aug/shiplepa.htm
391 Drezner JA. Exercises in the Treatment of Low- Back Pain. *Physician and Sportsmedicine* 2001; 29: physsportsmed.com/issues/2001/08_01/pa_drezner.htm
392 Kuritzky L, White J. Extend Yourself for Low-Back Pain Relief. *Physician and Sportsmedicine* 1997; 25: physsportsmed.com/issues/1997/01jan/back_pa.htm
393 "This suggests that ankle taping partly corrects impaired proprioception caused by modern athletic footwear and exercise." Robbins S, Waked E, Rappel R. Ankle taping improves proprioception before and after exercise in young men. *Br J Sports Med.* 1995 Dec;29(4):242-7
394 "We concluded that increased cutaneous sensory feedback provided by strips of athletic tape applied across the ankle joint of healthy individuals can help improve ankle joint position perception in nonweightbearing, especially for a midrange plantar-flexed ankle position." Simoneau GG, Degner RM, Kramper CA, Kittleson KH. Changes in Ankle Joint Proprioception Resulting From Strips of Athletic Tape Applied Over the Skin. *J Athl Train.* 1997 Apr;32(2):141-147 pubmedcentral.nih.gov
395 Callaghan MJ, Selfe J, Bagley PJ, Oldham JA. The Effects of Patellar Taping on Knee Joint Proprioception. *J Athl Train.* 2002 Mar;37(1):19-24 pubmedcentral.nih.gov/
396 "Application of stretch to the skin over VMO via the tape can increase VMO activity, suggesting that cutaneous stimulation may be one mechanism by which patella taping produces a clinical effect." Macgregor et al.Cutaneous stimulation from patella tape causes differential increase in vasti muscle activity in people with patellofemoral pain. *J Orthop Res* 2005;23:351-8

widespread realization that patients with chronic joint pain and recurrent injuries have proprioceptive defects is a paradigm shift of its own right, and it obviously sheds new light on therapy and prevention of musculoskeletal pain and recurrent injuries. **Spinal manipulation, skin taping,** and **specific exercises** have all been shown to improve sensorimotor coordination. Very interestingly, **vitamin D supplementation** also improves sensorimotor coordination and thereby helps prevent falls and subsequent musculoskeletal injuries, particularly in the elderly.[397] Vitamin D3 supplementation helps prevent fractures (especially in elderly patients) by at least three different mechanisms: ❶ Vitamin D3 increases calcium absorption in the gut and helps preserve bone strength, ❷ it improves balance and coordination so that falls are avoided, and ❸ vitamin D further protects bone and defends against osteoporosis via a systemic anti-inflammatory effect that reduces the catabolic effect of inflammation on bone.

- o The clinical importance of vitamin D: a paradigm shift with implications for all healthcare providers (*Altern Ther Health Med* 2004 Sep[398]): "Given the depth and breadth of the peer-reviewed research documenting the frequency and consequences of hypovitaminosis D, failure to diagnose and treat this disorder is ethically questionable and is inconsistent with the delivery of quality, science-based healthcare. ... Until proven otherwise, the balance of the research clearly indicates that oral supplementation in the range of 1,000 IU/day for infants, 2,000 IU/day for children, and 4,000 IU/day for adults is safe and reasonable to meet physiologic requirements, to promote optimal health, and to reduce the risk of several serious diseases. Safety and effectiveness of supplementation are assured by periodic monitoring of serum 25(OH)D and serum calcium."

- o Effects of vitamin D on the musculoskeletal system and the prevention of falls (*J Am Osteopath Assoc* 2012 Jan[399]): "Vitamin D supplementation helps prevent falls not only because of its effect on bone density and the regulation of calcium and phosphate metabolism, but also because of its effect on muscle and nervous system function. ... One study demonstrated that vitamin D supplementation improves muscle strength and postural equilibrium, which may in turn reduce the risk of falling."

---

[397] Dhesi JK, et al. Vitamin D supplementation improves neuromuscular function in older people who fall. *Age Ageing.* 2004 Nov;33(6):589-95
[398] Vasquez A, et al. Clinical importance of vitamin D: paradigm shift with implications for all healthcare providers. *Altern Ther Health Med* 2004 Sep ICHNFM.org/pdf
[399] Fraix M. Role of the musculoskeletal system and the prevention of falls. *J Am Osteopath Assoc.* 2012 Jan;112(1):17-21

Introduction to Injection Therapies: Trigger Points, Anesthetics, Viscous Agents, Prolotherapy

Injection therapies will be detailed and demonstrated in much greater detail in the next edition of *Integrative Orthopedics* (i.e., 4th Edition) and are overviewed here for the sake of introduction; their clinical application requires relevant review of anatomy, pharmacology, and clinical procedures is thus best contextualized in chapters that focus on musculoskeletal regions and specific disorders.

- <u>Trigger point and tender point injections</u>: Muscles can be injected with anesthetic such as lidocaine for pain relief; interestingly, many patients achieve lasting pain relief that extends far beyond the time anticipated by the drug's half-life. Injected normal saline and vitamin B-12 are also used frequently for muscular pain relief.

- <u>Intraarticular injection of anesthetics and viscous agents</u>: This is a particularly gratifying in-office procedure that often provides pain relieve and improved functional status in patients not sufficiently helped by oral and topical pain relievers; while anesthetics and steroids can be injected into any joint (or ligament or muscle for that matter), viscous agents are most specifically used in the knee.

- <u>Prolotherapy (***proliferative therapy***)</u>: "Finally, in 1939, I arrived at the conclusion that relaxation of the articular ligaments was responsible for a considerable number of low back disabilities. I decided to attempt strengthening the ligaments by the injection of a proliferating solution within the fibrous bands to stimulate the production of fibrous tissue. The treatment proved to be satisfactory almost from the beginning, and it was cautiously extended until now articular ligaments of the entire spine and pelvis and some other joints are treated with great satisfaction both to the patient and to me. ... A joint is only as strong as its weakest ligament."[400] Due to its ability to promote proliferation of connective tissue, dextrose prolotherapy may provide benefit for patients with ligamentous laxity and disc degeneration, as demonstrated in studies of patients with back pain, knee pain, and hand osteoarthritis.[401,402,403,404,405]

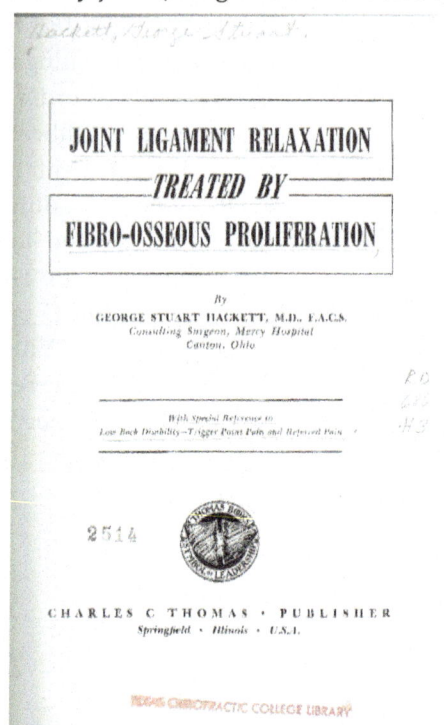

- <u>Intravenous colchicine</u>: Michael Rask MD has been the strongest advocate of the use of intravenous colchicine for the treatment of herniated spinal discs, and his monograph "*Colchicine use in 6,000 patients with disk disease and other related resistantly-painful spinal disorders*"[406] is required reading for any physician interested in using this technique clinically—the details of his protocol are much too extensive to review here, and clinicians will be better served by reading the original article. Notably, as part of the protocol for patients with disc herniation, in addition to intravenous colchicine, Rask advocates 1) treatment of myofascial trigger points, 2) weight loss, 3) cessation of alcohol, tobacco, and caffeine, 4) avoidance of *Solanaceae* plants such as eggplant, potato, tomato, and green and red peppers, 5) avoidance of sugars and junk foods, and 6) a strict vegan diet, especially for patients who are overweight. Although Rask (op cit 1989) notes that colchicine is "extremely effective" and "an exceedingly safe medication", other authors[407] have been less optimistic noting that the benefit was "often of short duration." Given that intravenous colchicine has been

[400] Hackett GS. *Joint Ligament Relaxation Treated by Fibro-Osseous Proliferation*. Springfield Illinois, Charles C Thomas Publishers, 1956

[401] "Prolotherapy injection with 10% dextrose resulted in clinically and statistically significant improvements in knee osteoarthritis. Preliminary blinded radiographic readings (1-year films, with 3-year total follow-up period planned) demonstrated improvement in several measures of osteoarthritis severity. ACL laxity, when present in these osteoarthritic patients, improved." Reeves KD, Hassanein K. Randomized prospective double-blind placebo-controlled study of dextrose prolotherapy for knee osteoarthritis with or without ACL laxity. *Altern Ther Health Med* 2000 Mar;6(2):68-74, 77-80

[402] Mooney V. Prolotherapy at the fringe of medical care, or is it the frontier? *Spine J.* 2003 Jul-Aug;3(4):253-4

[403] This study used intradiscal injection therapy with glucosamine, chondroitin sulfate, hypertonic dextrose and DMSO. "Although the results were statistically significant for the 30 patients as a whole, 17 of the 30 patients (57%) improved markedly with an average of 72% improvement in disability scores and 76% in visual analogue scores. The other 13 patients (43%) had little or no improvement." Klein RG, et al. Biochemical injection treatment for discogenic low back pain: a pilot study. *Spine J.* 2003 May-Jun;3(3):220-6

[404] "Dextrose prolotherapy was clinically effective and safe in the treatment of pain with joint movement and range limitation in osteoarthritic finger joints." Reeves KD, Hassanein K. Randomized, prospective, placebo-controlled double-blind study of dextrose prolotherapy for osteoarthritic thumb and finger (DIP, PIP, and trapeziometacarpal) joints: evidence of clinical efficacy. *J Altern Complement Med.* 2000 Aug;6(4):311-20

[405] "RESULTS: Each patient was injected an average of 3.5 times. Overall, 43.4% of patients fell into the sustained improvement group with an average improvement in numeric pain scores of 71%, comparing pretreatment and 18 month measurements." Miller MR, Mathews RS, Reeves KD. Treatment of painful advanced internal lumbar disc derangement with intradiscal injection of hypertonic dextrose. *Pain Physician.* 2006 Apr;9(2):115-21 painphysicianjournal.com/linkout_vw.php?issn=1533-3159&vol=9&page=115

[406] Rask MR. Colchicine use in 6,000 patients with disk disease and other related resistantly-painful spinal disorders. *J Neurological Orthopaedic Med Surgery* 1989; 10: 291-298

[407] "Results indicate a significant difference between the two groups, the intravenous colchicine group showing improvement in symptoms for a few hours or days over a 3-week course of treatment. However, the relief was often of short duration." Simmons et al. Intravenous colchicine for low back pain: a double-blind study. *Spine.* 1990 Jul;15(7):716-7

associated with complications such as pancytopenia, organ failure, and death[408], it is not a treatment to be taken lightly nor should inexperienced physicians administer it. Colchicine can be administered orally, but its low therapeutic efficacy in relation to its moderate gastrointestinal toxicity limits its applicability. In a poorly designed study by Schnebel and Simmons[409], orally administered colchicine was no better yet was more toxic than placebo; this study appears to have been designed specifically to show inefficacy and toxicity of colchicine since the patients were either given *no treatment* alternating with a *gastroirritative toxic dose* of colchicine.

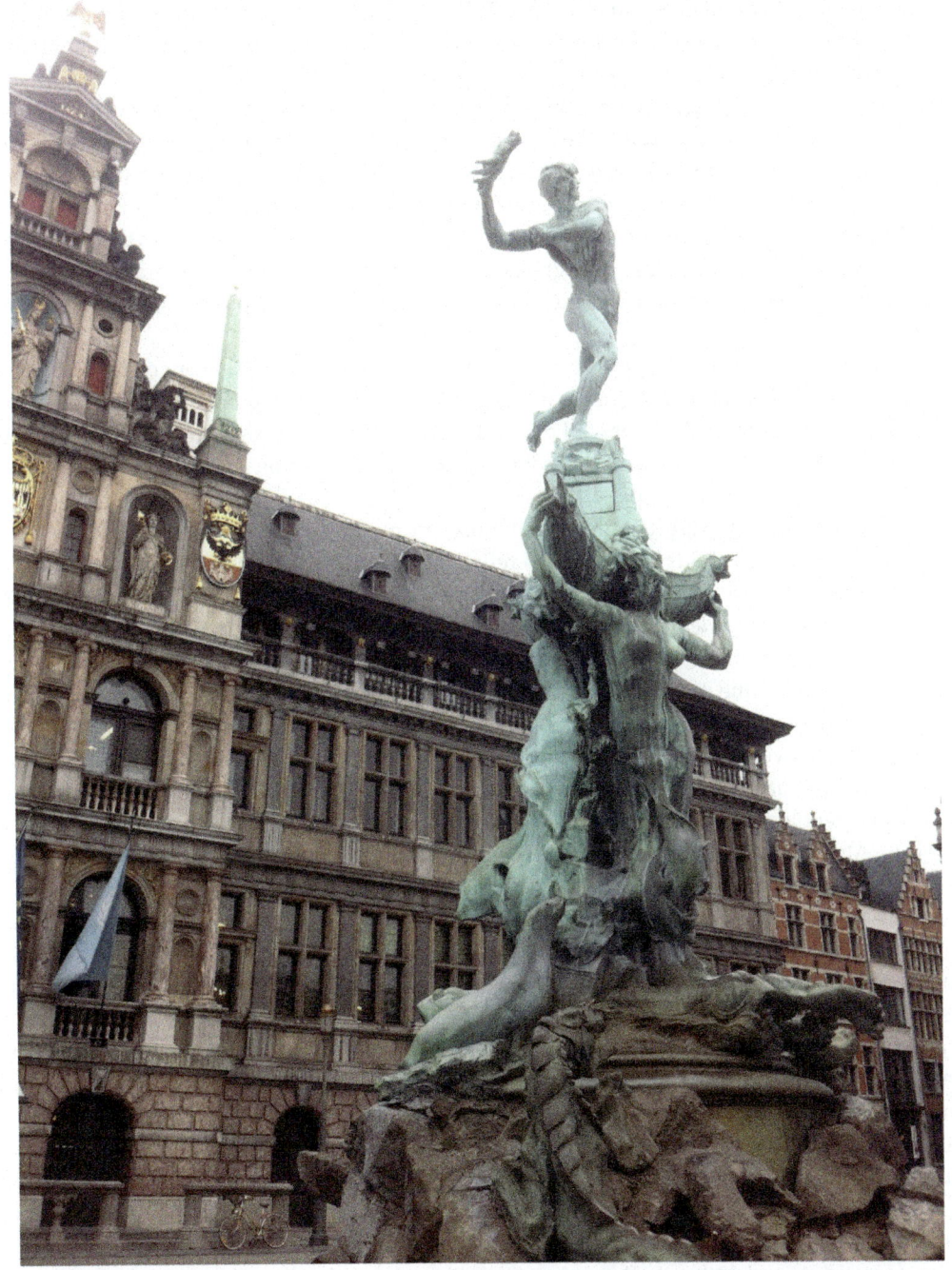

Statue of Silvius Brabo, a mythical Roman soldier who is said to have killed a giant and thrown his hand into the river, hence the name of the city Antwerp, which translates to "hand throwing." Photo at Antwerp City Hall, Belgium 2012 by DrV.

---

[408] "Bone marrow depression has been reported, primarily in cases of acute colchicine intoxication, and intravenous administration of the drug has been associated with severe pancytopenia and death." Levy M, Spino M, Read SE. Colchicine: a state-of-the-art review. *Pharmacotherapy*. 1991;11(3):196-211
[409] Schnebel BE, Simmons JW. The use of oral colchicine for low back pain. A double-blind study. *Spine*. 1988 Mar;13(3):354-7 Use of colchicine in this study varied from abstinence for 3 days followed by a toxic dose on day 4; therefore patients in the treatment group were subjected to no treatment for 75% of the time, followed by a dose that caused gastrointestinal toxicity—vomiting and diarrhea—the other 25% of the time. At neither phase of the study were patients exposed to a treatment that had any possibility of being effective in relation to the potential toxicity. This study was so poorly designed that its publication brings into question the editorial quality of *Spine* during this era.

Another Clinically Useful Acronym: "B.e.n.d. S.t.e.m.s."

"B.e.n.d. s.t.e.m.s." is aesthetically more appealing than the previously mentioned "p.r.i.c.e. a. t.u.r.n." acronym, though it is less complete. The goal, of course, is to have a useful memory key available when formulating the treatment plan. Just as all doctors are familiar with the *s.o.a.p.* format for writing chart notes to ensure their inclusion of *subjective, objective, assessment,* and *plan* for each visit, when arriving to the "p" portion of the note, integrative clinicians can use *price a turn* and/or *bend stems* to help remember key components to integrative and holistic care.

B **Botanical**: Numerous botanical medicines are available for a wide range of indications. Among the botanical medicines with the best research support for the treatment of musculoskeletal pain and inflammation are willow bark, *Boswellia, Harpagophytum, Uncaria,* ginger, and *Capsicum.*

E **Ergonomics/posture and Exercise**: Patients can improve their ergonomics at home, at work, and (occasionally) in the car. Likewise, attention to posture—the "style" with which one holds one's body—is important in the prevention of repetitive strain injuries, particularly to the shoulders and neck region. Most patients are overweight, out of shape, weak, and neuromuscularly uncoordinated; problems correctible with exercise.

N **Nutrition**: Nutritional supplements are extremely valuable in the treatment and prevention of a wide range of mild and serious health problems. Use of high-dose "supranutritional" levels of vitamins can be used to help patients overcome their enzyme and receptor defects to facilitate improved physiological function and improved overall health.[410]

D **Diet**: In order to remain consistent with the time-proven wisdom of the *Hierarchy of Therapeutics* (discussed in Chapter 2) and to avoid becoming an aimless horde of drug-pushing symptom-suppressors, holistic integrative clinicians must always attend to the basics—the foundational influences which powerfully affect metabolism and thus overall health. Clearly, diet is one of those basics, along with emotions and lifestyle—exercise, work, stress management, outlook, and relationships.

S **Stretching, strengthening, and stabilization**: Tight muscles can be stretched in the office, where the doctor is able to teach the patient proper methods and is able to refine the diagnosis and specificity of the stretch to ensure that targeted muscles are effectively addressed. Thereafter, the patient *must* continue these stretches at home—both physically and mentally. *Physical stretching* involves the therapeutic lengthening of muscles and fascia to maintain or restore ease of myofascial motion and to alleviate adhesions or restrictions that impair function. *Mental stretching* involves the patient's active use of reframing and discipline in order to attain a higher level of functioning and effectiveness in his/her relationships, lifestyle, work situation, mental outlook, habits and other phenomena in order to overcome the external or internal *adhesions* or *restrictions* that are impairing and preventing optimal function *of the patient as a whole*. Exercise and proproceptive rehabilitation for spinal and peripheral joint stabilization are essential requirements for neuromusculoskeletal health.

T **Trigger points**: Always remember to address the trigger point component (discussed previously in this chapter) when working with musculoskeletal pain. Seek and ye shall find; treat and the patient will improve. Think outside the region. A trigger point in the low-back or gluteal region may cause the patient to assume an antalgic posture that results in altered biomechanics and leads to a clinical presentation of shoulder or neck pain with chronic tension headaches; direct treatment of the painful shoulders or neck will provide improvement, but cure will not be effected until the cause—often distant from the region of complaint—is effectively addressed.[411]

E **Educate and Ensure return**: Educate the patient about the condition, its cause and solutions. Educate about PAR-B—procedures, risks, alternatives, and benefits of treatment. Also, educate the patient *in writing* about the importance of follow-up visits and time limitations on treatments; failure to ensure that the patient was educated to return for follow-up visits is grounds for malpractice if the patient's condition changes or deteriorates due to complications associated with the presenting complaint at the last office visit.

M **Manual medicine—mobilization, manipulation, massage**: Treat the problem effectively and directly with the skilled use of your hands. Practice produces proficiency.

S **Spirituality (emotions, psychology)**: Perceptions create our emotional and mental realities, and from these subjective realities do we engage the world. Inaccurate perceptions skew and misshape one's interactions with the world. Creating more accurate perceptions—a process that requires intentionality and hard work—enhances *effectiveness* and ultimately *enjoyment* of one's life experience.

---

[410] Ames BN, Elson-Schwab I, Silver EA. High-dose vitamin therapy stimulates variant enzymes. *Am J Clin Nutr.* 2002 Apr;75(4):616-58 ajcn.org/cgi/content/full/75/4/616
[411] "This patient seemed to respond favorably to conservative care that included regions of spine not traditionally associated with headache pain." Stude DE, Sweere JJ. A holistic approach to severe headache symptoms in a patient unresponsive to regional manual therapy. *J Manipulative Physiol Ther.* 1996 Mar-Apr;19(3):202-7

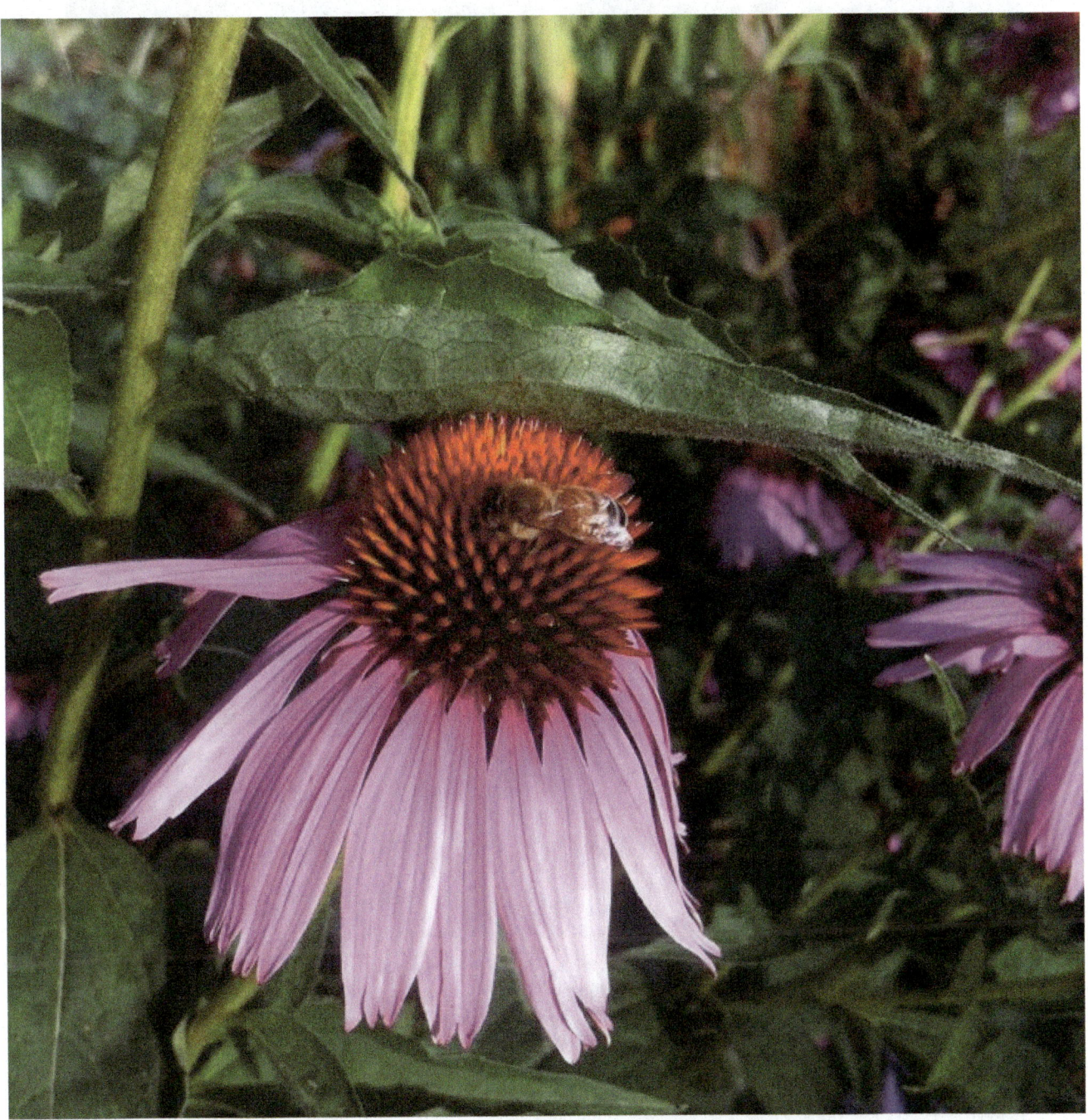

Purple coneflower (*Echinacea purpurea*) with honey bee (*Apis* genus): Portland Oregon 2011, photo by DrV

Progressive awakening

"**Only that day dawns to which we are awake.**"

Henry David Thoreau, *Walden*[412]

"In virtually all of the great spiritual and philosophical traditions of the world there appears some form of the idea that most human beings are sleepwalking through their own existence. **Enlightenment is identified with waking up.** Evolution and progress are identified with an expansion of consciousness."

Nathaniel Branden, *Six Pillars of Self-Esteem*[413]

"**And once you are awake, then shall you ever remain awake.**"

Friedrich Nietzsche, *Thus Spoke Zarathustra*[414]

---

[412] Thoreau HD. (Owen Thomas, Ed). *Walden and Civil Disobedience*. New York; WW Norton and Company: 1966, page 221
[413] Nathaniel Branden *The Six Pillars of Self-Esteem*, p. 67
[414] Nietzsche FW. *Thus Spoke Zarathustra*.

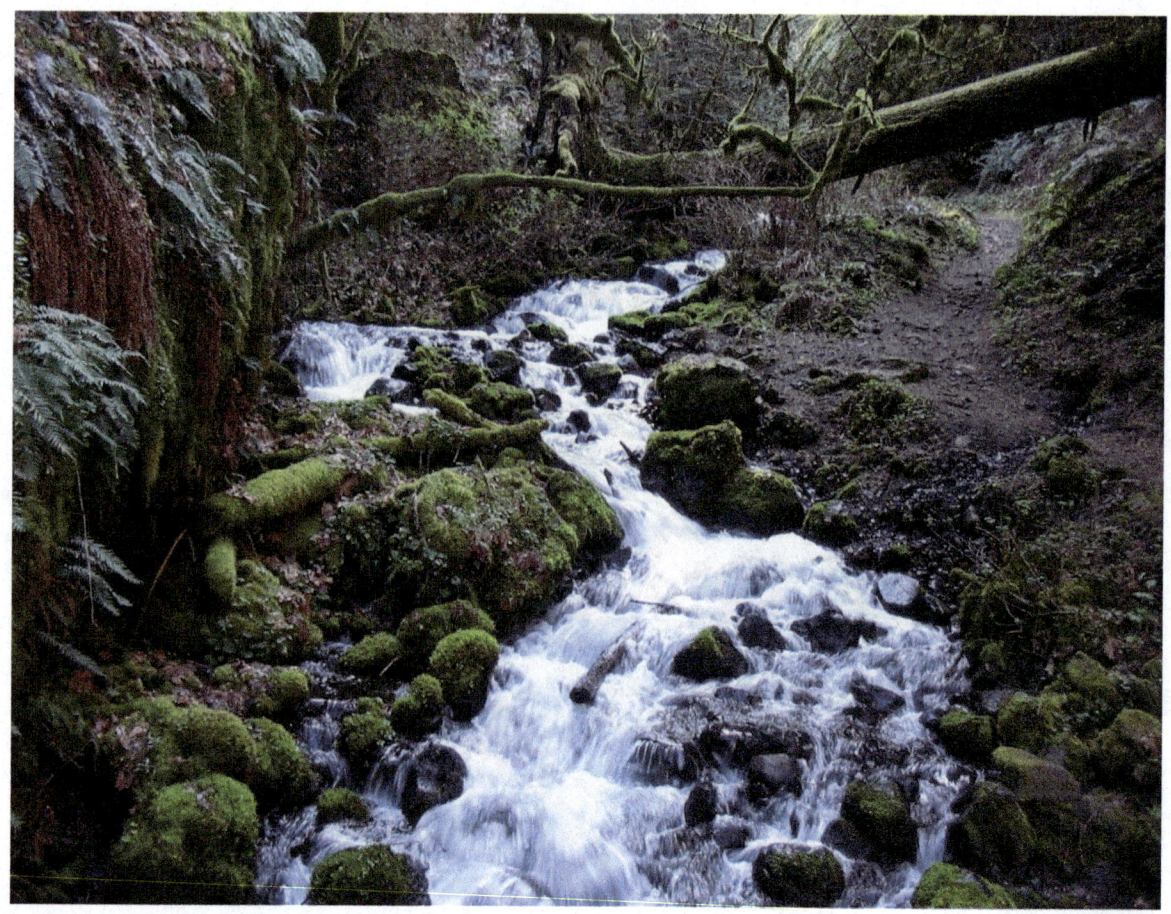

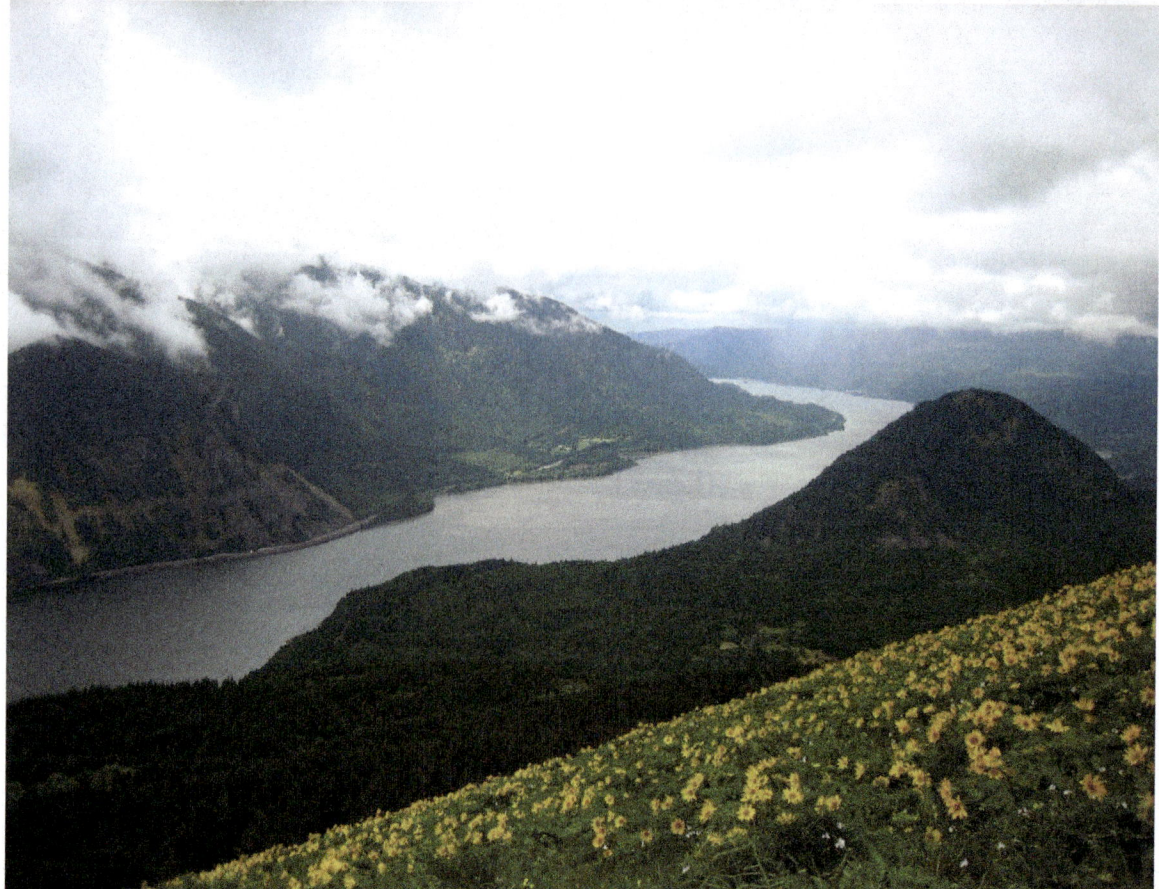

<u>Columbia River Gorge</u>: Wahkeena Falls, Oregon *above*, Dog Mountain, Washington *below*. Photos DrV

Chapter 4:

Introduction to DrV's Functional Inflammology Protocol: The Seven Major Modifiable Factors in Systemic Inflammation, Allergy, and Autoimmunity

---

Major Modifiable Influences on Immune and Inflammatory Balance

This section reviews clinically-relevant information related to the pathogenesis and etiology of inflammatory/allergic/autoimmune conditions. Following extensive reviews of the research literature in conjunction with the author's impressively successful clinical experience with patients with "idiopathic" and inflammatory/autoimmune disorders, the original version of this information was published in the first edition of *Integrative Rheumatology* (2006). This section is a distillation of thousands of research articles, abstracts, seminar notes, conversations with colleagues, one-on-one patient encounters and the author's own considerations and reflections.

Following my review and perusal of thousands of research articles in addition to the attentive application of my interest in these conditions throughout three doctoral programs, I have come to appreciate seven major modifiable factors that are chiefly relevant for the initial and long-term management of patients with inflammatory conditions and rheumatic diseases. These 7 factors are:

1. <u>Food intake and nutritional status</u>: The pro/anti-inflammatory effects of diet, including food allergies and intolerances, nutrient deficiencies and dependencies,
2. <u>Infections and dysbiosis</u>: Chronic exposure to microbial effectors/effects,
3. <u>Nutritional modulation of the immune system</u>: Nutrigenomic modification of immunocyte phenotype,
4. <u>Dysmetabolism and Dysfunctional organelles, most notably mitochondria</u>: Especially the pro-inflammatory, pro-oxidant, and anti-apoptotic consequences of dysfunctional mitochondria (DysMito or MitoDys); more recently the conversation has extended beyond mitochondrial dysfunction to include endoplasmic reticulum stress/dysfunction (ERS) and resultant unfolded protein response (UPR),
5. <u>Stress, sleep deprivation vs sleep sufficiency, spinal health, social and psychological considerations</u>: Included in this section is a collection of important considerations which—in the first draft of this acronym—started with stress management, sleep hygiene, and pSychological and social factors. Later versions have included spinal health (chiropractic model), somatic dysfunction (osteopathic model), surgery, specialized supplementation, and "stamp your passport"—sometimes we all just need to vacate for a while and implement some *geographic cure* for the sake of inspiration, life enhancement, exposure to new ideas and lifestyles, and the breaking of (dysfunctional) thought patterns and routines,
6. <u>Endocrine imbalances</u>: Hormones can promote or retard the genesis and perpetuation of inflammation/allergy/autoimmunity; therapeutic correction with prescription or nonprescription interventions can have a profound anti-inflammatory benefit.
7. <u>Xenobiotic immunotoxicity</u>: Exposure to and accumulation of toxic chemicals and/or toxic metals can alter immune responses toward allergy and autoimmunity and away from immunosurveillance against infections and cancer.

Common diseases such as psoriasis and rheumatoid arthritis are greater public health concerns and are more commonly encountered in clinical practice than are the more rare conditions; proportionate mention is made in the following section. Importantly, readers should appreciate that the information in various sections likely applies either conceptually or specifically to conditions described in other sections and that therefore the best way to understand inflammatory/allergic/autoimmune disorders in their totality is to appreciate the nuances of each and the common themes among all.

I am quite pleased to see that the original five variables that I defined in the first two editions of *Integrative Rheumatology* (2006, 2007) have stood the tests of time, science, and clinical practice: in fact, all have been strengthened in the intervening years.

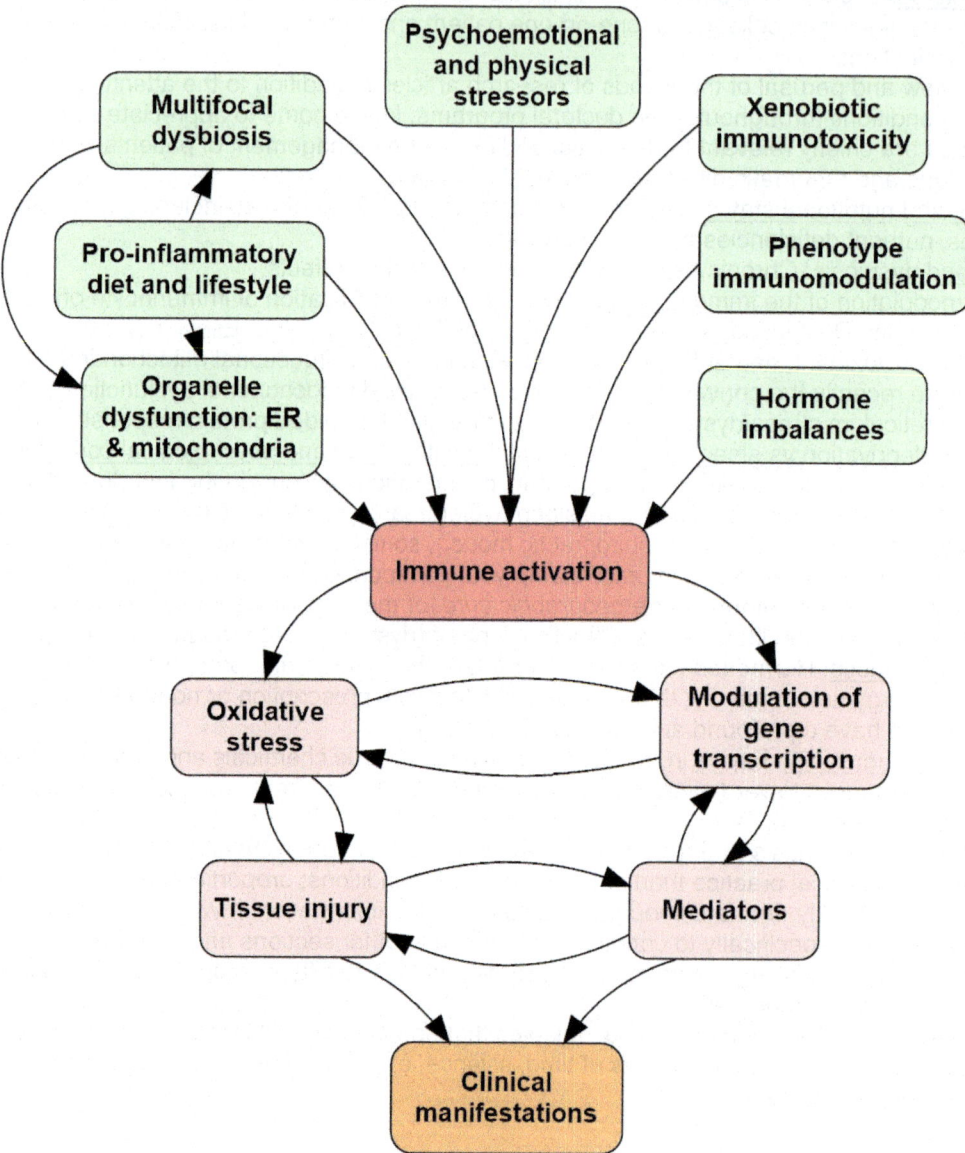

Inflammation in a simple cause-and-effect diagram: The major causative factors amenable to clinical implementation are represented, along with the pathophysiologic consequences and clinical effects. Molecular details, clinical assessments, and therapeutic interventions are introduced/reviewed in this chapter; in later volumes of this work, clinical protocols detail the drugs and doses, etc.

Nutrition & FxMed for chronic immune-inflammatory disorders

Causes of Inflammation-Immune-Metabolic Imbalance:

1. Food, Lifestyle

2. Infection, Dysbiosis

3. Nutritional Immunomodulation

4. Dysfunctional mitochondria

5. Stress, Emotions, Psychology, Sociology, Lifestyle

6. Endocrine, Hormones

7. Xenobiotics, Toxins

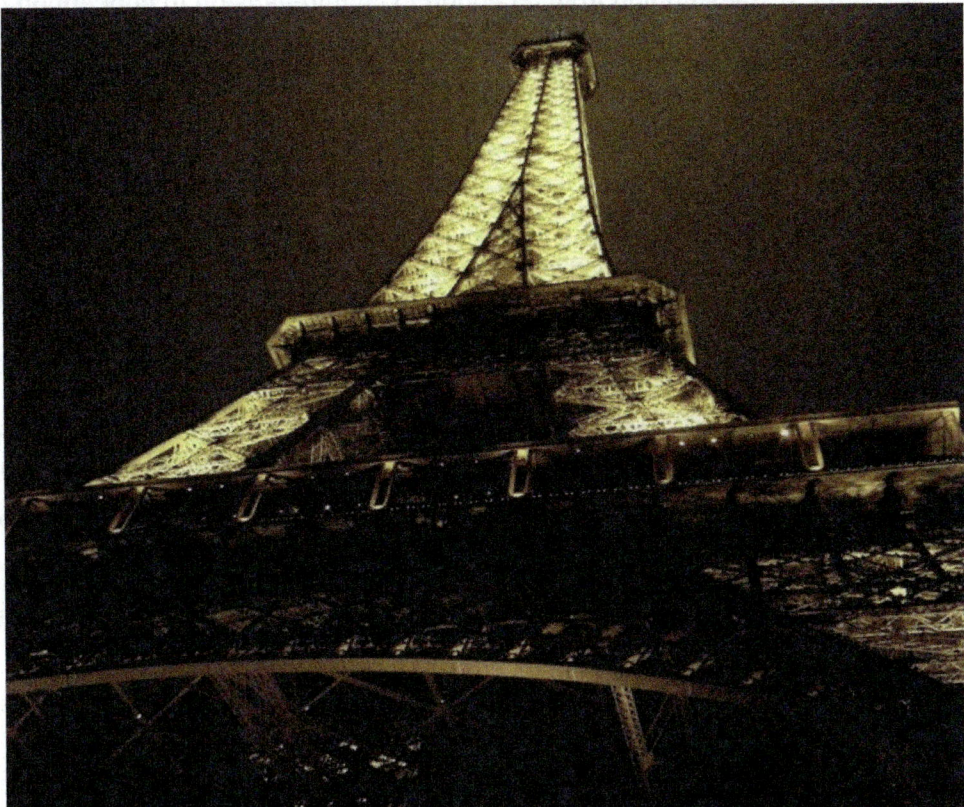

Notice that these 7 factors can be remembered by the acronym: **F.I.N.D. S.E.X.**

♥ First presented in Paris in 2012 ♥

The "Functional Inflammology Protocol" and FINDSEX® acronym: As the clinical protocol expanded from five components (diet, dysbiosis, xenobiotics, hormones, and stress) published in 2006 and 2007 to seven components (adding nutritional immunomodulation and mitochondrial dysfunction) in 2012, I realized that the time had come to attempt an acronym in order to facilitate student memorization and clinician application. I applied some priority to the sequence of the categories, and then experimented with a few acronyms. The rest, as is said, is history. This occurred just before a series of presentations in France (starting in Paris), Holland, and Belgium in March of 2012. The FINDSEX acronym is a registered trademark (e.g., ® and ™) in association with *Functional Immunology and Nutritional Immunomodulation*[1], *F.I.N.D.S.E.X. The Easily Remembered Acronym for the Functional Inflammology Protocol*[2], *Integrative Rheumatology and Inflammation Mastery, Third Edition*[3], and other books, videos[4], audios[5], and presentations by Dr Vasquez since 2012. One of the more recent introductions to this protocol was delivered at the International Conference on Human Nutrition and Functional Medicine in Portland Oregon in September 2013 and is posted here vimeo.com/ichnfm/drv-functional-inflammology-intro2013 and accessed with the password "DrVprotocol"; any changes to passwords, as well as access to new videos, book updates, and articles are periodically distributed by email newsletter from ICHNFM.ORG. Purchasers of this book can attend several hours of video introduction/review of this protocol via the access provided in the links below.[6]

[1] Published Jun 2012, ISBN-10: 1477603859, ISBN-13: 978-1477603857
[2] Published Apr 2013, ISBN-10: 1484046765, ISBN-13: 978-1484046760
[3] Published Jan 2014, ISBN-10: 1495272621, ISBN-13: 978-1495272622
[4] vimeo.com/drvasquez and vimeo.com/ichnfm
[5] itunes.apple.com/us/artist/dr-alex-vasquez/id475526413 and cdbaby.com/Artist/DrAlexVasquez
[6] Vasquez A. "Introduction to Functional Inflammology Protocol" presented at International Conference on Human Nutrition and Functional Medicine in Portland, Oregon September 25-29, 2013. More than eight hours of video introducing the functional inflammology protocol—to be used with the printed slides in the final section of this book—is available online: vimeo.com/album/2943155. Password: **DrVprotocol_volume1**

"The fact that today I still stand by these ideas, **that in the intervening time they themselves have constantly become more strongly associated with one another, even to the point of growing into each other, intertwining, and becoming** *one*, that has reinforced in me the joyful confidence that they may not have originally developed in me as single, random, or sporadic ideas, but up out of common roots, from some fundamental *will for knowledge* ruling from deep within, always speaking with greater clarity, always demanding greater clarity.

In fact, this is the only thing appropriate and proper for a philosopher. **We have no right to be isolated in any way: we are not permitted to make isolated mistakes or to run into isolated truths**. Our ideas, our values, our affirmations and denials, our *if*s and *but*s—these rather grow out of us from the same necessity which makes a tree bear its fruit—totally related and interlinked amongst each other: witnesses of one will, one health, one soil, one sun."

Nietzsche FW. *On the Genealogy of Morals*, 1887, Preface essay #2

"In order for a particular species to maintain itself and increase its power, **its conception of reality must comprehend enough of the calculable and constant** for it to **base a scheme of behavior on it**."

Nietzsche FW. *Will to Power*,1901, #480

Functional Inflammology
F.I.N.D.S.E.X.® acronym

"enough of the calculable and constant to base a scheme of behavior"

- Infection, dysbiosis
- Nutritional immunomodulation
- Food, Nutrition
- Dysmetabolism, dysfunctional mitochondria
- Style of living (lifestyle): psychology, sociology, politics, sweat/exercise, stress, sleep, special considerations such as surgery
- Xenobiotic load
- Endocrine

© ICHNFM.org

"If this book is incomprehensible to anyone and jars on his ears, the fault, it seems to me, is not necessarily mine. It is clear enough, assuming, as I do assume, that one has first read my earlier writings and has not spared some trouble in doing so: for they are, indeed, not easy to penetrate. Regarding my *Zarathustra*, for example, I do not allow that anyone knows the book who has not at some time been profoundly wounded and at some time profoundly delighted by every word in it; for only then may he enjoy the privilege of reverentially sharing in the halcyon element out of which that book was born and in its sunlight clarity, remoteness, breadth, and certainty. In other cases, people find difficulty with the aphoristic form: this arises from the fact that today this form is not taken seriously enough. An aphorism, properly stamped and molded, has not been "deciphered" when it has simply been read; rather, one has then to begin its exegesis—its explanation, its extraction, for which is required an art of searching, deciphering. To be sure, one thing is necessary above all if one is to practice reading as an art in this way, something that has been unlearned most thoroughly nowadays—something for which one has almost to be a cow and in any case not a "modern man": *rumination*—taking time to pause, to reflect, to consider..."

Friedrich Nietzsche, *On the Genealogy of Morals*, Preface, Section #8
Sils-Maria, Upper Engadine, July 1887

❶ <u>Food</u>: Diet and Basic Nutritional Supplementation

Major Concepts in this Section

"Food" is the first part of the protocol and the foundation of the overall plan, not simply for improving nutritional status, but for setting the biochemical stage for more profound improvements in immune balance, mitochondrial function, et al. Patients can and should appreciate that they have near complete control over what they consume; unfortunately and conversely, however, in countries such as the United States where much of the food supply is contaminated with pesticide residues and genetically manipulated food-type (GMO) products, consuming a health-promoting diet can present unique challenges.

<u>Contents of this section:</u>
1. Introduction to Nutrigenomics: Gene-Expression Effects of Foods and Nutrients
2. Basic Concepts and Practical Applications via Previously Published Articles
   a. A Five-Part Nutritional Wellness Protocol That Produces Consistently Positive Results: Brief Review of Scientific Rationale
   b. Implementing the Five-Part Nutritional Wellness Protocol for the Treatment of Various Health Problems
   c. Common Oversights and Shortcomings in the Study and Implementation of Nutritional Supplementation
   d. Revisiting the Five-Part Nutritional Wellness Protocol: The Supplemented Paleo-Mediterranean Diet
3. Diet Details, Biochemical Concepts, and Clinical Pearls
   a. Macronutrients and "The Big Picture": Protein, Carbohydrates, Lipids, Fiber, pH Balance
   b. Micronutrients and Nutritional Supplementation—Overview and Concepts: Vitamins, Minerals, Combination Fatty Acids, Probiotics
   c. Additional Considerations: GMO (Genetically Manipulated Organisms/Foods) and related toxins, Gluten, Fructose, TLR, AGE/RAGE, food-induced hypothalamic inflammation, GPR-120
4. Additional Details and Mini-Monographs:
   a. The Major Fatty Acids and End-products of Clinical Significance
   b. NFkB and Its Phytonutritional Modulation
   c. Food Allergy and Adverse Food Reactions: A few considerations and perspectives

---

<u>Introduction to Nutrigenomics: Pro-Inflammatory and Anti-Inflammatory Effects of Foods and Nutrients</u>

We must look beyond the nutritional properties of foods to appreciate that dietary patterns and the consumption of specific foods can influence genetic expression and either promote or retard the development of inflammation and related clinical disorders. The purpose of this section is to help clinicians attain a more profound understanding of the value of nutrition and its critical role as a foundational component in the treatment plan of patients with inflammatory disorders. The "correct" diet for the vast majority of patients with inflammatory disorders is the "supplemented Paleo-Mediterranean diet" which I have described in several other publications. The diet is modified for the specific exclusion of allergenic foods; it is implemented on a rotation basis, and it allows for periodic fasting and vegetarianism/veganism. The implementation of health-promoting dietary modifications is an *absolutely mandatory* component of the treatment plan, upon which other treatments depend for their success. The study of how dietary components and nutritional supplements influence genetic expression is referred to as *nutrigenomics* or *nutritional genomics* and has been described as "the next frontier in the postgenomic era."[7] Various nutrients have been shown to modulate genetic expression and thus alter phenotypic manifestations of disease by upregulating or downregulating specific genes, interacting with nuclear receptors, altering hormone receptors, and modifying the influence of transcription factors, such as pro-inflammatory NFkB (NFkB) and the anti-inflammatory peroxisome-proliferator activated receptors (PPARs).[8,9,10,11] **The previous view that nutrients only interact with human physiology at the metabolic/post-transcriptional level must be updated in light of current research showing that nutrients can, in fact, modify human physiology and phenotype at the genetic/pre-transcriptional**

---

[7] Kaput J, Rodriguez RL. Nutritional genomics: the next frontier in the postgenomic era. *Physiol Genomics.* 2004 Jan 15;16(2):166-77. Very important article.
[8] Vamecq J, Latruffe N. Medical significance of peroxisome proliferator-activated receptors. *Lancet.* 1999;354:141-8
[9] Ehrmann et al. Peroxisome proliferator-activated receptors (PPARs) in health and disease. *Biomed Pap Med Fac Univ Palacky Olomouc Czech Repub.* 2002 Dec;146(2):11-4
[10] Kliewer SA, Xu HE, Lambert MH, Willson TM. Peroxisome proliferator-activated receptors: from genes to physiology. *Recent Prog Horm Res.* 2001;56:239-63
[11] Delerive P, Fruchart JC, Staels B. Peroxisome proliferator-activated receptors in inflammation control. *J Endocrinol.* 2001;169(3):453-9

level. Fatty acids and their *eicosanoid, leukotriene,* and *isoprostane* intermediates and end-products modulate genetic expression in several ways. In general, n-3 fatty acids decrease inflammation and promote health while n-6 fatty acids (except for GLA, which is generally health-promoting) increase inflammation, oxidative stress, and the manifestation of disease. Corn oil, probably as a result of its high n-6 LA (linoleic acid) content, rapidly activates NFkB and thus promotes tumor development, atherosclerosis, and elaboration of proinflammatory mediators such as TNFa.[12,13,14] Similarly n-6 arachidonic acid increases production of the free radical *superoxide* approximately 4-fold when added to isolated Kupffer cells *in vitro*. Prostaglandin-E2 is produced from arachidonic acid by cyclooxygenase and increases genetic expression of cyclooxygenase and IL-6; thus, an increase in PG-E2 leads to additive expression of cyclooxygenase, which further increases inflammation and elevates C-reactive protein.[15] Some of the unique health-promoting effects of GLA are nutrigenomically mediated via activation of PPAR-gamma, resultant inhibition of NFkB, and impairment of estrogen receptor function.[16,17] Supplementation with ALA leads to a dramatic reduction of prostaglandin formation in humans[18], and this effect is probably mediated by downregulation of proinflammatory gene transcription, as evidenced by reductions in CRP, IL-6, and serum amyloid A.[19] EPA appears to exert much of its anti-inflammatory benefit by suppressing NFkB activation and thus reducing elaboration of proinflammatory mediators.[20,21] EPA also indirectly modifies gene expression and cell growth by reducing intracellular calcium levels and thus activating protein kinase R which impairs eukaryotic initiation factor-2alpha and inhibits protein synthesis at the level of translation initiation, thereby mediating an anti-cancer benefit.[22] DHA is the precursor to docosatrienes and resolvins which downregulate gene expression for IL-1, inhibit TNFa, and reduce neutrophil entry to sites of inflammation.[23] Oxidized EPA activates PPAR-alpha and thereby suppresses NFkB.[24,25] Other nutrients that inhibit the activation of NFkB include vitamin D[26,27], lipoic acid[28], green tea[29], rosemary[30], grape seed extract[31], resveratrol[32,33], caffeic acid phenethyl ester (CAPE) from bee propolis[34], indole-3-carbinol[35], N-acetyl-L-cysteine[36], selenium[37], and zinc.[38] Therefore, we see that fatty acids and nutrients

[12] Rusyn I, et al. Corn oil rapidly activates nuclear factor-kappaB in hepatic Kupffer cells by oxidant-dependent mechanisms. *Carcinogenesis.* 1999 Nov;20(11):2095-100

[13] Rose DP, et al. Effect of diets containing different levels of linoleic acid on human breast cancer growth and lung metastasis in nude mice. *Cancer Res* 1993;53:4686-90

[14] Dichtl et al. Linoleic acid-stimulated vascular adhesion molecule-1 expression in endothelial cells depends on nuclear factor-kappaB. *Metabolism* 2002;51:327-33

[15] Bagga et al. Differential effects of prostaglandin from n-6 and n-3 polyunsaturated fatty acids on COX-2 expression and IL-6 secretion. *Proc Natl Acad Sci.* 2003 Feb:1751-6.

[16] Menendez JA, Colomer R, Lupu R. Omega-6 polyunsaturated fatty acid gamma-linolenic acid (18:3n-6) is a selective estrogen-response modulator in human breast cancer cells: gamma-linolenic acid antagonizes estrogen receptor-dependent transcriptional activity, transcriptionally represses estrogen receptor expression and synergistically enhances tamoxifen and ICI 182,780 (Faslodex) efficacy in human breast cancer cells. *Int J Cancer.* 2004 May 10;109(6):949-54

[17] Jiang WG, Redfern A, Bryce RP, Mansel RE. Peroxisome proliferator activated receptor-gamma (PPAR-gamma) mediates the action of gamma linolenic acid in breast cancer cells. *Prostaglandins Leukot Essent Fatty Acids.* 2000 Feb;62(2):119-27

[18] Adam O, et al. Effect of alpha-linolenic acid in the human diet on linoleic acid metabolism and prostaglandin biosynthesis. *J Lipid Res.* 1986 Apr;27(4):421-6

[19] Rallidis et al. Dietary alpha-linolenic acid decreases C-reactive protein, serum amyloid A and interleukin-6 in dyslipidaemic patients. *Atherosclerosis.* 2003;167:237-42

[20] Zhao et al. Eicosapentaenoic acid prevents LPS-induced TNF-alpha expression by preventing NFkB activation. *J Am Coll Nutr.* 2004 Feb;23(1):71-8

[21] Mishra et al. Oxidized omega-3 fatty acids inhibit NFkB activation via a PPARalpha-dependent pathway. *Arterioscler Thromb Vasc Biol.* 2004 Sep;24:1621-7

[22] Palakurthi et al. Inhibition of translation initiation mediates the anti-cancer effect of the n-3 polyunsaturated fatty acid EPA. *Cancer Res.* 2000 Jun 1;60(11):2919-25

[23] "These results indicate that DHA is the precursor to potent protective mediators generated via enzymatic oxygenations to novel docosatrienes and 17S series resolvins that each regulate events of interest in inflammation and resolution." Hong S, Gronert K, Devchand PR, Moussignac RL, Serhan CN. Novel docosatrienes and 17S-resolvins generated from docosahexaenoic acid in murine brain, human blood, and glial cells. Autacoids in anti-inflammation. *J Biol Chem.* 2003 Apr 25;278(17):14677-87

[24] Mishra et al. Oxidized omega-3 fatty acids inhibit NFkB activation via a PPARalpha-dependent pathway. *Arterioscler Thromb Vasc Biol.* 2004 Sep;24:1621-7

[25] Delerive P, Fruchart JC, Staels B. Peroxisome proliferator-activated receptors in inflammation control. *J Endocrinol.* 2001;169(3):453-9

[26] "1Alpha,25-dihydroxyvitamin D3 (1,25-(OH)2-D3), the active metabolite of vitamin D, can inhibit NFkB activity in human MRC-5 fibroblasts, targeting DNA binding of NFkB ..." Harant et al. 1Alpha,25-dihydroxyvitamin D3 decreases DNA binding of nuclear factor-kappaB in human fibroblasts. *FEBS Lett.* 1998 Oct 9;436(3):329-34

[27] "Thus, 1,25(OH)2D3 may negatively regulate IL-12 production by downregulation of NF-kB activation and binding to the p40-kB sequence." D'Ambrosio D, et al. Inhibition of IL-12 production by 1,25-dihydroxyvitamin D3. Involvement of NFkB downregulation. *J Clin Invest.* 1998 Jan 1;101(1):252-62

[28] "ALA reduced TNF-alpha-stimulated ICAM-1 expression in a dose-dependent manner, to levels observed in unstimulated cells. Alpha-lipoic acid also reduced NFkB activity in a dose-dependent manner." Lee et al. Alpha-lipoic acid modulates NFkB activity in human monocytic cells by direct interaction with DNA. *Exp Gerontol.* 2002 Jan:401-10

[29] "In conclusion, EGCG is an effective inhibitor of IKK activity. This may explain, at least in part, some of the reported anti-inflammatory and anti-cancer effects of green tea." Yang et al. The green tea polyphenol (-)-epigallocatechin-3-gallate blocks nuclear factor-kappa B activation by inhibiting I kappa B kinase activity in the intestinal epithelial cell line IEC-6. *Mol Pharmacol.* 2001 Sep;60(3):528-33

[30] "These results suggest that carnosol suppresses the NO production and iNOS gene expression by inhibiting NFkB activation, and provide possible mechanisms for its anti-inflammatory and chemopreventive action." Lo AH, Liang YC, Lin-Shiau SY, Ho CT, Lin JK. Carnosol, an antioxidant in rosemary, suppresses inducible nitric oxide synthase through down-regulating nuclear factor-kappaB in mouse macrophages. *Carcinogenesis.* 2002 Jun;23(6):983-91

[31] "Constitutive and TNFalpha-induced NFkB DNA binding activity was inhibited by GSE at doses > or =50 microg/ml and treatments for > or =12 h." Dhanalakshmi et al. Inhibition of NFkB pathway in grape seed extract-induced apoptotic death of human prostate carcinoma DU145 cells. *Int J Oncol.* 2003 Sep;23(3):721-7

[32] "Resveratrol's anticarcinogenic, anti-inflammatory, and growth-modulatory effects may thus be partially ascribed to the inhibition of activation of NFkB and AP-1 and the associated kinases." Manna SK, Mukhopadhyay A, Aggarwal BB. Resveratrol suppresses TNF-induced activation of nuclear transcription factors NF-kappa B, activator protein-1, and apoptosis: potential role of reactive oxygen intermediates and lipid peroxidation. *J Immunol.* 2000 Jun 15;164(12):6509-19

[33] "Both resveratrol and quercetin inhibited NFkB-, AP-1- and CREB-dependent transcription to a greater extent than the glucocorticosteroid, dexamethasone." Donnelly LE, et al. Anti-inflammatory Effects of Resveratrol in Lung Epithelial Cells. *Am J Physiol Lung Cell Mol Physiol.* 2004 Oct;287(4):L774-83

[34] "Caffeic acid phenethyl ester (CAPE) is an anti-inflammatory component of propolis (honeybee resin). CAPE is reportedly a specific inhibitor of nuclear factor-kappaB (NFkB)." Fitzpatrick LR, Wang J, Le T. Caffeic acid phenethyl ester, an inhibitor of nuclear factor-kappaB, attenuates bacterial peptidoglycan polysaccharide-induced colitis in rats. *J Pharmacol Exp Ther.* 2001 Dec;299(3):915-20

[35] Takada Y, Andreeff M, Aggarwal BB. Indole-3-carbinol suppresses NF-{kappa}B and I{kappa}B{alpha} kinase activation causing inhibition of expression of NF-{kappa}B-regulated antiapoptotic and metastatic gene products and enhancement of apoptosis in myeloid and leukemia cells. *Blood.* 2005 Apr 5; [Epub ahead of print]

[36] Paterson RL, Galley HF, Webster NR. The effect of N-acetylcysteine on nuclear factor-kappa B activation, interleukin-6, interleukin-8, and intercellular adhesion molecule-1 expression in patients with sepsis. *Crit Care Med.* 2003 Nov;31(11):2574-8

[37] Faure et al. Selenium supplementation decreases nuclear factor-kappa B activity in blood mononuclear cells from type 2 diabetic patients. *Eur J Clin Invest.* 2004;34(7):475-81

[38] Uzzo et al. Zinc inhibits nuclear factor-kappa B activation and sensitizes prostate cancer cells to cytotoxic agents. *Clin Cancer Res.* 2002;8(11):3579-83

directly affect gene expression by complex and multiple mechanisms, as graphically illustrated in the accompanying diagram, and the synergism and potency of these anti-inflammatory nutraceuticals supports the rationale for the use of nutrition and select botanicals for the safe and effective treatment of inflammatory disorders.

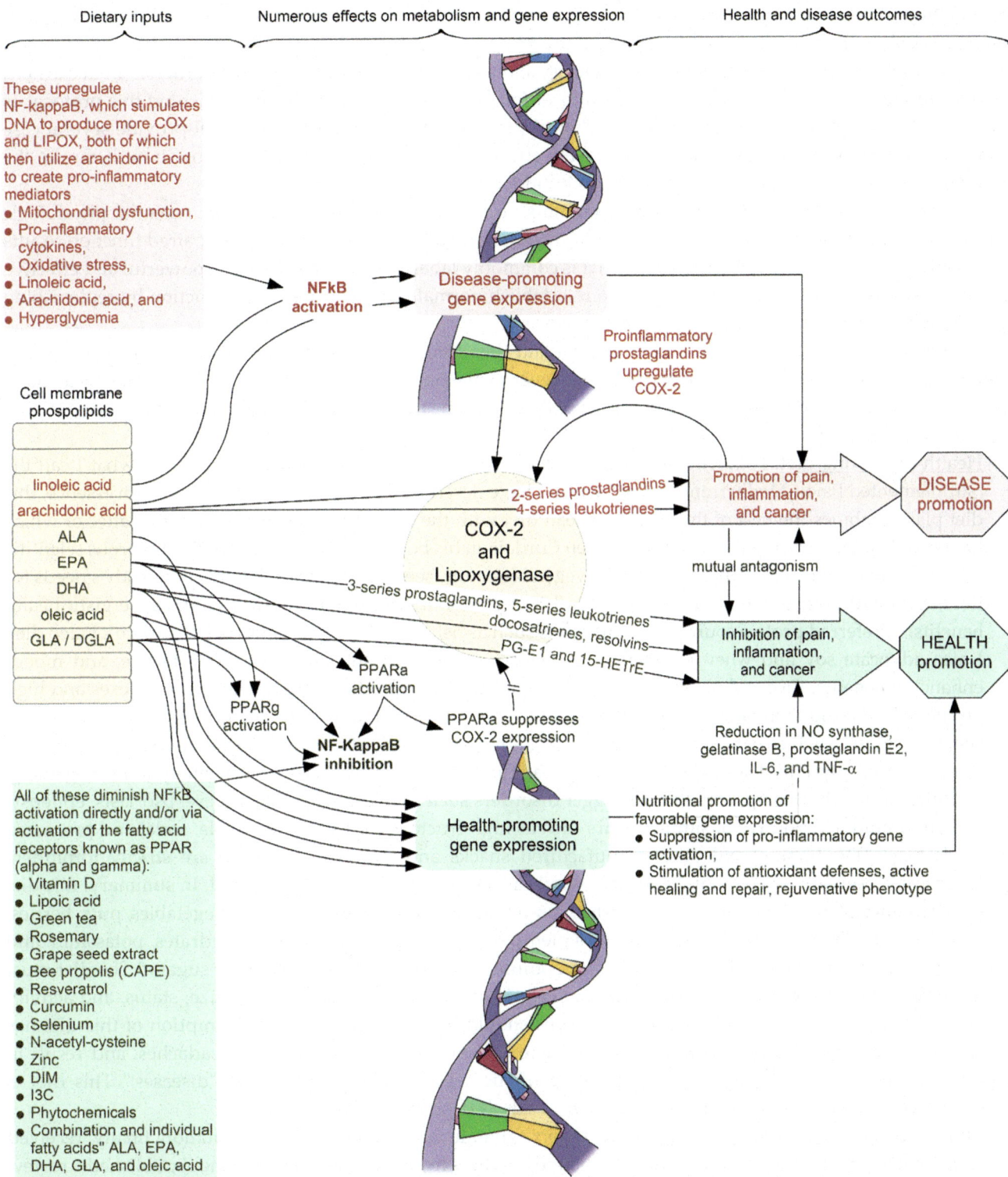

Schematic Representation of Simultaneous Nutrigenomic and Metabolic Effects of Nutrients: Although conceptually accurate, this diagram is highly simplified and not all-inclusive; rather, this diagram focuses exclusively on nutrients that affect the NFkB pathway. Updated from Vasquez 2005.[39]

---

[39] Vasquez A. New Insights into Fatty Acid Supplementation and Its Effect on Eicosanoid Production and Genetic Expression. *Nutritional Perspectives* 2005; Jan: 5-16

A Five-Part Nutritional Wellness Protocol That Produces Consistently Positive Results: Brief Review of Scientific Rationale

This article was originally published in *Nutritional Wellness*
nutritionalwellness.com/archives/2005/sep/09_vasquez.php

Introduction: When I am lecturing here in the U.S., as well as in Europe, doctors often ask if I will share the details of my protocols with them. Thus, in 2004, I published a 486-page textbook for doctors that includes several protocols and important concepts for the promotion of wellness and treatment of musculoskeletal disorders.[40] In this article, I will share with you what I consider a basic protocol for wellness promotion. I've implemented this protocol as part of the treatment plan for a wide range of clinical problems. In my next column, I will provide several case reports of patients from my office to exemplify the effectiveness of this program and show how it can be the foundation upon which additional treatments can be added as necessary.

Nutrients are required in the proper amounts, forms, and approximate ratios for essential physiologic function; if nutrients are lacking, the body cannot function normally, let alone optimally. Impaired function results in subjective and objective manifestations of what is commonly labeled as "disease." Thus, a powerful and effective alternative to treating diseases with drugs is to re-establish normal/optimal physiologic function by replenishing the body with essential nutrients.

Of course, many diseases are multifactorial and therefore require multicomponent treatment plans, and some diseases actually require the use of drugs. However, while only a relatively small portion of patients actually need drugs for their problems, I am sure we all agree that everyone needs a foundational nutrition plan, as outlined and substantiated below.

1. <u>Health-promoting diet</u>: Following an extensive review of the research literature, I developed what I call the "supplemented Paleo-Mediterranean diet," which I have described in greater detail elsewhere.[41] In essence, this diet plan combines the best of the Mediterranean diet with the best of the Paleolithic diet, the latter of which has been detailed and popularized by Dr. Loren Cordain in his book, *The Paleo Diet*, and his numerous scientific articles.[42] This diet places emphasis on fruits, vegetables, nuts, seeds, and berries that meet the body's needs for fiber, carbohydrates, and most importantly, the 8,000+ phytonutrients that have additive and synergistic health benefits.[43] Preferred protein sources are lean meats such as fish and poultry. In contrast to Cordain's Paleo diet, I also advocate soy and whey for their high-quality protein and anticancer, cardioprotective, and mood-enhancing benefits. Rice and potatoes are discouraged due to their relatively high glycemic indexes and high glycemic loads, and their lack of fiber and phytonutrients (compared to other fruits and vegetables). Generally speaking, grains such as barley, rye, and wheat (e.g., the "toxic triad" of inflammatory gluten) are discouraged due to the high glycemic loads/indexes of most breads and pastries, as well as the allergenicity/immunogenicity of gluten, a protein that appears to help trigger disorders such as migraine, celiac disease, psoriasis, epilepsy, and autoimmunity. Sources of simple sugars such as high-fructose corn syrup (e.g., cola, soda) and processed foods (e.g., "TV dinners" and other manufactured snacks and convenience foods) are strictly forbidden. Chemical preservatives, colorants, sweeteners and carrageenan are likewise prohibited. In summary, this diet plan provides plenty of variety, as most dishes comprised of poultry, fish, soy, fruits, vegetables, nuts, berries, and seeds are allowed. The diet also provides plenty of fiber, phytonutrients, carbohydrates, potassium, and protein, while simultaneously being low in fat, sodium, arachidonic acid, and "simple sugars." The diet must be customized with regard to total protein and calorie intake, as determined by the size, status, and activity level of the patient, and individual food allergens should be avoided. Regular consumption of this diet has shown the ability to reduce hypertension, alleviate diabetes, ameliorate migraine headaches, and result in improvement of overall health and a lessening of the severity of many common "diseases." This diet is supplemented with vitamins, minerals, and fatty acids as described below.

2. <u>Multivitamin and multimineral supplementation</u>: Vitamin and mineral supplementation finally received endorsement from "mainstream" medicine when researchers from Harvard Medical School published a review

---

[40] Vasquez A. *Integrative Orthopedics: The Art of Creating Wellness While Managing Acute and Chronic Musculoskeletal Disorders*. 2004, 2007, 2012

[41] Vasquez A. The Importance of Integrative Chiropractic Health Care in Treating Musculoskeletal Pain and Reducing the Nationwide Burden of Medical Expenses and Iatrogenic Injury and Death: Concise Review of Current Research and Implications for Clinical Practice and Healthcare Policy. *The Original Internist* 2005; 12(4): 159-182

[42] Cordain L. *The Paleo Diet*. (John Wiley and Sons, 2002). Also: Cordain L. Cereal grains: humanity's double edged sword. *World Rev Nutr Diet* 1999;84:19-73 Access to most of Dr Cordain's articles is available at thepaleodiet.com/

[43] Liu RH. Health benefits of fruit and vegetables are from additive and synergistic combinations of phytochemicals. *Am J Clin Nutr* 2003;78(3 Suppl):517S-520S

article in *Journal of the American Medical Association* that concluded, "Most people do not consume an optimal amount of all vitamins by diet alone. ...It appears prudent for all adults to take vitamin supplements."[44] Long-term nutritional insufficiencies experienced by the majority of the population promote the development of "long-latency deficiency diseases" such as cancer, neuroemotional deterioration, and cardiovascular disease.[45] Impressively, the benefits of multivitamin/multimineral supplementation have been demonstrated in numerous clinical trials. Multivitamin/multimineral supplementation has been shown to improve nutritional status and reduce the risk for chronic diseases[46], improve mood[47], potentiate antidepressant drug treatment[48], alleviate migraine headaches (when used with diet improvement and fatty acids[49]), improve immune function and infectious disease outcomes in the elderly[50] (especially diabetics[51]), reduce morbidity and mortality in patients with HIV infection[52,53] alleviate premenstrual syndrome[54,55] and bipolar disorder[56], reduce violence and antisocial behavior in children[57] and incarcerated young adults (when used with essential fatty acids[58]), and improve scores of intelligence in children.[59] Vitamin supplementation has anti-inflammatory benefits, as evidenced by significant reduction in C-reactive protein, (CRP) in a double-blind, placebo-controlled trial.[60] The ability to safely and affordably deliver these benefits makes multimineral-multivitamin supplementation and essential component of any and all health-promoting and disease-prevention strategies. Vitamin A can result in liver damage with chronic consumption of 25,000 IU or more, and intake should generally not exceed 10,000 IU per day in women of childbearing age. Iron should not be supplemented except in patients diagnosed with iron deficiency by the blood test ferritin. Additional vitamin D should be used, as described in the next section.

3. <u>Physiologic doses of vitamin D3</u>: The prevalence of vitamin D deficiency varies from 40 percent (general population) to almost 100 percent (patients with musculoskeletal pain) in the American population. I described the many benefits of vitamin D3 supplementation in the previous issue of *Nutritional Wellness* and in the major monograph published in 2004.[61] In summary, vitamin D deficiency causes or contributes to depression, hypertension, seizures, migraine, polycystic ovary syndrome, inflammation, autoimmunity, and musculoskeletal pain such as low-back pain. Clinical trials using vitamin D supplementation have proven the cause-and-effect relationship between vitamin D deficiency and these conditions by showing that each of these could be cured or alleviated with vitamin D supplementation. In our review of the literature, we concluded that daily vitamin D doses should be 1,000 IU for infants, 2,000 IU for children, and 4,000 IU for adults. Cautions and contraindications include the use of thiazide diuretics (e.g., hydrochlorothiazide) or any other medications that can promote hypercalcemia, as well as granulomatous diseases such as sarcoidosis, tuberculosis, and certain types of cancer, especially lymphoma. Effectiveness is monitored by measuring serum 25-OH-vitamin D, and safety is monitored by measuring serum calcium.

4. <u>Balanced and complete fatty acid supplementation</u>: A detailed survey of the literature reveals five major health-promoting anti-inflammatory fatty acids found in the human diet.[62] These are alpha-linolenic acid (ALA; omega-3, from flaxseed oil), eicosapentaenoic acid (EPA; omega-3, from fish oil), docosahexaenoic acid (DHA; omega-3, from fish oil and algae), gamma-linolenic acid (GLA; omega-6, most concentrated in borage oil), and oleic acid (omega-9, mainly from olive oil, also found in flaxseed and borage oils). Each of these fatty acids has health benefits that cannot be fully attained from supplementing a different fatty acid. The benefits of GLA

[44] Fletcher RH, Fairfield KM. Vitamins for chronic disease prevention in adults: clinical applications. *JAMA* 2002;287:3127-9
[45] Heaney RP. Long-latency deficiency disease: insights from calcium and vitamin D. *Am J Clin Nutr* 2003;78:912-9
[46] McKay DL, Perrone G, Rasmussen H, Dallal G, Hartman W, Cao G, Prior RL, Roubenoff R, Blumberg JB. The effects of a multivitamin/mineral supplement on micronutrient status, antioxidant capacity and cytokine production in healthy older adults consuming a fortified diet. *J Am Coll Nutr* 2000;19(5):613-21
[47] Benton D, Haller J, Fordy J. Vitamin supplementation for 1 year improves mood. *Neuropsychobiology* 1995;32(2):98-105
[48] Coppen A, Bailey J. Enhancement of the antidepressant action of fluoxetine by folic acid: a randomised, placebo controlled trial. *J Affect Disord* 2000;60:121-30
[49] Wagner W, Nootbaar-Wagner U. Prophylactic treatment of migraine with gamma-linolenic and alpha-linolenic acids. *Cephalalgia* 1997;17:127-30
[50] Langkamp-Henken et al. Nutritional formula enhanced immune function and reduced days of symptoms of URI in seniors. *J Am Geriatr Soc* 2004;52:3-12
[51] Barringer TA, et al. Effect of a multivitamin and mineral supplement on infection and quality of life. *Ann Intern Med* 2003;138:365-71
[52] Fawzi WW, Msamanga GI, et al. A randomized trial of multivitamin supplements and HIV disease progression and mortality. *N Engl J Med* 2004;351:23-32
[53] Burbano X, et al. Impact of a selenium chemoprevention clinical trial on hospital admissions of HIV-infected participants. *HIV Clin Trials* 2002;3:483-91
[54] Abraham GE. Nutritional factors in the etiology of the premenstrual tension syndromes. *J Reprod Med* 1983;28(7):446-64
[55] Stewart A. Clinical and biochemical effects of nutritional supplementation on the premenstrual syndrome. *J Reprod Med* 1987;32:435-41
[56] Kaplan BJ, et al. Effective mood stabilization with a chelated mineral supplement: an open-label trial in bipolar disorder. *J Clin Psychiatry* 2001;62:936-44
[57] Kaplan BJ, et al. Treatment of mood lability and explosive rage with minerals and vitamins: two case studies. *J Child Adolesc Psychopharmacol* 2002;12(3):205-19
[58] Gesch et al. Influence of supplementary vitamins, minerals and essential fatty acids on the antisocial behaviour of young adult prisoners. *Br J Psychiatry* 2002;181:22-8
[59] Benton D. Micro-nutrient supplementation and the intelligence of children. *Neurosci Biobehav Rev* 2001;25:297-309
[60] Church TS, Earnest CP, Wood KA, Kampert JB. Reduction of C-reactive protein levels through use of a multivitamin. *Am J Med* 2003;115:702-7
[61] Vasquez A, Manso G, Cannell J. The clinical importance of vitamin D (cholecalciferol): a paradigm shift. *Alternative Therapies in Health and Medicine* 2004;10:28-37
[62] Vasquez A. New Insights into Fatty Acid Supplementation and Its Effect on Eicosanoid Production and Genetic Expression. *Nutritional Perspectives* 2005; Jan: 5-16

(borage oil) are not attained by consumption of EPA and DHA (fish oil); in fact, consumption of fish oil can actually promote a deficiency of GLA.[63] Likewise, consumption of GLA alone can reduce EPA levels while increasing levels of proinflammatory arachidonic acid; both of these problems are avoided with co-administration of fish oil any time borage oil is used. Using ALA (flaxseed oil) alone only slightly increases EPA but generally leads to no improvement in DHA status and can lead to a reduction of oleic acid; thus, fish oil, olive oil (and borage oil) should be supplemented when flaxseed oil is used.[64] Obviously, the goal here is a balanced intake of all of the health-promoting fatty acids; using only one or two sources of fatty acids is not balanced and results in suboptimal improvement, at best. In clinical practice, I routinely use combination fatty acid therapy comprised of ALA, EPA, DHA, and GLA for essentially all patients. The product also contains a modest amount of oleic acid, and I encourage use of olive oil for salads and cooking. This approach results in complete and balanced fatty acid intake, and the clinical benefits are impressive.

5. Probiotics /gut flora modification: Proper levels of good bacteria promote intestinal health, proper immune function, and support overall health. Excess bacteria or yeast, or the presence of harmful bacteria, yeast, or "parasites" such as amoebas and protozoans, can cause "leaky gut," systemic inflammation, and a wide range of clinical problems. Intestinal flora can become imbalanced by poor diets, excess stress, immunosuppressive drugs, antibiotics, or exposure to contaminated food or water, all of which are common among American patients. Thus, as a rule, I reinstate the good bacteria by the use of probiotics (good bacteria and yeast), prebiotics (fiber, arabinogalactan, and inulin), and the use of fermented foods such as kefir (in patients not allergic to milk). Harmful yeast, bacteria, and other "parasites" can be eradicated with the combination of dietary change, drugs, and/or herbal extracts. For example, oregano oil in an emulsified, time-released form has proven safe and effective for the elimination of various parasites encountered in clinical practice.[65] Likewise, the herb *Artemisia annua* (sweet wormwood) commonly is used to eradicate specific bacteria and has been used for thousands of years in Asia for the treatment and prevention of infectious diseases, including malaria.[66]

Conclusion: In this brief review, I have outlined and scientifically substantiated a fundamental protocol that can serve as effective therapy for patients with a wide range of "diseases." Customizing the Paleo-Mediterranean diet to avoid food allergens, using vitamin-mineral supplements along with physiologic doses of vitamin D and broad-spectrum balanced fatty acid supplementation, and ensuring gastrointestinal health with the skillful use of probiotics, prebiotics, and antimicrobial treatments provides an excellent health-

Ayurvedic proverb
"When the diet is wrong, medicine is of no use. When the diet is correct, medicine is of no need."

promoting and disease-eliminating foundation and lifestyle for many patients. Often, this simple protocol is all that is needed for the effective treatment of a wide range of clinical problems. For other patients with more complex illnesses, of course, additional interventions and laboratory assessments can be used to customize the treatment plan. However, we must always remember that the attainment and preservation of health requires that we meet the body's basic nutritional needs. This five-step protocol begins the process of meeting those needs. In my next article, I'll give you some examples from my clinical practice and additional references to show this protocol's safety and effectiveness.

Implementing the Five-Part Nutritional Wellness Protocol for the Treatment of Various Health Problems

This article was originally published in *Nutritional Wellness*
nutritionalwellness.com/archives/2005/nov/11_vasquez.php

Introduction: In my last article in *Nutritional Wellness* I described a 5-part nutritional protocol that can be used in the vast majority of patients without adverse effects and with major benefits. For many patients, the basic protocol consisting of 1) the Paleo-Mediterranean diet, 2) multivitamin/multimineral supplementation, 3) additional vitamin D3, 4) combination fatty acid therapy with an optimal balance of ALA, GLA, EPA, DHA, and oleic acid, and 5) probiotics (including the identification and eradication of harmful yeast, bacteria, and other "parasites") is all the

[63] Cleland LG, Gibson RA, Neumann M, French JK. The effect of dietary fish oil supplement upon the content of dihomo-gammalinolenic acid in human plasma phospholipids. *Prostaglandins Leukot Essent Fatty Acids* 1990 May;40(1):9-12
[64] Jantti J, Nikkari T, Solakivi T, et al. Evening primrose oil in rheumatoid arthritis: changes in serum lipids and fatty acids. *Ann Rheum Dis* 1989;48(2):124-7
[65] Force M, Sparks WS, Ronzio RA. Inhibition of enteric parasites by emulsified oil of oregano in vivo. *Phytother Res* 2000;14:213-4
[66] Schuster BG. Demonstrating the validity of natural products as anti-infective drugs. *J Altern Complement Med* 2001;7 Suppl 1:S73-82

treatment that they need. For patients who need additional treatment, this foundational plan still serves as the core of the biochemical aspect of their intervention. Of course, in some cases, we have to use other lifestyle modifications (such as exercise), additional supplements (such as policosanol or antimicrobial herbs), manual treatments (including spinal manipulation) and occasionally select medications (such has hormone modulators) to obtain our goal of maximum improvement.

The following examples show how the 5-part protocol serves to benefit patients with a wide range of conditions. For the sake of saving space, I will use only highly specific citations to the research literature, since I have provided the other references in the previous issue of *Nutritional Wellness* and elsewhere.[67]

- A Man with High Cholesterol: This patient is a 41-year-old slightly overweight man with very high cholesterol. His total cholesterol was 290 (normal < 200), LDL cholesterol was 212 (normal <130), and his triglycerides were 148 (optimal <100). I am quite certain that nearly every medical doctor would have put this man on cholesterol-lowering statin drugs for life. *Treatment*: In contrast, I advised a low-carb Paleo-Mediterranean diet because such diets have been shown to reduce cardiovascular mortality more powerfully that "statin" cholesterol-lowing drugs in older patients.[68] Likewise, fatty acid supplementation is more effective than statin drugs for reducing cardiac and all-cause mortality.[69] We added probiotics, because supplementation with *Lactobacillus* and *Bifidobacterium* has been shown to lower cholesterol levels in humans with high cholesterol.[70] Finally, I also prescribed 20 mg of policosanol for its well-known ability to favorably modify cholesterol levels.[71] *Results*: Within *one month* the patient had lost weight, felt better, and his total cholesterol had dropped to normal at 196 (from 290!), LDL was reduced to 141, and triglycerides were reduced to 80. Basically, this treatment plan was "the protocol + policosanol." Drug treatment of this patient would have been more expensive, more risky, and would not have resulted in global health improvements.

- A Child with Intractable Seizures: This is a 4-year-old nonverbal boy with 3-5 seizures per day despite being on two anti-seizure medications and having previously had several other "last resort" medical and surgical procedures. He also had a history of food allergies. *Treatment*: Obviously, there was no room for error in this case. We implemented a moderately low-carb hypoallergenic diet since both carbohydrate restriction[72] and allergy avoidance[73] can reduce the frequency and severity of seizures. Since many "anti-seizure" medications actually cause seizures by causing vitamin D deficiency[74], I added 800 IU per day of emulsified vitamin D3 for its antiseizure benefit.[75] We used 1 tsp per day of a combination fatty acid supplement that provides balanced amounts of ALA, GLA, EPA, and DHA, since fatty acids appear to have potential antiseizure benefits.[76] Vitamin B-6 (250 mg of P5P) and magnesium (bowel tolerance) were also added to reduce brain hyperexcitability.[77] Stool testing showed an absence of *Bifidobacteria* and *Lactobacillus*; probiotics were added for their anti-allergy benefits.[78] *Results*: Within about 2 months seizure frequency reduced from 3-5 per day to one seizure every other day: *an 87% reduction in seizure frequency*. Patient was able to discontinue one of the anti-seizure medications. His parents also noted several global improvements: the boy started making eye contact with people, he was learning again, and intellectually he was "making gains every day." His parents considered this an "amazing difference." Going from 30 seizures per week to 4 seizures per week while reducing medication use by 50% is a major achievement. Notice that we simply used the basic wellness protocol with some additional B6 and magnesium. It is highly unlikely that B6 and magnesium alone would have produced such a favorable response.

- A Young Woman with Full-Body Psoriasis Unresponsive to Drug Treatment: This is a 17-year-old woman with head-to-toe psoriasis since childhood. She wears long pants and long-sleeved shirts year-round, and the

---

[67] Vasquez A. *Integrative Orthopedics*. By now of course, this book has been surpassed in content of nutritional information, particularly in books printed past 2009.
[68] Knoops KT, et al. Mediterranean diet, lifestyle factors, and 10-year mortality in elderly European men and women. *JAMA*. 2004 Sep 22;292(12):1433-9
[69] Studer M, et al. Effect of different antilipidemic agents and diets on mortality: a systematic review. *Arch Intern Med*. 2005;165:725-30
[70] Xiao JZ, et al. Effects of milk products fermented by Bifidobacterium longum on blood lipids in rats and healthy adult male volunteers. *J Dairy Sci*. 2003;86:2452-61
[71] Cholesterol-lowering action of policosanol compares well to that of pravastatin and lovastatin. *Cardiovasc J S Afr*. 2003;14(3):161
[72] Freeman JM, et al. The efficacy of the ketogenic diet-1998: a prospective evaluation of intervention in 150 children. *Pediatrics*. 1998;102:1358-63
[73] Egger J, Carter CM, Soothill JF, Wilson J. Oligoantigenic diet treatment of children with epilepsy and migraine. *J Pediatr*. 1989;114:51-8
[74] Ali FE, Al-Bustan MA, Al-Busairi WA, Al-Mulla FA. Loss of seizure control due to anticonvulsant-induced hypocalcemia. *Ann Pharmacother*. 2004;38:1002-5
[75] Christiansen C, Rodbro P, Sjo O."Anticonvulsant action" of vitamin D in epileptic patients? A controlled pilot study. *Br Med J*. 1974 May 4;2(913):258-9
[76] Yuen AW, et al. Omega-3 fatty acid supplementation in patients with chronic epilepsy: A randomized trial. *Epilepsy Behav*. 2005 Sep;7(2):253-8
[77] Mousain-Bosc M, et al. Magnesium VitB6 intake reduces central nervous system hyperexcitability in children. *J Am Coll Nutr*. 2004;23(5):545S-548S
[78] Majaama H, Isolauri E.Probiotics: a novel approach in the management of food allergy. *J Allergy Clin Immunol*. 1997 Feb;99(2):179-85

psoriasis is a major interference to her social life. Medications have ceased to help. **Treatment**: The Paleo-Mediterranean diet was implemented with an emphasis on food allergy identification.[1] We used a multivitamin-mineral supplement with 200 mcg selenium to compensate for the nutritional insufficiencies and selenium deficiency that are common in patients with psoriasis; likewise 10 mg of folic acid was added to address the relative vitamin deficiencies and elevated homocysteine that are common in these patients.[79] Combination fatty acid therapy with EPA and DHA from fish oil and GLA from borage oil was used for the anti-inflammatory and skin-healing benefits.[80] Vitamin E (1200 IU of mixed tocopherols) and lipoic acid (1,000 mg per day) were added for their anti-inflammatory benefits and to combat the oxidative stress that is characteristic of psoriasis.[81] Of course, probiotics were used to modify gut flora, which is commonly deranged in patients with psoriasis.[82] **Results**: Within a few weeks, this patient's "lifelong psoriasis" was essentially gone. Food allergy identification and avoidance played a major role in the success of this case. When I saw the patient again 9 months later for her second visit, she had no visible evidence of psoriasis. Her "medically untreatable" condition was essentially cured by the use of my basic protocol, with the addition of a few extra nutrients.

- <u>A Man with Fatigue and Recurrent Numbness in Hands and Feet</u>. This 40-year-old man had seen numerous neurologists and had spent tens of thousands of dollars on MRIs, CT scans, lumbar punctures, and other diagnostic procedures. No diagnosis had been found, and no effective treatment had been rendered by medical specialists. **Assessments**: We performed a modest battery of lab tests which revealed elevations of fibrinogen and C-reactive protein (CRP), two markers of acute inflammation. Assessment of intestinal permeability with the lactulose-mannitol assay showed major intestinal damage ("leaky gut"). Follow-up parasite testing on different occasions showed dysbiosis caused by *Proteus, Enterobacter, Klebsiella, Citrobacter*, and *Pseudomonas aeruginosa*—of course, these are gram-negative bacteria that can induce immune dysfunction and autoimmunity, as described elsewhere.[1] Specifically, *Pseudomonas aeruginosa* has been linked to the development of nervous system autoimmunity, such as multiple sclerosis.[83] **Treatment**: We implemented a plan of diet modification, vitamins, minerals, fatty acids, and probiotics. The dysbiosis was further addressed with specific antimicrobial herbs (including caprylic acid and emulsified oregano oil[84]) and drugs (such as tetracycline, Bactrim, and Augmentin). The antibiotic drugs proved to be ineffective based on repeat stool testing. **Results**: Within one month we witnessed impressive improvements, both subjectively and objectively. Subjectively, the patient reported that the numbness and tingling almost completely resolved. Fatigue was reduced, and energy was improved. Objectively, the patient's elevated CRP plummeted from abnormally high at 11 down to completely normal at 1. Eighteen months later, the patient's CRP had dropped to less than 1 and fatigue and numbness were no longer problematic. Notice that this treatment plan was basically "the protocol" with additional attention to eradicating the dysbiosis we found with specialized stool testing.

- <u>A 50-year-old Man with Rheumatoid Arthritis</u>. This patient presented with a 3-year history of rheumatoid arthritis that had been treated unsuccessfully with drugs (methotrexate and intravenous Remicade). The first time I tested his hsCRP level, it was astronomically high at 124 mg/L (normal is <3). Because of the severe inflammation and other risk factors for sudden cardiac death, I referred this patient to an osteopathic internist for immune-suppressing drugs; the patient refused, stating that he was no longer willing to rely on immune-suppressing chemical medications. His treatment was entirely up to me. **Assessments and Treatments**: We implemented the Paleo-Mediterranean diet and a program of vitamins, minerals, optimal combination fatty acid therapy (providing ALA, GLA, EPA, DHA, and oleic acid), and 4000 IU of vitamin D in emulsified form to overcome defects in absorption that are seen in older patients and those with gastrointestinal problems.[85] Hormone testing showed abnormally low DHEA, low testosterone, and slightly elevated estrogen; these problems were corrected with DHEA supplementation and the use of a hormone-modulating drug (Arimidex) that lowers estrogen and raises testosterone. Specialized stool testing showed absence of *Lactobacillus* and *Bifidobacteria* and intestinal overgrowth of *Citrobacter* and *Enterobacter* which was corrected with probiotics and antimicrobial treatments including undecylenic acid and emulsified oregano oil. Importantly, I also decided to

[79] Vanizor Kural B, et al. Plasma homocysteine and its relationships with atherothrombotic markers in psoriatic patients. *Clin Chim Acta*. 2003 Jun;332(1-2):23-3

[80] Vasquez A. New Insights into Fatty Acid Supplementation and Its Effect on Eicosanoid Production and Genetic Expression. *Nutritional Perspectives* 2005; January: 5-16

[81] Kokcam I, Naziroglu M. Antioxidants and lipid peroxidation status in the blood of patients with psoriasis. *Clin Chim Acta*. 1999 Nov;289(1-2):23-31

[82] Waldman A, et al. Incidence of Candida in psoriasis--a study on the fungal flora of psoriatic patients. *Mycoses*. 2001 May;44(3-4):77-81

[83] Hughes LE, et al. Antibody responses to Acinetobacter spp. and Pseudomonas aeruginosa in multiple sclerosis. *Clin Diagn Lab Immunol*. 2001;8(6):1181-8

[84] Force M, Sparks WS, Ronzio RA. Inhibition of enteric parasites by emulsified oil of oregano in vivo. *Phytother Res*. 2000 May;14(3):213-4

[85] Vasquez A. Subphysiologic Doses of Vitamin D are Subtherapeutic: Comment on the Study by The Record Trial Group. *TheLancet.com* Accessed June 16, 2005

inhibit NFkB (the primary transcription factor that upregulates the pro-inflammatory response[86]) by using a combination botanical formula that contains curcumin, piperine, lipoic acid, green tea extract, propolis, rosemary, resveratrol, ginger, and Phytolens™ (an antioxidant extract from lentils that may inhibit autoimmunity[87])—all of these herbs and nutrients have been shown to inhibit NFkB and to thus downregulate inflammatory responses.[88] ***Results***: Within 6 weeks, this patient had happily lost 10 lbs of excess weight and was able to work without pain for the first time in years. **Follow-up testing showed that his hsCRP had dropped from 124 to 7 mg/L—a drop of 114 points—95%!—in less than one month: better than had ever been achieved even with the use of intravenous immune-suppressing drugs!** This patient continues to make significant progress. Obviously this case was complex, and we needed to do more than the basic protocol. Nonetheless, the basic protocol still served as the foundation for the treatment plan. Note that vitamin D has significant anti-inflammatory benefits and can cause major reductions in inflammation measured by CRP.[89] The correction of the hormonal abnormalities and the dysbiosis, and downregulating NFkB with several botanical extracts were also critical components of this successful treatment plan.

Summary and Conclusions: These examples show how the nutritional wellness protocol that I described in the September issue of *Nutritional Wellness* can be used as the foundational treatment for a wide range of health problems. In many cases, implementation of the basic protocol is all that is needed. In more complex situations, we use the basic protocol and then add more specific treatments to address dysbiosis and hormonal problems, and we can add additional nutrients as needed. However, nothing will ever replace a healthy diet, sufficiencies of vitamin D and all five of the health-promoting fatty acids (i.e., ALA, GLA, EPA, DHA, and oleic acid), and normalization of gastrointestinal flora. Without these basics, survival and the appearance of health are possible, but true health and recovery from "untreatable" illnesses is not possible. In order to attain optimal health, we have to create the conditions that allow for health to be attained, and we start this process by supplying the body with the nutrients that it needs to function optimally. In the words of naturopathic physician Jared Zeff from the *Journal of Naturopathic Medicine*, "The work of the naturopathic physician is to elicit healing by helping patients to create or recreate the conditions for health to exist within them. Health will occur where the conditions for health exist. Disease is the product of the conditions which allow for it."[90]

Common Oversights and Shortcomings in the Study and Implementation of Nutritional Supplementation
This article was originally published in *Naturopathy Digest* naturopathydigest.com/archives/2007/jun/vasquez.php

Introduction: An impressive discrepancy often exists between the low efficacy of nutritional interventions reported in the research literature and the higher efficacy achieved in the clinical practices of clinicians trained in the use of interventional nutrition (i.e., naturopathic physicians). This discrepancy is dangerous for at least two reasons. First, it results in an undervaluation of the efficacy of nutritional supplementation, which ultimately leaves otherwise treatable patients untreated. Second, such untreated and undertreated patients are often then forced to use dangerous and expensive pharmaceutical drugs and surgical interventions to treat conditions that could have otherwise been easily and safely treated with nutritional supplementation and diet modification. Consequently, the burden of suffering, disease, and healthcare expense in the US is higher than it would be if nutritionally-trained clinicians were more fully integrated into the healthcare system.

Obstacles to Efficacy in the Use of Nutritional Supplementation: Below are listed some of the most common causes for the underachievement of nutritional supplementation in practice and in published research. While this list is not all-inclusive, it will serve as a review for clinicians and an introduction for chiropractic/naturopathic

[86] Tak PP, Firestein GS. NFkB: a key role in inflammatory diseases. *J Clin Invest*. 2001 Jan;107(1):7-11

[87] Sandoval M, et al. Peroxynitrite-induced apoptosis in epithelial (T84) and macrophage (RAW 264.7) cell lines: effect of legume-derived polyphenols (phytolens). *Nitric Oxide*. 1997;1(6):476-83

[88] Vasquez A. Nutritional and Botanical Inhibition of NFkB, the Major Intracellular Amplifier of the Inflammatory Cascade. A Practical Clinical Strategy Exemplifying Anti-Inflammatory Nutrigenomics. *Nutritional Perspectives* 2005;July: 5-12

[89] Timms PM, et al. Circulating MMP9, vitamin D and variation in the TIMP-1 response with VDR genotype. *QJM*. 2002 Dec;95(12):787-96

[90] Zeff JL. The process of healing: a unifying theory of naturopathic medicine. *Journal of Naturopathic Medicine* 1997; 7: 122-5

students. In both practice and research, the problems listed below often overlap and function synergistically to reduce the efficacy of nutritional supplementation.

1. <u>Inadequate dosing (quantity)</u>: Many clinical trials published in major journals and many doctors in clinical practice have used inadequate doses of vitamins (and other natural therapeutics) and have thus failed to achieve the results that would have easily been obtained had they implemented their protocol with the proper physiologic or supraphysiologic dose of intervention. The best example in my experience centers on vitamin D, where so many of the studies are performed with doses of 400-800 IU per day only to conclude that vitamin supplementation is ineffective for the condition being treated. The problem here is that the researchers failed to appreciate that the physiologic requirement for vitamin D3 in adults is approximately 3,000-5,000 IU per day[91] and that therefore their supplemental dose of 400-800 IU is only 10-20% of what is required. Subphysiologic doses are generally subtherapeutic. In this regard, I have had to correct journals such as *The Lancet*[92], *JAMA*[93], and *British Medical Journal*[94] from misleading their readers (many of whom are major policymakers) from concluding that nutritional supplementation is impotent; rather, their researchers and editors were not sufficiently educated in the design and review of studies using nutritional interventions. These journals should hire chiropractic and naturopathic physicians so that they have staff trained in natural treatments and who can thus provide an educated review of studies on these topics.[95]

2. <u>Inadequate dosing (duration)</u>: Often the effects of long-term nutritional deficiency are not fully reversible and/or may require a treatment period of months or years to achieve maximal clinical response. For example, full replacement of fatty acids in human brain phospholipids is an ongoing process that occurs over a period of several years; thus studies using fatty acid supplements for a period of weeks or 2-3 months generally underestimate the enhanced effectiveness that can be obtained with administration over many months or several years of treatment. Relatedly, recovery from vitamin D deficiency takes several weeks of high-dose supplementation in order to achieve tissue saturation and subsequent cellular replenishment; studies of short duration are destined to underestimate the results that could have been achieved with supplementation carried out over several months.[96]

3. <u>Failure to use proper forms of nutrients (quality)</u>: Nutrients are often available in different forms, not the least of which are "active" versus "inactive" and "natural" versus "unnatural." Most vitamin supplements, particularly high-potency B vitamins, are manufactured synthetically and are not from "natural sources" despite the marketing hype promulgated by companies that, for example, mix their synthetic vitamins with a vegetable powder and then call their vitamin supplements "natural." The simple fact is that production of high-potency supplements from purely natural sources would be prohibitively wasteful, inefficient, and expensive. Thus, while it is not necessary for vitamins to be "natural" in order to be useful, it is necessary that the vitamins are useable and preferably not "unnatural." The best example of the use of unnatural supplements is the use of synthetic DL-tocopherol in the so-called "vitamin E" studies; DL-tocopherol is 50% comprised of the L-isomer of tocopherol which is not only unusable by the human body but is actually harmful in that it interferes with normal metabolism and can exacerbate hypertension and cause symptomatic complications (e.g., headaches). Further, tocopherols exist within the body in relationship with the individual forms of the vitamin, such that supplementation with one form (e.g., alpha-tocopherol) can result in a relative deficiency of another form (e.g., gamma-tocopherol). One final example of the failure to use proper forms of nutrients is in the use of pyridoxine HCl as a form of vitamin B6; while this practice itself is not harmful, clinicians need to remember that pyridoxine HCl is ineffective until converted to the more active forms of the vitamin including pyridoxal-5-phosphate. Since this conversion requires co-nutrients such as magnesium and zinc, we can easily see that the reputed failure of B6 supplementation when administered in the form of pyridoxine HCl might actually be due to untreated insufficiencies of required co-nutrients, as discussed in the following section.

4. <u>Failure to ensure adequacy of co-nutrients</u>: Vitamins, minerals, amino acids, and fatty acids work together in an intricately choreographed and delicately orchestrated dance that culminates in the successful completion of

---

[91] Heaney RP, et al. Human serum 25-hydroxycholecalciferol response to extended oral dosing with cholecalciferol. *Am J Clin Nutr.* 2003 Jan;77(1):204-10

[92] Vasquez A. Subphysiologic Doses of Vitamin D are Subtherapeutic: Comment on the Study by The Record Trial Group. *The Lancet* 2005 Published on-line May 6

[93] Muanza DN, Vasquez A, Cannell J, Grant WB. Isoflavones and Postmenopausal Women. [letter] *JAMA* 2004; 292: 2337

[94] Vasquez A, Cannell J. Calcium and vitamin D in preventing fractures: data are not sufficient to show inefficacy. [letter] *BMJ: British Medical Journal* 2005;331:108-9

[95] Vasquez A. Allopathic Usurpation of Natural Medicine. *Naturopathy Digest* 2006 Feb naturopathydigest.com/archives/2006/feb/vasquez.php

[96] Vasquez A, Manso G, Cannell J. The clinical importance of vitamin D (cholecalciferol): a paradigm shift. *Altern Ther Health Med.* 2004 Sep-Oct;10(5):28-36

interconnected physiologic functions. If any of the performers in this event are missing (i.e., nutritional deficiency) or if successive interconversions are impaired due to lack of enzyme function, then the show cannot go on, or—if it does go on—impaired metabolism and defective function will result. So, if we take a patient with "vitamin B6 deficiency" and give him vitamin B6 in the absence of other co-nutrients needed for the proper activation and metabolic utilization of vitamin B6, we cannot honestly expect the "nutritional supplementation" to work in this case; rather, we might see a marginal benefit or perhaps even a negative outcome as an imbalanced system is pushed into a different state of imbalance despite supplementation with the "correct" vitamin. In the case of vitamin B6, necessary co-nutrients include zinc, magnesium, and riboflavin; deficiency of any of these will result in a relative "failure" of B6 supplementation even if a patient has a B6-responsive condition. Notably, overt magnesium deficiency is alarmingly common among patients and citizens in industrialized nations[97,98,99], and this epidemic of magnesium deficiency is due not only to insufficient intake but also to excessive excretion caused by consumption of high-glycemic foods, caffeine, and a diet that promotes chronic metabolic acidosis with resultant urinary acidification.

5. <u>Failure to achieve urinary alkalinization</u>: Western/American-style diets typified by overconsumption of grains, dairy, sugar, and salt result in a state of subclinical chronic metabolic acidosis which results in urinary acidification, relative hypercortisolemia, and consequent hyperexcretion of minerals such as calcium and magnesium.[100] [101] Thus, the common conundrum of magnesium replenishment requires not only magnesium supplementation but also dietary interventions to change the internal climate to one that is conducive to bodily retention and cellular uptake of magnesium.[102]

6. <u>Use of mislabeled supplements</u>: Even in the professional arena of nutritional supplement manufacturers, some companies habitually underdose their products either in an attempt to spend less in the manufacture of their products or as a consequence of poor quality control. If a product is labeled to contain 1,000 IU of vitamin D but only contains 836 IU of the nutrient, then obviously full clinical efficacy will not be achieved; this was a problem in a recent clinical trial involving vitamin D.[103] The problem for clinicians is in trusting the companies that supply nutritional supplements; some companies do "in house" testing which lacks independent review, while other companies use questionable "independent testing" which is not infrequently performed by a laboratory that is a wholly owned subsidiary of the parent nutritional company. Manufacturing regulations that are sweeping through the industry will cleanse the nutritional supplement world of poorly made products, and these same regulations will sweep some unprepared companies right out the door when they are unable to meet the regulatory requirements.

7. <u>Failure to ensure/assess bioavailability and optimal serum/cellular levels</u>: Clinical trials with nutritional therapies need to monitor serum or cellular levels to ensure absorption, product bioavailability, and the attainment of optimal serum levels. This is particularly relevant in the treatment of chronic disorders such as the autoimmune diseases, wherein so many of these patients have gastrointestinal dysbiosis and often have concomitant nutrient malabsorption.[104] Simply dosing these patients with supplements is not always efficacious; often the gut must be cleared of dysbiosis so that the mucosal lining can be repaired and optimal nutrient absorption can be reestablished.

8. <u>Coadministration of food with nutritional supplements (sometimes right, sometimes wrong)</u>: Food can help or hinder the absorption of nutritional supplements. Phytate and tannins in grains and teas, respectively, are notorious for inhibiting mineral absorption. Some supplements, like coenzyme Q10, should be administered with fatty food to enhance absorption. Other supplements, like amino acids, should be administered away from

---

[97] "Altogether 43% of 113 trauma patients had low magnesium levels compared to 30% of noninjured cohorts." Frankel H, Haskell R, Lee SY, Miller D, Rotondo M, Schwab CW. Hypomagnesemia in trauma patients. *World J Surg.* 1999 Sep;23(9):966-9

[98] "There was a 20% overall prevalence of hypomagnesemia among this predominantly female, African American population." Fox CH, Ramsoomair D, Mahoney MC, Carter C, Young B, Graham R. An investigation of hypomagnesemia among ambulatory urban African Americans. *J Fam Pract.* 1999 Aug;48(8):636-9

[99] "Suboptimal levels were detected in 33.7 per cent of the population under study. These data clearly demonstrate that the Mg supply of the German population needs increased attention." Schimatschek et al. Prevalence of hypomagnesemia in an unselected German population of 16,000 individuals. *Magnes Res.* 2001 Dec;14(4):283-90

[100] Cordain L, et al. Origins and evolution of the Western diet: health implications for the 21st century. *Am J Clin Nutr.* 2005 Feb;81(2):341-54

[101] Maurer M, Riesen W, Muser J, Hulter HN, Krapf R. Neutralization of Western diet inhibits bone resorption independently of K intake and reduces cortisol secretion in humans. *Am J Physiol Renal Physiol.* 2003 Jan;284(1):F32-40

[102] Vormann J, et al. Supplementation with alkaline minerals reduces symptoms in patients with chronic low back pain. *J Trace Elem Med Biol.* 2001;15(2-3):179-83

[103] Heaney RP, et al. Human serum 25-hydroxycholecalciferol response to extended oral dosing with cholecalciferol. *Am J Clin Nutr.* 2003 Jan;77(1):204-10

[104] Vasquez A. Nutritional and Botanical Treatments Against "Silent Infections" and Gastrointestinal Dysbiosis. *Nutritional Perspectives* 2006; January

protein-rich foods and are often better administered with simple carbohydrate to enhance cellular uptake; this is especially true with tryptophan.

9. <u>Correction of gross dietary imbalances enhances supplement effectiveness</u>: If the diet is grossly imbalanced, then nutritional supplementation is less likely to be effective. The best example of this is in the use of fatty acid supplements, particularly in the treatment of inflammatory disorders. If the diet is laden with dairy, beef, and other sources of arachidonate, then fatty acid supplementation with EPA, DHA, and GLA is much less likely to be effective, or much higher doses of the supplements will need to be used in order to help restore fatty acid balance. Generally speaking, the diet needs to be optimized to enhance the efficacy of nutritional supplementation.

Conclusion: In this brief review, I have listed and discussed some of the most common impediments to the success of nutritional supplementation. I hope that naturopathic students, clinicians, and researchers will find these points helpful in their design of clinical treatment protocols.

Revisiting the Five-Part Nutritional Wellness Protocol: Supplemented Paleo-Mediterranean Diet
This article was originally published in the January 2011 issue of *Nutritional Perspectives*

Abstract: This article reviews the five-part nutritional protocol that incorporates a health-promoting nutrient-dense diet and essential supplementation with vitamins/minerals, specific fatty acids, probiotics, and physiologic doses of vitamin D3. This foundational nutritional protocol has proven benefits for disease treatment, disease prevention, and health maintenance and restoration. Additional treatments such as botanical medicines, additional nutritional supplements, and pharmaceutical drugs can be used atop this foundational protocol to further optimize clinical effectiveness. The rationale for this five-part protocol is presented, and consideration is given to adding iodine-iodide as the sixth component of the protocol.

Introduction: In 2004 and 2005 I first published a "five-part nutrition protocol"[105,106] that provides the foundational treatment plan for a wide range of health disorders. This protocol served and continues to serve as the foundation upon which other treatments are commonly added, and without which those other treatments are likely to fail, or attain suboptimal results at best.[107] Now as then, I will share with you what I consider a basic foundational protocol for wellness promotion and disease treatment. I have used this protocol in my own self-care for many years and have used it in the treatment of a wide range of health-disease conditions in clinical practice.

This nutritional protocol is validated by biochemistry, physiology, experimental research, peer-reviewed human trials, and the clinical application of common sense. It is the most nutrient-dense diet available, satisfying nutritional needs and thereby optimizing metabolic processes while promoting satiety and weight loss/optimization. Nutrients are required in the proper amounts, forms, and approximate ratios for critical and innumerable physiologic functions; if nutrients are lacking, the body cannot function *normally*, let alone *optimally*. Impaired function results in subjective and objective manifestations of what is eventually labeled as "disease." Thus, a powerful and effective alternative to treating diseases with drugs is to re-establish normal/optimal physiologic function by replenishing the body with essential nutrients, reestablishing hormonal balance ("orthoendocrinology"), promoting detoxification of environmental toxins, and by reestablishing the optimal microbial milieu, especially the eradication of (multifocal) dysbiosis; this multifaceted approach can be applied to several diseases, especially those of the inflammatory and autoimmune varieties.[108]

Of course, most diseases are multifactorial and therefore require multicomponent treatment plans, and some diseases actually require the use of drugs in conjunction with assertive interventional nutrition. However, while only a smaller portion of patients actually need drugs for the long-term management their problems, all clinicians should agree that everyone needs a foundational nutrition plan because nutrients—not drugs—are universally required for life and health. This five-part nutrition protocol is briefly outlined below; a much more detailed substantiation of the underlying science and clinical application of this protocol was recently published in a review of more than 650 pages and approximately 3,500 citations.[109]

---

[105] Vasquez A. *Integrative Orthopedics: The Art of Creating Wellness While Managing Acute and Chronic Musculoskeletal Disorders*. 2004, 2007, 2012

[106] Vasquez A.Five-Part Nutritional Protocol that Produces Consistently Positive Results.*NutrWellness*2005Sep nutritionalwellness.com/archives/2005/sep/09_vasquez.php

[107] Vasquez A. Common Oversights and Shortcomings in the Study and Implementation of Nutritional Supplementation. *Naturopathy Digest* 2007 June.

[108] Vasquez A. Integrative Rheumatology. IBMRC: 2006, 2009.

[109] Vasquez A. *Chiropractic and Naturopathic Mastery of Common Clinical Disorders*. IBMRC: 2009

1. <u>Health-promoting Paleo-Mediterranean diet</u>: Following an extensive review of the research literature, I developed what I call the "supplemented Paleo-Mediterranean diet." In essence, this diet plan combines the best of the Mediterranean diet with the best of the Paleolithic diet, the latter of which has been best distilled by Dr. Loren Cordain in his book "The Paleo Diet"[110] and his numerous scientific articles.[111,112,113] The Paleolithic diet is superior to the Mediterranean diet in nutrient density for promoting satiety, weight loss, and improvements/normalization in overall metabolic function.[114,115] This diet places emphasis on fruits, vegetables, nuts, seeds, and berries that meet the body's needs for fiber, carbohydrates, and most importantly, the 8,000+ phytonutrients that have additive and synergistic health effects[116]—including immunomodulating, antioxidant, anti-inflammatory, and anti-cancer benefits. High-quality protein sources such as fish, poultry, eggs, and grass-fed meats are emphasized. Slightly modifying Cordain's Paleo diet, I also advocate soy and whey protein isolates for their high-quality protein and their anticancer, cardioprotective, and mood-enhancing (due to the high tryptophan content) benefits. Potatoes and other starchy vegetables, wheat and other grains including rice are discouraged due to their high glycemic indexes and high glycemic loads, and their relative insufficiency of fiber and phytonutrients compared to fruits and vegetables. Grains such as wheat, barley, and rye are discouraged due to the high glycemic loads/indexes of most breads, pastries, and other grain-derived products, as well as due to the immunogenicity of constituents such as gluten, a protein composite (consisting of a prolamin and a glutelin) that can contribute to disorders such as migraine, epilepsy, eczema, arthritis, celiac disease, psoriasis and other types of autoimmunity. Sources of simple sugars and foreign chemicals such as colas/sodas (which contain artificial colors, flavors, and high-fructose corn syrup, which contains mercury[117] and which can cause the hypertensive-diabetic metabolic syndrome[118]) and processed foods (e.g., "TV dinners" and other manufactured snacks and convenience foods) are strictly forbidden. Chemical preservatives, colorants, sweeteners, flavor-enhancers such as monosodium glutamate and carrageenan are likewise avoided. In summary, this diet plan provides plenty of variety, as most dishes comprised of poultry, fish, lean meats, soy, eggs, fruits, vegetables, nuts, berries, and seeds are allowed. The diet provides an abundance of fiber, phytonutrients, carbohydrates, potassium, and protein, while simultaneously being low in fat, sodium, arachidonic acid, and "simple sugars." The diet must be customized with regard to total protein and calorie intake, as determined by the size, status, and activity level of the patient; individual per-patient food allergens should be avoided. Regular consumption of this diet has shown the ability to reduce hypertension, alleviate diabetes, ameliorate migraine headaches, and result in improvement of overall health and a lessening of the severity of many common "diseases", particularly those with an autoimmune or inflammatory component. This Paleo-Mediterranean diet is supplemented with vitamins, minerals, fatty acids, and probiotics—making it the "supplemented Paleo-Mediterranean diet" as described below. The main considerations/contraindications to recommending increased intake of fruits and vegetables are 1) increased intake of vitamin K in the few patients taking warfarin for anticoagulation, and 2) increased intake of potassium in patients with pre-existing renal insufficiency as discussed in this video tutorial: vimeo.com/152296851 also at vimeo.com/152293616.

2. <u>Multivitamin and multimineral supplementation</u>: Vitamin and mineral supplementation has been advocated for decades by the chiropractic/naturopathic professions while being scorned by so-called "mainstream

---

[110] Cordain L. *The Paleo Diet*. John Wiley and Sons, 2002

[111] O'Keefe JH Jr, Cordain L. Cardiovascular disease resulting from a diet and lifestyle at odds with our Paleolithic genome. *Mayo Clin Proc.* 2004 Jan;79(1):101-8

[112] Cordain L. Cereal grains: humanity's double edged sword. *World Rev Nutr Diet* 1999;84:19-73

[113] Cordain L, et al. Origins and evolution of the Western diet: health implications for the 21st century. *Am J Clin Nutr.* 2005 Feb;81(2):341-54

[114] "A high micronutrient density diet mitigates the unpleasant aspects of the experience of hunger even though it is lower in calories. Hunger is one of the major impediments to successful weight loss. Our findings suggest that it is not simply the caloric content, but more importantly, the micronutrient density of a diet that influences the experience of hunger. It appears that a high nutrient density diet, after an initial phase of adjustment during which a person experiences "toxic hunger" due to withdrawal from pro-inflammatory foods, can result in a sustainable eating pattern that leads to weight loss and improved health." Fuhrman J, Sarter B, Glaser D, Acocella S. Changing perceptions of hunger on a high nutrient density diet. *Nutr J.* 2010 Nov 7;9:51 nutritionj.com/content/9/1/51

[115] "The Paleolithic group were as satiated as the Mediterranean group but consumed less energy per day (5.8 MJ/day vs. 7.6 MJ/day, Paleolithic vs. Mediterranean, p=0.04). Consequently, the quotients of mean change in satiety during meal and mean consumed energy from food and drink were higher in the Paleolithic group (p=0.03). Also, there was a strong trend for greater Satiety Quotient for energy in the Paleolithic group (p=0.057). Leptin decreased by 31% in the Paleolithic and by 18% in the Mediterranean group with a trend for greater relative decrease of leptin in the Paleolithic group." Jonsson T, Granfeldt Y, Erlansson-Albertsson C, Ahren B, Lindeberg S. A Paleolithic diet is more satiating per calorie than a Mediterranean-like diet in individuals with ischemic heart disease. *Nutr Metab* (Lond). 2010 Nov 30;7(1):85.

[116] Liu RH. Health benefits of fruit and vegetables are from additive and synergistic combinations of phytochemicals. *Am J Clin Nutr* 2003;78(3 Suppl):517S-520S

[117] "With daily per capita consumption of HFCS in the US averaging about 50 grams and daily mercury intakes from HFCS ranging up to 28 µg, this potential source of mercury may exceed other major sources of mercury especially in high-end consumers of beverages sweetened with HFCS." Dufault R, et al. Mercury from chlor-alkali plants: measured concentrations in food product sugar. *Environ Health.* 2009 Jan 26;8:2 ehjournal.net/content/8/1/2

[118] Vasquez A. *Integrative Medicine and Functional Medicine for Chronic Hypertension: An Evidence-based Patient-Centered Monograph for Advanced Clinicians*. IBMRC; 2011. See also: Reungjui S, et al. Thiazide diuretics exacerbate fructose-induced metabolic syndrome. *J Am Soc Nephrol.* 2007 Oct;18(10):2724-31

medicine." Vitamin and mineral supplementation finally received bipartisan endorsement when researchers from Harvard Medical School published a review article in *Journal of the American Medical Association* that concluded, "Most people do not consume an optimal amount of all vitamins by diet alone. ...it appears prudent for all adults to take vitamin supplements."[119] Long-term nutritional insufficiencies experienced by "most people" promote the development of "long-latency deficiency diseases"[120] such as cancer, neuroemotional deterioration, and cardiovascular disease. Impressively, the benefits of multivitamin/multimineral supplementation have been demonstrated in numerous clinical trials. Multivitamin/multimineral supplementation has been shown to improve nutritional status and reduce the risk for chronic diseases[121], improve mood[122], potentiate antidepressant drug treatment[123], alleviate migraine headaches (when used with diet improvement and fatty acids[124]), improve immune function and infectious disease outcomes in the elderly[125] (especially diabetics[126]), reduce morbidity and mortality in patients with HIV infection[127,128], alleviate premenstrual syndrome[129,130] and bipolar disorder[131], reduce violence and antisocial behavior in children[132] and incarcerated young adults (when used with essential fatty acids[133]), and improve scores of intelligence in children.[134] Multivitamin and multimineral supplementation provides anti-inflammatory benefits, as evidenced by significant reduction in C-reactive protein (CRP) in a double-blind, placebo-controlled trial.[135] The ability to safely and affordably deliver these benefits makes multimineral-multivitamin supplementation an essential component of any and all health-promoting and disease-prevention strategies. A few cautions need to be observed; for example, vitamin A can (rarely) result in liver damage with chronic consumption of 25,000 IU or more, and intake should generally not exceed 10,000 IU per day in women of childbearing age. Also, iron should not be supplemented except in patients diagnosed with iron deficiency by a blood test (serum ferritin).

3. <u>Physiologic doses of vitamin D3</u>: The prevalence of vitamin D deficiency varies from 40-80 percent (general population) to almost 100 percent (patients with musculoskeletal pain) among Americans and Europeans. Vasquez, Manso, and Cannell described the many benefits of vitamin D3 supplementation in a "paradigm-shifting" review published in 2004.[136]

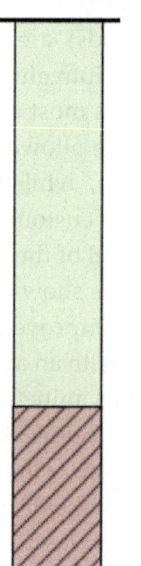

Excess vitamin D
> 100 ng/mL (250 nmol/L) with hypercalcemia

Optimal range
50 - 100 ng/mL (125 - 250 nmol/L)

Insufficiency range
< 20- 40 ng/mL (50 - 100 nmol/L)

Deficiency
< 20 ng/mL (50 nmol/L)

Image right: Interpretation of serum 25(OH) vitamin D levels: Updated from Vasquez et al, *Alternative Therapies in Health and Medicine* 2004 Sep

[119] Fletcher RH, Fairfield KM. Vitamins for chronic disease prevention in adults: clinical applications. *JAMA* 2002;287:3127-9
[120] Heaney RP. Long-latency deficiency disease: insights from calcium and vitamin D. *Am J Clin Nutr* 2003;78:912-9
[121] McKay et al. The effects of a multivitamin/mineral supplement on micronutrient status, antioxidant capacity and cytokine production in healthy older adults consuming a fortified diet. *J Am Coll Nutr* 2000;19(5):613-21
[122] Benton D, Haller J, Fordy J. Vitamin supplementation for 1 year improves mood. *Neuropsychobiology* 1995;32(2):98-105
[123] Coppen A, Bailey J. Enhancement of the antidepressant action of fluoxetine by folic acid: a randomised, placebo controlled trial. *J Affect Disord* 2000;60:121-30
[124] Wagner W, Nootbaar-Wagner U. Prophylactic treatment of migraine with gamma-linolenic and alpha-linolenic acids. *Cephalalgia* 1997;17:127-30
[125] Langkamp-Henken et al. Nutritional formula enhanced immune function and reduced days of symptoms upper respiratory tract infection in seniors. *J Am Geriatr Soc* 2004:3-12
[126] Barringer TA, et al. Effect of a multivitamin and mineral supplement on infection and quality of life. *Ann Intern Med* 2003;138:365-71
[127] Fawzi WW, Msamanga GI, et al. A randomized trial of multivitamin supplements and HIV disease progression and mortality. *N Engl J Med* 2004;351:23-32
[128] Burbano X, et al. Impact of a selenium chemoprevention clinical trial on hospital admissions of HIV-infected participants. *HIV Clin Trials* 2002;3:483-91
[129] Abraham GE. Nutritional factors in the etiology of the premenstrual tension syndromes. *J Reprod Med* 1983;28(7):446-64
[130] Stewart A. Clinical and biochemical effects of nutritional supplementation on the premenstrual syndrome. *J Reprod Med* 1987;32:435-41
[131] Kaplan BJ, et al. Effective mood stabilization with a chelated mineral supplement: an open-label trial in bipolar disorder. *J Clin Psychiatry* 2001;62:936-44
[132] Kaplan et al. Treatment of mood lability and explosive rage with minerals and vitamins: two case studies in children. *J Child Adolesc Psychopharmacol* 2002;12(3):205-19
[133] Gesch et al. Influence of supplementary vitamins, minerals and essential fatty acids on the antisocial behaviour of young adult prisoners. *Br J Psychiatry* 2002;181:22-8
[134] Benton D. Micro-nutrient supplementation and the intelligence of children. *Neurosci Biobehav Rev* 2001;25:297-309
[135] Church TS, Earnest CP, Wood KA, Kampert JB. Reduction of C-reactive protein levels through use of a multivitamin. *Am J Med* 2003;115:702-7
[136] Vasquez A, Manso G, Cannell J. The clinical importance of vitamin D (cholecalciferol). *Alternative Therapies in Health and Medicine* 2004;10:28-37

Our review showed that vitamin D deficiency causes or contributes to depression, hypertension, seizures, migraine, polycystic ovary syndrome, inflammation, autoimmunity, and musculoskeletal pain, particularly low-back pain. Clinical trials using vitamin D supplementation have proven the cause-and-effect relationship between vitamin D deficiency and most of these conditions by showing that each could be cured or alleviated with vitamin D supplementation. Per our review, daily vitamin D doses should be 1,000 IU for infants, 2,000 IU for children, and 4,000 IU for adults, although some adults respond better to higher doses of 10,000 IU per day. Cautions/contraindications include the use of thiazide diuretics (e.g., hydrochlorothiazide) or any other medications that promote hypercalcemia, as well as granulomatous diseases such as sarcoidosis, tuberculosis, and certain types of cancer, especially lymphoma. Effectiveness is monitored by measuring serum 25-OH-vitamin D, and safety is monitored by measuring serum calcium. Dosing should be tailored for the attainment of optimal serum levels of 25-hydroxy-vitamin D3, generally 50-100 ng/ml (125-250 nmol/l) as illustrated.

4. <u>Balanced and complete fatty acid supplementation</u>: A detailed survey of the literature shows that five fatty acids have major health-promoting disease-preventing benefits and should therefore be incorporated into the daily diet and/or regularly consumed as dietary supplements.[137] These are alpha-linolenic acid (ALA; omega-3, from flaxseed oil), eicosapentaenoic acid (EPA; omega-3, from fish oil), docosahexaenoic acid (DHA; omega-3, from fish oil and algae), gamma-linolenic acid (GLA; omega-6, most concentrated in borage oil but also present in evening primrose oil, hemp seed oil, black currant seed oil), and oleic acid (omega-9, most concentrated in olive oil, which contains in addition to oleic acid many anti-inflammatory, antioxidant, and anticancer phytonutrients). Supplementing with one fatty acid can exacerbate an insufficiency of other fatty acids; hence the importance of balanced combination supplementation. Each of these fatty acids has health benefits that cannot be fully attained from supplementing a different fatty acid; hence, again, the importance of balanced combination supplementation. The benefits of GLA are not attained by consumption of EPA and DHA; in fact, consumption of fish oil can actually promote a deficiency of GLA.[138] Likewise, consumption of GLA alone can reduce EPA levels while increasing levels of proinflammatory arachidonic acid; both of these problems are avoided with co-administration of EPA any time GLA is used because EPA inhibits delta-5-desaturase, which converts dihomo-GLA into arachidonic acid. Using ALA alone only slightly increases EPA but generally leads to no improvement in DHA status and can lead to a reduction of oleic acid; thus, DHA and oleic acid should be supplemented when flaxseed oil is used.[139] Obviously, the goal here is physiologically-optimal (i.e., "balanced") intake of all of the health-promoting fatty acids; using only one or two sources of fatty acids is not balanced and results in suboptimal improvement. In clinical practice, I routinely use combination fatty acid therapy comprised of ALA, EPA, DHA, and GLA for essentially all patients; when one appreciates that the average daily Paleolithic intake of n-3 fatty acids was 7 grams per day contrasted to the average daily American intake of 1 gram per day, we can see that—by using combination fatty acid therapy emphasizing n-3 fatty acids—we are simply meeting physiologic expectations via supplementation, rather than performing an act of recklessness or heroism. The product I use also contains a modest amount of oleic acid that occurs naturally in flax and borage seed oils, and I encourage use of olive oil for salads and cooking. This approach results in complete and balanced fatty acid intake, and the clinical benefits are impressive. Benefits are to be expected in the treatment of premenstrual syndrome, diabetic neuropathy, respiratory distress syndrome, Crohn's disease, lupus, rheumatoid arthritis, cardiovascular disease, hypertension, psoriasis, eczema, migraine headaches, bipolar disorder, borderline personality disorder, mental depression, schizophrenia, osteoporosis, polycystic ovary syndrome, multiple sclerosis, and musculoskeletal pain. The discovery in September 2010 that the G protein-coupled receptor 120 (GPR120) functions as an n-3 fatty acid receptor that, when stimulated with EPA or DHA, exerts broad anti-inflammatory effects (in cell experiments) and enhances systemic insulin sensitivity (in animal study) confirms a new mechanism of action of fatty acid supplementation and shows that we as clinician-researchers are still learning the details of the beneficial effects of commonly used treatments.[140]

---

[137] Vasquez A. New Insights into Fatty Acid Biochemistry and the Influence of Diet. *Nutritional Perspectives* 2004; October: 5, 7-10, 12, 14
[138] Cleland LG, Gibson RA, Neumann M, French JK. The effect of dietary fish oil supplement upon the content of dihomo-gammalinolenic acid in human plasma phospholipids. *Prostaglandins Leukot Essent Fatty Acids* 1990 May;40(1):9-12
[139] Jantti J, Nikkari T, Solakivi T, et al. Evening primrose oil in rheumatoid arthritis: changes in serum lipids and fatty acids. *Ann Rheum Dis* 1989;48(2):124-7
[140] Oh da Y, et al. GPR120 is an omega-3 fatty acid receptor mediating potent anti-inflammatory and insulin-sensitizing effects. Cell. 2010 Sep 3;142(5):687-98

5. <u>Probiotics /gut flora modification</u>: Proper levels of good bacteria promote intestinal health, support proper immune function, and encourage overall health. Excess bacteria or yeast, or the presence of harmful bacteria, yeast, or "parasites" such as amoebas and protozoans, can cause "leaky gut," systemic inflammation, and a wide range of clinical problems, especially autoimmunity. Intestinal flora can become imbalanced by poor diets, excess stress, immunosuppressive drugs, and antibiotics, and all of these factors are common among American patients. Thus, as a rule, I reinstate the good bacteria by the use of probiotics (good bacteria and yeast), prebiotics (fiber, arabinogalactan, and inulin), and the use of fermented foods such as kefir and yogurt for patients not allergic to milk. Harmful yeast, bacteria, and other "parasites" can be eradicated with the combination of dietary change, antimicrobial drugs, and/or herbal extracts. For example, oregano oil in an emulsified, time-released form has proven safe and effective for the elimination of various parasites encountered in clinical practice.[141] Likewise, the herb *Artemisia annua* (sweet wormwood) commonly is used to eradicate specific bacteria and has been used for thousands of years in Asia for the treatment and prevention of infectious diseases, including drug-resistant malaria.[142] Restoring microbial balance by providing probiotics, restoring immune function (immunorestoration) and eliminating sources of dysbiosis, especially in the gastrointestinal tract, genitourinary tract, and oropharynx, is a very important component in the treatment plan of autoimmunity and systemic inflammation.[143]

<u>Should combinations of iodine and iodide be the sixth component of the Protocol?*</u>: Both iodine and iodide have biological activity in humans. An increasing number of clinicians are using combination iodine-iodide products to provide approximately 3-6 mg/d [changed/corrected*]. Collectively, iodine and iodide provide antioxidant, antimicrobial, mucolytic, immunosupportive, antiestrogen, and anticancer benefits that extend far beyond the mere incorporation of iodine into thyroid hormones.[5] Benefits of iodine/iodide in the treatment of asthma[144,145] and systemic fungal infections[146,147] have been documented, and many clinicians use combination iodine/iodide supplementation for the treatment of estrogen-driven conditions such as fibrocystic breast disease.[148] While additional research is needed and already underway to further establish the role of iodine-iodide as a routine component of clinical care, clinicians can reasonably begin incorporating this nutrient into their protocols based on the above-mentioned physiologic roles and clinical benefits. *See update/addendum following this reprint.*

<u>Summary and Conclusions</u>: In this brief review, I have described and substantiated a fundamental protocol that can serve as effective therapy for patients with a wide range of diseases and health disorders. Customizing the Paleo-Mediterranean diet to avoid patient-specific food allergens, using vitamin-mineral supplements along with physiologic doses of vitamin D and broad-spectrum balanced fatty acid supplementation, and ensuring "immunomicrobial" health with the skillful use of probiotics, prebiotics, immunorestoration, and antimicrobial treatments provides an excellent health-promoting and disease-eliminating foundation and lifestyle for many patients. Often, this simple protocol is all that is needed for the effective treatment of a wide range of clinical problems, even those that have been "medical failures" for many years. For other patients with more complex illnesses, of course, additional interventions and laboratory assessments can be used to optimize and further customize the treatment plan. Clinicians should avoid seeking "silver bullet" treatments that ignore overall metabolism, immune function, and inflammatory balance, and we must always remember that the attainment and preservation of health requires that we first meet the body's basic nutritional and physiologic needs. This five-step protocol begins the process of meeting those needs. With it, health can be restored and the need for disease-specific treatment is obviated or reduced; without it, fundamental physiologic needs are not met, and health cannot be obtained and maintained. Addressing core physiologic needs empowers doctors to deliver the most effective healthcare possible, and it allows patients to benefit from such treatment.

[141] Force M, Sparks WS, Ronzio RA. Inhibition of enteric parasites by emulsified oil of oregano in vivo. *Phytother Res* 2000;14:213-4
[142] Schuster BG. Demonstrating the validity of natural products as anti-infective drugs. *J Altern Complement Med* 2001;7 Suppl 1:S73-82
[143] Vasquez A. Integrative Rheumatology. IBMRC: 2006, 2009.
[144] Tuft L. Iodides in bronchial asthma. *J Allergy Clin Immunol.* 1981 Jun;67(6):497
[145] Falliers CJ, McCann WP, Chai H, Ellis EF, Yazdi N. Controlled study of iodotherapy for childhood asthma. *J Allergy.* 1966 Sep;38(3):183-92
[146] Tripathy S, et al. Rhinofacial zygomycosis successfully treated with oral saturated solution of potassium iodide. *J Eur Acad Dermatol Venereol.* 2007 Jan;21(1):117-9
[147] Bonifaz A, et al. Sporotrichosis in childhood: clinical and therapeutic experience in 25 patients. *Pediatr Dermatol.* 2007 Jul-Aug;24(4):369-72
[148] Ghent WR, Eskin BA, Low DA, Hill LP. Iodine replacement in fibrocystic disease of the breast. *Can J Surg.* 1993 Oct;36(5):453-60

<mark>*Update and addendum to information on iodine and iodide</mark>:

- <u>Authoritative enthusiasm for high-dose iodine-iodide</u>: Several authoritative articles/authors stated that an advisable level of intake for iodine-iodide for the prevention and treatment of various conditions is approximately 12 mg/d. Because of these well-referenced and apparently authoritative publications, many clinicians and nutrition professionals began using higher doses iodine-iodide with patients and clients, quite often with benefit and nearly always with the absence of serious adverse effects. Several popular nutritional supplements used by clinicians and nutritionists contain both iodi<u>ne</u> (the <u>n</u>atural, diatomic form) and iodi<u>de</u> (the <u>d</u>ivided/ionic form most commonly consumed in <u>d</u>ietary supplements, such as potassium iodi<u>de</u>); both forms of this volatile metal have biologic properties in humans. Benefits of iodine-iodide supplementation focus mostly on the mucolytic, antimicrobial, and anti-estrogen effects.

  - <u>Dr Jonathan V Wright (*Nutrition and Healing* 2002 Nov and 2005 May)</u>: In *Nutrition and Healing* (2002 Nov), well-respected nutrition expert, pioneer, and clinician Jonathan V. Wright MD advocated high-dose iodine-iodide for a wide range of conditions, particularly those related to inflammation, excess estrogen, and microbial infections. In another issue of *Nutrition and Healing* (2005 May) Dr Wright wrote "12.5 milligrams (that's 12,500 micrograms) is the optimal daily amount of iodine, not only for your thyroid but for the rest of your body, too." In that same article, Dr Wright stated, "The Japanese have traditionally consumed more iodine, mostly from seaweed, than any other population. The average daily intake of iodine in Japan [is] 13.8 milligrams…", and throughout the article Dr Wright advocates that 12.5 mg/d is "the optimal daily dose" of combined iodine-iodine.

  - <u>Extrathyroidal benefits of iodine (*Journal of American Physicians and Surgeons* 2006 Winter)</u>: Independently and in a peer-reviewed publication, Donald Miller MD (Professor of Surgery, Division of Cardiothoracic Surgery, University of Washington School of Medicine) supported the daily intake of 12.5 mg/d in *Journal of American Physicians and Surgeons* and even supported higher doses with the statement "More than 4,000 patients in this project [Iodine Project] take iodine in daily doses ranging from 12.5 to 50 mg, and those with diabetes can take up to 100 mg /day." Miller also noted that dermatologists "treat inflammatory dermatoses, like nodular vasculitis and pyoderma gangrenosum, with SSKI (supersaturated potassium iodide), beginning with an iodine dose of 900 mg/day, followed by weekly increases of up to 6 g/day as tolerated. Fungal eruptions, like sporotrichosis, are treated initially in gram amounts with great effect."

  - <u>Iodine deficiency and therapeutic considerations (*Alternative Medicine Review* 2008 Jun)</u>: In 2008, Patrick wrote "Estimates of the average daily Japanese iodine consumption vary from 5,280 mcg to 13,800 mcg…" and this again supported and reinforced enthusiasm for doses of approximately 12 mg/d of iodine-iodine. However, in this article, Patrick did not advocate any specific daily dosage, citing 3-6 mg/d as beneficial and without adverse effect.

- <u>Review, reanalysis, and caution</u>: Soon after these enthusiastic publications, Alan Gaby MD published in several magazines, presented in post-graduate educational events, and discussed in his book *Nutritional Medicine* a review and reanalysis of the original data and concluded that the estimated average daily intake of iodine-iodine in Japan had been *overestimated* by a mathematical error (mistakenly interchanging wet and dry weights of seaweed and thus overestimating the daily Japanese intake of iodine-iodine). Per Gaby (*Nutritional Medicine*, page 175), the true intake of iodine-iodide in Japan averages 330-500 mcg/d, which is 25-fold lower than the estimate of 13.8 mg/d, upon which rested much of the rationale for implementing high-dose iodine-iodide supplementation empirically and routinely.

- <u>Benefits, perspectives, and additional research</u>: Many clinicians including the current author have used high-dose iodine-iodide ranging from approximately 12-48 mg/d for variable periods of time without personally experiencing or clinically observing apparent adverse effects; that statement does not imply endorsement of routine universal high-dose iodine-iodide supplementation. Some degree of caution is advised in consideration of the risks of inducing thyroid dysfunction (hyperthyroidism, hypothyroidism), intestinal hemorrhage[149], and

---

[149] Kinoshita et al. Severe duodenal hemorrhage induced by Lugol's solution administered for thyroid crisis treatment. *Intern Med.* 2010;49(8):759-61

anaphylaxis-like reactions.[150] Topical and systemic antimicrobial benefits of iodine-iodide are well known and well documented; oral high-dose iodine-iodide has been used to treat drug-resistant fungal infections (cited below). When applied for sufficient concentrations and durations, both diatomic iodine and ionic iodide possess potent broad-spectrum antimicrobial properties; essentially no "drug resistance" against iodine-iodide exists for bacteria, fungi, viruses, and protozoans. Iodine also has documented molecular and clinical anti-estrogen effects, thus providing scientific explanation for its ability to treat and prevent estrogen-related disorders ranging from fibrocystic breast disease to cancer. Indeed, iodine treatment of breast cancer cells has been shown to increase the mRNA levels of several genes involved in estrogen metabolism and "detoxification" such as cytochrome p450-1A1 while also decreasing the levels of estrogen responsive genes such as TFF1 and WISP2; also noted following iodine treatment is upregulation of gene expression for the enzyme glutathione peroxidase, an important selenium-dependent component of antioxidant defense mechanisms.[151]

- o Ultra-high dose iodide for sporotrichosis in childhood (*Pediatric Dermatology* 2007 Jul-Aug): Nineteen pediatric patients with proven sporotrichosis were successfully treated with potassium iodide per the following quoted protocol: "All patients were initially treated with potassium iodide (KI), and only those who were unresponsive or who developed side effects were given itraconazole. The dose of KI used was 1–3 g/day, starting at 1 g/day and increasing until the dose of 3 g/day was reached. ... Treatments were sustained until remission was reached, which ranged from 3 to 6 months."[152] Per the review by Miller[153] cited previously, KI 1g (1,000 mg) contains 770 mg of iodide. Thus, the pediatric patients in this case series were treated with 770-2,310 mg/d of iodide for successful antimycotic treatment. Two patients from the original group of 23 patients experienced nausea and vomiting from the KI and were switched to itraconazole; two other patients were lost to follow-up. The authors note that, "Side effects occur in 5% to 10% of patients, mainly presenting as gastrointestinal symptoms as well as headache and rhinorrhea to a lesser extent."

- o Ultra-high dose iodide for rhinofacial zygomycosis—case report (*Journal of European Academy of Dermatology and Venereology* 2007 Jan): A 19-year-old male "was put on oral SSKI at an initial dose of 0.5 mL three times daily. This was gradually increased by 0.1 mL/dose/day until a dose of 5 mL three times daily was reached."[154] Generic formulation of "saturated solution of potassium iodide" (SSKI) contains 1000 mg of KI per mL of solution, which provides roughly 750 mg iodide; thus, SSKI dosed at 5 mL thrice daily = 15 mL/d = 11,250 mg/d (slightly more than 11 grams per day) of iodide for this adult patient with rhinofacial zygomycosis. Treatment was continued for at least 12 months without report of adverse effect.

- o Modest dose iodine replacement in fibrocystic disease of the breast (*Canadian Journal of Surgery* 1993 Oct): Ghent and colleagues[155] sought to determine the response of patients with fibrocystic breast disease to "iodine replacement therapy" and reviewed three clinical studies of different design containing 233, 145 (later up to 1365), and 23 subjects; overall, subjective alleviation of pain and objective alleviation of breast fibrosis was seen in approximately 70% of patients. Consistent with other reports and impressions, the authors noted that, "Molecular iodine is nonthyrotropic and was the most beneficial." The dose of molecular iodine averaged 0.08 mg/kg body weight, which for an average 140-lb (63-kg) patient equates to approximately 5 mg/d.

- o Modest dose iodine in patients with cyclic mastalgia (*Breast Journal* 2004 Jul-Aug): Kessler[156] reports a randomized, double-blind, placebo-controlled, multicenter clinical trial was conducted with 111 otherwise healthy euthyroid women with a history of breast pain and fibrosis; subjects received molecular iodine for 6 months. Physicians assessed breast pain, tenderness, and nodularity each cycle; patients assessed breast pain and tenderness with the Lewin breast pain scale at 3-month intervals and with a VAS at each cycle. All iodine-treated subjects improved compared to no improvement seen in

---

[150] Indraccolo et al. Anaphylactic-like reaction to Lugol solution during colposcopy. *South Med J* 2009 Jan;102(1):96-7

[151] "Quantitative RT-PCR confirmed the array data demonstrating that iodine/iodide treatment increased the mRNA levels of several genes involved in estrogen metabolism (CYP1A1, CYP1B1, and AKR1C1) while decreasing the levels of the estrogen responsive genes TFF1 and WISP2." Stoddard FR 2nd, et al. Iodine alters gene expression in the MCF7 breast cancer cell line: evidence for an anti-estrogen effect of iodine. *Int J Med Sci.* 2008 Jul 8;5(4):189-96

[152] Bonifaz A, et al. Sporotrichosis in childhood: clinical and therapeutic experience in 25 patients. *Pediatr Dermatol.* 2007 Jul-Aug;24(4):369-72

[153] Said of KI, "The standard dose was 1g, which contains 770 mg of iodine." Miller DW. Extrathyroidal benefits of iodine. *J Am Physicians Surgeons* 2006;Winter,106-10

[154] Tripathy et al. Rhinofacial zygomycosis successfully treated with oral saturated solution of potassium iodide. *J Eur Acad Dermatol Venereol.* 2007;21:117-9

[155] Ghent et al. Iodine replacement in fibrocystic disease of the breast. *Can J Surg.* 1993 Oct;36(5):453-60

[156] Kessler JH. The effect of supraphysiologic levels of iodine on patients with cyclic mastalgia. *Breast J.* 2004 Jul-Aug;10(4):328-36

the placebo group. "Reductions in all three physician assessments were observed in patients after 5 months of therapy in the 3.0 mg/day (7/28; 25%) and 6.0 mg/day (15/27; 18.5%) treatment groups, but not the 1.5 mg/day or placebo group. ==Patients recorded statistically significant decreases in pain by month 3 in the 3.0 and 6.0 mg/day treatment groups==, but not the 1.5 mg/day or placebo group; more than 50% of the 6.0 mg/day treatment group recorded a clinically significant reduction in overall pain. All doses were associated with an acceptable safety profile. No dose-related increase in any adverse event was observed." Notably, the failure of the 1.5 mg/day dose implies that this dose is inadequate and thereby justifies higher routine dosing.

- <u>Clinical implementation and the author's perspective</u>: Iodide has a stronger effect on thyroid function and provides tissue-penetrating antimicrobial benefits from oral administration. Molecular iodine has anti-estrogen effects that correlate with the clinical alleviation of cyclic breast pain and fibrocystic breast disease; other anti-estrogen benefits such as an anti-cancer benefit are reasonably anticipated from supplemental iodine. Products with combined iodine and iodide are available and reasonable for clinical use, and a daily dose range of 3-6 mg does not appear unreasonable and has been shown to be beneficial in human studies. Iodine and iodide are impressively well tolerated. Nicely summarized in a personal email from Michael Gonzalez DSc PhD in November 2012, an overview of iodine-iodine's clinical applications may be stated as follows:

"Different tissues of the body respond to different forms of iodine. The Iodide form is believed to be particularly useful for the thyroid. But the supplement of choice for the breast is "iodine" not "iodide." Lugol's formula is Iodine 5% + Potassium iodide (KI) 10% in distilled water. Because different tissues concentrate different forms of iodine, using a supplement that contains both iodine and iodide is preferable to using a supplement that contains only one form. With different tissues responding to different forms of iodine, it would make common sense that a greater therapeutic benefit from iodine will be achieved by using a combination of iodide and iodine. ... The most frequent adverse reactions to potassium iodide are stomach upset, diarrhea, nausea, vomiting, stomach pain, salivary gland swelling/tenderness, acne and skin rash."

Antioxidant support in general and supplementation with selenium in particular are recommended always, and particularly when iodine-iodide doses greater than 1-3 mg/d are used. Selenium 200 mcg/d has been shown in several studies to have an ameliorating effect on thyroid autoimmunity and a supportive effect on peripheral thyroid hormone metabolism. Although iod<u>in</u>e is generally considered <u>n</u>onthyrotropic, periodic assessment of thyroid function and for thyroid autoimmunity is reasonable for patients taking long-term high-dose treatment. ==Clinicians should take advantage of iodine-iodide's safe and effective mucolytic, antimicrobial, and anti-estrogen benefits.==

Distinguishing iodiNe from iodiDe

iodiNe
- **Natural** elemental form—diatomic.
- **Nonthyrotropic**—no immediate adverse effects on thyroid function.
- **Nuclear**—affects gene expression, for example by promoting estrogen detoxification and reducing estrogen responsiveness.
- **Nixes microbes**, antimicrobial—very broad spectrum; povidone iodine is one of the most widely used topical antimicrobials in the history of microbiology and medicine.

iodiDe
- **Divided**—ionic, nondiatomic.
- **Dietary** form, such as in iodized salt which typically contains potassium iodate, potassium iodide, sodium iodate, or sodium iodide.
- **Dissolves mucus**—mucolytic benefits advantageous in the treatment of asthma, bronchitis and respiratory tract infections. Potassium iodide is thought to act as an expectorant by increasing respiratory tract secretions and thereby decreasing the viscosity of mucus; iodide levels increase in respiratory secretions within approximately 15 minutes after oral administration.
- **Directly thyrotropic**—necessary for thyroid hormone production; high doses can cause thyroid dysfunction, which may be problematic (exacerbation of thyroid autoimmunity, hypothyroidism, or hyperthyroidism) or therapeutic (inhibition of thyroid hormone production during hyperthyroidism).
- **Deals death to microbes**, antimicrobial—very broad spectrum, used in the form of potassium iodide (KI, SSKI) for the treatment of microbial infections such as zygomycosis and sporotrichosis.

Reply to "Role of Western Diet in Inflammatory Autoimmune Diseases" by Manzel et al. in *Current Allergy and Asthma Reports*, Volume 14, Issue 1, 2014 January

The short version of this letter was originally published in digital/online and printed formats in
Current Allergy and Asthma Reports 2014 Aug[157]

Interested readers should access ICHNFM.org/publications/ to see if
the full version of this letter has been published in digital/online open-access format in
International Journal of Human Nutrition and Functional Medicine[158]

I think the original article by Manzel et al[159] is/was a disservice to science, to clinicians, and to the *Journal* that published their intellectually impoverished 8-page 100-citation review. The full version of my original reply—as short as I could make it consistent with most *Letters to the Editor*—was approximately 1,500 words and 21 citations; the version accepted and published by the *Journal* was approximately 450 words and 4 citations, and it notably excluded my five main concluding statements, which I have included here:

"In sum, the review by Manzel et al is characterized by:
1) Questionable and/or erroneous statements presented as matter of fact without any citation,
2) Failure to include important research showing significant and replicated clinical data in humans,
3) Inappropriate promotion of drug treatments over nutritional treatments,
4) Apparent failure to disclose financial relationships with drug companies[160], and
5) Inaccurate, denigrating, and sweeping generalizations misrepresenting the (in)efficacy of nutritional supplements."

Out of respect and appreciation for the (new) editorial team at the *Journal*, and because of this book's space limitation (printing limit of 630 pages) and my own overscheduled schedule, I have chosen to not make the full version of my reply public yet, but may do so later in *International Journal of Human Nutrition and Functional Medicine* available at ICHNFM.org/publications/. While I honestly think the original article by Manzel et al is a horrid (mis)representation of the current state of the science, I do appreciate the modest-yet-significant show of integrity by the *Journal* editors in their acceptance and publication of my *Reply*; anything less would have warranted a potent response in defense of science, intellectual integrity, and the clinicians and patients dependent on the integrity of science for pain-alleviating and life-saving decisions.

---

[157] Vasquez A. Reply to "role of Western diet in inflammatory autoimmune diseases" by Manzel et Al. In *Current Allergy and Asthma Reports* (volume 14, issue 1, January 2014). *Curr Allergy Asthma Rep*. 2014 Aug;14(8):454. Published online 20 Jun 2014 link.springer.com/article/10.1007%2Fs11882-014-0454-4

[158] Vasquez A. Rebuttal to "Role of Western Diet in Inflammatory Autoimmune Diseases" by Manzel et al in Current Allergy Asthma Reports 2014 January. *International Journal of Human Nutrition and Functional Medicine* ® 2014:2(2);2 https://ichnfm.academia.edu/AlexVasquez

[159] Manzel A, Muller DN, Hafler DA, et al. Role of "Western diet" in inflammatory autoimmune diseases. *Curr Allergy Asthma Rep*. 2014 Jan;14(1):404

[160] "Dr. Linker has received personal compensation for activities with BayerVital, Biogen Idec, NovartisPharma, Merck Serono, and TEVA Pharma. Dr. Linker has received research support from BayerVital, Biogen Idec, NovartisPharma, Merck Serono, and TEVA Pharma. Dr. Kleinewietfeld has received royalty payments from Stemcell-Technologies. Dr. Hafler has received personal compensation for activities with Wyeth, Beckman Coulter, and Novartis." S50 Multiple Sclerosis: Novel Mechanisms of Action High Dietary Salt Aggravates Experimental Neuroinflammation in Mice via Induction of Th17 Cells. *Neurology* February 12, 2013 neurology.org/cgi/content/meeting_abstract/80/1_MeetingAbstracts/S50.003

Curr Allergy Asthma Rep (2014) 14:454
DOI 10.1007/s11882-014-0454-4

AUTOIMMUNITY (TK TARRANT, SECTION EDITOR)

Reply to "Role of Western Diet in Inflammatory Autoimmune Diseases" by Manzel et al. in *Current Allergy and Asthma Reports* (Volume 14, Issue 1, January 2014)

Alex Vasquez

Published online: 20 June 2014
© Springer Science+Business Media New York 2014

To the Editor,

Regarding the recent review "Role of Western Diet in Inflammatory Autoimmune Diseases" [1], while I appreciate the importance of this topic and the authors' review, I noted several shortcomings in this review and have questions about the omission of certain information. The authors failed to include relevant and important human data while instead relying on animal studies (their Table 1). The authors also include erroneous information, without appropriate citation.

The authors state that "a high-fat diet is a prominent factor in promoting obesity" but failed to provide citation for this. Importantly, other researchers have shown that high-fat ketogenic diets promote weight loss rather than obesity.

I found the reliance on animal data (especially their Table 1) and the exclusion of human data inappropriate for a review article of this nature and at this time in biomedical history. Several clinical trials have already documented the effectiveness of dietary intervention in human autoimmune diseases. For example, diets which emphasize increased consumption of plant foods (excluding gluten-containing grains) and dietary alteration of gastrointestinal flora have already shown clinical benefits [2]. Exclusion of gluten is of critical importance for some patients, and well established is gluten's role in inflammation, alteration of gastrointestinal flora, increasing intestinal permeability, and direct stimulation of inflammatory pathways. The authors mentioned hypertension four times in their review but failed to mention the remarkable efficacy of therapeutic fasting for this condition [3]. Clinical trials showing the safety and efficacy of dietary fatty acid supplementation were also excluded from the review, despite showing remarkable clinical safety and antirheumatic efficacy [4]. Antiinflammatory mechanisms of dietary intervention not mentioned in their review include alleviation of oxidative stress, alleviation of dysbiosis, reduced reactivity to dietary antigens, normalization of intestinal hyperpermeability, and alleviation of proinflammatory mitochondrial dysfunction [5].

This article is part of the Topical Collection on *Autoimmunity*

A. Vasquez (✉)
International College of Human Nutrition and Functional Medicine in Barcelona, Barcelona, Spain
e-mail: ichnfm@gmail.com

A. Vasquez
Biotics Research Corporation in Rosenberg, Rosenberg, TX, USA

References

1. Manzel A, Muller DN, Hafler DA, Erdman SE, Linker RA, Kleinewietfeld M. Role of "Western diet" in inflammatory autoimmune diseases. Curr Allergy Asthma Rep. 2014;14(1):404.
2. Peltonen R, Nenonen M, Helve T, et al. Faecal microbial flora and disease activity in rheumatoid arthritis during a vegan diet. Br J Rheumatol. 1997;36(1):64–8.
3. Goldhamer A, Lisle D, Parpia B, Anderson SV, Campbell TC. Medically supervised water-only fasting in the treatment of hypertension. J Manip Physiol Ther. 2001;24(5):335–9.
4. Belch JJ, Ansell D, Madhok R, O'Dowd A, Sturrock RD. Effects of altering dietary essential fatty acids on requirements for non-steroidal anti-inflammatory drugs in patients with rheumatoid arthritis: a double blind placebo controlled study. Ann Rheum Dis. 1988;47(2):96–104.
5. Vasquez A. Integrative rheumatology and inflammation mastery, Third Edition. Create Space Publishers; 2014.

Springer

Diet—Details, Biochemical Concepts, and Clinical Pearls

- **Macronutrients and "The Big Picture":** The following section balances details with practicality to review necessary "real world" information for clinicians who aspire to efficacy en route to excellence in the realm of nutritional medicine.

  o **Protein:** As with all nutrients, we can begin the conversation by breaking-down a large topic into its components, the main two of which are consumption and utilization, with the former obviously preceding the latter; realistically, those are preceded by availability, affordability, and selection.

    ▪ **Protein acquisition:** Challenges to dietary protein acquisition include: availability, cost, knowledge of need, social/political norms, and frequency of utilization. In famished countries and regions, carbohydrate-sufficient protein malnutrition (*kwashiorkor*) is noted, while a milder form of "subclinical protein malnutrition" is impressively common among vegetarians, vegans, and persons who simply do not consume sufficient dietary protein due to habit or ignorance. As my teacher Dr Jeffrey Bland wisely said in his lecture series on *Nutritional Biochemistry* several decades ago, "You can do no better than the food that you eat, but you can do a whole lot worse." As such, the minimum requirement for proper protein nutriture begins with consumption of the proper amount of high-quality dietary protein per age, size/weight, activity and physiologic needs; the following table provides excellent objective guidance:

Recommended <u>Grams of Protein</u> per <u>Patient Profile</u> and <u>Body Weight</u> Per Day		
<u>Patient Profile</u>	*Per* <u>**pound**</u> of weight[161]	*Per* <u>**kilogram**</u> of weight
Adult recreational exerciser	**0.5-0.75**	**1.1-1.65**
Adult competitive athlete	0.6-0.9	1.32-1.98
Adult building muscle mass	0.7-0.9	1.54-1.98
Dieting athlete	0.7-1.0	1.54-2.2
Growing teenage athlete	0.9-1.0	1.98-2.2

Sufficient dietary protein is essential for patients with musculoskeletal injuries because tissue healing relies on the constant availability of amino acids and micronutrients[162], which should be supplied by a healthy, balanced, whole-foods diet that may be supplemented with specific vitamins, minerals, and phytonutrients. Increased protein intake does not adversely affect bone health as long as dietary calcium intake is adequate[163]; acid-base balance, and intakes of vitamin D3, magnesium, anti-inflammatory fatty acids, and other nutrients such as vitamin K and phytonutrients are also clinically important. Per the excellent review by Lemon[164], "Those involved in strength training might need to consume as much as …1.7 g protein x kg(-1) x day(-1)…while those undergoing endurance training might need about 1.2 to 1.6 g x kg(-1) x day(-1)… …**there is no evidence that protein intakes in the range suggested will have adverse effects in healthy individuals.**" To calculate protein requirements for patients who are completely sedentary, multiply body weight in pounds by 0.4 and this will give the number of grams of protein that should be eaten each day.[165] For patients who are very active (frequent weight lifting, or competitive athlete), multiply body weight in pounds by 0.7-0.9 and this will give the number of grams of protein that should be eaten each day. Again, compared with *sedentary* people, those who are *sick, injured*, and *athletic* **need more dietary protein** to maintain weight, fight infections, repair injuries, and build and maintain muscle mass. Low-

---

[161] Slightly modified from Nancy Clark, MS, RD. Protein Power. *The Physician and Sportsmedicine* 1996, volume 24, number 4

[162] "Supplementation with protein and vitamins, specifically arginine and vitamins A, B, and C, provides optimum nutrient support of the healing wound." Meyer NA, Muller MJ, Herndon DN. Nutrient support of the healing wound. *New Horiz* 1994 May;2(2):202-14

[163] Heaney RP. Excess dietary protein may not adversely affect bone. *J Nutr* 1998 Jun;128(6):1054-7

[164] Lemon PW. Effects of exercise on dietary protein requirements. *Int J Sport Nutr* 1998 Dec;8(4):426-47

[165] Pellet PL. Protein requirements in humans. *Am J Clin Nutr* 1990 May;51(5):723-37

protein diets suppress immune function, reduce muscle mass, and impair healing[166,167] whereas intakes of higher amounts of protein safely facilitate healing and the maintenance of muscle mass.

- Carbohydrates, CHO: Carbohydrate intake should be sufficient but otherwise minimal because carbohydrates—much more so than proteins and lipids and in many cases exclusively—promote dyslipidemia, immunosuppression, mitochondrial impairment, hunger, tumorigenesis, inflammation, oxidative stress and antioxidant depletion. Importantly, carbohydrate intake is the most important macronutrient *inverse* determinant of endogenous bHB production; excessive carbohydrate intake suppresses bHB production and therefore leads to direct/relative mitochondrial impairment, oxidative stress, and an aging (rather than rejuvenative) phenotype. Excess carbohydrate intake—notably fermentable carbohydrates such as from wheat and potatoes—is also the most important dietary cause of small intestinal bacterial overgrowth (SIBO), which is the primary cause the majority of cases of fibromyalgia (FM)[168], gastroesophageal reflux[169], irritable bowel syndrome (IBS)[170], and restless leg syndrome (RLS)[171], especially when accompanied by IBS or FM. Benefits of carbohydrate intake include maintenance of glucose/glycogen stores and relative elevation of serum tryptophan (depression of other amino acid levels) for enhanced serotonergic cerebral neurotransmission. Although patients and doctors alike have been conditioned to believe that carbohydrate intake is necessary at every meal and via snacks and sugared beverages throughout the day, the more profound truths are that ❶ carbohydrate-rich foods are better avoided, ❷ carbohydrate intake should be minimized to meet physiologic requirements (e.g., recovery from exercise, maintenance of desired weight), and ❸ constant intake of carbohydrates produces what I term *carbohydrate-mediated carbohydrate dependence*—excessive physiologic dependence on carbohydrates via adaptation to this fuel source (for example in part via dietary modification of

Adverse effects of dietary carbohydrates (general) and processed fructose (specific)

- Adipogenesis
- Hyperphagia (absolute or relative)
- Immunosuppression
- Oxidative stress
- Antioxidant nutrient depletion
- Endogenous antimetabolites: Promotion of palmitate and ceramide production, with resultant insulin resistance.
- Hyperinsulinemia: Stimulation of sodium retention (promoting HTN) and HMG-CoA reductase (promoting hypercholesterolemia).
- Loss of endogenous bHB: Inhibition of bHB (beta-hydroxy-butyrate) production; loss of bHB causes a relative increase in oxidant stress and loss of mitochondrial function.
- GI microbial overgrowth: Residual and fermentable carbohydrates in the gastrointestinal tract directly promote microbial overgrowth in gut, promoting systemic inflammation (e.g., via LPS, increased intestinal permeability, and immune complexes), fibromyalgia, GERD, RLS.
- Problems specific to fructose: Induction of bacterial dysbiosis and increased intestinal permeability leading to endotoxinemia; induction of AGE / Maillard reaction / glycosylation glycation; rapid influx of processed/acellular fructose causes ATP depletion at fructokinase, activates inflammatory pathways, leads to increase in serum urate which causes endothelial dysfunction and insulin resistance—proof of this comes from inhibition of fructose-induced metabolic syndrome via allopurinol and avoidance of fructose-induced metabolic syndrome and weight gain when fructose is consumed with antioxidant/anti-inflammatory phytochemicals and citrate, the latter of which promotes urinary alkalinization for efficient urate excretion and thereby avoidance of problems induced by relative/absolute hyperuricaemia.

---

[166] Castaneda et al. Elderly women accommodate to a low-protein diet with losses of body cell mass, muscle function, and immune response. *Am J Clin Nutr* 1995;62:30-9

[167] [No author listed]. Vegetarians and healing. *JAMA* 1995; 273: 910

[168] Pimentel M, Wallace D, Hallegua D, Chow E, Kong Y, Park S, Lin HC. A link between irritable bowel syndrome and fibromyalgia may be related to findings on lactulose breath testing. *Ann Rheum Dis.* 2004 Apr;63(4):450-2. For much greater detail and explanation, see my later works/books/chapters on fibromyalgia which integrate this research with the secondary problems such as microbial mitochondriopathy; my most recent update to the fibromyalgia model was published in *Integrative Rheumatology and Inflammation Mastery* (2014); visit InflammationMastery.com for additional publications and updated publications and videos.

[169] Austin GL, Thiny MT, Westman EC, Yancy WS Jr, Shaheen NJ. A very low-carbohydrate diet improves gastroesophageal reflux and its symptoms. *Dig Dis Sci.* 2006 Aug;51(8):1307-12. Yancy WS Jr, Provenzale D, Westman EC. Improvement of gastroesophageal reflux disease after initiation of a low-carbohydrate diet: five brief case reports. *Altern Ther Health Med.* 2001 Nov-Dec;7(6):120, 116-9. Piche T, des Varannes SB, Sacher-Huvelin S, Holst JJ, Cuber JC, Galmiche JP. Colonic fermentation influences lower esophageal sphincter function in gastroesophageal reflux disease. *Gastroenterology.* 2003 Apr;124(4):894-902

[170] Lin HC. Small intestinal bacterial overgrowth: a framework for understanding irritable bowel syndrome. *JAMA.* 2004 Aug 18;292(7):852-8

[171] Weinstock et al. Restless legs syndrome in patients with irritable bowel syndrome: response to SIBO therapy. *Dig Dis Sci.* 2008 May;53(5):1252-6

electron transport chain supercomplex assembly[172]). Dietary carbohydrate sources can be selected based on their ability to promote or inhibit intestinal microbial growth; this is the basis for the specific carbohydrate diet (SCD)[173] and variations on that theme to prevent microbial overgrowth in the intestines and its complications such as autobrewery syndrome.[174, 175]

- ○ Fats, lipids: Average Paleolithic intake of n3 fatty acids was approximately 7 grams per day; and modern (American diet) intake is 1 gram per day; therefore, relatively speaking and contrasting physiologic expectations with modern dietary intakes, persons/patients can be considered n3-deficient unless they are consuming n3 supplementation or what would be considered today "special" (or by the allopathic paradigm: "faddish") diets. What is commonly called fatty acid *supplementation* should more appropriately be called fatty acid *replacement* since generally all that is being done is *normalizing* intake of fatty acids, rather than doing anything heroic or unnatural. All of the main dietary n3 fatty acids (FA)—ALA, EPA, DHA—have clinically significant anti-inflammatory benefits; n6FA linolenic and arachidonic acids are both clearly pro-inflammatory and tumorigenic, while n6FA GLA is clearly anti-inflammatory and anti-tumorigenic. In the gastrointestinal tract, dietary long-chain saturated fats promote LPS absorption from the gastrointestinal tract via chylomicron formation; in this way "saturated fat promotes inflammation" *via a mechanism completely independent from the metabolic and adipogenic effects of fat*: by serving as a carrier/container for pro-inflammatory bacterial LPS.

- ○ Fiber: Basically—from the perspective of clinicians, "fibers" and indigestible carbohydrate from plants can be considered in three different ways: ❶ Soluble—think "absorbing", bulking, and fermentable: Best example is oat bran, absorbs and reduces absorption of cholesterol, serves as fermentable food source for bacteria and in this manner increases fecal bulk (along with water retention), not necessarily a good idea for patients with SIBO, ❷ Insoluble—think "binding", bulking, and mostly nonfermentable: Best example is wheat bran, but rice bran is also commercially available and avoids the problems of wheat's toxic gluten; vegetable fibers are mostly insoluble fiber; more likely to bind minerals such as zinc and iron, generally/relatively nonfermentable and thus increases fecal bulk via mass and some water retention (rather than promoting growth of bacteria); reasonable for patients with SIBO; vegetable matter in general and brown rice in particular have favorable effects on human gastrointestinal flora, promoting eubiosis; in regard to the latter, carrots are notable for their antimicrobial/eubiosis effect for which carrots have been used for the treatment of infectious diarrhea (and SIBO); ❸ Fermentable carbohydrates lacking physical bulking action: Best examples are inulin and fructooligosaccharides (FOS) which generally promote growth of beneficial bacteria excepting *Klebsiella pneumoniae* growth on FOS; no physical bulking action except via bacterial proliferation; no absorbing/binding action of clinical significance.

- ○ pH and acid-base balance: Given the body's inherent acid-forming tendency, alkalinizing measures must be available to prevent what would otherwise be inevitable metabolic acidosis resulting specifically from cellular metabolism and its attendant production of organic acids, carbon dioxide, ketoacids, and sulfuric acid, the last in this list from sulfur-containing amino acid catabolism. Both acute and long-term acid-base balance are *grossly* regulated by respiration and urination, while the more subtle fine-tuning occurs via dietary input. In accord with the concept of biochemical individuality and the truism that treatment must always be individualized, some people tend to be more or less *acidic* or *basic* than others as measured by urine pH, which is a reasonable measure of systemic acid-base status provided adequate renal function and which allows direct measurement of urine pH, which—per the position paper by Proudfoot et al—should be at least 7.5 to promote xenobiotic excretion. However, generally speaking for most of the population consuming a Western diet characterized by *gross* insufficiency of **plants** (thus lack of [potassium] **citrate** as an immediate precursor for alkalinizing **bicarbonate**) and a *relative* excess of animal/dairy/grain **protein** (thereby

[172] Lapuente-Brun et al. Supercomplex assembly determines electron flux in the mitochondrial electron transport chain. *Science*. 2013 Jun 28;340(6140):1567-70
[173] Gottschall EG. *Breaking the Vicious Cycle: Intestinal Health Through Diet*, 1994
[174] Dahshan et al. Auto-brewery syndrome in a child with short gut syndrome: case report and review of the literature. *J Pediatr Gastroenterol Nutr*. 2001 Aug;33(2):214-5
[175] Cordell et al. Case Study of Gut Fermentation Syndrome (Auto-Brewery) with Saccharomyces cerevisiae as the Causative Organism. *Int J Clin Med* 2013, 4, 309-312

promoting endogenous formation of sulfuric acid); in this manner, the Western diet is said to promote diet-induced metabolic acidosis, which promotes many long-term (not acute) health problems such as osteoporosis, insulin resistance, hypertension, and possibly malignant disease.[176] Urinary alkalinization can be maintained via *a personalized combination of* plant-based diets, regular deep-breathing and exercise to promote respiratory alkalosis, and supplemental potassium/magnesium citrate/bicarbonate (rarely sodium bicarbonate, which has the disadvantage of sodium but the advantage of greater public availability); benefits of alkalinization include enhanced detoxification/clearance of xenobiotics, thereby contributing to alleviation of current disease and reduced risk of future disease[177], ❶ increased endorphin production for alleviation of pain[178] and depression, possible lessening of (tobacco) addiction[179], ❷ reduced serum cortisol and bone loss[180] and likely reductions in hippocampal atrophy and insulin resistance also via reductions in serum cortisol, ❸ enhanced intracellular retention of magnesium by 11%[181], ❹ enhanced xenobiotic excretion (generally).[182]

o Micronutrients and nutritional supplementation with vitamins, minerals, combination fatty acids, and probiotics: Space, time, and scope do not allow an exhaustive review of all vitamins and minerals in this volume; my last outline of all major vitamins and minerals was printed in *Chiropractic and Naturopathic Mastery of Common Clinical Disorders* (2009) and the next version of such will be published in an upcoming volume in this *Inflammation Mastery* series and/or in an open-access review published in *International Journal of Human Nutrition and Functional Medicine*. Here, I will only discuss a few classic must-know topics while the nutrients relevant for the **functional inflammology protocol** are discussed within contexts of clinical application; the subject of routine nutritional supplementation is also addressed in my accompanying presentation from ICHNFM 2013.[183] **Combination fatty acid therapy** (CFAT) is discussed in the minimonograph in this chapter; additional applications are mentioned in the description of the protocol and in additional volumes detailing clinical applications for specific conditions. **Probiotics** should be pretty well known to most of my readers; additional details are provided elsewhere in the book and are not replicated here; my clinical approach to probiotic therapy emphasizes 1) dietary optimization since diet is the most important determinant of intestinal microbial ecology, 2) daily consumption of fermented/probiotic foods such as yogurt, kefir, miso, real sauerkraut, etc, 3) stress reduction and nutrient supplementation (e.g., vitamins A and D, along with zinc and glutamine) to improve intestinal immunity and thereby reduce dysbiosis and promote eubiosis, 4) use of probiotic and synbiotic supplements to further ensure intake of beneficial microbes. The subsections that follow detail some of the most important general concepts and specific *must know* information about vitamins and minerals—again see the accompanying presentation from the 2013 International Conference on

Net acid and base production from common foods

Acid-producing foods: Notice that these foods represent the majority of food intake for many people, thereby promoting population-wide diet-induced metabolic acidosis:
- Fish, shellfish, meat, poultry, eggs,
- Cheese, milk
- Cereal grains
- Chloride ion (added in the form of sodium chloride, table salt)

Base-producing foods:
- Fruit, vegetables, tubers, roots, and nuts

Neutral:
- Legumes
- Fats
- Refined sugars

Cordain et al. Origins and evolution of Western diet. *Am J Clin Nutr.* 2005

---

[176] "Even a very mild degree of metabolic acidosis induces skeletal muscle resistance to the insulin action and dietary acid load may be an important variable in predicting the metabolic abnormalities and the cardiovascular risk of the general population, the overweight and obese persons, and other patient populations including diabetes and chronic kidney failure. High dietary acid load is more likely to result in diabetes and systemic hypertension and may increase the cardiovascular risk." Adeva MM, Souto G. Diet-induced metabolic acidosis. *Clin Nutr.* 2011 Aug;30(4):416-21

[177] Minich DM, Bland JS. Acid-alkaline balance: role in chronic disease and detoxification. *Altern Ther Health Med.* 2007 Jul-Aug;13(4):62-5

[178] Vormann J, et al. Supplementation with alkaline minerals reduces symptoms in patients with chronic low back pain. *J Trace Elem Med Biol.* 2001;15(2-3):179-83

[179] This study showed a small initial trend toward less tobacco smoke use/inhalation following urinary alkalinization with sodium bicarbonate. Cherek DR, Mauroner RF, Brauchi JT. Effects of increasing urinary pH on cigarette smoking. *Clin Pharmacol Ther.* 1982 Aug;32(2):253-60

[180] Maurer M, Riesen W, Muser J, Hulter HN, Krapf R. Neutralization of Western diet inhibits bone resorption independently of K intake and reduces cortisol secretion in humans. *Am J Physiol Renal Physiol.* 2003 Jan;284(1):F32-40

[181] Vormann J, et al. Supplementation with alkaline minerals reduces symptoms in patients with chronic low back pain. *J Trace Elem Med Biol.* 2001;15(2-3):179-83

[182] Proudfoot AT, Krenzelok EP, Vale JA. Position Paper on urine alkalinization. *J Toxicol Clin Toxicol.* 2004;42(1):1-26

[183] Vasquez A. "Introduction to Functional Inflammology Protocol" presented at International Conference on Human Nutrition and Functional Medicine in Portland, Oregon September 25-29, 2013. More than eight hours of video introducing the functional inflammology protocol—to be used with the printed slides in the final section of this book—is available online: vimeo.com/album/2943155. Password: **DrVprotocol_volume1**

Human Nutrition and Functional Medicine (vimeo.com/ICHNFM) for additional details, rationale, and citations. Before reviewing the important articles summarized and cited immediately following, I'd like to offer one additional consideration: Per standard definitions, our whole idea of "nutritional deficiency" and therefore the need/rightness/wrongness of nutritional supplementation is wrong. Nutritional deficiency should be defined as "insufficient amount relative to individual need" – not absolute amount. We have two intellectually defensible options: 1) scientific but impractical: test all levels and functional parameters to determine month-by-month/year-by-year nutritional needs which change per diet, illness, medication, lifestyle, age, or 2) reasonable and practical: provide a reasonable dose of nutrients to "cover the bases" and meet biochemical needs to safely, inexpensively, and effectively avoid the problems caused by common and occult micronutrient deficiency. The third option which requires zero thought is to 3) deny reality to the detriment of the patient: ignore this data and pretend everything will work out fine on its own.

- General rationale for routine nutritional supplementation #1—Vitamins for chronic disease prevention in adults (JAMA 2002 Jun[184]): "However, suboptimal intake of some vitamins, above levels causing classic vitamin deficiency, is a risk factor for chronic diseases and common in the general population, especially the elderly. ...low levels of the antioxidant vitamins (vitamins A, E, and C) may increase risk for several chronic diseases. Most people do not consume an optimal amount of all vitamins by diet alone. Pending strong evidence of effectiveness from randomized trials, it appears prudent for all adults to take vitamin supplements. ... Physicians should make specific efforts to learn about their patients' use of vitamins to ensure that they are taking vitamins they should...."

- General rationale for routine nutritional supplementation #2—Prevention of long-latency deficiency disease: insights from calcium and vitamin D (Am J Clin Nutr 2003 Nov[185]): "Nutrient intake recommendations and national nutritional policies have focused primarily on prevention of short-latency deficiency diseases. Most nutrient intake recommendations today are based on prevention of the index disease only. However, inadequate intakes of many nutrients are now recognized as contributing to several of the major chronic diseases that affect the populations of the industrialized nations. Often taking many years to manifest themselves, these disease outcomes should be thought of as long-latency deficiency diseases."

- General rationale for routine nutritional supplementation #3—Promotion of optimal metabolism in lieu of the expense and unavailability of extensive laboratory testing for each patient (Am J Clin Nutr 2002 Apr[186]): "As many as one-third of mutations in a gene result in the corresponding enzyme having an increased Michaelis constant, or K(m), (decreased binding affinity) for a coenzyme, resulting in a lower rate of reaction. About 50 human genetic dis-eases due to defective enzymes can be remedied or ameliorated by the administration of high doses of the vitamin component of the corresponding coenzyme, which at least partially restores enzymatic activity. Several single-nucleotide polymorphisms, in which the variant amino acid reduces coenzyme binding and thus enzymatic activity, are likely to be remediable by raising cellular concentrations of the cofactor through high-dose vitamin therapy."

- General rationale for routine nutritional supplementation #4—Vitamin D deficiency is the most common and most clinically significant nutrient deficiency seen regularly in the practice of primary care medicine (Altern Ther Health Med 2004 Sep[187]): Beyond vitamin and mineral supplementation in general is the clinicians' need to focus on vitamin D3 supplementation, especially given that most multivitamin formulations do not meet the physiologic requirement in adults of approximately 4,000 IU/d; per my 2004 "paradigm shift with implications for all healthcare providers" all readers should know that vitamin D deficiency causes—in large percentages of patients per diagnosis—hypertension, migraine headaches, widespread body

[184] Fletcher RH, Fairfield KM. Vitamins for chronic disease prevention in adults: clinical applications. JAMA. 2002 Jun 19;287(23):3127-9
[185] Heaney RP. Long-latency deficiency disease: insights from calcium and vitamin D. Am J Clin Nutr. 2003 Nov;78(5):912-9
[186] Ames BN, et al. High-dose vitamin therapy stimulates variant enzymes with decreased coenzyme binding affinity (increased Km). Am J Clin Nutr 2002 Apr;75:616-58
[187] Vasquez A, Manso G, Cannell J. The clinical importance of vitamin D (cholecalciferol): a paradigm shift. Altern Ther Health Med. 2004 Sep-Oct;10(5):28-36

pain identical to fibromyalgia, local pain consistent with low-back pain, insulin resistance, systemic inflammation and autoimmunity.

- General rationale for routine nutritional supplementation #5—DNA damage from micronutrient deficiencies is likely to be a major cause of cancer (*Mutat Res.* 2001 Apr[188]): " A deficiency of any of the micronutrients: folic acid, Vitamin B12, Vitamin B6, niacin, Vitamin C, Vitamin E, iron, or zinc, mimics radiation in damaging DNA by causing single- and double-strand breaks, oxidative lesions, or both. For example, the percentage of the US population that has a low intake (<50% of the RDA) for each of these eight micronutrients ranges from 2 to >20%. ... Some evidence, and mechanistic considerations, suggest that Vitamin B12 (14% US elderly) and B6 (10% of US) deficiencies also cause high uracil and chromosome breaks. ...Common micronutrient deficiencies are likely to damage DNA by the same mechanism as radiation and many chemicals, appear to be orders of magnitude more important, and should be compared for perspective. Remedying micronutrient deficiencies should lead to a major improvement in health and an increase in longevity at low cost."

- Additional clinical details on iron: Necessary for formation of hemoglobin and dopamine, iron—when accumulated "too much and in the wrong location"—promotes ROS-mediated cellular toxicity, leading to cardiomyopathy, hypogonadism, hepatopathy, and diabetes mellitus; an insufficiency of iron causes immune impairment, mitochondrial dysfunction, anemia, and depression/fatigue/anhedonia due to insufficient CNS dopamine and norepinephrine.

  - Excess absorption and altered storage: Hereditary iron-accumulation disorders such as genetic hemochromatosis are among the most common hereditary diseases in the human population, occurring in all races, both genders, with a clinical presentation occurring at any age but typically in adulthood. Among Caucasians and Hispanics, genetic hemochromatosis has a homozygote frequency of approximately 1 per 200-250 and a heterozygote frequency of 1 per 7; among Africans and African Americans, the clinical phenotype of severe iron overload has been reported as high as 1 per 80 in hospital populations. Genotropic iron-accumulation disorders are quantitative (i.e., excess intestinal absorption of iron) and qualitative (i.e., parenchymal storage which is abnormal and more cytotoxic than the normal deposition of iron in the mononuclear phagocyte system (MPS, previously termed the reticuloendothelial system).

  - Defective/deficient blood-brain transport: A subset of the population has a defect in transport of iron from the blood into the brain can thus develop "brain-specific iron deficiency" with anticipated deficiencies in dopamine, norepinephrine, and mitochondrial function. Clinical consequences of "cerebral iron deficiency" would therefore be expected to include deficits in attention, hedonia/pleasure/mood, motor control, and migraine precipitated by mitochondrial dysfunction. In 2005 Mizuno et al[189] showed low brain iron concentrations in patients with restless leg syndrome (RLS) was due to "dysfunction of iron transportation from serum to CNS in patients with idiopathic RLS" while a more detailed study performed in 2011 by Connor et al[190] confirmed "alterations in the iron management protein profile in RLS compared with controls at the site of blood-brain interface" and also noted a consistent "decrease in transferrin receptor expression in the microvasculature in the presence of relative brain iron deficiency."

- Food consumption: Reviewed here are some clinically important facts about food preparation, consumption, digestion, and metabolism. Advancements in technology and our molecular biology understanding make a conversation about digestion and mastication seem comparatively primitive.

---

[188] Ames BN. DNA damage from micronutrient deficiencies is likely to be a major cause of cancer. *Mutat Res.* 2001 Apr 18;475(1-2):7-20
[189] "These results indicate low brain iron concentration caused by the dysfunction of iron transportation from serum to CNS in patients with idiopathic RLS." Mizuno S, Mihara T, Miyaoka T, Inagaki T, Horiguchi J. CSF iron, ferritin and transferrin levels in restless legs syndrome. *J Sleep Res.* 2005 Mar;14(1):43-7
[190] Connor JR, et al. Profile of altered brain iron acquisition in restless legs syndrome. *Brain.* 2011 Apr;134(Pt 4):959-68

But we all need to pause and reflect on the importance of basic digestion, mastication, salvation etc for proper digestion. Regardless of advances in technology, certain physiologic truths remain inviolable.

- Preparation: Many people lack basic cooking skills, and are thus dependent on processed/packaged/industrial food products; indeed, one of the most important medical consequences of the dissolution of social and familial structure is the pervasive loss of essential life skills—one of the most important of which is food selection and preparation. Fundamental courses in food preparation should be required for all healthcare professionals, who have the responsibility to educate their patients and model good health practices. Most protein-dense animal-based foods can be consumed raw if fresh and sourced from noninfected animals; social customs and concern about microbial contamination commonly prompt cooking, which—despite denaturing dietary proteins—often increases digestibility, palatability, and ease of mastication, thereby increasing total protein intake. The most notable concern with diet-induced parasitosis is cysticercosis and neurocysticercosis caused from consumption of pork which is both undercooked and infected, classically with the pork tapeworm *Taenia solium*.[191] Food-transmitted prion-induced spongiform encephalopathies have been very rarely reported in humans following consumption of deer, boar, elk, and—classically in the case of *kuru*—cultural cannibalism of human brain.

- Consumption: Desire is psychoepistimological, a translation of intellectual and emotional presuppositions into emotional/visceral/emotive responses and actions. Acquisition is motivated by desire, and either facilitate or restrained by social, cultural, and financial realities. Proper protein nutriture requires adequate protein consumption. Psychosocial stress, depression, zinc deficiency, and certain medications (especially stimulants) commonly contribute to anorexia (inadequate appetite and food consumption). Zinc deficiency causes anorexia (reduced appetite/intake), hypogeusia (reduced sense of taste), and hyposmia (reduced sense of smell): all of which contribute to reduced food consumption.

- Mastication: Generally and simplistically speaking, digestion is the break-down of food from animal and plant tissue/material to its component proteins and constituent amino acids and peptides for absorption and cellular uptake; the enzymatic/biochemical breakdown of foods is facilitated by mechanical degradation, allowing greater surface area and thus more enzyme-protein contact, resulting in better "digestion." Teeth (dentition) and time (patience) are needed for proper mastication; an insufficiency of either via dental disease or lack of time allowance/prioritization, respectively, will compromise mastication and thus digestion and thus protein nutriture.

- Digestion—gastric: An adequacy of gastric hydrochloric acid (HCl) is necessary, especially for digestion of proteins, ionization of minerals for enhanced absorption, and microbicidal actions. Production/function of HCl is compromised by antacid substances (e.g., bicarbonate, histamine-2 receptor antagonists, proton-pump antagonists), *Helicobacter pylori* infection/colonization, zinc deficiency, hypocortisolemia, hypothyroidism, hypogonadism, and various types of psychoemotional stress. Inadequate HCl production is noted with atrophic gastritis (such as due to alcoholism) and pernicious anemia; incidence of these is increased in patients with autoimmune thyroiditis and/or vitiligo. HCL replacement with capsules/tablets of betaine HCl can be helpful, and may only need to be maintained for a limited period of time (e.g., 6-12 months), after which endogenous production may return. HCl production can be assessed clinically, via response to HCl supplementation, or by Heidelberg radiotelemetry.

- Digestion—pancreatic: Production and function of pancreatic enzymes is notably zinc-dependent. With pancreatic insufficiency—as especially noted in patients with cystic fibrosis, postpancreatitis pancreatic insufficiency, or acne rosacea—oral supplementation with pancreatic/proteolytic enzymes from porcine/botanical sources can be highly beneficial.

---

[191] See cdc.gov/parasites/cysticercosis/ and cdc.gov/parasites/taeniasis/ for discussion and images. Accessed April 2014

- **Digestion—mucosal:** Mucosal proteases and peptidases contribute to protein digestion and peptide and amino acid absorption; these enzymes can be damaged/reduced by intestinal disorders such as celiac, Crohn's, and by degradation of mucosal enzymes by bacterial proteases as seen in SIBO—small intestine bacterial overgrowth.

- **Absorption:** Efficient nutrient absorption is dependent on mucosal/villous integrity, vascular and lymphatic integrity (e.g., impaired in congestive heart failure, which leads to bowel wall edema and reduced intestinal absorption), and all of the above previous steps. Mucosal integrity and absorption can be objectively and practically assessed by measuring urine levels of orally administered *L*actulose (increased with a *L*eaky gut and increased paracellular absorption) and *M*annitol (decreased with *M*alabsorption and reduced transcellular absorption); 24-hour fecal fat can also be measured, as steatorrhea can be seen with both pancreatic insufficiency (maldigestion) and mucosal injury (malabsorption). Mucosal injury is always an active and current problem, since the intestinal mucosa is otherwise and generally rapidly replicative and reparative; as expected, mucosal replication and repair is nutrient-dependent (especially zinc, vitamin A, and glutamine), and malnutrition and malabsorption can become a vicious cycle.

- **Transport, cellular uptake, reception:** Classic and clinically important considerations with nutrient transport, uptake, reception are as follows:
  - **All/many nutrients:** To promote the essential catalytic functions of enzymes to sustain organismal life, vitamins and minerals serve as coenzymes and cofactors, respectively. When genotropic amino acid substitutions, an example of single nucleotide polymorphisms (SNPs or "snips"), occur in enzyme structure, the result is a generally a subtle or gross alteration in enzyme function, generally reduced enzyme function, commonly due to reduced affinity for binding with the required coenzyme or cofactor. When enzymes are "slow" or "defective" due to alterations in structure due to altered amino acid composition due to SNPs, the provision of supradietary amounts of cofactors and coenzymes—vitamin and mineral supplementation—can be used to partly/completely restore enzymatic function and thus the biochemical reactions necessary for life and health. As this model is scientifically established, clinically proven, and generally irrefutable, these facts establish the scientific and intellectual basis for vitamin and mineral supplementation among "apparently healthy" and ill patients alike, which has been referred to as "orthomolecular medicine" (per Pauling[192], "use the right molecules") and "mega-nutrient" therapy.[193]
    - Review: High-dose vitamin therapy stimulates variant enzymes with decreased coenzyme binding affinity (*Am J Clin Nutr* 2002 Apr[194])—quite likely the most authoritative article ever written on this topic: "As many as one-third of mutations in a gene result in the corresponding enzyme having an increased Michaelis constant, or K(m), (decreased binding affinity) for a coenzyme, resulting in a lower rate of reaction. About 50 human genetic dis-eases due to defective enzymes can be remedied or ameliorated by the administration of high doses of the vitamin component of the corresponding coenzyme, which at least partially restores enzymatic activity. Several single-nucleotide polymorphisms, in which the variant amino acid reduces coenzyme binding and thus enzymatic activity, are likely to be remediable by raising cellular concentrations of the cofactor through high-dose vitamin therapy."

---

[192] Pauling L. Orthomolecular psychiatry. *Science*. 1968 Apr 19;160(3825):265-71

[193] Newbold HL. *Mega-nutrients for your nerves*. P. H. Wyden; First Edition edition 1975

[194] Ames BN, et al. High-dose vitamin therapy stimulates variant enzymes with decreased coenzyme binding affinity (increased Km). *Am J Clin Nutr* 2002 Apr;75:616-58

- Time deficiency: Most people do not have/make time to relax, consider, prepare and masticate a health-promoting diet. **Without time and the prioritization of that time for self-care, parasympathetic-mediated and rejuvenative activities, health will always have to be pursued artificially.** In America, approximately 15-21% of food consumed by young adults 20-40y is "fast food" (generally characterized by chemical/pesticide/herbicide residues, a collection of GMO toxins, excess fat, carbohydrates, salt; absence of phytonutrients) while a much larger proportion is processed and unhealthy food; thus, **most of the food eaten promotes *disease*, not health**.

- Information deficiency: Most people receive no education about nutrition; the information provided by television shows and governmental education programs is generally 1) of very low quality, 2) confusing, 3) unsophisticated, and/or 4) intentionally counterproductive to the generation and preservation of health because the information was formed by medical/pharmaceutical and other private interest groups that have intentionally swayed dietary guidelines toward disease-promotion in order to ensure and preserve a customer base of patients. I have discussed/substantiated this in my publications on diabetes and especially hypertension (2010, 2011, new edition pending)—with regard to the latter, one should note that the dietary guides, notably the recipes for "sunshine rice", "classic macaroni and cheese", "banana-nut bread", and "frosted cake" published by the U.S. Department of Health and Human Services, National Institutes of Health website (reviewed 2014 Dec) nhlbi.nih.gov/health/resources/heart/syah-html are guaranteed to promote obesity and insulin resistance.

- Prioritization deficiency: The generation and protection of optimal health is not a priority for most people and for most "healthcare organizations" whether hospitals, medical schools, insurers, or governmental organizations. The clear truth is that—in contrast to the interests of their citizens—some governments *via school policies* prefer to promote poor nutrition, perhaps as a form of social control/suppression. Public school lunches and nutrition programs in the United States—generally consumed by children in the poorer and more intellectually/educationally/socially vulnerable strata—are notoriously maleficent, providing a superabundance of sugar-rich and nutrient-poor foods, most famously symbolized by the substitution of real vegetables with processed bioremnants, famously attributed to US President Ronald Reagan as the "***ketchup is a vegetable controversy***" per en.wikipedia.org/wiki/Ketchup_as_a_vegetable. Ongoing manipulation of nutrition programs consistently favors "important victories" for the low-nutrition disease-promoting processed junk-food industry, per reuters.com/article/2011/11/18/us-usa-lunch-idUSTRE7AH00020111118. Per a 2004 report, 75% of beverages and 85% of snacks available in American schools are of poor nutritional value and promote obesity, per medscape.com/viewarticle/479970; these same pseudofoods would be expected to impair intellectual performance and development. Supporting this concept is an international study published in December 2014 (Horton and Hoddinott) showing that—in contrast to the devastating neurointellectual and social consequences of undernutrition/malnutrition—enhanced nutrition in early life actually promotes and protects future health and development in a manner that actually pays financial dividends; this research shows that "every dollar spent on nutrition during the first 1,000 days of a child's life—from conception to age two—can provide a country up to $166 in future earnings." Thus, restrictive government policies intended to deprive/punish lower socioeconomic strata actually impose greater burdens—financially, socially, nationally—than programs of appropriate maternal and childhood nutrition.

- Political blockade, access deficiency: Food deficiencies in "developing"/exploited/repressed nations are generally due to political encumbrances rather than any true deficiency or legitimate scarcity. A good example is seen in my country of Colombia—a nation rich in equatorial sun exposure, terrain variation, fertile soil, water, and a willing hard-working population—where undernutrition and hunger are common, where public lands that could be employed for public farms are held stagnant by private and governmental ownership, where the USA-Colombia misnamed "free-trade agreement" has further impaired the development and deployment of agriculture resources, for example by undercutting markets and by forcing indigenous farmers—*los campesinos*—to destroy their own seeds and methods and use GMO seeds and agrochemicals from American multinational corporations like DuPont and Monsanto, per Mejia 2013.

1. Horton S, Hoddinott J. *Food Security and Nutrition*. 2014 Dec. uwaterloo.ca/news/news/each-dollar-spent-kids-nutrition-can-yield-more-100-later. copenhagenconsensus.com/sites/default/files/food_security_and_nutrition_perspective_-_horton_hoddinott_0.pdf
2. Mejia P. Will Colombia's Farmers Get What They Want? Agricultural riots this summer challenged free trade agreement, genetically modified seeds. *Rolling Stone* 2013 Nov rollingstone.com/politics/news/will-colombias-farmers-get-what-they-want-20131118
3. Impact of the FTA with Colombia on Afro-Colombian and Indigenous Communities: youtube.com/watch?v=9Q7NOY8Axf4
4. Colombian National Farmers and Social Strike gets seeds control law 970 suspended: youtube.com/watch?v=9Vz0tiRKvD0
5. Colombia's exports to US drop 13% after US-Colombia Free-Trade Agreement: democraticunderground.com/1014482725

- <u>Processed foods and the Western/American diet—general description and bioclinical considerations</u>: The general pattern eating described as the Western diet or the American diet (the latter with a higher specific emphasis on consumption of genetically manipulated organisms [GMO]) includes overconsumption of carbohydrates in general and sucrose, high-fructose corn syrup, wheat, potatoes, dairy in particular; insufficiency of fiber and phytonutrient-dense foods such as fruits and vegetables; overconsumption of chemicals such as colorants and preservatives and "flavor enhancers" such as MSG (excitoneurotoxic) and carrageenan (immunosuppressive, inflammatory, carcinogenic); overconsumption of sodium and chloride and underconsumption of potassium, magnesium, citrate, and bicarbonate; rampant vitamin and mineral deficiencies despite the outward appearance of obesity/overweight; diet-induced hunger, metabolic impairment, endoplasmic reticulum stress, mitochondrial dysfunction, and hypothalamic inflammation.

○ GMO (genetically manipulated organisms and related toxins): introduction and survey of literature: GMO foods were released onto the commercial food market in America in 1996 without adequate safety testing on animals, humans, and the environment. Genetic *"modification"* is a euphemism for interspecies **manipulation** of gene sequence and content; "modification" is far too benign a term, considering the *manipulation* (of politics, science, public opinion), *mistreatment* (of people, including what has been described as a *suicide belt* and *GM genocide* resulting from farmers bankrupted after using GMO crops and the imposition of profiteering corporate policies[195]), *maleficence* (harming people, animals, environment) that actually occurs, and the *metastatic* nature of GMO plants which have now contaminated previously nonGMO crops internationally, even in countries that have banned GMO crops, thus suggesting that airborne cross-pollination/contamination is inevitable, threatening global food security.[196] Because (multi)gene manipulation is used in tandem with high-dose pesticides and herbicides (therefore, in the real world,

> **GMO toxins: all genes and chemicals related to GMO crops designed to kill insects, plants, and promote use of higher levels of other pesticides and herbicides**
>
> - 3-MPPA: 3-methylphosphinicopropionic acid, metabolite of gluphosinate herbicide
> - AMPA: aminomethyl phosphoric acid, metabolite of glyphosate herbicide
> - Bt: bacterial toxin bacillus thuringiensis
> - Cry1Ab protein: one of the Bt toxins
> - GLUF: gluphosinate herbicide
> - GLYP: glyphosate herbicide
> - Ht: Herbicide tolerant, plants genetically altered to tolerate otherwise poisonous levels of herbicides
> - "Inert" ingredients: Several of these have been found harmful at real-life levels, promoting direct or indirect toxicity
> - PAGMF: pesticides associated to genetically modified foods
> - "Stacked GMO": single plants with multiple genetic manipulations, such as combinations of Bt and Ht. For example, DK 42-88RRYGPL corn is a "triple stack of NK603, MON863 and MON810 genes" while Pannar 4E-705RR/Bt corn is a "double stack" of NK603 and MON810.

these are always used in complex synergistic combinations) and to reduce/avoid the ongoing problems that occur in science when these items are studied in isolation (note that doing so does *not* reflect the real world application and therefore such science is itself *unscientific* insofar as it is *unrealistic*), I use the term "GMO toxins" to include all genetic changes such as Bt and Ht and GMO-associated chemicals especially pesticides, herbicides, and the other falsely labeled "inert" chemicals in these formations; indeed, my use of the term GMO toxins is appropriate since virtually all of these gene changes and chemicals are designed to directly/indirectly kill life forms, in this case insects and plants, some of which are necessary for the cycle of life, parts of which include pollination of crops and the consumption/degradation of plant material for recovery of nutrients for reuse. I find the term "GMO toxins" less cumbersome than the alternative proposed elsewhere of "pesticides associated to genetically modified foods" (PAGMF), which is both longer and less inclusive. Human safety studies have not been performed on GMO foods and toxins despite the fact that in America (the country that produces and consumes the most GM food) citizens eat more than their weight in GM foods per year.[197]

- Bt toxin—insecticidal via intestinal cell toxicity; reported link to intestinal toxicity in animals: *Bacillus thuringiensis* (or Bt) is a Gram-positive, soil-dwelling bacterium that produces crystal proteins called δ-endotoxins (Delta endotoxins, pore-forming toxins, also called Cry and Cyt

---

[195] "Imagine a storm blows across your property – and that now, without your knowledge or consent, genetically manipulated seeds are present in the garden you have tended for years. A few days later, representatives of a multi-national corporation pay you a visit, demand that you surrender your produce - and simultaneously file a criminal complaint against you for the illegal use of patented, genetically-manipulated seeds. Around the world, this story represents the bitter truth. It's the real-life experience of Canadians Percy und Louise Schmeiser, who have been fighting chemical and seed manufacturer Monsanto since 1996. Today, nearly three-fourths of genetically manipulated plants harvested worldwide originated in Monsanto labs." Percy Schmeiser - David versus Monsanto, film by Bertram Verhaag. denkmalfilm.tv/index.php?l=en&page=percy-schmeiser-4 and amazon.com/David-vs-Monsanto-Percy-Schmeiser/dp/B004R14BZ8/. "So Shankara became one of an estimated 125,000 farmers to take their own life as a result of the ruthless drive to use India as a testing ground for genetically modified crops. The crisis, branded the 'GM Genocide' by campaigners, was highlighted recently when Prince Charles claimed that the issue of GM had become a 'global moral question' - and the time had come to end its unstoppable march." dailymail.co.uk/news/article-1082559/The-GM-genocide-Thousands-Indian-farmers-committing-suicide-using-genetically-modified-crops.html. "The highest acreage of Bt cotton is in Maharashtra and this is also where the highest farmer suicides are. Suicides increased after Bt cotton was introduced — Monsanto's royalty extraction, and the high costs of seed and chemicals have created a debt trap. According to Government of India data, nearly 75 per cent rural debt is due to purchase inputs. As Monsanto's profits grow, farmers' debt grows. It is in this systemic sense that Monsanto's seeds are seeds of suicide." globalresearch.ca/the-seeds-of-suicide-how-monsanto-destroys-farming/5329947.
[196] Quist D, Chapela IH. Transgenic DNA introgressed into traditional maize landraces in Oaxaca, Mexico. *Nature.* 2001 Nov 29;414(6863):541-3
[197] "Americans are eating their weight and more in genetically engineered food every year, a new Environmental Working Group analysis shows. On average, people eat an estimated 193 pounds of genetically engineered food in a 12-month period. The typical American adult weighs 179 pounds. ... Shockingly, virtually no long-term health studies have been done on consumption of genetically engineered food." Sharp R. Americans Eat Their Weight In Genetically Engineered Food. *Environmental Working Group's AgMag* 2012 Oct ewg.org/agmag/2012/10/americans-eat-their-weight-genetically-engineered-food

toxins), which have insecticide action via binding of the delta-endotoxin to gut epithelium, causing cell lysis and insect death; this has led to the commercialized and patented insertion of Bt genes into plant crops to produce one common type of "genetically modified food" that, as a plant, provides its own endogenously-produced pesticide, theoretically leading to crop protection but possibly harming nontarget insects, including those necessary for pollination and other important functions in the web of life. Variants of the Bt gene can be inserted into plants to target specific insects; again, this basically converts what was previously a food (e.g., corn) into an unnatural hybrid of food-producing-a-bacterial-toxin-to-kill-intestinal-epithelial-cells. The question as to whether GMO/Bt causes biochemical/functional intestinal injury in animals and humans has not been answered; gross visualization (used in the study by Carman et al described below) is likely too insensitive and should be superseded by histologic or biochemical assessments such as the well-established sucrose/lactulose/mannitol absorption tests that are clinically and commercially available.

- Long-term toxicology study on pigs fed a combined genetically modified (GM) soy and GM maize diet (*Journal of Organic Systems* 2013[198]): "The GM diet was associated with gastric and uterine differences in pigs. GM-fed pigs had uteri that were 25% heavier than non-GM fed pigs. GM-fed pigs had a higher rate of severe stomach inflammation with a rate of 32% of GM-fed pigs compared to 12% of non-GM-fed pigs. The severe stomach inflammation was worse in GM-fed males compared to non-GM fed males by a factor of 4.0, and GM-fed females compared to non-GM fed females by a factor of 2.2." Publicized reviews of this article followed professional or business interests. Coverage by the news service Reuters[199] reported the research as accurate and quoted commentary from the industry group CropLife International, a global federation representing the plant science industry, stating "more than 150 scientific studies have been done on animals fed biotech crops and to date, there is no scientific evidence of any detrimental impact"; this statement by CropLife International—whose website in 2014 Jun reads that the private-interest group

> **GMO foods (e.g., soy, corn, cotton, canola, sugar beet, alfalfa, papaya [Chinese and Hawaiian], zucchini, and yellow squash*): imposed on an unconsenting population, without their knowledge, and without proper safety testing**
>
> "Americans are eating their weight and more in genetically engineered food every year, a new Environmental Working Group analysis shows. On average, people eat an estimated 193 pounds of genetically engineered food in a 12-month period. The typical American adult weighs 179 pounds. ... Shockingly, virtually no long-term health studies have been done on consumption of genetically engineered food."**
>
> The whole situation is complicated by the fact that these patented food such as soy, corn, and alfalfa are used as major feed sources for farm-raised fish, cows, pigs, and poultry. This has three major implications:
> 1) People are eating GMO-sourced food and related proteins and chemicals even when they think they are eating fish, beef, milk, cheese, yogurt, pork, chicken, turkey, and eggs,
> 2) These toxins and chemicals can be expected to bioconcentrate in animal tissues as do other nutrients and chemicals,
> 3) **Whoever controls these patented plants controls the entire grown food supply *beyond the GMO foods themselves.***
>
> *Jeffrey Smith, personal communication, 2014 Jul.
> **Sharp, Environmental Working Group. *AgMag* 2012

"promotes agricultural technologies such as pesticides and plant biotechnology" and whose members include Dow, Monsanto, Syngenta and other multinational chemical corporations—is obviously a lie, given the multiple studies demonstrating abnormalities in GMO-fed animals, only a small sample of which is presented in these pages. Criticism of the original research published by *Business Insider*[200] described the research as

---

[198] Carman et al. A long-term toxicology study on pigs fed a combined genetically modified (GM) soy and GM maize diet. *Journal of Organic Systems* 2013; 8(1),38-54
[199] Gillam C. Scientists say new study shows pig health hurt by GMO feed. *Reuters* 2013 reuters.com/article/2013/06/11/us-gmo-pigs-study-idUSBRE95A14K20130611
[200] Welsh J. Scientists Shred Study That Says Genetically Modified Food Makes Pigs Sick. *BusinessInsider.com* 2013 Jun businessinsider.com/gm-pig-study-is-deeply-flawed-2013-6#ixzz36bYn2igT—an excellent example of the idiotic journalism that now pervades and perverts social dialogue in America.

"misleading and flawed" and thereafter barraged the article with innuendo, *argumentum ad hominem*, accurate criticism (an example of which is the lack of major differences between groups in the combination of moderate and severe stomach inflammation), and illogic (e.g., "The enlarged uterus finding, while statistically significant, is not likely to be clinically relevant."). My (DrV) personal reading of the article finds the uterine abnormalities more significant/reliable than the stomach abnormalities.

- Glyphosate—the widely used herbicide produced by Monsanto: Glyphosate (gly-FO-SATE) is a broad-spectrum systemic herbicide used to kill plants, especially annual broadleaf weeds and grasses known to compete with commercial crops; it was brought to market in the 1970s by the biotechnology company Monsanto under the trade name "Roundup®." Glyphosate-based herbicides are currently the most commonly used herbicides in the world despite evidence of toxicity; glyphosate-based herbicide mixtures are applied internationally to food, air, and water without demonstration of safety and increasing evidence of harm. Glyphosate's *designated but not solitary* mode of action is to inhibit an enzyme involved in the synthesis of the aromatic amino acids tyrosine, tryptophan and phenylalanine. Some patented crops have been genetically engineered to be resistant to glyphosate (i.e., "Roundup Ready", also created by Monsanto Company); soy was the first "Roundup Ready" crop, and in the United States 94% of soy is GMO[201]—some have suggested that this is evidence of a market monopoly. Many articles in the scientific literature note problems with the population-wide and world-wide application of this chemical mixture and the financial and political policies that commonly accompany. The most consistent and painful theme in the research literature is the combination of data showing that GMO toxins have been imposed on entire large populations of the world (e.g., the entire country of the United States, with a population of more than 318 million people who eat the largest portion of GMO foods in the world) without any reasonable safety data and very clear evidence of biological harm; adding salt to this wound is the fact that major health organizations such as the American Medical Association, which claims "To promote the art and science of medicine and the betterment of public health" and promises "Together, we can shape a better, healthier future – not just for patients and physicians, but for the country as a whole"[202] have been completely quiescent, allowing this uncontrolled experiment on the American population. Some people have suggested that this is a human rights offense, an almost-certain health hazard, and worldwide environmental threat; yet most Americans are eating GMO foods+chemicals every day.

  - Exposure to glyphosate-based herbicide alters aromatase levels in rat testis and sperm nuclear quality (*Environ Toxicol Pharmacol* 2014 May[203]): The authors of this report write, "Roundup is the major pesticide used in agriculture worldwide; it is a glyphosate-based herbicide. Its molecular effects are studied following an acute exposure (0.5%) of fifteen 60-day-old male rats during an 8-day period. ...The major disruption is an increase of aromatase mRNA levels at least by 50% in treated rats at all times, as well as the aromatase protein. ... A rise of abnormal sperm morphology and a decrease of the expression of protamine 1 and histone 1 testicular in epididymal sperm are observed despite a normal sperm concentration and motility."

  - Toxicity of a glyphosate-based herbicide on the Neotropical fish Prochilodus lineatus (*Comp Biochem Physiol C Toxicol Pharmacol* 2008 Mar[204]): The authors note, "However, toxic effects of Roundup at sub-lethal concentrations have now been demonstrated in fish. Sub-lethal concentrations of glyphosate, corresponding to less than 2% of the LC50, caused ultrastructural damage in the liver of *C. carpio*. Histological alterations were also

---

[201] Carman et al. A long-term toxicology study on pigs fed a combined genetically modified (GM) soy and GM maize diet. *Journal of Organic Systems* 2013; 8(1),38-54
[202] ama-assn.org/ama/pub/about-ama/our-mission.page 2014 Jul
[203] Cassault-Meyer et al. Acute exposure to glyphosate-based herbicide alters aromatase levels in testis, sperm nuclear quality. *Environ Toxicol Pharmacol* 2014;38:131-40
[204] Langiano Vdo et al. Toxicity of glyphosate-based herbicide on Neotropical fish Prochilodus lineatus. *Comp Biochem Physiol C Toxicol Pharmacol* 2008 Mar:222-31

observed in liver, gills and kidneys of Nile tilapia (*Oreochromis niloticus*) after acute and chronic exposure to sub-lethal concentrations of Roundup. Despite the fact that Roundup is widely used in Brazil, only a limited amount of information is available on its toxic effects to native freshwater fishes." This data on glyphosate/Roundup-induced fish toxicity is increasingly important given the impending *death of the oceans*[205] and extinction of salt-water fish as a food source.[206]

- Glyphosate and gluten intolerance (*Interdiscip Toxicol* 2013 Dec[207]): The authors propose that glyphosate, the active ingredient in the herbicide Roundup is the most important causal factor in the epidemics of celiac disease and gluten intolerance. "Glyphosate residues in wheat and other crops are likely increasing recently due to the growing practice of crop desiccation just prior to the harvest. We argue that the practice of "ripening" sugar cane with glyphosate may explain the recent surge in kidney failure among agricultural workers in Central America. We conclude with a plea to governments to reconsider policies regarding … glyphosate residues in foods."

- Glyphosate's suppression of cytochrome P450 enzymes and other pathways to modern diseases (*Entropy* 2013 Apr[208]): These researchers report that glyphosate/Roundup chemical residues are found in the main foods of the Western diet, comprised primarily of sugar, corn, soy and wheat. Glyphosate's inhibition of cytochrome P450 (CYP) enzymes is an overlooked component of its toxicity to mammals because CYP enzymes play crucial roles in biology, one of which is to detoxify xenobiotics. The researchers further note that glyphosate enhances the damaging effects of other chemical residues and environmental toxins. … "Consequences are most of the diseases and conditions associated with a Western diet, which include gastrointestinal disorders, obesity, diabetes, heart disease, depression, autism, infertility, cancer and Alzheimer's disease."

- **Additive and synergistic toxicities of mislabeled "inert" chemicals—reproductive toxicity**: Extremely low dilutions of chemical combinations show additive/synergistic toxicities—specifically affecting cells of the reproductive system; this is a very concerning finding given that GMO-related toxins have been detected in pregnant human women and human fetal tissue, giving us every reason to believe that the cytotoxicity induced by pesticide formulations is affecting human lives in real time.

> **"Inert" can be cytotoxic and disease-promoting**
>
> A chemical that is "inert" against insects and plants can be harmful for humans.
>
> A chemical that is "inert in isolation" can be devastating when combined with other toxic chemicals and/or other "inert" chemicals.

- Human cytotoxicity of pesticide additives (*Scientific American* 2009 Jun[209]): "One specific inert ingredient, polyethoxylated tallowamine, or POEA, was more deadly to human embryonic, placental and umbilical cord cells than the herbicide itself – a finding the researchers call "astonishing." "This clearly confirms that the [inert ingredients] in Roundup formulations are not inert," wrote the study authors from France's University of Caen. "Moreover, the proprietary mixtures available on the market could cause cell damage and even death [at the] residual levels" found on Roundup-treated crops, such as soybeans, alfalfa and corn, or lawns and gardens. The research team suspects that Roundup might cause pregnancy problems by interfering with hormone production, possibly leading to abnormal fetal development, low birth weights or miscarriages."

- Ethoxylated adjuvants of glyphosate-based herbicides are active principles of human cell toxicity (*Toxicology* 2013 Nov[210]): "Pesticides are always used in formulations as mixtures of an active principle with adjuvants. … Here we demonstrate that all formulations are more toxic than glyphosate [alone], … POE-15 [polyethoxylated tallowamine] clearly appears to be the most toxic principle against human cells, even if others are not excluded. It begins to be active with negative dose-dependent effects on

[205] Renton A. The Death of the Oceans. *Newsweek* 2014 Jul newsweek.com/2014/07/11/disaster-weve-wrought-worlds-oceans-may-be-irrevocable-256962.html
[206] DeNoon D. Salt-Water Fish Extinction Seen By 2048. *CBS News* 2006 Nov 2 cbsnews.com/news/salt-water-fish-extinction-seen-by-2048/
[207] Samsel et al. Glyphosate, pathways to modern diseases II: Celiac sprue and gluten intolerance. *Interdiscip Toxicol*. 2013 Dec;6(4):159-84
[208] Samsel et al. Glyphosate's Suppression of Cytochrome P450 Enzymes and Amino Acid Biosynthesis by the Gut Microbiome. *Entropy* 2013 Apr, 15(4), 1416-1463
[209] Gammon C et al. Weed-Whacking Herbicide Proves Deadly to Human Cells. *Scientific American* 2009 Jun scientificamerican.com/article/weed-whacking-herbicide-p/
[210] Mesnage et al. Ethoxylated adjuvants of glyphosate-based herbicides are active principles of human cell toxicity. *Toxicology*. 2013 Nov 16;313(2-3):122-8

cellular respiration and membrane integrity between 1 and 3ppm, at environmental/occupational doses. We demonstrate in addition that POE-15 induces necrosis when its first micellization process occurs, by contrast to glyphosate which is known to promote endocrine disrupting effects after entering cells. Altogether, these results challenge the establishment of guidance values such as the acceptable daily intake of glyphosate, when these are mostly based on a long term in vivo test of glyphosate alone. Since pesticides are always used with adjuvants that could change their toxicity, the necessity to assess their whole formulations as mixtures becomes obvious. This challenges the concept of active principle of pesticides for non-target species."

- <u>GMO toxins absorbed by humans</u>: One of the main arguments espoused by the chemical industry is that GMO toxins and pesticides do not reach human consumers because such chemicals are said to decompose with time, cooking (assuming that the foods are cooked rather than eaten raw as many foods are), digestion; data in humans with analysis of human tissue samples has proven this argument to be a lie: humans *indeed* accumulate GMO toxins—Bt toxin and associated pesticide chemicals.
    - <u>Maternal and fetal exposure to pesticides associated to genetically modified foods</u> (*Reprod Toxicol* 2011 May[211]): "Pesticides associated to genetically modified foods (PAGMF), are engineered to tolerate herbicides such as glyphosate (GLYP) and gluphosinate (GLUF) or insecticides such as the bacterial toxin bacillus thuringiensis (Bt). … Blood of thirty pregnant women (PW) and thirty-nine nonpregnant women (NPW) were studied. Serum GLYP and GLUF were detected in nonpregnant women and not detected in pregnant women. Serum 3-MPPA and CryAb1 toxin were detected in pregnant women, their fetuses and nonpregnant women. This is the first study to reveal the presence of circulating pesticides associated to genetically modified foods in women with and without pregnancy, …"
    - <u>Glyphosate in humans correlates with disease</u> (*J Environ Anal Toxicol* 2014 Jan[212]): "Glyphosate excretion in German dairy cows was significantly lower than Danish cows. Cows kept in genetically modified free area had significantly lower glyphosate concentrations in urine than conventional husbandry cows. Also glyphosate was detected in different organs of slaughtered cows as intestine, liver, muscles, spleen and kidney. Fattening rabbits showed significantly higher glyphosate residues in urine than hares. Moreover, glyphosate was significantly higher in urine of humans with conventional feeding [non-organic foods]. Furthermore, chronically ill humans showed significantly higher glyphosate residues in urine than healthy population. The presence of glyphosate residues in both humans and animals could haul the entire population towards numerous health hazards, studying the impact of glyphosate residues on health is warranted and the global regulations for the use of glyphosate may have to be re-evaluated. … Glyphosate residues can remain stable in foods for a year or more, even if the foods are frozen, dried or processed. … Exposure of mammals to glyphosate may cause loss of mitochondrial transmembrane potential and result in oxidative stress to liver and brain. Both apoptosis and autophagy are involved in glyphosate toxicity mechanisms."

- <u>Commercial influence of science and politics</u>: One of the most damning research articles documenting adverse effects of GMO foods and toxins was published by Séralini et al[213] in

GMO documentaries, social context, health effects

<u>Genetic Roulette</u>
  seedsofdeception.com
<u>David versus Monsanto</u>
  youtube.com and
  rclvideolibrary.com
<u>Scientists under Attack</u>
  scientistsunderattack.com
<u>GMO Food, Dr. Russell Blaylock</u>
  youtube.com
<u>Seeds of Death: Unveiling The Lies of GMO</u> youtube.com
<u>Confessions of an Economic Hitman</u> youtube.com
<u>Hoodwinked: An Economic Hit Man Reveals Why the Global Economy Imploded—and How to Fix It</u> economichitman.com
<u>GMO OMG</u> gmofilm.com

[211] Aris et al. Maternal and fetal exposure to pesticides associated to genetically modified foods in Eastern Townships of Quebec, Canada. *Reprod Toxicol.* 2011;31:528-33
[212] Krüger et al. Detection of Glyphosate Residues in Animals and Humans. *J Environ Anal Toxicol* 2014 Jan 4:2. This article is open-access: omicsonline.org
[213] Séralini et al. Long term toxicity of a Roundup herbicide and a Roundup-tolerant genetically modified maize. *Food Chem Toxicol.* 2012 Nov;50(11):4221-31

Food Chem Toxicol 2012 Nov; in this paper, the authors show massive tumorigenesis and multiple organ abnormalities in animals fed GMO foods and related GMO toxins, e.g., genetically manipulated proteins and –cidal chemicals. The original research was deemed properly conducted, and the original manuscript was accepted by the journal with minimal editorial input; in other words: this was deemed by the editors to be good research. Following publication of the article, a deluge of letters refuting the article was published, and many of these denigrations and refutations were written by authors affiliated with Monsanto, the agrichemical multinational corporation that sells and massively profits from GMO. In 2014 Jan, the Séralini article was retracted by the journal after it created a new editorial position and filled that position with a researcher who worked for Monsanto. This unprecedented retraction violates scientific publication standards by well-established bioethics criteria; if biomedical journals and their publishers are going to pander to corporate interests, then the entirety of science—of truth, of medicine and healthcare, of reality itself—is at risk. GMO foods and toxins will be seen as "safe" if corporate-funded studies are published and independently/academically-funded articles are blocked or retracted; at this rate, if we as educated healthcare professionals and policymakers responsible for public welfare are going to allow the disgrace of reality, then we are resigning our integrity, courage, and our intellects in favor of passive idiocy and might as well therefore agree that ketchup is a vegetable[214] and therefore that frozen pizza is a vegetable[215], that climate change and global warming and ocean acidification are not occurring and that the icecaps aren't melting[216], and that $2 + 2 = 5$.[217] If doctors, medical societies/associations, and public health groups do not stand for the truth and for the health of the public, if their only (conveniently self-chosen) professional tasks are **patient-by-patient micromanagement of public health** and the protection of their own professional niche, then they are no better than other private interest groups seeking their own aggrandizement and profitability.

- Betrayal of science by Elsevier and its journal *Food and Chemical Toxicology* (*Bioethics Forum* 2014 Jan[218]): "11 of the [13] authors of letters to the editor slamming Séralini's study had undisclosed financial relationships with Monsanto. In 2013, Paul Christou, the editor of *Transgenic Research*, coauthored an attack on Séralini and the FCT editors in his own journal, calling for a retraction of the study. Christou did not disclose his multiple conflicts of interest, including being an inventor on patents on GM crop technology, many of which Monsanto owns. Meanwhile, back at *Food and Chemical Toxicology*, a new position for an associate editor was filled by Richard E. Goodman, a University of Nebraska professor who previously worked for Monsanto, and who has a longstanding association with the industry-funded International Life Sciences Institute (ILSI). Months later, Elsevier, FCT's publisher, announced the retraction. ...

---

[214] "The New York Times (9-28-81) noted that "Democrats are still chortling at what they hail as 'the Emperor's New Condiments' -- the attempt to declare ketchup a school-lunch vegetable." Nestle M. Ketchup Is a Vegetable? Again? The Atlantic 2011 Nov theatlantic.com/health/archive/2011/11/ketchup-is-a-vegetable-again/248538/

[215] "If there were any lingering doubts as to whom our elected representatives really work for, they were put to rest Tuesday when Congress announced that frozen pizza was a vegetable. The United States Congress voted to rebuke new USDA guidelines for school lunches that would have increased the amount of fresh fruit and vegetables in school cafeterias and instead declared that the tomato paste on frozen pizza qualified it as a vegetable. For this we can thank large food companies -- in this case ConAgra and Schwan -- which pressured Congress to comply with their financial interests. It simply doesn't suit the makers of frozen pizza, chicken nuggets and tater tots for schools to offer real food in the form of fresh fruits and vegetables." Wartman K. Pizza Is a Vegetable? Congress Defies Logic, Betrays Our Children. *Huffington Post* 2011 Nov huffingtonpost.com/kristin-wartman/pizza-is-a-vegetable_b_1101433.html. "As long as a serving of pizza contains at least 2 tablespoons of tomato sauce, this allows it to squeak in as a vegetable under the current rules." Petri A. Move over, ketchup! Pizza is a vegetable. 2011 Nov *Washington Post* washingtonpost.com/blogs/compost/post/move-over-ketchup-pizza-is-a-vegetable/2011/11/16/gIQAk1okRN_blog.html

[216] Cohen N. Climate change deniers have won. *The Guardian* 2014 Mar theguardian.com/commentisfree/2014/mar/22/climate-change-deniers-have-won-global-warming

[217] Orwell G. *1984*. Also: Moustaki N (Author), Podehl N (Narrator). *CliffsNotes 1984*, cliffsnotes.com/literature/n/1984/book-summary amazon.com/1984-CliffsNotes/dp/B004S8NFZ2/. Also: Video SparkNotes: Orwell's 1984 video summary. youtube.com/watch?v=pTqIVvUPAjw

[218] Fugh-Berman A, Sherman TG. Rounding Up Scientific Journals. *Bioethics Forum* 2014 Jan thehastingscenter.org/Bioethicsforum/Post.aspx?id=6684

The retraction of the Séralini study is a black mark on medical publishing, a blow to science, and a win for corporate bullies."

□ The Goodman Affair: Monsanto Targets the Heart of Science (*Independent Science News* 2013 May[219]): "But just a few months later, in early 2013 the *FCT* editorial board acquired a new "Associate Editor for biotechnology", Richard E. Goodman. This was a new position, seemingly established especially for Goodman in the wake of the "Séralini affair". Richard E. Goodman is...a former Monsanto employee, who worked for the company between 1997 and 2004. While at Monsanto he assessed the allergenicity of the company's GM crops and published papers on its behalf on allergenicity and safety issues relating to GM food (Goodman and Leach 2004). Goodman had no documented connection to the journal until February 2013. His fast-tracked appointment, directly onto the upper editorial board raises urgent questions. Does Monsanto now effectively decide which papers on biotechnology are published in FCT? And is this part of an attempt by Monsanto and the life science industry to seize control of science? ... FCT took on Goodman, a former Monsanto employee and well-known supporter of industry viewpoints, immediately following the publication of a controversial paper that was critical of Monsanto's principal products."

□ Article by former Assistant Secretary of the US Treasury Dr Paul Craig Roberts—2013 Feb[220]): As a former Assistant Secretary of the US Treasury working with Ronald Reagan, and as former Associate Editor of the *Wall Street Journal*, Dr Roberts (PhD, Economics) can speak very authoritatively from experience on government politics; his 2013 article "America the Polluted: One Nation, Under Monsanto" is publicly available online and describes how Monsanto holds powerful influence in American politics and is able to influence political outcomes through key positions; examples of such influence and conflict of interest are as follows:

♦ **Tom Vilsack, appointed US Secretary of Agriculture** in 2009, is former "Biotech Governor (Iowa 2001) of the Year", an award bestowed by the Biotechnology Industry Organization, "the world's largest trade association representing biotechnology companies", a proGMO/pesticide/herbicide trade group supported by multinationals such as AstraZeneca, Genentech/Roche, DuPont, and Monsanto[221]

♦ **Michael Taylor, appointed to the newly created position of Deputy Commissioner for Foods and Veterinary Medicine** (aka, "US Food Czar"), is former outside attorney for Monsanto, then Deputy Commissioner of Policy at the US Food and Drug Administration, then VP of Government Affairs for Monsanto[222]

♦ **Clarence Thomas, US Supreme Court Justice**, is a former employed attorney for Monsanto[223]

Dr Roberts argues that the infiltration of US political positions by people intimately connected with the business interests of private corporations is powerfully influencing

---

The Responsibility of Intellectuals

"It is the responsibility of intellectuals to speak the truth and to expose lies."

Noam Chomsky PhD. *New York Review of Books*, 1967

Years of falsity have blinded people to accurate perception

"We have been poisoned on so much [falsity and lies] for so many years, when the truth comes along and it's right in your face, you don't know what to do with it... You wake up one morning with a footprint on your face... You have to look the lie right in the eye and not be afraid to see too clearly."

Rollins H. *One from None*, 1991, p106-144

---

[219] Robinson C, Latham J. The Goodman Affair: Monsanto Targets the Heart of Science. *Independent Science News* 2013 May independentsciencenews.org/science-media/the-goodman-affair-monsanto-targets-the-heart-of-science/

[220] Roberts PC. America the Polluted: One Nation, Under Monsanto. *CounterPunch.com* 2013 Feb counterpunch.org/2013/02/26/one-nation-under-monsanto/

[221] "September 20, 2001: The Biotechnology Industry Organization (BIO) today named Iowa Gov. Tom Vilsack as Governor of the Year for his support of the industry's economic growth and agricultural biotechnology research." bio.org/media/press-release/iowas-vilsack-named-bio-governor-year 2014 Jul. "Tom Vilsack serves as the Nation's 30th Secretary of Agriculture. As leader of the U.S. Department of Agriculture (USDA), Vilsack is working hard to strengthen the American agricultural economy,... USDA is promoting American agriculture by conducting cutting-edge research and expanding markets at home and abroad." usda.gov/wps/portal/usda/usdahome?contentidonly=true&contentid=bios_vilsack.xml 2014 Jul

[222] "Michael R. Taylor was named deputy commissioner for foods at the Food and Drug Administration (FDA) in January 2010. He is the first individual to hold the position, which was created along with a new Office of Foods in August 2009. Other positions held by Mr. Taylor include senior fellow, Resources for the Future; professor, School of Medicine, University of Maryland; partner, King & Spalding law firm; and vice president for public policy, Monsanto Company. fda.gov/aboutfda/centersoffices/officeoffoods/ucm196721.htm 2014 Jul. Michael R. Taylor, J.D. (1991-1994), Deputy Commissioner for Policy. fda.gov/AboutFDA/WhatWeDo/History/Leaders/DeputyCommissioners/default.htm 2014 Jul

[223] "Clarence Thomas, Associate Justice... an attorney with the Monsanto Company from 1977-1979" supremecourt.gov/about/biographies.aspx 2014 Jul

the quality and availability of biomedical research, legislative changes, legal decisions, and voters' perceptions of issues related to GMO and biotechnology. Dr Roberts concludes, "Monsanto is not only sufficiently powerful to prevent any research other than that which it purchases with its funding, but also Monsanto succeeded last year in blocking with money and propaganda the GMO labeling law in California. I would tell you to be careful what you eat as it can make you ill and infertile, but you can't even find out what you are eating."

- Allergenicity, immunogenicity, inflammatory effects: The article cited below carries devastating implications for connecting GMO foods with autism, allergy, autoimmunity, obesity, and other inflammatory disorders. The finding that GMO corn—but not natural corn—lead to increases in IL-6 (which promotes Th-17 cell development, as well as cardiometabolic disease) and gamma-delta T cells is sufficient to mechanistically connect GMO foods with inflammatory and dysmetabolic disease in humans.

  - Intestinal and peripheral immune response to MON810 maize ingestion in weaning and old mice (*J Agric Food Chem* 2008 Dec[224]): The authors' abstract understates the importance of their findings, noting immune system abnormalities and an increase in the pro-inflammatory cytokine IL-6 following consumption of GMO corn compared with natural corn. The increase in IL-6 is by itself significant, given the role of inflammation in essentially all human diseases and the ability of IL-6 to induce Th-17 phenotype characteristic of more severe allergic and autoimmune diseases. However, per my reading of the full text of the article, I find this article to sound the alarm on GMO foods per the authors' report, "One of the more recurrent alterations in lymphocyte phenotypes observed in this study was an increase in the TCRγδ+ (gamma-delta T-cells) population. A high percentage of these lymphocytes are localized in the gut and ... γδT cells seem to be important regulatory elements of the immune system, being capable of modulating inflammatory response associated with infectious agents and autoantigens. Higher numbers of γδT cells have been observed in humans with asthma, in intraepithelial lymphocytes (IELs) of children with untreated food allergy, and in the duodenum of children with juvenile idiopathic arthritis or connective tissue disease with gastrointestinal symptoms." Further, gamma-delta T-cells are known to secrete IL-17, the cytokine responsible for the massive tissue damage seen in autoimmune diseases such as multiple sclerosis, rheumatoid arthritis, and psoriasis, and which is also elevated in autism.[225]

GMO-induced increase in IL-6 and gamma-delta Tcells + induction of mitochondrial dysfunction by GMO toxins: possible (synergistic) explanation to GMO connection to a wide range of human health problems

1. GMO-induced gamma-delta T cells: Rats fed GMO corn showed important increases in IL-6 (pro-inflammatory cytokine associated with many and perhaps nearly all human diseases) and in gamma-delta T cells (known to contribute to human allergic and autoimmune disease and to promote inflammatory damage and induction of pathogenic Th-17 cells). If GMO toxins cause the same inflammatory changes in humans, then this would be sufficient to explain the dramatic increases in autoimmunity, autism, and inflammatory and allergic diseases.

2. Induction of mitochondrial dysfunction by GMO toxins, especially glyphosate and associated (pseudo)inert chemicals: Mitochondrial dysfunction is known to contribute to inflammatory diseases, allergy, autoimmunity, Alzheimer's disease, Parkinson's disease, hypertension, diabetes mellitus type-2, and many other diseases; additionally, mitochondrial dysfunction promotes increased secretion of and sensitivity to inflammatory cytokines. If GMO toxins cause mitochondrial dysfunction in humans, then this would be sufficient to explain the marked increases in inflammatory diseases, allergy, autoimmunity, Alzheimer's disease, Parkinson's disease, hypertension, diabetes mellitus type-2, and many other diseases. Glyphosate's reported ability to inhibit cytochrome p450 activity, combined with its genotoxic and mitochondriopathic effects, is synergistically sufficient to promote disease; in a straightforward model, the chemical—especially in its complete formulation—inhibits is own clearance/detoxification, promotes disease, and progressively accumulates.

3. Potential additive and synergistic effects: Researchers should look for evidence of additive and synergistic effects of IL-6, IL-17, Th-17 cells, gamma-delta T-cells, and mitochondrial dysfunction in human patients, especially those with inflammatory disorders ranging from obesity to autoimmunity.

---

[224] Finamore et al. Intestinal and peripheral immune response to MON810 maize ingestion in weaning and old mice. *J Agric Food Chem*. 2008 Dec 10;56(23):11533-9
[225] Al-Ayadhi LY, Mostafa GA. Elevated serum levels of interleukin-17A in children with autism. *J Neuroinflammation*. 2012 Jul 2;9:158

- o **Grains with "toxic gluten"—barley, wheat, rye**: Many grains including corn and rice contain variants of "gluten", but from a clinical and immunologic standpoint our main consideration is on "toxic gluten" (differentiated by its adverse immunologic/histologic/clinical effect rather than its general categorization); the most immunogenic forms of gluten are found in wheat, rye, barley and their related processed products ranging from bread to beer. Thus, when we talk about "gluten" from a clinical standpoint, the implication is that we are talking about "toxic gluten" found in barley, wheat, rye.

  - ▪ **Specificity of tissue transglutaminase explains cereal toxicity in celiac disease** (*J Exp Med*. 2002 Mar[226]): In this important article, the authors note that celiac disease is caused immunogenic inflammation triggered by gluten, a complex mixture of storage proteins found in wheat, and that tissue transglutaminase (tTG) is involved in the generation of T-cell stimulatory gluten peptides through deamidation of glutamine. "Only particular glutamine residues, however, are modified by tTG. Here we provide evidence that the spacing between glutamine and proline, the second most abundant amino acid in gluten, plays an essential role in the specificity of deamidation. … Strikingly, these algorithms [developed in this study] identified many similar peptides in the gluten-like hordeins from barley and secalins from rye but not in the avenins from oats. The avenins contain significantly lower percentages of proline residues, which offers a likely explanation for the lack of toxicity of oats. Thus, the unique amino acid composition of gluten and related proteins in barley and rye favors the generation of toxic T cell stimulatory gluten peptides by tTG."

  Beyond acute/subacute prevention of starvation, no medical need exists for the consumption of wheat (nor rye, nor barley); the few nutrients available in wheat are better acquired in other foods that have less carbohydrate, more protein (e.g., meat) or phytonutrients (egg, fruits and vegetables). Wheat contains indigestible polysaccharides and therefore promotes small intestinal bacterial/microbial overgrowth (SIBO), especially when overconsumed; many people have wheat with breakfast (e.g., bread, toast, cereal, pancakes/waffles, donuts), lunch (sandwich, pizza), dinner (pasta in its various forms, bread as the international side-dish) and dessert (cake, pie). The proper term for the allergy, sensitivity, and intolerance associated with wheat and gluten is "gluten-related disorders." My judgment is that most organizations advocating "whole grains" and "whole wheat" as healthy food have basically sold their souls and resigned their consciousness to grain industry propaganda and "research" showing that whole grains are a healthier option than fiber-free hyperprocessed grain products which are essentially the nutritional equivalent of table sugar; whole oats, brown rice, and the inclusion of a few other relatively rare/primitive/nonGMO/organic grains is reasonable, again in contrast to blanket endorsements of "whole grains" which allows patients to eventually feel good about eating bread, pastries, and other sugar-laden, AGE-loaded, phytonutrient-depleted, carbohydrate-rich and SIBO-promoting foods. In concise summation, reasons to avoid wheat include the following:

  1. **Nutrient-poor**: Wheat is very low in nutrients compared with fruits and especially vegetables. When wheat is consumed, the opportunity is lost to have consumed a food with greater nutritional quantity and quality and (generally) of lower immunogenicity.

  2. **Phytonutrient-poor**: Wheat is very low in health-promoting phytonutrients when compared to fruits (e.g., antioxidant flavonoids) and vegetables (I3C/DIM).

  3. **High fermentation**: As demonstrated in three clinical trials in humans, wheat promotes microbial overgrowth of the small bowel due to its content of indigestible polysaccharides. The resulting microbial overgrowth promotes increased intestinal permeability and a pro-inflammatory state via low-grade endotoxinemia, which also promotes the development of chronic pain via inflammatory/immunogenic mechanisms and peripheral and central sensitization.[227]

---

[226] Vader et al. Specificity of tissue transglutaminase explains cereal toxicity in celiac disease. *J Exp Med*. 2002 Mar 4;195(5):643-9

[227] Yamaguchi et al. Low rather than high dose lipopolysaccharide 'priming' of muscle provides an animal model of persistent elevated mechanical sensitivity for study of chronic pain. *Eur J Pain*. 2011 Aug;724-31.Amaral et al.Commensal microbiota is fundamental for development of inflammatory pain.*Proc Natl Acad Sci* 2008 Feb:2193-7

4. Increased intestinal permeability: Recent research has shown that wheat/gluten triggers increased intestinal permeability—leaky gut—in essentially everyone; this finding is consistent with the finding that wheat triggers immune complex formation in apparently healthy patients (i.e., those considered to be without wheat allergy, celiac disease, or other gluten-related disorder).

5. Wheat/gluten/gliadin promotes formation of circulating immune complexes (CIC): These are formed even in health people; pathogenically, CIC contribute to vasculitis, nephritis, arthritis, and dermatitis.
   ▫ Gliadin IgG antibodies and circulating immune complexes (*Scand J Gastroenterol* 2009 Jan[228]): "Circulating immune complexes (CICs) in blood are associated with autoimmune-diseases such as systemic lupus erythematosus, immune complex glomerulonephritis, rheumatoid arthritis and vasculitis. ... 352 (265 F, 87 M), so far, healthy individuals were tested for CICs containing C1q and immunoglobulin G (IgG) as well as for gliadin IgG antibodies using the ELISA technique. ... In our study, 15.3% (54/352) of the patients presented with elevated CIC concentrations (above 50 microg/ml) and 6.5% (23/352) of the study population were positive for gliadin IgG antibodies (above 20 U/ml). CIC concentration levels were significantly higher in the group with elevated gliadin IgG antibodies (CIC median: 49.0 microg/ml) compared with the group with normal levels of gliadin IgG antibodies (CIC median: 30.0 microg/ml). ... The results of this study indicate that certain food antigens (e.g. gluten) could play a role in the formation of CICs."

6. Celiac disease is common: 1 per 141 people in USA (per *Am J Gastroenterol* 2012 Oct). Factors proposed to enhance the development of celiac disease are *Candida albicans* and glyphosate.

7. Inherently proinflammatory: In vitro, gliadin stimulates human monocytes to produce of IL-8 and TNF-alpha through a mechanism involving NF-kappaB (per *FEBS Lett* 2004 Jul); in this manner, wheat proteins can be said to be directly pro-inflammatory *independently from any allergy/intolerance/sensitivity*.

8. Wheat/gluten can trigger an assortment of health problems which "necessitate" medical/drug treatment if the underling dietary cause is not addressed: Gluten-induced disorders can include gluten ataxia, dermatitis herpetiformis, acne, skin rashes, migraine headache, somatic pain, Meniere's disease, infertility, IgA nephropathy, thyroid disease; these are commonly (mis)diagnosed as other problems and are "medically managed" with drugs—skin creams, analgesics, anti-inflammatory drugs, steroid pills and creams, etc—while the dietary origin under the guise of a "healthy whole grain" remains in place for years or the patient's lifetime. Avoidance of the "toxic glutens" in wheat, rye, barley along with a program of intestinal healing (discussed elsewhere in this book) and nutritional immunomodulation (detailed in this book with complete protocol) should be used in all patients with gluten-related disorders.
   ▫ Gluten sensitivity masquerading as systemic lupus erythematosus (*Ann Rheum Dis* 2004 Nov[229]): "Three patients are described whose original presentation and immunological profile led to the erroneous diagnosis of systemic lupus erythematosus (SLE). The correct diagnosis of gluten sensitivity was made after years of treatment with steroids and other immunosuppressive drugs."
   ▫ Celiac disease (CD) increases risk of SLE (*J Rheumatol.* 2012 Oct[230]): "Individuals with CD were at a 3-fold increased risk of SLE compared to the general population."
   ▫ Remission without insulin therapy on gluten-free diet in type 1 diabetes mellitus (*BMJ Case Rep.* 2012 Jun[231]): "A 5-year and 10-month old boy was diagnosed with classical type 1 diabetes mellitus (T1DM) without celiac disease. ... At 16 months after diagnosis the fasting blood glucose was 4.1 mmol/l and after 20 months he is still without daily insulin

[228] Eisenmann et al. Gliadin IgG antibodies and circulating immune complexes. *Scand J Gastroenterol.* 2009 Jan;44(2):168-71
[229] Hadjivassiliou et al. Gluten sensitivity masquerading as systemic lupus erythematosus. *Ann Rheum Dis.* 2004 Nov;63(11):1501-3
[230] Ludvigsson et al. Increased risk of systemic lupus erythematosus in 29,000 patients with biopsy-verified celiac disease. *J Rheumatol.* 2012 Oct;39(10):1964-70
[231] Sildorf et al. Remission without insulin therapy on gluten-free diet in a 6-year old boy with type 1 diabetes mellitus. *BMJ Case Rep.* 2012 Jun 21;2012. pii: bcr0220125878

therapy. ...The authors propose that the gluten-free diet has prolonged remission in this patient with T1DM and that further trials are indicated."

9. <u>Chronic pain and cognitive dysfunction</u>: Two contemporary studies showed that wheat consumption contributes to cognitive impairment in patients *with* celiac disease[232] and pain and fatigue in IBS patients *without* celiac disease—this second study is summarized below:

- <u>Gluten causes gastrointestinal symptoms in subjects without celiac disease</u> (*Am J Gastroenterol* 2011 Mar[233]): This is a double-blind, randomized, placebo-controlled rechallenge trial undertaken in patients with IBS in whom celiac disease was excluded and who were symptomatically controlled on a gluten-free diet. "Participants received either gluten or placebo in the form of two bread slices plus one muffin per day with a gluten-free diet for up to 6 weeks. ... On a visual analog scale, patients were significantly worse with gluten within 1 week for overall symptoms, pain, bloating, satisfaction with stool consistency, and tiredness." Noteworthy is the fact that all of these adverse clinical manifestations are directly attributable to wheat-induced SIBO regardless of any antigenicity of or immunosensitivity to wheat or gluten.

10. <u>Net acid load</u>: As noted previously, "fish, meat, poultry, eggs, shellfish, cheese, milk, and cereal grains are net acid producing, whereas fresh fruit, vegetables, tubers, roots, and nuts are net base producing."[234] Given the space limitations of the stomach and time and financial limitations of most humans, consuming wheat and other acid-forming foods by definition means that fewer base-forming foods will be consumed; this imbalance promotes/perpetuates diet-induced/maintained low-grade metabolic acidosis.[235]

11. <u>Wheat as a dietary—and environmental—Trojan horse for genotoxic, cyp450-inhibiting mitochondriotoxic glyphosate/Roundup®</u>: Glyphosate is very clearly applied to innumerable wheat crops internationally, and may have a role in the near-vertical increase in a wide range of diseases via its genotoxic[236] cyp450-inhibiting[237] mitochondriopathic[238] adverse effects; not surprisingly, glyphosate use, which can be reasonably described as "skyrocketing" particularly after the introduction of genetically manipulated foods, shows "dose-dependent" (implying causality) associations with various diseases in humans—on an international scale, humans *notably including women of childbearing age*[239] are showing glyphosate accumulation in body

---

[232] Biesiekierski et al. Gluten causes gastrointestinal symptoms in subjects without celiac disease. *Am J Gastroenterol*. 2011 Mar;106(3):508-14

[233] "In newly diagnosed coeliac disease, cognitive performance improves with adherence to the gluten-free diet in parallel to mucosal healing." Lichtwark et al. Cognitive impairment in celiac disease improves on a gluten-free diet and correlates with histological and serological indices of disease severity. *Aliment Pharmacol Ther* 2014 Jul;40:160-70

[234] Cordain et al. Origins and evolution of the Western diet. *Am J Clin Nutr*. 2005 Feb;81(2):341-54

[235] "The modern Western-type diet is deficient in fruits and vegetables and contains excessive animal products, generating the accumulation of non-metabolizable anions and a lifespan state of overlooked metabolic acidosis, whose magnitude increases progressively with aging due to the physiological decline in kidney function. ... Even a very mild degree of metabolic acidosis induces skeletal muscle resistance to the insulin action and dietary acid load may be an important variable in predicting the metabolic abnormalities and the cardiovascular risk of the general population, the overweight and obese persons, and other patient populations including diabetes and chronic kidney failure." Adeva MM, Souto G. Diet-induced metabolic acidosis. *Clin Nutr*. 2011 Aug;30(4):416-21

[236] "Glyphosate (G) is the largest selling herbicide worldwide; the most common formulations (Roundup, R) contain polyoxyethyleneamine as main surfactant. ... R was under all conditions more active than its [declared] active principle (G). ...Since we found genotoxic effects after short exposure to concentrations that correspond to a 450-fold dilution of spraying used in agriculture, our findings indicate that inhalation may cause DNA damage in exposed individuals." Koller et al. Cytotoxic and DNA-damaging properties of glyphosate and Roundup in human-derived buccal epithelial cells. *Arch Toxicol*. 2012 May;86(5):805-13. See also: Gammon C. Weed-Whacking Herbicide Proves Deadly to Human Cells: Used in gardens, farms, and parks around the world, the weed killer Roundup contains an ingredient that can suffocate human cells in a laboratory, researchers say. *Scientific American* 2009 Jun scientificamerican.com/article/weed-whacking-herbicide-p

[237] Samsel A, Seneff S. Glyphosate's Suppression of Cytochrome P450 Enzymes and Amino Acid Biosynthesis by the Gut Microbiome: Pathways to Modern Diseases. *Entropy* 2013, 15, 1416-1463 mdpi.com/1099-4300/15/4/1416

[238] "Caspase activity increased and mitochondrial membrane potential decreased only when the cells were exposed to a mixture of both TN-20 and glyphosate, but not after exposure to either one of these compounds. The results support the possibility that mixtures of glyphosate and TN-20 aggravate mitochondrial damage and induce apoptosis and necrosis. Throughout this process, TN-20 seems to disrupt the integrity of the cellular barrier to glyphosate uptake, promoting glyphosate-mediated toxicity." Kim et al. Mixtures of glyphosate and surfactant TN20 accelerate cell death via mitochondrial damage-induced apoptosis and necrosis. *Toxicol In Vitro*. 2013 Feb;27(1):191-7. "At the same time, we showed that the glyphosate-induced mitochondrial membrane potential disruption could be a cause of apoptosis in keratinocyte cultures." Heu et al. A step further toward glyphosate-induced epidermal cell death: involvement of mitochondrial and oxidative mechanisms. *Environ Toxicol Pharmacol*. 2012 Sep;34(2):144-53. "Therefore, the uncoupling of oxidative phosphorylation is also related to the non-specific membrane permeabilization induced by Roundup. Glyphosate alone does not show any relevant effect on the mitochondrial bioenergetics, in opposition to Roundup formulation products. The differences in the toxicity observed could be either attributed to some products of Roundup or to a synergic effect of glyphosate and formulation products. Bearing in mind that mitochondria is provided with a variety of bioenergetic functions mandatory for the regulation of intracellular aerobic energy production and electrolyte homeostasis, these results question the safety of Roundup on animal health." Peixoto F. Comparative effects of the Roundup and glyphosate on mitochondrial oxidative phosphorylation. *Chemosphere*. 2005 Dec;61(8):1115-22

[239] "Serum glyphosate (GLYP) and gluphosinate (GLUF) were detected in nonpregnant women (NPW) and not detected in PW." Aris A, Leblanc S. Maternal and fetal exposure to pesticides associated to genetically modified foods in Eastern Townships of Quebec, Canada. *Reprod Toxicol*. 2011 May;31(4):528-33

tissues and fluids.[240,241,242] These findings clearly indicate 1) international overuse of this chemical/formulation, and 2) failure of governmental regulation; population-wide exposures to glyphosate are population-wide toxic chemical exposures, analogous to population-wide tobacco cigarette smoking while the medical community self-servingly "waits for definitive evidence" just as it did with tobacco cigarette smoking.[243]

- □ Widespread glyphosate contamination of American air and water: herbicides and pesticides in Mississippi air and rain (*Environ Toxicol Chem*. 2014 Jun[244]): "Atrazine, metolachlor, and propanil were detected in ≥50% of the air and rain samples in both years. Glyphosate and its degradation product, aminomethyl-phosphonic acid (AMPA), were detected in ≥75% of air and rain samples in 2007 but were not measured in 1995. ... Total herbicide flux in 2007 was slightly greater than in 1995 and was dominated by glyphosate."

- □ Cytotoxic and DNA-damaging properties of glyphosate and Roundup in human epithelial cells. (*Arch Toxicol*. 2012 May[245]): "Glyphosate (G) is the largest selling herbicide worldwide; the most common formulations (Roundup, R) contain polyoxyethyleneamine as main surfactant. Recent findings indicate that G exposure may cause DNA damage and cancer in humans. ... R induced acute cytotoxic effects at concentrations > 40 mg/l after 20 min, which were due to membrane damage and impairment of mitochondrial functions. ... Furthermore, an increase of nuclear aberrations that reflect DNA damage was observed. The frequencies of micronuclei and nuclear buds were elevated after 20-min exposure to 10-20 mg/l, while nucleoplasmatic bridges were only enhanced by R at the highest dose (20 mg/l). R was under all conditions more active than its [declared] active principle (G). ...Since we found genotoxic effects after short exposure to concentrations that correspond to a 450-fold dilution of spraying used in agriculture, our findings indicate that inhalation may cause DNA damage in exposed individuals."

Glyphosate residues are found in humans internationally, notably among city-dwellers, indicating that the exposure is *not* from direct agricultural/occupational exposure in farming[246] and therefore must be from water and air (noting that more than 75% of water and air samples from Mississippi USA are contaminated with glyphosate[247]), and/or food, with the latter—food—likely being quantitatively most important. While Americans would be expected to have the greatest exposure to glyphosate/Roundup® because of the rampant *unlabeled* infiltration of their food supply with "Roundup-Ready" genetically manipulated foods (the average American eats more than his/her bodyweight each year in transgenic and multimanipulated foods[248]), glyphosate/Roundup® is also used on nontransgenic foods, forests and fields internationally.[249] The American chemoagricultural procedure known as "desiccation"[250] involves spraying supra-normal amounts of glyphosate/Roundup® onto crops in order to kill them (thus promoting

[240] Samsel A, Seneff S. Glyphosate, pathways to modern diseases II: Celiac sprue and gluten intolerance. *Interdiscip Toxicol*. 2013 Dec;6(4):159-84

[241] Swanson NL, Leu A, Abrahamson J, Wallet B. Genetically engineered crops, glyphosate, and the detrioration of health in the United States of America. *Journal of Organic Systems* 2014; 9: 6-37 organic-systems.org/journal/92/JOS_Volume-9_Number-2_Nov_2014-Swanson-et-al.pdf

[242] Krüger M, Schledorn P, Schrödl W, et al. Detection of Glyphosate Residues in Animals and Humans. *J Environ Anal Toxicol* 2014, 4:2 omicsonline.org/open-access/

[243] Wolinsky H, Brune T. *The Serpent on the Staff: The Unhealthy Politics of the American Medical Association*. GP Putnam and Sons, New York, 1994

[244] Majewski et al. Pesticides in Mississippi air and rain: a comparison between 1995 and 2007. *Environ Toxicol Chem*. 2014 Jun;33(6):1283-93

[245] Koller et al. Cytotoxic and DNA-damaging properties of glyphosate and Roundup in human-derived buccal epithelial cells. *Arch Toxicol*. 2012 May;86(5):805-13

[246] "...there have been virtually no studies undertaken in the US to assess glyphosate levels in human blood or urine. However, a recent study involving multiple countries in Europe provides disturbing confirmation that glyphosate residues are prevalent in the Western diet (Hoppe, 2013). This study involved exclusively city dwellers, who are unlikely to be exposed to glyphosate except through food sources. Despite Europe's more aggressive campaign against GMO foods than that in the Americas, 44% of the urine samples contained quantifiable amounts of glyphosate. Diet seems to be the main source of exposure. One can predict that, if a study were undertaken in the U.S., the percentage of affected population would be much larger." Samsel A, Seneff S. Glyphosate, pathways to modern diseases II: Celiac sprue and gluten intolerance. *Interdiscip Toxicol* 2013;6:159-84

[247] "Glyphosate and its degradation product, aminomethyl-phosphonic acid (AMPA), were detected in ≥75% of air and rain samples in 2007..." Majewski et al. Pesticides in Mississippi air and rain: a comparison between 1995 and 2007. *Environ Toxicol Chem*. 2014 Jun;33(6):1283-93

[248] "Americans are eating their weight and more in genetically engineered food every year, a new Environmental Working Group analysis shows. On average, people eat an estimated 193 pounds of genetically engineered food in a 12-month period. The typical American adult weighs 179 pounds." Sharp R. Americans Eat Their Weight In Genetically Engineered Food. *AgMag* 2012 Oct ewg.org/agmag/2012/10/americans-eat-their-weight-genetically-engineered-food

[249] Kogan M, Alister C. Glyphosate use in forest plantations. *Chilean Journal of Agricultural Research* 2010; 70: 652-666

[250] "Glyphosate residues in wheat and other crops are likely increasing recently due to the growing practice of crop desiccation just prior to the harvest. We argue that the practice of "ripening" sugar cane with glyphosate may explain the recent surge in kidney failure among agricultural workers in Central America." Samsel A, Seneff S. Glyphosate, pathways to modern diseases II: Celiac sprue and gluten intolerance. *Interdiscip Toxicol*. 2013 Dec;6(4):159-84

drying of the plant material) meanwhile triggering a response in the plant that causes it to "go to seed" and increase production of wheat grain (slightly increasing harvest) while drying/desiccating the plant eases the burden on harvesting machinery. Although logistically desirable for increased production and ease of harvest, the environmental and human consequences are conveniently ignored by commercial profiteers and (anti)regulatory sycophants; the factual result is deplorable contamination of the public's air and water with glyphosate. Therefore, wheat chemoagriculture contaminates wheat, air and water with glyphosate/Roundup®, and wheat consumption directly contributes to glyphosate/Roundup® exposure via residual glyphosate/Roundup® mixed within the grain. The table below shows US regulatory "tolerances for residues" for glyphosate in grains/wheat and other sample foods; this data needs to be interpreted with at least three real-world considerations: 1) Firstly, with the rampant—virtually malignant—deregulation of polluting/petroleum/chemical industries in the US, any reasonable and responsible concerned citizen might question whether violations of these tolerance levels are being monitored, let alone enforced, let alone enforced to any meaningful effect. 2) Secondly, wheat deserves special consideration in this conversation even though it is not allowed the highest level of glyphosate tolerance/contamination due to the fact that wheat is consumed so much more frequently than the other foodstuffs—wheat is a major staple in the American diet. Americans are encouraged by government and industry campaigns to increase their consumption of grains—especially so-called "whole grains"—and wheat is clearly the grain of choice in the American diet. Americans consume an average of 6-7 ounces of grains per day, mostly in the form of refined grains, with 40% consumed at breakfast (e.g., cereal, pancakes, waffles, toast, bagels, biscuits, croissants), 23% consumed at lunch (e.g., sandwiches, pita, plain bread, pasta, pizza, cake and pie), 17% consumed at dinner (e.g., bread, pasta, pizza, cake and pie) and the remaining 20% consumed in the form of snack foods throughout the day.[251] 3) Thirdly, although wheat chemoagriculture is likely an important contributor to air and water contamination (thus contaminating people regardless of their diet) and wheat consumption is likely a contributor to total body burden of glyphosate and other chemical toxins, clearly glyphosate/Roundup® is used on other foods—including natural plants as well as genetically manipulated pseudoplants—and is applied to parks, fields, forests, and private yards and gardens. In sum, wheat chemoagriculture and wheat consumption both contribute to environment-wide exposure and population-wide (bio)accumulation of glyphosate/Roundup®; reducing/avoiding wheat consumption reduces these problems.

Glyphosate allowances in US foods[252]—examples		US EPA "Crop Group 15": Cereal Grains
Food	**Parts per million**	Barley (*Hordeum* spp.)
Barley, bran	30	Buckwheat (*Fagopyrum esculentum*)
Beet, sugar, roots	10	Corn (*Zea mays*)
Canola, seed	20	Millet, pearl (*Pennisetum glaucum*)
Flax, meal	8.0	Millet, proso (*Panicum milliaceum*)
Grain, cereal, group 15 *except field corn, popcorn, rice, sweet corn, wild rice*	30	Oats (*Avena* spp.)
		Popcorn (*Zea mays* var. everta)
Peppermint, tops	200	Rice (*Oryza sativa*)
Spearmint, tops	200	Rye (*Secale cereale*)
Sugarcane, cane	2.0	Sorghum (milo) (*Sorghum* spp.)
Sugarcane, molasses	30	Triticale (*Triticum-Secale* hybrids)
Sunflower, seed	85	**Wheat (*Triticum* spp.)**
Tea, instant	7.0	Wild rice (*Zizania aquatica*)

[251] Lin et al. U.S. Grain Consumption Landscape. Economic Research Service, US Department of Agriculture.2007 Nov ers.usda.gov/media/216644/err50_reportsummary_1_.pdf
[252] US government printing office (GPO): Protection of Environment, Title 40, 180.364 Glyphosate; tolerances for residues. gpo.gov/fdsys/pkg/CFR-2012-title40-vol25/xml/CFR-2012-title40-vol25-part180.xml and Samsel A, Seneff S in Interdiscip Toxicol. 2013 Dec. US EPA Crop Group 15: Cereal Grains (ir4.rutgers.edu/Other/FederalCropGroups.htm) and US GPO Protection of Environment, Title 40 CFR 180.41, page 438 (gpo.gov/fdsys/granule/CFR-2012-title40-vol25/CFR-2012-title40-vol25-sec180-41)

- High fructose corn syrup (HFCS)—nonnutritive calories, ATP depletion, mercury: In the United States, much/most HFCS is sourced from GMO corn; the process of producing this nonphysiologic unnatural nutrient-depleted carbohydrate source introduces mercury—a toxic metal famous for its causation of hypertension and psychosis/neurotoxicity—in clinically meaningful amounts.[253] Initial metabolic processing of fructose occurs via fructokinase and causes ATP depletion leading to activation of inflammatory pathways and resultant production of uric acid which causes insulin resistance and clinical manifestations of weight gain, hypertension, and dyslipidemia and dysglycemia—the metabolic syndrome.[254] Fructose promotes urate formation, and urate formation stimulates fructokinase activity; in this manner a vicious cycle is established promoting the development of fructose-induced urate-mediated diseases such as fatty liver.[255] Fructose consumption from whole foods such as fruits does not cause the same problems noted with HFCS because 1) *cellular* carbohydrates—sugars within the context of fibers and other (phyto)nutrients—do not cause the same adverse physiologic affects noted with *acellular* carbohydrate sources, 2) lower carbohydrate:fiber ratio, 3) fruits contain ant inflammatory and antioxidant phytonutrients that offset and physiologically "balance" the adverse effects of the sugars, 4) plants generally have an alkalinizing effect via their content of citrates such as potassium citrate—this promotes urinary excretion of the fructose-induced urate via urinary alkalinization—in contrast to the acidifying effect of many "soft drinks" and "sodas" which are acidic due to the carbonation process that introduces carbon dioxide and subsequently carbonic acid—systemic/urinary acidification promotes retention of uric acid and thereby promotes exacerbation of fructose-induced and urate-mediated insulin resistance.
- Pasteurization, Maillard reaction, polyol pathway, advanced glycation end-products (AGE) and their receptor (RAGE): The nonenzymatic reaction wherein sugars such as glucose/fructose/lactose are bound to proteins in general and the amino acid lysine (also tryptophan and arginine) in particular to form amino sugars; this process is called glycation, glycosylation, or the Maillard reaction, and as with most nonenzymatic reactions, it occurs slowly over time, is dose/substrate-dependent, and is expedited by heat. The sequence below is slightly modified from Gaby[256]; in this diagram AGE = advanced glycation end product, which—as discussed below, interacts with its receptor, RAGE.

Reducing Sugar + Amino Acid + Heat/time → N-Glycosylamine → Amadori rearrangement → AGE/RAGE

Other pathways and several other AGEs and RAGE ligands exist. Methylglyoxal, also called pyruvaldehyde or 2-oxopropanal, is formed by the nonenzymatic degradation of the glycolytic intermediates, including dihydoxyacetone phosphate and glyceraldehyde-3-phosphate; its production is increased during sustained hyperglycemia, and methylglyoxal can be converted into AGE via reaction with free amino groups of lysine and arginine and with thiol groups of cysteine. Methylglyoxal is degraded/detoxified by the enzyme glyoxalase-1 (Glo1); however, GLo1 is downregulated by RAGE, and in this manner RAGE activation leads to additional RAGE activation via increased ligand availability.

Excess glycolytic intermediates → Methylglyoxal + lysine/arginine/cysteine → AGE → RAGE activation

Fructose is the most reactive of the reducing sugars, promoting hemoglobin glycosylation, protein cross-linking, and (lipid) peroxidation much more rapidly than does glucose. Glycosylated proteins can be further modified ultimately to advanced glycation end-products (AGE), which bind to DNA

---

[253] "Mercury contamination of food products as a result of the use of mercury contaminated HFCS seems like a very real possibility. With daily per capita consumption of HFCS in the US averaging about 50 grams and daily mercury intakes from HFCS ranging up to 28 μg, this potential source of mercury may exceed other major sources of mercury especially in high-end consumers of beverages sweetened with HFCS." Dufault et al. Mercury from chlor-alkali plants: measured concentrations in food product sugar. *Environ Health.* 2009 Jan 26;8:2

[254] "High doses of fructose raise the BP and cause the features of metabolic syndrome. Lowering the uric acid level prevents the increase in mean arterial blood pressure. Excessive intake of fructose may have a role in the current epidemics of obesity and diabetes." Perez-Pozo et al. Excessive fructose intake induces the features of metabolic syndrome in healthy adult men: role of uric acid in the hypertensive response. *Int J Obes* 2010 Mar;34(3):454-61

[255] "In conclusion, present study shows that metabolism of fructose by fructokinase results in the intracellular production of uric acid that feeds back to up-regulate fructokinase and increase sensitivity of the cell to the triglyceride-raising effects of fructose. Of interest, blockade of intracellular uric acid with allopurinol could inhibit the effect of fructose to increase fat accumulation." Lanaspa et al. Uric acid stimulates fructokinase and accelerates fructose metabolism in the development of fatty liver. *PLoS One.* 2012;7(10):e47948

[256] Gaby AR. Adverse effects of dietary fructose. *Altern Med Rev.* 2005 Dec;10(4):294-306

and also promote chronic pain and inflammation at least in part via interaction with the receptor for AGE (RAGE) which, as part of the innate immune system, is a pattern-recognition receptor predominantly involved in the recognition of endogenous molecules released in the context of infection, physiological stress or chronic/sustained inflammation.[257] AGE levels are increased in patients who are diabetic, fibromyalgic, elderly, and those with renal insufficiency; readers should appreciate that AGE levels reflect endogenous production (obviously exacerbated by hyperglycemia) and exogenous consumption (consumption of a diet high in processed foods, especially aged/cooked milk products and baked items such as pastries). As expected, the use of heat to reduce the bacterial load of cow's milk greatly increases the quantity of amino sugars in comparison with non-heated milk; in this manner, pasteurization changes the way these milk proteins are digested and thereafter perceived/processed by the intestinal immune system in a manner that promotes allergic sensitization.[258] The clinical significance of RAGE activation is its vicious contribution to inflammation, as perfectly summarized by Lee and Parker[259], "Interestingly, unlike other receptors, expression of RAGE is positively regulated by its ligand stimulation, which means that increasing concentration of ligands leads to up-regulation of RAGE. So, RAGE signals are accelerated more and more by the accumulation of signal stimulants. RAGE is found on the cell surface of various immune cells, and most of its ligands are mainly secreted by immune cells, including macrophages and dendritic cells; therefore one of the major roles of RAGE is involved in inflammation. Stimulation of RAGE by its ligands activates the proinflammatory transcription factor nuclear factor kappa B (NFkB)..." AGEs are excreted by the kidneys, which are also damaged by AGEs; thus a vicious cycle of AGE exposure, intrarenal AGE retention, renal injury, upregulation of RAGE receptors can culminate in renal failure, particularly due to diabetic nephropathy.

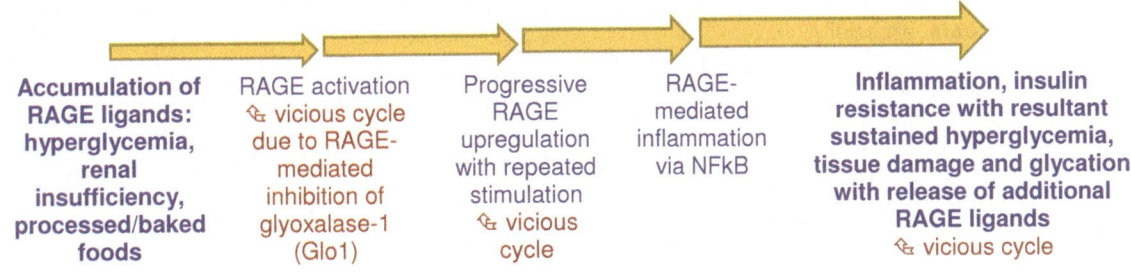

| Accumulation of RAGE ligands: hyperglycemia, renal insufficiency, processed/baked foods | RAGE activation ⚷ vicious cycle due to RAGE-mediated inhibition of glyoxalase-1 (Glo1) | Progressive RAGE upregulation with repeated stimulation ⚷ vicious cycle | RAGE-mediated inflammation via NFkB | Inflammation, insulin resistance with resultant sustained hyperglycemia, tissue damage and glycation with release of additional RAGE ligands ⚷ vicious cycle |

The polyol pathway, also called the sorbitol-aldose reductase pathway, is implicated in diabetic complications, especially in microvascular damage to the retina, kidney, and nerves. From a clinical perspective, the conversion of glucose to sorbitol via aldose reductase is important due to the resulting osmotic and oxidative stresses (and possible AGE production via sorbitol-amino binding), while the formation of fructose from sorbitol via sorbitol dehydrogenase is less consequential. Because the retina, kidney, and nervous tissues are insulin-independent, glucose enters in a dose-dependent manner per serum glucose levels, which reflect the balance between glucose intake (i.e., diet) and peripheral glucose uptake. In a hyperglycemic state, the affinity of aldose reductase for glucose rises, causing an escalating/disproportionate accumulation of sorbitol while also causing an escalating/disproportionate depletion of NADPH, resulting in tissue-specific glucose-induced oxidative stress. In these ways (osmotic stress, oxidative stress, AGE formation, inhibition nitric oxide and thus vasodilation and mitochondrial biogenesis), the polyol pathway is a major contributor to hyperglycemia-induced cellular/tissue damage and oxidative stress seen with sustained hyperglycemia, leading to the classic complications of diabetes: cataract, renal injury, neuropathy[260], and -more rarely and to a lesser extent- diabetic cerebral edema.

[257] Ibrahim et al. RAGE and TLRs: relatives, friends or neighbours? *Mol Immunol.* 2013 Dec;56(4):739-44
[258] Roth-Walter et al. Pasteurization of milk proteins promotes allergic sensitization by enhancing uptake through Peyer's patches. *Allergy.* 2008 Jul;63(7):882-90
[259] Lee EJ, Park JH. Receptor for Advanced Glycation Endproducts (RAGE), Its Ligands, and Soluble RAGE. *Genomics Inform.* 2013 Dec;11(4):224-9
[260] Chung et al. Contribution of polyol pathway to diabetes-induced oxidative stress. *J Am Soc Nephrol.* 2003 Aug;14(8 Suppl 3):S233-6

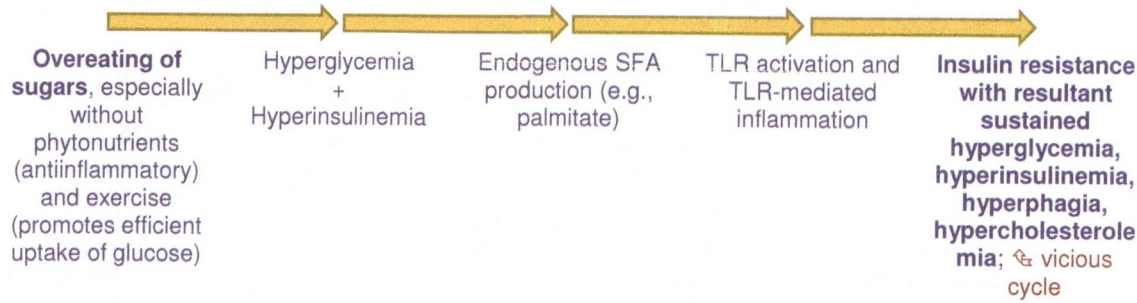

Glucose excess	Sorbitol formation via aldose reductase and depletion of NADPH: consequences are ❶ intracellular osmotic stress (e.g., diabetic cataractogenesis), ❷ reduced ability to reduce/regenerate glutathione (GSH), ❸ reduced ability to produce nitric oxide, ❹ formation of AGEs	Limited formation of fructose of via sorbitol dehydrogenase; fructose contributes to AGE formation and thus RAGE activation

o Dietary activation and modulation of Toll-like receptors (TLR): Toll-like receptors (TLR), especially TLR-2 and TLR-4, are part of the innate immune system activated by microbial motifs (pathogen-associated molecular patterns, PAMPs) and saturated fatty acids (SFA) to induce inflammation generally via NFkB-mediated pathways. As components of the innate immune system, TLR and RAGE can be seen as pro-inflammatory receptors with somewhat of an *outward* and *inward* focus, respectively, and for which some overlap in activation is likely to exist; TLR-2/4 are sensitive to PAMPS (hence an *outward* focus on external invaders) and saturated fatty acids while RAGE are predominantly sensitive to endogenous physiological/metabolic insults (e.g., resulting from hyperglycemia) or inflammation (hence an *inward* focus on homeodynamic balance). TLR activation by microbes and saturated fatty acids is of particular relevance for the development of insulin resistance and diabetes mellitus type-2 and the associated problems of obesity, hypertension, and appetite insatiation. The most simple model for understanding the sequence of events is as follows; this model of "metabolic inflammation" will be developed further in a following section in this book:

Overeating of sugars, especially without phytonutrients (antiinflammatory) and exercise (promotes efficient uptake of glucose)	Hyperglycemia + Hyperinsulinemia	Endogenous SFA production (e.g., palmitate)	TLR activation and TLR-mediated inflammation	Insulin resistance with resultant sustained hyperglycemia, hyperinsulinemia, hyperphagia, hypercholesterolemia; ↺ vicious cycle

TLR activation is *primarily* abrogated by treatment of causative dysglycemia/diabetes, dysbiosis, and dietary recklessness, *secondarily* mitigated via olive oil and fish oil which modulate intracellular TLR signaling, and *tertiarily* modulated by phytonutritional NFkB inhibitors.

o Processed food/fuel overload (PFO)—excess carbohydrates, excess (saturated and n6) fatty acids: Quantitative and persistent excess of calories in the form of dietary sugars and fats (dietary fat in the Western diet is typically unprecedentedly high in n6 fatty acids [notably linoleic acid and arachidonic acid, both of which are notably inflammatory], long-chain saturated fatty acids, and hydrogenated oils); the general and obvious descriptive term for this caloric excess is "fuel overload." The metabolic consequence of diet-induced hyperglycemia is hyperinsulinemia, which promotes increased production of ceramide, which is itself a mediator of insulin resistance; one of the most logical explanations for this glucose-induced insulin resistance via insulin-induced ceramide production is that it is a self-regulatory and self-protective mechanism whereby cells are able to protect themselves from fuel overload. Notably, the medical/pharmacologic/allopathic interpretation of this phenomenon is that the insulin resistance is a problem that needs to be "cured" with drugs that override this self-regulatory mechanism to enhance insulin sensitivity; in the end, this overriding of physiologic insulin resistance leads to exacerbation of pathologic intracellular fuel overload. The consequences of intracellular fuel overload due to excess dietary carbohydrates and fats include ❶ excess intracellular lipid (e.g., palmitate, ceramide) accumulation, which leads to ER stress, mitochondrial dysfunction, and the activation of oxidant and inflammatory pathways, ❷ suppression of mitochondrial ATP production at the level of ETC oxidative phosphorylation, ❸ intracellular accumulation of lipids that have physiologic consequences, notably palmitate and ceramide and their ability to mediate insulin resistance, ❹ intracellular accumulation of lipids that are biochemically altered (e.g., modified by LOX-mediated hydroperoxidation), ❺ fuel-induced activation of pro-inflammatory enzymes such as lipoxygenase (LOX) which promotes inflammatory macrophage recruitment, hydroperoxidation of unsaturated fatty acids, insulin resistance, mitochondrial dysfunction, ER stress and the subsequent UPR, ❻ hyperglycemia caused by dietary excess of carbohydrates and the above-mentioned complications leads to oxidative stress, activation of inflammatory pathways such as NFkB, and results in formation of endogenous AGEs which promote biological aging, inflammation, and pain perception/sensitization, ❼ the activation of inflammatory pathways causes suppression of endothelial nitric oxide synthase (eNOS), and the resultant decrease in nitric oxide (NO) production impairs vasodilation (promoting hypertension and erectile dysfunction) and mitochondrial biogenesis (promoting mitopenia which results in overwork and excess ROS production from remaining mitochondria, while also reducing ATP production and fatty acid oxidation/clearance). An efficient quote from the 2013 article by Mabalirajan and Ghosh[261] provides an excellent summary of many of these concepts: "It is a surprising paradox that high nutrient [carbohydrate and lipid] intake can lead to decreased oxidative phosphorylation. The imbalance between nutrient intake and its utilization leads to store abnormal lipid in adipocytes and obesity. This accumulated lipid induces various stress pathways and activates various lipid oxidative enzymes. It has been demonstrated that mice which were fed either high fat or western diet had shown the increased expression of 12/15-lipoxygenase (12/15-LOX), a nonheme iron dioxygenase, which catalyzes the hydroperoxidation of polyunsaturated fatty acids, in adipocytes." Mabalirajan and Ghosh should have specified overconsumption of *lipids* and *carbohydrates* since this is the real problem—not "high nutrient intake" since this is misleading.

o Food-induced hypothalamic inflammation, dietary activation of Toll-like receptors: As described in an excellent article by Milanski et al[262], ❶ long-chain saturated fatty acids produce an inflammatory response predominantly through the activation of TLR4 in hypothalamus with resultant local release of cytokines, and ❷ the physiologic consequences of diet-induced hypothalamic inflammation include local endoplasmic reticulum stress, systemic inflammation, adiposity, insulin resistance, and enhanced hunger, the latter via inhibited reception/function of anorexigenic (hunger-suppressing; the roots *orexi-, orex-, -orexia* are Greek with the denotation of hunger, desire, searching) hormones insulin and leptin. Inflammation in the hypothalamic region of the brain, which can occur following TLR activation secondary to glucose, saturated long-chain fatty acids, or exposure to microbial motifs (e.g., bacterial or viral). In the CNS, TLR4 are found in the microglia. Of additional note regarding brain inflammation, "…recent studies in the brain provide in vivo evidence supporting the model that both ER stress and inflammation are able to activate each other and to inhibit normal cellular metabolism."[263] Toll-like receptors (TLR, e.g., TLR2 and TLR4) are upregulated and activated by microbial motifs such as bacterial endotoxin/LPS as well as by glucose (hyperglycemia), long-chain saturated fatty acids, free fatty acids and "vegetable oil" (term used but undefined by Milanski et al, presumably n6 PUFA especially linoleic acid, known for its proinflammatory effects). The endoplasmic reticulum (ER) functions to synthesize and process proteins, whether used intracellularly, within the cell membrane, or secreted from the cell. In certain adverse situations—notably exposure to viruses,

> **Saturated fatty acids produce an inflammatory response through the activation of TLR4 in the hypothalamus, promoting obesity**
>
> "… the activation of an inflammatory response in the hypothalamus leads to the molecular and functional resistance to the adipostatic hormones, leptin and insulin, resulting in a defective control of food intake and energy expenditure. … In conclusion, saturated fatty acids activate TLR2 and TLR4 signaling and ER stress in hypothalamus. … The presence of a functional TLR4 signaling is required for the development of hyperlipidic dietary obesity."
> Milanski et al. *J Neurosci.* 2009 Jan

[261] Mabalirajan U, Ghosh B. Mitochondrial dysfunction in metabolic syndrome and asthma. *J Allergy* (Cairo). 2013;2013:340476
[262] Milanski et al. Saturated fatty acids produce an inflammatory response predominantly through activation of TLR4 signaling in hypothalamus.*J Neurosci.* 2009 Jan;29:359-70
[263] Hotamisligil GS. Endoplasmic reticulum stress and the inflammatory basis of metabolic disease. *Cell.* 2010 Mar 19;140(6):900-17

bacteria, hyperglycemia and hyper(long-chain saturated)lipidosis, disruption of ER function leads to accumulation of unfolded/misfolded proteins within the ER lumen; this *ER stress* (ERS) leads to a complex adaptive cellular response termed the *unfolded protein response* (UPR), which increases production and release of proteins and cytokines needed for immune surveillance. Induction of ERS-UPR occurs following stimulation of TLR2 or TRL4, leading to activation of the NFkB pathway; the linear flow can be depicted as follows:

Long-chain saturated fatty acids → TLR4 → NFkB → ERS+UPR → orexia, insulin resistance

ERS is obviously an adaptive mechanism, which most likely developed for sensing microbes, and which becomes maladaptive when chronically stimulated by overconsumption of carbohydrates and saturated fats; the sequel UPR is notably appropriate for response to microbes, and notably harmful when activated by habitual dietary excess. When ERS-UPR activation is sustained, the result is excess inflammation and immune system hypervigilance (e.g., pathophysiologic priming for disorders of metabolic/allergic/autoimmune inflammation); more intense activation of ERS may result in apoptosis.

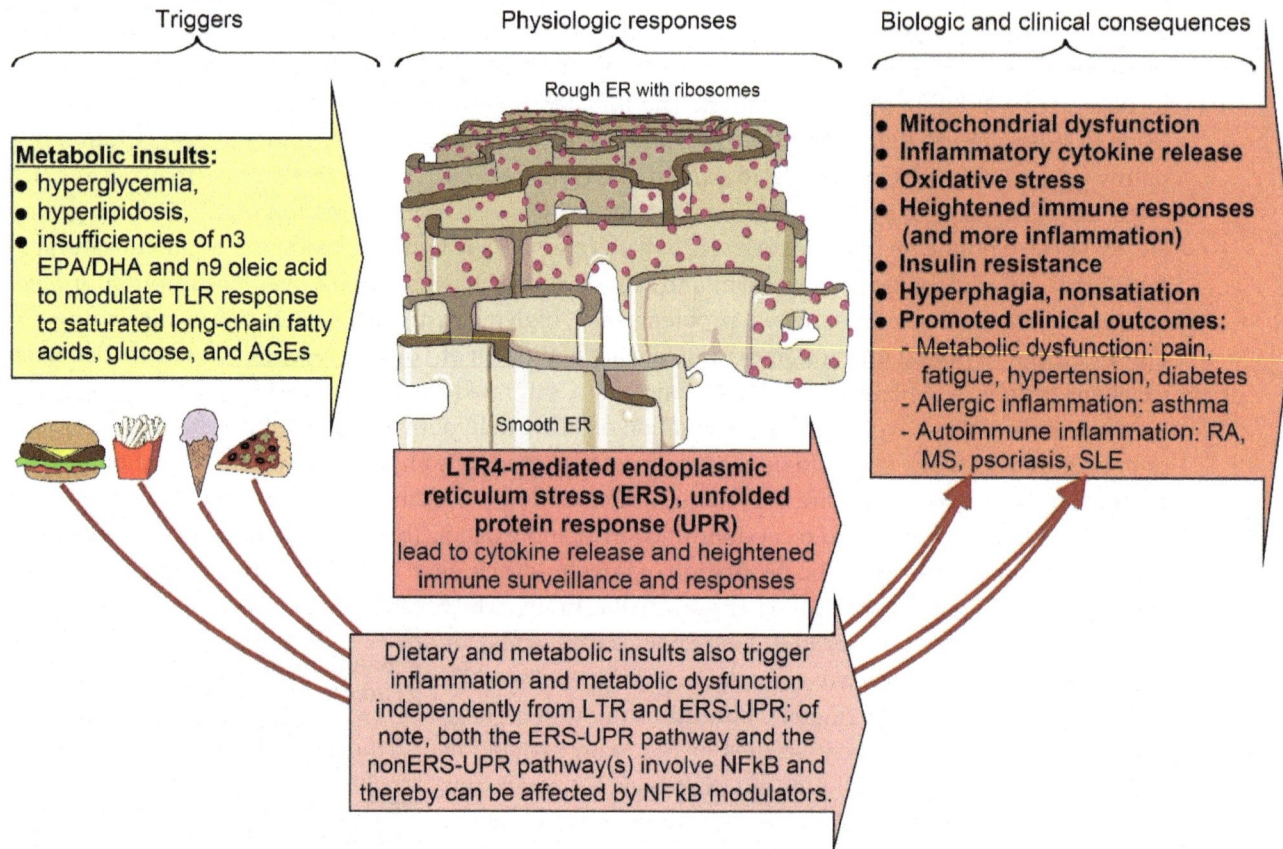

Dysnutrition/dysmetabolism causes TLR4-mediated ERS and proinflammatory UPR: Dietary and metabolic insults cause endoplasmic reticulum stress (largely but not entirely) mediated by TLR4 and lead to the UPR, which primes the immune system and leads to enhanced pro-inflammatory cytokine release.

Endoplasmic reticulum stress is somewhat analogous to a "traffic jam" inside the ER, and the unfolded protein response is a pro-inflammatory "traffic alert" in response; another more creative analogy would be that of an origami artist forced to fold and produce more than possible, with the resultant emotional breakdown/outrage analogous to the inflammatory UPR. Without the metabolic insults of excess glucose and excess saturated fatty acids—both of which are overpresent in Americanized/Westernized diets but which would have been absent for the vast majority of human history—the main expected stressors for induction of ERS would have been of microbial origin, and thus the resultant "alarms" and amplification of immune responses would have clearly been a positive and meaningful response; now that industrialized societies have essentially codified hyperglycemia and higher intakes of saturated fat, this ERS-UPR pathway is maintained in a higher state (quantitatively more) of sustained activation (longer duration). Saturated long-chain fatty acids activate TLR4 and induce NFkB-mediated inflammation via ERS-UPR and routes that are independent from ERS-UPR. While the ERS-UPR pathway effects elaboration of pro-inflammatory cytokines in an NFkB-dependent manner, the opposite is also true: NFkB activation causes ERS-UPR. Therefore, one would reasonably expect that inhibitors/modulators of the NFkB pathway (detailed elsewhere in this chapter) would be of therapeutic value in conditions of ERS-UPR; however, the clinical focus should always remain on identifying and eliminating the *origin* of the ERS-UPR/NFkB activation.

o <u>Conveniently and consistently overlooked social causes and medical consequences of obesity, insulin resistance, and medical management thereof</u>: I wish to make an extra effort to point out a few items here to underscore their importance; in this paragraph, I will restate and reframe a few ideas to ensure that readers fully grasp the realization I am trying to impart. Readers, of course, have the option to bypass these particular perspectives, but let's at least consider them *before* making that decision. ❶ <u>The medical-pharmaceutical goal of using drugs to "enhance insulin sensitivity" is simple-minded, noncurative, and self-serving</u>: Pharmacologic enhancement of insulin sensitivity *in lieu* of actually correcting the causes (mostly dietary, microbial, xenobiotic, and lifestyle) of insulin resistance increasingly occurs to me as a stupid idea (i.e., a forced pharmacologic override of normal physiology), leveraged by drug companies via drug-promotional journal articles and advertisements upon uninformed doctors and patients, who are purposefully kept ignorant by medical school and public education, respectively. The drug treatments for long-term management of insulin resistance offer no chance for curing the disease and simply keep patients in a state of perpetual drug dependency while medical doctors have basically become enslaved to the pharmaceutical industry. Many of these facts also apply to the long-term management of so-called chronic hypertension, which is likewise nearly always readily curable (not merely treatable) with nonpharmacologic means; some of this data was reviewed in my earlier books and articles covering diabetes and hypertension and will be revisited and expanded in Volume 2 of the *Inflammation Mastery* series. ❷ <u>Insulin resistance is cytoprotective</u>: The idea that the human body could be an infinite repository for glucose and other high-energy fuel substrates—storing these reactive molecules endlessly and without consequence—is among the feeblest ideas to permeate and be absorbed into the clinical practice of medicine in general and the treatment of diabetes mellitus type-2 in particular. Fuel overload—caused solely by an excess of glucose+fructose with variable amounts of lipid and sodium and an insufficiency of nutrients and physical exercise—causes numerous consequential intracellular and organism-damaging events including oxidative damage, immune impairment, antioxidant depletion, mitochondrial dysfunction, endoplasmic reticulum dysfunction, and systemic inflammation; faced with an excess intake of glucose+fructose and fatty acids sourced from processed and nutrient-depleted foods, the body's only way of blocking these intracellular events is by blocking cellular uptake of fuel in general and glucose in particular, and by this innate self-protective wisdom of the body do we have "insulin resistance" formerly called by a more accurate name of "glucose intolerance." Very importantly, note that the term "glucose intolerance" implies a problem with glucose (consumption) and therefore suggests a low-cost low-carbohydrate dietary remedy, while the term "insulin resistance" is much more ambiguous and suggests a problem with insulin and the "need" for "insulin-sensitizing drugs", or simply more insulin (pharmaceutical grade, via injection). ❸ <u>Insulin resistance is the predictable outcome of an unnatural diet and physically-constrained lifestyle</u>: The overconsumption of processed foods is the primary cause of insulin resistance via nutrient deficiencies (e.g., chromium, cholecalciferol, magnesium, fiber and phytonutrients), substrate overload (e.g., glucose, n6 fatty acids, fructose, and pro-inflammatory sodium), and accumulation of dysmetabolic intermediates such as palmitate and ceramide; adding dysbiotic microbial exposures (natural) and xenobiotic exposures (artifactual from corporate-government irresponsibility) synergizes with modern malnutrition (fuel overload with nutrient deficiency) to create the perfect storm for insulin resistance, obesity, metabolic syndrome and hypertension. ❹ <u>Insulin resistance and related inflammatory and cardiometabolic consequences can be</u>

produced on a population-wide basis: Making nutrient-poor fuel-rich foods less expensive than health-promoting foods, excising nutrition education and physical education (formerly "P.E." from when I was a grade-school student) from public and private schools, allowing xenobiotics to be distributed among the population at levels severe enough to cause endocrinologic (e.g., metabolic and reproductive) impairment, limiting opportunities and incentives for public recreation and exercise (e.g., making car-ownership mandatory in many communities while blocking access to parks, bikeways, etc) is a perfect way to make an entire population obese and diabetic—witness the trends in the United States (images below). ❺ Obesity and related inflammatory and cardiometabolic consequences are expensive (to the benefit of pharmaceutical-medical interests) and are unequally distributed among social/racial/economic groups: According to the US CDC[264] in 2014, "More than one-third of U.S. adults (34.9%) are obese and obesity-related conditions include heart disease, stroke, type 2 diabetes and certain types of cancer, some of the leading causes of preventable death. The estimated annual medical cost of obesity in the U.S. was $147 billion in 2008 U.S. dollars; the medical costs for people who are obese were $1,429 higher than those of normal weight. Obesity affects some groups more than others: Non-Hispanic blacks have the highest age-adjusted rates of obesity (47.8%) followed by Hispanics (42.5%), non-Hispanic whites (32.6%), and non-Hispanic Asians." ❻ Obesity trends (in America) follow very clear changes in governmental, social and economic policy—when people are insecure/scared about their personal finances and the stability of their society, they eat more: In a brilliant Op-Ed article titled "The Political Roots of American Obesity", Kihn describes what he calls "the American syndrome" as having started most clearly with changes in America's political climate in 1980; before this time, obesity trends had been both low and consistent for decades. Starting in 1980, economic insecurity started to skyrocket in the United States, and the obesity epidemic was initiated on a population-wide level.

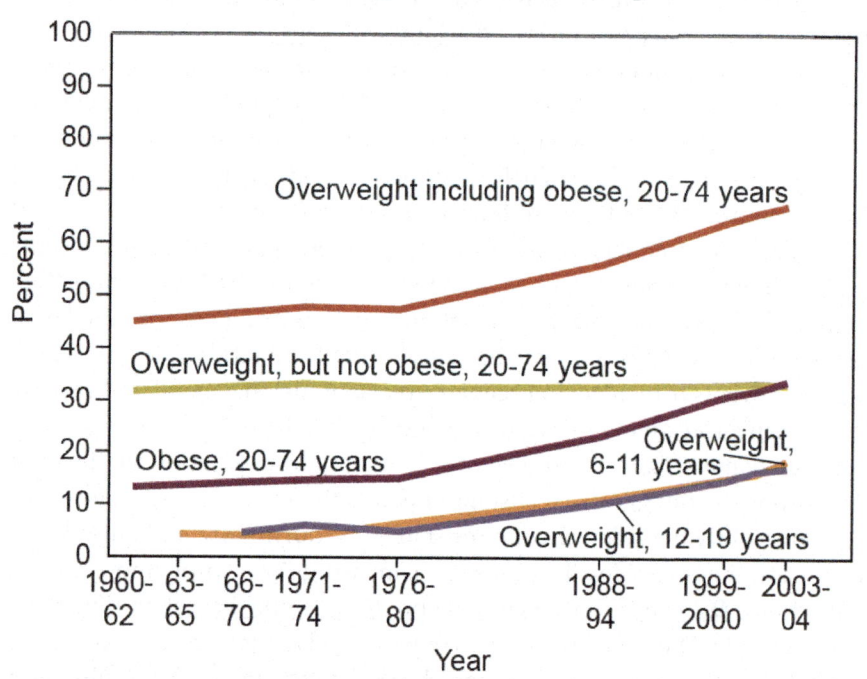

Overweight and obesity

SOURCES: Centers for Disease Control and Prevention, National Center for Health Statistics, *Health, United States, 2006*, Figure 13. Data from the National Health and Nutrition Examination Survey.

> **Who benefits from the obesity epidemic?**
> **What forces contribute to its perpetuation?**
>
> "The obesity epidemic helps American capitalism in two ways. On one side of the coin, **it creates a population that is more compliant, tired, sick,** self-hating and resigned to its misery. The last thing those sitting at the top want to see is a lean, clean and mean population. On the other side of the coin, **obese and overweight Americans bring in enormous profits for many vital industries** - agribusiness, food processing and transportation, food stores, restaurants, the medical industry, the diet industry and the pharmaceutical industry."
>
> Kihn. Political Roots of American Obesity. *Truthout* 2013

Obesity trends in the United States: Rapid obesification of Americans cannot be attributed to genetic causes; however it follows economic and political trends. "Obesity is the toxic consequence of economic insecurity and a failing economic environment." Image from cdc.gov/nchs/data/hus/hus06.pdf; quote from Drewnowski, *Nutr Rev* 2009.

---

[264] cdc.gov/obesity/data/adult.html 2014 Jul

According to Kihn, starting in 1980, new government policies acted quickly to dismantle unionized worker protections *and thus quality of work life—where people spend much or most of their adult lives, job security, worker safety, and quality pay with living wages*; the most obvious single event (which had a ripple effect throughout the country and clearly indicated the change in America's social contract) was the President-authorized firing of more than 11,000 unionized air traffic controllers which was followed by nation-wide "union busting", the marked declines in job/income security, and the now famous processes of "out-sourcing" jobs to temporary and part-time workers and "off-shoring" jobs to low-paying countries with no worker protections and no sustainable environmental policies. Kihn argues very cogently that while obesity may result from overeating fats and sugars, ==the drive to overeat has an emotional basis== in survival and resource insecurity; this trend of society-wide insecurity and anxiety has its origins in national policies that make people fearful for their survival—namely, job and income insecurity.

- "American Syndrome" and "The Political Roots of American Obesity" (*Truthout* 2013 May[265]): "When we [look at the trends and causes of obesity], we will discover that ==the obesity epidemic in America is essentially a mental health problem==, whose underlying causes are economic and political. ... As more and more Americans have seen their standard of living sink and their stress factors increase, they have taken to the all-purpose, all-American sedative—food—in a big way."

- Obesity, diets, and social inequalities (*Nutr Rev* 2009 May[266]): "Obesity and type-2 diabetes follow a socioeconomic gradient. Highest rates are observed among groups with the lowest levels of education and income and in the most deprived areas. ... This article discusses obesity as an economic phenomenon. ==Obesity is the toxic consequence of economic insecurity and a failing economic environment==."

- Poverty is obesogenic (*Nutr Hosp* 2013 Sep[267]): "Many studies have shown an overall socio-economic gradient in obesity in modern industrialized societies. Rates tend to decrease progressively with increasing socio-economic status."

- Economic security and "scientifically educated individualism" are protective against obesity (*BMJ Open* 2014 May[268]): "This might suggest that economically secure, scientifically educated individualism may therefore be protective against obesity."

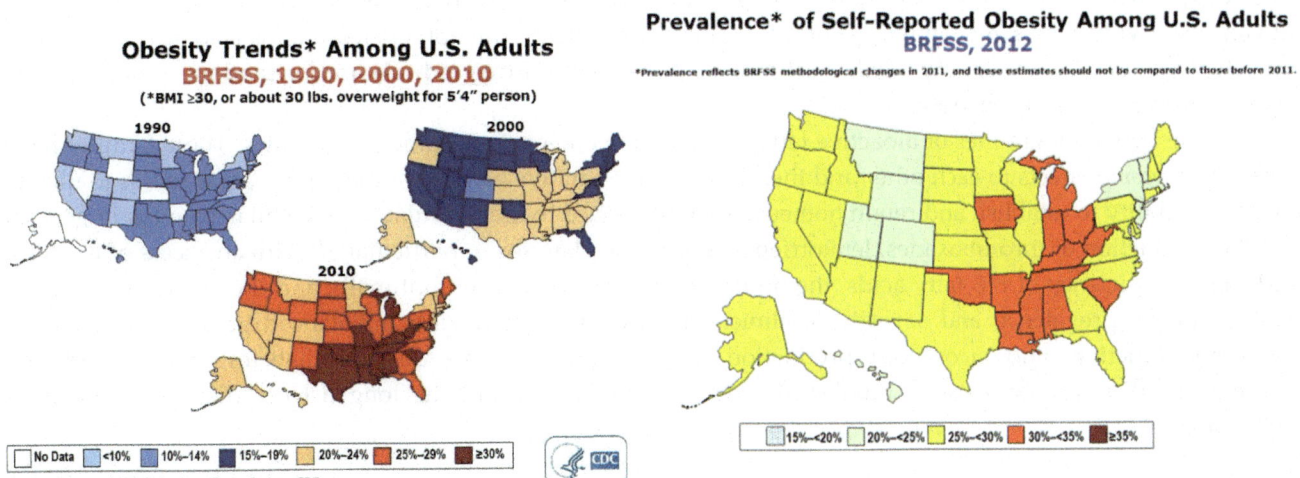

Obesity trends in the United States: The rapid obesification of the American population cannot be attributed to genetic causes; however it follows racial, economic, and political trends. Images from cdc.gov/obesity/data/adult.html 2014 Jul.

---

[265] Kihn ED. The Political Roots of American Obesity. *Truthout* 2013 May truth-out.org/opinion/item/16149-the-political-roots-of-american-obesity
[266] Drewnowski A. Obesity, diets, and social inequalities. *Nutr Rev*. 2009 May;67 Suppl 1:S36-9
[267] Pérez Rodrigo C. Current mapping of obesity. *Nutr Hosp*. 2013 Sep;28 Suppl 5:21-31
[268] Ulijaszek SJ. Do adult obesity rates in England vary by insecurity as well as by inequality? *BMJ Open*. 2014 May 13;4(5):e004430

Mini-Monograph: The Major Fatty Acids and End-products of Clinical Significance

The fatty acids of major importance and the ones discussed here are all polyunsaturated fatty acids, meaning that they have *several* carbon-to-carbon double bonds (i.e., C=C), which are vulnerable to oxidation, rancidification, and/or hydrogenation. Therefore, these fatty acids must be protected from oxygen, heat, light, and prolonged storage. Once structurally altered by oxygen, heat, or light, these fatty acids lose some or all of their biologic value, and they take on disease-promoting properties by interfering with fatty acid metabolism, altering cell membrane dynamics, and/or by having direct/indirect inflammatory and carcinogenic actions.

Fatty acids serve three primary biologic functions: 1) as cell membrane components that modulate membrane pliability and receptor sensitivity, 2) as precursors to potent biologic regulators such as prostaglandins and leukotrienes, and 3) as modulators of gene expression. Each fatty acid must be either provided by diet or manufactured from enzymatic conversion of its predecessor in order to carry out its physiologic role. Deficiency of any fatty acid results in impairment of physiologic function. These impairments begin subtly and often go unrecognized by clinicians who may then erroneously employ pharmacologic and surgical interventions to alleviate *diseases* that originate from *deficiencies* of fatty acids and other nutrients.

Polyunsaturated fatty acids (PUFA) are categorized based on the location of the first carbon-to-carbon double bond from the methyl group, which is located at the opposite end from the carboxyl carbon.[269] The major categories from a biological and nutritional standpoint are the omega-3 fatty acids (having the first carbon-to-carbon double bond starting at the third carbon from the methyl group) and the omega-6 fatty acids (having the first carbon-to-carbon double bond starting at the sixth carbon from the methyl group). The most commonly known member of the omega-9 group is oleic acid from olive oil; but it is of lesser biologic importance than the omega-3 and omega-6 fatty acids, which are the key determinants of the biologically powerful thromboxanes, leukotrienes, prostaglandins, and isoprostanes. The term "omega" is commonly represented as either "Ω" or "w" or "ω" or "n". For the sake of consistency and readability, I will use either the word "omega" or the symbol "n" in this text.

The general term "eicosanoids" is used to describe the various metabolic end products of 20-carbon fatty acid metabolism, including thromboxanes (TX), leukotrienes (LT), and prostaglandins (PG). Produced in minute quantities of approximately 1 milligram per day[270], prostaglandins are produced by nearly all mammalian cells; their production is not confined to leukocytes even though they are often associated with immune activation. Since they are produced and act locally at the site of metabolic activation, they are autocrine and paracrine rather than endocrine.[271] These chemicals have short half-lives, with thromboxanes existing only for a few seconds after production[272] while leukotrienes persist for as long as four hours.[273] While specific enzymes transform one fatty acid into another (within the same family, n-3 or n-6, respectively), the production of eicosanoids is *initiated by enzymes* but often *completed by non-specific, random interactions* dependent on free radicals and/or random conformational changes in enzymes and substrates.[274]

The two main families of bioactive fatty acids are the omega-3 and omega-6 families. These families have generally *opposing* effects to each other and therefore the quantitative balance of these fatty acids serves to dictate the body's ability to establish and retain homeostasis with regard to the modulation of cellular function in general and the production of thromboxanes, leukotrienes, and prostaglandins in particular.[275] With an excess of n-6 fatty acids and a deficiency of n-3 fatty acids, the human body fails to function optimally and the clinical result is an increase in the prevalence and severity of clinical diseases associated with imbalanced gene expression, cell membrane function, and eicosanoid production—namely cancer, heart disease, diabetes, arthritis, allergy, autoimmune diseases, depression, bipolar disorder, schizophrenia, and the long list of "diseases of Western civilization."[276]

[269] Erasmus U. *Fats that heal, fats that kill*. British Columbia Canada: Alive Books, 1993 Page 15-16
[270] Delvin TM. *Textbook of Biochemistry with Clinical Correlations*. New York: Wiley-Liss, 1997. Pages 431-441
[271] McGlivery RW. *Biochemistry: A Functional Approach. Third Edition*. Philadelphia: WB Saunders, 1983. Pages 747-750
[272] McGlivery RW. *Biochemistry: A Functional Approach. Third Edition*. Philadelphia: WB Saunders, 1983. Pages 747-750
[273] Delvin TM. *Textbook of Biochemistry with Clinical Correlations*. New York: Wiley-Liss, 1997. Pages 431-441
[274] Thuresson ED, Lakkides KM, Smith WL. Different catalytically competent arrangements of arachidonic acid within the cyclooxygenase active site of prostaglandin endoperoxide H synthase-1 lead to the formation of different oxygenated products. *J Biol Chem*. 2000 Mar 24;275(12):8501-7 jbc.org/cgi/reprint/275/12/8501
[275] Tapiero et al. Polyunsaturated fatty acids (PUFA) and eicosanoids in human health and pathologies. *Biomed Pharmacother*. 2002;56(5):215-22
[276] Price WA. *Nutrition and Physical Degeneration*. Santa Monica: Price-Pottinger Nutrition Foundation, 1945

Omega-3 fatty acids:

- **General properties**
  - The first double bond is at third carbon from the methyl group
  - **Primarily from flax seed and cold-water aquatic animals ("antifreeze" for deep water fish, seal, whale) and game animals, also from some leafy green vegetables in small amounts**.
  - Maintain cell membrane fluidity and tissue flexibility and elasticity due to markedly curved structure (maintains space between molecules) compared to saturated fatty acids (straight molecules are closely packed with less room for motion)
  - N-3 fatty acids consistently lower serum triglycerides levels in contrast to n-6 fatty acids, which generally cause serum triglycerides to increase.[277]
  - **Causes of n-3 deficiency include:**
    1. Low-fat diets (in general)
    2. Decreased intake of omega-3 (specifically)
    3. Increased intake of omega-6 (such as "to lower cholesterol")
    4. Intake of unnatural *trans*-fatty acids versus natural *cis*-fatty acids. *Trans*-fatty acids are found in hydrogenated oils (hydrogenation makes oil thicker, prevents oxidation, and "improves" taste), fried foods. *Trans*-PUFA increase LDL and reduce HDL.[278]
    5. Alteration of feed for farm animals (substitution of grasses, plants, insects with grains, which are high in n-6 FA), this is why wild game animals have more n-3
    6. High-fat diets if fats are imbalanced with excess of n-6 and trans-FA's
    7. Maldigestion and/or malabsorption
    8. Primary or secondary defects in enzyme function for the conversion of dietary precursors to the end-stage biologically-active fatty acids
  - **Clinical manifestations of deficiency of omega-3 fats are far more subtle than those associated with omega-6 deficiency: (in animal studies) reduced learning, impaired vision, polydypsia.** Given the importance of n-3 fatty acids in health and disease and the relative deficiency state which is the norm in America, we could also argue that deficiency of n-3 fatty acids predispose to the chronic degenerative diseases of cancer, diabetes, cardiovascular disease and to the more subtle functional problems of dermatitis and the epidemic of neurocognitive and neuropsychiatric disorders.
  - **Tissue levels are measurably changed within one week of supplementation and are restored to constant levels in 12 weeks of supplementation (per animal studies).** Not all manifestations of deficiency are corrected with supplementation, indicating that fatty acid deficiencies may leave permanent residual effects, particularly if deficiency occurs early in life during the time of rapid growth and development, especially of the brain.
- **Alpha-linolenic acid, linolenic acid, ALA, α-LNA, ALNA, 18:3n3**
  - **Essential fatty acid:** ALA is the parent fatty acid of the omega-3 class; it is the "first in line."
  - Sources include **flax seed oil (57% ALA)** and canola (rape seed) oil (9% ALA), soy oil, breast milk, English/black walnuts, soybeans, pine nuts, green vegetables, and beans.
  - ALA may theoretically be converted to EPA and DHA but this should not be expected to occur sufficiently in all patients at all times due to interindividual variations in enzyme activity and inadequate nutritional/cofactor status. To attain a measurable increase in EPA from ALA supplementation, approximately eleven-times (11x) the amount of ALA must be consumed to achieve a proportional response to that which can be achieved with direct supplementation of

---

[277] Simopoulos AP. Essential fatty acids in health and chronic disease. *Am J Clin Nutr.* 1999 Sep;70(3 Suppl):560S-569S
[278] Tapiero H, et al. Polyunsaturated fatty acids (PUFA) and eicosanoids in human health and pathologies. *Biomed Pharmacother.* 2002;56(5):215-22

EPA.[279] No increase in DHA has been observed in humans after supplementation of ALA; in fact, supplementation with flax seed oil has actually been shown to reduce DHA levels in humans.[280,281]

- o Lipid-lowering effects are not seen with ALA supplementation and are only attained with the use of EPA and DHA; however ALA can reduce blood pressure.[282]
- o ALA has potent anti-inflammatory benefits independent of its conversion to EPA or DHA.[283] The mechanism of action appears to be downregulation of NFkB rather than the direct modulation of eicosanoid biosynthesis. One study using flax oil as a source of ALA to treat rheumatoid arthritis found no clinical or biochemical benefit (i.e., no change in Hgb, CRP, ESR).[284]

- **Stearidonic acid, 18:4n3, octadecatetraenoic acid**
  - o Small amount found in black currant oil
  - o Human studies have found that stearidonic acid increases EPA 2x more efficiently than does ALA but does not increase DHA.[285]
  - o Inhibits 5-lipoxygenase.[286]

- **N-3 Eicosatetraenoic acid, 20:4n3**
  - o 20:4n-3 is eicosatetraenoic acid.[287,288]
  - o The term "eicosatetraenoic acid" applies to both 20:4n6 (arachidonic acid) of the omega-6 fatty acid family[289] and 20:4n3 of the omega-3 fatty acid family.[290,291] Therefore, to avoid the confusion that would result from the use of the term "eicosatetraenoic acid" by itself, "n-6 eicosatetraenoic acid" should be used when referring to 20:4n6 (arachidonic acid) and "n-3 eicosatetraenoic acid" should be used when referring to 20:4n3.

- **Eicosapentaenoic acid, EPA, 20:5n3**
  - o Effectively absent in vegan diets; the major dietary source is fish oil.
  - o EPA can decrease production of DGLA.[292]
  - o EPA doses of at least 4 grams per day are needed to increase bleeding time.[293]
  - o EPA–derived eicosanoids have anti-inflammatory properties, including a reduction in the production of pro-inflammatory eicosanoids such as LT-B4, PAFs, and cytokines such as TNF-alpha and IL-1, and a large reduction in PG-E2 and TX-B2.[294]
  - o Animal studies suggest that vitamin B-6 deficiency can reduce the function of delta-6-desaturase by 64% and lead to a reduction in EPA and DHA.[295]
  - o Children with allergies show altered fatty acid metabolism[296] that is not caused by impaired delta-6-desaturase activity and which results reduced EPA levels.[297]

[279] "Indu and Ghafoorunissa showed that while keeping the amount of dietary LA constant, 3.7 g ALA appears to have biological effects similar to those of 0.3 g long-chain n-3 PUFA with conversion of 11 g ALA to 1 g long-chain n-3 PUFA." Simopoulos AP. Essential fatty acids in health and chronic disease. *Am J Clin Nutr.* 1999 Sep;70(3 Suppl):560S-569S

[280] Saldeen T. *Health Effects of Fish Oil with a Focus on Natural, Stable, Fish Oil.* Buxton Road, New Mills, High Peak: Nutri Ltd. [Date unknown] page 33

[281] "Linear relationships were found between dietary alpha-LA and EPA in plasma fractions and in cellular phospholipids. … There was an inverse relationship between dietary alpha-LA and docosahexaenoic acid concentrations in the phospholipids of plasma, neutrophils, mononuclear cells, and platelets." Mantzioris E, et al. Differences exist in the relationships between dietary linoleic and alpha-linolenic acids and their respective long-chain metabolites. *Am J Clin Nutr.* 1995 Feb;61(2):320-4

[282] Simopoulos AP. Essential fatty acids in health and chronic disease. *Am J Clin Nutr.* 1999 Sep;70(3 Suppl):560S-569S

[283] "CONCLUSIONS: Dietary supplementation with ALA for 3 months decreases significantly CRP, SAA and IL-6 levels in dyslipidaemic patients. This anti-inflammatory effect may provide a possible additional mechanism for the beneficial effect of plant n-3 polyunsaturated fatty acids in primary and secondary prevention of coronary artery disease." Rallidis LS, Paschos G, Liakos GK, Velissaridou AH, Anastasiadis G, Zampelas A. Dietary alpha-linolenic acid decreases C-reactive protein, serum amyloid A and interleukin-6 in dyslipidaemic patients. *Atherosclerosis.* 2003 Apr;167(2):237-42

[284] "Thus, 3-month's supplementation with alpha-LNA did not prove to be beneficial in rheumatoid arthritis." Nordstrom DC, et al. Alpha-linolenic acid in the treatment of rheumatoid arthritis. A double-blind, placebo-controlled and randomized study: flaxseed vs. safflower seed. *Rheumatol Int.* 1995;14(6):231-4

[285] "RESULTS: Dietary SDA increased EPA and docosapentaenoic acid concentrations but not DHA concentrations in erythrocyte and in plasma phospholipids. The relative effectiveness of the tested dietary fatty acids in increasing tissue EPA was 1:0.3:0.07 for EPA:SDA:ALA." James MJ, Ursin VM, Cleland LG. Metabolism of stearidonic acid in human subjects: comparison with the metabolism of other n-3 fatty acids. *Am J Clin Nutr.* 2003 May;77(5):1140-5

[286] Guichardant M, Traitler H, Spielmann D, Sprecher H, Finot PA. Stearidonic acid, an inhibitor of the 5-lipoxygenase pathway. *Lipids.* 1993 Apr;28(4):321-4

[287] Tapiero H, et al. Polyunsaturated fatty acids (PUFA) and eicosanoids in human health and pathologies. *Biomed Pharmacother.* 2002;56(5):215-22

[288] Erasmus U. *Fats that heal, fats that kill.* Alive Books, 1993 Page 276

[289] "5,8,11,14-eicosatetraenoic (20:4(n-6))" Mimouni V, Christiansen EN, Blond JP, Ulmann L, Poisson JP, Bezard J. Elongation and desaturation of arachidonic and eicosapentaenoic acids in rat liver. Effect of clofibrate feeding. *Biochim Biophys Acta.* 1991 Nov 27;1086(3):349-53

[290] Tapiero H, et al. Polyunsaturated fatty acids (PUFA) and eicosanoids in human health and pathologies. *Biomed Pharmacother.* 2002 Jul;56(5):215-22

[291] Erasmus U. *Fats that heal, fats that kill.* British Columbia Canada: Alive Books, 1993 Page 276

[292] Horrobin DF. Interactions between n-3 and n-6 essential fatty acids (EFAs) in the regulation of cardiovascular disorders and inflammation. *Prostaglandins Leukot Essent Fatty Acids.* 1991 Oct;44(2):127-31

[293] "A dose of 1.8 g EPA/d did not result in any prolongation in bleeding time, but 4 g/d increased bleeding time and decreased platelet count with no adverse effects. In human studies, there has never been a case of clinical bleeding…" Simopoulos AP. Essential fatty acids in health and chronic disease. *Am J Clin Nutr.* 1999 Sep;70(3 Suppl):560S-569S

[294] Tapiero H, et al. Polyunsaturated fatty acids (PUFA) and eicosanoids in human health and pathologies. *Biomed Pharmacother.* 2002 Jul;56(5):215-22

[295] Tsuge H, Hotta N, Hayakawa T. Effects of vitamin B-6 on (n-3) polyunsaturated fatty acid metabolism. *J Nutr.* 2000 Feb;130(2S Suppl):333S-334S

[296] Yu G, Bjorksten B. Serum levels of phospholipid fatty acids in mothers and their babies in relation to allergic disease. *Eur J Pediatr.* 1998 Apr;157(4):298-303

[297] Yu G, Bjorksten B. Polyunsaturated fatty acids in school children in relation to allergy and serum IgE levels. *Pediatr Allergy Immunol.* 1998 Aug;9(3):133-8

- N-6 fatty acids facilitate elongation of EPA to n-3 DPA.[298] Thus, anti-inflammatory EPA is depleted by consumption of proinflammatory n-6 fatty acids.
- Evidence suggests that EPA must be incorporated into cell membrane phospholipids for its beneficial effects on eicosanoid metabolism to be realized. Administration of n-6 fatty acids removes EPA from cell membranes and relocates EPA from phospholipids into triacylglycerols. Therefore the benefits of EPA are mitigated by n-6 fatty acids, and thus "...dietary therapies designed to increase the EPA content of tissue phospholipids may need to focus on limiting n-6 fatty acid intake in addition to increasing EPA intake." [299]

- **DPA: n-3 docosapentaenoic acid, 22:5n3**
  - Production is increased slightly with consumption of the n-3 precursor ALA.[300]
  - Production can be increased with consumption of n-6 fatty acids.[301] The clinical implications of this finding are significant, because it implies that concomitant administration of n-6 fatty acids such as ALA and arachidonate with EPA would preferentially shuttle EPA to DPA, and therefore the formation of the beneficial EPA-derived eicosanoids would be reduced.
  - The term "docosapentaenoic acid" can apply to both 22:5n3 of the omega-3 fatty acid family[302,303] and 22:5n6 of the omega-6 fatty acid family.[304,305,306] Because to use the term "docosapentaenoic acid" may be ambiguous, the terms "n-3 docosapentaenoic acid" should be used when discussing 22:5n3 and "n-6 docosapentaenoic acid" should be used when discussing 22:5n6.

- **DHA: docosahexaenoic acid, 22:6n-3**
  - Found only in plants of the sea, phytoplankton/microalgae, and consumers of microalgae (such as fish)
  - Essential for neural function, effectively absent in vegan diets, present in breast milk (low in vegetarians); major n-3 in tissues; component of phosphatidylethanolamine and phosphatidylserine; deficiency is associated with inadequate intake of DHA and/or deficient conversion from ALA or EPA.
  - Animal studies have shown that induction of DHA deficiency causes memory deficits and a reduction in hippocampal cell size.[307]
  - DHA is an important component of cell membranes and generally appears to improve cell membrane function via improving receptor function and signal transduction.
  - DHA levels are reduced by ethanol consumption.[308]
  - Animal studies suggest that vitamin B-6 deficiency can reduce the function of delta-6-desaturase by 64% and lead to a reduction in EPA and DHA.[309]
  - Supplementation with EPA+DHA is generally safe and reduces all-cause mortality.[310]

---

[298] "The major findings of this study were: 1) n-6 fatty acids markedly stimulated the elongation of EPA to 22:5..." Rubin D, Laposata M. Cellular interactions between n-6 and n-3 fatty acids: a mass analysis of fatty acid elongation/desaturation, distribution among complex lipids, and conversion to eicosanoids. *J Lipid Res.* 1992 Oct;33(10):1431-40

[299] Rubin D, Laposata M. Cellular interactions between n-6 and n-3 fatty acids: a mass analysis of fatty acid elongation/desaturation, distribution among complex lipids, and conversion to eicosanoids. *J Lipid Res.* 1992 Oct;33(10):1431-40

[300] Tarpila, et al, Adlercreutz H. The effect of flaxseed supplementation in processed foods on serum fatty acids and enterolactone. *Eur J Clin Nutr.* 2002 Feb;56(2):157-65

[301] Rubin D, Laposata M. Cellular interactions between n-6 and n-3 fatty acids: a mass analysis of fatty acid elongation/desaturation, distribution among complex lipids, and conversion to eicosanoids. *J Lipid Res.* 1992 Oct;33(10):1431-40

[302] "docosapentaenoic acid (22:5n-3)" Williard DE, Harmon SD, Kaduce TL, Preuss M, Moore SA, Robbins ME, Spector AA. Docosahexaenoic acid synthesis from n-3 polyunsaturated fatty acids in differentiated rat brain astrocytes. *J Lipid Res.* 2001 Sep;42(9):1368-76

[303] "...docosapentaenoic acid (22:5n-3)..." Takahashi R, Nassar BA, Huang YS, Begin ME, Horrobin DF. Effect of different ratios of dietary N-6 and N-3 fatty acids on fatty acid composition, prostaglandin formation and platelet aggregation in the rat. *Thromb Res.* 1987 Jul 15;47(2):135-46

[304] Retterstol K, Haugen TB, Christophersen BO. The pathway from arachidonic to docosapentaenoic acid (20:4n-6 to 22:5n-6) and from eicosapentaenoic to docosahexaenoic acid (20:5n-3 to 22:6n-3) studied in testicular cells from immature rats. *Biochim Biophys Acta.* 2000 Jan 3;1483(1):119-31

[305] "docosapentaenoic acid (DPAn-6)" Ahmad A,et al.A decrease in cell size accompanies a loss of docosahexaenoate in the rat hippocampus.*Nutr Neurosci* 2002;5:103-13

[306] "The desaturation of adrenic acid to n-6 docosapentaenoic acid was decreased in the normo- and hyperglycemic diabetic rats." Mimouni V, Narce M, Huang YS, Horrobin DF, Poisson JP. Adrenic acid delta 4 desaturation and fatty acid composition in liver microsomes of spontaneously diabetic Wistar BB rats. *Prostaglandins Leukot Essent Fatty Acids.* 1994 Jan;50(1):43-7

[307] Ahmad A, et al. A decrease in cell size accompanies a loss of docosahexaenoate in the rat hippocampus. *Nutr Neurosci.* 2002 Apr;5(2):103-13

[308] Pawlosky RJ, Bacher J, Salem N Jr. Ethanol consumption alters electroretinograms and depletes neural tissues of docosahexaenoic acid in rhesus monkeys: nutritional consequences of a low n-3 fatty acid diet. *Alcohol Clin Exp Res.* 2001 Dec;25(12):1758-65

[309] Tsuge H, Hotta N, Hayakawa T. Effects of vitamin B-6 on (n-3) polyunsaturated fatty acid metabolism. *J Nutr.* 2000 Feb;130(2S Suppl):333S-334S

[310] "The recent GISSI (Gruppo Italiano per lo Studio della Sopravvivenza nell'Infarto miocardico)-Prevention study of 11,324 patients showed a 45% decrease in risk of sudden cardiac death and a 20% reduction in all-cause mortality in the group taking 850 mg/d of omega-3 fatty acids." O'Keefe JH Jr, Harris WS. From Inuit to implementation: omega-3 fatty acids come of age. *Mayo Clin Proc.* 2000 Jun;75(6):607-14

- In late 2003, bioactive metabolites of DHA were discovered. Previous to the publication of this research, production of bioactive metabolites of DHA via lipoxygenase and cyclooxygenase was unsuspected and/or unproved, and the anti-inflammatory biochemical and clinical effects of DHA were mostly thought to be due to alterations in membrane/receptor function and retroconversion to EPA. We now know that DHA is converted by several mechanisms (lipoxygenase, cyclooxygenase, random reactions, and cell-to-cell interactions) into docosatrienes and resolvins, which are described below.[311]

Bioactive and Clinically Significant End-products of Omega-3 Fatty Acids

End-products from n-3 fatty acids generally have what are considered "health-promoting effects" which are generally weaker than and opposite to the end-products of the major n-6 fatty acid, arachidonate. Additionally, since n-3 fatty acids compete with the same metabolizing enzymes as do the n-6 family of fatty acids, a major portion of the "clinical effectiveness" of n-3 fatty acids comes not from the production of n-3 end-products but rather from the *impairment of the n-6 cascade.*

- **Prostaglandin E-3 (PG-E3)**
  - PG-E3 and EPA both reduce formation of arachidonate-derived eicosanoids[312]
- **Prostaglandin G-3 (PG-G3)**
  - Formed from EPA by cyclooxygenase (COX)
- **Prostaglandin H-3 (PG-H3)**
  - Formed from PG-G3 by peroxidase
- **Prostaglandin I-3 (PG-I3)**
  - Decreases platelet aggregation[313]
  - Promotes vasodilation[314]
  - Possibly antiarrhythmic
  - Probably contributes to the hypotensive effect of fish oil[315]
- **Thromboxane A-3 (TX-A3)**
  - Biologically inert
- **Leukotriene B-5 (LT-B5)**
  - Significantly weaker than LT-B4; "functionally attenuated"[316]
  - May possess mild anti-inflammatory activity either directly or by reducing production of the more powerful arachidonate-derived LT-B4.[317]
- **Plasminogen activator inhibitor-1 (PAI-1)**
  - Increased with fish oil supplementation to maintain hemostasis
- <mark>**Docosatrienes**</mark>
  - Formed by (12-, 15-, 17-) lipoxygenase and cyclooxygenase-2 from DHA
  - Potent inhibitors of TNFa
  - Downregulate gene expression for proinflammatory IL-1
  - Reduce neutrophil entry to sites of inflammation

---

[311] "These results indicate that DHA is the precursor to potent protective mediators generated via enzymatic oxygenations to novel docosatrienes and 17S series resolvins that each regulate events of interest in inflammation and resolution." Hong S, Gronert K, Devchand PR, Moussignac RL, Serhan CN. Novel docosatrienes and 17S-resolvins generated from docosahexaenoic acid in murine brain, human blood, and glial cells. Autacoids in anti-inflammation. *J Biol Chem.* 2003 Apr 25;278(17):14677-87

[312] Erasmus U. *Fats that heal, fats that kill.* British Columbia Canada: Alive Books, 1993 Page 278

[313] Horrobin DF. Ascorbic acid and prostaglandin synthesis. *Subcell Biochem.* 1996;25:109-15

[314] Horrobin DF. Ascorbic acid and prostaglandin synthesis. *Subcell Biochem.* 1996;25:109-15

[315] Du Plooy WJ, Venter CP, Muntingh GM, et al. The cumulative dose response effect of eicosapentaenoic and docosahexaenoic acid on blood pressure, plasma lipid profile and diet pattern in mild to moderate essential hypertensive black patients. *Prostaglandins Leukot Essent Fatty Acids* 1992 Aug;46(4):315-21

[316] Rubin D, Laposata M. Cellular interactions between n-6 and n-3 fatty acids: a mass analysis of fatty acid elongation/desaturation, distribution among complex lipids, and conversion to eicosanoids. *J Lipid Res.* 1992 Oct;33(10):1431-40

[317] Rubin D, Laposata M. Cellular interactions between n-6 and n-3 fatty acids. *J Lipid Res.* 1992 Oct;33(10):1431-40

- **Resolvins**
  - Derived from EPA and DHA via the COX-2 enzyme with production notably increased in the presence of low-dose aspirin
  - Downregulate cytokine expression, reduce neutrophil entry to sites of inflammation, and reduce inflammation-related pain
- **Neuroprotectin**
  - Neuroprotectin D1 (NPD1) is derived from DHA and exerts potent anti-inflammatory and anti-apoptotic/neuroprotective bioactivity
  - Other forms include Neuroprotectins A and B
- **Maresins**
  - Discovered in 2009 and generated by the 14-lipoxygenase pathway[318]
  - The term *maresins* is coined from **Ma**crophage-derived **res**olution of **in**flammation
  - Potent anti-inflammatory and proresolving properties similar to Resolvin E1
  - Maresin 1, MaR1, proved to be a potent mediator, stopping PMN infiltration and stimulating macrophage phagocytosis of apoptotic cells—*efferocytosis*.[319]
- **GPR-120—a fatty acid receptor mediating some of the anti-inflammatory and insulin-sensitizing benefits of n3 fatty acids**
  - As indicated by the title of the original research supervised by Olefsky[320] in 2010, G protein-coupled receptor 120 (GPR120) is an omega-3 fatty acid receptor mediating potent anti-inflammatory and insulin-sensitizing effects.

Beyond "anti-inflammation" to and understanding of the *active resolution of inflammation*
What began to be appreciated by the discovery of the docosatrienes, resolvins, and maresins is that resolution of inflammation is and can be an active process, not merely the fading of a proinflammatory response. The identification of these mediators as stimulators of active pro-resolution agents gives a new perspective on the resolution of inflammation and injury—that it can be actively stimulated rather than merely passively awaited.

---

[318] Serhan CN et al. Maresins: novel macrophage mediators with potent antiinflammatory and proresolving actions. *J Exp Med*. 2009 Jan 16;206(1):15-23
[319] "In cell biology, efferocytosis (from efferre, Latin for 'to take to the grave', 'to bury') is the process by which dying/dead cells (e.g. apoptotic or necrotic) are removed by phagocytic cells. It can be regarded as the 'burying of dead cells'. en.wikipedia.org/wiki/Efferocytosis 2014 May
[320] Oh DY, Talukdar S, Bae EJ, Imamura T, Morinaga H, Fan W, Li P, Lu WJ, Watkins SM, Olefsky JM. GPR120 is an omega-3 fatty acid receptor mediating potent anti-inflammatory and insulin-sensitizing effects. *Cell*. 2010 Sep 3;142(5):687-98

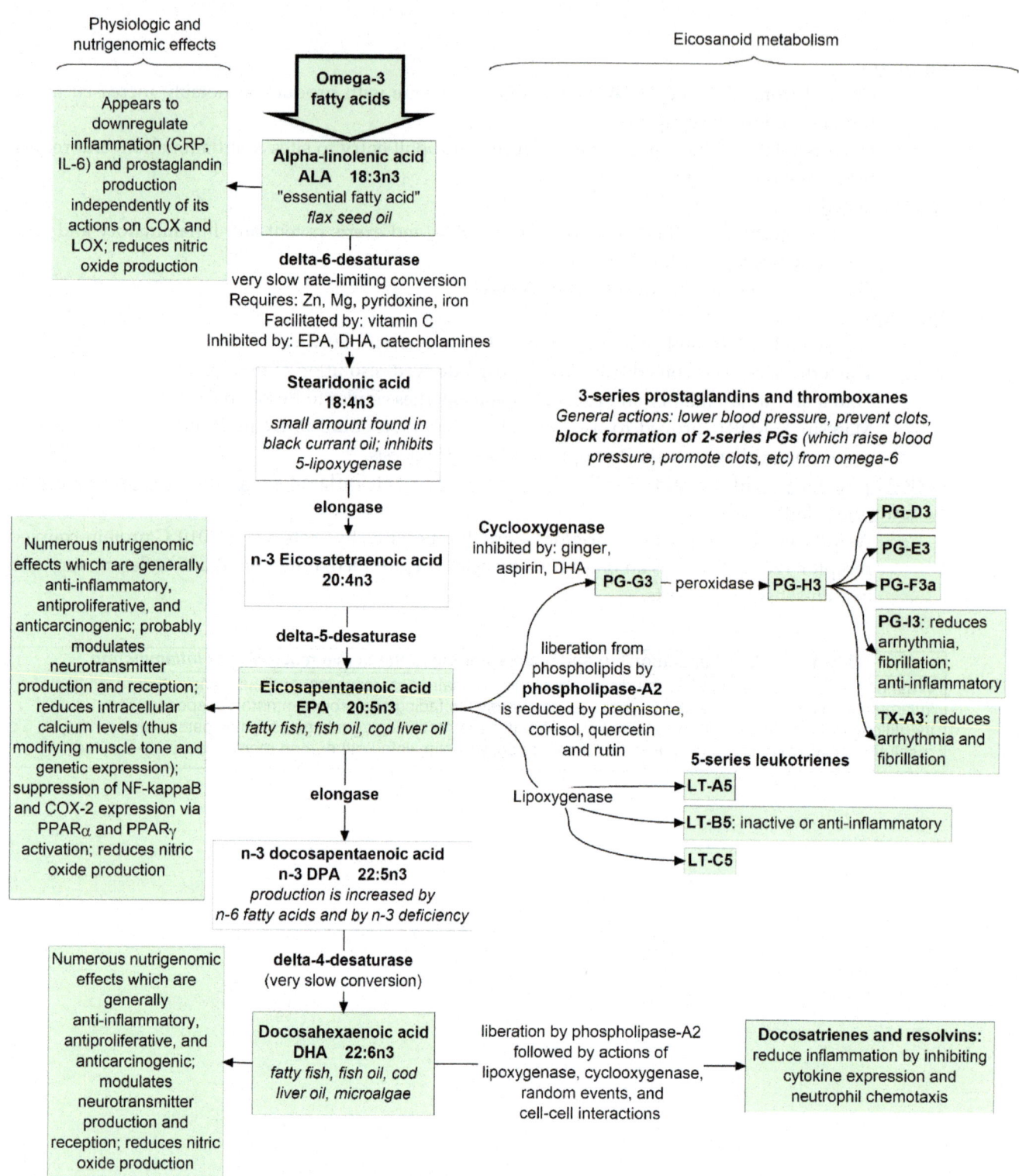

Metabolism of Omega-3 Fatty Acids and Related Eicosanoids: Health-promoting (i.e., either beneficial or neutral/blocking) fatty acids and metabolites are emphasized in the above diagram by the color green; obviously, n3 fatty acids are predominantly positive in their metabolic effects and associated health outcomes.

OMEGA-6—first double bond at 6th carbon from the methyl group

- **Linoleic acid, LA, 18:2n6, linoleate**
    - Essential fatty acid from nut, seed, and vegetable oils, especially safflower oil, sunflower oil, corn oil, walnut oil, sesame seed oil, LA is the parent fatty acid of the omega-6 class,
    - EPA and DHA decrease conversion of linoleate to arachidonate; high doses of LA inhibit conversion of alpha-LNA to EPA and DHA due to competition for delta-6 desaturase
    - Hydrogenated "trans" forms are common in processed and fried foods,
    - LA favors oxidative modification of LDL cholesterol, increases platelet response to aggregation, and suppresses the immune system.[321] Adipose LA levels are positively correlated with CVD.
    - Promotes metastasis and inflammation.
    - LA is the predominant PUFA in US diets. Daily intake of linoleic acid is approximately 10 grams, only a small amount of which is converted to arachidonate.[322]
    - LA effectively lowers cholesterol, but otherwise this fatty acid is consistently associated with exacerbation of cancer and inflammation and thus should be avoided.
    - LA undergoes oxidative metabolism by 15-lipoxygenase-1 to form 13-S-HODE[323], and this is discussed in greater detail later in this section
- **gamma (γ)-linolenic acid, GLA, 18:3n6, gamma-linolenate**
    - Formation is increased from linoleic acid by vitamin C[324]
    - Found in evening primrose oil, borage seed oil, hemp seed oil, and black currant seed oil
    - GLA restores action of delta-6-desaturase (D6D) in aging animals, suggesting that GLA intake should increase in older rats and humans
    - Useful in eczema for improvement in skin health and in diabetes especially for improvement in nerve function
    - GLA may facilitate the conversion of ALA to EPA and perhaps to DHA.
    - In patients who respond to GLA supplementation, we can reasonably hypothesize that they have impaired D-6-desaturase activity since most patients have adequate dietary intake of LA. Therefore, by extension, we can suppose that their conversion of ALA to EPA is likewise impaired and that they may benefit from EPA supplementation.
    - Formation of GLA from LA is inhibited by EPA and other n-3 EFAs[325]
    - Two publications have now documented induction/exacerbation of temporal lobe epilepsy with GLA[326,327] therefore warranting some caution
    - Overall, the weight of the research suggests that supplementation with GLA *does* lead to modest increases in arachidonate, despite the slow conversion of DGLA to arachidonate by delta-5 desaturase. Coadministration of EPA with GLA prevents any rise in arachidonate, as discussed later in this section.
- **Dihomo-gamma-linolenic acid, 20:3n6, DGLA, eicosatrienoic acid, eicosatrienoate**
    - DGLA eicosanoids have benefits for the cardiovascular system and have anti-inflammatory effects
    - Generally speaking, metabolites of DGLA are fewer in number and weaker in physiologic effect than the metabolites of arachidonic acid.
    - Vitamin C "has a significant effect in stimulating the conversion of DGLA into its metabolites…" at doses which are "…clinically relevant."[328]
    - DGLA levels are 34% lower than normal in patients with magnesium deficiency.[329]

---

[321] Simopoulos AP. Essential fatty acids in health and chronic disease. *Am J Clin Nutr.* 1999 Sep;70(3 Suppl):560S-569S

[322] Delvin TM. *Textbook of Biochemistry with Clinical Correlations*. New York: Wiley-Liss, 1997. Pages 431-441

[323] Shureiqi I, Lippman SM. Lipoxygenase modulation to reverse carcinogenesis. *Cancer Res.* 2001 Sep 1;61(17):6307-12

[324] Horrobin DF. Ascorbic acid and prostaglandin synthesis. *Subcell Biochem* 1996;25:109-15

[325] Horrobin DF. Interactions between n-3 and n-6 essential fatty acids (EFAs) in the regulation of cardiovascular disorders and inflammation. *Prostaglandins Leukot Essent Fatty Acids* 1991 Oct;44(2):127-31

[326] Vaddadi KS. The use of gamma-linolenic acid and linoleic acid to differentiate between temporal lobe epilepsy and schizophrenia. *Prostaglandins Med.* 1981 Apr;6(4):375-9

[327] Al-Khamees et al. Status epilepticus associated with borage oil ingestion. *J Med Toxicol.* 2011 Jun;7(2):154-7

[328] Horrobin DF. Ascorbic acid and prostaglandin synthesis. *Subcell Biochem.* 1996;25:109-15

[329] "…dihomogamma linoleic acid (20:3 n-6) was 34% lower…" Galland L. Impaired essential fatty acid metabolism in latent tetany. *Magnesium* 1985;4(5-6):333-8

- Production is decreased with supplementation of ALA[330] and EPA and other n-3 EFAs except when GLA is provided directly[331]
- Low levels of DGLA are associated with increased risk for stroke and myocardial infarction.[332] We could speculate that low levels of DGLA may be associated with pyridoxine or magnesium deficiency, of which are associated with cardiovascular disease.
- DGLA metabolites reduce the formation of the arachidonate-derived 2-series prostaglandins, 4-series leukotrienes and platelet-activating factor.[333]

- **Arachidonic acid, 20:4n6, n-6 eicosatetraenoic acid, AA, ARA**
  - Arachidonic acid is the predominant fatty acid in most tissues (diet-dependent!) acted upon by cyclooxygenase (to form prostaglandins and thromboxanes) and lipoxygenase (to form leukotrienes); it is the major n-6 in cell membranes and body tissues
  - Liberated from phospholipids by phospholipase enzymes, most notably phospholipase A2.
  - Most end-products of arachidonate metabolism are pro-inflammatory and are "in general harmful"[334] although arachidonate itself is a necessary component of phospholipids and sphingolipids in cell membranes.
  - Arachidonate and its metabolites are referred to as eicosanoids.[335] Arachidonic acid is the predominant fatty acid in membrane phospholipids and is the preferred substrate for eicosanoid production relative to EPA.[336] Given that arachidonate's eicosanoids are biologically more powerful than those of EPA, we can accurately generalize that arachidonate and its respective prostaglandins and leukotrienes dominate the fatty acid and eicosanoid playground in both *quantitative* and *qualitative* respects. Therefore, successful intervention against arachidonate metabolism must consider 1) the quantity of arachidonate, 2) the balance of n-3 to n-6, and also 3) specific measures to hinder the production of the harmful arachidonate metabolites.
  - Arachidonic acid is the direct precursor to the isoprostanes 8-iso prostaglandin-E2 (8-iso-PG-E2) and 8-iso prostaglandin-F2-alpha (8-iso-PG-F2-alpha), mediators that possess **inflammatory and hyperalgesic** properties and which are produced by the radical-mediated non-enzymatic peroxidation of arachidonate.[337] Inhibition of cyclooxygenase and/or lipoxygenase does not decrease the inflammatory and pain-producing effects of isoprostanes. Production of 8-iso-PG-F2-alpha is increased by and is a marker of oxidative stress. Obviously, inhibition of isoprostane formation is part of the biochemical and therefore clinical justification for antioxidant therapy in the treatment of painful orthopedic and rheumatic disorders. Supplemental ascorbic acid, tocopherols, and EPA have been shown to lower isoprostane levels in humans.
  - Formation of arachidonate from DGLA is inhibited by EPA.[338]
  - Formation of arachidonic metabolites is not increased by vitamin C.[339]
  - The term "eicosatetraenoic acid" can apply to both 20:4n6 (arachidonic acid) of the omega-6 fatty acid family[340] and to 20:4n3 of the omega-3 fatty acid family.[341,342] Therefore, to avoid the confusion that would result from the use of the term "eicosatetraenoic acid" by itself, "n-6 eicosatetraenoic acid" should be used when referring to 20:4n6 (arachidonic acid) and "n-3 eicosatetraenoic acid" should be used when referring to 20:4n3.

---

[330] Simopoulos AP. Essential fatty acids in health and chronic disease. *Am J Clin Nutr*. 1999 Sep;70(3 Suppl):560S-569S

[331] Horrobin DF. Interactions between n-3 and n-6 essential fatty acids (EFAs) in the regulation of cardiovascular disorders and inflammation. *Prostaglandins Leukot Essent Fatty Acids*. 1991 Oct;44(2):127-31

[332] Horrobin DF. Interactions between n-3 and n-6 essential fatty acids (EFAs) in the regulation of cardiovascular disorders and inflammation. *Prostaglandins Leukot Essent Fatty Acids* 1991 Oct;44(2):127-31

[333] Fan YY, Chapkin RS. Importance of dietary gamma-linolenic acid in human health and nutrition. *J Nutr*. 1998 Sep;128(9):1411-4

[334] Horrobin DF. Ascorbic acid and prostaglandin synthesis. *Subcell Biochem*. 1996;25:109-15

[335] Delvin TM. *Textbook of Biochemistry with Clinical Correlations*. New York: Wiley-Liss, 1997. Pages 431-441

[336] Rubin D, Laposata M. Cellular interactions between n-6 and n-3 fatty acids. *J Lipid Res*. 1992 Oct;33(10):1431-40

[337] Evans AR, et al. Isoprostanes, novel eicosanoids that produce nociception and sensitize rat sensory neurons. *J Pharmacol Exp Ther*. 2000 Jun;293(3):912-20

[338] Horrobin DF. Interactions between n-3 and n-6 essential fatty acids (EFAs) in the regulation of cardiovascular disorders and inflammation. *Prostaglandins Leukot Essent Fatty Acids* 1991 Oct;44(2):127-31

[339] Horrobin DF. Ascorbic acid and prostaglandin synthesis. *Subcell Biochem*. 1996;25:109-15

[340] "5,8,11,14-eicosatetraenoic (20:4(n-6))" Mimouni V, Christiansen EN, Blond JP, Ulmann L, Poisson JP, Bezard J. Elongation and desaturation of arachidonic and eicosapentaenoic acids in rat liver. Effect of clofibrate feeding. *Biochim Biophys Acta*. 1991 Nov 27;1086(3):349-53

[341] Tapiero H, et al. Polyunsaturated fatty acids (PUFA) and eicosanoids in human health and pathologies. *Biomed Pharmacother*. 2002 Jul;56(5):215-22

[342] Erasmus U. *Fats that heal, fats that kill*. British Columbia Canada: Alive Books, 1993 Page 276

- o Liberation of arachidonic acid from membrane phospholipids phosphatidylcholine and phosphatidylinositol is increased by contact with IgE.[343] This finding presumably helps explain why inflammatory conditions are generally exacerbated by allergen exposure and why allergy elimination and anti-allergy immunomodulatory treatments result in a reduction in pain and inflammation.
- o Elevated ARA may lead to altered binding of hormones, growth factors, neurotransmitters, and common food antigen peptides.
- o Dietary ARA works synergistically with proinflammatory genotypes such as the variant 5-lipoxygenase alleles which are common in the general population: Africans (24%), Asians and Pacific Islanders (19.4%), other racial/ethnic groups (18.2%), Hispanics (3.6%), whites (3.1%), and the atherogenic effect of dietary arachidonic acid in these patients can be mitigated by dietary EPA.[344]

- **Adrenic acid, 22:4n6, docosatetraenoic acid**
  - o Little is known about this fatty acid.
  - o Concentrated in and may have a regulatory role in the adrenal glands.[345]
- **N-6 docosapentaenoic acid, 22:5n6**
  - o 22:5n6 is increased by n-3 fatty acid deficiency, especially in the brain cortex.[346]
  - o The term "docosapentaenoic acid" can apply to both 22:5n3 of the omega-3 fatty acid family[347,348] and to 22:5n6 of the omega-6 fatty acid family.[349,350,351] Therefore, because to use the term "docosapentaenoic acid" may be ambiguous, the terms "n-3 docosapentaenoic acid" should be used when discussing 22:5n3 and "n-6 docosapentaenoic acid" should be used when discussing 22:5n6.

DGLA metabolites formed by cyclooxygenase

- **Prostaglandin E-1 (PG-E1)**
  - o The main metabolite from DGLA.[352]
  - o Production is increased by vitamin C.[353]
  - o Decreases platelet aggregation.[354]
  - o Causes vasodilation.[355]
  - o Lowers blood pressure.[356]
  - o Inhibits cholesterol biosynthesis and lowers cholesterol levels in animals.[357]
  - o "A potent anti-inflammatory agent." [358]
  - o Probably the most potent PG with respect to bronchodilation.[359]

---

[343] McGlivery RW. *Biochemistry: A Functional Approach. Third Edition*. Philadelphia: WB Saunders, 1983. Pages 747-750

[344] Dwyer JH, et al. Arachidonate 5-lipoxygenase promoter genotype, dietary arachidonic acid, and atherosclerosis. *N Engl J Med*. 2004 Jan 1;350(1):29-37

[345] Horrobin DF. Ascorbic acid and prostaglandin synthesis. *Subcell Biochem*. 1996;25:109-15

[346] Retterstol K, et al. The metabolism of 22:5(-6) and of docosahexaenoic acid [22:6(-3)] compared in rat hepatocytes. *Biochim Biophys Acta*. 1996 Oct 18;1303(3):180-6

[347] "docosapentaenoic acid (22:5n-3)" Williard DE, et al. Docosahexaenoic acid synthesis from n-3 polyunsaturated fatty acids in differentiated rat brain astrocytes. *J Lipid Res*. 2001 Sep;42(9):1368-76

[348] "...docosapentaenoic acid (22:5n-3)..." Takahashi R, et al. Effect of different ratios of dietary N-6 and N-3 fatty acids on fatty acid composition, prostaglandin formation and platelet aggregation in the rat. *Thromb Res*. 1987 Jul 15;47(2):135-46

[349] Retterstol K, Haugen TB, Christophersen BO. The pathway from arachidonic to docosapentaenoic acid (20:4n-6 to 22:5n-6) and from eicosapentaenoic to docosahexaenoic acid (20:5n-3 to 22:6n-3) studied in testicular cells from immature rats. *Biochim Biophys Acta*. 2000 Jan 3;1483(1):119-31

[350] "docosapentaenoic acid (DPAn-6)" Ahmad A, Murthy M, Greiner RS, Moriguchi T, Salem N Jr. A decrease in cell size accompanies a loss of docosahexaenoate in the rat hippocampus. *Nutr Neurosci*. 2002 Apr;5(2):103-13

[351] "The desaturation of adrenic acid to n-6 docosapentaenoic acid was decreased in the normo- and hyperglycemic diabetic rats." Mimouni V, et al. Adrenic acid delta 4 desaturation and fatty acid composition in liver microsomes of spontaneously diabetic Wistar BB rats. *Prostaglandins Leukot Essent Fatty Acids*. 1994 Jan;50(1):43-7

[352] Horrobin DF. Ascorbic acid and prostaglandin synthesis. *Subcell Biochem* 1996;25:109-15

[353] Horrobin DF. Ascorbic acid and prostaglandin synthesis. *Subcell Biochem*. 1996;25:109-15

[354] Horrobin DF. Interactions between n-3 and n-6 essential fatty acids (EFAs) in the regulation of cardiovascular disorders and inflammation. *Prostaglandins Leukot Essent Fatty Acids* 1991 Oct;44(2):127-31

[355] Tapiero H, et al. Polyunsaturated fatty acids (PUFA) and eicosanoids in human health and pathologies. *Biomed Pharmacother*. 2002 Jul;56(5):215-22

[356] Horrobin DF. Interactions between n-3 and n-6 essential fatty acids (EFAs) in the regulation of cardiovascular disorders and inflammation. *Prostaglandins Leukot Essent Fatty Acids* 1991 Oct;44(2):127-31

[357] Horrobin DF. Interactions between n-3 and n-6 essential fatty acids (EFAs) in the regulation of cardiovascular disorders and inflammation. *Prostaglandins Leukot Essent Fatty Acids* 1991 Oct;44(2):127-31

[358] Horrobin DF. Ascorbic acid and prostaglandin synthesis. *Subcell Biochem*. 1996;25:109-15

[359] Horrobin DF. Ascorbic acid and prostaglandin synthesis. *Subcell Biochem*. 1996;25:109-15

- o Production is decreased by n-3 fatty acids.[360]
- o May have a mood elevating effect insofar as levels are elevated in patients with mania, reduced in patients with depression, and are elevated by ethanol intake.[361]
- o Certain biological properties of PG-E1 are 20 times stronger than those of PG-E2.[362]
- o PG-E1 inhibits vascular smooth muscle cell proliferation in vitro.[363]

DGLA metabolites formed by 15-lipoxygenase
- **15-hydroxy-eicosatrienoic acid, 15-OH-DGLA, 15-OH-20:3n-6, 15-HETrE**
    - o Potent anti-inflammatory action and inhibition of arachidonic acid cascade via inhibition of 5-lipoxygenase and 12-lipoxygenase.[364,365]

Arachidonic acid metabolites formed by cyclooxygenase
- **Thromboxane A-2 (TX-A2)**
    - o Causes platelet aggregation[366] and vasoconstriction.[367]
    - o Promotes cardiac arrhythmias and hypertension.
    - o Considered much more powerful than the thromboxanes derived from EPA and DGLA.
    - o Precursor to TX-B2.
- **Thromboxane B2**
    - o Inactive[368]
- **Prostaglandin I2,PG-I2, prostacyclin**
    - o Commonly considered one of the only desirable/beneficial end-products of arachidonic acid metabolism[369] despite the little known fact that increases nociception and thus promotes hyperalgesia.[370]
    - o Production is increased by vitamin C.[371]
    - o Decreases platelet aggregation.
    - o Causes vasodilation[372] and lowers blood pressure.[373,374]
    - o Formed from PG-H2 via prostacyclin synthase.[375]
- **Prostaglandin D2, PG-D2**
    - o Causes bronchoconstriction, smooth muscle contraction, and hypotension and is the major arachidonate-cyclooxygenase product produced in mast cells.[376]
    - o Accentuates production of histamine and can trigger release of histamine from mast cells in the absence of IgE binding.
- **Prostaglandin E2, PG-E2**
    - o Produced from arachidonic acid by cyclooxygenase. PG-E2 increases expression of cyclooxygenase and IL-6; thus inflammation manifested by an increase in PG-E2 leads to additive expression of cyclooxygenase, which further increases inflammation.[377]

---

[360] Rubin D, Laposata M. Cellular interactions between n-6 and n-3 fatty acids: a mass analysis of fatty acid elongation/desaturation, distribution among complex lipids, and conversion to eicosanoids. *J Lipid Res*. 1992 Oct;33(10):1431-40

[361] Horrobin DF, Manku MS. Possible role of prostaglandin E1 in the affective disorders and in alcoholism. *Br Med J*. 1980 Jun 7;280(6228):1363-6

[362] Fan YY, Chapkin RS. Importance of dietary gamma-linolenic acid in human health and nutrition. *J Nutr*. 1998 Sep;128(9):1411-4

[363] Fan YY, Chapkin RS. Importance of dietary gamma-linolenic acid in human health and nutrition. *J Nutr*. 1998 Sep;128(9):1411-4

[364] Horrobin DF. Interactions between n-3 and n-6 essential fatty acids (EFAs) in the regulation of cardiovascular disorders and inflammation. *Prostaglandins Leukot Essent Fatty Acids* 1991 Oct;44(2):127-31

[365] Fan YY, Chapkin RS. Importance of dietary gamma-linolenic acid in human health and nutrition. *J Nutr*. 1998 Sep;128(9):1411-4

[366] Delvin TM. *Textbook of Biochemistry with Clinical Correlations*. New York: Wiley-Liss, 1997. Pages 431-441

[367] Horrobin DF. Ascorbic acid and prostaglandin synthesis. *Subcell Biochem* 1996;25:109-15

[368] Delvin TM. *Textbook of Biochemistry with Clinical Correlations*. New York: Wiley-Liss, 1997. Pages 431-441

[369] Horrobin DF. Ascorbic acid and prostaglandin synthesis. *Subcell Biochem*. 1996;25:109-15

[370] Evans AR, et al. Isoprostanes, novel eicosanoids that produce nociception and sensitize rat sensory neurons. *J Pharmacol Exp Ther*. 2000 Jun;293(3):912-20

[371] Horrobin DF. Ascorbic acid and prostaglandin synthesis. *Subcell Biochem*. 1996;25:109-15

[372] Horrobin DF. Ascorbic acid and prostaglandin synthesis. *Subcell Biochem* 1996;25:109-15

[373] Delvin TM. *Textbook of Biochemistry with Clinical Correlations*. New York: Wiley-Liss, 1997. Pages 431-441

[374] Tapiero H, et al. Polyunsaturated fatty acids (PUFA) and eicosanoids in human health and pathologies. *Biomed Pharmacother*. 2002 Jul;56(5):215-22

[375] "Prostacyclin synthase catalyzes an intramolecular redox reaction in which prostaglandin endoperoxide, PGH2, is converted to prostacyclin." oxfordbiomed.com/pg61prossyn.html on September 6, 2006

[376] Peters SP, et al. The role of prostaglandin D2 in IgE-mediated reactions in man. *Trans Assoc Am Physicians*. 1982;95:221-8

[377] Bagga D, Wang L, Farias-Eisner R, Glaspy JA, Reddy ST. Differential effects of prostaglandin derived from omega-6 and omega-3 polyunsaturated fatty acids on COX-2 expression and IL-6 secretion. *Proc Natl Acad Sci* U S A. 2003 Feb 18;100(4):1751-6 pnas.org/cgi/reprint/100/4/1751.pdf

- o Suppresses lymphocyte proliferation and natural killer cell activity[378]; appears to cause stimulation of "suppressor cells"
- o Released by tumor cells and suppressor cells; promotes chemotaxis; increases platelet aggregation
- o Causes relaxation of bronchus and uterus smooth muscle in nonpregnant animals and uterine contractions in pregnant animals[379]
- o PG-E2 causes pain and also but increases the intensity and duration of pain sensations that are mediated by other triggers such as histamine and bradykinin[380]
- o Increases IgE production[381]
- o Increases vascular permeability and vasodilation thus enhancing edema[382]
- o Promotes action of epidermal growth factor[383]
- o Production is decreased by n-3 fatty acids[384]

- **Prostaglandin F2-alpha, PG-F2a, PG-F2α**
  - o Promotes bronchoconstriction and uterine contractions
  - o Increased levels associated with dysmenorrhea
  - o Increased production with vitamin C deficiency, formation is reduced by vitamin C, and low levels of vitamin C are seen in women with dysmenorrhea.[385]
  - o Promotes formation of MMP-2 and other collagenases that promote joint destruction in various types of arthritis and are required by metastasizing cancer cells to penetrate basement membranes

- **Prostaglandin G2 (PG-G2)**
  - o Induces rapid and irreversible platelet aggregation[386]

- **Prostaglandin H2 (PG-H2)**
  - o Induces rapid and irreversible platelet aggregation[387]

Linoleic acid metabolites formed by lipoxygenases

- **13-S-HODE, 13-S-hydroxyoctadecadienoic acid**
  - o 13-S-HODE is formed from linolenic acid by 15-LOX-1 and is generally considered to have anticancer actions[388]; 13-S-HODE inhibits ornithine decarboxylase[389]
  - o "12/15-LOX may cause mitochondrial dysfunction through its metabolites such as 13-S-hydroxyoctadecadienoic acid (13-S-HODE) and 12-S-hydroxyeicosatetraenoic acid (12-S-HETE) which can cause mitochondrial degradation."[390]

Arachidonic acid metabolites formed by lipoxygenases

- **5-hydroperoxyeicosatetraenoic acid, 5-HPETE**
  - o HPETEs are converted to their respective HETEs either spontaneously or by peroxidases.[391]
  - o 5-hydroxyeicosatetraenoic acid is known to reduce the depolarization threshold of primary afferent neurons and may thus lead to pain
  - o Reinforces activation of 5-lipoxygenase
  - o May be directly cytotoxic
  - o Necessary for the formation of MMP-2 and other collagenases that promote joint destruction in various types of arthritis and are required by metastasizing cancer cells to penetrate basement membranes; formation is inhibited by the lipoxygenase inhibitors esculetin and caffeic acid[392]

---

[378] Calder PC. Long-chain n-3 fatty acids and inflammation: potential application in surgical and trauma patients. *Braz J Med Biol Res*. 2003 Apr;36(4):433-46

[379] McGlivery RW. *Biochemistry: A Functional Approach. Third Edition*. Philadelphia: WB Saunders, 1983. Pages 747-750

[380] Calder PC. Long-chain n-3 fatty acids and inflammation: potential application in surgical and trauma patients. *Braz J Med Biol Res*. 2003 Apr;36(4):433-46

[381] Calder PC. Long-chain n-3 fatty acids and inflammation: potential application in surgical and trauma patients. *Braz J Med Biol Res*. 2003 Apr;36(4):433-46

[382] Calder PC. Long-chain n-3 fatty acids and inflammation: potential application in surgical and trauma patients. *Braz J Med Biol Res*. 2003 Apr;36(4):433-46

[383] Tapiero H, et al. Polyunsaturated fatty acids (PUFA) and eicosanoids in human health and pathologies. *Biomed Pharmacother*. 2002;56(5):215-22

[384] Rubin D, Laposata M. Cellular interactions between n-6 and n-3 fatty acids: a mass analysis of fatty acid elongation/desaturation, distribution among complex lipids, and conversion to eicosanoids. *J Lipid Res*. 1992 Oct;33(10):1431-40

[385] Horrobin DF. Ascorbic acid and prostaglandin synthesis. *Subcell Biochem* 1996;25:109-15

[386] McGlivery RW. *Biochemistry: A Functional Approach. Third Edition*. Philadelphia: WB Saunders, 1983. Pages 747-750

[387] McGlivery RW. *Biochemistry: A Functional Approach. Third Edition*. Philadelphia: WB Saunders, 1983. Pages 747-750

[388] Shureiqi I, Lippman SM. Lipoxygenase modulation to reverse carcinogenesis. *Cancer Res*. 2001 Sep 1;61(17):6307-12

[389] Shureiqi I, Lippman SM. Lipoxygenase modulation to reverse carcinogenesis. *Cancer Res*. 2001 Sep 1;61(17):6307-12

[390] Mabalirajan U, Ghosh B. Mitochondrial dysfunction in metabolic syndrome and asthma. *J Allergy* (Cairo). 2013;2013:340476

[391] Delvin TM. *Textbook of Biochemistry with Clinical Correlations*. New York: Wiley-Liss, 1997. Pages 431-441

[392] Reich R, et al. Identification of arachidonic acid pathways required for the invasive and metastatic activity of malignant tumor cells. *Prostaglandins* 1996 Jan;51:1-17

- - 5-HPETE is the major lipoxygenase product in inflamed tissues and promotes chemotaxis and neutrophil degranulation of lysosomal hydrolytic enzymes[393]
  - 5-HPETE is considered to have pro-cancer actions and facilitates production of proteolytic enzymes that promote joint destruction and tumor invasiveness[394]
- **5-HETE, 5-S-HETE**
  - 5-HETE is considered to have pro-cancer actions by blocking apoptosis and promoting tumor growth[395]
- **8-S-HETE**
  - 8-S-HETE is genotoxic and promotes cancer development[396]
- **12-HPETE, 12-hydroperoxyeicosatetraenoic acid, 12-hydroperoxyeicosatetraenoate,**
  - 12-HPETE is the major lipoxygenase product in platelets and the pancreas[397]
- **12-R-HETE**
  - 12-R-HETE is produced by 12-R-LOX and promotes proliferation of colon cancer cells[398]
- **12-S-HETE**
  - 12-S-HETE promotes tumor growth by several mechanisms, including 1) "up-regulating adhesion molecules and increasing the adhesion of tumor cells to the microvessel endothelium," 2) "...promoting tumor spread,"" and 3) inhibiting apoptosis[399]
  - Expression of 12-S-LOX and presumably therefore production of 12-S-HETE is directly correlated with aggressiveness, stage, and grade in human prostate cancer[400]
  - "12/15-LOX may cause mitochondrial dysfunction through its metabolites such as 13-S-hydroxyoctadecadienoic acid (13-S-HODE) and 12-Shydroxyeicosatetraenoic acid (12-S-HETE) which can cause mitochondrial degradation."[401]
- **15-hydroperoxyeicosatetraenoic acid, 15-HPETE, 15-hydroperoxyeicosatetraenoate**
  - 15-HPETE is the major lipoxygenase product in eosinophils, T-lymphocytes, and the trachea[402]
- **15-S-HETE**
  - 15-S-HETE is formed from arachidonic acid by the action of 15-LOX-2 and appears to have anticancer action, yet the data on this are conflicting[403]
- **Leukotriene B4: LT-B4**
  - Promotes immunosuppression via inhibition of CD4 cells and promotion of proliferation of CD8 cells.[404]
  - Promotes edema: increases vascular permeability, enhances local blood flow, is a potent chemotactic agent for leukocytes,
  - Exacerbates tissue damage: induces release of lysosomal enzymes, increases production of reactive oxygen species, TNF-a, IL-1, and IL-6[405]
  - Associated with accelerated atherosclerosis in patients with proinflammatory variants of 5-lipoxygenase[406]
  - Production is increased by dietary arachidonic acid and production is reduced by EPA.[407]
  - LT-B4 inhibits apoptosis in cancer cells and is generally considered procarcinogenic.[408]
- **LT-C4 and LT-D4 and LT-E4:**
  - Promote muscle contraction, bronchoconstriction, intestinal muscle contraction,
  - Promote increased capillary permeability which results in edema
  - More powerful than histamine in promotion of "allergic" symptoms[409]
  - Patients with severe asthma have elevated levels of LT-E4 that are not reduced with steroid treatment.[410]

---

[393] Delvin TM. *Textbook of Biochemistry with Clinical Correlations*. New York: Wiley-Liss, 1997. Pages 431-441

[394] "Specific metabolites of each pathway, i.e. PGF2 alpha and 5-HPETE, are able to transcend the block and restore collagenase production, invasiveness in vitro and metastatic activity in vivo." Reich et al. Identification of arachidonic acid pathways required for the invasive and metastatic activity of malignant tumor cells. *Prostaglandins* 1996 Jan;5:1-17

[395] Shureiqi I, Lippman SM. Lipoxygenase modulation to reverse carcinogenesis. *Cancer Res*. 2001 Sep 1;61(17):6307-12

[396] Shureiqi I, Lippman SM. Lipoxygenase modulation to reverse carcinogenesis. *Cancer Res*. 2001 Sep 1;61(17):6307-12

[397] Delvin TM. *Textbook of Biochemistry with Clinical Correlations*. New York: Wiley-Liss, 1997. Pages 431-441

[398] Shureiqi I, Lippman SM. Lipoxygenase modulation to reverse carcinogenesis. *Cancer Res*. 2001 Sep 1;61(17):6307-12

[399] Shureiqi I, Lippman SM. Lipoxygenase modulation to reverse carcinogenesis. *Cancer Res*. 2001 Sep 1;61(17):6307-12

[400] Shureiqi I, Lippman SM. Lipoxygenase modulation to reverse carcinogenesis. *Cancer Res*. 2001 Sep 1;61(17):6307-12

[401] Mabalirajan U, Ghosh B. Mitochondrial dysfunction in metabolic syndrome and asthma. *J Allergy* (Cairo). 2013;2013:340476

[402] Delvin TM. *Textbook of Biochemistry with Clinical Correlations*. New York: Wiley-Liss, 1997. Pages 431-441

[403] Shureiqi I, Lippman SM. Lipoxygenase modulation to reverse carcinogenesis. *Cancer Res*. 2001 Sep 1;61(17):6307-12

[404] Delvin TM. *Textbook of Biochemistry with Clinical Correlations*. New York: Wiley-Liss, 1997. Pages 431-441

[405] Calder PC. Long-chain n-3 fatty acids and inflammation: potential application in surgical and trauma patients. *Braz J Med Biol Res*. 2003 Apr;36(4):433-46

[406] Dwyer JH, et al. Arachidonate 5-lipoxygenase promoter genotype, dietary arachidonic acid, and atherosclerosis. *N Engl J Med*. 2004 Jan 1;350(1):29-37

[407] Dwyer JH, et al. Arachidonate 5-lipoxygenase promoter genotype, dietary arachidonic acid, and atherosclerosis. *N Engl J Med*. 2004 Jan 1;350(1):29-37

[408] Shureiqi I, Lippman SM. Lipoxygenase modulation to reverse carcinogenesis. *Cancer Res*. 2001 Sep 1;61(17):6307-12

[409] Delvin TM. *Textbook of Biochemistry with Clinical Correlations*. New York: Wiley-Liss, 1997. Pages 431-441

[410] Vachier I, et al. High levels of urinary leukotriene E4 excretion in steroid treated patients with severe asthma. *Respir Med*. 2003 Nov;97(11):1225-9

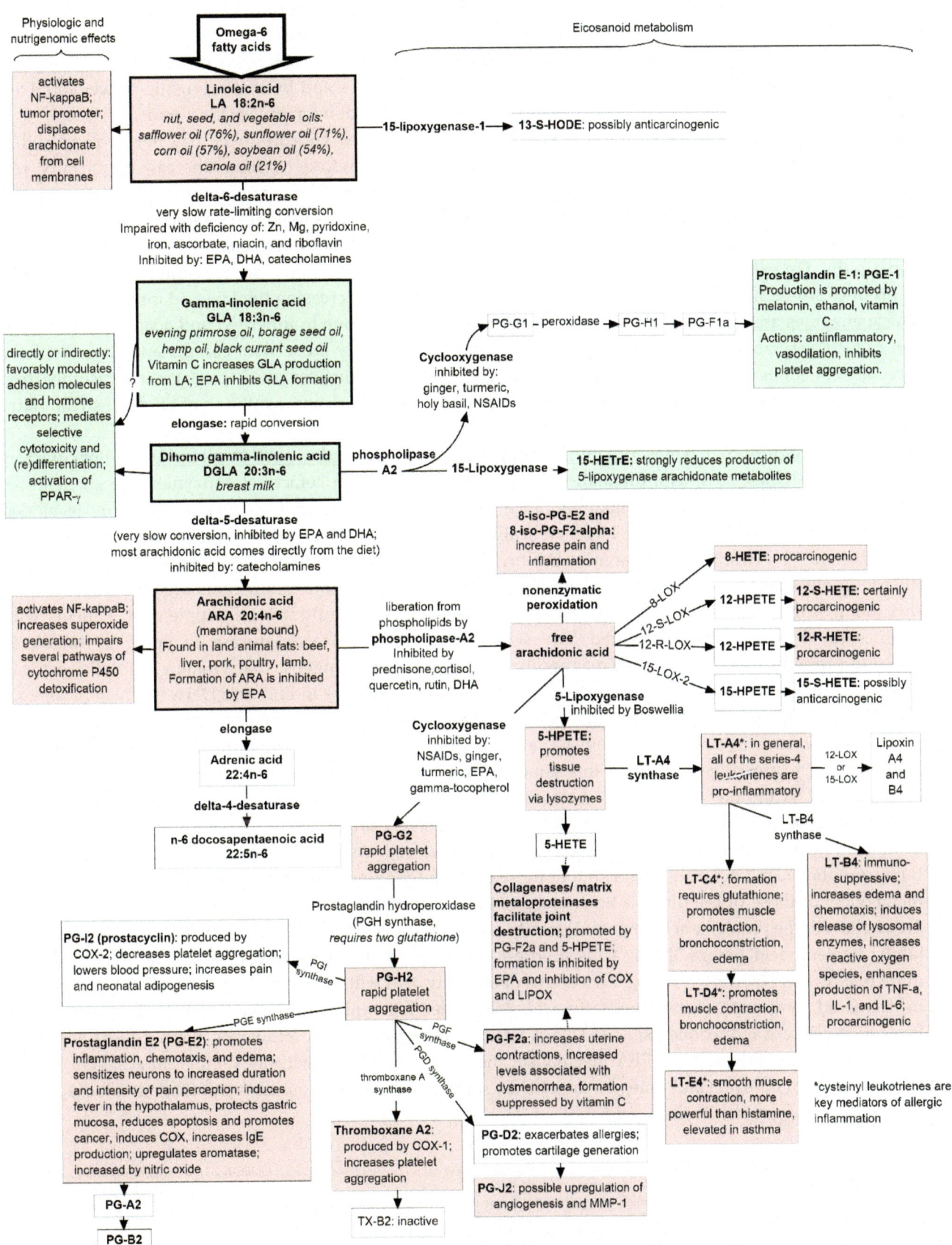

Metabolism of Omega-6 Fatty Acids and Related Eicosanoids: Health-promoting n6FA/derivatives are indicated by green, while inflammatory and disease-promoting n6FA/derivatives are indicated by red.

Important Enzymes in Fatty Acid Metabolism

Fatty acids are converted to other fatty acids in the same family by the desaturase and elongase enzymes. The major "direction" of these reactions is depicted in the diagrams; however these reactions, like nearly all enzymatic reactions, are reversible to a limited extent. Fatty acids are converted to biologically active end-products by enzymes such as the cyclooxygenases, lipoxygenases, cytochrome P-450 enzymes and by nonenzymatic conversion. Four important concepts need to be understood in relation to the enzymes that interconvert fatty acids:

1) **These enzymes do not work with equal efficiency**, and thus their end-products may not be produced in sufficient amounts to be biologically or clinically significant. Therefore, *on paper*, the cascade of fatty acid metabolism appears to flow easily from one fatty acid to its downstream progeny; in reality however, this process is often slow and therefore not immediately reliable when one is looking for rapid and reliable clinical results. The desaturase enzymes are slow and rate limiting, whereas the elongase enzymes function efficiently and rapidly. For example, Horrobin noted, "Because the 6-desaturation step is so rate-limiting, it is impossible to produce any significant elevation of DGLA levels in humans by increasing linoleic acid intake."[411]

2) **These enzymes are subject to significant interpatient variability** due to inherited and acquired factors that can reduce enzyme activity. For example, many patients (especially those with eczema and diabetes) have extreme reductions in the activity of delta-6-desaturase, the rate-limiting enzyme in the fatty acid cascades from ALA and LA. When delta-6-desaturase is slow to perform its conversions, synthesis of all downstream fatty acids is greatly reduced.

3) **All enzymes require coenzymes (organic [carbon-containing] molecules, such as vitamins) and/or cofactors (inorganic molcules, such as minerals).** If the patient is deficient in cofactors/coenzymes, the efficiency of enzymatic conversions is greatly impaired. Since micronutrient deficiencies are common even in developed countries, and since people can have clinically significant micronutrient deficiencies (i.e., "marginal malnutrition"[412]) yet still be "apparently healthy", a wise clinical strategy is to ensure that the patient's micronutrient status is adequate by encouraging the patient to consume a nutritious organic[413] whole-foods diet along with a high-potency broad-spectrum multivitamin and multimineral supplement. Patients with magnesium deficiency show impaired fatty acid metabolism because desaturase enzymes are unable to function properly without sufficient magnesium.[414] Animal studies suggest that vitamin B-6 deficiency can reduce the function of delta-6-desaturase by 64% and lead to reductions in EPA and DHA.[415]

4) **Substrates compete for enzymatic conversion.** In several instances, the same enzyme must act upon two different fatty acids in two different omega families. For example, delta-6-desaturase converts the omega-3 linolenic acid to stearidonic acid, yet this same enzyme also converts the omega-6 linoleic acid to gamma-linolenic acid. If the diet contains an absolute or relative excess of linoleic acid, then on a molecular and functional level, this excess linoleic acid will disproportionately utilize delta-6-desaturase and conversion of available linoleic acid to gamma-linolenic acid will be reduced. As reviewed by Dupont[416], "A competitive interaction between fatty acids exists so that those of the [alpha-linolenic acid, omega-3] family suppress the metabolism of those of the [linoleic acid, omega-6] family, and the [linoleic acid, omega-6] family suppress metabolism of the [linolenic acid, omega-3] family although less strongly. Both the [linoleic acid, omega-6] and [alpha-linolenic acid, omega-3] fatty acids suppress metabolism of the [oleic acid, omega-9] fatty acids." Stated more plainly by Pizzorno[417], "...a relative excess of one fatty acid will tend to hog an enzyme system, resulting in decreased conversion of the other fatty acids." In reviewing clinical evidence that EPA supplementation leads to significant reductions (50%) in DGLA levels, Horrobin[418] noted, "However, the n-3 EFAs are much more effective in inhibiting n-6 EFA metabolism than vice versa." A practical example: in a patient who is deficient in both omega-3 and omega-6 fatty acids, supplementation exclusively with flax oil will exacerbate the deficiency of gamma-linolenic acid.

[411] Horrobin DF. Interactions between n-3 and n-6 essential fatty acids (EFAs) in the regulation of cardiovascular disorders and inflammation. *Prostaglandins Leukot Essent Fatty Acids.* 1991 Oct;44(2):127-31

[412] Allen LH. The nutrition CRSP: what is marginal malnutrition, and does it affect human function? *Nutr Rev.* 1993 Sep;51(9):255-67

[413] Bob Smith. *Journal of Applied Nutrition* 1993; 45: 35-39

[414] Galland L. Impaired essential fatty acid metabolism in latent tetany. *Magnesium.* 1985;4(5-6):333-8

[415] Tsuge H, Hotta N, Hayakawa T. Effects of vitamin B-6 on (n-3) polyunsaturated fatty acid metabolism. *J Nutr.* 2000 Feb;130(2S Suppl):333S-334S

[416] Dupont J. Lipids. In: Brown ML (ed). *Present Knowledge in Nutrition. Sixth Edition.* Washington DC: International Life Sciences Institute;1990 page 62

[417] Pizzorno JE. *Total Wellness.* Rocklin: Prima; 1996 page 170

[418] Horrobin DF. Interactions between n-3 and n-6 essential fatty acids (EFAs) in the regulation of cardiovascular disorders and inflammation. *Prostaglandins Leukot Essent Fatty Acids.* 1991 Oct;44(2):127-31

- **Delta-6-desaturase (D6D):**
  - In omega-3 fatty acid metabolism, D6D converts linolenic acid to stearidonic acid. In omega-6 fatty acid metabolism, D6D converts linoleic acid to gamma-linolenic acid. D6D is the rate-limiting enzyme in fatty acid metabolism, meaning that it is the slowest functioning enzyme in the cascade of fatty acid conversions. Recall that in biochemistry the first enzyme in a series of biochemical reactions tends to be the rate-limiting enzyme for the sake of avoiding unnecessary downstream conversions. D6D is inhibited by trans fatty acids.[419] Action of this enzyme is increased during essential fatty acid deficiency.[420] Patients with eczema and diabetes have been noted to have defects in the function of D6D.[421]
  - Efficient function of D6D requires iron, magnesium, zinc, pyridoxine, niacin, and riboflavin. Administration of supraphysiologic doses of enzyme cofactors can improve function of defective or mutated enzymes.[422]
  - The catecholamines epinephrine and norepinephrine inhibit D5D and D6D.[423]
- **Delta-5-desaturase (D5D):**
  - In omega-6 fatty acid metabolism, D5D converts DGLA to arachidonic acid. However, this enzyme is slow, so that virtually all arachidonic acid found in body tissues originated from the consumption of land animal fats/meats[424] such as beef, liver, pork, lamb, and poultry. Additionally, some people (such as those with X-linked retinitis pigmentosa[425]) have reduced action of D5D and therefore have low levels of DHA. D5D is inhibited by EPA.[426] Released in increased amounts during stress and anxiety, the catecholamines epinephrine and norepinephrine inhibit D5D and D6D.[427]
- **Delta-4-desaturase**
  - Action of this enzyme is increased during essential fatty acid deficiency.[428]
- **Elongase:** These enzymes efficiently add carbon groups to the fatty acid chain.
- **Prostaglandin synthase complex (PGS):** This is the major enzyme system that is responsible for prostaglandin biosynthesis. PGS includes phospholipase A2 and cyclooxygenase.[429]
- **Phospholipase-A2**
  - Crucial to the arachidonic acid cascade since cyclooxygenase can act only on free arachidonate (i.e., after arachidonate has been liberated from membrane phospholipids); this is the rate-limiting step in the formation of arachidonate-derived prostaglandins.[430]
  - Contact of IgE with mast cells stimulates the release of arachidonate, which must occur via phospholipase A2[431]
  - Inhibited by adrenal steroids (cortisol) and prednisone
- **Cyclooxygenase (COX) (also called "prostaglandin synthase" or "PGS" or "prostaglandin endoperoxide synthase")**
  - COX-1 is "constitutive" and is found in all cells, while COX-2 is inducible by stimulation from monocytes/macrophages following stimulation by PAF, IL-1, or bacterial lipopolysaccharide; its induction is inhibited by glucocorticoids.[432]

---

[419] Simopoulos AP. Essential fatty acids in health and chronic disease. *Am J Clin Nutr*. 1999 Sep;70(3 Suppl):560S-569S

[420] "The delta 4 desaturase activity is increased in essential fatty acid deficiency similar to delta 6 desaturase." Christophersen BO, Hagve TA, Christensen E, Johansen Y, Tverdal S. Eicosapentaenoic- and arachidonic acid metabolism in isolated liver cells. *Scand J Clin Lab Invest Suppl*. 1986;184:55-60

[421] "This concept is illustrated by atopic eczema and diabetes, which may represent inherited and acquired examples of inadequate delta-6-desaturation." Horrobin DF. Fatty acid metabolism in health and disease: the role of delta-6-desaturase. *Am J Clin Nutr*. 1993 May;57(5 Suppl):732S-736S

[422] Ames BN, et al. High-dose vitamin therapy stimulates variant enzymes with decreased coenzyme binding affinity (increased K(m)). *Am J Clin Nutr* 2002 Apr;75:616-58

[423] Mamalakis G, et al. Anxiety and adipose essential fatty acid precursors for prostaglandin E1 and E2. *J Am Coll Nutr*. 1998 Jun;17(3):239-43

[424] Pizzorno JE. *Total Wellness*. Rocklin: Prima; 1996 page 169

[425] Hoffman DR, et al. Impaired synthesis of DHA in patients with X-linked retinitis pigmentosa. *J Lipid Res* 2001 Sep;42(9):1395-401

[426] Barham JB, Edens MB, Fonteh AN, Johnson MM, Easter L, Chilton FH. Addition of eicosapentaenoic acid to gamma-linolenic acid-supplemented diets prevents serum arachidonic acid accumulation in humans. *J Nutr*. 2000 Aug;130(8):1925-31

[427] Mamalakis G, et al. Anxiety and adipose essential fatty acid precursors for prostaglandin E1 and E2. *J Am Coll Nutr*. 1998 Jun;17(3):239-43

[428] "The delta 4 desaturase activity is increased in essential fatty acid deficiency similar to delta 6 desaturase." Christophersen BO, et al. Eicosapentaenoic- and arachidonic acid metabolism in isolated liver cells. *Scand J Clin Lab Invest Suppl*. 1986;184:55-60

[429] Delvin TM. *Textbook of Biochemistry with Clinical Correlations*. New York: Wiley-Liss, 1997. Pages 431-441

[430] Delvin TM. *Textbook of Biochemistry with Clinical Correlations*. New York: Wiley-Liss, 1997. Pages 431-441

[431] McGlivery RW. *Biochemistry: A Functional Approach. Third Edition*. Philadelphia: WB Saunders, 1983. Pages 747-750

[432] Delvin TM. *Textbook of Biochemistry with Clinical Correlations*. New York: Wiley-Liss, 1997. Pages 431-441

- COX is irreversibly inhibited following acetylation by aspirin.
- The expression of COX is inhibited by glucocorticoids,[433] which also inhibit phospholipase A2.
- **COX forms TXs and PGs, while LIPOX form LTs.**
- The COX metabolite PG-F2alpha is necessary for the formation of matrix metalloproteinase-2 and other collagenases which are utilized for the destruction of connective tissue[434]
- **COX is apparently activated by either n-6 fatty acids or the oxidized metabolites of n-6 fatty acids.[435] Therefore, consumption of n-6 fatty acids alone—*without trauma or inflammatory stimuli*—is sufficient for the increased production of the harmful arachidonate-derived prostaglandins and leukotrienes.** Thus, by definition, a diet high in n-6 fatty acids may subtly yet significantly promote pain, inflammation, joint destruction, and cancer.
- A well-established consequence of inhibiting COX is that of increasing LIPOX metabolites. Inhibiting COX will decrease COX metabolites, yet will cause an increase in LIPOX metabolites because of increased substrate levels; i.e., the liberated arachidonate that is not metabolized by COX is now available to be metabolized by LIPOX. Thus, inhibiting COX produces a "metabolic shunt" effect that increases production of inflammatory mediators such as HETE and the leukotrienes. Additionally, inhibition of COX inhibits formation of the beneficial anti-inflammatory DGLA metabolites.
- Arachidonate metabolites from COX function for the most part to increase inflammation and pain.[436]
- Increased expression of COX-2 increases production of PG-E2 and has been associated with increased production of anti-apoptotic proteins and a reduction in pro-apoptotic proteins in cultured rat intestinal cells.[437]
- The activity of lipoxygenase and cyclooxygenase produces reactive oxygen species (ROS) intermediates.
- The paradox of how a single enzyme such as cyclooxygenase can produce such a wide array of metabolites from a single substrate such as arachidonic acid is solved by recognizing that arachidonate is three-dimensionally rearranged once within the cyclooxygenase enzyme and that these random arrangements favor the production of different metabolites by the preferential molecular modification of the original arachidonate.[438] Additionally, cyclooxygenase may become slightly rearranged as well, thus further promoting the heterogeneity of progeny.

- **Lipoxygenases**: a family of enzymes that form leukotrienes
  - Corneal lipoxygenase is inhibited by vitamin C[439]
  - The activity of lipoxygenase and cyclooxygenase produce ROS intermediates
  - **5-lipoxygenase, 5-LOX**
    - This is a pro-inflammatory enzyme that has different basal levels of activity in different people and in different disease conditions. Proinflammatory variances of this enzyme are seen in Africans (24%), Asians and Pacific Islanders (19.4%), other racial/ethnic groups (18.2%), Hispanics (3.6%) and whites (3.1%) and are associated with accelerated atherosclerosis and elevations in CRP especially when the diet is high in arachidonic acid and low in EPA[440]

---

[433] Tapiero H, et al. Polyunsaturated fatty acids (PUFA) and eicosanoids in human health and pathologies. *Biomed Pharmacother.* 2002;56(5):215-22

[434] "Specific metabolites of each pathway, i.e. PGF2 alpha and 5-HPETE, are able to transcend the block and restore collagenase production, invasiveness in vitro and metastatic activity in vivo." Reich R, Martin GR. Identification of arachidonic acid pathways required for the invasive and metastatic activity of malignant tumor cells. *Prostaglandins* 1996 Jan;51(1):1-17

[435] " …due to activation of cyclooxygenase either by oxygenated metabolites of n-6 fatty acids or by the n-6 fatty acids themselves." Rubin D, Laposata M. Cellular interactions between n-6 and n-3 fatty acids: a mass analysis of fatty acid elongation/desaturation, distribution among complex lipids, and conversion to eicosanoids. *J Lipid Res.* 1992 Oct;33(10):1431-40

[436] Tapiero H, et al. Polyunsaturated fatty acids (PUFA) and eicosanoids in human health and pathologies. *Biomed Pharmacother.* 2002;56(5):215-22

[437] Tapiero H, et al. Polyunsaturated fatty acids (PUFA) and eicosanoids in human health and pathologies. *Biomed Pharmacother.* 2002;56(5):215-22

[438] Thuresson ED, Lakkides KM, Smith WL. Different catalytically competent arrangements of arachidonic acid within the cyclooxygenase active site of prostaglandin endoperoxide H synthase-1 lead to the formation of different oxygenated products. *J Biol Chem.* 2000 Mar 24;275(12):8501-7 jbc.org/cgi/reprint/275/12/8501

[439] Horrobin DF. Ascorbic acid and prostaglandin synthesis. *Subcell Biochem* 1996;25:109-15

[440] Dwyer JH, et al. Arachidonate 5-lipoxygenase promoter genotype, dietary arachidonic acid, and atherosclerosis. *N Engl J Med.* 2004 Jan 1;350(1):29-37

- 5-LOX has been described as "procarcinogenic" due to its role in producing LT-B4 which has mitogenic and anti-apoptotic actions[441]
- The 5-LOX metabolite 5-HPETE is necessary for the formation of matrix metalloproteinase-2 and other collagenases which are utilized for the destruction of connective tissue[442]
  - **8-lipoxygenase, 8-LOX**
    - 8-LOX is upregulated in animal models of cancer and has been described as "procarcinogenic" due to its role in producing 8-HETE, which has genotoxic effects and which is found in humans[443]
  - **12-R-lipoxygenase, 12-R-LOX**
    - 12-R-LOX has been described as "procarcinogenic" due to its role in producing 12-R-HETE[444]
  - **12-S-lipoxygenase, 12-S-LOX**
    - 12-S-LOX has been described as "procarcinogenic" due to its role in producing 12-S-HETE[445]
    - Expression of 12-S-LOX is directly correlated with aggressiveness, stage, and grade in human prostate cancer[446]
  - **15-lipoxygenase-1, 15-LOX-1**
    - 15-LOX-1 metabolizes n-6 linoleic acid into 13-S-HODE, which appears to have *anti*cancer actions[447]
  - **15-lipoxygenase-2, 15-LOX-2**
    - 15-LOX-2 metabolizes n-6 arachidonic acid into 15-S-HETE, which appears to have *anti*cancer actions[448]
  - **12/15-lipoxygenase, 12/15-LOX**
    - Earlier works cited previously described 12 LOX and 15 LOX separately; more recent reviews have described "12/15-LOX" as a single enzyme; in this moment, whether this term is being used to describe the 12 and 15 forms *separately yet in conjunction* or as a different enzyme from the other 12 and 15 forms is not clear, and the differentiation may not be of practical clinical importance at this time. However, what is relevant is the connection between Western high-fat diets, LOX activity, and mitochondrial dysfunction as contributors to insulin resistance; an impressive review article published in 2013 by Mabalirajan and Ghosh[449] noted that high-fat Western diets (in animal models) lead to activation of 12/15-LOX and resulted in oxidative modification of fatty acids and sequential mitochondrial impairment, ER stress, UPR, and insulin resistance. Beyond the intellectual gratification of enhanced understanding, this data suggests that LOX inhibition—such as for example via ginger or bioavailable curcumin—might be an additional therapeutic strategy against organelle (e.g., mito and ER) dysfunction and subsequent pathoclinical complications.

---

[441] "These targets include procarcinogenic lipoxygenases (LOXs), including 5-, 8-, and 12-LOX, and anticarcinogenic LOXs, including 15-LOX-1 and possibly 15-LOX-2." Shureiqi I, Lippman SM. Lipoxygenase modulation to reverse carcinogenesis. *Cancer Res.* 2001 Sep 1;61(17):6307-12

[442] "Specific metabolites of each pathway, i.e. PGF2 alpha and 5-HPETE, are able to transcend the block and restore collagenase production, invasiveness in vitro and metastatic activity in vivo." Reich R, Martin GR. Identification of arachidonic acid pathways required for the invasive and metastatic activity of malignant tumor cells. *Prostaglandins* 1996 Jan;51(1):1-17

[443] Shureiqi I, Lippman SM. Lipoxygenase modulation to reverse carcinogenesis. *Cancer Res.* 2001 Sep 1;61(17):6307-12

[444] Shureiqi I, Lippman SM. Lipoxygenase modulation to reverse carcinogenesis. *Cancer Res.* 2001 Sep 1;61(17):6307-12

[445] Shureiqi I, Lippman SM. Lipoxygenase modulation to reverse carcinogenesis. *Cancer Res.* 2001 Sep 1;61(17):6307-12

[446] Reich R, et al. Identification of arachidonic acid pathways required for the invasive and metastatic activity of malignant tumor cells. *Prostaglandins* 1996 Jan;51(1):1-17

[447] Shureiqi I, Lippman SM. Lipoxygenase modulation to reverse carcinogenesis. *Cancer Res.* 2001 Sep 1;61(17):6307-12

[448] Shureiqi I, Lippman SM. Lipoxygenase modulation to reverse carcinogenesis. *Cancer Res.* 2001 Sep 1;61(17):6307-12

[449] Mabalirajan U, Ghosh B. Mitochondrial dysfunction in metabolic syndrome and asthma. *J Allergy* (Cairo). 2013;2013:340476

Nuclear transcription factor kappaB (NFkB, NFkB) is one of several transcription factors which act as "facilitators" for the elaboration and amplification of specific gene products. In the case of NFkB, most of the genes that appear to be influenced are those that increase the production of pro-inflammatory mediators such as IL-2 (which increases production of collagen-digesting proteases), IL-6 (which then increases production of C-reactive protein), cyclooxygenase-2 (which then increases production of prostaglandins), lipoxygenase (which produces leukotrienes), and inducible nitric oxide synthase (for the production of nitric oxide), etc. Inhibition of NFkB is increasingly considered a major therapeutic goal in the treatment and prevention of a wide range of illnesses, including cancer, arthritis, autoimmune diseases, neurologic illnesses such as Alzheimer's and Parkinson's disease, and other "inflammatory" diseases.[450][451] While we as holistic clinicians work to address the underlying cause of the problem in a given patient, I believe that some degree of "suppression" of NFkB is therapeutically appropriate for at least two reasons: 1) it helps to limit tissue damage and to improve patient outcomes, and 2) suppression of NFkB helps to *break the vicious cycle* of positive feedback wherein *inflammation promotes more inflammation* by the NFkB stimulating effect of several of the products of NFkB activation: NFkB increases the production of IL-1, PG-E2, oxidative stress, TNF-a, and CRP—all of which work additively and synergistically to increase activation of NFkB. Therefore, regardless of the underlying cause, which may have already been addressed and eradicated, it is conceivable that some patients will suffer from inflammatory disorders simply because of the positive feedback that mediators have on the activation of NFkB, which then promotes more inflammation.

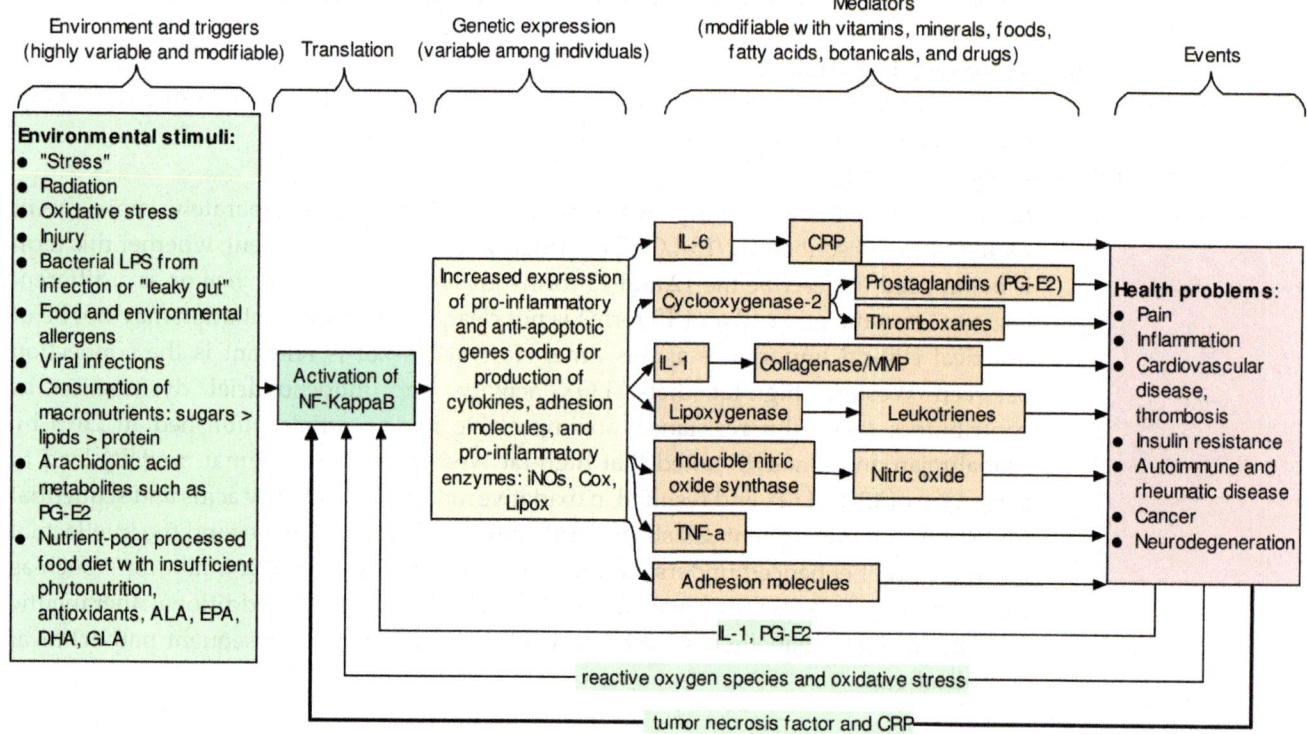

Schema of the NFkB pathway—from environmental triggers to clinical presentations: Notice the self-perpetuating cycle wherein inflammatory mediators activate NFkB for the formation of additional inflammatory mediators. From Vasquez 2005.[452]

Pharmaceutical companies are scrambling to develop clinically useful synthetic inhibitors of NFkB. These companies will eventually be successful in this endeavor, and we can also confidently predict that the pharmaceutical version of NFkB suppression will arrive with a plethora of adverse effects, most likely *because of the potency and specificity* of the drug. NFkB plays an important role in a wide range of normal, healthy physiologic processes, including the immune response to infectious diseases. We should therefore seek to *modulate* its function

[450] D'Acquisto F, May MJ, Ghosh S. Inhibition of Nuclear Factor Kappa B (NF-kB): An Emerging Theme in Anti-Inflammatory Therapies. *Mol Interv.* 2002 Feb;2:22-35
[451] Tak PP, Firestein GS. NFkB: a key role in inflammatory diseases. *J Clin Invest.* 2001 Jan;107(1):7-11 jci.org/cgi/content/full/107/1/7
[452] Vasquez A. Nutritional and Botanical Inhibition of NFkB, the Major Intracellular Amplifier of the Inflammatory Cascade. *Nutritional Perspectives* 2005;Jul:5-12

rather than sophomorically *suppress* its function. Fortunately, we can do this with several natural interventions, not the least of which are vitamin D[453,454], curcumin[455] (requires piperine for absorption[456]), lipoic acid[457], green tea[458], rosemary[459], grape seed extract[460], propolis[461], zinc[462], high-dose selenium[463], indole-3-carbinol[464,465], N-acetyl-L-cysteine[466], and resveratrol.[467,468] Other nutrients such as isohumulones from *Humulus lupulus*[469] and fatty acids inhibit NFkB *indirectly* via activation of peroxisome proliferator-activated receptors alpha (PPAR–α)and gamma (PPAR–γ). GLA activates PPAR-gamma and thereby inhibits NFkB[470], while (oxidized) EPA activates PPAR-alpha and thus inhibits NFkB[471]; these latter findings reflect a quantum leap in our understanding of the mechanisms of diet-induced anti-inflammation (i.e., anti-inflammatory nutrigenomics, or anti-inflammatory immunonutrigenomics) since they show that food constituents modify human physiology and phenotype at the genetic/pre-transcriptional level and not only at the metabolic/post-transcriptional level as was previously thought.

Almost certainly, many of the anti-inflammatory benefits of plant-based diets are partially resultant from the downregulation of NFkB by dietary phytonutrients, of which more than several thousand exist in complex and additive/synergistic combinations.[472] Notice that the above-mentioned suppressors of NFkB are mostly phenolic compounds that are naturally occurring in fruits, vegetables, herbs, and spices. A diet based upon fruits and vegetables would be naturally high in these compounds and would be likely to provide an anti-inflammatory influence on genetic expression. Indeed, this dietary and phytonutritional environment would be consistent with that in which human physiology evolved, to which it adapted, and upon which it thereby became dependent.[473,474]

[453] "1Alpha,25-dihydroxyvitamin D3 (1,25-(OH)2-D3), active metabolite of vitamin D, can inhibit NFkB activity in human MRC-5 fibroblasts, targeting DNA binding of NFkB but not translocation of its subunits p50 and p65." Harant et al. 1Alpha,25-dihydroxyvitamin D3 decreases DNA binding of nuclear factor-kappaB. *FEBS Lett*. 1998;436:329-34

[454] "Thus, 1,25(OH)$_2$D$_3$ may negatively regulate IL-12 production by downregulation of NF-kB activation and binding to the p40-kB sequence." D'Ambrosio D, et al. Inhibition of IL-12 production by 1,25-dihydroxyvitamin D3. *J Clin Invest*. 1998 Jan 1;101(1):252-62

[455] "Curcumin, EGCG and resveratrol have been shown to suppress activation of NF-kappa B." Surh et al. Molecular mechanisms underlying chemopreventive activities of anti-inflammatory phytochemicals: down-regulation of COX-2 and iNOS through suppression of NF-kappa B activation. *Mutat Res*. 2001 Sep 1;480-481:243-68

[456] Shoba G, et al. Influence of piperine on the pharmacokinetics of curcumin in animals and human volunteers. *Planta Med*. 1998 May;64(4):353-6

[457] "ALA reduced the TNF-alpha-stimulated ICAM-1 expression in a dose-dependent manner, to levels observed in unstimulated cells. Alpha-lipoic acid also reduced NFkB activity in these cells in a dose-dependent manner." Lee HA, Hughes DA. Alpha-lipoic acid modulates NFkB activity in human monocytic cells by direct interaction with DNA. *Exp Gerontol*. 2002 Jan-Mar;37(2-3):401-10

[458] "In conclusion, EGCG is an effective inhibitor of IKK activity. This may explain, at least in part, some of the reported anti-inflammatory and anticancer effects of green tea." Yang F, Oz HS, Barve S, de Villiers WJ, McClain CJ, Varilek GW. The green tea polyphenol (-)-epigallocatechin-3-gallate blocks nuclear factor-kappa B activation by inhibiting I kappa B kinase activity in the intestinal epithelial cell line IEC-6. *Mol Pharmacol*. 2001 Sep;60(3):528-33

[459] "These results suggest that carnosol suppresses the NO production and iNOS gene expression by inhibiting NFkB activation, and provide possible mechanisms for its anti-inflammatory and chemopreventive action." Lo AH, Liang YC, Lin-Shiau SY, Ho CT, Lin JK. Carnosol, an antioxidant in rosemary, suppresses inducible nitric oxide synthase through down-regulating nuclear factor-kappaB in mouse macrophages. *Carcinogenesis*. 2002 Jun;23(6):983-91

[460] "Constitutive and TNFalpha-induced NFkB DNA binding activity was inhibited by GSE at doses > or =50 microg/ml and treatments for > or =12 h." Dhanalakshmi et al. Inhibition of NFkB pathway in grape seed extract-induced apoptotic death of human prostate carcinoma DU145 cells. *Int J Oncol*. 2003;23:721-7

[461] "Caffeic acid phenethyl ester (CAPE) is an anti-inflammatory component of propolis (honeybee resin). CAPE is reportedly a specific inhibitor of nuclear factor-kappaB (NFkB)." Fitzpatrick LR, Wang J, Le T. Caffeic acid phenethyl ester, an inhibitor of nuclear factor-kappaB, attenuates bacterial peptidoglycan polysaccharide-induced colitis in rats. *J Pharmacol Exp Ther*. 2001 Dec;299(3):915-20

[462] "Our results suggest that zinc supplementation may lead to downregulation of the inflammatory cytokines through upregulation of the negative feedback loop A20 to inhibit induced NFkB activation." Prasad AS, et al. Antioxidant effect of zinc in humans. *Free Radic Biol Med*. 2004 Oct 15;37(8):1182-90

[463] Note that the patients in this study received a very high dose of selenium: 960 micrograms per day. This is at the top—and some would say over the top—of the safe and reasonable dose for long-term supplementation. This study lasted for three months. "In patients receiving selenium supplementation, selenium NFkB activity was significantly reduced, reaching the same level as the nondiabetic control group. CONCLUSION: In type 2 diabetic patients, activation of NFkB measured in peripheral blood monocytes can be reduced by selenium supplementation, confirming its importance in the prevention of cardiovascular diseases." Faure P, et al. Selenium supplementation decreases nuclear factor-kappa B activity in peripheral blood mononuclear cells from type 2 diabetic patients. *Eur J Clin Invest*. 2004 Jul;34:475-81

[464] Takada Y, Andreeff M, Aggarwal BB. Indole-3-carbinol suppresses NF-{kappa}B and I{kappa}B{alpha} kinase activation causing inhibition of expression of NF-{kappa}B-regulated antiapoptotic and metastatic gene products and enhancement of apoptosis in myeloid and leukemia cells. *Blood*. 2005 Apr 5; [Epub ahead of print]

[465] "Overall, our results indicated that indole-3-carbinol inhibits NFkB and NFkB-regulated gene expression and that this mechanism may provide the molecular basis for its ability to suppress tumorigenesis." Takada Y, et al. Indole-3-carbinol suppresses NFkB and IkappaBalpha kinase activation, causing inhibition of expression of NFkB-regulated antiapoptotic and metastatic gene products and enhancement of apoptosis in myeloid and leukemia cells. *Blood*. 2005 Jul 15;106:641-9

[466] "CONCLUSIONS: Administration of N-acetylcysteine results in decreased nuclear factor-kappa B activation in patients with sepsis, associated with decreases in interleukin-8 but not interleukin-6 or soluble intercellular adhesion molecule-1. These pilot data suggest that antioxidant therapy with N-acetylcysteine may be useful in blunting the inflammatory response to sepsis." Paterson RL, Galley HF, Webster NR. The effect of N-acetylcysteine on nuclear factor-kappa B activation, interleukin-6, interleukin-8, and intercellular adhesion molecule-1 expression in patients with sepsis. *Crit Care Med*. 2003 Nov;31(11):2574-8

[467] "Resveratrol's anticarcinogenic, anti-inflammatory, and growth-modulatory effects may thus be partially ascribed to the inhibition of activation of NFkB and AP-1 and the associated kinases." Manna SK, Mukhopadhyay A, Aggarwal BB. Resveratrol suppresses TNF-induced activation of nuclear transcription factors NF-kappa B, activator protein-1, and apoptosis: potential role of reactive oxygen intermediates and lipid peroxidation. *J Immunol*. 2000 Jun 15;164(12):6509-19

[468] "Both resveratrol and quercetin inhibited NFkB-, AP-1- and CREB-dependent transcription to a greater extent than the glucocorticosteroid, dexamethasone." Donnelly LE, et al. Anti-inflammatory Effects of Resveratrol in Lung Epithelial Cells. *Am J Physiol Lung Cell Mol Physiol*. 2004 Oct;287(4):L774-83

[469] Yajima H, et al. Isohumulones, bitter acids derived from hops, activate both peroxisome proliferator-activated receptor alpha and gamma and reduce insulin resistance. *J Biol Chem*. 2004 Aug 6;279(32):33456-62. Epub 2004 Jun 3. jbc.org/cgi/content/full/279/32/33456

[470] "Thus, PPAR gamma serves as the receptor for GLA in the regulation of gene expression in breast cancer cells." Jiang WG, et al. Peroxisome proliferator activated receptor-gamma (PPAR-gamma) mediates the action of gamma linolenic acid in breast cancer cells. *Prostaglandins Leukot Essent Fatty Acids*. 2000 Feb;62(2):119-27

[471] "...EPA requires PPARalpha for its inhibitory effects on NFkB." Mishra A, Chaudhary A, Sethi S. Oxidized omega-3 fatty acids inhibit NFkB activation via a PPARalpha-dependent pathway. *Arterioscler Thromb Vasc Biol*. 2004 Sep;24(9):1621-7. Epub 2004 Jul 1. atvb.ahajournals.org/cgi/content/full/24/9/1621

[472] "We propose that the additive and synergistic effects of phytochemicals in fruit and vegetables are responsible for their potent antioxidant and anticancer activities, and that the benefit of a diet rich in fruit and vegetables is attributed to the complex mixture of phytochemicals present in whole foods." Liu RH. Health benefits of fruit and vegetables are from additive and synergistic combinations of phytochemicals. *Am J Clin Nutr*. 2003 Sep;78(3 Suppl):517S-520S

[473] Heaney RP. Long-latency deficiency disease: insights from calcium and vitamin D. *Am J Clin Nutr*. 2003 Nov;78(5):912-9

[474] O'Keefe JH Jr, Cordain L. Cardiovascular disease resulting from a diet and lifestyle at odds with our Paleolithic genome. *Mayo Clin Proc*. 2004 Jan;79(1):101-8

Relatedly, our epidemic of vitamin D deficiency[475] resultant from our artificial, indoor, clothed lifestyles unquestionably contributes to our modern pro-inflammatory tendency, and vitamin D supplementation has already proven to be immunomodulating and anti-inflammatory in human clinical trials.[476,477,478]

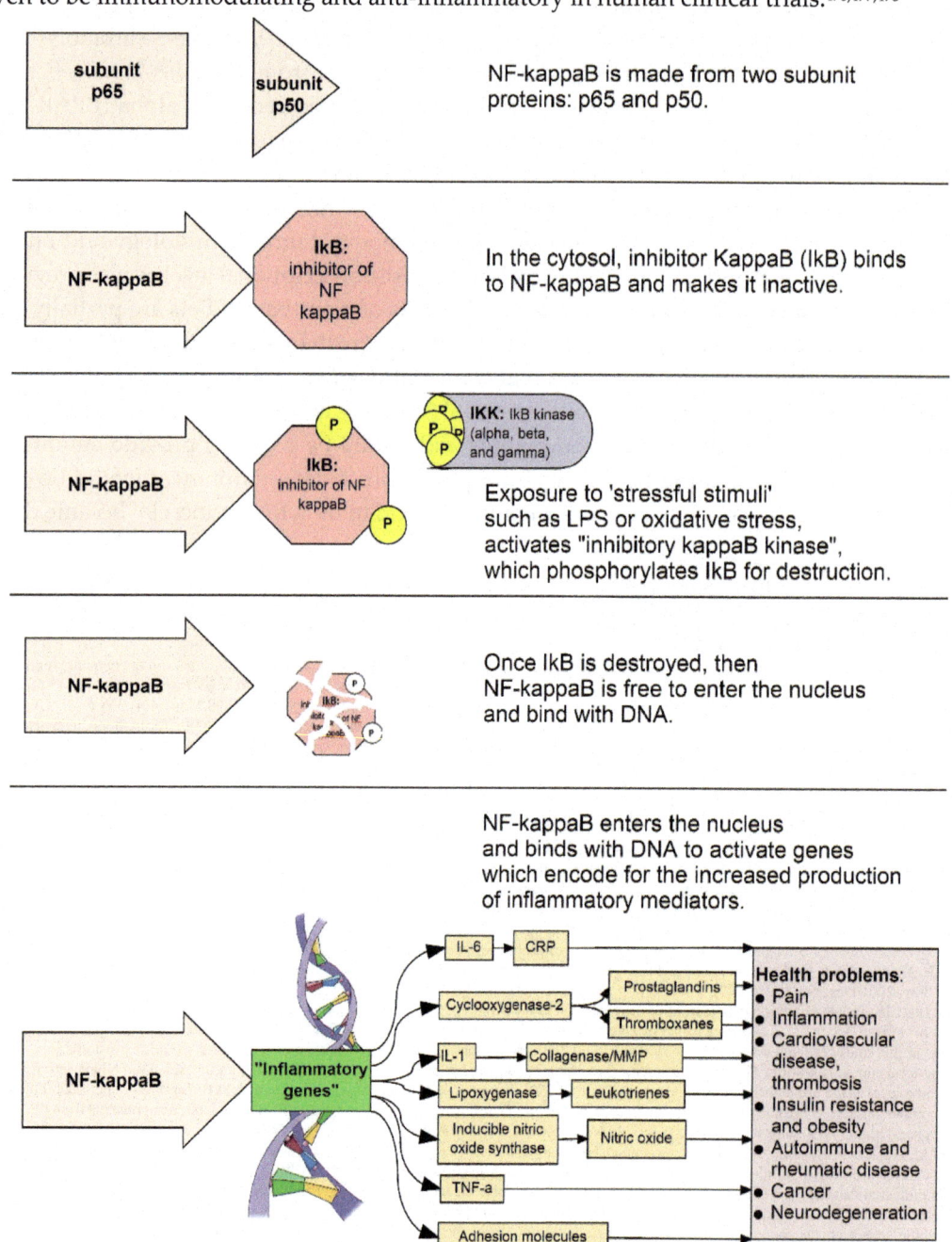

NF-kappaB is made from two subunit proteins: p65 and p50.

In the cytosol, inhibitor KappaB (IkB) binds to NF-kappaB and makes it inactive.

Exposure to 'stressful stimuli' such as LPS or oxidative stress, activates "inhibitory kappaB kinase", which phosphorylates IkB for destruction.

Once IkB is destroyed, then NF-kappaB is free to enter the nucleus and bind with DNA.

NF-kappaB enters the nucleus and binds with DNA to activate genes which encode for the increased production of inflammatory mediators.

Increased production of inflammatory mediators - such as cytokines, prostaglandins, leukotrienes - promotes cellular dysfunction and tissue destruction. Further, many vicious cycles of oxidant stress, mitochondrial dysfunction, and activation of DAMP receptors are initiated.

Basic Physiology of NFkB: A Simplified Conceptual Model: "Indeed, the previous view that nutrients only interact with human physiology at the metabolic/post-transcriptional level must be updated in light of current research showing that nutrients can, in fact, modify human physiology and phenotype at the genetic/pre-transcriptional level." Quote and updated image from Vasquez A. Nutritional and Botanical Inhibition of NFkB, the Major Intracellular Amplifier of the Inflammatory Cascade. A Practical Clinical Strategy Exemplifying Anti-Inflammatory Nutrigenomics. *Nutritional Perspectives* 2005;July: 5-12

[475] Thomas MK, et al. Hypovitaminosis D in medical inpatients. *N Engl J Med.* 1998 Mar 19;338(12):777-83
[476] Van den Berghe G, et al. Bone turnover in prolonged critical illness: effect of vitamin D. *J Clin Endocrinol Metab.* 2003 Oct;88(10):4623-32
[477] Hypponen E, et al. Intake of vitamin D and risk of type 1 diabetes: a birth-cohort study. *Lancet.* 2001 Nov 3;358(9292):1500-3
[478] Mahon BD, et al. Cytokine profile in patients with multiple sclerosis following vitamin D supplementation. *J Neuroimmunol.* 2003;134(1-2):128-32

Mini-Monograph: Food Allergy and Adverse Food Reactions—considerations, perspectives

"Adverse food reactions" is a broad and general category that includes food allergy, food sensitivity, and food intolerance. The term "food" here means anything that is ingested other than drugs and medications and includes food, drink, food additives, preservatives, and food dyes. Many studies in the medical literature underestimate the high prevalence and clinical importance of food allergies because of inconsistent terminology, imperfect laboratory assessments[479], and the assumption that an "apparently healthy" person would only be allergic/sensitive to one or two foods—this is an erroneous assumption considering that many patients with food allergy/sensitivity/intolerance must avoid several (common range 3-10) commonly eaten foods to obtain clinical response and maximal improvement.[480,481] Clinical practice differs from basic research in that we as clinicians must often do what is effective while having neither the need nor the luxury for determining the molecular and physiologic basis for the effectiveness of each treatment in each patient. Clinical research has scientifically proven that adverse food reactions, regardless of the underlying mechanism(s) or classification of allergy, intolerance, or sensitivity, can exacerbate a wide range of human illnesses, including thyroid disease[482], mental depression[483,484], asthma, rhinitis,[485] recurrent otitis media[486], migraine[487,488,489], attention deficit and hyperactivity disorders[490], epilepsy[491,492,493], gastrointestinal inflammation[494], hypertension[495], joint pain[496,497,498,499,500,501,502,] and other health problems.

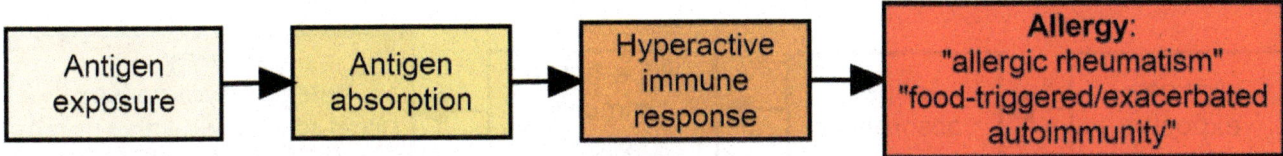

The common view of allergic phenomena: This model is incomplete and therefore inaccurate because it fails to include the prerequisite immune dysfunction and complex physiologic interconnections

"Food allergy" generally refers to adverse food reactions that are specifically immunoglobulin-mediated. Classically, food allergy is seen with immediate-onset allergy mediated via IgE antibodies which initiate mast cell degranulation and histamine release. The classic symptoms of immediate-onset allergies are skin rash, abdominal pain, angioedema, and bronchoconstriction. However, many doctors recognize the possibility of IgG-mediated allergies and suggest that these might be responsible for the delayed-onset or "hidden" food allergies which are clinically significant but more subtle and difficult to diagnose than the classic IgE-mediated allergies. The binding of antigens with immunoglobulins forms immune complexes that can deposit in parenchymal and synovial tissues where a localized immune response causes inflammation and organ dysfunction. **"Food sensitivity"** refers to immune-mediated adverse food reactions that are not antibody-mediated but are mediated by some other aspect

[479] Bindslev-Jensen C, Skov PS, Madsen F, Poulsen LK. Food allergy and food intolerance--what is the difference? *Ann Allergy.* 1994 Apr;72(4):317-20

[480] Grant EC. Food allergies and migraine. *Lancet.* 1979 May 5;1(8123):966-9

[481] Speer F. Multiple food allergy. *Ann Allergy.* 1975 Feb;34(2):71-6

[482] Sategna-Guidetti C, et al. Prevalence of thyroid disorders in untreated adult celiac disease patients and effect of gluten withdrawal. *Am J Gastroenterol.* 2001;96:751-7

[483] Mills N. Depression and food intolerance: a single case study. *Hum Nutr Appl Nutr.* 1986 Apr;40(2):141-5

[484] Parker G, Watkins T. Treatment-resistant depression: when antidepressant drug intolerance may indicate food intolerance. *Aust N Z J Psychiatry.* 2002 Apr;36(2):263-5

[485] Speer F. The allergic child. *Am Fam Physician.* 1975 Feb;11(2):88-94

[486] Juntti H, Tikkanen S, Kokkonen J, et al. Cow's milk allergy is associated with recurrent otitis media during childhood. *Acta Otolaryngol.* 1999;119(8):867-73

[487] Monro J, Carini C, Brostoff J. Migraine is a food-allergic disease. *Lancet.* 1984 Sep 29;2(8405):719-21

[488] Egger J, Carter CM, Wilson J,et al. Is migraine food allergy? A double-blind controlled trial of oligoantigenic diet treatment. *Lancet.* 1983 Oct 15;2(8355):865-9

[489] Monro J, Brostoff J, Carini C, Zilkha K. Food allergy in migraine. Study of dietary exclusion and RAST. *Lancet.* 1980 Jul 5;2(8184):1-4

[490] Boris M, Mandel FS. Foods and additives are common causes of the attention deficit hyperactive disorder in children. *Ann Allergy.* 1994 May;72(5):462-8

[491] Egger J, Carter CM, Soothill JF, Wilson J. Oligoantigenic diet treatment of children with epilepsy and migraine. *J Pediatr.* 1989;114(1):51-8

[492] Pelliccia A, et al. Partial cryptogenetic epilepsy and food allergy/intolerance. Reflections on three clinical cases. *Minerva Pediatr.* 1999 May;51(5):153-7

[493] Frediani T, Lucarelli S, Pelliccia A, et al. Allergy and childhood epilepsy: a close relationship? *Acta Neurol Scand.* 2001 Dec;104(6):349-52

[494] Marr HY, Chen WC, Lin LH. Food protein-induced enterocolitis syndrome: report of one case. *Acta Paediatr Taiwan.* 2001;42(1):49-52

[495] Grant EC. Food allergies and migraine. *Lancet.* 1979 May 5;1(8123):966-9

[496] Golding DN. Is there an allergic synovitis? *J R Soc Med.* 1990 May;83(5):312-4

[497] Panush RS. Food induced ("allergic") arthritis: clinical and serologic studies. *J Rheumatol.* 1990 Mar;17(3):291-4

[498] Pacor ML, Lunardi C, Di Lorenzo G, Biasi D, Corrocher R. Food allergy and seronegative arthritis: report of two cases. *Clin Rheumatol.* 2001;20(4):279-81

[499] Schrander JJ, Marcelis C, de Vries MP, van Santen-Hoeufft HM. Does food intolerance play a role in juvenile chronic arthritis? *Br J Rheumatol.* 1997;36(8):905-8

[500] van de Laar MA, van der Korst JK. Food intolerance in rheumatoid arthritis. I. A double blind, controlled trial. *Ann Rheum Dis.* 1992 Mar;51(3):298-302

[501] Haugen MA, et al. A pilot study of the effect of an elemental diet in the management of rheumatoid arthritis. *Clin Exp Rheumatol.* 1994 May-Jun;12(3):275-9

[502] van de Laar MA, et al. Food intolerance in rheumatoid arthritis. II. Clinical and histological aspects. *Ann Rheum Dis.* 1992 Mar;51(3):303-6

of the immune/inflammatory system. An example of this is the increased production of specific prostaglandins in food-induced irritable bowel syndrome.[503] **"Food intolerance"** refers to adverse food reactions which are associated with poor nutritional status and/or impaired hepatic detoxification and which are *not* immune-mediated. Classic and well-known examples of this category of adverse food reaction include MSG sensitivity (associated with deficiency of vitamin B-6 and subsequent defects in hepatic transamination), tyramine intolerance that can result in hypertension and headaches, and histamine intolerance that can result in bronchoconstriction.[504] From a practical clinical standpoint, the following facts are self-evident for any doctor working in the field of nutrition:

1. Some people have adverse food reactions from the foods that they eat.

2. Food-induced reactions may be either immediate-onset (i.e., within minutes) or delayed-onset (within days) of eating the triggering food.

3. The same patient might have immediate-onset reactions to food X with symptoms A and B and simultaneously have a delayed-onset reaction to food Y with symptom C.

4. Food X might cause symptoms D and E in one patient and symptoms F and G in another patient.

5. By avoiding allergens and/or improving immune function, many "diseases" go away without direct treatment and the patient experiences an improved state of health.

6. Failure to identify and avoid problematic foods combined with failure to correct the underlying immune dysfunction often makes the "disease" recalcitrant to remediation even with "generally effective" treatment. This has been demonstrated in migraine, hypertension[505], and drug-resistant mental depression.[506]

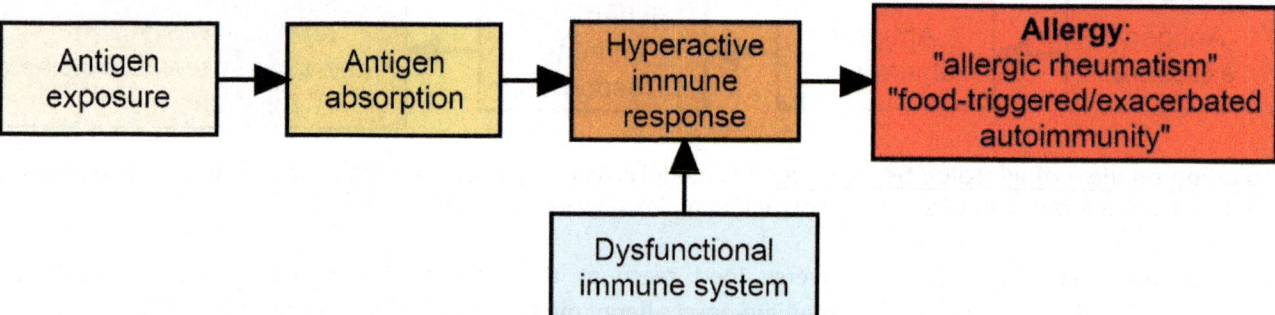

Approaching a more complete understanding of "allergy" in general and the "allergic" contribution to systemic inflammation and autoimmunity in particular: Simple and obvious though it may appear, the addition and acknowledgement of immune dysfunction to the schema of clinical allergy/inflammation contains a gateway for accessing more effective understandings and treatments for this common group of problems.

Food allergy both *results from* and *contributes to* immune dysfunction and a systemic proinflammatory state. Food allergy contributes to "autoimmunity" and musculoskeletal inflammation via several mechanisms, including but not limited to the following:

1. Stimulation of cytokine release: As will be discussed later, the term "superantigen" classically refers to microbial—viral, bacterial, or fungal—antigens which have the ability to induce production of excessive levels of cytokines and other inflammatory effectors[507], and superantigens appear to be involved in the

---

[503] "Food intolerance associated with prostaglandin production is an important factor in the pathogenesis of IBS." Jones VA, McLaughlan P, Shorthouse M, Workman E, Hunter JO. Food intolerance: a major factor in the pathogenesis of irritable bowel syndrome. *Lancet*. 1982 Nov 20;2(8308):1115-7

[504] Wantke F, Hemmer W, Haglmuller T, Gotz M, Jarisch R. Histamine in wine. Bronchoconstriction after a double-blind placebo-controlled red wine provocation test. *Int Arch Allergy Immunol*. 1996 Aug;110(4):397-400

[505] "When an average of ten common foods were avoided there was a dramatic fall in the number of headaches per month, 85% of patients becoming headache-free. The 25% of patients with hypertension became normotensive." Grant EC. Food allergies and migraine. *Lancet*. 1979 May 5;1(8123):966-9

[506] "The prevalence of food intolerance as a contributing factor to depressive disorders requires clarification. Clinicians should be aware of the possible syndrome and that it may be worsened by psychotropic medication." Parker G, Watkins T. Treatment-resistant depression: when antidepressant drug intolerance may indicate food intolerance. *Aust N Z J Psychiatry*. 2002 Apr;36(2):263-5

[507] "The basis of autoimmune disorders due to superantigen is due to greater stimulation of T-lymphocytes and elaborate cytokine production." Hemalatha V, Srikanth P, Mallika M. Superantigens - Concepts, clinical disease and therapy. *Indian J Med Microbiol* 2004;22:204-211

pathogenesis of inflammatory musculoskeletal disorders such as rheumatoid arthritis.[508,509] **In this section I propose that since food allergens appear capable of inducing cytokine production, they should in certain circumstances be considered "dietary superantigens"** since they invoke cytokine release similarly as do microbial superantigens. An important distinction here, however, is that microbial superantigens generally stimulate cytokine release as an inherent property in *all* patients, whereas **the production of cytokines by dietary (super)antigens is dependent on previous sensitization**; thus cytokine production by allergens is patient-dependent and not an inherent property of the allergen itself. **Mononuclear cells from egg-allergic patients produce much more proinflammatory cytokine (interferon) than do those from nonallergic patients.**[510] Similarly, **in children with autism, who commonly demonstrate immune dysfunction and neuroautoimmunity[511], exposure to food allergens greatly increases cytokine release compared to controls.**[512] Food allergy, NFkB activation, cytokine release, and increased intestinal permeability form a self-perpetuating vicious cycle because consumption of dietary allergens causes damage to the intestinal mucosa and stimulates NFkB activation and cytokine release which then increases intestinal permeability, thus allowing for increased absorption of dietary and microbial immunogens for the perpetuation and exacerbation of allergy and immune dysfunction.[513] Proinflammatory cytokines would be expected to contribute to autoimmune disease induction via mechanisms such as bystander activation and increased autoantigen processing regardless of their original stimuli.

2. <u>Immune complex formation and deposition</u>: **Dietary antigen-antibody immune complexes are formed following the consumption of allergenic foods by patients with allergy to those foods[514,515]** and these anti-food and anti-IgE immune complexes contribute to allergic symptomatology by a mechanism that has been described as "chronic serum sickness."[516] These immune complexes are then deposited in the joints to localize the resultant proinflammatory response. In the study by Carini et al[517], the authors found that **patients with food-induced joint pain and inflammation had anti-IgE IgG antibodies which formed large immune complexes that were detectable in synovial fluid and which probably contributed to the arthritis.** Anti-IgE IgG antibodies are commonly elevated in patients with allergic/inflammatory diseases such as eczema[518], asthma[519], and Crohn's disease[520] and thus tissue damage in these conditions appears mediated at least in part by anti-immunoglobulin immune complexes (i.e., anti-IgE IgG complexed with IgE) rather than the classic antigen-antibody immune complexes. In this way, food allergies cause joint pain and inflammation by the deposition of immune complexes into the synovium and joint cartilage.[521] Conversely, the consumption of a relatively hypoallergenic diet reduces intake of food antigens and helps

---

[508] "They also suggest that the etiology of RA may involve initial activation of V beta 14+ T cells by a V beta 14-specific superantigen with subsequent recruitment of a few activated autoreactive v beta 14+ T cell clones to the joints while the majority of other V beta 14+ T cells disappear." Paliard X, West SG, Lafferty JA, Clements JR, Kappler JW, Marrack P, Kotzin BL. Evidence for the effects of a superantigen in rheumatoid arthritis. *Science*. 1991 Jul 19;253(5017):325-9

[509] "Given that binding sites for superantigens have been mapped to the CDR4s of TCR beta chains, the synovial localization of T cells bearing V beta s with significant CDR4 homology indicates that V beta-specific T-cell activation by superantigen may play a role in RA." Howell MD, et al. Limited T-cell receptor beta-chain heterogeneity among interleukin 2 receptor-positive synovial T cells suggests a role for superantigen in rheumatoid arthritis. *Proc Natl Acad Sci*. 1991 Dec 1;88:10921-5

[510] "The levels of IFN-gamma production of only IL-2-stimulated or both ovalbumin-stimulated and IL-2-stimulated peripheral blood mononuclear cells from egg-sensitive patients with atopic dermatitis was significantly higher than that of healthy children and that of egg-sensitive patients with immediate allergic symptoms." Shinbara M, et al. Interferon-gamma and interleukin-4 production of ovalbumin-stimulated lymphocytes in egg-sensitive children. *Ann Allergy Asthma Immunol*. 1996;77(1):60-6

[511] "Autistic children, but not normal children, had antibodies to caudate nucleus (49% positive sera), cerebral cortex (18% positive sera) and cerebellum (9% positive sera)." Singh VK, Rivas WH. Prevalence of serum antibodies to caudate nucleus in autistic children. *Neurosci Lett*. 2004 Jan 23;355(1-2):53-6

[512] Jyonouchi H, Sun S, Itokazu N. Innate immunity associated with inflammatory responses and cytokine production against common dietary proteins in patients with autism spectrum disorder. *Neuropsychobiology*. 2002;46(2):76-84

[513] Ma TY, Iwamoto GK, Hoa NT, Akotia V, Pedram A, Boivin MA, Said HM. TNF-alpha-induced increase in intestinal epithelial tight junction permeability requires NF-kappa B activation. *Am J Physiol Gastrointest Liver Physiol*. 2004 Mar;286(3):G367-76 ajpgi.physiology.org/cgi/content/full/286/3/G367

[514] "Antigen entry and the formation of immune complexes occur in atopic subjects after food ingestion. ...Food allergic subjects showed, after food challenge, the presence of IgE and IgG immune complexes, which correlates with the subsequent occurrence of symptoms." Carini C, Brostoff J. Evidence for circulating IgE complexes in food allergy. *Ric Clin Lab*. 1987 Oct-Dec;17(4):309-22

[515] "Following challenge, immune complexes containing IgE, IgG, and antigen are detectable in the circulation. Their appearance correlates with the production of symptoms." Carini C, Brostoff J, Wraith DG. IgE complexes in food allergy. *Ann Allergy*. 1987 Aug;59(2):110-7

[516] Marinkovich V. "Immunology and Food Allergy" in "Applying Functional Medicine in Clinical Practice." Institute for Functional Medicine. Seattle, Washington: March 2005

[517] "In three food-allergic patients IgG anti-IgE was detectable in a complexed form in the serum samples examined before and after food challenge. The finding of IgG anti-IgE autoantibody in a group of patients with allergic arthralgia is quite exciting." Carini et al. Immune complexes in food-induced arthralgia. *Ann Allergy*. 1987 Dec;59(6):422-8

[518] "An IgG type of antibody directed against IgE has been studied in serum from healthy and allergic individuals. ... Significantly raised levels of anti-IgE autoantibody were found in patients suffering from atopic disorders in comparison to the controls." Carini et al. IgG autoantibody to IgE in atopic patients. *Ann Allergy*. 1988 Jan;60(1):48-52

[519] "Significantly enhanced levels of IgE/anti-IgE IC were detected in children with asthma." Ritter C, Battig M, Kraemer R, Stadler BM. IgE hidden in immune complexes with anti-IgE autoantibodies in children with asthma. *J Allergy Clin Immunol*. 1991 Nov;88(5):793-801

[520] "In CD sera no food-specific IgE could be detected, but levels of immune complexes of IgE and IgG anti-IgE autoantibodies were statistically significantly increased compared to healthy controls." Huber A, Genser D, Spitzauer S, Scheiner O, Jensen-Jarolim E. IgE/anti-IgE immune complexes in sera from patients with Crohn's disease do not contain food-specific IgE. *Int Arch Allergy Immunol*. 1998 Jan;115(1):67-72

[521] Inman RD. Antigens, the gastrointestinal tract, and arthritis. *Rheum Dis Clin North Am*. 1991 May;17(2):309-21

reduce IgE levels. This explains, in part, the success of hypoallergenic diets in the treatment of immune-complex-mediated diseases such as mixed cryoglobulinemia[522,523], hypersensitivity vasculitis[524], and leukocystoclastic vasculitis with arthritis.[525] In patients with rheumatoid arthritis, the symptomatic and clinical improvement induced by hypoallergenic diets correlates with reductions in antibodies to food antigens.[526]

3. Damage to the intestinal mucosa with resultant increased absorption of dietary and microbial antigens: Consumption of food allergens increases intestinal permeability[527] and thus amplifies the absorption of intestinal contents—dietary and microbial antigens. Patients with food allergy have "leaky gut" that is exacerbated by consumption of allergenic foods; thus lactulose-mannitol assays can be used to assist the diagnosis of food allergy.[528,529] By increasing intestinal permeability, consumption of dietary antigens serves to exacerbate the adverse effects of gastrointestinal dysbiosis by increasing antigen and (anti)metabolite absorption. Since both dietary allergens and bacterial endotoxin stimulate production of cytokines[530], **concomitant exposure to both allergens and intra-intestinal endotoxin leads to an additive increase in proinflammatory cytokine production.[531]** Thus, **consumption of allergenic foods in the presence of gastrointestinal dysbiosis would be expected to lead to more severe and more diverse adverse physiologic and clinical consequences than would be experienced following exposure to either allergens or dysbiosis alone.**

4. Dietary haptenization: **Dietary antigens can complex with human tissues to form *neoantigens* that are immunostimulatory.** The best example of this appears to be the induction of autoimmunity by wheat-derived gliadin which haptenizes with intestinal tissue transglutaminase and other extracellular matrix proteins and results in the allergic-autoimmune disease celiac disease.[532,533] **The finding that gliadin proteins haptenize with collagen and can induce the formation of anti-collagen antibodies in humans[534] makes clear the pathomechanism by which "wheat allergy" can directly precipitate systemic musculoskeletal autoimmunity.** Once initiated and perpetuated by dietary gliadin from wheat, additional autoimmunity ensues (perhaps mediated directly by epitope spreading and/or indirectly by deposition of immune complexes) which is directed against various tissues, most notably the thyroid gland[535], brain[536],

---

[522] "CONCLUSION: These data show that an LAC diet decreases the amount of circulating immune complexes in MC and can modify certain signs and symptoms of the disease." Ferri C, Pietrogrande M, Cecchetti R, et al. Low-antigen-content diet in the treatment of patients with mixed cryoglobulinemia. *Am J Med*. 1989 Nov;87:519-24

[523] Pietrogrande M, Cefalo A, Nicora F, Marchesini D. Dietetic treatment of essential mixed cryoglobulinemia. *Ric Clin Lab*. 1986 Apr-Jun;16(2):413-6

[524] "In three cases the vasculitis relapsed following the introduction of food additives; in one case with the addition of potatoes and green vegetables (i.e., beans and green peas) and in the last case with the addition of eggs to the diet." Lunardi C, Bambara LM, Biasi D, Zagni P, Caramaschi P, Pacor ML. Elimination diet in the treatment of selected patients with hypersensitivity vasculitis. *Clin Exp Rheumatol*. 1992 Mar-Apr;10(2):131-5

[525] "Described in this report are two children with severe vasculitis caused by specific foods." Businco L, Falconieri P, Bellioni-Businco B, Bahna SL. Severe food-induced vasculitis in two children. *Pediatr Allergy Immunol*. 2002 Feb;13(1):68-71

[526] Hafstrom I, et al. A vegan diet free of gluten improves the signs and symptoms of rheumatoid arthritis: the effects on arthritis correlate with a reduction in antibodies to food antigens. *Rheumatology* (Oxford). 2001 Oct;40(10):1175-9 rheumatology.oxfordjournals.org/cgi/content/full/40/10/1175

[527] "When compared to the control group, the 11 patients of the allergic group presented a normal mannitol urinary excretion (16.5 +/- 13.4%, p = NS, Student's t-test) and an increase in the lactulose excretion (1.36 +/- 0.92%, p < 0.001). Moreover, the allergic group showed a lactulose/mannitol ratio that was significantly different (0.105 +/- 0.071, p < 0.001)." Laudat A, et al. The intestinal permeability test applied to the diagnosis of food allergy in paediatrics. *West Indian Med J*. 1994 Sep;43(3):87-8

[528] "After ingestion of food allergens by the patients, mean mannitol recovery fell to 11.57% and mean recovery of lactulose rose to 1.04%, both values being significantly different from those obtained in the fasting patients." Andre C, Andre F, Colin L, Cavagna S. Measurement of intestinal permeability to mannitol and lactulose as a means of diagnosing food allergy and evaluating therapeutic effectiveness of disodium cromoglycate. *Ann Allergy*. 1987 Nov;59(5 Pt 2):127-30

[529] "A provocation IPT with food induced significant L/M ratio changes only in the group in which the food was proved to be responsible for the exacerbation of skin lesions." Dupont C, Barau E, Molkhou P, Raynaud F, Barbet JP, Dehennin L. Food-induced alterations of intestinal permeability in children with cow's milk-sensitive enteropathy and atopic dermatitis. *J Pediatr Gastroenterol Nutr*. 1989 May;8(4):459-65

[530] Jyonouchi H, Sun S, Itokazu N. Innate immunity associated with inflammatory responses and cytokine production against common dietary proteins in patients with autism spectrum disorder. *Neuropsychobiology*. 2002;46(2):76-84

[531] "Thus, endotoxin and allergen acting together could play a role in up-regulating the response of the human asthmatic airway to adenosine. However, our data suggest that the interaction would be additive rather than synergistic." Karmouty Quintana H, Mazzoni L, Fozard JR. Effects of endotoxin and allergen alone and in combination on the sensitivity of the rat airways to adenosine. *Auton Autacoid Pharmacol*. 2005 Oct;25(4):167-70

[532] "Our findings firstly demonstrated that gliadin was directly bound to tTG in duodenal mucosa of coeliacs and controls, and the ability of circulating tTG-autoantibodies to recognize and immunoprecipitate the tTG-gliadin complexes." Ciccocioppo R, Di Sabatino A, Ara C, Biagi F, Perilli M, Amicosante G, Cifone MG, Corazza GR. Gliadin and tissue transglutaminase complexes in normal and coeliac duodenal mucosa. *Clin Exp Immunol*. 2003 Dec;134(3):516-24

[533] "Thus, modification of gluten peptides by tTG, especially deamidation of certain glutamine residues, can enhance their binding to HLA-DQ2 or -DQ8 and potentiate T cell stimulation. Furthermore, tTG-catalyzed cross-linking and consequent haptenization of gluten with extracellular matrix proteins allows for storage and extended availability of gluten in the mucosa." Dieterich W, Esslinger B, Schuppan D. Pathomechanisms in celiac disease. *Int Arch Allergy Immunol*. 2003 Oct;132(2):98-108

[534] "Gliadins alpha1-alpha11, gamma1- gamma6, omega1-omega3, and omega5 were substrates for tTG. tTG catalyzed the crosslinking of gliadin peptides with interstitial collagens type I, III and VI. Coeliac patients showed increased antibody titers against the collagens I, III, V and VI." Dieterich W, Esslinger B, Trapp D, Hahn E, Huff T, Seilmeier W, Wieser H, Schuppan D. Crosslinking to tissue transglutaminase and collagen favours gliadin toxicity in coeliac disease. *Gut*. 2005 Sep 27

[535] "Elevated titres of antithyroid antibodies observed in children with coeliac disease (41.1%) in comparison to control group (3.56%) indicate the need for performing the screening tests for antithyroid antibodies in children with CD." Kowalska E, Wasowska-Krolikowska K, Toporowska-Kowalska E. Estimation of antithyroid antibodies occurrence in children with coeliac disease. *Med Sci Monit*. 2000 Jul-Aug;6(4):719-2 medscimonit.com/pub/vol_6/no_4/1240.pdf

[536] Kieslich M, Errazuriz G, Posselt HG, Moeller-Hartmann W, Zanella F, Boehles H. Brain white-matter lesions in celiac disease: a prospective study of 75 diet-treated patients. *Pediatrics*. 2001 Aug;108(2):E21 pediatrics.aappublications.org/cgi/content/full/108/2/e21

and musculoskeletal system.[537] Given the association between lupus and celiac disease[538,539,540], we may speculate that allergy becomes systemic autoimmunity in certain circumstances and in susceptible patients.

- Review and proposal: Hapten exposure might predispose to atopic disease—the hapten-atopy hypothesis (*Trends Immunol* 2009 Feb[541] and SkinAndAllergyNews.com 2010 Oct[542]): Dr McFadden and his colleagues propose that **orally-consumed chemicals—commonly consumed as processed foods—bind to and alter endogenous proteins to result in hapten-protein neoantigens that stimulate immunologic disease, particularly allergic conditions** such as atopic dermatitis (eczema), asthma and seasonal respiratory allergies. Per an interview with Jancin, McFadden explained that "Haptens are low-molecular-weight organic chemicals that aren't allergenic on their own but can bind to a peptide or protein, thereby altering its configuration and rendering it foreign and allergenic. Examples of haptens include antibiotics and some other drugs, as well as chemicals present in toiletries, processed foods, powdered milk, preservatives used in vaccines, and metal jewelry. ... **Various brands of powdered milk contain a mean of 12 haptens each.** ... Also, epidemiologic studies show that certain maternal occupations predispose to the birth of atopic children. Among these occupations are hairdresser, beautician, cleaner, electroplater, bar staff, dental assistant, confectionary maker, and book binder. What these diverse occupations have in common is increased environmental exposure to haptens."

5. Dietary molecular mimicry: Just as microbes produce structures similar to human molecules which then incite a cross-reacting immune response—**molecular mimicry** (discussed elsewhere in this chapter in the section on dysbiosis)—certain dietary antigens appear capable of inducing cross reactions. For example, Vojdani et al[543] recently demonstrated **cross-reactivity between anti-gliadin antibodies and anti-cerebellar antibodies in an experimental model that may partly explain the anti-brain autoimmunity seen in autism.** Further expanding this concept of dietary molecular mimicry is the finding that "the virulence factor of C albicans-hyphal wall protein 1 (HWP1)-contains amino acid sequences that are identical or highly homologous to known coeliac disease-related alpha-gliadin and gamma-gliadin T-cell epitopes."[544] This raises three interrelated possibilities: 1) that gastrointestinal overgrowth of *Candida albicans* and the resultant elaboration of HWP1 and immunostimulation may result in sensitivity to gluten, particularly as HWP1 and gliadin are both substrates for transglutaminase, 2) that consumption of wheat gluten may trigger sensitivity to *Candida albicans*, and 3) that wheat gluten and *Candida albicans* must both be present for the development of celiac disease and the ensuant autoimmunity. Additional details on the ability of *C. albicans* to contribute to autoimmunity are discussed in the section on dysbiosis.

6. Enhanced processing of autoantigens: Food-allergic patients may produce autoimmunity-stimulating autoantigens following exposure to foods to which they are sensitized. This has been demonstrated in autistic children, **exposure of lymphocytes from autistic patients to dietary antigens (gliadin and casein peptides) stimulates production of autoantigens that presumably incite and perpetuate autoimmunity.**[545] Thus, at least in autistic patients, we have evidence that food allergy can segue into

---

[537] "JIA children have an increased prevalence of autoimmune thyroiditis, subclinical hypothyroidism and coeliac disease." Stagi S, Giani T, Simonini G, Falcini F. Thyroid function, autoimmune thyroiditis and coeliac disease in juvenile idiopathic arthritis. *Rheumatology* (Oxford). 2005 Apr;44(4):517-2

[538] Zitouni M, Daoud W, Kallel M, Makni S. Systemic lupus erythematosus with celiac disease: a report of five cases. *Joint Bone Spine.* 2004 Jul;71(4):344-6

[539] Komatireddy GR, Marshall JB, Aqel R, Spollen LE, Sharp GC. Association of systemic lupus erythematosus and gluten enteropathy. *South Med J.* 1995 Jun;88:673-6

[540] Rustgi AK, Peppercorn MA. Gluten-sensitive enteropathy and systemic lupus erythematosus. *Arch Intern Med.* 1988 Jul;148(7):1583-4

[541] McFadden JP, et al. Does hapten exposure predispose to atopic disease? The hapten-atopy hypothesis. *Trends Immunol.* 2009 Feb;30(2):67-74

[542] Article by Bruce Jancin of the Skin & Allergy News Digital Network; interview with Dr. John P. McFadden. Expert Analysis from the Annual Congress of the European Academy of Dermatology and Venereology: Exploring the Hapten Hypothesis of Atopic Disease. skinandallergynews.com/news/medical-dermatology/single-article/eadv-exploring-the-hapten-hypothesis-of-atopic-disease/e7df2851ed.html Posted 10/26/10 and accessed May 31, 2011.

[543] "This cross-reaction was further confirmed by DOT-immunoblot and inhibition studies. We conclude that a subgroup of patients with autism produce antibodies against Purkinje cells and gliadin peptides, which may be responsible for some of the neurological symptoms in autism." Vojdani A, O'Bryan T, Green JA, Mccandless J, Woeller KN, Vojdani E, Nourian AA, Cooper EL. Immune response to dietary proteins, gliadin and cerebellar peptides in children with autism. *Nutr Neurosci.* 2004 Jun;7:151-61

[544] "Subsequently, C albicans might function as an adjuvant that stimulates antibody formation against HWP1 and gluten, and formation of autoreactive antibodies against tissue transglutaminase and endomysium." Nieuwenhuizen WF, et al. Is Candida albicans a trigger in the onset of coeliac disease? *Lancet.* 2003;361(9375):2152-4

[545] Vojdani A, Pangborn JB, Vojdani E, Cooper EL. Infections, toxic chemicals and dietary peptides binding to lymphocyte receptors and tissue enzymes are major instigators of autoimmunity in autism. *Int J Immunopathol Pharmacol.* 2003 Sep-Dec;16(3):189-99

autoimmunity. This phenomenon is probably not restricted only to autistic patients, as suggested by the association between celiac disease and the systemic autoimmune disease lupus.[546,547,548]

7. <u>Diet-derived xenobiotic immunotoxicity</u>: Foods commonly contain trace amounts of xenobiotics such as pesticides, fungicides, fumigants, fertilizers, preservatives, military propellants such as perchlorate[549], and toxic metals such as mercury. Some of these xenobiotics have been insufficiently studied in humans, while others such as mercury are well-known immunotoxins capable of inducing immune dysfunction which may contribute to autoimmunity. **Mercury poisoning/accumulation can occur in humans as a result of consumption of contaminated foods—especially seafood such as shark, swordfish, king mackerel, tilefish, and albacore ("white") tuna**[550], and the immunologic effects of organic and/or inorganic mercury include immunosuppression, immunostimulation, formation of antinucleolar antibodies targeting fibrillarin, and formation and deposition of immune-complexes, resulting in a syndrome called "mercury-induced autoimmunity" which can be induced by exposure of susceptible animals to mercury.[551] Mercury/"silver" amalgam dental fillings rank highly among the most significant source of mercury exposure in humans, and **implantation of mercury-silver dental amalgams in susceptible animals causes chronic stimulation of the immune system with induction of systemic autoimmunity.**[552] Besides being **a neurotoxin with no safe exposure limit**[553]**, mercury is known to modify/antigenize endogenous proteins to promote autoimmunity**[554], and **mercury may also promote autoimmunity by contributing to a pro-inflammatory environment that awakens quiescent autoreactive immunocytes via bystander activation**[555] (detailed later). For example, administration of mercury to "susceptible" mice induces autoimmunity via modification of the nucleolar protein *fibrillarin*[556]; noteworthy in this regard is the fact that antifibrillarin antibodies are characteristic of the autoimmune disease **scleroderma**.[557] Mercury toxicity is commonly encountered in clinical practice (diagnosis and treatment are discussed later), and a recent study published in *JAMA* showed that 8% of American women of childbearing age have sufficient levels of mercury in their bodies to produce neurologic damage in their children.[558] **The mercury-based preservative thimerosol is a type-IV (delayed hypersensitivity) sensitizing agent**[559]**, and recent research implicates mercury as an important contributor to the clinical manifestations of autism**[560,561] **and eczema.**[562] Preliminary clinical evidence shows that removal of mercury amalgams, particularly along with

---

[546] Zitouni M, Daoud W, Kallel M, Makni S. Systemic lupus erythematosus with celiac disease: a report of five cases. *Joint Bone Spine*. 2004 Jul;71(4):344-6

[547] Komatireddy GR, Marshall JB, Aqel R, Spollen LE, Sharp GC. Association of systemic lupus erythematosus and gluten enteropathy. *South Med J*. 1995 Jun;88:673-6

[548] Rustgi AK, Peppercorn MA. Gluten-sensitive enteropathy and systemic lupus erythematosus. *Arch Intern Med*. 1988 Jul;148(7):1583-4

[549] "The Bush administration has imposed a gag order on the U.S. Environmental Protection Agency from publicly discussing perchlorate pollution, even as two new studies reveal high levels of the rocket-fuel component may be contaminating the nation's lettuce supply." Peter Waldman. Rocket Fuel Residues Found in Lettuce: Bush administration issues gag order on EPA discussions of possible rocket fuel tainted lettuce. *Wall Street Journal*. See organicconsumers.org/toxic/lettuce042903.cfm, rhinoed.com/epa's_gag_order.htm, peer.org/press/508.html yubanet.com/artman/publish/article_13637.shtml

[550] Note cfsan.fda.gov/~dms/admehg3.html for the white-washed version; see ewg.org/issues/mercury/20040319/index.php for a more accurate and complete perspective.

[551] Havarinasab S, Hultman P. Organic mercury compounds and autoimmunity. *Autoimmun Rev*. 2005;4(5):270-5 generationrescue.org/pdf/havarinasab.pdf

[552] "We hypothesize that under appropriate conditions of genetic susceptibility and adequate body burden, heavy metal exposure from dental amalgam may contribute to immunological aberrations, which could lead to overt autoimmunity." Hultman P, Johansson U, Turley SJ, Lindh U, Enestrom S, Pollard KM. Adverse immunological effects and autoimmunity induced by dental amalgam and alloy in mice. *FASEB J*. 1994 Nov;8(14):1183-90 fasebj.org/cgi/reprint/8/14/1183

[553] University of Calgary Faculty of Medicine. How Mercury Causes Brain Neuron Degeneration commons.ucalgary.ca/mercury/

[554] Havarinasab S, Hultman P. Organic mercury compounds and autoimmunity. *Autoimmun Rev*. 2005 Jun;4(5):270-5

[555] "It is therefore theoretically possible that compounds present in vaccines such as thiomersal or aluminium hydroxyde can trigger autoimmune reactions through bystander effects." Fournie GJ, et al. Induction of autoimmunity through bystander effects: immunological disorders induced by heavy metals. *J Autoimmun*. 2001 May;16(3):319-26

[556] Nielsen JB, Hultman P. Mercury-induced autoimmunity in mice. *Environ Health Perspect*. 2002 Oct;110 Suppl 5:877-81

[557] "Since anti-fibrillarin antibodies are specific markers of scleroderma, the present animal model may be valuable for studies of the immunological aberrations which are likely to induce this autoimmune response." Hultman P, Enestrom S, Pollard KM, Tan EM. Anti-fibrillarin autoantibodies in mercury-treated mice. *Clin Exp Immunol*. 1989 Dec;78:470-7

[558] "However, approximately 8% of women had concentrations higher than the US Environmental Protection Agency's recommended reference dose (5.8 microg/L), below which exposures are considered to be without adverse effects. Women who are pregnant or who intend to become pregnant should follow federal and state advisories on consumption of fish." Schober SE, et al. Blood mercury levels in US children and women of childbearing age, 1999-2000. *JAMA*. 2003 Apr 2;289(13):1667-74

[559] "Thimerosal is an important preservative in vaccines and ophthalmologic preparations. The substance is known to be a type IV sensitizing agent. High sensitization rates were observed in contact-allergic patients and in health care workers who had been exposed to thimerosal-preserved vaccines." Westphal GA, et al. Homozygous gene deletions of the glutathione S-transferases M1 and T1 are associated with thimerosal sensitization. *Int Arch Occup Environ Health*. 2000 Aug;73(6):384-8

[560] Vojdani A, Pangborn JB, Vojdani E, Cooper EL. Infections, toxic chemicals and dietary peptides binding to lymphocyte receptors and tissue enzymes are major instigators of autoimmunity in autism. *Int J Immunopathol Pharmacol*. 2003 Sep-Dec;16(3):189-99

[561] Geier DA, Geier MR. A comparative evaluation of the effects of MMR immunization and mercury doses from thimerosal-containing childhood vaccines on the population prevalence of autism. *Med Sci Monit*. 2004 Mar;10(3):PI33-9. Epub 2004 Mar 1. medscimonit.com/pub/vol_10/no_3/3986.pdf

[562] Weidinger S, Kramer U, Dunemann L, Mohrenschlager M, Ring J, Behrendt H. Body burden of mercury is associated with acute atopic eczema and total IgE in children from southern Germany. *J Allergy Clin Immunol*. 2004 Aug;114(2):457-9

implementation of antioxidant therapy and/or mercury chelation, benefits the biochemical status and/or clinical course of autoimmune disease.[563,564]

8. <u>Diet-derived dysbiosis</u>: Induction and exacerbation of dysbiosis following chronic consumption of allergenic foods has been reported to occur in humans. Raw vegetables and salad greens are thoroughly contaminated with bacteria and occasionally other microbes. Food can be contaminated with pathogenic microbes via improper preparation, storage, or handling by chefs with contagious diseases and poor hygiene. An inflammatory "reactive" arthritis can result from consumption of food that is contaminated by microorganisms, most commonly *Salmonella*[565,566,567] and *Campylobacter* species.[568] Long-term autoimmune/inflammatory complications of gastrointestinal infections/colonization sourced from food include Reiter's syndrome, Guillian-Barre syndrome (peripheral nerve autoimmunity), uveitis, sacroiliitis, and ankylosing spondylitis.

9. <u>Diet-derived immunodysregulation</u>: Certain foods contain constituents that cause immune dysfunction and the induction or exacerbation of autoimmunity. L-Canavanine sulfate is a non-protein amino acid found in alfalfa sprouts which triggers a condition similar to systemic lupus erythematosus in monkeys[569,570] and which may exacerbate SLE in humans.

10. <u>Dietary xenobiotics</u>: Artificial sweeteners, thickeners, flavor enhancers, emulsifiers, and plasticizers can be found in foods, particularly those which are manufactured and processed. Some of these chemicals have the potential to alter immune mechanisms in favor of autoimmunity. These dietary xenobiotics may be particularly relevant for initiating and promoting Crohn's disease.[571]

11. <u>Immunogenicity induced by cooking—the Maillard reaction (non-enzymatic glycosylation)</u>: Heated exposure of lysine, arginine, and tryptophan to reducing sugars such as fructose and lactose results in the non-enzymatic binding (glycosylation) of the sugar with the amino acid. If the amino acid is a component of a protein, then the structure and antigenicity of the protein is altered as it is now a glycoprotein, which may either serve as a neoantigen or may increase the allergenicity of a protein that was previously hypoallergenic, as seen with the roasting of peanuts.[572,573] Glycoproteins formed from the baking and browning of foods are also called ***glycotoxins*** and are capable of exacerbating inflammation in patients with diabetes.[574] Similar to the formation of **glycotoxins** is the formation of **acrylamide**, a possible carcinogen, in fried and baked foods.

[563] Prochazkova J, Sterzl I, Kucerova H, Bartova J, Stejskal VD. The beneficial effect of amalgam replacement on health in patients with autoimmunity. *Neuro Endocrinol Lett.* 2004 Jun;25(3):211-8. See also: "The MELISA Test is reproducible, sensitive, specific, and reliable for detecting metal sensitivity in metal-sensitive patients." Valentine-Thon E, Schiwara HW. Validity of MELISA for metal sensitivity testing. *Neuro Endocrinol Lett.* 2003 Feb-Apr;24(1-2):57-64. See also: "The hypothesis that metal exposure from dental amalgam can cause ill health in a susceptible part of the exposed population was supported." Lindh U, et al. Removal of dental amalgam and other metal alloys supported by antioxidant therapy alleviates symptoms and improves quality of life in patients with amalgam-associated ill health. *Neuro Endocrinol Lett.* 2002 Oct-Dec;23(5-6):459-82 nel.edu/23_56/NEL235602A12_Lindh.htm and nel.edu/pdf_w/23_56/NEL235602A12_Lindh_wr.pdf

[564] "This study documents objective biochemical changes following the removal of these fillings along with other dental materials, utilizing a new health care model of multidisciplinary planning and treatment." Huggins HA, Levy TE. Cerebrospinal fluid protein changes in multiple sclerosis after dental amalgam removal. *Altern Med Rev.* 1998 Aug;3(4):295-300 thorne.com/altmedrev/.fulltext/3/4/295.pdf

[565] "We describe the case of a patient who became ill with Salmonella Blockley food poisoning while working in Cyprus in August 1994. As his diarrhoea resolved he began to suffer from lower limb joint pains which were diagnosed as acute salmonella reactive arthritis." Wilson IG, Whitehead E. Long-term post-Salmonella reactive arthritis due to Salmonella Blockley. *Jpn J Infect Dis.* 2004 Oct;57(5):210-1

[566] "Reactive joint symptoms after food-borne Salmonella infection may be more frequent than previously thought. The duration of diarrhea is strongly correlated with the occurrence of joint symptoms." Locht H, et al. High frequency of reactive joint symptoms after an outbreak of Salmonella enteritidis. *J Rheumatol.* 2002 Apr;29(4):767-71

[567] Leirisalo-Repo M, et al. Long-term prognosis of reactive salmonella arthritis. *Ann Rheum Dis.* 1997 Sep;56(9):516-20

[568] "Campylobacter jejuni is the most commonly reported bacterial cause of foodborne infection in the United States. Adding to the human and economic costs are chronic sequelae associated with C. jejuni infection--Guillian-Barre syndrome and reactive arthritis." Altekruse SF, Stern NJ, Fields PI, Swerdlow DL. Campylobacter jejuni--an emerging foodborne pathogen. *Emerg Infect Dis.* 1999 Jan-Feb;5(1):28-35

[569] "L-Canavanine sulfate, a constituent of alfalfa sprouts, was incorporated into the diet and reactivated the syndrome in monkeys in which an SLE-like syndrome had previously been induced by the ingestion of alfalfa seeds or sprouts." Malinow MR, Bardana EJ Jr, Pirofsky B, Craig S, McLaughlin P. Systemic lupus erythematosus-like syndrome in monkeys fed alfalfa sprouts: role of a nonprotein amino acid. *Science.* 1982 Apr 23;216(4544):415-7

[570] "Occurrence of autoimmune hemolytic anemia and exacerbation of SLE have been linked to ingestion of alfalfa tablets containing L-canavanine." Alcocer-Varela J, et al. Effects of L-canavanine on T cells may explain the induction of systemic lupus erythematosus by alfalfa. *Arthritis Rheum.* 1985 Jan;28(1):52-7

[571] "Various food additives, especially emulsifiants, thickeners, surface-finishing agents and contaminants like plasticizers share structural domains with mycobacterial lipids. It is therefore hypothesized, that these compounds are able to stimulate by molecular mimicry the CD1 system in the gastrointestinal mucosa and to trigger the pro-inflammatory cytokine cascade." Traunmuller F. Etiology of Crohn's disease: Do certain food additives cause intestinal inflammation by molecular mimicry of mycobacterial lipids? *Med Hypotheses.* 2005;65(5):859-64

[572] "Roasted peanuts exhibited a higher level of IgE binding, which was correlated with a higher level of AGE adducts. We concluded that there is an association between AGE adducts and increased IgE binding (i.e., allergenicity) of roasted peanuts." Chung SY, Champagne ET. Association of end-product adducts with increased IgE binding of roasted peanuts. *J Agric Food Chem.* 2001 Aug;49(8):3911-6

[573] "The data presented here indicate that thermal processing may play an important role in enhancing the allergenic properties of peanuts and that the protein modifications made by the Maillard reaction contribute to this effect." Maleki SJ, Chung SY, Champagne ET, Raufman JP.The effects of roasting on the allergenic properties of peanut proteins. *J Allergy Clin Immunol.* 2000 Oct;106(4):763-8

[574] "A study now reveals that the consumption of foods rich in browned and oxidized products (so-called glycotoxins) induces a chronic inflammatory state in diabetic individuals." Monnier VM, Obrenovich ME. Wake up and smell the maillard reaction. *Sci Aging Knowledge Environ.* 2002 Dec 18;2002(50):pe21

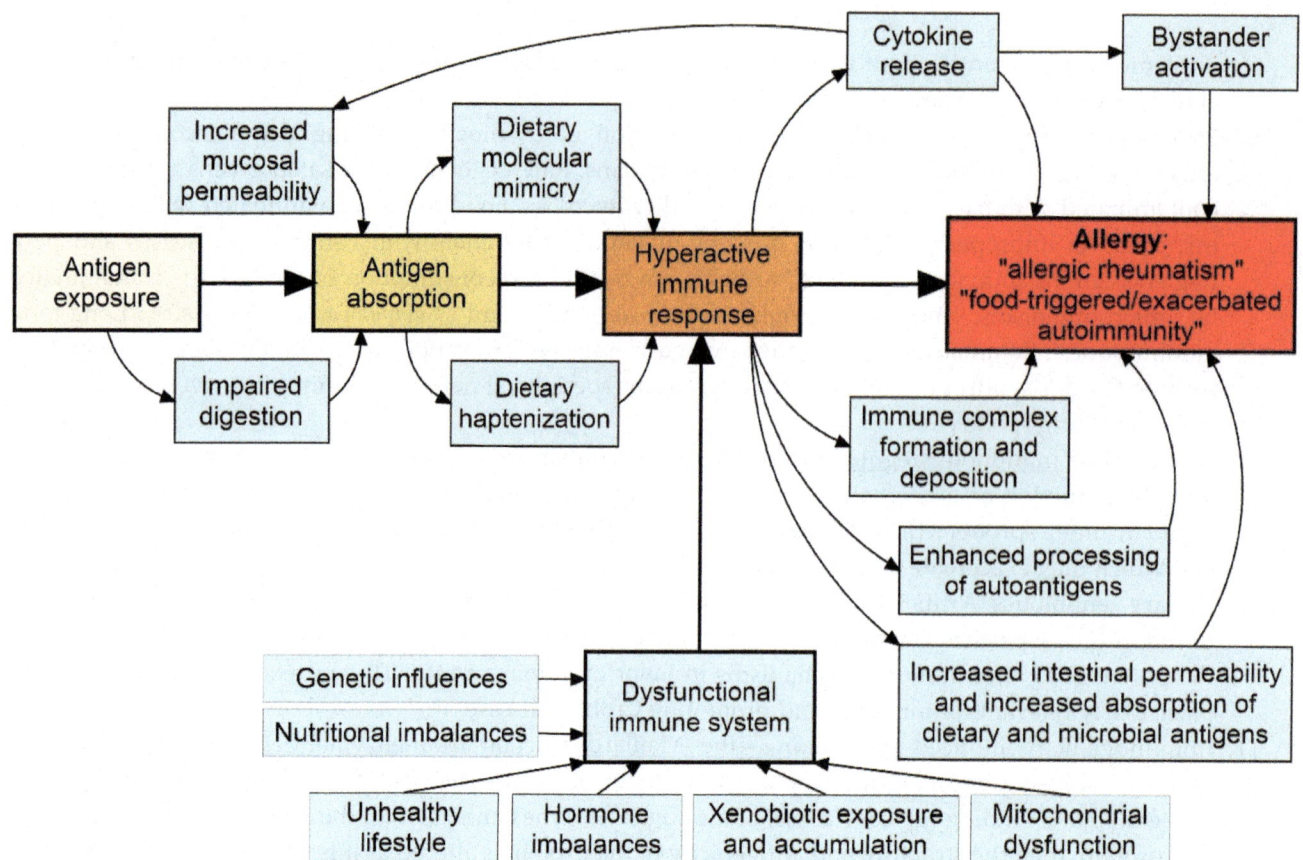

Approaching a More Comprehensive Understanding of "Food Allergy" and Its Contribution to Immune Dysfunction and Musculoskeletal Inflammation: Useful as an example of a more profound understanding of "allergy", this diagram is self-explanatory.

Common allergy treatments advocated by the pharmaceutical industry create an overly simplistic and inaccurate view of the allergic process which obfuscates the identification and correction of the underlying processes, only two of which are antigen exposure and histamine release. Nutritionally-oriented doctors, too, often emphasize the identification and elimination of allergen exposure as the sole means of addressing allergic diathesis with the presumption that allergen avoidance cures the allergy. These simplistic models and the incomplete treatments based upon them fail to address the underlying cause of the allergic phenomenon: immune dysfunction. Allergic manifestations always require at least two factors: 1) exposure of the antigen to the immune system (antigen absorption) and 2) a dysfunctional immune system that "overreacts" to the otherwise benign antigen. Allergy treatment that fails to address the underlying immune dysfunction is incomplete. Allergy treatment that addresses the underlying immune dysfunction has the opportunity to correct the *total problem*, rather than merely reducing the manifestations of the problem. Therefore, treatment of the allergic diathesis must always address issues of antigen exposure, antigen absorption, *and the dysfunctional immune system* that results in the hyperactive immune response that we call "allergy." Elimination of either antigen exposure or antigen absorption eliminates allergic manifestations, but does not necessarily correct the underlying immune defect(s). Complete correction of the underlying immune defect obviates the need for the identification and avoidance of the allergen. In clinical practice, a combination of both approaches—allergen avoidance and immune modulation—is the most effective approach, affording relatively high effectiveness in symptom reduction even with only modest compliance.

Orthomolecular Immunomodulation: The Author's Approach to Alleviating Allergy
My clinical approach to improving immune function in patients with allergy begins with supplementation of vitamin E, CoQ-10, vitamin B-12, vitamin C, bioflavonoids, honey, and fish oil. Thereafter, I look at hormones, particularly DHEA, estrogen (quantitative and qualitative), testosterone, and cortisol. I also look at diet and bowel health with respect to putrefaction and intestinal permeability. Although rarely powerful when used in isolation,

these treatments when used in combinations tailored to the individual patient often result in an impressive reduction in allergic manifestations even when allergen avoidance is either not pursued or not feasible. The process of alleviating allergic disorders is, however, arduous and time-consuming unless the doctor uses a group of protocols such as those described herein which address the most common contributing factors to allergic problems. Here I extend my previous three-step process[575] into a four-tiered approach, with the fourth step including selected pharmaceutical drugs.

Step 1: From initial patient assessment to the first phase of treatment

In a patient with presumed "allergy" who is in otherwise good health, following a basic health assessment and exclusion of significant disease, I begin by correcting problems that are common to patients with allergy. Minor improvements in allergy symptoms as a result of a low-cost low-risk interventions can be multiplied with a specified group of interventions; we aim for a modest improvement with several treatments rather than a "silver bullet" miracle cure with a single intervention. For example, 10% improvement in symptoms may be insignificant in itself; however a 10% improvement from six interventions results in a 60% improvement and enhances patient confidence long enough for other interventions and assessments to be implemented, if necessary. The goal with the first step of treatment is to correct the most common and most likely problems, namely fatty acid imbalances, micronutrient deficiencies, phytonutrient insufficiencies, and dysbiosis.

- Avoidance of suspected food allergens: The most common allergens are wheat, cow's milk, and eggs; however any patient can be allergic to any food. It is not uncommon for patients to have to avoid up to 10 foods before attaining maximal improvement, and up to 85% of migraine patients can be cured of their headaches by the use of allergy avoidance alone.[576] Food allergy avoidance for 1 month helps achieve symptomatic relief and allows the gut to heal and the immune system to recalibrate. The diet should emphasize consumption of lean meats, fruits, vegetables, nuts, seeds, and berries to ensure a systemic anti-inflammatory effect and increased consumption of anti-inflammatory phytonutrients, especially flavonoids. High-glycemic foods are avoided as are "food additives" such as tartrazine, which is known to exacerbate allergic asthma. Some foods like tuna, certain cheeses and wines are high in histamine; frequent consumption of these foods by an allergic individual is analogous to adding fuel to a fire that the patient is simultaneously trying to extinguish. Recall that in breast-feeding infants, the mother will have to consume a hypoallergenic diet to prevent passage of allergens[577] and allergen-antibody immune complexes[578] in breast milk.
- Rotation diet: While select foods should be completely avoided, the remaining foods that are consumed should be rotated in and out of the diet with a periodicity of 3-5 days. Patients should avoid "dietary monotony"[579] by consuming a variety of foods. By rotating different foods in and out of the diet, patients are more likely to consume a nutritious diet and are less likely to develop or perpetuate food allergies.
- Probiotics: Supplementation with probiotics (beneficial strains of bacteria and yeast) appears to improve intestinal barrier function, promote microecological balance in the gastrointestinal tract, modulate immune function—specifically by inducing the Treg phenotype, and thus reduce manifestations of allergic disease.[580,581,582]

---

[575] Vasquez A. Improving neuromusculoskeletal health by optimizing immune function and reducing allergic reactions. *Nutritional Perspectives* 2005; October: 27-35, 40

[576] Grant EC. Food allergies and migraine. *Lancet*. 1979 May 5;1(8123):966-9

[577] "In all, clinical disappearance of symptoms was observed after removal of milk from the mother's diet and/or elimination from the child's diet of any cow's-milk-based hypoallergenic formula." Barau E, Dupont C. Allergy to cow's milk proteins in mother's milk or in hydrolyzed cow's milk infant formulas as assessed by intestinal permeability measurements. *Allergy*. 1994 Apr;49(4):295-8

[578] The finding of egg-allergen immune complex in breast milk inplies 1) egg protein escapes complete digestion/degradation in the gastrointestinal tract, 2) egg protein is absorbed intact through the mucosa, 3) egg protein escapes filtration by the liver, 4) egg protein stimulates formation IgA immune complexes, and 5) egg-IgA immune complexes are secreted in milk which would then expose the infant to both allergen and immune complex, possibly resulting in clinical disease. Hirose J, et al. Occurrence of the major food allergen, ovomucoid, in human breast milk as an immune complex. *Biosci Biotechnol Biochem*. 2001 Jun;65(6):1438-40

[579] Pelchat ML, Schaefer S. Dietary monotony and food cravings in young and elderly adults. *Physiol Behav*. 2000 Jan;68(3):353-9

[580] Majamaa H, Isolauri E. Probiotics: a novel approach in the management of food allergy. *J Allergy Clin Immunol* 1997 Feb;99(2):179-85

[581] von der Weid T, Ibnou-Zekri N, Pfeifer A. Novel probiotics for the management of allergic inflammation. *Dig Liver Dis*. 2002 Sep;34 Suppl 2:S25-8

[582] "The administration of probiotics, strains of bacteria from the healthy human gut microbiota, have been shown to stimulate antiinflammatory, tolerogenic immune responses, the lack of which has been implied in the development of atopic disorders. Thus probiotics may prove beneficial in the prevention and alleviation of allergic disease." Rautava S, Isolauri E. The development of gut immune responses and gut microbiota: effects of probiotics in prevention and treatment of allergic disease. *Curr Issues Intest Microbiol*. 2002 Mar;3(1):15-22

- Vitamin C: A recent clinical trial showed that 2 grams per day of ascorbic acid reduced blood histamine levels by 38%.[583] Cathcart hypothesized that high doses of vitamin C (i.e., bowel tolerance) may impair the adsorption of IgE with allergens and thus retard the allergic cascade from being initiated.[584] Either of these two mechanisms, perhaps in addition to other mechanisms, may explain the anti-allergy effects of ascorbic acid.[585]

- CoQ-10: CoQ-10 levels are low in approximately 40% of patients with allergies, according to a small study conducted by Folkers and Pfeiffer.[586] Asthmatics also have lower levels of CoQ-10 compared to healthy people.[587] In my experience, clinical improvement is commonly seen in allergic patients after supplementation with CoQ-10. I generally prescribe 100-300mg/day of CoQ-10 for adults.

> **CoQ-10 for allergy treatment**
> The mechanisms involved with this benefit are likely mediated primarily via improved mitochondrial function which ultimately manifests as reduced inflammation, oxidant stress, and enhanced Treg formation, as well as direct inhibition of NFkB by CoQ-10.

- Vitamin E: Vitamin E has been shown to reduce IgE levels in humans and to reduce the manifestations of allergy-related disease.[588] I commonly prescribe 800-2,000 IU per day of mixed tocopherols with approximately 40% gamma tocopherol for patients with allergy.

- Bioflavonoids: Bioflavonoids stabilize mast cell membranes and thus reduce the liberation of histamine. Additionally, quercetin and catechin inhibit the action of histidine decarboxylase, which converts histidine into histamine. Many fruits, vegetables, and herbal teas are excellent sources of flavonoids, which can also be consumed in the form of tablets and capsules.

- Vitamin B-12: Vitamin B-12 has been shown to reduce physiologic manifestations of allergy in ovalbumin-sensitized mice.[589] Since vitamin B-12 is safe, non-toxic, and bioavailable when administered orally in large doses to humans, I commonly prescribe 2,500-5,000 mcg per day for allergic patients for a one-month trial. Although the benefit of vitamin B-12 in patients with sulfite-sensitive asthma is biochemically mediated rather than immunologically mediated[590], this research adds tangential support to the use of high-dose vitamin B-12 in selected patients with allergy (particularly asthma), at least for a short-term clinical trial. Hydroxocobalamin and methylcobalamin are preferred over cyanocobalamin due to the content of cyanide in the latter.[591]

Step 2: Additional interventions for moderate or unresponsive allergies: For patients who do not respond sufficiently to the first phase of treatment, the following interventions can be considered.

- Pancreatic and proteolytic enzymes: Pancreatic enzymes have been shown to alleviate symptoms of food allergy in a controlled clinical trial.[592] Administration of enzyme preparations can alleviate intestinal and extra-intestinal manifestations of food allergy.[593] Proteolytic enzymes are safe and effective for the relief of musculoskeletal pain, as reviewed later in this text and elsewhere.[594] When taken with food, pancreatic/proteolytic enzymes facilitate hydrolysis of proteins, fats, and carbohydrates and are then absorbed into the systemic circulation for an anti-inflammatory effect. Although individual enzymes may be used in isolation, enzyme therapy is generally delivered in the form of polyenzyme preparations containing pancreatin, bromelain, papain, amylase, lipase, trypsin and alpha-chymotrypsin.

- NFkB inhibitors: The clinical significance of NFkB and its phytonutritional modulation is detailed later in this book and elsewhere.[595] Nutrients that can be used to downregulate inflammatory responses are vitamin

[583] "Chemotaxis was inversely correlated to blood histamine (r = -0.32, p = 0.045), and, compared to baseline and withdrawal values, histamine levels were depressed 38% following VC supplementation. ... These data indicate that VC may indirectly enhance chemotaxis by detoxifying histamine in vivo." Johnston CS, Martin LJ, Cai X. Antihistamine effect of supplemental ascorbic acid and neutrophil chemotaxis. *J Am Coll Nutr*. 1992 Apr;11(2):172-6

[584] "Allergic and sensitivity reactions are frequently ameliorated and sometimes completely blocked by massive doses of ascorbate. I now hypothesize that one mechanism in blocking of allergic symptoms is the reducing of the disulfide bonds between the chains in antibody molecules making their bonding antigen impossible." Cathcart RF 3rd. The vitamin C treatment of allergy and the normally unprimed state of antibodies. *Med Hypotheses*. 1986 Nov;21(3):307-21

[585] Bucca C, Rolla G, Oliva A, Farina JC. Effect of vitamin C on histamine bronchial responsiveness of patients with allergic rhinitis. *Ann Allergy*. 1990 Oct;65(4):311-4

[586] Ye CQ, et al. A modified determination of coenzyme Q10 in human blood and CoQ10 blood levels in diverse patients with allergies. *Biofactors*. 1988 Dec;1(4):303-6

[587] Gazdik F, et al. Decreased levels of coenzyme Q(10) in patients with bronchial asthma. *Allergy*. 2002 Sep;57(9):811-4

[588] Tsoureli-Nikita E, et al. Evaluation of dietary intake of vitamin E in the treatment of atopic dermatitis. *Int J Dermatol*. 2002 Mar;41(3):146-50

[589] "We infer that Cbl administration significantly reduced the IL-2 concentration, and secondarily the IL-4, IgE and histamine concentrations." Funada U, Wada M, Kawata T, Tanaka N, Tadokoro T, Maekawa A. Effect of cobalamin on the allergic response in mice. *Biosci Biotechnol Biochem* 2000 Oct;64(10):2053-8

[590] Anibarro B, et al. Asthma with sulfite intolerance in children: a blocking study with cyanocobalamin. *J Allergy Clin Immunol*. 1992 Jul;90(1):103-9

[591] Freeman AG. Cyanocobalamin--a case for withdrawal: discussion paper. *J R Soc Med*. 1992 Nov;85(11):686-7

[592] Raithel M, Weidenhiller M, Schwab D, Winterkamp S, Hahn EG. Pancreatic enzymes: a new group of antiallergic drugs? *Inflamm Res*. 2002 Apr;51 Suppl 1:S13-4

[593] Gaby AR. Pancreatic enzymes block food allergy reactions. *Townsend Letter for Doctors and Patients* townsendletter.com/Nov_2002/gabyliteraturereview1102.htm

[594] Vasquez A. Improving overall health while safely and effectively treating musculoskeletal pain. *Nutritional Perspectives* 2005; 28: 34-38, 40-42

[595] Vasquez A. Nutritional and botanical inhibition of NFkB, the major intracellular amplifier of the inflammatory cascade. *Nutritional Perspectives*, July 2005:5-12.

D, curcumin (requires piperine for absorption), lipoic acid, green tea, rosemary, grape seed extract, propolis, resveratrol, selenium, zinc, and N-acetyl-cysteine.

- <u>Eradication of harmful intestinal yeast, bacteria, and other "parasites"</u>: I have seen several patients become cured of their "allergies" once we eradicated the dysbiotic bacteria, yeast, amoebas, or other microorganisms from their gastrointestinal tract. Intestinal colonization with harmful bacteria/yeast/protozoa/amebas can cause mucosal injury and result in macromolecular absorption and thus promotes immune sensitization to dietary antigens; in these situations, correction of dysbiosis via eradication of harmful microorganisms can lead to an impressive reduction in food-associated allergic phenomena. Although many indirect mechanisms will be discussed later, the most direct means by which dysbiosis may contribute to "allergy" is via endogenous formation of histamine via bacterial histidine decarboxylase. Galland and Lee[596] reported that eradication of *Giardia lamblia* in patients with chronic digestive complaints lessened the severity of food intolerance/allergy in 54% of patients. The supremely important topic of gastrointestinal dysbiosis is detailed later in this chapter.

<u>Step 3: Treatment for severe allergies</u>: For some patients with severe allergies, we start with selected treatments from Step 2 or Step 3 on the first visit *in addition to* the treatments included in Step 1. Implementation is customized based on history, examination, laboratory findings, and the doctor's experience and good judgment.

- <u>Calcium and magnesium butyrate</u>: Butyrate is a short-chain fatty acid which can be obtained from 1) a limited number of foods, namely butter, 2) intestinal fermentation of carbohydrates by probiotic bacteria, and 3) use of nutritional supplements. It is increasingly well-established that probiotic bacteria have immune-normalizing and "anti-allergy" effects, and this benefit is probably mediated at least in part by probiotic production of butyrate. The mechanisms of the anti-allergy effect of butyrate are manifold, and as a fatty acid butyrate activates peroxisome-proliferator activated receptor-alpha (PPAR-alpha) and thereby results in an immunomodulatory action and a suppressive effect on NFkB.[597,598] Butyrate is also a primary fuel for enterocytes and may improve enterocyte metabolism for the normalization of intestinal permeability. In the treatment of patients with inflammatory bowel disease, 4 grams per day of orally administered butyrate salts safely improves the action of mesalamine[599] as does topical application of butyrate in distal ulcerative colitis.[600] As a normal dietary component and product of the gastrointestinal tract, supplemental calcium and magnesium salts of butyrate are safe and effective for human consumption at doses of 1,000 – 4,500 mg butyrate per day for the alleviation of allergic diseases.[601,602]
- <u>Purified chondroitin sulfate and glucosamine sulfate</u>: Doctors and patients everywhere should already know that chondroitin sulfate and glucosamine sulfate are safe and effective for the treatment of osteoarthritis. Furthermore, purified chondroitin sulfate is cardioprotective and that it helps to reduce the vessel occlusion characteristic of atherosclerosis.[603] Additionally, new experimental evidence shows that chondroitin sulfate and glucosamine sulfate can inhibit allergic reactions.[604] With this in mind, it is reasonable to speculate that many arthritic patients who respond to glucosamine and chondroitin may actually be responding to the anti-allergy benefits of chondroitin and glucosamine *rather than* or *in addition to* the "cartilage building" properties of these supplements. Furthermore, there is evidence that purified chondroitin sulfate can act as a "decoy" and reduce adhesion of harmful bacteria; the role of harmful gastrointestinal bacteria in the genesis and perpetuation of joint pain and inflammation will be discussed in the next article in this series. For now, it will suffice to say that occult gastrointestinal infections (i.e., gastrointestinal dysbiosis) are a major contributor to the systemic pain and inflammation seen in conditions such as rheumatoid arthritis and ankylosing spondylitis.

[596] Galland L, Lee M. Abstract #170 High frequency of giardiasis in patients with chronic digestive complaints. *Am J Gastroenterol* 1989;84:1181
[597] Zapolska-Downar D, Siennicka A, Kaczmarczyk M, Kolodziej B, Naruszewicz M. Butyrate inhibits cytokine-induced VCAM-1 and ICAM-1 expression in cultured endothelial cells: the role of NFkB and PPARalpha. *J Nutr Biochem.* 2004 Apr;15(4):220-8
[598] Luhrs H, et al. Butyrate inhibits NFkB activation in lamina propria macrophages of patients with ulcerative colitis. *Scand J Gastroenterol.* 2002 Apr;37(4):458-66
[599] Vernia P, et al. Combined oral sodium butyrate and mesalazine treatment compared to oral mesalazine alone in ulcerative colitis. *Dig Dis Sci.* 2000 May;45:976-81
[600] Vernia P, et al. Topical butyrate improves efficacy of 5-ASA in refractory distal ulcerative colitis: results of a multicentre trial. *Eur J Clin Invest.* 2003 Mar;33(3):244-8
[601] Neesby TE. Method for desensitizing the gastrointestinal tract from food allergies. United States Patent 4,721,716. January 26, 1988
[602] Neesby TE. Method for desensitizing the gastrointestinal tract from food allergies. United States Patent 4,735,967. April 5, 1988
[603] Morrison LM, Enrick N. Coronary heart disease: reduction of death rate by chondroitin sulfate A. *Angiology.* 1973 May;24(5):269-87
[604] Theoharides TC, Bielory L. Mast cells and mast cell mediators as targets of dietary supplements. *Ann Allergy Asthma Immunol.* 2004 Aug;93(2 Suppl 1):S24-34

- **Hormones**: DHEA, progesterone, testosterone, and cortisol tend to be lower in allergic/autoimmune individuals than in healthy controls. I use either serum testing and/or 24-hour urine samples before prescribing hormones, though I will empirically use progesterone in a woman or a 3-month trial of DHEA in a man with allergies if I find sufficient indications and no contraindications. Treatment is customized per patient. I discuss the hormonal contributions to autoimmunity later in this chapter under the heading of "orthoendocrinology." As I have noted previously[605], much of what applies to "allergy" also applies to "autoimmunity" and *vice versa*; they are both manifestations of immune dysfunction.

Step 4: Drug treatments: We must acknowledge a place for drug therapy in patients with recalcitrant or severe allergies.

- **Prednisone**: For patients with allergies that are inconsolable, prednisone becomes a reasonable consideration. The lowest effective dose should be used for the shortest possible period of time. Discontinuation of treatment that has lasted longer than 4 days must be gradual in order to avoid adrenal insufficiency. Topical rather than systemic therapy should be used when appropriate.

- **Sodium cromoglycate**: Cromoglycate is a mast cell stabilizer which can be applied nasally for allergic rhinitis (Nasalcrom) or taken orally (Gastrocrom) by patients with food allergy to inhibit the local response to type-1 allergies.[606] The drug is poorly absorbed; therefore its anti-allergy effect is mediated at the gastrointestinal mucosa even though the benefits are systemic. Although not officially "approved" in the US for the treatment of food allergy, numerous studies support its use for this purpose.[607] Cromoglycate has been shown to reduce allergy-induced migraine[608] and eczema[609] and prevent the formation of immune complexes following the consumption of allergenic foods. In addition to preventing the allergic phenomena related directly to the consumption of allergenic foods, an additional mechanism of action of sodium cromoglycate is probably that it reduces the allergy-induced increase in intestinal permeability[610] and thereby prohibits absorption of bacterial and other microbial antigens and metabolites; stated differently, some of the manifestations attributed to "food allergy" are probably not mediated by the response to food allergens directly but result from the adverse immunologic and metabolic responses toward gut-derived microbial antigens and metabolites which are absorbed in increased amounts following the consumption of allergenic foods which increase intestinal permeability and absorption of "foreign" and "toxic" intraluminal contents which would have otherwise been excluded. Common doses for children are 100 mg 30 minutes before food (up to 400 mg per day) and 100-200 mg qid for adults 30 minutes before meals. Capsules or ampules should be mixed in plain water before consumption.

- **Leukotriene antagonists**: Montelukast (Singulair®, Merck) is an orally active leukotriene receptor antagonist that blocks leukotriene D4 from the cysteinyl leukotriene CysLT-1 receptor and thereby reduces

[605] Vasquez A. "Inflammation and Autoimmunity: A Functional Medicine Approach." David S. Jones, MD (Editor-in-Chief). *Textbook of Functional Medicine*. Gig Harbor, WA; Institute for Functional Medicine: 2006, pages 409-417. These ideas have been further developed in my own books and presentations.

[606] drugs.com/MMX/Cromolyn_Sodium.html Accessed November 24, 2005

[607] "Both the clinician's and patient's preferences and the clinician's evaluation of the specific response to challenge showed a significant benefit from SCG." Dannaeus A, Foucard T, Johansson SG. The effect of orally administered sodium cromoglycate on symptoms of food allergy. *Clin Allergy*. 1977 Mar;7(2):109-15

[608] "Immune complexes were not produced in those patients who were protected by sodium cromoglycate. These observations confirm that a food-allergic reaction is the cause of migraine in this group of patients." Monro J, Carini C, Brostoff J. Migraine is a food-allergic disease. *Lancet*. 1984 Sep 29;2(8405):719-21

[609] "The same atopic patients pretreated with oral sodium cromoglycate had less antigen entry, diminished immune-complex formation, and no atopic symptoms." Paganelli R, Levinsky RJ, Brostoff J, Wraith DG. Immune complexes containing food proteins in normal and atopic subjects after oral challenge and effect of sodium cromoglycate on antigen absorption. *Lancet*. 1979 Jun 16;1(8129):1270-2

[610] "It is suggested that a local IgE-mediated mechanism acts as a "trigger" for the entry of antigen and the formation of immune complexes by altering the permeability of the gut mucosa. The resulting delayed onset symptoms could be viewed as a form of serum sickness with few or many target organs affected." Carini C, Brostoff J, Wraith DG. IgE complexes in food allergy. *Ann Allergy*. 1987 Aug;59(2):110-7

vasodilation, eosinophilic inflammation, and vascular hyperpermeability. Montelukast is used in the medical treatment of asthma, rhinitis, and eczema.

<u>Objective means for the identification of allergens: skin-prick testing, serum IgE and IgG assays, double-blind placebo-controlled food challenges, and the elimination and challenge technique</u>

- <u>Skin prick testing</u>: IgE-dependent immediate-onset allergies as assessed with a skin-prick test are indicative of immediate-onset allergy to the particular allergen, and provide the identity of the allergen, quantification of the severity of the allergic response, *and evidence of underlying immune dysfunction*. Skin-prick testing does not assess for delayed-onset allergies, thus leaving at least one class of adverse food reactions literally unassessed.

- <u>Allergen-specific serum levels of IgE and IgG</u>: Elevated serum levels of IgE and IgG, which are identified as specific for certain foods, also provide the identity of the allergen *and evidence of underlying immune dysfunction*. These "objective" tools are part of the clinician's repertoire for identifying food allergens, while keeping in mind that both skin-prick testing and serum testing are prone to both false positives and false negatives. Serum IgE testing does not assess IgG-mediated allergies, nor does it assess for sensitivity (immune but not immunoglobulin-mediated responses) or intolerance, which tends to be biochemical rather than immunologic. IgG assays and the subclasses of IgG-4 assays have not gained acceptance for their sensitivity or specificity, even though clinicians order them and patients pay for them.

- <u>Double-blind placebo-controlled food challenge</u>: Another commonly mentioned objective means for identifying food allergens is the "double-blind placebo-controlled food challenge" (DBPCFC) wherein food is administered a double-blind fashion with placebo control generally via either capsules or nasogastric tube. Unfortunately, DBPCFC is commonly considered the gold standard for the identification of particular allergens and the establishment of an allergic diathesis. This is unfortunate because the hospital admission and associated costs are expensive, cumbersome and therefore inaccessible for most patients. Some patients will have a false-negative response when challenged with isolated foods because of the lack of "accessory antigens", "accomplice antigens", or "bystander antigens."[611] Some patients will have adverse food reactions only when foods are eaten either with *high frequency* or in *specific combinations* or when *gastrointestinal problems* (e.g., dysbiosis or increased intestinal permeability) are present at the same time as the food challenge. For example, while the patient may tolerate eggs alone and wheat alone without the manifestation of allergic symptoms, the additive insult of the combination of both eggs and wheat may cause sufficient intestinal damage and/or immune activation that clinical manifestations become apparent. With single food challenges given with **DBPCFC**, "real life" situations are not reproduced, and false negative results may erroneously suggest that either the patient has no allergies or that a particular food is not offensive.

- <u>Elimination and challenge</u>: The "**elimination and challenge**" technique (more accurately described as "avoidance and challenge") requires that the patient first clear the diet of all possible offending foods, either by **fasting** or by **consuming a simple diet of unlikely-to-be-allergenic foods**, such as the classic triad of rice, lamb, and pears or a relatively hypoallergenic hydrolyzed formula such as Vivonex. After 7-14 days of elimination (i.e., avoidance) *and the clearing of symptoms thought to be allergy-mediated*, an offending food is reintroduced by intense consumption (i.e., eaten with every meal) for a period of up to two days. Every two to four days, a new food is added back into the diet, and a correlation is searched for between consumption of a given food and the exacerbation of symptoms. If the symptoms do not abate or disappear with the fasting/elimination phase, then confirming the nature of the disorder as allergic is more difficult and determining the identity of the allergen is additionally unlikely. However, in some cases, clinical signs and symptoms that are indeed allergy-mediated will fail to regress significantly during the brief washout period. This is because the underlying tissue damage is too great to be healed in such a short time. A good example is the thyroid disease induced by gluten-containing grains in people with the severe gluten allergy called

---

[611] "The mechanisms of enhanced permeability to specific and bystander antigens have been delineated as well as the molecular events involved in the sequential phases of allergic reactions." Heyman M. Gut barrier dysfunction in food allergy. *Eur J Gastroenterol Hepatol*. 2005 Dec;17(12):1279-1285

celiac disease; simply avoiding gluten for 1-2 weeks does not restore endocrine function because the body needs more time to reacquire homeostasis and to heal injured tissues. A common scenario is one in which symptoms remit during fasting/elimination and then return *gradually* rather than *immediately* when the offending food is eaten. In these situations, the most likely explanations are either 1) a threshold of time was necessary for physiologic abnormalities (e.g., immune complex deposition, increased intestinal permeability, dysbiosis, accumulative immune stimulation) to culminate in the reproduction of symptoms, or 2) synergistic factors may have to be combined in order to produce the symptoms of allergy, such as the induction of IgE-mediated increased intestinal permeability by food R which then leads to the increased absorption of food S, to which the peripheral immune system then responds with an IgG-mediated reaction with resultant clinical manifestations. In the latter case, food R or food S *when eaten alone or on a rotation basis* may be insufficient to produce allergic manifestations, but the combination of R+S, which would not be identified with skin-prick testing, serum tests, or one-at-a-time DBPCFC, may produce allergic manifestations. Since, in real life, foods are eaten in combination when they cause allergic disease (e.g. a headache or joint pain after eating a hamburger with wheat/gluten, cheese/milk, mayonnaise/egg, and pickle/tartrazine/yeast), a reasonable conclusion is that foods will have to be avoided in specific combinations to attain maximal improvement in allergic symptoms since complex foods probably work synergistically to produce allergic manifestations in affected people. Creating chronological distance between the consumption of allergenic foods explains the success of the **rotation diets** in alleviating allergic manifestations, but it does little to address the underlying immune dysfunction other than to reduce the total allergenic load to which the immune system is exposed. **Intestinal dysbiosis** can also increase intestinal permeability and result in increased absorption of food antigens and depletion of detoxification co-factors, which can mimic or perpetuate immune-mediated food allergies; correction of the dysbiosis can (*begin to* or *immediately*) normalize immune function and eliminate symptoms *attributed to* or *triggered by* the consumption of specific foods.

Objective Assessments for Adverse Food Reactions—A Quick Clinical Guide

	Advantages	Disadvantages
Skin-prick testing	<ul><li>Proves presence of allergic diathesis.</li><li>Identifies allergen that is being responded to by IgE-mediated reaction.</li><li>Can be used for both food and inhalant allergies.</li></ul>	<ul><li>Numerically impossible to test for all probable allergens due to method of testing, which can be quite painful</li><li>Allergen preparations may not contain full spectrum of immunogenic epitopes that are present in "real food" thus patient may not respond to offensive food, resulting in clinically relevant false negative results.</li><li>Subcutaneous injection is not the natural or physiologic route of allergen exposure.</li><li>Does not assess for IgG or other delayed-onset allergies, thus resulting in clinically relevant false negative results.</li><li>Does not assess for reactions that are mediated by immune complexes, thus resulting in clinically relevant false negative results.</li><li>Procedure is moderately expensive.</li><li>Does not assess for intolerances or biochemical perturbations, thus resulting in clinically relevant false negative results.</li></ul>
Serum IgE assay	<ul><li>Identifies allergen that is being responded to by IgE-mediated reaction.</li><li>Can be used for both food and inhalant allergies.</li><li>Procedure is relatively painless and provides "objective evidence" of food allergies.</li></ul>	<ul><li>Numerically impossible to test for all probable allergens due to method of testing.</li><li>Allergen preparations may not contain full spectrum of immunogenic epitopes that are present in "real food" thus patient may not respond to offensive food, resulting in clinically relevant false negative results.</li><li>Does not assess for IgG or other delayed-onset allergies, thus resulting in clinically relevant false negative results.</li><li>Does not assess for reactions that are mediated by IgG, IgM, or IgA immune complexes, thus resulting in clinically relevant false-negative results.</li><li>Does not assess for intolerances or biochemical perturbations, thus resulting in clinically relevant false negative results.</li></ul>
Serum IgG4 assay	<ul><li>Identifies allergen that is being responded to by IgG-mediated reaction.</li><li>Mostly used in an attempt to identify delayed-onset food allergies.</li><li>Procedure is relatively painless.</li><li>Procedure provides "objective evidence" of food allergies.</li></ul>	<ul><li>Numerically impossible to test for all probable allergens due to method of testing.</li><li>Allergen preparations may not contain full spectrum of immunogenic epitopes that are present in "real food" thus patient may not respond to offensive food, resulting in clinically relevant false negative results.</li><li>Does not assess for IgE or other immediate-onset allergies, thus resulting in clinically relevant false negative results.</li><li>Does not assess for reactions that are mediated by immune complexes, thus resulting in clinically relevant false negative results.</li><li>Procedure is moderately expensive.</li><li>Does not assess for intolerances or biochemical perturbations, thus resulting in clinically relevant false negative results.</li><li>The clinical relevance of IgG4 antibodies to food is controversial.[612]</li></ul>

---

[612] "...it seems unlikely that increased IgG4 antibody levels against egg white is a cause of egg hypersensitivity, and one should pay much attention to IgG1 antibodies ...it is possible that increased IgG4 may reduce the effect of complement-fixing antibodies like IgG1 and/or interfere the action of IgE antibodies." Nakagawa T. Egg white-specific IgE and IgG subclass antibodies and their associations with clinical egg hypersensitivity. *N Engl Reg Allergy Proc.* 1988 Jan-Feb;9(1):67-73

Objective Assessments for Adverse Food Reactions—A Quick Clinical Guide *continued*

	Advantages	Disadvantages
Double-blind placebo-controlled food challenges	• Allows for control of interfering factors. • Removes psychological cues and triggers that can be mistakenly interpreted as adverse food reactions. • Procedure provides "objective evidence" of food allergies.	• Setting and experiment are artificial and not representative of the real environment in which the patient lives and is exposed to allergen(s). • Testing of single antigens alone is not reflective of real life wherein antigens are consumed in combination. • Numerically impossible to test for all probable allergens due to method of testing. • Allergen preparations may not contain full spectrum of immunogenic epitopes that are present in "real food" thus patient may not respond to offensive food, resulting in clinically relevant false negative results. • Procedure is time-consuming and cumbersome and requires the preparation of both food challenge and placebo, which are administered either by capsules or by nasogastric tube. • Due to small quantity of allergen and limited time of observation, does not assess for reactions that are quantity-dependent, delayed-onset, or mediated by immune complexes, thus resulting in clinically relevant false negative results. • Procedure is moderately expensive. • Does not assess for intolerances or biochemical perturbations, thus resulting in clinically relevant false negative results.
Elimination and challenge	• Represents "real life" situations with psychological influences, daily stress, and combinations of foods. • No financial cost. • Easy to implement for motivated patients. • Trains patients to be active in their healthcare and to learn how to diagnose and treat themselves—the true goals of wellness promotion. • Allows patients and clinicians to assess for dysbiotic food reactions secondary to nonspecific SIBO (e.g., bloating and flatulence), H2S toxicity secondary to sulfur-reducing bacteria (e.g., myalgia, dyscognition, hypothermia), or D-lactate toxicity (e.g., headache and dyscognition).	• Compliance is a challenge for unmotivated or undisciplined patients. • Identification of offending allergen may take time and repeated cycles of elimination and challenge before the allergen is conclusively identified.

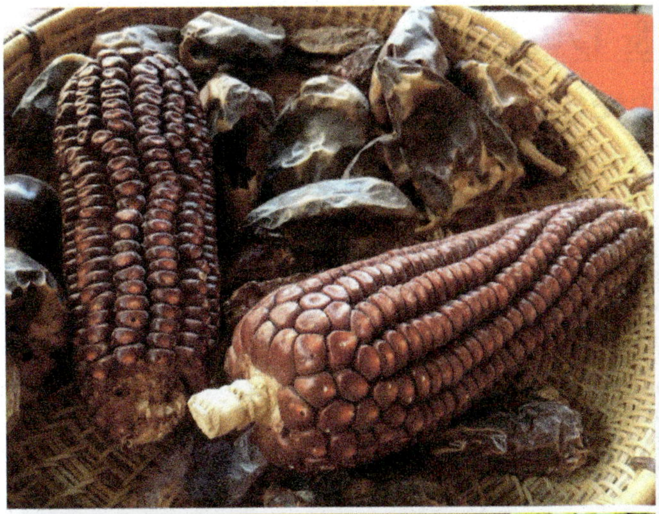

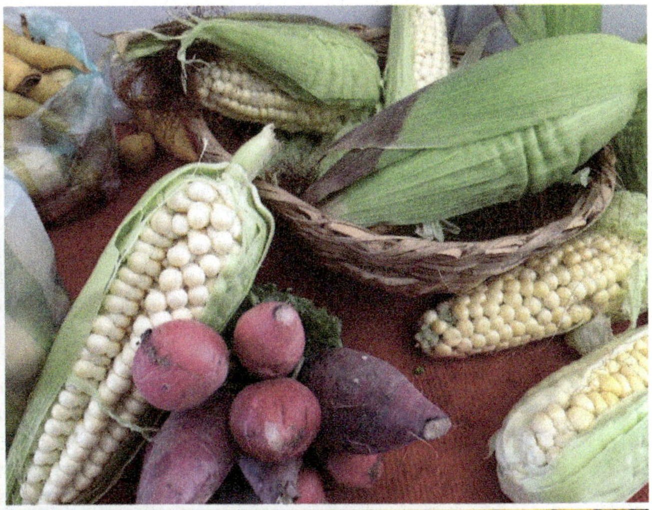

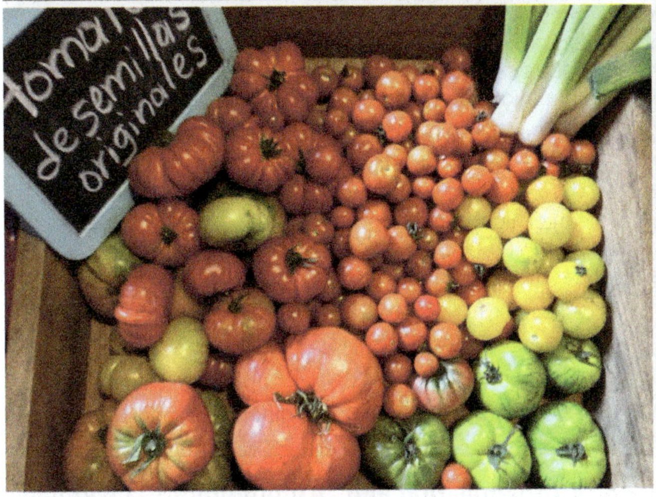

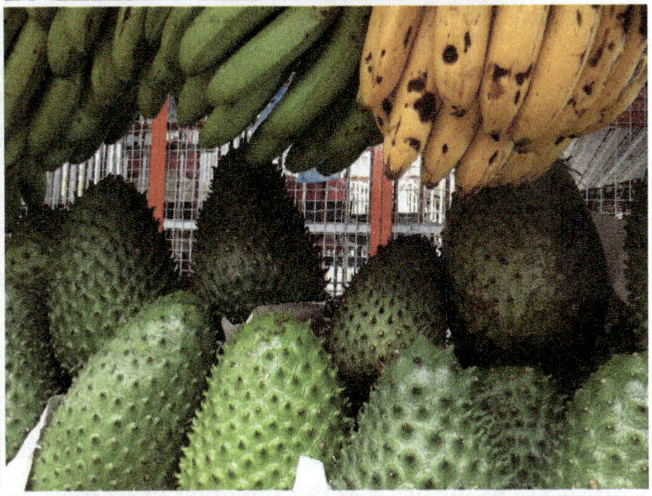

Real natural food is a human right: Corporate profiteers state that food and water are not human rights, but—in contrast to historical precident and social interests—corporate property. In this manner, private corporations become stronger than governments, when they control access to food, water, and thus very foundation of daily life and and thus national stability. When multinational corporations control the grain and water supply, then they also control the supply of poultry, cattle/livestock, and—increasingly—farm-raised fish.Corporations that control a society's food/water supply have control over that society, and they have the wealth to buy politicians, laws, and selective enforcement.

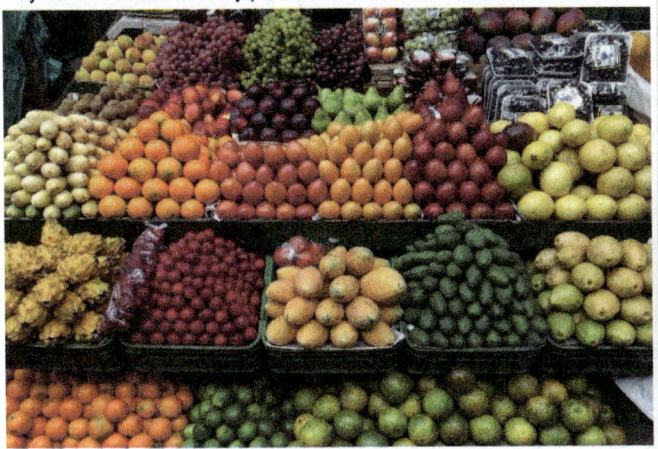

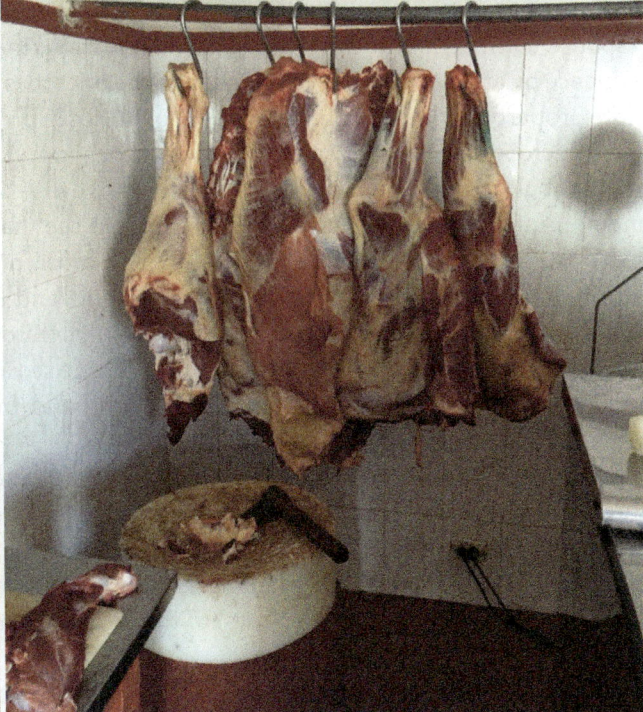

❷ Infections & Dysbiosis:
Subclinical Infections & Persistent Microbial Colonization

Major Concepts in this Section

This section reviews in detail the mechanisms by which dysbiosis—also described as multifocal polydysbiosis, subclinical infection(s), microbial colonization—contributes to immune, metabolic, and neurologic dysfunction and resultant clinical disorders; understanding this section and taking appropriate clinical action is of the highest importance in the successful treatment of these conditions. Readers of this section must attain ❶ an appreciation of the mechanisms by which microbes and their molecular effects contribute to pro-inflammatory immune dysfunction, and ❷ an appreciation that exclusive therapeutic focus on the eradication of microbes is fraught with inefficacy if it fails to address the intrinsic patient-specific imbalances that allowed that individual patient to be susceptible to microbe-induced inflammation and dysmetabolism.

"Dysbiosis" is not simply about the effects of microbes in inflammatory disease, and the clinical approach therefore should not focus exclusively on the detection and eradication of those microbes. Although this section focuses on microbes and their effects, detection, and eradication, the complete treatment of dysbiosis needs to contain three major components: ❶ microbe-specific treatment (e.g., antimicrobial botanicals and pharmaceuticals), ❷ restoration of immune function and other means by which to make the human host less hospitable to (re)colonization (e.g., stress avoidance, sleep optimization, and nutritional immunorestoration, especially with zinc, glutamine, and vitamins A and D), and ❸ promotion of immune and inflammatory tolerance (e.g., nutritional immunomodulation protocol[1]). This introductory section on dysbiosis emphasizes bacteria, with some mention of yeast/fungi and other microbes such as amoeba and other eukaryotes; viruses are introduced but detailed elsewhere in separate works/sections. Rheumatic/autoimmune consequences are emphasized.

Topics in my conversation on the 2nd section detailing "Infections and Dysbiosis" of my Functional Inflammology Protocol[2] are currently divided into the following major subsections:
1. Molecules from microbes that promote disease (and health)
2. Mechanisms of bacterial and fungal dysbiosis/colonization effects in clinical disease
3. Prototypic microbe-disease clinical presentations
4. Locations of dysbiosis, introduction to the viral microbiome (viruses and anti-viral strategies are discussed separately)
5. Survey of dysbiotic microbes seen in general practice
6. Therapy 1—Immunorestoration
7. Therapy 2—Immunotolerance (detailed in Chapter 4, section 3)
8. Therapy 3—Antimicrobial agents
9. Viruses and antiviral strategies—discussed separately[3] due to the volume of information and different clinical approach
10. Disease-dysbiosis patterns: appreciation for clinical intervention

---

Multifocal Dysbiosis: A Major Promoter of ~~Chronic~~ *Sustained* Inflammation and "Autoimmunity" Overview:
Because of their tissue-damaging and disease-promoting effects, microbial molecules generally incite an immune response consistent with what we call inflammation; in cognitive and grammatic shorthand, we abbreviate this sequence by attributing the inflammation to the microbes (e.g., "microbes cause inflammation") whereas we should more properly attribute the inflammation to the host's physiologic response, which is variable and thus modifiable. Most microbes can thus be said to be pro-inflammatory and contributory to acute and chronic inflammatory and dysmetabolic diseases and disorders. However, we also respect a few microbes for the salutary, health-promoting, and anti-inflammatory benefits; from this we can see that the host's total microbial load (TML) contributes to the host's total inflammatory load, and that the TML must include consideration of both the pro-inflammatory and the anti-inflammatory microbes *in balance and imbalance* and the resulting immunologic consequences and phenotypic outcomes. Given that most microbes are pro-inflammatory and that inflammation itself contributes to essentially all of the chronic/sustained clinical disorders that we see as clinicians and study as researchers, the focus of this text will be mostly that of elucidating the molecular and immunologic mechanisms and thereafter and ultimately providing clinically useful solutions.

Microbes contribute to noninfectious human diseases—including chronic/sustained inflammation and autoimmunity—by mechanisms which are singular/numerous, simple/complex, and additive/synergistic. For the purposes of this discussion, I will use my own broad definition of dysbiosis that implies "a relationship of non-acute host-microorganism interaction that adversely affects the human host." The subtype of dysbiosis can be distinguished based on the location(s) of the dysbiotic foci/focus, as well as per the dominant adverse effect, i.e.,

---

[1] Vasquez A. *Inflammation and Autoimmune Solutions: The Seven Keys of the Updated F.I.N.D.S.E.X.® Protocol, 2nd Edition*. ICHNFM, 2014

[2] Vasquez A. *Functional Inflammology: Volume 1*. International College of Human Nutrition and Functional Medicine, 2014. ISBN 0990620409 / 978-0990620402

[3] Vasquez A. *Antiviral Nutrition: Against Colds, Flu, Herpes, AIDS, Hepatitis, Ebola, Dengue, and Autoimmunity*. International College of Human Nutrition and Functional Medicine, 2014. (ASIN: B00OPDQG4W) amazon.com/dp/B00OPDQG4W. Book format: Vasquez A. *Antiviral Strategies and Immune Nutrition*, 2014. (ISBN: 1502894890)

the dominant pattern of immune/inflammatory response, degree and specificity of metabolic dysfunction, and the clinical disorder that results.

I have come to categorize inflammation into three subtypes, based on the predominant phenotypic presentation; very clearly, overlap exists among these subtypes. Generally, we can identify that most inflammatory disorders have a predominant manifestation, whether ❶ **metabolic inflammation**, e.g., the dysbiotic components of diabetes mellitus, insulin resistance, mitochondrial dysfunction, and neuropsychiatric disorders, ❷ **allergic inflammation**, e.g., the dysbiotic component of atopic dermatitis, eczema, or ❸ **autoimmune inflammation**, e.g., the powerful dysbiotic contributions to conditions such as rheumatoid arthritis and psoriasis. In the study of clinical disease and the practice of clinical medicine, we commonly see the overlaps of these types of inflammation within the same patients and disorders. For example, patients with systemic inflammation commonly have a metabolic components (e.g., insulin resistance, obesity, depression) and allergic components (e.g., asthma); further we see that these types of inflammation are additive/synergistic in that—for example—obese and insulin resistant patients tend to have allergic disorders that are more severe and difficult to treat. Likewise, we also note overlap between allergy (e.g., immunologic hypersensitivity to exogenous molecules) and autoimmunity (e.g., immunologic hypersensitivity to endogenous molecules).[4] Also, we see that rheumatic/autoimmune patients fare worse if they are obese and insulin resistant rather than *eu*metabolic, otherwise healthy and lean. Therefore and clearly, these subtypes of inflammation can be seen simultaneously as separate, interconnected, and additive/synergistic.

My system of dysbiosis categorization appreciates and distinguishes the following locations, most of which are self-explanatory and all of which are detailed following this introduction: ❶ **gastrointestinal**—prototype and largest contributor, ❷ **orodental**, ❸ **sinorespiratory**, ❹ **genitourinary**, ❺ **dermal**, ❻ **tissue/parenchymal/blood**—involving bacteria (noteworthy in chronic low back pain) and viruses (noteworthy in Alzheimer's disease, SLE, Sjogren's disease, and scleroderma), ❼ **environmental**—adverse physiologic effect from microbes not located within the human body, but in the surrounding environment, and ❽ **microbial**—microbial colonization of other microbes,

---

Dysbiosis: definitions, descriptions, mechanisms

Dysbiosis: A relationship of non-acute non-infectious host-microorganism interaction that adversely affects the host.

Dysbiosis subtypes (based on location): ❶ Orodental, ❷ Sinorespiratory, ❸ Gastrointestinal, ❹ Genitourinary, ❺ Parenchymal, tissue, blood—including mostly bacteria and viruses, ❻ Cutaneous, ❼ Environmental, ❽ Microbial.

Multifocal dysbiosis: A clinical condition characterized by a patient's having more than one foci/location of dysbiosis; generally the adverse physiologic and clinical consequences are additive and synergistic.

Polydysbiosis: Concurrent dysbiosis with different microbes

Combinatorial dysbiosis: The phenotypic sum total of the additive, synergistic, and neutralizing effects of the various components of the patient's "total dysbiotic load" (TDL) and "total microbial load" (TML), the latter term must also include the total viral load (TVL) which includes exogenous viruses, endogenous viruses, and bacteriophages.

Microbial molecules, mechanisms, morphology:
1. Gram-negative bacterial products, LPS
2. Gram-positive bacterial products
3. L-form, pleomorphic, "cell wall-deficient" bacteria
4. Immunostimulation by bacterial DNA, viral DNA and bacteriophage DNA
5. Superantigens
6. Antimetabolites
7. Beneficial metabolites and molecular signatures

Pathophysiologic responses:
1. Damage to the intestinal mucosa
2. Activation of inflammatory pathways—Toll-like receptors (TLR), NFkB, DAMP and PAMP, inflammasome
3. Mitochondrial hyperpolarization, mTOR activation
4. Molecular mimicry, cross-reactivity
5. Enhanced presentation of autoantigens
6. Bystander activation
7. Haptenization and the formation of neoautoantigens
8. Immune complex formation and deposition
9. Insufficiency dysbiosis
10. Microbial allergy, hypersensitivity
11. Inhibition of detoxification
12. Bacterial and fungal proteases impair immune defenses
13. Immunosuppression via gliotoxins
14. Mold toxins—mycotoxins
15. Biofilms
16. Impairment of mucosal digestion
17. Central sensitization, microbiome-gut-brain axis
18. Dysbiosis-induced endocrine dysfunction
19. Microbe-induced epigenetic changes
20. Altered vitamin D metabolism and reception

Prototypic clinical manifestations:
1. Autointoxication, auto-brewery syndrome, encephalopathy
2. Syndromes of pain, fatigue, depression
3. Dysbiotic arthropathy, dermatitis, vasculitis
4. Reactive arthritis

---

[4] Valenta et al. Linking allergy to autoimmune disease. *Trends Immunol.* 2009 Mar;30(3):109-16

with the clearest example being the infection/colonization of intestinal bacteria with the bacteria-specific viruses known as bacteriophages, with noted aberrations in Crohn's disease.

In approximately 2006, I coined and published the phrase "multifocal dysbiosis"[5] which—by logical extension per appreciation that microbes will vary in different locations—implies the existence of "multifocal polydysbiosis." Indeed, patients may have more than one dysbiotic locus at a time with microbes from more than one kingdom, i.e., bacteria, archaea (e.g., noted in dental infections and prosthetic joint colonizations), and eukaryote (e.g., fungi and protozoa); students of Biology will recall that viruses have always presented a classification conundrum, due to their dependence on other life forms for their own replication. One condition that serves as an example of multifocal polydysbiosis is the multisystem inflammatory disease Behcet's syndrome, characterized by subclinical pulmonary infection (sinorespiratory dysbiosis) with *Chlamydia pneumoniae*[6], cutaneous colonization (dermal dysbiosis) with *Staphylococcus aureus*[7], and orodental dysbiosis with *Streptococcus sanguis*[8]; one could easily opine that each microbial focus could be "statistically insignificant" while the combination of all three could easily be additively/synergistically pathogenic, particularly with an inflammation-prone immunophenotype, whether due to genetic predisposition(s), nutritional deficiencies, xenobiotic accumulation, or all of these together.

The additive/synergistic effect of multiple microbial colonizations/infections must be appreciated; extending this appreciation to different patterns of metabolic/allergic/autoimmune responses per microbe provides the basis for my concept of combinatorial multifocal polydysbiosis, roughly defined as the *phenotypic expression / clinical presentation* of the additive, synergistic, and/or neutralizing effects of various microbial colonizations/infections on the patient's overall metabolism/physiology and immune status/reactivity. Stated differently, combinatorial multifocal polydysbiosis is the summarized microbial effect of the total microbial load, including symbionts, pathobionts, pathogens, and including bacteria, fungi, viruses, etc. These are components of the total inflammatory load (the subject of Chapter 4 in its entirety), which together with other factors including genetics and epigenetics, amalgamate to produce the patient's/disease phenotype, studied in its totality as combinatorial inflammology, a concept developed throughout my functional inflammology model and FINDSEX® protocol. Readers should appreciate that the total dysbiotic load (TDL) is part of the total microbial load (TML) and contributes to the total inflammatory load (TIL).

As a simple exercise, we can imaginatively combine multifocal dysbiosis a few pro-rheumatic genetic traits (especially HLA-B27) and pro-inflammatory dietary imbalances[9]; even with only these three components we can already see why rheumatic diseases are generally still considered "idiopathic" when reviewed from a reductionistic medical paradigm that fails to appreciate the interconnected and "holistic" web of influences that synergize to produce systemic inflammation.[10] For the majority of patients in outpatient clinical practice, the location of their "dominant" (i.e., most important) dysbiosis is the gut, which is easily assessed with specialized stool testing and microbiology/parasitology examinations, and which is easily treated with oral botanical/pharmaceutical antimicrobials and dietary modification. In my own clinical practice, I have long considered stool testing extremely valuable and have estimated that 80% of microbiology/parasitology examinations return with at least one clinically-relevant abnormality. Obviously, the stool testing needs to be performed by a competent laboratory[11] that can provide broad-spectrum microbial identification along with analysis of gastrointestinal inflammatory, metabolic, and functional markers. I will demonstrate in this section that testing for and treating dysbiosis is absolutely essential in patients with chronic fatigue, fibromyalgia, autoimmunity, and any type of so-called "chronic inflammatory disease"—the latter is more wisely termed *sustained inflammatory response*.

---

[5] Vasquez A. Multifocal Dysbiosis. *Naturopathy Digest* 2006 Jun naturopathydigest.com/archives/2006/jun/vasquez.php

[6] "These finding provide serological evidence of chronic C. pneumoniae infection in association with Behcet's disease." Ayaslioglu E, Duzgun N, Erkek E, Inal A. Evidence of chronic Chlamydia pneumoniae infection in patients with Behcet's disease. *Scand J Infect Dis*. 2004;36(6-7):428-30

[7] "Staphylococcus aureus (41/70, 58.6%, p = 0.008) and Prevotella spp (17/70, 24.3%, p = 0.002) were significantly more common in pustules from BS patients..." Hatemi G, et al. The pustular skin lesions in Behcet's syndrome are not sterile. *Ann Rheum Dis*. 2004 Nov;63(11):1450-2

[8] "These data indicate that the BD patients are infected with IgA protease-producing S. sanguis strains, which cause an increase of IgA titer against these organisms and IgA protease antigen." Yokota K, Oguma K. IgA protease produced by Streptococcus sanguis and antibody production against IgA protease in patients with Behcet's disease. *Microbiol Immunol*. 1997;41(12):925-31

[9] Seaman DR. The diet-induced proinflammatory state: a cause of chronic pain and other degenerative diseases? *J Manipulative Physiol Ther*. 2002 Mar-Apr;25:168-79

[10] Vasquez A. Web-like interconnections of physiological factors. *Integrative Medicine* 2006; April/May: 32-7 InflammationMastery.com/reprints

[11] Unfortunately, one particular laboratory in the functional medicine community used bogus analytical methods for many years, obviously thereby deceiving/defrauding doctors and patients of millions of dollars in addition to wasting time and resources and directly compromising physician care and patient outcomes.Gingras et al. Assessment of diagnostic accuracy of recently introduced DNA stool screening test. *Int J Hum Nutr Funct Med* 2014:2(1);1 ichnfm.org/publications/IJHNFM_2014_review.pdf

Clinical Implications—Clearing Obfuscations, Outdated Information, and Misteachings:

A problem that plagues many healthcare providers of all professions is that most of them are still under the spell of the Pasteurian paradigm of infectious disease, namely that pathogenic microorganisms cause *a specific disease* by causing *a specific infection*. Relatedly, Koch's postulates first published in 1884 held that "the organism must be found in all animals suffering from the disease, but not in healthy animals" and "the cultured organism should cause disease when introduced into a healthy animal."[12] Such contributions by Pasteur, Koch, and other researchers were essential in providing a preliminary understanding of the role of microorganisms in the genesis of human disease; however, we must appreciate that these simplistic, linear, and rather primitive models do not suffice for explaining all microbe-induced disorders. The major problems with the paradigms proposed by Pasteur and Koch are that both of these models fail to appreciate 1) adverse microbe-host interactions which may not *result in* nor *result from* a true "infection" (thus refuting the Pasteurian paradigm), and 2) the importance of the patient's biochemical individuality and genetic uniqueness which influence the clinical manifestations of dysbiosis-induced disease such that a) not all patients exposed to a pathogenic microbe will express the stereotypic disease, and b) some patients exposed to microorganisms that are generally considered benign commensals will produce a dramatic inflammatory response which results in clinical disease (thus refuting Koch's postulates). Supported amply by the research reviewed herein, healthcare providers have an obligation to move beyond these simplistic "pathogenic" "infection-based" models of microorganism-induced disease to apprehend the more common "functional" disorders that can result from exposure to microbes. Readers will note that these new concepts and ideas are amply supported by the references to the biomedical research that are included in the footnotes.[13,14]

The distinction between colonization and infection might be made as follows: "colonization" implies the presence (and thus the allowance of) microbes living in/on host tissues—generally for an extended period of time—without directly appreciatively damaging cells and tissues (e.g., gastrointestinal dysbiosis, bacterial colonization of intervertebral discs in low-back pain[15,16]), while "infection" implies infiltration that results in tissue damage and acute/subacute inflammation (e.g., infectious hemorrhagic diarrhea, acute bacterial discitis and vertebral osteomyelitis). Colonization, dysbiosis, and infection are detailed in the following table for clarity.

Microbial presence	Duration	Local tissue damage	Local inflammatory response	Systemic consequences	Examples
Colonization	Long-term	None, minimal	None, minimal	None or disease-specific, opportunistic	Nares/sinus colonization with *Staph. Aureus* in ANCA vasculitis and atopic dermatitis
Dysbiosis (colonization with systemic consequences)	Long-term	None, minimal	None, minimal	Generally important, predominant	D-lactate dysbiosis with fatigue and dyscognition in the absence of major GI complaints
Infection	Acute, subacute	Pathologic	Severe	Secondary to inflammatory response	Suppurative pharyngitis

Distinguishing colonization, dysbiosis, and infection: All of these conditions are characterized by microbial presence resulting in pathophysiologic consequences; the distinctions in onset, duration, local and systemic effects are important.

At least 70% of patients with chronic arthritis are carriers of "silent infections", according to a 1992 article published in the peer-reviewed medical journal *Annals of the Rheumatic Diseases*.[17] A 2001 article in this same journal which focused exclusively on five bacteria showed that 56% of patients with idiopathic inflammatory arthritis had gastrointestinal or genitourinary dysbiosis.[18] Indeed, published research strongly and consistently indicates that bacteria, yeast/fungi, amebas, protozoa, and other "parasites" (rarely including helminths/worms) are

---

[12] Koch's Postulates. encyclopedia.thefreedictionary.com/Koch%27s+postulates Accessed October 4, 2005
[13] Noah PW. The role of microorganisms in psoriasis. *Semin Dermatol*. 1990 Dec;9(4):269-76
[14] Samarkos M, Vaiopoulos G. The role of infections in the pathogenesis of autoimmune diseases. *Curr Drug Targets Inflamm Allergy*. 2005 Feb;4(1):99-10
[15] Sample I. Antibiotics could cure 40% of chronic back pain patients. theguardian.com/society/2013/may/07/antibiotics-cure-back-pain-patients
[16] Albert et al. Does nuclear tissue infected with bacteria following disc herniations lead to Modic changes in the adjacent vertebrae? *Eur Spine J*. 2013 Apr;22(4):690-6
[17] "At the time of initial evaluation, 57 (69%) of the patients with oligoarthritis and 4/20 (20%) of the control subjects were carriers of clinically silent infections." Weyand CM, Goronzy JJ. Clinically silent infections in patients with oligoarthritis: results of a prospective study. *Ann Rheum Dis*. 1992 Feb;51(2):253-8
[18] Fendler et al. Frequency of triggering bacteria in patients with reactive arthritis…and the relative importance of tests used for diagnosis. *Ann Rheum Dis*. 2001 Apr;60(4):337-43

underappreciated causes of neuromusculoskeletal inflammation. This section will explain the mechanisms by which **silent infections**, *noninfectious* **microbial colonization**, and **dysbiosis** can cause and perpetuate numerous health problems, and I will also discuss basic assessment and treatment measures that can be used clinically to help patients with microbe-induced musculoskeletal inflammation.

One of the rhetorical positions espoused by skeptics is, "If infections caused autoimmunity, then antibiotics would cure autoimmune disease." This *reductio ad absurdum* is irrelevant for several reasons:

1. First, autoimmunity may be incited by microbes and then persist in the absence of those same microbes: Analogy: when a hammer breaks a window, removing the hammer does not repair the window. Autoimmunity—whether induced by xenobiotics or microorganisms—has a tendency to persist due to the immune sensitization toward autoantigens that have been haptenized, exposed, or otherwise immunogenized (for example via epitope spreading), and due to the secondary endocrinologic changes and xenobiotic accumulation that have been induced by the disease process and which perpetuate the dysregulated pro-inflammatory state. Increasingly per new research, we appreciate the self-perpetuating cycles of inflammation including the components of persistent NFkB and mTOR activation in concert with mitochondrial dysfunction/hyperpolarization; as discussed in a later section, mTOR activation by microbes (or dietary stress or xenobiotics) leads directly to a vicious cycle of inflammation, tissue damage, and immunophenotype, (i.e., Treg/Th17) imbalance. The autoimmune "reactive arthritis" that follows microbial infection responds only partially to early antibiotic treatment[19], thus indicating that microbe-induced musculoskeletal inflammation—once induced—may persist despite [supposedly] effective antimicrobial treatment. Pro-inflammatory antigens can persist in synoviocytes and immunocytes for years following an *acute* bacterial infection that results in *chronic* inflammatory arthritis.[20] Conversely, the observation that antimicrobial intervention, particularly with more powerful treatments, can significantly reduce (not eliminate) the development of "autoimmune" phenomena in patients following bacterial infection[21] supports the perception that 1) microorganisms/bacteria contribute directly to the genesis of inflammatory/autoimmune disorders, and that 2) antimicrobial treatment of autoimmune disorders is warranted although not universally effective. The failure of antimicrobial treatment should not be confused with the failure of the microbe-rheumatic model; we note clinically and in the research that oftentimes the "correct" antimicrobial therapy is inefficacious, but later *empiric* treatment has antimicrobial effectiveness resulting in clinical improvement or cure. As demonstrated clinically (for example, among patients with fibromyalgia treated with antimicrobial drugs[22]), antimicrobial therapy *per se* has no value; what has value is *effective* antimicrobial therapy.

> **Microbes can induce autoimmunity**
> "Infectious agents can cause autoimmune disease by different mechanisms, which fall into two categories: *antigen specific* in which pathogen products or elements have a central role e.g. **superantigens** or epitope **(molecular) mimicry**, and *antigen non-specific* in which the pathogen provides the appropriate inflammatory setting for **bystander activation**."
>
> Samarkos, Vaiopoulos. *Curr Drug Targets Inflamm Allergy.* 2005 Feb

2. Second, all clinicians are aware that no antimicrobial treatment eradicates *all* microbes from *all* surfaces. For example, an orally administered broad-spectrum antibiotic is not appropriate for eradicating a fungal infection located in the sinuses. Microbial drug resistance is an increasingly large problem in outpatient and hospital-based medicine[23] where antimicrobial drug therapies are the mainstay treatment of bacterial infections and no consideration is given to effective botanical antimicrobials (reviewed later) and to strengthening host defenses (described throughout this text and particularly in sections on diet and immunonutrition). Except—and even this exception may be erroneous—in clear cases of reactive arthritis wherein *one* infection/microbe is leading to the inflammatory rheumatic response, what we appreciate clinically and in the research literature is that patients with dysbiosis-induced inflammation—in addition to having multiple metabolic/nutritional/hormonal liabilities—almost always have *multifocal poly*dysbiosis; hence, treatment with a *single* course of a *single* antimicrobial agent is the clinical manifestation of simplistic/wishful thinking that—although occasionally successful—is generally discordant with the documented scientific facts.

[19] Laasila K, Laasonen L, Leirisalo-Repo M. Antibiotic treatment and long term prognosis of reactive arthritis. *Ann Rheum Dis.* 2003 Jul;62(7):655-8
[20] "Extensive bacterial cultures of the synovial fluid were negative…We conclude that in patients with reactive arthritis after yersinia infection, microbial antigens can be found in synovial-fluid cells from affected joints." Granfors et al. Yersinia antigens in synovial-fluid cells from patients with reactive arthritis. *N Engl J Med* 1989;320:216-2
[21] Yli-Kerttula et al. Effect of a three month course of ciprofloxacin on the late prognosis of reactive arthritis. *Ann Rheum Dis.* 2003 Sep;62:880-4
[22] Wallace DJ, Hallegua DS. Fibromyalgia: the gastrointestinal link. *Curr Pain Headache Rep.* 2004 Oct;8(5):364-8
[23] Sharma R, Sharma CL, Kapoor B. Antibacterial resistance: Current problems and possible solutions. *Indian J Med Sci* 2005 Dec 27;59:120-129

3. <u>Third, the administration of antimicrobial therapeutics of a *limited scope/effectiveness* for a *limited time* may allow the dysbiosis to return when the antimicrobials are discontinued</u>. The autoimmune condition problem may continue or recur despite even "appropriate" antimicrobial treatment if the duration of treatment is too brief, thereby allowing for suppression without eradication, and/or if the host "milieu"—the biological terrain, the patient's overall health—is not improved. Oftentimes, clinicians will have to use antimicrobial strategies different from those learned in medical school and residency training wherein these concepts are generally not taught; likewise, therapeutic strategies *beyond the administration of antimicrobials*—such as correction of faulty diet, nutritional deficiencies, immune (in)competence, mitochondrial dysfunction, immunophenotype imbalance, hormonal imbalances—are often needed for these patients to achieve optimal improvement.

4. <u>Fourth, even when the microbe is eradicated, its antigens may persist</u>. Microbial antigens can persist within the human body for years following clearance of the primary infection.[24,25,26] Relatedly and of high clinical importance, microbial antigens from vaccinations/immunizations may also persist for extended durations—culminating in severe systemic inflammation and/or lethal consequences—due to the effects of adjuvants (e.g., aluminum) in promoting an exaggerated immune response and antigen/immunogen persistence.[27]

5. <u>Fifth, the microbe-autoimmunity model of autoimmune disease induction does not state that microbes are the *sole cause* of autoimmunity</u>. What I have documented here with an abundance of research is that microbes are a major contributor to autoimmunity and that dysbiosis works in concert with hormonal abnormalities, xenobiotic immunotoxicity, food intolerances, and a proinflammatory lifestyle (etc.) which synergize to create pro-inflammatory immune dysfunction that happens to destroy body tissues in a phenomenon that gets anthropocentrically and phenomenonistically labeled "autoimmunity." Generally, these autoimmune patients have *multiple* physiologic predispositions, and we can visualize a model in which a microbial trigger would initiate an inflammatory cascade that could persist even after the clearance/eradication of the offending microbe following the commencement of various pathophysiologic process, such as inflammation-mediated elaboration of autoantigens and various danger/damage-associated molecular patterns (DAMPs). Those factors that I consider to be most important are the ones integrated into my "functional inflammology protocol" as detailed in *Functional Inflammology, Volume 1* and *Inflammation and Autoimmune Solutions, 2nd Edition* and outlined below.

Despite the ability of autoimmunity/inflammation to persist following the eradication of causative microorganisms, clinicians (and patients) will be pleased to learn that effective oligo/poly-microbial eradication can result in dramatic clinical improvements in patients with autoimmunity. This observation is not merely anecdote from practicing clinicians; **published research and relatively large clinical trials (cited and discussed later) are increasingly documenting that comprehensive antimicrobial treatments do indeed *promote regression* and *initiate cure* in a growing list of previously "untreatable" autoimmune diseases.**

While everyone acknowledges that autoimmune and inflammatory disorders are "multifactorial", hardly anyone has taken the time to determine what these factors are and how to remediate each; I began this work when teaching Rheumatology at Bastyr University starting in 2001, published the first book on the topic—*Integrative Rheumatology*—in 2006, and then completed the model in 2012 with my presentation and publication of the "functional inflammology protocol", organized and recalled by the FINDSEX® acronym which represents the following seven components: ❶ **F**ood and nutrition, ❷ **I**nfections and dysbiosis, ❸ **N**utritional immunomodulation of Treg/Th17 phenotype, ❹ **D**ysmetabolism and dysfunctional mitochondria (also now including endoplasmic reticulum stress and mTOR activation), ❺ **S**tress, sleep, style of living, and other supplemental considerations, ❻ **E**ndocrine imbalances, and ❼ **X**enobiotic immunotoxicity. An exemplary case report is provided on the following page, and the introduction to the functional inflammology protocol is available in video format online: vimeo.com/100089988 with password DrVprotocol_volume1.

[24] Inman RD. Antigens, the gastrointestinal tract, and arthritis. *Rheum Dis Clin North Am.* 1991 May;17(2):309-21

[25] "These samples were studied by immunochemical techniques for the presence of Yersinia antigens at the beginning of infection and up to 4 years thereafter... This study has, for the first time, directly demonstrated that bacterial antigens persist for a long time in patients who develop ReA after Y. enterocolitica O:3 infection." Granfors et al. Persistence of Yersinia antigens in peripheral blood cells from patients with Yersinia enterocolitica O:3 infection with or without reactive arthritis. *Arthritis Rheum.* 1998 May;41(5):855-62

[26] "Extensive bacterial cultures of the synovial fluid were negative...We conclude that in patients with reactive arthritis after yersinia infection, microbial antigens can be found in synovial-fluid cells from affected joints." Granfors et al. Yersinia antigens in synovial-fluid cells from patients with reactive arthritis. *N Engl J Med* 1989;320:216-2

[27] Lee SH. Detection of human papillomavirus L1 gene DNA fragments in postmortem blood and spleen after Gardasil vaccination. *Advances Biosci Biotech* 2012:3,1214-1224

Clinical Case Exemplary case of clinical and laboratory evidence of reversal of "severe, aggressive, drug-resistant" rheumatoid arthritis in a 51yoWF following implementation of the Functional Inflammology Protocol: This summarizes the 13-month clinical outcome of the first patient treated with the updated functional inflammology protocol after its revision and expansion in March 2012.[28] After being diagnosed accurately by a rheumatologist—for this patient very clearly met diagnostic criteria—this patient presented for care following notably inefficacious treatment with the full medicopharmaceutical antirheumatic protocol comprised of NSAIDs, prednisone (she had only minimal response to prednisone >60mg/d), methotrexate, hydroxychloroquine, and "biologics" including etanercept/Enbrel; she was now being recommended to start newer "experimental" drugs. Following the failure of medical treatment, the patient was treated at the teaching clinic of a naturopathic college where her treatments included a clinician-supervised 26-day water-only fast, which resulted in the loss of 30 pounds (13.6 kilograms) but provided no clinical benefit for the rheumatoid arthritis. Of note, the treatment protocol for this patient was determined mostly via background research and the clinician's pattern recognition, rather than on extensive and expensive batteries of tests; stool microbiologic testing was "remarkably unremarkable" excepting a slight above-normal elevation in sIgA and no yeast or dysbiotic microbes identified.

March 2012—severe symptoms and CCP >250: Patient reports suffering significantly with joint pain and lower extremity edema; foundational nutritional protocol[29] is implemented with antidysbiotic/antimicrobial intervention limited to emulsified oregano oil 600mg/d, mitochondrial support and the nutritional immunomodulation protocol. CCP level at this time is beyond laboratory testing limits, measured simply as "greater than" 250 units.

CCP Antibodies IgG/IgA	>250	High	units	0 – 19
			Negative	<20
			Weak positive	20 – 39
			Moderate positive	40 – 59
			Strong positive	>59

January 2013—mild symptoms and CCP 195: Few modifications are made for the first 9 months and patient feels progressively better, but wants to "move to the next level of improvement" because—despite feeling and functioning significantly better solely with dietary and nutritional interventions—patient still notes exacerbations of pain, particularly following extended manual farm labor. At this time, labs are drawn showing an impressive reduction in CCP levels from "greater than" 250 units to 195 units, correlating with a reduction of at least 22%. At this time, patient was commenced on additional treatments including cabergoline (despite normal serum prolactin), oral vancomycin (despite absence of gastrointestinal complaints; treatment aimed at presumptive colonization with segmented filamentous bacteria), and azithromycin (for systemic absorption, antimicrobial effectiveness, and effectiveness against other inflammatory/autoimmune disorders [e.g., reactive arthritis and psoriasis]).

CCP Antibodies IgG/IgA	195	High	units	0 – 19
			Negative	<20
			Weak positive	20 – 39
			Moderate positive	40 – 59
			Strong positive	>59

April 2013—virtually normal, CCP 54: Patient continues to improve clinically; her subjective and objective clinical improvements (including additional loss of 30 pounds [13.6 kilograms] and reduction in hand swelling necessitating resizing of wedding ring) correlate nicely with the reduction in CCP levels, which have reduced from >250 units to 54 units, for a reduction of more than 78%.Thus, by objective physical and laboratory criteria, this patient appears to be experiencing authentic reversal—cure—of her disease due to the functional inflammology protocol.

CCP Antibodies IgG/IgA	54	High	units	0 – 19
			Negative	<20
			Weak positive	20 – 39
			Moderate positive	40 – 59
			Strong positive	>59

---

[28] Vasquez A. *Functional Immunology and Nutritional Immunomodulation*, 2012 updated as *F.I.N.D. S.E.X® The Easily Remembered Acronym for the Functional Inflammology Protocol*, 2013 and completely revised in *Functional Inflammology, Volume 1*, 2014 and *Inflammation and Autoimmune Solutions, 2nd Edition*, 2014.
[29] Vasquez A. Revisiting the Five-Part Nutritional Wellness Protocol: Supplemented Paleo-Mediterranean Diet. *Nutr Perspect* 2011 Jan ichnfm.org/faculty/vasquez/profile.html

Microbial Induction of Noninfectious Systemic Disease

I have compiled the following ever-growing list of mechanisms by which microorganisms can cause immune dysfunction that promotes neuromusculoskeletal inflammation/pain, which has been the main focus of my work in musculoskeletal medicine, starting with my teaching of Orthopedics and Rheumatology for the Naturopathic Medicine program at Bastyr University in 2000 and 2001 and eventuating as my first three books *Integrative Orthopedics* (2004), *Integrative Rheumatology* (2006), and *Musculoskeletal Pain* (2008) . Each of the following exemplifies a mechanism by which microbes can cause "disease" without causing an "infection." Such mechanisms include but are not limited to those listed in the following numbered section and subsections. Microbial molecules are listed and described as the molecule itself *and then again* if it has an additional category and/or if it activates a particular receptor or inflammatory response; in this manner, clinicians have an opportunity to understand each component in detail and then see how to "connect the dots" to better understand how the dots coalesce to make the whole, the clinical presentation, the pathologic phenomenon, to which they are now being provided the decipherative tools. I refer to this first section as "*Microbial Morphology, Molecules, Metabolites, and Pathophysiologic Mechanisms*"—it lays most of the conceptual and information framework that will support the later conversations in clinical applications.

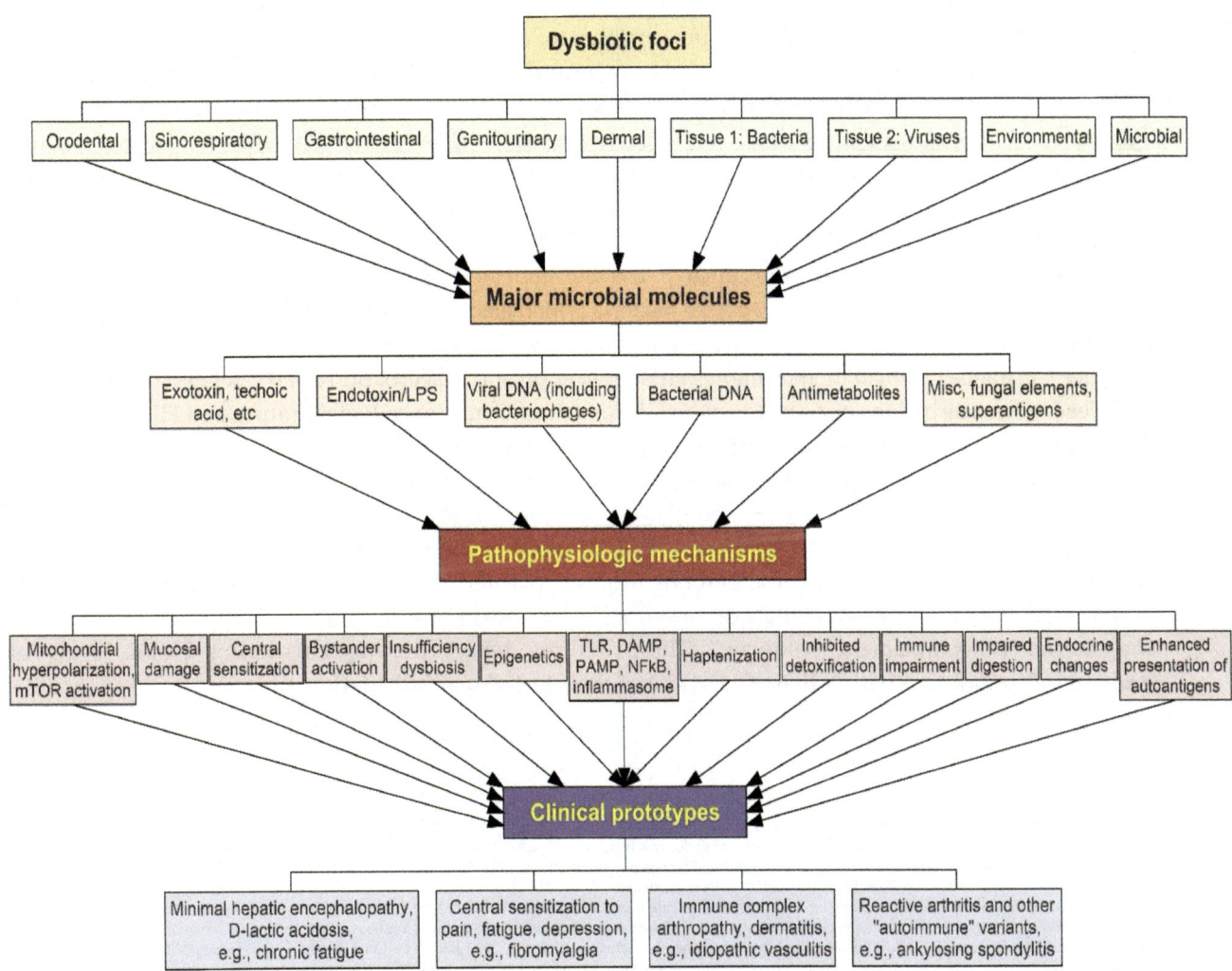

Clinical pathophysiology of dysbiosis-induced disease: The total microbial load communicates to the human body in general and the innate/adaptive immune systems specifically from various locations via specific molecules, which then are "combinatorially summarized" in conjunction with the patient's physiologic profile—including genetic makeup, nutritional status, xenobiotic load, sleep and stress status—to produce a ***pattern*** of clinical manifestations.

Microbial molecules and the three major morphologic types of bacteria: Gram-negative, Gram-positive, and wall-free bacteria: We begin with a short section on the major categories of microbial debris and metabolites.

1. <u>Endotoxins (lipopolysaccharide, LPS) from Gram-negative bacteria</u>: Gram-negative bacteria are defined by their presence an external surrounding membrane comprised of lipopolysaccharide (LPS, comprised of lipid and polysaccharide described as "O-antigen") which fails to "take up" or receive a specific dye called Gram's stain; because LPS is a primary mediator of pathogenic or "toxic" inflammatory responses, and because it is intrinsic or endogenous to the bacterial membrane itself, it is also called endotoxin. In the past, early microbiologists thought that release of endotoxin occurred only with death of the microorganism while exotoxins were actively secreted into the bacteria's surrounding environment; today we appreciate that various endotoxins are secreted at a basal level as a normal part of bacterial trafficking/communication via vesicles and that their release can be increased by stressors, such as antibiotic exposure, and by population death/turnover which occurs constantly. Even in the absence of viable bacteria, the exposure of humans to endotoxin, say for example by intravenous administration for the purpose of experimentation, produces a wide range of adverse physiologic consequences, including 1) triggering an acute proinflammatory response resembling febrile illness or sepsis, 2) increasing intestinal permeability, causing "leaky gut"[30] (via tissue irritation, inflammation, and zonulin[31]), 3) inhibiting hepatic detoxification[32], 4) disrupting the blood-brain barrier and promoting neurodegeneration via neuroinflammation.[33,34,35] The pathophysiologic effects of endotoxin/LPS are often *similar to* and *synergistic with* those of superantigens to effect altered tissue function and widespread inflammation. **LPS and antigens from gram-negative bacteria (in the absence of viable bacteria) exacerbate arthritis in experimental models[36] and trigger inflammatory arthropathy (reactive arthritis) in humans**.[37]

   - <u>Psoriasis and lipopolysaccharide from Gram-negative bacteria—Proposed explanation for the exacerbation of psoriasis in AIDS with a discussion of substance P and gram-negative bacteria</u> (*Autoimmunity* 2004 Feb[38]): The author of this paper proposes that the well-known induction or exacerbation of psoriasis by HIV infection may be due to a variety of factors, including ❶ increased colonization of skin by *Staphylococcus aureus*, ❷ increased release of substance P by immunocytes rather than neurons, and ❸ increased infections/colonization with Gram-negative bacteria which elaborate endotoxin/lipopolysaccharide, which is potently pro-inflammatory. Also proposed is the model of a vicious cycle wherein psoriatic lesions produce substance P, which then promotes HIV replication and exacerbation of HIV-related disease, which then leads to exacerbations of psoriasis, which leads to more substance P elaboration and HIV replication. Other researchers have noted that psoriatic lesions show increased nerve growth and increased elaboration from nerves of substance P, which is a pro-inflammatory neuropeptide.[39]

   - <u>Psoriasis—6 of 11 (54%) patients were shown to have endotoxinemia</u> (*Archives of Dermatology* 1982 Mar[40]): The authors introduce their letter by stating, "Our interest in the possibility of endotoxemia in psoriasis followed recent demonstrations of alterations in levels of alternative complement pathway components and of circulating IgA immune complexes in psoriasis. Endotoxin and immune IgA complexes each activate the alternative complement pathway." These authors report finding **circulating blood levels of endotoxin/lipopolysaccharide in 6 of 11 (54%) of their tested psoriatic patients.**

---

[30] "After endotoxin administration systemic absorption and excretion of lactulose increased almost two-fold... These data suggest that a brief exposure to circulating endotoxin increases the permeability of the normal gut." O'Dwyer et al. A single dose of endotoxin increases intestinal permeability in healthy humans. *Arch Surg*. 1988 Dec;123:1459-64

[31] Fasano A. Intestinal permeability and its regulation by zonulin: diagnostic and therapeutic implications. *Clin Gastroenterol Hepatol*. 2012 Oct;10(10):1096-100

[32] Shedlofsky SI, et al, Blouin RA. Endotoxin depresses hepatic cytochrome P450-mediated drug metabolism in women. *Br J Clin Pharmacol*. 1997 Jun;43(6):627-32

[33] "Following administration of lipopolysaccharide to immunized mice, antibodies gain access to the brain. They bind preferentially to hippocampal neurons and cause neuronal death with resulting cognitive dysfunction and altered hippocampal metabolism..." Kowal et al. Cognition and immunity; antibody impairs memory. *Immunity* 2004 Aug:179-88

[34] Fassbender K, et al . The LPS receptor (CD14) links innate immunity with Alzheimer's disease. *FASEB J*. 2004 Jan;18(1):203-5. fasebj.org/cgi/reprint/03-0364fjev1

[35] Laflamme N, Rivest S. Toll-like receptor 4: the missing link of the cerebral innate immune response triggered by circulating gram-negative bacterial cell wall components. *FASEB J*. 2001 Jan;15(1):155-163 fasebj.org/cgi/reprint/15/1/155.pdf

[36] "The results showed that administration of LPS was followed by reactivation of AIA in a dose-related fashion." Yoshino S, Yamaki K, Taneda S, Yanagisawa R, Takano H. Reactivation of antigen-induced arthritis in mice by oral administration of lipopolysaccharide. *Scand J Immunol*. 2005 Aug;62(2):117-22

[37] "Extensive bacterial cultures of synovial fluid were negative...We conclude that in patients with reactive arthritis after yersinia infection, microbial antigens can be found in synovial-fluid cells from affected joints."Granfors et al.Yersinia antigens in synovial-fluid cells from patients with reactive arthritis. *N Engl J Med* 1989;320:216-2

[38] Namazi. Paradoxical exacerbation of psoriasis in AIDS: proposed explanations including potential roles of substance P, gram-negative bacteria. *Autoimmunity* 2004 Feb:67-71

[39] "Indeed, we have noted marked proliferation of nerve fibers in transplanted psoriatic plaques compared with the few nerves in transplanted normal human skin. By double label immunofluorescence staining, we have further demonstrated that in these terminal cutaneous nerves there is a marked upregulation of neuropeptides, such as substance P and calcitonin gene-related protein." Raychaudhuri SP, Raychaudhuri SK. Role of NGF and neurogenic inflammation in the pathogenesis of psoriasis. *Prog Brain Res*. 2004;146:433-7

[40] Belew PW, Rosenberg EW, Skinner RB Jr, Marley WM. Endotoxemia in psoriasis [letter]. *Arch Dermatol* 1982 Mar;118(3):142-3

- Psoriasis and endotoxin/LPS from Gram-negative bacteria—Improvement of psoriasis with cholestyramine (*Arch Dermatol* 1982 Mar[41]): In this letter to the editor, the authors report the <mark>rapid improvement of psoriasis after the oral administration of cholestyramine resin in five patients with psoriasis.</mark> The rationale for this intervention is to reduce the patient's total inflammatory load by reducing the amount of bacterial endotoxin/LPS absorbed from the gastrointestinal tract. Five patients were treated with oral cholestyramine 4 grams 4 times daily and topical chlorhexidine soap.

- Psoriasis—Endotoxin/lipopolysaccharide (LPS) from intestinal Gram-negative bacteria and the effect of binding with orally administered bile acids (*Pathophysiology* 2003 Dec[42]): This is an impressively large and innovative study. The authors tested the hypothesis that an insufficiency in bile acid production by the liver results in increased bacterial endotoxin absorption from the intestines and that this endotoxin contributes to the immune dysfunction and systemic inflammation of psoriasis. The authors note that, under normal conditions, bile acids secreted from the hepatobiliary system act as detergents by degrading intestinal endotoxins and thereby protecting the host from their pathophysiologic sequelae. Bile acids thereby participate in "physico-chemical defense" by splitting endotoxin/lipopolysaccharide into nontoxic fragments and thus preventing the consequent release of inflammatory cytokines. In this clinical trial, a total of 800 psoriasis patients participated in the study and <mark>551 were treated with oral bile acid (dehydrocholic acid) supplementation for 1-8 weeks</mark>. Treatment efficacy was evaluated clinically and by use of the standard Psoriasis Area Severity Index (PASI) score. The authors note remarkable improvement; "During this treatment, 434 patients (78.8%) became asymptomatic. Of 249 psoriatics receiving the conventional therapy, only 62 (24.9%) showed clinical recovery during the same period of time (P<0.05)." Patients with more acute and short-term psoriasis showed very high rates of improvement; 95% of these patients had resolution of their psoriasis. After two years of treatment, 319 of 551 (57.9%) psoriasis patients treated with bile acids were asymptomatic, compared to only 15 of 249 (6.0%) patients receiving the standard drug treatment. As for the subset of patients with acute psoriasis, at the end of two years, 147 of 184 (79.9%) of psoriatic patients treated with bile acids were asymptomatic; only 10 of 139 (7.2%) acute psoriasis patients receiving standard drug treatment were cured. The authors summarize, "To conclude, the results obtained suggest that <mark>psoriasis can be treated with success by oral bile acid supplementation presumably affecting the microflora and endotoxins released and their uptake in the gut.</mark>" These findings are consistent with the facts that ❶ psoriasis manifests most obviously as dermal hyperproliferation induced by cytokines and that ❷ endotoxin/LPS is one of the most powerful inducers of cytokine release.

- Psoriasis—Use of cholestyramine to bind intestinal endotoxin, and nutrient treatment of severe psoriasis in alcoholics (*J Drugs Dermatol* 2010 Apr[43]): Alcoholism increases the risk of initiation/exacerbation of psoriasis by as much as 800%, with the effect being strongest in men. Of course, alcoholism causes other health problems, too; notable for this discussion are ❶ increased intestinal permeability leading to bacterial endotoxin absorption, and ❷ vitamin and mineral deficiencies commonly causing elevated homocysteine levels and hypomagnesemia, respectively. The two patients in this 2-case report and brief review were treated with magnesium 600 mg, folic acid 5 mg, pyridoxine 100 mg, and cobalamin 1 mg in addition to routine topical and oral medications for psoriasis, acute infections (one patient was treated with Bactrim for MRSA); one patient was treated with cholestyramine 4 grams 4 times per day for 5 days repeated for 3 courses. In the discussion section of the article, the authors review that alcoholism causes increased intestinal permeability and resultant increased absorption of endotoxin with immunogenic/inflammatory consequences. Additionally, cholestyramine while being appropriate for alcoholics to bind endotoxin might exacerbate magnesium deficiency via reduced intestinal absorption (i.e., binding) and by increased urinary excretion, perhaps due to vitamin D deficiency, according to an animal study.[44] As has been noted elsewhere, the authors of this report note that both psoriatics and alcoholics tend to have higher levels of

---

[41] Skinner RB, Rosenberg EW, Belew PW, Marley WM. Improvement of psoriasis with cholestyramine [letter]. *Arch Dermatol*. 1982 Mar;118(3):144

[42] Gyurcsovics K, Bertók L. Pathophysiology of psoriasis: coping endotoxins with bile acid therapy. *Pathophysiology*. 2003 Dec;10(1):57-61

[43] Aronson PJ, Malick F. Towards rational treatment of severe psoriasis in alcoholics: report of two cases. *J Drugs Dermatol*. 2010 Apr;9(4):405-8

[44] "Cholestyramine-fed rats had a net negative balance for calcium and a lower net positive balance for magnesium, iron, and zinc than the controls. Other effects of cholestyramine were an increased urinary excretion of calcium and magnesium, a decreased urinary zinc, and an alkalinization of urine." Watkins et al. Alterations in calcium, magnesium, iron, and zinc metabolism by dietary cholestyramine. *Dig Dis Sci*. 1985 May;30(5):477-82

homocysteine; less widely appreciated is the fact that homocysteine primes neutrophils for inflammatory responses, tissue homing, and induction of increased oxidative stress and tissue damage, some of which is relevant and somewhat specific for the pathogenesis of psoriasis. A separate publication cited by these authors noted that homocysteine levels correlated positively and folate levels correlated negatively with the severity and extent of psoriasis. Homocysteine causes intracellular depletion of magnesium; this problem is ameliorated by supplementation with magnesium, folate, pyridoxine, cobalamin, cholecalciferol and the promotion of systemic/urinary alkalinization. Not mentioned in this report is the possibility that hypomagnesemia contributes to psoriasis via enhancement of neurogenic inflammation, and that folate and other coenzymes are necessary for the epigenetic modifications (most obviously, DNA methylation) that might favorably influence the psoriatic and proinflammatory phenotype.

2. Peptidoglycans, teichoic acid, and exotoxins from Gram-positive bacteria: Exotoxins are toxic inflammation-inducing molecules secreted by bacteria into their surrounding environment by viable bacteria and can also be released upon death/lysis of the bacteria. Teichoic acids (TAs, including the variants of wall teichoic acids, [WTA] and lipoteichoic acids [LTA]) are glycopolymers that function in bacterial shape, division, and antibiotic resistance; upon receipt by the innate immune response, TAs trigger inflammatory responses. Peptidoglycan (PG) is a major cell-wall component of Gram-positive bacteria. Peptidoglycans from gram-positive bacteria such as group-A streptococci can cause malaise, fever, dermatosis, tenosynovitis, cryoglobulinemia (an immune complex disease), and arthritis.[45]

> **PROPOSED MECHANISM OF DISEASE**
>
> Rudzki et al[65] stated that "undisputed" positive correlation between bacterial allergy and skin disease exists if the three conditions of *provocation, focal reaction,* and *isomorph effect* are present after skin testing with bacterial antigens. Provoca-
>
> **Gram-positive bacteria and peptidoglycan promote inflammatory disease by several mechanisms**
>
> 1. Bacterial allergy
> 2. Stimulated formation of immune complexes
> 3. Stimulation of sensitization and cross-reactivity to other microbes for additive and synergistic and perpetually maintained microbe-induced inflammation, even after clearance of the original Gram-positive microbe
> 4. Stimulation of the innate immune system
>
> Ely PH. Bowel bypass syndrome: response to bacterial peptidoglycans. *J Am Acad Dermatol* 1980 Jun

Experimental arthritis can be induced in animals by exposing them to group-B streptococci isolated from the nasopharynx of human patients with rheumatoid arthritis.[46] *Staphylococcus aureus* is a gram-positive bacterium, certain strains of which produce the toxic shock syndrome toxin-1 (TSST-1) that causes scalded skin syndrome, toxic shock syndrome, and food poisoning; other strains of *Staphylococcus aureus* that do not produce TSST-1 are also capable of causing toxic shock syndrome from colonization of bone, vagina, wounds, or rectum.[47] Experimental evidence has shown that peptidoglycan-polysaccharide complexes from "good" and "normal" bacteria such as Bifidobacteria and *Lactobacillus casei* can also induce an inflammatory arthritis; this speaks against the "more is better" approach to probiotic supplementation and also demonstrates how **bacterial overgrowth of the small bowel (detailed later) can induce joint pain and inflammation even in the absence of so-called "pathogens."**[48,49]

- Lipoteichoic acid in infection and inflammation. (*Lancet Infect Dis.* 2002 Mar[50]): "Lipoteichoic acid (LTA)...binds to target cells either non-specifically, to membrane phospholipids, or specifically, to CD14 and to Toll-like receptors...[and] triggers the release from neutrophils and macrophages of reactive oxygen and nitrogen species, acid hydrolases, highly cationic proteinases, bactericidal cationic peptides, growth factors, and cytotoxic cytokines, which may act in synergy to amplify cell damage. Thus, LTA shares with endotoxin (lipopolysaccharide) many of its pathogenetic properties. In animal studies, LTA has induced arthritis, nephritis, uveitis, encephalomyelitis, meningeal inflammation, and periodontal lesions, and also triggered cascades resulting in septic shock and multiorgan failure."

---

[45] "A characteristic intermittent neutrophilic dermatosis, associated with polyarthritis, tenosynovitis, malaise, fever, and cryoglobulinemia, occurs in 20% of patients who undergo ileojejunal bypass surgery for the treatment of morbid obesity... Peptidoglycans from numerous intestinal bacteria...are suggested as causative of the toxic and immunologic features of this syndrome." Ely PH. The bowel bypass syndrome: a response to bacterial peptidoglycans. *J Am Acad Dermatol*. 1980 Jun;2(6):473-87

[46] "The origin of rheumatoid arthritis (RA) is in our opinion a bacterial infection." Svartz N. The origin of rheumatoid arthritis. *Rheumatology*. 1975;6:322-8

[47] Shandera, Moran. "Infectious diseases: viral and rickettsial." Tierney, McPhee, Papadakis (eds). *Current Medical Diagnosis and Treatment. 44th Edition*. 2005, 1356-8

[48] Simelyte E, et al. Bacterial cell wall-induced arthritis: chemical composition and tissue distribution of four Lactobacillus strains. *Infect Immun*. 2000 Jun;68(6):3535-40

[49] Toivanen P. Normal intestinal microbiota in the aetiopathogenesis of rheumatoid arthritis. *Ann Rheum Dis*. 2003;62:807-11 ard.bmjjournals.com/cgi/reprint/62/9/807

[50] Ginsburg I. Role of lipoteichoic acid in infection and inflammation. *Lancet Infect Dis*. 2002 Mar;2(3):171-9

- Peptidoglycan appears to be a major causative factor for psoriasis (*Trends Immunol* 2006 Dec[51]): Peptidoglycan is a major cell-wall component of Gram-positive bacteria and has been detected within antigen-presenting cells of patients with psoriasis. Furthermore, the skin of patients with psoriasis shows Th1 cells that are specifically responsive to streptococcal and/or staphylococcal peptidoglycans; this indicates that peptidoglycan is probably an important T-cell stimulator which contributes to psoriasis. Additionally, patients with psoriasis appear to be genetically predisposed to disorders associated with peptidoglycans because their immune cells are altered in such a way as to allow for enhanced T-cell response to the bacterial antigens such as peptidoglycans. The authors conclude, "These observations suggest that peptidoglycan is a major etiological factor for psoriasis and emphasize the importance of peptidoglycan in bacterial-infection-induced inflammatory disease."

- Patients with cutaneous and arthritic psoriasis have elevated IgA antibodies against streptococcal peptidoglycan-polysaccharide (*Clin Exp Rheumatol* 1997 Jul-Aug[52]): Patients with psoriasis and psoriatic arthritis have elevated IgA levels specific to streptococcal peptidoglycan-polysaccharide (PG-PS); antibody levels do not vary with disease severity. Very remarkably, the authors concluded by stating, "The results suggest chronic mucosal stimulation of lymphocytes by long-lived streptococcal antigens in patients with psoriasis..." Readers should appreciate that the evidence linking psoriasis with mucosal infections with the streptococcal bacteria is consistent and very strong. The mucosal surfaces of the nose, sinuses, and throat are the most common locations for chronic streptococcal bacteria colonization/dysbiosis.

- Rheumatoid arthritis and peptidoglycans: Normal intestinal bacteria appear to contribute to rheumatoid arthritis and other inflammatory diseases (*Ann Rheum Dis* 2003 Sep[53]): In this article Professor Toivanen reviews 61 published articles to advance the model of inflammatory disease induction by bacteria, particularly what might generally be considered normal intestinal bacteria. Professor Toivanen notes several interesting items of fact: ❶ bacteria that are genetically identical per PCR testing can have subtle differences in their peptidoglycan structure, and these minute differences in peptidoglycan structure [perhaps due to epigenetic factors] can effect profound differences in pathophysiologic responses, i.e., either promoting or suppressing inflammatory responses by the immune system, ❷ bacterial peptidoglycan can stimulate the production of the autoantibody **rheumatoid factor**, which for many decades was considered the primary serologic diagnostic marker for rheumatoid arthritis (80% positivity), and which is present in other autoimmune disorders such as Sjogren's syndrome (70% positivity), and which contributes directly to joint and tissue injury and inflammation via direct deposition, particularly in the form of immune complexes, and ❸ peptidoglycans induce inflammatory responses following binding with Toll-like receptor 2 (TLR-2). Three successive sentences are particularly worthy of quotation:

    "The ability of bacterial cell walls to induce chronic, erosive arthritis was first described in the rat by using *Streptococcus pyogenes*. Self-perpetuating arthritis, closely resembling human rheumatoid arthritis by histological criteria, develops in susceptible rat strains after a single intraperitoneal injection of the bacterial cell wall. In addition to *Streptococcus pyogenes*, several bacterial species representing *Lactobacillus*, *Bifidobacterium*, *Eubacterium*, *Collinsella*, and *Clostridium* have been observed to have a similar ability."

    The important observation that, in experimental models with genetically susceptible animals, chronic inflammatory arthritis can be induced by a one-time exposure to commonly encountered bacteria provides clear objective proof that bacteria and—importantly—their nonviable cell wall fragments can induce chronic inflammatory disease. Readers should note that *Streptococcus pyogenes* can contribute to inflammatory *arthritis* in certain models, while contributing to inflammatory *dermatitis* in others.

- Contribution of *Staphylococcus aureus* cell wall products teichoic acid and peptidoglycan to immunoglobulin (IgE, IgA, IgG) synthesis in patients with atopic dermatitis (*Immunology* 1992 Jan[54]): Patients with atopic dermatitis (eczema) have increased skin and nasal colonization with *Staphylococcus aureus*, and the immune response induced by living or dead *Staphylococcus aureus* differs in eczema patients from that seen in normal

[51] Baker BS, Powles A, Fry L. Peptidoglycan: a major aetiological factor for psoriasis? *Trends Immunol*. 2006 Dec;27(12):545-51
[52] Rantakokko K, et al. Antibodies to streptococcal cell wall in psoriatic arthritis and cutaneous psoriasis. *Clin Exp Rheumatol*. 1997 Jul-Aug;15(4):399-404
[53] Toivanen P. Normal intestinal microbiota in the aetiopathogenesis of rheumatoid arthritis. *Ann Rheum Dis*. 2003 Sep;62(9):807-11
[54] Neuber K, König K. Effects of Staphylococcus aureus cell wall products (teichoic acid, peptidoglycan) and enterotoxin B on immunoglobulin (IgE, IgA, IgG) synthesis and CD23 expression in patients with atopic dermatitis. *Immunology*. 1992 January; 75(1): 23–28 ncbi.nlm.nih.gov/pmc/articles/PMC1384797/

healthy patients; in patients with eczema, exposure to fragments of *Staphylococcus aureus* actually causes immunosuppression (reductions in IgA and IgG) rather than the expected immune upregulation that should occur following exposure to a pathogenic microbe. Furthermore, in patients with eczema, exposure to *Staphylococcus aureus* cell wall fragments increases production of IgE and histamine, two pathophysiologic factors inextricably associated with the skin inflammation and discomfort/itchiness of eczema. The finding that bacterial cell wall fragments can lead to *reduced* production of IgA and IgG implies that mucous membrane and/or skin colonization with *Staphylococcus aureus* (and perhaps *Bordetella pertussis*, *Haemophilus influenzae* and Gram-negative bacteria which produce lipopolysaccharide [LPS]) can promote local and systemic immune suppression which favors (poly)microbial colonization and persistence while also contributing to skin inflammation and irritation via enhanced production of IgE and histamine. Relatedly, psoriatic patients also have increased nasal and skin colonization with *Staphylococcus aureus*; thus, *Staphylococcus aureus* probably acts via similar molecular mechanisms to contribute to these two disorders, which differ from each other yet at the same time can be seen as variants on the theme of microorganism-triggered "patterns of inflammation."

- Skin disorders and peptidoglycans (*Brain Behav Immun* 2008 Jan[55]): The authors of this paper note that many inflammatory diseases such as psoriasis, atopic dermatitis, lichen planus, and vitiligo have also been associated with emotional stress and local alterations of the sympathetic (adrenergic) nervous system. Using a unique experimental model, the authors show that peptidoglycan from Gram-positive bacteria—but not lipopolysaccharide from Gram-negative bacteria—promoted a Th1-type inflammation.

3. L-form, pleomorphic, "cell wall-deficient" bacteria: Long-term metabolic and inflammatory complications: Classically, in science and medicine, we have divided bacteria into two gross categories depending on their ability to take-up or repel a chemical dye referred to as Gram's stain; Gram-positive bacteria stain either strongly or weakly, while Gram-negative bacteria resist the stain via the lipophilic exterior membrane which is the endotoxin or lipopolysaccharide/LPS that defines Gram-negative bacteria. (A few of us actually performed these laboratory techniques in doctorate-level coursework, but these days most medical students just study books.) This is quite often of critical clinical importance since many antibiotics target the bacterial wall directly, and therefore the physician must know whether to use an antibiotic agent that targets Gram-positive or Gram-negative bacteria. A third category exists: these are L-form or "cell wall-deficient" bacteria (CWDB or L-forms, named after the Lister Institute where they were discovered in 1935) that are neither Gram-negative nor Gram-positive in the true sense because they have no exterior wall. Many common Gram-positive and Gram-negative bacteria, including many clinically important pathogens, have the ability to assume a wall-less phenotype and to compensate via production of additional interior cell membrane; *Staphylococcus aureus* and *Bacillus subtilis* are classic and pathogenic Gram-positive bacteria that can

> **Wall-less bacteria: difficult to see, understand, culture and kill, but nonetheless present and relevant**
>
> "Although many free-living mycobacteria can be cultured from the human intestinal tract, no cell wall-defective mycobacteria were found in 27 controls but they were found in 12% of patients with Crohn's disease and in 16% with ulcerative colitis. Pleomorphic, variably acid-fast bacteria were found in 52% of ulcerative colitis patients and only 7% of controls."
>
> Domingue et al. Bacterial persistence and expression of disease. *Clin Microbiol Rev* 1997.

assume a wall-less L-form.[56,57] Without cell walls to target with drugs (or an effective immune response), and without walls to identify microscopically, these bacteria are difficult to comprehend and are thereby easily ignored/forgotten by doctors and pathologists/microbiologists, respectively; complicating manners further is that these wall-less bacteria are difficult and often impossible to culture. Wall-less bacteria are thereby exceedingly difficult to identify, understand, kill, and culture; therefore people are more likely to think about concrete items than to ponder them. Domingue[58] reviewed his work spanning 30 years (1967-1997) in a 2010 review published in *Discovery Medicine* and noted the presence of "considerable circumstantial evidence linking tissue pleomorphic forms of unknown origin with idiopathic chronic inflammatory, collagen, lymphoproliferative, nephro-urological (including interstitial cystitis and prostatodynia), and neoplastic

[55] Manni M, Maestroni GJ. Sympathetic nervous modulation of the skin innate and adaptive immune response to peptidoglycan but not lipopolysaccharide: involvement of beta-adrenoceptors and relevance in inflammatory diseases. *Brain Behav Immun*. 2008 Jan;22(1):80-8

[56] Claessen D, van Wezel GP. Off the wall. *Elife*. 2014 Nov 26;3 elifesciences.org/content/3/e05427 ncbi.nlm.nih.gov/pmc/articles/PMC4244568/

[57] Errington J. L-form bacteria, cell walls and the origins of life. *Open Biol* 2013 Jan:3; 120143

[58] Domingue GJ. Demystifying pleomorphic forms in persistence and expression of disease. *Discov Med.* 2010 Sep;10(52):234-46

diseases" and that "these altered forms created in vivo take up intracellular and/or extracellular residence; possibly establishing a sort of immune protected parasitic relationship, resisting/surviving phagocytic action, and creating subtle pathologic changes in the host during a prolonged period of tissue persistence. This might translate into an etiology for chronic inflammatory diseases, when the stressed bacteria increase in numbers and overwhelm the normal biological functions of the host." He further proposes that "in vivo persistence of these bacterial elements escape immune surveillance partially, completely, or may integrate with host cell organelles to create bacteria-host-cell-antigen complexes which could provoke immunopathologic consequences... in a wide spectrum of diagnostically troublesome human diseases." In an earlier 1997 review in *Clinical Microbiology Reviews* published by the American Society for Microbiology, Domingue and Woody[59] detail CWDB, and connect these enigmatic life forms with several clinical diseases, including idiopathic urinary tract diseases, aphthous stomatitis, Whipple's disease, and Crohn's disease. Of high clinical relevance is that the uniquely prolonged and occult existence of these wall-less bacteria enables them to incite low-level immune activation and to produce metabolites and immunogens; this can be described as a hidden internal impairment/agitation/battle that can promote stimulation of the innate immune system and promote all forms of inflammation—metabolic, allergic, and autoimmune.

- Cell-wall-deficient bacteria in psoriasis (*Chin Med J* 2009 Dec[60]): "CWDB were isolated from 74.2% of psoriasis patients, 23.5% of chronic tonsillitis patients and only 6.3% of controls. Antibiotic therapy was appropriate for approximately 80% of psoriasis patients with CWDB infection, and in only 8.9% psoriasis patients CWDB infection was detected after antibiotic therapy. Meanwhile, our study showed that CWDB and wide-type bacteria did remarkably enhance the production of IFN-gamma, in vitro, and PBMC proliferation."

- Variably acid-fast bacteria in a necropsied case of systemic lupus erythematosus (*Cutis* 1984 Jun[61]): "In a necropsy of a 41-yoF with systemic lupus erythematosus (SLE) who died of acute myocardial infarction (AMI), Cantwell and Cove found "Variably acid-fast coccoid forms, suggestive of CWDB, were observed in specially-stained (intensified Kinyoun acid-fast stain) microscopic sections of the heart, lungs, kidney, adrenal glands, brain, connective tissue, and other organs."

- Histologic observations of cell wall deficient bacteria in cutaneous in systemic lupus erythematosus. (*Int J Dermatol.* 1982 Nov[62]): "The cutaneous lesions of seven consecutive patients with cutaneous lupus erythematosus (LE), two patients with systemic LE, and a patient with both dermatomyositis and cutaneous LE, were studied bacteriologically and microscopically for the presence of bacteria. ... Basophilic- and eosinophilic-stained coccoid forms, suggestive of CWD bacteria, were identified in the microscopic sections of all the cases, as were non-acid-fast coccoid forms. ... The complex bacteriology of LE is discussed, as well as the possibility that variably acid-fast CWD microbes might be the long sought-after etiologic agent or agents in the production of LE."

> **Practical applications and paradigm shift in antibiotic drug prescribing**
>
> One of the implications of acknowledging wall-less bacteria is that we as clinicians cannot prescribe antimicrobial drugs based on Gram-positivity/negativity as we most commonly do. Importantly, the administration of antimicrobials that interfere with cell wall formation is one of the triggers for bacteria to switch to the wall-less phenotype. Clinicians should anticipate the need to use different antimicrobial (bactericidal) agents than those to which they are accustomed; antimicrobial therapy is discussed later in this work/series.

4. Bacterial DNA, viral DNA and bacteriophage DNA: **Bacterial DNA stimulates a proinflammatory response that is comparable to that induced by endotoxin/LPS.** Exposure to single-stranded *bacterial* DNA induces formation of antibodies against single-stranded *mammalian* DNA. These findings may be particularly relevant to patients with systemic lupus erythematosus—a disorder for which the pathogenic hallmark is the formation of anti-DNA antibodies—since these patients have an impaired ability to clear bacterial DNA from the serum

[59] Domingue GJ Sr, Woody HB Bacterial persistence and expression of disease. *Clin Microbiol Rev.* 1997 Apr;10(2):320-44
[60] Wang GL et al. Cell-wall-deficient bacteria: a major etiological factor for psoriasis? *Chin Med J* (Engl). 2009 Dec 20;122(24):3011-6
[61] Cantwell AR Jr, Cove JK. Variably acid-fast bacteria in a necropsied case of systemic lupus erythematosus with acute myocardial infarction. *Cutis.* 1984 Jun;33(6):560-7
[62] Cantwell et al. Histologic observations of coccoid forms suggestive of cell wall deficient bacteria in cutaneous/systemic lupus erythematosus. *Int J Dermatol.* 1982 Nov:526-37

and therefore experience prolonged pro-inflammatory stimulation when exposed to bacterial DNA.[63] Chronic exposure to microbial immunogens is a recognized means for the induction of autoimmunity in animal models.

- Antibodies to DNA: "idiopathic" or infection? (*Lupus* 2009 Nov[64]): "Antibodies to DNA (anti-DNA) are the serological hallmark of systemic lupus erythematosus (SLE) and unique markers of the immunological disturbances critical to disease pathogenesis. In the form of immune complexes, anti-DNA autoantibodies can deposit in the tissue to incite inflammation and damage; in addition, these complexes can induce cytokine production, most prominently, type 1 interferon. … Because bacterial DNA is a potent stimulant of innate immunity by both toll-like receptor (TLR) and non-TLR signaling pathways, foreign DNA introduced during the course of bacterial or viral infection could have a dual role in antibody induction. This DNA could serve as an adjuvant to activate innate immunity as well as an immunogen to drive an antigen-specific antibody response. In this scenario, the generation of cross-reactive autoantibodies, in contrast to highly specific antibodies to bacterial DNA, most likely depends on genetically determined abnormalities in the B-cell repertoire in patients with SLE. Given the universal expression of DNA, this model suggests that many different kinds of infections could trigger pathogenic autoantibody responses in SLE, as well as induce flare."

- Bacterial DNA (bactDNA) in the peripheral blood of patients with active psoriasis (*JAMA Dermatol* 2015 Mar[65]): "Blood bactDNA was present in 16 patients with psoriasis, all of whom showed the phenotype of plaque psoriasis (16 of 45 [35.5%]), whereas 6 patients with guttate psoriasis, 3 with inverse psoriasis, and all 27 controls did not have bactDNA in the blood. Species identification corresponded to *Escherichia coli* (n=9), *Klebsiella pneumoniae* (n=2), *Enterococcus faecalis* (n=2), *Proteus mirabilis* (n=1), *Streptococcus pyogenes* (n=1), and *Shigella fresneli* (n=1). … The systemic inflammatory response was significantly higher in patients with bactDNA compared with other patients and controls." Inflammatory markers correlated with bactDNA included IL-1, IL-6, IL-12, TNF, and IFN-gamma. At first look, the one-bacteria-per-patient appearance is somewhat misleading; obviously other microbial colonizations, including those without DNA present in the blood and other types of colonizations—especially yeast—would be expected to be present but were not searched for in this investigation.

- Enhanced immune activation in psoriasis vulgaris mediated by combination of streptococcal antigen with bacterial DNA (*J Invest Dermatol* 2009 Nov[66]): These researchers investigated the effect of streptococcal DNA on lymphocyte proliferation and activation as well as cytokine secretion in psoriasis. As has been previously reported by other researchers, the authors of this paper also found that peripheral blood mononuclear cells (PBMCs) from psoriatic patients had higher proliferative responses upon stimulation by streptococcal antigens (SA) when compared with those from healthy individuals. Pretreatment of the streptococcal antigens with an enzyme that degrades DNA (DNase-1) reduced the amount of immune stimulation elicited following exposure of immune cells to streptococcal antigens, thus implicating streptococcal DNA as having an important role in the induction of the pro-inflammatory response elicited by streptococcal antigens in psoriatic immune cells. The authors conclude, "This study demonstrates the integral function of SA, particularly streptococcal DNA, in the pathogenesis of psoriasis."

- Antigen DNA isolated from immune complexes in plasma of patients with systemic lupus erythematosus hybridizes with the Escherichia coli lac Z gene (*Clin Exp Immunol* 1991 Jul[67]): "These data strongly suggest that the antigen DNA obtained from three patients [with active systemic lupus erythematosus (SLE)] is of bacterial origin."

- Extrinsic DNA in immune complexes in systemic lupus erythematosus (*Biochem Biophys Res Commun* 1991 Jan[68]): Antigen DNA isolated from immune complexes in patients with active systemic lupus erythematosus was found to have regions from *E. coli* (metK gene) and bacteriophage f1. Both of these

[63] "The immunostimulatory activities of bacterial DNA are varied and encompass the mitogenicity of B cells and the induction of cytokines including IFN-α/β, IFN-γ, tumor necrosis factor alpha, interleukin 6 (IL-6), and IL-12 (17, 21, 23). Together, these activities resemble those of endotoxin…" Pisetsky DS. Antibody responses to DNA in normal immunity and aberrant immunity. *Clin Diagn Lab Immunol.* 1998 Jan;5(1):1-6 cvi.asm.org/cgi/reprint/5/1/1
[64] Pisetsky DS, Vrabie IA. Antibodies to DNA: infection or genetics? *Lupus.* 2009 Nov;18(13):1176-80
[65] Ramírez-Boscá et al. Identification of bacterial DNA in the peripheral blood of patients with active psoriasis. *JAMA Dermatol.* 2015 Mar [Epub ahead of print]
[66] Cai YH, Lu ZY, Shi RF, Xue F, Chen XY, Pan M, Yuan WR, Xu H, Li WP, Zheng J. Enhanced proliferation and activation of peripheral blood mononuclear cells in patients with psoriasis vulgaris mediated by streptococcal antigen with bacterial DNA. *J Invest Dermatol.* 2009 Nov;129:2653-60
[67] Terada et al. Antigen DNA isolated from immune complexes in plasma of patients with systemic lupus erythematosus hybridizes with the Escherichia coli lac Z gene. *Clin Exp Immunol.* 1991 Jul;85(1):66-9
[68] Terada et al. Demonstration of extrinsic DNA from immune complexes in plasma of patient with systemic lupus erythematosus. *Biochem Biophys Res Commun* 1991 Jan:323-30

microbial DNA fragments interacted with the patient's IgG fraction to form immune complexes. The authors showed that the "antigen DNA was proved to be originated from bacteria or bacteriophage."

- SLE and reduced colonization resistance (*Epidemiol Infect* 1994 Apr[69]): "Anti-ds-DNA antibodies may be pathogenic in SLE by forming immune complexes with DNA. Foreign bacteria in the intestines could constitute the stimulus for anti-ds-DNA antibody production in SLE. Colonization Resistance (CR) is the defense capacity of the indigenous microflora against colonization of the intestines by foreign bacteria. A low CR implies increase of translocation of bacteria and a higher chance of subsequent, possibly DNA-cross-reacting antibacterial antibody production. We measured CR by a comprehensive biotyping technique in healthy individuals and patients with inactive and active SLE. CR tended to be lower in active SLE patients than in healthy individuals. This could indicate that in SLE more and different bacteria translocate across the gut wall due to a lower CR. Some of these may serve as polyclonal B cell activators or as antigens cross-reacting with DNA." Obviously the clinical implications are clear and profound; for most of medical history, SLE was considered an idiopathic "autoimmune" condition, but now we have consistent data showing that a highly significant part of lupus pathophysiology is microbe-triggered and a *misdirected immune response* against commensal bacteria, resulting in the formation of pathogenic disease-causing immune complexes that contain microbial—not human—DNA. Combining this with the pro-inflammatory immunophenotype induced by mitochondrial hyperpolarization[70] and mTOR activation[71] provides not simply insight into the pathology of the disease but legitimate breakthrough opportunities for improved treatment, which is safe, effective, affordable, and readily available.[72]

5. Superantigens: Many viral, bacterial, and fungal microbes produce superantigens—molecules which are capable of causing widespread, nonspecific, and unregulated proinflammatory immune activation. One of the hallmarks of superantigens is their ability to induce polyclonal T- and B-lymphocyte activation and the production of excessive levels of cytokines and other inflammatory effectors.[73] Solanki et al[74] described superantigens as "microbial or viral toxins" which behave as "immunostimulatory molecules" and "extremely potent polyclonal T-cell mitogens" which "bind major histocompatibility complex (MHC) class-II molecules without any prior processing and stimulate large numbers of T cells (up to 20% of all T cells)" due to "their **unique ability to cross-link MHC class II [found on antigen-presenting cells] and the T-cell receptor (TCR)**, forming a trimolecular complex"; these authors concisely note that superantigens "activate antigen-presenting dendritic cells by producing increased expression of HLA-DR antigen and co-stimulatory molecules (CD54, CD83 and CD86) and the production of tumor necrosis factor TNF-alpha [as well as TNF-beta, IL-2, and gamma-interferon]." Obviously, when the body is in such a state of unregulated inflammation *combined with simultaneous bacterial antigen presentation,* inevitably some of this inflammation will affect the structures of the musculoskeletal system especially because articular tissues are predisposed to immune attack due to their proclivity to retain antigens and immune complexes[75,76]; the resulting inflammatory response is further exaggerated/exacerbated by superantigen-driven immunostimulation. Several research groups have found evidence of superantigen involvement in the pathogenesis of rheumatoid arthritis.[77,78] Superantigens can be categorized as ❶ **endogenous superantigens**—these are encoded by viruses such as Epstein-Barr virus, ❷

[69] Apperloo-Renkema et al. Host-microflora interaction in systemic lupus erythematosus (SLE): colonization resistance of the indigenous bacteria of the intestinal tract. *Epidemiol Infect.* 1994 Apr;112(2):367-73

[70] Vasquez A. *Mitochondrial Nutrition and Endoplasmic Reticulum Stress in Primary Care, Second Edition,* 2014. [ISBN 1502952505]

[71] Vasquez A. *Mastering mTOR.* International College of Human Nutrition and Functional Medicine (February 21, 2015). [ASIN B00TVT5YK2]

[72] Vasquez A. *Functional Inflammology: Volume 1, Naturopathic Rheumatology v3.*5. International College of Human Nutrition and Functional Medicine, 2014

[73] "The basis of autoimmune disorders due to superantigen is due to greater stimulation of T-lymphocytes and elaborate cytokine production." Hemalatha V, Srikanth P, Mallika M. Superantigens - Concepts, clinical disease and therapy. *Indian J Med Microbiol* 2004;22:204-211

[74] Solanki LS, Srivastava N, Singh S. Superantigens: a brief review with special emphasis on dermatologic diseases. *Dermatology Online Journal* 2008 Feb 28;14(2):3

[75] Inman RD. Antigens, the gastrointestinal tract, and arthritis. *Rheum Dis Clin North Am.* 1991 May;17(2):309-21

[76] "Other factors, like the specific properties of synovial vessels and the adhesion molecules responsible for synovium-specific homing, will contribute to the guiding of the monocytes from the mucosal areas into the joints." Wuorela M, Tohka S, Granfors K, Jalkanen S. Monocytes that have ingested Yersinia enterocolitica serotype O:3 acquire enhanced capacity to bind to nonstimulated vascular endothelial cells via P-selectin. *Infect Immun.* 1999 Feb;67(2):726-32 iai.asm.org/cgi/content/full/67/2/726

[77] "They also suggest that the etiology of RA may involve initial activation of V beta 14+ T cells by a V beta 14-specific superantigen with subsequent recruitment of a few activated autoreactive v beta 14+ T cell clones to the joints while the majority of other V beta 14+ T cells disappear." Paliard X, West SG, Lafferty JA, Clements JR, Kappler JW, Marrack P, Kotzin BL. Evidence for the effects of a superantigen in rheumatoid arthritis. *Science.* 1991 Jul 19;253(5017):325-9

[78] "Given that binding sites for superantigens have been mapped to the CDR4s of TCR beta chains, the synovial localization of T cells bearing V beta s with significant CDR4 homology indicates that V beta-specific T-cell activation by superantigen may play a role in RA." Howell MD, Diveley JP, Lundeen KA, Esty A, Winters ST, Carlo DJ, Brostoff SW. Limited T-cell receptor beta-chain heterogeneity among interleukin 2 receptor-positive synovial T cells suggests a role for superantigen in rheumatoid arthritis. *Proc Natl Acad Sci* U S A. 1991 Dec 1;88(23):10921-5

exogenous superantigens—these are elaborated by bacteria and include staphylococcal enterotoxins and streptococcal pyrogenic exotoxins, and ❸ B-cell superantigens—these predominantly stimulate B-cells to produce antibodies/immunoglobulins; an example of a B-cell superantigen is staphylococcal proteins A and Fv. Very noteworthy is the fact that superantigens, which are directly immunologically active at very low concentrations, are resistant to degradation by protein-digesting enzymes (proteases) and that they are absorbed intact directly through the skin and mucosal surfaces; therefore, a direct positive relationship is likely to exist between microbial production and physiologic effects of superantigens.

> **Important concepts about superantigens**
> Bacteria and other microorganisms (microbes) can each produce several—not just one—superantigens. The implications are that 1) one single microbe can promote inflammation and immune dysfunction via elaboration of several different superantigens, and that 2) researchers have to test for several superantigens per microbe per patient per disease in order to fully appreciate the role of a microbe's superantigen repertoire in association with a particular disease. Further adding to the complexity of these associations is the fact that other molecules—beside and beyond the classic/known/prototypic superantigens—can also contribute to pro-inflammatory immune dysfunction; bacterial DNA is known to be immunostimulatory.

- Superantigens in dermatologic diseases. (*Dermatology Online Journal* 2008 Feb[79]): In this excellent review of molecular biology and clinical disorders, the authors note that microbial superantigens are associated with many important clinical disease that affect the skin, including staphylococcal toxic shock syndrome, staphylococcal scalded skin syndrome, guttate psoriasis, psoriasis vulgaris (chronic plaque psoriasis), Kawasaki syndrome, atopic dermatitis, cutaneous T-cell lymphoma, and acute juvenile pityriasis rubra pilaris. The authors state, "Evidence shows that T-cells in psoriasis are triggered by conventional antigens and superantigens. It is suggested that although **the process is initiated by bacterial superantigens, molecular mimicry between the bacterial antigens and keratin 17 leads to activation of autoreactive T-cells and persistence of disease.**" The authors note that all streptococci secrete SPEC, a superantigen known to stimulate marked expansion of T-cells which display a particular marker "Vβ2"; these Vβ2 T-cells are found in increased quantities in acute skin lesions of patients with guttate psoriasis.

- High prevalence of *Staphylococcus aureus* cultivation and superantigen production in patients with psoriasis. (*Eur J Dermatol* 2009 May[80]): This excellent research—conducted by assessing the skin and nasal cavities (nostrils, nares) of 50 psoriatics and 50 healthy controls—demonstrates the following associations between psoriasis and active colonization with the bacteria *Staphylococcus aureus*:

  1) Psoriatic skin lesions have more *Staphylococcus aureus* than does nearby unaffected skin: In patients with psoriasis, skin lesions are more likely to culture *Staphylococcus aureus* (64%) than is the unaffected non-lesional skin (14%).

  2) Psoriatic patients are more likely to harbor *Staphylococcus aureus* in their nares/nostrils than are healthy people: "*Staphylococcus aureus* was cultivated from the nares in 25 (50%) of 50 patients with psoriasis and in 17 (34%) of 50 healthy controls."

  3) The *Staphylococcus aureus* found at the site of psoriatic lesions is more likely to be a strain of bacteria that produces distinct toxins: "In psoriasis patients, 31 (96.8%) out of the 32 strains isolated from the lesional skin and 3 (42.3%) out of the 7 strains isolated from the non-lesional skin were toxigenic (p = 0.01)." This means that psoriasis is quantitatively (more bacteria) and qualitatively (more toxin-producing bacteria) linked with *Staphylococcus aureus*. A very important contribution of this study is the finding that *Staphylococcus aureus* produces numerous—not only one—superantigens capable of inducing a significant part of the pathophysiology of psoriasis; these superantigens can be described as "non-classical superantigens" such as methicillin resistance gene (*mecA*), *etb*, *eta* and *see* as well as classical superantigens such as *sea*, *seb*, *sec*, *sed* and *tst*.

  4) The *Staphylococcus aureus* found in the nares/nostrils of psoriatic patients is more likely to be a strain of bacteria that produces distinct toxins: "Isolated strains from the nares were toxigenic in 96% (24/25) for patients with psoriasis and in 41.2% (7/17) for healthy controls, respectively (p = 0.006)." A strong correlation of approximately 70% was found between the *Staphylococcus aureus* in the nares and on the skin of patients with psoriasis; this suggests bidirectional contamination.

[79] Solanki LS, Srivastava N, Singh S. Superantigens: a brief review with special emphasis on dermatologic diseases. *Dermatology Online Journal* 2008 Feb 28;14(2):3
[80] Balci et al. High prevalence of Staphylococcus aureus cultivation and superantigen production in patients with psoriasis. *Eur J Dermatol*. 2009 May-Jun;19(3):238-42

5) <u>Psoriatic patients with lesions that culture positive for *Staphylococcus aureus* have worse disease activity than psoriatic patients with negative cultures</u>: "Patients with cultivation-positive in lesional skin had a significantly higher PASI score than patients who were cultivation-negative in lesional skin (8.28 +/- 3.97 vs. 5.89 +/- 2.98, p = 0.031)." More *Staphylococcus aureus* in psoriasis lesions could be cause (i.e., the *Staphylococcus aureus* are directly contributing to the psoriatic lesions) or effect (i.e., the psoriatic lesions are more likely to become colonized with *Staphylococcus aureus*). However, given the established molecular role of superantigens in two primary hallmarks of psoriasis—inflammation and cytokine-induced cellular hyperproliferation—the most logical interpretation is that the association between *Staphylococcus aureus* and psoriasis is causal rather than casual.

The authors conclude by stating, "Our results confirm that *S. aureus* colonization and its toxigenic-strains are associated with psoriasis. According to our findings, non-classical superantigens such as methicillin resistance gene (*mecA*), *see* and *etb* may also be associated with psoriasis."

6. <u>Antimetabolites</u>: Yeast and bacteria can produce certain molecules which *jam up, monkey wrench*, or otherwise interfere with normal human cellular metabolism. The best example is **D-lactic acid**, which impairs human metabolic pathways that are designed to work with the "human" form of this metabolite—the levo isomer—L-lactic acid. Commonly resulting in headache, fatigue, depression, and sometimes death, D-lactic acidosis is extensively well documented in the medical research literature and commonly occurs in association with bacterial overgrowth of the intestine, particularly following intestinal bypass surgery.[81] Other antimetabolites produced from (intestinal) microbes which are associated with human disease and dysfunction include **ammonia, tryptamine, tyramine, octopamine, mercaptates, aldehydes, alcohol (ethanol), tartaric acid, indolepropionic acid, indoleacetic acid, skatole, indole, putrescine**, and **cadaverine**. Many of these metabolites are seen in higher amounts in patients with migraine, depression, weakness, confusion, schizophrenia, agitation, hepatic encephalopathy, chronic arthritis and rheumatoid arthritis. **Gut-derived neurotoxins** from bacteria and yeast may contribute to autistic symptomatology[82,83], and case reports have consistently demonstrated that excess absorption of bacterial metabolites can alter behavior in humans and result in acute neurocognitive decline and behavioral abnormalities in children.[84] **Hydrogen sulfide (H2S)**, produced by intestinal bacteria such as *Citrobacter freundii*[85], is a mitochondrial poison[86] and is strongly associated with disease activity in ulcerative colitis.[87] Degradation of tryptophan by bacterial tryptophanase predisposes the host to a "functional tryptophan deficiency" and may result in insufficiency of serotonin which would contribute to hyperalgesia, depression, impaired adrenal responsiveness[88] ("hypoadrenalism"), and insomnia; **indole** and **skatole**, which are gut-derived bacterial degradation products of tryptophan, produce an inflammatory arthritis identical to rheumatoid arthritis in animal models.[89,90]

- <u>Increased D-lactic acid intestinal bacteria in chronic fatigue syndrome</u> (*In Vivo* 2009 Jul[91]): These researchers begin by noting that the symptoms of cognitive dysfunction and neurological impairment which are commonly seen in patients with chronic fatigue syndrome (CFS) are also classic presenting complaints in

[81] "D-Lactic acidosis is a potentially fatal clinical condition seen in patients with a short small intestine and an intact colon. Excessive production of D-lactate by abnormal bowel flora overwhelms normal metabolism of D-lactate and leads to an accumulation of this enantiomer in the blood." Vella A, Farrugia G. D-lactic acidosis: pathologic consequence of saprophytism. *Mayo Clin Proc.* 1998 May;73(5):451-6

[82] Sandler RH, Finegold SM, Bolte ER, et al. Short-term benefit from oral vancomycin treatment of regressive-onset autism. *J Child Neurol.* 2000 Jul;15(7):429-35

[83] Shaw et al. Increased urinary excretion of analogs of Krebs cycle metabolites and arabinose in two brothers with autistic features. *Clin Chem* 1995;41(8Pt1):1094-104

[84] "The neurological features consisted of a depressed conscious state, confusion, aggressive behaviour, slurred speech and ataxia. The organic acid profile of urine demonstrated increased amounts of lactic, 3-hydroxypropionic, 3-hydroxyisobutyric, 2-hydroxyisocaproic, phenyllactic, 4-hydroxyphenylacetic and 4-hydroxyphenyllactic acids. Of the lactic acid 99% was D-lactic acid." Haan et al. Severe illness caused by products of bacterial metabolism in child with short gut. *Eur J Pediatr.* 1985;144:63-5

[85] Lennette EH (editor in chief). *Manual of Clinical Microbiology. Fourth Edition.* Washington DC; American Society for Microbiology: 1985, page 269. See also web.indstate.edu/thcme/micro/GI/general/sld038.htm Accessed 10/27/2005

[86] "Treatment of H2S poisoning may benefit from interventions aimed at minimizing ROS-induced damage and reducing mitochondrial damage." Eghbal MA, Pennefather PS, O'Brien PJ. H2S cytotoxicity mechanism involves reactive oxygen species formation and mitochondrial depolarisation. *Toxicology.* 2004 Oct 15;203(1-3):69-76

[87] "CONCLUSIONS: Metabolic effects of sodium hydrogen sulfide on butyrate oxidation along the length of the colon closely mirror metabolic abnormalities observed in active ulcerative colitis, and increased production of sulfide in ulcerative colitis suggests that the action of mercaptides may be involved in the genesis of ulcerative colitis." Roediger WE, et al. Reducing sulfur compounds of the colon impair colonocyte nutrition: implications for ulcerative colitis. *Gastroenterology* 1993 Mar;104:802-9

[88] "This hypothesis is supported by the findings in chronic MS patients of a significantly diminished adrenal cortisol reactivity to insulin-induced hypoglycemia which is considered a stress response mediated through the 5-HT system. Consequently, since patients with MS exhibit an abnormal response to stress it follows that increased tryptophan availability through dietary supplementation would diminish their vulnerability to psychological stress." Sandyk R. Tryptophan availability and the susceptibility to stress in multiple sclerosis: a hypothesis. *Int J Neurosci.* 1996 Jul;86(1-2):47-53

[89] Nakoneczna I, Forbes JC, Rogers KS. The arthritogenic effect of indole, skatole and other tryptophan metabolites in rabbits. *Am J Pathol.* 1969 Dec;57(3):523-38

[90] Rogers KS, Forbes JC, Nakoneczna I. Arthritogenic properties of lipophilic, aryl molecules. *Proc Soc Exp Biol Med.* 1969 Jun;131(2):670-2

[91] Sheedy JR, et al. Increased d-lactic acid intestinal bacteria in patients with chronic fatigue syndrome. *In Vivo.* 2009 Jul-Aug;23(4):621-8

patients with D-lactic acidosis, which is always caused by bacterial overgrowth of the small bowel and/or (more rarely) by the patient's inability to metabolize/detoxify products of bacterial metabolism produced in the small and/or large bowel. The authors report finding a **significant increase of Gram-positive facultative anaerobic fecal microorganisms** in 108 CFS patients as compared to 177 control subjects. Specifically, they report, "The viable count of D-lactic acid producing *Enterococcus* and *Streptococcus* spp. in the fecal samples from the CFS group (3.5 x 10(7) cfu/L and 9.8 x 10(7) cfu/L respectively) were significantly higher than those for the control group (5.0 x 10(6) cfu/L and 8.9 x 10(4) cfu/L respectively). **Readers should note that this is approximately a 10-fold increase in *Enterococcus* and a 1,000-fold increase in *Streptococcus* in the CFS group compared with the control group. These Gram-positive bacteria produced not only more lactic acid in general but specifically they produced more of the dextro isomer D-lactic acid** than the Gram negative *Escherichia coli*. The authors correctly conclude that these findings "might explain not only neurocognitive dysfunction in CFS patients but also mitochondrial dysfunction, these findings may have important clinical implications." A note of personal experience: the current author (Dr Vasquez) had one event of severe headache and dyscognition following consumption of a prebiotic (FOS) supplement during my 6-year bout with a CFS-related condition; from this experience, I furthered my understanding of dysbiosis and continued to do so *via personal experience* for the following 10 years. Of further note, based on my personal experience and review of the biomedical literature, I proposed in my CME monograph *Musculoskeletal Pain: Expanded Clinical Strategies* (2008, Institute for Functional Medicine) that D-lactic acidosis was one of the pathophysiologic mechanisms by which microbial overgrowth of the intestines causes fibromyalgia; I was therefore gratified to see this article—published in 2009, nearly 2 years after I had proposed this mechanism—verifying my hypothesis.

> **D-lactate triad: SIBO, CHO, and IP— bacterial overgrowth, carbohydrate, and increased permeability; the solutions are to reduce SIBO, reduce/modify CHO, heal gut, promote motility**
>
> "D-lactate is usually produced in excess when small bowel resection allows delivery of a high carbohydrate load to the colon. Elevation of D-lactate in plasma may also occur after other types of abdominal surgery, as a result of increased intestinal permeability and bacterial translocation across the intestinal mucosal barrier. Nonsurgical causes of intestinal hyperpermeability also increase absorption of D-lactate from the intestinal lumen."
>
> Galland L. Gut microbiome and the brain. *J Med Food.* 2014 Dec

- Short bowel syndrome and D-lactic acidosis (*Arch Dis Child* 1980 Oct[92]): The three-sentence abstract of this case report reads, "Metabolic acidosis in a 3-year-old child with short bowel syndrome led to the discovery of massive D-lactic aciduria. After normalization of the intestinal bacterial flora, D-lactate disappeared together with the acidosis. Dysbacteriosis with excessive production of D-lactate by intestinal bacteria (unidentified) and subsequent absorption explains this unusual cause of metabolic acidosis." Note the use of "dysbacteriosis" which is more commonly abbreviated to "dysbiosis", with the latter being more accurate in its nonspecificity since the disease-producing microbes may be from several different kingdoms and thus not exclusive to bacteria. The young boy in this case report underwent bowel resection secondary to multiple congenital malformations and complications from infection, i.e., mesenteric thrombosis tertiary to dehydration secondary to infectious diarrhea. After several episodes of neurocognitive dysfunction including weakness and dyspnea, the child was eventually diagnosed with multiple nutritional deficiencies, malabsorption, and lactic acidosis secondary to intestinal overgrowth of Gram-positive D-lactate-producing bacteria and an insufficiency of Gram-negative bacteria. The child was treated only with probiotic supplementation—no antibiotics were given—and D-lactate levels fell quickly within 4 days and were virtually undetectable by day 11. Thus, probiotic therapy alone may be sufficient treatment for some cases of D-lactic acidosis, particularly when an "insufficiency dysbiosis" of beneficial bacteria and a relative or absolute "overgrowth dysbiosis" of harmful bacteria coexist.

- Propionic acid is a dysbiotic neuro/psycho-toxic antimetabolite (*Glob Adv Health Med* 2013 Nov[93]): Propionic acid is found in some foods such as wheat and dairy products and is also produced endogenously by gut bacteria; in elevated amounts, it alters brain function, mitochondrial function, carnitine metabolism, fatty acid synthesis while it induces oxidative stress, glutathione depletion, and microglial activation. Elevated

---

[92] Schoorel EP, Giesberts MA, Blom W, van Gelderen HH. D-Lactic acidosis in a boy with short bowel syndrome. *Arch Dis Child.* 1980 Oct;55(10):810-2
[93] Macfabe D. Autism: metabolism, mitochondria, and the microbiome. *Glob Adv Health Med.* 2013 Nov;2(6):52-66. doi: 10.7453/gahmj.2013.089

amounts of propionic acid are noted in children with autism, and propionic acid induces autistic-like behavioral changes when administered to rats. Some bacterial groups, such as *Desulfovibrio* and *Clostridia*, are able to produce more than one neurotoxic antimetabolite; thus, appreciating the combinatorial effects of microbes and their metabolites is clearly more clinically accurate and will therefore produce the best interventions when translated into clinical care.

- P-cresol (and related metabolites) is a dysbiotic neuro/psycho-toxic antimetabolite (*Neurotoxicol Teratol* 2013 Mar[94]): P-cresol (4-methylphenol) is found in some foods in small amounts and is produced by dysbiotic gut bacteria. "Urinary p-cresol and its conjugated derivative p-cresylsulfate have been found elevated in an initial sample and recently in a replica sample of autistic children below 8 years of age, where it is associated with female sex, greater clinical severity regardless of sex, and history of behavioral regression." P-cresol and/or its metabolites impair hepatic function and detoxification, promote inflammation, promote membrane depolarization and seizure activity, and inhibit conversion of dopamine to norepinephrine. P-cresylsulfate is said to "share conformational features with myelin basic protein (MBP) so that it cross-reacts with antibodies targeted against MBP peptide"; this molecular mimicry and resultant cross-reactivity are particularly relevant for autism, multiple sclerosis, and schizophrenia—all of which are neuro/psych diseases with dysbiotic and autoimmune components. Clinicians must appreciate the clinical relevance of p-cresol's inhibition of dopamine beta-hydroxylase[95] and synergism with HPHPA (discussed elsewhere) which does the same; both promote excess dopamine and insufficient norepinephrine.

7. Beneficial metabolites and molecular signatures: For most of the study of microbiologic means of disease causation, we in the basic and health sciences have focused on the disease-promoting effects of pathogenic bacteria rather than the health-promoting effects of beneficial bacteria; this disease-oriented model appears appropriate, given the conditions under which the discipline of microbiology developed and the historical context. However, in these modern times we increasingly appreciate the value of beneficial bacteria which when present have an anti-inflammatory effect and when absent are not available to provide health-promoting input into the mix of molecular signals and substrates. This "insufficiency dysbiosis" is discussed in a later section. Butyrate stands preeminent as a beneficial microbial metabolite; butyrate shows clear anti-inflammatory, mitochondrial-supportive, and immunomodulatory/epigenetic benefits.

8. Biofilms—brief introduction: In this now-ended section on microbial molecules and morphology, I could have included discussion of biofilms, since this could be considered a particular type of microbial morphology. While this is true from the perspective of Microbiology (ie, bacteria and fungi form biofilms) and inpatient Hospital Medicine (ie, biofilms form on catheters and endotracheal tubes), I do not deem it accurate from the perspective of outpatient Clinical Medicine, wherein our concern is not with biofilms from a microbiologic or nosocomaial perspective, but rather as a host-microbe interaction wherein biofilms are constructed with host immune cells and host proteins and nuclear material and thereby contribute to inflammation/autoimmunity. As such, I have decided to describe biofilms in the following section on pathophysiologic responses.

Active learning and reflection

Use the limited space below to consider a few of the clinical implications of each of the following, as if you were explaining dysbiosis to a medical student or educated patient:

1. Gram-negative bacterial products, LPS
2. Gram-positive bacterial products
3. L-form, pleomorphic, "cell wall-deficient" bacteria
4. Immunostimulation by bacterial DNA, viral DNA and bacteriophage DNA
5. Superantigens
6. Antimetabolites
7. Beneficial metabolites and molecular signatures—note that these are generally anti-inflammatory

---

[94] Persico AM, Napolioni V. Urinary p-cresol in autism spectrum disorder. *Neurotoxicol Teratol.* 2013 Mar-Apr;36:82-90
[95] "p-Cresol binds DBH by a mechanism that is kinetically indistinguishable from normal dopamine substrate binding. ... p-Cresol is shown to be a rapid mechanism-based inactivator of DBH. This inactivation exhibits pseudo-first-order kinetics, is irreversible, is prevented by tyramine substrate or competitive inhibitor..." Goodhart et al. Mechanism-based inactivation of dopamine beta-hydroxylase by p-cresol and related alkylphenols. *Biochemistry.* 1987 May 5;26(9):2576-83

Pathophysiologic responses: In the following sections, we transition from simple microbial molecules to the human-microbe interface—the reception of and response to those microbial markers and metabolites.

1. <mark>Damage to the intestinal mucosa, increased intestinal permeability (IP)</mark>: One of the indirect ways by which gastrointestinal microbes can cause non-infectious disease is by damaging the intestinal mucosa, a situation which results in "leaky gut." The increased absorption of molecular debris from the gut—"antigen overload" from otherwise benign yeast, bacteria, and foods—results in "systemic inflammation"[96] and "immune activation"[97], which contribute to enhanced autoantigen processing and bystander activation. Exacerbations and relapse of ulcerative colitis and Crohn's disease are preceded by increases in intestinal permeability; this is direct evidence of "leaky gut" preceding clinical disease.[98] Evidence of "leaky gut" is seen in several systemic inflammatory disorders, including asthma[99], eczema[100], psoriasis[101], Behcet's disease[102], seronegative spondyloarthritis[103] and ankylosing spondylitis[104] and nearly all of the so-called "idiopathic" juvenile arthropathies such as enteropathic spondyloarthropathy and oligoarticular juvenile idiopathic arthritis.[105] A "leaky gut" type of intestinal disease (protein-losing enteropathy) occurs in some patients with lupus.[106]

   - Increased intestinal permeability in patients with <mark>fibromyalgia</mark> and patients with <mark>complex regional pain syndrome</mark> (*Rheumatology* 2008 Aug[107]): The authors of this paper, which I have cited in several locations in this text as a testament to its inclusiveness and importance, state early in their introduction an excellent summary of the points made in the preceding paragraph, "<mark>In several disorders, SIBO is known to cause an increased intestinal permeability (IP) that is an increased degree of leakiness of the intestinal epithelial layer to luminal products. Such increased leakiness has direct pathophysiological relevance as luminal products passing through the epithelial layer gain abnormal access to both the intestinal and extraintestinal immune systems. Upon contact these products may stimulate immunocompetent cells to play a role in causing the systemic disease such as in inflammatory bowel disease, allergies and arthritides.</mark>"

   - Intestinal permeability in patients with psoriasis (*J Dermatol Sci* 1991 Jul[108]): In this study of 15 psoriatic patients and 15 healthy volunteers, intestinal permeability was evaluated using the 51Cr-labeled EDTA absorption test. 24-h urine excretion of 51Cr-EDTA from psoriatic patients was 2.46% which was significantly higher than the results from controls at 1.95% and therefore indicated <mark>increased intestinal permeability among patients with psoriasis</mark>. Clinical implications of these results include 1) that psoriasis is not merely a skin condition—it affects other vital structures, in this instance, the gastrointestinal tract, and 2) that enhanced intestinal absorption of food antigens and microbial metabolites and immunogenic debris is ensured among psoriatic patients and would be expected to contribute to systemic inflammation and immunologic sensitization. This study was published in 1991 and used urinary measurement of orally administered 51Cr-EDTA to determine intestinal permeability; today most practicing clinicians use the lactulose:mannitol assay as a more sensitive/reliable indicator of mucosal permeability status.

   - Small intestinal permeability in dermatological disease (*Quarterly Journal of Medicine* 1985 Sep[109]): The authors of this study assessed small intestinal permeability using the cellobiose/mannitol differential sugar absorption test (using urinary excretion of absorbed cellobiose and mannitol to determine intestinal permeability). Test subjects included 62 patients with atopic eczema, 29 with psoriasis, and 18 with

[96] Campbell DI, Elia M, Lunn PG. Growth faltering in rural Gambian infants is associated with impaired small intestinal barrier function, leading to endotoxemia and systemic inflammation. *J Nutr*. 2003 May;133(5):1332-8

[97] "Altered gastrointestinal motility and sensation, changed activity of the central nervous system, and increased sympathetic drive and immune activation may be understood as consequences of the host response to SIBO." Lin HC. Small intestinal bacterial overgrowth: a framework for understanding irritable bowel syndrome. *JAMA*. 2004 Aug:852-8

[98] Wyatt J, Vogelsang H, Hubl W, Waldhoer T, Lochs H. Intestinal permeability and the prediction of relapse in Crohn's disease. *Lancet*. 1993 Jun 5;341(8858):1437-9

[99] Hijazi Z, et al. Intestinal permeability is increased in bronchial asthma. *Arch Dis Child*. 2004 Mar;89(3):227-9

[100] Ukabam SO, Mann RJ, Cooper BT. Small intestinal permeability to sugars in patients with atopic eczema. *Br J Dermatol*. 1984 Jun;110(6):649-52

[101] "The 24-h urine excretion of 51Cr-EDTA from psoriatic patients was 2.46 +/- 0.81%. These results differed significantly from controls (1.95 +/- 0.36%; P less than 0.05)." Humbert P, Bidet A, Treffel P, Drobacheff C, Agache P. Intestinal permeability in patients with psoriasis. *J Dermatol Sci*. 1991 Jul;2(4):324-6

[102] Fresko I, et al. Intestinal permeability in Behcet's syndrome. *Ann Rheum Dis*. 2001 Jan;60(1):65-6

[103] Di Leo V, D'Inca R, Bettini MB, Podswiadek M, Punzi L, Mastropaolo G, Sturniolo GC. Effect of Helicobacter pylori and eradication therapy on gastrointestinal permeability. Implications for patients with seronegative spondyloarthritis. *J Rheumatol*. 2005 Feb;32(2):295-300

[104] "Patients with AS have altered small intestinal, but not gastric, permeability. NSAID use cannot explain all the abnormality. Bowel permeability abnormalities, possibly genetically determined, may antedate development of bowel or joint symptoms." Vaile JH, Meddings JB, Yacyshyn BR, Russell AS, Maksymowych WP. Bowel permeability and CD45RO expression on circulating CD20+ B cells in patients with ankylosing spondylitis and their relatives. *J Rheumatol*. 1999 Jan;26(1):128-35

[105] Picco P, et al. Increased gut permeability in juvenile chronic arthritides. A multivariate analysis of diagnostic parameters. *Clin Exp Rheumatol*. 2000 Nov-Dec;18:773-8

[106] "Fourteen cases of primary lupus-associated protein-losing enteropathy have now been reported in the English-language literature." Perednia DA, Curosh NA. Lupus-associated protein-losing enteropathy. *Arch Intern Med*. 1990 Sep;150(9):1806-10

[107] Goebel et al. Altered intestinal permeability in patients with primary fibromyalgia and in patients with complex regional pain syndrome. *Rheumatology*. 2008 Aug;47(8):1223-7

[108] Humbert P, Bidet A, Treffel P, Drobacheff C, Agache P. Intestinal permeability in patients with psoriasis. *J Dermatol Sci*. 1991 Jul;2(4):324-6

[109] Hamilton I, Fairris GM, Rothwell J, Cunliffe WJ, Dixon MF, Axon AT. Small intestinal permeability in dermatological disease. *Q J Med*. 1985 Sep;56(221):559-67

dermatitis herpetiformis. Results of testing were *generally* unremarkable among *most* psoriatics and eczema patients when compared to the control population. However, some patients showed distinct abnormalities. Among the 62 patients with eczema, 7 (11%) had abnormal cellobiose/mannitol absorption as measured by urinary excretion; 6 of these patients underwent jejunal biopsy, and one patient was found to have celiac disease. Among the 29 patients with psoriasis, 7 (24%) had abnormal cellobiose/mannitol recovery. Among the 18 patients with dermatitis herpetiformis, 11 (61%) had abnormal cellobiose/mannitol recovery; this is not surprising given the intimate causative association between celiac disease and dermatitis herpetiformis. Thus, reasonable interpretations of this data are that ❶ a clinically significant number of patients with eczema, psoriasis, and dermatitis herpetiformis have abnormal intestinal permeability, ❷ that these "skin conditions" and apparent "dermatological diseases" are systemic disorders which commonly occur with gastrointestinal components, and ❸ given the important role of intestinal mucosa integrity as a barometer of health and as a determinant of systemic inflammation and immune responses, attention to gastrointestinal (dys)function in these patients is worthy of additional investigation by researchers and attention by clinicians. This study was published in 1985 and used urinary measurement of orally administered cellobiose and mannitol to determine intestinal permeability; today most practicing clinicians use the lactulose:mannitol assay as a more sensitive/reliable indicator of mucosal permeability status.

2. <u>Activation of inflammatory pathways of innate immunity—Toll-like receptors (TLR), NFkB, DAMP and PAMP, Inflammasome</u>: The following subsections describe some of the means by which molecular patterns are perceived/received for eventual translation into inflammatory responses. What we see in inflammatory diseases are "too many inflammatory signals"; the medical/drug approach is to use drugs to block the formation/reception of these signals (i.e., what I have called "the endless game of trying to intercept the inflammatory football") while the naturopathic/functional approach is to address and remove the causes of the inflammatory responses (i.e., "stopping the game", aiming to cure—not endlessly "manage"—the disease).

   - <u>Pattern recognition receptors—PRRs</u>: Pattern recognition receptors (PRRs) are a "primitive" part of the innate immune system; as the name implies, PRRs recognize molecular patterns that correlate with microbes (pathogen-associated molecular patterns [PAMPs]) and/or tissue damage (damage-associated molecular patterns [DAMPs]).

   - <u>Pathogen-associated molecular patterns—PAMP—receptors</u>: PAMP receptors recognize bacterial carbohydrates (such as lipopolysaccharide or LPS, mannose), nucleic acids (such as bacterial or viral DNA or RNA), bacterial peptides (flagellin), peptidoglycans and lipoteichoic acids (from Gram-positive bacteria), N-formylmethionine, lipoproteins and fungal glucans and chitin. Microbial products such as peptidoglycans and endotoxins (as well as others) promote inflammation and arthritogenesis by activating receptors and nuclear transcription factors with the resultant non-specific upregulation of pro-inflammatory genetic expression.

   - <u>Danger/damage-associated molecular patterns—DAMP—receptors</u>: DAMPs include uric acid (an indicator of cell death, oxidative stress), mitochondrial fragments, DNA, and extracellular ATP.
     - Circulating mitochondrial DAMPs cause inflammatory responses (*Nature* 2010 Mar[110]): "Here we show that injury releases mitochondrial DAMPs (MTDs) into the circulation with functionally important immune consequences. MTDs include formyl peptides and mitochondrial DNA. These activate human polymorphonuclear neutrophils (PMNs) through formyl peptide receptor-1 and Toll-like receptor (TLR) 9, respectively. MTDs promote PMN Ca(2+) flux and phosphorylation of mitogen-activated protein (MAP) kinases, thus leading to PMN migration and degranulation in vitro and in vivo. Circulating MTDs can elicit neutrophil-mediated organ injury. Cellular disruption by trauma releases mitochondrial DAMPs with evolutionarily conserved similarities to bacterial PAMPs into the circulation. These signal through innate immune pathways identical to those activated in sepsis to create a sepsis-like state. The release of such mitochondrial 'enemies within' by cellular injury is a key link between trauma, inflammation and SIRS."

---

[110] Zhang et al. Circulating mitochondrial DAMPs cause inflammatory responses to injury. *Nature*. 2010 Mar 4;464(7285):104-7

- <u>Toll-like receptors—TLR</u>: TLRs are transmembrane proteins that trigger innate immune responses (e.g., nonspecific inflammation) upon activation with substances such as bacterial endotoxin/LPS. Mammalian TLRs are numbered 1 to 11, with TLR4 being the most famous for its reception of LPS and subsequent activation of NFkB. Interestingly, TLR4 is also activated by hyperglycemia/obesity-associated saturated fatty acids and mediates hypothalamic inflammation which reduces satiety (thereby perpetuating obesity) and induces systemic inflammation and insulin resistance. **A well-known function of TLRs is, via their transmembrane domain and a cytoplasmic tail domain that is homologous to the interleukin-1 receptor, the initiation of various intracellular signaling cascades, including activation of nuclear factor-kB (NFkB), which is a key transcription factor that promotes transcription of genes coding for pro-inflammatory molecules** such as cytokines, chemokines, co-stimulatory molecules (needed for immune responsiveness), and adhesion molecules (needed for the homing of immunocytes to inflamed/damaged tissue). Nuclear transcription factor kappaB (NFkB) is considered one of the most important nuclear transcription factors for stimulating genetic expression of proinflammatory genes, and NFkB is activated by microbes and their structures including viruses and endotoxins[111]; generally speaking, activation of TLR leads to activation of NFkB. In this manner, we can discuss TLR and NFkB as existing along a continuum, while also appreciating that TRL activates additional inflammatory pathways (independent from NFkB) and NFkB can be activated by additional inflammatory stimuli (independent from TLR). Toll-like receptors (TLRs, especially TLR-2 and even more so with TLR-4) promote an inflammatory response by NFKB-dependent and NFKB-independent pathways following exposure to microbial structures including but not limited to peptidoglycans and lipopolysaccharides.[112] About a dozen different TLRs have been identified, and these play an important role in the joint destruction seen in the classic example of dysbiotic arthropathy—rheumatoid arthritis.[113] From a nutritional perspective, we see that **Toll-like receptor activity is stimulated by saturated fatty acids and inhibited by polyunsaturated fatty acids, especially the omega-3 fatty acid docosahexaenoic acid.**[114] Likewise, NFkB activity can be modulated by numerous nutrients as I have reviewed later in this text and elsewhere.[115] Of course, nutritional, botanical, or pharmacologic modulation of inflammation should not supersede investigation and correction of the underlying cause(s) of inflammation.

  - <u>Psoriasis and bacterial activation of TLRs and NFkB</u> (*Adv Dermatol* 2008 Nov[116]): Keratinocytes in **psoriatic lesions have increased levels of TLRs 1, 2, 4, 5 and 9 compared with normal skin**; this suggests the probability of enhanced responsiveness to microbial immunogens. Whether this upregulated expression of TLRs is a nonspecific response to inflammation or a specific response to the presence of microorganisms is not clear; however what is very obvious is that the presence of microbe-sensing TLRs with the presence of additional bacteria on the skin of psoriatic patients certainly provides a well-set stage for dermatologic inflammation. "Thus," the author notes, "TLR activation may also play a role in the pathophysiology of psoriasis by exacerbating the disease process." Also noted is the very important observation that **the antimicrobial peptide cathelicidin (LL-37), which is found at high levels in psoriatic skin, can convert non-stimulatory self-DNA into a potent activator of TLR-9** on dendritic cells (plasmacytoid DCs) resulting in production of IFN-alpha, leading to the conclusion that "This may be one important mechanism of how **TLRs can promote autoimmunity in psoriasis.**" Per review by Lamphier et al[117], TLR-9 is expressed intracellularly and is activated in response to DNA, in particular DNA containing unmethylated CpG motifs that are more prevalent in microbial than in mammalian DNA; however, under certain conditions, TLR-9 can recognize self-DNA and this may promote immune responses against DNA such as noted in the autoimmune disease systemic lupus erythematosus (SLE) particularly as TLR-9 binds rather indiscriminately to a broad range of DNAs. Notice the implications and four-step stream of probable events: ❶ microbe-induced skin inflammation and tissue injury → ❷ upregulation of TLRs (esp. TLR-9) and antimicrobial

[111] Tak PP, Firestein GS. NFkB: a key role in inflammatory diseases. *J Clin Invest*. 2001;107(1):7-11 jci.org/cgi/content/full/107/1/7

[112] Armant MA, Fenton MJ. Toll-like receptors: a family of pattern-recognition receptors in mammals. *Genome Biol*. 2002 Jul 29;3(8):REVIEWS3011

[113] Ospelt C, et al. Toll-like receptors in rheumatoid arthritis joint destruction mediated by two distinct pathways. *Ann Rheum Dis*. 2004 Nov;63 Suppl 2:ii90-ii91

[114] Lee et al. Saturated fatty acids, but not unsaturated fatty acids, induce expression of cyclooxygenase-2 mediated through Toll-like receptor 4. *J Biol Chem*. 2001 May:16683-9

[115] Vasquez A. Nutritional and botanical inhibition of NFkB. *Nutr Perspectives* 2005 Jul:5-12 InflammationMastery.com/reprints

[116] Miller LS. Toll-like receptors in skin. *Adv Dermatol*. 2008;24:71-87

[117] Lamphier MS, Sirois CM, Verma A, Golenbock DT, Latz E. TLR9 and the recognition of self and non-self nucleic acids. *Ann N Y Acad Sci*. 2006 Oct;1082:31-43

peptides (esp. cathelicidin) ➔ ❸ cathelicidin-induced conversion of nonoffensive self-DNA into an autoinflammatory immunogen, which then potently activates the already upregulated TLR-9 ➔ ❹ thereby, microbial inflammation results in autoimmunity/autoinflammation (to self-DNA).

- <u>NOD-like receptors (NLR)</u>: NOD (nucleotide-binding oligomerization domain) proteins bind DAMPs such as extracellular ATP to activate inflammatory responses. A related group of primitive PRRs, NLRs are a group of approximately 20 cytoplasmic proteins that regulate inflammatory and apoptotic responses. These receptors are activated by exogenous/microbial and endogenous/damage-related molecular patterns to trigger nonspecific innate immune responses. NOD1 recognizes meso-DAP, a peptidoglycan constituent of Gram-negative bacteria. NOD2 proteins recognize intracellular MDP (muramyl dipeptide), a peptidoglycan constituent of both Gram-positive and Gram-negative bacteria.

- <u>Nuclear transcription factor kappa beta—NFkB</u>: Most inflammatory stimuli such as those which activate receptors for PRR, PAMP, DAMP, TLR, and NLR essentially always lead to NFkB activation, but NFkB can be activated by other means. Refer to minimonograph on NFkB in Chapter 1 for details and interventions.

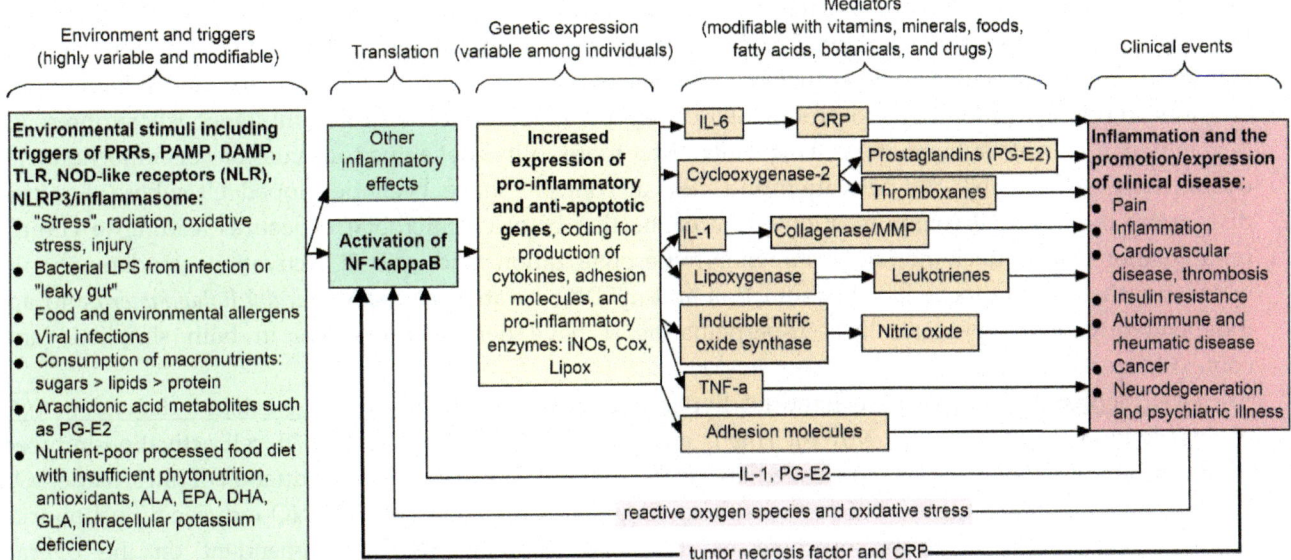

Schema of the NFkB pathway—from environmental triggers to clinical presentations: Notice the self-perpetuating cycle wherein inflammatory mediators activate NFkB for the formation of additional inflammatory mediators. From Vasquez 2005.[118]

- <u>Inflammasome</u>: The inflammasome is a multiprotein oligomer consisting of receptors and enzymes; variations on the same theme lead to descriptions using singular (inflammasome) and plural (inflammasomes) descriptions. Discovered in 2002, inflammasomes are assemblies or "platforms" for reception of molecules such as DAMP and PAMP and the translation of that pattern into an appropriate immune/inflammatory response via the recruitment of enzymes which, for example, perform the final modifications on pro-cytokines to create the active effector cytokines. The exact composition of an inflammasome depends on the activator which initiates inflammasome assembly. PRRs such as TLRs and NLRs are on the receiving end, while enzymes such as caspases are on the effector end, inducing final modification for the activation of cytokines (e.g., pro-IL-1 to IL-1, pro-IL-18 to IL-18) or initiating induction of programmed cell death via pyroptosis. As an example, the NLRP3 inflammasome is activated by a large number of stimuli, including low intracellular potassium concentrations, viruses such as influenza A, *Neisseria gonorrhoeae,* bacterial toxins e.g. nigericin and maitotoxin, liposomes, urban particulate matter, and crystallized endogenous molecules such as cholesterol crystals and monosodium urate (MSU) crystals.

  □ <u>NLRP3 inflammasome is activated in fibromyalgia and reduced by coenzyme Q10</u> (*Antioxid Redox Signal* 2014 Mar[119]): "Mitochondrial dysfunction was accompanied by increased protein expression of

[118] Vasquez A. Nutritional and Botanical Inhibition of NFkB. *Nutr Perspectives* 2005 Jul:5-12 InflammationMastery.com/reprints
[119] Cordero et al. NLRP3 inflammasome is activated in fibromyalgia: the effect of coenzyme Q10. *Antioxid Redox Signal.* 2014 Mar 10;20(8):1169-80

interleukin (IL)-1, NLRP3 (NOD-like receptor family, pyrin domain containing 3) and caspase-1 activation, and an increase of serum levels of proinflammatory cytokines (IL-1 and IL-18). CoQ10 deficiency induced by p-aminobenzoate treatment in blood mononuclear cells and mice showed NLRP3 inflammasome activation with marked algesia. A placebo-controlled trial of CoQ10 in FM patients has shown a reduced NLRP3 inflammasome activation and IL-1 and IL-18 serum levels. …CONCLUSION: These findings provide new insights into the pathogenesis of FM and suggest that NLRP3 inflammasome inhibition represents a new therapeutic intervention for the disease. … After CoQ10 supplementation [300 mg/day CoQ10 divided into three doses], NLRP3 and IL-1 gene were downregulated. … IL-1 and IL-18 serum levels were significantly reduced with respect to placebo." The most complete/consistent model of FMS is that it is caused by SIBO, leading to mitochondrial dysfunction, central sensitization, tryptophan/serotonin/melatonin deficiencies; these interconnections are illustrated later in this chapter and detailed elsewhere.[120]

3. **Mitochondrial dysfunction and mTOR activation**: Dysbiosis and microbial overabundance promote inflammation and autoimmunity by triggering mitochondrial hyperpolarization which subsequently promotes mTOR activation; additively or synergistically, the increased oxidative stress from the mitochondrial hyperpolarization would add to the inflammatory load by promoting activation of NFkB and DAMP/PAMP/inflammasome. Activation of mTOR directly promotes inflammation in general and autoimmunity in particular by accentuating the polarity between pro-inflammatory and anti-inflammatory effectors; mTOR activation leads to promotion of TH17 inflammatory cells while simultaneously suppressing development of anti-inflammatory Treg cells. My more fully developed discussion of mitochondrial dysfunction[121,122] and mTOR's activation and clinical control[123] have been developed elsewhere. For this discussion, the essential communication is the connection between microbial exposures leading to clinical inflammation via mitochondrial dysfunction/hyperpolarization and mTOR activation; readers should appreciate that both mitochondrial dysfunction and mTOR activation are *pathologically inflammatory* and are independently and synergistically self-perpetuating. I have demonstrated this in both simplistic and contextualized illustrations.

   - **T-cell activation induces mitochondrial hyperpolarization** via ROI/ROS- and calcium-dependent NO production (*J Immunol* 2003 Nov[124]): This is an excellent article showing that "T cell activation-induced mitochondrial hyperpolarization is mediated by Ca2- and redox-dependent production of nitric oxide." On the final page of the full-text article, the authors diagram the three fates of NOS/NO-induced mitochondrial hyperpolarization, with the outcome of this final common pathway dependent on the overall mitochondrial milieu; this provides fascinating insight into the understanding of the paradoxical effects of various effectors (in this case, nitric oxide) with the ultimate outcome dependent *not on the molecule* but on the contextualized microenvironment, particularly in this case the microbial, nutritional, and preexisting mitochondrial status of the host. CD3/CD28 co-stimulation, by either ROS production or calcium (Ca) release, leads to increased nitric oxide (NO) production and hyperpolarization, with the ultimate fate and outcome as follows:

     ❶ Nitric oxide → mitochondrial hyperpolarization → mitochondrial biogenesis → robustness, cell proliferation

     ❷ Nitric oxide → mitochondrial hyperpolarization → ATP depletion → necrosis → inflammation/autoimmunity

     ❸ Nitric oxide → mitochondrial hyperpolarization → mitochondrial depolarization → apoptosis

     Readers should appreciate the self-perpetuating nature of mitochondrial hyperpolarization with inflammation, particularly the type of inflammation that manifests clinically as autoimmunity: mitochondrial hyperpolarization activates NFkB for generalized inflammation and mTOR for autoimmune-type inflammation; thereafter, immune activation promotes additional mitochondrial hyperpolarization to perpetuate the cycle *in a suitable environment*. Further, the model presented here helps

[120] Vasquez A. *Naturopathic Rheumatology and Integrative Inflammology v3.5*, 2014 and *Fibromyalgia in a Nutshell*, 2012

[121] Vasquez A. *Mitochondrial Nutrition and Endoplasmic Reticulum Stress in Primary Care, Second Edition*, 2014. [ISBN 1502952505]

[122] Vasquez A. *Functional Inflammology: Volume 1: Introduction to Clinical Nutrition, Functional Medicine, and Integrative Pain Management for Disorders of Susustained Inflammation*. International College of Human Nutrition and Functional Medicine, 2014

[123] Vasquez A. *Mastering mTOR: Resveratrol, Reductive (Antioxidant) Therapies, and Restrictive Diets especially Relevant for Rheumatology*. International College of Human Nutrition and Functional Medicine (February 21, 2015). [ASIN B00TVT5YK2]

[124] Nagy et al. T cell activation-induced mitochondrial hyperpolarization is mediated by Ca2+- and redox-dependent production of nitric oxide. *J Immunol*. 2003 Nov;171:5188-97

us understand/reconcile other data, and helps us shift our focus from mitochondrial hyperpolarization per se to the environment of that polarization. Further, we should appreciate that transient mitochondrial hyperpolarization is normal, and essential for processes such as pancreatic insulin secretion in response to hyperglycemia; the distinction of pathogenic mitochondrial hyperpolarization is its distribution, duration/permanence/inflexibility, and its outcome.

- <u>LPS triggers TRL4 to activate mitochondrial hyperpolarization</u> via a combination of NFkB and NADPH oxidase (*J Cell Physiol* 2010 May[125]): "The stimulation of TLR4 by LPS induced a time- and dose-dependent contractile dysfunction, which was associated with a decrease of TLR2 messenger, a rearrangement of microfilament cytoskeleton and an oxidative imbalance, i.e., the formation of reactive oxygen species (ROS) together with the depletion of GSH content. An alteration of mitochondria, namely a hyperpolarization of their membrane potential, was also detected. Most of these effects were partially prevented by the NADPH oxidase inhibitor apocynin or the NFkappaB inhibitor MG132."

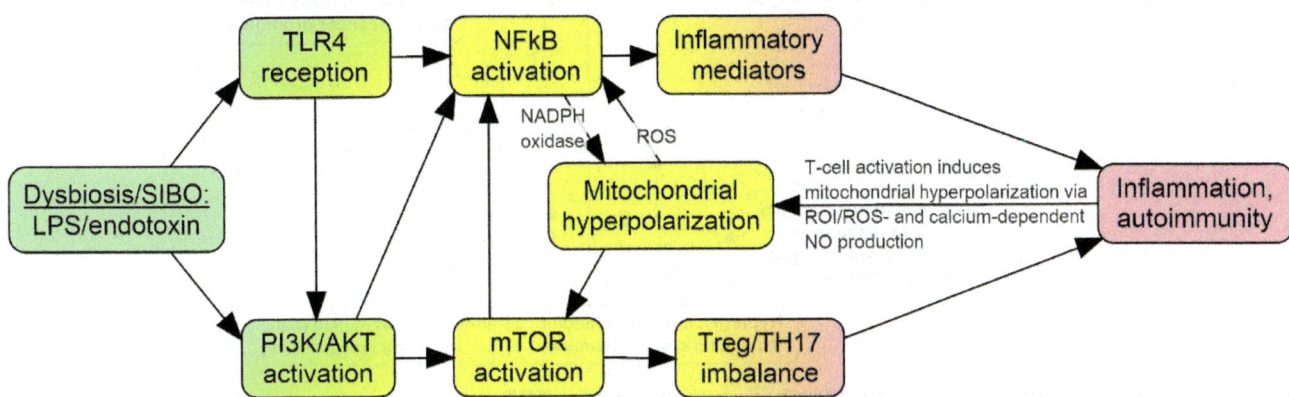

The simplified connection between microbes, mitochondria, mTOR, and inflammatory damage: Endotoxin/LPS from Gram-negative bacteria activates TLR4 which then induces mitochondrial hyperpolarization via either of two pathways: NFkB and NADPH oxidase. The observation that mitochondrial hyperpolarization induced by LPS/TLR4 can be blocked by inhibition of either NFkB or NADPH oxidase indicates that both are necessary for LPS/TLR4-induced induction of mitochondrial hyperpolarization. Endotoxin/LPS activates mTOR, directly via AKT and indirectly via mitochondrial hyperpolarization. mTOR promotes activation of NFkB for additional and direct inflammation. Note that NFkB, mTOR, and mitochondrial hyperpolarization form a vicious cycle. Per Figure 5 ("Proposed model" clearly showing that LPS activates PI3K/mTOR independently from activation of NFkB) of Hou et al, *Am J Physiol Lung Cell Mol Physiol* 2012 Jan, activation of PI3K/AKT directly activates NFkB; "LPS administration activated PI3K/AKT pathway and then stimulated mTOR and NFkB signaling..." Data also from Scirocco et al, *J Cell Physiol* 2010 May and Yue et al, *J Endocrinol* 2015 Jan.

- <u>LPS administration activates PI3K/AKT pathway and stimulates mTOR</u> and NFkB signaling, increasing the expression of cytokines IL-1, TNFa, IL-6 (*J Endocrinol.* 2015 Jan[126]): "In this study, we showed that LPS stimulates the mTOR signaling pathway through the enhanced phosphorylation of mTOR(Ser2448) and p70S6K(Thr389). We also showed that LPS administration increased the phosphorylation of FOXO1, the p65 subunit of nuclear factor kappa B, and FOXO1/3a. Blocking the mTOR pathway significantly attenuated the LPS-induced anorexia by decreasing the phosphorylation of p70S6K, FOXO1, and FOXO1/3a."

- <u>LPS administration activates mTOR</u> (*Nat Commun.* 2013 Nov[127]): "Interestingly, stimulation of bone marrow derived macrophages (BMDMs) with IL-4 or LPS resulted in mTORC1 activation as indicated by increased phosphorylation of the downstream targets S6K1 and 4E-BP1 (Fig. 1a), suggesting that the mTORC1 pathway may coordinate metabolic changes during macrophage activation."

- <u>TLR activates PI3K/Akt to activate mTOR</u> (*Eur J Immunol* 2008 Nov[128]): "Here we demonstrate that TLR activate mTOR via phosphoinositide 3-kinase/Akt." The authors also state, "PI3K/Akt signaling represents a key pathway for mTOR activation" and "First we show that membrane bound TLR directly activate mTOR via the PI3K/Akt axis."

125 Scirocco A et al. Exposure of Toll-like receptors 4 to bacterial lipopolysaccharide impairs human colonic smooth muscle cell function. *J Cell Physiol.* 2010 May:442-50
126 Yue et al. A central role for the mammalian target of rapamycin in LPS-induced anorexia in mice. *J Endocrinol.* 2015 Jan;224(1):37-47
127 Byles et al. The TSC-mTOR pathway regulates macrophage polarization. *Nat Commun.* 2013 Nov;4:2834
128 Schmitz et al. Mammalian target of rapamycin (mTOR) orchestrates the defense program of innate immune cells.*Eur J Immunol.* 2008 Nov;38(11):2981-92

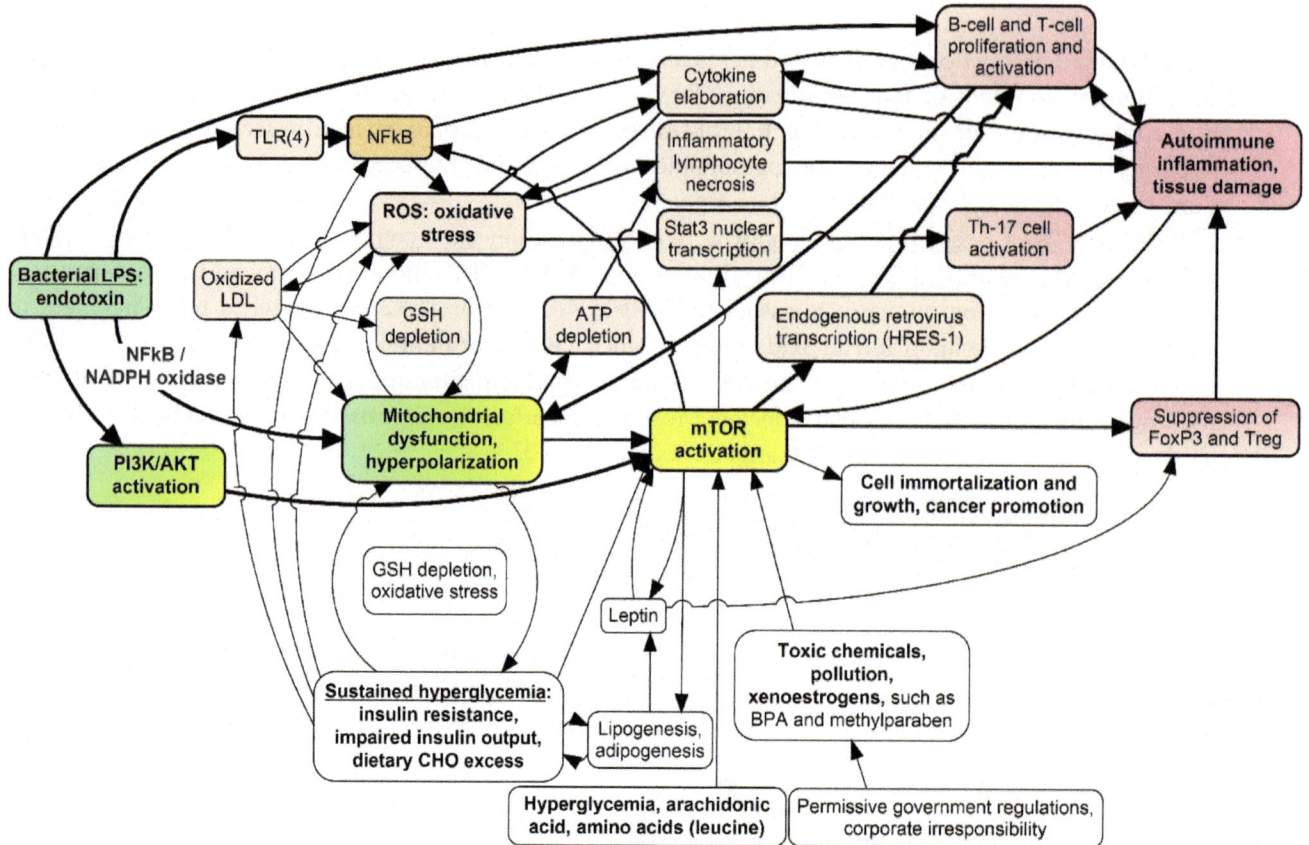

The contextualized connection between microbes, mitochondria, mTOR, and inflammatory damage: This streamlined illustration provides emphasis on the microbe→mitochondria→mTOR→inflammation pathway while also including the most important contextual components. LPS administration activates PI3K/AKT pathway and stimulates mTOR and NFkB signaling, increasing the expression of cytokines IL1, TNFα, IL-6 per Yue et al, *J Endocrinol* 2015 Jan. Illustration modified from © 2015 Vasquez A. *Mastering mTOR: Resveratrol, Reductive (Antioxidant) Therapies, and Restrictive Diets especially Relevant for Rheumatology*. International College of Human Nutrition and Functional Medicine (February 21, 2015). [ASIN B00TVT5YK2].

- LPS activates NF-kB via the Akt/mTOR pathway (*Am J Physiol Lung Cell Mol Physiol*. 2012 Jan[129]): This is among the most eloquently written basic science articles that I have read (among thousands); the expressed thought is clear and easily transferred. "Inhibition of mTOR represses LPS-induced production of inflammatory cytokines and phosphorylation of NFkB in neutrophils", implying that LPS activates mTOR which then in-turn activates NFkB. This fascinating investigation showed that "administration of GLN improved cell viability subjected to LPS stimulation, inhibited NFkB activation through the PI3K/Akt/mTOR pathway, and suppressed NFkB DNA-binding activity, which led to repression of the expression of NFkB-targeted genes." In the LPS→PI3K/Akt/mTOR→NFkB inflammatory pathway, glutamine appears to block inflammation at the level of both PI3K/Akt/mTOR and NFkB; paradoxically, low levels of glutamine appear to support basal mTOR activity but the overall effect is modulatory/balancing and ultimately anti-inflammatory following exposure to inflammatory/LPS stimuli. The finding that "Upon activation of PI3K/Akt signaling, Akt phosphorylates mTOR and promotes IKK-dependent activation of NFkB" provides two critically important insights that 1) LPS stimulation activates PI3K/Akt/mTOR to activate NFkB, and because we already know that 2) LPS activates NFkB, and that 3) LPS promotes oxidative stress and mitochondrial hyperpolarization, both of which promote activation of mTOR, we can then appreciate that 4) LPS-promoted inflammation is sustained by bidirectional activation of NFkB→mTOR and mTOR→NFkB along with LPS→hyperpolarization→mTOR and LPS→ROS/inflammation. Experienced clinicians—or at least those who are aware of the clinical use of glutamine (generally 3-9 grams orally thrice daily, powder preferred for adults)—should find this

---

[129] Hou YC1, Chiu WC, Yeh CL, Yeh SL. Glutamine modulates lipopolysaccharide-induced activation of NF-κB via the Akt/mTOR pathway in lung epithelial cells. *Am J Physiol Lung Cell Mol Physiol*. 2012 Jan 1;302(1):L174-83—A really excellent article, written to the point of eloquence.

information fascinating because the "dual action blockade" of NFkB along with mTOR likely explains a large part of the immunomodulating, anti-inflammatory, anti-infection, and anti-cancer benefits that are clinically appreciated.

4. Molecular mimicry, cross-reactivity: Molecular mimicry is the sharing of amino acid sequences between humans and microbes, while cross-reactivity is the resultant immunologic responses aimed at microbial sequences that also targets the human sequences; the former can occur without the latter but the latter is dependent on the former. Such molecules are also called "mimotopes" (similar/mimicking epitopes) or "homologs" because of the similar/homologous sequences that mimic each other, either by direct sequence or by availability of a similar sequence via three-dimensional conformation/shape. Several microbes have peptides and other structures that resemble or "mimic" the peptides and cell structures found in human tissues. Thus, when the immune system fights against the microbe, the antibodies and T-cells can "cross-react" with the tissues of the human host. In this way, the immune system begins attacking the human body, which is otherwise an innocent bystander—the victim of "friendly fire."[130] As reviewed by Ringrose[131], evidence clearly indicates that specific microbial proteins have amino acid homology with human proteins and/or that homologous bacterial peptides appear to stimulate (auto)immunity toward similar neighboring human peptides. Therefore the two underlying bases for autoimmune induction by molecular mimicry—namely 1) homology between human and microbial amino acid sequences, and 2) stimulation of immunity against human peptides—do indeed occur *in vivo*. **Molecular mimicry is strongly implicated in the pathogenesis of reactive arthritis and ankylosing spondylitis.**[132,133]

> **Molecular mimicry in psoriatic skin and bacterial proteins**
>
> These amino acid sequences are found both in human keratin and M-protein from the bacteria *Streptococcus pyogenes*.
> 1. ALEEAN
> 2. LRR-LD
> 3. AKLEA
> 4. AKLEAE
>
> Gudmundsdottir et al. *Clin Exp Immunol.* 1999 Sep

- Cross-reactivity between sequences in *Acinetobacter* sp., *Pseudomonas aeruginosa*, myelin basic protein and myelin oligodendrocyte glycoprotein in multiple sclerosis. (*J Neuroimmunol*. 2003 Nov[134]): "Antibodies to mimicry peptides from *Acinetobacter*, *P. aeruginosa*, myelin basic protein (MBP) and myelin oligodendrocyte glycoprotein (MOG) were significantly elevated in MS patients compared to controls. Antisera against MBP (residues 110-124) reacted with both *Acinetobacter* and *Pseudomonas* peptides from 4- and gamma-carboxymuconolactone decarboxylase, respectively. MOG (residues 43-57) antisera reacted with *Acinetobacter* peptide from 3-oxo-adipate-CoA-transferase subunit A. ... suggesting bacterial infections could play a role in MS pathogenesis."

- Antibody responses to Acinetobacter spp. and Pseudomonas aeruginosa in multiple sclerosis. (*Clin Diagn Lab Immunol*. 2001 Nov[135]): "In MS patients, elevated levels of antibodies against all strains of *Acinetobacter* tested were present, as well as antibodies against *P. aeruginosa*, MBP, and neurofilaments, but not antibodies to *E. coli*, compared to the CVA group and controls. The myelin-*Acinetobacter*-neurofilament antibody index appears to distinguish MS patients from patients with CVAs or healthy controls."

- Psoriasis and molecular mimicry—Ex vivo experimental study using human T-cells (*Clin Exp Immunol* 1999 Sep[136]): The authors of this paper introduce their topic by noting that psoriasis is an inflammatory disease mediated largely by T-cells in the skin and that psoriasis has a strong association with infections by group-A beta-hemolytic streptococci bacteria, also known as *Streptococcus pyogenes*. The authors cite their previous work which showed that patients with active psoriasis have Th1-like cells that respond to a 20 amino acid (AA) sequence shared between a protein made by streptococcal bacteria (M protein) that has the same AA

---

[130] Wucherpfennig KW. Mechanisms for the induction of autoimmunity by infectious agents. *J Clin Invest*. 2001 Oct;108(8):1097-104 jci.org/cgi/reprint/108/8/1097

[131] Ringrose JH. HLA-B27 associated spondyloarthropathy, an autoimmune disease based on crossreactivity between bacteria and HLA-B27? *Ann Rheum Dis*. 1999 Oct;58(10):598-610 ard.bmjjournals.com/cgi/content/full/58/10/598

[132] "HLA-B27 and proteins from enteric bacteria are structurally related, in a manner that may affect T cell response to enteric pathogens." Inman RD, Scofield RH. Etiopathogenesis of ankylosing spondylitis and reactive arthritis. *Curr Opin Rheumatol*. 1994 Jul;6(4):360-70

[133] "With respect to bacterial infection, recent findings in bacterial antigenicity, host response through interactions of antigen-presenting cells, T cells, and cytokines are providing new understanding of host-pathogen interactions and the pathogenesis of arthritis." Kim TH, Uhm WS, Inman RD. Pathogenesis of ankylosing spondylitis and reactive arthritis. *Curr Opin Rheumatol*. 2005 Jul;17(4):400-5

[134] Hughes et al. Cross-reactivity between related sequences found in Acinetobacter sp., Pseudomonas aeruginosa, myelin basic protein and myelin oligodendrocyte glycoprotein in multiple sclerosis. *J Neuroimmunol*. 2003 Nov;144(1-2):105-15

[135] Hughes et al. Antibody responses to Acinetobacter spp. and Pseudomonas aeruginosa in multiple sclerosis: prospects for diagnosis using the myelin-acinetobacter-neurofilament antibody index. *Clin Diagn Lab Immunol*. 2001 Nov;8(6):1181-8

[136] Gudmundsdottir AS, et al. Is an epitope on keratin 17 a major target for autoreactive T lymphocytes in psoriasis? *Clin Exp Immunol*. 1999 Sep;117(3):580-6

sequence as the human protein found in the skin named keratin, specifically keratin 17. "Keratin" is a group of fibrous structural proteins forming the key structural material of the outer layer of human skin; keratin is also the key structural component of hair and nails. Keratin 17 is not expressed in normal skin except for hair follicles, sweat/sebaceous glands, and basal cells in the scalp; however, keratin 17 is expressed in suprabasal keratinocytes in lesional psoriatic skin, thus making its presence in skin a unique feature of psoriasis lesions. Increased production of keratin 17 can be induced by the pro-inflammatory cytokines gamma-interferon, which plays a key role as a mediator of psoriatic inflammation, and IL-6, which is abundant in psoriatic lesions. Langerhans cells are the dendritic cells of the epidermis; as such, they function as antigen-presenting cells (APC). Given that keratin within skin cells exists as an intracellular structural (cytoskeletal) protein, its ability to be exposed to the immune system is required for it to function as an autoantigen, a target of self-induced immunologic attack. The authors of this paper note that "cytoplasmic processes of Langerhans cells can extend into the cytoplasm of adjacent keratinocytes with frequent absence of intervening plasma membranes at the apices of these processes"; thus these epidermal APCs can uptake and present antigen via MHC class 1 and class 2 molecules to CD8 and CD4 T-cells, respectively. These same Th1-like cells are deleted following treatment with ultraviolet B (UVB) radiation that induces clinical remission; the fact that the disappearance of these cells correlates with clinical improvement following treatment implies that these cells may have a direct causative role in the skin inflammation of psoriasis. In the ex vivo experiment, the authors took T-cells from the blood of 17 psoriatic patients and 17 healthy controls and then challenged these T-cells with keratin peptides and M-peptides to monitor for increased production of gamma-interferon [IFNg]), which implies specificity for the corresponding amino acid sequences.

Peptide identification and source	Peptide amino acid (AA) sequence
Peptide 146-M from *Streptococcus pyogenes*	**AKKQVEKALEEANSKLAALE**
Peptide 146-M49 from *Streptococcus pyogenes*	AKKKVEADLAEANSKLQALE
Peptide 146-K17* from human keratin subtypes 14 and 17	**SYLDKVRALEEANADLEVK**
Peptide 146-K9 from human keratin	SYLDKVQALEEANNDLENKI

Results of the investigation showed that the most frequent and strongest responses were observed to a peptide from keratin 17 that shares a specific AA sequence with M-protein: T-cell responses to the ALEEAN sequence were stronger than to the corresponding M-peptide containing the ALEEAN sequence; this implies that sensitized T-cells preferentially attack keratin rather than the bacterial peptide. *Data from Figure 1 and Table 1 of Gudmundsdottir et al, *Clin Exp Immunol* 1999 Sep;117(3):580-6. Based on the frequency of IFN-g-producing T-cells of patients and controls after stimulation with M- and keratin peptides sharing the ALEEAN sequence, peptide 146-K17 is the only peptide which elicited significantly stronger responses in psoriatic patients than in healthy controls.

The ALEEAN sequence present in keratin 17 is also found in keratin subtype 14, which is overexpressed in psoriatic skin; thus, for T-cells already primed to respond to ALEEAN following exposure to *Streptococcus pyogenes*, the dual exposure to ALEEAN in keratins 14 and 17—both of which are uniquely present in psoriatic skin—may promote localized attack by T-cells against keratinocytes, i.e., immune cross-reactivity via molecular mimicry. UVB treatment abolished T-cell responses to keratin and M protein, while responses to other bacterial antigens (streptokinase [SK] and streptodornase [SD]) were not affected. The authors conclude, "These findings are consistent with the notion that AA sequences which keratin has in common with M-protein may be a major target for autoreactive T cells in psoriasis." Per Table 2 of their article, 13 of 17 psoriatic patients demonstrated a T-cell response to peptide 146-K17 (from human keratins subtypes 14 and 17) contrasted to only 4 of 17 healthy controls; interestingly, three patients and eight controls showed no responses to either keratin or M protein. This lack of perfect concordance indicates that molecular mimicry and the resulting immune cross-reaction does not account for the entirety of the pathogenesis of psoriasis, or that ❶ the research methods employed in the study were imperfect resulting in a few false negatives and/or false positives, or ❷ seasonal variation in streptococcal infections caused varying intensities of immune responsiveness, ❸ seasonal vitamin D fluctuations caused varying intensities of immune responsiveness, ❹ that a variable unaccounted for (e.g., sun exposure, medication use, etc) influenced these results, or that ❺ other nonstreptococcal infections/microbes—as very well documented by Rosenberg, Noah and colleagues[137]—and dysbiotic microbial relationships may have been causative in some cases of psoriasis. The ALEEAN sequence is not the only sequence shared between human keratin and staphylococcal M-protein; other homologous sequences include LRR-LD, AKLEA, and AKLEAE.

- Psoriasis is an autoimmune disease caused in whole or in part by molecular mimicry. (*Trends Immunol* 2009 Oct[138]): The authors of this paper note that T cells in psoriatic lesions are oligoclonal and that these T-cells recognize amino acid sequences (determinants) common to streptococcal M-protein and human skin keratin; they propose that CD8(+) T cells in psoriatic epidermis respond mainly to such determinants. Further, they note that streptococcal peptidoglycan may act as an adjuvant for this immune response and that, likewise, a streptococcal superantigen may promote an inflammatory/cytokine milieu that advances skin-homing of tonsillar T cells. They conclude their abstract/summary by stating that if the above bases are correct, then "tonsillectomy should be associated with fewer T cells that recognize keratin and streptococcal determinants." These conclusions are conceptually consistent with previously published literature, in particular the work of Noah and colleagues[139], which has also emphasized the microbial link to psoriasis and has noted the documented benefit of tonsillectomy. I included citation to this article for the additional reason that it is one of the first articles to boldly state *in its title*—"Psoriasis—as an autoimmune disease caused by molecular mimicry"—that molecular mimicry is a defining pathoetiologic aspect of psoriasis, thus emphasizing the role of this mechanism and the relationship to the triggering/mimicking bacteria in this condition previously acquiesced by the medical profession to the realms of esotericity and idiopathicity in order to justify perpetual pharmaceuticalization of these patients.[140]

5. Enhanced production/processing/presentation of autoantigens: When the immune system perceives the presence of microbial molecules, mechanisms are enhanced which facilitate the processing and presentation of preexistent antigens to the immune system, which then targets these antigens for destruction. Of course, this is beneficial when fighting a true infection; but recent evidence shows that chronic/silent/sustained infections can facilitate the processing and presentation of the body's own antigens (autoantigens) which are then attacked. Clinically, we see the immune system attacking the body, and we call this an "autoimmune disease" even though the original cause of the problem may have been an occult infection or exposure to specific microbial molecules. This process is also described as "Aberrant MHC [major histocompatibility complex] class 2 expression: Aberrant class-2 MHC expression on non-antigen presenting cells [APC] may lead to presentations of autoantigens to autoreactive T-cells."[141] Ringrose et al[142] showed that infecting HLA-B27-positive human cells with *Salmonella typhimurium* and *Shigella flexneri* caused these cells to express autoantigens, namely human histone H3, human ribosomal protein S17 (two separate amino acid sequences) and the heavy chain of HLA-B27. A similar phenomenon has been demonstrated in autistic children wherein patients exposed to bacterial antigens (streptokinase), toxic chemicals (Thimerosal, ethyl-mercury), and dietary antigens (gliadin and casein peptides) produce autoantigens that appear capable of inciting and perpetuating autoimmunity.[143] In two separate reports, Zhu wrote that experimental cytomegalovirus (CMV) infection induced cell-surface presentation of intracellular autoantigen[144]; CMV infection with exposure to ultraviolet (UV) radiation produced a synergistic effect, resulting in an increased level of autoantigen exposure.[145] Therefore, we have

---

[137] Rosenberg EW, Noah PW, Skinner RB Jr. Microorganisms and psoriasis. *J Natl Med Assoc.* 1994 Apr;86(4):305-10

[138] Valdimarsson et al. Psoriasis—as an autoimmune disease caused by molecular mimicry. *Trends Immunol.* 2009 Oct;30(10):494-501

[139] Rosenberg EW, Noah PW, Skinner RB Jr. Microorganisms and psoriasis. *J Natl Med Assoc.* 1994 Apr;86(4):305-10

[140] Vasquez A. Twilight of the Idiopathic Era and the Dawn of New Possibilities in Health and Healthcare. *Naturopathy Digest* 2006 Mar

[141] George J, Levy Y, Kallenberg CG, Shoenfeld Y. Infections and Wegener's granulomatosis--a cause and effect relationship? *QJM.* 1997 May;90(5):367-73

[142] Ringrose et al. Influence of infection of cells with bacteria with reactive arthritis on peptide repertoire presented by HLA-B27. *J Med Microbiol* 2001 Apr:385-9

[143] Vojdani et al. Infections, toxic chemicals and dietary peptides binding to lymphocyte receptors and tissue enzymes are major instigators of autoimmunity in autism. *Int J Immunopathol Pharmacol.* 2003 Sep-Dec;16(3):189-99

[144] "Specific but ubiquitous cytoplasmic proteins are the targets of autoantibodies such as anti-Ro/SS-A, anti-La/SS-B, and anti-calreticulin. These antibodies may be pathogenic in systemic lupus erythematosus (SLE) and Sjogren's syndrome (SS). ... Enhanced expression of class I MHC was detected on the cell surface in response to the virus infection. ... Viral infection was found to alter the distribution of host cell proteins, including autoantigens. Cell surface expression of calreticulin could provide a target for circulating autoantibody and contribute to the autoimmune process." Zhu J, Newkirk MM. Viral induction of the human autoantigen calreticulin. *Clin Invest Med.* 1994 Jun;17(3):196-205

[145] "Using a fixed-cell ELISA to detect autoantigen expression, a synergistic effect between ultraviolet B (UVB) exposure and CMV infection on the surface expression of 52-kD/Ro antigen, but not 60-kD/Ro or calreticulin, was observed. ... Immunofluorescence studies confirmed these findings and indicated that cells expressed 52-kD/Ro protein on their surface at 24 h after a combined UVB and CMV treatment. These studies provide evidence that synergy between UVB irradiation and CMV infection may play a role in the induction of cell surface expression of the human autoantigen, 52-kD/Ro." Zhu J. Ultraviolet B irradiation and cytomegalovirus infection synergize to induce the cell surface expression of 52-kD/Ro antigen. *Clin Exp Immunol.* 1996 Jan;103(1):47-53

experimental evidence with human cells *in vitro* which demonstrates that *enhanced processing/presenting of autoantigens* occurs following exposure to bacterial antigens, dietary allergens, and xenobiotics.

- Psoriasis and microbially-evoked autoantigens (see especially *Clin Exp Immunol* 1999 Sep[146]): Amino acid sequences in skin keratin subtypes 14 and 17 have homology with peptides from the bacterium *Streptococcus pyogenes*, thereby establishing the basis for molecular mimicry and subsequent cross-reactivity in chronic human disease. Evidence has shown that psoriatic patients have T-cells which specifically target keratin 17 thereby indicating that keratin 17 serves as an autoantigen in psoriasis; Johnston et al[147] wrote, "…psoriatic individuals have CD8(+) T cells that recognize keratin self-antigens." As noted earlier in this chapter, increased production of keratin 17 can be induced by the pro-inflammatory cytokines gamma-interferon, which plays a key role as a mediator of psoriatic inflammation, and IL-6, which is abundant in psoriatic lesions. Factors that can increase IFN-g and/or IL-6 production are numerous and include infection, injury, obesity, and consumption of a pro-inflammatory diet; increased production of IFN-g and IL-6 is characteristic of nearly any immune response and is certainly not specific to psoriasis or any other rheumatic condition. The ALEEAN sequence present in keratin 17 is also found in keratin subtype 14, which is overexpressed in psoriatic skin; thus, for T-cells already primed to respond to ALEEAN following exposure to *Streptococcus pyogenes*, the dual exposure to ALEEAN in keratins 14 and 17—both of which are uniquely present in psoriatic skin—may promote localized attack by T-cells against keratinocytes, i.e., immune cross-reactivity via molecular mimicry. The data demonstrate the following:

1) Exposure to microbes induces IFNg and/or IL-6: IFN-g and IL-6 production is increased during overt or occult infection/colonization/dysbiosis, such as with *Streptococcus pyogenes*.

2) Increased production of IFN-g and IL-6 increases production of keratin-17: Increased production of IFN-g and IL-6 increases production of keratin-17.

3) Keratin-17 is an autoantigen in psoriatic skin: Keratin-17 is a clinically-important autoantigen in psoriasis based on its location, molecular homology with proteins made by *Streptococcus pyogenes* which is a known trigger in psoriasis, and the identification of T-cells specifically responsive to keratin-17.

4) Therefore, microbial exposure → IFN-g and IL-6 → increased keratin-17 = increased autoantigen production induced by pro-inflammatory cytokines induced by microbial exposure.

5) Furthermore, increased production of autoantigen keratin-17 by IFN-g and IL-6 is not uniquely microbe-dependent. Obesity in general and visceral adipose tissue in particular are causally associated with increased production of these inflammatory cytokines. If non-microbial induction of IFN-g and IL-6 can stimulate increased production of autoantigen keratin-17, then we would expect conditions such as obesity/hyperadiposity to be associated with more severe psoriasis; indeed this is the situation, as recently shown in studies showing that obese young women are at increased risk for severe psoriasis[148] and that weight loss treatments can improve psoriasis.[149]

Combination effects—microbe-induced inflammation-driven exposure of cryptic antigens with simultaneous molecular mimicry and cross-reactivity: Antiphospholipid antibody syndrome (APAS, Hughes syndrome) is best modeled as a four-step or four-component autoimmune disease comprised of ❶ genetic predisposition, including amino acid sequences of target proteins and HLA subtypes, ❷ excess exposure to bacterial endotoxin from a pro-inflammatory gut dysbiosis, leading to a three-dimensional conformational change in the structure of endogenous proteins such as beta2-glycoprotein, leading to exposure of otherwise hidden/cryptic amino acid sequences that pair with various microorganisms and vaccine components, ❸ various microorganisms (*Haemophilus influenzae, Neisseria gonorrhoeae*) and vaccine components (tetanus toxoid) share amino acid homology with human protein sequences, thereby allowing for cross-reactive immune responses, ❹ an inflammation-predisposed immune system, see discussions on immunophenotype (Treg/Th17) imbalance and total inflammatory load in *Functional Inflammology, Vol 1 / Naturopathic Rheumatology v3.5* and later.

---

[146] Gudmundsdottir AS, et al. Is an epitope on keratin 17 a major target for autoreactive T lymphocytes in psoriasis? *Clin Exp Immunol*. 1999 Sep;117(3):580-6

[147] Johnston A, et al. Peripheral blood T cell responses to keratin peptides that share sequences with streptococcal M proteins are largely restricted to skin-homing CD8(+) T cells. *Clin Exp Immunol*. 2004 Oct;138(1):83-93 ncbi.nlm.nih.gov/pmc/articles/PMC1809187/pdf/cei0138-0083.pdf

[148] "Multivariate analysis demonstrated an association between excess increase in body mass index and psoriasis in females only." Bryld LE, et al. High body mass index in adolescent girls precedes psoriasis hospitalization. *Acta Derm Venereol*. 2010 Sep;90(5):488-93

[149] "…two recent reports of chronic severe psoriasis improving with weight loss after Roux-en-Y gastric bypass surgery. …two patients with body mass indices greater than 50 kg/m(2) who had marked improvement in their psoriasis after gastric bypass surgery." Hossler et al. Gastric bypass surgery improves psoriasis. *J Am Acad Dermatol*. 2010 Jul

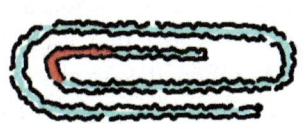 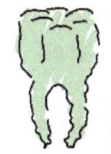 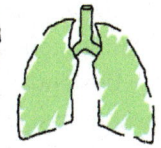 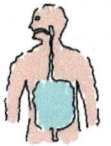 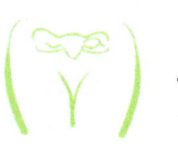

| Depiction of a human protein (blue) with a circular structure and a protected antigenic sequence (red) | Exposure to bacterial endotoxin/LPS, such as from ❶ overt infection, ❷ persistent SIBO, or mucosal breach (❸ "leaky gut" or ❹ "leaky gums") or a combination of each of these, leads to conformational change in protein structure | Cross-reactive antigen is revealed following exposure to microbial immunogens (e.g., LPS), allowing immune cross-reaction to occur |

A "double hit" model of microbe synergism for autoimmunity induction—one microbial exposure changes the structure of the protein with the second exposure stimulates immune cross-reactivity: In antiphospholipid antibody syndrome, the best current model holds that in genetically predisposed persons, ❶ exposure to bacterial endotoxin (or other binding agent) leads to a conformational change in beta2-glycoprotein I (β2GPI), exposing a previously hidden/protected amino acid sequence, which shares homology (molecular mimicry) with proteins from various microorganisms and/or vaccine components. Following ❷ exposure to specific microbial homologs—such as from *Haemophilus influenzae*, *Neisseria gonorrhoeae*, and tetanus toxoid—which may occur during infection/colonization, increased exposure due to permeable mucosae, and/or tetanus vaccination[150]), the immune response against the microbial peptides cross-reacts with the endogenous protein, leading to autoimmunity and pathology. While this model applies to specifically to antiphospholipid antibody syndrome, similar models of infection/inflammation-induced exposure or enhanced processing of endogenous antigens plus molecular-mimicry leading to cross-reactivity are noted in the clinical research literature, most notably with psoriasis. These processes would be exacerbated in a nutrient-deficient and inflammation-prone patient with insufficiency dysbiosis, xenobiotic overload, hormonal imbalances mitochondrial dysfunction and mTOR activation, (etc[151]) or possibly/likely with concomitant exposure to vaccine media/adjuvants/allergens/immunogens such as aluminum, mercury, formaldehyde, neomycin, monkey kidney cells, glutaraldehyde, human diploid cells, yeast (etc[152]).

- Role of the gut microbiota in antiphospholipid syndrome (*Curr Rheumatol Rep* 2015 Jan[153]): "Commensal bacteria within an individual are estimated to outnumber human cells ten to one; on average, the human gut is colonized by ~160 bacterial species, and more than 1000 species in total can be found across the human population. ... While a variety of autoantigens are identified in APS, β2-glycoprotein I (β2GPI) is the most commonly detected in patients. ... β2GPI is a common serum protein with pleiotropic functions including anticoagulant properties, scavenging lipopolysaccharide (LPS), mediating apoptotic cell clearance, and limiting oxidative stress during apoptosis. ... Binding of β2GPI to LPS or phospholipids that are exposed on the surface of apoptotic cells changes its conformation from a closed, circular state to an open, hook-like structure, which is thought to contribute to antigenicity by exposing cryptic epitopes... In addition, the anatomical localization of β2GPI in the body is another variable. β2GPI coats in the open conformation the endothelial cells of the uterus and the trophoblast during pregnancy, which is likely why miscarriages and pre-eclampsia are such a frequent complication in APS." Clinicians should take note that "the gram-positive anaerobic commensal *Roseburia intestinalis*, is particularly abundant in the human gut and stimulatory to lymphocytes from APS patients."
- Bacterial induction of autoantibodies to beta2-glycoprotein-I accounts for the infectious etiology of antiphospholipid syndrome (*J Clin Invest* 2002 Mar[154]): In a mouse model of antiphospholipid antibody syndrome, cross-reactivity between endogenous β2GPI and the microbial homologs/mimotopes from *Haemophilus influenzae*, *Neisseria gonorrhoeae*, or tetanus toxoid induce *pathogenic* antiphospholipid antibody formation. Other microbes capable of inducing autoantibody formation (including *nonpathogenic* antibodies) and/or those with a high degree of molecular mimicry include *C. albicans, Streptococcus pneumoniae, Shigella dysenteriae*, and *Staphylococcus aureus* (protein Sbi). One can easily and reasonably picture a clinical scenario and subsequent effects of *poly*microbial colonization and epitope spreading.

---

[150] Meyer et al. Antiphospholipid syndrome following a diphtheria-tetanus vaccination: coincidence vs. causality. *Isr Med Assoc J*. 2010 Oct;12(10):638-9
[151] Protocol components detailed in Vasquez A. *Functional Inflammology, Vol 1* (2014) or *Naturopathic Rheumatology v3.5* (2014) and later versions.
[152] Vaccine Excipient & Media Summary: Excipients Included in U.S. Vaccines. cdc.gov/vaccines/pubs/pinkbook/downloads/appendices/B/excipient-table-2.pdf 2015 May
[153] Ruff et al. The role of the gut microbiota in the pathogenesis of antiphospholipid syndrome. *Curr Rheumatol Rep*. 2015 Jan;17(1):472
[154] Blank et al. Bacterial induction of autoantibodies to beta2-glycoprotein-I accounts for infectious etiology of antiphospholipid syndrome. *J Clin Invest*. 2002 Mar;109:797-804

6. <mark>Bystander activation</mark>: Evidence suggests that we all have immunocytes capable of attacking our body tissues, and thus we all have the potential to develop autoimmune disease. Normally, these autoreactive cells are kept anergic, dormant, quiescent, and otherwise inactive through various mechanisms that regulate the immune system; in this way, such (potentially) autoreactive cells can be considered "bystanders" because they are not really doing anything and are basically "standing by." Bystander activation occurs when these cells are awakened by the cascade of inflammatory processes that occur as a result of superantigen exposure, molecular mimicry, immune complex deposition, or xenobiotic immunotoxicity. Bystander activation appears to contribute to the development of certain **autoimmune conditions, such as drug-induced lupus**[155], and it may be a contributing pathogenic mechanism in **heavy/toxic metal-induced autoimmunity**.[156]

- Psoriasis and bystander activation—Keratinocytes are immunologically active cells that present bacterial-derived superantigens to T lymphocytes. (*J Dermatol Sci* 1993 Oct[157]): Most doctors and researchers have believed that epidermal keratinocytes were relatively passive components of the outer layers of the skin where these cells form a mechanical barrier against injury and infection; likewise, their role in skin diseases was considered passive, with keratinocytes acting as passive targets and "**innocent bystanders**." However, newer research mandates that we reclassify keratinocytes from passive barrier cells to "fully fledged members of the immune system (i.e. immunocytes)" based on the findings that keratinocytes produce important cytokines, adhesion molecules, and mononuclear cell chemotactic factors. Activated keratinocytes "can initiate and perpetuate the inflammatory and immunological reactions in the skin which contribute to the pathobiology of psoriasis." Specifically, cytokine-activated keratinocytes can present bacterial superantigens to T-cells, resulting in activation and proliferation of these effectors of psoriasis.

- Thyroid autoimmunity induced by hepatitis C virus via bystander activation—Binding of hepatitis C virus E2 protein to thyroid cells may cause thyroid autoimmunity via bystander activation (*J Autoimmun* 2008 Dec[158]): Hepatitis C virus (HCV) infection is well-known to be causally associated with thyroid autoimmunity (e.g., Hashimoto's thyroiditis) but the molecular mechanism by which this association manifests has not been previously elucidated. In this study, researchers Akeno, Blackard, and Tomer showed that thyroid cells express a surface receptor called CD81, which is a binding site for the HCV protein E2. When HCV E2 binds to CD81, the proinflammatory cytokine IL-8 is produced. These authors concluded, "In summary, we have shown that CD81 is expressed in thyroid cells and can bind HCV envelope protein E2 leading to IL-8 production. These data suggest that local effects of HCV proteins can induce thyroiditis by bystander activation mechanisms." Although their conclusion might be premature insofar as their data showed deductive probability rather than objective certainty, it may be considered pragmatically sufficient.

7. <mark>Haptenization and the formation of neoantigens/neoautoantigens</mark>: A nonantigenic microbial molecule may bind to a nonantigenic human molecule and result in the formation of a new hybridized or "haptenized" molecule—neoantigen—which stimulates immunologic attack. Haptenization may be the underlying mechanism by which viruses induce autoimmunity[159] and appears to be a primary mechanism by which *Staphylococcus aureus* contributes to autoimmune vasculitis in <mark>ANCA-associated vasculitis</mark> (also called "granulomatosis with polyangiitis", formerly <mark>Wegener's granulomatosis</mark>[160], and most succinctly as "ANCA vasculitis"), namely by producing an antigenic acid phosphatase enzyme which binds with human endothelial cells by a charge interaction—the resultant hybrid/hapten/neoantigen formed by the antigen-endothelium complex becomes the target of immune attack, thus creating the phenomenon of "autoimmunity" and the clinical consequences of vasculitis.[161] Similarly, <mark>Hwp1 (Hyphal wall protein-1)</mark> of *Candida albicans* is a substrate

---

155 "…induction of autoimmunity will be discussed, including bystander activation of autoreactive lymphocytes due to drug-specific immunity or to non-specific activation of lymphocytes, direct cytotoxicity with **release of autoantigens** and disruption of central T-cell tolerance." Rubin RL. Drug-induced lupus. *Toxicology*. 2005 Apr 15;209(2):135-47

156 "It is therefore theoretically possible that compounds present in **vaccines such as thiomersal or aluminium hydroxide can trigger autoimmune reactions** through bystander effects." Fournie GJ, et al. Induction of autoimmunity through bystander effects. *J Autoimmun*. 2001 May;16(3):319-26

157 Nickoloff BJ, et al. Activated keratinocytes present bacterial-derived superantigens to T lymphocytes: relevance to psoriasis. *J Dermatol Sci*. 1993 Oct;6(2):127-33

158 Akeno et al. HCV E2 protein binds directly to thyroid cells and induces IL-8 production: mechanism for HCV induced thyroid autoimmunity. *J Autoimmun*. 2008 Dec:339-44

159 Van Ghelue M, et al. Autoimmunity to nucleosomes related to viral infection: a focus on hapten-carrier complex formation. *J Autoimmun*. 2003;20(2):171-82

160 Reiter and Wegener were both actively involved in Nazi atrocities during World War 2, and they have both been stripped of their eponymic recognition. Reiter's syndrome is now "reactive arthritis, and Wegener's granulomatosus is now "ANCA-associated vasculitis" or "granulomatosis with polyangiitis." Scheinberg MA. Nazi past and changes in disease names. *Rev Bras Reumatol*. 2012 Mar:300-1. Panush et al. Retraction of suggestion to use "Reiter's syndrome" sixty-five years later. *Arthritis Rheum*. 2007 Feb:693-4

161 Brons RH, Bakker HI, Van Wijk RT, et al. Staphylococcal acid phosphatase binds to endothelial cells via charge interaction; a pathogenic role in Wegener's granulomatosis? *Clin Exp Immunol*. 2000 Mar;119(3):566-73 blackwell-synergy.com/doi/abs/10.1046/j.1365-2249.2000.01172.x

for the tissue transglutaminase enzyme and cross-links with proteins in the mammalian mucosa[162]; the resultant neoantigen from this microbe-human haptenization would be a prime candidate to incite autoimmunity, as has been demonstrated by the transglutaminase-mediated haptenization of gliadin with human collagen *in vivo*.[163,164] In fact, since both Hwp1 and gliadin are substrates for tissue transglutaminase, *Candida albicans* may be synergistic with gluten/gliadin in the production of the systemic inflammatory/autoimmune/allergic condition known as celiac disease[165]; this may exemplify the interrelated nature of dysbiosis, food allergy, and autoimmunity. Lastly, since many toxic metals, xenobiotics, and drugs appear to trigger autoimmunity via haptenization[166,167,168], the adverse effects of these toxicants will be enhanced by microbe-induced alterations in xenobiotic detoxification and/or the proinflammatory effects of peptidoglycans, exotoxins, endotoxins, lipoteichoic acid, and other antigens and superantigens. In a recent animal study, exposure to bacterial endotoxin exacerbated metal-induced autoimmunity.[169] Endotoxin from gram-negative bacteria impairs detoxification by inhibiting the first cytochrome-p450-mediated step of detoxification[170]; this inhibition of detoxification increases the risk for drug toxicity and chemical accumulation. Bacteria can also adversely affect detoxification by elaborating beta-glucuronidase in the lumen of the intestine which cleaves bile-secreted toxins from their water-soluble conjugation moieties, resulting in increased "enterohepatic recycling"[171] or "enterohepatic recirculation"[172] as discussed below; increased re-exposure to previously detoxified endogenous and exogenous toxins can result in an upregulation of Phase 1 (cytochrome-p450-mediated biotransformation) leading to the formation of reactive intermediates and a condition commonly described by clinicians as "imbalanced detoxification" or "pathological detoxification."

- ANCA-associated vasculitis (also called "granulomatosis with polyangiitis", formerly Wegener's granulomatosis[173]) and bacterial enzyme haptenization—Staphylococcal enzyme acid phosphatase binds to (i.e., haptenizes) endothelial cells via charge interaction in ANCA-associated vasculitis (*Clin Exp Immunol* 2000 Mar[174]): ANCA-associated vasculitis is an autoimmune vasculitic condition with a high mortality; the majority of untreated patients die an average of 5 months following diagnosis, and 2-year survival without treatment is 10%. Histologically, the condition demonstrates focal accumulations of inflammation and immune cell activity (i.e., granulomas); however, the main clinical concern is the vasculitis in general and in particular the vasculitis affecting the kidneys and which commonly leads to kidney failure, a leading cause of death in affected patients. This excellent study by Brons and coworkers shows that the bacterium *Staphylococcus aureus* produces an enzyme—acid phosphatase—which binds to endothelial cells, the cells

---

[162] "By serving as a microbial substrate for epithelial cell transglutaminase, Hwp1 (Hyphal wall protein 1) of Candida albicans participates in cross-links with proteins on the mammalian mucosa." Staab JF, et al. Expression of transglutaminase substrate activity on Candida albicans germ tubes through a coiled, disulfide-bonded N-terminal domain of Hwp1 requires C-terminal glycosylphosphatidylinositol modification. *J Biol Chem.* 2004 Sep 24;279(39):40737-47 jbc.org/cgi/content/full/279/39/40737

[163] "Our findings firstly demonstrated that gliadin was directly bound to tTG in duodenal mucosa of coeliacs and controls, and the ability of circulating tTG-autoantibodies to recognize and immunoprecipitate the tTG-gliadin complexes." Ciccocioppo R, Di Sabatino A, Ara C, Biagi F, Perilli M, Amicosante G, Cifone MG, Corazza GR. Gliadin and tissue transglutaminase complexes in normal and coeliac duodenal mucosa. *Clin Exp Immunol.* 2003 Dec;134(3):516-24

[164] "Thus, modification of gluten peptides by tTG, especially deamidation of certain glutamine residues, can enhance their binding to HLA-DQ2 or -DQ8 and potentiate T cell stimulation. Furthermore, tTG-catalyzed cross-linking and consequent haptenization of gluten with extracellular matrix proteins allows for storage and extended availability of gluten in the mucosa." Dieterich W, Esslinger B, Schuppan D. Pathomechanisms in celiac disease. *Int Arch Allergy Immunol.* 2003 Oct;132(2):98-108

[165] "Subsequently, C albicans might function as an adjuvant that stimulates antibody formation against HWP1 and gluten, and formation of autoreactive antibodies against tissue transglutaminase and endomysium." Nieuwenhuizen WF, et al. Is Candida albicans a trigger in the onset of coeliac disease? *Lancet.* 2003;361(9375):2152-4

[166] Rao T, Richardson B. Environmentally induced autoimmune diseases: potential mechanisms. *Environ Health Perspect.* 1999 Oct;107 Suppl 5:737-42

[167] "Here, Peter Griem and colleagues focus on several aspects of neoantigen formation by xenobiotics: metabolism of xenobiotics into reactive, haptenic metabolites; polymorphisms of metabolizing enzymes; induction of costimulatory signals; and sensitization of T cells." Griem P, Wulferink M, Sachs B, Gonzalez JB, Gleichmann E. Allergic and autoimmune reactions to xenobiotics: how do they arise? *Immunol Today.* 1998 Mar;19(3):133-4

[168] "It appears that the patients' antibodies recognize epitopes consisting of the TFA group plus associated structural features of the protein carriers (100 kDa, 76 kDa, 59 kDa, 57 kDa and 54 kDa), not the TFA hapten alone." Kenna JG, et al. Metabolic basis for a drug hypersensitivity: antibodies in sera from patients with halothane hepatitis recognize liver neoantigens that contain the trifluoroacetyl group derived from halothane. *J Pharmacol Exp Ther.* 1988 Jun;245(3):1103-9 As an extension of this work, also see: "These investigations have further revealed that the antibodies are directed against distinct polypeptide fractions (100 kDa, 76 kDa, 59 kDa, 57 kDa, 54 kDa) that have been covalently modified by the reactive trifluoroacetyl halide metabolite of halothane." Satoh H, et al. Human anti-endoplasmic reticulum antibodies in sera of patients with halothane-induced hepatitis are directed against a trifluoroacetylated carboxylesterase. *Proc Natl Acad Sci* 1989 Jan;86(1):322-6 pnas.org/cgi/reprint/86/1/322

[169] Abedi-Valugerdi M, Nilsson C, Zargari A, Gharibdoost F, DePierre JW, Hassan M. Bacterial lipopolysaccharide both renders resistant mice susceptible to mercury-induced autoimmunity and exacerbates such autoimmunity in susceptible mice. *Clin Exp Immunol.* 2005 Aug;141(2):238-47

[170] Shedlofsky SI, et al, Blouin RA. Endotoxin administration to humans inhibits hepatic cytochrome P450-mediated drug metabolism. *J Clin Invest.* 1994 Dec;94:2209-14

[171] "Enterohepatic recycling occurs by biliary excretion and intestinal reabsorption of a solute, sometimes with hepatic conjugation and intestinal deconjugation. ... Of particular importance is the potential amplifying effect of enterohepatic variability in defining differences in the bioavailability, apparent volume of distribution and clearance of a given compound." Roberts et al. Enterohepatic circulation: physiological, pharmacokinetic and clinical implications. *Clin Pharmacokinet* 2002;41:751-90

[172] Liska DJ. The detoxification enzyme systems. *Altern Med Rev.* 1998 Jun;3(3):187-98

[173] Reiter and Wegener were both actively involved in Nazi atrocities during World War 2, and they have both been stripped of their eponymic recognition. Reiter's syndrome is now "reactive arthrtitis, and Wegener's granulomatosus is now "ANCA-associated vasculitis" or "granulomatosis with polyangiitis." Scheinberg MA. Nazi past and changes in disease names. *Rev Bras Reumatol.* 2012 Mar:300-1. Panush et al. Retraction of suggestion to use "Reiter's syndrome" sixty-five years later. *Arthritis Rheum.* 2007 Feb:693-4

[174] Brons et al. Staphylococcal acid phosphatase binds to endothelial cells via charge interaction; pathogenic role in Wegener granulomatosis? *Clin Exp Immunol* 2000 Mar:566-73

that form the inner linings of arteries and all blood vessels. This positively-charged enzyme has also been shown to bind to the renal basement membrane, a target of immune attack in inflammatory/autoimmune renal diseases described as crescentic glomerulonephritis, a type of immune-mediated renal disease seen in several autoimmune conditions such as Goodpasture syndrome, IgA nephropathy, and systemic lupus erythematosus. Because the staphylococcal acid phosphatase is a foreign non-self protein, the human immune system forms antibodies against it; these antibodies are measurable in the blood of patients with ANCA-associated vasculitis. Thus, when the staphylococcal acid phosphatase binds to endothelial cells, the antibodies directed against the acid phosphatase induce a vigorous immune response and inflammatory reaction on the surface of the vessel wall—this is the hallmark of vasculitis. The authors conclude that "Since antibodies directed against staphylococcal acid phosphatase are present in patients with WG and these antibodies recognize endothelial cell-bound staphylococcal acid phosphatase, we suggest that the results published in this study support the hypothesis that staphylococcal acid phosphatase may play a role in the initiation of vasculitis and glomerulonephritis in patients with WG by acting as a planted antigen." For this discussion, "planted antigen" and "hapten" are synonymous and interchangeable.

> **The molecular evidence**
>
> Immune complexes in intestinal bypass arthritis contain IgG, IgM, and IgA antibodies directed against bacterial antigens from *E. coli*, *Bacteroides*, *Lactobacilli*, and Group D (gamma) streptococcus.
>
> Ross e al. *Baillieres Clin Rheumatol.* 1989 Aug

8. <u>Immune complex formation and deposition</u>: What we can reasonably describe as "chronic infection of the dysbiosis type" generally results in the increased production of immune complexes, which are polymeric antigen-antibody combinations. Antigen-antibody combinations are formed almost anytime the humoral immune system is fighting against a virus, bacteria, yeast, or food allergen; immune complexes are simply combinations of antigens and antibodies connected to each other to form a chain-like structure. Because each antibody/immunoglobulin has two "heads"—two antigen-binding sites—each immunoglobulin can bind two antigens; as such, a consecutive chain of antigens and immunoglobulins can be formed, as illustrated in the following diagram. Although essential for the destruction and clearance of pathogenic antigens, immune complexes pose a problem for the body due to 1) the difficulty in clearing them from the systemic circulation, and 2) their proclivity for deposition in the skin and joints.[175] **Indeed, immune complexes are significant contributors to most "autoimmune" diseases; immune complex deposition is responsible for triggering joint inflammation in rheumatoid arthritis[176] and for the facial rash and many of the other clinical manifestations which characterize systemic lupus erythematosus (SLE, lupus).** Immune complex deposition directly contributes to the renal disease and vasculitis common in patients with autoimmune disease. Patients with autoimmune disease commonly have circulating IgM and IgA antibodies against bacteria from the gastrointestinal and genitourinary tracts[177] clearly indicating an active immune response against these bacteria and also suggesting breaches in mucosal integrity. Since IgA-containing immune complexes are cleared from the serum by hepatocytes and are secreted intact into the bile[178,179,180], hepatobiliary phytostimulation may thereby produce an anti-rheumatic benefit; however, this hypothesis requires serologic and outcomes-based validation in a clinical trial.[181]

- IgA immune complexes in psoriasis (*J Invest Dermatol* 1983 Jun[182]): Using a sensitive and specific Raji cell radioimmunoassay, authors of this study analyzed the sera of 35 patients with psoriatic arthritis for IgA-containing circulating immune complexes (IgA-CIC). Additionally, measurements for circulating immune complexes (CIC) containing IgG or IgM were performed using the 125I-Clq binding assay and the Raji IgG radio-immunoassay. Results showed that, "**Twenty-eight of thirty five (80%) patients with PsA were**

---

[175] Inman RD. Antigens, the gastrointestinal tract, and arthritis. *Rheum Dis Clin North Am.* 1991 May;17(2):309-21

[176] Abramson SB. Mediators of inflammation, tissue destruction, repair: cellular constituents. In Klippel JH. *Primer on rheumatic diseases. 11th Ed.* Arthritis Foundation;1997,39

[177] "IgM and IgA anti-Proteus antibodies were significantly higher in patients with RF-positive RA compared with all other patient groups." Newkirk et al. Elevated levels of IgM and IgA antibodies to Proteus mirabilis and IgM antibodies to Escherichia coli are associated with early RF-positive rheumatoid arthritis. *Rheumatology* 2005;44:1433-41

[178] "Clearance of IgA immune complexes was delayed after bile duct ligation." Harmatz PR, Kleinman RE, Bunnell BW, McClenathan DT, Walker WA, Bloch KJ. The effect of bile duct obstruction on the clearance of circulating IgA immune complexes. *Hepatology.* 1984 Jan-Feb;4(1):96-100

[179] Lemaitre-Coelho I, et al. High levels of secretory IgA and free secretory component in the serum of rats with bile duct obstruction. *J Exp Med.* 1978 Mar 1;147(3):934-9

[180] "CONCLUSIONS: Biliary obstruction secondary to both calculus or malignancy of the hepatobiliary system causes suppression of bile IgA secretion and elevated serum level of secretory IgA. Bile secretory IgA secretion recovers with endoscopic drainage of the obstructed system." Sung JJ, Leung JC, Tsui CP, Chung SS, Lai KN. Biliary IgA secretion in obstructive jaundice: the effects of endoscopic drainage. *Gastrointest Endosc* 1995 Nov;42:439-44

[181] Vasquez A. Do Benefits of Botanical and Physiotherapeutic Hepatobiliary Stimulation Result from Enhanced Excretion of IgA Immune Complexes? *Naturo Digest* 2006; Jan

[182] Hall RP, Peck GL, Lawley TJ. Circulating IgA immune complexes in patients with psoriasis. *J Invest Dermatol.* 1983 Jun;80(6):465-8

found to have IgA-containing circulating immune complexes. In contrast, only 13 of 35 (37%) had IgG-containing circulating immune complexes detected using the Raji IgG assay and 10 of 33 (33%) had IgG- or IgM-containing immune complexes detected using the 125I-Clq binding assay." Frequency, level, or subclass of immune complexes did not correlate with different types or severities of cutaneous psoriasis. However, **the level of IgA-CIC did significantly correlate with the severity of psoriatic arthritis**—higher levels of IgA-CIC corresponded with more severe psoriatic arthritis. The authors concluded, "The finding of IgA-containing circulating immune complexes in 80% of patients with psoriatic arthritis as well as the significantly higher levels of these complexes in the patients with more severe arthritis suggests that IgA-containing circulating immune complexes may play a role in the pathogenesis of psoriatic arthritis." Because IgA is the subclass of antibody/immunoglobulin that is used to defend mucosal surfaces such as the mouth, throat, respiratory tract, and the gastrointestinal and genitourinary tracts, elevations of IgA and IgA-CIC naturally encourage physicians to consider microbial colonization of one or more mucosal surfaces. Additionally, since IgA-CIC are cleared by the liver for excretion into the bile and therefore into the intestines, additional attention (phytotherapeutic and physiologic) to ensuring optimal hepatobiliary and intestinal functions is likely to be of clinical benefit.[183]

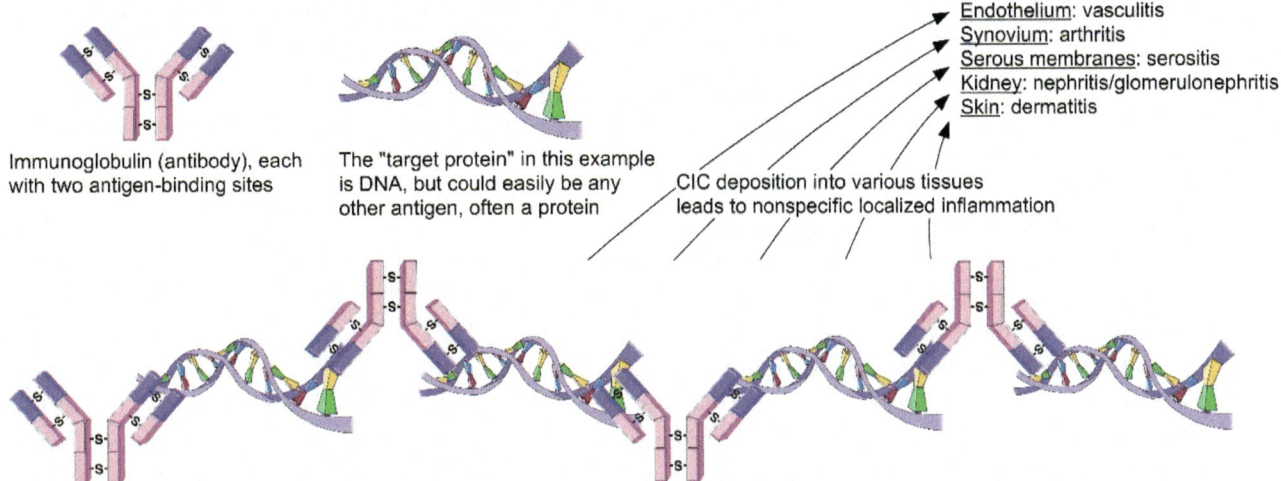

Immunoglobulin (antibody), each with two antigen-binding sites

The "target protein" in this example is DNA, but could easily be any other antigen, often a protein

CIC deposition into various tissues leads to nonspecific localized inflammation

Endothelium: vasculitis
Synovium: arthritis
Serous membranes: serositis
Kidney: nephritis/glomerulonephritis
Skin: dermatitis

Illustration of the formation of immune complexes: Because each immunoglobulin (antibody) can bind with two antigens, these combinations have the potential to form interconnected linear chain-like structures called immune complexes (IC), which when in circulation are called circulating immune complexes (CIC). CIC are problematic in that they are difficult to clear from systemic circulation and have predilection for deposition in certain tissues, specifically those which serve as "bypasses" or "filters" for fluids and other, generally smaller molecules. Such tissues include the endothelium, synovium, pleura/serosa, kidneys, and skin. Deposition of CIC in such tissues leads to a localized inflammatory response, including activation of the complement cascade. Clinical presentations can therefore include vasculitis, arthritis, serositis, nephritis/glomerulonephritis, and dermatitis, respectively. Chain-like combinations of antibodies and antigens trigger localized inflammation in various tissues, even though the origin of the antigens and antibodies is almost always from a distant site. For example, food/bacterial/viral antigens absorbed from the gastrointestinal tract can form circulating immune complexes (CIC) that are later deposited in the joints, skin, or vasculature to induce the clinical presentation of arthritis, dermatitis, or vasculitis, respectively.

- Psoriasis and immune complexes—IgA-containing immune complexes in patients with psoriatic arthritis (*Clin Exp Rheumatol* 1984 Jul[184]): In this study, blood samples from 21 patients with psoriasis were examined for the presence of IgA-CIC using the Raji IgA radioimmunoassay. Further, the Raji IgG radioimmunoassay and 125I-Clq binding assay were used to detect IgG-CIC and IgM-CIC. Results from the patients with psoriatic arthritis were contrasted against results from 25 patients with various nonpsoriatic hyperkeratotic skin disorders. Patients were given systemic therapy with etretinate (20 patients) or 13-cis-retinoic acid (1 patient)[Note 185]; blood from 15 patients treated with etretinate was studied before, during, and after therapy.

---

[183] Vasquez A. Do Benefits of Botanical/Physiotherapeutic Hepatobiliary Stimulation Result From Enhanced Excretion of IgA Immune Complexes? *Naturopathy Digest* 2006 Jan

[184] Hall RP, Gerber LH, Lawley TJ. IgA-containing immune complexes in patients with psoriatic arthritis. *Clin Exp Rheumatol*. 1984 Jul-Sep;2(3):221-5

[185] Of note, etretinate is an aromatic retinoid which was approved for severe psoriasis in 1986 and removed from the Canadian market in 1996 and the United States market in 1998 due to the high risk of birth defects; it has been somewhat replaced by acitretin, a safer metabolite of etretinate. 13-cis-retinoic acid is more commonly known as isotretinoin and is available by prescription; like other synthetic variants of vitamin A, it is highly teratogenic (i.e.,isotretinoin causes severe birth defects.).

Whereas 14 of 21 (67%) patients with psoriasis had evidence of IgA-CIC during the course of their disease, only 1 of 25 patients (4%) with other hyperkeratotic skin disorders showed this finding. Among the psoriatic patients, only 2 of 19 (11%) had evidence of IgG-CIC using the Raji IgG assay, and only 1 of 19 (5%) had evidence of IgG-CIC or IgM-CIC using the 125I-Clq binding assay. As was found in their previous study[186], these authors again showed a positive correlation between the extent of *psoriatic* disease and the level of IgA-CIC. Among 15 patients followed during therapy, results showed that levels of IgA-CIC did not change in response to positive response to treatment. Thus,

> ### The three most important consequences of (gastrointestinal) insufficiency dysbiosis—the lack of beneficial bacteria ("probiotics") in the gut
>
> 1. <u>Lack of anti-inflammatory benefit, especially including maximal induction of Treg cells</u>: Via metabolic and molecular molecules, "good bacteria" induce local and systemic tolerance. Systemically, this is effected by Treg cells that are induced in the GALT via epigenetic changes, maximally induced by the combination of nutrients such as vitamins A and D as well as probiotics. Lack of these good bacteria leads to the opposite immunophenotype (excess of inflammatory Th1, Th2, and Th17 cells) and the resulting predispositions toward metabolic, allergic, and autoimmune inflammatory disorders.
> 2. <u>Increased probability of infection, reduced colonization resistance (CR)</u>: Probiotic bacteria produce antimicrobial substances, promote mucosal immunity, and occupy receptor sites—all of these effects synergize to reduce intestinal colonization with pathogens and pathobionts (potential pathogens). Without this colonization resistance against pathogens and pathobionts, the gut is vulnerable to colonization or overpopulation with harmful inflammation-inducing and mucosa-damaging bacteria. Consider this along with the synergy of #1 above and you will note that even with these very basic mechanisms, the scales are tilted strongly in favor of "idiopathic systemic inflammation" simply by lack of beneficial probiotic-type bacteria in the gut.
> 3. <u>Increased intestinal permeability ("leaky gut") and increased bacterial translocation</u>: Metabolites such as butyrate have a trophic effect on gut mucosa; lack of such microbe-derived metabolic support predisposes toward failure to maintain a high-integrity/-fidelity mucosal barrier. A well-known consequence of reduced CR (#2 above) is increased translocation of intestinal bacteria into the GALT and portal circulation, wherein bacterial DNA and LPS famously promote hepatic damage and systemic inflammation, including with a high degree of certainty the formation of an immune response against bacterial DNA and other cross-reacting immune responses.
>
> Note the synergism of these three very well established effects of probiotic insufficiency dysbiosis: ❶ lack of immunotolerance and increased systemic inflammation, ❷ additional inflammation induced by pro-inflammatory bacteria and increased absorption of antigens, with ❸ direct absorption of bacteria, microbial DNA, and pro-inflammatory structures such as LPS.

given the correlation of IgA-CIC with the severity of psoriatic arthritis, the lack of correlation of IgA-CIC with improvement, and the lack of correlation of IgG-CIC and IgM-CIC with psoriasis, the authors concluded that, "…IgA-containing CIC are not directly related to the cutaneous manifestations of psoriasis, but may be important in the modification of immune or inflammatory responses in these patients." Another more likely explanation in the opinion of the current author (Dr Vasquez) is that IgA-CIC contribute to and represent the underlying pathophysiology of psoriasis (i.e., mucosal colonization with antigenic microbes and/or exposure to dietary antigens) which exists in proportion to the severity of the illness (i.e., serving as a reflection of both antigenic stimulation and abnormally increased mucosal permeability) and which persists despite clearance of skin lesions (i.e., the most superficial manifestation of the illness).

9. <mark>Insufficiency dysbiosis—an absolute or relative lack of beneficial bacteria—promotes inflammatory dysbiosis, systemic inflammation, immune dysregulation, and intestinal hyperpermeability</mark>: Clinicians performing stool tests on a regular basis—current author included—commonly find that patients simultaneously have—in addition to other problems—"too many bad bacteria and not enough good bacteria", as is commonly explained to patients. An <mark>insufficiency of beneficial bacteria</mark> leads to increased bacterial translocation, reduced <mark>colonization resistance, and failure to induce regulatory T-cells; all of these contribute to systemic inflammation.</mark> Beneficial bacteria in general exert many positive benefits for the host which might be summarized as follows: ❶ maintaining the health and permeability integrity of the mucosa, ❷ providing fuel—butyrate—for enterocytes and specifically colonocytes, ❸ maintaining a slightly acidic pH due to elaboration of metabolic acids, ❹ blocking colonization by harmful yeasts and bacteria via several mechanisms such as by *directly* producing antimicrobial factors and *indirectly* inducing enhanced secretion of secretory IgA from mucosal plasma cells, ❺ metabolism/processing of phytonutrients for absorption and enhanced physiologic function, ❻ co-feeding other probiotic bacteria, for example, Bifidobacteria convert carbohydrate substrate to

---

[186] Hall RP, Gerber LH, Lawley TJ. IgA-containing immune complexes in patients with psoriatic arthritis. *Clin Exp Rheumatol.* 1984 Jul-Sep;2(3):221-5

lactate and acetate which are then further metabolized by *Lactobacillus* into butyrate; in this way, probiotic bacteria "support each other" and are dependent/interdependent, ❼ maintaining a favorable biochemical and immunologic milieu for other beneficial bacteria, ❽ promoting elaboration of anti-inflammatory cytokines and suppression of pro-inflammatory cytokines, specifically inducing tolerogenic DCs producing lowered amounts of pro-inflammatory IFN-gamma and elevated amounts of anti-inflammatory IL-10, ❾ helping to ameliorate allergy in general and food allergy in particular by the above mechanisms, and ❿ promoting maturation of undifferentiated/naïve T-cells into regulatory T-cells (Treg) for the suppression/modulation of pro-inflammatory Th17-cells which are some of the primary pathologic effectors of autoimmune-mediated tissue damage, particularly in multiple sclerosis. Induction of Foxp3+ Treg from mature Th2-type memory T-cells by use of combination treatment including retinoic acid (an active form of vitamin A) has been performed experimentally[187], probably occurs in vivo in humans, and is reviewed elsewhere in this book. Several of these aforementioned mechanisms are well-known and/or self-evident; however, induction of Treg by probiotics is a relatively new concept and is of supreme clinical importance and will be given additional detail here:

- SLE and colonization resistance of the intestinal tract (*Epidemiol Infect.* 1994 Apr[188]): "Anti-ds-DNA antibodies may be pathogenic in SLE by forming immune complexes with DNA. Foreign bacteria in the intestines could constitute the stimulus for anti-ds-DNA antibody production in SLE. Colonization Resistance (CR) is the defense capacity of the indigenous microflora against colonization of the intestines by foreign bacteria. A low CR implies increase of translocation of bacteria and a higher chance of subsequent, possibly DNA-cross-reacting antibacterial antibody production. We measured CR by a comprehensive biotyping technique in healthy individuals and patients with inactive and active SLE. CR tended to be lower in active SLE patients than in healthy individuals. This could indicate that in SLE more and different bacteria translocate across the gut wall due to a lower CR. Some of these may serve as polyclonal B cell activators or as antigens cross-reacting with DNA."

- Probiotic induction of Treg and DCreg: Generation of regulatory dendritic cells and CD4+Foxp3+ T cells by probiotics administration suppresses immune disorders (*Proc Natl Acad Sci USA* 2010 Feb[189]): The authors used a probiotic mixture which was found to achieve several very important goals: ❶ up-regulation of CD4(+)Foxp3(+) regulatory T cells (Tregs) from the CD4(+)CD25(-) population, ❷ induction of both T-cell and B-cell hyporesponsiveness, ❸ down-regulation of T helper (Th) 1, Th2, and Th17 cytokines without apoptosis induction—the significance here is that the goal is to regulate and modulate the immune system, not induce death in key elements, and ❹ increase in the suppressor activity of naturally occurring CD4(+)CD25(+) Tregs. The authors note that conversion of T-cells into Foxp3(+) Tregs is directly mediated by regulatory dendritic cells (DCreg) that express high levels of IL-10, TGF-beta, COX-2, and indoleamine 2,3-dioxygenase (IDO)—an enzyme involved in tryptophan degradation and the expression of which is very important for the formation of DCregs and therefore Tregs—and they also note that therapeutic benefits in animal models of experimental inflammatory bowel disease, atopic dermatitis, and rheumatoid arthritis is associated with and likely directly due to the enrichment of CD4 Foxp3 Tregs in the inflamed regions, following their maturation/promotion in the environment of the gut-associated lymphoid tissue.

- Probiotic induction of anti-inflammatory IL-10: Oral probiotic administration induces interleukin-10 production and prevents spontaneous autoimmune diabetes in the NOD mouse (*Diabetologia* 2005 Aug[190]): Researchers used the probiotic supplement VSL#3 on diabetes-prone mice (the non-obese diabetic [NOD] mouse develops a spontaneous form of autoimmune diabetes similar to the human disease). Results showed that probiotic administration prevented diabetes development in NOD mice and that the mice treated with the probiotic "showed reduced insulitis and a decreased rate of beta cell destruction. Prevention was associated with an increased production of IL-10 from Peyer's patches and the spleen and with increased IL-10 expression in the pancreas, where IL-10-positive islet-infiltrating mononuclear cells were detected." This is a very interesting experiment showing that marrow-derived immunocytes are re-

---

[187] Kim BS, et al. Conversion of Th2 memory cells into Foxp3+ regulatory T cells suppressing Th2-mediated allergic asthma. *Proc Natl Acad Sci* 2010 May 11;107:8742-7

[188] Apperloo-Renkema et al. Host-microflora interaction in SLE: colonization resistance of the indigenous bacteria of the intestinal tract. *Epidemiol Infect.* 1994 Apr;112(2):367-73

[189] Kwon et al. Generation of regulatory dendritic cells and CD4+Foxp3+ T cells by probiotics administration suppresses immune disorders. *Proc Natl Acad Sci.* 2010 Feb:2159-64

[190] Calcinaro et al. Oral probiotic administration induces interleukin-10 production and prevents spontaneous autoimmune diabetes in non-obese diabetic mouse. *Diabetologia.* 2005 Aug;48(8):1565-75

programmed in gut-associated lymphoid tissue (GALT) and subsequently redistribute to the periphery to effect cellular immunomodulation and thereby prevent autoimmune-mediated tissue injury.

- **Probiotic induction via IL-10 of Treg: Alleviation of experimental autoimmune encephalomyelitis by probiotics** (*PLoS One* 2010 Feb[191]): Experimental autoimmune encephalomyelitis (EAE) is the experimental animal model of the human disease multiple sclerosis (MS), a chronic inflammatory autoimmune disease of the central nervous system (CNS). The authors note that, "One potential therapeutic strategy for MS is to induce regulatory cells that mediate immunological tolerance." Probiotics, including lactobacilli, have been shown to have immunomodulatory activity. Accordingly, they tested various *Lactobacillus* strains for suppression of EAE; tested strains included *L. paracasei* DSM 13434, *L. plantarum* DSM 15312 and DSM 15313, each of which reduced inflammation in CNS and autoreactive T cell responses. The research showed that "***L. paracasei* and *L. plantarum* DSM 15312 induced CD4(+)CD25(+)Foxp3(+) regulatory T cells (Tregs)** in mesenteric lymph nodes (MLNs) and enhanced production of serum TGF-beta1, while *L. plantarum* **DSM 15313 increased serum IL-27 levels**." Work by other researchers has shown that IL-27 suppresses Th17 activity while apparently promoting Th1 activity. Very interestingly and of high clinical importance is the finding that "each monostrain probiotic failed to be therapeutic in diseased mice, while a mixture of the three lactobacilli strains suppressed the progression and reversed the clinical and histological signs of EAE." As would be expected in a classic scenario, *Lactobacillus*-induced suppressive activity "correlated with attenuation of pro-inflammatory Th1 and Th17 cytokines followed by IL-10 induction in MLNs, spleen and blood." In a separate experiment, the researchers showed **that IL-10-producing CD4(+)CD25(+) Tregs played the main role in the anti-inflammatory effects induced by probiotic administration.**

10. Microbial hypersensitivity, bacterial allergy: Microbes can illicit an immune response more typical of allergy than of the typical antimicrobial inflammatory response. The response may be cell-mediated and/or IgE-mediated; lack of elevation in specific or total IgE does not exclude the condition. This is noted with vulvovaginal candidiasis and in atopic dermatitis in response to *Staphylococcus aureus* (as discussed later). Very interestingly as noted with vulvovaginal Candida hypersensitivity[192], the lymphocyte-driven immune response against *Candida* is impaired by the macrophage-driven PGE2-mediated hypersensitivity response, thereby promoting chronicity of both the infection/colonization as well as the tissue irritation/inflammation. A very significant component of bowel-associated dermatitis-arthritis syndrome (BADAS) is an allergic-type response; thus "bacterial allergy" works in synergy with other types of inflammatory responses, including those mediate by exotoxins and immune complexes, thereby exacerbating the arthritis, dermatitis, and vasculitis.[193]

> **Bacteria can induce allergy-type immune responses**
>
> Rudzki et al[65] stated that "undisputed" positive correlation between bacterial allergy and skin disease exists if the three conditions of *provocation, focal reaction,* and *isomorph effect* are present after skin testing with bacterial antigens. Provoca-
>
> Ely PH. The bowel bypass syndrome: a response to bacterial peptidoglycans. *J Am Acad Dermatol.* 1980 Jun;2(6):473-87

11. Inhibition of detoxification: **All clinicians must appreciate that bioaccumulation of toxic chemicals can trigger/promote autoimmunity.**[194,195,196] Examples of this include the increased autoimmunity seen in humans exposed to pesticides[197,198], the scleroderma-like disease that results from exposure to vinyl chloride[199], the

---

[191] Lavasani et al. A novel probiotic mixture exerts a therapeutic effect on experimental autoimmune encephalomyelitis mediated by IL-10 producing regulatory T cells. *PLoS One.* 2010 Feb 2;5(2):e9009

[192] Bernstein JA, Seidu L. Chronic vulvovaginal Candida hypersensitivity: An underrecognized and undertreated disorder by allergists. *Allergy Rhinol.* 2015 Jan;6(1):44-9

[193] Ely PH. The bowel bypass syndrome: a response to bacterial peptidoglycans. *J Am Acad Dermatol.* 1980 Jun;2(6):473-87

[194] "Autoimmunity due to chemical exposure was evidenced by elevation of TA1 phenotype frequencies and presence of rheumatoid factor, immune complexes, ANA, and anti myelin basic protein antibodies. We conclude that chemical exposure may induce immune abnormalities including immune suppression and autoimmunity." Vojdani A, Ghoneum M, Brautbar N. Immune alteration associated with exposure to toxic chemicals. *Toxicol Ind Health* 1992;8:239-253

[195] Crinnion WJ. Results of a decade of naturopathic treatment for environmental illnesses. *J Naturophatic Med* 1994;17:21-27

[196] Crinnion WJ. Environmental medicine, part 1: the human burden of environmental toxins and their common health effects. *Altern Med Rev.* 2000 Feb;5(1):52-63 See also: Crinnion WJ. Environmental medicine, part 2 - health effects of and protection from ubiquitous airborne solvent exposure. *Altern Med Rev.* 2000 Apr;5(2):133-43

[197] "IgG levels decreased with increasing p,p'-DDE levels, with a statistically significant decrease of approximately 50% in the highest two categories of exposure. Sixteen (12%) were positive for antinuclear antibodies... These analyses provide evidence that p,p'-DDE modulates immune responses in humans." Cooper GS, et al. Associations between plasma DDE levels and immunologic measures in African-American farmers in North Carolina. *Environ Health Perspect.* 2004 Jul;112(10):1080-4

[198] "Twelve individuals who were exposed to chlorpyrifos were studied 1-4.5 y following exposure to determine changes in the peripheral immune system. The subjects were found to have a high rate of atopy and antibiotic sensitivities, elevated CD26 cells (p < .01), and a higher rate of autoimmunity, compared with two control groups." Thrasher JO, Madison R, Broughton A. Immunologic abnormalities in humans exposed to chlorpyrifos: preliminary observations. *Arch Environ Health* 1993;48:89-93

[199] "Vinyl chloride (VC) monomer can induce a scleroderma-like syndrome in a proportion of workers exposed to it during production of polyvinyl chloride." Black CM, Welsh KI, Walker AE, et al. Genetic susceptibility to scleroderma-like syndrome induced by vinyl chloride. *Lancet.* 1983 Jan 1;1(8314-5):53-5

association of mercury and pesticide exposure with lupus[200], and the well-recognized connection between drug and chemical exposure and various autoimmune syndromes such as drug-induced lupus.[201] Indeed, more than 40 pharmaceutical drugs are known to cause drug-induced lupus, and bystander activation appears to be one of the primary mechanisms involved.[202] Thus having established the general premise that chemical exposure can trigger autoimmune disease, it seems logical and probable that anything which would inhibit the body's ability to detoxify these chemicals would likewise increase the risk for autoimmunity. Stated differently, factors that inhibit detoxification and which therefore increase the body-burden of immunotoxic xenobiotics would serve to indirectly contribute to immunodysfunction and the resultant autoimmunity. Indeed, **patients with lupus and systemic sclerosis show defects in detoxification[203], and different detoxification defects have been documented in patients with ankylosing spondylitis.**[204] Surmounting detoxification defects and xenobiotic exposure by the use of comprehensive detoxification programs (discussed later) is clinically beneficial.[205,206,207,208] Dysbiotic bacterial overgrowth of the gastrointestinal tract directly impairs detoxification via the following four mechanisms:

> **Immune alteration associated with exposure to toxic chemicals; many chemicals activate mTOR to promote inflammation and autoimmunity**
>
> "Autoimmunity due to chemical exposure was evidenced by elevation of TA1 phenotype frequencies and presence of rheumatoid factor, immune complexes, ANA, and antimyelin basic protein antibodies. **We conclude that chemical exposure may induce immune abnormalities including immune suppression and autoimmunity.**"
>
> Vojdani et al. *Toxicol Ind Health.* 1992 Sep-Oct

1) <u>Cytochrome P450/phase-1 inhibition</u>: Bacterial lipopolysaccharide (endotoxin) has been shown to significantly impair Phase 1 of chemical detoxification.[209] Obviously when major cytochrome p450 pathways are inhibited by endotoxin, then detoxification/biotransformation of xenobiotics and drugs is greatly impaired.[210] The logical extrapolation is that these chemicals would accumulate in the body and promote immunologic and/or neurogenic sensitization.[211]

2) <u>Deconjugation and enterohepatic recirculation</u>: Several species of bacteria produce deconjugating enzymes (such as beta-glucuronidase) that cleave previously "detoxified" toxins from their water-soluble moieties thus allowing the toxin to be reabsorbed in a mechanism termed "enterohepatic recycling"[212] or "enterohepatic recirculation."[213]

3) <u>Increased intestinal permeability</u>: Damage to the intestinal mucosa increases absorption of intraluminal contents and thus increase the toxic load placed on the detoxification mechanisms, which are mostly located

---

[200] "...reported occupational exposure to mercury (OR 3.6), mixing pesticides for agricultural work (OR 7.4), and among dental workers (OR 7.1). ...these associations were fairly strong and statistically significant..." Cooper et al. Occupational risk factors for development of systemic lupus erythematosus. *J Rheumatol.* 2004 Oct;31:1928-33

[201] Hess EV. Environmental chemicals and autoimmune disease: cause and effect. *Toxicology.* 2002 Dec 27;181-182:65-70

[202] "Drug-induced lupus has been reported as a side-effect of long-term therapy with over 40 medications... Several mechanisms for induction of autoimmunity will be discussed, including bystander activation of autoreactive lymphocytes due to drug-specific immunity or to non-specific activation of lymphocytes, direct cytotoxicity with release of autoantigens ..." Rubin RL. Drug-induced lupus. *Toxicology.* 2005;209(2):135-47

[203] "The observed increased frequencies of the CYP1A1 mutant Val-allele and the slow actylator phenotype in idiopathic autoimmune disease support our concept that in slow acetylators non-acetylated xenobiotics may accumulate and are subsequently metabolized by other enzymes into reactive intermediates. Thus, enhanced formation of reactive metabolites could alter self-proteins..." von Schmiedeberg S, et al. Polymorphisms of the xenobiotic-metabolizing enzymes CYP1A1 and NAT-2 in systemic sclerosis and lupus erythematosus. *Adv Exp Med Biol.* 1999;455:147-52

[204] "Homozygosity for poor metabolizer alleles was found to be associated with AS... Significant within-family association of CYP2D6*4 alleles and AS was demonstrated. Weak linkage was also demonstrated between CYP2D6 and AS. We postulate that altered metabolism of a natural toxin or antigen by the CYP2D6 gene may increase susceptibility to AS." Brown MA, et al. Polymorphisms of the CYP2D6 gene increase susceptibility to ankylosing spondylitis. *Hum Mol Genet.* 2000 Jul 1;9(11):1563-6

[205] Crinnion WJ. Results of a decade of naturopathic treatment for environmental illnesses. *J Naturopathic Med* 1994;17:21-27

[206] Crinnion WJ. Environmental medicine, part 1: the human burden of environmental toxins and their common health effects. *Altern Med Rev.* 2000 Feb;5(1):52-63 See also: Crinnion WJ. Environmental medicine, part 2 - health effects of and protection from ubiquitous airborne solvent exposure. *Altern Med Rev.* 2000 Apr;5(2):133-43

[207] Krop J. Chemical sensitivity after intoxication at work with solvents: response to sauna therapy. *J Altern Complement Med.* 1998 Spring;4(1):77-86

[208] "Retesting following the detoxification program showed significantly improved scores on: three memory tests, block design, trails B, and embedded figures. Thus, there was significant reversibility of impairment after the detoxification interval." Kilburn KH, Warsaw RH, Shields MG. Neurobehavioral dysfunction in firemen exposed to polycholorinated biphenyls (PCBs): possible improvement after detoxification. *Arch Environ Health.* 1989 Nov-Dec;44(6):345-50

[209] Shedlofsky et al. Endotoxin administration to humans inhibits hepatic cytochrome P450-mediated drug metabolism. *J Clin Invest.* 1994 Dec;94(6):2209-14

[210] "CONCLUSIONS: These data show that endotoxin-induced inflammation decreases hepatic cytochrome P450-mediated metabolism of selected probe drugs in women as it does in men." Shedlofsky et al. Endotoxin depresses hepatic cytochrome P450-mediated drug metabolism in women. *Br J Clin Pharmacol.* 1997 Jun;43(6):627-32

[211] "The sick building syndrome and multiple chemical sensitivity syndrome have been defined as clinical entities in which exposure to chemical inhalants gives rise to disease. Current data on the existence of chemical irritant receptors in the airway and skin are discussed; neurogenic inflammation arising from stimulation of chemical irritant receptors is a possible model to explain many of the aspects of chemical sensitivities." Meggs WJ. Neurogenic inflammation and sensitivity to environmental chemicals. *Environ Health Perspect.* 1993 Aug;101(3):234-8

[212] "Enterohepatic recycling occurs by biliary excretion and intestinal reabsorption of a solute, sometimes with hepatic conjugation and intestinal deconjugation. ... Of particular importance is the potential amplifying effect of enterohepatic variability in defining differences in the bioavailability, apparent volume of distribution and clearance of a given compound." Roberts et al. Enterohepatic circulation: physiological, pharmacokinetic and clinical implications. *Clin Pharmacokinet.* 2002;41:751-90

[213] Liska DJ. The detoxification enzyme systems. *Altern Med Rev.* 1998 Jun;3(3):187-98

in the liver; eventually these pathways become depleted, rendering the host susceptible to the consequences of nutritional depletion and impaired detoxification.[214]

4) <u>Constipation</u>: Bacterial overgrowth can lead to excess production of methane which causes constipation[215] and thus increases the "toxic load" in the colon which then increases the load on the liver via the portal circulation. Likewise, hydrogen sulfide also promotes constipation; however, often, constipation leads to laxation/diarrhea once a sufficient amount of microbial toxins/debris/metabolites have accumulated. Clinicians can recall that microbial *hydr*ogen gas can be said to *hydr*ate the stool insofar as it increases intestinal motility and tends to promote diarrhea, while *methan*e *makes* people constipated and hydrogen *sulf*ide *stops* motility and electron transport.

Taken together, these enterometabolic mechanisms are consistent with the observance of increased risk for xenobiotic-associated diseases such as breast cancer[216,217] and Parkinson's disease[218,219] in patients with chronic constipation. With regard to Phase-1 acetylation, Evans[220] noted in a review published in 1984 that slow acetylation has been strongly noted in patients with Gilbert's disease and also bladder cancer, whereas the rapid acetylator phenotype is associated with diabetes mellitus. We would expect that patients with endotoxin-producing bacterial overgrowth of the small intestine would be more susceptible to the chemical accumulation that leads to multiple chemical sensitivity syndrome (MCS) and the xenobiotic-induced immune dysfunction that may result. In my own clinical practice, I have seen many patients with multiple chemical sensitivity respond very favorably to the eradication of their intestinal bacterial overgrowth, and I consider this treatment essential for all patients with autoimmune disease.

- <u>Psoriasis</u>—Genetic variants in drug metabolizing enzymes as risk factors for psoriasis (*Journal of Investigative Dermatology* 2003 May[221]): Foreign chemicals (xenobiotics) and drugs such as antimalarials and beta-blockers can trigger the onset or exacerbation of psoriasis; other exposures such as lithium, ACE inhibitors, nonsteroidal anti-inflammatory drugs, terbinafine, cigarette smoking, and heavy consumption of alcohol are also associated with the onset and exacerbation of psoriasis. Abnormalities in detoxification processes, such as different metabolic efficiencies caused by variant alleles of xenobiotic metabolizing enzymes, often leads to the accumulation of xenobiotics and/or their reactive metabolites. Accumulation of xenobiotics and/or their metabolites in tissues can result in the formation of neoantigens (i.e., haptens) and/or the exposure of cryptic peptides (e.g., autoantigens); these neoantigens and exposed autoantigens can then initiate and stimulate an aggressive T-cell response, resulting in tissue inflammation and injury. In this study, the authors analyzed xenobiotic-metabolizing enzymes in 327 Caucasian psoriasis patients and 235 control persons. Gene variants were tested for four phase I (oxidation) enzymes and three phase II (conjugation) enzymes. CYP1A1 alleles *2A and *2C were found more often in healthy controls, suggesting a protective role for these gene variants. The authors note that no significant difference between patients and controls could be found for the phase I alleles 1B1*1, 1B1*3, 2E1*1A, and 2E1*5B nor for the phase II enzymes GSTT1 or NQOR when considered in isolation. However, an increased risk for psoriasis was associated with genetic variations in GSTM1 and with heterozygosity for CYP2C19 alleles *1A and *2A. The combination of CYP1A1*1A (reduced enzyme activity) with CYP2C19*1A increased the odds ratio (OR) in favor of psoriasis by 3.3 (OR=3.3) while the combination of CYP1A1*1A with GSTM1 increased the OR to 4.84. CYP1A1*2C encodes for an enzyme of greater detoxification activity and reduces the risk for developing psoriasis (OR=0.44). The authors conclude, "This is the first large-scale study on these enzymes and the results obtained support the concept that **different activities of metabolizing enzymes can contribute to disease etiology and progression**." This article supports the concept that genetic/inheritable abnormalities in detoxification abilities can increase the risk for developing psoriasis; if the increased risk

[214] Lunn PG, Northrop-Clewes CA, Downes RM. Intestinal permeability, mucosal injury, and growth faltering in Gambian infants. *Lancet.* 1991 Oct 12;338(8772):907-1

[215] Lin HC. Small intestinal bacterial overgrowth: a framework for understanding irritable bowel syndrome. *JAMA.* 2004 Aug 18;292(7):852-8

[216] "These observations are consistent with an hypothesized association between constipation and increased risk of breast cancer." Micozzi MS, Carter CL, Albanes D, Taylor PR, Licitra LM. Bowel function and breast cancer in US women. *Am J Public Health.* 1989 Jan;79(1):73-5

[217] Petrakis NL, King EB. Cytological abnormalities in nipple aspirates of breast fluid from women with severe constipation. *Lancet.* 1981 Nov 28;2(8257):1203-4

[218] "...lower frequency bowel movements predict the future risk of PD. ...They also hypothesize that some yet undefined toxins break through the mucosal barrier of the intestine and are incorporated into the axon terminal of the vagus nerve and transported in a retrograde manner to the vagus nucleus." Ueki A, Otsuka M. Life style risks of Parkinson's disease: association between decreased water intake and constipation. *J Neurol.* 2004 Oct;251 Suppl 7:vII18-23

[219] "CONCLUSIONS: Findings indicate that infrequent bowel movements are associated with an elevated risk of future PD." Abbott RD, et al. Frequency of bowel movements and the future risk of Parkinson's disease. *Neurology.* 2001 Aug 14;57(3):456-62

[220] Evans DA. Survey of the human acetylator polymorphism in spontaneous disorders. *J Med Genet.* 1984 Aug;21(4):243-53

[221] Richter-Hintz D, et al. Allelic variants of drug metabolizing enzymes as risk factors in psoriasis. *J Investigative Dermatology.* 2003 May;120(5):765-70

is indeed due to the defective detoxification and not due to the gene products themselves per se, then any condition—importantly for this discussion the influence of bacteria—that alters detoxification could also increase the risk for psoriasis. The best singular example of this reality is the inhibition of CYP enzymes by bacterial endotoxin/lipopolysaccharide.

- Psoriasis—Evidence of impaired Phase-2 acetylation in psoriatics and psoriatics with psoriatic siblings (*Dermatologica* 1989 Oct[222]): Researchers conducting this study assessed acetylation ability using sulfamethazine as a probe in 64 psoriatic patients and in 157 control subjects. Among the 157 control subjects, 90 (57.3%) were slow acetylators. Among the 64 psoriatic patients, 40 (62.5%) were slow acetylators. Among the 27 psoriatic patients who had a sibling with psoriasis, 22 (81%) were slow acetylators (p < 0.05). Thus, a possible familial predisposition) increases the prevalence of an associated phase-2 acetylation defect from 62% to 81%, leading the authors to conclude, **"Slow acetylator phenotype may be a genetic risk factor for the development of psoriasis."** Interestingly, the slow acetylator phenotype noted above to be associated with psoriasis is also, per a 1984 review by Evans[223], associated with diabetes mellitus; clinical-epidemiologic research has consistently linked psoriasis and diabetes mellitus. The cause could be genetic (e.g., single nucleotide polymorphism [SNP]) and/or genetic predisposition to carriage of LPS-producing Cyp450-inhibiting microbes; an acetylation defect would be expected to increase the presence of reactive intermediates and to also impair xenobiotic clearance.

12. Bacterial and fungal proteases impair immune defenses: Microbial colonization of mucosal surfaces can result in impaired local immunity by causing loss of protective secretory IgA (e.g., loss of mucosal immunoglobulin defense) or by causing direct tissue damage that results in increased absorption of microbes and antigens (e.g., breach of mucosal barrier defense, allowing microbial debris absorption and bacterial translocation) as well as other dietary (e.g., peptides) and environmental (e.g., pollen) antigens. The combination of mucosal damage, destruction of sIgA, immunosuppression, and microbial overgrowth/colonization synergize to sensitize the systemic immune system toward allergic and proinflammatory disease.[224] Several microorganisms such as *Entamoeba histolytica*[225], *Streptococcus sanguis*[226], and *Candida albicans*[227] externalize protein-digesting enzymes (proteinases, proteases) that "digests" defensive immunoglobulins, including secretory IgA and humoral immunoglobulins. The proteinases produced by *Candida* are capable of lysing not only sIgA but also keratin and collagen[228], obviously providing for a breach of protection from other infections and antigens. In this way, mucosal microbial colonization with yeast/bacteria that secrete proteases/proteinases can "open the door" to previously excluded microbes or antigens to promote the resultant "infection" or "allergy", respectively. Furthermore, because IgA is destroyed by the protease, the infection is allowed to fester, resulting in on-going immune stimulation and its consequences such as bystander activation. This may explain why women with chronic vaginal candidiasis, which always implies chronic yeast overgrowth of the intestine[229], have nearly double the incidence of allergic rhinitis compared to patients without chronic yeast overgrowth.[230] Further supporting the link between yeast and allergy is another recent study showing that allergy/atopy is more common in patients with chronic yeast infections/colonizations.[231]

- Candida albicans protease degrades IgA, IgG, complement C3, alpha 2 macroglobulin and alpha 1 proteinase inhibitor (*Infect Immun* 1995 Mar[232]): "The ability of human polymorphonuclear leukocytes to kill Staphylococcus aureus was greatly reduced when the bacteria were opsonized with human serum

---

[222] Jiménez-Nieto LC, Ladero JM, Fernández-Gundín MJ, Robledo A. Acetylator phenotype in psoriasis. *Dermatologica*. 1989 Oct;178(3):136-7

[223] Evans DA. Survey of the human acetylator polymorphism in spontaneous disorders. *J Med Genet*. 1984 Aug;21(4):243-53

[224] "Studies performed in humans show that selective IgA deficiency, preterm delivery, intestinal helminth infection and type of feeding during the neonatal period may influence antigen uptake by the intestinal epithelium. These conditions...may cause increased absorption of intraluminal antigens and result in the triggering of allergic type responses." Reinhardt MC. Macromolecular absorption of food antigens in health and disease. *Ann Allergy*. 1984 Dec;53(6 Pt 2):597-601

[225] Kelsall BL, Ravdin JI. Degradation of human IgA by Entamoeba histolytica. *J Infect Dis*. 1993 Nov;168(5):1319-22

[226] "BD patients are infected with IgA protease-producing S. sanguis strains, which cause an increase of IgA titer against these organisms and IgA protease antigen." Yokota et al. IgA protease produced by Streptococcus sanguis and antibody production against IgA protease in patients with Behcet's disease. *Microbiol Immunol*. 1997;41(12):925-31

[227] Kaminishi H, Miyaguchi H, Tamaki T, et al. Degradation of humoral host defense by Candida albicans proteinase. *Infect Immun*. 1995 Mar;63(3):984-8

[228] "The enzymes produced by these yeasts are all carboxyl proteinases capable of degrading secretory IgA, the major immunoglobulin of mucous membranes. Some have keratino- or collagenolytic activity." Douglas LJ. Candida proteinases and candidosis. *Crit Rev Biotechnol*. 1988;8(2):121-9

[229] "The results showed that if C albicans was cultured from the vagina, it was always found in the stool... The gut-reservoir concept may well apply to other forms of candidiasis." Miles MR, Olsen L, Rogers A. Recurrent vaginal candidiasis. Importance of an intestinal reservoir. *JAMA*. 1977 Oct 24;238(17):1836-7

[230] Moraes PS. Recurrent vaginal candidiasis and allergic rhinitis: a common association. *Ann Allergy Asthma Immunol*. 1998 Aug;81(2):165-9

[231] Neves NA, Carvalho LP, De Oliveira MA, et al. Association between atopy and recurrent vaginal candidiasis. *Clin Exp Immunol*. 2005 Oct;142(1):167-71

[232] Kaminishi et al. Degradation of humoral host defense by Candida albicans proteinase. *Infect Immun*. 1995 Mar: 984-88

treated with the proteinase [from Candida albicans]. …The reduction of serum bactericidal activity was attributed to the degradation of complement C3 by proteolysis …the proteinase also degrades endogenous proteinase inhibitors, such as alpha 2 macroglobulin and alpha 1 proteinase inhibitor, which are involved in regulating inflammation. These results suggest that destruction of a host's defense-oriented or regulatory proteins facilitates debilitation of the infected host."

13. <u>Immunosuppression via gliotoxins</u>: *Candida albicans* produces a mycotoxin which functions as an immunotoxin named "gliotoxin", which suppresses human immunity.[233] Microbial proteases work synergistically with biofilm formation to nullify immunologic attack (via immunosuppression and cytokine inactivation) and are important for the establishment of chronic mucosal colonization.[234]

- <u>Aspergillus fumigatus' gliotoxin—at levels seen in patients with invasive aspergillosis—suppresses immunity/ phagocytosis</u> (*Microbes Infect.* 2007 Jan[235]): "Gliotoxin is a mycotoxin having a considerable number of immuno-suppressive actions and is produced by several molds such as *Aspergillus fumigatus*. In this study, we investigated its toxic effects on human neutrophils at concentrations corresponding to those found in the blood of patients with invasive aspergillosis. Incubation of the cells for 10min with 30-100ng/ml of gliotoxin inhibited phagocytosis of either zymosan or serum-opsonized zymosan without affecting superoxide production or the exocytosis of specific and azurophil granules." This research supports this mechanism of microbe-induced immune impairment, although the researcher's use of "concentrations corresponding to those found in the blood of patients with invasive aspergillosis" prohibits us from extending these findings to milder cases of colonization/dysbiosis except to say that local/mucosal immunity/phagocytosis might be impaired and might be achievable *locally not systemically* by a mucosal colonization such as the type seen in CRS. *Aspergillus fumigatus* can cause infection in immunocompetent humans but is much more commonly associated with invasive infections in immunocompromised hosts or chronic colonizations in patients with asthma or cystic fibrosis; however, *Aspergillus fumigatus* is common in ambient indoor environments, especially water-damaged buildings (WDB), and mycotoxin levels in indoor air can reach levels that are clinically significant.

14. <u>Mold toxins—mycotoxins—available from foods, environment, and endogenous/mucosal biofilms/colonizations</u>: Mycotoxins—toxic and carcinogenic metabolites produced by yeast/fungi—can be produced in situ (e.g., in the human body, on mucosal surfaces) or in foods especially grains which are consumed and the toxins thereby with absorbed; among various mycotoxins, aflatoxin is the best known by the general public and is the most common cause of acute or long-term mycotoxin-related illness. Adverse health effects of mycotoxins include esophageal cancer, liver cancer, gastroenteritis, child growth impairment, neural tube defects, acute toxicoses, immunotoxicity, and renal diseases.[236] Fungal colonization of the human sinuses is virtually universal, with colonization rates of as low as 92% but generally closer to 95-100% among people with and without chronic rhinosinusitis (CRS). Fungi in human sinuses can produce mycotoxins[237]; the possibility exists that fungal colonization of the sinuses can persist for years, especially if protected by microbial biofilms, and that mycotoxins could be absorbed systemically with immunosuppressive, pro-inflammatory, neuroinflammatory, neurotoxic, endocrinologic, oxidative, mitochondrial, or other dysmetabolic effects.[238] Mycotoxins, some of which are inflammatory and neurotoxic, such as from *Stachybotrys chartarum*, are

---

[233] "This study suggests a previously unrecognized potential virulence factor of C. albicans that could contribute to persistence of yeast colonization or recurrence of symptomatic infection through diminished host resistance." Shah et al. Effect of gliotoxin on human polymorphonuclear neutrophils. *Infect Dis Obstet Gynecol* 1998;6:168-75

[234] "The two proteases, alkaline protease and elastase, inhibit the function of the cells of the immune system (phagocytes, NK cells, T cells), inactivate several cytokines (IL-1, IL-2, IFN-r, TNF), cleave immunoglobulins and inactivate complement. Inhibition of the local immune response by bacterial proteases provides an environment for the colonization and establishment of chronic infection." Kharazmi A. Mechanisms involved in the evasion of the host defence by Pseudomonas aeruginosa. *Immunol Lett.* 1991 Oct;30(2):201-5

[235] Coméra et al. Gliotoxin from Aspergillus fumigatus affects phagocytosis and the organization of the actin cytoskeleton by distinct signalling pathways in human neutrophils. *Microbes Infect.* 2007 Jan;9(1):47-54

[236] Wu F, Groopman JD, Pestka JJ. Public health impacts of foodborne mycotoxins. *Annu Rev Food Sci Technol.* 2014;5:351-72

[237] Lieberman et al. Measurement of mycotoxins in patients with chronic rhinosinusitis. *Otolaryngol Head Neck Surg.* 2011 Aug;145(2):327-9

[238] Brewer JH, Thrasher JD, Hooper D. Chronic illness associated with mold and mycotoxins: is naso-sinus fungal biofilm the culprit? *Toxins* (Basel). 2013 Dec 24;6(1):66-80. I cannot say that I am completely pleased with this article, as I found some of their citations/attributions/conclusions to be inaccurate. Likewise with this separate paper—Dennis et al. Fungal exposure endocrinopathy in sinusitis with growth hormone deficiency: Dennis-Robertson syndrome. *Toxicol Ind Health.* 2009 Oct-Nov;25(9-10):669-80—these authors used the same laboratory company as Brewer et al, and I am concerned that—even though their conclusions may be correct—some misuse of information might be occurring based on the fact that they erroneously cited the Lieberman et al (whom I contacted) study and misrepresented the data therein. I do think that the overall proposal is both rational and likely—fungal colonization is known to occur, the fungi are known to produce mycotoxins—in this case in very close proximity to the brain, and the mycotoxins are known to be inflammatory, neurotoxic and to cause mitochondrial impairment. See also: Doi K, Uetsuka K. Mechanisms of mycotoxin-induced neurotoxicity through oxidative stress-associated pathways. *Int J Mol Sci.* 2011;12(8):5213-37

impressively manifold and complex[239], with some fungi strains being more or less toxigenic than other strains with the same name, and the complex mixtures of mycotoxins clearly need to be appreciated in context with each other, with other microbial (e.g., bacterial) products, and with other air contaminants in order to be evaluated to a higher level of sophistication and accuracy. Airborne microbial elements, including glucans, mycotoxins and volatile organic compounds will be discussed in more detail in the section on *Environmental Dysbiosis*.

> **Urine mycotoxin detection does not necessarily indicate mold-induced disease; higher levels of mycotoxins are suggestive of more exposure, but more research is needed here**
>
> "Mycotoxins are metabolites of some fungi that can cause illness in humans and animals, primarily after ingestion of contaminated foods. Low levels of mycotoxins are found in many foods; therefore, mycotoxins are found in the urine of healthy persons.
>
> "Antifungal medications are used to treat fungal infections, not illnesses caused by toxins produced by fungi."*
>
> Kawamoto M, Page E. Use of Unvalidated Urine Mycotoxin Tests for the Clinical Diagnosis of Illness — United States, 2014. *MMWR Morb Mortal Wkly Rep* 2015 Feb;64(06);157-158 *Obviously these are statements of fact, especially from a conservative standpoint; but in clinical reality, the fact remains that clinicians frequently target microbes to reduce the load of microbial toxins even when the microbes themselves are not causing a clinical infection.

- Water-damaged home and health of occupants—possible evidence of sinorespiratory colonization with neurotoxic mycotoxin-producing fungi (*J Environ Public Health.* 2012 Sep[240]): "A family of five and pet dog who rented a water-damaged home and developed multiple health problems. … The family had the following diagnosed conditions: chronic sinusitis, neurological deficits, coughing with wheeze, nose bleeds, and fatigue among other symptoms. … The mycotoxins were detected in bulk samples, urine and nasal secretions, breast milk, placenta, and umbilical cord. *Pseudomonas aueroginosa, Acinetobacter, Penicillium,* and *Aspergillus fumigatus* were cultured from nasal secretions (father and daughter). RT-PCR revealed *A. fumigatus* DNA in sinus tissues of the daughter."

- Adverse health effects of indoor molds. (*Arh Hig Rada Toksikol.* 2012 Dec[241]): "Regarding mycotoxins with rather well characterised toxicity (incl. carcino-, muta-, teratogenicity, cytotoxicity and immunosuppression) after ingestion or dermal exposure, an adverse biological effect can be caused by the inhalation of a dose at the minimum level of one tenth of the alimentary one."

15. Biofilms and quorum sensing: Many microbes—specifically bacteria and yeast/fungi—protect themselves with a surrounding matrix of extracellular polymeric substance (EPS); biofilms are more difficult to remove than would be "free floating" or independently adherent microbes, and biofilms also create a barrier against antimicrobial drug penetration and immune system access. While this does not require extensive conversation, a few additional details and nuances will be cited and annotated below; natural agents such as garlic and proteolytic/pancreatic enzymes have been suggested in the literature to promote biofilm dissolution, at least in vitro. Also relevant and worthy of inclusion in the conversation of biofilms, but not sufficiently robust to warrant a separate conversation, is the topic of quorum sensing, the process by which microbial communities are able to "sense and respond to their environment as a group" rather than as isolated and independent microbes. Emerging antimicrobial strategies—especially for hospitalized patients, those who have indwelling catheters or who are on long-term intubation, and those with dental appliances/implants—is searching for ways to disrupt biofilms and interfere with quorum sensing to provide therapeutic/preventive antimicrobial advantage. Of note, dental flossing—which most of us learn as children as a means to remove food from between teeth—functions by disrupting microbial biofilms, not simply by dislodging the occasional food particle. Antibiotic-induced antibiotic resistance is mediated in part by enhanced/responsive biofilm formation[242] as well as induction of the previously discussed L-form wall-less bacteria.

- Clinical effects of interdental cleansing on supragingival biofilm formation and development of experimental gingivitis (*Oral Health Prev Dent.* 2009[243]): "Toothbrushing alone yielded better outcomes than did any of the flossing [alone, without brushing] protocols. Interdental cleansing with a waxed floss had

---

[239] "Macrocyclic trichothecene mycotoxins, produced by one chemotype of this fungus, are potent translational inhibitors and stress kinase activators that appear to be a critical underlying cause for a number of adverse effects. Notably, these toxins form covalent protein adducts in vitro and in vivo and, furthermore, cause neurotoxicity and inflammation in the nose and brain of the mouse." Pestka JJ et al. Stachybotrys chartarum, trichothecene mycotoxins, and damp building-related illness. *Toxicol Sci.* 2008 Jul;104(1):4-26

[240] Thrasher JD et al. A water-damaged home and health of occupants: a case study. *J Environ Public Health.* 2012 Sep;2012:312836

[241] Piecková E. Adverse health effects of indoor moulds. *Arh Hig Rada Toksikol.* 2012 Dec;63(4):545-9

[242] "Exposure to subinhibitory concentrations of antibiotics can enhance biofilm formation and mutagenesis. Thus, a global response to cell stress seems to be responsible for antibiotic-induced biofilm formation." Jolivet-Gougeon A, Bonnaure-Mallet M. Biofilms as a mechanism of bacterial resistance. *Drug Discov Today Technol.* 2014 Mar;11:49-56

[243] Salvi et al. Clinical effects of interdental cleansing on supragingival biofilm formation and development of experimental gingivitis. *Oral Health Prev Dent.* 2009;7(4):383-91

better biofilm removal effects than with unwaxed floss. CONCLUSIONS: Toothbrushing without interdental cleansing using dental floss and interdental cleansing alone cannot prevent the development of gingivitis." In other words, flossing is mandatory for oral/dental health.

- ▪ Strategies for combating bacterial biofilm infections (*Journal of Oral Science*. 2014 Dec[244]): The authors of this paper provide a concise and well-written introduction to the topic of biofilms by stating, "Formation of biofilm is a survival strategy for bacteria and fungi to adapt to their living environment, especially in the hostile environment. Under the protection of biofilm, microbial cells in biofilm become tolerant and resistant to antibiotics and the immune responses, which increases the difficulties for the clinical treatment of biofilm infections. Clinical and laboratory investigations demonstrated a perspicuous correlation between biofilm infection and medical foreign bodies or indwelling devices. Clinical observations and experimental studies indicated clearly that antibiotic treatment alone is in most cases insufficient to eradicate biofilm infections."

- ▪ Clearance of apoptotic bodies, NETs, and biofilm DNA: Implications for autoimmunity (*Front Immunol.* 2014 Jul[245]): In yet another excellent article from the *Frontiers* journal group, Marko Radić—whose work I appreciate and cite in my work in *Rheumatology*—begins by contrasting the relatively clean and anti-inflammatory/noninflammatory death of apoptosis with that of the programmed cell death of NETosis, in which neutrophil extracellular traps (NETs) are formed from neutrophil nuclear chromatin, which forms a fibrous meshwork, adding to biofilm formation along with extracellular DNA from bacteria and fungi. In providing clinical perspective, he notes that "How apoptotic bodies, NETs, and biofilm DNA are safely cleared is of great interest, because incomplete clearance leads to systemic inflammation and autoantibody production." After additional description of this intermixing of human/host and microbial DNA, he goes on to note that this "tangle of bacteria and nuclear chromatin should be viewed as a "dangerous liaison" between lupus autoantigens and bacterial adjuvants that, by acting as a molecular complex, could trigger an adaptive immune response." In other words, microbe- and inflammation-triggered immunocyte activation leads to the intercombination of human/host DNA along with microbial DNA, thereby creating ripe opportunities for immune cross-reactivity and what I will call "persistence of immunogenic foci" that can mature overtime to initiate/promote autoreactivity. Fungal and bacterial DNA is extruded extracellularly for use in creating the structure and strength of microbial biofilms; this microbial DNA stimulates inflammatory responses via the previously mentioned PRRs (pattern recognition receptors) such as TLRs. The clinical implications of this excellent expert-level summary are that apoptosis should be supported for its promotion of tolerogenic immune responses, while necrosis and NETosis are not simply pro-inflammatory but specifically promotional of autoimmunity. Viewing microbial biofilms as a mesh of human/host plus microbial DNA (in addition to other structural components) will help clinicians appreciate the need to clear infections/colonizations as a means to eradicate biofilms and the reverse—clearance of biofilms to eradicate the housed microbes.

16. <mark>Impairment of mucosal digestion by microbial proteases and inflammation</mark>: Similar to the degradation of human IgA by microbial proteases/proteinases is the degradation of mucosal digestive enzymes such as the disaccharidases (sucrase, maltase, lactase, and isomaltase) and dipeptidases. First, impaired digestion of carbohydrates skews the intestinal milieu toward one favorable to bacterial/yeast overgrowth by increasing the levels of carbohydrate substrate upon which microbes feed. Impaired peptide breakdown promotes immune sensitization, protein malnutrition, and putrefaction. Second, inflammation resultant from intestinal dysbiosis further impairs carbohydrate digestion via downregulation of sucrase-isomaltase gene expression by inflammatory cytokines.[246] Third, destruction of microvilli exacerbates loss of mucosal enzymes and leads to additional malabsorption, maldigestion, and increased macromolecular absorption, such as seen in patients with intestinal giardiasis.[247] Impairment/reduction of disaccharidases and dipeptidases is also seen in patients with inflammatory bowel disease.[248]

---

[244] Wu H, Moser C, Wang HZ, Høiby N, Song ZJ. Strategies for combating bacterial biofilm infections. *Journal of Oral Science*. 2014 Dec [Epub ahead of print]

[245] Radic M. Clearance of Apoptotic Bodies, NETs, and Biofilm DNA: Implications for Autoimmunity. *Front Immunol*. 2014 Jul 30;5:365

[246] Ziambaras et al. Regulation of sucrase-isomaltase gene expression in human intestinal epithelial cells by inflammatory cytokines. *J Biol Chem*. 1996 Jan 12;271(2):1237-42

[247] Buret AG. Immunopathology of giardiasis. *Mem Inst Oswaldo Cruz*. 2005 Mar;100 Suppl 1:185-90 scielo.br/pdf/mioc/v100s1/v100ns1a31.pdf

[248] "A significant reduction of the specific activity of disaccharidases (lactase, sucrase and trehalase) in jejunal mucosal homogenate occurred in patients with inflammatory bowel disease. ... Several dipeptidases such as glycyl-leucine, leucyl-glycine, glycyl-glycine and valyl-proline hydrolase activities were lower in patients with inflammatory bowel disease than in controls." Arvanitakis C. Abnormalities of jejunal mucosal enzymes in ulcerative colitis and Crohn's disease. *Digestion*. 1979;19(4):259-66

17. <mark>Central sensitization to pain and depression; connection of gut microbes and intestinal permeability to depression, pain and fatigue syndromes:</mark> As the name implies, central sensitization describes a condition of heightened perception of / responsiveness to sensory stimuli, particularly pain. In an authoritative review by Woolf[249] in 2011, the following introduction provides both definition and description, "Nociceptor inputs can trigger a prolonged but reversible increase in the excitability and synaptic efficacy of neurons in central nociceptive pathways, the phenomenon of central sensitization. Central sensitization manifests as pain hypersensitivity, particularly dynamic tactile allodynia, secondary punctate or pressure hyperalgesia, aftersensations, and enhanced temporal summation." Woolf goes on to note that central sensitization (CS) can be elicited in humans by diverse experimental noxious stimuli to skin, muscles or viscera, and that CS "results in secondary changes in brain activity that can be detected by electrophysiological or imaging techniques." Clinical conditions in which CS plays a role include fibromyalgia, osteoarthritis, headache, temporomandibular joint disorders, chronic musculoskeletal pain, dental pain, neuropathic pain, visceral pain hypersensitivity disorders (such as irritable bowel syndrome, IBS), and post-surgical/traumatic pain. In essence, anything that causes pain (e.g., injury) or contributes to increased pain perception (e.g., sleep deprivation, magnesium deficiency, vitamin D deficiency) can contribute to central sensitization simply by virtue of neuronal plasticity, which makes repeatedly activated pathways—in this case the perception of and response to pain—become more permanent via synaptogenesis, e.g., pain chronification via activity/repetition-dependent synaptic plasticity. In experimental models, bacterial LPS has been shown to promote central sensitization via activation of microglial release of extracellular ATP which in turn triggers astrocytes to promote glutaminergic neurotransmission, thereby increasing neurocortical hyperexcitability and promoting pain, depression, central fatigue, and migraine/seizure. As paraphrased here and noted in the diagram from Béchade et al[250], <mark>LPS stimulates microglia to externalize the DAMP extracellular ATP, recruiting astrocytes to release glutamate leading to increased excitatory transmission via a glutamate, the major excitatory neurotransmitter. Clinicians should appreciate that LPS is a prototype agonist</mark> but certainly not the only "environmental factor" capable of <mark>triggering hyperglutaminergic neurotransmission</mark> (excess glutamate activating the glutamate-sensitive NMDA receptors) or what might be called glutamate-mediated hypertransmission (normal levels of glutamate triggering a hypersensitive receptor, or a hypersensitive or "loaded" or "primed" intracellular cascade). The clinical correlates of this model are relevant for chronic pain, depression, central fatigue, neurodegeneration, post-traumatic pain, post-traumatic stress disorder (PTSD), epilepsy and migraine. LPS is one of many "noxious stimuli" that can trigger microglia activation for eventual hyperglutaminergic neurocortical hyperexcitability and excitotoxicity; other factors include trauma and inflammatory cytokines and prostaglandins. <mark>LPS, other microbial immunogens, and other inflammatory triggers need not originate in the gut, as many long-term/chronic "dysbiotic-like" infections are localized within the brain and central nervous system, such as HSV[251], *Chlamydia pneumoniae*[252], and "algal" chlorovirus ATCV-1[253]; neuropathologic infections, antigens and neurotoxins such as the aluminum used in vaccines/immunizations as an adjuvant can be trafficked from the periphery into the brain by the immune system.[254]</mark> This author's perspective is that gut-derived microbial signals do indeed evoke central sensitization, most likely via direct CNS entry (via a "leaky" blood-brain barrier; perhaps trafficked by immunocytes), but at the very least indirectly by peripheral immune activation and the systemic proinflammatory state characterized by increased production of cytokines and prostaglandins which readily cross the blood-brain barrier to produce microglial activation and the subsequent hyperexcitation, excitotoxicity, and sickness behavior—including fatigue, depression, sensitivity. Microglial activation promotes neuronal hyperexcitation/excitotoxicity, and the reverse is also true: neuronal (hyper)activity promotes microglial activation; thereby forming a vicious cycle. Additionally, factors such as heightened

[249] Woolf CJ. Central sensitization: implications for the diagnosis and treatment of pain. *Pain*. 2011 Mar;152(3 Suppl):S2-15
[250] Béchade C, Cantaut-Belarif Y, Bessis A. Microglial control of neuronal activity. *Front Cell Neurosci*. 2013 Mar 28;7:32
[251] Ball et al. Intracerebral propagation of Alzheimer's disease: strengthening evidence of a herpes simplex virus etiology. *Alzheimers Dement*. 2013 Mar;9(2):169-75
[252] Hammond et al. Immunohistological detection of Chlamydia pneumoniae in the Alzheimer's disease brain. *BMC Neurosci*. 2010 Sep 23;11:121
[253] Yolken et al. Chlorovirus ATCV-1 is part human oropharyngeal virome associated changes in cognitive functions in humans and mice. *Proc Natl Acad Sci* 2014 Nov:16106-11
[254] "We previously showed that poorly biodegradable aluminum-coated particles injected into muscle are promptly phagocytosed in muscle and the draining lymph nodes, and can disseminate within phagocytic cells throughout the body and slowly accumulate in brain." Gherardi et al. Biopersistence and brain translocation of aluminum adjuvants of vaccines. *Front Neurol* 2015 Feb;6:4. See also: "Detection of Al(III) in tissues indicated presence of aluminum in the nervous tissue of experimental animals." Luján et al. Autoimmune/autoinflammatory syndrome induced by adjuvants (ASIA syndrome) in commercial sheep. *Immunol Res* 2013 Jul:317-24

glutamate/NMDA receptor sensitivity, depleted antioxidant defenses and specific nutrient deficiencies (e.g., pyridoxine, magnesium, zinc, vitamin D, n3 fatty acids), mitochondrial impairment, and an pro-inflammatory microenvironment combine additively/synergistically to promote the progressively accelerated pace of reciprocal microglial activation and neuronal hyperexcitation/excitotoxicity noted in several neurodegenerative states. This could be complicated by gut *Clostridia* production of 3-3-hydroxyphenyl-3-hydroxypropionic acid (HPHPA) and p-cresol causing neurotransmitter imbalance—elevated dopamine and reduced norepinephrine.

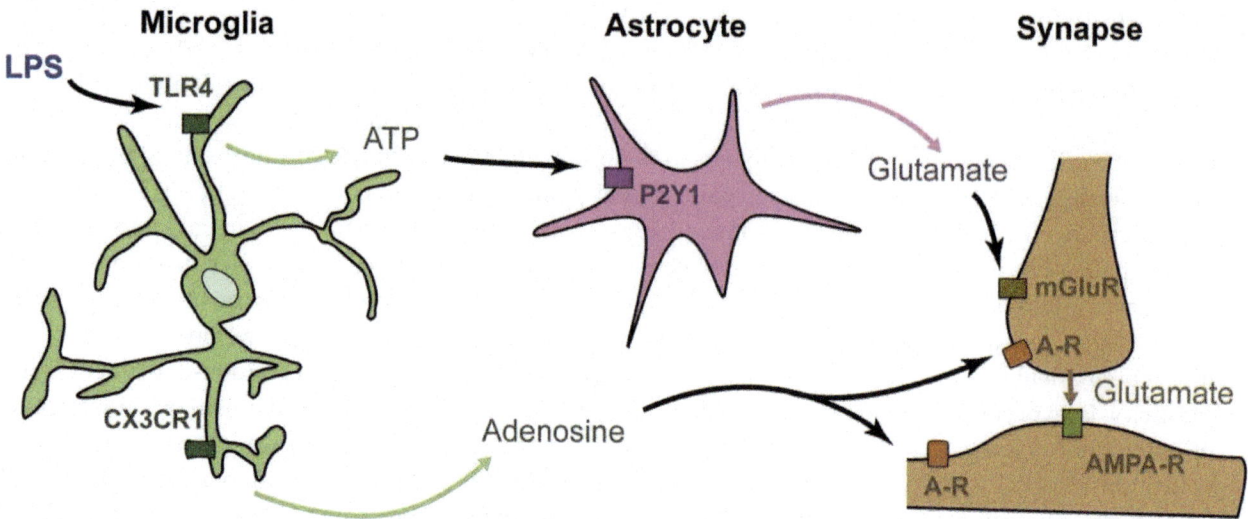

Microglial LPS reception leads to (extracellular) ATP elaboration, which stimulates astrocytes to produce glutamate, which increases glutaminergic neurotransmission: "Upon LPS stimulation, microglia rapidly produce ATP, which recruits astrocytes. Astrocytes subsequently release glutamate, and this leads to increased excitatory transmission via a metabotropic glutamate receptor-dependent mechanism." Illustration and quote from: Béchade C, Cantaut-Belarif Y, Bessis A. Microglial control of neuronal activity. *Front Cell Neurosci*. 2013 Mar 28;7:32[255]

Verified in animal models and likely contributory to clinical pain syndromes such as fibromyalgia is the observation that bacterial endotoxin/LPS can also contribute to central sensitization. This concept is introduced here and will be further substantiated in a following section on clinical pain syndromes and more so in separate writings, whether specific to fibromyalgia[256] or general to rheumatology.[257] The basic pathophysiology is quite simple and linear, as depicted below and itemized with citations thereafter.

Bacterial LPS ➔ microglial activation ➔ astrocyte hyperglutaminogenesis ➔ neurocortical hyperexcitation ➔ pain

However, the correlation of serum LPS (or its indirect marker, anti-LPS antibodies) with increased intestinal permeability provides another interpretation, wherein serum LPS activity is simply a correlate with increased IP which promotes pain via nonspecific and non-LPS mechanisms, as shown in the following sequence:

SIBO/LPS-induced mucosal damage ➔ absorption of gut-derived immunogens and toxins ➔ microglial activation ➔ astrocyte hyperglutaminogenesis ➔ neurocortical hyperexcitation ➔ pain/depression/fatigue and associated low-grade immune activation

- Endotoxemia induces visceral hypersensitivity and altered pain evaluation in healthy humans (*Pain*. 2012 Apr[258]): "…transient systemic immune activation results in decreased visceral sensory and pain thresholds and altered subjective pain ratings."
- LPS-induced hyperalgesia in healthy humans (*Brain Behav Immun* 2014 Oct[259]): "Our results revealed widespread increases in musculoskeletal pain sensitivity in response to a moderate dose of LPS (0.8 ng/kg), which correlate both with changes in IL-6 and negative mood."

[255] Béchade C, Cantaut-Belarif Y, Bessis A. Microglial control of neuronal activity. *Front Cell Neurosci*. 2013 Mar 28;7:32 doi: 10.3389/fncel.2013.00032 journal.frontiersin.org/article/10.3389/fncel.2013.00032/abstract. Copyright © 2013 Béchade, Cantaut-Belarif and Bessis. *Front Cell Neurosci* is an open-access journal distributed under terms of Creative Commons Attribution License, which permits use/distribution/reproduction in other forums, provided original authors/source are credited.
[256] Vasquez A. *Fibromyalgia in a Nutshell: A Safe and Effective Functional Medicine Strategy*. 2012, and later versions.
[257] Vasquez A. *Functional Medicine Rheumatology v3.5*. 2014, and later versions.
[258] Benson et al. Acute experimental endotoxemia induces visceral hypersensitivity and altered pain evaluation in healthy humans. *Pain*. 2012 Apr;153(4):794-9
[259] Wegner et al. Inflammation-induced hyperalgesia: timing, dosage, and negative affect on somatic pain in human endotoxemia. *Brain Behav Immun*. 2014 Oct;41:46-54

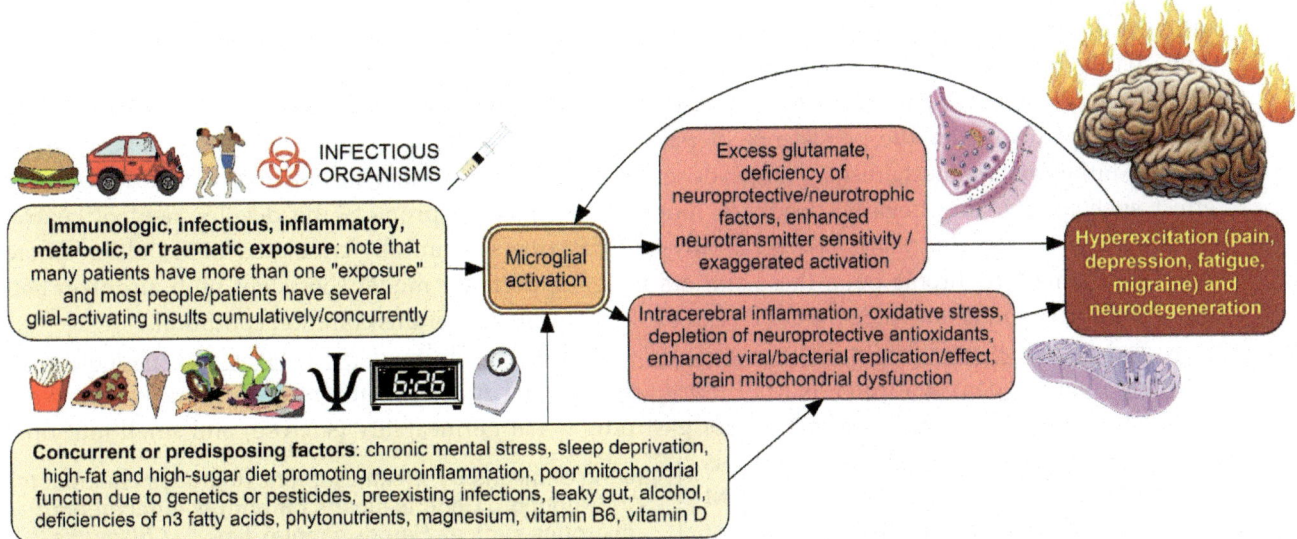

Numerous insults—immunologic, inflammatory, infectious, metabolic, traumatic, toxins—can "team up" or act individually to incite glial activation: Very importantly, glial activation can remain in an activated state promoting neurotransmitter imbalance, hyperexcitation, and neurodegeneration for several years after a single biochemical, infectious, or physical assault. High-fat foods, physical trauma from sports and accidents, psychological and mental stress, sleep deprivation, and the metabolic stress of hyperglycemia, insulin resistance, and obesity all contribute to brain inflammation—also called "the brain on fire" per Cohen, *Annals of Neurology* 1994—to promote pain, depression, migraine/seizure, and neurodegeneration.
Images and descriptions above by Dr Vasquez except for image of brain by isaacmao per Flickr.com via Creative Commons.

Gut bacteria also affect CNS/brain neurotransmission via vagal stimulation. According to a 2014 review by Galland, "Intrinsic primary afferent neurons (IPANs) are cellular targets of neuroactive bacteria and transmit microbial messages to the brain via the vagus nerve. Live bacteria may not be needed for these effects; in the case of *B. fragilis*, a lipid-free polysaccharide is both necessary and sufficient for IPAN activation. … Gut bacteria influence reactivity of the HPA axis and the induction and maintenance of nREM sleep. They may influence mood, pain sensitivity and normal brain development."[260]

> **Dysbiosis—SIBO and LPS—alter brain function, neurotransmission, to promote pain, fatigue, depression**
>
> "Structural bacterial components such as **lipopolysaccharides** provide low-grade tonic stimulation of the innate immune system. Excessive stimulation due to bacterial **dysbiosis, small intestinal bacterial overgrowth**, or increased intestinal permeability may produce systemic and/or central nervous system inflammation."
>
> Galland L. *J Med Food*. 2014 Dec

- Commemsal microbiota are necessary for the development of inflammatory pain (*Proc Natl Acad Sci.* 2008 Feb[261]): In this remarkably insightful article, the authors introduce their work by stating, "The sensation of pain can be enhanced by acute or chronic inflammation", and that in their experimental model using germ-free and "conventional" (colonized) mice, they "show that inflammatory hypernociception induced by carrageenan, lipopolysaccharide, TNF-alpha, IL-1beta, and the chemokine CXCL1 was reduced in germ-free mice" while hypernociception induced by prostaglandins and dopamine was not altered by the presence/absence of bacteria. However, "reposition of the microbiota" or systemic administration of LPS essentially restored the pain and inflammation that was absent in germ-free mice, which also produced more IL-10, which—via experiments using anti-IL-10 antibody—proved to mediate both anti-inflammation and anti-nociception. The authors concluded that, "Therefore, these results show that contact with commensal microbiota is necessary for mice to develop inflammatory hypernociception. … Therefore, these results show that contact with commensal microbiota [or LPS] is necessary for mice to develop inflammatory hypernociception possibly in a TLR-dependent manner. "

---

260 Galland L. The gut microbiome and the brain. *J Med Food*. 2014 Dec;17(12):1261-72
261 Amaral et al. Commensal microbiota is fundamental for the development of inflammatory pain. *Proc Natl Acad Sci U S A*. 2008 Feb 12;105(6):2193-7

- <u>Low-dose LPS 'priming' of muscle provides an animal model of persistent elevated mechanical sensitivity for the study of chronic pain</u> (*Eur J Pain* 2011 Aug[262]): In this experiment using intramuscular hypertonic saline with either high or low doses of LPS, the authors found that low-dose LPS exacerbated long-term pain, while high-dose LPS caused the expected acute inflammatory response but did not promote development of chronic pain; the authors speculate that the low dose of LPS "primed" inflammatory and neurologic pathways for the persistence of pain perception while the higher dose may have invoked counter-inflammatory mechanisms ("larger-dose of LPS in this experiment may have provoked a protective effect such as invoking negative feedback loops") that failed to promote the development of central sensitization. By showing that low-level locally-administered systemically-circulated LPS could promote the development of chronic pain, these authors have supported a model consistent with an integrated model of fibromyalgia, in which SIBO/LPS can explain the entirety of this common condition.
- <u>Increased intestinal permeability (IP) in patients with primary fibromyalgia (FM) and in patients with complex regional pain syndrome (CRPS)</u> (*Rheumatology* 2008 Aug[263]): Authors of this study used well-established tests of mucosal permeability for gastroduodenal permeability (sucrose) and small intestinal permeability (lactulose and mannitol, as discussed in Chapter 1) to find that both FM and CRPS patients show increased burden of intestinal involvement; they write, "Patients with FM had a significantly higher IP than healthy volunteers. Indeed, both FM and CRPS groups had significantly higher IP values than healthy volunteers for both gastroduodenal permeability and small bowel permeability. The difference in gastroduodenal permeability between the two patient groups did not reach significance. Gastroduodenal permeability, as measured with the sucrose test, was increased in 13 patients with FM (32.5%) and in six patients with CRPS (35.3%) and in one healthy volunteer. The small bowel permeability index [using lactulose and mannitol] was increased in 15 patients with FM (37.5%), three patients with CRPS (17.6%) and in none of the volunteers." A wonderful addition to / extension of this work would have been the measurement of serum LPS levels, but this was not performed in the current study and has not been performed as of early 2015—noted and summarized immediately below is one study (Maes et al, *J Affect Disord* 2007 Apr) that measured antibodies to LPS (not LPS directly) in patients with CFS—chronic fatigue syndrome. Notably, increased IP in FM did not correlate with GI symptoms; however increased IP did correlate with serologic positivity against *Helicobacter pylori*, *Yersinia enterocolitica* and *Campylobacter jejuni*.

Listing of means by which dysbiotic microbes can affect CNS function: General means for both ❶ intracerebral microbes such as Herpes simplex type 1, *Chlamydia pneumoniae* and ❷ remote/gut/noncerebral/all microbes
- Highly relevant clinical associations are indicated

1. Direct infection with atypical microbes (not encephalitis)—herpes simplex 1, algal virus
   - Alzheimer's disease, dementia, mental slowness
2. Inflammation, cytokines—direct microglial and immunocyte activation; local incitement of inflammatory cytokines; systemic cytokines readily cross the blood-brain barrier to change cognition and affect; increased absorption of food and microbial antigens via mucosal damage, leading to inflammation and immune responses; alteration in Treg/TH17 balance
   - Neurodegeneration, depression, and dementia via glial activation and excitotoxicity
3. Glial activation—resulting in glutaminergic excitotoxicity
   - Pain, seizure, vaccination encephalopathy
4. Mitochondrial/metabolic dysfunction, central fatigue, hypothalamic inflammation
   - DM, CFS/SEID, neurodegeneration, insatiability/hunger
5. Malnutrition—via malabsorption (e.g., B-12) seen with SIBO
   - Geriatric dementia, depression, neuropathy, anemia
6. Microbe-induced neuronal autoimmunity, neuroinflammation—cross-reactivity molecular mimicry, infection-induced neuropathologies
   - MS, sensory/motor peripheral neuropathy (Guillain-Barre), PANDAS, subacute sclerosing panencephalitis
7. Vagal nerve stimulation
   - Anti-inflammation
8. "Small molecule modification"— including epigenetic changes and other changes induced by metabolites such as acetate and butyrate
   - Obesity, DM, CVD, inflammation
9. Dopamine and norepinephrine alterations—via p-cresol and 3-3-hydroxyphenyl-3-hydroxypropionic acid (HPHPA)
   - Autism, schizophrenia
10. Deficiencies of tryptophan, serotonin, melatonin—via microbial intraluminal tryptophanase
    - Depression, anxiety, pain, fibromyalgia

[262] Yamaguchi et al. Low rather than high dose lipopolysaccharide 'priming' of muscle provides an animal model of persistent elevated mechanical sensitivity for the study of chronic pain. *Eur J Pain*. 2011 Aug;15(7):724-31
[263] Goebel et al. Altered intestinal permeability in patients with primary fibromyalgia and in patients with complex regional pain syndrome. *Rheumatology* 2008 Aug;47(8):1223-7

- Increased serum IgA and IgM against LPS of enterobacteria in chronic fatigue syndrome (CFS) shows involvement of gram-negative enterobacteria and increased gut-intestinal permeability in the etiology of CFS (*J Affect Disord* 2007 Apr[264]): These investigators measured IgA and IgM to LPS of the enterobacteria *Hafnia alvei, Pseudomonas aeruginosa, Morganella morganii, Proteus mirabilis, Pseudomonas putida, Citrobacter koseri,* and *Klebsiella pneumoniae* and "found that the prevalences and median values for serum IgA against the LPS of enterobacteria are significantly greater in patients with CFS than in normal volunteers and patients with partial CFS. Serum IgA levels were significantly correlated to the severity of illness, as measured by the FibroFatigue scale and to symptoms, such as irritable bowel, muscular tension, fatigue, concentration difficulties, and failing memory. The results show that enterobacteria are involved in the etiology of CFS and that an increased gut-intestinal permeability has caused an immune response to the LPS of gram-negative enterobacteria."

18. Dysbiosis-induced endocrine dysfunction: Although research in this area is less conclusive, the pattern of emerging research indicates that the multifaceted phenomenon of inflammation, particularly the elaboration of cytokines, alters endocrine function, and these inflammation-induced endocrine alterations further promote additional musculoskeletal inflammation. Endocrine changes induced by chronic inflammation include increased production of proinflammatory **prolactin**, and reduced production of anti-inflammatory and immunoregulatory **cortisol** and **androgens**. The link between dysbiosis and inflammation-induced changes in endocrine status has only recently begun to be documented, and some of these conclusions are logical though somewhat speculative. However, the nature of holistic healthcare requires us to consider *all* potentially significant contributions and interconnections, and thus microbe-endocrine links are briefly outlined here based on *highly suggestive*—yet not *wholly conclusive*—data. What is very clear is that autoimmune patients have alterations in hypothalamic-pituitary-adrenal/gonadal function. What is not yet clear is whether or not these are primary initiators of disease or secondary results of the disease process. Here I propose that both of these statements are true, namely that 1) endocrine dysfunction predisposes to the immune dysfunction that results in autoimmunity, and that 2) systemic inflammation further exacerbates endocrine dysfunction. Further, I speculate and add that 3) in some patients, chronic dysbiosis and subclinical inflammation and bacterial endotoxinemia/exotoxinemia can initiate the endocrine dysfunction and pro-inflammatory state that can eventually cross a diagnostic threshold to become overt clinical autoimmunity.

    - Altered hypothalamic responsiveness and circadian rhythm: The region of the basal hypothalamus is not protected by the blood-brain barrier and is sensitive and vulnerable to substances in the blood.[265] Because of this, hypothalamic and thus pituitary responses can be tuned to and/or altered by circulating prostaglandins, cytokines, and bacterial endotoxins and exotoxins. Patients with rheumatoid arthritis show hypothalamic/endocrine disturbances including blunted responsiveness to ACTH, abnormal circadian rhythm of prolactin and cortisol, and abnormalities in growth hormone secretion.[266] Furthermore, arginine vasopressin (AVP) is secreted from the hypothalamus in response to stress, is inherently pro-inflammatory, and is capable of augmenting prolactin secretion to further increase inflammation.[267]

        - Irritable bowel syndrome as a clinical model of intestinal bacterial overgrowth dysbiosis: Dysregulation of the hypothalamic-pituitary-adrenal (HPA) axis in irritable bowel syndrome (*Journal of Neurogastroenterology and Motility* 2009 Feb[268]): In order to utilize irritable bowel syndrome (IBS) as a model of dysbiosis (subtype: microbial overgrowth within the intestines) and to thereby describe the hypothalamic and neuro-endocrine alterations as exemplifications of dysbiosis-induced alterations in neuro-endocrine function, a brief review to (re)acquaint readers with the fundamental cause of IBS will be provided (part 1) which will be followed by a brief overview of the neuro-endocrine abnormalities caused by dysbiosis in this condition (part 2). ❶ IBS was erroneously assumed to be enigmatic and esoteric by clinicians well-versed in the idiopathic

---

[264] Maes et al. Increased serum IgA and IgM against LPS of enterobacteria in chronic fatigue syndrome (CFS): indication for the involvement of gram-negative enterobacteria in the etiology of CFS and for the presence of an increased gut-intestinal permeability. *J Affect Disord* 2007 Apr, 99:237–240

[265] Waxman SG. *Clinical Neuroanatomy 25th Edition*. McGraw Hill Medical, New York, 2003, p 160

[266] Anisman H, et al. Neuroimmune mechanisms in health and disease: 2. Disease. *CMAJ*. 1996 Oct 15;155(8):1075-82

[267] Chikanza et al. Hypothalamic-pituitary-mediated immunomodulation: arginine vasopressin is a neuroendocrine immune mediator. *Br J Rheumatol*. 1998 Feb;37:131-6

[268] Chang L, et al. Dysregulation of the hypothalamic-pituitary-adrenal (HPA) axis in irritable bowel syndrome. *Neurogastroenterol Motil*. 2009 Feb;21(2):149-59

ideology of allopathic/pharmacocentric medicine; meanwhile, the fact seemed quite obvious to the rest of us that so-called IBS was simply a manifestation of small intestine bacterial overgrowth (SIBO). Thankfully, the correct viewpoint—after years of clinical validation in integrative practices—has finally received widespread publication, although not necessarily widespread acceptance by scientific nihilists and therapeutic obstructionists. The masterful review by Lin[269] "Small intestinal bacterial overgrowth: a framework for understanding irritable bowel syndrome" published in *JAMA-Journal of the American Medical Association* in 2004 should have laid to rest the search for the major direct cause of IBS, particularly since follow-up studies using orally-administered nonabsorbable antibiotics[270,271,272,273] have shown consistent benefit despite the limited scope of the pharmacologic intervention, failure to perform microbial identification and sensitivity testing, and the general failure to use probiotic therapy and dietary improvements which are required to (re)establish and maintain eubiosis. Thus, having established IBS to be a manifestation of intestinal dysbiosis generally and SIBO—or more accurately SIMO for "small intestinal microbial overgrowth" since the microbes may be yeast/fungi, amoebas or protozoas[274] rather than exclusively bacteria—specifically, let us now look at the hypothalamic abnormalities seen in patients with "SIMO-induced IBS" (redundancy noted). ❷ Chang et al[275] in 2009 found evidence of HPA axis dysregulation in women with IBS without psychiatric comorbidity as evidenced by SIMO-IBS patients' significantly lower basal secretion of adrenocorticotrophic hormone (ACTH) with slightly elevated and asynchronic secretion of cortisol contrasted with the findings in the control group. FitzGerald et al[276] showed that "women with IBS display blunted ACTH and cortisol responses to the LP (lumbar puncture used as a psychological stressor) along with a profile of affective responsiveness suggestive of chronic psychosocial stress, although no CRF (corticotropin-releasing hormone in cerebrospinal fluid) differences between groups are observed." Whether these hypothalamic-pituitary dysfunctions are a contributing cause to or a result of SIMO-IBS could only be established by clinical trials with a 5-part protocol (i.e., 1. assessment of normal subjects, 2. intentional induction of SIMO-IBS, 3. reassessment, 4. successful treatment, 5. reassessment) which would be logistically cumbersome and ethically untenable.

- Increased production of prolactin: Prolactin is a highly proinflammatory hormone produced by the anterior pituitary gland as well as by peripheral lymphocytes. As a model of infection-induced inflammation, **sepsis is generally associated with increased prolactin production in humans.**[277] Prolactin levels increase due to chronic psychoemotional stress. **The classic exemplification of dysbiosis-induced musculoskeletal inflammation—reactive arthritis—is frequently associated with hyperprolactinemia.**[278]
  - Infection-induced arthritis: Elevated prolactin in reactive arthritis (*J Rheumatol* 1994 Jul[279]): Without any question whatsoever, reactive arthritis—formerly called Reiter's syndrome—is one of the prototypes of inflammatory arthritis and "autoimmunity" triggered by microorganisms, whether as an acute infection such as a urinary tract infection or gastroenteritis or as a chronic subclinical infection. This classic association—that between the microbe and the induction of arthritis and systemic inflammation—is discussed in all textbooks of pathology and all thorough textbooks of microbiology; it is therefore a matter of "medical fact." Therefore, the identification of hormonal abnormities in patients with this prototypic microbe-induced autoimmune/inflammatory syndrome would be supportive of either/both of the following: ❶ microbial infection or colonization can result in hormone imbalances, such as elevated prolactin, and/or ❷ hormone imbalances such as elevated

---

[269] Lin HC. Small intestinal bacterial overgrowth: a framework for understanding irritable bowel syndrome. *JAMA*. 2004 Aug 18;292(7):852-8

[270] Esposito I, de Leone A, Di Gregorio G, Giaquinto S, de Magistris L, Ferrieri A, Riegler G. Breath test for differential diagnosis between small intestinal bacterial overgrowth and irritable bowel disease: an observation on non-absorbable antibiotics. *World J Gastroenterol*. 2007 Dec 7;13(45):6016-21

[271] Peralta et al. Small intestine bacterial overgrowth and irritable bowel syndrome-related symptoms: experience with Rifaximin. *World J Gastroenterol*. 2009 Jun 7;15:2628-31

[272] Majewski et al. Results of small intestinal bacterial overgrowth testing in irritable bowel syndrome: clinical profiles and effects of antibiotic trial. *Adv Med Sci*. 2007;52:139-42

[273] Cuoco et al. Small intestine bacterial overgrowth in irritable bowel syndrome: a retrospective study with rifaximin. *Minerva Gastroenterol Dietol*. 2006 Mar;52(1):89-95

[274] Galland L, Lee M. #170 High frequency of giardiasis in patients with chronic digestive complaints. *Am J Gastroenterol* 1989;84:1181

[275] Chang L, et al. Dysregulation of the hypothalamic-pituitary-adrenal (HPA) axis in irritable bowel syndrome. *Neurogastroenterol Motil*. 2009 Feb;21(2):149-59

[276] FitzGerald LZ, Kehoe P, Sinha K. Hypothalamic--pituitary-- adrenal axis dysregulation in women with irritable bowel syndrome in response to acute physical stress. *West J Nurs Res*. 2009 Nov;31(7):818-36

[277] "Prolactin levels are regularly elevated in sepsis…" Dennhardt et al. Patterns of endocrine secretion during sepsis. *Prog Clin Biol Res*1989;308:751-6

[278] "Hyperprolactinemia (PRL > 20 ng/ml) was found in 9 of 25 (36%) patients with RS." Jara et al. Hyperprolactinemia in Reiter's syndrome. *J Rheumatol* 1994;21:1292-7

[279] Jara et al. Hyperprolactinemia in Reiter's syndrome. *J Rheumatol*. 1994 Jul;21(7):1292-7

prolactin function synergistically with microbial colonization to result in systemic inflammation and dysbiotic rheumatism. In this study, the authors measured serum prolactin (PRL) in patients with reactive arthritis and groups of other patients. Results showed that elevated PRL levels > 20 ng/ml were found in 9 of 25 (36%) patients with reactive arthritis but almost none of the other patients. Furthermore, a direct positive correlation between serum prolactin levels and the clinical intensity of conjunctivitis, urethritis, dysentery, and uveitis was noted.

- **Reduced production of cortisol:** Cortisol is an immunoregulatory hormone which tends to suppress excess immune activity, and relative reductions in cortisol production are commonly seen in patients with autoimmunity and allergic disorders.[280,281] **Cortisol production is reduced by chronic psychoemotional stress**[282], and the stress of chronic inflammation due to dysbiosis and the resultant disease, pain, disability, and disfigurement may impair normal endocrine function.

  - Allergies, autoimmunity, and fatigue-related syndromes—Mild adrenocortical deficiency and the work of Jefferies (*Med Hypotheses* 1994 Mar[283]): In his book *Safe Uses of Cortisol* and peer-reviewed articles, Jefferies has been the strongest proponent of the idea that patients with chronic allergies, autoimmune disorders, and chronic fatigue syndrome have mild adrenocortical deficiency resulting in low physiologic reserve and immune abnormalities that would be better treated with physiologic doses of bioidentical cortisol rather than high doses of synthetic cortisol mimetics. Dr Jefferies' approach—using physiologic amounts of cortisol at doses less than 20 mg per day—does not cause adrenal suppression or adverse effects which are commonly seen when synthetic cortisol mimetics such as prednisone are used. Allergies and autoimmune disorders are commonly treated with synthetic cortisol mimetics as part of standard medical practice; this can be viewed as appreciation for the role of cortisol in immunomodulation. Relatedly, a clinical trial by Cleare et al[284] among patients with chronic fatigue syndrome (CFS) showed that low-dose cortisol in amounts of 5-10 mg per day provided significant benefit.

- **Reduced production and bioavailability of androgens—testosterone and/or dehydroepiandrosterone (DHEA):** High-intensity stress associated with military training leads to 60-80% reductions in androgens[285]; the chronic stress and pain associated with musculoskeletal inflammation may contribute to a similar profile on a subacute and chronic basis. Hyperprolactinemia further complicates this problem by simulating hepatic production of sex hormone binding globulin (SHBG) which adsorbs androgens and reduces their bioavailability. Indeed, the clinical manifestations of hypogonadism—including probably inflammatory/rheumatic complications—can be seen despite adequate production of androgens when elevated prolactin stimulates increased SHBG production and results in reduced bioavailability of androgens.[286]

  - Inflammatory bowel disease and dysbiosis—Patients with chronic inflammatory bowel disease have low levels of DHEA (*Clin Exp Rheumatol* 1998 Sep-Oct[287]): Readers should note that both of the major forms of inflammatory bowel disease (IBD)—Crohn's disease (CD) and ulcerative colitis (UC)—are very closely associated with gastrointestinal dysbiosis; in fact, a very strong case can be made that IBD is one of the prototypic manifestations of gastrointestinal dysbiosis.[288] In this study,

---

280 "Yet evidence that patients with rheumatoid arthritis improved with small, physiologic dosages of cortisol or cortisone acetate was reported over 25 years ago, and that patients with chronic allergic disorders or unexplained chronic fatigue also improved with administration of such small dosages was reported over 15 years ago..." Jefferies WM. Mild adrenocortical deficiency, chronic allergies, autoimmune disorders and the chronic fatigue syndrome: a continuation of the cortisone story. *Med Hypotheses.* 1994 Mar;42(3):183-9

281 "The etiology of rheumatoid arthritis ...explained by a combination of three factors: (i) a relatively mild deficiency of cortisol, ..., (ii) a deficiency of DHEA, ...and (iii) infection by organisms such as mycoplasma,..." Jefferies WM. The etiology of rheumatoid arthritis. *Med Hypotheses.* 1998 Aug;51(2):111-4

282 "Prolonged psychological stress is associated with a transient suppression of the HPA axis, manifested by low morning cortisol and reduced cortisol response to ACTH. The reduction of cortisol response is sufficient to cause false diagnosis of HPA insufficiency." Zarkovic M, Stefanova E, Ciric J, Penezic Z, Kostic V, Sumarac-Dumanovic M, Macut D, Ivovic MS, Gligorovic PV. Prolonged psychological stress suppresses cortisol secretion. *Clin Endocrinol* (Oxf). 2003 Dec;59(6):811-6

283 Jefferies WM. Mild adrenocortical deficiency, chronic allergies, autoimmune disorders and the chronic fatigue syndrome. *Med Hypotheses.* 1994 Mar;42(3):183-9

284 Cleare AJ, et al. Low-dose hydrocortisone in chronic fatigue syndrome: a randomised crossover trial.*Lancet.* 1999 Feb 6;353(9151):455-8

285 "Plasma levels of testosterone, free testosterone, dehydroepiandrosterone, 17 alpha-hydroxyprogesterone, and androstenedione decreased by 60-80% during the course." Opstad PK. Androgenic hormones during prolonged physical stress, sleep, and energy deficiency. *J Clin Endocrinol Metab.* 1992 May;74(5):1176-83

286 "The pitfalls of measuring only total serum testosterone are illustrated by a 52 year old man whose hyperprolactinaemia was associated with normal total serum testosterone but a raised sex-hormone-binding globulin, giving a low free testosterone. Prolactin suppression with bromocriptine normalized sex-hormone-binding globulin and free testosterone..." Hardy KJ, Seckl JR. Endocrine assessment of impotence--pitfalls of measuring serum testosterone without sex-hormone-binding globulin. *Postgrad Med J.* 1994 Nov;70(829):836-7. This excellent article should have made the testing of free and total testosterone—rather than total testosterone alone—the standard of practice.

287 de la Torre et al. Blood and tissue dehydroepiandrosterone sulphate levels and their relationship to chronic inflammatory bowel disease. *Clin Exp Rheumatol.* 1998 Sep:579-82

288 Tamboli CP, Neut C, Desreumaux P, Colombel JF. Dysbiosis in inflammatory bowel disease. *Gut.* 2004 Jan;53(1):1-4

DHEA-sulfate (DHEA-s) levels were measured in blood from 112 patients with IBD (66 with CD and 46 with UC), and the levels were compared with those in 80 healthy controls. DHEA-s concentrations were measured in tissue samples from 40 patients (28 patients with IBD and 12 with other bowel disorders) who had undergone intestinal surgery. Results of these analyses showed that average blood DHEA-s were markedly lower in the two IBD groups (1350 nmol/l in UC and 1850 nmol/l in CD vs. 3300 nmol/l in controls); readers should note that the DHEA-s levels in the IBD patients were roughly half—50%—of normal. Andus et al[289] showed that DHEA 200mg/d provided important benefits for patients with treatment-resistant IBD.

◻ HIV/AIDS—Testosterone deficiency is common in men and women infected with HIV (*Clin Infect Dis* 2001 Sep[290]): The authors note, "Androgen deficiency is a common endocrine abnormality among men and women with human immunodeficiency virus (HIV) infection. … The most useful laboratory indicator is the serum bioavailable (free) **testosterone** concentration." Clinical benefits of the correction of hypoandrogenism—specifically serum free testosterone and/or serum total testosterone—include improvements in lean body mass, energy, quality of life, and mood-depression scores.

19. Epigenetic dysbiosis/eubiosis, microbial dysepigenetics, microbial epigenosis: Here and for the first time, "epigenetic dysbiosis" is defined as dysbiosis that mediates its clinical/physiologic effect via epigenetic alterations in the host.[291] The earliest publication related to the main concept of this section—here using the preferred terms "epigenetic dysbiosis" (to denote the epigenome-changing **microbial imbalance**) and "microbial epigenosis" (to denote the microbe-induced **epigenetic dysfunction** or adverse alteration)—appears to be the 2009 review by Minárovits, "Microbe-induced epigenetic alterations in host cells: the coming era of patho-epigenetics of microbial infections"[292] in which the following examples of microbe-induced genetic/epigenetic changes are reviewed:

> **Pathoepigenetics**
>
> "Elucidation of the epigenetic consequences of microbe-host interactions (the emerging new field of patho-epigenetics) may have important therapeutic implications because [microbe-induced] epigenetic processes can be reverted [reversed] and elimination of microbes inducing patho-epigenetic changes may prevent disease development."
>
> Minárovits. Microbe-induced epigenetic alterations in host cells. *Acta Microbiol Immunol Hung.* 2009 Mar

1) Direct integration of dsDNA viruses: Double-stranded DNA viruses incorporate viral DNA into human/host DNA. This is obviously a genetic (not an epigenetic) change because the actual DNA code is altered.

2) Retroviral integration: Retroviruses incorporate their single-stranded positive sense RNA into human DNA via viral reverse transcriptase which produces DNA from retroviral RNA; this new viral DNA is then incorporated into the host cell genome by integrase enzyme, creating retroviral DNA (provirus). In times of stress, nutritional deficiency, and activation of other viral infections (e.g., viral transactivation), these incorporated retroviruses can undergo enhanced transcription, with clear relevance for inflammatory and autoimmune diseases, as discussed later and more thoroughly detailed in the digital publication, *Antiviral Strategies and Immune Nutrition* which was first published in 2014 and is periodically updated (digital updates automatically delivered).[293] Again, as with #1 above, these viral integrations effect a *genetic* change, not an *epigenetic* change; actually, perhaps the term "**envirogenetics**" (phrase applied here and used in context; other uses of this term have been published previously) should be applied here to denote genetic coding changes induced by the environment (in this case, acquired and integrated viral infections) which are not endogenously genetic (arising from within the host) and neither are they epigenetic (changes in DNA-associated molecules that change gene expression).

[289] Andus T, et al. Patients with refractory Crohn's disease or ulcerative colitis respond to dehydroepiandrosterone. *Aliment Pharmacol Ther.* 2003 Feb;17(3):409-14

[290] Mylonakis et al. Diagnosis and treatment of androgen deficiency in human immunodeficiency virus-infected men and women. *Clin Infect Dis.* 2001 Sep 15;33:857-64

[291] Related terms can include "epigenetic eubiosis" for beneficial microbe-epigenome relationships and "microbial dysepigenetics" or "microbial epigenosis" for adverse epigenetic alterations induced in the human and mediated directly by or in response to microorganisms. The term "microbial epigenetics" is used widely to describe epigenetic mapping/characterization of microorganisms; the term "genetic dysbiosis" was characterized in 2014 by Nibali et al as encompassing "the role of human genetic variants affecting microbial recognition and host response in creating an environment conducive to changes in the normal microbiota." Nibali et al. Genetic dysbiosis: the role of microbial insults in chronic inflammatory diseases. *J Oral Microbiol.* 2014; 6: 10

[292] Minárovits J. Microbe-induced epigenetic alterations in host cells: coming era of patho-epigenetics of microbial infections. *Acta Microbiol Immunol Hung.* 2009 Mar;56:1-19

[293] Digital clinical protocol updated regularly: Vasquez A. *Antiviral Nutrition: Against Colds, Flu, Herpes, AIDS, Hepatitis, Ebola, Dengue, and Autoimmunity: A Concept-Based and Evidence-Based Handbook and Research Review for Practical Use.* International College of Human Nutrition and Functional Medicine, 2014. (ASIN: B00OPDQG4W) amazon.com/dp/B00OPDQG4W. Printed in book format: Vasquez A. *Antiviral Strategies and Immune Nutrition.* CreateSpace Publishing, 2014. (ISBN: 1502894890)

3) *In situ—localized—*microbe-induced alterations in DNA methylation and histone acetylation (along with other epigenetic modifications): For example and per Minárovits cited previously, *Campylobacter rectus* promotes pre-term birth in humans (verified[294]) by mechanisms likely including the hypermethylation of the placental IGF-2 promoter region, leading to reduced placental and hence fetal growth. Relatedly, *Helicobacter pylori,* which is phylogenetically related to the previously mentioned *Campylobacter rectus,* is the most important acquired risk factor for gastric cancer in humans and has been shown to induce aberrant DNA methylation in the gastric mucosa, leading to inactivation of expression of the tumor suppressor epithelial cadherin (E-cadherin), an adhesion molecule that retards tumor invasion and metastasis. The fact that Epstein-Barr virus (EBV), a very common human herpesvirus, also induces hypermethylation of the E-cadherin promoter and subsequent downregulation of E-cadherin gene expression suggests the possibility that simultaneous co-infection with EBV and *Helicobacter pylori* might have additive or synergistic consequences; attentive readers will notice that the clinical implications of EBV together with *Helicobacter pylori* are discussed later with regard to the pathogenesis of scleroderma (see my *Rheumatology v3.5* and later versions). Human papillomavirus (HPV) type 16-E1A alters both methyltransferase activity and histone deacetylase activity, with the later leading to increased histone acetylation, consistent with enhanced gene expression, possibly/likely contributing to cell growth and proliferation. Hepatitis B virus infection appears to induce the cancer-specific pattern of global DNA hypomethylation with regional hypermethylation, with the latter localized to specific tumor suppressor genes. Human immunodeficiency virus (HIV) increases DNA methyltransferase expression resulting in increased DNA methylation, specifically of the IFN-g promoter region, leading to dysregulation of cytokine gene expression. Readers should note that all of the above examples of microbial epigenetic changes are "in situ"—the epigenetic changes occur in the same cells that harbor the microbe or—in the case of viruses—the viral genome; while this documentation is important, it is not wholly surprising because we could reasonably anticipate that microbes, most especially those that are intracellular, would have an effect on gene expression, either somewhat randomly or as is more often the case for microbial advantage. Given this, the report by Kumar et al in late 2014—reviewed immediately below as example #4—is truly remarkable because they show that microbes in one location (the gut) could affect body-wide DNA methylation.

4) *At large—***systemic—**microbe-induced alterations in DNA methylation and histone acetylation (along with other epigenetic modifications): In late 2014, Kumar et al[295] published remarkable findings that appear to have surprised even the authors per their comments, "This is one of the first studies that highlights the association of the predominant bacterial phyla in the gut with methylation patterns. ... Intriguingly, we found that blood DNA methylation patterns were associated with gut microbiota profiles. ... For the first time, we report here a position of the predominant gut microbiota in epigenetic profiling, suggesting one potential mechanism in obesity with comorbidities..." Quite impressively, the authors start their article with this assertive first sentence in their abstract, "The core human gut microbiota contributes to the developmental origin of diseases by modifying metabolic pathways."; the importance of this statement is that it opens to us a new way of thinking about the means by which microbes can affect human health and disease patterns—via epigenetic modulation, rather than by inflammation or direct invasion. The researchers profiled the gut flora of eight pregnant women to find strong correlation between gut microbial phylal dominance (categorized as either *Bacteroidetes, Firmicutes,* [*Actinobacteria,* one of the top-three dominant phyla, was not noted] or the quantitatively smaller *Proteobacteria*) and peripheral *extraintestinal* epigenetic patterns. Dominance by *Firmicutes* (contrasted with dominance by *Bacteroidetes*) in the gut was distinguished by gene expression patterns consistent with increased risk for cardiovascular disease, altered lipid metabolism, obesity, and inflammation. Clearly, this association does not imply causality; put in context with other data, the relationship is most likely bidirectional (not necessarily equivalently), given that both physical phenotype and gut flora appear capable of changing each other. Clinicians should note

---

[294] "Campylobacter species (C. jejuni, C. fetus) are enteric abortifacient bacteria in humans and ungulates. Campylobacter rectus is a periodontal pathogen associated with human fetal exposure and adverse pregnancy outcomes including preterm delivery." Arce et al. Characterization of the invasive and inflammatory traits of oral Campylobacter rectus in a murine model of fetoplacental growth restriction and in trophoblast cultures. *J Reprod Immunol.* 2010 Mar;84(2):145-53

[295] Kumar et al. Gut microbiota as an epigenetic regulator: pilot study based on whole-genome methylation analysis. *MBio.* 2014 Dec 16;5(6). pii: e02113-14

that this effect is quantitatively impressive; changes in gastrointestinal flora correlate with patterned changes in gene expression affecting at least 813 genes: "...the promoters of a total of 568 genes were more methylated and the promoter of 245 genes were less methylated in mothers with higher levels of Firmicutes (HighFirm group) than in mothers with higher levels of Bacteroidetes and Proteobacteria (HighBact group)." Additionally and importantly, besides DNA methylation changes, gut microflora influence histone acetylation via elaboration of the short-chain fatty acids (SCFA) acetate, propionate, and butyrate, which suppress activity of histone deacetylases (HDACs), resulting in enhanced/maintained histone acetylation, which is one of the mechanisms by which beneficial probiotic-type microbes promote the development and maintenance of Treg cells and hence immunotolerance and thereby protection from metabolic, allergic, and autoimmune inflammatory disorders, as discussed in the immediately following section and reviewed in much more detail in Chapter 4 section 3 which contains the "nutritional immunomodulation protocol." Again, suppressed activity of histone deacetylase promotes retention of histone acetylation, which is generally considered beneficial, associated with a "rejuvenative phenotype" and improved mental function.

> **Epigenetic dysbiosis, microbial epigenosis: more than 800 genes affected**
>
> "Intriguingly, we found that blood DNA methylation patterns were associated with gut microbiota profiles. ... "To evaluate the predominant microbiota as an epigenetic modifier, we classified 8 pregnant women into two groups based on their dominant microbiota, i.e., Bacteroidetes, Firmicutes, and Proteobacteria. Deep sequencing of DNA methylomes revealed a clear association between bacterial predominance and epigenetic profiles. The genes with differentially methylated promoters in the group in which Firmicutes was dominant were linked to risk of disease, predominantly to cardiovascular disease and specifically to lipid metabolism, obesity, and the inflammatory response. ... "...the promoters of a total of **568 genes were more methylated and the promoter of 245 genes were less methylated** in mothers with higher levels of Firmicutes (HighFirm group) than in mothers with higher levels of Bacteroidetes and Proteobacteria (HighBact group)."
>
> Kumar et al. Gut microbiota as an epigenetic regulator. *MBio: American Society for Microbiology*. 2014 Dec

5) <u>Epigenetic modulation of peripheral immunocyte phenotype by intestinal flora</u>: Cells that eventually become effector T-cells originate in the bone marrow, circulate to the thymus for maturation and selective deletion, then undergo further maturation and differentiation in the peripheral immune system, most of which is located in the gut associated lymphoid tissue (GALT) in anatomic proximity and functional contact to the gastrointestinal microflora[296], and these intestinal microbes have a decisive effect on immunocyte differentiation and the resultant balance of immune effector cells. Bacteria generally categorized as beneficial and commonly found in probiotic formulations induce via epigenetic modifications the tolerogenic regulatory T-cell phenotype (Treg) characterized by the transcription factor FoxP3; conversely, pathogenetic bacteria in general and segmented filamentous bacteria (SFB) in particular induce via epigenetic mechanisms the pro-inflammatory Th17 T-cell phenotype (Th17 cells) characterized by the transcription factor retinoic-acid-receptor-related orphan receptor gamma (RORγ).[297] This fifth category of microbe-induced epigenetic modifications has immediate clinical implications and supports the use of gut flora modification in the treatment of inflammatory, allergic, and autoimmune diseases and disorders; this entire protocol with at least 14 components in the 2015 version is termed "nutritional immunomodulation" detailed in Chapter 4 section 3 (4.3) and is a subprotocol within the entire "functional inflammology protocol" applied via the FI<u>N</u>DSEX® acronym. Epigenetic modulation of nucleated blood cells via gastrointestinal flora is a proven occurrence; immunocytes have close proximity and occasionally direct contact with antigens and metabolites from gut microflora and then circulate systemically, carrying the effects of that molecular modification. The extent to which gut flora profiles affect epigenetic profiles of peripheral tissues such as liver, muscle, and brain requires correlational studies with tissue biopsies and cannot rely on the testing of blood samples.

20. <u>Vitamin D benefits, discussion and controversial/erroneous "deficiency induction protocol"</u>: Vitamin D3 functions via the vitamin D receptor (VDR) to support innate and acquired immune responses via several mechanisms including ❶ regulating inflammation via mechanisms that include suppression of NFkB, ❷ inhibiting viral replication and enhancing anti-viral defenses via elaboration of antimicrobial peptides (AMP),

---

[296] Rogers AW. *Cells and Tissues: An Introduction to Histology and Cell Biology*. Academic Press; 1979, 112
[297] Furusawa Y, Obata Y, Hase K. Commensal microbiota regulates T cell fate decision in the gut. *Semin Immunopathol*. 2015 Jan;37(1):17-25

❸ via the aforementioned AMP, enhancing innate immunity against cancer, bacteria, fungi, and other microbes, ❹ assisting in the maintenance of gastrointestinal integrity, helping prevent intestinal hyperpermeability (per studies showing that VDR-knockout animals have "leaky gut" whereas wildtype animals do not), and others.

Marshall and Waterhouse (*Ann N Y Acad Sci* 2009 Sep, reviewed below) from have claimed that microbes usurp vitamin D metabolism and produce vitamin D analogs that interfere with VDR function; they further advocate the use of a multicomponent treatment plan for microbe-induced autoimmunity, including the following three main characteristics: ❶ antimicrobial agents to promote clearance of the disease-inducing microbes, ❷ pharmacologic activation of the VDR with olmesartan, and ❸ intentional iatrogenic induction of vitamin D deficiency by eliminating all dietary and environmental vitamin D sources (e.g., foods and nutritional supplements containing vitamin D, sunlight exposure [patients are to use long pants, long-sleeved shirts, hats, sunglasses and sunscreen to deplete themselves of vitamin D over the course of ~3 years in order to—according to this controversial protocol—deplete the body of vitamin D to thereby deplete substrate from microbes so that—again theoretically—the microbes will not be able to produce VDR-blocking metabolites that impair immune function. Of the three components

Purported microbial interference with VDR-mediated immunity: agreeable and disagreeable components of this model
☺ **Agreeable**: Microbes directly contribute to long-term inflammatory diseases, especially autoimmunity.
☺ **Agreeable**: Combination antibacterial drugs may be used to reduce/eliminate the pro-inflammatory microbial load to alleviate the resulting microbe-triggered illness.
☺ **Agreeable**: The inflammatory response to immunogenic triggers can precipitate the formation of granulomatous tissue, which is known to expedite conversion of 25-OH-D to 1,25-dihydroxyvitamin D, thereby causing so-called "vitamin D hypersensitivity" and increasing risk for hypercalcemia; sarcoidosis is the classic example of this phenomenon.
☺ **Agreeable**: Microbes may produce substances that interfere with the VDR—vitamin D receptor; this is a reasonable proposal but needs further substantiation.
☺ **Agreeable**: Therapeutic activation of the VDR with a VDR-activating agent (assuming this occurs to a meaningful level in vivo) such as olmesartan is reasonable per the assumption that the VDR is being blocked by microbial metabolites; obviously the agent—such as the proposed olmesartan—would have to be dosed appropriately.
☹ Not agreeable, not consistent with the bulk of research and clinical practice: The proposed intentional induction of iatrogenic vitamin D deficiency via deprivation of sunlight and dietary vitamin D is not at all consistent with the weight of research and clinical practice.

above, #1 is reasonable, #2 is possible but unproven, and #3 is contrary to the bulk of research supporting the importance of vitamin D3 in human physiology, particularly defense from microbial infections and protection from inflammatory and autoimmune diseases. While a small number of viruses (EBV, HIV), bacteria (*Mycobacterium tuberculosis, M leprae*), and fungi (*Aspergillus fumigatus*) appear able to interfere with VDR function[298]—and presumably thereby cause impaired immune responsiveness via lack of VDR stimulation resulting in lack of AMP elaboration and other immune defects thereby promoting persistent infection and inflammation—microbial VDR blockade argues for *additional* vitamin D supplementation (not for induction of vitamin D deficiency) to support/salvage VDR activity in microbe-impaired cells and to support normal function in noninfected cells; for example, the benefit of vitamin D3 supplementation was demonstrated clinically in a 2015 study that showed lowering of EBV activity in MS patients.[299] As such the Marshall-Waterhouse protocol is one of the most poorly articulated and weakly justified/defended interventions in nutritional medicine, and in my opinion has gained a foothold only because of the patient desperation, fear-mongering, and clinician ignorance and power- and profit-seeking. Note that I am not stating that all patients should receive vitamin D at all times; clearly, all clinical decisions need to be made per individual case, condition, and tolerance as consistent with good clinical care, exactly as I stated in the 2004 "vitamin D paradigm shift" monograph, "Until proven otherwise, the balance of the research clearly indicates that oral supplementation in the range of 1,000 IU/day for infants, 2,000 IU/day for children, and 4,000 IU/day for adults is safe and reasonable to meet physiologic requirements, to promote optimal health, and to reduce the risk of several serious diseases. Safety and effectiveness of supplementation are assured by periodic monitoring of

---

[298] Mangin et al. Inflammation and vitamin D: the infection connection. *Inflamm Res.* 2014 Oct;63(10):803-19
[299] Najafipoor et al. The beneficial effects of vitamin D3 on reducing antibody titers against Epstein-Barr virus in multiple sclerosis patients. *Cell Immunol.* 2015 Mar;294:9-12

serum 25(OH)D and serum calcium." However, the rote withholding of vitamin D3 from all patients with autoimmune and inflammatory diseases is incompatible with the bulk of research to the point of being irresponsible and unethical.

- <u>Cited but controversial paper: Reversing bacteria-induced vitamin D receptor dysfunction is key to autoimmune disease (*Ann N Y Acad Sci* 2009 Sep[300]):</u> The authors state that in autoimmunity, intracellular bacteria cause vitamin D receptor (VDR) dysfunction within phagocytes leading to a decline in innate immune function that causes susceptibility to additional infections that contribute to inflammatory/autoimmune disease progression. The authors propose treatment aimed at "gradually restoring VDR function with the VDR agonist olmesartan and subinhibitory dosages of certain bacteriostatic antibiotics." They state that with this approach, "Diseases showing favorable responses to treatment so far include systemic lupus erythematosus, rheumatoid arthritis, scleroderma, sarcoidosis, Sjogren's syndrome, autoimmune thyroid disease, psoriasis, ankylosing spondylitis, [reactive arthritis], type I and II diabetes mellitus, and uveitis." The most controversial part of this strategy is the iatrogenic induction of vitamin D deficiency; the authors state, "Disease reversal using this approach requires limitation of vitamin D in order to avoid contributing to dysfunction of nuclear receptors…" They also state that, "The existence of communities of multiple bacterial species, like those occurring in biofilms, means that combinations of antibiotics are likely to be necessary to fully target all species."

Articles and videos by this same group/organization[301], along with the so-called "Marshall protocol", present a confusing mix of scientific accuracy with profound misunderstandings on behalf of the authors/advocates; the good components of this concept are ❶ affirming the role of microbes in autoimmunity and sustained inflammation, and ❷ raising the possibility of microbial interference with the VDR and the possibility of therapeutic stimulation of the VDR with olmesartan—these authors have failed to substantiate this important component of their model, and their first eight citations are self-referential, mostly conference abstracts/presentations from their own group unavailable for legitimate peer-review. Lastly, I agree with the statement and concept, ❸ The first two components of this model and

On Sat, Jul 26, 2014 at 1:20 AM, ▮▮▮▮▮▮▮, MD <▮▮▮▮▮@gmail.com> wrote:

Yes, Alex Vitamin D has an anti-inflammatory effect, in the same way prednisone also has an anti-inflammatory effect, but suppressing inflammation when the body is trying to fight a stealth infection might not be a good idea.   sort of like giving prednisone to a patient with TB

http://www.sciencedaily.com/releases/2008/01/080125223302.htm

http://www.townsendletter.com/Jan2009/vitaminD0109.htm

Example of ongoing clinical confusion about vitamin D, per the proposal by Marshall, Waterhouse, et al: To demonstrate how severe/profound and acute/current is the effect of this erroneous information about vitamin D, I have included here an excerpt from a group conversation among—to my astonishment—several "functional medicine" practitioners and presenters, including several with prominent leadership and administrative roles. The author of the above message, part of an email group discussion, is a medical doctor, board certified in Internal Medicine; notice that he directly cites the Waterhouse and Marshall publications. That a doctorate-level clinician, an internist, with years of additional training in functional medicine would state that vitamin D "suppresses inflammation" and that its use is "like giving prednisone to a patient with TB" is appalling; although painful, this conversation and the confusion it represents demonstrates the need to address this topic, both in this textbook as well as in peer-reviewed publications.

"protocol" are reasonable or possibly reasonable; however, per the overwhelming data showing the benefit of vitamin D, their notion and advocacy of iatrogenic vitamin D deficiency is, per my perception, unscientific at best, ridiculous or harmful at worst. As noted above, among the most controversial and poorly defended interventions advocated by some authors and used by some clinicians is the intentional induction of vitamin D deficiency supposedly to reduce microbial metabolites that interfere with function of the VDR; my opinion—after a reasonable literature review and perusal of conversations with several clinicians who advocate this position or unnecessary confusion[302,303]—is that this position, the resulting clinical confusion, and therapeutic

---

[300] Waterhouse et al. Reversing bacteria-induced vitamin D receptor dysfunction is key to autoimmune disease. *Ann N Y Acad Sci*. 2009 Sep;1173:757-65

[301] Waterhouse JC. Reversing Bacteria-Induced Vitamin D Receptor Dysfunction to Treat Chronic Disease: Why Vitamin D Supplementation Can Be Immunosuppressive, Potentially Leading to Pathogen Increase. *Townsend Letter for Doctors & Patients* 2009 Jan townsendletter.com/Jan2009/vitaminD0109.htm

[302] Brady D, et al, "TAP Experts": Vitamin D Testing. TAP Integrative. Feb 18, 2015 youtube.com/watch?v=ww_DLRU-27s. Also, email group discussion among several faculty/members of Institute for Functional Medicine, July 25-29, 2014

[303] Mercola J. Clearing Up Confusion on Vitamin D: Why I Don't Recommend the Marshall Protocol. Mercola.com 2009 March 14. articles.mercola.com/sites/articles/archive/2009/03/14/clearing-up-confusion-on-vitamin-d--why-i-dont-recommend-the-marshall-protocol.aspx

452   INFLAMMATION MASTERY & FUNCTIONAL INFLAMMOLOGY   © ICHNFM.ORG

inertia are unreasonable, easily dismantled by the most plain line of questioning and scientific probing. I will define the argument and its counterarguments in the following paragraphs, but I will also state that the "anti-vitamin D" position occurs to me as a simpleminded* countercurrent against the overwhelmingly positive research data and clinical benefits supporting the routine use of vitamin D in clinical practice.[304] A consistent failing by proponents of this iatrogenic "intervention" is noted in their descriptions and explanations of therapeutic responses, for example, stating 1) that patients should feel ill if the treatment is working, 2) that if patients don't feel ill then they are not improving (note the no-win situations here) and 3) that any clinical improvement with vitamin D is factitious; in this model, patients and clinicians alike are confused and rendered impotent to interpret events, make decisions, take action, and think clearly. A more reasonable approach—as I stated very clearly in my 2004 "paradigm-shift" monograph—is to ❶ begin with a patient assessment, including assessment of renal function, vitamin D status, and serum calcium, (increasingly we test 1,25-dihydroxyvitamin D3 as well), then ❷ implement vitamin D replacement/supplementation as needed to optimize serum levels, and ❸ then monitor clinical response and serum calcium and other laboratory results/responses as indicated clinically. This is a logical, safe, methodological approach to clinical action and decision-making; this is the same logic used for nearly all clinical decisions and is not specific to the issues of vitamin D, inflammation, infectious disease: ❶ assess, ❷ treat carefully, and ❸ monitor response to treatment. *The reasons for my somewhat harsh description of this proposed intervention as "simpleminded" is that not only is easily deflated with minimal effort, but that the arguments espoused by its proponents also—very tellingly—lack internal consistency; for example, when they note that patients benefit from vitamin D supplementation they countermeasure not with fact but with additional unsupported supposition; Albert, Proal, and Marshall[305] of the "Marshall *iatrogenic hypovitaminosis D* protocol" state "...symptomatic improvements among those administered vitamin D is the result of 25-D's ability to temper bacterial-induced inflammation by slowing VDR activity. While this results in short-term palliation, persistent pathogens that may influence disease progression, proliferate over the long-term." Thus, when faced with evidence showing that patients have less inflammation and fewer symptoms after receiving vitamin D, the authors superstitiously attribute this to an analgesic/anti-inflammatory drug-like effect, suppressing symptoms while allowing the disease to fester—their proposal is unsupported by science. Furthermore, if this proposal were true, then vitamin D *deficiency* would *reduce* disease and mortality, and this is contrary to the bulk of the science, which consistently shows improved clinical and population-wide health benefits with improved vitamin D nutriture. The landmark 1999 review of "Vitamin D supplementation, 25-hydroxyvitamin D concentrations, and safety" by Vieth[306] already laid to rest most of the concerns raised by Marshall's group, leaving one to wonder if the latter has read the former; Vieth's article is one of the most powerful ever published in the medical nutrition literature and his clear statements such as "Except in those with conditions causing hypersensitivity, there is no evidence of adverse effects with serum 25(OH)D concentrations <140 nmol/L, which require a total vitamin D supply of 250 microg (10000 IU)/d to attain" demonstrated clear authority of the literature and paved the way for our "paradigm shift" paper that followed after (Vasquez et al, *Altern Ther Health Med* 2004 Sep, op cit).

- Argument in favor of iatrogenic vitamin D deficiency: Some authors and clinicians state that, in autoimmunity and chronic illnesses, vitamin D is being converted by microbes into metabolites that actually cause immunosuppression by interfering with VDR function, thereby leading to the perpetuation of microbial colonization, which promotes illness; they have notably failed to substantiate this position. While it may be true, the real controversy arrives when the authors advocate vitamin D depletion as part of the treatment protocol. They state that induction of vitamin D deficiency is necessary to deprive microbes of the vitamin D that the microbes will use to create these immunosuppressive VDR antagonists.

- Counterargument #1—Lack of risk-benefit analysis: Even if the argument were true, the risk-to-benefit ratio would have to be evaluated. Iatrogenic induction of vitamin D deficiency for the supposed purpose of liberating the VDR from microbial metabolites would have to be justified by being proven superior to the

[304] **Vasquez A, Manso G, Cannell J. The clinical importance of vitamin D (cholecalciferol): a paradigm shift with implications for all healthcare providers.** *Altern Ther Health Med.* **2004 Sep.** See also: Vasquez A, Cannell J. Calcium and vitamin D in preventing fractures. *BMJ.* 2005 Jul 9 Article archive: InflammationMastery.com/reprints
[305] Albert PJ, Proal AD, Marshall TG. Vitamin D: the alternative hypothesis. *Autoimmun Rev.* 2009 Jul;8(8):639-44
[306] Vieth R. Vitamin D supplementation, 25-hydroxyvitamin D concentrations, and safety. *Am J Clin Nutr.* 1999 May;69(5):842-56

known and likely effects of vitamin D deficiency, including immunoimpairment, leaky gut, depression, migraine/seizure, pain, increased risk for cancer, autoimmunity, hypertension and cardiovascular disease. Proponents of iatrogenic hypovitaminosis D have failed to substantiate a favorable risk-to-benefit ratio for their intervention.

- **Counterargument #2—Lack of consideration for repletion or supranutritional supplementation of vitamin D to overcome VDR impairment**: A more logical or equally logical argument could be made that increasing vitamin D nutriture would help overcome the VDR impairment, even more so considering that serum 25-hydroxyvitamin D, which is directly affected by dietary supplementation, indeed has biological activity, albeit less than that of 1,25-dihydroxyvitamin D. Why not allow vitamin D itself to serve as its own VDR agonist by raising the levels of 25-OH-D and/or 1,25-dihydroxy-D to overcome the microbial monkeywrench?

- **Counterargument #3—Per the proposed hypothesis, vitamin D supplementation should be harmful and vitamin D deficiency is beneficial in these prototypic autoimmune diseases**: If, as the authors state, microbes are converting vitamin D into an immunosuppressive metabolite, then providing vitamin D supplementation should itself be immunosuppressive; not only has this not been shown, but the opposite has been consistently demonstrated. Providing vitamin D supplementation to autoimmune and chronically ill patients provides benefit. The ultimate proof is shown—as always—in clinical trials, a representative sample of which are provided here:

  □ Vitamin D supplementation benefits patients with **back pain** ("despite" the high prevalence of bacterial infection reported in this condition[307,308,309]): ❶ "This article reviews **6 selected cases of improvement/resolution of chronic back pain or failed back surgery after vitamin D repletion**... This case series supports information that has recently become apparent in the literature about vitamin D deficiency and its influence on back pain, muscle pain, and failed back surgery. Doses in the range of 4000 to 5000 IU of vitamin D3/day may be needed for an adequate response."[310] ❷ "Findings showed that 83% of the study patients (n = 299) had an abnormally low level of vitamin D before treatment with vitamin D supplements. **After treatment, clinical improvement in symptoms was seen in all the groups that had a low level of vitamin D, and in 95% of all the patients (n = 341)**. CONCLUSIONS: Vitamin D deficiency is a major contributor to chronic low back pain in areas where vitamin D deficiency is endemic. Screening for vitamin D deficiency and treatment with supplements should be mandatory in this setting. Measurement of serum 25-OH cholecalciferol is sensitive and specific for detection of vitamin D deficiency, and hence for presumed osteomalacia in patients with chronic low back pain."[311]

  □ Vitamin D supplementation benefits patients with **lupus/SLE**: Cholecalciferol 100,000 IU per week for 4 weeks followed by 100,000 IU of cholecalciferol per month for 6 months in 20 SLE patients with hypovitaminosis D increased serum 25(OH)D levels from 18 ng/mL to 51 ng/mL at 2 months and to 41 ng/mL. "Vitamin D was well tolerated and induced a preferential increase of naïve CD4+ T cells, an increase of regulatory T cells and a decrease of effector Th1 and Th17 cells. **Vitamin D also induced a decrease of memory B cells and anti-DNA antibodies**."[312] *Comment*: Anti-DNA antibodies are **the** defining laboratory and pathologic hallmark of SLE; their reduction is worthy of interpretation as a clear indication in reduced disease activity by vitamin D.

  □ Vitamin D supplementation benefits patients with **viral hepatitis**: ❶ "Cases treated with vitamin D [vitamin D3 2000 IU/d orally] showed significant higher early (P<0.04) and sustained (P<0.05) virological response. There was a high frequency of vitamin D deficiency among the Egyptian HCV children, with significant decrease in bone density. The vitamin D level should be assessed before the start of antiviral treatment with the correction of any detected deficiency. Adding vitamin D to conventional Peg/RBV

---

[307] Sample I. Antibiotics could cure 40% of chronic back pain patients. theguardian.com/society/2013/may/07/antibiotics-cure-back-pain-patients

[308] "In total, microbiological cultures were positive in 28 (46 %) patients. Anaerobic cultures were positive in 26 (43 %) patients, and of these 4 (7 %) had dual microbial infections, containing both one aerobic and one anaerobic culture." Albert HB, Lambert P, Rollason J, et al. Does nuclear tissue infected with bacteria following disc herniations lead to Modic changes in the adjacent vertebrae? *Eur Spine J*. 2013 Apr;22(4):690-6

[309] Albert HB, Sorensen JS, Christensen BS, Manniche C. Antibiotic treatment in patients with chronic low back pain and vertebral bone edema (Modic type 1 changes): a double-blind randomized clinical controlled trial of efficacy. *Eur Spine J*. 2013 Apr;22(4):697-707

[310] Schwalfenberg G. Improvement of chronic back pain or failed back surgery with vitamin D repletion: a case series. *J Am Board Fam Med*. 2009 Jan-Feb;22(1):69-74

[311] Al Faraj S, Al Mutairi K. Vitamin D deficiency and chronic low back pain in Saudi Arabia. *Spine* (Phila Pa 1976). 2003 Jan 15;28(2):177-9

[312] Terrier B et al. Restoration of regulatory and effector T cell balance and B cell homeostasis in systemic lupus erythematosus patients through vitamin D supplementation. *Arthritis Res Ther*. 2012 Oct 17;14(5):R221

therapy significantly improved the virological response and helped to prevent the risk of emerging bone fragility."[313] ❷ "Low vitamin D levels predicts negative treatment outcome, and adding vitamin D [oral vitamin D3 2000 IU/d] to conventional Peg/RBV therapy for patients with HCV genotype 2-3 significantly improves viral response."[314]

- Counterargument #4—Failures in microbiology: 1) failure to identify the specific bacteria that produce the supposed VDR agonists, 2) failure to establish that those particular bacteria are present in human patients and are causative for the corresponding diseases, 3) failure to establish that those bacteria are responsive/sensitive to the proposed "subinhibitory dosages of certain bacteriostatic antibiotics."

- Counterargument #5—The Marshall Protocol claims that vitamin D supplementation is harmful despite the fact that essentially all studies have shown clinical benefit and reduced mortality and disease incidence with improved vitamin D nutriture: My conclusion is that the Marshall Protocol's inclusion of iatrogenic vitamin D deficiency is almost certainly harmful and clearly not beneficial, neither in the long-term nor the short-term. Several studies and metaanalyses involving tens of thousands of patients have shown dose-dependent and therefore causal protective benefits of vitamin D supplementation.

  □ Meta-analysis of randomized controlled trials: Vitamin D supplementation and total mortality (*Arch Intern Med.* 2007 Sep[315]): "Intake of ordinary doses of vitamin D supplements seems to be associated with decreases in total mortality rates." Most of the studies reviewed in this meta-analysis used subphysiologic doses of vitamin D; yet they still produced benefit in reduced total mortality, some of which is likely attributable to reductions in the incidence and severity of infections and autoimmunity.

  □ Vitamin D supplementation in first year of life reduces risk of type 1 diabetes by at least 78%. (*Lancet.* 2001 Nov[316]): In this pioneering and prophetic study—amazingly started in 1966 and ended in 1997— the authors assessed the effect of vitamin D supplementation in more than 10,000 infants (n = 10366) to find that "Vitamin D supplementation was associated with a decreased frequency of type 1 diabetes when adjusted for neonatal, anthropometric, and social characteristics (rate ratio [RR] for regular vs no supplementation 0.12, 95% CI 0.03-0.51, and irregular vs no supplementation 0.16, 0.04-0.74. Children who regularly took the recommended dose of vitamin D (2000 IU daily) had a RR of 0.22 (0.05-0.89) compared with those who regularly received less than the recommended amount. Children suspected of having rickets during the first year of life had a RR of 3.0 (1.0-9.0) compared with those without such a suspicion. Interpretation: Dietary vitamin D supplementation is associated with reduced risk of type 1 diabetes. Ensuring adequate vitamin D supplementation for infants could help to reverse the increasing trend in the incidence of type 1 diabetes." This is a landmark study that should have resulted in routine implementation of vitamin D supplementation in all children because the cost is minimal, the health benefits (including and beyond diabetes) are massive, and the risks are truly almost negligible— in this study of more than 10,000 infants, not a single adverse effect was reported. Note the very clear dose-response relationship and the fact that severe vitamin D deficiency rickets was associated with a 300% increased risk for diabetes.

  □ Estimated benefits in reduction in economic burden and premature deaths due to vitamin D deficiency in Canada. (*Mol Nutr Food Res.* 2010 Aug[317]): "Vitamin D deficiency has been linked to many diseases and conditions in addition to bone diseases, including many types of cancer, several bacterial and viral infections, autoimmune diseases, cardiovascular diseases, and adverse pregnancy outcomes. ... It is estimated that the death rate could fall by 37,000 deaths (22,300-52,300 deaths), representing 16.1% (9.7-22.7%) of annuals deaths and the economic burden by 6.9% (3.8-10.0%) or $14.4 billion ($8.0 billion-$20.1 billion) less the cost of the program. It is recommended that Canadian health policy leaders consider measures to increase serum 25(OH)D levels for all Canadians."

  □ Vitamin D reduces risk of multiple sclerosis: ❶ Estimated vitamin D intake and serum 25-hydroxyvitamin D (25[OH]D) during pregnancy were assessed in 35,794 mothers and correlated with

[313] Eltayeb et al. Vitamin D status and viral response to therapy in hepatitis C infected children. *World J Gastroenterol.* 2015 Jan 28;21(4):1284-91
[314] Nimer A, Mouch A. Vitamin D improves viral response in hepatitis C genotype 2-3 naïve patients. *World J Gastroenterol.* 2012 Feb 28;18(8):800-5
[315] Autier P, Gandini S. Vitamin D supplementation and total mortality: a meta-analysis of randomized controlled trials. *Arch Intern Med.* 2007 Sep;167(16):1730-7
[316] Hyppönen et al. Intake of vitamin D and risk of type 1 diabetes: a birth-cohort study. *Lancet.* 2001 Nov 3;358(9292):1500-3
[317] Grant WB, Schwalfenberg et al. An estimate of the economic burden and premature deaths due to vitamin D deficiency in Canada. *Mol Nutr Food Res.* 2010 Aug;54:1172-81

offspring incidence of developing MS. "The relative risk of MS was lower among women born to mothers with high milk or vitamin D intake during pregnancy. ... The predicted 25[OH]D level in the pregnant mothers was also inversely associated with the risk of MS in their daughters. Comparing extreme quintiles, the adjusted RR was 0.59; (95% CI, 0.37-0.92; p trend = 0.002). *INTERPRETATION*: Higher maternal milk and vitamin D intake during pregnancy may be associated with a lower risk of developing MS in offspring."[318] ❷ "METHODS: Dietary vitamin D intake was examined directly in relation to risk of MS in two large cohorts of women: the Nurses' Health Study (NHS; 92,253 women followed from 1980 to 2000) and Nurses' Health Study II (NHS II; 95,310 women followed from 1991 to 2001). ... The pooled age-adjusted relative risk (RR) comparing women in the highest quintile of total vitamin D intake at baseline with those in the lowest was 0.67. Intake of vitamin D from supplements was also inversely associated with risk of MS; the RR comparing women with intake of >or=400 IU/day with women with no supplemental vitamin D intake was 0.59. ... CONCLUSION: These results support a protective effect of vitamin D intake on risk of developing MS."[319]

Proven benefits based on multiple studies of vitamin D3 supplementation include excellent risk:benefit in the prevention and treatment of many conditions*	Faults needing remediation in favor of "iatrogenic induction of vitamin D deficiency as therapy against infections and infection-induced inflammatory disease" per Marshall, Waterhouse, et al
1. Alleviation of depression (strong) and improved neurologic function (weak-modest)—antidepressant benefit shown in at least 5 trials; reduced risk for schizophrenia; improved neuromuscular coordination and reduced falls; benefit suggested in neurodegenerative/neuroinflammatory disorders 2. Prevention/alleviation of diabetes types 1 (strong) and 2 (modest)—major reductions in risk; improvements in glycemic control, reduced comorbidities such as depression, hypertension, infection 3. Reduction of cardiovascular risk (modest)—mechanisms include reduction in inflammation and hypertension 4. Prevention/alleviation of nearly all autoimmune diseases (strong)—specifically multiple sclerosis, autoimmune diabetes, and rheumatoid arthritis 5. Reduction musculoskeletal pain (very strong)—back pain, migraine, limb pain, fibromyalgia-like presentations, opioid requirements 6. Normalization of Treg:Th17 ratios; anti-inflammatory benefits (strong)—important for changing the immune imbalance that underlies many inflammatory conditions, including metabolic syndrome and autoimmunity 7. Reduced incidence of various cancers, including breast, colon, and prostate (strong)—vitamin D supplementation shown to delay progression of prostate cancer, mechanisms include gene regulation, anti-inflammation, and anti-estrogen 8. Excellent safety, affordability, availability, risk:benefit and cost:effectiveness characteristics: 9. Reduced all-cause mortality (strong)—consistent with above	1. Microbes not identified, model is too nonspecific—molecular mechanisms weakly explained, 2. Lack of peer-reviewed citations in the primary supporting document—many of the citations in *Ann N Y Acad Sci* 2009 Sep are not available for legitimate peer-review and scientific evaluation; having their first 8 citations referenced to their own group and their own impressively-unavailable conference presentations is highly suspect and is actually unprofessional and not in accord with journal publication standards, which require that sources are peer-reviewed and available for evaluation. 3. No risk:benefit analysis provided—benefit not shown to outweigh risks for nontreatment of conditions that respond to vitamin D supplementation; benefit of proposed reduction in VDR-impairing microbial metabolites not shown to outweigh the anticipated increases in depression, diabetes, autoimmunity, migraine, back pain, cancers and all-cause mortality 4. Numerous inconsistencies in their model—for example repeatedly stating that vitamin D is immunosuppressive is erroneous to the point of being illogical given the available data; implying that patients will suffer in the long-term despite proven short-term *and long-term* benefits demonstrated in studies ranging from 3 months to 30 years is inconsistent with current literature at best, illogical fear-mongering at worst
*Data strength casually ranked as strong/moderate/weak per literature perusal and prior publications on this topic, especially Vasquez et al. The clinical importance of vitamin D. *Altern Ther Health Med* 2004 Sep ICHNFM.ORG/reprints	

In concluding this section, the table above casually yet accurately outlines the arguments against the proposal espoused by Marshall, Waterhouse, and colleagues. Their proposal carries clear risks with no established benefit(s)

---

[318] Mirzaei et al. Gestational vitamin D and the risk of multiple sclerosis in offspring. *Ann Neurol.* 2011 Jul;70(1):30-40
[319] Munger et al. Vitamin D intake and incidence of multiple sclerosis. *Neurology.* 2004 Jan 13;62(1):60-5

and as such, this particular component of the so-called "Marshall protocol" is not scientific, nor is it scientifically supported. Ethical questions and medicolegal concerns stemming from the intentional withholding of an essential nutrient with numerous physiological roles and clinical benefits are obvious and are not supportive of this intervention. In order to test and externally validate my critique, I organized my arguments and submitted them for peer-review in *International Journal of Human Nutrition and Functional Medicine;* the argument underwent peer-review within the journal by the IJHNFM Board of Editors and Reviewers and was also submitted via social media to more than 12,000 people including several groups of healthcare professionals (receiving more than 400 views within the first 24 hours) for feedback, correction, criticism, support, or counterarguments. The final version of my paper was posted scientific/academic websites in April 2015 for additional critique by the international community. Readers are invited to review my peer-reviewed critique[320] and any resulting discussions/responses posted at IntJHumNutrFunctMed.org and ICHNFM.org.

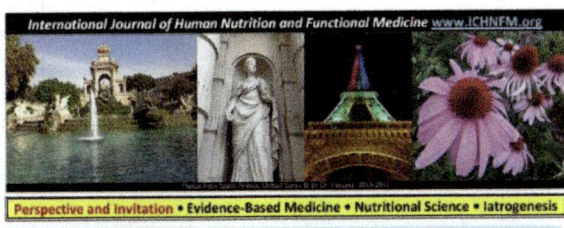

Conclusion to this section: As this "*Microbial Morphology, Molecules, Metabolites, and Pathophysiologic Mechanisms*" section now closes, clinicians should have a better appreciation for the means by which microbes profoundly affect human physiology—and ultimately—the clinical presentation of diseases and disorders, many of which are commonly assigned the label of "idiopathic" and relegated to endless (psychoactive/analgesic) drug "management." The more than 200 articles previously cited in this introduction are sufficient to establish the pathophysiologic basis and understanding for the concept of microbe-induced inflammation in the absence of overt clinical "infection."

On the following page, I have placed a diagram worthy of study so that clinicians can appreciate the *flow*, the *confluence* of events and pathways. In the study of the so-called basic sciences leading up to the study of Pathology before the clinical work of our doctorate programs (I've been through this sequence three times for each of my doctorate degrees), we are mostly taught short linear sequences, as if our human physiology could only take short steps before pausing or bringing the relevant pathway to completion. This is not a realistic view of the (patho)physiology we are tasked to mend, and thus "trained" we as doctors have been given abbreviated and horrendously linear misperceptions—the perfect teaching plan for creating doctors who cannot see the forest for the trees nor the "simple complexity" that sits before them. But these abbreviated and disconnected "understandings" are perfect for ensuring that patients will be treated with polypharmacy—"a pill for every ill"—and will need a cadre of "specialists" to manage each head of the hydra-like interconnected physiologic disruption that might otherwise respond to an orchestrated and intelligent healthcare plan. In contrast to the previous much more linear diagram placed at the start of this chapter/subsection, the diagram on the following page has more of a flow, and the overlapping and interconnected pathways provide options for different clinical outcomes. For sure, in the worst-case-scenario, everything results in fatigue, pain, depression, and inflammation/autoimmunity; but most patients are somewhere on the map, short of the final scenario, a bit to one side or the other, and with other covariables influencing the clinical presentation. Understanding the pattern of "dysbiotic contribution" intermixed with other contributions—social, psychological, metabolic, hormonal—will help clinicians address that particular and very important component, while continuing to deconstruct the other overlapping illusions of apparent complexity so that the patient's true health and potential can be freed from the burden of illness.

---

[320] Vasquez A. Iatrogenic induction of vitamin D deficiency: The position against this potentially harmful practice and open invitation for its proponents to articulate substantiation. *Int J Hum Nutr Funct Med* 2015;v3(q1):p1

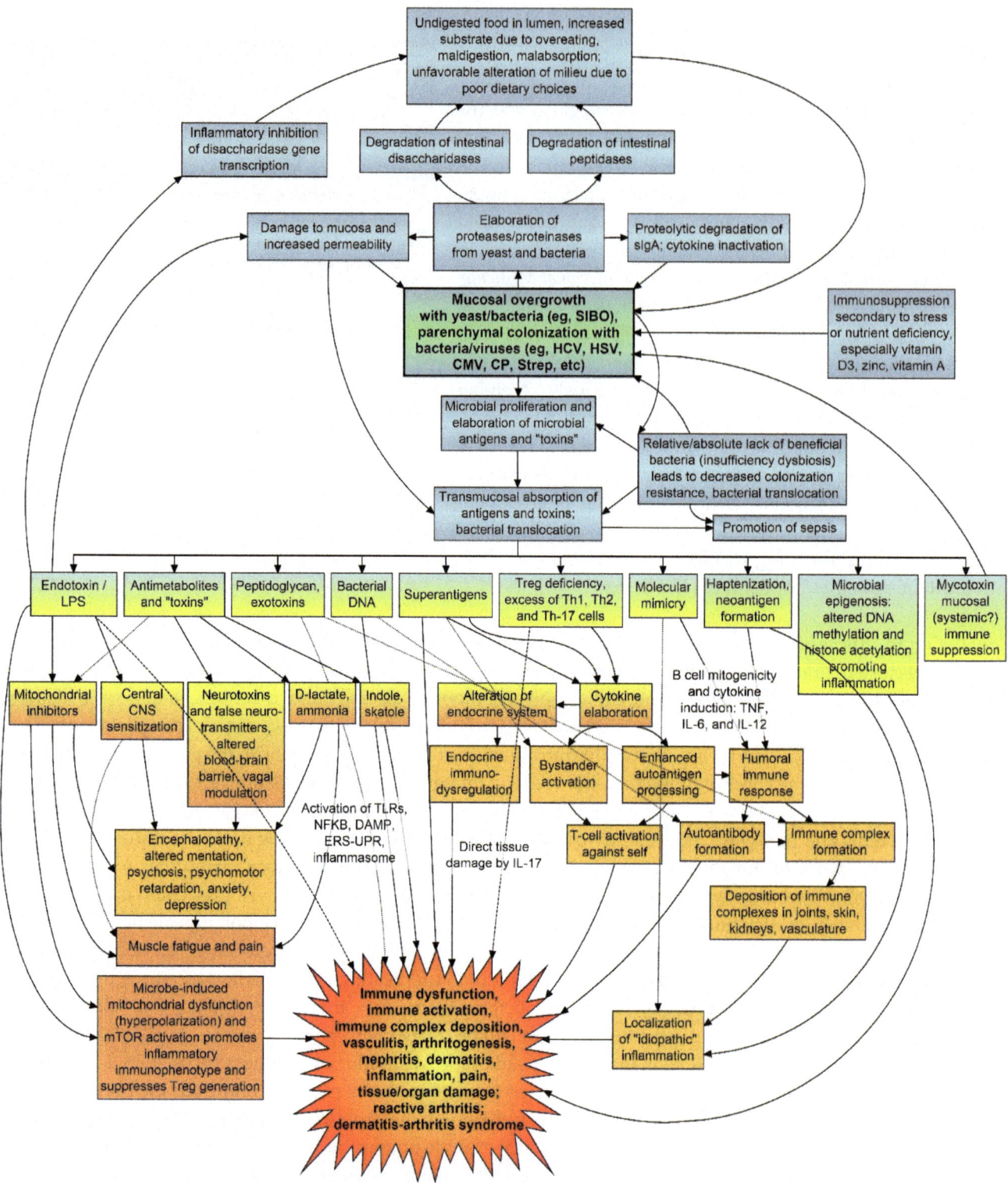

Interconnected pathways involved in dysbiosis-induced mitochondrial and mental impairment, immune dysfunction, and musculoskeletal inflammation/autoimmunity: "What I talk about is only what I have lived through. If you have not lived through something, it is just not true." Kabir (1440-1518), Indian poet

Physiology and pathophysiology are interconnected confluences
"Whoever writes in blood and proverbs does not want to be read, but to be learned by heart. In the mountains the shortest way is from peak to peak, but for that one must have long legs. Proverbs should be peaks, and those who are addressed should be great and tall."   Nietzsche FW. *Thus Spoke Zarathustra, On Reading and Writing*

Prototypic clinical manifestations: This section on "mechanisms of dysbiosis" concludes with discussion of three different prototypic clinical manifestations of dysbiosis, with the first clearly localized to the gut, the second less dependent on a gut reservoir, and the third inclusive of and at times completely independent from gut microbiota.

1. Autointoxication, auto-brewery syndrome, hepatic encephalopathy *in the absence of liver disease*: The term "autointoxication" fell out of favor among American allopaths in the 1940s despite the recognition and objective documentation that systemically absorbed microbial metabolites/toxins from the colon could adversely affect systemic health, particularly neurocognitive function.[321] Recognition that excess or abnormal microbes in the gut could cause neuropsychiatric symptoms contributed to the rationale for the use of colonic irrigation in clinical practice which was fully endorsed by the American Medical Association in a position paper published in 1932.[322] Concurrently, an article published in the *New England Journal of Medicine*[323] in this same year documented the clinical benefits of colonic irrigation in patients with mental disease; the treatment was deemed effective against most cases of dementia, depression, neurosis and many cases of irritability, headaches, and hypertension. Enemas and colonics, which promote hepatobiliary detoxification[324,325] and cleanse the bowel of harmful microbes, were valued by clinicians as a cure or adjunctive treatment for numerous systemic diseases.[326] Although the term "autointoxication" is eschewed as "unscientific", all medical professionals recognize that gastrointestinal dysbiosis—particularly generalized overgrowth of yeast and bacteria—can cause clinical conditions characterized by inflammatory vasculitis, dermatitis, arthritis as well as neurological symptoms ranging from confusion and disorientation to somnolence and death. "Hepatic encephalopathy"—classically characterized by elevated serum ammonia which is a direct and surrogate marker for putrefactive dysbiosis overwhelming hepatic detoxification capacity and impaired neurotransmission, respectively—seems to be one of the currently acceptable terms for this phenomenon of "gastrointestinal microflora-induced altered mental status", and probably the condition exists among some outpatients to a milder degree than that which is classically seen in patients with fulminant liver failure; I first published that sentence in early 2006[327], and in 2014-2015 I worked with a patient who proved this to be true—see accompanying Clinical Case.

> **Minimal hepatic encephalopathy**
>
> "Minimal hepatic encephalopathy (MHE) is the earliest form of hepatic encephalopathy and can affect up to 80% of cirrhotic patients. By definition, it has no obvious clinical manifestation and is characterized by neurocognitive impairment in attention, vigilance and integrative function. Although often not considered to be clinically relevant and, therefore, not diagnosed or treated, MHE has been shown to affect daily functioning, quality of life, driving and overall mortality."
>
> Stinton LM, Jayakumar S. Minimal hepatic encephalopathy. *Can J Gastroenterol.* 2013 Oct;27(10):572-4

On a less dramatic but much more frequent note, bacterial overgrowth of the small bowel is also a cause of gastroesophageal reflux disease (GERD) because products of bacterial fermentation relax the lower esophageal sphincter[328] and retard intestinal transit[329]; ameliorating the intestinal bacterial overgrowth by simply "starving" the bacteria of carbohydrate by implementation of a **low-carbohydrate diet** alleviates GERD symptoms and substantiates the cause-and-effect relationship.[330,331]

One of the liver's chief functions is that of "detoxifying" environmentally ingested and endogenously produced metabolites and toxins, including those of microbial origin produced de novo within the gastrointestinal tract. The metabolic activity of the microbial population within the intestinal lumen is

---

[321] Person JR, Bernhard JD. Autointoxication revisited. *J Am Acad Dermatol.* 1986;15(3):559-63

[322] Bastedo WA. Colon irrigations: their administration therapeutic applications and dangers. *Journal of the American Medical Association* 1932;98:734-6

[323] Marshall HK, Thomson CR. Colon irrigation in the treatment of mental disease. *N Engl J Med* 1932; 207 (Sept 8): 454-7

[324] Garbat, AL, Jacobi, HG: Secretion of Bile in Response to Rectal Installations. *Arch Intern Med* 1929; 44: 455-462

[325] "Caffeine enemas cause dilation of bile ducts, which facilitates excretion of toxic cancer breakdown products by the liver and dialysis of toxic products from blood across the colonic wall. The therapy must be used as an integrated whole." Gerson M. The cure of advanced cancer by diet therapy. *Physiol Chem Phys.* 1978;10(5):449-64

[326] Snyder RG. The value of colonic irrigations in countering auto-intoxication of intestinal origin. *Medical Clinics of North America* 1939; May:781-788

[327] Vasquez A. Nutritional and Botanical Treatments against "Silent Infections" and Gastrointestinal Dysbiosis. *Nutr Perspectives* 2006; Jan InflammationMastery.com/reprints

[328] "In summary, we have shown that colonic fermentation, through the production of SCFAs, exerts a controlled feedback on LES motor function." Piche T, et al. Modulation by colonic fermentation of LES function in humans. *Am J Physiol Gastrointest Liver Physiol.* 2000 Apr;278(4):G578-84

[329] "Altered gastrointestinal motility and sensation, changed activity of the central nervous system, and increased sympathetic drive and immune activation may be understood as consequences of the host response to SIBO." Lin HC. Small intestinal bacterial overgrowth: a framework for irritable bowel syndrome. *JAMA.* 2004 Aug 18;292(7):852-8

[330] "These data suggest that a very low-carbohydrate diet in obese individuals with GERD significantly reduces distal esophageal acid exposure and improves symptoms." Austin GL, et al. A very low-carbohydrate diet improves gastroesophageal reflux and its symptoms. *Dig Dis Sci.* 2006 Aug;51(8):1307-12

[331] "The 5 individuals described in these case reports experienced resolution of GERD symptoms after self-initiation of a low-carbohydrate diet." Yancy WS Jr, et al. Improvement of gastroesophageal reflux disease after initiation of a low-carbohydrate diet: five brief case reports. *Altern Ther Health Med.* 2001 Nov-Dec;7(6):120, 116-9

quantitatively enormous, physiologically important, and clinically significant; an estimated ten trillion microorganisms reside within the intestinal lumen of each human. Being very small of course creates very large surface-to-volume ratios for microorganisms; if we take as given that an average bacterium of spherical shape has surface area of approximately 12 micrometers squared, then multiplying this surface area by 10 trillion in order to give some appreciation of the mass of lipopolysaccharide and peptidoglycan mass yields a surface area of 120 trillion micrometers squared or 120 billion meters squared, equal to approximately 29,652,645 acres or 12,000,000 hectares. Given that the total surface of the bacterial community is constantly being shed and replaced by individual microbes throughout each unit of time and also per death of each microbe, then the "functional surface area" of the microbial population is massive beyond comprehension, leaving unquantifiable debris to be either physically excluded or immunologically processed. In addition to this "physical debris", microbes secrete even more metabolic molecules, some of which are intentionally and directly toxic and all of which have to be processed/detoxified/eliminated if and when they are absorbed systemically. As stated previously in this chapter, readers should appreciate that the "total dysbiotic load" (TDL) from all sources—skin, gastrointestinal tract, genitourinary tract, sinorespiratory tract, orodental cavity, environment, and any subclinical parenchymal foci—contributes to the total inflammatory load (TIL) and total xenobiotic load (TXL) which the immune system must process and which the hepatobiliary system must detoxify. In a review article[332] published in 2010 which applies specifically to the gastrointestinal subtype of dysbiosis, the authors start their paper by stating, "Detoxification of gut-derived toxins and microbial products from gut-derived microbes is a major role of the liver. While the full repertoire of gut-derived microbial products that reach the liver in health and disease is yet to be explored, the levels of bacterial lipopolysaccharide (LPS), a component of Gram-negative bacteria, is increased in the portal and/or systemic circulation in several types of chronic liver diseases." The total metabolic and toxic load from the microbes in the gut can be of such a volume that the body's ability to detoxify/metabolize these toxins is overwhelmed.

- Child with ethanol intoxication secondary to bacterial/fungal overgrowth of the intestines (*J Pediatr Gastroenterol Nutr* 2001 Aug[333]): In this case report and review of the literature, the authors begin their article by noting that, "The term **auto-brewery syndrome** has been used to describe patients who become repeatedly inebriated after ingestion of food of high carbohydrate nature in the presence of abnormal yeast proliferation, particularly of *Candida* species." The case report centers on a 13-year-old girl who had bowel resection for important reasons when a neonate and who later had "recurrent episodes of bizarre behavior, somnolence, disorientation, and a fruity odor of her breath and was suspected to be abusing alcohol." **The young girl was diagnosed with alcohol intoxication when ethanol blood levels were repeatedly elevated in the range of 250 mg/dL to 350 mg/dL**; she persistently denied any intake of alcoholic beverages. Readers should note that in most states in the United States, a blood alcohol concentration (BAC) of or greater than 100 mg/dL is the legal definition of intoxication and drunkenness.[334] The young girl's father—a physician—began testing the girl's breath alcohol level at home and noticed a strong correlation between her elevated ethanol levels and the intake of carbohydrate-rich meals or fructose-containing drinks, such as fruit juices.

The girl was treated empirically for bacterial overgrowth of the intestines with courses of the anti-bacterial drugs Bactrim, Flagyl, and Augmentin and attained zero benefit. The girl then underwent upper gastrointestinal endoscopy study to obtain aspirates for microbial analysis; the aspirate grew abundant *Candida glabrata* and *Saccharomyces cerevisiae*. **Sensitivity-directed treatment with fluconazole resolved all symptoms and prevented recurrence of the elevated ethanol levels**. The combination of bacterial with fungal overgrowth was likely synergistic; bacterial LPS blocked Cyp450 detoxification and thereby heightened sensitivity to the fungally-produced ethanol.

> **Dysbiotic encephalopathy**
>
> "**Ammonia** is a well-known neurotoxin, produced in the intestinal tract from urea by the action of bacterial ureases. ... In addition to direct neurotoxic injury, ammonia alters function of the blood–brain barrier, impairing intracerebral synthesis of serotonin and dopamine and producing **abnormal neurotransmitters such as octopamine**."
>
> Galland L. *J Med Food*. 2014 Dec

---

[332] Szabo G, Bala S, Petrasek J, Gattu A. Gut-liver axis and sensing microbes. *Dig Dis.* 2010;28(6):737-44

[333] Dahshan et al. Auto-brewery syndrome in a child with short gut syndrome: case report and review of the literature. *J Pediatr Gastroenterol Nutr.* 2001 Aug;33:214-5

[334] Cohen JS. (Plantz SH, Talavera F, Anker A, editors). Alcohol Intoxication. emedicinehealth.com/alcohol_intoxication/page2_em.htm June 9, 2011

Clinical Case Elevated plasma ammonia in the absence of liver disease in a 45yo male with SIBO, neurologic symptoms, muscle fasciculation: These laboratory results from 2014-2015 show elevated plasma/serum ammonia in a 45yo previously athletic male suffering with a 2-year history of debilitating fatigue and neuromuscular disorder; the patient has no history of liver disease, and all other laboratory testing is remarkably normal. Iron overload was excluded (ferritin level ranging from 49-81 ng/ml on several occasions); copper overload was excluded (normal ceruloplasmin and serum copper). Other testing showed a remarkably elevated urine DHPPA (3,4 dihydroxyphenylpropionic acid), which is produced by various bacteria from dietary chlorogenic acid, sourced from a wide variety of fruits, vegetables, tea and coffee; elevated DHPPA is an objective marker consistent with SIBO—small intestine bacterial overgrowth. Tartaric acid is found in small/modest amounts in fruits such as grapes, bananas, and tamarinds but elevated levels in urine generally correlate with fungal/yeast overgrowth of the intestines. Of additional note, this patient was unlikely to be biotin deficient per daily supplementation of approximately 2 mg/d; nevertheless, we increased biotin intake to 5 mg/d while treating with laxative doses of ascorbic acid each morning followed later in the day by berberine 1500 mg/d, time-released emulsified oregano oil 600 mg/d, rifaxamin 550 mg QD-TID, and low-fermentation diet. These treatments and especially the addition of azithromycin 250 mg/d per high antibody titers against *Chlamydophila pneumoniae* (discussed in Chapters 1 [laboratory assessments] and 4 [dysbiosis]) led to important clinical improvements; this patient has improved markedly, but we are still working toward a total cure as of early 2015 and have recently added tinidazole 2g/d.

Results dated 2014 Apr

Test Name: AMMONIA (P)

Analyte Name	Units	Ref Range	04/11/14
AMMONIA (P)	UMOL/L	< OR = 47	58 (H)

Results dated 2013 Aug

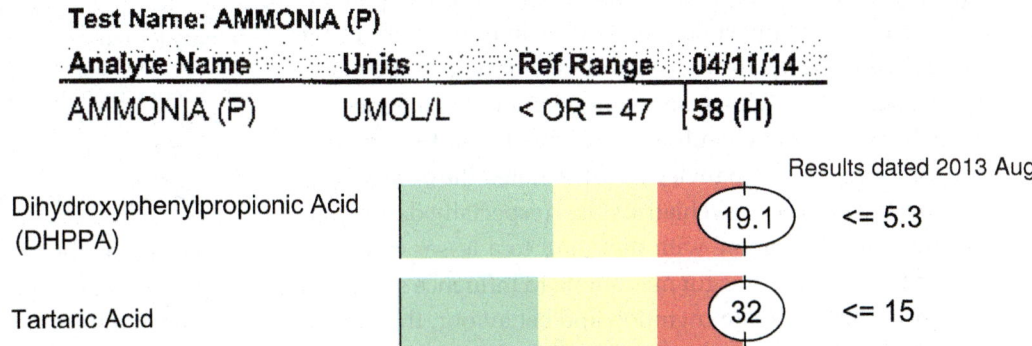

Dihydroxyphenylpropionic Acid (DHPPA)	19.1	<= 5.3
Tartaric Acid	32	<= 15

Results dated 2015 Jan

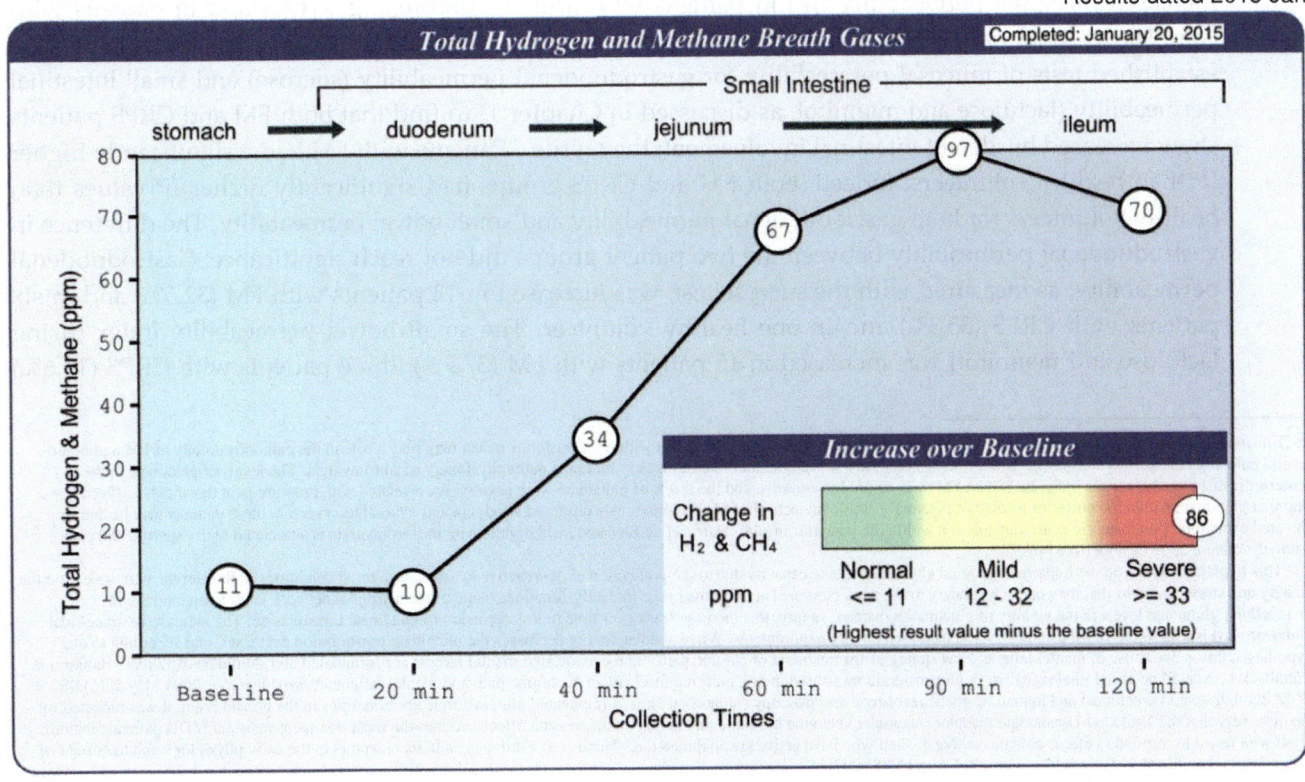

Total Hydrogen and Methane Breath Gases — Completed: January 20, 2015

2. <mark>Syndromes of pain, fatigue, depression—all of which correlate with low-grade inflammation, increased intestinal permeability, and increased CNS glutaminergic neurotransmission</mark>: Many clinical syndromes chiefly characterized by <mark>pain</mark>, <mark>fatigue</mark>, and <mark>depression</mark> all commonly have associated ❶ low-grade inflammation, ❷ increased intestinal permeability (indicating localized gut-specific involvement), and ❸ increased CNS glutaminergic neurotransmission. Of these, the first is well-established and does not need substantiation here; the second is supported previously and in a following summary (Goebel et al. *Rheumatology* 2008 Aug), leaving the third to be developed and interconnected here. <mark>Increased CNS—specifically the brain—glutaminergic neurotransmission is seen in chronic pain (e.g., fibromyalgia[335]), mental fatigue[336], and depression (notably responsive to the glutamate receptor agonist, ketamine[337])</mark>; my proposal is that the increased glutaminergic neurotransmission is triggered at least in part by microbe/LPS-triggered CNS microglial activation which in turn leads to astrocyte release of glutamate, an excitatory neurotransmitter that contributes to the central aspects of pain, fatigue, and depression. Along with the low-grade inflammation triggered by dysbiosis in general and LPS in particular comes the release of cytokines and prostaglandins which—independently yet synergistically with glia/astrocyte-induced cerebral hyperglutaminosis—also contribute to pain sensitization, fatigue, depression, memory impairment and other cognitive/emotional aspects of the commonly reported "brain fog" or "fibro fog" commonly reported by affected patients. Biochemical and physiological cocontributors—within this model—to these syndromes include primary and secondary nutritional deficiencies (especially vitamin D, magnesium, and n3FA) and mitochondrial impairment, just to name two categories. In their 2015 review, Dash[338] noted the bidirectional relationship between psychiatric states (especially depression)

> **Administration of low-dose LPS to humans causes fatigue, depression, pain, central sensitization, memory impairment**
>
> "Parenteral administration of LPS to humans in nanogram quantities... depressed mood, increased anxiety, and impaired long-term memory for emotional stimuli. In addition, visceral pain sensitivity thresholds are reduced and visceral pain (provoked by rectal distension) is rated as more unpleasant after administration of low-dose LPS."
>
> Galland. Gut microbiome and brain. *J Med Food* 2014

and the gut microbiome with diet (and to a lesser extent, exercise) serving as the intermediaries and stated, "Given the ability of the gut microbiota to influence serotonin and its precursor, tryptophan, regulate the stress response, and modulate cognition and behaviour, the potential importance of the gut microbiota to psychiatry in general and to depression specifically is apparent."

- Increased intestinal permeability (IP) in patients with primary fibromyalgia (FM) and in patients with complex regional pain syndrome (CRPS) (*Rheumatology* 2008 Aug[339]): Authors of this study used well-established tests of mucosal permeability for gastroduodenal permeability (sucrose) and small intestinal permeability (lactulose and mannitol, as discussed in Chapter 1) to find that both FM and CRPS patients show increased burden of intestinal involvement; they write, "<mark>Patients with FM had a significantly higher IP than healthy volunteers. Indeed, both FM and CRPS groups had significantly higher IP values than healthy volunteers for both gastroduodenal permeability and small bowel permeability.</mark> The difference in gastroduodenal permeability between the two patient groups did not reach significance. <mark>Gastroduodenal permeability, as measured with the sucrose test, was increased in 13 patients with FM (32.5%) and in six patients with CRPS (35.3%) and in one healthy volunteer. The small bowel permeability index [using lactulose and mannitol] was increased in 15 patients with FM (37.5%), three patients with CRPS (17.6%)</mark>

[335] "Enhanced glutamatergic neurotransmission resulting from higher concentrations of Glu within the posterior insula may play a role in the pathophysiology of FM and other central pain augmentation syndromes.... These findings point towards a potential role of insular Glu in the pathophysiology of fibromyalgia. The levels of glutamate in the posterior insula were higher for individuals with FM as compared to controls, and the levels of glutamate were negatively correlated with pressure pain thresholds.... Overall we find that glutamate within the posterior insula is a potential pathologic factor in FM. The previously observed allodynia and hyperalgesia seen in these patients may be due to elevated excitatory glutamatergic neurotransmission within the posterior insula." Harris et al. Elevated insular glutamate in fibromyalgia is associated with experimental pain. *Arthritis Rheum.* 2009 Oct;60(10):3146-52

[336] "This hypothesis relies on the impaired astroglial glutamate uptake capacity due to the production of neuroactive substances, altered conditions in the chronic pain state, and the anxiety and stress reactions that may occur secondary to the pain. Neuronal activity over time in the dysfunctional state of the astroglial network leads to an increase in extracellular glutamate levels in the vicinity of glutamate synapses. In turn, this increase leads over time to less precision in glutamate transmission. The increased extracellular glutamate levels lead to increased excitability and increased energy requirements. When cellular energy decreases the glutamate transmission decreases, and according to our hypothesis, this is one cause of mental fatigue. New strategies for treatment of chronic pain and the associated mental fatigue are formulated and should be explored." Hansson E, Rönnbäck L. Altered neuronal-glial signaling in glutamatergic transmission as a unifying mechanism in chronic pain and mental fatigue. *Neurochem Res.* 2004 May;29(5):989-96

[337] "Although several preclinical and human magnetic resonance spectroscopy studies had already implicated glutamatergic abnormalities in the human brain, it was rocketed by the discovery that the N-methyl-D-aspartate receptor antagonist ketamine has rapid and potent antidepressant effects in even the most treatment-resistant MDD patients, including those who failed to respond to electroconvulsive therapy and who have active suicidal ideation." Niciu et al. Glutamate and its receptors in the pathophysiology and treatment of major depressive disorder. *J Neural Transm.* 2014 Aug;121(8):907-24

[338] Dash S, Clarke G, Berk M, Jacka FN. The gut microbiome and diet in psychiatry: focus on depression. *Curr Opin Psychiatry.* 2015 Jan;28(1):1-6

[339] Goebel et al. Altered intestinal permeability in patients with primary fibromyalgia and in patients with complex regional pain syndrome. *Rheumatology* 2008 Aug;47(8):1223-7

and in none of the volunteers." A wonderful addition to / extension of this work would have been the measurement of serum LPS levels, but this was not performed in the current study and has not been performed as of early 2015—noted and summarized immediately below is one study (Maes et al. *J Affect Disord* 2007 Apr) that measured antibodies to LPS (not LPS directly) in patients with CFS—chronic fatigue syndrome. Notably, increased IP in FM did not correlate with GI symptoms; however increased IP did correlate with serologic positivity against *Helicobacter pylori*, *Yersinia enterocolitica* and *Campylobacter jejuni*.

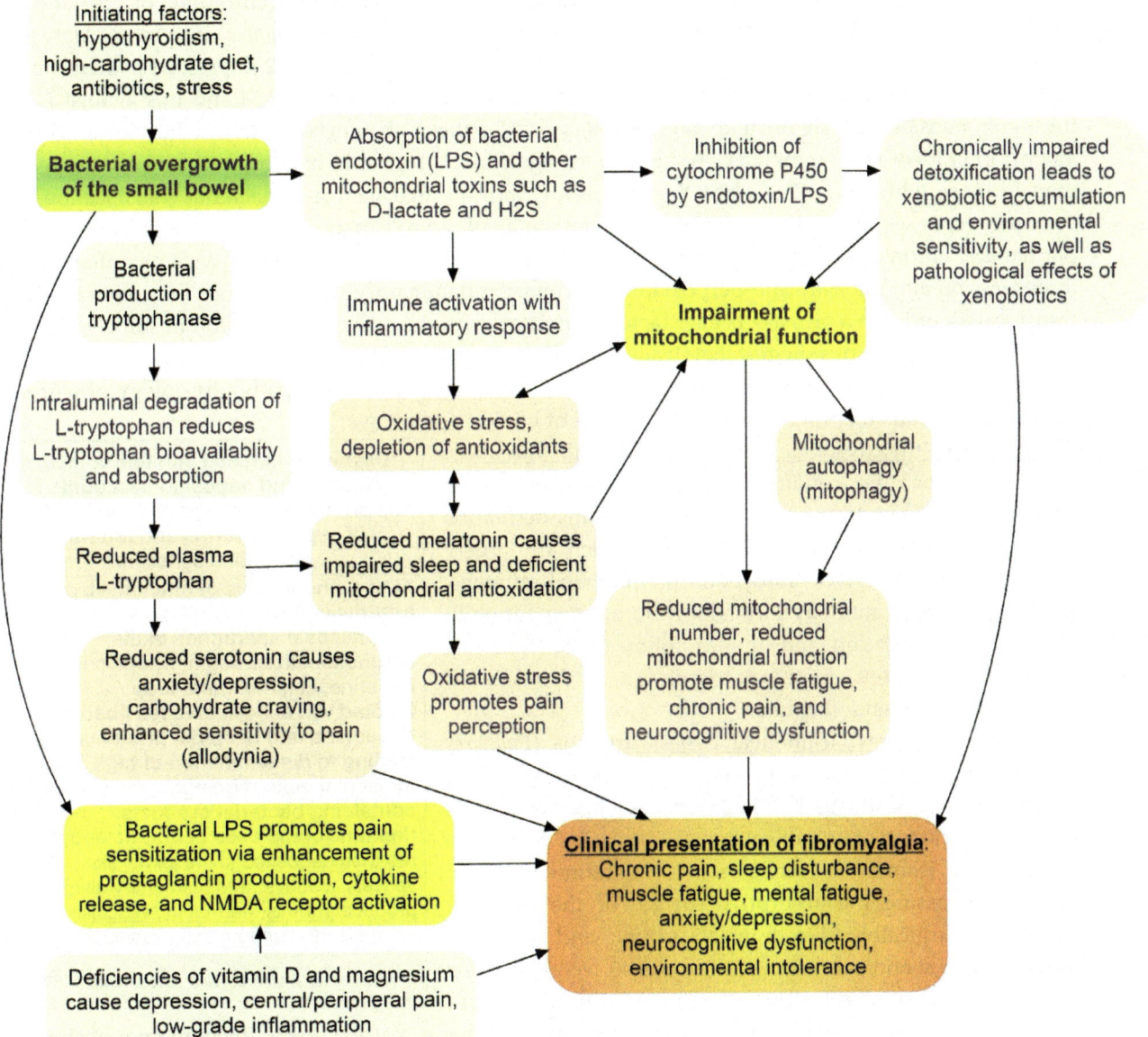

Representative clinical example—fibromyalgia initiated by dysbiosis (SIBO): As a prototypic pain syndrome, fibromyalgia can be explained entirely from its etiologic pathogenesis in the gut. Diagram from Vasquez.[340]

- Increased IgA responses to the LPS of commensal bacteria is associated with inflammation and symptomatology in chronic fatigue syndrome (*J Affect Disord* 2012 Feb[341]): Patients with chronic fatigue syndrome (CFS) have low-grade inflammation characterized by significant increases in serum levels of IL-1, TNF-alpha, neopterin (marker of immune activation and oxidative stress), and elastase; all of these are

---

[340] Vasquez A. *Fibromyalgia in a Nutshell*. 2012, and later versions. Vasquez A. *Functional Medicine Rheumatology v3.5*. 2014, and later versions.
[341] Maes et al. Increased IgA responses to the LPS of commensal bacteria is associated with inflammation and activation of cell-mediated immunity in chronic fatigue syndrome. *J Affect Disord*. 2012 Feb;136(3):909-17

positively correlated with heightened IgA responses to LPS. Furthermore "serum IL-1, TNFα and neopterin are significantly related to fatigue, a flu-like malaise, autonomic symptoms, neurocognitive disorders, sadness and irritability. CONCLUSIONS: The findings show that increased IgA responses to commensal bacteria in ME/CFS are associated with inflammation and cell-mediated immunity (CMI) activation, which are associated with symptom severity. It is concluded that increased translocation of commensal bacteria may be responsible for the disease activity in some ME/CFS patients."

- Increased IgA and IgM responses against gut commensals in chronic depression (*J Affect Disord* 2012 Dec[342]): After discovering that clinical depression is accompanied by increased IgM and IgA responses directed against gram negative gut commensals, these authors measured serum concentrations of IgM and IgA against the LPS of gram-negative enterobacteria, i.e. *Hafnia alvei, Pseudomonas aeruginosa, Morganella morganii, Pseudomonas putida, Citrobacter koseri*, and *Klebsiella pneumoniae* in 112 depressed patients and 28 normal controls to find that "The prevalences and median values of serum IgM and IgA against LPS of these commensals were significantly higher in depressed patients than in controls. The IgM levels directed against the LPS of these commensal bacteria were significantly higher in patients with chronic depression than in those without. ... DISCUSSION: The results indicate that increased bacterial translocation with immune responses to the LPS of commensal bacteria may play a role in the pathophysiology of depression, particularly chronic depression. Bacterial translocation may a) occur secondary to systemic inflammation in depression and intensify and perpetuate the primary inflammatory response once the commensals are translocated; or b) be a primary trigger factor associated with the onset of depression in some vulnerable individuals. The findings suggest that "translocated" gut commensal bacteria activate immune cells to elicit IgA and IgM responses and that this phenomenon may play a role in the pathophysiology of (chronic) depression by causing progressive amplifications of immune pathways."

3. **Dysbiotic arthropathy, dysbiotic dermatitis, dysbiotic vasculitis**: Current terms for this condition include "bowel-associated dermatosis-arthritis syndrome"[343], "intestinal arthritis-dermatitis syndrome"[344], and "bypass disease"[345]—all of which are largely mediated by the gut-derived absorption of microbial antigens, mucosal and systemic antibody formation, and antigen-antibody binding in the circulation and tissues followed by systemic deposition of circulating immune complexes in skin, joints, kidneys, and vascular endothelium.

> **Dysbiosis-induced immune complex formation and deposition accounts for the primary underlying pathophysiology of bypass arthritis and arthritis-dermatitis syndrome**
>
> "The pathogenesis of intestinal bypass arthritis involves bacterial overgrowth and mucosal alterations in the defunctionalized segment of small intestine, i.e., the 'blind loop'. ... "The blunted villi allow increased absorption of bacteria and bacterial products, leading to dissemination of high molecular weight immune complexes containing bacterial products." These "immune complexes of enteric antigens" are then deposited in the joints, skin, vessels, kidneys, and pulmonary alveoli to produce arthritis, dermatitis, vasculitis, nephritis, and pneumonitis, respectively.
>
> Ross et al. *Baillieres Clin Rheumatol.* 1989 Aug

- Authoritative review: Jejunoileal bypass arthritis (*Baillieres Clin Rheumatol* 1989 Aug[346]): In this 17-page review chapter, authors Ross, Scott, and Pincus discuss the allopathic medicosurgical use of jejunoileal bypass, a surgical procedure wherein the jejunum is connected to the terminal ileum, thereby bypassing the absorptive surface of the jejunum, causing a surgically-induced malabsorption and diarrhea-induced nausea and anorexia which results in weight loss for the "treatment" of obesity. The procedure was used on more than 100,000 patients between the years 1954-1983, when it was discarded due to the high rates of clinically important post-operative complications, noted in up to 58% of patients. Interestingly, studying the rheumatologic complications of jejunoileal bypass contributed to scientific knowledge about the relationship of microbial dysbiosis and inflammatory diseases, particularly skin inflammation and joint inflammation; the authors write, "However, important advances in the understanding of inflammatory joint disease emerged from studies of the prominent rheumatologic complication of intestinal bypass known as the **arthritis-dermatitis syndrome**. Furthermore, the symptoms of "**bypass arthritis**" have been

---

[342] Maes et al. Increased IgA/IgM responses against gut commensals in chronic depression: evidence for bacterial translocation or leaky gut. *J Affect Disord* 2012 Dec:55-62

[343] Jorizzo JL, et al. Bowel-bypass syndrome without bowel bypass. Bowel-associated dermatosis-arthritis syndrome. *Arch Intern Med.* 1983 Mar;143(3):457-61

[344] Stein HB, Schlappner OL, Boyko W, Gourlay RH, Reeve CE. The intestinal bypass: arthritis-dermatitis syndrome. *Arthritis Rheum.* 1981 May;24(5):684-90

[345] Utsinger PD. Systemic immune complex disease following intestinal bypass surgery: bypass disease. *J Am Acad Dermatol.* 1980 Jun;2(6):488-95

[346] Ross CB, Scott HW, Pincus T. Jejunoileal bypass arthritis. *Baillieres Clin Rheumatol.* 1989 Aug;3(2):339-55

recognized in individuals who have not undergone intestinal bypass, but who had perturbations of intestinal anatomy secondary to postoperative, inflammatory or diverticular conditions." The pathophysiology of bypass arthritis-dermatitis syndrome is straightforward and linear and easy to understand: ❶ altered intestinal structure and function leads to bacterial overgrowth and compromise of the intestinal mucosa, ❷ bacterial overgrowth and compromise of the intestinal mucosa leads to increased absorption of bacteria and bacterial antigens, perhaps as well as food antigens, ❸ increased absorption of bacteria and bacterial antigens leads to antibody formation, ❹ combination of bacterial antigens with antibodies leads to immune complex formation, ❺ immune complexes have a biologic proclivity for deposition in the joints, vessels, kidneys, skin, alveoli, and serosal surfaces, ❻ deposition of immune complexes in any tissue results in a localized immune response with resultant inflammation regardless of the primary origin of the antigens from the overgrowth/overcolonization of bacteria. Per the authors, "The pathogenesis of intestinal bypass arthritis involves bacterial overgrowth and mucosal alterations in the defunctionalized segment of small intestine, i.e., the 'blind loop'. ... "The blunted villi allow increased absorption of bacteria and bacterial products, leading to dissemination of high molecular weight immune complexes containing bacterial products." These "immune complexes of enteric antigens" are then deposited in the joints, skin, vessels, kidneys, and pulmonary alveoli to respectively produce arthritis, dermatitis, vasculitis, nephritis, and pneumonitis.

New-onset inflammatory joint symptoms are noted in 6-52% of patients following jejunoileal bypass. Most commonly the inflammatory arthritis is seen in females, and the presentation "mimics early rheumatoid arthritis" with

Intestinal arthritis-dermatitis syndrome: rheumatic-inflammatory complications of SIBO-induced systemic inflammation and immune complex deposition

1. **Arthritis***‡—Most commonly of the peripheral joints but may also include the spine and sacroiliac joints; may be destructive or nondestructive, with or without RF and serologic evidence of immune complex mediation such as hypocomplementemia
2. **Dermatitis***‡—"The most common non-articular inflammatory findings in patients with intestinal bypass arthritis involve the skin, reported in as many as 77% of patients." Rashes may be urticarial, maculopapular, papulovesicular or vesiculopustular affecting any part of the face, trunk or extremities
3. Myalgia
4. Myositis, polymyositis‡
5. Pleuritis‡
6. Pericarditis‡
7. Raynaud's phenomenon
8. Vasculitis, leukocytoclastic angiitis*‡
9. Oral ulceration‡
10. Tenosynovitis
11. Paresthesias, peripheral neuropathy*
12. Carpal tunnel syndrome

* Note that these are common clinical manifestations of underlying immune complex pathophysiology.
‡ Note that many of these clinical manifestations of bypass-induced intestinal dysbiosis are clinical manifestations of—and indeed components of the diagnostic criteria for—prototypic autoimmune diseases such as systemic lupus erythematosus.

Ross et al. *Baillieres Clin Rheumatol.* 1989

involvement of the hands, wrists, and knees and less commonly the spine and sacroiliac joints. Morning stiffness—a finding classic for inflammatory joint disease—is common. The arthritis is generally nondestructive; however, some post-bypass patients will develop periarticular erosions and sclerosis—findings common to rheumatoid arthritis. Tests for antinuclear antibodies (ANA), rheumatoid factor (RF), and serum complement are generally normal, but some patients will develop cryoglobulinemia due to immune complex formation and others positive for HLA-B27 will develop spondylitis. "Therefore", the authors note in 1989, "the diagnosis of intestinal bypass arthritis remains primarily clinical." Very interestingly, one patient developed "classic rheumatoid arthritis with erosions and rheumatoid factors following jejunoileal bypass. ... ...the patient experienced complete remission of musculoskeletal disease soon after revision [surgical reversal] of the bypass..." The vast majority (up to 77%) of patients with bypass-induced dysbiotic arthritis develop skin inflammation alongside; "The most common non-articular inflammatory findings in patients with intestinal bypass arthritis involve the skin, reported in as many as 77% of patients. ... Typical rashes may be urticarial, maculopapular, papulovesicular or vesiculopustular... Any part of the face, trunk or extremities may be involved."

Beside and beyond the merely symptomatic treatments such as NSAIDs—which notoriously increase intestinal permeability and may therefore contribute to the pathophysiology of intestinal dysbiosis—ultimate treatments for bypass dermatitis-arthritis syndrome are either antimicrobial therapy to eradicate the intestinal bacterial overgrowth or surgical restoration of the original intestinal anatomy. Impressively, surgical restoration of normal anatomy can completely resolve the condition within 48 hours, thereby proving the cause-and-effect relationship. **Broad-spectrum antimicrobial drugs are used empirically: tetracycline, metronidazole, trimethoprim/sulfamethoxazole, and clindamycin.** Oral corticosteroids may be used to help control the inflammation; adverse effects including exacerbation of diabetes and hypertension, as well as promotion of additional bacterial overgrowth due to intestinal immunosuppression are well-known. Importantly, "bowel bypass disease without bowel bypass" can occur secondary to any condition that promotes bacterial overgrowth of the intestines and the resultant immune complex formation; the term used to describe this phenomenon is "bowel-associated dermatitis and arthritis."

- Pro-inflammatory effect of *Lactobacillus rhamnosus Lcr35 (PLoS One* 2011 Apr[347])： This experimental study suggests that some intestinal bacteria—in this case, a specific strain of *Lactobacillus* identified as *Lactobacillus rhamnosus Lcr35*—can incite a proinflammatory effect. The possibility exists that the physiologic consequences of an individual bacterium might be different *in vivo* when intermixed with the effects of other microbes; however, a reasonable interpretation of these data is that *Lactobacillus rhamnosus* promotes inflammation and should therefore be avoided in patients already experiencing excessive inflammation. The authors introduce their paper appropriately by stating, "Some [probiotic] strains modulate the cytokine production of dendritic cells (DCs) in vitro and induce a regulatory response, while others induce conversely a pro-inflammatory response." Results of this experiment showed that, by use of DNA microarray and qRT-PCR analysis, the probiotic induced a large-scale change in gene expression (nearly 1,700 modulated genes, with 3-fold changes), but only with high doses. Cytokine measurements showed strong dose-dependent increases in pro-Th1/Th17 cytokine levels (TNFα, IL-1β, IL-12p70, IL-12p40 and IL-23) contrasted with only a slight increase in anti-inflammatory IL-10. Very importantly, the bacteria were killed prior to cell exposure ("Before being added to the DC samples, the bacterial cells were inactivated by exposure to UV for 40 min. Successful inactivation of bacteria was assessed by plating the final suspension on agar plates.) and the significance of this is that the pro-inflammatory effects of the bacteria were not offset by the anti-inflammatory effects of the microbial metabolites This article is noteworthy for showing the molecular evidence of dose-dependent inflammation induction by a bacterium generally considered to be among a group of beneficial bacteria; many people consider *"Lactobacillus"* as a group to be exclusively beneficial while this evidence demonstrates pro-inflammatory effects. Bacterial overgrowth of the small bowel (aka, small intestine bacterial overgrowth [SIBO]) commonly includes a mix of Gram-negatives with Gram-positives, anaerobes with aerobes, and so-called "beneficial" bacteria along with pathogens and potential pathogens.

4. <mark>Reactive arthritis (ReA)</mark>: **Reactive arthritis is defined as an inflammatory arthritis secondary to an *identified* infection;** the distribution is generally symmetrical and peripheral, however, axial variants—spondyloarthropathy or (preferred) spondyloarthritis—can exist independently or in conjunction with peripheral arthritis, tenosynovitis, and enthesitis. An earlier eponym was Reiter's syndrome, but this term has been formally retracted from the biomedical literature because Hans Reiter for whom this was named was "a Nazi war criminal responsible for heinous atrocities that violated the precepts of humanity, ethics, and professionalism."[348] Attentive readers are invited to re-read the definition and note the anthropocentric (physician-centric) component—namely that this disease only formally exists to the extent that the physician encounters the

Reactive arthritis—defined and described
"Reactive arthritis is a painful form of inflammatory arthritis that develops in reaction to an infection by bacteria."
• Can affect the heels, toes, fingers, palms, soles, eyes (conjunctivitis, iritis, uveitis), low back (spondylitis, sacroiliitis), and joints, especially of the knees or ankles,
• Triggering infection is usually GU (*Chlamydia trachomatis* urethritis) or GI (*Campylobacter, Salmonella, Shigella* and *Yersinia*)
• Most commonly affected are men 20-50y
• Self-resolving or chronic
• HLA-B27 is associated with more acute, severe, and durable disease
• Treatment mainstays are NSAIDs, DMARDs and steroids
• "New research suggests that a prolonged course of two or more antibiotics might be effective in patients with chronic Chlamydia-induced reactive arthritis. However, more studies are needed."
American College of Rheumatology. Reactive arthritis. February 2013. rheumatology.org/Practice/Clinical/Patients/Diseases_And_Conditions/Reactive_Arthritis

[347] Evrard B, et al. Dose-Dependent Immunomodulation of Human Dendritic Cells by the Probiotic Lactobacillus rhamnosus Lcr35. *PLoS One*. 2011 Apr 18;6(4):e18735
[348] Panush RS, Wallace DJ, Dorff RE, Engleman EP. Retraction of the suggestion to use the term "Reiter's syndrome" sixty-five years later. *Arthritis Rheum*. 2007 Feb;56(2):693-4

infection; this, in turn, is dependent upon the physician's vigilance, skill, and available technology. The condition is also commonly described as "seronegative" because—specifically—blood tests for rheumatoid factor are negative; seronegative is a misnomer because the term implies that *all* blood tests are negative. Other forms of seronegative/reactive arthritis include psoriatic arthritis, ankylosing spondylitis, and enteropathic arthritis/spondylitis[349]; this should lead physicians to appreciate that these latter conditions are also infection/microbe-triggered, but alas this has not taken effect. By acceptance of the first premise, the others follow by logical extension:

1) **Defined prototype—Reactive arthritis is a microbe-triggered inflammatory musculoskeletal condition**: ReA is commonly noted to have extra-articular inflammatory manifestations affecting the eyes and skin; the condition may be mild or severe, acute or subacute, and either self-resolving, relapsing, or chronic. Molecular mimicry and immune cross-reactivity are the interconnections between the commonly noted HLA-B27 and microbial infections; several microbial proteins share amino acid homology with HLA-B27.

2) **Given that the microbe alone is not sufficient, enhancing host resistance/tolerance becomes a major clinical goal**: Given that **the triggering infection is "necessary but not sufficient"**, clinicians should consider the factors that make some individuals susceptible and others resistant; by identifying these nonmicrobial host factors, clinicians can implement these variables as therapeutics when possible.

3) **One major "infection" could be molecularly mimicked by several milder colonizations**: If one major microbial trigger can cause "full-blown" reactive arthritis, then a combination of minor microbial triggers would be capable of triggering milder or otherwise different variants of the same. Overt infections can trigger objective/real pathologically-defined musculoskeletal inflammation and extraskeletal inflammation of the eyes and skin; therefore, subclinical/mild/occult infections/colonizations/dysbiosis are capable of inducing milder or otherwise different variants of the same. Hence, the importance of the concept of *multi*focal *poly*dysbiosis which could be summarily equivalent and/or sufficiently similar from molecular and immunologic standpoints to *mono*focal *uni*dysbiosis.

4) **Persistence of inflammation following resolution or antimicrobial clearance of infection suggests retention of the microbial trigger (failure of clearance or retained antigen), microbe-independent epitope spreading, bystander activation, or other perpetuating factor—none of which are "idiopathic"**: Microbe-triggered inflammation/autoimmunity can persist following antimicrobial treatment for the following reasons: ❶ failure of clearance of the microbe despite quantitative reduction, i.e., the microbe is diminished but not eradicated, leading to a "smoldering" colonization despite the disappearance of the "flaming" symptomatic infection, ❷ microbial antigens can persist in synovial fluid for years following a triggering infection, ❸ epitope spreading occurs when inflammation triggers elaboration of previously occult self-antigens and/or immune responses toward previously tolerated self-antigens, ❹ bystander activation can occur during acute inflammation and can incite tissue damage that then becomes self-perpetuating via release of inflammatory mediators and DAMP/PAMP receptor agonists, ❺ the possibility exists that factors such as antibiotic-induced mitochondrial dysfunction or infection/inflammation-induced increased intestinal permeability might be sufficient to perpetuate bystander activation and immune cross-reactivity to epitopes (microbial or human) which were previously tolerated.

Microbes known to trigger systemic inflammation and reactive arthritis are common

1. *Shigella* spp.
2. *Salmonella* spp.
3. *Yersinia* spp.
4. *Campylobacter jejuni*
5. *Klebsiella pneumoniae**
6. *Brucella* spp.
7. *Clostridium difficile*
8. *Giardia lamblia*
9. *Entamoeba* spp.
10. *Blastocystis hominis*
11. *Cryptosporidia*
12. *Chlamydia trachomatis*
13. *Chlamydophila pneumoniae**
14. *Ureoplasma ureolyticum**
15. *Mycoplasma hominis*
16. *Neisseria gonorrhoea*
17. *Streptococci**
18. *Staphylococci**
19. *Leptospira*
20. *Borrelia*
21. *Mycobacterium tuberculosis*
22. *Gardenella vaginalis*

Int J Prev Med. 2013 Jul

* Note that some of these microbes are considered "normal" flora, and they are therefore **commonly overlooked causes of persistent inflammation and autoimmunity**.

---

[349] National Institute of Arthritis and Musculoskeletal and Skin Diseases. Questions and Answers about Reactive Arthritis. 2013 Oct. niams.nih.gov/health_info/reactive_arthritis/

In conclusion, **this survey of the literature has supported the concept that dysbiosis can contribute to pain, systemic inflammation, immune activation, and various forms of clinical symptomatology by numerous mechanisms**. Clinical experience has demonstrated repeatedly that eradicating dysbiosis helps normalize immune function, alleviate autoimmunity and allergy, reduce inflammation, improve detoxification, and to help improve and frequently "cure" people of their previously "incurable" multiple chemical sensitivity, environmental illness, and inflammatory disorders, whether metabolic, allergic, or autoimmune.

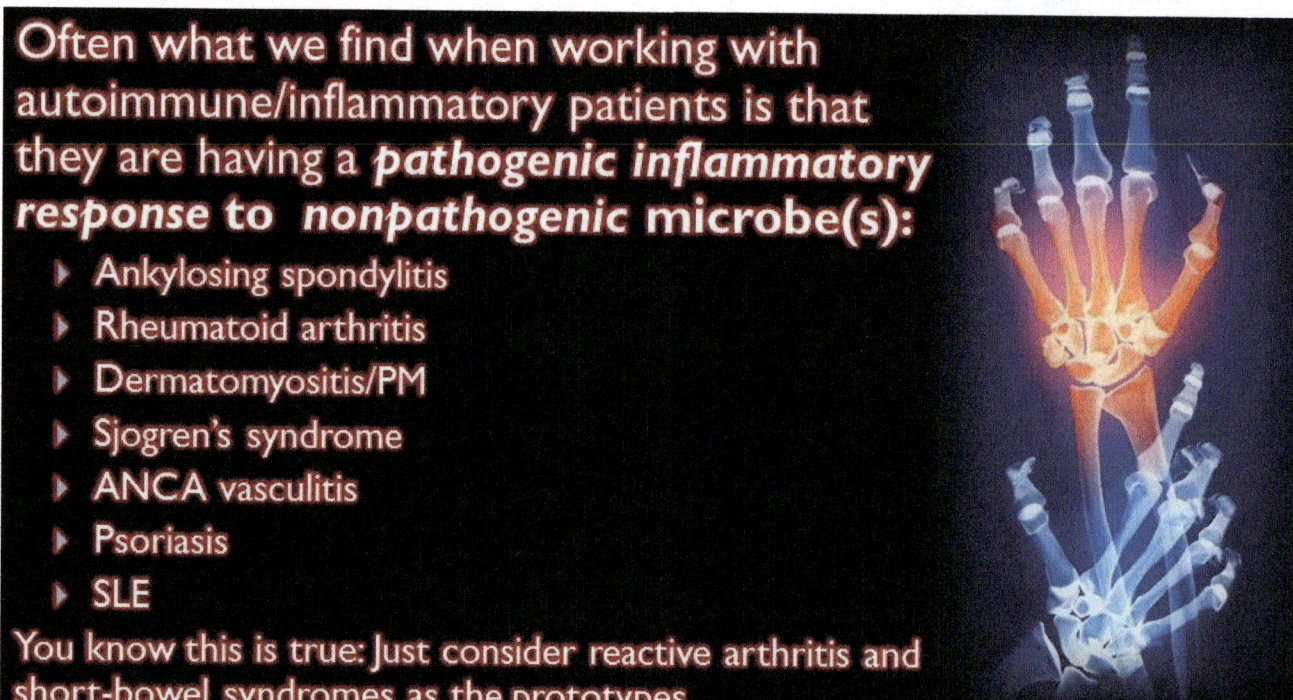

Often what we find when working with autoimmune/inflammatory patients is that they are having a *pathogenic inflammatory response to nonpathogenic microbe(s)*:

▸ Ankylosing spondylitis
▸ Rheumatoid arthritis
▸ Dermatomyositis/PM
▸ Sjogren's syndrome
▸ ANCA vasculitis
▸ Psoriasis
▸ SLE

You know this is true: Just consider reactive arthritis and short-bowel syndromes as the prototypes.

Dysbiotic inflammation—beyond the microbe: "Often what we find when working with autoimmune/inflammatory patients is that they are having a pathogenic inflammatory response to a nonpathogenic microbe"—I had been saying this for many years in presentations and my writings; finally in 2013, a near-quote made headlines "inflammation triggered by an immune response to otherwise harmless microorganisms" and "The inflammatory response and the resulting damage from the prolonged inflammation are caused by the body's own immune response to harmless microbiota."[350] Remember, we are not looking for classic "infection" here; we are looking to determine which underlying disruptions may be exacerbating inflammation and the patient's symptomatology. We have to look beyond the disease-associated characteristics of the microbe to see the patient's individualized response to the microbe. Dysbiosis in one patient may present with dermatitis, while [what appears to be] the same microbial imbalance in another patient can present as peripheral neuropathy or inflammatory arthritis. For one of my more recent conversations on these ideas and this particular image, access my 2015 presentation at London's Royal Society of Medicine: https://vimeo.com/123715277 / https://vimeo.com/ichnfm/2015rsm.

---

[350] Harmless Members of Microbiome Spark Immune Reaction. sciencedaily.com/releases/2013/12/131219134455.htm Dec. 19, 2013. Original source: With Sinus Study, SLU Investigators Add Immune System Dimension to Discussion of Microbiota and Disease. slu.edu/x89847.xml

Active learning and reflection

Use the space below to list as many of the previously detailed mechanisms as possible:

1.
2.
3.
4.
5.
6.
7.
8.
9.
10.
11.
12.
13.
14.
15.
16.
17.
18.
19.
20.

Use the space below to describe—in narrative format— to an educated patient or professional colleague how bacteria can contribute to non-infectious metabolic/inflammatory disease:

Autointoxication, auto-brewery syndrome

Syndromes of pain, fatigue, depression

Dysbiotic arthropathy, dysbiotic dermatitis, dysbiotic vasculitis

Reactive arthritis (ReA)

Diabetes, insulin resistance via systemic inflammation

The Seven Main Loci of Dysbiosis

For a microorganism to induce a systemic proinflammatory immunodysregulatory response in a human, the microbe or its metabolic products must be exposed to a susceptible host. Non-infectious microbial overgrowth can occur inside the body (gastrointestinal, sinus, respiratory tract and lungs, genitourinary, or orodental), on the surface of the body (dermal), or outside of the body (environmental). The adverse physiologic and clinical effects can be similar regardless of the location of the microorganism. The term "dysbiosis" is classically applied to harmful, non-infectious relationships between the human host and yeast, bacteria, protozoans, amoebas, or other "parasites" located specifically in the gastrointestinal tract, and "dysbiosis" is now an accepted term in the medical literature.[351] However, we must also appreciate that harmful, noninfectious microbe-host interactions can also occur when microbes are localized in the sinuses, oral cavity, genitourinary tract, skin, and in the external environment. I prefer to use a broad definition of dysbiosis that implies "a relationship of non-infectious host-microorganism interaction that adversely affects the human host" and then to specify the subtype based on the location: gastrointestinal, oral, sinus, genitourinary, dermatologic, or environmental. Gastrointestinal dysbiosis is clearly the prototype for understanding other types of dysbiosis; this is because it seems to be the most common form of dysbiosis, perhaps due to the large numbers and types of microbes in the gut and the extensive surface area of the gastrointestinal tract. Clinicians must appreciate the anatomical interconnections that can segue one type of loci of dysbiosis into another. Orodental dysbiosis may result in gastrointestinal dysbiosis if the microbes can survive in the gastrointestinal tract. Sinus dysbiosis could likewise drain into the lungs and gastrointestinal tract. In women, close relationships between gastrointestinal dysbiosis and vaginal dysbiosis are well documented.[352] Bacterial and fungal superantigens from the surrounding environment can contribute to a proinflammatory response in the lungs and on the skin and which becomes systemic, leading to autoimmunity.[353,354]

Correlation of dysbiotic locations with inflammatory (especially autoimmune and rheumatic) diseases: a rough guide showing relative contributions and strength of research; rheumatoid arthritis, reactive arthritis, and psoriasis have the greatest association with multiple sites of dysbiosis with multiple microbes (multifocal polydysbiosis)

Disease & dysbiosis	Gastro-intestinal	Orodental	Sino-respiratory	Genito-urinary	Tissue (including viruses)	Cutaneous	Environ-mental
SLE	✓		✓		✓ HERV		
RA	✓	✓	✓	✓	✓ (osteomyel: one case)		
ReA	✓		✓	✓	✓ pneumon		✓
Psor	✓	✓	✓	✓	✓	✓	
PM-DM			✓				
Spond-AS	✓			✓			
Sclerod	✓				✓		
ANCA-v	✓		✓				
Vasc	✓				✓ viral hep		
Behc		✓	✓			✓	
Neuro	✓			✓			✓
DM	✓	✓			✓		
MS	✓				✓		
✓ = **Positive research and clinical evidence in humans**; SLE = lupus; RA = rheumatoid arthritis; ReA = reactive arthritis; Psor = Psoriasis or psoriatic arthritis; PM-DM = polymyositis/dermatomyositis; PMR = polymyalgia rheumatica; Sjo = Sjogren's syndrome; Spond-AS = spondyloarthropathy and ankylosing spondylitis; Sclerod = scleroderma; ANCA-v= ANCA-associated vasculitis; Vasc = vasculitis; Behc = Behcet's syndrome; Neuro = neurologic autoimmunity; DM = diabetes mellitus; MS = multiple sclerosis; Osteomyel = osteomyelitis; Pneumon = pneumonia.							

[351] Tamboli CP, Neut C, Desreumaux P, Colombel JF. Dysbiosis in inflammatory bowel disease. *Gut.* 2004 Jan;53(1):1-4
[352] "The results showed that if C albicans was cultured from the vagina, it was always found in the stool... The gut-reservoir concept may well apply to other forms of candidiasis." Miles MR, Olsen L, Rogers A. Recurrent vaginal candidiasis. Importance of an intestinal reservoir. *JAMA.* 1977 Oct 24;238(17):1836-7
[353] Campbell et al. Neural autoantibodies and neurophysiologic abnormalities in patients exposed to molds in water-damaged buildings. *Arch Environ Health.* 2003 Aug;58:464-74
[354] Gray et al. Mixed mold mycotoxicosis: immunological changes in humans following exposure in water-damaged buildings. *Arch Environ Health* 2003 Jul;58:410-20

Gastrointestinal dysbiosis: Overview of the prototype of all forms of dysbiosis

We all have bacteria and occasionally small quantities of yeast in our intestines, and this is normal and generally healthy. However, problems arise when these yeast/bacteria become imbalanced or when *harmful* yeast, bacteria, parasites take up residence within the gut. Particularly in the European research literature, this condition has been more widely researched and described as "dysbacteriosis" or "dysbacterosis."[355] These latter terms are somewhat unfortunate because they imply that the problem has a *bacterial* origin, which is partially (and therefore significantly) misleading since dysbiosis commonly involves bacteria *and yeast* (including but not limited to *Candida albicans*) and commonly other harmful non-bacterial microbes such as *Giardia lamblia, Blastocystis hominis, Endolimax nana, Entamoeba histolytica* and a cast of other malcontents that adversely affect the overall health of their human host.[356] "Candidiasis" and yeast-related problems have been described in the research literature and general press.[357] Dysbiosis is probably a major aspect of the phenomenon that was previously referred to in the medical literature as "autointoxication" and which was effectively treated with dietary modifications, nutritional supplementation, and colonic irrigation.[358] **Given that endotoxin/lipopolysaccharide is one of the major activators of nuclear factor kappa-B (NFkB)[359], and that NFkB activation is a major rate-limiting step in the production of**

> **The gut microbiome orchestrates human metabolism, immunity, gene expression**
>
> "The hundred trillion bacteria in the body of an adult human contain about 4 million distinct bacterial genes, with **more than 95% of them located in the large intestine**. Since most of these genes encode for enzymes and structural proteins that influence the functioning of mammalian cells, **the gut microbiome can be viewed as an anaerobic bioreactor programmed to synthesize molecules which direct the mammalian immune system, modify the mammalian epigenome, and regulate host metabolism**."
>
> Galland L. Gut microbiome and brain. *J Med Food*. 2014

proinflammatory cytokines and in the induction of proinflammatory enzymes such as cyclooxygenase, lipoxygenase, and inducible nitric oxide synthase,[360] then the link between dysbiosis and systemic inflammation becomes clear: gastrointestinal bacterial overgrowth leads to excess production and absorption of endotoxin, which then initiates immune dysfunction and a systemic proinflammatory response. Intestinal overgrowth of gram-negative bacteria is, in this author's opinion, highly problematic since endotoxin/lipopolysaccharide can cause intestinal inflammation, leaky gut, inhibition of hepatic detoxification, hyperalgesia[361], brain dysfunction[362] and immune dysfunction by acting as superantigen(s).[363] **Indeed, many of the systemic manifestations associated with dysbiosis are clearly not mediated by the infecting organism but are mediated by the host response to microbial debris/metabolites/"toxins" and to the systemic dysfunction induced by increased intestinal permeability and subsequent alterations in hepatic and immune function. Thus, the sequelae of dysbiosis are mediated by alterations in human metabolic/immunologic physiology rather than being directly caused by the microbe.** Different microbes are classically linked with respective human autoimmune/inflammatory diseases, for example *Entamoeba histolytica* with Henoch Schonlein purpura[364], *Klebsiella pneumoniae* with ankylosing spondylitis[365], *Proteus mirabilis* with rheumatoid arthritis[366,367] and ankylosing spondylitis[368], *Pseudomonas aeruginosa* with multiple sclerosis[369], and *Helicobacter pylori* with reactive arthritis.[370]

[355] Lizko NN. Problems of microbial ecology in man space mission. *Acta Astronaut*. 1991;23:163-9

[356] Galland L. Intestinal protozoan infection is a common unsuspected cause of chronic illness. *J Advancement Med*. 1989;2: 539-552

[357] Crook W. *The Yeast Connection*. Professional Books. Jackson. Tennessee. 1983

[358] "The writer has observed numerous cases suffering from such conditions as chronic arthritis, hypertension, coronary disease, chronic abdominal distention, constipation, and colitis, in which the element of constipation, auto-intoxication and possible colon infection seemed to play a prominent part, which responded very satisfactorily to colonic irrigations after failure to improve following the usual forms of medical treatment." Snyder RG. The value of colonic irrigations in countering auto-intoxication of intestinal origin. *Medl Clin North America* 1939; May: 781-788

[359] D'Acquisto F, May MJ, Ghosh S. Inhibition of Nuclear Factor Kappa B (NF-B). *Mol Interv*. 2002 Feb;2(1):22-35 molinterv.aspetjournals.org/cgi/content/full/2/1/22

[360] Tak PP, Firestein GS. NFkB: a key role in inflammatory diseases. *J Clin Invest*. 2001 Jan;107(1):7-1 jci.org/cgi/content/full/107/1/7

[361] "We have recently shown that 'illness'-inducing agents, such as intraperitoneally administered lipopolysaccharide (LPS; bacterial endotoxin), can produce prolonged hyperalgesia." Watkins et al. Illness-induced hyperalgesia is mediated by spinal neuropeptides and excitatory amino acids. *Brain Res*. 1994 Nov 21;664(1-2):17-24

[362] "The immunogen E. coli lipopolysaccharide (LPS, endotoxin) has been widely used to stimulate immune/inflammatory responses both systemically and in the CNS... LPS appears to release glutamate, which then acts at non-NMDA receptors to remove the voltage-sensitive Mg2+ block of NMDA receptors, thus permitting NMDA receptors to be activated..." Wang et al. The bacterial endotoxin lipopolysaccharide causes rapid inappropriate excitation in rat cortex. *J Neurochem*. 1999 Feb;72:652-60

[363] "Superantigens are potent activators of CD4+ T cells, causing rapid and massive proliferation of cells and cytokine production... Superantigens have also been implicated in acute diseases such as food poisoning and TSS, and in chronic diseases such as psoriasis and rheumatoid arthritis." Torres et al. Superantigens. *Exp Biol Med*. 2001 Mar:164-76

[364] Demircin G, Oner A, Erdogan O, Bulbul M, Memis L. Henoch Schonlein purpura and amebiasis. *Acta Paediatr Jpn*. 1998 Oct; 40(5): 489-91

[365] Ahmadi K, et al. Antibodies to Klebsiella pneumoniae lipopolysaccharide in patients with ankylosing spondylitis. *Br J Rheumatol*. 1998 Dec;37(12):1330-3

[366] Ebringer A, Rashid T, Wilson C. Rheumatoid arthritis: proposal for the use of anti-microbial therapy in early cases. *Scand J Rheumatol* 2003;32(1):2-11

[367] Rashid T, et al. Proteus IgG antibodies and C-reactive protein in English, Norwegian and Spanish patients with rheumatoid arthritis. *Clin Rheumatol* 1999;18(3):190-5

[368] Wilson C, et al. Cytotoxicity responses to Peptide antigens in rheumatoid arthritis and ankylosing spondylitis. *J Rheumatol* 2003 May;30(5):972-8

[369] Hughes LE, et al. Antibody responses to Acinetobacter spp. and Pseudomonas aeruginosa in multiple sclerosis. *Clin Diagn Lab Immunol*. 2001 Nov;8(6):1181-8

[370] "... HP may be included in the list of possible arthritis triggering microbes."Melby et al.Helicobacter pylori--a trigger of reactive arthritis?*Infection*.1999;27:252-5

Gastrointestinal dysbiosis: Subtypes and categorization

Building upon a previous four-subtype categorization proposed by Galland[371], here I describe eight different types of gastrointestinal dysbiosis:

<table>
<tr><td colspan="2">Major (nonexclusive) types of dysbiosis</td></tr>
<tr><td>1.</td><td>Insufficiency dysbiosis</td></tr>
<tr><td>2.</td><td>Bacterial overgrowth, small intestinal bacterial/microbial overgrowth (SIBO/SIMO)</td></tr>
<tr><td>3.</td><td>Immunosuppressive dysbiosis</td></tr>
<tr><td>4.</td><td>Hypersensitivity/allergic dysbiosis</td></tr>
<tr><td>5.</td><td>Inflammatory dysbiosis</td></tr>
<tr><td>6.</td><td>Amoebas, cysts, protozoas, and other parasites</td></tr>
<tr><td>7.</td><td>Metabolic/dysmetabolic dysbiosis</td></tr>
<tr><td>8.</td><td>Neurotoxic dysbiosis</td></tr>
</table>

1. <u>Insufficiency dysbiosis</u>: Beneficial bacteria in the intestines helps to normalize systemic immune response and promote proper digestion, elimination and nutrient absorption. Absence of "good bacteria" such as *Bifidobacteria* and *Lactobacillus* ❶ leaves the gastrointestinal tract vulnerable to colonization with pathogens (reduced colonization resistance [CR]) which allows/growth of pathogens and the potential pathogens (pathobionts) and to the development of SIBO, ❷ promotes increased bacterial translocation (with important inflammatory [e.g., NFkB and TLR] and immunologic [e.g., ANA] consequences) and ❸ impairs optimal development of Treg. Numerous studies have documented the powerful benefits of supplementing with good bacteria (probiotics), supporting their growth with fermentable carbohydrates such as inulin and fructooligosaccharides (prebiotics), and by co-administering probiotics with prebiotics (synbiotics). An excellent narrative review by Velasquez-Manoff in *Nature* (2015 Feb)[372] provides a succinct and contemporary understanding of insufficiency dysbiosis including and beyond what we have appreciated previously and what is readily noted on stool culture results—see sample stool test results that follow in this section. What we have come to realize over the past few years and—*importantly*—what we can now observe with modern stool testing is that the presence of the beneficial "clostridial cluster" is important for promoting immunomodulation, clinically beneficial by its promotion of a tolerogenic, anti-inflammatory, anti-allergy, and anti-autoimmune phenotype. Clinicians must distinguish between the harmful *Clostridium difficile* which is notorious for causing recalcitrant life-threatening diarrhea from the beneficial clostridial groups IV (4), IX (9), XIVa (14a) and XVIII (18); within clostridial cluster 4 is *Faecalibacterium prausnitzii,* which appears prominent with regard to anti-inflammatory and anti-obesity benefits. At least 46 different Clostridial species exist as part of the gastrointestinal microbiome. Velasquez-Manoff clarifies, "Dubbed 'clostridial clusters', these microbes are distantly related to *Clostridium difficile*, a scourge of hospitals and an all-too-frequent cause of death by diarrhea. But where *C. difficile* prompts endless inflammation, bleeding and potentially catastrophic loss of fluids, the clostridial clusters do just the opposite—they keep the gut barrier tight and healthy, and they soothe the immune system."; he also describes *Faecalibacterium prausnitzii* as "powerfully anti-inflammatory" and a "peacekeeping microbe", notably absent in patients with IBD, especially Crohn's disease. Species of the genus Clostridium are all Gram-positive spore-formers; they can be killed by antibacterial drugs, including vancomycin (discussed later); beneficial clostridial clusters induce anti-inflammatory benefits specifically but not exclusively via induction of regulatory T-cells (Treg) and a robust protective mucus barrier in the gut. Again per Velasquez-Manoff, "Mucus serves both as an antimicrobial repellent and a growth medium for friendly bacteria. ...these clostridial clusters may promote gut health and a balanced immune system by ensuring a healthy flow of mucus. ...these microbes may favorably shape the greater gut ecosystem by stimulating secretion of the sugars other friendly microbes graze on." In humans, dietary inclusion of *fermented foods* such as Chinese yam and bitter melon and *fermentable carbohydrates* (e.g., soluble fiber, inulin, fructooligosaccharides) can promote growth of *Faecalibacterium prausnitzii*, which in one impressive case report involving the aforementioned dietary changes "increased from an undetectable percentage to 14.5% of total gut bacteria."[373]; of additional note from this same article is the observation that the plant alkaloid berberine (discussed later) helps to offset the obesogenic effect of a high-fat diet via favorable modulation of the gut microbiome. Clinicians should seek to optimize—generally by numeric force except in cases of SIBO—the keystone microbes such as *Faecalibacterium prausnitzii* and the other more commonly known probiotic bacteria such as Bifidobacteria Lactobacillus, and Streptococcus thermophilus; these bacteria provide

---

[371] Attributed to Galland L. "Fire in the belly: update on gut fermentation." Presented to Great Lakes Association of Clinical Medicine, circa 1996. Also, personal email from Leo Galland dated October 28, 2005: "I have used the concept of 4 types of dysbiosis (putrefaction, fermentation, depletion and immune activation forms) in several presentations and in one written document."
[372] Velasquez-Manoff M. Gut microbiome: the peacekeepers. *Nature*. 2015 Feb 26;518(7540):S3-11
[373] Hvistendahl M. My microbiome and me. *Science*. 2012 Jun 8;336(6086):1248-50

important benefits directly (e.g., colonization resistance, metabolites such as short-chain fatty acids [SCFA]) but perhaps even more importantly shape the ecosystem of the gut and its trillions of microbes.

2. <u>Bacterial overgrowth, small intestinal bacterial/microbial overgrowth (SIBO/SIMO)</u>: This is a quantitative excess bacteria—commonly accompanied by excess or abnormal yeast—in the gut. Bacterial overgrowth of the small bowel is a well-established medical problem that is particularly common in patients who are diabetic (with gastroparesis), elderly (with atrophic gastritis), immunosuppressed (such as with corticosteroids/prednisone[374,375]), naturally hypochlorhydric or iatrogenically hypochlorhydric due to acid-blocking drugs.[376,377] SIBO/SIMO commonly results in gas, bloating, malabsorption, constipation and/or diarrhea, "irritable bowel syndrome" (IBS), as well as myalgias and systemic immune activation.[378] **Animal studies have proven that peripheral arthritis can activated/reactivated by inducing bacterial overgrowth of the small bowel; endotoxins and other microbial products stimulate a systemic proinflammatory state which re-activates inflammation of joints and periarticular structures.**[379] Bacterial overgrowth of the small intestine is seen in 84% of patients with irritable bowel syndrome[380] and in **100% of patients with fibromyalgia**.[381] Endotoxin causes impairment of muscle function (lowered lactate threshold[382]) and promotes pain sensitization (at the levels of peripheral tissues/nerves, spinal cord, and brain[383]) thereby adding mechanistic explanation to the link between intestinal dysbiosis and chronic neuromusculoskeletal pain, especially fibromyalgia and complex regional pain syndrome.[384] Drs Over and Bucknall[385] describe a patient with **systemic sclerosis** who achieved **long-term remission** of her disease following **antibiotic treatment for**

> **Clinical pearl: Dietary sulfur intolerance and dysbiosis**
>
> Some patients with dysbiosis clearly do not tolerate high-sulfur foods and nutritional supplements such as dairy/milk/cheese, eggs, poultry (including chicken broth), sulfited wines (and perhaps drugs), cruciferous vegetables, NAC and lipoic acid. The reasons for this are categorized as ❶ <u>sulfur-stimulated microbial growth</u>—dietary sulfur contributes to the growth of some yeast and several sulfur-reducing bacteria, and ❷ <u>conversion of dietary sulfur to H2S</u>—resulting mitochondrial dysfunction and intestinal stasis. When patients experience a "bloom" of sulfur-reducing bacteria and/or overproduction of H2S, they will note very distinct episodes of dyscognition, fatigue, sulphurous flatus, lower body temperature, and/or headache and myalgia.

intestinal bacterial overgrowth. Bacterial overgrowth generally leads to pathologically synergistic clinical effects mediated by fermentation, putrefaction, constipation, increased enterohepatic recycling, bile acid deconjugation, malabsorption (particularly fat-soluble nutrients and vitamin B-12), nutritional deficiencies, sugar cravings (likely secondary to bacterial tryptophanase-induced tryptophan deficiency), increased intestinal permeability, immune complex formation, and induction of a systemic proinflammatory response with immune complexes that is particularly prone to manifest as vasculitis and arthritis.[386,387,388] SIBO is generally anticipated to result in increased intestinal permeability due to microbial elaboration of proteases,

---

[374] "A 63-year-old man with systemic lupus erythematosus and selective IgA deficiency developed intractable diarrhoea the day after treatment with prednisone, 50 mg daily, was started. The diarrhoea was considered to be caused by bacterial overgrowth and was later successfully treated with doxycycline." Denison H, Wallerstedt S. Bacterial overgrowth after high-dose corticosteroid treatment. *Scand J Gastroenterol.* 1989 Jun;24(5):561-4

[375] "These bacteria also translocated to the mesenteric lymph nodes in mice injected with cyclophosphamide or prednisone." Berg RD, Wommack E, Deitch EA. Immunosuppression and intestinal bacterial overgrowth synergistically promote bacterial translocation. *Arch Surg.* 1988 Nov;123(11):1359-64

[376] "SIBO, assessed by GHBT, occurs significantly more frequently among long term PPI users than patients with IBS or control subjects. High dose therapy with rifaximin eradicated 87%-91% of cases of SIBO in patients who continued PPI therapy." Lombardo et al. Increased incidence of small intestinal bacterial overgrowth during proton pump inhibitor therapy. *Clin Gastroenterol Hepatol.* 2010 Jun;8(6):504-8

[377] Saltzman JR, Russell RM. Nutritional consequences of intestinal bacterial overgrowth. *Compr Ther.* 1994;20(9):523-30

[378] Lin HC. Small intestinal bacterial overgrowth: a framework for understanding irritable bowel syndrome. *JAMA.* 2004 Aug 18;292(7):852-8

[379] Lichtman et al. Reactivation of arthritis induced by small bowel bacterial overgrowth in rats: role of cytokines, bacteria, bacterial polymers. *Infect Immun* 1995 Jun;63:2295-301

[380] Lin HC. Small intestinal bacterial overgrowth: a framework for understanding irritable bowel syndrome. *JAMA.* 2004 Aug 18;292(7):852-8

[381] Pimentel et al. A link between irritable bowel syndrome and fibromyalgia may be related to findings on lactulose breath testing. *Ann Rheum Dis.* 2004 Apr;63(4):450-2

[382] Bundgaard H, Kjeldsen K, Suarez Krabbe K, et al. Endotoxemia stimulates skeletal muscle Na+-K+-ATPase and raises blood lactate under aerobic conditions in humans. *Am J Physiol Heart Circ Physiol.* 2003 Mar;284(3):H1028-34. ajpheart.physiology.org/cgi/reprint/284/3/H1028

[383] For perspectives and mechanisms on how bacterial components contribute to pain, see the previous discussion under the header of "central sensitization" and the following: Amaral et al. Commensal microbiota is fundamental for the development of inflammatory pain. *Proc Natl Acad Sci U S A.* 2008 Feb 12;105(6):2193-7. Yamaguchi et al. Low rather than high dose lipopolysaccharide 'priming' of muscle provides an animal model of persistent elevated mechanical sensitivity for the study of chronic pain. *Eur J Pain.* 2011 Aug;15(7):724-31. Hains et al. Pain intensity and duration can be enhanced by prior challenge: initial evidence suggestive of a role of microglial priming. *J Pain.* 2010 Oct;11(10):1004-14

[384] Goebel et al. Altered intestinal permeability in patients with primary fibromyalgia and in patients with complex regional pain syndrome. *Rheumatology.* 2008 Aug;47(8):1223-7

[385] Over et al. Regression of skin changes in patient with systemic sclerosis following treatment for bacterial overgrowth with ciprofloxacin. *Br J Rheumatol* 1998;37:696

[386] Lin HC. Small intestinal bacterial overgrowth: a framework for understanding irritable bowel syndrome. *JAMA.* 2004 Aug 18;292(7):852-8. Excellent article.

[387] Zaidel O, Lin HC. Uninvited guests: the impact of small intestinal bacterial overgrowth on nutrition. *Practical Gastroenterology* 2003; 27(7):27-34

[388] "The initial skin changes were frankly vasculitic with "target' lesions, whilst older lesions showed a psoriasiform scale and a tendency to central clearing. The illness was associated with raised levels of IgM and IgG containing circulating immune complexes and deposition of IgM and IgG in the dermis." Fairris GM, Ashworth J, Cotterill JA. A dermatosis associated with bacterial overgrowth in jejunal diverticula. *Br J Dermatol.* 1985 Jun;112(6):709-13

LPS and nonspecific irritation of mucosa and neutralization of defenses; we can reasonably state that intestinal hyperpermeability is *part and parcel*—an intrinsic component—of SIBO/SIMO. Increased intestinal permeability increases the nonselective absorption of microbial and dietary antigens and is generally associated with (clinically) and expected to result in (pathophysiologically) progressive inflammation, debility, central sensitization, environmental sensitivity, and immune reactivity—including food allergies—among affected patients.

Microbial metabolites affect bowel transit and systemic health and thereby allow the clinician to intuit the pattern of SIBO/SIMO via history in *lieu of* or *prior to*

> ### SIBO/SIMO = intestinal damage
> **"A major pathophysiologic consequence of SIBO relates to the inflammatory epithelial changes that subsequently occur in the gut.** The degree of mucosal inflammation can vary considerably both grossly and microscopically. The inflammation that occurs in the setting of SIBO is nonspecific and is likely due to the overgrowth of more invasive strains of bacteria. This inflammatory process may result in a variety of epithelial changes including the blunting of the villi... Facultative anaerobes cause epithelial injury by direct adherence and production of enterotoxins, while aerobes produce enzymes and metabolic products that result in injury."
>
> DiBaise JK. Nutritional consequences of small intestinal bacterial overgrowth. *Practical Gastroenterology* 2008 Dec

laboratory testing; included here after the main metabolites is repeated mention of intestinal hyperpermeability ("leaky gut") because this is commonly caused by SIBO/SIMO: Hydrogen—Post-prandial gas and bloating, flatulence with minimal odor, tendency toward diarrhea. Methane—Post-prandial gas and bloating, flatulence with minimal odor, tendency toward constipation. Hydrogen sulfide—Post-prandial gas and bloating, flatulence with strong sulfurous odor, tendency toward constipation; with microbial blooms, patient experiences occasional muscle aches, mental impairment, and low body temperature due to mitochondrial ETC impairment and poisoning of glutamate dehydrogenase conversion of glutamate to alpha-ketoglutarate, with the latter components contributing to the clinical pictures of FMS and CFS. LPS—If not overt inflammation, then chemical sensitivity and environmental intolerance due to inhibition of Cyp450; particularly noteworthy with *Klebsiella pneumoniae*.

3. Immunosuppressive dysbiosis: Some microbes, particularly yeast, produce toxins that suppress immune function; in other cases, the induction of a hypersensitivity-type immune response retards killing/clearance of the microbe via impaired lymphocyte-mediated immune defenses. ❶ Immunosuppressive toxins: The immunosuppressive mycotoxin produced by *Candia albicans* is called gliotoxin[389], and it is produced at the site of yeast overgrowth, thus suppressing local—and possibly, systemic—immune function.[390] ❷ Immunoglobulin proteases: Since secretory IgA is the first line of defense against allergens and infections in the gastrointestinal tract, its destruction by microbes such as *Candida albicans* and *Entamoeba histolytica* via IgA-specific proteases retards this immune barrier, and this can be considered a form of local immunosuppression. ❸ Paradoxical hypersensitivity immunosuppression: Very interestingly as noted with vulvovaginal *Candida* hypersensitivity, the macrophage-driven PGE2-mediated hypersensitivity response impairs the lymphocyte-driven immune response against *Candida*; per Bernstein and Seidu in 2015, "This observation led to speculation that a vaginal hypersensitivity response to *C albicans* may be associated with increased levels of prostaglandin E2, which is capable of suppressing localized vaginal cell-mediated immune responses. The loss of this localized vaginal defense mechanism can result in colonization by yeast leading to repetitive infections."[391]

4. Hypersensitivity/allergic dysbiosis: **Some people have an exaggerated immune response to otherwise "normal" yeast and bacteria. In this situation, we have to eradicate their "normal" yeast/bacteria—and/or improve immunotolerance—in order to alleviate their hypersensitivity reaction.** The best example of this is the **severe intestinal inflammation that some patients develop in response to intestinal colonization with *Candida albicans***, which is generally considered "nonpathogenic" in small amounts. In susceptible patients, *Candida* can induce a severe local inflammatory reaction, such as colitis, that only remits with antifungal treatment.[392] **Gastrointestinal overgrowth of *Candida albicans* and *C. glabrata* caused near-fatal**

---

[389] "Candida albicans is known to produce gliotoxin, which has several prominent biological effects, including immunosuppression." Shah DT, Jackman S, Engle J, Larsen B. Effect of gliotoxin on human polymorphonuclear neutrophils. *Infect Dis Obstet Gynecol.* 1998;6(4):168-75

[390] "Based on the recent finding that C. albicans is able to produce an immunosuppressive mycotoxin, gliotoxin, we analyzed vaginal samples of 3 women severely symptomatic for vaginal candidiasis and found that they contained significant levels of gliotoxin." Shah DT, Glover DD, Larsen B. In situ mycotoxin production by Candida albicans in women with vaginitis. *Gynecol Obstet Invest.* 1995;39(1):67-9

[391] Bernstein JA, Seidu L. Chronic vulvovaginal Candida hypersensitivity: An underrecognized and undertreated disorder by allergists. *Allergy Rhinol.* 2015 Jan;6(1):44-9

[392] Doby T. Monilial esophagitis and colitis. *J Maine Med Assoc.* 1971 May;62(5):109-14

hypersensitivity alveolitis that remitted with eradication of gastrointestinal candidiasis.[393] Some women become "allergic" to their own vaginal *Candida albicans*[394]; surely some men are likewise allergic to their own intestinal yeast. In patients with lupus, gastrointestinal bacteria are abnormal (decreased colonization resistance[395]), and gastrointestinal bacteria in these patients may translocate into the systemic circulation to induce formation of antibodies that cross-react with double-stranded DNA to produce the clinical manifestations of the disease.[396,397] **Most (57%) of patients with atopic dermatitis show evidence of IgE-mediated histamine release (i.e., "allergy") to exotoxins secreted from *Staphylococcus aureus*,** which commonly colonizes eczematous skin[398]; in other words: most eczema patients are allergic to their own dermal bacteria and can thus be said to have *hypersensitivity dermal dysbiosis*.

5. Inflammatory dysbiosis: People with specific genotypes and HLA markers are susceptible to a proinflammatory "autoimmune" syndrome that occurs following exposure to specific microbial molecules that are structurally similar to human body tissues; this is classically understood as molecular mimicry with resulting immunologic cross-reactivity. The best-known example of systemic musculoskeletal inflammation caused by microbial exposure is reactive arthritis, which is classically seen in patients with the genotype HLA-B27 following urogenital exposure to *Chlamydia trachomatis* or other gastrointestinal or genitourinary infection as previously described among the prototypic diseases resulting from dysbiosis. Likewise, short bowel syndrome and arthritis-dermatitis syndrome, both of which result primarily from SIBO-induced hyperpermeability, antigen excess, and immune complex formation and deposition, were also detailed in a previous section on dysbiotic clinical prototypes.

Nonexclusive types of inflammatory dysbiosis		
Mechanism(s)	**Microbes**	**Prototype(s)**
Molecular mimicry, cross-reactivity	*Campylobacter, Salmonella, Shigella, Yersinia*	Reactive arthritis, spondyloarthritis
Epigenetic induction of Th17 over Treg	Segmented filamentous bacteria (SFB), generalized gut inflammation	Systemic and gastrointestinal autoimmunity
Overproduction of bacterial cell wall debris with resulting immune complex deposition	SIBO, generally with mucosal hyperpermeability	Short bowel syndrome, arthritis-dermatitis syndrome, vasculitis
Bacterial translocation, sensitivity to bactDNA; exacerbated in animal models via SFB-Th17 mechanism described previously	Likely nonspecific, possibly exacerbated by intermixing of bacterial and human DNA in biofilms; E coli is notable in human DNA-specific immune complexes	Systemic lupus erythematosus (SLE), systemic sclerosis
Neuronal autoimmunity, glial activation	Group A Streptococcus, Pseudomonas aeruginosa, and others linked with Guillain-Barre syndrome	Pediatric Autoimmune Neuropsychiatric Disorders Associated with Streptococcal infections (PANDAS)

Inflammatory bowel diseases (IBD)—Crohn's disease and ulcerative colitis—are notoriously associated with gastrointestinal dysbiosis[399]; the questions that remain are those of defining the microbial imbalances, microbial correction, and promotion of tolerance. An important new development in the study of dysbiosis in IBD is that the microbial alterations may not appear in per normal/routine stool testing; some of the abnormalities are present only on biopsy samples, with the microbes and their associated/altered communities and quorums likely embedded in tissue-adherent biofilms. Further, clinicians should know that IBD is *more than dysbiosis* and more than the gut; these patients have systemic pro-inflammatory imbalances

[393] "We conclude that the disease was induced by C.a.-antigen reaching the lungs from the intestinal tract via the bloodstream." Schreiber J, Struben C, Rosahl W, Amthor M. Hypersensitivity alveolitis induced by endogenous candida species. *Eur J Med Res*. 2000 Mar 27;5(3):126

[394] Ramirez De Knott HM, et al. Cutaneous hypersensitivity to Candida albicans in idiopathic vulvodynia. *Contact Dermatitis*. 2005 Oct;53(4):214-8

[395] "Colonization Resistance (CR)...tended to be lower in active SLE patients than in healthy individuals. This could indicate that in SLE more and different bacteria translocate across the gut wall due to a lower CR. Some of these may serve as polyclonal B cell activators or as antigens cross-reacting with DNA." Apperloo-Renkema et al. Host-microflora interaction in systemic lupus erythematosus (SLE): colonization resistance of the indigenous bacteria of the intestinal tract. *Epidemiol Infect*. 1994;112(2):367-73

[396] "The lower IgG antibacterial antibody titres in active SLE might possibly result from sequestration of these IgG antibodies in immune complexes, indicating a possible role for antibacterial antibodies in exacerbations of SLE." Apperloo-Renkema HZ, Bootsma H, Mulder BI, Kallenberg CG, van der Waaij D. Host-microflora interaction in systemic lupus erythematosus (SLE): circulating antibodies to the indigenous bacteria of the intestinal tract. *Epidemiol Infect*. 1995 Feb;114(1):133-41

[397] Pisetsky DS. Antibody responses to DNA in normal immunity and aberrant immunity. *Clin Diagn Lab Immunol* 1998;5:1-6

[398] "These data indicate that a subset of patients with AD mount an IgE response to SEs that can be grown from their skin." Leung DY, et al. Presence of IgE antibodies to staphylococcal exotoxins on the skin of patients with atopic dermatitis. Evidence for a new group of allergens. *J Clin Invest*. 1993 Sep;92(3):1374-80

[399] deVrieze J. Crohn's disease...dramatic changes in gut bacteria. *Science* 2014 Mar news.sciencemag.org/biology/2014/03/crohns-disease-marked-dramatic-changes-gut-bacteria

and responses *triggered by microbes* and *localized to the gut* but with a complex pathophysiology that extends beyond the dysbiotic trigger and gut localization. Gastrointestinal dysbiosis can be pro-inflammatory independently from the simple and well-accepted models of molecular mimicry, cross-reactivity, and reactive arthritis; what we appreciate now is that gut microbes play a major role in determining immunophenotype balance, most specifically exemplified by the ratio between regulatory T-cells (Treg) and proinflammatory effectors, especially Th17 cells but also including Th-1 and Th-2 cells, among others. Optimization of this balance is achieved via my "nutritional immunomodulation" protocol detailed in Chapter 4, section 3.

- Microbial colitis induced by the Gram-negative *Aeromonas* species: ❶ "We describe a 40-yr-old woman who presented with abdominal pain and diarrhea, and who was found to have segmental colitis involving the cecum and ascending colon. *Aeromonas hydrophila* was isolated from the stool, and her symptoms responded to appropriate antibiotic therapy. Follow-up colonoscopy confirmed complete endoscopic and histologic resolution of her colitis."[400] ❷ "We describe a 67-yr-old woman who presented with abdominal pain and bloody diarrhea and was diagnosed with left-sided, segmental colitis due to *Aeromonas sobria*, which was proven by stool culture. Extensive work-up for ischemic colitis was unremarkable, and after treatment with antibiotics, the patient's symptoms resolved, and follow-up colonoscopy failed to reveal any evidence of residual colitis or inflammatory bowel disease. Our report supports the view that *Aeromonas* species need to be considered in the differential diagnosis of colitis, and we believe it to be the first report of left-sided, segmental colitis secondary to *Aeromonas sobria* infection."[401] ❸ "Three patients with an acute colitis in which the only pathogen detected was either *Aeromonas hydrophila* or *A sobria* progressed to a chronic phase after the infection had been eliminated by antibiotic treatment in two and had resolved spontaneously in the third. The final diagnosis in each case was ulcerative colitis. ... The sequence of symptoms and observations in these cases, as well as in others from the literature involving more familiar pathogens, suggests that bacterial infection may contribute to the development of chronic colitis."[402] Obviously, if one offending microbe can induce acute colitis, we would by reasonable extension consider that multiple microbial imbalances might also contribute to other clinical phenotypes and durations of inflammatory bowel disease.

- Dysbiosis in IBD—Crohn's disease (CD) and ulcerative colitis (UC) (*Microb Ecol Health Dis*. 2015 Feb[403]): The 2015 review by Carding et al has been chosen to serve as a representative review on the topic of dysbiosis and IBD. The connection between dysbiosis and IBD is intuitively obvious by this time, and previous articles have supported the association, so what is needed now is a better, more defined microbial/molecular understanding; this review by Carding et al sufficiently serves that purpose and represents the general trends in thought on the dysbiosis-IBD connection. "Overall, patients exhibit a decrease in microbial population and functional diversity and stability of their intestinal microbiota with decreases in specific *Firmicutes* and a concomitant increase in *Bacteroidetes* and facultative anaerobes such as *Enterobacteriaceae*. ... In CD, the predominant dysbiosis has been described to be associated with five bacterial species amongst which alterations in the abundance of *Faecalibacterium prausnitzii* is associated with the prolongation of disease remission, with this bacterium having a therapeutic effect in experimental models of colitis. ... Indeed, up to now, it is still unclear whether intestinal microbial dysbiosis is a direct cause for the inflammation in IBD, or merely the result of a disturbed environment in the GI-tract. ... Gevers et al (*Cell Host Microbe* 2014)...analysed the microbiota of a large cohort of newly diagnosed pediatric CD patients and found clear differences in bacterial populations between CD and healthy control patients. CD patients had increased abundance of *Enterobacteriaceae*, *Pasteurellaceae*, *Veillonellaceae*, and *Fusobacteriaceae*, and decreased abundance in *Erysipelotrichales*, *Bacteroidales*, and *Clostridiales* compared to healthy control patients. Interestingly, these differences were only revealed when analyzing mucosal samples (rather than faecal samples), indicating that the bacteria resident in the mucosal layer may be more significant for disease etiology." With due appreciation for their concision and listing of microbial aberrancies, again noting that mucosal rather than stool samples appear to reveal the most important differences, I suspect that what we are heading toward is the realization—as with sinusitis—that the microbial imbalance plus

[400] Farraye et al. Segmental colitis associated with Aeromonas hydrophila. *Am J Gastroenterol*. 1989 Apr;84(4):436-8
[401] Deutsch et al. Aeromonas sobria-associated left-sided segmental colitis. *Am J Gastroenterol*. 1997 Nov;92(11):2104-6
[402] Willoughby et al. Chronic colitis after Aeromonas infection. *Gut*. 1989 May;30(5):686-90
[403] Carding S, Verbeke K, Vipond DT, Corfe BM, Owen LJ. Dysbiosis of the gut microbiota in disease. *Microb Ecol Health Dis*. 2015 Feb 2;26:26191

the overzealous immune response is the problem, rather than the microbial imbalance per se. By now, this should be the accepted bipartite model, and these conditions should be treated as such while we await refinement of these approaches per additional research.

<table>
<tr><td>

Systemic immune balance is powerfully influenced by microbial balance in the gut

"Recent studies have demonstrated that bacterial components, as well as their metabolites, play a central role in regulating TH cell development. Furthermore, these metabolites can elicit changes in histone posttranslational modification to modify the expression of critical regulators of T cell fate."

Furusawa et al. Commensal microbiota regulates T cell fate decision in the gut. *Semin Immunopathol.* 2015 Jan

</td></tr>
</table>

- <u>Multiple sclerosis and the gut microbiome (*Medscape Family Medicine* 2014 Oct[404])</u>:"...we wanted to determine what the constituents of the gut microbiome are in MS patients compared with non-MS patients. We studied 105 patients and recently expanded our cohort to 250. The preliminary data show that there are at least a couple of different genera of bacteria that are different in the gut of MS patients compared with healthy controls. We found that a [bacterium] called *Methanobrevibacteriaceae* is enriched in the gut of MS patients and seems to have immunoproliferative properties that drive inflammation. We also found that the population of *Butyricimonas* bacteria is low in MS patients compared with healthy controls."

- <u>Fecal microbiota in early rheumatoid arthritis (*J Rheumatol* 2008 Aug[405])</u>: Fecal bacterial composition was analyzed from patients with rheumatoid arthritis (RA, n=51) or fibromyalgia (FM, n=50) with flow cytometry, 16S rRNA hybridization, DNA-staining and oligonucleotide probes. "RESULTS: In comparison to patients with FM, the RA patients had significantly less *Bifidobacteria* and bacteria of the *Bacteroides-Porphyromonas-Prevotella* group, *Bacteroides fragilis* subgroup, and *Eubacterium rectale--Clostridium coccoides* group. Results from the 8 probes showed a significant overall difference between the 2 patient groups, indicating widespread microbial differences. CONCLUSION: These findings support the hypothesis that intestinal microbes participate in the etiopathogenesis of RA."

- <u>Intestinal flora of patients with rheumatoid arthritis: induction of chronic arthritis in rats by cell wall fragments from isolated *Eubacterium aerofaciens* strains (*Br J Rheumatol.* 1990 Dec[406])</u>: "Cell wall fragments from four *E. aerofaciens* strains (two from RA, two from healthy subjects [HS]) were tested for arthritis induction in rats. All four strains induced chronic arthritis which was histologically confirmed. We concluded that in the normal intestinal flora of RA patients *Eubacterium* species are present in high numbers (i.e. greater than 10(9)/g feces); cell walls from isolated E. aerofaciens strains had arthropathic properties." This is an important study, showing that debris from gut microbes is arthritogenic and readily available biologically; all that appears necessary is a leaky/hyperpermeable gut mucosa.

What must be appreciated these days is the combined effect of multiple microbes, and the differential effect that these variations of microbes (again, relevant here are my concepts of "multifocal polydysbiosis" and "total microbial load [TML]") can have when combined with a pro-inflammatory genotype, phenotype, and "xenobiophenotype", used and defined here for the first time as the patient's pattern of accumulated organic and nonorganic/metallic xenobiotics and the effect that those xenobiotics have on the patient's phenotype.[407] Very clear now is that gut microbial determination of Treg/Th17 balance sets the inflammatory stage for "chronic"/sustained/long-term specific microbe-disease induction.

- <u>Commensal microbiota influence systemic autoimmune responses via regulation of systemic T-cell phenotype</u>: ❶ "Antinuclear antibodies are a hallmark feature of generalized autoimmune diseases, including systemic lupus erythematosus and systemic sclerosis. ...We further demonstrate antinuclear antibody production is influenced by the presence of commensal gut flora, in particular increased colonization with segmented filamentous bacteria, and IL-17 receptor signaling. Together, these data

[404] Stetka BS. Multiple Sclerosis and the Microbiome: What's the Connection? An Expert Interview with Sushrut Jangi, MD. *Medscape Family Medicine* 2014 Oct www.medscape.com/viewarticle/832385. Cited to: Gandhi R, Glehn FV, Mazzola MA, et al. Gut microbiome is linked to immune cell phenotype in multiple sclerosis. Program and abstracts of the 2014 Joint ACTRI MS-ECTRI MS Meeting; September 10-13, 2014; Boston, Massachusetts. Poster 616.
[405] Vaahtovuo et al. Fecal microbiota in early rheumatoid arthritis. *J Rheumatol.* 2008 Aug;35(8):1500-5
[406] Severijnen et al. Intestinal flora of patients with rheumatoid arthritis: induction of chronic arthritis in rats by cell wall fragments from isolated Eubacterium aerofaciens strains. *Br J Rheumatol.* 1990 Dec;29(6):433-9
[407] I coined "xenobiophenotype" to indicate the physical/actual pattern of xenobiotics within and their effect upon the clinical phenotype of the patient. This word does not exist per Google or Medline/Pubmed in 2015 Apr.

indicate that neonatal colonization of gut microbiota influences generalized autoimmunity in adult life."[408] This is a nice article, based on multifaceted animal experiments with immunologic and microbial variables, interconnecting the pathophysiology of anti-DNA autoimmunity with SFB; most previous articles had not mentioned SFB specifically with anti-DNA autoimmunity and rather connected the latter with bacterial translocation. Merging these models together, we immediately see the potential synergy with SFB-mediated Th17-induction with bacterial (e.g., *E coli*) translocation thereby, respectively, providing inflammatory immunophenotype "priming" with a microbial target of DNA. ❷ "Segmented filamentous bacteria and Clostridium species belonging to clusters XIVa and IV induce the accumulation of Th17 cells in the small intestine and Foxp3(+) regulatory T cells in the large intestine, respectively. The immune cells induced by the gut microbiota likely contribute to intestinal homeostasis and influence systemic immunity in the host."[409] This previous quote succinctly summarizes what is well represented in many articles; other probiotic-type bacteria have also been shown to promote induction of Treg. ❸ "Commensal microbiota shapes the intestinal immune system by regulating T helper (TH) cell lineage differentiation. For example, *Bacteroides fragilis* colonization not only optimizes the systemic TH1/TH2 balance, but also can induce regulatory T (Treg) cell differentiation in the gut. In addition, segmented filamentous bacteria (SFB) facilitate the development of TH17 cells in the small intestine. The 17 strains within clusters IV, XIVa, and XVIII of Clostridiales found in human feces can also induce the differentiation and expansion of Treg cells in the colon."[410]

Segmented filamentous bacteria in small intestine ➔ pro-inflammatory Th17 cells

SIBO, molecular mimicry, immune complexes ➔ systemic inflammation with(out) "targeted" tissue inflammation

Probiotic bacteria in the small and large intestine ➔ anti-inflammatory Foxp3(+)Treg cells

Clostridium clusters XIVa and IV in the large intestine ➔ anti-inflammatory Foxp3(+)Treg cells

Any effective and accurate model of clinical pathophysiologic reality must accept and integrate if not all then at least a manageable amount of relevant information. In the following table, I separate the effects of dysbiosis as ❶ "mechanistic" (e.g., SIBO, immune complex disease, molecular mimicry with HLA-B27 and various microbes) from the ❷ "immunodysregulatory" pro-inflammatory and autoimmunity-promoting induction of Th17 cells and reciprocal suppression of Tregs; a third component is ❸ systemic inflammation. With only these three variables, we can see seven combinatorial variations and proposed clinical expectations.

Major variables in the model and concept of "combinatorial inflammology": Ingredients and the overlap create the final pattern; a medical extension of Euclidean geometry

- Genes—cytokine SNP, VDR mutations
- Genes—HLA-B27 + molecular mimicry
- Diet: processed food + AGE intake
- Hyperglycemia
- TML—total microbial load
- TXL—total xenobiotic load, including the mitochondrial, estrogenic and antibiotic effects of glyphosate and other pervasive corporate chemicals
- Vitamin D status (AMP, Treg, mucosal permeability)
- Mitochondrial (dys)function
- Adiposity/adipokines/estrogen
- Hormonal balance
- Phenotypic immune balance
- Stress, sleep, and psychosocial health
- Structural/spinal integrity

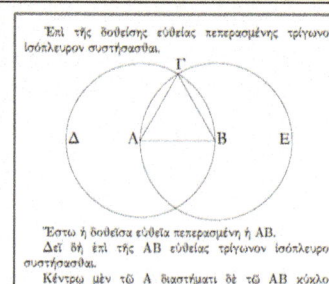

Com•bi•na•to•ri•al: *adjective.* 1. of, pertaining to, or involving the **combination of elements**, as in phonetics or music. 2. of or pertaining to the enumeration of the number of ways of arranging items in a specific configuration. 3. of or pertaining to **combination, or the modes, properties, etc., of combinations. In•flam•mol•o•gy:** *noun.* 1. the study of the causes of and various contributors to the (patho)physiologic processes, molecular mechanisms, and clinical and societal consequences of inflammation and inflammatory diseases.

---

[408] Van Praet et al. Commensal microbiota influence systemic autoimmune responses. *EMBO J.* 2015 Feb 12;34(4):466-74
[409] Nishio J, Honda K. Immunoregulation by the gut microbiota. *Cell Mol Life Sci.* 2012 Nov;69(21):3635-50
[410] Furusawa et al. Commensal microbiota regulates T cell fate decision in the gut. *Semin Immunopathol.* 2015 Jan;37(1):17-25

❶ "Mechanistic dysbiosis"— triggering microbe with "mechanistic" pathophysiologic effects—*transient or persistent depending on microbial persistence*	❷ "Immunodysregulatory dysbiosis"— immunophenotype (e.g., Treg/Th17) imbalance via SFB and other microbes	❸ Total inflammatory load (TIL) and total microbial load (TML)— dysbiotic pattern and/or systemic inflammation	Proposed/prototypical clinical outcome
Microbe-induced "mechanistic" inflammation			"**Reactive** inflammation" until microbe is cleared
	Th17-promoted auto-inflammation		**Mild** inflammatory tendency/disease
		Systemic inflammation	**Mild** inflammatory tendency/disease
Microbe-induced "mechanistic" inflammation	Th17-promoted autoinflammation		**Moderate-severe** inflammatory disease
Microbe-induced "mechanistic" inflammation		Systemic inflammation	**Moderate-severe** inflammatory disease
	Th17-promoted autoinflammation	Systemic inflammation	**Moderate-severe** inflammatory disease
Microbe-induced "mechanistic" inflammation	Th17-promoted autoinflammation	Systemic inflammation	**Very severe**: worst case scenario
Mechanistic pathophysiology: such as antigen overload, molecular mimicry, immune complex deposition. SFB: segmented filamentous bacteria, notorious for their induction of Th17 cells. TIL: also includes pro-inflammatory genome/SNP (single nucleotide polymorphisms), pro-inflammatory diet, obesity, mTOR, mitochondrial (dys)function, stress/sleep/social factors, endocrine (im)balance, xenobiotic load.			

Dysbiosis can take three main forms, and these forms can exist in separately, additively, and synergistically: Better than the perception of "dysbiosis as a microbe" is the view that "dysbiosis is always a pattern" which can occur via ❶ a single microbe or mechanism, ❷ a systemic immunophenotype imbalance, ❸ a dysbiotic pattern or pro-inflammatory pattern, per Haller "It would appear that *some combinations of bacteria are 'dysbiotic'*…"[411]

6. Amoebas, cysts, protozoas, and other parasites: In this case when we use the term "parasites'" we are not talking about worms/helminths, *per se*, although these are occasionally found with parasitology examinations. Certain microorganisms are not consistent with optimal health and should be eliminated even though the microbe is not classically identified as a "pathogen." Interestingly, 97% of patients severely infected with the gastrointestinal "parasite" *Entamoeba histolytica* develop the autoreactive ANCA antibody[412], suggesting the possibility that this microbe or infections in general can induce or sustain autoimmunity.

    ▪ Parasitic rheumatism with the ameba *Endolimax nana* presenting as rheumatoid arthritis (*J Rheumatol.* 1983 Jun[413]): "A symmetrical polyarthritis with low titer positive rheumatoid factor occurred in a young man who also complained of chronic diarrhea after returning from Vietnam. *Endolimax nana* grew on stool culture. Both the patient's diarrhea and arthritis responded effectively to therapy with metronidazole. The diagnosis of parasitic rheumatism was made in retrospect." This is a classic case of what can be described as ameba-induced reactive arthritis or, as the authors stated, parasitic rheumatism.

7. Metabolic/dysmetabolic dysbiosis: I consider "metabolic dysbiosis" to have two major clinical manifestations which of course are interrelated but also sufficiently distinct and compartmentalized to be distinguished; these will be introduced differently and then substantiated in combination as ❶ metabolic dysbiosis resulting in mitochondrial dysfunction, with particular relevance for fibromyalgia (FM) and chronic fatigue syndrome (CFS, recently renamed systemic exertion intolerance disease [SEID[414]]), and ❷ metabolic dysbiosis resulting in systemic inflammation and insulin resistance. The origin of both is classically the gut, namely SIBO as detailed in several previous sections including this selfsame section. Mitochondrial dysfunction and low-grade systemic inflammation commonly occur together and contribute to end-organ dysfunction—such as either the insulin

[411] Technische Universität München. Bacterial communities cause inflammation of the gut. 2015 Apr tum.de/en/about-tum/news/press-releases/short/article/32365/ related to Schaubeck et al. Dysbiotic gut microbiota causes transmissible Crohn's disease-like ileitis independent of failure in antimicrobial defence. *Gut.* 2015 Apr. pii: gutjnl-2015-309333
[412] George J, Levy Y, Kallenberg CG, Shoenfeld Y. Infections and Wegener's granulomatosis--a cause and effect relationship? *QJM.* 1997 May;90(5):367-73
[413] Burnstein SL, Liakos S. Parasitic rheumatism presenting as rheumatoid arthritis. *J Rheumatol.* 1983 Jun;10(3):514-5
[414] Crawford C. Chronic Fatigue Syndrome: Renamed and Redefined. *AAFP.org* 2015 Mar aafp.org/news/health-of-the-public/20150302newchronicfatigue.html. Institute of Medicine. Beyond myalgic encephalomyelitis / chronic fatigue syndrome: redefining an illness. iom.edu/~/media/Files/Report%20Files/2015/MECFS/MECFScliniciansguide.pdf

resistance of diabetes type-2 or the muscular pain and cognitive impairment of fibromyalgia and CFS/SEID; the first two—triggered by microbial molecules—strongly appear to contribute to the third—the clinical phenotypes. Demonstration of the third in causative connection with dysbiosis—preferably via positive clinical response to eradication of dysbiosis—supports/substantiates the existence of the prior two.

- Pain/fatigue syndromes and SIBO—fibromyalgia (*Current Pain and Headache Reports* 2004 Oct[415]): This article discusses the results of two experiments using antibiotics in the treatment of FM: ❶ 96 patients with SIBO diagnosed by lactulose hydrogen breath testing (LHBT) were offered antibiotic treatment for the reduction of gastrointestinal bacteria; 25 of the 96 patients returned for a follow-up LHBT. Neomycin was the most commonly used antibiotic. Eleven of the 25 patients achieved complete transient eradication of SIBO after antibiotic treatment and experienced better improvement in more of their FM symptom scores when compared with the patients who did not achieve complete eradication. This indicates that **a direct relationship exists between the presence of SIBO and intestinal and extraintestinal symptoms in fibromyalgia, and that FM can be alleviated by effective antimicrobial/antibiotic treatment.** ❷ In this double-blind trial of eradication of SIBO in fibromyalgia, 46 patients fulfilling the established criteria for FM were tested for SIBO using LHBT. Forty-two of the 46 patients (91.3%) were positive for SIBO and were randomized to receive placebo or 500 mg of liquid neomycin (a minimally-absorbed gastrointestinal-specific antibiotic drug) twice daily for 10 days. Only six of the 20 patients (30%) in the neomycin group achieved eradication (indicating inefficacy of treatment); thus, no statistically significant difference between groups was available for analysis. Thereafter, 28 patients in the double-blind study testing positive for SIBO went on to receive open-label antibiotic treatment to eradicate SIBO, and this time 17 of the 28 patients (60.7%) achieved eradication of SIBO. When these 23 patients were compared with the 15 patients who failed to eradicate or did not undergo open-label treatment, significant improvement attributable to antibiotic treatment in the FM scores was detected. **Results show that eradication of SIBO results in a clinically significant alleviation of FM symptoms, thereby substantiating that FM is caused largely by SIBO.** Additional components of FM are also explained by SIBO, as detailed in *Rheumatology 3.5* and later.

- Pain/fatigue syndromes and SIBO—excess neurotoxic and mitochondriotoxic D-lactate production—CFS/SEID (*In Vivo* 2009 Jul-Aug[416]): This excellent clinical research fully supports the pathoetiologic (disease causation) model presented in this chapter, which is derived and updated from a previous publication by this author: Vasquez A. *Musculoskeletal Pain: Expanded Clinical Strategies* published by the Institute for Functional Medicine in 2008. The authors of this 2009 study state in the summary of their research, "Patients with chronic fatigue syndrome (CFS) are affected by symptoms of cognitive dysfunction and neurological impairment, the cause of which has yet to be elucidated. However, these symptoms are strikingly similar to those of patients presented with D-lactic acidosis. A significant increase of Gram-positive facultative anaerobic fecal microorganisms in 108 CFS patients as compared to 177 control subjects is presented in this report. The viable count of D-lactic acid producing *Enterococcus* and *Streptococcus* spp. in the fecal samples from the CFS group (3.5 x 10(7) cfu [colony forming units]/L and 9.8 x 10(7) cfu/L respectively) were significantly higher than those for the control group (5.0 x 10(6) cfu/L and 8.9 x 10(4) cfu/L respectively). **[Note: This is approximately a 7x increase in D-lactate producing *Enterococcus* and 1,100x increase in D-lactate producing *Streptococcus*.]** Analysis of exometabolic profiles of *Enterococcus faecalis* and *Streptococcus sanguinis*, representatives of *Enterococcus* and *Streptococcus* spp. respectively, by NMR and HPLC showed that these organisms produced significantly more lactic acid from (13)C-labeled glucose, than the Gram negative *Escherichia coli*. Further, **both *E. faecalis* and *S. sanguinis* secrete more D-lactic acid than *E. coli*.** This study suggests a probable link between intestinal colonization of Gram-positive facultative anaerobic D-lactic acid bacteria and symptom expressions in a subgroup of patients with CFS. Given the fact that **this might explain not only neurocognitive dysfunction in CFS patients but also mitochondrial dysfunction, these findings may have important clinical implications.**" D-lactate competes with physiologic L-lactate and pyruvate; thus via substrate competition, D-lactate reduces mitochondrial ATP production.[417]

[415] Wallace DJ, Hallegua DS. Fibromyalgia: the gastrointestinal link. *Curr Pain Headache Rep*. 2004 Oct;8(5):364-8

[416] Sheedy JR, Wettenhall RE, Scanlon D, et al. Increased d-lactic acid intestinal bacteria in patients with chronic fatigue syndrome. *In Vivo*. 2009 Jul-Aug;23(4):621-8

[417] Ling et al. D-Lactate altered mitochondrial energy production in rat brain and heart but not liver. *Nutr Metab* (Lond). 2012 Feb 1;9(1):6

- **Insulin resistance and gut dysbiosis**—the antidiabetic drug metformin functions in part by modulating gut bacteria (*Gut.* 2014 May[418]): "High-fat diet (HFD)-fed mice treated with metformin showed a higher abundance of the mucin-degrading bacterium *Akkermansia* than HFD-fed control mice. In addition, the number of mucin-producing goblet cells was significantly increased by metformin treatment (p<0.0001). Oral administration of *Akkermansia muciniphila* to HFD-fed mice without metformin significantly enhanced glucose tolerance and attenuated adipose tissue inflammation by inducing Foxp3 regulatory T cells (Tregs) in the visceral adipose tissue (VAT). *CONCLUSIONS*: Modulation of the gut microbiota (by an increase in the *Akkermansia* spp. population) may contribute to the antidiabetic effects of metformin, thereby providing a new mechanism for the therapeutic effect of metformin in patients with T2D. This suggests that pharmacological manipulation of the gut microbiota in favor of *Akkermansia* may be a potential treatment for T2D." While the antidiabetic drug metformin produces its benefit via several different *including "off-target"* mechanisms, per this data, metformin achieves some of its anti-diabetic benefits via favorable modulation of gut flora, specifically increases in *Akkermansia muciniphila*.

- **Insulin resistance and gut dysbiosis**—modification of gut flora improves tolerance and effectiveness of metformin (*J Diabetes Sci Technol.* 2015 Mar[419]): Metformin induces gastrointestinal upset, particularly diarrhea, in ~20% of diabetic patients. This study in diabetic humans used metformin along with a GI microbiome modulator (GIMM) to assess improved metformin tolerance and diabetic control. The GIMM known as NM504 is designed to shift the gut microbiota; it contains "concentrated bioactive food ingredients: inulin, a fiber; beta-glucan and polyphenolic antioxidant compounds."[420] "The combination of metformin and GIMM treatment produced a significantly better tolerance score to metformin than the placebo combination (6.78 ± 0.65 [mean ± SEM] versus 4.45 ± 0.69, P = .0006). Mean fasting glucose levels were significantly (P < .02) lower with the metformin-GIMM combination (121.3 ± 7.8 mg/dl) than with metformin-placebo (151.9 ± 7.8 mg/dl). *CONCLUSION*: Combining a GI microbiome modulator with metformin might allow the greater use of metformin in T2D patients and improve treatment of the disease. While this study shows that dietary modification of the gut microbiome improves metformin tolerance and anti-diabetic effect, the mechanisms might include 1) enhanced drug absorption due to reduction in microbe-mediated inflammation, and/or 2) additive/synergistic benefit of the combination of metformin along with metabolic improvements directly derived from favorable modulation of gut flora (i.e., reduced systemic inflammation.

- **Insulin resistance and microbe excess, presumably from the gut**—antidiabetic effect of antimicrobial berberine in experimental diabetes in rats (*PLoS One.* 2012 Aug[421]): "Berberine, a major pharmacological component of the Chinese herb Coptis chinensis, which was originally used to treat bacterial diarrhea, has recently been demonstrated to be clinically effective in alleviating type 2 diabetes. In this study, we revealed that berberine effectively prevented the development of obesity and insulin resistance in high-fat diet (HFD)-fed rats... Bar-coded pyrosequencing of the V3 region of 16S rRNA genes revealed a significant reduction in the gut microbiota diversity of berberine-treated rats. ... Taken together, our findings suggest that the prevention of obesity and insulin resistance by berberine in HFD-fed rats is at least partially mediated by structural modulation of the gut microbiota, which may help to alleviate inflammation by reducing the exogenous antigen load in the host and elevating SCFA levels in the intestine." Berberine is poorly absorbed from the gut and is an antimicrobial agent effective against various yeast, amebas, and bacteria, especially Gram-positives; one could consider berberine to be a natural version of vancomycin, a nonabsorbed antibiotic drug with specificity for Gram-positive bacteria. The finding of anti-diabetic effects from berberine is supportive of the model that insulin resistance results partly and significantly from excess exposure to gut-derived microbial molecules.

[418] Shin et al. An increase in the Akkermansia spp. induced by metformin treatment improves glucose homeostasis in diet-induced obese mice. *Gut.* 2014 May;63(5):727-35
[419] Burton et al. Addition of a Gastrointestinal Microbiome Modulator to Metformin Improves Metformin Tolerance and Fasting Glucose Levels. *J Diabetes Sci Technol.* 2015 Mar 23. pii: 1932296815577425
[420] Endocrine Society. Blood sugar improves with first gastrointestinal microbiome modulator, NM504. 2014 Jun. sciencedaily.com/releases/2014/06/140623120414.htm
[421] Zhang et al. Structural changes of gut microbiota during berberine-mediated prevention of obesity and insulin resistance in high-fat diet-fed rats. *PLoS One.* 2012;7(8):e42529

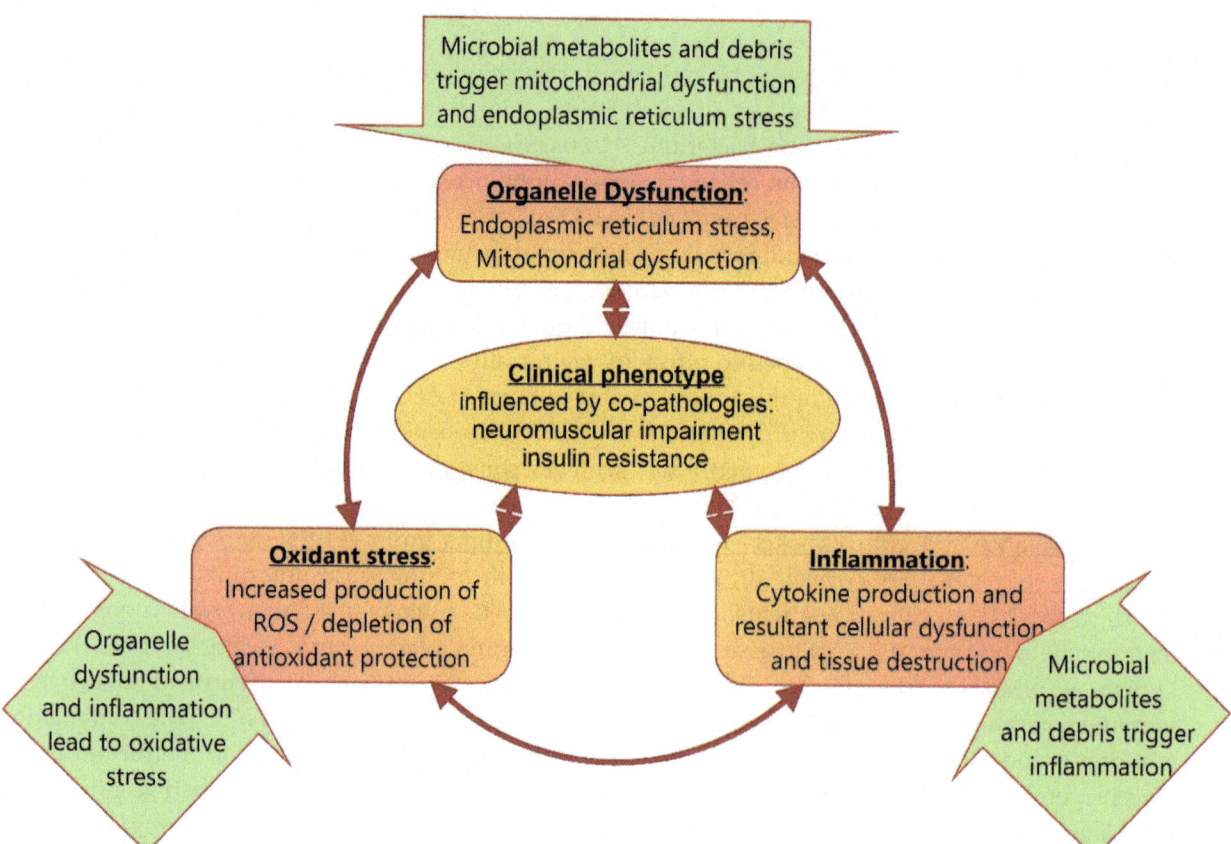

Dysmetabolic dysbiosis: Microbial metabolites and debris cause inflammation and promote mitochondrial dysfunction and endoplasmic reticulum stress, all of which lead to oxidant stress; clinical manifestations beyond inflammation include impairment of muscle and neurologic function as noted in the clinical syndromes of FM and CFS/SEID, and induction of insulin resistance, the hallmark of metabolic syndrome and diabetes type-2. While each of these conditions has additional factors, the microbial factors are of high pathophysiologic/clinical/therapeutic relevance.[422]

- <u>Insulin resistance and microbe excess, presumably from the gut—berberine's antidiabetic benefit may be derived significantly from modification of gut bacteria</u> (*Med Sci Monit.* 2011 Jul[423]): Berberine's antidiabetic and antihypercholesterolemic benefits are well established; here the authors speculate that part of the mechanism of benefit is via favorable modification/reduction in gut dysbiosis. "The protective effect against diabetes of gut microbiota modulation with probiotics or antibiotics has been confirmed in recent observations. Berberine has significant antimicrobial activity against several microbes through inhibiting the assembly function of FtsZ and halting the bacteria cell division. Because berberine acts topically in the gastrointestinal tract and it is poorly absorbed, berberine might modulate gut microbiota without systemic anti-infective activity. Our hypothesis is that gut microbiota modulation may be one mechanism of the antidiabetic effect of berberine."

- <u>Gut dysbiosis in rosacea</u>—Small intestinal bacterial overgrowth in rosacea (*Clin Gastroenterol Hepatol.* 2008 Jul[424]): "We enrolled 113 consecutive rosacea ambulatory patients (31 M/82 F; mean age, 52 +/- 15 years) and 60 healthy controls who were sex- and age-matched. ... Patients positive for SIBO were randomized to receive rifaximin therapy (1200 mg/day for 10 days) or placebo. ... The prevalence of SIBO was higher in patients than controls (52/113 vs 3/60, P < .001). After eradication, cutaneous lesions cleared in 20 of 28 and greatly improved in 6 of 28 patients, whereas patients treated with placebo remained unchanged (18/20) or worsened (2/20) (P < .001). Placebo patients were subsequently switched to rifaximin therapy, and SIBO was eradicated in 17 of 20 cases. Fifteen had a complete resolution of rosacea. After antibiotic therapy, 13 of 16 patients with negative BTs for SIBO remained unchanged, and this result differed from SIBO-positive

---

[422] These concepts are developed in my *Functional Inflammology, Volume 1* and *Mitochondrial Nutrition and Endoplasmic Reticulum Stress in Primary Care, Second Edition* and will continue to be developed in subsequent works; my *Fibromyalgia in a Nutshell* substantiates this model and provides corresponding treatment protocol for that condition (FM).
[423] Han et al. Modulating gut microbiota as an anti-diabetic mechanism of berberine. *Med Sci Monit.* 2011 Jul;17(7):RA164-7
[424] Parodi et al. Small intestinal bacterial overgrowth in rosacea: clinical effectiveness of its eradication. *Clin Gastroenterol Hepatol.* 2008 Jul;6(7):759-64

cases (P < .001). CONCLUSIONS: This study demonstrated that rosacea patients have a significantly higher SIBO prevalence than controls. Moreover, eradication of SIBO induced an almost complete regression of their cutaneous lesions and maintained this excellent result for at least 9 months." This research and its clinical implications—that rosacea patients should receive *effective* treatment for SIBO—are crystal clear; other data has shown that rosacea patients have pancreatic exocrine insufficiency and that they respond to orally administered pancreatic/proteolytic enzymes.

- Gut dysbiosis in rosacea—Helicobacter pylori infection but not small intestinal bacterial overgrowth may play a pathogenic role in rosacea (*United European Gastroenterol J.* 2015 Feb[425]): "...90 patients with rosacea... We used the (13)C Urea Breath Test and *H. pylori* stool antigen (HpSA) test to assess *H. pylori* infection and the glucose breath test to assess SIBO. Patients infected by H. pylori were treated with clarithromycin-containing sequential therapy. Patients positive for SIBO were treated with rifaximin. RESULTS: We found that 44/90 (48.9%) patients with rosacea and 24/90 (26.7%) control subjects were infected with *H. pylori* (p = 0.003). Moreover, 9/90 (10%) patients with rosacea and 7/90 (7.8%) subjects in the control group had SIBO (p = 0.6). Within 10 weeks from the end of antibiotic therapy, the skin lesions of rosacea disappeared or decreased markedly in 35/36 (97.2%) patients after eradication of *H. pylori* and in 3/8 (37.5%) patients who did not eradicate the infection (p < 0.0001). Rosacea skin lesions decreased markedly in 6/7 (85.7%) after eradication of SIBO whereas of the two patients who did not eradicate SIBO, one (50%) showed an improvement in rosacea (p = 0.284). CONCLUSIONS: Prevalence of *H. pylori* infection was significantly higher in patients with rosacea than control group, whereas SIBO prevalence was comparable between the two groups. Eradication of *H. pylori* infection led to a significant improvement of skin symptoms in rosacea patients."

Unhealthy diets promote diabetes via microbial mechanisms, not simply nutrient intake		
What is becoming clear is that diets that enhance the development of diabetes and obesity—especially high-carbohydrate, low-fiber, high-fat, high-fructose, and high-artificial sweetener diets—do so via by means that strongly include the gut microbiome.		
Dietary factor	**Simple idea**	**Microbial understanding**
High-carbohydrate diet	Excess calories	SIBO, microbe-induced inflammation
Low-fiber diet	Excess sugar absorption	Gut dysbiosis
High-fat diet (HFD)	Excess calories	Gut dysbiosis, increased bacterial translocation, endotoxinemia
High-fructose diet	Excess calories	Gut dysbiosis, along with elevated urate
Artificial sweeteners	Increased diabetes risk despite lower caloric intake	Gut dysbiosis
Alcohol	Behaves as sugar since it is a fuel source and promotes lipogenesis	Damages intestinal mucosa; allows increased absorption of microbial inflammogens

8. Neurotoxic dysbiosis: A third subtype of metabolic dysbiosis is that of neurotoxic dysbiosis, the most obvious and accepted versions of which are D-lactic acidosis and hepatic encephalopathy; this dysbiotic neurotoxicity is probably mediated by a combination of ❶ mitochondrial dysfunction, ❷ false neurotransmitters (e.g., ammonia, tyramine), ❸ altered neurotransmission (e.g., dopamine and norepinephrine imbalances via HPHPA and p-cresol), and ❹ neuronal autoimmunity and glial activation (i.e., neuroinflammation).

- Gut microbiome alterations in autism—benefit from oral vancomycin treatment of regressive-onset autism (*J Child Neurol* 2000 Jul[426]): "Many parents of children with "regressive"-onset autism have noted antecedent antibiotic exposure followed by chronic diarrhea. We speculated that, in a subgroup of children, disruption of indigenous gut flora might promote colonization by one or more neurotoxin-producing bacteria, contributing, at least in part, to their autistic symptomatology. To help test this hypothesis, 11 children with regressive-onset autism were recruited for an intervention trial using a minimally absorbed oral antibiotic. Entry criteria included antecedent broad-spectrum antimicrobial exposure followed by chronic persistent

---

[425] Gravina et al. Helicobacter pylori infection not small intestinal bacterial overgrowth may play pathogenic role in rosacea. *United European Gastroenterol J.* 2015 Feb;3:17-24
[426] Sandler RH, Finegold SM, Bolte ER, et al. Short-term benefit from oral vancomycin treatment of regressive-onset autism. *J Child Neurol.* 2000 Jul;15(7):429-35

diarrhea, deterioration of previously acquired skills, and then autistic features. Short-term improvement was noted using multiple pre- and post-therapy evaluations. ... these results indicate that a possible gut flora-brain connection warrants further investigation, as it might lead to greater pathophysiologic insight and meaningful prevention or treatment in a subset of children with autism. ... The vancomycin dose was 500mg/day given orally as a liquid (500mg/6mL), divided 2mL three times per day for 8 weeks. This was followed by 4 weeks of oral treatment with a probiotic mixture of *Lactobacillus acidophilus*, *L bulgaricus*, and *Bifidobacterium bifidum* (40×10^9 [40,000,000,000 = 40 billion] colony-forming units/mL). " The gut microbiome contributes to autism via combined effects from metabolic neurotoxicity, inflammation (including cytokines and glial activation) and induction/promotion of neuronal autoimmunity.

> **Three major types of gastrointestinal Clostridia of major clinical relevance**
>
> ❶ *Clostridium difficile* diarrhea—famous antibiotic-induced and antibiotic-resistant diarrhea
> ❷ Beneficial Clostridial clusters—eumetabolic and anti-inflammatory, such as *Faecalibacterium prausnitzii*
> ❸ Neurotoxic Clostridia—associated with schizophrenia, autism, and other nonspecific clinical syndromes of neuropathology. Classic examples of neurotoxin-producing Clostridia are *Clostridium tetani* and *Clostridium botulinum* (also *Clostridium butyricum* and *Clostridium baratii*), which cause the paralytic conditions tetanus and botulism, respectively; nonclassic examples include those Clostridia that produce psychopathic HPHPA, p-cresol, and propionic acid

- Microbiome alterations in autism—N = 1 study of dramatic improvement in autism following amoxicillin administration (*Microb Ecol Health Dis*. 2015 Mar[427]): "....a physician confirmed strep via a rapid strep test and prescribed a 10-day course of amoxicillin... Neither had received an antibiotic before ...Earlier that year our son had been diagnosed with moderate-to-severe autism by a team of clinicians and practitioners at Children's Medical Center in Dallas, Texas. On day four of his 10-day course of amoxicillin, we began noticing changes in his autism symptoms: he began making eye contact, which he had previously avoided; his speech, which was severely delayed, began to improve markedly; he became less 'rigid' in his insistence for sameness and routine; and he also displayed an uncharacteristic level of energy, which he had historically lacked." Given the broad spectrum and systemic absorption of amoxicillin, objective improvements in autistic manifestations—unlikely due to a psychopharmacologic effect of the drug itself—do not localize the site of antimicrobial effectiveness; however, the most likely locales are the gut and nasopharynx. Doctorate-level clinicians are well aware of post-pharyngitis encephalitis/encephalopathy and related psychiatric and psychomotor disorders (e.g., PANDAS—pediatric autoimmune neuropsychiatric disorders associated with streptococcal infections); hence, the observation of microbe-induced neuronal autoimmunity and mood-altering glial activation are well established and accepted.

- Gut microbiome alterations in autism—Gastrointestinal microflora studies in late-onset autism (*Clin Infect Dis* 2002 Sep[428]): "Fecal flora of children with regressive autism was compared with that of control children, and clostridial counts were higher. The number of clostridial species found in the stools of children with autism was greater than in the stools of control children. Children with autism had 9 species of Clostridium not found in controls, whereas controls yielded only 3 species not found in children with autism. In all, there were 25 different clostridial species found. In gastric and duodenal specimens, the most striking finding was total absence of non-spore-forming anaerobes and microaerophilic bacteria from control children and significant numbers of such bacteria from children with autism. These studies demonstrate significant alterations in the upper and lower intestinal flora of children with late-onset autism and may provide insights into the nature of this disorder."

- Gut microbiome alterations in autism and schizophrenia—Gastrointestinal microflora studies in late-onset autism (*Nutr Neurosci*. 2010 Jun[429]): "A compound identified as 3-(3-hydroxyphenyl)-3-hydroxypropionic acid (HPHPA) was found in higher concentrations in urine samples of children with autism compared to age and sex appropriate controls and in an adult with recurrent diarrhea due to Clostridium difficile infections. The highest value measured in urine samples was 7500 mmol/mol creatinine, a value 300 times the median normal adult value, in a patient with acute schizophrenia during an acute psychotic episode. The psychosis remitted after treatment with oral vancomycin with a concomitant marked decrease in

[427] Rodakis J. An n=1 case report of a child with autism improving on antibiotics and a father's quest to understand what it may mean. *Microb Ecol Health Dis*. 2015 Mar;26:26382
[428] Finegold et al. Gastrointestinal microflora studies in late-onset autism. *Clin Infect Dis*. 2002 Sep 1;35(Suppl 1):S6-S16
[429] Shaw W. Increased urinary excretion of a 3-(3-hydroxyphenyl)-3-hydroxypropionic acid (HPHPA), an abnormal phenylalanine metabolite of Clostridia spp. in the gastrointestinal tract, in urine samples from patients with autism and schizophrenia. *Nutr Neurosci*. 2010 Jun;13(3):135-43

HPHPA. The source of this compound appears to be multiple species of anaerobic bacteria of the Clostridium genus. The significance of this compound is that it is a probable metabolite of m-tyrosine (3-hydroxyphenylalanine), a tyrosine analog which depletes brain catecholamines and causes symptoms of autism (stereotypical behavior, hyperactivity, and hyper-reactivity) in experimental animals."

- Real-time PCR quantitation of clostridia in feces of autistic children (*Appl Environ Microbiol.* 2004 Nov[430]): "Based on the hypothesis that intestinal clostridia play a role in late-onset autism, we have been characterizing clostridia from stools of autistic and control children. We applied the TaqMan real-time PCR procedure to detect and quantitate three *Clostridium* clusters and one *Clostridium* species, *C. bolteae*, in stool specimens. ... The assay showed high sensitivity: as few as 2 cells of members of cluster I, 6 cells of cluster XI, 4 cells of cluster XIVab, and 0.6 cell of *C. bolteae* could be detected per PCR. Analysis of the real-

> **Psycho(mind)pathic(disease) dysbiosis—a model of excess dopamine (psychosis) and glutamate (hyperexcitation) with a deficiency of norepinephrine (attentiveness)**
>
> One model for the contribution of gut dysbiosis to autism and other neuropsychiatric disorders is as follows: intestinal overgrowth of *Clostridia* species leads to microbial production and subsequent intestinal-to-systemic absorption of the phenylalanine metabolite 3-3-hydroxyphenyl-3-hydroxypropionic acid (HPHPA), which—like p-cresol—inhibits the dopamine beta-hydroxylase enzyme which would otherwise convert dopamine to norepinephrine. Therefore, in this model, *Clostridial* HPHPA blocks conversion of dopamine (leading to excess CNS dopamine) to norepinephrine (leading to insufficient CNS norepinephrine), the neurotransmitter responsible for vigilance and attention. In the allopathic medical model of psychosis, increased dopaminergic neurotransmission is causative, hence the reliance on anti-dopaminergic anti-psychotic drugs. Other microbial products and the cytokines elaborated in response to microbes would be expected to contribute to glial activation and the resulting excess in glutaminergic neurotransmission. The dopamine beta-hydroxylase enzyme requires ascorbate and copper for its function, while CNS glutaminergic neurotransmission is suppressed/modulated with pyridoxine, zinc, magnesium, and vitamin D.

time PCR data indicated that the cell count differences between autistic and control children for *C. bolteae* and the following *Clostridium* groups were statistically significant: mean counts of *C. bolteae* and clusters I and XI in autistic children were 46-fold ($P = 0.01$), 9.0-fold ($P = 0.014$), and 3.5-fold ($P = 0.004$) greater than those in control children, respectively, but not for cluster XIVab (2.6 x 10(8) CFU/g in autistic children and 4.8 x 10(8) CFU/g in controls; respectively)."

- Anaerobic clostridium and autism (*J Immunoassay Immunochem* 2014 Sep[431]): "3-(3-hydroxy phenyl)-3-hydroxypropionic acid (HPHPA) excretion rates which is a metabolic product of the genus *Clostridium*, were measured via mass spectrometry-gas chromatography (MS-GC) method from urine samples. When the assayed average HPHPA values compared with each group, a statistically significant difference was found ($p < 0.05$). Data obtained from this study support the existence of a significant correlation between autism etiology and anaerobic bacteria. ... The average HPHPA values in the [autism] patient group was 245 mmol/mol creatinine, while the control group's value was 84 mmol/mol creatinine. The average HPHPA values of the patient group and the control group were significantly different ($p<0.05$)."

- Gastrointestinal disorders and the microbiome in schizophrenia (*Schizophr Res.* 2014 Jul[432]): The authors of this paper do a fine job of herding various concepts and studies into a single document; overall, the model that is proposed is one of high but not unmanageable complexity, emphasizing the contribution of various factors that culminate in schizophrenia. The major initiating factors and physiologic responses are exposure to immunogens (*immune* response *gen*erating substances) and inflammogens (*inflamm*ation *gen*erating substances) such as gluten, microbes in general and the *Toxoplasma gondii* in particular, the exorphins (neuroactive food antigen/peptides resembling endorphins, with capacity to bind to opioid receptors) such as gluten-related peptides and bovine milk casein, HERV-induced neurologic autoimmunity, increased intestinal inflammation and resultant zonulin-mediated increases in gut and blood-brain-barrier (BBB) permeability. The authors propose—and I concur—that the future medical management of schizophrenia and autism will certainly consider factors *beyond neurotransmitters* and locations *outside of the brain* for optimal treatment.

[430] Song et al. Real-time PCR quantitation of clostridia in feces of autistic children. *Appl Environ Microbiol.* 2004 Nov;70(11):6459-65

[431] Keşli et al. Investigation of the relation between anaerobic bacteria genus clostridium and late-onset autism etiology in children. *J Immunoassay Immunochem.* 2014;35:101-9

[432] Severance et al. Autoimmune diseases, gastrointestinal disorders and the microbiome in schizophrenia. *Schizophr Res.* 2014 Jul 14. pii: S0920-9964(14)00319-3

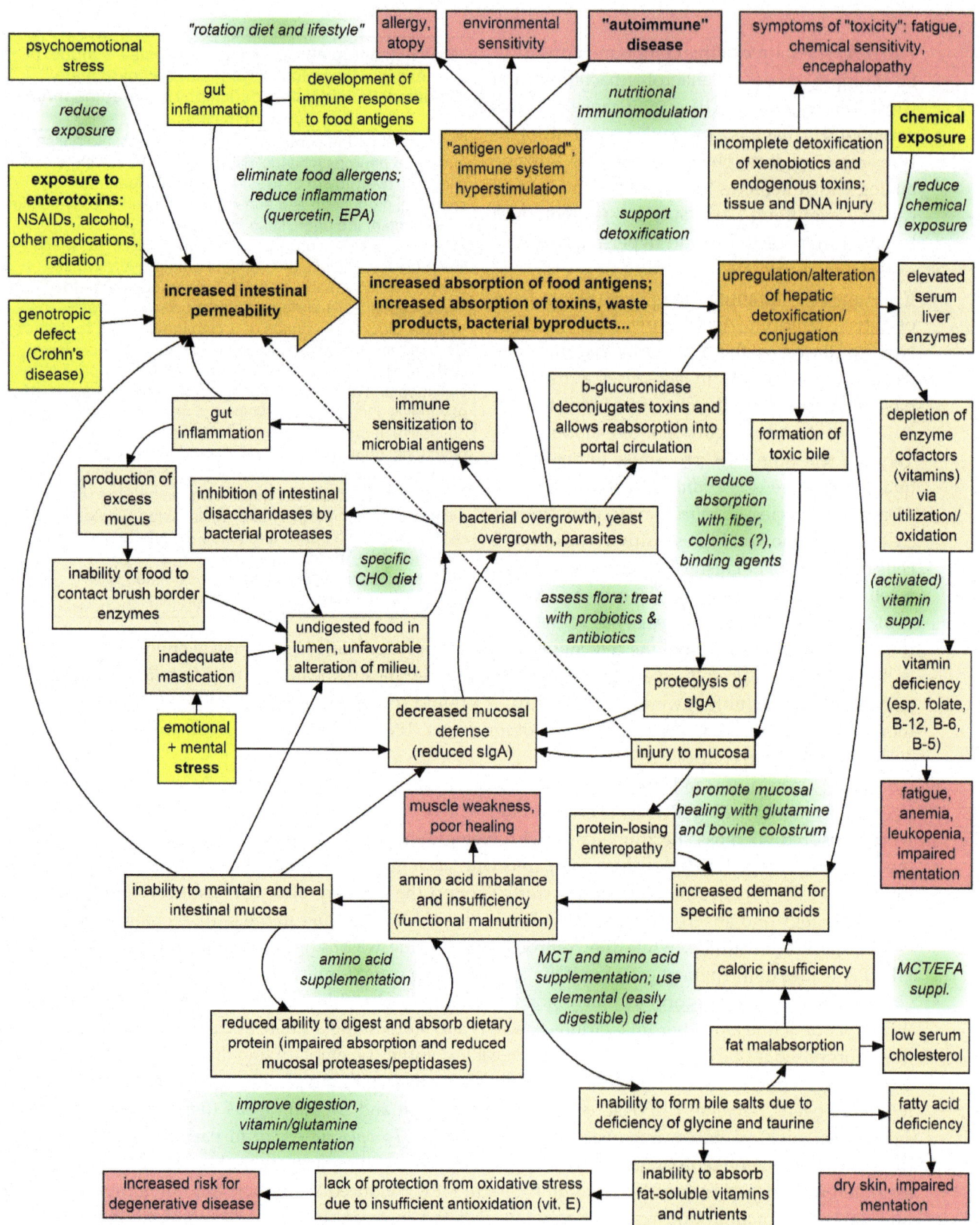

Gastrointestinal dysbiosis, "leaky gut" and impaired detoxification—interconnected scenarios: Therapeutic considerations are italicized and highlighted in green while "entry points" are colored in yellow, and clinical manifestations are mostly colored in red. This diagram—made by Dr Vasquez at age 28y after several years of chronic fatigue and dysbiosis—was published for the first time in _Integrative Orthopedics_ 2004 and is presented here virtually without change, excepting colorization. "And when a person goes through fire for his teaching [education], what does that prove? It is more meaningful—truly—when out of one's own burning cometh one's own teaching!" Nietzsche FW. _Thus Spoke Zarathustra_. Part 26

Gastrointestinal dysbiosis: Assessments

- **History**: Clinicians should suspect gastrointestinal dysbiosis in their patients with gas, bloating, alternating constipation/diarrhea, irritable bowel syndrome, fibromyalgia, chronic fatigue syndrome, multiple chemical sensitivity, severe allergies, and autoimmunity, especially Crohn's disease, ulcerative colitis, rheumatoid arthritis, and ankylosing spondylitis. Frequent gas and bloating indicates excess gastrointestinal fermentation by yeast and/or overgrowth of aerobic bacteria. Abdominal pain, chronic constipation, and/or diarrhea are clear indications for stool testing; however, clinicians must remember that **many very heavily colonized patients will have no gastrointestinal symptoms**. Thus, **assessment and treatment for gastrointestinal dysbiosis is *not unnecessary simply because the patient lacks gastrointestinal symptoms**.

- **Breath testing**: Bacterial overgrowth of the small bowel can be objectively documented with measurement of a **post-carbohydrate hydrogen/methane breath test**, but I consider a history of postprandial gas and bloating to be sufficiently diagnostic.

- **Lactulose-mannitol assay:** The intestinal wall should function as a tightly regulated barrier that accomplishes two tasks: 1) **efficient absorption** of nutrients, and 2) **selective exclusion** of antigens, foreign debris, microbes and microbial antigens, and indigestible food residues. Compromise of the intestinal barrier results in impairments in nutrient absorption and/or toxin exclusion. Impaired nutrient absorption predisposes to and commonly results in micro- or macro-nutrient deficiencies. Impaired exclusion results in increased absorption of microbes, antigens, waste products, and debris into the systemic circulation.[433,434] In many patients this injury is occult, and **they commonly have no gastrointestinal symptoms whatsoever**; other patients may have nonspecific manifestations including diarrhea, constipation, abdominal pain, fatigue, general malaise, dyscognition, and an increase in number/severity of food allergies/sensitivities/intolerances. The **lactulose and mannitol assay** evaluates paracellular (pathologic) and transcellular (physiologic) absorption, respectively; increased lactulose:mannitol ratio is a non-specific finding that indicates gastrointestinal damage, generally due to 1) enterotoxin consumption such as with alcohol or NSAIDs, 2) malnutrition, 3) food allergy including celiac disease, 4) inflammatory bowel disease, 5) major trauma, and/or 6) dysbiosis. **Recall that "leaky gut" is always a manifestation of another, larger problem**.

- **Comprehensive stool analysis and comprehensive parasitology**: The single best test for the assessment of gastrointestinal dysbiosis is a comprehensive stool analysis and comprehensive parasitology examination performed by a specialty laboratory that provides bacterial culture, yeast culture, microscopic exam, and measurement of sIgA to assess mucosal immune response, along with markers of inflammation such as lactoferrin, calprotectin, and/or lysozyme. Comprehensive parasitology examinations (x3) to assess for bacteria, yeast, and parasites should be followed by culture and sensitivity to fine-tune the identification of the microbes and to guide treatment. These tests should be performed by a specialty laboratory rather than a regular medical or hospital laboratory. Additional markers can help put microbiological findings into the proper context; for example, in a patient with no "pathogens" other than normal *Candida albicans*, the finding of an exaggerated inflammatory response suggests a hypersensitivity/allergic dysbiosis that should be eradicated. **Stool testing must be performed by a specialty laboratory** because the quality of testing provided by most standard "medical labs" and hospitals is completely inadequate. Initial samples should be collected on three separate occasions by the patient and each sample should be analyzed separately by the laboratory. Important qualitative and quantitative markers include the following:
  - Beneficial bacteria ("probiotics"): Microbiological testing should quantify and identify various beneficial bacteria, which should be present at "+4" levels on a 0-4 scale.
  - Harmful and potentially harmful bacteria, protozoans, amebas, etc.: Questionable or harmful microbes should be eradicated even if they are not identified as true pathogens in the Pasteurian/Kochian sense.
  - Yeast and mycology: At least two tests must be performed for a complete assessment: 1) yeast culture, and 2) microscopic examination for yeast elements. Per Galland and Gaby, I learned many years ago from their extensive experience, the patients that tend to have the most significant yeast-induced illness (and

[433] Hollander D. Intestinal permeability, leaky gut, and intestinal disorders. *Curr Gastroenterol Rep.* 1999 Oct;1(5):410-6

[434] Keshavarzian A, Holmes EW, Patel M, Iber F, Fields JZ, Pethkar S. Leaky gut in alcoholic cirrhosis. *Am J Gastroenterol.* 1999 Jan;94(1):200-7

thus the greatest possibility of clinical improvement following yeast eradication) are the patients whose intestinal yeast does not grow on culture but is visible microscopically (i.e., "negative culture, positive microscopic exam").

- o Microbial sensitivity testing: Sensitivity testing with natural/pharmacologic agents helps guide therapy.

- o Secretory IgA: SIgA levels are elevated in patients who are having an immune response to either food or microbial antigens.[435] Thus, in a patient with minimal dysbiosis, say for example with *Candida albicans*, an elevated sIgA can indicate that the patient is having a hypersensitivity reaction to an otherwise benign microbe—in this case, eradication of the microbe is warranted and may result in a positive clinical response. Low sIgA suggests either primary or secondary immune defect such as selective sIgA deficiency[436] or malnutrition, stress, prednisone/corticosteroids, or possibly mycotoxicosis (immunosuppression due to fungal immunotoxins).

- o Short-chain fatty acids (SCFA): These are produced by intestinal bacteria. Quantitative excess indicates bacterial overgrowth of the intestines, while insufficiency indicates a lack of probiotics or an insufficiency of dietary substrate, i.e., soluble fiber. Abnormal patterns of individual short-chain fatty acids indicate qualitative/quantitative abnormalities in gastrointestinal microflora, particularly anaerobic bacteria that cannot be identified with routine bacterial cultures. While SCFA have been appreciated for decades for their function as a ❶ fuel source for enterocytes, more recently we have come to appreciate that SCFA serve ❷ anti-inflammatory roles and also function as ❸ epigenetic regulators, notably for the Th immunocytes that are programmed in the gut associated lymphoid tissue (GALT); with appreciation of these diverse and beneficial roles of SCFA, clinicians are able to appreciate the impact of a lack of SCFA-producing bacteria and/or lack of dietary substrate such as soluble fiber, namely enterocyte fragility, mucosal inflammation, and failure of immune regulation, respectively.

- o Beta-glucuronidase: This is an enzyme produced by several different intestinal bacteria. High levels of beta-glucuronidase in the intestinal lumen serve to nullify the benefits of detoxification (specifically glucuronidation) by cleaving the toxicant from its glucuronide conjugate. This can result in re-absorption of the toxicant through the intestinal mucosa which then re-exposes the patient to the toxin that was previously detoxified ("enterohepatic recirculation" or "enterohepatic recycling"). This is an exemplary aspect of "auto-intoxication" that results in chronic fatigue and upregulation of Phase 1 detoxification systems.

- o Lactoferrin: The iron-binding glycoprotein lactoferrin is an inflammatory marker that helps distinguish functional disorders (i.e., IBS) from more serious diseases (i.e., IBD).

- o Lysozyme: Elevated in proportion to intestinal inflammation in dysbiosis and IBD. A very interesting study published in 2015 showed that the inoculation of IBD-prone mice with a combination of dysbiotic bacteria could lead to Paneth cell dysfunction and subsequent loss of protective lysozyme; the authors conclude their summary by stating, "We provide clear experimental evidence for the causal role of gut bacterial dysbiosis in the development of chronic ileal inflammation with subsequent failure of Paneth cell function."[437] The clinical significance of this, beyond its provision of yet another confirmation of the link between dysbiosis and IBD, is the possibility that clinically significant dysbiosis may paradoxically present without elevations in lysozyme due to the dysbiosis-induced Paneth cell dysfunction.

- o Other markers: Other markers of digestion, inflammation, and absorption are reported with the more comprehensive test panels, are not always necessary, are helpful when working with complex patients, and are relatively self-explanatory and/or are described in the laboratory's interpretive guide.

[435] Quig DW, Higley M. Noninvasive assessment of intestinal inflammation: IBD vs. IBS. *Townsend Letter for Doctors and Patients* 2006;Jan:74-5

[436] "Selective IgA deficiency is most common form of immunodeficiency. Certain select populations, including allergic individuals, patients with autoimmune and gastrointestinal tract disease and patients with recurrent upper respiratory tract illnesses, have an increased incidence." Burks et al. Selective IgA deficiency. *Ann Allergy*. 1986;57:3-13

[437] Schaubeck et al. Dysbiotic gut microbiota causes transmissible Crohn's disease-like ileitis independent of failure in antimicrobial defence. *Gut* 2015 Apr.pii:gutjnl-2015-309333

Gastrointestinal dysbiosis: Interventions

- The "antidysbiotic lifestyle" as key to addressing persistent microbial incongruity: Two of the key distinguishing characteristics of my dysbiosis model and my anti-dysbiosis protocols are their level of comprehensiveness and detail, and my broadening of the focus beyond the microbe(s) to emphasize the importance of immune defenses, immune tolerance, and the modification of the host milieu to make a less hospitable to persistent problematic colonization, respectively. Nonmicrobial methods of changing "dysbiotic relationships" are sampled in the following table but can really be understood only within the comprehensive totality of the model that I have developed, most recently in *Functional Inflammology, volume 1* and—by adding a section on clinical applications for inflammatory disease—*Naturopathic Rheumatology v3.5*; anything less than the complete model, including the contextualizing information in Chapters 2 and 3, is by definition partial and incomplete and therefore less effective, less potent. As Hollingdale[438] accurately stated in his classic compilation of Nietzsche's philosophical writings, "no selection can do justice to the work as a whole, and any selection must to a greater or less extent be a simplification and thus to some extent a falsification of it."

Anti-dysbiotic lifestyle	Mechanisms against dysbiosis-related diseases and microbial incongruity
Diet optimization	Avoidance of the dysbiosis-inducing American/Western diet; diet should be plant-based protein-adequate and supplemented with appropriate nutrients per 5pSPMD
Vigorous exercise	Often includes periodic "fasting" periods anticipated to promote microbial diversity while also increasing endogenous production of bHB which inhibits inflammasome activity while enhancing antioxidant defenses and mitochondrial ETC function, reinforces healthy diet and other lifestyle factors including those that affect work/personal relationships and self-esteem; promotes intestinal peristalsis to reduce intestinal and thus whole-body microbial load; induction of a more "athletic phenotype" including minimization of adiposity changes (gut) microflora
Immunonutrition, nutritional immunorestoration, nutritional immunomodulation for Treg:Th17 optimization (Chapter 4, section 3)	Most people and especially those with "chronic diseases" and persistent "infections" are in a vicious cycle of nutrient insufficiency, immunoimpairment, and persistent microbial colonization and activation; so-called "immuonutrients" such as zinc, selenium, glutamine, arginine, vitamin A, cholecalciferol commonly need to be supplemented in order to "break the cycle" of infection-disease-deficiency-immunosuppression; nutritional immunomodulation protocol is implemented to promote elaboration of Treg and suppression of Th1, Th2, and Th17
Sleep optimization, stress avoidance/management (Chapter 2)	Antioxidant and immune-stimulating effects of melatonin are well documented; modulation of stress responses is important since microbes sense catecholamines (microbial endocrinology) and respond to exploit their host's stress by becoming increasingly virulent; circadian rhythm disruption promotes dysbiosis[439]
Hormonal optimization (thyroid assessment detailed in Chapter 1; others in Chapter 4, section 6)	Hormonal status and function must be optimized if inflammatory tolerance is likewise to be optimized; all hormones affect inflammatory balance and tolerance. Serum testing of prolactin, estradiol, insulin, DHEA-S, cortisol (preferably with ACTH challenge), free and total testosterones. Thyroid status is optimized per Chapter 1; hypothyroidism promotes SIBO via hypochlorhydria and hypoperistalsis.
For details and citations and clinical implementation, see *Naturopathic Rheumatology v3.5* or later versions and *Antiviral Strategies and Immune Nutrition*, available in print and digital versions.	

Simple samples of anti-dysbiotic lifestyle components: Clinicians must, if they want intellectual accuracy and clinical efficacy, expand their conception of dysbiosis beyond the microbe and—likewise—of anti-dysbiotic treatments beyond antimicrobial interventions. Antibiotic interventions against dysbiosis-induced disease are occasionally "therapeutically miraculous" but remain rare due to failure to optimize inherent inflammatory tolerance and defensive immune functions.

- Diet optimization for immunorestoration and anti-fermentation: The 5-part "supplemented Paleo-Mediterranean diet" (5pSPMD or SPMD—reviewed in Chapter 4, Section 1, and in online article and compilation[440]) consists of ❶ plant-based low-carbohydrate diet of fruits, vegetables, nuts, seeds, berries and

[438] Hollingdale RJ (ed). *Nietzsche Reader*. Penguin Books, page 4

[439] Voigt et al. (2014) Circadian Disorganization Alters Intestinal Microbiota. *PLoS ONE* 9(5): e97500

[440] Vasquez A. Revisiting the five-part nutritional wellness protocol: the supplemented Paleo Mediterranean diet. *Nutritional Perspectives* 2011 Jan. For the original PDF of this article and additional notes and excerpts, see folder at InflammationMastery.com/reprints

lean sources of protein: the plant-based diet optimizes antioxidant and phytonutrient intake[441] while promoting favorable modification of gastrointestinal flora for a systemic anti-inflammatory benefit[442]; carbohydrate intake is minimized and tailored per individual need for weight maintenance and exercise recovery/compensation; maintaining mild ketosis via low carbohydrate intake helps maintain optimal body weight, mitochondrial efficiency, bHB's antioxidant function and a rejuvenative phenotype via histone acetylation[443]; plant-based diets promote alkalinization and counteract the Western diet's promotion of diet-induced acidosis[444]; fermentable carbohydrates from soluble fibers, inulin, and fructooligosaccharides promote the growth of beneficial bacteria (caution with Klebsiella pneumoniae and Proteus species) and elaboration of their metabolites and enhanced production of mucus which simultaneously protects enterocytes and provides additional carbohydrates to beneficial bacteria; intake of cruciferous vegetables provides aryl-hydrocarbon receptor ligands which optimize mucosal immunity[445]; renal insufficiency mandates vigilance for hyperkalemia, especially when considering implementation of a potassium-rich diet ❷ multivitamin and multimineral supplementation: this component serves to correct pandemic nutritional deficiencies[446], prevent long-latency deficiency diseases[447], improve mood[448], reduce systemic inflammation[449], and provide some/partial/complete compensation for genotropic metabolic defects[450], ❸ physiologic doses of vitamin D3 (range 2,000-10,000 IU/d): vitamin D3 supplementation[451] alleviates pain, improves mood, reduces inflammation, enhances immunity, normalizes hypertension, ❹ combination fatty acid therapy (CFAT) with n3-ALA, n6-GLA, n3-EPA, n3-DHA, and phytochemical-rich olive oil which contains n9-oleate: anti-inflammatory, mood-enhancing, and cardioprotective benefits are conclusively documented, ❺ probiotics: probiotics promote immunotolerance via several mechanisms including induction of Treg; probiotic supplementation helps prevent and treat insufficiency dysbiosis, which causes 1) decreased colonization resistance, 2) increased bacterial translocation, and 3) failure of optimal Treg induction. Per "Expert consensus document: The International Scientific Association for Probiotics and Prebiotics consensus statement" published in *Nature Reviews Gastroenterology and Hepatology* 2014 Aug[452], probiotics—by definition—require administration of at least one billion (1,000,000,000 or 1x10^9) colony forming units (CFU); many probiotic nutritional supplements in the form of powders and capsules contain 1-20 billion organisms yet not all organisms are viable at time of consumption and not all viable organisms become CFU. Importantly, some benefits of probiotic supplementation are not dependent on viable microorganisms but rather on the molecular signature of the microbe; other—and obviously more complete—benefits require microbial viability and are mediated via metabolites, which are themselves interdependent on microbes and the host's diet. Bertazzoni et al[453] extensively reviewed the issue of microbial/CFU count number and concluded that the appropriate dose is patient-dependent, disease-dependent, and strain-dependent and thus cannot be generalized; their review included several studies that safely and effectively used varying doses, e.g., 1, 30, 70, 300 billion CFU/d. Per expert clinical opinion[454], a clinician might use one billion [units = microbes or CFU] for a small or young child, and a starting dose of 10 billion scaling up to 90 billion per day for adults. Prebiotic carbohydrate sources such as inulin, fructans, and fructooligosaccharides can lead to clear exacerbations of D-lactate overproduction specifically and SIBO in general; otherwise their judicious and persistent utilization promotes the growth of beneficial bacteria generally

---

[441] Liu RH. Health benefits of fruit and vegetables are from additive and synergistic combinations of phytochemicals. *Am J Clin Nutr*. 2003 Sep;78(3 Suppl):517S-520S

[442] Peltonen R et al. Faecal microbial flora and disease activity in rheumatoid arthritis during a vegan diet. *Br J Rheumatol*. 1997 Jan;36(1):64-8

[443] Shimazu T, Hirschey MD, et al. Suppression of oxidative stress by β-hydroxybutyrate, an endogenous histone deacetylase inhibitor. *Science* 2013 Jan;339:211-4. To access more of Dr Matt Hirschey's work and video presentations, please see ichnfm.org/events/MitochondrialMedicine. For additional information on the rejuvenative effect of histone acetylation, see: Matuoka et al. Rapid reversion of aging phenotypes by nicotinamide through possible modulation of histone acetylation. *Cell Mol Life Sci*. 2001 Dec;58:2108-16

[444] Adeva et al. Diet-induced metabolic acidosis. *Clin Nutr*. 2011 Aug;30:416-21. Cordain et al. Origins and evolution of the Western diet. *Am J Clin Nutr*. 2005 Feb;81(2):341-54

[445] Hooper LV. You AhR what you eat: linking diet and immunity. *Cell*. 2011 Oct 28;147(3):489-91

[446] Fletcher RH, Fairfield KM. Vitamins for chronic disease prevention in adults: clinical applications. *JAMA*. 2002 Jun 19;287(23):3127-9

[447] Heaney RP. Long-latency deficiency disease: insights from calcium and vitamin D. *Am J Clin Nutr*. 2003 Nov;78(5):912-9

[448] Benton D, Haller J, Fordy J. Vitamin supplementation for 1 year improves mood. *Neuropsychobiology*. 1995;32(2):98-105

[449] Church TS, Earnest CP, Wood KA, Kampert JB. Reduction of C-reactive protein levels through use of a multivitamin. *Am J Med*. 2003 Dec 15;115(9):702-7

[450] Ames BN, et al. High-dose vitamin therapy stimulates variant enzymes with decreased coenzyme binding affinity (increased Km). *Am J Clin Nutr*. 2002 Apr;75(4):616-58

[451] See discussion and citaitons throughout Chapter 4. Vasquez A, Manso G, Cannell J. The clinical importance of vitamin D (cholecalciferol): a paradigm shift with implications for all healthcare providers. *Altern Ther Health Med*. 2004 Sep-Oct;10(5):28-36 inflammationmastery.com/reprints/

[452] Hill et al. Expert consensus document: The International Scientific Association for Probiotics and Prebiotics consensus statement on the scope and appropriate use of the term probiotic. *Nat Rev Gastroenterol Hepatol*. 2014 Aug;11(8):506-14

[453] Bertazzoni et al. Probiotics and clinical effects: is the number what counts? *J Chemother*. 2013 Aug;25(4):193-212

[454] Conversation and personal communication 2014 Aug with my friend and colleague Mike Ash DO ND, an international expert on probiotics and mucosal immunology, "But some studies suggest 1 billion is the number needed to generate an effect (of clinical relevance), and this may suit a small or young child. I tend to start at 10 billion and rarely ever exceed 90 billion in a day [for adults]."

speaking (with *Klebsiella pneumoniae* and *Proteus* species being the noted exceptions[455]), promotes elaboration of metabolites such as short-chain fatty acids (SCFA) which serve as fuel sources for enterocytes, acidifying agents for the stool pH, indirect antioxidants, and epigenetic modulators which change gene expression and immunophenotype (e.g., Treg versus Th17 induction), and can deliver microbe-independent direct antioxidant benefits to the intestinal lumen, thereby protecting enterocytes.[456]

o Additional details—implementation of the "low-carbohydrate (low fermentation) supplemented Paleo-Mediterranean diet" ("low-carb SPMD"): The diet should be plant-based, but not necessarily vegan or vegetarian; I refer to this diet at "plant-based Paleo" since "the Paleo diet" as commonly discussed is simply a diet of whole natural foods which can generally be consumed without cooking or processing. For purposes of meeting physiologic expectations and attaining the highest satiety, weight optimization, and nutrient density with a phytonutrient-dense low-fermentation diet, the diet should primarily consist of fruits, vegetables, nuts, seeds, berries, and lean sources of protein; carbohydrate intake is modulated per caloric and carbohydrate needs while protein intake is tailored to lean body mass, exercise and healing/recuperation needs. Preferred sources of protein are grass-fed land animals as well as wild-caught cold-water fish, both of which are low in total fat and high in the anti-inflammatory and immunomodulatory omega-3 fatty acids, especially EPA and DHA. Whey protein isolate can also be used as it is an inexpensive convenient source of high-quality protein well-tolerated for most patients and as it also contains many functional components such as glutathione precursors, tryptophan, immunoglobulins, and growth factors anti-gastrin effects which help to heal/protect damaged intestinal mucosa. Plant-based diets, which can be further phyto-supplemented with food concentrates and fruit/vegetable smoothies/juices, provide the greatest dietary density and diversity of phytonutrients which generally have antioxidant and anti-inflammatory effects; also very important is the highly important modulation of gastrointestinal flora by plant-based diets which serves as a major mechanism by which such diets exert their clinically significant systemic anti-inflammatory benefits. I have detailed this diet—"the Supplemented Paleo-Mediterranean diet" as a combination of the "Paleolithic" or "Paleo diet" and the well-known "Mediterranean diet", both of which are well described in peer-reviewed journals and the lay press. (See Chapter 2 and my other publications[457,458] for details). This diet is the most nutrient-dense diet available, and its benefits are further enhanced by supplementation with vitamins, minerals, and the health-promoting fatty acids: ALA, GLA, EPA, DHA, and oleic acid. Vitamin and mineral supplementation is warranted in the general population and even more so among patients[459], who are more likely to be nutrient deficient due to their disease processes, mediations, and concomitant problems such as mild metabolic acidosis, malabsorption, and drug-induced nutrient depletions. Beyond routine vitamin-mineral supplementation, additional vitamin D3 supplementation is generally needed to meet the physiologic requirement of approximately 4,000 IU per day and to achieve the physiologic and clinical benefits including prevention/alleviation of depression, chronic pain, diabetes mellitus, hypertension, immunosuppression, immune activation, and cancer.[460] Likewise, absolute or relative deficiencies/insufficiencies of health-promoting anti-inflammatory fatty acids—namely: ALA, GLA, EPA, DHA, and oleic acid—are common and clinically consequential insofar as these deficiencies/insufficiencies promote chronic/sustained inflammation, pain, and neuroemotional impairment; thus, combination fatty acid therapy/replacement/supplementation (CFAT) is indicated based on its physiological effects and clinical benefits. Probiotics, especially when consumed in conjunction with a plant-based diet which promotes an enhanced milieu for their growth and effect, provide clear clinical benefits which are both local to the gut (e.g., reduced incidence of opportunistic infections/colonizations, prevention/amelioration of increased intestinal permeability) and systemic via the anti-inflammatory

---

[455] Hartemink et al. Growth of enterobacteria on fructo-oligosaccharides. *J Appl Microbiol*. 1997 Sep;83(3):367-74

[456] Franco-Robles E, López MG. Implication of Fructans in Health: Immunomodulatory and Antioxidant Mechanisms. *Scientific World Journal* 2015 Mar Article ID 289267

[457] Vasquez A. A Five-Part Nutritional Protocol that Produces Consistently Positive Results. *Nutritional Wellness* 2005 September

[458] Vasquez A. Implementing the Five-Part Nutritional Wellness Protocol for the Treatment of Various Health Problems. *Nutritional Wellness* 2005 November

[459] "However, suboptimal intake of some vitamins, above levels causing classic vitamin deficiency, is a risk factor for chronic diseases and common in the general population, especially the elderly. ... Most people do not consume an optimal amount of all vitamins by diet alone. Pending strong evidence of effectiveness from randomized trials, it appears prudent for all adults to take vitamin supplements. ... Physicians should make specific efforts to learn about their patients' use of vitamins to ensure that they are taking vitamins they should, ..." Fletcher RH, Fairfield KM. Vitamins for chronic disease prevention in adults: clinical applications. *JAMA*. 2002 Jun 19;287(23):3127-9

[460] Vasquez et al. The clinical importance of vitamin D (cholecalciferol): a paradigm shift. *Altern Ther Health Med*. 2004 Sep-Oct;10(5):28-36 InflammationMastery.com/reprints

benefits of enhanced induction of Treg cells at the reciprocal expense of Th17 cells. This "supplemented Paleo-Mediterranean diet" obviates overconsumption of chemical preservatives, artificial sweeteners, and carbohydrate-dominant foods such as candies, pastries, breads, potatoes, grains, and other foods with a high glycemic load and high glycemic index (from a practical and conceptual standpoint: glycemic load x glycemic index = glycemic impact = more oxidative stress, antioxidant depletion, immunosuppression, and mitochondrial impairment).

- Supplemented Paleo-Mediterranean diet / Specific Carbohydrate Diet: The specifications of the *specific carbohydrate diet* (SCD) detailed by Gottschall[461] are met with adherence to the Paleo diet by Cordain.[462] The combination of both approaches and books will give patients an excellent combination of informational understanding and culinary versatility.

- The use of a low starch diet in the treatment of patients suffering from ankylosing spondylitis: alleviation of dysbiosis and immune complex formation via nutritional intervention (*Clin Rheumatol* 1996 Jan[463]): "The majority of ankylosing spondylitis (AS) patients not only possess HLA-B27, but during active phases of the disease have elevated levels of total serum IgA, suggesting that a microbe from the bowel flora is acting across the gut mucosa. .... Furthermore AS patients from 10 different countries have been found to have elevated levels of specific antibodies against Klebsiella bacteria. It has been suggested that these Klebsiella microbes, found in the bowel flora, might be the trigger factors in this disease and therefore reduction in the size of the bowel flora could be of benefit in the treatment of AS patients. Microbes from the bowel flora depend on dietary starch for their growth and therefore a reduction in starch intake might be beneficial in AS patients. A "low starch diet" involving a reduced intake of "bread, potatoes, cakes and pasta" has been devised and tested in healthy control subjects and AS patients. The "low starch diet" leads to a reduction of total serum IgA in both healthy controls as well as patients, and furthermore to a decrease in inflammation and symptoms in the AS patients."

- Celiac disease and autoimmunity (*J Gastroenterol Hepatol* 2013 Jan[464]): 356 patients with CD participated in this study. "Autoimmune thyroiditis (10.6% vs 0.4%), insulin dependent diabetes mellitus (IDDM) (2.2% vs 1.7%), systemic lupus erythematosus (SLE) (1.1% vs 0), and psoriasis (12.9% vs 5.5%) occurred more frequently in CD patients."

- *Saccharomyces boulardii*: A non-colonizing, non-pathogenic yeast that increases sIgA production and can aid in the elimination of pathogenic/dysbiotic yeast, bacteria, and parasites. It is particularly useful during antibiotic treatment to help prevent secondary *Candida* and *Clostridium difficile* infections. Common dose is 250 mg thrice daily for adults and twice daily for children.

- Gastrointestinal antimicrobial interventions for isolated and combined use: Treatment for nonspecific dysbiosis and SIBO is empiric with the use of a variety of agents; when pharmaceutical agents are used, empiric selection and occasional rotation of agents (to theoretically/actually reduce the incidence of resistance) is standard medical practice—cited here are two of the best articles ever written on this topic, both freely available.[465,466]

  - Berberine (generally available as generic berberine hydrochloride or as a plant-based standardized extract with synergistic phytochemicals[467]) 1,000-1,500 mg/d in divided doses PO for up to 3 months: Berberine is a botanical alkaloid extracted from plants such as *Berberis vulgaris*, and *Hydrastis canadensis* with millennia of clinical use for various conditions and also specifically for the

> **Empiric treatment is standard for SIBO**
>
> "The bacterial species involved in inducing SIBO are diverse; preference is given to antibiotics effective against Gram-negative and anaerobic bacteria. ... At our institution, empirical treatment for moderate-risk patients (defined as those with no radiological or clinical evidence of dysmotility) comprises a seven-day treatment of rotating oral gentamicin and metronidazole, followed by no antibiotics for seven days and then restarting the cycle again."
>
> Malik et al. Diagnosis and pharmacological management of small intestinal bacterial overgrowth in children with intestinal failure. *Can J Gastroenterol* 2011 Jan

---

[461] Gotschall E. *Breaking the Vicious Cycle: Intestinal health though diet*. Kirkton Press; Rev edition (August, 1994) scdiet.com/

[462] Cordain L. *The Paleo Diet*. John Wiley & Sons Inc., New York 2002 thepaleodiet.com/

[463] Ebringer A, Wilson C. The use of a low starch diet in the treatment of patients suffering from ankylosing spondylitis. *Clin Rheumatol*. 1996 Jan;15 Suppl 1:62-66

[464] Iqbal et al. Celiac disease arthropathy and autoimmunity study. *J Gastroenterol Hepatol*. 2013 Jan;28(1):99-105

[465] DiBaise JK. Nutritional consequences of small intestinal bacterial overgrowth. *Practical Gastroenterology* 2008 Dec; 15-28

[466] Malik et al. Diagnosis and pharmacological management of small intestinal bacterial overgrowth in children with intestinal failure. *Can J Gastroenterol* 2011;25(1):41-45

[467] Stermitz FR, Lorenz P, Tawara JN, Zenewicz LA, Lewis K. Synergy in a medicinal plant: antimicrobial action of berberine potentiated by 5'-methoxyhydnocarpin, a multidrug pump inhibitor. *Proc Natl Acad Sci U S A*. 2000 Feb 15;97(4):1433-7

treatment of infectious diseases, such as those caused by *E coli*, *Giardia lamblia* (comparable to metronidazole), *Entamoeba histolytica*, *Streptococcus* and *Chlamydia trachomatis*.[468] Many clinicians use berberine as a standard treatment for gastrointestinal dysbiosis due to bacteria, yeast, and/or other microbes; it is very safe and has a wide range of antimicrobial action with no appreciated drug interactions, other than possible potentiation of hypoglycemia with metformin given that berberine is dose-for-dose at least if not more effective than metformin. Oral dose of 400 mg per day has been traditionally common for adults[469]; however newer clinical research has shown that berberine 1,000-1,5000 mg/d for three months provides major clinical benefits and is effective treatment for dyslipidemia, insulin resistance, diabetes mellitus type-2 (comparable to metformin), and overweight/obesity.[470,471,472,473] Berberine is available in a "generic" form from many nutraceutical companies, either as pure berberine HCl or as whole-plant extracts with synergists.

> **Emulsified time-released oil of oregano against gastrointestinal dysbiosis: one of the only agents (besides berberine) with human clinical data supporting efficacy and safety**
>
> "After 6 weeks of supplementation with 600 mg emulsified oil of oregano daily, there was complete disappearance of *Entamoeba hartmanni* (four cases), *Endolimax nana* (one case), and *Blastocystis hominis* in eight cases. Also, *Blastocystis hominis* scores declined in three additional cases. Gastrointestinal symptoms improved in seven of the 11 patients who had tested positive for *Blastocystis hominis*."
>
> Force et al. Inhibition of enteric parasites by emulsified oil of oregano in vivo. *Phytother Res.* 2000 May

o Oregano oil (time-released emulsified preparation named "ADP" from Biotics Research Corporation) 600 mg/d generally given as 200 mg/d PO TID for 6 weeks: Oil of Mediterranean oregano *Oreganum vulgare* was orally administered to 14 adult patients whose stools tested positive for enteric parasites, *Blastocystis hominis*, *Entamoeba hartmanni* and *Endolimax nana*. Six weeks of supplementation with 600 mg emulsified oil of oregano daily resulted in complete disappearance of *Entamoeba hartmanni* (four cases), *Endolimax nana* (one case), and *Blastocystis hominis* in eight cases. *Blastocystis hominis* scores declined in three additional cases.[474] An *in vitro* study[475] and clinical experience support the use of emulsified oregano against *Candida albicans* and various gastrointestinal microbes. Many clinicians use ADP as a standard treatment for gastrointestinal dysbiosis due to bacteria, yeast, and/or other microbes; it is very safe and has a wide range of antimicrobial action with no appreciated drug interactions. Emulsification increases dispersal and surface area/coverage; delayed release ensures/promotes coverage throughout more of the gastrointestinal tract rather than allowing immediate release and absorption.

o Undecylenic acid (also known as 10-undecenoic acid, available as "Formula SF722" from Thorne Research, each gelcap contains 10-undecenoic acid 50 mg) dosed at "450-750 mg undecylenic acid daily in three divided doses"[476] equates to 10-15 capsules per day, or 5 capsules 2-3 times per day: An eleven-carbon monounsaturated fatty acid found naturally in the body (occurring in sweat) and produced commercially by the vacuum distillation of castor bean oil, undecylenate shows laboratory and limited clinical human-trial effectiveness against *Herpes simplex*, *Candida albicans*, and tinea pedis caused by *Trychophyton rubrumor* and *Trychophyton mentagrophytes*.

---

[468] [No authors listed]. Berberine. *Altern Med Rev.* 2000 Apr;5(2):175-7

[469] Berberine. *Altern Med Rev.* 2000 Apr;5(2):175-7 thorne.com/altmedrev/.fulltext/5/2/175.pdf

[470] Kong et al. Berberine is a novel cholesterol-lowering drug working through a unique mechanism distinct from statins. *Nat Med.* 2004 Dec;10(12):1344-51

[471] "...bese human subjects (Caucasian) were given 500 mg berberine orally 3 times a day for 12 weeks. Efficacy and safety of berberine treatment was determined by measurements of body weight, comprehensive metabolic panel, blood lipid and hormone levels, expression levels of inflammatory factors, complete blood count, and electrocardiograph. Sprague-Dawley rat experiment was also performed to identify anti-obesity effects of berberine treatment. Results demonstrate that berberine treatment produced mild weight loss (average 5 lb/subject) in obese human subjects. But more interestingly, treatment significantly reduced blood lipid levels (23% decrease of triglyceride and 12.2% decrease of cholesterol levels) in human subjects." Hu et al. Lipid-lowering effect of berberine in human subjects and rats. *Phytomedicine* 2012 Jul;19:861-7

[472] "In study A, 36 adults with newly diagnosed type 2 diabetes mellitus were randomly assigned to treatment with berberine or metformin (0.5 g 3 times a day) in a 3-month trial. The hypoglycemic effect of berberine was similar to that of metformin. Significant decreases in hemoglobin A1c (from 9.5%+/-0.5% to 7.5%+/-0.4%, P<.01), fasting blood glucose (from 10.6+/-0.9 mmol/L to 6.9+/-0.5 mmol/L, P<.01), postprandial blood glucose (from 19.8+/-1.7 to 11.1+/-0.9 mmol/L, P<.01), and plasma triglycerides (from 1.13+/-0.13 to 0.89+/-0.03 mmol/L, P<.05) were observed in the berberine group. In study B, 48 adults with poorly controlled type 2 diabetes mellitus were treated supplemented with berberine in a 3-month trial. Berberine acted by lowering fasting blood glucose and postprandial blood glucose from 1 week to the end of the trial. Hemoglobin A1c decreased from 8.1%+/-0.2% to 7.3%+/-0.3% (P<.001)." Yin J, Xing H, Ye J.Efficacy of berberine in patients with type 2 diabetes mellitus. *Metabolism.* 2008 May;57(5):712-7

[473] "One hundred sixteen patients with type 2 diabetes and dyslipidemia were randomly allocated to receive berberine (1.0 g daily) and the placebo for 3 months. ... In the berberine group, fasting and postload plasma glucose decreased from 7.0 +/- 0.8 to 5.6 +/- 0.9 and from 12.0 +/- 2.7 to 8.9 +/- 2.8 mm/liter, HbA1c from 7.5 +/- 1.0% to 6.6 +/- 0.7%, triglyceride from 2.51 +/- 2.04 to 1.61 +/- 1.10 mm/liter, total cholesterol from 5.31 +/- 0.98 to 4.35 +/- 0.96 mm/liter, and low-density lipoprotein-cholesterol from 3.23 +/- 0.81 to 2.55 +/- 0.77 mm/liter,..." Zhang et al. Treatment of type 2 diabetes and dyslipidemia with the natural plant alkaloid berberine. *J Clin Endocrinol Metab.* 2008 Jul;93(7):2559-65

[474] Force M, Sparks WS, Ronzio RA. Inhibition of enteric parasites by emulsified oil of oregano in vivo. *Phytother Res.* 2000 May;14(3):213-4

[475] Stiles JC, Sparks W, Ronzio RA. The inhibition of Candida albicans by oregano. *J Applied Nutr* 1995;47:96–102

[476] [No authors listed] Undecylenic acid. Monograph. *Altern Med Rev.* 2002 Feb;7(1):68-70

o Combination botanical antimicrobials ("Tricycline" from Allergy Research Group): Contains black walnut, artemesinin, berberine, and citrus seed extract; in the early days of my clinical practice, I used this product routinely with a standard dosing of "2 capsules twice per day until the bottle [n=90] is empty."

o *Artemisia annua*: Artemisinin has been safely used for centuries in Asia for the treatment of malaria, and it also has effectiveness against anaerobic bacteria due to the pro-oxidative sesquiterpene endoperoxide.[477,478] This author has commonly used artemisinin at 200 mg per day in divided doses for adults with dysbiosis. Given its pro-oxidative mechanism, treatment should probably be of limited duration, i.e., 1-2 months; concomitant neuroprotection with CoQ-10 and NAC (et al) would be reasonable.

o St. John's Wort (*Hypericum perforatum*): Hyperforin from *Hypericum perforatum* shows impressive antibacterial action *in vitro*, particularly against gram-positive bacteria such as *Staphylococcus aureus*, *Streptococcus pyogenes*, *Streptococcus agalactiae*[479] and perhaps gram-negative *Helicobacter pylori*.[480] Up to 600 mg three times per day of a 3% hyperforin standardized extract is customary in the treatment of depression.

o Bismuth: Bismuth is commonly used in the empiric treatment of diarrhea (e.g., "Pepto-Bismol") and is commonly combined with other antimicrobial agents to reduce drug resistance and increase antibiotic effectiveness.[481]

o Peppermint (*Mentha piperita*): Peppermint shows antimicrobial and antispasmodic actions and has demonstrated clinical effectiveness in patients with bacterial overgrowth of the small bowel.

o DrV's (in)famous "vitamin C purge"—the author's perspective and rationale: Generally when I lecture on the topic of dysbiosis to post-graduate audiences, I mention one of my preferred treatments for GI dysbiosis, for which I seem to be either famous or infamous, namely my "vitamin C purge." The application is essentially as straightforward as the underlying logic: the *per os* use of vitamin C (20-60 grams in 1 liter of water, preferably with two cups of coffee) for its osmotic laxative effect to rapidly reduce the quantity of bacteria/microorganisms throughout the gut by introduction of a cleansing water bolus; while the vitamin C and water serve as an osmotic nonstimulant laxative (perhaps with some antimicrobial effect), the coffee/caffeine serves as a bowel stimulant. I have used this treatment empirically with great success in achieving rapid quantitative reductions in gastrointestinal microbes. For many years plain ascorbic acid was used at doses of 20-60 grams 20,000-60,000 mg) to induce therapeutic laxation (occasionally described as "do-it-yourself top-to-bottom gastrointestinal lavage") with onset of action generally within 30-60 minutes following consumption of powered ascorbate in approximately one liter of water, preferably *and often necessarily* with a bowel peristalsis stimulant such as coffee. The goal and purpose are to achieve a cleansing "water bolus" that purges the bowels of dysbiotic microbes and their pro-inflammatory debris and mitochondria-impairing metabolites. The use of therapeutic laxatives for the treatment of intestinal parasitic disease is well represented in the Infectous Disease and Tropical Medicine literature; in this instance, we are using ascorbic acid as an osmotic laxative and the coffee as a bowel stimulant. In high concentrations, ascorbic acid is directly microbicidal, at least against *E coli* (per Gaby, c 1993). The vitamin C can be administered as ascorbic acid—perfectly fine but very acidic, Ca/Mg/K buffered ascorbate—same laxative effect with the additional nutritive or laxative effect of minerals, or as home-made buffered ascorbate by mixing—per my own use—one heaping teaspoon or tablespoon of ascorbic acid with 1/2-one teaspoon baking soda (sodium bicarbonate). Additional agents can be ingested simultaneously for additional antimicrobial effect (e.g., iodine-iodide 12-48 mg [given that the standard antimicrobial dose for systemic/dermal infections usually starts at 1,000mg/d]) or intraluminal adsorption (e.g., activated charcoal). Patient selection excludes those who are generally frail and those with renal impairment, cardiac arrhythmia, bowel obstruction, electrolyte imbalance, dementia/psychosis, postural instability and/or reduced mobility to attend the toilet promptly, etc; patients with iron overload are reasonably be excluded— thus serum ferritin should be tested as described in Chapter 1—given that oral vitamin C administration

[477] Dien et al. Effect of food intake on pharmacokinetics of oral artemisinin in healthy Vietnamese subjects. *Antimicrob Agents Chemother*. 1997 May;41(5):1069-72

[478] Giao et al. Artemisinin for treatment of uncomplicated falciparum malaria: is there a place for monotherapy? *Am J Trop Med Hyg*. 2001 Dec;65(6):690-5

[479] Schempp CM, Pelz K, Wittmer A, Schopf E, Simon JC. Antibacterial activity of hyperforin from St John's wort, against multiresistant Staphylococcus aureus and gram-positive bacteria. *Lancet*. 1999 Jun 19;353(9170):2129

[480] "A butanol fraction of St. John's Wort revealed anti-Helicobacter pylori activity with MIC values ranging between 15.6 and 31.2 microg/ml." Reichling J, Weseler A, Saller R. A current review of the antimicrobial activity of Hypericum perforatum L. *Pharmacopsychiatry*. 2001 Jul;34 Suppl 1:S116-8

[481] Veldhuyzen van Zanten SJ, Sherman PM, Hunt RH. Helicobacter pylori: new developments and treatments. *CMAJ*. 1997;156(11):1565-74 cmaj.ca/cgi/reprint/156/11/1565.pdf

may lead to clinical deterioration in patients with hemochromatosis, per a single case report.[482] As a general rule, the vitamin C purge is initiated only in the morning 1-2 hours before the first meal and is followed later in the day—especially when used for several days consecutively—some effective form of electrolyte replacement, whether in supplemental pill/powder form or as salted vegetable juice; patients can use this treatment PRN, at the beginning of antimicrobial therapy especially to break the vicious cycle of SIBO and resultant GI stasis resulting from microbial methane and H2S, or consecutively; when the latter, periodic assessment of serum electrolytes is reasonable, with one standard interval for monitoring dietary intervention being weekly.

Coffee as a gastrointestinal stimulant

"Coffee stimulates gastrin release and gastric acid secretion... Coffee induces cholecystokinin release and gallbladder contraction... **Coffee increases rectosigmoid motor activity within 4 min after ingestion** in some people. ... Coffee promotes gastro-esophageal reflux, but is not associated with dyspepsia. Coffee stimulates gallbladder contraction and colonic motor activity.
Boekema et al. Coffee and gastrointestinal function: facts and fiction. *Scand J Gastroenterol.* 1999;230:35-9

"**Caffeinated coffee stimulates colonic motor activity.** Its magnitude is similar to a meal, 60% stronger than water and 23% stronger than decaffeinated coffee."
Rao et al. Is coffee a colonic stimulant? *Eur J Gastroenterol Hepatol.* 1998 Feb;10(2):113-8

Laxatives promote eradication of intestinal microbes; notably useful in patients with stasis/constipation

"Our case shows that although the dose of praziquantel is an important issue, **supportive care, including the optimal use of an oral laxative and enemas** to ensure smooth evacuation of the worm, is also important. This is especially true for young patients who are usually constipated or who cannot evacuate feces intentionally.
Fujita et al. A 2-year-old girl with Diphyllobothrium nihonkaiense infection treated with oral praziquantel and a laxative. *J Nippon Med Sch.* 2008 Aug;75:225-7

For irritable bowel syndrome with constipation: "Treatment with osmotic laxatives (milk of magnesia or polyethylene glycol) may increase stool frequency, improve stool consistency, and reduce straining."
Papadakis M, McPhee SJ, Rabow MW (eds). *Current Medical Diagnosis and Treatment 2014*

- o Commonly used antibiotic/antifungal drugs: Some commonly employed drugs for intestinal bacterial overgrowth are listed below; numerous reviews are available.[483,484,485] Antimicrobial drug selection can be based on ❶ microbiology: culture and sensitivity results if available, ❷ practicality and empiricism: patient response and tolerance, and ❸ evidence-based medicine: representative-correlational drug regimens described in the research literature. Treatment duration is generally at least 2 weeks, up to 8 weeks, and occasionally "indefinitely" depending on clinical response and the severity and diversity of the intestinal overgrowth. Drug dose is selected per normal indications, with a tendency to use *lower doses for longer durations* rather than higher doses for shorter durations. With all anti*bacterial* treatments, empiric anti*fungal* treatment to prevent yeast overgrowth is customary; some patients benefit from antifungal treatment that is continued for *months* and occasionally *years*. Probiotic yeast and bacteria are generally appropriate except in patients with hypersensitivity, severe immunosuppression, or extreme or recalcitrant bacterial overgrowth of the intestines. Drugs can generally be co-administered with natural antibiotics/antifungals for improved efficacy. Examples of doses are provided below, but clinicians must choose dose and duration per their judgment, experience, and the patient's situation, comorbidity, age, hepatic and renal function, accompanying polypharmacy; use of dosing and drug-interaction data (e.g., *Epocrates.com*) is recommended.
  - ▪ Metronidazole, tinidazole: 250-500 mg BID-QID (generally limit to 1.5-2 g/d); metronidazole has systemic bioavailability and effectiveness against a wide range of dysbiotic microbes, including protozoans, amebas/Giardia, *H. pylori*, *Clostridium difficile* and most anaerobic gram-negative bacilli.[486] Adverse effects are generally limited to stomatitis, nausea, diarrhea, and—rarely and/or with long-term use—peripheral neuropathy, dizziness, and metallic taste; the drug must not be consumed with alcohol. Metronidazole

[482] "We describe rapidly fatal cardiomyopathy in a young man. He had for twelve months ingested large amounts of ascorbic acid and was admitted with severe heart failure having been symptomatic for two months. He died after eight days. Idiopathic haemochromatosis was diagnosed at autopsy." McLaran et al. Congestive cardiomyopathy and haemochromatosis--rapid progression possibly accelerated by excessive ingestion of ascorbic acid. *Aust N Z J Med.* 1982 Apr;12(2):187-8
[483] Saltzman JR, Russell RM. Nutritional consequences of intestinal bacterial overgrowth. *Compr Ther.* 1994;20(9):523-30
[484] DiBaise JK. Nutritional consequences of small intestinal bacterial overgrowth. *Prac Gastroenterol.* 2008;69:15–28—one of my favorite articles on this topic.
[485] Malik et al. Diagnosis and pharmacological management of SIBO in children with intestinal failure. *Can J Gastroenterol.* 2011 Jan;25:41-5—excellent article.
[486] Tierney ML. McPhee SJ, Papadakis MA. *Current Medical Diagnosis and Treatment 2006. 45th edition*. New York; Lange Medical Books: 2006, pages 1578-1577

resistance by *Blastocystis hominis* and other parasites has been noted. Tinidazole and metronidazole are equally effective for bacterial vaginosis[487]; tinidazole may be superior for gastrointestinal infections.[488]

- **Rifaxamin/Xifaxan**: Rifaxamin is a standard drug for SIBO and IBS with a dose range of 800 mg QD up to 550 mg TID po for 2-8 weeks; it is generally considered to be nonabsorbed and thus gut-specific. Most doctors would probably describe it as an "excellent and safe gut-specific antibiotic with a prohibitive price" since a single reasonable course of the drug could easily cost €/$1,500.

- **Amoxicillin, Augmentin**: These are nice drugs with systemic absorption and tissue penetration following oral administration; specific for Gram-positive bacteria; caution with penicillin-sensitive patients.

- **Azithromycin**: Nice alternative for penicillin-sensitive patients; systemic absorption; generally not used specifically for GI infections but listed here for completeness/convenience; will be detailed in following sections on disease-specific applications for use in psoriasis in general and against *Chlamydia/Chlamydophila pneumoniae* in particular.

- **Oral vancomycin**: One of my favorite treatments for many years for recalcitrant autoimmunity; one of the only therapeutics effective against the previously mentioned SFB, which by now should be at the forefront of considerations when autoimmunity is addressed. I have seen patients respond very well to low-dose oral vancomycin 125 mg/d—total dose per day of 125 mg; in 2013, Tabibian et al[489] corroborated my experience by showing that low-dose oral vancomycin 125 mg QID (total dose 500 mg/d) was superior to higher dose vancomycin or metronidazole for primary sclerosing cholangitis.

- **Erythromycin**: 250-500 mg TID-QID; this drug is a widely used antibiotic that also has intestinal promotility benefits (thus making it an ideal treatment for intestinal bacterial overgrowth associated with or caused by intestinal dysmotility/hypomotility such as seen in scleroderma[490,491]). Do not combine erythromycin with the promotility drug **cisapride** due to risk for serious cardiac arrhythmia.

- **Prescription antifungal agents—Nystatin**: Nystatin 500,000 units BID-TID with food; duration of treatment begins with a minimum duration of 2-4 weeks and may continue as long as the patient is deriving benefit; low absorption and high safety give this "drug" one of the highest safety profiles seen in pharmacology. For gastrointestinal yeast, a combination of ADP and nystatin is highly safe and effective; if necessary, the addition of undecylenic acid as a third treatment should eradicate even the more recalcitrant GI yeast before needing to up the pharmacologic ante. Fluconazole/Diflucan: Available PO as 50,100,150,200 mg tablets; very effective drug for mild and life-threatening fungal infections and therefore dose intensity depends on clinical intensity. For dysbiotic indications, such as vulvovaginal or oroesophageal candidiasis, 150-200 mg with a frequency ranging from one dose or one dose each 72 hours for two doses total (mild-severe vulvovaginal candidiasis) or daily for 2 weeks (esophageal candidiasis) provides some perspective on clinical use. Serious cardiac, allergic, and idiosyncratic reactions can occur, so the drug—unlike nystatin—needs to be used with some degree of caution.

- Miscellaneous—other drugs, comments:
  - **Minocycline**: Minocycline 200 mg/day[492] has received the most attention in the treatment of rheumatoid arthritis due to its superior response (65%) over placebo (13%)[493]; in addition to its antibacterial action, the drug is also immunomodulatory and anti-inflammatory, including inhibition

---

[487] Schwebke JR1, Desmond RA. Tinidazole vs metronidazole for the treatment of bacterial vaginosis. *Am J Obstet Gynecol.* 2011 Mar;204(3):211.e1-6

[488] "The results indicate that tinidazole is more effective and better tolerated than metronidazole when given as a short course in single daily doses for symptomatic intestinal amoebiasis and amoebic liver abscess and as a single dose in symptomatic giardiasis." Bakshi JS, Ghiara JM, Nanivadekar AS. How does tinidazole compare with metronidazole? A summary report of Indian trials in amoebiasis and giardiasis. *Drugs.* 1978;15 Suppl 1:33-42

[489] "Thirty-five patients with PSC were randomised in a double-blind manner into four groups: vancomycin 125 mg or 250 mg four times/day, or metronidazole 250 mg or 500 mg three times/day for 12 weeks. The primary endpoint was decrease in alkaline phosphatase (ALK) at 12 weeks. ... The primary endpoint was reached in the low-dose (-43% change in ALK, P = 0.03) and high-dose (-40%, P = 0.02) vancomycin groups, with two patients in the former experiencing ALK normalisation. ... Mayo PSC risk score decreased significantly in the low-dose vancomycin (-0.55, P = 0.02) and low-dose metronidazole group (-0.16, P = 0.03). ...Both vancomycin and metronidazole demonstrated efficacy; however, only patients in the vancomycin groups reached the primary endpoint, and with less adverse effects. Larger, longer-term studies are needed to further examine the safety and efficacy of antibiotics as a potential treatment for patients with primary sclerosing cholangitis." Tabibian et al. Randomised clinical trial: vancomycin or metronidazole in patients with primary sclerosing cholangitis - a pilot study. *Aliment Pharmacol Ther.* 2013 Mar;37(6):604-12

[490] "Prokinetic agents effective in pseudoobstruction include metoclopramide, domperidone, cisapride, octreotide, and erythromycin. ... The combination of octreotide and erythromycin may be particularly effective in systemic sclerosis." Sjogren RW. Gastrointestinal features of scleroderma. *Curr Opin Rheumatol.* 1996 Nov;8(6):569-75

[491] "Erythromycin accelerates gastric and gallbladder emptying in scleroderma patients and might be helpful in the treatment of gastrointestinal motor abnormalities in these patients." Fiorucci et al. Effect of erythromycin administration on upper gastrointestinal motility in scleroderma patients. *Scand J Gastroenterol* 1994 Sep:807-13

[492] "...48-week trial of oral minocycline (200 mg/d) or placebo." Tilley et al. Minocycline in rheumatoid arthritis. A 48-week, double-blind, placebo-controlled trial. MIRA Trial Group. *Ann Intern Med.* 1995 Jan 15;122(2):81-9

[493] "In patients with early seropositive RA, therapy with minocycline is superior to placebo." O'Dell et al. Treatment of early rheumatoid arthritis with minocycline or placebo: results of a randomized, double-blind, placebo-controlled trial. *Arthritis Rheum.* 1997 May;40(5):842-8

496 INFLAMMATION MASTERY & FUNCTIONAL INFLAMMOLOGY © ICHNFM.ORG

of microglial activation. Ironically, minocycline can cause drug-induced autoimmunity, especially lupus.[494],[495]

- Tetracycline, and related drugs: 250-500 mg QID; commonly used in isolation or in combination with other drugs in various regimens. Two characteristics that I like about tetracyclines is the targeting of ribosomal function (protein synthesis) rather than cell wall provides effectiveness against L-form bacteria detailed previously, and tetracycline has low mitochondrial toxicity compared to the commonly used ciprofloxacin as well as the rarely used ampicillin and kanamycin.[496]

- Ciprofloxacin: 500 mg BID is common. Caution: tendinopathy and rupture can occur within 48 hours of quinolone use. Most doctors are avoiding quinolones as much as possible these days. Ciprofloxacin should be used with NAC to reduce mitochondrial toxicity.

- Cephalexin/Keflex: 250 mg QID; useful for *Klebsiella* and *Staphylococcus*.

> **Empiric treatment is the standard for SIBO**
>
> "The goal when treating SIBO should not be to sterilize the gastrointestinal tract but rather to reduce the numbers of pathogenic bacteria present. ... a trial-and-error approach to antibiotic therapy is often used with success being judged on improvement in gas-related symptoms, reduction in stool output and/or weight gain. Given the diversity of organisms present in SIBO, antimicrobial therapy should provide coverage for both aerobic and anaerobic organisms; monotherapy directed against anaerobes should be avoided. ... A variety of antibiotics have been reported to be effective in SIBO, but little objective evidence exists to favor one agent over another."
>
> DiBaise JK. *Practical Gastroenterology* 2008 Dec

- Fecal transplant: Fecal transplants have been used in medicine for centuries—the first literary record appears to be a fourth century Chinese handbook of emergency medicine *Zhou Hou Bei Ji Fang* (or *Handy Therapy for Emergencies*)[497]— and have been described in many editions of *The Merck Manual*, generally considered one of the standard books in clinical medicine. The treatment is notably simple (stool "donation" from a healthy donor is generally homogenized and filtered, but one might wonder if this is simply superfluous processing to "medicalize" what would otherwise be simple and obviously straightforward) and administered per mouth, rectum, or nasogastric/enteroscope procedure. This is a lifesaving treatment for many patients infected with drug-resistant *Clostridium difficile*. Whereas probiotic administration supplies a few bacteria, fecal transplant essentially provides an entire ecosystem, inclusive of the partnering bacteria that use and provide the probiotic/eubacteria mutualism that promotes healthy and complex microbial communities that provide sought-after diversity and durability.

- Bacteriophage therapy: An emerging therapy that still requires more clinical data and experience before widespread use, reliance, and safety are established is the administration of presumably safe and selective bacterial viruses—bacteriophages—to infect and lyse/destroy dysbiotic bacteria, effectively behaving as "viral antibiotics." As discussed in my *Antiviral Strategies and Immune Nutrition* work, I have some concern about bacteriophages due to what appears *per balance of the data* to be their involvement in Crohn's disease and lupus/SLE; further, quantitative overabundance of bacteriophages is likely to contribute to the total viral load (TVL) and provoke nonspecific immune responses that promote inflammation. As with all emerging therapies and proposed pathologic mechanisms, what will be necessary here is continued review of new research, contextualized within a multiperspective model from various disciplines.

Conclusion to this section reviewing the "basic and clinical sciences of dysbiosis"—microbiology, pathophysiology, pharmacology: Before a few sample clinical cases that follow, I have outlined a reasonable and progressively tiered clinical approach in the table below. Clinicians should begin to implement treatment on the first visit in which GI dysbiosis especially SIBO is suspected; delaying therapy for lab tests is generally sophomoric and inefficient when safe and effective interventions can be used with a low threshold due to their excellent risk:benefit ratios and low cost.

---

[494] "...many cases of drug-induced lupus related to minocycline have been reported. Some of those reports included pulmonary lupus..." Christodoulou et al. Respiratory distress due to minocycline-induced pulmonary lupus. *Chest*. 1999 May;115(5):1471-3 chestjournal.org/cgi/content/full/115/5/1471

[495] Lawson TM, Amos N, Bulgen D, Williams BD. Minocycline-induced lupus: clinical features and response to rechallenge. *Rheumatology* (Oxford). 2001 Mar;40(3):329-35

[496] Kalghatgi et al. Bactericidal antibiotics induce mitochondrial dysfunction and oxidative damage in Mammalian cells. *Sci Transl Med*. 2013 Jul 3;5(192):192ra85

[497] Zhang F, Luo W, Shi Y, Fan Z, Ji G. Should we standardize the 1,700-year-old fecal microbiota transplantation? *Am J Gastroenterol*. 2012 Nov;107(11):1755

Foundational interventions	Intermediate interventions	Agressive interventions
• Diet optimization, 5pSPMD, obviously this includes probiotics and fibers • Antidysbiotic lifestyle: stress reduction, sleep optimization, exercise • Nutritional repletion, early immunonutrition • Full thyroid assessment and empiric treatment, preferably with T3 as discussed in Chapter 1; hypothyroidism clearly promotes SIBO/dysbiosis via hyposecretion and hypoperistalsis • Seek elimination of causative drugs, e.g., PPI and H2 blockers, prednisone (caution with tapering[498]), opioids • Stool softening with magnesium and ascorbate • Empiric course of emulsified time-released oregano up to 600 mg/d and/or berberine 1,500 mg/d in divided doses	All previous treatments, with progressive addition of the following: • First-morning ascorbate-coffee cleanse • Undecylenic acid or caprylic acid • Nystatin if yeast suspected; low threshold for implementation given high safety and low cost • Rifaximin 800 mg QD up to 550 mg BID-TID per financial tolerance • Revisit and rotate probiotics • Strengthen immunonutrition program and add/increase glutamine, vitamin A, vitamin D, zinc, and *Saccharomyces* if not already done	All previous treatments, with progressive addition of the following: • Pharmaceutical antibiotics, used alone, in combination, and/or on rotational basis • Fluconazole if recalcitrant or extraintestinal yeast is documented or strongly suspected • Consider fecal transplant • Consider—metaphorically or literally—getting a dog[499], working on a farm, playing in dirt, gardening, or other means of enhanced microbial exposure to promote microbial diversity

Conceptual and practical application of a reasonable three-tiered protocol against gastrointestinal dysbiosis: The above table outlines the general clinical approach I have used since the start of my clinical practice in 2000. While the step-wise progression is obviously logical, what is not intuitive per this diagram is that some of the more "severe" clinical cases will respond immediately and permanently to the foundational interventions and will not need more aggressive treatments. As demonstrated in the following case of autoimmune peripheral neuropathy, some cases that have existed for years will *durably* clear within the first month.

Active learning and reflection

Name at least eight interventions for gastrointestinal dysbiosis (e.g., SIBO) that can be implemented with a low threshold for use due to excellent safety and effectiveness; write the dose/administration for each:

1. _____
2. _____
3. _____
4. _____
5. _____
6. _____
7. _____
8. _____

Name any contraindications to the above.

---

[498] Immunosuppressive/anti-inflammatory "steroids" such as prednisone must be tapered slowly if they have been used for long periods of time and/or at high doses; adrenal suppression with high-dose oral and parenteral steroids begins as soon as day #5 of treatment. Steroid-induced adrenal suppression is dose- and time-dependent but difficult to predict clinically. Only clinicians with appropriate prescriptive authority should manage steroid tapering; rapid cessation can cause fatalities. See any standard pharmacology/clinical textbook for review; one available review is available online: Liu et al. A practical guide to the monitoring and management of the complications of systemic corticosteroid therapy. *Allergy Asthma Clin Immunol.* 2013 Aug 15;9(1):30 aacijournal.com/content/9/1/30

[499] "Early-life exposure to dogs is protective against allergic disease development, and dog ownership is associated with a distinct milieu of house dust microbial exposures. Here, we show that mice exposed to dog-associated house dust are protected against airway allergen challenge. These animals exhibit reduced Th2 cytokine production, fewer activated T cells, and a distinct gut microbiome composition, highly enriched for Lactobacillus johnsonii, which itself can confer airway protection when orally supplemented as a single species." Fujimura et al. House dust exposure mediates gut microbiome Lactobacillus enrichment and airway immune defense against allergens and virus infection. *Proc Natl Acad Sci U S A.* 2014 Jan 14;111(2):805-10

Clinical Case **Abnormal lactulose-mannitol ratio in a patient with idiopathic peripheral neuropathy prior to comprehensive stool analysis and parasitology showing intestinal dysbiosis**: 40-yo man presented with multiyear history of periodic febrile exacerbations of mixed sensory-motor peripheral neuropathy. Neuropathic exacerbations were triggered by shellfish consumption and accompanied by severe paresthesias and motor deficits. Patient had been evaluated by several board-certified medical neurologists to no avail. Laboratory, imaging, electrodiagnostic studies, and cerebrospinal fluid (CSF) analysis revealed nonspecific abnormalities that did not lead to any diagnosis. From my naturopathic/functional medicine perspective, food allergy combined with intestinal dysbiosis were the most obvious probable etiologies; the most likely and obvious pathophysiology is that of shellfish-triggered IgE-mediated intestinal hyperpermeability leading to absorption of cross-reactive microbial antigens and the resulting immunologic attack on the patient's peripheral neurons.

Patient:	Completed: April 24, 2003	ALEX VASQUEZ DC ND
Age: 40	Received: April 22, 2003	
Sex: M	Collected: April 21, 2003	Houston, TX 77098
MRN:		

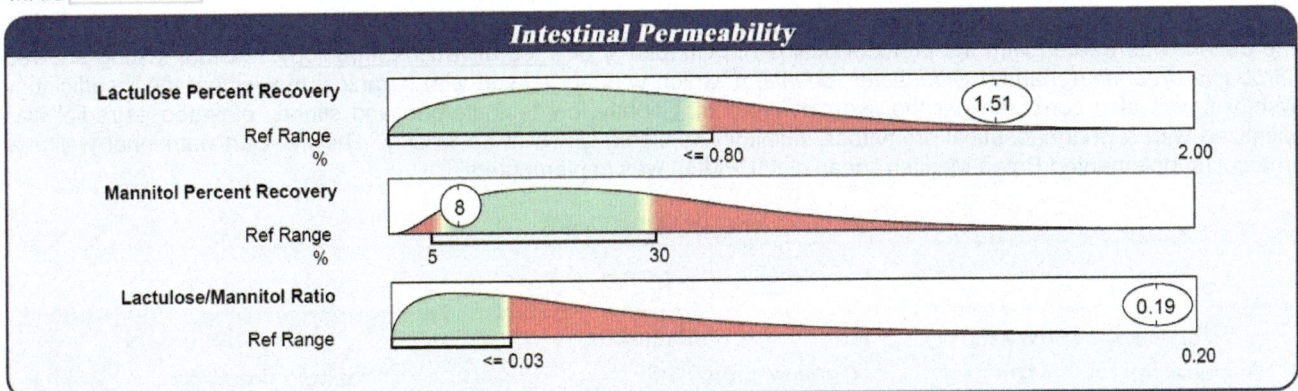

Stool testing showed dysbiosis: insufficiency of *Lactobacillus* and presence of *Psuedomonas* and abnormal yeast. *Psuedomonas aeruginosa* shows molecular mimicry with human neuronal tissues and is associated with human neuronal autoimmunity.[500],[501] Eradication of the dysbiotic condition with antimicrobial drugs and herbs and dietary improvement, nutritional supplementation, hormonal optimization, lead to rapid and sustained remission of this "idiopathic peripheral neuropathy" which had defied standard medical diagnosis and treatment for many years.

Comprehensive Stool Analysis / Parasitology x3

MICROBIOLOGY

Bacteriology Culture

Beneficial flora		Imbalances		Dysbiotic flora	
Bifidobacter	4+	Haemolytic E. coli	4+	Pseudomonas sp.	4+
E. coli	4+	Gamma strep	2+		
Lactobacillus	2+				

Mycology (Yeast) Culture

Normal flora		Dysbiotic flora
Candida glabrata	1+	
Rhodotorula sp.	1+	

---

[500] Hughes LE, Bonell S, Natt RS, et al. Antibody responses to Acinetobacter spp. and Pseudomonas aeruginosa in multiple sclerosis: prospects for diagnosis using the myelin-acinetobacter-neurofilament antibody index. *Clin Diagn Lab Immunol*. 2001 Nov;8(6):1181-8 cvi.asm.org/content/8/6/1181.full.pdf

[501] Hughes LE, Smith PA, Bonell S, Natt RS, Wilson C, Rashid T, Amor S, Thompson EJ, Croker J, Ebringer A. Cross-reactivity between related sequences found in Acinetobacter sp., Pseudomonas aeruginosa, myelin basic protein and myelin oligodendrocyte glycoprotein in multiple sclerosis. *J Neuroimmunol*. 2003 Nov;144(1-2):105-15

Clinical Case Elevated hsCRP (high-sensitivity c-reactive protein) in a male patient with metabolic syndrome and rheumatoid arthritis—response to treatment protocol in *Integrative Rheumatology*: This 52-year-old male patient presented with a 4-year history of rheumatoid arthritis which was unresponsive to prednisone and anti-TNF (tumor necrosis factor alpha) drugs, ie, "biologics." As expected, the prednisone exacerbated the patient's insulin resistance and hypertension; the drug failed to produce an anti-inflammatory benefit for this patient. At a cost of several thousand dollars per treatment, the anti-TNF "biologic" drugs failed to provide any benefit. At the intial visit in July 2005, the hsCRP level was 124 mg/L (normal range 0-3 mg/L), as shown in these lab results.

DATE OF SPECIMEN	TIME	DATE RECEIVED	DATE REPORTED	TIME		Houston	TX	77036-0000
7/08/2005	16:19	7/08/2005	7/11/2005	7:38	419	ACCOUNT NUMBER:	42407150	

TEST	RESULT	LIMITS	LAB
C-Reactive Protein, Cardiac			
> C-Reactive Protein, Cardiac	124.00H mg/L	0.00 - 3.00	HD
	Relative Risk for Future Cardiovascular Event		
	Low	<1.00	
	Average	1.00 - 3.00	
	High	>3.00	

The patient was treated with the protocol outlined in Chapter 4 of *Integrative Rheumatology*.[502] Stool testing showed *Citrobacter freundii* (renamed *Citrobacter rodentium*) which was addressed with botanical medicines; the insufficiency dysbiosis was also corrected per the five-part protocol. Slightly low testosterone and slightly elevated estradiol was optimized with a pharmaceutical aromatase inhibitor (Arimidex) given twice weekly. The five-part nutritional wellness protocol (supplemented Paleo-Mediterranean diet [SPMD]) was implemented.[503]

MICROBIOLOGY

Bacteriology Culture

Beneficial flora		Imbalances		Dysbiotic flora	
Bifidobacter	0+	Gamma strep	1+	Citrobacter freundii	1+
E. coli	2+	Enterobacter sp.	1+		
Lactobacillus	0+				

Mycology (Yeast) Culture

Normal flora	Dysbiotic flora
No yeast isolated	

PARASITOLOGY

	Sample 1		Sample 2
No	Ova or Parasites	No	Ova or Parasites

No anti-inflammatory drugs or botanicals were used. Within five weeks of treatment, the patient's hsCRP dropped from 124 mg/L to 7.58 mg/L—a reduction of approximately 95%—far superior to any previoius response to corticosteroid and biologic drugs. Patient experienced significant alleviation of pain and improved mobility.

8/17/2005	11:06	8/18/2005	8/18/2005	12:32	738	ACCOUNT NUMBER:	42407150	

TEST	RESULT	LIMITS	LAB
C-Reactive Protein, Cardiac			
C-Reactive Protein, Cardiac	7.58H mg/L	0.00 - 3.00	HD

---

[502] Vasquez A. *Integrative Rheumatology*. See InflammationMastery.com for newest edition, which in 2014 is *Naturopathic Rheumatology v3.5*.
[503] Vasquez A. Revisiting the Five-Part Nutritional Wellness Protocol. *Nutritional Perspectives* 2011 Jan Reprinted and updated in Chapter 4.

Clinical Case 45yo HLA-B27+ woman with recurrent UTIs and a 7-year history of ankylosing spondylitis treated with anti-TNF drugs: Positive urine culture and positive stool culture demonstrating bacteria (*Escherichia coli* and *Klebsiella pneumoniae*) known to share molecular mimicry and cross-reactivity with HLA-B27: The Gram-negative bacterium *E. coli* produces a protein named "hypothetical protein 168" (Protein Identification Resource [PIR] data bank access code #jp0612) which shares the amino acid sequence "**RRYLE**" with HLA-B27, which contains the sequence "EWL**RRYLE**IGKETLQRVDP."[504] Per the same citation, *Klebsiella pneumoniae*'s protein (PIR s01840) nitrogenase (reductase) molybdenum-iron protein NifN contains the sequence "EWLRR." This amino acid homology confers validation to the phenomenon of molecular mimicry and thus that immune system components such as immunoglobulins and activated T-cells can cross-react between microbial peptides and human tissue antigens.[505] This patient was treated with the combination pharmaceutical antibiotic trimethoprim and sulfamethoxazole commonly referred to as "Bactrim DS" in addition to dietary optimization, hormonal optimization, and nutritional supplementation. Antimicrobial treatment with amoxicillin-clavulanate would have been reasonable, too, except for this patient's prior allergic reaction to the drug.

Urine Culture, Routine

```
Urine Culture, Routine        Final Report
Result 1
      Escherichia coli
      50,000-100,000 colony forming units per mL
Antimicrobial Susceptibility
      ***** S = Susceptible; I = Intermediate; R = Resistant *****
                 P = Positive; N = Negative
           MICS are expressed in micrograms per mL
```

Antibiotic	RSLT#1
Amoxicillin/Clavulanic Acid	S
Ampicillin	S
Cefazolin	S
Cefepime	S
Ceftriaxone	S
Cefuroxime	S
Cephalothin	I
Ciprofloxacin	R
ESBL	N
Ertapenem	S
Gentamicin	S
Imipenem	S
Levofloxacin	R
Nitrofurantoin	S
Piperacillin	S
Tetracycline	S
Tobramycin	S
Trimethoprim/Sulfa	S

Comprehensive Stool Analysis / Parasitology x3

BACTERIOLOGY CULTURE		
Expected/Beneficial flora	**Commensal (Imbalanced) flora**	**Dysbiotic flora**
4+ Bacteroides fragilis group	3+ Alpha hemolytic strep	3+ Klebsiella pneumoniae ssp pneumoniae
3+ Bifidobacterium spp.		
4+ Escherichia coli		
3+ Lactobacillus spp.		
NG Enterococcus spp.		
2+ Clostridium spp.		
NG = No Growth		

PRESCRIPTIVE AGENTS				
	Resistant	**Intermediate**	**Susceptible**	
Amoxicillin-Clavulanic Acid			S	Susceptible results imply that an infection due to the bacteria may be appropriately treated when the recommended dosage of the tested antimicrobial agent is used. **Intermediate** results imply that response rates may be lower than for susceptible bacteria when the tested antimicrobial agent is used. **Resistant** results imply that the bacteria will not be inhibited by normal dosage levels of the tested antimicrobial agent.
Ampicillin	R			
Cefazolin			S	
Ceftazidime			S	
Ciprofloxacin			S	
Trimeth-sulfa			S	

[504] Scofield RH, Warren WL, Koelsch G, Harley JB. A hypothesis for the HLA-B27 immune dysregulation in spondyloarthropathy: contributions from enteric organisms, B27 structure, peptides bound by B27, and convergent evolution. *Proc Natl Acad Sci U S A*. 1993 Oct 15;90(20):9330-4

[505] Rashid T, Ebringer A. Ankylosing spondylitis is linked to Klebsiella—the evidence. *Clin Rheumatol*. 2007 Jun;26(6):858-64

Name the various types of gastrointestinal dysbiosis and provide distinguishing features:

Name the various clinical conditions associated with or known to be caused (in large part) by gastrointestinal dysbiosis:

Name the treatments that are safe and effective enough to justify a low threshold of use for a patient suspected of having SIBO on the first day of treatment without confirmatory/laboratory/objective testing; also, name the two most studied botanical medicines for gastrointestinal dysbiosis along with their dosage and duration:

- Diet and nutrition:

- Botanicals:

- Safe/nonabsorbed antimicrobial agents:

- Additional treatments:

How does hypothyroidism contribute to SIBO? How is hypothyroidism assessed and treated?

- History (at least 6 items):

- Physical exam (at least 3 objective findings that are specific to hypothyroidism):

- Laboratory (name the 6 lab tests):

- Empiric treatment and response to treatment (define treatment and dosages—give 3 prescription options):

- Contraindications to treatment with thyroid hormone:

Orodental dysbiosis

- **Dysbiosis-disease causation**: The human oral cavity is heavily populated by microbes, and these microbes and their products such as endotoxin can enter the bloodstream to induce a proinflammatory response via "metastatic infection" and **"metastatic inflammation"**, respectively.[506] The systemic inflammatory response triggered by mild oral/dental "infections" is now appreciated to exacerbate/promote conditions such as atherosclerotic disease and diabetes mellitus[507] and is also important in the more severe inflammatory/autoimmune conditions. **Patients with rheumatoid arthritis have heightened antibody levels against common oral bacteria. IgG levels against** *Porphyromonas gingivalis, Prevotella melaninogenica, Bacteroides forsythus,* **and** *Prevotella intermedia* **were found to be significantly higher in RA patients when compared with those of controls.**[508] In the first human clinical trial to test the hypothesis that treatment of orodental dysbiosis would provide subjective and objective clinical benefits for patients with RA, Al-Katma et al (*J Clin Rheumatol* 2007 Jun—summarized below) showed that **periodontal treatment consisting of scaling/root planing and oral hygiene instruction reduced symptom scores and inflammatory markers in patients with RA.** Obviously, if the mouth and teeth are heavily colonized by bacteria and yeast—which by their very existence produce cell wall debris, DNA, proteins, enzymes, and other immunogens—then this immunogenic material will either be absorbed/translocated locally or will be ingested, where it will either be partly destroyed, absorbed, or serve to alter quorum sensing and the microbial-inflammatory milieu, suggested here to have systemic consequences. Gingivitis is polymicrobial, not only of bacteria and yeast, but also of viruses such as Epstein-Barr and cytomegalovirus herpesviruses, according to Contreras et al[509]; therefore use of a structured antiviral protocol might also be included in the optimization of orodental health.
    - Control of periodontal infection reduces the severity of active rheumatoid arthritis (*J Clin Rheumatol.* 2007 Jun[510]): "Seventeen subjects completing the study received periodontal treatment consisting of scaling/root planing and oral hygiene instruction; 12 subjects completing the study received no treatment. Participants continued their usual disease-modifying medications for RA without any changes in DMARD therapy during the study period. ... Ten of 17 subjects (58.8%) in the treated group and 2 of 12 subjects (16.7%) in the untreated group showed improvement in RA scores. There was a statistically significant difference in DAS28 (4.3 vs. 5.1) and erythrocyte sedimentation rate (31.4 vs. 42.7) between the treatment and the control groups. CONCLUSION: Control of periodontal infection and gingival inflammation by scaling/root planing and plaque control in subjects with periodontal disease may reduce the severity of RA. This notion is supported by reported subjective improvement in treated patients."
    - Periodontal therapy reduces the severity of active rheumatoid arthritis (*J Periodontol.* 2009 Apr[511]): "Forty participants diagnosed with moderate/severe RA (under treatment for RA) and severe periodontitis were randomly assigned to receive initial non-surgical periodontal therapy with scaling/root planing and oral hygiene instructions (n = 20) or no periodontal therapy (n = 20). To control RA, all participants had been using disease-modifying anti-rheumatic drugs, and 20 had also been using anti-TNF-alpha before randomization. Probing depth (PD), clinical attachment level (CAL), bleeding on probing (BOP), gingival index (GI), plaque index (PI), RA disease activity score 28 (DAS28), and erythrocyte sedimentation rate (ESR) were measured at baseline and 6 weeks later. ...Patients receiving periodontal treatment showed a significant decrease in the mean DAS28, ESR ($P < 0.001$), and serum TNF-alpha ($P < 0.05$). There was no statistically significant decrease in these parameters in patients not receiving periodontal treatment. ... CONCLUSIONS: Non-surgical periodontal therapy had a beneficial effect on the signs and symptoms of RA, regardless of the medications used to treat this condition. Anti-TNF-alpha therapy without periodontal treatment had no significant effect on the periodontal condition."

[506] Li X, Kolltveit KM, Tronstad L, Olsen I. Systemic diseases caused by oral infection. *Clin Microbiol Rev.* 2000 Oct;13(4):547-58 cmr.asm.org/cgi/content/full/13/4/547
[507] Amar S, Han X. The impact of periodontal infection on systemic diseases. *Med Sci Monit.* 2003 Dec;9(12):RA291-9 medscimonit.com/pub/vol_9/no_12/3776.pdf
[508] Ogrendik M, Kokino S, Ozdemir F, et al. Serum antibodies to oral anaerobic bacteria in patients with rheumatoid arthritis. *MedGenMed.* 2005 Jun 16;7(2):2
[509] "The results indicate that subgingival EBV-1, HCMV, and viral coinfections are associated with the subgingival presence of some periodontal pathogens and periodontitis. Herpesviruses may exert periodontopathic potential by decreasing the host resistance against subgingival colonization and multiplication of periodontal pathogens." Contreras et al. Relationship between herpesviruses and adult periodontitis and periodontopathic bacteria. *J Periodontol.* 1999 May;70(5):478-84
[510] Al-Katma et al. Control of periodontal infection reduces the severity of active rheumatoid arthritis. *J Clin Rheumatol.* 2007 Jun;13:134-7
[511] Ortiz et al. Periodontal therapy reduces severity of active rheumatoid arthritis in patients treated with/without tumor necrosis factor inhibitors. *J Periodontol.* 2009 Apr:535-40

The two main concerns with regard to oral-dental health are ❶ dental carries, also called cavities—these are holes formed in dental enamel via the solubilization of calcium phosphate by microbial acids derived from the metabolism of dietary sugars, ❷ gum disease, gingivitis—heavy colonization of gums and teeth promotes inflammation and recession of the gums and microbial disintegration of the teeth, respectively. Tooth loss and mandibular bone infection (osteomyelitis) can follow, but are generally preceded by items 1 and 2 above and thus the interventional and health-maintenance focus for most patients and physicians needs to remain on these primary lesions, both of which are necessarily preceded by formation of biofilms, which were discussed previously in the section on *Microbial Morphology, Molecules, Metabolites, and Pathophysiologic Mechanisms.* Formation of biofilms is dependent on microbial growth, which is itself dependent on a supportive environment of ❶ dietary sugar, ❷ lack of dental cleaning / microbial removal, either via lack of dental hygiene and/or for example lack of saliva in Sjogren's syndrome, and ❸ a permissive immune response, appreciating that the latter might be insufficient even if perfectly robust if overwhelmed by sugar and lack of microbial removal. From the perspective of my focus on inflammation, the concerns with orodental dysbiosis are primarily of induction of systemic inflammation via absorption of bacterial molecules, most notably the exquisitely proinflammatory endotoxin/LPS and also direct bacterial translocation via inflamed "leaky gums."

| Hospitable oral environment: ❶ dietary sugar, ❷ lack of microbial removal, ❸ immune allowance. | → | Microbial proliferation | → | Establishment of biofilms | → | Carries, gingivitis, can lead to tooth loss; dental work generally includes immunotoxins such as mercury and BPA | → | Absorption of microbial molecules and metabolites, bacterial translocation, promotion of systemic inflammation |

Important but not detailed here are the contributions of dental amalgam "fillings"—via mercury—to systemic mercury load, neurotoxicity, induction of autoimmunity and immunosensitization, and promotion of drug-resistant bacteria; synthetic dental fillings/sealants/resins are notoriously potent long-term sources of toxic BPA, now known to activate mTOR, induce mitochondrial dysfunction, promote inflammatory and allergic diseases including food allergy and asthma, and function as an endocrine disruptor (with notable relevance for infertility and diabetes) with an economic healthcare impact quantified in billions of dollars internationally and an incomprehensible personal health impact in suffering, disease burden, and early death.[512]

- **Assessments**: Obviously, any major microbial infestations of the mouth, such as gingivitis or thrush, need to be treated regardless of the presence or absence of systemic inflammatory disease. **Culture of mouth, throat, dentures for yeast and bacteria can be performed** (see Noah[513]). Palpation/provocation of the gums and teeth should not cause pain and bleeding; the presence of pain/bleeding suggests underlying inflammation, which in turn indicates underlying infection. If flossing causes bleeding and pain, this is indicative of unhealthy gums due to an overgrowth of bacteria below the gum line. Mild gum regression and the development of deep dental pockets is an indication for intervention with fastidious oral hygiene and professional dental care. Patients with systemic disease may have asymptomatic infections of the mandible that can only be detected with non-standard imaging techniques such as computer-enhanced mandibular ultrasound.[514]

- **Specific treatment considerations**: A professional cleaning by a dentist or oral hygienist is a reasonable start. Thereafter, twice-daily brushing, daily/weekly flossing, and the use of an antiseptic mouthwash and a plaque-removing solution should be employed. To improve understanding and compliance, clinicians should instruct patients that the purpose of flossing is not to remove (visible) food *per se* but to disrupt (invisible) microbial biofilms. Natural toothpastes with antimicrobial botanical oils such as from *Salvia officinalis* (sage) and

---

[512] For discussion of BPA consider the following free/open-access sources: Małkiewicz et al. Release of bisphenol A and its derivatives from orthodontic adhesive systems available on the European market as a potential health risk factor. *Ann Agric Environ Med.* 2015 Feb 24;22(1):172-7. Konieczna et al. Health risk of exposure to Bisphenol A (BPA). *Rocz Panstw Zakl Hig.* 2015;66(1):5-11. Fillon M. Getting it right: BPA and the difficulty proving environmental cancer risks. *J Natl Cancer Inst.* 2012 May 2;104:652-5. "The use of bisphenol A, or BPA, in food and beverage containers, according to the study, is responsible for an estimated $3 billion a year in costs associated with childhood obesity and adult heart disease." Peeples L. BPA among Toxic Chemicals Driving Up Health Care Costs. huffingtonpost.com/2014/01/22/bpa-health-care-costs_n_4644372.html
[513] Noah PW. The role of microorganisms in psoriasis. *Semin Dermatol.* 1990 Dec;9(4):269-76
[514] "Through-transmission alveolar ultrasonography (TAU) is a novel imaging modality in dental medicine. A brief introduction to through-transmission ultrasonography (TTU) is followed by a description of the first commercially available TAU device, the Cavitat CAV 4000 (Cavitat Medical Technologies, Inc., Alba, TX)." Imbeau J. Introduction to through-transmission alveolar ultrasonography (TAU) in dental medicine. *Cranio.* 2005 Apr;23(2):100-12. Cavitat Medical Technologies appears to have been involved in some litigation and regulatory issues and may have closed per internet information and fda.gov/ohrms/dockets/dailys/01/aug01/080801/cp0001.pdf surveyed 2014 Jan. "A 21-year-old female presented to the ED with chin swelling and 'boils.' Although her visual examination was benign, CPUS of her facial swelling quickly established a more concerning disease process, which was eventually confirmed by aspiration and bone biopsy to be mandibular osteomyelitis. The causative organism, Serratia odorifera, is rarely associated with infections, and we are aware of no previously reported cases of osteomyelitis due to this species." Hayden et al. Ultrasound-guided diagnosis of occult mandibular osteomyelitis. *J Emerg Med.* 2014 Nov;47(5):557-60

Rosmarinus officinalis (rosemary) should be used for their natural, safe, effective antibacterial, antifungal, and anti-inflammatory benefits.[515] Toothbrushes should be periodically disinfected (e.g., iodine/iodide, H2O2, diluted bleach) and replaced. Electric toothbrushes are more efficient than manual toothbrushes, and three-dimensional and ultrasound toothbrushes can cleanse below the gum line. Avoiding sucrose and refined carbohydrates is essential. Sugar-free chewing gums help to reduce bacterial loads at least in part by stimulating saliva production, and chewing gums with xylitol significantly reduce bacterial colonization of the oral cavity.[516,517] Immunonutrition as described later should be used to improve overall systemic defenses; particular consideration should be given to glutamine, bovine colostrum and IgG, zinc, and thymus extract—the latter per an animal study of experimental dental disease showing administration of thymus extract normalized immune function and reduced orodental dysbiosis.[518] Some patients will require administration of antimicrobial drugs—500-1,000 mg amoxicillin, for example—with dental cleaning to avoid exacerbations of gingivitis and/or to reduce the risk of endocarditis in patients predisposed by valvulopathy. The following annotated bibliography provides examples of the connection between orodental dysbiosis and systemic inflammation, with a few citations also specific to oil pulling/swishing, which gained popularity in the western world in 2014/2015 after being practiced in other countries for many centuries. Biofilm control has several components, including *microbial* (replacing/changing/discouraging cariogenic microbes via dietary and environmental means, as well as direct antimicrobial means), *chemical* dissolution and *physical* disruption; plant and petroleum oils disrupt dental biofilms.[519] Oil swishing is effective against bacterial biofilms via *antimicrobial* (direct killing with lauric acid), *chemical* (proposed detergent action following saponification), and *physical* (vigorous swishing) means.

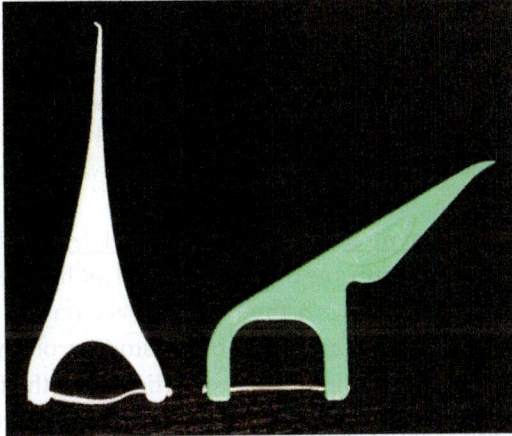

Floss-picks pictured above: Easier to use and avoids the "finger tournequet" effect induced by string-type dental floss, thereby increasing comfort and compliance

Interventions *contra* orodental dysbiosis
1. Professional dental care—start with a professional cleaning and assessment
2. Avoid sugars
3. Treat any salivary insufficiency, e.g., Sjogren's syndrome per protocol in *Rheumatology v3.5* or later
4. Treat immunodeficiencies
5. Treat nutrient deficiencies, especially CoQ10, methylfolate/folinic acid, vitamins A and D3
6. Gum chewing, saliva substitutes
7. Brushing, use of electronic toothbrush; replace or disinfect periodically
8. Flossing, including use of "floss picks"—encouraging the use of flossing on at least a once-weekly basis rather than a daily basis might improve compliance; floss picks avoid tourniquet effect
9. Oil pulling/swishing
10. Antiseptic mouthwash
11. Avoid to the extent possible dental fillers/finishes with mercury and BPA

For oil pulling/swishing, a tablespoon (teaspoon for young children) of sesame/coconut/olive/other oil is taken in the mouth, sipped, sucked, and pulled between the teeth for 10-15 min.[520] The viscous oil turns thin and milky white, indicating saponification. This oil should not be swallowed; it should be spit out of the mouth following the procedure and thereafter followed by rinsing of the mouth, flossing, tooth brushing, and other components such as use of an antimicrobial rinse. Of available oils, coconut oil which is ~50% lauric acid has the best direct antimicrobial effectiveness against bacteria and yeast, both of which are cariogenic. Beyond the

515 "The results suggest that the extracts of R. officianalis L. and S. officianalis L. may be useful as antiplaque agents." Narayanan N, Thangavelu L. Salvia officinalis in dentistry. *Dent Hypotheses* 2015;6:27-30
516 "Chewing 100% xylitol gum caused significant reductions on salivary MS scores (p < 0.025) which was little different from the 55% xylitol group. The results suggest that the use of xylitol chewing gum can reduce the levels of MS in plaque and saliva." Thaweboon S, Thaweboon B, Soo-Ampon S. The effect of xylitol chewing gum on mutans streptococci in saliva and dental plaque. *Southeast Asian J Trop Med Public Health.* 2004 Dec;35(4):1024-7
517 "Especially xylitol-containing chewing gum may significantly reduce the growth of mutans streptococci and dental plaque which may be associated with dental caries." Makinen et al. Six-month polyol chewing-gum programme in kindergarten-age children. *Int Dent J.* 2005 Apr;55(2):81-8
518 Manti etal.Effects of immunomodulating agent on peripheral blood lymphocytes and subgingivalmicroflora in ligature-induced periodontitis.*Infect Immun*1984;45:172-9
519 Filogônio et al. Effect of vegetable oil (Brazil nut oil) and mineral oil (liquid petrolatum) on dental biofilm control. *Braz Oral Res.* 2011 Nov-Dec;25(6):556-61
520 Asokan S. Oil pulling therapy. *Indian J Dent Res* 2008;19:169

direct antimicrobial effect of some oils, oil pulling/swishing results in saponification of the oils that allows the "deconstruction" of microbial biofilms via either/both killing of microbes and/or physical removal via detergent action as well as the physical action of the vigorously "swished" mixture.[521]

- o Oil pulling versus chlorhexidine on oral malodor: a randomized controlled trial. (*J Clin Diagn Res*. 2014 Nov[522]): "Oil pulling with sesame oil is equally efficacious as chlorhexidine in reducing oral malodor and microbes causing it. It should be promoted as a preventive home care therapy."

- o Effect of coconut oil in plaque-related gingivitis (*Niger Med J*. 2015 Mar[523]): "Oil pulling or oil swishing therapy is a traditional procedure in which the practitioners rinse or swish oil in their mouth. It is supposed to cure oral and systemic diseases but the evidence is minimal. Oil pulling with sesame oil and sunflower oil was found to reduce plaque related gingivitis. Coconut oil is an easily available edible oil. It is unique because it contains predominantly medium chain fatty acids of which 45-50 percent is lauric acid. Lauric acid has proven anti-inflammatory and antimicrobial effects. ... 60 age matched adolescent boys and girls in the age-group of 16-18 years with plaque induced gingivitis were included in the study and oil pulling was included in their oral hygiene routine. The study period was 30 days. Plaque and gingival indices of the subjects were assessed at baseline days 1,7,15 and 30. ... A statistically significant decrease in the plaque and gingival indices was noticed from day 7 and the scores continued to decrease during the period of study. CONCLUSION: Oil pulling using coconut oil could be an effective adjuvant procedure in decreasing plaque formation and plaque induced gingivitis."

- o Effect of oil pulling on plaque induced gingivitis: a randomized, controlled, triple-blind study (*Indian J Dent Res*. 2009 Jan[524]): "The oil pulling therapy showed a reduction in the plaque index, modified gingival scores, and total colony count of aerobic microorganisms in the plaque of adolescents with plaque-induced gingivitis."

- o Oil pulling on Streptococcus mutans count in plaque and saliva: a randomized, controlled, triple-blind study (*J Indian Soc Pedod Prev Dent*. 2008 Mar[525]): "The study group [n=10] practiced oil pulling with sesame oil and the control group [n=10] used chlorhexidine mouthwash for 10 min every day in the morning before brushing. ... The reduction in the S. mutans count in the plaque of the study group was statistically significant after 1 and 2 weeks; the control group showed significant reduction at all the four time points (24 h, 48 h, 1 week, and 2 weeks). ... CONCLUSION: Oil pulling can be used as an effective preventive adjunct in maintaining and improving oral health."

- ▪ Treat nutritional deficiencies: Nutrients particularly worthy of consideration and supplementation are vitamin A, vitamin D, systemic/topical folic acid[526] (as methylfolate or folinic acid), CoQ10[527], and of course vitamin C.

- ▪ Hypotheses/proposals—implications of microbe-induced trigeminal activation: I am curious about the effects of oral/dental microbial immunogens on the inflammatory activation of the trigeminal nerve (peripherally and

[521] Thaweboon S, Nakaparksin J, Thaweboon B. Effect of oil-pulling on oral microorganisms in biofilm models. *Asia J Public Health* 2011;2:62-6

[522] Sood et al. Comparative efficacy of oil pulling and chlorhexidine on oral malodor: a randomized controlled trial. *J Clin Diagn Res*. 2014 Nov;8(11):ZC18-21

[523] Peedikayil et al. Effect of coconut oil in plaque related gingivitis - A preliminary report. *Niger Med J*. 2015 Mar-Apr;56(2):143-7

[524] Asokan et al. Effect of oil pulling on plaque induced gingivitis: a randomized, controlled, triple-blind study. *Indian J Dent Res*. 2009 Jan-Mar;20(1):47-51

[525] Asokan et al. Effect of oil pulling on Streptococcus mutans count in plaque and saliva using Dentocult SM Strip mutans test: a randomized, controlled, triple-blind study. *J Indian Soc Pedod Prev Dent*. 2008 Mar;26(1):12-7

[526] "On days 0 and 30 of a double blind study, two groups of 15 subjects each were evaluated using a plaque index, a gingival index, a gingival exudate flow and fasting plasma folic acid levels. Group I received 2 mg of folic acid twice daily for 30 days while Group II received a placebo. Results of the study seem to indicate that folic acid supplemented to the diet may increase the resistance of the gingiva to local irritants and thus lead to a reduction in inflammation." Vogel et al. The effect of folic acid on gingival health. *J Periodontol*. 1976 Nov;47(11):667-8. "A double blind study was designed to determine the effects of folate mouthwash (MW) on established gingivitis in non-pregnant adults. ... Subjects used 5 ml of MW twice daily for 4 weeks, rinsing for 1 min before expectorating. Experimental MW contained 5 mg folate per 5 ml. ... Initially, groups were similar except that the experimental group exhibited more bleeding sites at the outset, but after 4 weeks, the experimental group showed a significant decrease in mean number of colour change sites (from 70.17 +/- 12.89 to 56.62 +/- 17.42) and in bleeding sites (from 48.59 +/- 24.28 to 29.28 +/- 19.64) compared with control group (colour: from 66.93 +/- 15.27 to 66.20 +/- 18.83; bleeding: from 36.93 +/- 16.96 to 39.47 +/- 16.67) p less than 0.001. ... Folate MW appears to have an influence on gingival health through local rather than systemic influence." Pack AR. Folate mouthwash: effects on established gingivitis in periodontal patients. *J Clin Periodontol*. 1984 Oct;11(9):619-28

[527] "About 60% of the 40 diseased gingival tissues showed a deficiency of coenzyme Q(10) at its site in this succinate-coenzyme Q(10) enzyme. Of the 24 control tissues, 20% showed deficiencies of coenzyme Q(10)." Nakamura et al. Study of CoQ10-enzymes in gingiva from patients with periodontal disease and evidence for a deficiency of coenzyme Q10. *Proc Natl Acad Sci* 1974 Apr;71(4):1456-60

centrally), which might—in addition to promoting inflammatory oral pain[528]—result in sensitization of the trigeminal nucleus and thereby contribute to pain, perhaps including migraine and head pain (supported[529]), and might contribute to inflammatory transactivation of intra-CNS herpes and other virus replication.

- <u>Hypotheses and proposals—gut seeding/alteration by orodental and sinorespiratory microbes</u>: For many years I have proposed that microbes in the mouth might contribute to gastrointestinal dysbiosis by direct seeding (thereby accounting in part for the persistence of gastrointestinal dysbiosis) or perhaps by altering the inflammatory or microbial milieu via molecules, alteration in quorum sensing, or other more-or-less direct means.

Active learning and reflection

Name the signs of mild "subclinical" gingivitis:

_____

_____

_____

_____

_____

Name at least 10 treatments for gingivitis:

1.	2.
3.	4.
5.	6.
7.	8.
9.	10.

Given that "sensitive teeth" and/or gums that bleed when flossed or provoked are indications of gum disease and the resultant odontogenic inflammation and bacterial translocation and endotoxemia, write your plan for assessing this in your patients and managing the problem clinically:

_____

_____

_____

_____

_____

_____

---

[528] "These findings are consistent with the hypothesis that trigeminal neurons are capable of detecting pathogenic bacterial components leading to sensitization of TRPV1, possibly contributing to the inflammatory pain often observed in bacterial infections." Diogenes et al. LPS sensitizes TRPV1 via activation of TLR4 in trigeminal sensory neurons. *J Dent Res.* 2011 Jun;90(6):759-64. "Collectively, these data demonstrate for the first time that LPS from P. gingivalis, at concentrations found in infected canal systems, significantly sensitizes TRPV1 responses in trigeminal neurons. These findings have clear scientific and clinical implications and may shed light on the mechanism by which bacteria can directly sensitize trigeminal nociceptors." Ferraz et al. Lipopolysaccharide from Porphyromonas gingivalis sensitizes capsaicin-sensitive nociceptors. *J Endod.* 2011 Jan;37:45-8
[529] "Ipsilateral intraoral tenderness and increased local temperature were consistently observed during unilateral migraine and tension-type headache, suggesting local inflammation. Intraoral chilling and topical application of a nonsteroidal anti-inflammatory drug were highly effective for the treatment of migraine and tension-type headache, both in the acute phase and for headache prevention. These results suggest that a local intraoral inflammation may be associated with the pathogenesis of these common headaches." Friedman MH. Local inflammation as a mediator of migraine and tension-type headache. *Headache.* 2004 Sep;44(8):767-71

- **Dysbiosis-disease causation**: Sinorespiratory dysbiosis refers to adverse health consequences resultant from noninfectious colonization of the respiratory tract. Patients with acute and chronic rhinosinusitis (CRS) commonly display a rich mixture of bacteria and fungi in their sinuses. Regarding bacteria, both anaerobic and aerobic bacteria are seen, as are Gram-positives such as *Staphylococcus aureus, Streptococcus* sp, Peptococcus/Peptostreptococcus, and Gram-negative (endotoxin-producing) species including *Klebsiella pneumoniae, Proteus mirabilis, Bacteroides, Haemophilus parainfluenzae,* and *Haemophilus influenzae*.[530,531] Regarding fungi, **almost all patients with chronic sinus congestion have occult fungal sinus infections**, as shown in a landmark article wherein the authors concluded, "Fungal cultures of nasal secretions were positive in 202 (96%) of 210 consecutive chronic rhinosinusitis patients."[532] As anticipated, the bacteria and fungi colonizing the sinuses are characteristically embedded in and protected by complex biofilms; interestingly a report in *Frontiers Microbiol* 2015 Mar[533] suggested that "bacterial community diversity was significantly lower in CRS...whereas bacterial load was not associated with disease status" thereby implying that "imbalance or dysbiosis in community structure" was the main problem, not microbial overload and commonly and simply presumed. Per the data from Saint Louis University in 2013, immunologic intolerance to benign bacteria appears to be the

> **DrV's favorite way of explaining dysbiosis: "Often what we find when working with autoimmune/inflammatory patients is that they are having a pathogenic inflammatory response to *nonpathogenic* microbes."**
>
> Research that exemplifies this concept:
> - "Saint Louis University researchers have analyzed the microbiomes of people with chronic rhinosinusitis and healthy volunteers and found evidence that **some chronic sinus issues may be the result of inflammation triggered by an immune response to otherwise harmless microorganisms in the sinus membranes**.
> - "Further study findings suggested that bacteria and fungi are not causing an infection in the sinuses, but rather, that the **immune system was responding to commensals, microorganisms that, themselves, do not harm the human body**.
> - "When the immune system reacts in a hyper-responsive way, unnecessarily fighting off a harmless microorganism, it can initiate an immune response like inflammation. The body can then get locked into a cycle where inflammation generates more inflammation, causing a chronic condition.
> - "Patients with CRS are hyper-responsive to normal microbiota," said Aurora. "Our take-home message is that the problem doesn't lie in the microbiota. The inflammatory response and the resulting damage from the prolonged inflammation are caused by the body's own immune response to harmless microbiota."
>
> Harmless Members of Microbiome Spark Immune Reaction. sciencedaily.com/releases/2013/12/131219134455.htm Dec. 19, 2013. Original source: With Sinus Study, SLU Investigators Add Immune System Dimension to Discussion of Microbiota and Disease. slu.edu/x89847.xml

problem, rather than a normal response to pathogenic bacteria.[534] What I started to appreciate about microbial diversity per these articles is that microbial diversity prevents a single pattern of microbial messages from becoming dominant and thereby pushing a specific immune response from *physiology* to *pathophysiology* and then to *pathology*; using a musical metaphor, with diversity the microbial orchestra hums in unison rather than having a few isolated screamers.

Reactive arthritis and cutaneous vasculitis have been reported in an HLA-B27-negative patient with *Chlamydia pneumoniae* pneumonia.[535] Perhaps the best current exemplification of the link between sinus infections and chronic inflammatory disease is seen in patients with ANCA-associated vasculitis, who have a high incidence of sinus colonization with *Staphylococcus aureus*. In these patients, *Staphylococcus aureus* produces a superantigen as well as an antigenic acid phosphatase which induces autoimmune vasculitis, nephritis, the production of antineutrophil anticytoplasmic antibody (ANCA), and the formation of immune complexes. **Antimicrobial treatment to eradicate *Staphylococcus aureus* results in clinical remission of the**

---

[530] "Aspirates of 72 chronically inflamed maxillary sinuses were processed for aerobic and anaerobic bacteria. Bacterial growth was present in 66 of the 72 specimens (92%).... The predominant anaerobic organisms were anaerobic cocci and Bacteroides sp, and the predominant aerobes or facultatives were Streptococcus sp and Staphylococcus aureus." Brook I. Bacteriology of chronic maxillary sinusitis in adults. *Ann Otol Rhinol Laryngol.* 1989 Jun;98(6):426-8
[531] "The most frequently isolated bacteria were Streptococcus viridans, Klebsiella pneumoniae, Proteus mirabilis, and Hemophilus parainfluenzae." Jiang RS, Hsu CY, Leu JF. Bacteriology of ethmoid sinus in chronic sinusitis. *Am J Rhinol.* 1997 Mar-Apr;11(2):133-7
[532] Ponikau JU, et al. The diagnosis and incidence of allergic fungal sinusitis. *Mayo Clin Proc.* 1999 Sep;74(9):877-84
[533] Biswas et al. The nasal microbiota in health and disease: variation within and between subjects. *Front Microbiol.* 2015 Mar 2;9:134
[534] Harmless Members of Microbiome Spark Immune Reaction. sciencedaily.com/releases/2013/12/131219134455.htm Dec. 19, 2013. Original source: With Sinus Study, SLU Investigators Add Immune System Dimension to Discussion of Microbiota and Disease. slu.edu/x89847.xml
[535] "Here we present the case history of a patient with C. pneumoniae community acquired pneumonia (CAP) who subsequently developed a ReA and a cutaneous vasculitis." Cascina et al. Cutaneous vasculitis and reactive arthritis following respiratory infection due to Chlamydia pneumoniae. *Clin Exp Rheumatol.* 2002;20(6):845-7

"autoimmune" disease[536], thus proving the microbe-autoimmune link. Increased nasal colonization with *Staphylococcus aureus* has also been documented in other inflammatory/autoimmune diseases, including systemic lupus erythematosus[537] and psoriasis.[538] The nose/nares is commonly a repository for *Staphylococcus aureus* and allows microbial dispersal directly to the skin to promote eczema and surgical infections, while the absorbent sinorespiratory mucosa translocates microbial toxins and antigens, notably the pathogenic acid phosphatase enzyme. As a very powerful example of dysbiosis/infection-induced neuronal autoimmunity, we note Pediatric Autoimmune Neuropsychiatric Disorders Associated with Streptococcal infections (PANDAS) as one of several "post-streptococcal autoimmune disorders of the central nervous system"; per review by Dale[539], "Group A Streptococcus can induce autoimmune disease in humans with particular involvement of the heart, joints, and brain. The spectrum of post-streptococcal disease of the central nervous system (CNS) has been widened recently and includes movement disorders (chorea, tics, dystonia, and Parkinsonism), psychiatric disorders (particularly emotional disorders), and associated sleep disorders."

> **Sinus dysbiosis: reduced diversity, not increased load**
>
> "Chronic rhinosinusitis (CRS) affects approximately 5% of the adult population in Western societies and severely reduces the patient's quality of life. The role of bacteria in the pathogenesis of this condition has not yet been established with certainty. However, recent reports of **bacterial and fungal biofilms** in CRS highlight a potential role for these microorganisms. ... In addition, **bacterial community diversity was significantly lower in CRS samples** compared to those from healthy subjects, whereas **bacterial load was not associated with disease status.** Although members of the genera Corynebacterium and Staphylococcus were prevalent in the majority of samples (including healthy subjects), the large amount of variation observed between individuals, particularly within the CRS cohort, suggests that an **imbalance or dysbiosis in community structure** could be the driving force behind the disease."
>
> Biswas et al. The nasal microbiota in health and disease. *Front Microbiol.* 2015 Mar

- **Assessments**: Several studies documenting fungal and bacterial colonization of the sinuses have used diagnostic/surgical techniques that are not routinely available to clinicians working in outpatient settings. **Nasal swab and culture, throat culture for bacteria and yeasts can be performed** per Noah[540] in her excellent discussion of the dysbiosis-psoriasis causation. Accessing the sinuses is generally not feasible on a clinical/nonsurgical basis. Response to antimicrobial treatment implies cure of the occult infection. In severe cases, MRI or CT can be used to assess for occult infectious sinusitis.
  - Culturome of the human nose reveals bacterial fingerprint patterns (*Environ Microbiol* 2015 Apr[541]): "Samples [n=34] were collected systematically during surgery and examined by an extensive culture-based approach and, for a subset, by 16S rRNA gene community profiling. Cultivation yielded 141 taxa with members of *Staphylococcus*, *Corynebacterium* and *Propionibacterium* as most common isolates comprising the nasal core culturome together with *Finegoldia magna* [formerly *Peptostreptococcus magnus*]. *S.aureus* was most frequently found in association with *Staphylococcus epidermidis* and *Propionibacterium acnes* and the posterior vestibules were redefined as *S.aureus'* principle habitat. Culturome analysis revealed host-specific bacterial "fingerprints" irrespective of host-driven factors or intranasal sites."

- **Specific treatment considerations**: Systemic antibiotics are commonly used when treating sinus infections. Nasal lavage with saline is highly efficacious for relieving sinus congestion.[542] The basic solution is approximately one cup of warm water with one-half teaspoon of salt (sodium chloride) and one-half teaspoon baking soda (sodium bicarbonate). Distilled, bottled, or otherwise filtered and purified water may be preferred to avoid the microbial contaminants that are found in municipal tap water. To this can be added antimicrobial

---

[536] Popa et al. Staphylococcus aureus and Wegener's granulomatosis. *Arthritis Res.* 2002;4(2):77-9 arthritis-research.com/content/4/2/077

[537] Medline abstract from Polish research: "In 9 from 14 patients with (64.3%) a.b. very massive growth of Staphylococcus aureus in culture from vestibulae of the nose swab was, in other cultures very massive growth of physiological flora was seen. ...clinical significance of asymptomatic bacteriuria and pathogenic bacteria colonisation of nostrils as a precedence to symptomatic infections needs further investigations." Koseda-Dragan M, Hebanowski M, Galinski J, Krzywinska E, Bakowska A. [Asymptomatic bacteriuria in women diagnosed with systemic lupus erythematosus (SLE)] *Pol Arch Med Wewn.* 1998 Oct;100(4):321-30.

[538] "The nasal carriage rate of Staphylococcus aureus in psoriatics was higher ...." Singh G, Rao DJ. Bacteriology of psoriatic plaques. *Dermatologica.* 1978;157(1):21-7

[539] Dale RC. Post-streptococcal autoimmune disorders of the central nervous system. *Dev Med Child Neurol.* 2005 Nov;47(11):785-91

[540] Noah PW. The role of microorganisms in psoriasis. *Semin Dermatol.* 1990 Dec;9(4):269-76. Utterly brilliant work.

[541] Kaspar et al. The Culturome of the Human Nose Habitats Reveals Individual Bacterial Fingerprint Patterns. *Environ Microbiol.* 2015 Apr 28. [Epub ahead of print]

[542] "Endonasal irrigations with salt solutions are effective in the treatment of chronic sinusitis..." Bachmann G, Hommel G, Michel O. Effect of irrigation of the nose with isotonic salt solution on adult patients with chronic paranasal sinus disease. *Eur Arch Otorhinolaryngol.* 2000 Dec;257(10):537-41

botanicals such as berberine, hyperforin (highly effective against *Staphylococcus aureus*[543]), artemisinin, and others (discussed later) as well as diluted iodine[544] and powdered Nystatin (sugar-free only.) Compounding pharmacists can customize antimicrobial nasal sprays that include amphotericin B. Irrigation with a bulb syringe (such as used to clear an infant's nostrils) or Neti lota pot (aka: Neti pot, or Jala neti pot) can be performed by the patient while leaning over the sink. In the author's experience, 10-15 drops of povidone iodine 10% solution can be added to one cup of nasal lavage; higher amounts of iodine cause a burning sensation. Intranasal mupirocin can be used to target *Staphylococcus aureus* (described for the treatment of eczema in the section on *dermal dysbiosis*); however, 5% iodine—specifically but not exclusively 3M™ "Skin and Nasal Antiseptic" (Povidone-Iodine Solution 5% w/w [0.5% available iodine] USP)—is less expensive, not susceptible to microbial resistance, polyantimicrobial, and much faster to achieve microbial eradication.[545,546] Irrigating while kneeling with the head on the floor is the most effective technique for irrigating the maxillary sinuses and frontal recess; however most techniques are inefficient for accessing the sphenoid and frontal sinuses.[547] Nasal sprays and nebulizers with saline and/or antimicrobial herbs and medications can also be utilized.[548] However, clinicians and patients must remember that the creation of microbial imbalance is possible in the sinuses just as it is in the gastrointestinal tract; thus, the use of an antibacterial agent may result in fungal overgrowth or proliferation of resistant microbes. Patients with sinus dysbiosis can integrate antimicrobial sinus lavage into their daily hygiene routine, e.g., as at the same time they brush their teeth in the morning and evening. The data over many years and from many different centers using different methods has proven that the sinuses are colonized by Gram-positives, Gram-negatives, and fungi.

In the first edition of *Integrative Rheumatology* (2006), I concluded this section with the sentence "Perhaps we will find that many cases of recalcitrant gastrointestinal dysbiosis have recurred because of the gastrointestinal 'seeding' of microbes from the sinorespiratory tract", and in 2015 I found the study by Yang et al stating "Rhinosinusitis derived *Staphylococcal* enterotoxin B possibly associates with pathogenesis of ulcerative colitis" (*BMC Gastroenterol* 2005 Sep).

Active learning and reflection

Given that chronic sinusitis is common and is associated with an exaggerated immune response to benign bacteria/fungi, name at least two examples of interventions for each of the following 3 categories of treatments against sinus dysbiosis:

- Antimicrobial:

- Immunorestorative:

- Tolerogenic:

---

[543] Schempp et al. Antibacterial activity of hyperforin from St John's wort, against multiresistant Staphylococcus aureus and gram-positive bacteria. *Lancet.* 1999 Jun 19;353(9170):2129

[544] "Gargling with povidone-iodine before oral intubation reduces the transport of bacteria into the trachea." Ogata J, Minami K, Miyamoto H, Horishita T, Ogawa M, Sata T, Taniguchi H. Gargling with povidone-iodine reduces the transport of bacteria during oral intubation. *Can J Anaesth.* 2004 Nov;51(9):932-6 cja-jca.org/cgi/content/full/51/9/932 See also: "...a technique with facial, nasal vestibule and nasal cavity disinfection with a povidone-iodine solution followed by a cleansing of the nasal cavity (N = 87 patients and 166 samples)." Rombaux et al. The role of nasal cavity disinfection in the bacteriology of chronic sinusitis. *Rhinology.* 2005 Jun;43(2):125-9

[545] Hill RL, Wade JJ; Interscience Conference on Antimicrobial Agents and Chemotherapy. Elimination of Nasal Carriage of S. aureus with 5% Povidone-Iodine Cream: a Double-Blind Placebo-Controlled Trial. *Abstr Intersci Conf Antimicrob Agents Chemother Intersci Conf Antimicrob Agents Chemother.* 2000 Sep 17-20; 40: 483 gateway.nlm.nih.gov

[546] Anderson et al. Efficacy of Skin and Nasal Povidone-Iodine Preparation against mupirocin resistant MRSA and Staphylococcus aureus within the anterior nares. *Antimicrob Agents Chemother.* 2015 Mar 2. pii: AAC.04624-14

[547] "...nasal douching while kneeling with the head on the floor...Nasal douches are more effective in distributing irrigation solution to the maxillary sinus and frontal recess.This should be the method of choice for irrigating these areas." Wormald et al.Comparative study of three methods of nasal irrigation.*Laryngoscope* 2004;114:2224-7

[548] "Therapy with a 4-week course of large-particle nebulized aerosol therapy improves symptomatology and objective parameters of rhinosinusitis in patients refractory to surgical and medical therapies. Addition of tobramycin appears of minimal benefit." Desrosiers MY, Salas-Prato M. Treatment of chronic rhinosinusitis refractory to other treatments with topical antibiotic therapy delivered by means of a large-particle nebulizer: results of a controlled trial. *Otolaryngol Head Neck Surg.* 2001 Sep;125(3):265-9

Tissue/Parenchymal/Blood Dysbiosis—part 1: Occult bacterial colonizations

- **Dysbiosis-disease causation**: True "infections" and microbial colonization of internal organs is generally incompatible with life and unlikely to be a silent/asymptomatic locus of inflammatory stimuli due to the appropriate febrile response that typically characterizes such infections. However, exceptions to these rules do exist, and infections of parenchymal tissue—especially of liver or bone—have been reported as initiators/mimickers of systemic rheumatic/inflammatory disease. **Viral hepatitis may present with polyarthropathy while the hepatitis is asymptomatic and serum levels of liver enzymes are within normal limits**; in these cases, the underlying dysbiosis/infection is identified with the use of specific serologic testing.[549] **Polyarteritis nodosa** is an autoimmune/inflammatory vasculitic syndrome strongly associated with hepatitis B infection, and 90% of patients with the immune complex vasculitis cryoglobulinemia have hepatitis C.[550] Robertson and Hickling[551] describe the case of a young girl who was **tentatively diagnosed with juvenile rheumatoid arthritis before being more accurately diagnosed with "recurrent multifocal osteomyelitis."** Dysbiosis (characterized by the acute nature of the microbial colonization) can segue into a true "infection." An advantage to the term *dysbiosis* in this situation is that it encourages clinicians to search for inflammation-generating microbial foci that may exist despite the absence of organ failure or classic/standard characteristics associated with parenchymal infection. "Blood dysbiosis" may at first appear to be a novel or awkward term, but it is a term used in the peer-reviewed biomedical literature; those of us who have studied histology will recall that blood is a type of connective tissue—living cells embedded within a nonliving matrix. For so-called "blood dysbiosis", the question of whether or not the bacteria are actually living in the blood is somewhat irrelevant; we are obviously not dealing with sepsis in this conversation, but perhaps a low-grade bacteremia. Physicians should appreciate that *culturable* low-grade bacteremia is a common daily experience, for example after teeth-brushing[552]; the variables worth considering therefore obviously become those of magnitude, combination, specific microbial type(s), and patient tolerance. Further, and perhaps equally obvious, the finding of bacterial DNA in the blood does not necessarily imply that all represented bacteria are living in the blood; more likely is that the bacterial DNA are being circulated from other foci/reservoirs, the largest of course being that of the gastrointestinal tract. The most common sources of bacterial DNA in the blood are ❶ the oral cavity, ❷ gastrointestinal tract (including bacterial translocation of living bacteria[553] and absorption of DNA and other inflammatory debris from dead bacteria, obviously quantitatively exacerbated by SIBO, increased intestinal permeability ["leaky gut"], intestinal obstruction, surgical manipulation, and major trauma/burns), and ❸ any foci of active infection, such as the skin or genitourinary tract.

> **"Blood microbiota dysbiosis" is associated with the onset of cardiovascular events in a large population**
>
> "The main finding of the study is that a **dysbiosis in blood microbiota**, defined by a decrease in blood bacterial DNA content and an increase in the proportion of Proteobacteria phylum within **blood microbiota**, predicts long-term cardiovascular prognosis."
>
> Amar J, et al. *PLoS ONE* 2013:8(1); e54461

- **Assessments**: Given the increasing prevalence of viral hepatitis and its protean manifestations, specific serologic testing for viral hepatitis is warranted in patients with constitutional symptoms and inflammatory/idiopathic arthralgia. Likewise, occult osteomyelitis—particularly of the mandible—is increasingly appreciated, particularly as newer imaging techniques are facilitating detection. Bone scans can detect clinically occult bone infections.

- **Specific clinical considerations**: Listed below are several of the most consistent representations of "tissue dysbiosis and human disease" in the clinical literature. Of these, multiple sclerosis has the longest history of association with microbial colonization; the best model appears to be that of—as readers should expect by now—multifocal polydysbiosis, with *Chlamydia pneumoniae* seeming to take the lead both in terms of

[549] "HCV arthritis should be considered in the differential diagnosis of seronegative arthritis of undetermined etiology even in the setting of normal liver chemistries." Akhtar AJ, Funnye AS. Hepatitis C virus associated arthritis in absence of clinical, biochemical and histological evidence of liver disease--responding to interferon therapy. *Med Sci Monit.* 2005 Jul;11(7):CS37-9 medscimonit.com/pub/vol_11/no_7/6300.pdf

[550] Tierney ML. McPhee SJ, Papadakis MA (eds). *Current Medical Diagnosis and Treatment 2006. 45th edition.* New York; Lange Medical Books: 2006, pages 844-850

[551] Robertson LP, Hickling P. Chronic recurrent multifocal osteomyelitis is a differential diagnosis of juvenile idiopathic arthritis. *Ann Rheum Dis.* 2001 Sep;60(9):828-31

[552] "Positive blood cultures were detected in 29.6% of patients after dental extraction, in 10.8% of patients after tooth brushing and in no patients after chewing. ... Our study confirmed that bacteraemia occurs after tooth brushing." Maharaj et al. An investigation of the frequency of bacteraemia following dental extraction, tooth brushing and chewing. *Cardiovasc J Afr.* 2012 Jul;23(6):340-4

[553] MacFie J. Current status of bacterial translocation as a cause of surgical sepsis. *Br Med Bull.* 2004 Dec 13;71:1-11

importance as well as its localization within the brain. Excellent data on diabetes has been accumulating, as represented by the literature sample below, and the microbe-diabetes link may explain at least in part the efficacy of therapeutics such as berberine, which is highly effective for diabetes, likely working via an antimicrobial mechanism.[554] Finally, the connection between intervertebral disc infections and chronic low back pain appeared rapidly in 2013 and was immediately validated by identification of microbes in the spinal disc material and confirmed via a stunningly fast and significant clinical response to antimicrobial therapy; hence the research was immediately touted as "worthy of a Nobel Prize."[555]

> **Bacterial translocation from the gut**
>
> "...bacteria could migrate from the gastrointestinal tract into the portal circulation in the absence of an infective process in humans. Subsequently it has become clear that, in addition to Gram-negative bacteria, endotoxin, Gram-positive bacteria and fungi can pass through the mucosal barrier. ... The term 'bacterial translocation' is used to describe the passage of viable resident bacteria from the gastrointestinal tract to normally sterile tissues such as the mesenteric lymph nodes and other internal organs. The term also applies to the passage of inert particles and other macromolecules, such as lipopolysaccharide endotoxin, across the intestinal mucosal barrier."
>
> MacFie J. Current status of bacterial translocation as a cause of surgical sepsis. *Br Med Bull.* 2004 Dec 13;71:1-11

- **Dormant blood microbiome in chronic, inflammatory diseases** (*FEMS Microbiol Rev* 2015 May[556]): **Blood is not sterile**—especially in Parkinson's/Alzheimer's diseases—but contaminated with bacteria in a dormant state. The authors propose that *dysbiosis* (e.g., in mouth/gut) promotes *microbial translocation* and *"atopobiosis"*—relocated bacteria (e.g., in blood), from which inflammatory diseases are promoted.

- **Psoriasis and blood dysbiosis:** Bacterial DNA (bactDNA) in the peripheral blood of patients with active psoriasis (*JAMA Dermatol.* 2015 Mar[557]): "Blood bactDNA was present in 16 patients with psoriasis, all of whom showed the phenotype of plaque psoriasis (16 of 45 [35.5%]), whereas 6 patients with guttate psoriasis, 3 with inverse psoriasis, and all 27 controls did not have bactDNA in the blood. Species identification corresponded to *Escherichia coli* (n=9), *Klebsiella pneumoniae* (n=2), *Enterococcus faecalis* (n=2), *Proteus mirabilis* (n=1), *Streptococcus pyogenes* (n=1), and *Shigella flexneri* (n=1). ... The systemic inflammatory response was significantly higher in patients with bactDNA compared with other patients and controls." Inflammatory markers correlated with bactDNA included IL-1, IL-6, IL-12, TNF, and IFN-gamma. At first look, the one-bacteria-per-patient appearance is somewhat misleading; obviously other microbial colonizations, including those without DNA present in the blood and other types of colonizations—especially yeast—would be expected to be present but were not searched for in this investigation.

- **Insulin resistance and tissue dysbiosis:** Acute infections are known to induce long-term insulin resistance in humans (*J Clin Endocrinol Metab.* 1989 Aug[558]): "Acute infections provoke insulin resistance. ... We conclude that acute infections induce severe and long-lasting insulin resistance, which is localized to glucose-utilizing pathways. The rate of carbohydrate oxidation is normal during infections, whereas the rate of nonoxidative glucose disposal, as determined by indirect calorimetry, is nearly zero." Obviously, if an acute infection can induce acute/subacute insulin resistance, then low-grade long-term dysbiosis/dysbioses/colonizations—via identical mechanisms simply at a lower level and longer duration—would be expected to effect the same.

- **Diabetes and tissue dysbiosis:** Involvement of tissue bacteria in the onset of diabetes in humans (*Diabetologia* 2011 Dec[559]): "RESULTS: We analysed 3,280 participants without diabetes or obesity at baseline. **The 16S rDNA concentration was higher [in the blood] in those destined to have diabetes.** No difference was observed regarding obesity. However, the 16S rDNA concentration was higher in those who had abdominal adiposity at the end of follow-up. The adjusted OR for incident diabetes and for abdominal adiposity were 1.35 and 1.18, respectively. Moreover, pyrosequencing analyses showed that participants destined to have diabetes and the controls shared a core blood microbiota, mostly

554 "Because berberine acts topically in the gastrointestinal tract and it is poorly absorbed, berberine might modulate gut microbiota without systemic anti-infective activity. Our hypothesis is that gut microbiota modulation may be one mechanism of the antidiabetic effect of berberine." Han et al. Modulating gut microbiota as an anti-diabetic mechanism of berberine. *Med Sci Monit.* 2011 Jul;17(7):RA164-7

555 Sample I. Antibiotics could cure 40% of chronic back pain patients. theguardian.com/society/2013/may/07/antibiotics-cure-back-pain-patients

556 Potgieter et al. The dormant blood microbiome in chronic, inflammatory diseases. *FEMS Microbiol Rev.* 2015 May 3. pii: fuv013

557 Ramírez-Boscá et al. Identification of bacterial DNA in the peripheral blood of patients with active psoriasis. *JAMA Dermatol.* 2015 Mar [Epub ahead of print]

558 Yki-Järvinen et a. Severity, duration, and mechanisms of insulin resistance during acute infections. *J Clin Endocrinol Metab.* 1989 Aug;69(2):317-23

559 Amar et al. Involvement of tissue bacteria in the onset of diabetes in humans: evidence for a concept. *Diabetologia.* 2011 Dec;54(12):3055-61

composed of the Proteobacteria phylum (85-90%). "*CONCLUSIONS/INTERPRETATION*: 16S rDNA was shown to be an independent marker of the risk of diabetes. These findings are **evidence for the concept that tissue bacteria are involved in the onset of diabetes in humans**."

- *How do we reconcile microbial inputs with what we know about diabetes etiology including xenobiotic exposure and mitochondrial dysfunction[560]?*—This question is easy to answer because both microbes and xenobiotics contribute to mitochondrial dysfunction, with resulting impairments in insulin secretion and peripheral reception. Production of LPS from Gram-negative bacteria from the gut would be expected to impair cytochrome p450 and result in progressive xenobiotic accumulation, thereby exacerbating mitochondrial dysfunction. Also, infections and microbial colonization add to the total inflammatory load (TIL) and could thereby indirectly exacerbate/uncover xenobiotic-induced mitochondria-mediated insulin resistance and diabetes.

  o **Low-back pain** and tissue dysbiosis: Chronic bacterial infections/dysbiosis in the intervertebral discs of patients with chronic low back pain and disc herniation: Research published in 2013 showed that 46% of patients with chronic low back pain and lumbar disc herniations harbored chronic microbial infections within their intervertebral discs; these infections/colonizations were most commonly and significantly due to anaerobic bacteria (predominantly *Propionibacterium acnes*) while fewer patients carried aerobic bacteria in their disc material and these aerobic infections/colonizations appeared to be of lesser significance with regard to induction of pain and bone edema.[561] Antibiotic treatment (amoxicillin with clavulanic acid for 100 days) of patients with chronic low back pain was shown to provide important dose-dependent clinical benefit at the end of 100 days of treatment with benefits durable and progressive for one year[562]; impressive clinical response—approximately 50% reductions in pain and disability—following antimicrobial therapy was seen in 80% of patients.

    - *How do we reconcile the new data showing bacterial infection as a cause of chronic low-back pain with previous data showing efficacy of spinal manipulation and exercise[563] for low-back pain?*—Spinal manipulation and exercise alleviate low-back pain by several mechanisms including reduced nociceptive input and enhanced neuromuscular coordination; one might also speculate that motion-induced promotion of flow of interstitial fluid through the disc (recall that intervertebral discs have no direct blood supply, but receive nutrition via diffusion from the surrounding vertebrae) might dissipate inflammatory mediators that cause pain or might dissipate the microbes themselves to either reduce the local microbial load or enhance recognition by the immune system. Additionally, exercise and manipulation, including proprioceptive retraining, may simply address the neuromusculoskeletal component of low-back pain to reduce the total afferent input to a level lower than that required to cross the perceptible pain threshold. Thereby, these two seemingly different paradigms/models of back pain—simultaneously responsive to manual/physical and antimicrobial therapies—are reconcilable. Conceptually, we could reframe the perception of numerous disease states from that of *a point on a line, which when passed signifies the crossing of a diagnostic threshold*, to one of *perception of sound or the raising of a level of water wherein the culminated total of a variety of inputs and influences effects the crossing of a line, or the raising to a level of perceptible and distinct change*. The linear model promotes the (mis)perception of a corresponding singular cause, whereas the volume-related model of either water or sound encourages us to appreciate—and therefore search for and address—each of the contributors to this change in

[560] Lim S, Cho YM, Park KS, Lee HK. Persistent organic pollutants, mitochondrial dysfunction, and metabolic syndrome. *Ann N Y Acad Sci.* 2010 Jul;1201:166-76. See also: Lee HK, Vasquez A. Dr Hong Lee's Personal and Educational Path: Interview with endocrinologist and mitochondrial toxicologist Dr Hong Kyu Lee by Dr Alex Vasquez. *Int J Hum Nutr Funct Med* 2015;v3(q1):p3 available from IntJHumNutrFunctMed.org

[561] "In total, microbiological cultures were positive in 28 (46 %) patients. Anaerobic cultures were positive in 26 (43 %) patients, and of these 4 (7 %) had dual microbial infections, containing both one aerobic and one anaerobic culture." Albert HB, Lambert P, Rollason J, et al. Does nuclear tissue infected with bacteria following disc herniations lead to Modic changes in the adjacent vertebrae? *Eur Spine J.* 2013 Apr;22(4):690-6

[562] Albert HB, Sorensen JS, Christensen BS, Manniche C. Antibiotic treatment in patients with chronic low back pain and vertebral bone edema (Modic type 1 changes): a double-blind randomized clinical controlled trial of efficacy. *Eur Spine J.* 2013 Apr;22(4):697-707

[563] Among the many studies and reports available, these are sufficient to support the view that chiropractic manipulative therapy is effective for low-back pain. Meade TW, Dyer S, Browne W, Townsend J, Frank AO. Low-back pain of mechanical origin: randomised comparison of chiropractic and hospital outpatient treatment. *BMJ.* 1990;300(6737):1431-7. Meade TW, Dyer S, Browne W, Frank AO. Randomised comparison of chiropractic and hospital outpatient management for low-back pain: results from extended follow up. *BMJ.* 1995;311(7001):349-5. Manga P, Angus D, Papadopoulos C, et al. The Effectiveness and Cost-Effectiveness of Chiropractic Management of Low-Back Pain. Richmond Hill, Ontario: Kenilworth Publishing; 1993

volume/load of physiologic variables that when skewed in concert eventually tip the scales from health to disease.

- *How do we reconcile the new data showing bacterial infection as a cause of chronic low-back pain with previous data showing efficacy of vitamin D3[564] for low-back pain?*—Vitamin D replenishment alleviates ❶ peripheral pain, ❷ central pain, ❸ systemic inflammation while ❹ improving neuromuscular coordination (noted to alleviate low-back pain) and ❺ enhancing immune effectiveness by promoting the elaboration of the body's natural endogenous antibiotics—the antimicrobial peptides (AMP) such as beta-defensin and cathelicidin LL-37. Thereby, these two seemingly different paradigms/models of back pain—simultaneously responsive to vitamin D and antimicrobial therapies—are very reconcilable, given that both converge in antimicrobial effects.

- **Multiple sclerosis (MS) and tissue dysbiosis: Role of multiple pathogens** (*Int Rev Immunol.* 2014 Jul[565]): "Infectious pathogens are the likely environmental factors involved in the development of MS. Pathogens associated with the development or exacerbation of MS include bacteria, such as *Mycoplasma pneumoniae* and *Chlamydia pneumoniae*, the *Staphylococcus aureus*-produced enterotoxins that function as superantigens, viruses of the herpes virus (Epstein-Barr virus and human herpesvirus 6) and human endogenous retrovirus (HERV) families and the protozoa *Acanthamoeba castellanii*." Mechanisms for the connection between microbes and MS include molecular mimicry, epitope spreading, bystander activation and microglial activation.

- **Multiple sclerosis (MS) and tissue dysbiosis: Chlamydia pneumoniae-specific intrathecal oligoclonal antibody response is detected in a subset of multiple sclerosis patients with progressive forms** (*J Neurovirol* 2009 Sep[566]): "These findings suggest that an intrathecal production of anti-C. pneumoniae IgG is part of humoral polyreactivity driven by MS chronic brain inflammation. However, an intrathecal release of C. pneumoniae-specific oligoclonal IgG can occur in a subset of patients with MS progressive forms in whom a C. pneumoniae-persistent brain infection may play a pathogenetic role."

- **Multiple sclerosis (MS) and tissue dysbiosis: Cerebrospinal fluid molecular demonstration of Chlamydia pneumoniae DNA correlates with relapsing-remitting multiple sclerosis** (*Mult Scler.* 2004 Aug[567]): "The analysis of CSF expression of each single C. pneumoniae-specific gene revealed that detectable levels of major outer membrane protein (MOMP) were significantly more frequent in MS patients with relapse (P < 0.05), whereas PCR positivity for MOMP and 16S rRNA genes were more represented in MS patients with clinical and MRI evidence of disease activity (P < 0.05). …These findings confirm that the C. pneumoniae detection within the central nervous system (CNS) is not selectively restricted to MS, but accounts in a variety of neurological diseases. In addition, our results suggest that CSF C. pneumoniae-specific DNA detection can occur in a subset of MS patients with clinical and MRI active RR form in whom a C. pneumoniae brain chronic persistent infection may play a significant role in the development of disease."

- **Multiple sclerosis (MS) and tissue dysbiosis: Increased prevalence of and gene transcription by Chlamydia pneumoniae in cerebrospinal fluid of patients with relapsing-remitting multiple sclerosis.** (*J Neurol.* 2004 May[568]): "C. pneumoniae-specific DNA was more often detected in MS patients (50 %) than in all OND patients combined (28.1%, p = 0.003)… In MS patients (n = 20), chlamydial heat shock protein 60-mRNA (75%) and 16S-rRNA (70%) were more often detected than in OND patients (n = 16; 18.8%; p < 0.005). Although more often detected in remitting-relapsing MS, C. pneumoniae DNA in CSF is not specific for MS owing to its high prevalence in OND controls. However, the higher rate of gene transcription suggests a more active metabolism of C. pneumoniae in MS patients."

[564] Schwalfenberg G. Improvement of chronic back pain or failed back surgery with vitamin D repletion. *J Am Board Fam Med.* 2009 Jan-Feb;22(1):69-74. Al Faraj S, Al Mutairi K. Vitamin D deficiency and chronic low back pain in Saudi Arabia. *Spine* (Phila Pa 1976). 2003 Jan 15;28(2):177-9

[565] Libbey JE, Cusick MF, Fujinami RS. Role of pathogens in multiple sclerosis. *Int Rev Immunol.* 2014 Jul-Aug;33(4):266-83

[566] Fainardi et al. Chlamydia pneumoniae-specific intrathecal oligoclonal antibody response is predominantly detected in a subset of multiple sclerosis patients with progressive forms. *J Neurovirol.* 2009 Sep;15(5-6):425-33

[567] Contini et al. Cerebrospinal fluid molecular demonstration of Chlamydia pneumoniae DNA is associated to clinical and brain magnetic resonance imaging activity in a subset of patients with relapsing-remitting multiple sclerosis. *Mult Scler.* 2004 Aug;10(4):360-9

[568] Dong-Si et al. Increased prevalence of and gene transcription by Chlamydia pneumoniae in cerebrospinal fluid of patients with relapsing-remitting multiple sclerosis. *J Neurol.* 2004 May;251(5):542-7

Cutaneous Dysbiosis, Dermal Dysbiosis

- **Dysbiosis-disease causation**: Microorganisms from dermal infections such as acne can incite systemic inflammation either by dermal absorption of bacterial[569] and fungal[570] (super)antigens and by serving as loci for metastatic infections which produce septic arthritis.[571] **Patients with the autoimmune vasculitic syndrome known as Behcet's disease are more likely to develop arthritis if their skin lesions are infected, thus implicating absorption of an inflammatory immunogen.**[572] Most (57%) of patients with atopic dermatitis show evidence of IgE-mediated histamine release (i.e., "allergy") to exotoxins secreted from *Staphylococcus aureus*, which commonly colonizes eczematous skin[573]; in other words: most eczema patients are allergic to their own dermal bacteria and can thus be said to have *hypersensitivity dermal dysbiosis*.

- **Assessments**: Routine physical examination of the skin and scalp is generally sufficient to screen for obvious infections and any lesions that may be presumed to be colonized. Dermal scrapings and swabs are taken for bacterial, viral, and fungal cultures and microscopic examination. Skin/nail culture, Giemsa staining, culture of lesioned skin on blood agar, MacConkey agar, Sabouraud plates can be performed; see the review by Noah[574] for additional details. For many patients, especially those with atopic dermatitis, treatment can be empiric, per the protocol that follows, and clinically effective antimicrobial and immunorestorative treatment confirms the diagnosis of dysbiosis retrospectively; in other words, a successful clinical intervention — *therapeutic trial* — can provide diagnostic data — *diagnostic trial*.

> **Skin, nares, and nails: components for cyclic contamination and persistent colonization**
>
> Skin to nares, nares to nails, nails to skin: recurrent infection/colonization is highly likely unless all areas are treated simultaneously.
>
> Riley et al. Finger nails as a reservoir for Candida albicans in recurrence of vaginal candidosis. *Genitourin Med.* 1986 Oct;358

- **Specific treatment considerations**: Topical and/or systemic antimicrobial treatment along with immunonutrition (detailed later) may be necessary for complete treatment of patients with inflammation perpetuated by dermal dysbiosis. Topical *Mahonia/Berberis aquifolium* is effective for dermal psoriasis[575] via its combined anti-inflammatory and antimicrobial benefits. Other botanical antimicrobials available in topical creams, gels, and soaps include grape seed extract, artemesinin from *Artemisia annua*, and tea tree oil. A complete outline of therapeutic interventions is as follows:

  1. Orally administered antimicrobial drugs to reduce total microbial load (TML), especially targeting *Staphylococcus aureus*: For example, cephalexin 50 mg/kg per day (maximum of 2 g/day), divided into 3 daily doses, for 2 weeks.[576]

  2. Intranasal antimicrobial treatment: Topical 5% povidone iodine is the fastest, most broadly antimicrobial, and least expensive; mupirocin ointment has been used in several studies. Patients and their household members are instructed to apply intranasal treatment twice daily for five consecutive days of each month.

  3. Diluted bleach bath to reduce the total microbial load (TML) on the skin: Detailed in the accompanying textbox and in the following summaries:

     o Efficacy and safety of sodium hypochlorite (bleach) baths in patients with moderate to severe atopic dermatitis (*J Dermatol* 2013 Sep[577]): "*Staphylococcus aureus* on skin and in nares contributes to disease pathogenesis in atopic dermatitis (AD). Patients between 2 and 30 years old with moderate to severe AD were enrolled in a prospective, randomized, placebo-controlled study. Patients soaked in diluted bleach (treatment) or distilled water baths (placebo) for 10 min, twice a week for 2 months. Patients in the treatment group showed significant reductions in Eczema Area and

---

[569] Delyle et al. Chronic destructive oligoarthritis associated with Propionibacterium acnes in a female patient with acne vulgaris: septic-reactive arthritis? *Arthritis Rheum.* 2000 Dec;43(12):2843-7

[570] Hemalatha V, Srikanth P, Mallika M. Superantigens - Concepts, clinical disease and therapy. *Indian J Med Microbiol* 2004;22:204-211

[571] Schaeverbeke et al. Propionibacterium acnes isolated from synovial tissue and fluid in a patient with oligoarthritis associated with acne and pustulosis. *Arthritis Rheum.* 1998 Oct;41(10):1889-93

[572] Diri et al. Papulopustular skin lesions are seen more frequently in patients with Behcet's syndrome who have arthritis. *Ann Rheum Dis.* 2001 Nov;60(11):1074-6

[573] "These data indicate that a subset of patients with AD mount an IgE response to SEs that can be grown from their skin." Leung DY, et al. Presence of IgE antibodies to staphylococcal exotoxins on the skin of patients with atopic dermatitis. *J Clin Invest.* 1993 Sep;92(3):1374-80

[574] Noah PW. The role of microorganisms in psoriasis. *Semin Dermatol.* 1990 Dec;9(4):269-76

[575] "Taken together, these clinical studies conducted by several investigators in several countries indicate that Mahonia aquifolium is a safe and effective treatment of patients with mild to moderate psoriasis." Gulliver WP, Donsky HJ. A report on three recent clinical trials using Mahonia aquifolium 10% topical cream and a review of the worldwide clinical experience with Mahonia aquifolium for the treatment of plaque psoriasis. *Am J Ther.* 2005 Sep-Oct;12(5):398-406

[576] Huang JT et al. Treatment of Staphylococcus aureus colonization in atopic dermatitis decreases disease severity. *Pediatrics.* 2009 May;123(5):e808-14

[577] Wong SM, et al R. Efficacy and safety of sodium hypochlorite (bleach) baths in patients with moderate to severe atopic dermatitis in Malaysia. *J Dermatol.* 2013 Sep 20

Severity Index (EASI) scores. **A 41.9% reduction in S. aureus density from baseline was seen at 1 month further reducing to 53.3% at 2 months.** Equal numbers of patients in both groups experienced mild side-effects. This study demonstrates that diluted bleach baths clinically improved AD in as little as 1 month. No patient withdrew from the treatment arm because of intolerance to the baths."

- o Treatment of Staphylococcus aureus colonization in atopic dermatitis decreases disease severity (_Pediatrics_ 2009 May[578]): "METHODS: A randomized, investigator-blinded, placebo-controlled study was conducted with 31 patients, 6 months to 17 years of age, with moderate to severe atopic dermatitis and clinical signs of secondary bacterial infections. All patients received **orally administered** cephalexin **for 14 days** and were assigned randomly to receive intranasal mupirocin ointment treatment and sodium hypochlorite (bleach) baths (treatment arm) or intranasal petrolatum ointment treatment and plain water baths (placebo arm) for 3 months. The primary outcome measure was the Eczema Area and Severity Index score. RESULTS: The prevalence of community-acquired methicillin-resistant S aureus in our study (7.4% of our S aureus-positive skin cultures and 4% of our S aureus-positive nasal cultures) was much lower than that in the general population with cultures at Children's Memorial Hospital (75%-85%). **Patients in the group that received both the dilute bleach baths and intranasal mupirocin treatment showed significantly greater mean reductions from baseline in Eczema Area and Severity Index scores,** compared with the placebo group, at the 1-month and 3-month visits. The mean Eczema Area and Severity Index scores for the head and neck did not decrease for patients in the treatment group, whereas scores for other body sites (submerged in the dilute bleach baths) decreased at 1 and 3 months, in comparison with placebo-treated patients.

4. Nutritional immunorestoration: Patient-appropriate doses of vitamin A (not beta-carotene), zinc, vitamin D3, glutamine, arginine, etc.

5. Environmental decontamination: For example, bed sheets, towels, clothing, and furniture should all be cleaned thoroughly, preferably with an antimicrobial agent (as appropriate) such as bleach, alcohol, or povidone iodine. Clothes, bedding, and the environments in the car, home, and work should be disinfected and/or routinely washed; see section on _environmental dysbiosis_.

"Bleach bath" treatment for dermal dysbiosis

- Fill the bathtub with lukewarm water: approximately 40 gallons of water,
- Stir in one-quarter to one-half cup of common bleach (sodium hypochlorite 5-6% solution) solution to the bath water; the goal is to make a modified Dakin's solution with a final concentration of about 0.005%,
- Have patients soak in the chlorinated water for 5 to 10 minutes,
- Rinse thoroughly and pat (not rub) dry; use skin creams and emollients/moisturizers (if any) as usual,
- Perform bleach baths 2–3 times a week or as prescribed by the physician.
- Do not apply nondiluted bleach to skin; diluted bleach solution is generally well tolerated (same hypochlorite concentration as swimming pool water) but may likewise cause dryness and irritation, especially at skin lesions; avoid use or use extra caution in patients with contact allergy to chlorine.

Krakowski AC, et al. Management of atopic dermatitis in the pediatric population. _Pediatrics._ 2008 Oct

---

Active learning and reflection

Name 5 treatments for cutaneous/dermal dysbiosis and instructions for implementation:

1. _____

2. _____

3. _____

4. _____

5. _____

---

[578] Huang JT, et al. Treatment of Staphylococcus aureus colonization in atopic dermatitis decreases disease severity. _Pediatrics._ 2009 May;123(5):e808-14

Environmental dysbiosis

- **Dysbiosis-disease causation**: Microbes in the patient's environment may trigger simple atopic allergic reactions such as asthma and eczema and may also trigger systemic inflammation and neurologic dysfunction. Patients may develop inflammation/autoimmunity from exposures to microbial toxins from their home, work, or recreational environments. Many microorganisms, particularly yeasts/molds, defend themselves via elaboration of toxins to fend off other microbes that might otherwise invade their territory. Environmental and occupational researchers appreciate that yeast/mold commonly elaborate immunomodulating bioaerosols, while gram-negative bacteria exude endotoxin, which is a common contaminant of house dust. We may reasonably speculate that a susceptible person might have a systemic inflammatory response from the inhalation of bioaerosols and/or endotoxin in the air of their home and/or work environments. Airborne immunogens include fungi, bacteria, actinomycetes, endotoxin, ß(1,3)-glucans, peptidoglycans, microbial volatile organic compounds (MVOC), and mycotoxins.[579] "Toxic mold syndrome" and more recently "mixed mold mycotoxicosis"[580] describes patients with systemic health problems resultant from exposure to fungal bioaerosols, classically associated with mold-contaminated buildings following water damage. Such individuals may develop systemic autoimmunity that resembles multiple sclerosis and chronic inflammatory polyneuropathy mediated in part by antibodies against endogenous neuronal structures.[581] Additional evidence shows that mold exposure can lead to proinflammatory immune activation and resultant multisystem (especially neurologic) autoimmunity.[582] This is yet another example of how microorganisms can cause human disease without causing "infection." Obviously, patients with inflammatory lung disorders such as asthma, idiopathic pulmonary fibrosis, and especially acute pulmonary hemorrhage in infants[583] are candidates for environmental evaluation and intervention. Patients with Crohn's disease are well-known to have exquisite sensitivity to the yeast *Saccharomyces cerevisiae,* and a few doctors have reported improvement in Crohn's patients following environmental disinfection. Of related interest is the finding that intraperitoneal exposure of autoimmune-prone mice to fungal components stimulates autoimmune arthritis resembling rheumatoid arthritis.[584] To explain the persistence of "mold-induced illness" for long periods of time even after remediation of the building and/or after the patient has left the offending location, some authors have proposed that the offending molds have taken residence in the sinuses of the patients, are protected by biofilms, and produce myco-neurotoxins that are absorbed via the mucosa, either systemically or locally via direct transfer via the nervous system (e.g., olfactory, trigeminal, vagal nerve uptake and retrograde transmission). While this idea is certainly biologically plausible, the reviewed literature is not sufficiently supportive to establish its clinical existence.[585]

  - <u>Chlamydophila pneumoniae antibodies in office workers with and without inflammatory rheumatic diseases in a moisture-damaged building</u> (*Eur J Clin Microbiol Infect Dis* 2005 Mar[586]): "In the study reported here, we evaluated the serum samples obtained from 18 of the office workers, both at work and

---

[579] Douwes J, et al. Bioaerosol health effects and exposure assessment: progress and prospects. *Ann Occup Hyg.* 2003 Apr;47(3):187-200

[580] Gray MR, et al. Mixed mold mycotoxicosis: immunological changes in humans following exposure in water-damaged buildings. *Arch Environ Health.* 2003;58:410-20

[581] "The authors concluded that exposure to molds in water-damaged buildings increased the risk for development of neural autoantibodies, peripheral neuropathy, and neurophysiologic abnormalities in exposed individuals." Campbell AW, Thrasher JD, Madison RA, Vojdani A, Gray MR, Johnson A. Neural autoantibodies and neurophysiologic abnormalities in patients exposed to molds in water-damaged buildings. *Arch Environ Health.* 2003 Aug;58(8):464-74

[582] "Abnormally high levels of ANA, ASM, and CNS myelin (immunoglobulins [Ig]G, IgM, IgA) and PNS myelin (IgG, IgM, IgA)... showing an increased risk for autoimmunity. ...exposure to mixed molds and their associated mycotoxins in water-damaged buildings leads to multiple health problems involving the CNS and the immune system... Mold exposure also initiates inflammatory processes." Gray MR, Thrasher JD, Crago R, Madison RA, Arnold L, Campbell AW, Vojdani A. Mixed mold mycotoxicosis: immunological changes in humans following exposure in water-damaged buildings. *Arch Environ Health.* 2003 Jul;58(7):410-20

[583] "Mean colony counts for all fungi averaged 29227 colony-forming units (CFU)/m3 in homes of patients and 707 CFU/m3 in homes of controls... Conclusion Infants with pulmonary hemorrhage and hemosiderosis were more likely than controls to live in homes with toxigenic S atra and other fungi in the indoor air." Etzel RA, et al. Acute pulmonary hemorrhage in infants associated with exposure to Stachybotrys atra and other fungi. *Arch Pediatr Adolesc Med.* 1998 Aug;152(8):757-62

[584] Yoshitomi H, Sakaguchi N, Kobayashi K, et al. A role for fungal {beta}-glucans and their receptor Dectin-1 in the induction of autoimmune arthritis in genetically susceptible mice. *J Exp Med.* 2005 Mar 21;201(6):949-60 jem.org/cgi/content/full/201/6/949

[585] Brewer JH, Thrasher JD, Hooper D. Chronic illness associated with mold and mycotoxins: is naso-sinus fungal biofilm the culprit? *Toxins* (Basel). 2013 Dec 24;6(1):66-80. I cannot say that I am completely pleased with this article, as I found some of their citations/attributions/conclusions to be inaccurate. Likewise with this separate paper—Dennis et al. Fungal exposure endocrinopathy in sinusitis with growth hormone deficiency: Dennis-Robertson syndrome. *Toxicol Ind Health.* 2009 Oct-Nov;25(9-10):669-80—these authors used the same laboratory company as Brewer et al, and I am concerned that—even though their conclusions may be correct—some misuse of information might be occurring based on the fact that they erroneously cited the Lieberman et al (whom I contacted) study. I do think that the overall proposal is both rational and likely—fungal colonization is known to occur, the fungi are known to produce mycotoxins—in this case in very close proximity to the brain, and the mycotoxins are known to be inflammatory, neurotoxic and to cause mitochondrial impairment. See also: Doi K, Uetsuka K. Mechanisms of mycotoxin-induced neurotoxicity through oxidative stress-associated pathways. *Int J Mol Sci.* 2011;12(8):5213-37

[586] Seuri M, Paldanius M, Leinonen M, Roponen M, Hirvonen MR, Saikku P. Chlamydophila pneumoniae antibodies in office workers with and without inflammatory rheumatic diseases in a moisture-damaged building. *Eur J Clin Microbiol Infect Dis.* 2005 Mar;24(3):236-7

following a vacation period of 2–4 weeks' duration. Among the 18 employees, seven had rheumatic diseases and two had upper and lower respiratory symptoms, while nine employees had no diseases or prolonged respiratory symptoms. All of the subjects were female and their mean age at the time of the study was about 50 years. ... The elevated antibody levels in the employees we tested might have been caused by prolonged exposure to *C. pneumoniae* or some immunologically active part(s) of the microbe. The clustering of inflammatory rheumatic diseases among individuals in moisture damaged buildings is rare and its causes are not known. We suggest that *C. pneumoniae* or some other microbe(s) capable of producing similar antibody reactions and living possibly within amoebae potentially cause these clusters."

- Changes in pro-inflammatory cytokines in association with exposure to moisture-damaged building microbes (*Eur Respir J* 2001 Dec[587]): "In the present study, the authors compared the respiratory symptoms, the production of inflammatory mediators interleukin (IL)-1, IL-4, IL-6, tumor necrosis factor-alpha (TNF-alpha) and cell count in nasal lavage fluid and induced sputum samples of subjects working in moisture-damaged and control school buildings. ... The authors found a significant elevation of IL-1, TNF-alpha and IL-6 in nasal lavage fluid and IL-6 in induced sputum during the spring term in the subjects from the moisture-damaged school building compared to the subjects from the control building. The exposed workers reported sore throat, phlegm, eye irritation, rhinitis, nasal obstruction and cough in parallel with these findings. The present data suggests an association between microbial exposure, and symptoms as well as changes in pro-inflammatory mediators detected from both the upper and lower airways."

- Building-associated neurological damage modeled in human cells (*Mycopathologia* 2010 Dec[588]): "Damage to human neurological system cells resulting from exposure to mycotoxins confirms a previously controversial public health threat for occupants of water-damaged buildings. ... Damage to the neurological system can result from exposure to trichothecene mycotoxins in the indoor environment. This study demonstrates that neurological system cell damage can occur from satratoxin H exposure to neurological cells at exposure levels that can be found in water-damaged buildings contaminated with fungal growth. The constant activation of inflammatory and apoptotic pathways at low levels of exposure in human brain capillary endothelial cells, astrocytes, and neural progenitor cells may amplify devastation to neurological tissues and lead to neurological system cell damage from indirect events triggered by the presence of trichothecenes."

- Co-cultivated damp building related microbes *Streptomyces californicus* and *Stachybotrys chartarum* induce immunotoxic and genotoxic responses via oxidative stress (*Inhal Toxicol* 2009 Aug[589]): "Oxidative stress has been proposed to be one mechanism behind the adverse health outcomes associated with living in a damp indoor environment. In the present study, the capability of damp building-related microbes *Streptomyces californicus* and *Stachybotrys chartarum* to induce oxidative stress was evaluated in vitro. In addition, the role of oxidative stress in provoking the detected cytotoxic, genotoxic, and inflammatory responses was studied by inhibiting the production of reactive oxygen species (ROS) using N-acetyl-l-cysteine (NAC). RAW264.7 macrophages were exposed in a dose- and time-dependent manner to the spores of co-cultivated *S. californicus* and *S. chartarum*, to their separately cultivated spore-mixture, or to the spores of these microbes alone. ... **All the studied microbial exposures triggered oxidative stress and subsequent cellular damage in RAW264.7 macrophages**. The ROS scavenger, NAC, prevented growth arrest, apoptosis, DNA damage, and cytokine production induced by the co-culture since it reduced the intracellular level of ROS within macrophages. In contrast, the DNA damage and cell cycle arrest induced by the spores of *S. californicus* alone could not be prevented by NAC. Bioaerosol-induced oxidative stress in macrophages may be an important mechanism behind the frequent respiratory symptoms and diseases suffered by residents of moisture damaged buildings. Furthermore, microbial

[587] Purokivi et al. Changes in pro-inflammatory cytokines in association with exposure to moisture-damaged building microbes. *Eur Respir J*. 2001 Dec;18(6):951-8
[588] Karunasena E, Larrañaga MD, Simoni JS, Douglas DR, Straus DC. Building-associated neurological damage modeled in human cells: a mechanism of neurotoxic effects by exposure to mycotoxins in the indoor environment. *Mycopathologia*. 2010 Dec;170(6):377-90
[589] Markkanen Penttinen P, Pelkonen J, Tapanainen M, Mäki-Paakkanen J, Jalava PI, Hirvonen MR. Co-cultivated damp building related microbes Streptomyces californicus and Stachybotrys chartarum induce immunotoxic and genotoxic responses via oxidative stress. *Inhal Toxicol*. 2009 Aug;21(10):857-67

interactions during co-cultivation stimulate the production of highly toxic compound(s) which may significantly increase oxidative damage."

- **Assessments**: Location-specific exacerbation of symptoms is an important historical indicator. Home, work, and recreational environments can be surveyed for microbial contamination, particularly mold. Pier-and-beam homes should be inspected for mold and water in the crawlspace; likewise, attics should be inspected for occult leaks and mold. Mold plates, Petri dishes, and filter cartridges can be used to identify airborne microbes. *Fusarium, Trichoderma,* and *Stachybotrys* produce mycotoxins.[590] Thorough cleaning/sanitization of wigs, shoes, furniture, whirlpool/pool water should be implemented; again, see the review by Noah.[591]

- **Specific treatment considerations**: Treatment has to be tailored to the specific nuances of the problems in the building/environment and the specific microbes involved. Walls, windows, utility closets, bathrooms, and under-sink cabinets should be assessed for mold and thoroughly cleaned. High-efficiency air filters can be used in the HVAC system; stand-alone air purifiers and dehumidifiers can be used. Bedding, sheets, blankets, pillows, carpets, furniture and drapes should be inspected for contamination and thoroughly cleaned. Eucalyptus oil can be added to washing detergent to kill dust mites[592], as described in the following section. Buildings may have to be professionally and thoroughly remediated; on occasion, people will need to change to different work areas (i.e., new office space, work from home, change jobs) or—if the home is affected—relocate to a new living space.

  - **Inflammatory mediators in nasal lavage, induced sputum and serum of employees with rheumatic and respiratory disorders** (*Eur Respir J* 2001 Sep[593]): "Exposure to microbes present in mold-damaged buildings has been linked to increased frequency of various inflammatory diseases. The current study examined differences in inflammatory mediators in nasal lavage (NAL), induced sputum (IS) and serum of occupants with rheumatic or respiratory disorders and their controls, all working in the same moisture-damaged building. ... Concentrations of NO, interleukin (IL)-1, IL-4, IL-6 and tumor necrosis factor-alpha in NAL, IS and serum (excluding NO and IL-1) of the subjects were measured during an occupational exposure period and the vacation period without such exposure. The concentrations of IL-4 in NAL fluid were significantly higher among all occupants during the working period (geometric mean 8.5 microg x mL(-1), range 0-206.5 microg x mL(-1)), as compared to that during vacation (0.4 microng x mL(-1) range 0-3.7 pg x mL(-1)) (p = 0.008). Absence from the work environment also significantly diminished reporting of symptoms. IL-4 levels in the serum of case subjects were significantly higher than in controls. Moreover, employees with respiratory symptoms had markedly higher exhaled NO values than their controls (p = 0.028). In summary, these data suggest that mediators in nasal lavage samples reflect the occupational exposure to molds, whereas possible indicators of existing disorders are detectable in serum."

  - **Joint symptoms and diseases associated with moisture damage in a health center** (*Clin Rheumatol* 2003 Dec[594]): "Rheumatic diseases do not usually cluster in time and space. It has been proposed that environmental exposures may initiate autoimmune responses. We describe a cluster of rheumatic diseases among a group of health center employees who began to complain of symptoms typically related to moldy houses, including mucocutaneous symptoms, nausea and fatigue, within a year of moving into a new building. Dampness was found in the insulation space of the concrete floor below ground level. Microbes indicating mold damage and actinobacteria were found in the flooring material and in the outer wall insulation. ... All 34 subjects working at the health center had at least some rheumatic complaints. Two fell ill with a typical rheumatoid factor (RF)-positive rheumatoid arthritis (RA), and 10 had arthritis that did not conform to any definite arthritic syndrome (three met the classification criteria for RA). Prior to moving into the problem building one subject had suffered reactive arthritis, which had then recurred. Another employee had undiagnosed ankylosing spondylitis and later developed psoriatic arthritis, and another developed undifferentiated vasculitis. A total of 16 subjects developed joint pains, 11 of these

[590] Am Acad Pediatrics.Toxic effects of indoor molds. Committee on Environ Health. *Pediatrics* 1998;101(4p1):712-4

[591] Noah PW. The role of microorganisms in psoriasis. *Semin Dermatol.* 1990 Dec;9(4):269-76

[592] Tovey et al. Simple washing procedure with eucalyptus oil for controlling house dust mites and allergens in clothing bedding. *J Allergy Clin Immunol* 1997;100:464-6

[593] Roponen et al. Inflammatory mediators in nasal lavage, induced sputum and serum of employees with rheumatic and respiratory disorders. *Eur Respir J* 2001;18:542-8

[594] Luosujärvi RA, et al. Joint symptoms and diseases associated with moisture damage in a health center. *Clin Rheumatol.* 2003 Dec;22(6):381-5

after beginning work at the health center. Three subjects developed Raynaud's symptom. Fourteen cases had elevated levels of circulating immune complexes in 1998, 17 in 1999, but there were only three cases in 2001, when the health center had been closed for 18 months. The high incidence of joint problems among these employees suggests a common triggering factor for most of the cases. As some of the symptoms had tended to subside while the health center was closed, the underlying causes are probably related to the building itself and possibly to the abnormal microbial growth in its structures."

- Sick building syndrome (SBS) and exposure to water-damaged buildings: time series study, clinical trial and mechanisms (*Neurotoxicol Teratol* 2006 Sep[595]): "Studies have demonstrated that the indoor air of water-damaged buildings (WDBs) often contains a complex mixture of fungi, mycotoxins, bacteria, endotoxins, antigens, lipopolysaccharides, and biologically produced volatile compounds. A case-series study with medical assessments at five time points was conducted to characterize the syndrome after a double-blinded, placebo-controlled clinical trial conducted among a group of study participants investigated the efficacy of cholestyramine (CSM) therapy. ... Data from Time Point 1 indicated a group-mean of 23 out of 37 symptoms evaluated; and visual contrast sensitivity (VCS), an indicator of neurological function, was abnormally low in all participants. Measurements of matrix metalloproteinase 9 (MMP9), leptin, alpha melanocyte stimulating hormone (MSH), vascular endothelial growth factor (VEGF), immunoglobulin E (IgE), and pulmonary function were abnormal in 22, 13, 25, 14, 1, and 7 participants, respectively. Following 2 weeks of CSM therapy to enhance toxin elimination rates, measurements at Time Point 2 indicated group-means of 4 symptoms with 65% improvement in VCS at mid-spatial frequency-both statistically significant improvements relative to Time Point 1. Moderate improvements were seen in MMP9, leptin, and VEGF serum levels. ... High levels of MMP9 indicated that exposure to the complex mixture of substances in the indoor air of the WDBs triggered a pro-inflammatory cytokine response. ... Because the only known benefit of CSM therapy is to enhance the elimination rates of substances that accumulate in bile by preventing re-absorption during enterohepatic re-circulation, results from the clinical trial also supported the general study hypothesis that SBS is associated with exposure to WDBs because the only relevant function of CSM is to bind and remove toxigenic compounds."

- Sick building syndrome: chronic, biotoxin-associated illness from exposure to water-damaged buildings (*Neurotoxicol Teratol* 2005 Jan[596]): Assessment = visual contrast sensitivity (VCS); treatment = cholestyramine (CSM); n = 19. "The results indicated that CSM was an effective therapeutic agent, that VCS was a sensitive and specific indicator of neurologic function, and that illness involved systemic and hypothalamic processes. Although the results supported the general hypothesis that illness was associated with exposure to the WDBs, this conclusion was tempered by several study limitations."

- Estuary-associated syndrome (*Environ Health Perspect*. 2001 Oct [597]): "Evidence suggests that the estuarine dinoflagellates, Pfiesteria piscicida Steidinger & Burkholder and P. shumwayae Glasgow & Burkholder, members of the toxic Pfiesteria complex (TPC), may release one or more toxins that kill fish and adversely affect human health. In the current study we investigated the potential for undiagnosed cases of possible estuary-associated syndrome (PEAS), as termed by the Centers for Disease Control and Prevention (CDC)... The VCS improved and symptoms abated after 2 weeks of treatment with cholestyramine. Cholestyramine, the original drug approved for treatment of hypercholesterolemia, has previously been reported to enhance the elimination rates of a variety of toxins, presumably by interruption of enterohepatic recirculation through toxin entrapment in its polymeric structure and/or anion-exchange process."

- Learning and memory difficulties after environmental exposure to waterways containing toxin-producing Pfiesteria or Pfiesteria-like dinoflagellates (*Lancet*. 1998 Aug[598]): "At the beginning of autumn,

---

[595] Shoemaker RC, House DE. Sick building syndrome (SBS) and exposure to water-damaged buildings: time series study, clinical trial and mechanisms. *Neurotoxicol Teratol*. 2006 Sep-Oct;28(5):573-88

[596] Shoemaker RC, House DE. A time-series study of sick building syndrome: chronic, biotoxin-associated illness from exposure to water-damaged buildings. *Neurotoxicol Teratol*. 2005 Jan-Feb;27(1):29-46

[597] Shoemaker RC. Residential and recreational acquisition of possible estuary-associated syndrome: a new approach to successful diagnosis and treatment. *Environ Health Perspect*. 2001 Oct;109 Suppl 5:791-6

[598] Grattan et al. Learning and memory difficulties after environmental exposure to waterways containing toxin-producing Pfiesteria or Pfiesteria-like dinoflagellates. *Lancet*. 1998 Aug 15;352(9127):532-9

1996, fish with "punched-out" skin lesions and erratic behaviour associated with exposure to toxins produced by Pfiesteria piscicida or Pfiesteria-like dinoflagellate species were seen in the Pocomoke River and adjacent waterways on the eastern shore of the Chesapeake Bay in Maryland, USA. In August, 1997, fish kills associated with Pfiesteria occurred in these same areas. People who had had contact with affected waterways reported symptoms, including memory difficulties, which raises questions about the human-health impact of environmental exposure to Pfiesteria toxins. ... People with environmental exposure to waterways in which Pfiesteria toxins are present are at risk of developing a reversible clinical syndrome characterised by difficulties with learning and higher cognitive functions. Risk of illness is directly related to degree of exposure, with the most prominent symptoms and signs occurring among people with chronic daily exposure to affected waterways."

Cleaning the home/work/recreational environment of microbial contaminants—summary of interventional strategies with some specificity for helping alleviate asthma and atopic dermatitis

Household "dust" is actually a complex mixture of microscopic particles such as fabric fragments (from bedding, carpet, clothing, etc.), pollen (from outdoor plants), dirt (which has settled from the air), dead skin cells (from humans and pets), bacteria and mold, and the feces of dust mites and other insects. Since dust, especially the feces from dust mites, is very allergenic, particularly for patients with eczema. Reducing the amount of "dust" in a home environment involves 3 general steps:

1. **Dust, mold, and chemical removal**
   - Cleaning: Periodically, use a damp cloth on furniture to remove dust that accumulates.
   - Vacuuming: Vacuum the floors/carpet and ensure that the vacuum is equipped with an *allergy filter* or HEPA filter to ensure that the dust is not simply transposed from the floor back into the air and onto furniture, bedding, and clothes. In severe cases, patients with inflammatory disorders, allergies/eczema, and environmental sensitivity may choose to have carpets removed and replaced either with a low-offgassing/outgassing flooring such as bamboo hardwoods or ceramic tile.
   - Exclude pollen/mold: Close doors and windows on days the pollen/mold count is high.
   - Pet control: If you have pets, it is often helpful to 1) wash them regularly, 2) keep them off the bedding, and/or 3) allow them to stay outdoors as much as is possible and practical.
   - Using air filters for the central cooling/heating unit: Consider the "Filterete Allergen Reducing Filter" from 3M (comes with a purple label); more expensive and effective options are available for complicated cases.
   - Vinyl/hypoallergenic mattress cover: Buy and use a simple hypoallergenic or vinyl mattress cover to eliminate exposure to years of accumulated dust inside the mattress which is slept on for 8 hours each night. The goal is create an airtight seal around the mattress to contain the dust and antigens. Vinyl mattress covers are inexpensive and widely available.
2. **Reducing the amount of moisture in the air**. Ideally, the steam from bathing and cooking areas should be vented outdoors so that moisture does not accumulate inside the living area. Moisture is necessary for dust mites and mold to live and to create allergens; if the air is very moist then the inflammation-producing activities of the dust mites and mold are stimulated. Conversely, by reducing the humidity in the air, we are able to impair the microbes and thus reduce the amount of antigens. Reducing the amount of moisture in the air by use of an electric dehumidifier may be necessary to help reduce the amount of both dust allergen and mold in a home.
3. **Wash clothes/linens with eucalyptus oil to eliminate dust mites:** The combination of 1) hot water, 2) detergent, and 3) eucalyptus oil is an effective and natural way to get rid of dust mites and dust allergens. As validated by research published in *Journal of Allergy and Clinical Immunology*[599], this is an effective technique for killing and eliminating dust mites from clothing and bed sheets. "Bi-O-Klean Hand Dishwashing Liquid" available at Whole Foods Market or "Kit liquid dishwashing detergent concentrate" meet the criteria for the selection of a detergent for this purpose. Eucalyptus oil must never be applied to the skin or taken internally.

Metric measurements from the original study	"American" unit translation	One-half recipe
1. **Eucalyptus oil**: 100 mL	6 tablespoons or 3.4 oz.	3 tablespoons or 1½ oz.
2. **Detergent**: 25 mL liquid concentrated dishwashing detergent	1 ½ tablespoons or 0.8 oz.	¾ tablespoons or 0.4 oz.
3. **Warm water** (30°C): 50 Liters	86°F water: 13 gallons	86°F water: 6 gallons
4. **Soak clothing/bedding in hot detergent-eucalyptus solution for 15-30 minutes, then wash in machine as usual.**		

---

[599] 1) When mixed, the oil-detergent mixture should dissolve to form a clear homogenous solution, and 2) five mL (1 teaspoon) of the mixture stirred with 200 mL (6 oz.) of water should form a "milky, opaque solution that is stable (does not "break oil") for at least 10 minutes." Tovey ER, McDonald LG. A simple washing procedure with eucalyptus oil for controlling house dust mites and their allergens in clothing and bedding. *J Allergy Clin Immunol*. 1997 Oct;100(4):464-6

Dysbiosis—definition:

Dysbiosis subtypes (based on location)—name each location following each of the prompts:
1. SR:
2. OD:
3. GI:
4. GU:
5. Derm:
6. Tissue:
7. Environment:

Multifocal dysbiosis—definition:

Polydysbiosis—definition:

Combinatorial dysbiosis—definition:

Microbial molecules, mechanisms, morphology—describe mechanisms/consequences of each:
1. Gram-negative bacterial products, LPS:

2. Gram-positive bacterial products:

3. L-form, pleomorphic, "cell wall-deficient" bacteria:

4. Immunostimulation by bacterial DNA, viral DNA and bacteriophage DNA:

5. Superantigens:

6. Antimetabolites:
   a) D-lactate:
   b) H2S:
   c) Propionic acid:
   d) Ammonia:
   e) P-cresol:
   f) HPHPA:

7. Beneficial metabolites and molecular signatures—name at least one:

Pathophysiologic responses—describe mechanisms/consequences of each:

1. Damage to the intestinal mucosa—what is the cause, and what is the effect?
   What is zonulin, and what two specific items trigger its release?

2. Activation of inflammatory pathways—define each and name one agonist:
   a) Toll-like receptors (TLR):
   b) NFkB:
   c) DAMP:
   d) PAMP:
   e) Inflammasome:

3. Mitochondrial hyperpolarization—name 1 cause and 1 consequence:

   mTOR activation—name 1 cause and 1 consequence:

4. Molecular mimicry, cross-reactivity—give 2 examples of diseases with the associated microbes/molecules:

5. Enhanced presentation of autoantigens—name 1 trigger:

6. Bystander activation—name 1 trigger:

7. Haptenization and the formation of neoautoantigens—name the classic disease association:

8. Immune complex formation and deposition—name 3 conditions:

9. Microbial allergy, hypersensitivity—name 3 conditions:

10. Insufficiency dysbiosis—name 3 consequences:

11. Inhibition of detoxification—name one cause beyond genetics/SNP and medications:

12. Vitamin D metabolism and reception—name the two human antimicrobial peptides:

13. Bacterial and fungal proteases impair immune defenses—what is the consequence of IgA protease?

14. Immunosuppression, gliotoxins—name one microbe that produces local immunosuppression:

15. Mold toxins—mycotoxins—name two treatments for environmental toxin exposure:

16. Biofilms—how are dental biofilms removed?

17. What causes impairment of mucosal digestion? Name 2 causes and 1 consequence:

18. What is central sensitization? Name 2 causes and 1 consquence of glial activation:

19. Dysbiosis-induced endocrine dysfunction—which 3 hormones are elevated? Which 3 are suppressed?

20. Microbe-induced epigenetic changes—what are "HERVs"?

Prototypic clinical manifestations:

1. Autointoxication, auto-brewery syndrome, encephalopathy:

    a) Evaluations:

    b) Treatments:

2. Syndromes of pain, fatigue, depression (e.g., fibromyalgia) caused by dysbiosis:

    a) Evaluations:

    b) Treatments:

    c) Name one microbial molecule that can cause mitochondrial dysfunction and glial activation:

3. Dysbiotic arthropathy, dermatitis, vasculitis

    a) Evaluations:

    b) Treatments:

    c) What are immune complexes, and what are the clinical consequences?

4. Reactive arthritis

    a) Evaluations:

    b) Treatments:

    c) Name two microbes that share amino acid homology with HLA-B27:

Problematic Bacteria, Yeast, and Parasites: A Listing of Commonly Encountered Dysbiotic Microorganisms

All of the following yeast, bacteria, and "parasites" have been observed in various patients in my private practice of chiropractic and naturopathic medicine. Even though several of these microbes are considered nonpathogenic by outdated medical paradigms[600,601,602] that are still hypnotized by Pasteur and Koch (i.e., the "external invader paradigm"), their presence is generally inconsistent with optimal health and their eradication is rewarding for both doctor and patient. In other words, **even if a microbe is not a true pathogen and is thus not a therapeutic target from a *disease-oriented paradigm*, we as clinicians are still justified in eradicating it from our chronically ill patient from a *wellness-oriented paradigm* because we know that 1) eradicating potentially harmful bacteria will do no harm to the patient, and 2) in many cases—indeed *the majority* of cases—patients experience a significant and sustained clinical improvement regardless of their presenting complaint, thus implying a causal relationship between the microbe and the non-infectious illness.**

The following microbes are commonly detected with stool testing performed by a specialty laboratory. **One of the benefits of specialized stool testing is that it allows the presence of microbes to be determined within a context that evaluates the patient's individualized response.** For example, the finding of a mild degree of *Candida albicans* ("+1" on a 0-4 scale) might be considered insignificant; however if no other pathogens are identified, and the secretory IgA, lactoferrin, and lysozyme levels are elevated, then the clinician is justified in determining that the patient is having a hypersensitivity reaction to an otherwise "benign" yeast. **Remember, we are not looking for classic "infection" here; we are looking to determine which underlying disruptions may be exacerbating inflammation and the patient's symptomatology.** We have to look beyond the *disease-associated characteristics of the microbe* to see *the patient's individualized response to the microbe*. **Often what we find when working with autoimmune/inflammatory patients is that they are having a *pathogenic inflammatory response* to a *nonpathogenic* microbe.** When reading the following table, rather than focusing on the details, readers should read the information with due diligence with the final goal being not the memorization of microbe-disease associations but rather the concept that microbial colonization is a sufficient trigger for induction of inflammation and the clinical appearance of many "autoimmune disorders." The distinguishing characteristic that differentiates "an idiopathic autoimmune disease" from "microbe-triggered reactive arthritis" is not the biochemistry of the inflammatory cascade nor the pathohistologic findings; but rather, the defining characteristic of reactive arthritis is the presence of an identified microbial exposure. Therefore, the practical distinction is made by the clinician—not the disease entity itself. If the physician searches for and empirically treats the microbial triggers for most "idiopathic inflammatory disorders" and "autoimmune diseases", then that clinician will—in the words of Henry David Thoreau in *Walden*—"meet with a success unexpected in common hours."

Commonly Encountered Dysbiotic Microorganisms—*alphabetized listing*

Dysbiotic microbe	Pathophysiology and clinical manifestations
Aeromonas hydrophila	• *Aeromonas hydrophila* can cause colitis and should therefore be eradicated immediately upon detection.[603]
Blastocystis hominis	• Commonly asymptomatic; can cause abdominal pain, nausea, vomiting, diarrhea, weight loss[604,605], fever, chills, malaise, anorexia, flatus, eosinophilia[606] • Fecal leukocytes are occasionally seen[607]; can cause colitis[608]

600 "...standard of care in developed countries is to maintain schizophrenia patients on neuroleptics, this practice is not supported by the 50-year research record for the drugs. ...this paradigm of care worsens long-term outcomes, ... 40% of all schizophrenia patients would fare better if they were not so medicated." Whitaker R. The case against antipsychotic drugs: a 50-year record of doing more harm than good. *Med Hypotheses*. 2004;62:5-1 psychrights.org/Research/Digest/Chronicity/50yearecord.pdf
601 Hyman M. Paradigm shift: the end of "normal science" in medicine understanding function in nutrition, health, and disease. *Altern Ther Health Med*. 2004;10:10-5,90-4
602 Heaney RP. Vitamin D, nutritional deficiency, and the medical paradigm. *J Clin Endocrinol Metab* 2003;88:5107-8 jcem.endojournals.org/cgi/content/full/88/11/5107
603 Farraye FA, Peppercorn MA, Ciano PS, Kavesh WN. Charles A. Segmental colitis associated with Aeromonas hydrophila. *Am J Gastroenterol*. 1989 Apr;84(4):436-8
604 O'Gorman MA, et al. Prevalence and characteristics of Blastocystis hominis infection in children. *Clin Pediatr* (Phila) 1993 Feb;32(2):91-6
605 Telalbasic S, Pikula ZP, Kapidzic M. Blastocystis hominis may be a potential cause of intestinal disease. *Scand J Infect Dis* 1991;23(3):389-90
606 Sheehan DJ, Raucher BG, McKitrick JC. Association of Blastocystis hominis with signs and symptoms of human disease. *J Clin Microbiol*. 1986;24(4):548-50
607 Diaczok BJ, Rival J. Diarrhea due to Blastocystis hominis: an old organism revisited. *South Med J* 1987 Jul;80(7):931-2
608 Russo AR, Stone SL, Taplin ME, Snapper HJ, Doern GV. Presumptive evidence for Blastocystis hominis as a cause of colitis. *Arch Intern Med*. 1988 May;148(5):1064

Microbe	Pathophysiology and clinical manifestations
Candida albicans and other yeasts	• Although normal in small amounts ("+1"), excess *Candida* in the intestines is never a sign of optimal health. Patients may have mild general symptoms such as fatigue and dyscognition ("brain fog"); gas and intestinal bloating following consumption of carbohydrates are common. • *Candida* produces an immunosuppressive myotoxin called gliotoxin as well as an IgA-destroying protease and can cause watery diarrhea, particularly in elderly, ill, and immunosuppressed patients.[609] • *Candida* is always present in the gastrointestinal tract of women with recurrent yeast vaginitis.[610] • Some people have an inflammatory hypersensitivity to *Candida,* as it can cause **local allergic dermatitis/mucositis**[611], **colitis**[612], and **pulmonary inflammation** (**hypersensitivity alveolitis** from gastrointestinal colonization).[613] • Other yeasts such as *Candida parapsilosis* and *Geotrichum capitatum* are occasionally seen and should be eradicated.
Citrobacter rodentium *Citrobacter freundii*	• *Citrobacter freundii* is a gram-negative anaerobe; it produces pro-inflammatory endotoxin. • *Citrobacter* species may cause **gastroenteritis** in humans[614] • Most strains of *Citrobacter freundii* produce hydrogen sulfide[615] which interferes with mitochondrial function and energy production and may be a major causative molecule in **ulcerative colitis**.[616] • Animal studies have shown that this bacterium can induce an intense inflammatory response in the gastrointestinal tract that resembles **inflammatory bowel disease**.[617] • Gastrointestinal dysbiosis with *Citrobacter freundii* may be causative in so-called "rheumatoid arthritis" in some patients.[author's experience]
Dientamoeba fragilis	• *Dientamoeba fragilis* is a flagellate protozoan that can cause **diarrhea, abdominal pain, nausea, vomiting, fatigue, malaise, eosinophilia, urticaria, pruritus and/or weight loss**. It is commonly associated with pinworm infection and may produce a clinical picture that mimics **food allergy, colitis, or eosinophilic enteritis**.[618]

[609] Gupta TP, Ehrinpreis MN. Candida-associated diarrhea in hospitalized patients. *Gastroenterology* 1990 Mar;98(3):780-5

[610] Miles MR, Olsen L, Rogers A. Recurrent vaginal candidiasis. Importance of an intestinal reservoir. *JAMA*. 1977 Oct 24;238(17):1836-7

[611] Ramirez De Knott HM, McCormick TS, et al. Cutaneous hypersensitivity to Candida albicans in idiopathic vulvodynia. *Contact Dermatitis*. 2005 Oct;53(4):214-8

[612] Doby T. Monilial esophagitis and colitis. *J Maine Med Assoc*. 1971 May;62(5):109-14

[613] "We conclude that the disease was induced by C.a.-antigen reaching the lungs from the intestinal tract via the bloodstream." Schreiber J, Struben C, Rosahl W, Amthor M. Hypersensitivity alveolitis induced by endogenous candida species. *Eur J Med Res*. 2000 Mar 27;5(3):126 Stunningly brilliant article.

[614] "Members of this genus can cause neonatal meningitis and, perhaps, gastroenteritis in both children and adults." Lipsky BA, Hook EW 3rd, Smith AA, Plorde JJ. Citrobacter infections in humans: experience at the Seattle Veterans Administration Medical Center and a review of the literature. *Rev Infect Dis*. 1980 Sep-Oct;2:746-60

[615] Lennette EH (editor in chief). *Manual of Clinical Microbiology. Fourth Edition*. Washington DC; American Society for Microbiology: 1985, page 269. See also web.indstate.edu/thcme/micro/GI/general/sld038.htm Accessed 10/27/2005

[616] "CONCLUSIONS: Metabolic effects of sodium hydrogen sulfide on butyrate oxidation along the length of the colon closely mirror metabolic abnormalities observed in active ulcerative colitis, and the increased production of sulfide in ulcerative colitis suggests that the action of mercaptides may be involved in the genesis of ulcerative colitis." Roediger et al. Reducing sulfur compounds of the colon impair colonocyte nutrition: implications for ulcerative colitis. *Gastroenterology*. 1993 Mar;104(3):802-9

[617] Higgins LM, Frankel G, Douce G, Dougan G, MacDonald TT. Citrobacter rodentium infection in mice elicits a mucosal Th1 cytokine response and lesions similar to those in murine inflammatory bowel disease. *Infect Immun*. 1999 Jun;67(6):3031-9 iai.asm.org/cgi/reprint/67/6/3031.pdf

[618] Cuffari C, Oligny L, Seidman EG. Dientamoeba fragilis masquerading as allergic colitis. *J Pediatr Gastroenterol Nutr*. 1998 Jan;26(1):16-20

Commonly Encountered Dysbiotic Microorganisms—*alphabetized listing,* *continued*

Microbe	Pathophysiology and clinical manifestations
Endolimax nana	• *Endolimax nana*, a protozoa, has a world-wide distribution and is commonly considered an harmless commensal of the intestine.[619] • Intestinal infection with *Endolimax nana* can cause a **peripheral arthropathy** that is clinically similar to **rheumatoid arthritis** and which remits with effective parasite eradication.[620] • In my own clinical practice, I have seen several cases of intestinal colonization with *Endolimax nana* in patients who presented with **chronic fatigue, myalgia, eczema**, and especially refractory **chronic vaginitis.**
Entamoeba histolytica	• Induces tissue damage, **amebic colitis**, and **liver abscess.**[621] • Associated with **Henoch Schonlein purpura** in a single case report[622] • **Amebic colitis** may be misdiagnosed as **ulcerative colitis.**[623] • May contribute to **irritable bowel syndrome, rheumatoid arthritis, fibromyalgia, food allergy,** or **multiple chemical sensitivity** and can **exacerbate HIV infection.**[624] • Hepatic infection is associated with induction of antineutrophil cytoplasmic antibodies (ANCA) such as seen with ANCA-associated vasculitis.[625]
Gamma *strep* **Enterococcus**	• "Gamma strep", *Enterococcus faecalis*, and *Streptococcus faecalis* are somewhat interchangeable terms.[626,627,628] These terms refer to gram-positive *Enterococcus* species such as *Enterococcus faecalis*, which cause **urinary tract infections, bacteremia, intra-abdominal infections, and endocarditis.** • Enterococci produce **lipoteichoic acid** which is proinflammatory in a manner similar to endotoxin from gram-negative bacteria, and these gram-positive bacteria also appear to produce a superantigen.[629] • "Gamma strep" is commonly identified in stool tests of patients with **chronic unwellness and fatigue.**
Giardia lamblia **"Beaver fever"**	• Causatively associated with **abdominal pain, diarrhea, constipation, bloating, chronic fatigue, and food allergy/intolerance.**[630] • May contribute to **irritable bowel syndrome, rheumatoid arthritis, food allergy, or multiple chemical sensitivity.**[631] • Extraintestinal symptoms of gastrointestinal *Giardia* infection can include **fever, maculopapular rashes, geographic tongue, pulmonary infiltrates, lymphadenopathy, polyarthritis, aphthous ulcers, and urticaria.**[632]

[619] Information available at www2.provlab.ab.ca/bugs/webbug/parasite/artifact/enana.htm as of December 26, 2003

[620] "Endolimax nana grew on stool culture. Both the patient's diarrhea and arthritis responded effectively to therapy with metronidazole. The diagnosis of parasitic rheumatism was made in retrospect." Burnstein SL, Liakos S. Parasitic rheumatism presenting as rheumatoid arthritis. *J Rheumatol.* 1983 Jun;10(3):514-5

[621] Huston CD. Parasite and host contributions to the pathogenesis of amebic colitis. *Trends Parasitol.* 2004 Jan; 20(1): 23-6

[622] Demircin G, Oner A, Erdogan O, Bulbul M, Memis L. Henoch Schonlein purpura and amebiasis. *Acta Paediatr Jpn.* 1998 Oct; 40(5): 489-91

[623] Galland L. Intestinal protozoan infection is a common unsuspected cause of chronic illness. *J Advancement Med.* 1989;2: 539-552

[624] Galland L. Intestinal protozoan infection is a common unsuspected cause of chronic illness. *J Advancement Med.* 1989;2: 539-552

[625] George J, et al. Infections and Wegener's granulomatosis--a cause and effect relationship? *QJM.* 1997 May;90(5):367-73 qjmed.oxfordjournals.org/cgi/reprint/90/5/367

[626] "Figure 38: "Gamma *Streptococcus*" : *Enterococcus faecalis*" and "The genus *Enterococcus* was once a part of the *Streptococcus* genus, was considered a "gamma *Streptococcus* species." microbelibrary.org/asmonly/details_print.asp?id=1986&lang

[627] "Enterococcus faecalis. Synonyms: group D strep, Streptococcus faecalis. Classification: facultative anaerobic, gram+ bacteria, cocci." medinfo.ufl.edu/year2/mmid/bms5300/bugs/strfaeca.html

[628] "Microscopically, Gram-positive cocci occurring in chains or pairs with individual cells being somewhat elongated can be presumed to be streptococci or enterococci." members.tripod.com/piece_de_resistance/SAARS/bugs/menteroc.htm

[629] Lynn E. Hancock and Michael S. Gilmore. Department of Microbiology and Immunology, University of Oklahoma Health Sciences Center. Pathogenicity of Enterococci published in "Gram-Positive Pathogens" edited by Fischetti V et al. w3.ouhsc.edu/enterococcus/lynn_revirew.asp

[630] Galland L, Lee M. #170 High frequency of giardiasis in patients with chronic digestive complaints. *Am J Gastroenterol* 1989;84:1181

[631] Galland L. Intestinal protozoan infection is a common unsuspected cause of chronic illness. *J Advancement Med.* 1989;2: 539-552

[632] Corsi A, et al. Ocular changes associated with Giardia lamblia infection in children. *Br J Ophthalmol.* 1998 Jan;82:59-62 bjo.bmjjournals.com/cgi/content/full/82/1/59

Microbe	Pathophysiology and clinical manifestations
Giardia lamblia [continued from previous page]	• **Ocular complications** from gastrointestinal infection include iridocyclitis, choroiditis, retinal hemorrhages, anterior and posterior uveitis, retinal vasculitis, and "salt and pepper" retinal degeneration. These complications are most likely due to deposition of **immune complexes** in the retinal epithelium.[633] • Reported to have caused numerous cases of **reactive arthritis (peripheral arthritis and/or sacroiliitis)** in patients who are either positive or negative for HLA-B27[634]; "beaver fever" is a cause of reactive arthritis.[635] • Antigen detection appears superior to microscopic examination for detection.[636]
Hafnia alvei	• *Hafnia alvei* is a gram-negative bacterium capable of causing **reactive arthritis** from gastrointestinal infection; the reactive arthritis associated with *Hafnia alvei* occurs without association with HLA-B27.[637]
Helicobacter pylori	• *H. pylori* is a gram-negative endotoxin-producing rod that causes stomach ulcers and appears to cause **reactive arthritis** in some patients.[638] • *H. pylori* colonization is increased in patients with **scleroderma.**[639] • *H. pylori* is commonly found in the middle ear of patients with acute otitis media.[640] • Strongly and causatively associated with Raynaud's syndrome/phenomenon.
Klebsiella pneumoniae	• Many cases of gastrointestinal colonization with this microorganism produce no acute gastrointestinal symptoms such as nausea, vomiting, constipation, or diarrhea. Patients may have mild general symptoms such as fatigue and dyscognition ("brain fog"). • Can cause **diarrhea**[641] and **acute gastroenteritis.**[642] • Associated with **reactive arthritis** such as **ankylosing spondylitis.**[643] • Gram-negative bacteria, produces endotoxin/lipopolysaccharide that is capable of impairing cytochrome p-450 and **reducing hepatic clearance and urinary/biliary excretion of drugs.**[644]

[633] "The retinal changes associated with giardiasis are more than likely caused by immune mechanisms. Wania reported that circulating immune complexes were found in all of the patients with ocular complications he examined." Corsi A, Nucci C, Knafelz D, Bulgarini D, Di Iorio L, Polito A, De Risi F, Ardenti Morini F, Paone FM. Ocular changes associated with Giardia lamblia infection in children. *Br J Ophthalmol*. 1998 Jan;82(1):59-62 bjo.bmjjournals.com/cgi/content/full/82/1/59

[634] Layton et al. Sacroiliitis in an HLA B27-negative patient following giardiasis. *Br J Rheumatol*. 1998;37:581-3 rheumatology.oxfordjournals.org/cgi/reprint/37/5/581

[635] "Giardia lamblia infection is rarely associated with adult reactive arthritis. We report first North American case and review pediatric and adult literature. Antimicrobial treatment is essential to eradicate the parasite and control the arthritis." Tupchong et al. Beaver fever—a rare cause of reactive arthritis. *J Rheumatol* 1999;26:2701-2

[636] "For all patients, microscopy was uniformly negative, but 6 of 13 patients were antigen positive... Giardiasis, an increasing problem in family practice, should be considered early in patients with GI disturbances. New, sensitive immunodiagnostic tests that usually require a single specimen are more useful than microscopy." Chappell CL, Matson CC. Giardia antigen detection in patients with chronic gastrointestinal disturbances. *J Fam Pract*. 1992 Jul;35(1):49-53

[637] Toivanen P, Toivanen A. Two forms of reactive arthritis? *Ann Rheum Dis*. 1999 Dec;58(12):737-41 ard.bmjjournals.com/cgi/content/full/58/12/737 See also: Newmark JJ, Hobbs WN, Wilson BE. Reactive arthritis associated with Hafnia alvei enteritis. *Arthritis Rheum*. 1994 Jun;37(6):960

[638] "Our findings suggest that HP may be included in the list of possible arthritis triggering microbes." Melby KK, Kvien TK, Glennas A. Helicobacter pylori—a trigger of reactive arthritis? *Infection*. 1999;27(4-5):252-5

[639] "Patients with SSc have H. pylori infection at a higher prevalence than the general population." Yazawa N, Fujimoto M, Kikuchi K, et al. High seroprevalence of Helicobacter pylori infection in patients with systemic sclerosis: association with esophageal involvement. *J Rheumatol*. 1998 Apr;25(4):650-3

[640] "Twelve of 15 smears for MEE were positive for HP by immunohistochemistry and 14 by Giemsa that were Gram-negative." Morinaka S, Tominaga M, Nakamura H. Detection of Helicobacter pylori in the middle ear fluid of patients with otitis media with effusion. *Otolaryngol Head Neck Surg*. 2005 Nov;133(5):791-4

[641] Niyogi SK, Pal A, Mitra U, Dutta P. Enteroaggregative Klebsiella pneumoniae in association with childhood diarrhoea. *Indian J Med Res* 2000 Oct;112:133-4

[642] Ananthan et al. Enterotoxigenicity of Klebsiella pneumoniae associated with childhood gastroenteritis in Madras, India. *Jpn J Infect Dis* 1999 Feb;52(1):16-7

[643] Ahmadi et al. Antibodies to Klebsiella pneumoniae lipopolysaccharide in patients with ankylosing spondylitis. *Br J Rheumatol*. 1998 Dec;37(12):1330-3

[644] Hasegawa T, Takagi K, Kitaichi K. Effects of bacterial endotoxin on drug pharmacokinetics. *Nagoya J Med Sci* 1999 May;62(1-2):11-28

Commonly encountered dysbiotic microorganisms—*alphabetized listing, continued*

Microbe	Pathophysiology and clinical manifestations
Proteus mirabilis	• Gram-negative bacteria, produces endotoxin/lipopolysaccharide.[645] • Gastrointestinal and urinary tract colonization is associated with **rheumatoid arthritis**[646,647] and **ankylosing spondylitis**.[648] • In one of my patients, GI dysbiosis with *Proteus* incited "**idiopathic inflammatory polyneuropathy**" that disappeared within one month of parasite eradication and which coincided with normalization of hsCRP.
Pseudomonas aeruginosa	• *Pseudomonas aeruginosa* is a gram-negative bacterium, produces endotoxin[649] and can cause antibiotic-associated diarrhea.[650,651] • Many cases of gastrointestinal colonization with this microorganism produce no acute gastrointestinal symptoms such as nausea, vomiting, constipation, or diarrhea. Patients may have mild general symptoms such as fatigue and dyscognition ("brain fog"). • Patients with **multiple sclerosis** show evidence of a heightened immune response against *Pseudomonas aeruginosa*, consistent with cross-reactivity.[652]

Comprehensive Stool Analysis / Parasitology x3

MICROBIOLOGY

Bacteriology Culture

Beneficial flora		Imbalances		Dysbiotic flora	
Bifidobacter	4+	Haemolytic E. coli	4+	Pseudomonas sp.	4+
E. coli	4+	Gamma strep	2+		
Lactobacillus	2+				

Mycology (Yeast) Culture

Normal flora		Dysbiotic flora
Candida glabrata	1+	
Rhodotorula sp.	1+	

Stool culture results showing overgrowth of *Pseudomonas* in a patient with sensorimotor peripheral neuropathy—immunorestoration, immunomodulation, and antimicrobial therapy resulted in sustained remission of fatigue, periodic fever, and neuropathy: *Psuedomonas aeruginosa* shows cross-reactivity with human neuronal tissues.[653,654] Note also the abnormal yeast, consistent with GI immunosuppression.

---

[645] Kondakova et al. Structural and serological studies of the O-antigen of Proteus mirabilis O-9. *Carbohydr Res* 2003 May 23;338(11):1191-6

[646] Ebringer A, Rashid T, Wilson C. Rheumatoid arthritis: proposal for the use of anti-microbial therapy in early cases. *Scand J Rheumatol* 2003;32(1):2-11

[647] Rashid T, et al. Proteus IgG antibodies and C-reactive protein in English, Norwegian and Spanish patients with rheumatoid arthritis. *Clin Rheumatol* 1999;18(3):190-5

[648] Wilson C, Rashid T, Tiwana H, et al. Cytotoxicity responses to Peptide antigens in rheumatoid arthritis and ankylosing spondylitis. *J Rheumatol* 2003 May;30(5):972-8

[649] Bergan T. Pathogenetic factors of Pseudomonas aeruginosa. *Scand J Infect Dis Suppl.* 1981;29:7-12

[650] Kim et al. Pseudomonas aeruginosa as a potential cause of antibiotic-associated diarrhea. *J Korean Med Sci.* 2001 Dec;16(6):742-4

[651] Porco et al. Pseudomonas aeruginosa as a cause of infectious diarrhea successfully treated with oral ciprofloxacin. *Ann Pharmacother.* 1995 Nov;29(11):1122-3

[652] Hughes LE, Bonell S, Natt RS, et al. Antibody responses to Acinetobacter spp. and Pseudomonas aeruginosa in multiple sclerosis: prospects for diagnosis using the myelin-acinetobacter-neurofilament antibody index. *Clin Diagn Lab Immunol.* 2001 Nov;8(6):1181-8

[653] Hughes LE, Bonell S, Natt RS, et al. Antibody responses to Acinetobacter spp. and Pseudomonas aeruginosa in multiple sclerosis: prospects for diagnosis using the myelin-acinetobacter-neurofilament antibody index. *Clin Diagn Lab Immunol.* 2001 Nov;8(6):1181-8 cvi.asm.org/content/8/6/1181.full.pdf

[654] Hughes LE, Smith PA, Bonell S, Natt RS, Wilson C, Rashid T, Amor S, Thompson EJ, Croker J, Ebringer A. Cross-reactivity between related sequences found in Acinetobacter sp., Pseudomonas aeruginosa, myelin basic protein and myelin oligodendrocyte glycoprotein in multiple sclerosis. *J Neuroimmunol.* 2003 Nov;144:105-15

Microbe	Pathophysiology and clinical manifestations
Segmented filamentous bacteria (SFB)	• **Segmented filamentous bacteria (SFB) are *uncluturable* Gram-positive** spore-forming rods most closely related to the genus Clostridium; within a short period of time, SFB rapidly took the spotlight of microbial fame when several articles were published showing the ability of SFB to induce highly pathogenic Th17 cells[655,656], known for their involvement in diabetes mellitus and especially their prime role in **autoimmune diseases such as rheumatoid arthritis, multiple sclerosis, and psoriasis.** SFB are present in the human gastrointestinal tract per research by Caselli et al[657] who documented SFB-like organisms in histological slides of ileo-cecal valves in patients with ulcerative colitis; in their small study of 18 patients, they noted " SFB-like organisms are more often seen and in much greater density in patients with UC than in control cases without bowel inflammation, while they are never found in CD patients. … As both **antibiotics and probiotics have previously proved to be active against SFB in mice**, we suggest that therapeutic manipulation of SFB might be tried in UC patients." Also in 2013, Jonsson[658] reported the "presence of a human variant of SFB" by analyzing ileostomy samples from 10 human subjects (4 samples each) who had been protocolectomized for UC; only 2 of 40 samples contained SFB, and both were from the same person during consumption of a high-fiber diet. Jonsson's SFB variants lead him to suggest "more than one type of SFB could be present in humans." • Orally administered vancomycin is one of the only and quite likely the best of anti-SFB antimicrobial agents suitable for human clinical outpatient use; in my recent clinical experience with this agent, I have found that low-modest doses —even as low as 125 mg/d for months at a time— promote notable benefit (e.g., major clinical improvement and reduction in serum CCP) with no detectable adverse effect. Empiric use (i.e., without laboratory identification of SFB in particular or a targeted bacterium in general) of oral vancomycin has shown noteworthy benefit in autism[659] and primary sclerosing cholangitis (PSC)[660]—in PSC, highly noteworthy and consistent with my own clinical experience is the fact that lower-dose oral vancomycin appears to be safer and more clinically effective than a higher dose. Oral vancomycin generally has zero-low intestinal absorption and systemic bioavailability.[661] However, several case reports of adverse effects (including allergy/hypersensitivity, anaphylaxis, red man syndrome) following oral vancomycin make clear the fact that some patients absorb an amount worthy of clinical consideration; absorption is increased in patients with bowel inflammation, and clearance is reduced (thus serum levels and risk for adverse effects are higher) in patients with renal insufficiency.[662] Quite obviously, any plan to change gastrointestinal microbial flora must also ❶ aim for the eradication of multiple disease-inducing agents (i.e., rarely only one microbial offender is responsible; often multiple antimicrobial agents will have to be used), ❷ unfailingly include and emphasize a plant-based gluten-free diet (which generally does not have to be and in many cases should not be vegan or completely vegetarian), ❸ generally include probiotic therapy via direct supplementation, and ❹ generally be implemented for many months (some clinical cases will respond brilliantly to only a few days or weeks of treatment, while all cases will require long-term preservation of eubiosis for maintenance of optimal immunoinflammatory outcomes). Since berberine is also effective against Gram-positive microbes, one might consider using berberine additionally or alternatively against SFB despite the lack of supporting evidence from a microbiologic standpoint; the clinical efficacy and safety of berberine (500 mg BID-TID for 3 months) is well documented in recent clinical trials in patients with dyslipidemia and diabetes mellitus type-2.

[655] Ivanov II, Littman DR. Segmented filamentous bacteria take the stage. *Mucosal Immunol.* 2010 May;3(3):209-12

[656] Ivanov II, Atarashi K, Manel N et al. Induction of intestinal Th17 cells by segmented filamentous bacteria. *Cell.* 2009 Oct 30;139(3):485-98

[657] Caselli et al. Segmented filamentous bacteria-like organisms in histological slides of ileo-cecal valves in patients with UC. *Am J Gastroenterol.* 2013 May;108(5):860-1

[658] "In this study, ileostomy samples from 10 human subjects were screened with PCR, using primers derived from sequences of SFB from rat and mouse. PCR products were obtained from samples taken from one individual at two time points. Sequencing revealed the presence of a 16S rRNA gene with high similarity (98%) to the corresponding genes from SFB of mouse and rat origin, thus indicating the presence of a human variant of SFB." Jonsson H. Segmented filamentous bacteria in human ileostomy samples after high-fiber intake. *FEMS Microbiol Lett.* 2013 May;342(1):24-9

[659] "The vancomycin dose was 500 mg/day…" Sandler et al. Short-term benefit from oral vancomycin treatment of regressive-onset autism. *J Child Neurol* 2000 Jul:429-35

[660] Oral vancomycin 125mg or 250 mg QID. Tabibian et al. Vancomycin metronidazole patients primary sclerosing cholangitis. *Aliment Pharmacol Ther* 2013 Mar;604-1

[661] "Orally administered vancomycin at 125 mg 4 times daily was not absorbed from the gastrointestinal tract." Rao et al. Systemic absorption of oral vancomycin in patients with Clostridium difficile infection. *Scand J Infect Dis.* 2011 May;43(5):386-8

[662] Osawa R, Kaka AS. Maculopapular rash induced by oral vancomycin. *Clin Infect Dis.* 2008 Sep 15;47(6):860-1

Commonly encountered dysbiotic microorganisms—*alphabetized listing*, *continued*

Microbe	Pathophysiology and clinical manifestations
Staphylococcus aureus ***Staphylococcus epidermidis***	• **Any and all *Staphylococcus aureus* should be eradicated immediately due to the well-known inflammatory consequences of the toxins and superantigens this bacterium produces.** *Staphylococcus aureus* is a gram-positive bacterium, certain strains of which produce the toxic shock syndrome toxin-1 (TSST-1) that produces scalded skin syndrome, toxic shock syndrome, and food poisoning; other strains of *Staphylococcus aureus* that do not produce TSST-1 are also capable of causing toxic shock syndrome from colonization of bone, vagina, wounds, or rectum.[663] • Gastrointestinal colonization with *Staphylococcus aureus* is a known cause of **acute colitis**[664], and nasal carriage of this bacterium is documented in patients with several autoimmune disorders, including **ANCA-associated vasculitis**[665], **systemic lupus erythematosus**[666] and **psoriasis.**[667, 668] • *Staphylococcus aureus* can trigger **reactive arthritis.**[669] • *Staphylococcus epidermidis* can trigger **reactive arthritis and sacroiliitis.**[670] • Patients with **Behcet's syndrome** commonly have skin lesions that are colonized by *Staphylococcus aureus.*[671] • Most (57%) of patients with **atopic dermatitis** show evidence of IgE-mediated histamine release (i.e., "allergy") to exotoxins secreted from *Staphylococcus aureus*, which commonly colonizes eczematous skin[672]; in other words: most eczema patients are allergic to their own dermal bacteria and can thus be said to have *hypersensitivity dermal dysbiosis.*
Streptococcus pyogenes **Group A streptococci**	• Intestinal overgrowth of this bacterium, which produces peptidoglycans, can cause **dermatosis, <u>inflammatory polyarthritis</u>, tenosynovitis, malaise, fever, and cryoglobulinemia.**[673] • Non-infectious manifestations precipitated by infection with *S. pyogenes* include **autoimmune neuropsychiatric disorders** (including obsessive-compulsive disorder and Sydenham's chorea), **dystonia, glomerulonephritis, and reactive arthritis.**[674] • Group A streptococci can cause **reactive arthritis** in humans.[675] • *Streptococcus pyogenes* is a very likely trigger of **psoriasis**[676]; chronic penicillin treatment leads to clinical improvement of recalcitrant psoriasis.[677] • Certain strains of *S. pyogenes* produce an exotoxin that can cause toxic shock syndrome.[678]

[663] Shandera WX, Moran A. "Infectious diseases: viral and rickettsial." In Tierney et al (eds). Current Medical Diagnosis and Treatment. 44th edition. 2005, page 1356-8
[664] Watanabe H, Masaki H, Asoh N, Watanabe K, Oishi K, Kobayashi S, Sato A, Nagatake T. Enterocolitis caused by methicillin-resistant Staphylococcus aureus: molecular characterization of respiratory and digestive tract isolates. *Microbiol Immunol.* 2001;45(9):629-34 jstage.jst.go.jp/article/mandi/45/9/629/_pdf
[665] Popa ER, et al. Staphylococcus aureus and Wegener's granulomatosis. *Arthritis Res.* 2002;4(2):77-9 arthritis-research.com/content/4/2/077
[666] Medline abstract from Polish research: "In 9 from 14 patients with (64.3%) a.b. very massive growth of Staphylococcus aureus in culture from vestibulae of the nose swab was, in other cultures very massive growth of physiological flora was seen. ...clinical significance of asymptomatic bacteriuria and pathogenic bacteria colonisation of nostrils as a precedence to symptomatic infections needs further investigations." Koseda-Dragan M, Hebanowski M, Galinski J, Krzywinska E, Bakowska A. [Asymptomatic bacteriuria in women diagnosed with systemic lupus erythematosus (SLE)] *Pol Arch Med Wewn.* 1998 Oct;100(4):321-30.
[667] "Nasal carriage rate of Staphylococcus aureus in psoriatics was higher than control groups."Singh et al. Bacteriology of psoriatic plaques. *Dermatologica* 1978;157:21-7
[668] "S aureus was present in more than 50% of patients with AD and PS. ...the severity of AD and PS significantly correlated to enterotoxin production of the isolated S aureus strains." Tomi et al. Staphylococcal toxins in psoriasis, atopic dermatitis, and erythroderma, and in healthy control subjects. *J Am Acad Dermatol.* 2005 Jul;53(1):67-72
[669] "CONCLUSION—Reactive arthritis may rarely follow Staph aureus infection. HLA-B27 negativity may be associated with a self limited arthritis in these cases." Siam AR, Hammoudeh M. Staphylococcus aureus triggered reactive arthritis. *Ann Rheum Dis.* 1995 Feb;54(2):131-3
[670] "We report an unusual case of a patient with SE bacteriaemia, who developed elbow arthritis, asymmetrical sacroiliitis, keratoderma and restrictive cardiomyopathy." Giordano et al. Reactive arthritis by staphylococcus epidermidis: report of an unusual case. *Clin Rheumatol.* 1996;15(1):59-61
[671] "At least one type of microorganism was grown from each pustule. Staphylococcus aureus (41/70, 58.6%, p = 0.008) and Prevotella spp (17/70, 24.3%, p = 0.002) were significantly more common in pustules from BS patients, and coagulase negative staphylococci (17/37, 45.9%, p = 0.007) in pustules from acne patients. CONCLUSIONS: The pustular lesions of BS are not usually sterile." Hatemi et al. The pustular skin lesions in Behcet's syndrome are not sterile. *Ann Rheum Dis.* 2004 Nov;63(11):1450-2
[672] "These data indicate that a subset of patients with AD mount an IgE response to SEs that can be grown from their skin." Leung et al. Presence of IgE antibodies to staphylococcal exotoxins on the skin of patients with atopic dermatitis. Evidence for a new group of allergens. *J Clin Invest.* 1993 Sep;92(3):1374-80
[673] Ely PH. The bowel bypass syndrome: a response to bacterial peptidoglycans. *J Am Acad Dermatol.* 1980 Jun;2(6):473-87
[674] Hahn RG, Knox LM, Forman TA. Evaluation of poststreptococcal illness. *Am Fam Physician.* 2005 May 15;71(10):1949-54 aafp.org/afp/20050515/1949.pdf
[675] "We present a patient whose clinical features are more consistent with post-streptococcal reactive arthritis than acute rheumatic fever." Howell EE, Bathon J. A case of post-streptococcal reactive arthritis. *Md Med J.* 1999 Nov-Dec;48(6):292-4
[676] "These findings justify the hypothesis that S pyogenes infections are more important in the pathogenesis of chronic plaque psoriasis than has previously been recognized, and indicate the need for further controlled therapeutic trials of antibacterial measures in this common skin disease." El-Rachkidy et al. Increased Blood Levels of IgG Reactive with Secreted Streptococcus pyogenes Proteins in Chronic Plaque Psoriasis. *J Invest Dermatol.* 2007 Mar 8
[677] "Total duration of the study was two years. Initially benzathine penicillin 1.2 million units, was given I.M. AST fortnightly. After 24 weeks benzathine penicillin was reduced to 1.2 million units once a month... Significant improvement in the PASI score was noted from 12 weeks onwards. All patients showed excellent improvement at 2 years." Saxena VN, Dogra J. Long-term use of penicillin for the treatment of chronic plaque psoriasis. *Eur J Dermatol.* 2005 Sep-Oct;15(5):359-62
[678] Chikkamuniyappa S. Streptococcal toxic shock syndrome and sepsis manifesting in a patient with chronic rheumatoid arthritis. *Dermatol Online J.* 2004 Jul 15;10(1):7

Clinical Benefits of Identifying and Eradicating Dysbiosis

In the previous section, I described the biochemical/physiologic mechanisms by which microorganisms can contribute to disease *without causing a classic "infection"* and promote systemic inflammation and human disease. Thus having developed the precept that **microorganisms can cause inflammatory disease by noninfectious means**, I will (re)state here that the cure of human disease by eradication of harmful microbes is not a requirement to prove the validity of this thesis. Inflammation and autoimmunity are self-perpetuating phenomena that can persist despite the effective eradication of the principle cause, and research has demonstrated that microbial antigens can remain present in synovial fluid for several years after the eradication of the primary infection.[679] With that said, we are fortunate to observe that **many patients with autoimmunity are indeed benefited and occasionally "cured" by removal of instigating microbes**. I have seen this on numerous occasions in my clinical practice, and this phenomenon has also been documented in the research literature. Examples published in the research include the amelioration of one patient's scleroderma with the eradication of intestinal bacterial overgrowth[680], the amelioration of ANCA-associated vasculitis with antimicrobial therapy against *Staphylococcus aureus*[681,682], and the alleviation of inflammatory arthritis following the use of antibiotics against genitourinary *Chlamydia trachomatis* and gastrointestinal *Salmonella enteritidis, Yersinia enterocolitica, Shigella flexneri* or *Campylobacter jejuni.*[683] Treatments for addressing dysbiosis and its numerous sequelae are described in the pages/sections that follow.

> **Landmark work by Dr Patricia Noah**
>
> "We have repeatedly observed psoriatic flares associated with microbial infection, sequestered antigen, and colonization. **Removal of these microbial foci results in clearing of the disease.**"
>
> Patricia Noah PhD from University of Tennessee College of Medicine. *Semin Dermatol.* 1990

Natural Treatments for the Eradication of Dysbiosis and Related Immune-Complex Diseases

Although antimicrobial drugs may be used, these are not universally curative and are not necessarily "more powerful" or "more effective" than natural treatments. Treatments for gastrointestinal dysbiosis may be somewhat summarized as follows: *"Starve, Poison, Crowd, Purge, and Support Immunity."* The following concepts and therapeutics are particularly—though not exclusively—relevant for the treatment of *gastrointestinal* dysbiosis.

1. **Diet modifications (*"starve the microbes"*)**: The diet plan should ensure **avoidance of sugar**, grains, soluble fiber, gums, prebiotics, and dairy products since these contain **fermentable carbohydrates that promote overgrowth of bacteria and other microorganisms in the gut**. Short-term **fasting** starves intestinal microbes, temporarily eliminates dietary antigens, alleviates "autointoxication", and stimulates the humoral immune system in the gut to more effectively destroy local microbes.[684,685] Thus, implementation of the **"specific carbohydrate diet"** popularized by Gottschall[686] along with periodic fasting, which has obvious anti-inflammatory benefits[687], can be used therapeutically in patients with conditions associated with dysbiosis-induced inflammation. Plant-based low-carbohydrate diets can lead to favorable changes in the quality and quantity of intestinal microflora. Hypoallergenic diets are proven beneficial for the treatment of the **immune complex disease** called mixed cryoglobulinemia.[688,689]

2. **Antimicrobial treatments (*"poison the microbes, not the patient"*)**: Anti-microbial herbs can be used which directly kill or strongly inhibit the intestinal microbes. The most commonly used and well-documented botanicals in this regard are listed in the section below. Antimicrobial treatment is frequently continued for 1-3 months, and co-administration of drugs can be utilized when appropriate. Sometimes antimicrobial drugs are necessary, especially for acute and severe infections; often nutritional and botanical interventions are safer and more effective. Although these herbs are generally taken orally, some of them can also be applied topically

[679] "Extensive bacterial cultures of synovial fluid were negative... We conclude that in patients with reactive arthritis after yersinia infection, microbial antigens can be found in synovial-fluid cells from affected joints."Granfors et al.Yersinia antigens in synovial-fluid cells from patients with reactive arthritis. *N Engl J Med* 1989;320:216-2

[680] Over et al. Regression of skin changes in patient with systemic sclerosis following treatment for bacterial overgrowth with ciprofloxacin. *Br J Rheumatol* 1998;37:696

[681] Popa et al. Staphylococcus aureus and Wegener's granulomatosis. *Arthritis Res.* 2002;4(2):77-9 arthritis-research.com/content/4/2/077

[682] George J, Levy Y, Kallenberg CG, Shoenfeld Y. Infections and Wegener's granulomatosis--a cause and effect relationship? *QJM.* 1997 May;90(5):367-73

[683] Kobayashi et al. Reactive arthritis: recent advances and clinical manifestations. *Intern Med.* 2005 May;44:408-12 jstage.jst.go.jp/article/internalmedicine/44/5/408/_pdf

[684] Trollmo C, Verdrengh M, Tarkowski A. Fasting enhances mucosal antigen specific B cell responses in rheumatoid arthritis. *Ann Rheum Dis.* 1997 Feb;56(2):130-4

[685] Ramakrishnan T, Stokes P. Beneficial effects of fasting and low carbohydrate diet in D-lactic acidosis associated with short-bowel syndrome. *JPEN J Parenter Enteral Nutr.* 1985 May-Jun;9(3):361-3

[686] Gottschall E. *Breaking the Vicious Cycle: Intestinal Health Through Diet.* Kirkton Press; Rev edition (August 1, 1994)

[687] "The pooling of these studies showed a statistically and clinically significant beneficial long-term effect." Muller H, de Toledo FW, Resch KL. Fasting followed by vegetarian diet in patients with rheumatoid arthritis: a systematic review. *Scand J Rheumatol.* 2001;30(1):1-10

[688] "CONCLUSION: These data show that an LAC diet decreases the amount of circulating immune complexes in MC and can modify certain signs and symptoms of the disease." Ferri C, Pietrogrande M, Cecchetti R, et al. Low-antigen-content diet in the treatment of patients with mixed cryoglobulinemia. *Am J Med.* 1989 Nov;87:519-24

[689] Pietrogrande M, Cefalo A, Nicora F, Marchesini D. Dietetic treatment of essential mixed cryoglobulinemia. *Ric Clin Lab.* 1986 Apr-Jun;16(2):413-6

(in a cream or lotion), and nasally (in a saline water lavage, as detailed previously). Botanical medicines are generally used in combination, and lower doses of each can be used when used in combination compared to the doses that are necessary when the herbs are used in isolation.

- **<u>Oregano oil in an emulsified and time-released tablet</u>**: Botanical oils that are not emulsified do not attain maximal dispersion in the gastrointestinal tract; products that are not time-released may be absorbed before reaching the colon in sufficient concentrations. Emulsified oil of oregano in a time-released tablet is proven effective in the eradication of harmful gastrointestinal microbes, including *Blastocystis hominis, Entamoeba hartmanni,* and *Endolimax nana.*[690] An in vitro study[691] and clinical experience support the use of emulsified oregano against *Candida albicans.* The common dose is 600 mg per day in divided doses for at least 6 weeks.[692]

- **<u>Berberine</u>**: Berberine is an alkaloid extracted from plant such as *Berberis vulgaris,* and *Hydrastis canadensis,* and it shows effectiveness against *Giardia, Candida,* and *Streptococcus* in addition to its direct anti-inflammatory and antidiarrheal actions. Oral dose of 400 mg/d had been common for adults[693] until newer research showed that berberine 1,000-1,500 mg/d for 3 months was safe and impressively effective for the treatment of dyslipidemia, dysglycemia, metabolic syndrome, diabetes type-2; berberine is more effective dose-for-dose than is metformin.[694] Topical *Mahonia/Berberis aquifolium* is effective for dermal psoriasis[695] via its combined anti-inflammatory and antimicrobial benefits.

- ***<u>Artemisia annua</u>***: Artemisinin has been safely used for centuries in Asia for the treatment of malaria[696,697], and it also has **effectiveness against anaerobic bacteria** due to the pro-oxidative sesquiterpene endoperoxide. In a recent study treating patients with malaria, "the adult artemisinin dose was 500 mg; children aged < 15 years received 10 mg/kg per dose" and thus the dose for an 80-lb child would be 363 mg per day by these criteria.[698] I commonly use **artemisinin at 100 mg twice per day (with other antimicrobial botanicals such as berberine) in divided doses for adults with dysbiosis**. One of the additional benefits of artemisinin is its systemic bioavailability.

- **<u>St. John's Wort (*Hypericum perforatum*)</u>**: Best known for its antidepressant action, **hyperforin from *Hypericum perforatum* also shows impressive antibacterial action, particularly against gram-positive bacteria such as *Staphylococcus aureus, Streptococcus pyogenes* and *Streptococcus agalactiae*.** According to in vitro studies, the lowest effective hyperforin concentration is 0.1 mcg/mL against *Corynebacterium diphtheriae* with increasing effectiveness against multiresistant *Staphylococcus aureus* at higher concentrations of 100 mcg/mL.[699] Since oral dosing with hyperforin can result in serum levels of 500 nanogram /mL (equivalent to 0.5 microgram/mL) then it is possible that high-dose hyperforin will have systemic antibacterial action. Regardless of its possible systemic antibacterial effectiveness, **hyperforin should clearly have antibacterial action when applied "topically" such as when it is taken orally against gastric and upper intestinal colonization.** Extracts from St. John's Wort hold particular promise against multidrug-resistant *Staphylococcus aureus*[700] and perhaps *Helicobacter pylori.*[701]

- **<u>Myrrh (*Commiphora molmol*)</u>**: Myrrh is remarkably effective against parasitic infections.[702] A recent clinical trial against **schistosomiasis**[703] showed "The parasitological cure rate after three months was 97.4%

---

[690] Force M, Sparks WS, Ronzio RA. Inhibition of enteric parasites by emulsified oil of oregano in vivo. *Phytother Res.* 2000 May;14(3):213-4

[691] Stiles JC, Sparks W, Ronzio RA. The inhibition of Candida albicans by oregano. *J Applied Nutr* 1995;47:96–102

[692] Force M, Sparks WS, Ronzio RA. Inhibition of enteric parasites by emulsified oil of oregano in vivo. *Phytother Res.* 2000 May;14(3):213-4

[693] Berberine. *Altern Med Rev.* 2000 Apr;5(2):175-7 thorne.com/altmedrev/.fulltext/5/2/175.pdf

[694] Yin et al. Efficacy of berberine in patients with type 2 diabetes mellitus. *Metabolism.* 2008 May;57(5):712-7. See also Kong et al. Berberine is a novel cholesterol-lowering drug working through a unique mechanism distinct from statins. *Nat Med.* 2004 Dec;10(12):1344-51

[695] "Taken together, these clinical studies conducted by several investigators in several countries indicate that Mahonia aquifolium is a safe and effective treatment of patients with mild to moderate psoriasis." Gulliver WP, Donsky HJ. A report on three recent clinical trials using Mahonia aquifolium 10% topical cream and a review of the worldwide clinical experience with Mahonia aquifolium for the treatment of plaque psoriasis. *Am J Ther.* 2005 Sep-Oct;12(5):398-406

[696] Dien TK, et al. Effect of food intake on pharmacokinetics of oral artemisinin in healthy Vietnamese subjects. *Antimicrob Agents Chemother.* 1997 May;41(5):1069-72

[697] Giao PT, et al. Artemisinin for treatment of uncomplicated falciparum malaria: is there a place for monotherapy? *Am J Trop Med Hyg.* 2001 Dec;65(6):690-5

[698] Giao PT, Binh TQ, Kager PA, Long HP, Van Thang N, Van Nam N, de Vries PJ. Artemisinin for treatment of uncomplicated falciparum malaria: is there a place for monotherapy? *Am J Trop Med Hyg.* 2001 Dec;65(6):690-5 ajtmh.org/cgi/reprint/65/6/690

[699] Schempp et al. Antibacterial activity of hyperforin from St John's wort, against multiresistant Staphylococcus aureus and gram-positive bacteria. *Lancet.* 1999;353:2129

[700] Gibbons S, Ohlendorf B, Johnsen I. The genus Hypericum--a valuable resource of anti-Staphylococcal leads. *Fitoterapia.* 2002 Jul;73(4):300-4

[701] "A butanol fraction of St. John's Wort revealed anti-Helicobacter pylori activity with MIC values ranging between 15.6 and 31.2 microg/ml." Reichling J, Weseler A, Saller R. A current review of the antimicrobial activity of Hypericum perforatum L. *Pharmacopsychiatry.* 2001 Jul;34 Suppl 1:S116-8

[702] El Baz, et al. Clinical and parasitological studies on efficacy of Mirazid in treatment of schistosomiasis haematobium in Tatoon. *J Egypt Soc Parasitol* 2003;33:761-76

[703] Schistosomiasis. dpd.cdc.gov/dpdx/HTML/Schistosomiasis.htm

and 96.2% for *S. haematobium* and *S. mansoni* cases with the marvelous clinical cure without any side-effects."[704]

- **<u>Bismuth</u>**: Bismuth is commonly used in the empiric treatment of diarrhea (e.g., "Pepto-<u>Bismol</u>") and is commonly combined with other antimicrobial agents to reduce drug resistance and increase antibiotic effectiveness.[705]

- **<u>Peppermint</u> (*Mentha piperita*)**: Peppermint shows antimicrobial and antispasmodic actions and has demonstrated clinical effectiveness in patients with bacterial overgrowth of the small bowel.

- **<u>Uva Ursi</u>**: Uva ursi can be used against gastrointestinal pathogens on a limited basis per culture and sensitivity findings; its primary historical and modern use is as a urinary antiseptic which is effective only when the urine pH is alkaline.[706] Components of uva ursi potentiate antibiotics.[707] **This herb has some ocular and neurologic toxicity and should be used with professional supervision for low-dose and/or short-term administration only.**[708]

- **<u>Garlic</u>**: Garlic shows *in vitro* antimicrobial action against numerous microorganisms, including *H. pylori, Pseudomonas aeruginosa,* and *Candida albicans*, and this effect is mediated *directly* via microbicidal actions as well as *indirectly* via dissolution of microbial biofilms[709] and inhibition of quorum sensing.[710] However, since the antimicrobial components of garlic are likely absorbed in the upper gastrointestinal tract, I propose that it is unlikely that garlic can exert a clinically significant anti-dysbiotic effect in the lower small intestine and colon. In fact, two studies in humans have shown that—despite its *in vitro* effectiveness against *H. pylori*—garlic is ineffective in the treatment of gastric *H. pylori* colonization.[711,712] While these studies argue against the use of garlic as antimicrobial monotherapy, the possibility remains that garlic may enhance the clinical effectiveness of other antimicrobial therapeutics via its aforementioned ability to weaken microbial biofilms and to impair quorum sensing, which otherwise serve to protect yeast/bacteria from immune attack and from antibacterial/antifungal therapeutics.

- **<u>Cranberry</u>**: Particularly effective for the prevention and adjunctive treatment of urinary tract infections, mostly by inhibiting adherence of *E. coli* to epithelial cells.[713]

- **<u>Thyme</u> (*Thymus vulgaris*)**: Thyme extracts have direct antimicrobial actions and also potentiate the effectiveness of tetracycline against drug-resistant *Staphylococcus aureus*.[714] Thyme also appears effective against *Aeromonas hydrophila*.[715]

- **<u>Clove</u> (*Syzygium* species)**: Clove's eugenol has been shown in animal studies to have a potent antifungal effect.[716]

- **<u>Anise</u>**: Although it has weak antibacterial action when used alone, anise does show in vitro activity against molds.[717]

- **<u>Buchu/betulina</u>**: Buchu has a long history of use against urinary tract infections and systemic infections.[718]

---

[704] Abo-Madyan AA, Morsy TA, Motawea SM. Efficacy of Myrrh in the treatment of schistosomiasis (haematobium and mansoni) in Ezbet El-Bakly, Tamyia Center, El-Fayoum Governorate, Egypt. *J Egypt Soc Parasitol.* 2004 Aug;34(2):423-46

[705] Veldhuyzen van Zanten SJ, Sherman PM, Hunt RH. Helicobacter pylori: new developments and treatments. *CMAJ.* 1997;156(11):1565-74

[706] Yarnell E. Botanical medicines for the urinary tract. *World J Urol.* 2002 Nov;20(5):285-93

[707] Shimizu M, Shiota S, Mizushima T, Ito H, Hatano T, Yoshida T, Tsuchiya T. Marked potentiation of activity of beta-lactams against methicillin-resistant Staphylococcus aureus by corilagin. *Antimicrob Agents Chemother.* 2001 Nov;45(11):3198-201 aac.asm.org/cgi/reprint/45/11/3198

[708] "A 56-year-old woman who ingested uva ursi for 3 years noted a decrease in visual acuity within the past year. Ocular examination including fluorescein angiography revealed a typical bull's-eye maculopathy bilaterally." Wang L, Del Priore LV. Bull's-eye maculopathy secondary to herbal toxicity from uva ursi. *Am J Ophthalmol.* 2004 Jun;137:1135-7

[709] "Sub-MICs of allicin also diminished the biofilm formations by S. epidermidis." Perez-Giraldo C, et al. In vitro activity of allicin against Staphylococcus epidermidis and influence of subinhibitory concentrations on biofilm formation. *J Appl Microbiol.* 2003;95(4):709-11

[710] "The results indicate that a QS-inhibitory extract of garlic renders P. aeruginosa sensitive to tobramycin, respiratory burst and phagocytosis by PMNs, as well as leading to an improved outcome of pulmonary infections." Bjarnsholt T, et al. Garlic blocks quorum sensing and promotes rapid clearing of pulmonary Pseudomonas aeruginosa infections. *Microbiology.* 2005 Dec;151(Pt 12):3873-80. The in vivo portion of this study was performed in lab animals, not humans.

[711] "This study did not support a role for either garlic or jalapenos in the treatment of H. pylori infection. Caution must be used when attempting to extrapolate data from in vitro studies to the in vivo condition." Graham et al. Garlic or jalapeno peppers for treatment of Helicobacter pylori infection. *Am J Gastroenterol.* 1999 May;94(5):1200-2

[712] "Five patients completed the study. There was no evidence of garlic eradication or suppression of H. pylori or symptom improvement whilst taking garlic oil." McNulty CA, et al. A pilot study to determine the effectiveness of garlic oil capsules in the treatment of dyspeptic patients with Helicobacter pylori. *Helicobacter.* 2001;6(3):249-53

[713] Lynch DM. Cranberry for prevention of urinary tract infections. *Am Fam Physician.* 2004 Dec 1;70(11):2175-7 aafp.org/afp/20041201/2175.pdf

[714] Fujita M, Shiota S, Kuroda T, Hatano T, Yoshida T, Mizushima T, Tsuchiya T. Remarkable synergies between baicalein and tetracycline, and baicalein and beta-lactams against methicillin-resistant Staphylococcus aureus. *Microbiol Immunol.* 2005;49(4):391-6

[715] "...thyme essential oil showed the greatest inhibition against A. hydrophila." Fabio A, Corona A, Forte E, Quaglio P. Inhibitory activity of spices and essential oils on psychrotrophic bacteria. *New Microbiol.* 2003 Jan;26(1):115-20

[716] Chami N, et al. Antifungal treatment with carvacrol and eugenol of oral candidiasis in immunosuppressed rats. *Braz J Infect Dis.* 2004 Jun;8(3):217-26

[717] "Anise oil was not particularly inhibitory to bacteria (inhibition zone, approximately 25 mm); however, anise oil was highly inhibitory to molds." Elgayyar M, et al. Antimicrobial activity of essential oils from plants against selected pathogenic and saprophytic microorganisms. *J Food Prot.* 2001 Jul;64(7):1019-24

[718] "Buchu preparations are now used as a diuretic and for a wide range of conditions including stomach aches, rheumatism, bladder and kidney infections and coughs and colds." Simpson D. Buchu--South Africa's amazing herbal remedy. *Scott Med J* 1998 Dec;43(6):189-91

- **Caprylic acid and undecylenic acid**: Caprylic acid is a medium chain fatty acid that is commonly used in patients with dysbiosis, particularly that which has a fungal/yeast component. Beside empiric use, caprylic acid may be indicated by culture-sensitivity results provided with comprehensive parasitology. When bacterial/fungal sensitivity tests indicate caprylic acid, many clinicians prefer to use undecylenic acid which is reportedly up to six times more powerful than caprylic acid.[719] Commercial preparations delivering 50 mg undecylenic acid per gelcap can be taken orally in doses of 3-5 gelcaps three times per day. Anti-candidal action has been reported[720], and my impression is that undecylenic acid is among the more valuable therapeutics in the treatment of gastrointestinal dysbiosis.
- **Dill (*Anethum graveolens*)**: Dill shows activity against several types of mold and yeast.[721]
- *Brucea javanica*: Extract from *Brucea javanica* fruit shows *in vitro* activity against *Babesia gibsoni*, *Plasmodium falciparum*[722], *Entamoeba histolytica*[723] and *Blastocystis hominis*.[724,725]
- *Acacia catechu*: *Acacia catechu* shows moderate *in vitro* activity against *Salmonella typhi*.[726]

3. *Oral administration of proteolytic enzymes*: The use of polyenzyme therapy in patients with dysbiotic inflammation is justified for at least four reasons. First, orally administered proteolytic enzymes are efficiently absorbed by the gastrointestinal tract into the systemic circulation[727] to then provide a **clinically significant anti-inflammatory benefit** as I reviewed recently.[728] Second and more specifically, oral administration of proteolytic enzymes is generally believed to effect a **reduction in immune complexes and their clinical consequences**[729], and immune complexes are probably a major mechanism of dysbiosis-induced disease and are pathogenic in rheumatoid arthritis[730] and many other autoimmune diseases such as systemic lupus erythematosus, dermatomyositis, Sjogren's syndrome, and polyarteritis nodosa.[731] Third, proteolytic enzymes have been shown to **stimulate immune function**[732] and may thereby promote clearance of occult infections. Fourth, **proteolytic enzymes inhibit formation of microbial biofilms** and increase immune penetration and the effectiveness of antimicrobial therapeutics.[733] Although individual enzymes may be used in isolation, enzyme therapy is generally delivered in the form of polyenzyme preparations containing pancreatin, bromelain, papain, amylase, lipase, trypsin and alpha-chymotrypsin.[734]

4. **Probiotic supplementation (*"crowd out the bad with the good"*)**: Given that "healthy" intestinal bacteria can alleviate disease and promote normal immune function[735], then it is conversely true that a condition of harmful or suboptimal intestinal bacteria could promote disease and lead to immune dysfunction. For patients with gastrointestinal and genitourinary dysbiosis, supplementation with *Bifidobacteria*, *Lactobacillus*, and perhaps *Saccharomyces* and other beneficial strains is mandatory. The wide-ranging and well-documented benefits seen with probiotic supplementation provide direct support for the importance of microbial balance in health and

[719] Undecylenic acid. Monograph. *Altern Med Rev*. 2002 Feb;7(1):68-70 thorne.com/altmedrev/.fulltext/7/1/68.pdf

[720] McLain N, et al. Undecylenic acid inhibits morphogenesis of Candida albicans. *Antimicrob Agents Chemother*. 2000 Oct;44(10):2873-5

[721] "Antimicrobial testings showed high activity of the essential A. graveolens oil against the mold Aspergillus niger and the yeasts Saccharomyces cerevisiae and Candida albicans." Jirovetz L, Buchbauer G, Stoyanova AS, Georgiev EV, Damianova ST. Composition, quality control, and antimicrobial activity of the essential oil of long-time stored dill (Anethum graveolens L.) seeds from Bulgaria. *J Agric Food Chem*. 2003 Jun 18;51(13):3854-7

[722] Murnigsih T, Subeki, Matsuura H, et al. Evaluation of the inhibitory activities of the extracts of Indonesian traditional medicinal plants against Plasmodium falciparum and Babesia gibsoni. *J Vet Med Sci*. 2005 Aug;67(8):829-31 jstage.jst.go.jp/article/jvms/67/8/829/_pdf

[723] Wright CW, O'Neill MJ, Phillipson JD, Warhurst DC. Use of microdilution to assess in vitro antiamoebic activities of Brucea javanica fruits, Simarouba amara stem, and a number of quassinoids. *Antimicrob Agents Chemother*. 1988 Nov;32(11):1725-9

[724] "Dichloromethane and methanol extracts from the Brucea javanica seed and a methanol extract from Quercus infectoria nut gall showed the highest activity." Sawangjaroen N, Sawangjaroen K. The effects of extracts from anti-diarrheic Thai medicinal plants on the in vitro growth of the intestinal protozoa parasite: Blastocystis hominis. *J Ethnopharmacol*. 2005 Apr 8;98(1-2):67-72

[725] "The crude extracts of Coptis chinensis (CC) and Brucea javanica (BJ) were found to be most active against B. hominis." Yang LQ, et al. In vitro response of Blastocystis hominis against traditional Chinese medicine. *J Ethnopharmacol*. 1996 Dec;55(1):35-42

[726] "Moderate antimicrobial activity was shown by Picorhiza kurroa, Acacia catechu, ..." Rani P, Khullar N. Antimicrobial evaluation of some medicinal plants for their anti-enteric potential against multi-drug resistant Salmonella typhi. *Phytother Res*. 2004 Aug;18(8):670-3

[727] Liebow C, Rothman SS. Enteropancreatic Circulation of Digestive Enzymes. *Science* 1975; 189(4201): 472-474

[728] Vasquez A. Improving overall health while safely and effectively treating musculoskeletal pain. *Nutr Perspectives* 2005; 28: 34-38, 40-42 InflammationMastery.com/reprints

[729] Galebskaya LV, Ryumina EV, Niemerovsky VS, Matyukov AA. Human complement system state after wobenzyme intake. *VESTNIK MOSKOVSKOGO UNIVERSITETA. KHIMIYA*. 2000. Vol. 41, No. 6. Supplement. Pages 148-149

[730] Edwards JC, Cambridge G. Rheumatoid arthritis: the predictable effect of small immune complexes in which antibody is also antigen. *Br J Rheumatol*. 1998 Feb;37(2):126-30 rheumatology.oxfordjournals.org/cgi/reprint/37/2/126

[731] Jancar S, Sanchez Crespo M. Immune complex-mediated tissue injury: a multistep paradigm. *Trends Immunol*. 2005 Jan;26(1):48-55

[732] Zavadova E, Desser L, Mohr T. Stimulation of reactive oxygen species production and cytotoxicity in human neutrophils in vitro and after oral administration of a polyenzyme preparation. *Cancer Biother*. 1995 Summer;10(2):147-52

[733] "The enzymes were shown to inhibit the biofilm formation. When appplilied to the formed associations, the enzymes potentiated the effect of antibiotics on the bacteria located in them." Tets VV, et al. [Impact of exogenic proteolytic enzymes on bacteria][Quote from abstract; article in Russian] *Antibiot Khimioter*. 2004;49(12):9-13

[734] Vasquez A. Improving overall health while safely and effectively treating musculoskeletal pain. *Nutritional Perspect* 2005; 28: 34-38, 40-42 InflammationMastery.com/reprints

[735] Isolauri E, Sutas Y, Kankaanpaa P, Arvilommi H, Salminen S. Probiotics: effects on immunity. *Am J Clin Nutr*. 2001 Feb;73(2 Suppl):444S-450S

disease. Supplementation with probiotics (live bacteria) is the best option, however prebiotics (such as fructooligosaccharides), and synbiotics (probiotics + prebiotics) may also be used. Synbiotic supplementation has been shown to reduce endotoxinemia and clinical symptoms in 50% of patients with minimal hepatic encephalopathy[736], and probiotic supplementation safely ameliorated the adverse effects of bacterial overgrowth in a clinical study of patients with renal failure.[737]

5. **Immunonutrition**: Obviously, the diet should be nutritious and free of sugars and other "junk foods" that promote inflammation and suppress immune function.[738] Especially in patients with gastrointestinal dysbiosis, vitamin and mineral supplementation should be used to counteract the effects of malabsorption, maldigestion, and hypermetabolism

> **Probiotic mutualism via cross-feeding ultimately affects human gene expression, enterocyte health, and intestinal permeability**
>
> Oral supplementation with synbiotics provides inulin and fructooligosaccharides to *Bifidobacterium* and *Lactobacillus* which partially metabolize carbohydrate substrates to acetate and lactate which then serve as substrate for butyrogenic microbes such as *Roseburia intestinalis* and *Anaerostipes caccae* for the production of butyrate, which provides anti-inflammatory nutrigenomic benefits via suppression of NFkB, serves as a major fuel source for enterocytes especially colonocytes, and improves epithelial barrier integrity by modulating the expression of certain tight junction proteins such as cingulin, intercellular ZO (zonula occludens) proteins, and occludin. In this way, one can see how food intake influences/supports microbial mutualism for production of a metabolite that affects the tissue physiology and cellular molecular biology of the human host.
>
> Bosscher et al. Food-based strategies to modulate the composition of the intestinal microbiota and their associated health effects. *J Physiol Pharmacol.* 2009 Dec

that accompany immune activation. Additionally, oral glutamine in doses of six grams three times daily can help normalize intestinal permeability, enhance immune function, and improve clinical outcomes in severely ill patients.[739] Zinc and vitamin A supplementation are each well known to support immune function against infection. Selenium has anti-inflammatory and antiviral actions.[740] Vitamin D supplementation reduces inflammation, protects against autoimmunity, and promotes immunity against viral and bacterial infections.[741] Supplementation with IgG from bovine colostrum can also provide benefit against chronic and acute infections.[742,743] Extracts from bovine thymus are safe for clinical use in humans and have shown anti-infective and anti-inflammatory benefits in elderly patients[744] as well as antirheumatic/anti-inflammatory benefits in patients with autoimmune diseases[745,746,747]; in an animal study of experimental dental disease, administration of thymus extract was shown to normalize immune function and reduce orodental dysbiosis.[748]

6. **Hepatobiliary stimulation for IgA-complex removal**: The binding of immunoglobulin A (IgA) with antigen creates IgA immune complexes that contribute to tissue destruction by complement activation (alternate pathway) and other pathomechanisms in IgA nephropathy[749], Henoch-Schonlein purpura[750], rheumatoid vasculitis[751], lupus[752], and Sjogren's syndrome.[753] Autoreactive IgA antibodies are a characteristic of lupus and Sjogren's syndrome[754] and correlate strongly with disease activity in rheumatoid arthritis.[755] **Immune**

[736] Liu Q, et al. Synbiotic modulation of gut flora: effect on minimal hepatic encephalopathy in patients with cirrhosis. *Hepatology.* 2004 May;39(5):1441-9

[737] Simenhoff ML, Dunn SR, Zollner GP, Fitzpatrick ME, Emery SM, Sandine WE, Ayres JW. Biomodulation of the toxic and nutritional effects of small bowel bacterial overgrowth in end-stage kidney disease using freeze-dried Lactobacillus acidophilus. *Miner Electrolyte Metab.* 1996;22(1-3):92-6

[738] Seaman DR. The diet-induced proinflammatory state: a cause of chronic pain and other degenerative diseases? *J Manipulative Physiol Ther.* 2002 Mar-Apr;25:168-79.

[739] Miller AL. Therapeutic considerations of L-glutamine: a review of the literature. *Altern Med Rev.* 1999 Aug;4(4):239-48

[740] Beck MA. Nutritionally induced oxidative stress: effect on viral disease. *Am J Clin Nutr.* 2000 Jun;71(6 Suppl):1676S-81S

[741] Vasquez A, Manso G, Cannell J. The clinical importance of vitamin D (cholecalciferol). *Altern Ther Health Med.* 2004 Sep;10(5):28-36 InflammationMastery.com/reprints

[742] Mero A, Kahkonen J, Nykanen T, Parviainen T, Jokinen I, Takala T, Nikula T, Rasi S, Leppaluoto J. IGF-I, IgA, and IgG responses to bovine colostrum supplementation during training. *J Appl Physiol.* 2002 Aug;93(2):732-9 jap.physiology.org/cgi/content/full/93/2/732

[743] "The preparation has high antibacterial antibody titres, and a high capacity for the neutralization of bacterial toxins. It is well tolerated and highly effective in the treatment of severe diarrhoea, e.g. in AIDS patients." Stephan et al. Antibodies from colostrum in oral immunotherapy. *J Clin Chem Clin Biochem.* 1990 Jan;28(1):19-23

[744] Pandolfi et al. T-dependent immunity in aged humans.Clinical and immunological evaluation after three months of thymic extract. *Thymus* 1983;5:235-40

[745] Lavastida MT, Goldstein AL, Daniels JC. Thymosin administration in autoimmune disorders. *Thymus.* 1981 Feb;2(4-5):287-95

[746] Thrower PA, Doyle DV, Scott J, Huskisson EC. Thymopoietin in rheumatoid arthritis. *Rheumatol Rehabil.* 1982 May;21(2):72-7

[747] Malaise et al.Treatment of active rheumatoid arthritis with intravenous injections of thymopentin.*Lancet* 1985;1:832-6

[748] Manti F, Kornman K, Goldschneider I. Effects of an immunomodulating agent on peripheral blood lymphocytes and subgingival microflora in ligature-induced periodontitis. *Infect Immun.* 1984 Jul;45(1):172-9 pubmedcentral.gov/articlerender.fcgi?tool=pubmed&pubmedid=6234232

[749] "...it is likely that the usual instance of IgA-associated glomerulonephritis is due to deposition of circulating immune complexes containing IgA." McPhaul JJ Jr. IgA-associated glomerulonephritis. *Annu Rev Med.* 1977;28:37-42

[750] "... it is generally considered to be an immune complex-mediated disease characterized by the presence of polymeric IgA1 (pIgA1)-containing immune complexes predominantly in dermal, gastrointestinal, and glomerular capillaries. ...also been observed in the kidneys of patients with liver cirrhosis, dermatitis herpetiformis, celiac disease, and chronic inflammatory disease of the lung. " Rai A, Nast C, Adler S. Henoch-Schonlein purpura nephritis. *J Am Soc Nephrol.* 1999 Dec;10(12):2637-44

[751] Voskuyl AE, Hazes JM, Zwinderman AH, Paleolog EM, van der Meer FJ, Daha MR, Breedveld FC. Diagnostic strategy for the assessment of rheumatoid vasculitis. *Ann Rheum Dis.* 2003 May;62(5):407-13 ard.bmjjournals.com/cgi/reprint/62/5/407

[752] Sikander FF, Salgaonkar DS, Joshi VR. Cryoglobulin studies in systemic lupus erythematosus. *J Postgrad Med* 1989;35:139-43

[753] Pourmand N, Wahren-Herlenius M, Gunnarsson I, et al. Ro/SSA and La/SSB specific IgA autoantibodies in serum of patients with Sjogren's syndrome and systemic lupus erythematosus. *Ann Rheum Dis.* 1999 Oct;58(10):623-9 ard.bmjjournals.com/cgi/content/full/58/10/623

[754] Pourmand et al. Ro/SSA and La/SSB specific IgA autoantibodies in serum of patients with Sjogren's syndrome and systemic lupus erythematosus. *Ann Rheum Dis.* 1999 Oct;58(10):623-9

[755] Jonsson T, Valdimarsson H. What about IgA rheumatoid factor in rheumatoid arthritis? *Ann Rheum Dis.* 1998 Jan;57(1):63-4

complexes containing secretory IgA that has been reabsorbed from mucosal surfaces mediate many of the clinical phenomenon of dysbiosis-related musculoskeletal disease[756], and these same IgA-containing immune complexes are eliminated from the systemic circulation via the liver and biliary system[757,758], thus providing the rationale for the use of botanicals and physiotherapeutics that promote liver function and bile flow in the treatment of IgA-mediated inflammatory disorders. Numerous experimental studies in animals have shown that circulating IgA immune complexes are taken up by hepatocytes and then secreted into the bile for elimination.[759,760] The fact that bile duct obstruction retards systemic clearance of IgA immune complexes and that normalization/optimization of bile flow reduces serum IgA levels by enhancing biliary excretion in animals[761,762] and humans[763] proves the importance of ensuring optimal hepatobiliary function and supports the use of botanical and physiological therapeutics that facilitate bile flow. A 1929 clinical study with human patients published in *Archives of Internal Medicine* provided irrefutable radiographic documentation that therapeutic enemas safely and effectively stimulate bile flow for 45-60 minutes following administration[764], and this finding, along with the obvious quantitative reduction in intestinal microbes induced by such "cleansing", helps explain the reported benefits of colonics/enemas in patients with systemic illness[765,766,767,768] and other immune-complex associated diseases such as cancer.[769] Validation of this concept is demonstrated by the significant efficacy of immunoadsorption[770] and plasmapheresis[771,772] (techniques for removing immune complexes) in patients with lupus. Furthermore, this directly supports the naturopathic concept of "treating the liver" in patients with systemic disease by the use of dietary and botanical therapeutics that stimulate bile flow, such as beets, ginger[773], curcumin/turmeric[774], *Picrorhiza*[775], milk thistle[776], *Andrographis paniculata*[777], and *Boerhaavia diffusa*.[778] Investigation of an antirheumatic benefit from phytophysiotherapeutic hepatobiliary

[756] Inman RD. Antigens, the gastrointestinal tract, and arthritis. *Rheum Dis Clin North Am.* 1991 May;17(2):309-21

[757] Russell MW, Brown TA, Claflin JL, Schroer K, Mestecky J. Immunoglobulin A-mediated hepatobiliary transport constitutes a natural pathway for disposing of bacterial antigens. *Infect Immun.* 1983 Dec;42(3):1041-8 pubmedcentral.gov/articlerender.fcgi?tool=pubmed&pubmedid=6642659

[758] "The liver therefore appears to be singularly capable of transporting both free and complexed IgA into its secretion, the bile." Russell MW, Brown TA, Mestecky J. Preferential transport of IgA and IgA-immune complexes to bile compared with other external secretions. *Mol Immunol.* 1982 May;19(5):677-82

[759] "These results indicate that mouse hepatocytes are involved in the uptake and hepatobiliary transport of pIgA and pIgA-IC of low mol. wt." Phillips JO, Komiyama K, Epps JM, Russell MW, Mestecky J. Role of hepatocytes in the uptake of IgA and IgA-containing immune complexes in mice. *Mol Immunol.* 1988 Sep;25(9):873-9

[760] "Thus hepatobiliary transport appears to be the major pathway for the clearance of both IgA IC and free IgA from the circulation." Brown TA, Russell MW, Kulhavy R, Mestecky J. IgA-mediated elimination of antigens by the hepatobiliary route. *Fed Proc.* 1983 Dec;42(15):3218-21

[761] "Clearance of IgA immune complexes was delayed after bile duct ligation." Harmatz PR, Kleinman RE, Bunnell BW, McClenathan DT, Walker WA, Bloch KJ. The effect of bile duct obstruction on the clearance of circulating IgA immune complexes. *Hepatology.* 1984 Jan-Feb;4(1):96-100

[762] Lemaitre-Coelho I, et al. High levels of secretory IgA and free secretory component in the serum of rats with bile duct obstruction. *J Exp Med.* 1978 Mar 1;147:934-9

[763] "CONCLUSIONS: Biliary obstruction secondary to both calculus or malignancy of the hepatobiliary system causes suppression of bile IgA secretion and elevated serum level of secretory IgA. Bile secretory IgA secretion recovers with endoscopic drainage of the obstructed system." Sung JJ, Leung JC, Tsui CP, Chung SS, Lai KN. Biliary IgA secretion in obstructive jaundice: the effects of endoscopic drainage. *Gastrointest Endosc.* 1995 Nov;42(5):439-44

[764] Garbat AL, Jacobi HG. Secretion of Bile in Response to Rectal Installations. *Arch Intern Med* 1929; 44: 455-462

[765] Crinnion WJ. Results of a decade of naturopathic treatment for environmental illnesses. *J Naturopathic Med* 1994;17:21-27

[766] Snyder RG. The value of colonic irrigations in countering auto-intoxication of intestinal origin. *Medical Clinics of North America* 1939; May: 781-788

[767] Marshall HK, Thomson CR. Colon irrigation in the treatment of mental disease. *N Engl J Med* 1932; 207 (Sept 8): 454-7

[768] Bastedo WA. Colon irrigations: their administration, therapeutic applications, and dangers. *Journal of the American Medical Association* 1932; 98(9): 734-6

[769] Gonzalez NJ, Isaacs LL. Evaluation of pancreatic proteolytic enzyme treatment of adenocarcinoma of the pancreas, with nutrition and detoxification support. *Nutr Cancer.* 1999;33(2):117-24

[770] Braun N, Erley C, Klein R, Kotter I, Saal J, Risler T. Immunoadsorption onto protein A induces remission in severe systemic lupus erythematosus. *Nephrol Dial Transplant.* 2000 Sep;15(9):1367-72 ndt.oxfordjournals.org/cgi/reprint/15/9/1367

[771] Santos-Ocampo AS, Mandell BF, Fessler BJ. Alveolar hemorrhage in systemic lupus erythematosus: presentation and management. *Chest.* 2000 Oct;118(4):1083-90 chestjournal.org/cgi/content/full/118/4/1083

[772] Choi BG, Yoo WH. Successful treatment of pure red cell aplasia with plasmapheresis in a patient with systemic lupus erythematosus. *Yonsei Med J.* 2002 Apr;43(2):274-8 eymj.org/2002/pdf/04274.pdf

[773] "Further analyses for the active constituents of the acetone extracts through column chromatography indicated that [6]-gingerol and [10]-gingerol, which are the pungent principles, are mainly responsible for the cholagogic effect of ginger." Yamahara J, Miki K, Chisaka T, Sawada T, Fujimura H, Tomimatsu T, Nakano K, Nohara T. Cholagogic effect of ginger and its active constituents. *J Ethnopharmacol.* 1985;13(2):217-25

[774] "On the basis of the present findings, it appears that curcumin induces contraction of the human gall-bladder." Rasyid A, Lelo A. The effect of curcumin and placebo on human gall-bladder function: an ultrasound study. *Aliment Pharmacol Ther.* 1999 Feb;13(2):245-9

[775] "Significant anticholestatic activity was also observed against carbon tetrachloride induced cholestasis in conscious rat, anaesthetized guinea pig and cat. Picroliv was more active than the known hepatoprotective drug silymarin." Saraswat B, Visen PK, Patnaik GK, Dhawan BN. Anticholestatic effect of picroliv, active hepatoprotective principle of Picrorhiza kurrooa, against carbon tetrachloride induced cholestasis. *Indian J Exp Biol.* 1993 Apr;31(4):316-8

[776] "We conclude that SIL counteracts TLC-induced cholestasis by preventing the impairment in both the BS-dependent and -independent fractions of the bile flow." Crocenzi FA, Sanchez Pozzi EJ, Pellegrino JM, Rodriguez Garay EA, Mottino AD, Roma MG. Preventive effect of silymarin against taurolithocholate-induced cholestasis in the rat. *Biochem Pharmacol.* 2003 Jul 15;66(2):355-64

[777] "Andrographolide from the herb Andrographis paniculata (whole plant) per se produces a significant dose (1.5-12 mg/kg) dependent choleretic effect (4.8-73%) as evidenced by increase in bile flow, bile salt, and bile acids in conscious rats and anaesthetized guinea pigs." Shukla B, Visen PK, Patnaik GK, Dhawan BN. Choleretic effect of andrographolide in rats and guinea pigs. *Planta Med.* 1992 Apr;58(2):146-9

[778] "The extract also produced an increase in normal bile flow in rats suggesting a strong choleretic activity." Chandan BK, Sharma AK, Anand KK. Boerhaavia diffusa: a study of its hepatoprotective activity. *J Ethnopharmacol.* 1991 Mar;31(3):299-307

stimulation is worthy of clinical trials with pre- and post-intervention measurement of serum immune complexes and other clinical indexes.[779]

7. **Ensure generous bowel movements and consider therapeutic purgatives** (*purge: to free from impurities*): Dysbiotic patients should consume a low-fermentation fiber-rich diet that allows for 1-2 very generous bowel movements per day. Constipation must absolutely be eliminated—pun intended; for patients being treated for dysbiosis of any type, constipation is absolutely unacceptable, since the gastrointestinal tract provides the largest burden of pro-inflammatory (e.g., endotoxin, bacterial DNA) and anti-metabolic (e.g., D-lactate, H2S) microbial debris and metabolites. Patients with severe or recalcitrant dysbiosis can start the day with a laxative dose of ascorbic acid (e.g., 20-60 grams with 4 cups of water) and should expect liquid diarrhea within 30-60 minutes. The goal here is purgative physical removal of enteric microbes; in high concentrations, ascorbic acid has a direct antibacterial effect. Magnesium in elemental doses of 500-1,500 mg also helps soften stool and promote laxation. One-two cups of coffee promotes the laxative effect and provides some sense of pleasure to an otherwise not-so-pleasant experience; however, dysbiosis-affected patients often feel impressively better following therapeutic laxation. Rapid-acting antimicrobials, such as iodine/iodide, can be coadministered. Electrolyte replacement, for example with salted vegetable juice, is advisable for patients using therapeutic laxation on a regular basis.

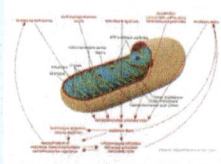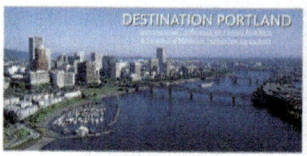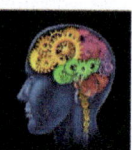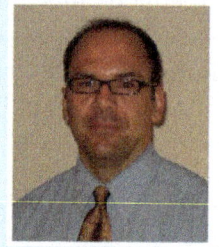

2013 INTERNATIONAL CONFERENCE ON HUMAN NUTRITION AND FUNCTIONAL MEDICINE

PORTLAND OREGON CONVENTION CENTER • SEPTEMBER 25-29, 2013

Antirheumatic Use of Antimicrobial Drugs with Neuroendocrine Interventions in the Treatment of Autoimmunity

Alex Vasquez D.C., N.D., D.O., F.A.C.N.

2013 presentation and slides:
- Presentation slides: CreateSpace.com/4478800
- Video access: vimeo.com/ichnfm/drv2013dysbiosisdrugs
- Password: DrV2013DysbiosisDrugs.

The clinical implementation of an anti-dysbiosis program must be tailored to the patient's overall condition and his/her willingness to implement the above-mentioned treatment options. Some patients are only willing to take a few treatments, while empowered autonomous nonmasochistic patients are more willing to do **whatever is necessary** in order to regain their health, even if it means taking numerous supplements, improving diet, starting/ending the day with enemas, and making appropriate changes in lifestyle and relationships to improve immune function. To the extent that we *first, do no harm*, all of the above-mentioned therapeutic interventions are reasonable "alternatives" to life-long medicalization, surgery, and immune-system destroying high-dose chemotherapy, which is astoundingly expensive, highly hazardous, and incompletely effective. **Patients with autoimmune diseases have numerous, largely untapped options for the treatment of their autoimmune diseases**; therefore, (pseudo)justifying lethal and expensive and devastating medical interventions on the basis of a "lack of other treatment alternatives"[780] when reasonable, safe, and effective options have not been implemented is scientifically inaccurate, ethically untenable, and medicolegally questionable.

---

[779] Vasquez A. Do the Benefits of Botanical and Physiotherapeutic Hepatobiliary Stimulation Result From Enhanced Excretion of IgA Immune Complexes? *Naturopathy Digest* 2006; January: naturopathydigest.com/archives/2006/jan/vasquez_immune.php

[780] Binks M, Passweg JR, Furst D, et al. Phase I/II trial of autologous stem cell transplantation in systemic sclerosis: procedure related mortality and impact on skin disease. *Ann Rheum Dis.* 2001 Jun;60(6):577-84 ard.bmjjournals.com/cgi/content/full/60/6/577

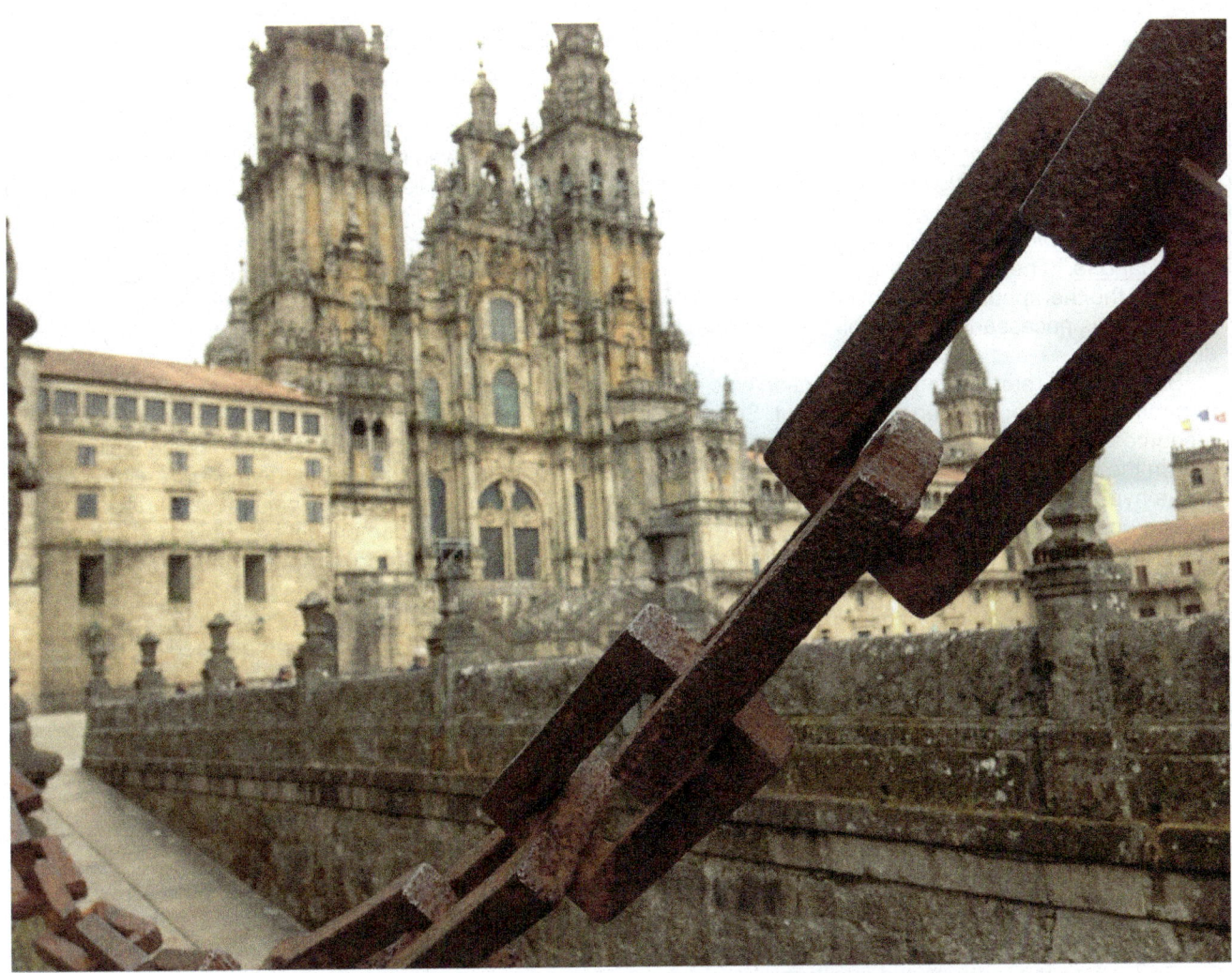

Santiago De Compostela: "Many chains have been laid upon man so that he should no longer behave like an animal, and he has in truth become gentler, more spiritual, more joyful, more reflective than any other animal is. Now, however, he suffers: from having worn his chains for so long, from being deprived for so long of clean air and free movement. These chains are those heavy and pregnant errors contained in the conceptions of morality, religion and metaphysics. Only when this sickness from one's chains has also been overcome will the first great goal have truly been attained: the separation of man from the animals. We stand now in the midst of our work of removing these chains, and we need to proceed with the greatest caution." Nietzsche FW. *Human, All Too Human*, Section: *The Wanderer and His Shadow*

❷ Infections & Dysbiosis—Part 2: Viral Dysbiosis & DrV's Antiviral Strategy

Introduction
The sections that follow detail and organize the four main components of my antiviral strategy. This section originated in _Mastery of Common Clinical Disorders_[1] in 2009; the work was refreshed and reformatted for publication in _Rheumatology v3.5_[2] in 2014 and immediately thereafter published as a separate book in print and digital formats— _Antiviral Strategies and Immune Nutrition: Against Colds, Flu, Herpes, AIDS, Hepatitis, Ebola, and Autoimmunity: A Concept-Based and Evidence-Based Handbook and Research Review for Practical Use._[3] The antiviral strategy described here differs from the FINDSEX ® protocol, although obviously many of the therapeutics overlap; clearly, both protocols can be used at the same time. The conceptual framework is necessarily different in treating specific viral infections from treating long-term inflammatory diseases. Because the reformatting of this section was stylized for _both_ print _and_ digital formats, the layout is different from other sections intended only for print. Specifically for the digital publication, hyperlinks to articles and other resources are included in body of the text rather than—as in the other chapters and sections—being included only in the footnotes. The obvious rationale for this difference is to facilitate access via the digital version's active hyperlinks to additional resources so that clinicians can make immediate POC (point of care) decisions. The goal of providing this antiviral strategy and the clinical protocols that comprise it is simply **to efficiently communicate in a practical and authoritative/cited manner antiviral protocols that can be understood and implemented in real time**; reflecting on my days as a hospital intern with no time to spare and yet no room for errors in the implementation of treatment decisions, I've striven to deliver these protocols in a manner that is brief and efficient, bordering on terse. Readers can (re)read the work and access the hyperlinks and resources for more details. This work is paradigm-shifting, and while the information is presented efficiently for point-of-care implementation, readers will need to spend time with the material and accompanying videos and hyperlinked materials in order to fully grasp the concepts and approach for clinical mastery. See video presentation: https://vimeo.com/album/3086248. Password: AntiViral_Nutrition_Strategy

Topics in Antiviral Strategies and Immune Nutrition:

1) Diagrams Explaining Viruses, Antiviral Strategies, and Viral Infections
2) Viral Infections and General Disease Patterns—Recent News and Important Concepts
   1. 2014—the year of new and impressively acute viral infections
   2. Vaccine cautions and questions
   3. Viral infections cause/contribute to autoimmune diseases
   4. Human endogenous retroviruses (HERVs) clearly play a role in autoimmune diseases
   5. Bacteriophages (viruses that infect bacteria) associated with autoimmune diseases
3) Common Viruses—Overview in Table Format
4) Four-part Plan of Interconnected and Overlapping AntiViral Strategies: Molecular Basis and Clinical Support
   1. Antiviral
   2. Antireplication
   3. Immunonutrition
   4. Cell-System Support

---

[1] Vasquez A. _Chiropractic and Naturopathic Mastery of Common Clinical Disorders_. www.createspace.com/3753564. See www.amazon.com/author/alexvasquez for any updates.
[2] Vasquez A. _Functional Medicine Rheumatology v3.5_. https://www.createspace.com/5014558. _Naturopathic Rheumatology v3.5_. See amazon.com/author/alexvasquez for updates.
[3] Vasquez A. _Antiviral Strategies and Immune Nutrition: Against Colds, Flu, Herpes, AIDS, Hepatitis, Ebola, and Autoimmunity: A Concept-Based and Evidence-Based Handbook and Research Review for Practical Use_. Print: createspace.com/5058779 Digital: amazon.com/dp/B00OPJXMTS

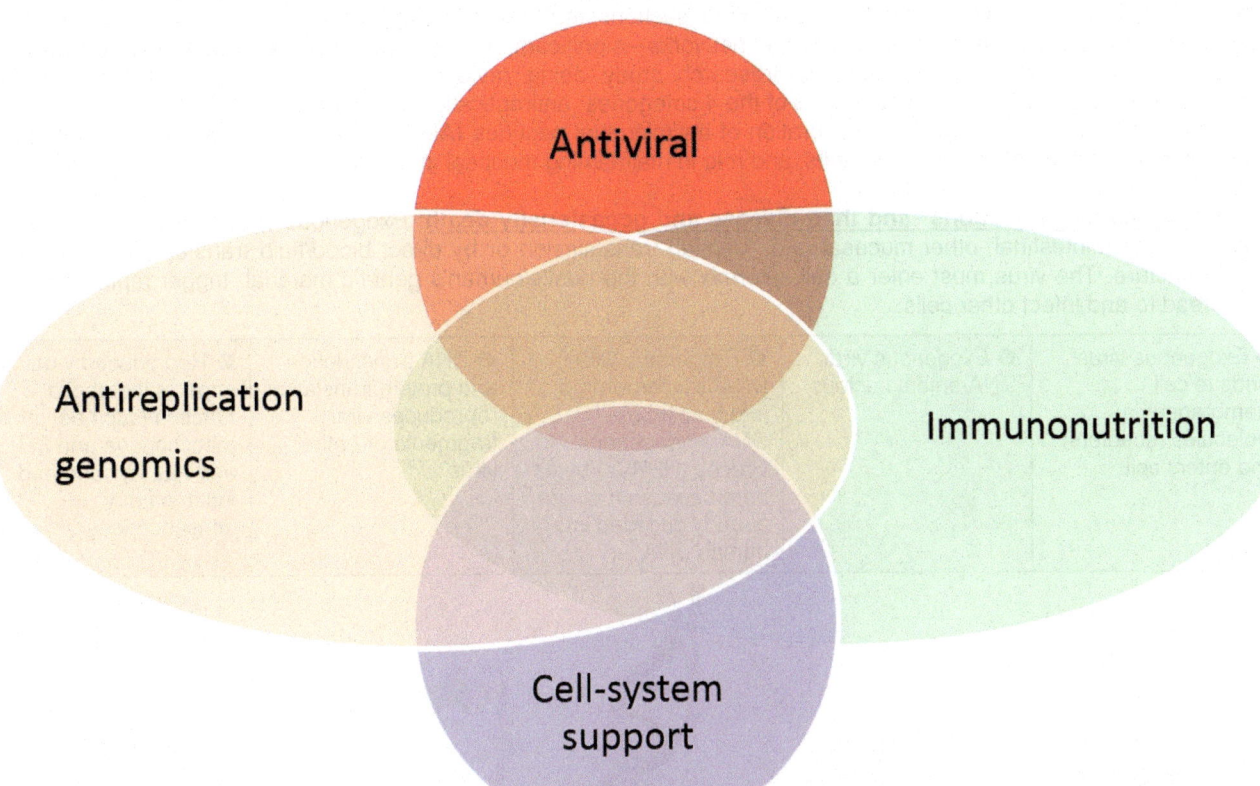

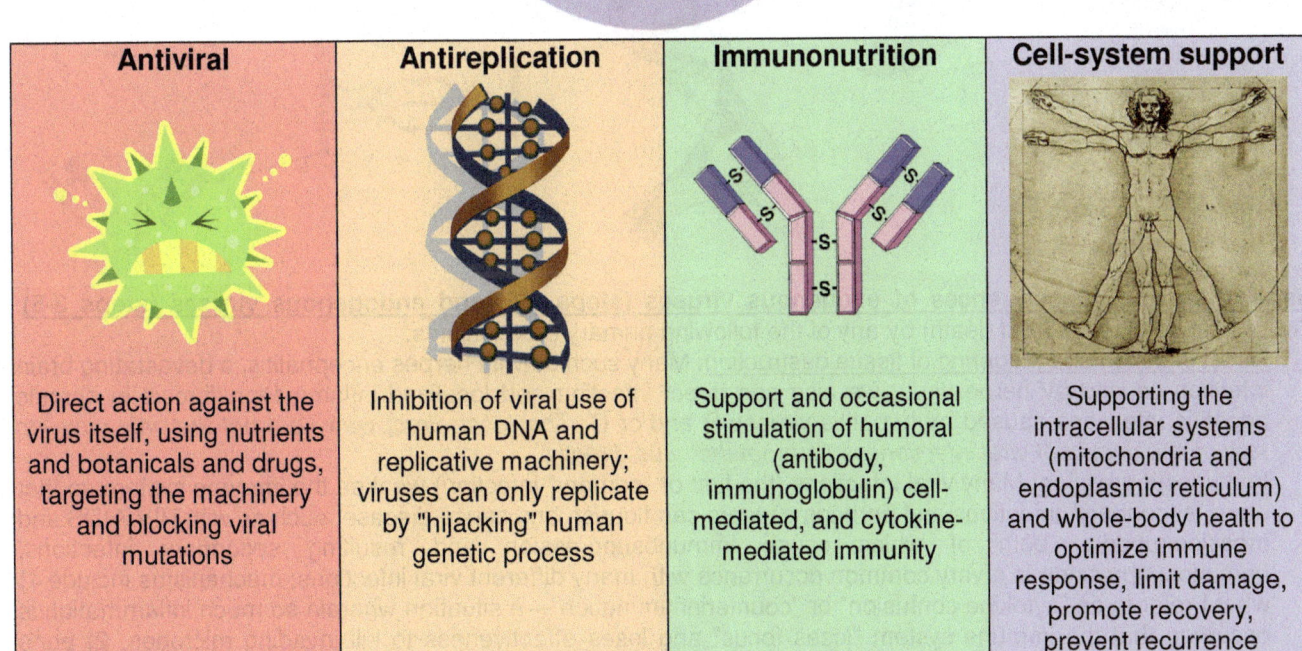

Antiviral	**Antireplication**	**Immunonutrition**	**Cell-system support**
Direct action against the virus itself, using nutrients and botanicals and drugs, targeting the machinery and blocking viral mutations	Inhibition of viral use of human DNA and replicative machinery; viruses can only replicate by "hijacking" human genetic process	Support and occasional stimulation of humoral (antibody, immunoglobulin) cell-mediated, and cytokine-mediated immunity	Supporting the intracellular systems (mitochondria and endoplasmic reticulum) and whole-body health to optimize immune response, limit damage, promote recovery, prevent recurrence

Antiviral strategies: Per this author's pattern recognition of the primary means to alleviate human suffering due to viral illness—acute, chronic, degenerative, autoimmune—therapeutic interventions and interventional therapeutics can be organized under the main headings of 1) antiviral—targeting the virus specifically, whether by eradication (using disinfectants, avoidance, hand-washing, etc) or direct anti-viral botanicals, nutrients, or pharmaceuticals, 2) antireplicative interventions—aimed at targeting the mechanisms of viral replication; most drugs work at this level, as do many nutrients, 3) immunonutrition and immune support—using interventions in general and nutrients in particular to support and occasionally stimulate immune function, and 4) cellular support and whole-systems biology, body-based approaches; integration; all too often, viral infections are viewed and treated as separate from the immune system; even more commonly viral infections are viewed and treated as separate from the body being infected, which must mount the immune response, and which is responsible for transcribing and therefore "making the virus." This fourth category includes cellular support—the reason for this should be increasingly obvious as clinicians appreciate that viral infections induce endoplasmic reticulum stress and mitochondrial dysfunction—and whole-systems body-based support. The following literature compilation is organized into the following four sections; readers should appreciate that—especially for nutrients since they always work on multiple pathways and networks—significant overlap exists and that organizational decisions were made per emphasis of the particular research study being reviewed; as such, for example, vitamin D3 (cholecalciferol) plays major roles in at least 3 of the 4 categories: antireplication via inhibition of NFkB and promotion of DNA methylation, immunonutrition via elaboration of antimicrobial peptides (AMP), and cell-system support via its anti-inflammatory effects, antidepressant benefits, and role in maintaining mucosal integrity.

How viruses cause "infections" and then disease and occasionally death: Exogenous viruses enter the body via respiratory, gastrointestinal, other mucosal (e.g., genital) transmission or by direct blood/fluid transfer via a wound or needle puncture. The virus must enter a cell, intermix with the host's/human's genetic material, trigger replication and then spread to and infect other cells.

❶ Exogenous virus binds to cell membrane (via molecules/receptors) and enters cell	❷ Exogenous viral DNA enters nucleus	❸ Exogenous viral DNA is incorporated into host (human) DNA; endogenous viruses (HERVs) begin here because they are already encoded into human DNA	❹ DNA transcription and protein translation reproduces viral fragments or entire virus	❺ Reproduced virus impacts metabolic function (such as mitochondria and ER) and has immune and inflammatory consequences

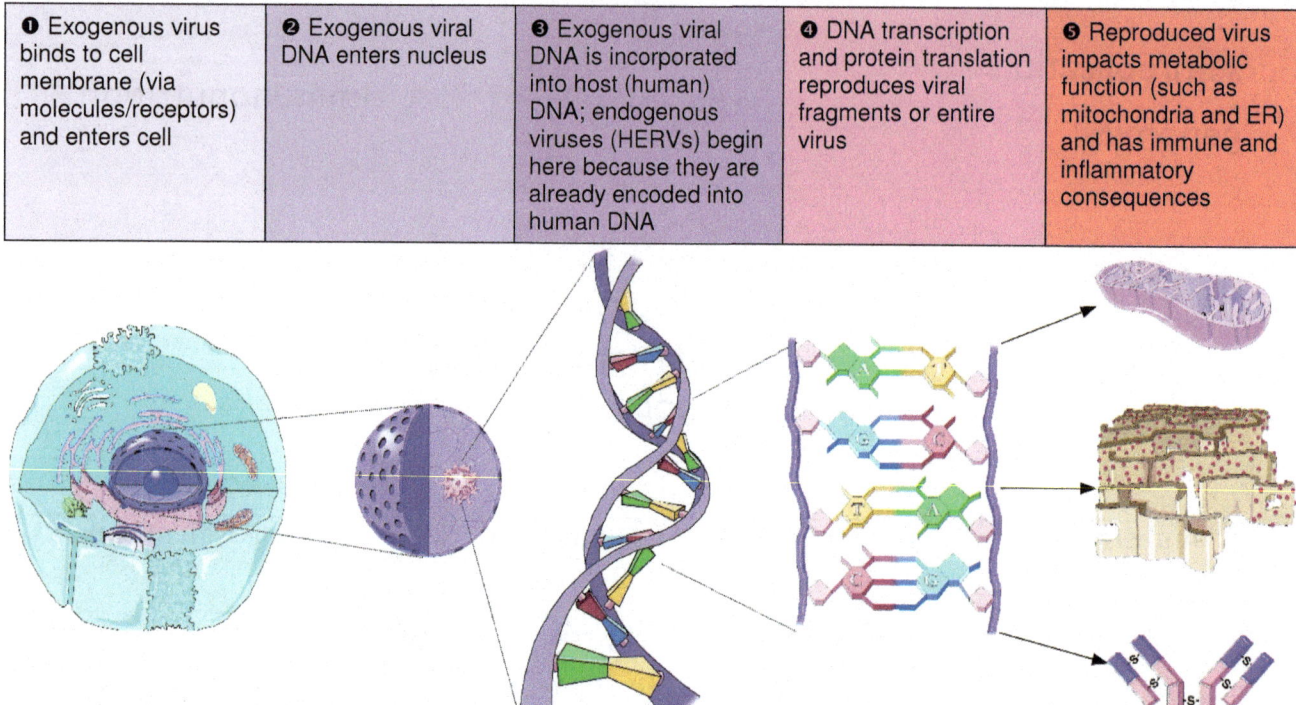

Replication and consequences of exogenous viruses (steps 1-5) and endogenous viruses (steps 3-5):
Viruses cause disease (and death) by any of the following primary mechanisms:

1) <u>Direct infection and triggering of tissue destruction</u>: Many such as with herpes encephalitis, a devastating brain infection caused by herpesvirus; we also see direct infection and localized inflammation/fibrosis in chronic hepatitis infections caused by hepatitis viruses B and/or C. *The most direct way—but not the only way—to reduce the impact of viral infections is to target the virus directly.*

2) <u>Immunosuppression</u>: Many viral infections (the first or "primary" infection) weaken the immune system so that other "secondary" infections and perhaps cancers can flourish and cause disease, such as with HIV/AIDS and measles/rubeola, both of which cause immunosuppression and resulting secondary infections. Immunosuppression is a very common occurrence with many different viral infections; mechanisms include 1) what I refer to as "cytokine confusion" or "counterinflammation"—a situation wherein so much inflammation is occurring that the immune system "loses focus" and loses effectiveness to kill invading microbes, 2) bone marrow suppression, leading to reduced numbers of immune cells (lymphocytes, lymphocytopenia), and 3) lymphocyte destruction (apoptosis, necrosis). *Thus, an important means by which to limit the impact of viral illnesses is to support the immune system to attack the virus and to avoid/counteract the immune suppression.*

3) <u>Sustained cellular dysfunction and "slow death"</u>: Viruses can trigger rapid cell death and tissue destruction as mentioned previously; in other situations, the progression of cellular death is much slower and occurs via process of protracted cellular impairment, such as mitochondrial dysfunction or endoplasmic reticulum stress, both of which cause cellular dysfunction and inflammation. For example, herpes simplex virus type-1 causes recurrent oral/mucosal lesions (painful blisters) in its acute form, and this same virus appears capable of causing protracted "slow infections" that contribute to Alzheimer's disease and dementia as well. *Thus, an important means by which to limit the impact of viral illnesses is to support cellular functions such as mitochondrial function in order to limit excess damage and inflammation and to promote more rapid recovery.*

4) <u>Cytokine storm, shock, hemorrhage</u>: Some viruses trigger cellular/tissue damage and a massive inflammatory response that causes hemodynamic instability and shock (loss of blood volume and blood pressure), which can cause death. Loss of blood volume can occur via damage to blood vessels that allows fluid (plasma) to leak into the tissues (vascular leak); loss of blood volume can also occur via bleeding/hemorrhage if the blood cannot clot/coagulate due to loss of platelets and/or loss of clotting proteins due to inflammation-induced liver damage. Platelet count can be reduced via anti-platelet antibodies, by inflammation-induced impairment of bone marrow function, and by destruction of platelets in the spleen (hypersplenism). Cytokine storm is one of the mechanisms noted with Ebola infection. *Thus, an important means by which to limit the impact of viral illnesses is to modulate—control or limit—the excessive immune response since much of the damage is cause by excess inflammation and not by the virus itself.*

5) <u>Autoimmunity</u>: Somewhat related to the cytokine storm mentioned previously is the induction of severe and sustained systemic inflammation, generally accompanied by other factors such as molecular mimicry and immune-complex deposition, which appears to be particularly relevant for rheumatologic conditions such as systemic lupus erythematosus (SLE, lupus), Sjogren's syndrome, scleroderma and systemic sclerosis. Very importantly, patients can have multiple viral and bacterial infections at the same time, thus leading to and accounting for the different "patterns of inflammation" that we see clinically with "different" so-called autoimmune diseases. *Thus, we need to address the viral component of many "chronic" and "degenerative" and "autoimmune" diseases.*

Within each cell (except RBC), the nucleus contains DNA, from which viruses (either endogenous or exogenous) are replicated, depending on epigenetic modifications such as DNA methylation and inflammatory/dietary activation of transcription factors such as NF-kappaB, with the viral products affecting function and responses of the mitochondria (e.g., mitoinflammation, destruction of mitochondrial DNA and thus the ETC), endoplasmic reticulum (e.g., endoplasmic reticulum stress and the resultant unfolded protein response), and immune system (e.g., inflammatory responses [e.g., NFkB], cytokine release [e.g., interferon], antibody generation and immune complex formation). Patients with autoimmune conditions such as lupus, scleroderma, and Sjogren's show heightened immunoinflammatory responses against numerous endogenous and exogenous viruses—clear examples of viral polydysbiosis, or polyviral dysbiosis. Nutrients such as folinic acid / methylfolate and betaine can supply and transfer the methyl groups necessary for the epigenetic silencing of viral sequences, suppression of viral replication and the promotion of viral latency; other nutrients such as vitamin D3 help coordinate the pattern of DNA methylation away from inflammation and viral replication and toward stabilized homeodynamics. Viral infections can themselves alter epigenetic control of DNA transcription and in this way—along with other transactivating mechanisms such as NFkB activation—promote additional viral replication; likewise, other proinflammatory dietary (e.g., hyperglycemia), microbial (e.g., bacteria, SIBO), xenobiotic and pharmaceutical (e.g., hydralazine [antihypertensive vasodilator], procainamide [antiarrhythmic]) can promote viral replication via epigenetic and inflammatory mechanisms. Epigenetic modifications induced by microbes[4] can be termed "microbial epigenetic dysregulation" or "microbe-induced reversible epigenetic reprogramming." Appreciating the 5-part sequence of viral infections (depicted above) is important for forming rational strategies against *the clinical consequences of viral infections* because each step implies specific preventive and/or therapeutic options. For steps 1-3, the goal is prevention of contact/spread, promoting immunologic recognition with vaccinations to prevent severe acute primary illness, and the "herd immunity" concept; related to these first steps is the concept of immunonutrition which serves to optimize immune function so that when/if a viral agent is encountered it will be well controlled (ie, the immunonutritional equivalent of immunopreparation via vaccination). At step #4, we suddenly have an impressive array of interventions at our immediate disposal because by using nutrients (including botanicals) we can significantly modify DNA expression and viral replication; this area of intervention is the main focus of the antiviral nutritional strategy. Area #5 deals with supporting metabolic/physiologic functions so that the consequences of viral infections are minimized; for example, mitochondria-specific nutrients such as co-enzyme Q10 can be used to protect mitochondrial from virus-induced or inflammation-mediated mitochondrial dysfunction. Similarly, nutrients and botanicals might be used—along with dietary interventions—to alleviate endoplasmic reticulum stress and—specifically per my nutritional immunomodulation protocol described in Chapter 4 of *Functional Inflammology, volume 1* and/or *Naturopathic Rheumatology v3.5*—to alleviate the immunohyperreactivity that commonly complicates otherwise mild or benign microbial colonizations (dysbiosis). Further, nutritional and botanical interventions provide many options for direct anti-viral, virus-killing or virus-inactivating interventions—such as the use of ionized zinc, iodine/iodide, licorice extract, and the use of antioxidants such as vitamin E (generally speaking) and selenium to reduce the rate of viral mutations, which would otherwise allow viruses to change their behavior and molecular appearance and to thereby escape immune-mediated destruction.

---

[4] "This may result in epigenetic dysregulation and subsequent cellular dysfunctions that may manifest in or contribute to the development of pathological changes (e.g. initiation and progression of malignant neoplasms; immunodeficiency). Bacteria infecting mammals may cause diseases in a similar manner, by causing hypermethylation of key cellular promoters at CpG dinucleotides (promoter silencing, e.g. by Campylobacter rectus in the placenta or by Helicobacter pylori in gastric mucosa)." Minárovits J. Microbe-induced epigenetic alterations in host cells: the coming era of patho-epigenetics of microbial infections. *Acta Microbiol Immunol Hung.* 2009 Mar;56(1):1-19

Viral Infections and General Disease Patterns:
Recent News and Important Concepts

Topics for this section:
1) 2014—the year of new and impressively acute viral infections
2) Antiviral drugs and vaccines: cautions and questions
3) Viral infections cause/contribute to autoimmune diseases
4) Human endogenous retroviruses (HERVs) play a role in autoimmune diseases
5) Bacteriophages (viruses that infect bacteria) gain attention in clinical care

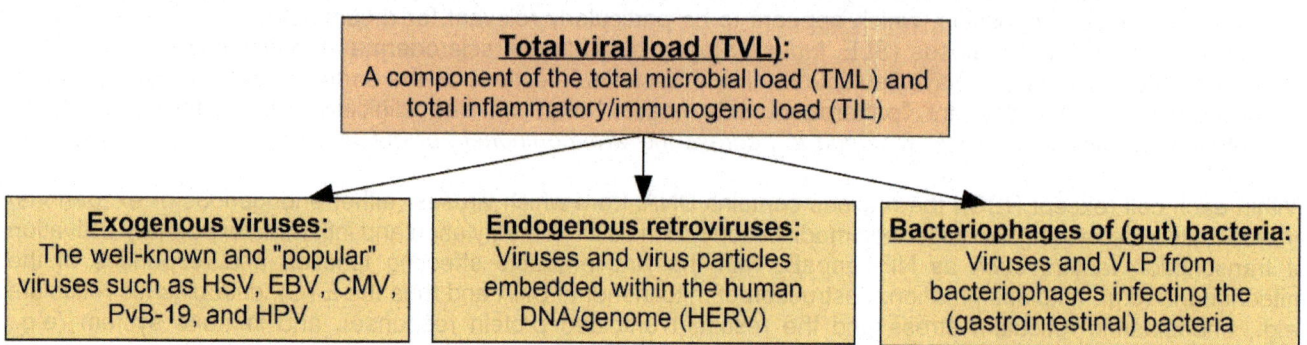

The total viral load (TVL): TVL contributes to TML (total microbial load) and thus to the TIL (total inflammatory load), to which are added the TCL (total carbohydrate load) and TXL (total xenobiotic load). This concept is discussed relevant to the treatment of autoimmunity in *Rheumatology v3.5* and later versions.

==2014—the start of ongoing viral panic==: In 2014, viral infections started making the news on a daily basis, causing appropriate/inappropriate concern (occasional panic) worldwide. The hysteria surrounding Ebola and the other "newsworthy" viral infections of 2014 was just the start; we have seen the manipulation of science and public perception continue into 2016, now with ongoing and apparently nonstop hysteria about mandatory vaccines and Zika virus. Discovered more than 70 years ago, Zika was a relatively benign virus that was suddenly blamed for microcephaly in Brazil in 2016, exactly one year following the introduction of mandatory vaccines for pregnant women, the introduction of genetically modified mosquitoes, and Brazil's ongoing catastrophic overuse of pesticides, which have been consistently linked with microcephaly internationally for decades. Viruses are the perfect scapegoat for mandating vaccines, ignoring other social and biomedical causes of disease, and controlling and distracting the international population via fearmongering.

❶ ==2014—the year of "new" and impressively acute viral infections==: Strange, new and aggressive viral infections have been making international headlines and inspiring the appropriate/intended fear and social paralysis. This news is available widely through international news services; some important updates, links, and summaries are also posted here www.facebook.com/AntiviralNutrition on an ongoing basis.
   o Ebola: Ebola virus infections started becoming epidemic in parts of Africa—"The 2014 Ebola epidemic is the largest in history, affecting multiple countries in West Africa."[5]—causing thousands of deaths, contributed to by delays in healthcare delivery and rampant malnutrition in these regions. The infection soon spread to Europe and the United States via airline travel; healthcare workers (nurses and doctors) and aviation employees (pilots and flight attendants) are considered to be at particularly high risk of exposure.
   o Enterovirus D68—a rare viral infection causing several deaths across America: Enterovirus D68 (EV-D68) is one of more than 100 non-polio enteroviruses[6]; possible viral mutations or emergence of a new strain

---

[5] cdc.gov/vhf/ebola/outbreaks/2014-west-africa/index.html
[6] cdc.gov/non-polio-enterovirus/about/ev-d68.html

have caused hundreds of infections and several deaths.[7] In 2014, US CDC recommended consideration of D68 "as a possible cause of acute, unexplained severe respiratory illness, even if the patient does not have fever."[8]

- o Measles—return of a virus thought to be eliminated: "From January 1 to May 23, 2014, 288 confirmed cases were reported to the CDC, a figure that exceeds the highest reported annual total number of cases (220 cases in 2011) since measles was declared eliminated in the United States in 2000."[9] "This year the United States is experiencing a record number of measles cases. From January 1 to September 29, there have been 594 confirmed measles cases reported to CDC's National Center for Immunization and Respiratory Diseases (NCIRD). This is the highest number of cases since measles elimination was documented in the U.S. in 2000."[10]

- o Other viruses such as influenza, hepatitis B and C, and HIV/AIDs: At the same time the aforementioned "new" viral infections and recurrences are making headlines, the "older" viruses have not ceased making their mortal impact; other viruses such as influenza, hepatitis B and C, and HIV/AIDs continue to kill tens-hundreds of thousands of people each year.

❷ **Antiviral drug costs and inefficacy; vaccine cautions and questions**: Vaccines and antiviral drugs are expensive, not readily accessible (especially internationally), and—particularly vaccines—are associated with numerous adverse effects, the vast majority of which are underreported. The problems with antiviral drugs are numerous, including:

1) Large financial burden to healthcare, state, national systems: High cost,

2) Antiviral drugs require frequent/consistent dosing: Need for frequent/uninterrupted daily dosing to prevent viral mutations or relapse.

3) Adverse metabolic effects: Numerous adverse effects, such as metabolic impairment (leading to, for example, diabetes and lipodystrophy),

4) Allergy and intolerance: Occasional allergy and intolerance,

5) Lack of ready availability: Lack of availability (in addition to lack of affordability) in many international populations,

6) Overspecificity prohibits general antiviral effectiveness: Of supreme importance—antiviral drugs' high specificity: antiviral drugs generally block *one* pathway/enzyme in one virus or a limited number of viruses within the same class; if the virus undergoes mutation *as viruses are notorious for doing* in a way that alters the drug target or bypasses the targeted pathway/enzyme, then the drug can immediately become ineffective,

7) Replication-inefficacy paradox: What I will call here the "viral-replication drug-inefficacy paradox": Antiviral drugs tend to be less effective or ineffective in viral diseases characterized by slow viral replication; if the drug is targeting a metabolic pathway, but the pathway is not used at a high rate, then the drug is not highly effective (example: herpes keratitis[11]). Conversely, if the virus has a high rate of replication, then it likely has a high/higher rate of mutation as well, and if targeted pathways/enzymes mutate or are bypassed, then the drug will lose effectiveness/efficacy,

8) Small window of opportunity: Antiviral drugs often have to be administered early in the course of the disease to be effective; this is actually true of many therapeutics—including nutrients and botanicals—and is because of the obvious: treatments are most effective when the number of viral replications/copies is still low and before the virus has had the opportunity to mutate and become resistant to the treatment.

9) Low clinical significance despite "statistical significance" in large studies: At their best, many antiviral drugs—such as for influenza—only reduce duration of illness by a couple/few days. In contrast, antiHIV drugs have a solid record of success in the long-term management of HIV infection, but with significant cost and very frequent adverse effects of the multidrug/polypharmacy regimens/cocktails that have to be

---

[7] washingtonpost.com/posttv/national/health-science/how-a-virus-like-enterovirus-d68-mutates/2014/10/14/5872ee28-53c1-11e4-b86d-184ac281388d_video.html

[8] cdc.gov/non-polio-enterovirus/hcp/EV-D68-hcp.html

[9] 2014 Oct emedicine.medscape.com/article/966220-overview

[10] 2014 Oct cdc.gov/measles/cases-outbreaks.html

[11] "HSV-1 multiplication rates have been shown to vary in different tissues and the rate of multiplication may correlate with susceptibility to antiviral chemotherapy. Herpetic stromal keratitis is a necrotizing condition refractive to antiviral therapy and this lack of antiviral efficacy in stromal disease may be the result of very low rates of viral replication in the corneal stromal keratocytes." Upadhyay et a. The effect of HSV multiplication rate on antiviral drug efficacy in vitro. *Antiviral Res.* 1991 Jan;15(1):67-76

used. For example, some antiviral drugs used for acute infections reduce the duration of illness only by a few days; on the one hand this is simply a convenience for most patients while on the other hand—especially for elderly or immune-suppressed patients, this small curtailment of the duration of illness can be quite important.

10) <u>Distraction from other measures, many of which provide enhanced overall health and collateral benefits</u>: Sole reliance and overemphasis on vaccinations distracts doctors and patients from other measures that can be taken to reduce the incidence and morbidity/mortality associated with infectious diseases; this is especially true for improvement in nutritional status and overall health, two areas where medical students/physicians are notoriously undertrained.

11) <u>Administration to malnourished patients impairs optimal response</u>: Antiviral drugs and vaccinations are generally administered in isolation (without other immune-supporting treatments) by medical doctors untrained in nutrition despite research showing enhanced immunological health and overall health when nutritional supplementation is provided. A much more successful approach would be to use these antiviral drugs along with nutritional therapies such as vitamin D, folic acid, betaine and SAMe, as will be discussed in following sections on therapeutics; for an immediate representative example of improved drug efficacy with the coadministration of nutritional therapy, please see the following sample research/hyperlinks—which will be reviewed/detailed later:

   - <u>Supplementation with zinc, but not vitamin A, improves seroconversion to vibriocidal antibody in children given an oral cholera vaccine</u> (*J Infect Dis*. 2003 Mar[12]):
     www.ncbi.nlm.nih.gov/pubmed/12660937
   - <u>SAMe and betaine improve antiviral drug response</u> (*PLoS One* 2010 Nov[13]):
     www.ncbi.nlm.nih.gov/pmc/articles/PMC2975710/

Nothing I state here nor elsewhere in this book is "anti-vaccination" nor "anti-drug" nor "anti-medicine"; in this first section, I am simply providing some discussion and a few samples of readily available research to contextualize and balance the pro-vaccination, pro-drug, and pro-medicine "news", television shows, advertisements (30 hours per year for the average American), and mandates to which we are daily exposed and which has resulted in the clear overuse of drug treatments and aggregation of the associated iatrogenic morbidity/mortality and disease-care costs.[14] The strengths and weaknesses of various approaches will be made plain in the following sections via quotes directly from research organized per topic; readers are encouraged to read and review the information and then arrive at their own conclusions. Regardless of any controversy on the

---

[12] Albert et al. Supplementation with zinc, but not vitamin A, improves seroconversion to vibriocidal antibody in children given an oral cholera vaccine. *J Infect Dis*. 2003 Mar 15;187(6):909-13

[13] Filipowicz et al. S-adenosyl-methionine and betaine improve early virological response in chronic hepatitis C patients with previous nonresponse. *PLoS One*. 2010 Nov 8;5(11):e15492 http://www.plosone.org/article/info%3Adoi%2F10.1371%2Fjournal.pone.0015492

[14] Substantiation of this point is readily available to anyone who wishes to access the facts; some familiar/notable/recent references are provided here: "Our findings suggest that Americans who watch average amounts of television may be exposed to more than 30 hours of direct-to-consumer drug advertisements each year, far surpassing their exposure to other forms of health communication." Brownfield et al. Direct-to-consumer drug advertisements on network television. *J Health Commun*. 2004 Nov-Dec;9(6):491-7 "Americans popped more pills than ever last year." Wile R. America Is More Medicated Than Ever. 2012 Sep http://www.businessinsider.com/america-is-more-medicated-than-ever-2012-9 "U.S. Centers for Disease Control and Prevention indicates: Americans buy much more medicine per person than any other country." Savoia S, AP. America: The land of the medicated? People in U.S. consuming more medicine than ever before. http://www.nbcnews.com/id/7503122/ns/health-health_care/t/america-land-medicated/#.VEGVXfldVS1 Also reported via http://www.cbsnews.com/news/america-the-medicated/. Barber C. The Medicated Americans: Antidepressant Prescriptions on the Rise: Close to 10 percent of men and women in America are now taking drugs to combat depression. http://www.scientificamerican.com/article/the-medicated-americans/ "Privately insured surgical patients who had a complication provided hospitals with a 330% higher profit margin than those without a complication, … Medicare patients with a complication produced a 190% higher margin. The findings mean that, for hospital managers, efforts to reduce surgical complications could result in substantially worsened financial performance." Harvard School of Public Health. For immediate release: April 16, 2013: Patients with surgical complications provide greater hospital profit-margins. http://www.hsph.harvard.edu/news/press-releases/patients-with-surgical-complications-provide-greater-hospital-profit-margins/ "Recent estimates suggest that each year more than 1 million patients are injured while in the hospital and approximately 180,000 die because of these injuries. Furthermore, drug-related morbidity and mortality are common and are estimated to cost more than $136 billion a year." Holland, Degruy. Drug-induced disorders. *Am Fam Physician*. 1997 Nov http://www.ncbi.nlm.nih.gov/pubmed/9371009 I find the situation very odd that this article appears to have been removed from the AAFP website, even though the associated Letter is still posted. http://www.aafp.org/afp/1998/0601/p2615.html "More than 4 billion prescriptions were written in 2011. That's the most ever. Everything from sleeping pills to drugs for anxiety and depression—you name it. … The question medical ethicists are asking is 'if we are taking entirely too many pills for our own good? Something changed in the 1990s, when it became legal for drug makers to advertise. And that's created a sense on the part of many patients who say 'I saw that ad on television. I think I should be on that medicine.' Demand for drugs skyrocketed." http://www.today.com/video/today/51490407/#51490407 America spends $60,000,000 per week on healthcare/diseasecare/drugcare. http://video.msnbc.msn.com/jansing-and-co/50906214#50906214 "These findings add to the weight of evidence that DTC advertising likely promotes unnecessary treatment, which in turn would lead to excessive prescription drug spending. By now, we are all familiar with the ubiquitous pharmaceutical advertisements that attract our attention during commercial breaks interspersed within our television programming. But now, we can be more certain that this advertising is, in fact, marketing—not public health service announcements—at that, at least in some circumstances, it is effectively getting someone to buy something that they do not need." Ross JS, Kravitz RL. Direct-to-consumer television advertising: time to turn off the tube? *J Gen Intern Med*. 2013 Jul;28(7):862-4 http://www.ncbi.nlm.nih.gov/pmc/articles/PMC3682047/ Smith R. Medical journals are an extension of the marketing arm of pharmaceutical companies. *PLoS Med*. 2005 May;2(5):e138 http://www.ncbi.nlm.nih.gov/pmc/articles/PMC1140949/ "China has fined the British pharmaceuticals giant GlaxoSmithKline (GSK) $488.8 million (3 billion Yuan) for a "massive bribery network" to get doctors and hospitals to use its products. Five former employees were sentenced to two to four years in jail, but ordered deported instead of imprisoned, according to state news agency Xinhua today." Xiao K. GlaxoSmithKline fined $488.8M for massive bribery network. 2014 Sep http://abc7chicago.com/news/glaxosmithkline-fined-$4888m-for-massive-bribery-network-/316390/ Connolly C. U.S. Patients Spend More but Don't Get More, Study Finds: Even in Advantaged Areas, Americans Often Receive Inadequate Health Care. *Washington Post*, May 5, 2004. Starfield B. Is US health really the best in the world? *JAMA*. 2000;284(4):483-5.

risks and inefficacy of vaccinations, undue reliance on vaccinations as the main antiviral strategy is unsafe and unwise for a variety of reasons. Forcing the population to rely on vaccinations—*or any singular treatment for that matter*—as the major/sole antiviral strategy is fraught with logistical encumbrances and opportunities for financial profiteering at the expense/burden of the healthcare system and individual payers; no-one, no healthcare system, no country, nor the global community should ever put all of its assets into one approach if the goal is sustainability and success. The conflict of interest presented when pharmaceutical companies present data on the safety and efficacy of the same drugs from which they profit is ridiculously obvious. The denial of adverse vaccination events and the denigration of parents and patients who report them demonstrates the lack of scientific objectivism that occurs when power, profit, and paradigm are at stake. Meanwhile, documented and reliable reports of adverse vaccine effects/events justify appropriate precaution and warrant updates to the informed consent process and further question and cast doubt upon the ethical appropriateness of mandatory vaccination enforcement for employees, children, and students. Optimal vaccination response requires proper nutritional adequacy (e.g., zinc and vitamin D) and hormonal balance (e.g., DHEA); these factors need to be considered if vaccines are to be used to full and appropriate benefit.

- o American Thoracic Society: "Children Who Get Flu Vaccine Have 3x Risk of Hospitalization for Flu: "They found that children who had received the flu vaccine had three times the risk of hospitalization, as compared to children who had not received the vaccine. In asthmatic children, there was a significantly higher risk of hospitalization in subjects who received the TIV, as compared to those who did not ($p= 0.006$). But no other measured factors—such as insurance plans or severity of asthma—appeared to affect risk of hospitalization."
    - www.sciencedaily.com/releases/2009/05/090519172045.htm
    - http://www.eurekalert.org/pub_releases/2009-05/ats-fsn051209.php
- o Spectrum of post-vaccination inflammatory CNS demyelinating syndromes. (*Autoimmun Rev.* 2014 Mar): "The most commonly reported vaccinations that were associated with CNS demyelinating diseases included influenza (21 cases), human papilloma virus (HPV) (9 cases), hepatitis A or B (8 cases), rabies (5 cases), measles (5 cases), rubella (5 cases), yellow fever (3 cases), anthrax (2 cases), meningococcus (2 cases) and tetanus (2 cases). ... Usually the symptoms of the CNS demyelinating syndrome appear few days following the immunization (mean: 14.2 days) but there are cases where the clinical presentation was delayed (more than 3 weeks or even up to 5 months post-vaccination) (approximately a third of all the reported cases). In terms of the clinical presentation and the affected CNS areas, there is a great diversity among the reported cases of post-vaccination acute demyelinating syndromes."
    - http://www.ncbi.nlm.nih.gov/pubmed/24514081
    - http://www.sciencedirect.com/science/article/pii/S156899721300178X
- o Acute disseminated encephalomyelitis with severe neurological outcomes following virosomal seasonal influenza vaccine. (*Hum Vaccin Immunother.* 2014 May): "Acute disseminated encephalomyelitis (ADEM) is an inflammatory, usually monophasic, immune mediate, demyelinating disease of the central nervous system which involves the white matter. ADEM is more frequent in children and usually occurs after viral infections, but may follow vaccinations, bacterial infections, or may occur without previous events. Only 5% of cases of ADEM are preceded by vaccination within one month prior to symptoms onset."
    - http://www.ncbi.nlm.nih.gov/pubmed/24785431
    - https://www.landesbioscience.com/journals/vaccines/article/28961/
- o Two cases of vasculitis following HPV immunization (*Rheumatology Oxford.* 2013 Mar): "we report two cases of vasculitis following HPV immunization, which has not previously been described. Case 1, a 15-year-old girl, presented with three small purpuric lesions on the lower left leg 3 days after the second dose of the HPV vaccine."
    - http://www.ncbi.nlm.nih.gov/pubmed/22879461
    - http://rheumatology.oxfordjournals.org/content/52/3/581.long
- o Post-vaccination encephalomyelitis: literature review and illustrative case. (*J Clin Neurosci.* 2008 Dec): "Acute disseminated encephalomyelitis (ADEM) is an inflammatory demyelinating disease of the central nervous system that is usually considered a monophasic disease. ADEM forms one of several categories of primary inflammatory demyelinating disorders of the central nervous system including multiple sclerosis, optic neuropathy, acute transverse myelitis, and neuromyelitis optica (Devic's disease). ... Post-

vaccination ADEM has been associated with several vaccines such as rabies, diphtheria-tetanus-polio, smallpox, measles, mumps, rubella, Japanese B encephalitis, pertussis, influenza, hepatitis B, and the Hog vaccine."

- http://www.ncbi.nlm.nih.gov/pubmed/18976924
- http://www.sciencedirect.com/science/article/pii/S0967586808001896

o Acute disseminated encephalomyelitis following 2009 H1N1 influenza vaccine. (*Pediatr Int.* 2012 Aug): "We describe a previously healthy 2-year-old boy with ADEM, who exhibited high fever, lethargy, and recurrent seizures at 25 days after H1N1 influenza vaccination."

- http://www.ncbi.nlm.nih.gov/pubmed/22830541
- http://onlinelibrary.wiley.com/doi/10.1111/j.1442-200X.2011.03501.x/abstract

o Influenza Vaccine-Induced CNS Demyelination in a 50-Year-Old Male. (*Am J Case Rep.* 2014 Aug): "We report a case of a 50-year-old Caucasian male with a course of progressive, focal, neurologic deficits within 24 h after receiving the influenza vaccine. Subsequent work-up revealed the possibility of an acute central nervous system (CNS) demyelinating episode secondary to the influenza vaccine, best described as either CIS or ADEM."

- http://www.ncbi.nlm.nih.gov/pubmed/25175754
- http://www.ncbi.nlm.nih.gov/pmc/articles/PMC4159247/
- http://www.amjcaserep.com/download/index/idArt/891416

o Acute disseminated encephalomyelitis with severe neurological outcomes following virosomal seasonal influenza vaccine. (*Hum Vaccin Immunother.* 2014 May): "We describe the first case of ADEM occurred few days after administration of virosomal seasonal influenza vaccine. The patient, a 59-year-old caucasic man with unremarkable past medical history presented at admission decreased alertness, 10 days after flu vaccination. During the 2 days following hospitalization, his clinical conditions deteriorated with drowsiness and fever until coma. The magnetic resonance imaging of the brain showed multiple and symmetrical white matter lesions in both cerebellar and cerebral hemispheres, suggesting demyelinating disease with inflammatory activity, compatible with ADEM. The patient was treated with high dose of steroids and intravenous immunoglobulin with relevant sequelae and severe neurological outcomes."

- http://www.ncbi.nlm.nih.gov/pubmed/24785431
- https://www.landesbioscience.com/journals/vaccines/article/28961/

❸ **Viral infections cause/contribute to autoimmune diseases**: I categorize as "known" and/or "popular" those viruses that we commonly consider, such as Epstein-Bar virus (EBV), parvovirus B-19 (PvB19), cytomegalovirus (CMV), human papilloma virus (HPV) and other such viruses as we generally consider clinically and/or studied in whatever medical school we as clinicians attended. These have been described as epigenomic and/or exogenous viruses because they are close to but not part of the human genome—"epi" is a Greek-derived prefix denoting "above, on, over, nearby, upon"; these *epigenomic* viruses are contrasted with the *endogenous* viruses that are integrally "built in" to the human DNA. All four viruses mentioned in the previous sentence have been associated with autoimmunity; more recently has arrived the data supporting our new appreciation that "autoimmune patients" *may well be* and *generally are* "actively infected" with many of these viruses simultaneously—this is well-documented now in scleroderma, patients with which show active and "ectopic" (unusual locations) infections simultaneously with EBV, PvB19, and CMV. *Helicobacter pylori* may play a powerful role as a synergistic bioagent via its ability to *simultaneously* and *paradoxically* cause immunosuppression (thereby allowing other microbes to flourish) and systemic inflammation[15]; in this manner, the bacterial infection is permissive to and perhaps necessary for the autoimmune-inducing vasculopathic and fibrogenic viral infections (see section on Scleroderma for pathology details). An important concept to remember is that viral infections promote other viral infections—transactivation—via direct genomic enhancement of viral replication, by promoting a favorable cytokine environment for viral replication, and/or by stimulating NFkB which is commonly "hijacked" by viruses to promote viral replication; therefore activation or suppression of any virus can be said to contribute *indirectly* to the activation or suppression, respectively, of other viral populations.[16] Relatedly and as will be discussed in the following section on endogenous viruses, replication of

---

[15] "Infectious agents such as Helicobacter pylori (Hp) may cause chronic inflammation and autoimmune reactivity in susceptible subjects. The results of in vitro experiments performed with lymphocytes from Hp infected patients indicate that Hp can cause immunosuppression which might be eliminated by successful eradication therapy." Hybenova et al. The role of environmental factors in autoimmune thyroiditis. *Neuro Endocrinol Lett.* 2010;31(3):283-9

[16] White et al. Reciprocal transactivation between HIV-1 and other human viruses. *Virology.* 2006 Aug 15;352(1):1-13

exogenous/epigenomic viruses—such as influenza virus and herpes simplex type-1—increases expression of endogenous viruses.

Autoimmune conditions such as systemic lupus erythematosus (SLE, lupus), scleroderma, and Sjogren's disease have long been thought to have an infectious—especially viral—etiology. This research-clinical link is now strong enough to warrant action, and my work (starting with *Rheumatology v3.5* in 2014) and the earlier work of others (notably Dreyfus, "Autoimmune disease: A role for new anti-viral therapies?" *Autoimmun Rev.* 2011 Dec) proposed the use of antiviral protocols as a part of the overall treatment plan for the aforementioned autoimmune conditions. My protocol in *Rheumatology v3.5* was the first to emphasize the use of combination antiviral nutrients as the basis of the protocol and also to provide a complete holographic understanding capable of capturing and convincing the consciousness of healthcare providers by presenting the information in a manner that was conceptually comprehensible and clinically manageable—both are necessary for clinicians to give attention to a subject. In support of this is a diagram on the following pages that shows how multiple microbial infections—both viral and bacterial—can explain and perpetuate the pathogenic process that manifest clinically as the "autoimmune" disease scleroderma (systemic sclerosis).

Academicians and clinicians tend to see autoimmune diseases as "chronic" and therefore nonurgent and thus "not an emergency" and often and comparatively/relatively "not so important"; but for the patient suffering with pain and disability (before despair and nihilism set in), each day is urgent, and each lost opportunity to engage fully in this short process and experience of life is its own tragedy, worthy of our immediate attention.

- o Epstein-Barr virus in the pathogenesis of some autoimmune disorders (*Eur J Microbiol Immunol* 2011 Dec[17]): "Moreover, many observations indicate that EBV contributes also to the pathomechanism of SLE. However, this contribution differs from the relationship between EBV and MS, as shown by the lack of any increase in the risk of SLE after IM [infectious mononucleosis]. In SLE, EBV serology is quantitatively and qualitatively different from the normal response - that is, EBV viral load is higher and a strong cross-reaction can be detected between certain EBV antigens and autoantigens of pathological importance."

- o Lupus and Epstein-Barr (*Curr Opin Rheumatol* 2012 Jul[18]): "SLE patients have a dysregulated immune response against EBV. EBV antigens exhibit structural molecular mimicry with common SLE antigens and functional molecular mimicry with critical immune-regulatory components. SLE patients, from a number of unique geographic regions, are shown to have higher rates of EBV seroconversion, especially against early EBV antigens, suggesting frequent viral reactivation. SLE patients also have increased EBV viral loads and impaired EBV-specific CD8 cytotoxic T cells, with impaired cytokine responses to EBV in lupus patients. ... Recent advances demonstrate SLE-specific serologic responses, gene expression, viral load, T-cell responses, humoral fine specificity, and molecular mimicry with EBV, further supporting potential roles for EBV in lupus etiology and pathogenesis."

- o HTLV (human T-lymphotropic virus) in SLE (*Clin Immunol.* 2002 Feb[19]): "SLE patients produce high titer antibodies to various retroviral proteins, including Gag, Env, and Nef of HIV and HTLV (human T-lymphotropic virus), in the absence of overt retroviral infection. ... In particular, we consider the role of HTLV-1-related endogenous sequence (HRES-1) in SLE. We propose that molecular mimicry between HRES-1 and the small ribonucleoprotein complex initiates the production of autoantibodies, leading to immune complex formation, complement fixation, and pathological tissue deposition."

- o **Cytomegalovirus**—Induction of vasculopathy via direction infection and induction of pro-inflammatory cytokines, molecular mimicry: CMV causes experimental vasculopathy resembling SSc; interestingly and consistent with my (DrV) model of dysbiosis which appreciates immunosuppression as (pre)requisite, experimental CMV-induced vasculopathy requires immunosuppression: "A viral agent known for its ability to damage vessel walls is cytomegalovirus (CMV). ... Infected immunocompetent animals exhibited only perivascular inflammation, suggesting that infection and immunosuppression were co-requisites of [vasculopathy] neointima formation. ... Induction of TGF-β1, the canonical pro-fibrotic cytokine, by human CMV (HCMV) was reported by other authors (16), implicating that a primary endothelial cell infection by HCMV may induce myofibroblast activation in the vessel wall under the

[17] Füst G. The role of the Epstein-Barr virus in the pathogenesis of some autoimmune disorders - Similarities and differences. *Eur J Microbiol Immunol* (Bp). 2011 Dec;1:267-78
[18] James JA, Robertson JM. Lupus and Epstein-Barr. *Curr Opin Rheumatol.* 2012 Jul;24(4):383-8
[19] Adelman MK, Marchalonis JJ. Endogenous retroviruses in systemic lupus erythematosus: candidate lupus viruses. *Clin Immunol.* 2002 Feb;102(2):107-16

effect of this cytokine."[20] "…higher prevalence of IgA antihuman cytomegalovirus antibodies in patients with SSc. … CMV infection may play a part in SSc pathogenesis due to its ability to infect both endothelial and monocyte/macrophage cells and through the upregulation of fibrogenic cytokines and induction of immune dysregulation. … association between increased serum levels of CMV-specific antibodies and the prevalence of SSc-related autoantibodies in patients with SSc. … Molecular mimicry is a mechanism that may explain the pathogenicity of antibodies against viral proteins in SSc. Infection with HCMV may generate a host-antiviral response that is self-reactive toward autoantigens and endothelial cells."[21] Vulnerably to CMV-induced SSc may include genetic factors and fetomaternal/transfusional microchimerism, noted to be more common in women with SSc.

- **Epstein-Barr virus**—Localized infection in skin fibroblasts and endothelial cells, upregulation of cytokine production: "Here we show that EBV establishes infection in the majority of fibroblasts and endothelial cells in the skin of SSc patients, characterized by the expression of the EBV noncoding small RNAs (EBERs) and the increased expression of immediate-early lytic and latency mRNAs and proteins. We report that EBV is able to persistently infect human SSc fibroblasts in vitro, inducing an aberrant innate immune response in infected cells. EBV-Toll-like receptor (TLR) aberrant activation induces the expression of selected IFN-regulatory factors (IRFs), IFN-stimulated genes (ISGs), transforming growth factor-$\beta1$ (TGF$\beta1$), and several markers of fibroblast activation, such as smooth muscle actin and Endothelin-1, and all of these genes play a key role in determining the profibrotic phenotype in SSc fibroblasts. These findings imply that EBV infection occurring in mesenchymal, endothelial, and immune cells of SSc patients may underlie the main pathological features of SSc including autoimmunity, vasculopathy, and fibrosis, and provide a unified disease mechanism represented by EBV reactivation."[22]

- **Parvovirus B19**—Induction of fibrosis: "The presence of parvovirus B19 DNA was demonstrated in a significant percentage of bone marrow biopsies from SSc patients and was never detected in the control group. … These patients showed the most severe active endothelial injury and perivascular inflammation. …incubation with parvovirus B19-containing serum induced an invasive phenotype in normal human synovial fibroblasts."[23] Note that bone marrow-derived fibrocytes are involved in the pathogenesis of SSC; therefore, the strong positive correlation between B19 positivity and SSc and the negative correlation seen with B19 negativity and health suggests a likelihood of direct cause and effect.

- Epstein-Barr virus in Sjögren's syndrome salivary glands drives local autoimmunity (*Nat Rev Rheumatol. 2014 Jul*[24]): Paraphrasing from the original article: "Ectopic lymphoid structures (ELS) within the salivary glands of patients with Sjögren's syndrome serve as niches for latency and reactivation of EBV and

---

CMV meets pathogenic criteria for SSc

- Direct infection of endothelial cells and immune cells
- Induction of pro-fibrotic cytokines
- Higher levels of CMV antibodies in SSc patients
- Exact molecular mimicry between HCMV late protein UL94 and human endothelial cell surface integrin–NAG-2 protein complex
- Cross-reacting CMV-endothelial antibodies kill endothelial cells and cause fibrosis
- Anti-UL94 antibodies bind to dermal fibroblasts and convert them to a scleroderma phenotype

Moroncini et al. *Clin Exp Rheumatol.* 2013 Mar

EBV meets pathogenic criteria for SSc

- Majority of SSc patients show active infection in vascular and dermal cells
- Virus-induced gene induction promotes the profibrotic scleroderma phenotype

Farina et al. *J Invest Dermatol.* 2014 Apr

PvB19 meets pathogenic criteria for SSc

- Direct infection of endothelial cells, immune cells, and dermal epithelial cells
- Induction of pro-fibrotic cytokines
- Bone marrow infection is seen in many SSc patients, correlates directly with disease severity, and is never noted in health patients; bone marrow fibrocytes contribute to SSc.
- PvB19 infection triggers formation of multiple autoantibodies: nuclear antigens (ANA), rheumatoid factor (RF), neutrophils cytoplasmic antigens, mitochondrial antigens (AMA), smooth muscle, gastric parietal antigens and phospholipids.

Moroncini et al. *Clin Exp Rheumatol.* 2013 Mar

---

[20] Moroncini et al. Role of viral infections in the etiopathogenesis of systemic sclerosis. *Clin Exp Rheumatol.* 2013 Mar-Apr;31(2 Suppl 76):3-7

[21] Radić et al. Infectious disease as aetiological factor in the pathogenesis of systemic sclerosis. *Neth J Med.* 2010 Nov;68(11):348-53

[22] Farina et al. Epstein-Barr virus infection induces aberrant TLR activation pathway and fibroblast-myofibroblast conversion in scleroderma. *J Invest Dermatol.* 2014 Apr:954-64

[23] Radić et al. Infectious disease as aetiological factor in the pathogenesis of systemic sclerosis. *Neth J Med.* 2010 Nov;68(11):348-53

[24] Onuora S. Connective tissue diseases: Epstein-Barr virus in Sjögren's syndrome salivary glands drives local autoimmunity. *Nat Rev Rheumatol.* 2014 Jul;10(7):384

contribute to the activation and differentiation of plasma cells. ... EBV is aberrantly expressed in the salivary glands of patients with Sjögren's syndrome, specifically in those glands that displayed ELS, as revealed by the presence of EBV-encoded small RNA (EBER) transcripts and EBER+ cells within infiltrating cells. ... EBV reactivation occurs in a substantial proportion of perifollicular plasma cells that produce anti-Ro52 antibodies."

- Epstein-Barr Virus Infection in Disease-Specific Autoreactive B Cell Activation in Ectopic Lymphoid Structures of Sjögren's Syndrome (*Arthritis Rheumatol.* 2014 Sep[25]): "Active EBV infection is selectively associated with ELS in the salivary glands of patients with SS and appears to contribute to local growth and differentiation of disease-specific autoreactive B cells."

- Epstein-Barr Virus Infection, Vitamin D Deficiency, and Steps to Autoimmunity: A Unifying Hypothesis (*Autoimmune Dis.* 2012[26]): Per this model, "Autoimmunity is postulated to evolve in the following steps: (1) CD8+ T-cell deficiency, (2) primary EBV infection, (3) decreased CD8+ T-cell control of EBV, (4) increased EBV load and increased anti-EBV antibodies, (5) EBV infection in the target organ, (6) clonal expansion of EBV-infected autoreactive B cells in the target organ, (7) infiltration of autoreactive T cells into the target organ, and (8) development of ectopic lymphoid follicles in the target organ [which drive the tissue damage and autoantibody production as recently demonstrated per *Nat Rev Rheumatol* 2014 Jul[27] and *Arthritis Rheumatol* 2014 Sep[28]]. It is also proposed that deprivation of sunlight and vitamin D at higher latitudes facilitates the development of autoimmune diseases by aggravating the CD8+ T-cell deficiency and thereby further impairing control of EBV." Congratulations to this author—Pender—for predicting two years in advance the research that would later support this model.

- Aryl hydrocarbon receptor-mediated induction of EBV reactivation as a risk factor for Sjögren's syndrome (*J Immunol* 2012 May[29]): This is very impressive research, connecting xenobiotic exposure with viral reactivation. "The aryl hydrocarbon receptor (AhR) is a ligand-activated transcription factor that mediates a variety of biological effects by binding to environmental pollutants, including 2,3,7,8-tetrachlorodibenzo-p-dioxin (TCDD or dioxin). ... This study evaluated the possibility that ligand-activated AhR reactivates EBV. ... TCDD enhanced BZLF1 transcription, which mediates the switch from the latent to the lytic form of EBV infection in EBV-positive B cell lines and in a salivary gland epithelial cell line. Moreover, TCDD-induced increases in BZLF1 mRNA and EBV genomic DNA levels were confirmed in the B cell lines. Saliva from SS patients activated the transcription of both CYP1A1 and BZLF1. Additionally, there was a positive correlation between CYP1A1 and BZLF1 promoter activities. AhR ligands elicited the reactivation of EBV in activated B cells and salivary epithelial cells, and these ligands are involved in SS." This is stunning research: it provides direct links between infections, xenobiotic exposure, and autoimmunity; further, by extension, this research also suggests that xenobiotic exposure could also enhance transcription of HERVs (directly, or indirectly via viral transactivation) which also contributes to autoimmunity.

- Reactive arthritis responding to antiretroviral therapy in an HIV-1-infected individual (*Int J STD AIDS.* 2012 May[30]): "Reactive arthritis (ReA) is an autoimmune seronegative spondyloarthropathy that occurs in response to a urogenital or enteric infection. Several studies have reported a link between ReA and HIV infection. We report a case of an HIV-1-infected patient diagnosed with a disabling ReA who failed to respond to conventional therapy but whose symptoms resolved rapidly after starting antiretroviral therapy (ART)."

- Human immunodeficiency virus associated spondyloarthropathy (*Ann Rheum Dis.* 2001 Jul[31]): "In this case report a patient is described with severe HIV associated reactive arthritis, who on magnetic resonance imaging and sonographic imaging of inflamed knees had extensive polyenthesitis and

[25] Croia et al. Implication of Epstein-Barr Virus Infection in Disease-Specific Autoreactive B Cell Activation in Ectopic Lymphoid Structures of Sjögren's Syndrome. *Arthritis Rheumatol.* 2014 Sep;66(9):2545-57

[26] Pender MP. CD8+ T-Cell Deficiency, Epstein-Barr Virus Infection, Vitamin D Deficiency, and Steps to Autoimmunity. *Autoimmune Dis.* 2012;2012:189096

[27] Onuora S. Connective tissue diseases: Epstein-Barr virus in Sjögren's syndrome salivary glands drives local autoimmunity. *Nat Rev Rheumatol.* 2014 Jul;10(7):384

[28] Croia et al. Implication of Epstein-Barr Virus Infection in Disease-Specific Autoreactive B Cell Activation in Ectopic Lymphoid Structures of Sjögren's Syndrome. *Arthritis Rheumatol.* 2014 Sep;66(9):2545-57

[29] Inoue et al. Aryl hydrocarbon receptor-mediated induction of EBV reactivation as a risk factor for Sjögren's syndrome. *J Immunol.* 2012 May 1;188(9):4654-62

[30] Scott et al. Reactive arthritis responding to antiretroviral therapy in an HIV-1-infected individual. *Int J STD AIDS.* 2012 May;23(5):373-4

[31] McGonagle et al. Human immunodeficiency virus associated spondyloarthropathy. *Ann Rheum Dis.* 2001 Jul;60(7):696-8

adjacent osteitis. The arthritis deteriorated despite conventional antirheumatic treatment, but improved dramatically after highly active antiretroviral treatment, which was accompanied by a significant rise in CD4 T lymphocyte counts."

Rationale for anti-viral therapy for treating autoimmunity

"Cited epidemiologic and experimental evidence suggests that increased replication of epigenomic viral pathogens such as Epstein-Barr Virus (EBV) in chronic human autoimmune diseases such as rheumatoid arthritis (RA), systemic lupus erythematosus (SLE), and multiple sclerosis (MS) may activate endogenous human retroviruses (HERV) as a pathologic mechanism."

Dreyfus DH. Autoimmune disease: A role for new anti-viral therapies? *Autoimmun Rev.* 2011 Dec

- Viral infections associated with Kawasaki disease (*J Formos Med Assoc.* 2014 Mar[32]): "We enrolled 226 children with KD and 226 age- and sex-matched healthy children from February 2004 to March 2010. Throat and nasopharyngeal swabs were taken for both viral isolation and polymerase chain reaction (PCR) for various viruses. …Cases of KD had a significantly higher positive rate of viral isolation in comparison with the control group (7.5% vs. 2.2%, p = 0.02). Compared with the control group, cases of KD were more likely to have overall positive rates of viral PCR (50.4% vs. 16.4%, p < 0.001) and for various viruses including enterovirus (16.8% vs. 4.4%, p < 0.001), adenovirus (8.0% vs. 1.8%, p = 0.007), human rhinovirus (26.5% vs. 9.7%, p < 0.001), and coronavirus (7.1% vs. 0.9%, p = 0.003)."

- Ischemic retinal vasculitis in an 18-year-old man with chickenpox infection (*Clin Ophthalmol.* 2014 Feb[33]): "We report a case of a healthy 18-year-old man who presented with unilateral ischemic retinal vasculitis 10 days after the onset of chickenpox. … Fundus imaging, optical coherence tomography, fundus fluorescence angiography, and electrophysiologic studies confirmed the diagnosis of retinal vasculitis, which led to generalized retinal ischemia."

- Antineutrophil cytoplasmic antibody-associated vasculitis associated with Epstein-Barr virus infection (*Infection* 2014 Jun[34]): "Although a previous study indicated that there was a high positive rate of ANCA in the sera positive for IgM antibodies to EBV and EBV infection might trigger the relapse of AAV, this is the first case of incipient AAV associated with acute EBV infection. One possible explanation might be that EBV infection stimulated the production of ANCA."

- Cytomegalovirus-related necrotizing vasculitis mimicking Henoch-Schönlein syndrome (*Clin Exp Rheumatol.* 2014 May[35]): "The causative role of viral infection was revealed by the presence of CMV DNA in patient's blood and positive IgG titer against the virus. … Our report suggests that CMV vasculitis is probably more frequent than previously thought, even in immunocompetent patients, with a protean clinical presentation, mimicking other types of vasculitides."

- Hepatitis C virus infection and its rheumatologic implications. *Gastroenterol Hepatol* 2014 May[36]): "Symptoms of HCV infection and rheumatic diseases may be similar and include arthralgia, myalgia, arthritis, and vasculitis. …It is imperative to distinguish whether symptoms such as arthralgia, myalgia, and arthritis occur in patients with HCV infection due to primary chronic HCV infection or to a newly developed rheumatologic disease process."

- Varicella zoster virus in the temporal artery of a patient with giant cell arteritis (*J Neurol Sci.* 2013 Dec[37]): "We recently detected varicella zoster virus (VZV) in the temporal arteries (TA) of 5/24 patients with clinically suspect giant cell arteritis (GCA) whose TAs were GCA-negative pathologically; in those GCA-negative, VZV+TAs, virus antigen predominated in the arterial adventitia, but without medial necrosis and multinucleated giant cells. During our continuing search for VZV antigen in GCA-negative TAs, in the TA of one subject, we found abundant VZV antigen, as well as VZV DNA, in multiple regions (skip areas) of the TA spanning 350 [micrometers], as well as in skeletal muscle adjacent to the infected TA."

- Is giant cell arteritis an infectious disease? (*Presse Med.* 2004 Nov[38]): "Simultaneous occurrence of peaks of GCA/PMR and respiratory infections have been observed in Denmark. Several viruses have been suspected as triggers and assessed by serological testing, PCR or immunostaining on temporal artery

[32] Chang et al. Viral infections associated with Kawasaki disease. *J Formos Med Assoc.* 2014 Mar;113(3):148-54
[33] Poonyathalang et al. Ischemic retinal vasculitis in an 18-year-old man with chickenpox infection. *Clin Ophthalmol.* 2014 Feb 24;8:441-3
[34] Xu et al. Antineutrophil cytoplasmic antibody-associated vasculitis associated with Epstein-Barr virus infection: a case report and review of the literature. *Infection.* 2014 Jun;42(3):591-4
[35] D'Alessandro et al. Cytomegalovirus-related necrotising vasculitis mimicking Henoch-Schönlein syndrome. *Clin Exp Rheumatol.* 2014 May-Jun;32(3 Suppl 82):S73-5
[36] Sayiner et al. Hepatitis C virus infection and its rheumatologic implications. *Gastroenterol Hepatol* 2014 May;10(5):287-93
[37] Nagel et al. Varicella zoster virus in the temporal artery of a patient with giant cell arteritis. *J Neurol Sci.* 2013 Dec 15;335(1-2):228-30
[38] Duhaut P, Bosshard S, Ducroix JP. Is giant cell arteritis an infectious disease? *Presse Med.* 2004 Nov 6;33(19 Pt 2):1403-8

biopsies, or both techniques: the hepatitis B virus can be ruled out, as well as Herpes simplex 1 and 2, Herpes varicellae, Epstein-Barr virus and cytomegalovirus. Recent studies focused on parainfluenza virus, Parvovirus B19 and Chlamydia pneumoniae. Immunological studies suggest, at the origin of the inflammatory reaction leading to the typical pathological features of giant cell arteritis, the existence of a triggering antigen of unknown nature activating T-cells in the artery wall."

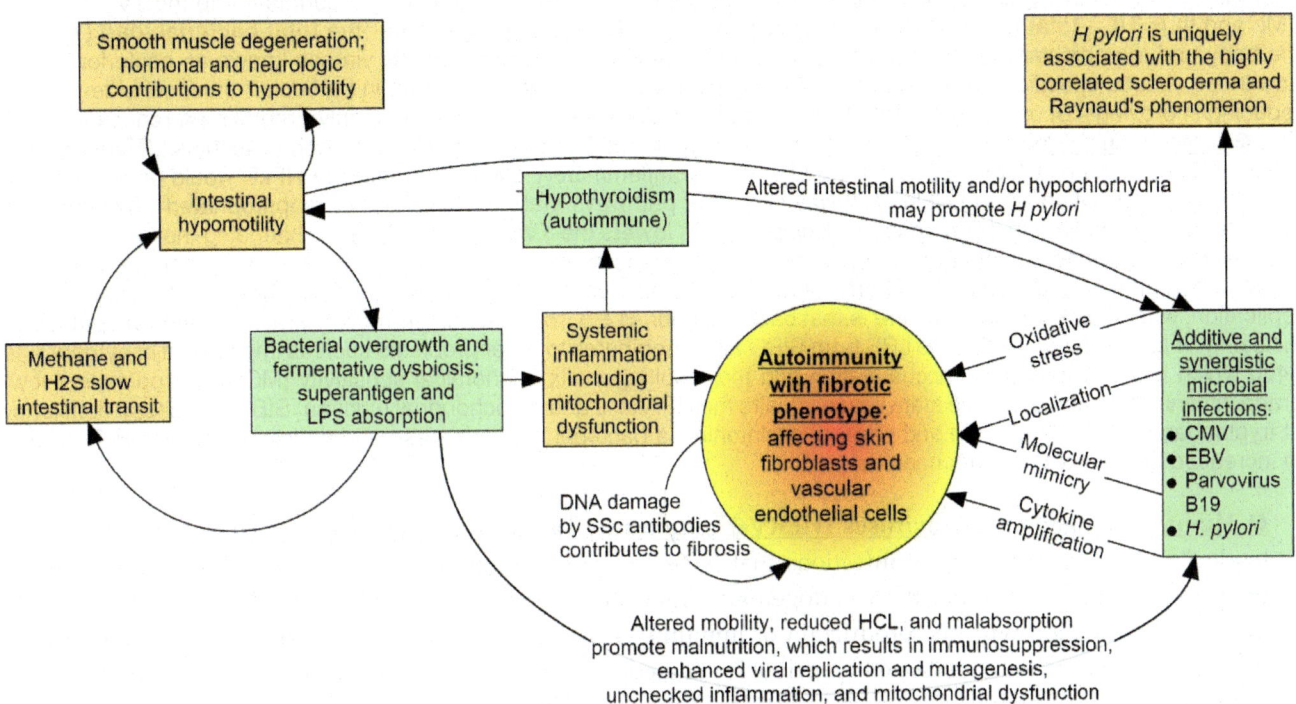

Clinical implications of polymicrobial dysbiosis in scleroderma: diagram by Vasquez; quotes from Radić et al and Svegliati et al: "Systemic sclerosis is an autoimmune disease characterized by vascular obliteration, excessive extracellular matrix deposition and fibrosis of the connective tissues of the skin, lungs, gastrointestinal tract, heart, and kidneys. The pathogenesis of systemic sclerosis is extremely complex; at present, no single unifying hypothesis explains all aspects. Over the last 20 years increasing evidence has accumulated to implicate infectious agents in the etiology of systemic sclerosis. Increased antibody titers, a preponderance of specific strains in patients with systemic sclerosis, and evidence of molecular mimicry inducing autoimmune responses suggest mechanisms by which infectious agents may contribute to the development and progression of systemic sclerosis."[39] "Trichostatin A, an HDAC inhibitor, prevented WIF-1 loss, β-catenin induction, and collagen accumulation in an experimental fibrosis model. Our findings suggest that oxidative DNA damage induced by SSc autoreactive antibodies enables Wnt activation that contributes to fibrosis."[40]

At the risk of redundancy and stating what should be obvious by now to readers who have studied the material in this book—especially chapter 4—here I will outline the implications of the information presented up to this point in this section on scleroderma/SSc. Quite obviously, the typical patient with scleroderma has multiple active microbial infections/colonizations and is therefore—by definition—demonstrating immunosuppression. Thus, two of the three components of my three-part dysbiosis model are established in SSC, and the third component—nutritional immunomodulation—is discussed in the following section. Given the solid data demonstrating polyviral activity for what I will describe as "popular viruses"—EBV, CMV, PvB19—we should reasonably assume that increased transcription of other viruses such as HSV (type-1 in 50% of the adult population; type-2 in 20% of the adult population) and the HERVs— human endogenous retroviruses—is also occurring. Serologic, newer generation PCR testing, and specialty tests—such as western blot for HSV infections—should ideally be performed to assess for the presence and severity/level of viral replication. Per previous discussions, clinicians must appreciate the **total microbial load (TML)** and not simply the presence/absence of these infections; bacterial quantifications—especially *H pylori*—must also be made if the initial laboratory evaluation is to be considered partly complete. Thereafter, the antimicrobial mission becomes on of search and destroy, using a combination of direct antiviral/antimicrobial agents as well as immunorestoration. My opinion and perspective is that antiviral pharmaceutic drugs—which by definition target single pathways in single viruses and are therefore easily bypassed by viral mutations and which have limited efficacy on the **total viral load (TVL)**, respectively— are of limited clinical value but may still be used if found efficacious in individual patients; any failure of pharmacologic antiviral intervention in autoimmunity does not refute the viral etiology of autoimmunity but is rather to be expected from

[39] Radić M, Martinović Kaliterna D, Radić J. Infectious disease as aetiological factor in the pathogenesis of systemic sclerosis. *Neth J Med.* 2010 Nov;68(11):348-53
[40] Svegliati et al. Oxidative DNA damage induces ATM-mediated transcriptional suppression of Wnt inhibitor WIF-1 in systemic sclerosis and fibrosis. *Sci Signal* 2014 Sept;ra84

the failure to effectively address the larger viral load and to restore various aspects of disturbed homeodynamics. Attention should be directed toward a global or generalized antiviral approach to reduce TVL for various categories of viruses *concretely* and TVL *conceptually*, reasonably described here as ❶ common/popular viruses—these are the common viruses most commonly considered by clinicians and patients and for which we have readily available diagnostic tests, namely HIV, HBV, HCV, HSV 1 and 2, CMV, EBV, PvB19; readers should note from the above that SSC patients show viral infections that are not simply *more active* but are *active in different locations* compared to nonSSC persons, ❷ human endogenous retroviruses—viruses permanently embedded in the human genome, for which laboratory assessments are generally not clinically available; clinicians should consider this category to be an occult contributor to the TVL and thus TML and thus TIL—total inflammatory/immunogenic load, ❸ bacteriophage load—the total bacterial load (TBL) of the body and in particular the biomass in the intestines houses the bacteria-specific viruses known as bacteriophages, and these viruses-specific-for-bacteria contribute significantly to the TML of the gut in particular; thus, consideration to reducing/improving TBL in the gut would be expected to reduce the TVL as well, benignly promoting a reduction in the TIL, ❹ other means of reducing TVL—reducing inflammation and bacterial load: Bacterial debris such as LPS/endotoxin, other viral infections (via "transactivation"), and any other inflammatory stimuli that activate NFkB would be expected to promote viral replication via the NFkB pathway and other pathways that are "hijacked" or reappropriated[41] by viruses to promote their replication. In this manner, reducing the TBL lowers the TVL and thus the TIL. Extending the understanding and implications: Understanding this helps clinicians and researchers make sense of the confusion seen particularly in the research on CFS [caused by SIBO and GI dysbiosis] which is commonly complicated by evidence of increased viral replication; what I think is occurring here is that bacterial debris/LPS from SIBO is promoting viral replication via pathways including NFkB. Problematically, the LPS from SIBO also contributes to other problems such as impairment of cytochrome p450 which leads to xenobiotic accumulation and the resulting multiple chemical sensitivity [MCS], the persistent low-grade inflammatory and oxidative state which impairs the HPA axis and mitochondrial function; SIBO can cause deficiency of tryptophan and thus serotonin and perhaps melatonin via bacterial tryptophanase and deficiency of vitamin B-12 due to increased binding of B-12 with bacterial H2S.

❹ **Human endogenous retroviruses (HERVs) play a role in autoimmune diseases**: Human DNA is "pre-loaded" with remnants of viral infections that have coursed through and been transmitted from parents to offspring for millions of years; these endogenous viral genomes implanted into human DNA are now known to undergo reactivation with the production of immunogenic viral remnants and the anticipated inflammatory immune response. As mentioned previously related to exogenous viral transactivation, replication of exogenous/epigenomic viruses—such as influenza virus and herpes simplex type-1—increases expression of endogenous viruses[42]; as such, one method to reduce/control activation of HERVs is to suppress replication of exogenous viruses. HERV activation is inhibited by DNA methylation; conversely, DNA hypomethylation is consistently associated with SLE in humans and animals.[43,44]

- Human endogenous retroviruses in the development of autoimmune diseases (*Int Rev Immunol* 2010 Aug[45]): In 2010, Balada et al provided a succinct and authoritative summary of HERVs and their relationship to the pathogenesis of autoimmunity: "Retroviruses can exist in an endogenous form, in which viral sequences are integrated into the human germ line and are vertically transmitted in a Mendelian fashion. Human endogenous retroviruses (HERVs), probably representing footprints of ancient germ-cell retroviral infections, occupy about 1% of the human genome. ... Although some of these elements show mutations and deletions, some HERVs are transcriptionally active and produce functional proteins. Some medical conditions, notably cancer and autoimmune diseases, are linked to the transcription of HERV genes, to the expression of HERV proteins (that may act as superantigens, for example), and/or to the development of antibodies against them that might cross-react with our own proteins. Their genetic sequences may also be, totally or partially, integrated into genes that regulate the immune response. These mechanisms could give rise to autoimmune diseases, such as lupus erythematosus, insulin-dependent diabetes mellitus, multiple sclerosis, Sjögren's syndrome, and rheumatoid arthritis, among others."

[41] "As viruses evolve under the highly selective pressures of the immune system, they acquire the capacity to target critical steps in the host cell life, hijacking vital cellular functions to promote viral pathogenesis. Many viruses have evolved mechanisms to target the NF-kB pathway to facilitate their replication, cell survival, and evasion of immune responses." Hiscott et al. Hostile takeovers: viral appropriation of the NF-kappaB pathway. *J Clin Invest.* 2001 Jan;107(2):143-51

[42] "Since viral infections have previously been reported to transactivate retroviral long terminal repeat regions we examined the basal expression of HERV-W elements and following infections by influenza A/WSN/33 and Herpes simplex 1 viruses in human cell-lines. ... Subsets of HERV-W elements were transactivated by viral infection in the different cell-lines. Transcriptional activation of these elements, including that encoding syncytin, was dependent on viral replication and was not induced by antiviral responses." Nellaker et al. Transactivation of elements in the human endogenous retrovirus W family by viral infection. *Retrovirology.* 2006 Jul 6;3:44

[43] "This raises the possibility that HERV demethylation participates in the pathogenesis of SLE." Renaudineau et al. Epigenetics and autoimmunity, with special emphasis on methylation. *Keio J Med.* 2011;60(1):10-6

[44] "Hypomethylation of HERV-E and HERV-K was also observed in SLE patients." Katoh et al. Association of endogenous retroviruses and long terminal repeats with human disorders. *Front Oncol.* 2013 Sep 11;3:234

[45] Balada E et al. Implication of human endogenous retroviruses in the development of autoimmune diseases. *Int Rev Immunol.* 2010 Aug;29(4):351-70

o Human endogenous retroviruses in the pathogenesis of autoimmune diseases (*Med Sci Monit.* 2012 Jun[46]): "This theory takes into account the existence in the human genome, since approximately 40 million years, of so-called human endogenous retroviruses (HERVs), which are transmitted to descendants vertically by the germ cells. It was recently established that these generally silent sequences perform some physiological roles, but occasionally become active and influence the development of some chronic diseases like diabetes, some neoplasms, chronic diseases of the nervous system (e.g., sclerosis multiplex), schizophrenia and autoimmune diseases."

o Endogenous retroviral pathogenesis in lupus (*Curr Opin Rheumatol.* 2010 Sep[47]: "ERV proteins may trigger lupus through structural and functional molecular mimicry, whereas the accumulation of ERV-derived nucleic acids stimulates interferon and anti-DNA antibody production in SLE."

o Autoimmune disease treatment with anti-viral therapies (*Autoimmun Rev* 2011 Dec[48]): "Cited epidemiologic and experimental evidence suggests that increased replication of epigenomic viral pathogens such as Epstein-Barr Virus (EBV) in chronic human autoimmune diseases such as rheumatoid arthritis (RA), systemic lupus Erythematosus (SLE), and multiple sclerosis (MS) may activate endogenous human retroviruses (HERV) as a pathologic mechanism. ... Other [drug] anti-viral therapies of chronic autoimmune diseases, such as retroviral integrase inhibitors, could be effective, although not without risk." This article provides support and rationale for using antiviral therapies in the treatment of autoimmunity; since anti-viral drugs nearly always have limited effectiveness and an excess of adverse effects and high cost while natural antiviral agents are safer and more broadly effective, the therapeutic choice is very clear.

o Role of endogenous retroviruses in murine SLE—an established animal model of human SLE[49] (*Autoimmun Rev.* 2010 Nov[50]): "Among the principal targets of the autoantibodies produced in murine SLE are nucleic acid-protein complexes and the envelope glycoprotein gp-70 of endogenous retroviruses. Recent studies have revealed that the innate receptor TLR-7 plays a pivotal role in the development of a wide variety of autoimmune responses against DNA- and RNA-containing nuclear antigens... Moreover, the demonstration that TLR-7 is involved in the acute phase expression of serum gp70 uncovers an additional pathogenic role of TLR7 in murine lupus nephritis by promoting the expression of nephritogenic gp-70 autoantigen." Thus this animal model proves with molecular detail the cause-and-effect relationship between ERVs and SLE and further points to TLR-7 as a necessary byway for nephritogenic autoantigen expression; parallels to human SLE and according therapeutic interventions are likely. While most readers should already appreciate that TLRs recognize pathogen-associated molecular patterns (PAMPs) expressed on infectious agents (and saturated fatty acids for TLR-4, as discussed in Chapter 4) and mediate the specific PAMP-TLR expression of inflammatory cytokines for immune defense responses, what is important to note here is that TLR-7 recognizes single-stranded RNA in endosomes, a common feature of viral genomes internalized within macrophages and dendritic cells;

HERV-autoimmunity associations

- Rheumatoid arthritis: expression of multiple ERVs detected in RA patients; HERV-K10 shows molecular mimicry
- Juvenile RA: HERV-K10
- Multiple sclerosis: MS-associated retroviral element (MRSV)-type HERV-W; increased expression of the env RNA and protein expression in the blood and brain cells of MS patients; also clear increase in HERV-H/F family HERV-Fc1 activity and RNA production; HERV-K18 on chromosome 1 is a risk factor for MS
- Psoriasis: Increased expression of HERV-W, K, E, and variant ERV-9/HERV-W
- Lupus: Hypomethylation of HERV-E & HERV-K

Mechanisms for HERV-induced autoimmune diseases:
- Molecular mimicry (HERV-K10)
- Superantigen production (HERV-K)
- LTR (long terminal repeat)-mediated alterations of gene expression
- Antigenicity and immune complex formation

Activation of HERVs:
- DNA hypomethylation
- Transactivation

---

[46] Brodziak et al. The role of human endogenous retroviruses in the pathogenesis of autoimmune diseases. *Med Sci Monit.* 2012 Jun;18(6):RA80-8

[47] Perl et al. Endogenous retroviral pathogenesis in lupus. *Curr Opin Rheumatol.* 2010 Sep;22(5):483-92

[48] Dreyfus DH. Autoimmune disease: A role for new anti-viral therapies? *Autoimmun Rev.* 2011 Dec;11(2):88-97

[49] "Murine models are useful tools for the study of the etiology of lupus. A multitude of models exist, each sharing a subset of attributes with SLE observed in humans. In addition, each model affords the study of different aspects of lupus pathogenesis." Perry et al. Murine Models of Systemic Lupus Erythematosus. *J Biomed Biotech* 2011; 271694

[50] Baudino et al. Role of endogenous retroviruses in murine SLE. *Autoimmun Rev.* 2010 Nov;10(1):27-34

in this manner, TLR-7 is poised to be the mediator of virus-induced HERV transactivation with resultant production of pathogenic autoantigens.

- o Selective antibody reactivity with peptides from human endogenous retroviruses—HERVs—and nonviral poly(amino acids) in patients with systemic lupus erythematosus (*Arthritis Rheum* 1996 Oct[51]): "Measurement by immunoassay revealed increased frequencies of antiretroviral antibodies against 2 peptides derived from the env gene of the type C-like class, which includes ERV-9 and HERV-H, and against 2 peptides from the gag region of human T-lymphotropic virus type I-related endogenous sequence 1, in patients with SLE. Antibodies to 2 nonviral peptides, polyhistidine and polyproline, were also overrepresented in patient sera. In 1 patient, longitudinal data obtained over a period of 12 years indicated that the concentrations of certain antiretroviral antibodies varied according to disease activity. CONCLUSION: Reactivity to certain type C HERV-derived antigens was found among patients with SLE. This reactivity could be explained by increased exposure to cross-reactive epitopes from essentially complete type C HERVs."

- o Endogenous retroviruses in systemic lupus erythematosus: candidate lupus viruses (*Clin Immunol.* 2002 Feb[52]): "SLE patients produce high titer antibodies to various retroviral proteins, including Gag, Env, and Nef of HIV and HTLV (human T-lymphotropic virus), in the absence of overt retroviral infection. … In particular, we consider the role of HTLV-1-related endogenous sequence (HRES-1) in SLE. We propose that molecular mimicry between HRES-1 and the small ribonucleoprotein complex initiates the production of autoantibodies, leading to immune complex formation, complement fixation, and pathological tissue deposition."

❺ **Bacteriophages (viruses that infect bacteria) gain attention in clinical care**: The fact that the lumen of the gastrointestinal tract is loaded with bacteria is well known; progressively, all healthcare providers and researchers are appreciating that bacterial imbalances (quantitative) and metabolic/behavioral disturbances (qualitative) contribute to various disease via multiple mechanisms, as reviewed in the section on dysbiosis in Chapter 4. The next step in our understanding of dysbiosis is what I have referred to previously as microbial dysbiosis—infections within microbes. Bacteriophages are viruses that infect bacteria, and the gastrointestinal bacteria, which are themselves susceptible to innumerable quantitative and qualitative imbalances, are susceptible to viral infections. Thus, any complete understanding of dysbiosis must also consider the role of bacteriophages; these will be reviewed via the following survey of the literature. *Samples—notably limited—of reliable data supporting/contextualizing this section:*

- o Dysbiosis in inflammatory bowel disease via bacteriophages (*Gut.* 2008 Mar[53]): In this excellent and brief report by Lepage et al, the authors propose that bacteriophage-mediated or bacteriophage-induced inflammatory dysbiosis may play a role in inflammatory bowel disease; and they note that bacteriophages outnumber bacteria 10-fold "in many natural ecosystems." Bacteriophages are diverse, with more than 1,200 genotypes found within the human gastrointestinal tract; per biopsy sample from the human gastrointestinal tract, an average of 1.2 billion (1.2×10^9) virus-like particles (VLP) are quantifiable and dominated by the families *Siphoviridae, Myoviridae* and *Podoviridae.* Patients with the "autoimmune disease" Crohn's disease (CD) harbor many more VLP per biopsy sample (2.1-4.1 billion) than do healthy controls (1.2 billion).

- o Human gut virome: inter-individual variation and response to diet (*Genome Res.* 2011 Oct[54]): "VLP sequences represent a minority of the total DNA from stool, in the range of from 4% to 17%"; while this may be a *numerical* minority the physiologic and immunogenic significance could be massive. This article provides technical information and demonstrates phage response to diet, but the clinical implications and the authors' presentation of data are not clear.

- o Bacteriophages in gut samples from pediatric Crohn's disease patients (*Inflamm Bowel Dis.* 2013 Jul[55]): "The largest number of viral hits was obtained from the CD gut wash samples (n = 691), followed by CD

---

[51] Bengtsson et al. Selective antibody reactivity with peptides from human endogenous retroviruses and nonviral poly(amino acids) in patients with systemic lupus erythematosus. *Arthritis Rheum.* 1996 Oct;39(10):1654-63

[52] Adelman MK, Marchalonis JJ. Endogenous retroviruses in systemic lupus erythematosus: candidate lupus viruses. *Clin Immunol.* 2002 Feb;102(2):107-16

[53] Lepage et al. Dysbiosis in inflammatory bowel disease: a role for bacteriophages? *Gut.* 2008 Mar;57(3):424-5

[54] Minot et al. The human gut virome: inter-individual variation and dynamic response to diet. *Genome Res.* 2011 Oct;21(10):1616-25

[55] Wagner et al. Bacteriophages in gut samples from pediatric Crohn's disease patients: metagenomic analysis using 454 pyrosequencing. *Inflamm Bowel Dis.* 2013 Jul:1598-608

ileal samples (n = 52), control ileum samples (n = 20), and CD colonic samples (n = 1). The most abundant virus sequences identified belonged to the Caudovirales phage. CONCLUSIONS: ... The large abundance of phages in CD ileum tissue and CD gut wash sample suggests a role of phage in CD development. The role of phage dysbiosis in CD is currently unknown but opens up a new area of research."

- o Viral and microbial communities associated with Crohn's disease: a metagenomic approach. (*Clin Transl Gastroenterol*. 2013 Jun[56]): "A lower diversity but more variability between the CD samples in both virome and microbiome was found, with a clear distinction between groups based on the microbiome. Only 5% of the differential viral biomarkers are more represented in the CD group (Synechococcus phage S CBS1 and Retroviridae family viruses), compared with 95% in the control group. ... Further characterization of Retroviridae viruses in the CD group could be of interest, given their links with immunodeficiency and the immune responses."

To be clear: The role of bacteriophages in inflammatory bowel disease and autoimmunity is not clear at this time; however, I can easily offer a few conceptual options to explain the association, namely that ❶ it is an unrelated association (this is least likely), ❷ these virus particles may be causing the tissue response and inflammation, such as via stimulation of the innate immune system that simply responds nonspecifically and nonselectively to the bacteriophage MAMPs/PAMPs—microbe/pathogen-associated molecular patterns, ❸ inflammatory bowel disease itself is the cause of the increased bacteriophage replication, such as the inflammation and/or associated oxidative stress promoting viral replication, and finally that ❹ the bacteriophages alter the physiologic (quorum-sensing[57]) or-pathogenic behavior of the bacteria[58] in such a way that the bacteria then become the mediators ("puppets") of the bacteriophages. My personal perspective favors associations #2-4, which form a vicious cycle, each interconnected component of which is supported by reason and/or scientific data.

Bacteriophages (also called "phages" or "virus-like particles" or VLP)

- Bacteriophages ("viruses that infect bacteria") are the most abundant biological entities on earth; they outnumber bacteria by 10x; more than 1,200 genotypes found within the human gastrointestinal tract
- The gut virome is dominated by these prokaryotic viruses that prey on gut bacteria; since the reproductive capability of all phage particles is unknown, describing them as "viruses" is discouraged in preference for "virus-like particles" (VLP)
- Bacteriophages influence bacterial diversity and "population structure" via "destabilization of bacterial communities"; the infectious and lytic nature of bacteriophages will obviously influence survival and death of specific populations of bacteria while the effects of lysogeny result directly in more viral particles and death of bacteria with release of bacterial and viral immunogens. Conversely, human gut bacteriophage populations do not change impressively with the corresponding bacterial colonizations (exception seen with *Faecalibacterium prausnitzii* which has a proportionate phage population) within physiologic norms (longitudinal stability); the majority of phages seem to correspond (34-41%) to the *Firmicutes* phylum of bacteria.
- Bacteriophages participate in gene transfer and genome reorganization; they also carry numerous antibiotic resistance genes: multidrug efflux transporters (n = 355), vancomycin resistance genes (n = 129), tetracycline resistance genes (n = 18), and beta-lactamases (n = 16).
- VLP sequences represent 4% to 17% of the total DNA from human stool; this quantitative minority of DNA material could have profound pathological implications for conditions characterized by anti-nuclear antibodies and the resulting immune complexes. Viral particles from intestinal bacteriophages are certainly absorbed and would thereafter contribute to 1) primary inflammation, and almost certainly to 2) transactivation of HERVs, 3) cross-reactivity to DNA (e.g., ANA), and 4) immune complex deposition.
- Patients with the "autoimmune disease" Crohn's disease harbor many more bacteriophages per biopsy sample (2.1-4.1 billion) than do healthy controls (1.2 billion).
- Phage populations are modified via dietary change (*Genome Res* 2012 Oct); but the implications are not clear.

---

[56] Pérez-Brocal et al. Study of the viral and microbial communities associated with Crohn's disease: a metagenomic approach. *Clin Transl Gastroenterol*. 2013 Jun 13;4:e36

[57] Hargreaves et al. What does the talking?: quorum sensing signalling genes discovered in a bacteriophage genome. *PLoS One*. 2014 Jan 24;9(1):e85131

[58] "Bacteriophages have an essential gene kit that enables their invasion, replication, and production. In addition to this "core" genome, they can carry "accessory" genes that dramatically impact bacterial biology, and presumably boost their own success." Hargreaves et al. Bacteriophage behavioral ecology: How phages alter their bacterial host's habits. *Bacteriophage*. 2014 Jul 8;4:e29866 "The transfer of novel genetic material into the genomes of bacterial viruses (phages) has been widely documented in several host-phage systems. Bacterial genes are incorporated into the phage genome and, if retained, subsequently evolve within them. The expression of these phage genes can subvert or bolster bacterial processes, including altering bacterial pathogenicity." Hargreaves et al. What does the talking?: quorum sensing signalling genes discovered in a bacteriophage genome. *PLoS One*. 2014 Jan 24;9(1):e85131

Common Viruses: Quick Overview in Table Format

Introduction: This chapter/book focuses on antiviral nutritional interventions and has no aspiration to be or function as a microbiology text. The focus of this work is on antiviral strategies in general with an obviously strong emphasis on nutritional and botanical interventions; both of these categories of interventions are notable for their safety and effectiveness as well as their nonpatentability and therefore ready availability and relatively low cost internationally. If the goals of healthcare truly include autonomy, beneficence, nonmaleficence, and distributive justice, then nutritional interventions should take prominence in the hands of primary care providers. The following table introduces and reviews the viruses that are either commonly encountered clinically and/or which are mentioned in the main section on therapeutics immediately hereafter.

Examples of commonly considered viruses of particular recent newsworthiness and/or noteworthiness

Virus: unique characteristics	Acute disease	Chronic disease causation/association
Cytomegalovirus (CMV): Double-stranded DNA herpes virus present in >60% of the US population; importantly, all herpesviruses are double-stranded (ds) DNA viruses with obvious implications for the prototypic dsDNA disease lupus/SLE	• CMV causes asymptomatic infection or mild flulike illness; can cause Guillain-Barré syndrome, meningoencephalitis, pericarditis, colitis and pneumonitis in immunosuppressed patients; myocarditis, thrombocytopenia, and hemolytic anemia; retinitis in immunosuppressed/HIV patients; can cause transient but severe immunosuppression; virus remains latent in leukocytes	• <u>Scleroderma</u>: CMV can cause many/most of the disease manifestations of the autoimmune diseases scleroderma (systemic sclerosis); CMV infects endothelial cells and immune cells and induces pro-fibrotic cytokines; likely functions in conjunction with other microbes to produce the inflammatory disease[59]
Epstein-Barr virus (EBV): All herpesviruses are double-stranded (ds) DNA viruses; pathodiagnostically famous for inducing formation of "heterophile antibodies" which are nonspecific and do not bind to EBV.	• <u>Acute infectious mononucleosis</u>: Viral infection typified by sore throat, significant fatigue, and splenomegaly; may have hepatitis and rash	• <u>Rheumatic/autoimmune diseases</u>: Autoimmune diseases, especially scleroderma[60] and Sjogren's syndrome[61] but also systemic lupus erythematosus (SLE, lupus) and multiple sclerosis (MS) • Chronic reactivation can lead to B-cell lymphoma or Burkitt lymphoma
Human immunodeficiency virus (HIV):	• Initial infection may be asymptomatic or similar to cold or flu	• Progressive immunosuppression with numerous complications including secondary infections, dementia, neuropathy, cancer

---

[59] Moroncini et al. Role of viral infections in the etiopathogenesis of systemic sclerosis. *Clin Exp Rheumatol.* 2013 Mar-Apr;31(2 Suppl 76):3-7
[60] Farina et al. Epstein-Barr virus infection induces aberrant TLR activation pathway and fibroblast-myofibroblast conversion in scleroderma. *J Invest Dermatol* 2014 Apr:954-64
[61] Onuora S. Connective tissue diseases: Epstein-Barr virus in Sjögren's syndrome salivary glands drives local autoimmunity. *Nat Rev Rheumatol.* 2014 Jul;10(7):384. See original data: Croia et al. Implication of Epstein-Barr Virus Infection in Disease-Specific Autoreactive B Cell Activation in Ectopic Lymphoid Structures of Sjögren's Syndrome. *Arthritis Rheumatol.* 2014 Sep;66(9):2545-57

Examples of commonly considered viruses—*continued*

Virus: unique characteristics	Acute disease	Chronic disease causation/association
Common "syndromic" viruses: Viral infections that typically cause an acute and self-limited infection or "viral syndrome"	• Rhinoviruses—estimated to cause 50% of common colds, may cause ear infections and asthma exacerbations • Rotaviruses ("stomach flu")—acute gastroenteritis with abdominal pain, vomiting, watery diarrhea • Influenza ("flu")—respiratory illness ranging from very mild to severe and possibly fatal • Measles (rubeola)—epidemic in US in 2014; RNA paramyxovirus initially replicates in respiratory epithelial cells then to lymphoid tissues and systemically; supremely contagious febrile respiratory infection with characteristic skin rash (14 days after exposure, spread from head to trunk) and intrabuccal mucosal lesions (Koplik spots); can cause immunosuppression during infection, blinding keratitis, severe pneumonia and croup, birth defects, infection/inflammation of any organ including brain/encephalitis (1 of every 1000, often results in permanent brain damage and is fatal in about 10% of patients) • Mumps (Rubulavirus of genus paramyxovirus)—acute, self-limited, systemic viral illness characterized by the swelling of one or more of the salivary glands due to inflammation and obstruction of salivary gland ducts; infection can also occur in testes/ovaries, and central nervous system (10%, most common extrasalivary site) • Rubella (togavirus)—generalized viral illness characterized by rash starting on head/face and moves to trunk/extremities within 1-5 days of onset.	• Influenza ("flu")—associated with increased risk of Parkinson's disease likely due to neuroinflammation and mitochondrial dysfunction rather than any ongoing infection • Measles (rubeola)—Subacute sclerosing panencephalitis (SSPE) is a degenerative CNS disease resulting from persistent measles infection, with behavioral and intellectual deterioration and seizures; average onset 11 years after an acute infection

<u>Virus</u>: unique characteristics	Acute disease	Chronic disease causation/association
<u>**Herpes simplex virus type-1 (HSV-1)**</u>: Noted in approximately 50% of adults worldwide; best test is Western blot but IgG testing is also very reliable; initial infection occurs in skin/mucosal cells and then spreads to nervous system with periodic reactivation and neurogenic viral replication/distribution manifesting dermatologically; importantly, all herpesviruses are double-stranded (ds) DNA viruses with obvious implications for the prototypic dsDNA disease lupus/SLE	• Initial infection may be asymptomatic or severe vesicular/blistering illness (typically oral/labial but can also be genital); brain infection (herpes encephalitis) is generally devastating/lethal; asymptomatic transmission is common; the leading cause of corneal blindness	• <u>Recurrent lesions</u>: Recurrent/periodic outbreaks of herpetic lesions with frequent viral shedding even when no symptoms or lesions are present • <u>Multiple sclerosis (MS)</u>: HSV1-MS association exists but is weaker with HSV-1 than with other herpes viruses and the bacteria *Chlamydophila/Chlamydia pneumoniae* • <u>Alzheimer's disease</u>: Impressively consistent pathologic and epidemiologic evidence[62] • <u>Giant cell arteritis, temporal arteritis (GCA-TA)</u>: HSV DNA is correlated with this vasculitic disease[63]
<u>**Herpes simplex virus type-2 (HSV-2)**</u>: Noted in approximately 20% of adults worldwide; see previous details for HSV-1 since these viruses are very similar	• Initial infection may be asymptomatic or severe vesicular/blistering illness (typically genital but can also be oral/labial); asymptomatic transmission is common	• <u>Recurrent lesions</u>: Recurrent/periodic outbreaks of herpetic lesions with frequent viral shedding even when no symptoms or lesions are present
<u>**Human herpesvirus 6 (HHV-6)**</u>: Occurs in two forms: Human herpesvirus 6A (HHV-6A) and Human herpesvirus 6B (HHV-6B); importantly, all herpesviruses are double-stranded (ds) DNA viruses with obvious implications for the prototypic dsDNA disease lupus/SLE	• HHV-6B primary infection causes the childhood illness exanthem subitum (also known as roseola infantum or sixth disease). • HHV-6B reactivation is common in transplant recipients and can cause encephalitis, bone marrow suppression, and pneumonitis.	• Chronic disease associations include multiple sclerosis (MS), chronic fatigue syndrome (CFS), Hashimoto's thyroiditis[64]

---

[62] "We reiterate convincing data from our own (and other) laboratories, reviewing the first anatomic foothold neurofibrillary tangles gain in brainstem and/or entorhinal cortex; the chronic immunosurveillance cellularity of the trigeminal ganglia wherein HSV-1 awakens from latency to reactivate; the inabilities of p-tau protein's physical properties to promote it to jump synapses; the amino acid homology between human p-tau and VP22, a key target for phosphorylation by HSV serine/threonine-protein kinase UL13; and the exosomic secretion of HSV-1-infected cells' L-particles, attesting to the cell-to-cell passage of microRNAs of herpesviruses." Ball et al. Intracerebral propagation of Alzheimer's disease: strengthening evidence of a herpes simplex virus etiology. *Alzheimers Dement.* 2013 Mar;9(2):169-75

[63] "HSV DNA was detected in 21 (88%) of 24 histologically positive and 8 (53%) of 15 histologically negative specimens (P = .027; Fisher exact test). Analysis of 10 renal artery samples from age-matched control subjects using the same assay showed no detectable HSV DNA. We conclude that detectable HSV DNA is correlated with histologically confirmed GCA in this patient population." Powers et al. High prevalence of herpes simplex virus DNA in temporal arteritis biopsy specimens. *Am J Clin Pathol.* 2005 Feb;123(2):261-4

[64] Broccolo et al. Possible role of human herpesvirus 6 as a trigger of autoimmune disease. *ScientificWorldJournal.* 2013 Oct 24;2013:867389

Examples of commonly considered viruses—*continued*

Virus: unique characteristics	Acute disease	Chronic disease causation/association
Human papilloma virus (HPV): Several different strains of HPV, generally of little or consequence except for warts and in rare cases epithelial cancer; most people clear or suppress the infection	• Warts: Skin warts are generally not "acute" but are generally the first and only manifestation of the infection • Invisible and asymptomatic and generally transitory ("self-limiting") skin/mucosal infection:	• Warts: May last for years, particularly problematic if genital or laryngeal • Epithelial cancer: Cervical cancer, throat/tonsillar cancer • Possible connection to "autoimmune" vasculitis, notably giant cell arteritis, temporal arteritis (GCA-TA): Patients with temporal arteritis show evidence of increased HPV DNA in their lesions according to one study[65]; relatedly, two cases of vasculitis have been reported following HPV vaccination[66]
Parvovirus B19 (PvB19): one of the smallest DNA viruses	• Classic acute infection is fifth disease or erythema infectiosum, or "slapped cheek syndrome" • Arthritis—transient or chronic • Aplastic crisis, reticulocytopenia—severe anemia, notably severe and dangerous in patients with sickle cell anemia or hereditary spherocytosis • Acute immune-complex-mediated vasculitis/glomerulonephritis: Rare and underdiagnosed; forms basis for virus-mediated chronic vasculitis/nephritis[67]	• Scleroderma (systemic sclerosis)[68]
Varicella zoster virus (VZV): importantly, all herpesviruses are double-stranded (ds) DNA viruses with obvious implications for the prototypic dsDNA disease lupus/SLE	• Chickenpox: can also cause interstitial pneumonia, encephalitis, transverse myelitis, and necrotizing visceral lesions	• Shingles, herpes zoster: Recurrent/periodic nerve inflammation, generally causing skin eruptions in a limited, dermatomal distribution • Giant cell arteritis, temporal arteritis (GCA-TA): VZV DNA is correlated with vasculitic disease[69]

[65] "HPV DNA was detected by PCR and genotyping in 16 of 22 (73%) histologically positive cases of GCA and in only five of 21 (24%) histologically negative temporal artery biopsies. Among the vascular margin controls, only three of 15 (20%) were positive for HPV DNA. ... Conclusions: The results of our study revealed a statistically significant association between HPV positivity and biopsy confirmed temporal giant cell arteritis GCA (p = 0.001). Further studies are necessary to elucidate the pathophysiology underlying this association." Mohammadi et al. Association between human papillomavirus DNA and temporal arteritis. *BMC Musculoskelet Disord.* 2012 Jul 25;13:132

[66] "Quite clearly and without any doubt whatsoever, adverse effects from vaccinations are horridly underreported by the medical profession and by international healthcare systems worldwide. The authors report two cases of vasculitis following HPV immunization, which has not previously been described. Melo Gomes S, et al. Vasculitis following HPV immunization. *Rheumatology* (Oxford). 2013 Mar;52(3):581-2

[67] "Here, we present the case of a 45-year-old female who showed acute glomerulonephritis induced by HPVB19 infection with various autoantibodies. She had proteinuria (175 mg/g creatinine) and hematuria (20-29 erythrocytes per high-power field) in a urinalysis, and various autoantibodies such as antinuclear antibodies, proteinase-3-antineutrophil cytoplasmic antibodies (PR3-ANCA), antiglomerular basement membrane (GBM) antibodies, and anticardiolipin antibodies in a blood examination. A renal biopsy showed that endocapillary proliferative glomerulonephritis comprised of mononuclear cell infiltration. By using immunofluorescence microscopy, IgG, IgA, IgM, C3, C4, and C1q deposits were detected mainly in glomerular capillaries. .. Our patient's case may provide a clue to the etiology of ANCA-associated vasculitis or lupus nephritis." Shimohata et al. Human parvovirus B19-induced acute glomerulonephritis: a case report. *Ren Fail.* 2013;35(1):159-62

[68] Radić et al. Infectious disease as aetiological factor in the pathogenesis of systemic sclerosis. *Neth J Med.* 2010 Nov;68(11):348-53

[69] "PCR was positive for VZV DNA in 9 (26%) temporal arteries tested that showed histologic evidence of GCA. The remaining 26 histologically positive temporal arteries and all 29 histologically negative arteries tested gave negative PCR results for VZV DNA. ... This study showed a significant association of VZV DNA to temporal artery biopsy samples positive for GCA compared with the negative specimens. The results support the hypothesis that VZV may play a role in the pathogenesis of some cases of GCA." Mitchell BM, Font RL. Detection of varicella zoster virus DNA in some patients with giant cell arteritis. *Invest Ophthalmol Vis Sci.* 2001 Oct;42(11):2572-7

Virus: unique characteristics	**Acute disease**	**Chronic disease causation/association**
Flaviviruses—West Nile virus, Dengue, yellow fever: Viruses transmitted by mosquitoes from birds	• <u>West Nile virus</u>: Lymphatic spread can lead to infection in CNS, liver, heart, pancreas; meningoencephalitis is 10% fatal and can cause permanent brain damage/impairment	• Not widely appreciated; not known
Hepatitis viruses B and C (HBV and HCV): HBV is a partly double-stranded DNA virus ("partially double-stranded, relaxed-circular DNA [rcDNA]"[70]); HCV is a single-stranded RNA virus ("positive-stranded viral RNA"[71]); both are difficult to clear and thus causes chronic active-destructive infection	• <u>Viral hepatitis</u>: Can present as acute illness but is generally a mild and insidious infection that progresses over many years; many patients have very few symptoms and minimal or no elevations in liver enzymes (most common indicator of liver damage); hepatic injury is due to inflammation not directly by virus.	• <u>Liver failure, liver cancer</u> • <u>Rheumatic/autoimmune diseases</u>: HBV and especially HCV can mimic or exacerbate SLE, rheumatoid arthritis (RA), vasculitis, nephritis, cryoglobulinemia
Ebola virus, and other viral hemorrhagic fevers including Marburg and Lassa: RNA viruses from different families; reservoir is other nonhuman animals and thus distribution is geographically limited; infection involves endothelial cells and thus when combined with thrombocytopenia can lead to hemorrhage; macrophage and dendritic cell infection leads to "cytokine storm"	• <u>Mild acute illness</u>: fever, headache, rash, myalgia, neutropenia and thrombocytopenia • <u>Severe acute illness</u>: hemorrhage, vascular leak and hypotension, seizure, DIC—disseminated intravascular coagulation, shock; commonly lethal (50-70%)	Not widely appreciated; not known
Endogenous retroviruses (human ERV, HERV): These are viral remnants permanently encoded in human DNA	• HERV activation likely contributes to symptoms of fatigue and viral illness but is not clinically appreciated and is generally ascribed to an exogenous virus, particularly one of the common syndromic viruses listed above	• <u>Autoimmune diseases, especially systemic lupus erythematosus (SLE, lupus)</u>: DNA demethylation and transactivation via other viral infections are known to increase activity of HERVs[72]

---

70 Seeger C, Mason WS. Hepatitis B virus biology. *Microbiol Mol Biol Rev.* 2000 Mar;64(1):51-68

71 Rosen HR. Clinical practice. Chronic hepatitis C infection. *N Engl J Med.* 2011 Jun 23;364(25):2429-38

72 For clinical review including interaction with other viral infections and bacterial infections especially *H pylori*, see Chapter 5 from Vasquez A. <u>Rheumatology v3.5</u> or later http://inflammationmastery.com. For citations supporting the connection between HERVs and autoimmunity, see the following examples: "This raises the possibility that HERV demethylation participates in the pathogenesis of SLE." Renaudineau et al. Epigenetics and autoimmunity, with special emphasis on methylation. *Keio J Med.* 2011;60(1):10-6. "Hypomethylation of HERV-E and HERV-K was also observed in SLE patients." Katoh et al. Association of endogenous retroviruses and long terminal repeats with human disorders. *Front Oncol.* 2013 Sep 11;3:234. Balada E et al. Implication of human endogenous retroviruses in the development of autoimmune diseases. *Int Rev Immunol.* 2010 Aug;29(4):351-70. Brodziak et al. The role of human endogenous retroviruses in the pathogenesis of autoimmune diseases. *Med Sci Monit.* 2012 Jun;18(6):RA80-8. Perl et al. Endogenous retroviral pathogenesis in lupus. *Curr Opin Rheumatol.* 2010 Sep;22(5):483-92

<u>Examples of commonly considered viruses</u>—*continued*

<u>Virus</u>: unique characteristics	Acute disease	Chronic disease causation/association
<u>Viruses that infect bacteria, bacteriophages</u>: These are viruses that infect bacteria; bacteriophages represent approximately 10-15% of microbial genetic material in the human gastrointestinal tract **Bacteriophages are the most prevalent form of life on Earth** "Bacteriophages or phages are the most abundant organisms in the biosphere and they are a ubiquitous feature of prokaryotic existence. A bacteriophage is a virus which infects a bacterium."[73]	• No acute human illness is appreciated from bacteriophage infection, but the possibility exists that bacteriophage viruses could promote pathogenic behavior/traits in infectious bacteria (either by phenotypic modification or gene transfer), and/or that a "bloom" of bacteriophages infecting gastrointestinal bacteria could produce viral immunogens that cause a systemic inflammatory response "of unknown origin"	• <u>Possible/probable connection with autoimmunity, especially Crohn's (inflammatory bowel) disease</u>: Bacteriophage-induced inflammatory responses may play a role in inflammatory disease, for example via systemic absorption of viral immunogens from the gastrointestinal tract. Patients with the "autoimmune disease" Crohn's disease (CD) harbor many more virus-like particles (VLP) per biopsy sample (2.1-4.1 billion) than do healthy controls (1.2 billion).[74]

---

[73] Clokie MRJ et al. Phages in nature. *Bacteriophage*. 2011 Jan-Feb; 1(1): 31–45 http://www.ncbi.nlm.nih.gov/pmc/articles/PMC3109452/
[74] Lepage et al. Dysbiosis in inflammatory bowel disease: a role for bacteriophages? *Gut*. 2008 Mar;57(3):424-5

Four-Part Plan of Interconnected and Overlapping AntiViral Strategies: Molecular and Clinical Support for a Dietary and Nutritional Antiviral and Immunosupportive Protocol

From concept ("antiviral <u>Clinical Mastery</u> protocol" in 2009[75]), to extended application in the treatment of autoimmunity (<u>Rheumatology v3.5</u> in 2014[76]) to urgent global need per the ongoing viral and Ebola outbreaks in latter 2014 and beyond

<u>Topics for this section</u>:
1) Antiviral
2) Antireplication
3) Immunonutrition
4) Cell-System Support

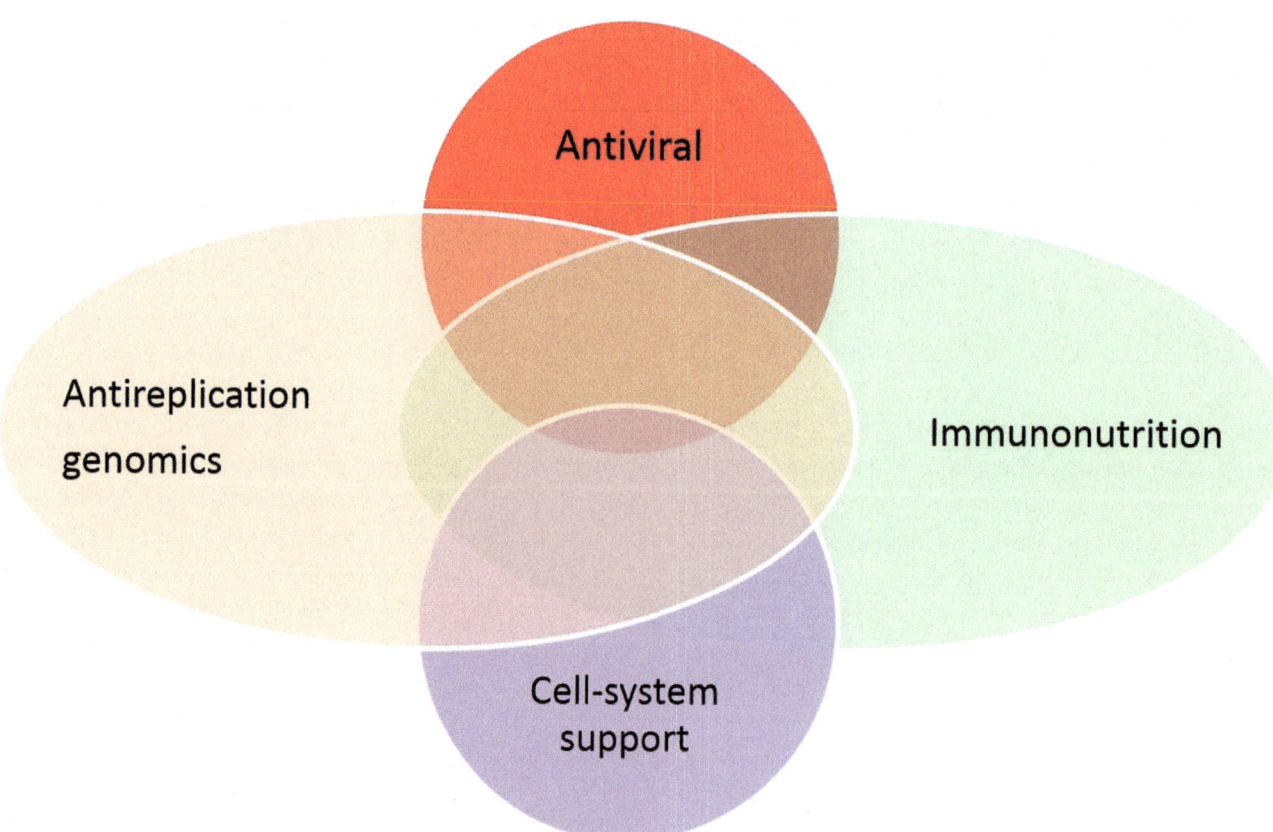

<u>**Sometimes, articulating the obvious is revolutionary**</u>: Having worked my way through three doctoral programs, dozens of medical textbooks, and thousands of research articles, I have never seen the clinical pathogenesis and treatment of viral infections explained in a way that actually helps clinicians understand how to treat—in a strategic manner—each of the core components of these common conditions. The consequence of this confusion, obfuscation, and phenomenalistic (ie, mostly or somewhat random) clinical approach has left clinicians somewhat retarded in their ability to treat virally-infected patients, which is all patients—everyone—at all times.

---

[75] Vasquez A. <u>*Chiropractic and Naturopathic Mastery of Common Clinical Disorders*</u>, 2009. createspace.com/3753564
[76] Vasquez A. <u>*Functional Medicine Rheumatology v3.5*</u> (ISBN: 9781502481368), <u>*Naturopathic Rheumatology v3.5*</u> (ISBN: 978-0990620426)

Strategy #1: Target the Virus Directly

Antiviral	Antireplication	Immunonutrition	Cell-system support
Best treatments are licorice, *Melissa*, zinc, selenium, and perhaps iodine/iodide; for herpesvirus infections, add lysine			

Emphasized in this section are interventions that act at the level of the virus itself—targeting metabolic and replicative machinery and molecular targets; most antiviral drugs work at this level. Drugs will not receive a major review here because clinicians who have access to and institutional mandates the prescription of these drugs will already have the prescribing information at hand per resource or institutional guidelines; for persons without such prescriptive authority, the information would be mostly superfluous. Furthermore, drug-based information is widely available from drug companies and is therefore not in need of review and recitation in this resource, the focus of which is to provide practical updates to strategies within the genre of alternative and complimentary medicines, ie, interventions that can replace (for example when drugs are too costly, unavailable, or are contraindicated per patient intolerance or treatment failure [per viral mutation or resistant strain, for example]) or to complement and enhance drug treatments (for example, betaine and SAMe are nutrients proven to enhance the effectiveness of drug-based treatments for HCV infection). Without further ado, let's get into it.

Antiviral botanicals

- **Licorice (*Glycyrrhiza glabra*)**: Licorice has been consumed by humans for thousands of years as a food spice, tea, and medicine. Ancient documents from China, India, and Greece all mention its use for symptoms of viral respiratory tract infections and hepatitis. Beyond its sweet taste used in the confectionary industry, licorice is best known medicinally for its use in soothing the gastrointestinal tract as well as for its potent broad-spectrum antiviral effects. The current author has worked with several patients plagued by recurrent, persistent, and pharmacorecalcitrant herpes simplex infections for whom drugs such as acyclovir failed and for whom licorice worked very satisfactorily. An articulate and accurate summary licorice's clinical value was provided by Ming and Yin AC in their 2013 review[77]: "Glycyrrhizic acid (GA), belonging to a class of triterpenes, is a conjugate of two molecules, namely glucuronic acid and glycyrrhetinic acid. It is naturally extracted from the roots of licorice plants. ... At low appropriate doses, anti-inflammatory, anti-diabetic, antioxidant, anti-tumor, antimicrobial and anti-viral properties have been reported by researchers worldwide." The pro-hypertensive sodium-retaining potassium-depleting pseudoaldosterone effect of licorice should be well appreciated by all clinicians with doctorate-level training. Less well known is the ability of licorice to potentiate cortisol and to impair testosterone biosynthesis, with the latter action useful for patients with excess testosterone or estradiol; the effect begins within four days as measured by reductions in serum testosterone (or estradiol).
  - In vitro research: Glycyrrhizic acid inhibits virus growth and inactivates virus particles (*Nature* 1979[78]): "...a component of Glycyrrhiza glabra roots, found to be glycyrrhizie acid, is active against viruses. We report here that this drug inhibits growth and cytopathology of several unrelated DNA and RNA viruses... In addition, glycyrrhizic acid inactivates herpes simplex virus particles irreversibly."
    - www.ncbi.nlm.nih.gov/pubmed/233133
    - www.InflammationMastery.com/antiviral/licorice_nature1979.pdf
  - Prevention of hepatitis C virus progression with licorice (*Oncology*. 2014 Jul[79]): "We analyzed stepwise progression rates from cirrhosis to hepatocellular carcinoma (HCC) and to death using a Markov model in 1,280 patients with HCV-related cirrhosis. During the observation period, 303 patients received

---

[77] Ming LJ, Yin AC. Therapeutic effects of glycyrrhizic acid. *Nat Prod Commun.* 2013 Mar;8(3):415-8
[78] Pompei et al. Glycyrrhizic acid inhibits virus growth and inactivates virus particles. *Nature*. 1979;281(5733):689-90
[79] Ikeda et al. Prevention of disease progression with anti-inflammatory therapy in patients with HCV-related cirrhosis: a Markov model. *Oncology*. 2014;86(5-6):295-302

interferon and 736 received glycyrrhizin injections as anti-inflammatory therapy. ... Glycyrrhizin injection therapy is useful in the prevention of disease progression in interferon-resistant or intolerant patients with HCV-related cirrhosis."

- http://www.ncbi.nlm.nih.gov/pubmed/24924385
- http://www.karger.com/Article/FullText/357713

o <u>Review: Antiviral effects of Glycyrrhiza species (Phytother Res. 2008 Feb[80])</u>: Clinical trials have demonstrated the Glycyrrhiza glabra derived compound glycyrrhizin and its derivatives are clinically beneficial in patients with chronic hepatitis B and C, including a reduction in the risk of hepatocellular carcinoma. Animal studies have shown benefit against herpes simplex virus encephalitis and influenza A virus pneumonia. In vitro studies show activity against HIV-1, SARS related coronavirus, respiratory syncytial virus, arboviruses, vaccinia virus and vesicular stomatitis virus. Numerous mechanisms are involved, including direct viral inactivation and blockade of cell entry (anti-viral effect) and enhancement of interferon gamma in T-cells (host-augmenting effect).

- www.ncbi.nlm.nih.gov/pubmed/17886224
- http://onlinelibrary.wiley.com/doi/10.1002/ptr.2295/abstract

o <u>Antiviral activity of glycyrrhizin against hepatitis C virus in vitro. (PLoS One. 2013 Jul[81])</u>: "Glycyrrhizin (GL) has been used in Japan to treat patients with chronic viral hepatitis, as an anti-inflammatory drug to reduce serum alanine aminotransferase levels. GL is also known to exhibit various biological activities, including anti-viral effects, but the anti-hepatitis C virus (HCV) effect of GL remains to be clarified. In this study, we demonstrated that GL treatment of HCV-infected Huh7 cells caused a reduction of infectious HCV production using cell culture-produced HCV (HCVcc). ... Taken together, these results suggest that GL inhibits release of infectious HCV particles. ... GL is identified as a novel anti-HCV agent that targets infectious virus particle release."

- http://www.plosone.org/article/info%3Adoi%2F10.1371%2Fjournal.pone.0068992
- http://www.ncbi.nlm.nih.gov/pmc/articles/PMC3715454/

o <u>Ex vivo study: Glycyrrhizin, an active component of licorice roots, and replication of SARS-associated coronavirus (Lancet. 2003 Jun[82])</u>: "We assessed the antiviral potential of ribavirin, 6-azauridine, pyrazofurin, mycophenolic acid, and glycyrrhizin against two clinical isolates of coronavirus (FFM-1 and FFM-2) from patients with SARS admitted to the clinical center of Frankfurt University. Of all the compounds, glycyrrhizin was the most active in inhibiting replication of the SARS-associated virus."

- www.thelancet.com/journals/lancet/article/PIIS0140-6736(03)13615-X/fulltext

o <u>Licorice has anti-viral activity against human respiratory syncytial virus (HRSV) in human respiratory tract cell lines (J Ethnopharmacol. 2013 Jul[83])</u>: "Anti-HRSV activities of hot water extracts of preparations of licorice, glycyrrhizin and 18beta-glycyrrhetinic acid (18beta-GA), the active constituents of licorice, were examined by plaque reduction assay in both human upper (HEp-2) and low (A549) respiratory tract cell lines. ... Radix Glycyrrhizae and Radix Glycyrrhizae Preparata dose-dependently inhibited HRSV-induced plaque formation in both HEp-2 and A549 cell lines (p<0.0001)." Very interestingly in this study, the authors noted that "glycyrrhizin was ineffective" and yet "18beta-GA showed a potent anti-HRSV activity." As expected, treatment was more effective when administered prior to viral inoculation, likely due to its inhibition of viral attachment and penetration. Licorice markedly decreased the viral load within the cells and appeared to promote secretion of IFN-Beta to counteract viral infection.

> **Broad-spectrum antiviral activity of licorice**
>
> "... a component of Glycyrrhiza glabra roots, found to be glycyrrhizie acid, is active against viruses. We report here that this drug inhibits growth and cytopathology of several unrelated DNA and RNA viruses... **In addition, glycyrrhizic acid inactivates herpes simplex virus particles irreversibly.**"
>
> Pompei et al. Glycyrrhizic acid inhibits virus growth and inactivates virus particles. *Nature.* 1979 Oct

- http://www.ncbi.nlm.nih.gov/pubmed/23643542
- http://www.sciencedirect.com/science/article/pii/S037887411300305X

---

[80] Fiore et al. Antiviral effects of Glycyrrhiza species. *Phytother Res.* 2008 Feb;22(2):141-8
[81] Matsumoto et al. Antiviral activity of glycyrrhizin against hepatitis C virus in vitro. *PLoS One.* 2013 Jul 18;8(7):e68992
[82] Cinatl et al. Glycyrrhizin, an active component of liquorice roots, and replication of SARS-associated coronavirus. *Lancet.* 2003 Jun 14;361(9374):2045-6
[83] Feng Yeh et al. Water extract of licorice had anti-viral activity against human respiratory syncytial virus in human respiratory tract cell lines. *J Ethnopharmacol.* 2013 Jul 9;148(2):466-73

- o Intravenous glycyrrhizin for the treatment of chronic hepatitis C: a double-blind, randomized, placebo-controlled phase I/II trial (*J Gastroenterol Hepatol* 1999 Nov[84]): In Japan, glycyrrhizin therapy is widely used for chronic hepatitis C and reportedly reduces the progression of liver disease to hepatocellular carcinoma. 57 patients with chronic hepatitis C, non-responders or unlikely to respond (genotype 1/cirrhosis) to interferon therapy, were randomized to one of the four dose groups: 240, 160 or 80 mg glycyrrhizin or placebo (0 mg glycyrrhizin). Medication was administered intravenously thrice weekly for 4 weeks; follow up also lasted for 4 weeks. "RESULTS: Within 2 days of start of therapy, serum ALT had dropped 15% below baseline in the three dosage groups (P < 0.02). The mean ALT decrease at the end of active treatment was 26%, significantly higher [greater reduction] than the placebo group (6%). A clear dose-response effect was not observed (29, 26, 23% ALT decrease for 240, 160 and 80 mg, respectively). Normalization of ALT at the end of treatment occurred in 10% (four of 41). The effect on ALT disappeared after cessation of therapy. During treatment, viral clearance was not observed: the mean decrease in plasma HCV-RNA after active treatment was 4.1 x 10(6) genome equivalents/mL (95% confidence interval, 0-8.2 x 10(6); P > 0.1). No major side-effects were noted. None of the patients withdrew from the study because of intolerance. CONCLUSIONS: Glycyrrhizin up to 240 mg, thrice weekly, lowers serum ALT during treatment, but has no effect on HCV-RNA levels. The drug appears to be safe and is well tolerated."
  - http://www.ncbi.nlm.nih.gov/pubmed/10574137
  - http://onlinelibrary.wiley.com/doi/10.1046/j.1440-1746.1999.02008.x/abstract
- o Review: The use of alternative medicine in the treatment of hepatitis C (*Am Clin Lab.* 2002 May[85]): "The active component of licorice root, glycyrrhizin, has been shown to reduce alanine transaminase and aspartate transaminase values in the serum. This protective function has recently been explained as the inhibitory effects of glycyrrhizin on immune-mediated cytotoxicity against hepatocytes and on nuclear factor (NF)-kappa B, …"
- **Carica papaya ("papaya")—juice from leaf, not fruit**: Numerous cases and peer-reviewed studies support the use of papaya leaf (not fruit) juice against viral infections, most notably *but not exclusively* dengue virus. The antiviral action is direct, via inhibition of viral assembly, as well as replication.
  - o Carica papaya leaves Juice Significantly Accelerates the Rate of Increase in Platelet Count among Patients with Dengue Fever and Dengue Hemorrhagic Fever. (*Evid Based Complement Alternat Med.* 2013[86]): "The study was conducted to investigate the platelet increasing property of Carica papaya leaves juice (CPLJ) in patients with dengue fever (DF). An open labeled randomized controlled trial was carried out on 228 patients with DF and dengue hemorrhagic fever (DHF). Approximately half the patients received the juice, for 3 consecutive days while the others remained as controls and received the standard management. Their full blood count was monitored 8 hours for 48 hours. Gene expression studies were conducted on the ALOX 12 and PTAFR genes. The mean increase in platelet counts were compared in both groups using repeated measure ANCOVA. There was a significant increase in mean platelet count observed in the intervention group (P < 0.001) but not in the control group 40 hours since the first dose of CPLJ. Comparison of mean platelet count between intervention and control group showed that mean platelet count in intervention group was significantly higher than control group after 40 and 48 hours of admission (P < 0.01). The ALOX 12 (FC = 15.00) and PTAFR (FC = 13.42) genes were highly expressed among those on the juice. It was concluded that CPLJ does significantly increase the platelet count in patients with DF and DHF."
    - http://www.ncbi.nlm.nih.gov/pmc/articles/PMC3638585/
    - http://www.hindawi.com/journals/ecam/2013/616737/
    - https://www.youtube.com/watch?v=3nVQL9t7kns (video on how to prepare juice)
    - https://www.youtube.com/watch?v=7yZgSZRoC3o (supporting video)

---

[84] van Rossum et al. Intravenous glycyrrhizin for the treatment of chronic hepatitis C: a double-blind, randomized, placebo-controlled phase I/II trial. *J Gastroenterol Hepatol.* 1999 Nov;14(11):1093-9
[85] Bean P. The use of alternative medicine in the treatment of hepatitis C. *Am Clin Lab.* 2002 May;21(4):19-21
[86] Subenthiran et al. Carica papaya Leaves Juice Significantly Accelerates the Rate of Increase in Platelet Count among Patients with Dengue Fever and Dengue Haemorrhagic Fever. *Evid Based Complement Alternat Med.* 2013;2013:616737

- o Flavonoid from Carica papaya inhibits NS2B-NS3 protease and prevents Dengue 2 viral assembly. (*Bioinformation*. 2013 Nov[87]): "We analysed the anti-dengue activities of the extracts from Carica papaya by using bioinformatics tools. Interestingly, we find the flavonoid quercetin with highest binding energy against NS2B-NS3 protease which is evident by the formation of six hydrogen bonds with the amino acid residues at the binding site of the receptor. Our results suggest that the flavonoids from Carica papaya have significant anti-dengue activities."
    - http://www.ncbi.nlm.nih.gov/pubmed/24307765
    - http://www.ncbi.nlm.nih.gov/pmc/articles/PMC3842573/
- o Effects of papaya leaves on thrombocyte counts in dengue—case report. (*J Pak Med Assoc*. 2014 Mar[88]): "Dengue fever is on the rise in developing nations like India, Pakistan, Sri Lanka and Bangladesh. There is no antiviral chemotherapy or vaccine for dengue virus and management of the disease is done on supportive measures. The decline in the thrombocyte count leads to dengue hemorrhagic fever accounting for complications and mortality. Oral administration of Carica papaya leaves extract is said to have a positive impact on thrombocyte count. A 23-year-old man was administered a calculated dose for five days. Blood samples were tested for complete blood count before and after the administration of the juice. Thrombocyte count had increased from 28000/micro liter to 138000/micro liter at the end of five days."
    - http://www.ncbi.nlm.nih.gov/pubmed/24864622
- o Dengue fever treatment with Carica papaya leaves extracts. (*Asian Pac J Trop Biomed*. 2011 Aug[89]): "Subsequently, the blood samples were rechecked after the administration of leaves extract. It was observed that the PLT count increased from 55×10(3)/μL to 168×10(3)/μL, WBC from 3.7×10(3)/μL to 7.7×10(3)/μL and NEUT from 46.0% to 78.3%. From the patient feelings and blood reports it showed that Carica papaya leaves aqueous extract exhibited potential activity against Dengue fever. Furthermore, the different parts of this valuable specie can be further used as a strong natural candidate against viral diseases."
    - http://www.ncbi.nlm.nih.gov/pmc/articles/PMC3614241/
    - http://www.ncbi.nlm.nih.gov/pubmed/23569787/
- **Lemon balm (*Melissa officinalis*)**: *Melissa officinalis* is available for oral (e.g., tea or tablets) and/or topical use. Like licorice, it has nonspecific antiviral benefits. Possible interference with thyroid function when *Melissa officinalis* is consumed in high doses internally/orally can be monitored via clinical and laboratory assessments. Aqueous extracts from lemon balm (*Melissa officinalis*), peppermint (*Mentha piperita*), prunella (*Prunella vulgaris*), rosemary (*Rosmarinus officinalis*), sage (*Salvia officinalis*) and thyme (*Thymus vulgaris*) exert a direct antiviral effect on free herpes simplex virus.[90]
    - o Topical application of *Melissa officinalis* L. leaves (70:1) for recurring herpes labialis (*Phytomedicine*. 1999 Oct[91]): A cream made from *Melissa officinalis* L. leaves (concentrated 70:1) was studied among 66 patients with herpes simplex labialis. Patients had at least four herpes episodes per year. Cream was applied to the affected area four times daily over five days. "The tested formulation is effective for the treatment of herpes simplex labialis." Benefits included shortening of the healing period, the prevention of a spreading of the infection, prolonged intervals between the periods with herpes outbreaks, and rapid reduction of typical symptoms: itching, tingling, burning, stabbing, swelling, tautness and erythema.

Antiviral nutrients

- **Zinc: up to 50 mg per day of elemental zinc for adults; limit duration and/or co-administer copper to avoid zinc-induced copper deficiency**: Zinc ions are directly antiviral, and this is the rationale behind the use of zinc throat lozenges, which generally show significant benefit in the prevention and treatment of respiratory tract infections, including influenza.[92] Zinc is also required for the proper production of thymulin, which is an immune-supporting peptide hormone made by the thymus gland required for maturation of T-helper cells; in

---

[87] Senthilvel et al. Flavonoid from Carica papaya inhibits NS2B-NS3 protease and prevents Dengue 2 viral assembly. *Bioinformation*. 2013 Nov 11;9(18):889-95
[88] Siddique et al. Effects of papaya leaves on thrombocyte counts in dengue--a case report. *J Pak Med Assoc*. 2014 Mar;64(3):364-6
[89] Ahmad et al. Dengue fever treatment with Carica papaya leaves extracts. *Asian Pac J Trop Biomed*. 2011 Aug;1(4):330-3
[90] Nolkemper et al. Antiviral effect of aqueous extracts from species of Lamiaceae family against Herpes simplex virus type 1 and 2 in vitro. *Planta Med*. 2006 Dec;72:1378-82
[91] Koytchev R, Alken RG, Dundarov S. Balm mint extract (Lo-701) for topical treatment of recurring herpes labialis. *Phytomedicine*. 1999 Oct;6(4):225-30
[92] Roxas M, Jurenka J. Colds and influenza: a review of diagnosis and conventional, botanical, and nutritional considerations. *Altern Med Rev*. 2007 Mar;12(1):25-4

zinc-depleted chronically infected patients, their undetectable levels of thymulin can be raised to the normal level following zinc supplementation with a corresponding restoration of immune function. Zinc has an important role in cell-mediated immune functions and also functions as anti-inflammatory and antioxidant agent[93]; thus, the state of zinc deficiency (which can be assessed by measuring serum zinc, among other methods) is a state of immunodysfunction/immunosuppression, and superfluous pro-inflammation and oxidative stress. Per the review by Hadden[94], the adverse effects on the immune system caused by zinc deficiency include but are not limited to thymic involution, thymocyte depletion in thymus, depression of serum thymopoietin and thymulin, depression of delayed type hypersensitivity, depressed peripheral T-lymphocyte and/or T-cell numbers, depressed T-cell mitogen responses, depressed primary and secondary responses to sheep red blood cells, depressed T-helper function, depressed natural killer function. Furthermore, per the review by Prasad[95], in zinc deficiency, the CD4+ to CD8+ ratio is decreased and Th-1 cytokines IL-2 and IFN-gamma are both decreased; this would obviously favor the acquisition and persistence of viral infections.

- o Clinical trial contrasting oral zinc (20 mg/d) plus multivitamin syrup or multivitamin syrup alone: Impact of zinc supplementation on subsequent growth and morbidity in Bangladeshi children with acute diarrhea (*Eur J Clin Nutr.* 1999 Jul[96]): "These results suggest that a short course of zinc supplementation (20 mg/d) to malnourished children during acute diarrhea reduces growth-faltering and diarrhea and respiratory [infection] morbidity during subsequent two months."
- o Double-blind, controlled trial: Zinc supplementation (10 mg/d) reduces the incidence of acute lower respiratory infections in infants and preschool children (n=298 vs 311 controls) (*Pediatrics* 1998 Jul[97]): "Zinc-supplemented children had 0.19 acute lower respiratory infection episodes/child/year compared with 0.35 episodes/child/year in the control children. After correction for correlation of data using generalized estimating equation regression methods, there was a reduction of 45% in the incidence of acute lower respiratory infections in zinc-supplemented children." These results are impressive for low-dose zinc monotherapy.
- o Clinical trial of zinc (10-20 mg/d) with or without a single large dose of vitamin A (100,000-200,000 IU): Effect of routine zinc supplementation on acute lower respiratory tract infections and pneumonia in children aged 6 months to 3 years: randomized controlled trial in an urban slum (*BMJ.* 2002 Jun[98]): "Zinc supplementation resulted in a lower incidence of pneumonia than placebo... CONCLUSIONS: Zinc supplementation substantially reduced the incidence of pneumonia in children who had received vitamin A."

- **Iodine/iodide—oral administration of pharmacologic doses**: Both iodine and iodide have biological activity in humans. Beyond thyroid hormone metabolism, iodine/iodide has important roles in estrogen metabolism—both in the modulation of estrogen subfractions as well as in the modulation (downregulation) of cellular estrogen receptors; these "anti-estrogen effects of iodine" contribute to its anticancer benefits. Relevant to this conversation is the antimicrobial effects of iodine/iodide; by their first or second year of professional education, all healthcare students who have had hand-on access to microbiology laboratory work are familiar with Lugol's solution. Lugol's solution is a broad-spectrum antiseptic introduced into medicine/microbiology in 1829 by the French physician Jean Lugol; it is an effective bactericide, fungicide, and virucide made by dissolving 10 parts of potassium iodide and 5 parts of iodine in 85 parts of water. By this time, clinicians should appreciate the potential benefits of routinely employing an essential nutrient with antiestrogen benefits, anticancer benefits, and antimicrobial (antibacterial, antiviral, and antifungal) effects. Human leukocytes preferentially concentrate iodide 1200-fold greater than do erythrocytes; experimental studies have shown that the combination of iodide with hydrogen peroxide and myeloperoxidase greatly increases the bactericidal activity over what is seen with myeloperoxidase alone.[99] The virucidal effect of 1% Lugol's solution against influenza was shown *in vitro* in 1944 by Dunham and MacNeal.[100] What is being proposed here is the *potential* for antiviral benefit from the

---

[93] Prasad AS. Zinc: mechanisms of host defense. *J Nutr.* 2007 May;137(5):1345-9
[94] Hadden JW. The treatment of zinc deficiency is an immunotherapy. *Int J Immunopharmacol.* 1995 Sep;17(9):697-701
[95] Prasad AS. Zinc: mechanisms of host defense. *J Nutr.* 2007 May;137(5):1345-9
[96] Roy et al. Impact of zinc supplementation on subsequent growth and morbidity in Bangladeshi children with acute diarrhoea. *Eur J Clin Nutr.* 1999 Jul;53(7):529-34
[97] Sazawal et al. Zinc supplementation reduces the incidence of acute lower respiratory infections in infants and preschool children. *Pediatrics.* 1998 Jul;102(1 Pt 1):1-5
[98] Bhandari et al. Effect of routine zinc supplementation on pneumonia in children aged 6 months to 3 years. *BMJ.* 2002 Jun 8;324(7350):1358
[99] Klebanoff SJ. Iodination of bacteria: a bactericidal mechanism. *J Exp Med.* 1967 Dec 1;126(6):1063-78
[100] Dunham WB, MacNeal WJ. Inactivation of Influenza Virus by Mild Antiseptics. *Journal of Immunology* 1944; 49: 123-128

supplemental use of this nutrient; of course, the recognition of this positive potentiality precedes the necessary clinical trials to validate this concept, but the safety and basic science are well established. At the very least, we could reasonably anticipate that Lugol's solution—whether consumed as liquid drops or in tablet form as is commercially available—would have activity against microbes in the upper gastrointestinal tract, namely *Helicobacter pylori*; again, clinical trials are needed here. Saturated solution of potassium iodide (SSKI) is also used in humans for nutritional and therapeutic purposes. Limited evidence does prove (*not merely suggest*) that orally administered iodine/iodide has systemic antimicrobial benefit in humans.

- o Case report: Rhinofacial zygomycosis (RFZ) successfully treated with oral saturated solution of potassium iodide: a case report (*J Eur Acad Dermatol Venereol.* 2007 Jan[101]): "A diagnosis of RFZ was made and the patient was put on oral SSKI at an initial dose of 0.5 mL three times daily. This was gradually increased by 0.1 mL/dose/day until a dose of 5 mL three times daily was reached." By the one year of treatment, an 80% reduction in facial swelling.
  - http://www.ncbi.nlm.nih.gov/pubmed/17207186
  - http://onlinelibrary.wiley.com/doi/10.1111/j.1468-3083.2006.01803.x/abstract
- o Case reports: Sporotrichosis in childhood: clinical and therapeutic experience in 25 patients (*Pediatr Dermatol.* 2007 Jul[102]): "*Sporothrix schenckii* was isolated in all patients… Nineteen patients were treated and cured clinically and mycologically with potassium iodide… The dose of KI used was 1–3 g/day, starting at 1 g/day and increasing until the dose of 3 g/day was reached." The authors write that the duration of treatment is generally 3 months, and that side-effects occur in 5% to 10% of patients, mainly consisting of gastrointestinal symptoms, headache, or rhinorrhea; these adverse effects are eliminated when treatment is discontinued or the dose is reduced.
  - http://www.ncbi.nlm.nih.gov/pubmed/17845157
  - http://onlinelibrary.wiley.com/doi/10.1111/j.1525-1470.2007.00452.x/abstract

- **Lysine**: Lysine as an amino acid supplement is most famous for its use in the suppression of herpes outbreaks. Herpes simplex virus (HSV) type-1 infects about 50% of the human population, while HSV type-2 infects about 20% of the human population. Many and perhaps most patients are either asymptomatic and/or are unaware that they carry the infection and can transmit it via close contact such as kissing or sexual intercourse. *Lack of a visible outbreak or symptoms in no way indicates lack of transmissibility.* On the other end of the symptomatic spectrum, some unfortunate patients live in perpetual cycles of painful blistering and weeping outbreaks; these patients generally suffer quietly as they receive no time off from work or other compensation during what can be very painful attacks. HSV infects close to 70% of adults worldwide. From a pathologic perspective, HSV-1 is notorious for causing herpes encephalitis, which is a commonly fatal or devastating infection of the brain, generally involving the temporal lobes; this infection is typically fatal when neonates are infected during travel through an *actively herpetic* birth canal. When used for its anti-HSV effects, lysine should be consumed between meals, with avoidance of arginine-containing foods, and in combination with other immunosupportive nutrients such as licorice and lipoic acid and other NFkB inhibitors within a context of improved overall nutrition and lifestyle. There is no "cure" in terms of eradication for herpes—it is a chronic life-long infection, whether symptomatic or asymptomatic, hence the adage, "Love can be fleeting, but herpes is forever."

  - o Double-blind, placebo-controlled, multicenter trial: Success of l-lysine therapy in frequently recurrent herpes simplex infection (*Dermatologica* 1987[103]): Twenty-seven patients were given L-Lysine monohydrochloride tablets (1,000 mg L-lysine per dose) 3 times a day for 6 months and their outcomes were compared to a placebo group. "The L-lysine treatment group had an average of 2.4 less HSV infections [during the 6-month period], symptoms were significantly diminished in severity and healing time was significantly reduced [i.e., faster healing]. L-Lysine appears to be an effective agent for reduction of occurrence, severity and healing time for recurrent HSV infection." The results of this study are comparable to if not better than the results obtained with several of the new anti-herpes drugs; however this treatment is inexpensive and does not carry the risks of chemical hepatitis and life-threatening drug reactions that are noted with the anti-herpes drugs.

---

[101] Tripathy et al. Rhinofacial zygomycosis successfully treated with oral saturated solution of potassium iodide. *J Eur Acad Dermatol Venereol.* 2007 Jan;21(1):117-9
[102] Bonifaz et al. Sporotrichosis in childhood: clinical and therapeutic experience in 25 patients. *Pediatr Dermatol.* 2007 Jul-Aug;24(4):369-72
[103] Griffith et al. Success of l-lysine therapy in frequently recurrent herpes simplex infection. Treatment and prophylaxis. *Dermatologica* 1987;175:183-90

- o <u>Double-blind, controlled crossover study: Lysine prophylaxis in recurrent herpes simplex labialis</u> (*Acta Derm Venereol.* 1980[104]): L-lysine has an inhibitory effect on the multiplication of herpes simplex virus in cell cultures. This study used only 1,000 mg L-lysine monohydrochloride daily to find little benefit within 12 weeks; note that the dose used in this study was only 33% of the dose used by Griffith et al[105] and that the duration was 3 months compared with 6 months. Nonetheless, the authors noted, "…significantly more patients were recurrence-free during lysine than during placebo treatment (p = 0.05), suggesting that certain patients may benefit from prophylactic lysine administration."

- o <u>Prospective, randomized, double-blind, placebo-controlled, cross-over study of forty-one patients: Treatment of recurrent herpes simplex infections with L-lysine monohydrochloride</u> (*Cutis.* 1984 Oct[106]): The authors report that oral ingestion of 1,248 mg a day of L-Lysine monohydrochloride shows evidence of decreasing the recurrence rate of herpes simplex attacks in their patient population of "nonimmunocompromised hosts", while a dose of 624 mg a day was not effective. Further, they report that "L-Lysine may also be capable of decreasing the severity of symptoms associated with recurrences."

- **Adenosine monophosphate (AMP)**: Based on published trials and clinical experience, Gaby[107] has been a proponent of AMP in the treatment of herpes simplex virus (HSV) infections, and he reviewed its supporting literature in 2006. Different dosage schemes have been published (see article by Gaby for review and procedure): one scheme involves using AMP administered in a series of intramuscular injections with each intramuscular injection containing AMP 1.5-2.0 mg per kg body weight are administered every other day for a total of 9-12 treatments; Gaby reports using intramuscular AMP injections (usually 100 mg per injection) for a series of 10 injections with good clinical effect. Patients with herpesvirus infections show low levels of AMP in their blood compared with uninfected controls. The antiviral mechanism of AMP is not specifically defined; it may involve modulation of the cyclic adenosine monophosphate-response element, which is a transcription factor complex that participates in the regulation of viral gene expression and virus-induced diseases. Although AMP is a constituent of the human body and is therefore generally safe and nontoxic when administered parenterally/intramuscularly, clinicians might use caution in asthmatic patients given that *inhaled* AMP induces airway obstruction in asthmatic patients (but not in healthy subjects).[108]

  - o <u>Herpes zoster. The treatment and prevention of neuralgia with adenosine monophosphate</u> (*JAMA.* 1985 Mar[109]): Thirty-two adults were treated with intramuscular injections of gel-sustained adenosine monophosphate (AMP) given three times a week for up to four weeks for acute herpes zoster. Patients reported a reduction in pain soon after the start of treatment; also noted were decreased desquamation time and faster healing of skin lesions. Duration of viral shedding was reduced; indicating both the healing of skin lesions, reduced viral replication, and reduced risk of infectivity. "At the end of the initial four-week treatment period, 88% of AMP-treated patients were pain free, as opposed to only 43% in the placebo group. … All these patients recovered from pain within three weeks after initiation of treatment. No recurrence of pain or lesions was experienced from three to 18 months after the end of treatment."[110] Adenosine monophosphate is a natural cellular metabolite, and thus showed no adverse effects or toxicity during or following the treatment. Thus, the anti-herpes effect of AMP is seen against both herpes zoster virus and herpes simplex virus.
    - http://www.ncbi.nlm.nih.gov/pubmed/3968773
    - http://jama.jamanetwork.com/article.aspx?articleid=397257

- <u>Grape seed extract (GSE)</u>: GSE has been safely used in humans mostly for its benefits as a botanical antioxidant; it also has anti-inflammatory, anticarcinogenic, and antimicrobial properties. One would reasonably expect it to have antiviral properties via its ability to block the NFkB pathway; direct antiviral—virucidal—activity appears to have been demonstrated by Su and D'Souza in 2011 in the study summarized and cited below:

---

[104]Milman N, Scheibel J, Jessen O. Lysine prophylaxis in recurrent herpes simplex labialis: a double-blind, controlled crossover study. *Acta Derm Venereol.* 1980;60(1):85-7
[105] Griffith et al. Success of l-lysine therapy in frequently recurrent herpes simplex infection. Treatment and prophylaxis. *Dermatologica* 1987;175:183-90
[106] McCune MA, Perry HO, Muller SA, O'Fallon WM. Treatment of recurrent herpes simplex infections with L-lysine monohydrochloride. *Cutis.* 1984 Oct;34(4):366-73
[107] Gaby AR. Natural remedies for Herpes simplex. *Altern Med Rev.* 2006 Jun;11(2):93-101
[108] "The mechanism of AMP is indirect and occurs via its decay product, adenosine. It stimulates mast cells through its low-affinity receptor A2B to release histamine, which ultimately leads to smooth muscle contraction." Vass et al. Adenosine and adenosine receptors in the pathomechanism and treatment of respiratory diseases. *Curr Med Chem.* 2008;15(9):917-22
[109] Sklar et al. Herpes zoster. The treatment and prevention of neuralgia with adenosine monophosphate. *JAMA.* 1985 Mar 8;253(10):1427-30
[110] Sklar et al. Herpes zoster. The treatment and prevention of neuralgia with adenosine monophosphate. *JAMA.* 1985 Mar 8;253(10):1427-30

- o Grape seed extract for control of human enteric viruses. (*Appl Environ Microbiol.* 2011 Jun[111]): "In the present study, the effect of commercial GSE, Gravinol-S, on the infectivity of human enteric virus surrogates (feline calicivirus, FCV-F9; murine norovirus, MNV-1; and bacteriophage MS2) and hepatitis A virus (HAV; strain HM175) was evaluated. ...At high titers (□7 log(10) PFU/ml), FCV-F9 was significantly reduced by 3.64, 4.10, and 4.61 log(10) PFU/ml; MNV-1 by 0.82, 1.35, and 1.73 log(10) PFU/ml; MS2 by 1.13, 1.43, and 1.60 log(10) PFU/ml; and HAV by 1.81, 2.66, and 3.20 log(10) PFU/ml after treatment at 37°C with 0.25, 0.50, and 1 mg/ml GSE, respectively (P < 0.05) in a dose-dependent manner. GSE treatment of low titers (□5 log(10) PFU/ml) at 37°C also showed viral reductions. ... Our results indicate that GSE shows promise for application in the food industry as an inexpensive novel natural alternative to reduce viral contamination and enhance food safety." Although this is an in vitro study and the authors used " human enteric virus surrogates", the findings of this study appear to indicate that GSE has direct virucidal properties; of particular note is the effectiveness against the bacteriophage which might—by a reasonably logical extension—help explain part of the beneficial effects of plant-based diets in the prevention and treatment of inflammatory disorders, per the assumption (mine) that gastrointestinal bacteriophages may promote stimulation of a systemic inflammatory response.

Novel antiviral drugs and prescription agents (and links to other medical treatments and resources)

The only antiviral drugs that are reviewed here are those which are unique/novel/off-label; physicians with prescriptive authority—especially those physicians specializing in the treatment of infectious diseases—are already well-versed in antiviral drug use, and any review here would be superfluous. Updated information about antiviral drugs is available per the following official, authoritative, and self-explanatory databases; the website hyperlinks provided in the following list serve as examples and gateways for additional information:

- Ebola: http://www.cdc.gov/vhf/ebola/treatment/index.html
- Enterovirus D68: http://www.cdc.gov/features/evd68/
- Flu: http://www.cdc.gov/flu/professionals/**antivirals**/summary-clinicians.htm
- Herpes: http://www.cdc.gov/std/Herpes/default.htm
- HIV: http://www.cdc.gov/hiv/guidelines/persons.html
- Antiviral Drugs for viruses other than human immunodeficiency virus. (*Mayo Clin Proc* 2011 Oct): This is a notably well-organized, thorough, and practical review available as full-text / open-access.
  - o http://www.ncbi.nlm.nih.gov/pmc/articles/PMC3184032/
  - o http://www.mayoclinicproceedings.org/article/S0025-6196(11)65243-9/abstract
- Novel antiviral applications for drugs:
  - o FDA-approved selective estrogen receptor modulators inhibit Ebola virus infection (*Sci Transl Med.* 2013 Jun[112]): This fascinating research found that two drugs inhibit Ebola virus infection; although both drugs mentioned are anti-estrogen drugs, their antiviral effect is independent of estrogen reception, signaling, or metabolism. "[W]e identified a set of selective estrogen receptor modulators (SERMs), including clomiphene and toremifene, which act as potent inhibitors of EBOV infection. Anti-EBOV activity was confirmed for both of these SERMs in an in vivo mouse infection model. This anti-EBOV activity occurred even in the absence of detectable estrogen receptor expression, and both SERMs inhibited virus entry after internalization, suggesting that clomiphene and toremifene are not working through classical pathways associated with the estrogen receptor."
    - ▪ http://stm.sciencemag.org/content/5/190/190ra79.long
    - ▪ http://www.ncbi.nlm.nih.gov/pmc/articles/PMC3955358/
  - o High-dose mannose-binding lectin therapy for Ebola virus infection. (*J Infect Dis.* 2011 Jan[113]): Mannose-binding lectin (MBL) is a protein made in the liver and which serves as part of the innate immune system by binding onto microorganisms (select bacteria and viruses with specific surface glycans) for destruction by phagocytosis and/or complement-mediated lysis. "Although recombinant human MBL (rhMBL) trials have focused on reconstitution therapy, safety studies have identified no barriers to its use at higher levels. Ebola viruses cause fatal hemorrhagic fevers for which no treatment exists and that are feared as

---

[111] Su X, D'Souza DH. Grape seed extract for control of human enteric viruses. *Appl Environ Microbiol.* 2011 Jun;77(12):3982-7
[112] Johansen et al. FDA-approved selective estrogen receptor modulators inhibit Ebola virus infection. *Sci Transl Med.* 2013 Jun 19;5(190):190ra79
[113] Michelow et al. High-dose mannose-binding lectin therapy for Ebola virus infection. *J Infect Dis.* 2011 Jan 15;203(2):175-9

potential biothreat agents. We found that mice whose rhMBL serum concentrations were increased ≥7-fold above average human levels survived otherwise fatal Ebola virus infections and became immune to virus rechallenge."

- http://www.ncbi.nlm.nih.gov/pmc/articles/PMC3071052/
- http://jid.oxfordjournals.org/content/203/2/175.full.html
- http://jid.oxfordjournals.org/content/203/2/175.full.pdf

Antimutagenesis as a direct antiviral strategy

An extension of the direct antiviral strategies is antimutagensis, because viruses "use" mutagenesis as a means to change behavior (becoming more pathogenic/virulent) and to escape immune detection/destruction (changing molecular surfaces, molecules, and "signatures" or "appearances" provides a constantly moving target to which the immune system must constantly adapt; in this way, viruses gain advantage and more time to continue replicating. According to the important work of Dr Melinda Beck, a major driver of viral mutagenesis—and thus pathogenicity and immune evasion—is the free radical burden and oxidant stress level of the host; more free radicals in the environment (the tissues and fluids of the human host are the external environment of the virus) promote DNA damage of the virus and thus mutations in that DNA which can provide the virus with a survival advantage.

> **Nutritional deficiencies impair host immune responses and mucosal defenses, and promote viral mutations that lead to more severe and recalcitrant infections**
>
> "Many viral infections, for example infections with rotavirus, measles, and parainfluenza virus, are much more severe in malnourished hosts as compared with well-nourished hosts. ... With the current interest in emerging infectious diseases, it would be important to consider the **host nutritional status as a driving force for viral mutations**."
>
> Beck MA. Antioxidants and viral infections: host immune response and viral pathogenicity. *J Am Coll Nutr.* 2001

- Selenium: 600-1,000 mcg per day, limit duration of highest doses:
  - Review: Antioxidants and viral infections: host immune response and viral pathogenicity (*J Am Coll Nutr.* 2001 Oct[114]): "Work in our laboratory has demonstrated that not only is the host affected by the nutritional deficiency, but the invading pathogen is as well. ... The immune system was altered in the Se-deficient animals, as was the viral pathogen itself." Dr Beck goes on to note that viral isolates recovered from Se-deficient mice demonstrated mutations in the viral genome of both coxsackievirus and influenza virus, and that these changes in the viral genome are associated with increased pathogenicity of the virus. Many of the antiviral/immunosupportive benefits of selenium appear to be mediated though the antioxidant selenoenzyme, glutathione peroxidase-1, given that glutathione peroxidase knockout mice developed myocarditis, similar to the Se-deficient mice, when infected with the benign strain of myocarditis.
  - Review: Nutritionally induced oxidative stress: effect on viral disease (*Am J Clin Nutr.* 2000 Jun[115]): "The nutritional status of the host can have a profound influence on a virus, so that a normally avirulent virus becomes virulent because of changes in the viral genome."
  - Review: Selenium and vitamin E status: impact on viral pathogenicity (*J Nutr.* 2007 May[116]): "Recent work has demonstrated that deficiencies in either Se or vitamin E result in increased viral pathogenicity and altered immune responses. Furthermore, deficiencies in either Se or vitamin E results in specific viral mutations, changing relatively benign viruses into virulent ones."
  - Review: Selenium and host defense towards viruses (*Proc Nutr Soc.* 1999 Aug[117]): Nutritional deficiencies cause immunosuppression—this point has been made very clear and is medically irrefutable, despite the fact that it is commonly medically ignored. In this review, Dr Beck again reminds us that the adverse alterations due to nutritional deficiency are not limited to the effect on the human host; when the human host is nutritionally deficient, the changes in the biochemical milieu also affect the replication and level of mutagenicity within the viral invader. Nutritional deficiency leads to increased oxidative stress; increased oxidative stress promotes additional mutations within the virus, and these additional mutations cause the virus to behave more aggressively, thereby increasing the severity of the viral

---

[114] Beck MA. Antioxidants and viral infections: host immune response and viral pathogenicity. *J Am Coll Nutr.* 2001 Oct;20(5 Suppl):384S-388S

[115] Beck MA. Nutritionally induced oxidative stress: effect on viral disease. *Am J Clin Nutr.* 2000 Jun;71(6 Suppl):1676S-81S

[116] Beck MA. Selenium and vitamin E status: impact on viral pathogenicity. *J Nutr.* 2007 May;137(5):1338-40

[117] Beck MA. Selenium and host defence towards viruses. *Proc Nutr Soc.* 1999 Aug;58(3):707-11

infection while also increasing the infectivity of the virus to include nutritionally-replete hosts. "Six nucleotide changes were found in the virus that replicated in the deficient mice, and once these mutations occurred, even mice with normal nutrition became susceptible to disease. Thus, the nutritional status of the host was able to transform an avirulent virus into a virulent one due to genomic changes in the virus."

o Double-blind, randomized, placebo-controlled trial clinical trial: Suppression of human immunodeficiency virus type 1 viral load with selenium supplementation: a randomized controlled trial (*Arch Intern Med.* 2007 Jan [118]): This study used "High selenium yeast supplementation (200 mcg/d)" to evaluate effect on HIV-1 viral load and CD4 count after 9 months of treatment among 262 HIV-positive men and women. Evidence of dose-response was noted, with higher selenium levels correlating with lower HIV viral load and higher CD4 count. The authors conclude that, "Daily selenium supplementation can suppress the progression of HIV-1 viral burden and provide indirect improvement of CD4 count. The results support the use of selenium as a simple, inexpensive, and safe adjunct therapy in HIV spectrum disease."
  - http://www.ncbi.nlm.nih.gov/pubmed/17242315
  - http://archinte.jamanetwork.com/article.aspx?articleid=411535

o Clinical trial: Selenium in Intensive Care (SIC): results of a prospective randomized, placebo-controlled, multiple-center study in patients with severe systemic inflammatory response syndrome, sepsis, and septic shock (*Crit Care Med.* 2007 Jan[119]): This trial took place among eleven intensive care units in Germany among 249 patients with severe systemic inflammatory response syndrome, sepsis, and septic shock. Acute Physiology and Chronic Health Evaluation (APACHE) III score was >70. Patients received 1000 microg of sodium-selenite as a 30-min bolus injection, followed by 14 daily continuous infusions of 1000 microg intravenously, or placebo. "The intention-to-treat analysis of the remaining 238 patients revealed a mortality rate of 50.0% in the placebo group and 39.7% in the selenium-treated group. ... the 28-day mortality rate was significantly reduced to 42.4% compared with 56.7% in 97 patients of the placebo group." No side effects were observed due to high-dose sodium-selenite treatment. Orally administered 1000 mcg of selenium is a reasonable dose for in-office use; duration can optionally be limited to a few days or a few weeks but should not extend for more than about two months unless professionally supervised and clinically indicated.

o Clinical trial: Effects of high doses of selenium, as sodium selenite, in septic shock: a placebo-controlled, randomized, double-blind, phase II study (*Crit Care.* 2007[120]): "CONCLUSION: Continuous infusion of selenium as sodium selenite (4,000 microg on the first day, 1,000 microg/day on the nine following days) had no obvious toxicity but did not improve the clinical outcome in septic shock patients." The importance of this study—beyond confirming the lack of toxicity of 4,000 mcg followed by 1,000 mcg of selenium—is that it suggests that 4,000 mcg is too much selenium to give as a loading dose; this appears to be the only protocol variable in the study that differentiates it from the more successful study listed previously that showed significant benefit when 1,000 mcg was used as the loading dose.

---

[118] Hurwitz et al. Suppression of human immunodeficiency virus type 1 viral load with selenium supplementation. *Arch Intern Med.* 2007 Jan 22;167(2):148-54
[119] Angstwurm et al. Selenium in Intensive Care (SIC): results of a prospective randomized, placebo-controlled, multiple-center study in patients with severe systemic inflammatory response syndrome, sepsis, and septic shock. *Crit Care Med.* 2007 Jan;35(1):118-26
[120] Forceville et al. Effects of high doses of selenium, as sodium selenite, in septic shock: a placebo-controlled, randomized, double-blind, phase II study. *Crit Care.* 2007;11:R73

Strategy #2: Block Viral Replication

Antiviral	Antireplication	Immunonutrition	Cell-system support
	Best natural treatments are methylators such as betaine and "folate", and the long list of NFkB inhibitors especially NAC, lipoate, selenium, zinc		

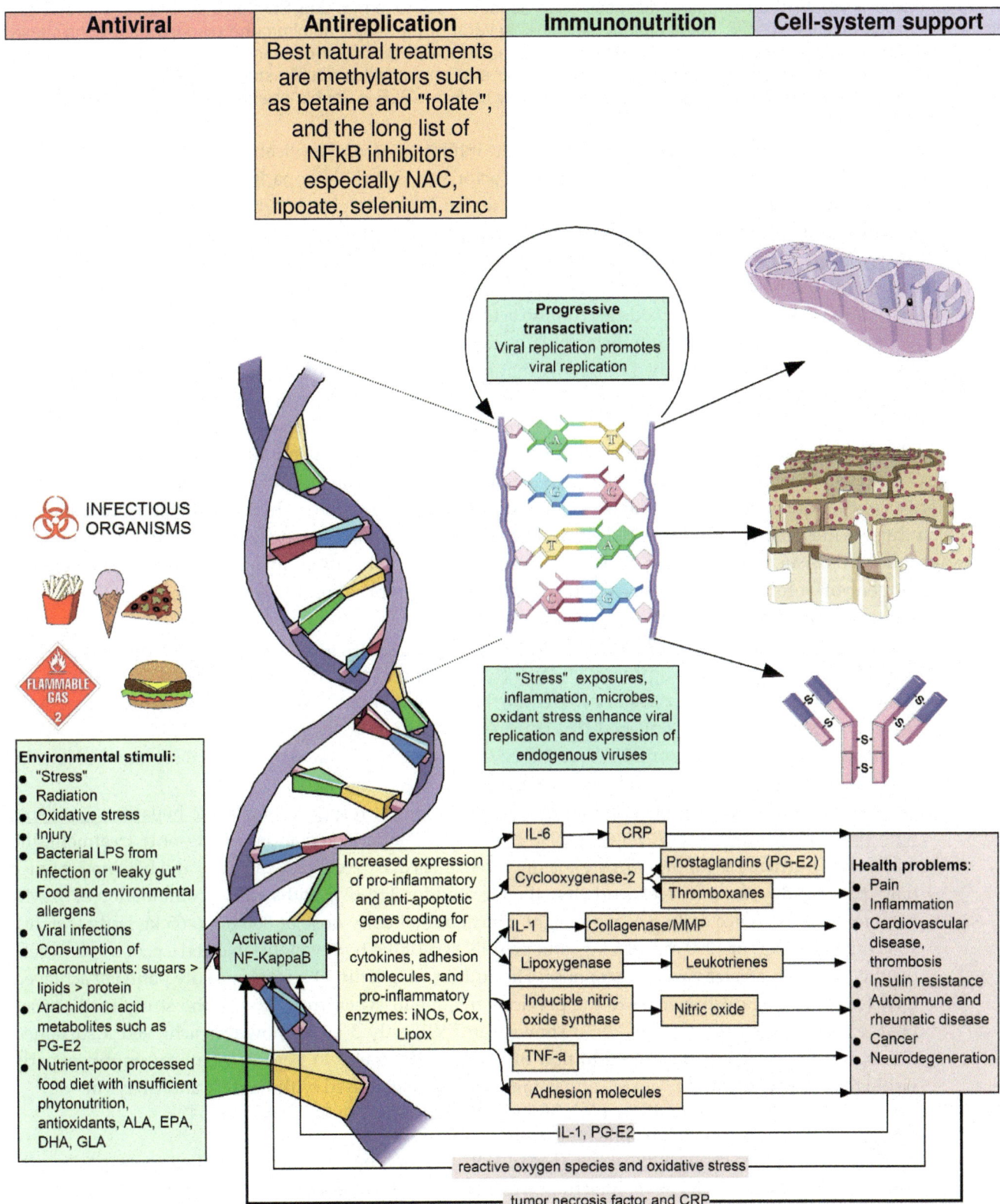

Progressive transactivation: Viral replication promotes viral replication

INFECTIOUS ORGANISMS

FLAMMABLE GAS 2

"Stress" exposures, inflammation, microbes, oxidant stress enhance viral replication and expression of endogenous viruses

Environmental stimuli:
- "Stress"
- Radiation
- Oxidative stress
- Injury
- Bacterial LPS from infection or "leaky gut"
- Food and environmental allergens
- Viral infections
- Consumption of macronutrients: sugars > lipids > protein
- Arachidonic acid metabolites such as PG-E2
- Nutrient-poor processed food diet with insufficient phytonutrition, antioxidants, ALA, EPA, DHA, GLA

Activation of NF-KappaB

Increased expression of pro-inflammatory and anti-apoptotic genes coding for production of cytokines, adhesion molecules, and pro-inflammatory enzymes: iNOs, Cox, Lipox

IL-6	→	CRP
Cyclooxygenase-2	→	Prostaglandins (PG-E2)
		Thromboxanes
IL-1	→	Collagenase/MMP
Lipoxygenase	→	Leukotrienes
Inducible nitric oxide synthase	→	Nitric oxide
TNF-a		
Adhesion molecules		

Health problems:
- Pain
- Inflammation
- Cardiovascular disease, thrombosis
- Insulin resistance
- Autoimmune and rheumatic disease
- Cancer
- Neurodegeneration

IL-1, PG-E2

reactive oxygen species and oxidative stress

tumor necrosis factor and CRP

__(De)Constructing the phenomena of viral replication and its contributory and reinforcing components__: Specific and nonspecific activators of stress responses such as mitochondrial dysfunction, endoplasmic reticulum stress, and NFkB activation promote viral replication and viral mutagenesis via mechanisms including transactivation (virus-stimulated viral replication), oxidative stress (promotes viral mutations leading to immune escape), epigenetic dysfunction (e.g., inappropriate demethylation), and NFkB activation which leads to enhanced viral replication. Via this diagram, readers can see how nonviral factors promote viral expression; this same concept applies to endogenous and exogenous viruses, which can then transactivate each other and lead to the progressive inflammation and immune complications (e.g., cytokine amplification and immune complex deposition with complement activation) that are characteristic of many of the so-called "idiopathic" autoimmune diseases such as lupus, scleroderma, and Sjogren's syndrome. As reviewed elsewhere in the disease-specific rheumatology sections, several of the major autoimmune diseases are consistently associated with enhanced viral activity and immunologic responses, with particular relevance for the induction of fibrosis and vasculitis; many of the viruses associated with systemic autoimmunity are double-stranded DNA viruses, which is noteworthy considering that the pathogenic hallmark antibody for lupus/SLE is double-stranded DNA antibodies.

The two main concepts which become clinical targets for the inhibition of viral replication are 1) promotion of DNA methylation, and 2) inhibition of Nuclear transcription Factor kappa-B (NF-kappa B, NFkB), which is generally considered a pro-inflammatory transcription factor but one that is also "highjacked/hijacked" by viral replication machinery to provide a vicious cycle of inflammation and viral replication.

- **DNA methylation as an antiviral antireplication strategy**: Viruses can only replicate after viral genetic "code" material is integrated into the host/human DNA and then read/transcribed (converted from DNA to RNA) and then translated (conversion of RNA code into amino acid sequence) into proteins that form structural molecules and enzymes. DNA sequences have to be actively accessed or "turned on" by transcription factors—such as NFkB—in order to be read/transcribed into RNA that provides the code for the assembly of amino acids into structural and functional/enzymatic proteins. Conversely, DNA sequences can be blocked or "turned off" by tagging them with a molecule called a methyl group; this is called DNA methylation. DNA methylation is generally stated to "silence" genes by blocking their transcription, and methylation is achieved via provision of methyl groups via nutrients (such as folinic acid, betaine, and SAMe) and then coordinating the methylation pattern via other nutrients (such as vitamin D3) and avoiding drugs such as hydralazine and procainamide which cause widespread/global DNA demethylation. DNA methylation can be used to reduce replication of exogenous viruses such as EBV, HPV, and HCV; likewise, DNA methylation can also be used as an adjunct in the treatment of autoimmune diseases via retarding/reducing replication of exogenous viruses as well as endogenous viruses (HERVs) as well.
  - DNA methyltransferases promote Epstein-Barr virus restricted latency (*J Virol* 2012 Jan[121]): "Establishment of persistent Epstein-Barr virus (EBV) infection requires transition from a program of full viral latency gene expression (latency III) to one that is highly restricted (latency I and 0) within memory B lymphocytes. It is well established that DNA methylation plays a critical role in EBV gene silencing, and recently the chromatin boundary protein CTCF has been implicated as a pivotal regulator of latency via its binding to several loci within the EBV genome."
  - S-adenosyl-methionine and betaine improve early virological response in chronic hepatitis C patients with previous nonresponse (*PLoS One*. 2010 Nov[122]): In comparison standard drug-only treatment, the addition of nutrients as follows "SAMe 400 mg three times daily p.o. (1200 mg/day) and betaine 3 g twice daily p.o. (6 g/day) for one week, and were then treated for 3 to 12 months with a combination of SAMe, betaine, ribavirin twice daily p.o. at a weight adjusted total daily dose of 800 mg (<65 kg body weight), 1000 mg (65–85 kg) or 1200 mg (>85 kg), and pegIFN (1.5 µg/kg bodyweight) injected s.c. once per week" resulted in much greater virologic response. The authors note "only 14% [of drug-only patients] achieved EVR [early virological response] to the previous treatment. When treated with the study medications [SAMe and betaine], 17 patients (59%) showed an EVR, only 3 (10%) however achieved a sustained virological response (SVR)... The addition of SAMe and betaine to pegIFN/ribavirin improves early virological response in CHC." SAMe and betaine are safe when used with PegIFN and ribavirin.
    - http://www.plosone.org/article/info%3Adoi%2F10.1371%2Fjournal.pone.0015492
    - http://www.ncbi.nlm.nih.gov/pmc/articles/PMC2975710/
  - Folate deficiency and cervical dysplasia. (*JAMA* 1992 Jan[123]): "The number of sexual partners, parity, oral contraceptive use, and HPV-16 infection were significantly associated with cervical dysplasia. ... However, red blood cell folate levels at or below 660 nmol/L interacted with HPV-16 infection. The

[121] Hughes et al. Contributions of CTCF and DNA methyltransferases DNMT1 and DNMT3B to Epstein-Barr virus restricted latency. *J Virol*. 2012 Jan;86(2):1034-45
[122] Filipowicz et al. S-adenosyl-methionine and betaine improve early virological response in chronic hepatitis C patients with previous nonresponse. *PLoS One*. 2010 Nov 8;5(11):e15492
[123] Butterworth et al. Folate deficiency and cervical dysplasia. *JAMA*. 1992 Jan 22-29;267(4):528-33

adjusted odds ratio for HPV-16 was 1.1 among women with folate levels above 660 nmol/L but 5.1 (95% confidence interval, 2.3 to 11) among women with lower levels."

Understanding DNA methylation and "folic acid"*

What DNA methylation does:
- It is a means of mostly "silencing" or "turning off" genes so that they are not expressed. In this manner, DNA methylation is of supreme importance in blocking viral expression/replication and (by antiviral and other means) cancer development. Generally, methylation is neither all good nor all bad, since too much (**hyper**methylation) is also associated with disease (such as cancer); however, the bigger problem is that of insufficient methylation—hypomethylation. Stated simply: we need "good genes" turned on and free for expression, while we need "bad genes"—such as cancer-promoting genes and virus-replicating genes—turned off. Lack of ability to methylate the "bad genes" leaves them in the "on" position to promote disease.

Problems associated with **HYPO**methylation:
- Increased risk for cancer, especially viral-induced cancer, particularly cervical cancer promoted by HPV—human papilloma virus
- Increased viral replication, especially EBV and HPV
- Greatly increased risk for the autoimmune disease lupus, SLE—widespread or "global" demethylation is a characteristic of the disease, and is known to be triggered by the two drugs most famous for triggering the disease (procainamide, hydralazine)

Why do so many doctors advocate testing and treatment for "methylation disorders":
- Methylation disorders: Genetic impairments in the enzymes that participate in this complex network of reactions) are very common and are clinically consequential.
- Nutritional deficiencies are common: Nutrient deficiencies of "folic acid"* and vitamin B12 are common and cause **hypo**methylation. The methyl groups are provided and carried by nutrients such as folic acid* and betaine and SAMe (S-adenosyl-methionine); if a person is deficient in these methyl-carrying nutrients then we can be almost certain that they will be "globally" hypomethylated.
- Profiteering: Many doctors are just trying to scare the public, create dependency, and the then profiteer by selling consultations, nutritional supplements, and lab tests (all generally overpriced). Regardless of the profiteering motive, the science is irrefutable on this topic; however, profiteering and intelligence are generally inversely associated and therefore some of the doctors who are the biggest advocates for treating and testing "methylation disorders" are the least informed and least effective.

Optimizing methylation—nutrition and beyond:
1. **Provision**—Provide optimal nutrition, particularly vegetables and supplements: Folic acid*, betaine, vitamin B12 (avoid the form cyano-cobalamin if you can use a different [hydroxo-, methyl-, adenosyl-] form), vitamin B6 (which requires magnesium), NAC, and lecithin.
2. **Coordination**—maintain the machinery and proper pattern: Lifestyle habits such as exercise[124] and other nutrients such as vitamin D3[125] help to reorganize the pattern of methylation and gene expression (via DNA methylation and also histone acetylation, etc); given that exercise and vitamin D3 are two of the most powerful means for enhancing immunity and avoiding disease according to innumerable studies, we can presumptively conclude that "nonmethylating" interventions such as exercise and vitamin D3 function in part by coordinating the overall pattern of methylation and by maintaining the "methylation machinery" that attaches, removes, and transfers methyl groups to the correct places on DNA.
3. **Retention**—Avoid chemical/pollution and unnecessary drug exposure: Some drugs—procainamide and hydralazine are most notorious—cause widespread/global DNA demethylation and are thus generally believed to promote aberrant gene expression—particularly of viruses and HERVs—which lead to a variant of lupus/SLE called "drug-induced lupus."

*What's the deal with "folic acid"?:
- Folic acid is the synthetic form of the vitamin, and even though it is helpful and well absorbed, it is also associated with long-term "toxicity" in the form of increased risk of some types of cancer because the conversion of synthetic folic acid into the active form causes production of free radicals which can cause DNA damage. For this reason, nearly all doctors have switched to either folinic acid or methyl-folate when using "folic acid" supplementation. For convenience and habit, we still use the term "folic acid", but in clinical practice we do not use this vitamin in this form; we use folinic acid or methyl-folate.

---

[124] Rönn et al. A Six Months Exercise Intervention Influences the Genome-wide DNA Methylation Pattern in Human Adipose Tissue. *PLoS Genet* 2013; 9(6): e1003572
[125] Zhu et al. A genome-wide methylation study of severe vitamin D deficiency in African American adolescents. *J Pediatr.* 2013 May;162(5):1004-9. Fetahu et al. Vitamin D and the epigenome. *Front Physiol.* 2014 Apr 29;5:164

- **NFkB inhibition as an antiviral antireplication strategy**: Blocking NFkB is easily accomplish with dietary interventions and nutritional supplementation. Many viruses responsible for human disease are dependent upon the NFkB pathway for their replication and thus survival and ability to create disease. Per the review by Hiscott et al[126], "...certain viruses, including human immunodeficiency virus type I (HIV-I), human T-cell leukemia virus type 1 (HTLV-1), Human herpesvirus 8 (HHV8) and Epstein–Barr virus (EBV), have incorporated aspects of NFkB signaling into their life cycle and pathogenicity, and thus induce NFkB activation." NFkB is also involved in the host defense system; so the paradox of NFkB is that it is necessary for *anti-viral defense* as well as for *viral replication*. Thus, at this time, the goal of intervention in this regard is toward one of NFKB *modulation*, rather than complete suppression or additional activation. Patients following the American/Western lifestyle are adept at activating NFkB through physical inactivity, sarcopenia, excess adiposity, widespread nutritional deficiencies, and overconsumption of dietary fats (especially saturated fats) and simple carbohydrates in large amounts. Phytonutritional modulation of NFkB is reviewed in Chapter 4.[127]

  - Clinical trial of combination antioxidant nutrients and antiviral botanicals: Treatment of chronic hepatitis C virus infection via [oral and intravenous] antioxidants: results of a phase I clinical trial (*J Clin Gastroenterol.* 2005 Sep[128]): The authors of this study correctly begin their introduction with an appreciation of host factors that are important in chronic hepatitis C virus infection when they state, "The pathogenesis of chronic hepatitis C virus (HCV) infection is associated with a defective host antiviral immune response and intrahepatic oxidative stress. Oxidative stress and lipid peroxidation play major roles in the fatty liver accumulation (steatosis) that leads to necro-inflammation and necrosis of hepatic cells." In this Phase-1 study, fifty chronic HCV patients were treated for 20 weeks with a combination of seven orally-administered nutritional supplements: glycyrrhizin, schisandra, silymarin, ascorbic acid, lipoic acid, L-glutathione, and alpha-tocopherol); they also received "four different intravenous preparations (glycyrrhizin, ascorbic acid, L-glutathione, B-complex) twice weekly for the first 10 weeks, and followed up for an additional 20 weeks." Assessments included HCV-RNA levels, liver enzymes, and liver histology, while quality of life was assessed using the SF-36 questionnaire. Results showed normalization of liver enzymes in 44% of patients who had elevated pretreatment ALT levels (15 of 34). "A decrease in viral load (one log or more) was observed in 25% of the patients. Histologic improvement (2-point reduction in the HAI score) was noted in 36.1% of the patients. The SF-36 score improved in 26 of 45 patients throughout the course of the trial (58% of the patients). Treatment was well tolerated by all patients. No major adverse reactions were noted." As may be expected with the use of licorice, hypokalemia was seen in 3 patients (10.7%) and hypertension was seen in 2 patients (3.6%); both problems were mild and were treated symptomatically. Clinicians with any experience in the management of patients with HCV should appreciate the value of these findings, given the debilitating and fatal course of the disease when untreated, and the frequently devastating effects of pharmaceutical drugs that are expensive, toxic, and poorly efficacious.

- **Lipoic acid: 400 mg 3-4 times per day, ensure coverage with multivitamin**: Some clinicians note that because lipoic acid and thiamine work together in certain biochemical pathways (e.g., the pyruvate dehydrogenase complex between glycolysis and the Kreb's cycle) that thiamine should be co-administered when high-dose lipoic acid is used. Integrative clinicians should always cover the nutritional basics with the Paleo-Mediterranean diet and a high-potency broad-spectrum multivitamin/multimineral, so that this concern does not require special attention. Lipoic acid plays important metabolic, antioxidant, and NFkB-inhibiting roles in human physiology; recently, its antiinflammatory actions—via elevation of cAMP and the resultant elevation of IL-10 and suppression of TNFa—have become clear (as reviewed in Chapter 4 in the section on nutritional immunomodulation).

  - Alpha-lipoic acid is a potent inhibitor of NF-kappa B activation in human T cells. (*Biochem Biophys Res Commun.* 1992 Dec[129]): "The long terminal repeat (LTR) region of HIV proviral DNA contains binding sites for nuclear factor kappa B (NF-kappa B), and this transcriptional activator appears to regulate HIV activation. Recent findings suggest an involvement of reactive oxygen species (ROS) in signal

---

[126] Hiscott et al. Manipulation of the nuclear factor-kappaB pathway and the innate immune response by viruses. *Oncogene.* 2006 Oct 30;25(51):6844-67

[127] Vasquez A. Nutritional and Botanical Inhibition of NF-kappaB, the Major Intracellular Amplifier of the Inflammatory Cascade. *Nutr Perspect* 2005;Jul: 5-12

[128] Melhem et al. Treatment of chronic hepatitis C virus infection via antioxidants: results of a phase I clinical trial. *J Clin Gastroenterol.* 2005 Sep;39(8):737-42

[129] Suzuki et al. Alpha-lipoic acid is a potent inhibitor of NF-kappa B activation in human T cells. *Biochem Biophys Res Commun.* 1992 Dec 30;189(3):1709-15

transduction pathways leading to NF-kappa B activation. ... The inhibitory action of alpha-lipoic acid was found to be very potent as only 4 mM was needed for a complete inhibition, whereas 20 mM was required for N-acetylcysteine. These results indicate that alpha-lipoic acid may be effective in AIDS therapeutics."

Nutrients that inhibit NFkB
1. 1,25-dihydroxyvitamin D3
2. Bee propolis (CAPE)
3. Boswellia serratia
4. CoQ-10
5. Curcumin
6. GLA via PPAR-gamma
7. Glycyrrhizin from licorice
8. Grape seed extract
9. Green tea
10. Indole-3-carbinol
11. Isohumulones
12. Lipoic acid
13. N-acetyl-L-cysteine
14. EPA via PPAR-alpha
15. Resveratrol
16. Rosemary
17. Selenium
18. Silibinin, Silymarin
19. Zinc

o Lipoate effects on blood redox state in human immunodeficiency virus infected patients. (*Arzneimittelforschung*. 1993 Dec[130]): "In an open and unblinded pilot study the short term effect of the natural antioxidant lipoate (Thioctacid) on blood antioxidants and peroxidation products was investigated in HIV positive patients (CDC IV). In the majority of the patients, lipoate increased plasma ascorbate (9 of 10 patients) total glutathione (7 of 7 patients), total plasma thiol groups (8 of 9 patients); T helper lymphocytes and T helper/suppressor cell ratio (6 of 10 patients), while the lipid peroxidation products malondialdehyde (8 of 9 patients) and 4-hydroxynonenal (7 of 9 patients) were decreased."

o Randomized, double-blinded, placebo-controlled trial conducted at two study sites: Restoration of blood total glutathione status and lymphocyte function following alpha-lipoic acid supplementation (300 mg thrice daily; 900 mg per day total) in patients with HIV infection (*J Altern Complement Med.* 2008 Mar[131]): This study involved 33 human immunodeficiency virus (HIV)-infected men and women with history of unresponsiveness (viral load >10,000 copies/ml) to highly active antiretroviral treatment (HAART). Results showed that mean blood total glutathione level in ALA-supplemented subjects was increased after 6 months from 0.81 to 1.34 mmol/L in contrast to no change in the placebo control group. Lymphocyte proliferation response was enhanced or stabilized after 6 months of ALA supplementation compared to progressive decline in the placebo group. No significant change was noted in either HIV RNA level or CD4 count. The authors concluded, "Supplementation with alpha-lipoic acid may positively impact patients with HIV and acquired immune deficiency syndrome by restoring blood total glutathione level and improving functional reactivity of lymphocytes to T-cell mitogens." Given that this group of patients had been previously unresponsive to HAART, we could reasonably expect a more severe level of oxidant stress and nutritional depletion; the mono-therapeutic intervention here with lipoate shows short-term safety and some biochemical efficacy; however, more impressive results would have been attained with a more comprehensive intervention.

o Alpha-lipoic acid is an effective inhibitor of human immuno-deficiency virus (HIV-1) replication (*Klin Wochenschr.* 1991 Oct[132]): "We observed a dose dependent inhibition of HIV-1-replication in CPE (Cytopathic effect) formation, reverse transcriptase activity and plaque formation on CD4-transformed HeLa-cells. An over 90% reduction of reverse transcriptase activity could be achieved with 70 micrograms alpha-lipoic acid/ml, a complete reduction of plaque-forming units at concentrations of greater than or equal to 35 micrograms alpha-lipoic acid/ml. An augmentation of the antiviral activity was seen by combination of zidovudine and low dose of alpha-lipoic acid (7 micrograms/ml)."

o Lipoic acid attenuates coxsackievirus B3-induced ectopic calcification in heart, pancreas, and lung. (*Biochem Biophys Res Commun.* 2013 Mar[133]): "In this study, coxsackievirus B3 (CVB3) infection in mice resulted in significant tissue injury, especially in the heart and pancreas. ... Intriguingly, we showed that α-lipoic acid diminished CVB3-mediated inflammatory and apoptotic tissue damage, subsequently ameliorating ectopic calcification via the suppression of osteogenic signals. Collectively, our data provide evidence that ectopic calcification induced by CVB3 infection is implicated in the induction of osteogenic propensity, and α-lipoic acid may be a potential therapeutic agent to ameliorate pathologic calcification."

[130] Fuchs et al. Studies on lipoate effects on blood redox state in human immunodeficiency virus infected patients. *Arzneimittelforschung*. 1993 Dec;43(12):1359-62
[131] Jariwalla et al. Restoration of blood total glutathione status and lymphocyte function following alpha-lipoic acid supplementation in patients with HIV infection. *J Altern Complement Med.* 2008 Mar;14(2):139-46
[132] Baur et al. Alpha-lipoic acid is an effective inhibitor of human immuno-deficiency virus (HIV-1) replication. *Klin Wochenschr.* 1991 Oct 2;69(15):722-4
[133] Kim et al. α-Lipoic acid attenuates coxsackievirus B3-induced ectopic calcification in heart, pancreas, and lung. *Biochem Biophys Res Commun.* 2013 Mar 8;432(2):378-83

- **N-acetyl-cysteine (NAC): 500-1,500 mg tid between meals**: NAC is commonly used in emergency medicine and outpatient integrative care alike. Relevant to the treatment of viral infections in general and respiratory infections in particular, we see that although most clinical trials have used monotherapy and doses that were probably too low to produce optimal efficacy[134], NAC does show benefit in the treatment and prevention of respiratory infections. Mechanisms of action include serving as a glutathione precursor and thus providing antioxidant protection, inhibiting viral replication—perhaps by potently suppressing NFkB, and thinning mucus to promote expectoration and prevent airway obstruction. In patients with acetaminophen overdose and the resulting hepatotoxicity and oxidative stress, Kelly[135] reported NAC doses as follows: "...loading dose of 140 mg oral NAC per kg of body weight, followed four hours later by 70 mg per kg given every four hours for an additional 17 doses." These doses are life-saving for a potentially fatal situation. Doses used clinically for routine and preventive purposes are more in the range of 500-600 mg thrice daily between meals; higher doses can be used when indicated.

> **Research Quote**
>
> "Administration of **N-acetylcysteine during the winter, thus, appears to provide a significant attenuation of influenza and influenza-like episodes**, especially in elderly high-risk individuals. N-acetylcysteine did not prevent A/H1N1 virus influenza infection but **significantly reduced the incidence of clinically apparent disease**."
>
> De Flora et al. Attenuation of influenza-like symptomatology and improvement of cell-mediated immunity with long-term N-acetylcysteine treatment. *Eur Respir J*. 1997 Jul;10(7):1535-41

  o Clinical trial: Effect of N-acetylcysteine (NAC) treatment on HIV-1 infection: a double-blind placebo-controlled trial (*Eur J Clin Pharmacol*. 1996[136]): Authors of this study used low-dose 800 mg/d of NAC in patients with HIV to find that "After treatment the low plasma cysteine level in the NAC group increased to normal, and the decline of the CD4+ lymphocyte count before the study start, was less steep in the NAC group than in the placebo group after treatment." These are the anticipated findings for an effective antiviral agent.

  o Randomized, double-blind trial involving 20 Italian Centers: Attenuation of influenza-like symptomatology and improvement of cell-mediated immunity with long-term N-acetylcysteine 600 mg twice daily (*Eur Respir J*. 1997 Jul[137]): "NAC treatment was well tolerated and resulted in a significant decrease in the frequency of influenza-like episodes, severity, and length of time confined to bed. Both local and systemic symptoms were sharply and significantly reduced in the NAC group."

  o Randomized, 8-week, double-blind, placebo-controlled trial of high-dose NAC (8,000 mg/d) followed by optional open-label trial: N-acetylcysteine replenishes glutathione in HIV infection (*Eur J Clin Invest*. 2000 Oct[138]): Eighty-one HIV-infected, low GSH, CD4 T cells < 500 micro L(-1) with no active opportunistic infections or other debilitation showed serologic increase in GSH following NAC supplementation. The authors concluded, "NAC treatment for 8 weeks safely replenishes whole blood GSH and T cell GSH in HIV-infected individuals. Thus, NAC offers useful adjunct therapy to increase protection against oxidative stress, improve immune system function..." Many clinicians will be impressed by the high dose of NAC used in this study: 8000 mg of NAC per day in divided doses; the average NAC intake was 7g/d. NAC should be consumed between meals, and if high doses are used for long periods of time, trace mineral supplementation, especially including copper, is advised. NAC has the ability to chelate minerals from the body; this can be used for life-saving benefit in patients with arsenic poisoning.

  o Review: N-acetylcysteine: a new approach to anti-HIV therapy (*AIDS Res Hum Retroviruses*. 1992 Feb[139]): Paralleling previous themes discussed earlier in this chapter in the topics of selenium and NFkB inhibition, authors of this review note that "NAC is different than many other antiviral drugs in that it inhibits host-mediated stimulation of viral replication arising in normal immune responses..." They go on to note that NAC "inhibits the action of inflammatory cytokines which may mediate cachexia, thereby raising the possibility that it may alleviate the deleterious wasting that accompanies late stage AIDS." This latter finding is important because the prevention of anorexia supports food intake which resists or

---

[134] Roxas M, Jurenka J. Colds and influenza: a review of diagnosis and conventional, botanical, and nutritional considerations. *Altern Med Rev*. 2007 Mar;12(1):25-4

[135] Kelly GS. Clinical applications of N-acetylcysteine. *Altern Med Rev*. 1998 Apr;3(2):114-27

[136] Akerlund et al. Effect of N-acetylcysteine (NAC) treatment on HIV-1 infection: a double-blind placebo-controlled trial. *Eur J Clin Pharmacol*. 1996;50(6):457-61

[137] De Flora et al. Attenuation of influenza-like symptomatology and improvement of cell-mediated immunity with long-term N-acetylcysteine treatment. *Eur Respir J*. 1997 Jul;10(7):1535-41

[138] De Rosa et al. N-acetylcysteine replenishes glutathione in HIV infection. *Eur J Clin Invest*. 2000 Oct;30(10):915-29

[139] Roederer M, Ela SW, Staal FJ, Herzenberg LA, Herzenberg LA. N-acetylcysteine: a new approach to anti-HIV therapy. *AIDS Res Hum Retroviruses*. 1992 Feb;8(2):209-17

reverses the nutrient depletion caused by chronic infection, and which, if left unchecked, causes a progressive decline in immune function and ever increasing susceptibility to progressive and additive infections.

- o Placebo-controlled double-blind multicenter study: Combination therapy with interferon-alpha plus N-acetyl cysteine for chronic hepatitis C (*J Med Virol.* 2000 Aug[140]): In this study, chronic hepatitis C patients (n=73) were treated with interferon-alpha plus NAC 600 mg thrice daily (IFN+NAC) or IFN alone (n=74) for 6 months with an additional 6-month follow-up. "Amongst patients receiving IFN plus NAC, sustained virological responses were observed in 5.5%, transient responses in 26% and non-response in 68.5%. The figures for patients receiving IFN only were 4.1%, 24.3% and 71.6% respectively." This study showed biochemical benefit to NAC+IFN therapy over IFN alone, but the benefits are only marginally better than not using NAC. The NAC dose of 600 mg/d is reasonable. Two problems with this study may have contributed to the inefficacy: ❶ In the Materials and Methods section of the full-text of the article, the authors make no mention of advising patients to consume the NAC between meals, on an empty stomach. This subtle yet important oversight may have retarded absorption and thus contributed to the negation of benefit. Clinicians untrained in nutrition would not be attentive to this level of detail, and details like this are clinically important. ❷ Also, the authors failed to test for changes in GSH levels. Such measurement would have provided objective data about the efficacy of the supplement being used, as well as about the compliance of each patient.

- o Two randomized trials: Improvement of immune functions in HIV infection by sulfur supplementation (*J Mol Med.* 2000[141]): The authors of this study randomized 40 patients on antiretroviral therapy (ART; study 1) and 29 patients without ART (study 2) to treatment for 7 months with NAC or placebo dosed at "an individually adjusted dose according to a defined scheme." The authors report that both studies consistently showed that NAC causes a marked increase in immune functions and plasma albumin concentrations. The effect of NAC on viral load was not consistent. Our findings suggest that the impairment of immunological functions in HIV+ patients results at least partly from cysteine deficiency. The authors conclude by advocating NAC as a means for "**immunoreconstituting**" HIV patients to counter the effect of "HIV-induced cysteine depletion" which is a novel pathogenic mechanism "by which a virus destroys the immune defense of the host and escapes immune elimination."

- **Polyphenolics and phytonutrients**: Phytonutrients and polyphenolics have immune-modulating and NFkB-suppressing actions that are generally beneficial. Patients should have an optimized foundational whole-foods diet, upon which nutritional supplements, possibly including phytonutrient supplements, are added.

  - o Double-blind, randomized, placebo-controlled trial: Immunity and Antioxidant Capacity in Humans Is Enhanced by Consumption of a Dried, Encapsulated Fruit and Vegetable Juice Concentrate (*J Nutr.* 2006 Oct[142]): This trial involved oral supplementation with a commercially available encapsulated fruit and vegetable juice powder concentrate (FVJC) to provide phytonutrients; test subjects included 59 healthy law students who consumed either FVJC or placebo capsules for 77 days. "The FVJC group tended to have fewer total symptoms than the placebo group (P < 0.076). ... FVJC consumption during this study period resulted in increased plasma nutrients and antioxidant capacity, reduction in DNA strand breaks, and an increase in circulating gammadelta-T cells." Plasma levels of vitamin C, beta-carotene, lycopene, and lutein increased significantly from baseline in the FVJC group as did plasma oxygen radical absorptive capacity (50% increase in ORAC).

  - o Study: Several indicators of oxidative stress, immunity, and illness improved in trained men consuming an encapsulated juice powder concentrate for 28 weeks (*J Nutr.* 2007 Dec[143]): Subjects for this study involving a commercially available encapsulated juice powder concentrate (JPC) included 41 trained men from a homogenous police Special Forces unit, randomly assigned in a double blind manner to either JPC (n = 21) or placebo (n = 20). Subjects consumed 3 capsules twice daily with food; capsules contained

[140] Grant et al. Combination therapy with interferon-alpha plus N-acetyl cysteine for chronic hepatitis C. *J Med Virol.* 2000 Aug;61(4):439-42

[141] Breitkreutz et al. Improvement of immune functions in HIV infection by sulfur supplementation: two randomized trials. *J Mol Med.* 2000;78(1):55-62

[142] Nantz et al. Immunity and Antioxidant Capacity in Humans Is Enhanced by Consumption of a Dried, Encapsulated Fruit and Vegetable Juice Concentrate. *J Nutr.* 2006 Oct;136(10):2606-10

[143] Lamprecht et al. Several indicators of oxidative stress, immunity, and illness improved in trained men consuming an encapsulated juice powder concentrate for 28 weeks. *J Nutr.* 2007 Dec;137(12):2737-41

dehydrated juice extracts from apple, beet, bilberry, blackberry, black currant, blueberry, broccoli, cabbage, carrot, cherry (acerola), Concord grape, cranberry, elderberry, kale, orange, peach, papaya, parsley, pineapple, raspberry, red currant, spinach, and tomato. Over 28 weeks of treatment, levels of carbonyl groups on protein and TNFalpha were lower in the JPC group. Importantly, "Over the final 20 wk of the study, the placebo group tended to have more days of illness than the JPC group. These data suggest beneficial JPC effects with regard to reduction of duty days lost due to illness..."

- o Clinical trial: Immune Function in Elderly Smokers and Nonsmokers Improves during Supplementation with Fruit and Vegetable Extracts (*Integrative Medicine* 1999[144]): "Conclusions: Fruit and vegetable extract supplementation significantly enhanced multiple measures of immune function in elderly subjects, and improved IL-2 levels in smokers. Fruit and vegetable extract supplementation offers a novel way to improve compliance with current nutritional recommendations and may potentially lower disease risk."

Reducing HERV replication/elaboration in autoimmunity via DNA methylation, antiinflammation, and antitransactivation—the "antiHERV" concept and approach

Given that HERVs are 100% pervasive among humans and give rise to active transcription to HERV proteins, superantigens and the resultant antibodies—noting that microbial proteins + superantigens + antibodies = the perfect recipe for immune complex disease, made even worse among persons (e.g., lupus patients) with an inability to clear immune complexes—the most important question then becomes *what steps can be taken to suppress/repress/hamper HERV replication? Can we use the same effective antiviral treatments which we already have available (in the previously listed antiviral protocol)?* Obviously, since we are not dealing with free viral particles, some of the previously mentioned antiviral treatments will have no effect because the mechanisms are irrelevant (such as selenium's prevention of immune-escape by reducing viral mutagenesis) or cannot reach within the nucleus to have effect (such as the virucidal activity of zinc ions, or the binding-inactivating effect of glycyrrhetinic acid to HSV particles). Given that "the virus" is already and permanently embedded/encoded within the human genome, the most immediate and obvious solutions would be those of promoting DNA methylation to silence **HERV long terminal repeats** (**LTR**, not to be confused with TLR for Toll-like receptors) and to prevent/reduce active transcription of those HERV LTR via transcription factors like NFkB and/or a pro-inflammatory cytokine milieu. This is to say, the means would most likely have to be ❶ *contra* DNA transcription, most notably via the promotion of DNA methylation, ❷ reducing any contribution of viral transactivation, ❸ reducing any contribution of inflammatory (e.g., TLR-7 pathway) and stress-induced (trans)activation. In partial and perhaps theoretical contradiction to my own statement above, we might actually be able to "attack" HERV codes in the same way we try to attack exogenous viral DNA because ❹ HERV genetic fragments relocate to different parts of the human DNA, and during this time of relocation/transposition, they might be vulnerable to "antiviral" therapeutics.

- AntiHERV via DNA methylation to address this component of autoimmunity, especially lupus/SLE: "There has been a reasonable prediction that aberrant LTR activation could trigger malignant disorders and autoimmune responses if epigenetic changes including DNA hypomethylation occur in somatic cells. ... Hypomethylation of HERV-E and HERV-K was also observed in SLE patients."[145]
  - o Clinical implementation of optimal DNA methylation: For optimization of DNA methylation, methyl-donating/transferring nutrients such as folate (used clinically as folinic acid and/or methylfolate), betaine, and (methyl)cobalamin are *necessary but not sufficient*. Other nutrients—particularly vitamin D3—play critical and complex roles, promoting methylation of some DNA regions and demethylation of others[146]; in the case of vitamin D, we note consistent epidemiologic and clinical experimental research showing that vitamin D3 protects against and treats inflammatory/autoimmune diseases. The complexity of nutrients, in this case vitamin D3, is demonstrated by the observation that vitamin D causes complex changes in gene expression at different locations and likely under different circumstances; vitamin D and activation of its receptor correlate with DNA methylation and the *conceptual opposite* DNA demethylation

---

[144] Inserra et al. Immune Function in Elderly Smokers and Nonsmokers Improves During Supplementation with Fruit and Vegetable Extracts. *Integrative Medicine* 1999: 2; 3-10
[145] Katoh et al. Association of endogenous retroviruses and long terminal repeats with human disorders. *Front Oncol.* 2013 Sep 11;3:234
[146] "In summary, alterations in DNA methylation lead to aberrant gene expression and disruptions of genomic integrity, which contribute to development and progression of diseases. Vitamin D can regulate these processes; the mechanisms behind need further investigations." Fetahu et al. Vitamin D and the epigenome. *Front Physiol.* 2014 Apr 29;5:164

(occurring at different DNA sites), while also promoting histone acetylation of some regions and histone deacetylation of others.[147] Lastly and very importantly, clinicians have to think beyond nutrients and methylating nutrients to fully appreciate and optimize DNA methylation, given that this process is potently impacted by numerous environmental factors, including xenobiotic/toxin exposure, ultraviolet (UV) light exposure, and drug exposure (e.g., procainamide, hydralazine); again noted is the fact that SLE patients show global hypomethylation of DNA[148] therefore suggesting that the patients need a combination of nutritional optimization (adding methyl-active nutrients such as folinic acid, cobalamin, and cholecalciferol) and environmental optimization (subtracting injurious agents such as UV light, xenobiotics and drugs) in order to optimize DNA methylation patterns and balance.

- AntiHERV via anti-virus: Blocking HERV transcription by blocking exogenous virus replication
  - Rationale for autoimmune disease treatment with anti-viral therapies: "Cited epidemiologic and experimental evidence suggests that increased replication of epigenomic viral pathogens such as Epstein-Barr virus (EBV) in chronic human autoimmune diseases such as rheumatoid arthritis (RA), systemic lupus Erythematosus (SLE), and multiple sclerosis (MS) may activate endogenous human retroviruses (HERV) as a pathologic mechanism."[149]
  - Blocking HERV transcription by blocking exogenous virus replication: "Herpes simplex viruses are known to transactivate retroviral regulatory LTR regions of both exogenous and endogenous human retroviruses..."[150]

- AntiHERV via anti-stress and anti-inflammation: Blocking HERV transcription by blocking nonspecific cellular stress and inflammation: "Induction of cellular stress responses through serum deprivation did however, to some extent, mimic the effects of virus infection in terms of transcription of HERV-W elements. ... Environmental stressors can modulate the transcriptional activities of certain HERV-W elements which could thereby be markers for such insults."[151]

- AntiHERV via anti-bacteria-induced inflammation: Blocking bacterial promotion of viral replication via inflammatory pathways: Bacterial debris such as DNA and LPS are known to trigger inflammatory responses via TLR and NFkB; activation of NFkB—the proinflammatory transcription factor often "hijacked" by viruses to promote their own replication—promotes viral replication. Thus, increased total bacterial load (TBL, such as SIBO) would be expected to promote viral replication.

- AntiHERV via anti-bacteria-induced immunosuppression—an extension of the previously mentioned counterinflammation model: Blocking HERV transcription increased by bacterial promotion of viral replication via immunosuppression: As a specific example, *Helicobacter pylori* may play a powerful role as a synergistic bioagent for the microbial promotion of autoimmunity via its ability to *simultaneously* and *paradoxically* cause immunosuppression (thereby allowing other microbes to flourish) and systemic inflammation[152]; in this manner, the bacterial infection is permissive to and perhaps necessary for the autoimmune-inducing vasculopathic and fibrogenic viral infections (see section on Scleroderma for pathology details).

---

[147] "These changes involve the methylation of genomic DNA and/or reversible post-translational modifications of histone proteins, such as acetylation or deacetylation at exposed lysine residues." Carlberg C. Genome-wide (over)view on the actions of vitamin D. *Front Physiol*. 2014 Apr 29;5:167

[148] "The mechanisms causing altered DNA methylation in autoimmunity, aging and carcinogenesis are incompletely characterized but include exposure to environmental agents and drugs, diet, altered signaling in pathways regulating DNA methyltransferase expression and changes in endogenous regulatory mechanisms. ... Initial studies demonstrated that T cells from patients with active lupus had globally hypomethylated DNA. ... Treating normal T cells with DNA methylation inhibitors is sufficient to cause a lupus-like disease in animal models, so exposure to exogenous DNA methylation inhibitors might similarly contribute to the development of autoimmunity. In support of this, the two drugs most frequently implicated in causing a lupus-like disease, procainamide and hydralazine, have been reported to inhibit DNA methylation...and induce autoreactivity in human and murine T lymphocytes." Richardson BC. Role of DNA methylation in the regulation of cell function: autoimmunity, aging and cancer. *J Nutr*. 2002 Aug;132(8 Sup):2401S-2405S

[149] Dreyfus DH. Autoimmune disease: A role for new anti-viral therapies? *Autoimmun Rev*. 2011 Dec;11(2):88-97

[150] Nellaker et al. Transactivation of elements in the human endogenous retrovirus W family by viral infection. *Retrovirology*. 2006 Jul 6;3:44

[151] Nellaker et al. Transactivation of elements in the human endogenous retrovirus W family by viral infection. *Retrovirology*. 2006 Jul 6;3:44

[152] "Infectious agents such as Helicobacter pylori (Hp) may cause chronic inflammation and autoimmune reactivity in susceptible subjects. The results of in vitro experiments performed with lymphocytes from Hp infected patients indicate that Hp can cause immunosuppression which might be eliminated by successful eradication therapy." Hybenova et al. The role of environmental factors in autoimmune thyroiditis. *Neuro Endocrinol Lett*. 2010;31(3):283-9

Date and Time Collected	Date Entered	Date and Time Reported	Physician Name	NPI	Physician ID
09/03/15 06:30	09/08/15	09/09/15 17:10ET			A

Tests Ordered
EBV Acute Infection Antibodies; Written Authorization

TESTS	RESULT	FLAG	UNITS	REFERENCE INTERVAL

EBV Acute Infection Antibodies

EBV Ab VCA, IgM	49.5	High	U/mL	0.0 - 35.9
			Negative	<36.0
			Equivocal	36.0 - 43.9
			Positive	>43.9
EBV Early Antigen Ab, IgG	14.7	High	U/mL	0.0 - 8.9

Hepatitis A, Hepatitis C and HIV antibodies may cross-react with this assay.

			Negative	< 9.0
			Equivocal	9.0 - 10.9
			Positive	>10.9
EBV Ab VCA, IgG	>600.0	High	U/mL	0.0 - 17.9
			Negative	<18.0
			Equivocal	18.0 - 21.9
			Positive	>21.9
EBV Nuclear Antigen Ab, IgG	>600.0	High	U/mL	0.0 - 17.9
			Negative	<18.0
			Equivocal	18.0 - 21.9
			Positive	>21.9

Interpretation:

EBV Interpretation Chart

Interpretation	EBV-IgM	EA(D)-IgG	VCA-IgG	EBNA-IgG
EBV Seronegative	−	−	−	−
Early Phase	+	−	−	−
Acute Primary Infection	+	+or−	+	−
Convalescence/Past Infection	−	+or−	+	+
Reactivated Infection	+or−	+	+	+

+ Antibody Present   − Antibody Absent

Homocysteine Assay - Plasma

Date of Report   03/04/2015

Methodology: Competitive Immunoassay

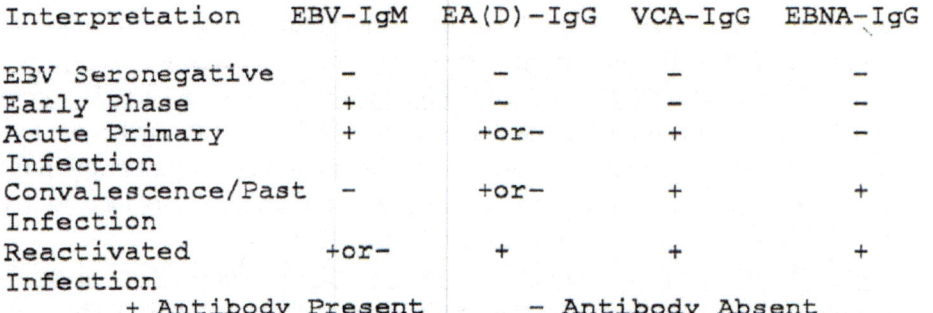

	Results nmol/mL	Quintile Ranking	95% Reference Range
1. Homocysteine	13.4 H		3.0-14.0

Laboratory results for a 51yoM patient with chronic exhaustion, tinnitus, headaches, and persistent sore throat, and cognitive difficulties: In this case, the elevated homocysteine suggests faulty methylation, and the actionable assumption is that the patient is deficient in methylation (co)factors. Lack of homocysteine methylation likely reflects a simultaneous lack of DNA methylation, which promotes viral replication. Agents such as methylfolate/folinate 5mg/d and NAC ~1,500 mg/d can be used to simultaneously lower homocysteine levels while also promoting DNA methylation and NFkB inhibition, respectively, to reduce viral replication. The serum B12 is clinically meaningless unless as 1) gut microbes can produce B12 analogs that are "laboratory positive but physiologically inactive"[153], and 2) this laboratory reference range is ridiculously wide; serum B12 levels should always be above 600 pg/mL *minimum*.[154] This patient clearly needs at least 6 months of cobalamin administration, e.g., 4,000 mcg/d PO; patients with recent-onset B12 deficiency respond quickly while those with long-term deficiency need at least 6 months of cobalamin replacement to promote neuroregeneration.

Non-Hemolytic Anemia Evaluation

Collected Date	06/17/2015
Collected Time	12:50:00

Procedure		Units	Ref Range
Vitamin B12	664	pg/mL	[211-946]

[153] Murphy et al. Megaloblastic anaemia due to vitamin B12 deficiency caused by small intestinal bacterial overgrowth: possible role of vitamin B12 analogues. *Br J Haematol.* 1986 Jan;62(1):7-12

[154] Catalano et al. Catatonia. Another neuropsychiatric presentation of vitamin B12 deficiency? *Psychosomatics.* 1998 Sep-Oct;39(5):456-60

<u>Strategy #3</u>: Support Immune Responses against the Virus

Antiviral	Antireplication	Immunonutrition	Cell-system support
		Emphasize low-carbohydrate diet, adequate protein (especially from whey protein isolate), zinc, vitamin D3, vitamin A	

- **Immunonutrition—common components and beneficial effects**: While the nonspecific term "immunonutrition" could probably be accurately applied to any nutrient (and therefore essentially all nutrients) that affect or benefit immune function, immunonutrition generally is relatively specific to the provision of glutamine, arginine, n-3 fatty acids such as EPA and DHA, and dietary nucleotides. These can be used alone, but their benefit, as expected by the interactive and synergistic activity of nutrients and physiological processes, is generally enhanced when used in combination. Numerous multi-site and international studies have consistently demonstrated significant benefit in terms of reduced infection rates, morbidity, mortality, duration of hospitalization, and hospital costs when immunonutrition intervention is utilized in patients with major trauma, burns, and sepsis.

  > **Perspective & Context**
  >
  > Although these interventional considerations are presented in the context of the treatment and prevention of acute and chronic viral infections, several of these treatments are also applicable to bacterial and fungal infections as well. Viral infections are chosen as the emphasis of this chapter because of their enigmatic nature, their high frequency, and the limited efficacy and high costs of many drug treatments. This review is also intended to be practical (rather than exhaustive, and exhausting) so that clinicians can focus on the most established and accessible treatments.

  o <u>Clinical trial and review: Immunonutrition in patients after multiple trauma (*Br J Nutr.* 2002 Jan[155])</u>: "In the recovery period after trauma (1-72 h after injury) a limitation of the inflammatory response of immunocompetent cells must be achieved as quickly as possible (<72 h). The only strategy available to clinicians caring for trauma patients is immunonutrition, and this should be strongly considered as a rational approach improving immune function and reducing septic complications in critically ill or injured patients."

  o <u>Clinical trial: Influence of arginine, omega-3 fatty acids and nucleotide-supplemented enteral support on systemic inflammatory response syndrome and multiple organ failure in patients after severe trauma (*Nutrition.* 1998 Feb[156])</u>: This study used an enteral diet supplemented with arginine, omega-3 fatty acids, and nucleotides (Impact, Sandoz Nutrition, Berne, Switzerland) in patients at high risk for systemic inflammatory response syndrome (SIRS) and multiple organ failure (MOF) after severe trauma. Thirty-two patients were enrolled in this prospective, randomized, double-blind, controlled study. "In the test group, significantly fewer SIRS days per patient were found… MOF score was significantly lower in the test group on d 3 and d 8-11. … The results of the study provide further support for beneficial effects of arginine, omega-3-fatty acids and nucleotide-supplemented enteral diet in critically ill patients." These benefits are counterbalanced by neutral findings of no significant differences in T-lymphocyte CD4/CD8 ratio, interleukin-2 receptor expression, infection rate, mortality (2/16 vs. 4/13), and hospital stay between supplemented and unsupplemented patients.

  o <u>Randomized, controlled, double-blind trial: Early enteral supplementation with key pharmaconutrients improves Sequential Organ Failure Assessment score in critically ill patients with sepsis (*Crit Care Med.* 2008 Jan[157])</u>: This study tested an "enteral pharmaconutrition supplement containing glutamine dipeptides, antioxidative vitamins and trace elements, and butyrate" [Intestamin, Fresenius Kabi] among

---

[155] Bastian L, Weimann A. Immunonutrition in patients after multiple trauma. *Br J Nutr.* 2002 Jan;87 Suppl 1:S133-4

[156] Weimann et al. Influence of arginine, omega-3 fatty acids and nucleotide-supplemented enteral support on systemic inflammatory response syndrome and multiple organ failure in patients after severe trauma. *Nutrition.* 1998 Feb;14(2):165-72

[157] Beale et al. Early enteral supplementation with key pharmaconutrients improves Sequential Organ Failure Assessment score in critically ill patients with sepsis: outcome of a randomized, controlled, double-blind trial. *Crit Care Med.* 2008 Jan;36(1):131-44

fifty critically ill, septic patients. Patients receiving the experimental supplement showed significantly faster improvement in daily SOFA [Sequential Organ Failure Assessment] score over time compared with control group, leading the authors to conclude, "In medical patients with sepsis, early enteral pharmaconutrition with glutamine dipeptides, vitamin C and E, beta-carotene, selenium, zinc, and butyrate in combination with an immunonutrition formula results in significantly faster recovery of organ function compared with control."

- o Review: Antioxidant supplementation in sepsis and systemic inflammatory response syndrome (*Crit Care Med.* 2007 Sep[158]): "Three antioxidant nutrients have demonstrated clinical benefits and reached level A evidence: a) selenium improves clinical outcome (infections, organ failure); b) glutamine reduces infectious complication in large-sized trials; and c) the association of eicosapentaenoic acid and micronutrients has significant anti-inflammatory effects."

- **Vitamin D3 (cholecalciferol, not ergocalciferol): 4,000-10,000 IU per day; for acute infections in deficient patients consider a one-time loading dose of 100,000-300,000 IU followed by a more conservative maintenance dose**: In our 2004 monograph by Vasquez, Manso, and Cannell, we fulfilled our promise of creating a "paradigm shift" that summarized new applications for the clinical use of vitamin D beyond its application in patients with osteoporosis or malabsorption to include the mandate of empiric treatment or laboratory assessment of all patients seen in clinical practice.[159] Vitamin D3 has a particularly relevant role in the prevention of viral infections, especially viral infections of the respiratory tract, including influenza. Daily doses generally average between 4,000-10,000 IU/d for adults, with an acceptable one-time loading dose of 100,000-300,000 IU in patients for whom it is advantageous and safe to raise serum 25-hydroxy-vitamin D levels quickly and without concern for compliance failure; the logistical goal with vitamin D supplementation is to maintain serum 25-hydroxy-vitamin D levels in the optimal range, as defined in the illustration; Dr V's articles and excerpts on vitamin D3 are available online in this website folder: www.InflammationMastery.com/D3

- o Review: Acute lower respiratory infections in childhood: opportunities for reducing the global burden through nutritional interventions (*Bull World Health Organ.* 2008 May[160]): "The active form of vitamin D affects a variety of immune functions, including the synthesis of endogenous antimicrobial peptides."

- o Review: Vitamin D for Treatment and Prevention of Infectious Diseases: A Systematic Review of Randomized Controlled Trials (*Endocr Pract.* 2009 Jun[161]): "Based on studies reviewed to date, the strongest evidence supports further research into adjunctive vitamin D therapy for tuberculosis, influenza, and viral upper respiratory illnesses."

- o Review: Vitamin D signaling, infectious diseases, and regulation of innate immunity (*Infect Immun.* 2008 Sep[162]): Evidence is accumulating that vitamin D sufficiency confers protection against tuberculosis and a wide range of other bacterial as well as viral infections. Studies support a role for vitamin D in protection against upper and lower respiratory tract infections, most of which are typically caused by viruses, and some of which are then later complicated by secondary bacterial infection (after the viral infection has exacerbated nutritional depletion and lead to damage of respiratory epithelium). Subclinical vitamin D deficiency increases the risk for severe pneumonia and was associated with a 13-fold-increased risk of pneumonia in Ethiopian children. Readers should revisit the illustrated optimal range in this section in light of the quote, "A Finnish study found that there was an association between serum 25D concentrations of less than 40 nM (16 ng/ml) and a range of acute respiratory infections (sinusitis, tonsillitis, otitis, bronchitis, pneumonia, pharyngitis, and laryngitis) in young army recruits."

- o Expert literature review: Epidemic influenza and vitamin D (*Epidemiol Infect.* 2006 Dec[163]): Vitamin D3 stimulates the expression of potent anti-microbial peptides from neutrophils, monocytes, natural killer cells, and in epithelial cells lining the respiratory tract. "An interventional study showed that vitamin D reduces the incidence of respiratory infections in children."

[158] Berger MM, Chioléro RL. Antioxidant supplementation in sepsis and systemic inflammatory response syndrome. *Crit Care Med.* 2007 Sep;35(9 Suppl):S584-90
[159] Vasquez A, Manso G, Cannell J. The clinical importance of vitamin D (cholecalciferol). *Altern Ther Health Med.* 2004 Sep-Oct;10(5):28-36
[160] Roth et al. Acute lower respiratory infections in childhood: reducing the global burden through nutritional interventions. *Bull World Health Organ.* 2008 May;86(5):356-64
[161] Yamshchikov et al. Vitamin D for Treatment and Prevention of Infectious Diseases: A Systematic Review of Randomized Controlled Trials. *Endocr Pract.* 2009 Jun 2:1-29
[162] White JH. Vitamin D signaling, infectious diseases, and regulation of innate immunity. *Infect Immun.* 2008 Sep;76(9):3837-43
[163] Cannell et al. Epidemic infleunza and vitamin D. *Epidemiol Infect.* 2006;134(6):1129-40

- o <u>Meta-analysis of randomized controlled trials: Vitamin D supplementation and total mortality</u> (*Arch Intern Med.* 2007 Sep[164]): "Intake of ordinary doses of vitamin D supplements seems to be associated with decreases in total mortality rates." Most of the studies reviewed in this meta-analysis used subphysiologic doses of vitamin D; yet they still produced benefit in terms of reduced total mortality, some of which is likely attributable to reductions in the incidence and severity of infections, including viral infections.

- o <u>Hypothesis—Ultraviolet-B irradiance and vitamin D reduce the risk of viral infections and thus their sequelae, including autoimmune diseases and some cancers</u> (*Photochem Photobiol.* 2008 Mar[165]): "Vitamin D, through induction of cathelicidin, which effectively combats both bacterial and viral infections, may reduce the risk of several autoimmune diseases and cancers by reducing the development of viral infections."

- **Vitamin C (ascorbic acid)**: Ascorbate as treatment for the common cold and other respiratory viral infections may not have lived up to Dr Pauling's high expectations, but the overall evidence suggests some efficacy when used in isolation.[166] We would tend to expect better results if this agent is used in an appropriate combination approach since this more accurately reflects the interconnected nature of nutritional biochemistry and immune physiology. The combination of modest efficacy and a near absence of adverse effects produces a sufficiently high benefit:risk ratio at low cost to make vitamin C worthy of clinical utilization.

> **Historical and Clinical Perspective**
> The most frequently studied nutritional interventions to reduce the clinical impact of respiratory infections in children *of developing nations* are ❶ breast-feeding (preferably from a well-nourished mother), ❷ vitamin A, ❸ zinc, ❹ folic acid, and ❺ iron.

- **Vitamin A: load with 300,000 IU per day for about 3-5 days (for adults, for acute infections only), then 25-000-50,000 IU per day until well; limit 2-4 weeks; monitor for toxicity (headaches, dry skin, cracked lips, bone pain)**: Vitamin A clearly shows immunosupportive benefits. Vitamin A stores are depleted by the stress of infection and injury because reduced hepatic production of retinol-binding protein paradoxically results in increased renal loss of retinol exactly at the time it is critically needed in order to support function of the immune system and maintenance/repair of epithelial tissue. In a patient with vitamin A sufficiency, whose tissue stores of this fat-soluble vitamin are well stocked, the reduced production of retinol binding protein serves to liberate retinol for uptake by cells; in patients with marginal or depleted vitamin A status, they do not have the *tissue nutrient reserve* to supply immune and epithelial cells at the same time that retinol is increasingly lost in the urine. Further, not all of the benefits of vitamin A for immune function are available on an acute basis; the maintenance of proper respiratory epithelial structure/function requires vitamin A, but in a vitamin A-deficient patient, acute administration of vitamin A does not immediately restore the respiratory epithelium to promote clearance of the infection, even though other aspects of immune function will recover more quickly. From a practical clinical perspective, consider giving 200,000-300,000 IU per day of retinol palmitate (the least toxic form) for 1-2 weeks, then taper; reduce dose or discontinue with onset of toxicity symptoms such as skin problems (dry skin, flaking skin, chapped or split lips, red skin rash, hair loss), joint pain, bone pain, headaches, anorexia (loss of appetite), edema (water retention, weight gain, swollen ankles, difficulty breathing), fatigue, and/or liver damage. Patients should be given written instructions that clearly delineate the time limit for high-dose vitamin A supplementation and advise them of the potential adverse effects. Women who are pregnant or might become pregnant and who are planning to carry the baby to full term delivery should not ingest more than 10,000 IU of vitamin A per day. Several studies are listed below documenting the precedent use of high-dose vitamin A; clinicians must be aware of the potential adverse effects, must monitor and select patients appropriately, and should generally not use these high doses for the durations listed in these clinical trials.

  - o <u>Vitamin A for all patients with measles.</u> (http://emedicine.medscape.com/article/966220-overview; Updated: Sep 29, 2014[167]): "The World Health Organization recommends vitamin A supplementation for all children diagnosed with measles, regardless of their country of residence, based on their age, as follows: Infants younger than 6 months: 50,000 IU/day PO for 2 doses; Age 6-11 months: 100,000 IU/day

---

[164] Autier P, Gandini S. Vitamin D supplementation and total mortality: a meta-analysis of randomized controlled trials. *Arch Intern Med.* 2007 Sep;167(16):1730-7
[165] Grant WB. Hypothesis—ultraviolet-B irradiance and vitamin D reduce the risk of viral infections and thus their sequelae, including autoimmune diseases and some cancers. *Photochem Photobiol.* 2008 Mar-Apr;84(2):356-65
[166] Roxas M, Jurenka J. Colds and influenza: a review of diagnosis and conventional, botanical, and nutritional considerations. *Altern Med Rev.* 2007 Mar;12(1):25-4
[167] Chen SSP, Steele RW (ed). Measles. Updated: Sep 29, 2014. http://emedicine.medscape.com/article/966220-overview

PO for 2 doses; Older than 1 year: 200,000 IU/day PO for 2 doses; Children with clinical signs of vitamin A deficiency: The first 2 doses as appropriate for age, then a third age-specific dose given 2-4 weeks later."

- o Documentation of the use and safety of high-dose vitamin A: Adjuvant treatment of stage I lung cancer with high-dose vitamin A (*J Clin Oncol.* 1993 Jul[168]): "…retinol palmitate administration (orally 300,000 IU daily for 12 months) … CONCLUSION: Daily oral administration of high-dose vitamin A is effective in reducing the number of new primary tumors related to tobacco consumption and may improve the disease-free interval in patients curatively resected for stage I lung cancer."

- o Documentation of the use and safety of high-dose vitamin A: Safety of high-dose vitamin A. Randomized trial on lung cancer chemoprevention (*Oncology.* 1991[169]): After administering retinol palmitate (300,000 IU daily for at least 12 months), the authors report their experience with the safety of such doses. "Skin dryness and desquamation were the most frequent symptoms, affecting 60% of all treated patients. Other symptoms such as dyspepsia, headache, nosebleeds and mild hair loss occurred in less than 10% of patients, and were self-terminating. Only in 4 patients (3%) was the treatment interrupted because of symptoms potentially related to vitamin A administration."

- o Documentation of the use and safety of high-dose vitamin A: Laboratory evaluation during high-dose vitamin A administration: a randomized study on lung cancer patients after surgical resection (*J Cancer Res Clin Oncol.* 1991[170]): Adverse effects of high-dose vitamin A in this report included elevations of serum gamma-glutamyltransferase (abnormally elevated in 69% of the treated patients compared to 39% of controls (mean values 149 vs 57 IU/l at 24 months)) and elevations of serum triglyceride concentrations (over 150 mg/dl seen in 74% of treated patients compared to 43% of controls at 12 months; the average concentration was 283 mg/dl compared to 179 mg/dl). "…there was no other laboratory evidence of toxicity attributable to vitamin A. … In our experience **300,000 IU/day of retinyl palmitate can be administered as a possible chemopreventive agent with reasonable safety for up to 2 years.**"

- **Fatty acids**: Fatty acids (FA) have many interconnected roles in human physiology, and these interactions are at their most critical importance during disorders of inflammation. An excess of pro-inflammatory FA and deficiency of anti-inflammatory FA may have been tolerated by the patient for decades without *obvious* adverse effect. However, during times of illness or injury, these fatty acid imbalances are made more apparent by the biological activation of these generally inert fatty acids into their biologically active—often inflammatory and painful—chemical mediators, including but not limited to prostaglandins, leukotrienes, isoprostanes, and (beneficially) the anti-inflammatory docosatrienes and resolvins. **Part of the benefit of fatty acid supplementation during infection is that it helps modulate inflammatory responses to prevent them from leading to excess tissue damage and vicious cycles of *inflammation-induced inflammation*. Extreme inflammatory responses actually cause immunosuppression (counterinflammation[171]) that can increase the susceptibility to or severity of infection.** "Fatty acid" supplementation in the context of acute illness, trauma, and sepsis generally means EPA and DHA from fish oil; however, some studies have used EPA without DHA, while others have used EPA with GLA.

  - o Clinical trial: Nutritional supplements [cod liver oil and a children's multivitamin-mineral with selenium] as adjunctive therapy for children with chronic/recurrent sinusitis: pilot research (*Int J Pediatr Otorhinolaryngol.* 2004 Jun[172]): "Four, six, and eight weeks after beginning study supplements, the responders had decreased sinus symptoms, fewer episodes of acute sinusitis, and fewer doctor visits for acute illnesses. Their parents reported that they had begun to recover from upper respiratory illnesses without complications, which was unusual for these children…"

  - o Clinical trial: Lemon-flavored cod liver oil and a multivitamin-mineral supplement for the secondary prevention of otitis media in young children (*Ann Otol Rhinol Laryngol.* 2002 Jul[173]): "…8 children received 1 teaspoon of lemon-flavored cod liver oil (containing both EPA and vitamin A) and 1 half-tablet of a selenium-containing children's chewable multivitamin-mineral tablet per day. During this OM season,

[168] Pastorino et al. Adjuvant treatment of stage I lung cancer with high-dose vitamin A. *J Clin Oncol.* 1993 Jul;11(7):1216-22
[169] Pastorino et al. Safety of high-dose vitamin A. Randomized trial on lung cancer chemoprevention. *Oncology.* 1991;48(2):131-7
[170] Infante et al. Laboratory evaluation during high-dose vitamin A administration. *J Cancer Res Clin Oncol.* 1991;117(2):156-62
[171] Bistrian BR. Practical recommendations for immune-enhancing diets. *J Nutr.* 2004;134(10 Sup):2868S-2872S jn.nutrition.org/cgi/content/full/134/10/2868S
[172] Linday et al. Nutritional supplements as adjunctive therapy for children with chronic/recurrent sinusitis: pilot research. *Int J Pediatr Otorhinolaryngol.* 2004 Jun;68(6):785-93
[173] Linday et al. Lemon-flavored cod liver oil and a multivitamin-mineral supplement for secondary prevention of otitis media in young children. *Ann Otol Rhinol Laryngol.* 2002 Jul;111(7 Pt 1):642-52

study subjects received antibiotics for OM for 12.3% fewer days during supplementation than before supplementation."

- o Clinical trial: Effect of daily cod liver oil and a multivitamin-mineral supplement with selenium on upper respiratory tract pediatric visits by young, inner-city, Latino children (*Ann Otol Rhinol Laryngol.* 2002 Jul[174]): "The supplementation group had a statistically significant decrease in the mean number of upper respiratory tract [infection] visits over time... Use of these nutritional supplements...was associated with a decrease in upper respiratory tract [infection] pediatric visits over time...."

- o Systematic review: Immunonutrition in critically ill patients: a systematic review and analysis of the literature (*Intensive Care Med.* 2008 Nov[175]): This systematic review compared studies with various combinations of arginine, glutamine, and/or fish oil and concluded that only fish oil supplementation provided consistent benefit in terms of mortality and length of stay [LOS]. "Mortality, infections and LOS were significantly lower only in the ICU patients receiving the FO [fish oil] IMD [immuno-modulating diets] (OR 0.42, 95% CI 0.26-0.68; OR 0.45, 95% CI 0.25-0.79 and WMD -6.28 days, 95% CI -9.92 to -2.64, respectively)." The benefits of fish oil across such a heterogeneous group of patients is due to the following: ❶ deficiency of EPA and DHA is essentially universal among patients consuming an American/Western diet, ❷ the provision of EPA and DHA provides potent anti-inflammatory effects, some of which such as activation of PPAR-alpha is enhanced when the fatty acid ligand (e.g., EPA) is in an oxidized state, and 3) oral consumption of lipid stimulates the vagus nerve, which then provides an anti-inflammatory effect via **neuroimmunomodulation.**

- **Glutamine: 3-9 grams x3 between meals (TID IC):** Glutamine (Gln) is a conditionally essential nutrient that is needed by immunocytes and enterocytes in increased amounts during times of trauma and infection. Insufficient glutamine availability is a compound problem resulting in immunosuppression and increased intestinal permeability; clinicians should appreciate that this is the perfect formula for gram-negative sepsis. Further, insufficiency of glutamine would also be expected to result in a deficiency of glutathione and the resultant increase in oxidative stress. All clinicians should know that glutathione (GSH) is a critically important antioxidant that has numerous functions for regulating cell cycle, DNA repair, and inflammatory responses, and that this antioxidant is formed endogenously from three amino acids: cysteine, glycine, and glutamine/glutamate. This explains the benefit of providing cysteine (generally in the form of N-acetyl-cysteine [which has additional benefits independent from its contribution to GSH], supported by many human trials) and glutamine (supported by animal research) to patients with toxic exposures, such as Tylenol/acetaminophen overdose. In clinical practice, 9-18 grams per day between meals (amino acids are generally administered between meals) is reasonable, although higher doses have been used and reported in clinical trials in specific situations. After administering glutamine 26 grams/d to severely burned patients, Garrel et al[176] concluded that glutamine reduced the risk of infection by 3-fold and that **oral glutamine "may be a life-saving intervention"** in patients with severe burns. A dose of 30 gm/d was used in a clinical trial showing hemodynamic benefit in patients with sickle cell anemia.[177] The highest glutamine dose that the current author is aware of is the study by Scheltinga et al[178] who used intravenous glutamine 0.57 gm/kg/day in cancer patients following chemotherapy administration; for a 220-lb-pt, this would be approximately 57 grams/d of glutamine.

  - o Ex vivo study: Glutamine-enhanced bacterial killing by neutrophils from postoperative patients (*Nutrition.* 1997 Oct[179]): Not all studies have replicated this finding of enhanced antibacterial action of neutrophils following the addition of glutamine; however, these findings provide an excellent *partial* explanation for the anti-infective and immunosupportive effects of glutamine administration to humans,

---

[174] Linday et al. Effect of daily cod liver oil and a multivitamin-mineral supplement with selenium on upper respiratory tract pediatric visits by young, inner-city, Latino children: randomized pediatric sites. *Ann Otol Rhinol Laryngol.* 2004 Nov;113(11):891-901

[175] Marik PE, Zaloga GP. Immunonutrition in critically ill patients: a systematic review and analysis of the literature. *Intensive Care Med.* 2008 Nov;34(11):1980-90

[176] The glutamine dose in this study was "a total of 26 g/day" administered in four divided doses. CONCLUSION: "The results of this prospective randomized clinical trial show that enteral G reduces blood culture positivity, particularly with P. aeruginosa, in adults with severe burns and may be a life-saving intervention." Garrel et al. Decreased mortality and infectious morbidity in adult burn patients given enteral glutamine supplements: a prospective, controlled, randomized clinical trial. *Crit Care Med.* 2003 Oct;31(10):2444-9

[177] Niihara et al. L-glutamine therapy reduces endothelial adhesion of sickle red blood cells to human umbilical vein endothelial cells. *BMC Blood Disord.* 2005 Jul 25;5:4

[178] "Subjects with hematologic malignancies in remission underwent a standard treatment of high-dose chemotherapy and total body irradiation before bone marrow transplantation. After completion of this regimen, they were randomized to receive either standard parenteral nutrition (STD, n = 10) or an isocaloric, isonitrogenous nutrient solution enriched with crystalline L-glutamine (0.57 g/kg/day, GLN, n = 10)." Scheltinga et al. Glutamine-enriched intravenous feedings attenuate extracellular fluid expansion after a standard stress. *Ann Surg.* 1991 Oct;214(4):385-93; discussion 393-5 For additional review, see Ziegler TR. Glutamine supplementation in cancer patients receiving bone marrow transplantation and high dose chemotherapy. *J Nutr.* 2001 Sep;131(9 Suppl):2578S-84S

[179] Furukawa et al. Glutamine-enhanced bacterial killing by neutrophils from postoperative patients. *Nutrition.* 1997 Oct;13(10):863-9

which has been documented in numerous trials. "This finding indicated that as plasma Gln fell, there was an enhancement of neutrophil E. coli-killing activity by neutrophils in *in vitro* tests when the Gln concentration was increased from 500 to 1000 nmol/mL. ... In conclusion, Gln supplementation enhanced the in vitro bactericidal function of neutrophils from postoperative patients."[180]

- o Clinical trial and documentation of hospital cost savings by the use of glutamine administration in critically ill patients (despite no reduction in mortality): Randomized clinical outcome study of critically ill patients given glutamine-supplemented enteral nutrition (*Nutrition*. 1999 Feb[181]): "However, there was a significant reduction in the median postintervention ICU and hospital patient costs in the glutamine recipients $23,000 versus $30,900 in the control patients (P 5 0.036). For patients given glutamine there was a reduced cost per survivor of 30%."Given the safety and low cost of glutamine, one might wonder why hospitals have not already started to implement glutamine therapy on a regular basis, based on this research and other supporting research which also points toward clinical efficacy and lack of adverse effects.

- o Randomized clinical trial: Benefits of early enteral nutrition with glutamine and probiotics in brain injury patients (*Clin Sci*. 2004 Mar[182]): This clinical trial of brain injury patients showed that an enteral formula containing glutamine and probiotics decreased the infection rate and shortened the stay in the intensive care unit; "The infection rate was higher in controls (100%) when compared with the study group (50%; P=0.03) and the median (range) number of infections per patient was significantly greater (P<0.01) in the control group compared with the study group."

- o Double-blind, randomized, controlled study of alanyl-glutamine dipeptide-supplemented parenteral nutrition in SICU patients requiring parenteral nutrition: Efficacy of parenteral nutrition supplemented with glutamine dipeptide to decrease hospital infections in critically ill surgical patients (*PEN J Parenter Enteral Nutr*. 2008 Jul[183]): This clinical trial in the surgical intensive care unit (SICU) compared ❶ standard hospital parenteral/intravenous nutrition (STD-PN) against ❷ alanyl-glutamine dipeptide-supplemented parenteral nutrition (GLN-PN) in two different patient populations: 1) SICU patients requiring parenteral nutrition and 2) SICU care after surgery for pancreatic necrosis, cardiac, vascular, or colonic surgery. Nutritional intake was isonitrogenous, either containing no glutamine (standard nutrition) or containing 0.5 g/kg/d glutamine dipeptide. GLN-PN did not alter the incidence of infection after pancreatic necrosis surgery; however, in nonpancreatic surgery patients, GLN-PN was associated with significantly decreased total nosocomial infections (STD-PN 36 vs GLN-PN 13), bloodstream infections (7 vs 0), pneumonias (16 vs 6), and infections attributed to *Staphylococcus aureus*, fungi, and enteric Gram-negative bacteria. The authors concluded, "Glutamine dipeptide-supplemented parenteral nutrition did not alter infection rates following pancreatic necrosis surgery but significantly decreased infections in SICU patients after cardiac, vascular, and colonic surgery."

- **Dietary nucleotides**: Especially during times of infection/immunoproliferation/immunoactivation and trauma/repair, rapidly proliferating tissues, such as the immune system or the intestine are not able to fulfill the needs of cell nucleotides exclusively by de novo synthesis; in these times, nutritional supplementation with dietary nucleotides can provide therapeutic value by promoting mucosal maintenance/repair and immune responses to infection. Dietary nucleotides have several effects on immune function, including beneficial influence on immunoglobulin response and lymphocyte maturation/activation/proliferation and enhancement of macrophage phagocytosis and (anti)tumor responses.[184] Similar to glutamine, arginine, EPA, DHA, and GLA, nucleotides appear to be conditionally-essential nutrients for the provision of an adequate supply of purines and pyrimidines for nucleic acid synthesis during times of growth/proliferation such as during infancy and in response to infection/trauma.

  - o Review: The role of nucleotides in adult nutrition (*J Nutr*. 1994 Jan[185]): The authors of this study review relevant literature and summarize that dietary RNA is required to maintain immune function, and to

---

[180] Furukawa et al. Glutamine-enhanced bacterial killing by neutrophils from postoperative patients. *Nutrition*. 1997 Oct;13(10):863-9

[181] Jones et al. Randomized clinical outcome study of critically ill patients given glutamine-supplemented enteral nutrition. *Nutrition*. 1999 Feb;15(2):108-15

[182] Falcão de Arruda et al. Benefits of early enteral nutrition with glutamine and probiotics in brain injury patients. *Clin Sci* (Lond). 2004 Mar;106(3):287-92

[183] Estívariz et al. Efficacy of parenteral nutrition supplemented with glutamine dipeptide to decrease hospital infections in critically ill surgical patients. *JPEN J Parenter Enteral Nutr*. 2008 Jul-Aug;32(4):389-402

[184] Gil A. Modulation of the immune response mediated by dietary nucleotides. *Eur J Clin Nutr*. 2002 Aug;56 Suppl 3:S1-4

[185] Van Buren et al. The role of nucleotides in adult nutrition. *J Nutr*. 1994 Jan;124(1 Suppl):160S-164S

restore lost immune function after protein deprivation, following which adequate calories and protein alone do not return immune function to normal. The authors proceed to note that dietary nucleotides can restore lost immune function even during protein starvation and weight loss. "In two separate double blind clinical studies the patients fed the enteral diet containing nucleotides had improved immune function compared with patients receiving a nucleotide free diet. In addition, infectious complications and length of hospital stay were reduced in postoperative cancer patients fed Impact [a commercial nucleotide-containing immunonutrition formula] compared with a control group."

- **Whey protein isolate**: Whey protein is a mixture of globular proteins isolated from whey, the liquid material created as a by-product of cheese production. The major protein fractions in whey are beta-lactoglobulin, alpha-lactalbumin, bovine serum albumin and immunoglobulins. Whey proteins are rich in cysteine as well as in the GSH-precursors (lactoferrin, beta-lactalbumin, bovine serum albumin, cystine [cysteine bonded to cysteine]). Whey protein isolates are processed to remove fat and lactose and are generally > 90% protein by weight. Although whey proteins are responsible for some "milk allergies", the major allergens in milk are caseins; many "milk allergic" patients can tolerate whey protein isolate even if they are intolerant of other milk/dairy products. Whey protein isolate provides high-quality easily digestible protein to meet body needs, either on an everyday basis or on a special needs basis, such as during infection or recovery from injury. Reviewed in the section below are supporting articles with specific reference to the use of whey protein supplementation in patients with infections. Whey protein isolate can easily be incorporated into even the most noncompliant patient's regimen, either in the form of smoothies or incorporated into raw-foods brownies or other treats; smoothies can be blended with whey protein isolate, fish oil, borage oil, fresh/frozen berries, and fiber sources such as wheat bran or flax seeds.

  o Prospective double-blind clinical trial: Oral supplementation with whey proteins increases plasma glutathione levels of HIV-infected patients (*Eur J Clin Invest*. 2001 Feb[186]): Authors of this study sought to restore glutathione (GSH) levels by providing the semi-essential amino acid cysteine via oral supplementation with two different cysteine-rich whey protein formulas: Protectamin (Fresenius Kabi, Bad Hamburg, Germany) or Immunocal (Immunotec, Vandreuil, Canada). One intervention included the addition of a daily dose of 45 g whey protein to either Protectamin or Immunocal for two weeks. "**Following two weeks of oral supplementation with whey proteins, plasma GSH levels increased in the Protectamin group by 44%** (2.79 microM, P = 0.004) while the difference in the Immunocal group did not reach significance (+ 24.5%, 2.51 microM, P = 0.43)." This study showed that while both whey protein supplements increased GSH levels, one product (Protectamin) significantly out-performed the other in terms of the difference in plasma GSH levels. This appears to be a significant biochemical difference, although the clinical significance in terms of patient outcomes (which would requires years of study in the same patient group) was not studied here.

  o Clinical trial: Effects of long-term supplementation with whey proteins on plasma glutathione levels of HIV-infected patients (*Eur J Nutr*. 2002 Feb[187]): This study reported again that Protectamin outperformed Immunocal insofar as Protectamin lead to higher levels of GSH when given at 45 g whey protein per day. Very interestingly, the biochemical benefits continued to accumulate over at least 6 months of treatment. "After six months, total GSH plasma levels were still significantly elevated compared to baseline (day 1: 1.95 microM vs. month 1: 2.18 microM; month 3: 2.39 microM; month 6: 2.47 microM)." The authors found that body weight, T-cell counts, and other clinical parameters did not change, and that the most common mild side effect was intestinal disturbance. No severe adverse events occurred. This study supports the importance of long-term adherence to dietary optimization and nutritional supplementation, with the benefits of whey protein supplementation (45 g/d) continuing to accumulate for at least 6 months after the initiation of treatment.

  o Prospective double-blind clinical trial: Features of whey protein concentrate supplementation in children with rapidly progressive HIV infection (*J Trop Pediatr*. 2006 Feb[188]): This trial lasted 4 months and included 18 vertically HIV-infected children (2-6 years of age), taking antiretroviral therapy, who had received

---

[186] Micke et al. Oral supplementation with whey proteins increases plasma glutathione levels of HIV-infected patients. *Eur J Clin Invest*. 2001 Feb;31(2):171-8
[187] Micke et al. Effects of long-term supplementation with whey proteins on plasma glutathione levels of HIV-infected patients. *Eur J Nutr*. 2002 Feb;41(1):12-8
[188] Moreno et al. Features of whey protein concentrate supplementation in children with rapidly progressive HIV infection. *J Trop Pediatr*. 2006 Feb;52(1):34-8

whey protein (treatment), maltodextrin (placebo) or none. "A significant median increase of 16.14 mg/dl (p = 0.018) in erythrocyte glutathione levels was observed in the whey protein-supplemented group; the TCD4/CD8 lymphocyte ratio showed a non-significant increase and **lower occurrence of associated co-infections was also observed.**"

- o Clinical trial: Beneficial effects of aggressive protein feeding with whey protein in severely burned children (*Ann Surg.* 1980[189]): Injured and infected patients are hypermetabolic; nutrient utilization is greatly increased due to physiologic hyperthermia, cell turnover, immune activation, and tissue repair. This hypermetabolic state depletes protein stores (i.e., tissue proteins, such as muscle) and vitamins (either due to metabolic utilization or oxidative destruction). In this study, 18 children with burns averaging 60% total surface area were randomized into two groups and studied for at least six weeks. The first group was given a normal diet with "a balanced nutritional supplement", while the second group was supplemented with milk whey protein. Details of their report were impressive: "The normal protein group received 87.1% of their desired caloric intake with 16.5% of calories from protein compared to 77.7% of desired caloric intake with 23.0% of calories from protein for the high protein group. Despite a higher caloric intake, the normal protein group had...lower levels of C3 (1371 vs. 1585 micrograms/ml), lower levels of IgG (805 vs. 975 micrograms/ml), lower levels of transferrin (200 vs. 283 mg/dl), lower levels of total serum protein (5.5 vs. 6.3 g/dl), more bacteremic days (11% vs. 8%) and worse survival (5/9--56% vs. 9/9--100%)." As expected, patients receiving the high protein diet had significantly higher plasma levels of amino acids. Plasma asparagine levels positively correlated with better neutrophil function. The authors conclude that, "These studies provide evidence that many immunologic functions are dependent upon optimal availability of specific amino acids, and that routine diets do not provide sufficient protein to satisfy the needs of seriously burned children."

- **Melatonin: 5-40 mg hs (*hora somni*—Latin: sleep hour)**: Melatonin has proven anti-infectious and immunosupportive properties; it must be taken only at night (within a few hours of sleep) in order to be beneficial.
  - o Clinical trial: Effects of melatonin treatment in septic newborns (*Pediatr Res.* 2001 Dec[190]): Immunostimulatory anti-infective action of melatonin was demonstrated in a small clinical trial wherein septic newborns administered 20 mg melatonin showed significantly increased survival over nontreated controls. "Three of 10 septic children who were not treated with melatonin died within 72 h after diagnosis of sepsis; none of the 10 septic newborns treated with melatonin died."
  - o Ebola virus disease—potential treatment with melatonin (*J Pineal Res.* 2014 Sep[191]): In this article, the authors review the rationale for the use of melatonin to interfere with multiple pathways in Ebola-induced pathophysiology and conclude by recommending at least 20 mg po as treatment, given the risk:benefit ratios and immediate and wide availability. In the full-text of the article, the authors conclude by recommending early intervention with melatonin "20 mg or more for a single dose; since there is no precedent for an effective melatonin dose, some upward adjustment of the dose may have greater efficacy; this dose should be given several times per day for a prolonged period."
    - http://www.ncbi.nlm.nih.gov/pubmed/25262626
  - o Review: Therapeutic potential of melatonin in immunodeficiency states, viral diseases, and cancer (*Adv Exp Med Biol.* 1999[192]): The clinical benefits of melatonin (MLT) administration have been well documented and consistently documented in patients with various forms of cancer receiving various forms of chemotherapy and/or radiation treatment. In this review, Maestroni provides a partial review of this research and also adds to clinicians' mechanistic understanding of the immunosupportive and immunostimulatory actions, summarized as, "T-helper cells bear G-protein-coupled MLT cell membrane receptors and, perhaps, MLT nuclear receptors. Activation of MLT receptors enhances the release of T-helper cell cytokines, such as gamma-interferon and interleukin-2 (IL-2), ... MLT has been reported also to enhance the production of interleukin-1, interleukin-6 and interleukin-12 in human monocytes. These mediators may counteract secondary immunodeficiencies, ..."

---

[189] Alexander et al. Beneficial effects of aggressive protein feeding in severely burned children. *Ann Surg.* 1980;192(4):505-17
[190] Gitto et al. Effects of melatonin treatment in septic newborns. *Pediatr Res.* 2001 Dec;50(6):756-60 pedresearch.org/cgi/content/full/50/6/756
[191] Tan DX, Reiter RJ, Manchester LC. Ebola virus disease: Potential use of melatonin as a treatment. *J Pineal Res.* 2014 Sep 27. doi: 10.1111/jpi.12186
[192] Maestroni GJ. Therapeutic potential of melatonin in immunodeficiency states, viral diseases, and cancer. *Adv Exp Med Biol.* 1999;467:217-26

- o Review: The potential of melatonin in reducing morbidity-mortality after craniocerebral trauma (*J Pineal Res.* 2007 Jan[193]): Actions that make melatonin a reasonable treatment after trauma such as craniocerebral trauma include ❶ neutralization of both oxygen-based and nitrogen-based free radicals, ❷ stimulation of the activities of a variety of antioxidative enzymes (e.g. superoxide dismutase, glutathione peroxidase, glutathione reductase and catalase), ❸ inhibition of pro-inflammatory cytokines and activation-adhesion molecules which consequently reduces lymphocytopenia and **reduces infections by opportunistic organisms**, ❹ reestablishment of the natural circadian rhythm of sleep and wakefulness, ❺ reduction in the toxicity of the drugs used in the treatment of craniocerebral trauma, ❻ enhanced function of drugs used in the treatment of craniocerebral trauma, ❼ reduction in brain contusion volume, and ❽ stabilization of cellular membranes preventing vasospasm and apoptosis of endothelial cells.

  - o Pharmacological utility of melatonin in the treatment of septic shock (*J Pharm Pharmacol.* 2006[194]): "Melatonin has well documented protective effects against the symptoms of severe sepsis/shock in both animals and in humans; its use for this condition significantly improves survival. Melatonin administration counteracts mtNOS induction and respiratory chain failure, restores cellular and mitochondrial redox status, and reduces proinflammatory cytokines. Melatonin clearly prevents multiple organ failure, circulatory failure, and mitochondrial damage in experimental sepsis, and reduces lipid peroxidation, indices of inflammation and mortality in septic human newborns. Considering these effects of melatonin and its virtual absence of toxicity, the use of melatonin (along with conventional therapy) to preserve mitochondrial bioenergetics as well as to limit inflammatory responses and oxidative damage should be seriously considered as a treatment option in both septic newborn and adult patients."
    - http://www.ncbi.nlm.nih.gov/pubmed/16945173
    - http://onlinelibrary.wiley.com/doi/10.1211/jpp.58.9.0001/abstract
    - http://onlinelibrary.wiley.com/doi/10.1211/jpp.58.9.0001/pdf
  - o Melatonin stimulates release of tissue factor pathway inhibitor from the vascular endothelium. (*Blood Coagul Fibrinolysis.* 2011[195]): "Our data indicate that melatonin stimulates vascular endothelial cells to secrete TFPI without altering transcription of the TFPI gene. If melatonin increases TFPI release in a similar fashion in vivo as in vitro, this could have potential clinical implications in both prophylaxis and treatment of thromboembolic events."
    - http://www.ncbi.nlm.nih.gov/pubmed/21297449

- **Silibinin/silybin from *Silymarin marianum*—special (but not exclusive) application for viral hepatitis**: In the world of botanical medicine, certainly most herbalists and naturopathic physicians would readily but not exclusively associate *Silymarin marianum* with the treatment of liver disorders, ranging from cirrhosis to cholestasis. Herbal preparations are safe, well standardized, and useful "beyond the liver" in support of general detoxification, cancer treatment, and renoprotection.

  - o Triple-blind, randomized, placebo-controlled trial: A randomized controlled trial to assess the safety and efficacy of Silymarin on symptoms, signs and biomarkers of acute hepatitis (*Phytomedicine.* 2009 May [196]): This study enrolled 105 patients with symptoms compatible with acute clinical hepatitis and serum alanine aminotransferase (ALT) levels >2.5 times the upper limit of normal. Per the authors' description, "The intervention consisted of three times daily ingestion of either a standard recommended dose of 140 mg of silymarin (Legalon, MADAUS GmbH, Cologne, Germany), or a vitamin placebo for four weeks with an additional four-week follow-up." No adverse events were noted. Results showed that, "Patients randomized to the silymarin group had quicker resolution of symptoms related to biliary retention: dark urine (p=0.013), jaundice (p=0.02) and scleral icterus (p=0.043). There was a reduction in indirect bilirubin among those assigned to silymarin (p=0.012), but other variables including direct bilirubin, ALT and aspartate aminotransferase (AST) were not significantly reduced."

[193] Maldonado et al. The potential of melatonin in reducing morbidity-mortality after craniocerebral trauma. *J Pineal Res.* 2007 Jan;42(1):1-11
[194] Escames et al. Pharmacological utility of melatonin in the treatment of septic shock: experimental and clinical evidence. *J Pharm Pharmacol.* 2006; 58: 1153-1165
[195] Kostovski et al. Melatonin stimulates release of tissue factor pathway inhibitor from the vascular endothelium. *Blood Coagul Fibrinolysis.* 2011; 22: 254-259
[196] El-Kamary et al. A randomized controlled trial to assess the safety and efficacy of silymarin on symptoms, signs and biomarkers of acute hepatitis. *Phytomedicine.* 2009 May;16(5):391-400

o Clinical trial of intravenous silibinin/silybin from *Silymarin marianum*: Silibinin is a potent antiviral agent in patients with chronic hepatitis C not responding to pegylated interferon/ribavirin therapy (*Gastroenterology*. 2008 Nov[197]): Silibinin, also known as silybin, is the major active constituent of silymarin, the mixture of flavonolignans extracted from milk thistle, *Silybum/Silymarin marianum*. Oral dosing of silibinin, like oral dosing of many nutrients, cannot achieve the high serum levels attainable with intravenous treatment. In this study, sixteen patients unresponsive to full-dose pegylated (Peg)-interferon/ribavirin (PegIFN/RBV) received 10 mg/kg/day SIL IV (Legalon Sil; Madaus, Köln, Germany) for 7 days. In a subsequent dose-finding study, 20 patients received 5, 10, 15, or 20 mg/kg/day SIL for 14 days. The authors report that subjects treated with SIL IV showed an "unexpected" temporary reduction in HCV-RNA which was dose dependent and which decreased further after 7 days combined SIL/PegIFN/RBV. In 7 patients on 15 or 20 mg/kg SIL, their viral load became undetectable at week 12 (despite previous nonresponse to PegIFN/RBV. Mild gastrointestinal symptoms were the only adverse effect attributed to IV SIL monotherapy. The authors conclude that, "IV SIL is well tolerated and shows a substantial antiviral effect against HCV in nonresponders."

> **Orally administered antioxidant nutrients and antiviral botanicals used in the study by Melhem et al**
> - Glycyrrhiza: 500 mg bid*
> - Schizandrae: 500 mg tid*
> - Ascorbate: 2,000 mg tid
> - Glutathione: 150 mg bid
> - Silymarin: 250 mg tid*
> - Lipoic acid: 150 mg bid
> - D-alpha-tocopherol: 800 IU/d
>
> *No data was provided about the standardization of the botanicals.
>
> Melhem et al. Treatment of chronic hepatitis C virus infection via antioxidants: results of a phase I clinical trial. *J Clin Gastroenterol.* 2005 Sep;39(8):737-42

o Review, and a word of caution in the use of silymarin in non-hepatitis viral infections: Immunosuppressive effect of silibinin in experimental autoimmune encephalomyelitis, and Silibinin polarizes Th1/Th2 immune responses through the inhibition of immunostimulatory function of dendritic cells (*Arch Pharm Res.* 2007 Oct[198]): Silymarin has beneficial effects in models (including human clinical trials) of liver disease; new research is promoting its use in anti-cancer protocols. Silymarin inhibits NFkB and this probably explains a good deal of its anti-inflammatory and anti-fibrotic effects. However, a few articles, such as by Min et al suggest that silymarin might impair antiviral Th-1 immune responses; they write, "...silibinin Ag-nonspecifically down-regulated the secretion of pro-inflammatory Th1 cytokines and up-regulated the anti-inflammatory Th2 cytokines in vitro. Silibinin also dose-dependently inhibited the production of Th1 cytokines ex vivo. These results indicate that silibinin is both immunosuppressive and immunomodulatory." Identically, Lee et al[199] found, in an experiment involving dendritic cells (DC) that, "...silibinin-treated DCs evidenced an **impaired induction of Th1 response**, and a normal cell-mediated immune response."

- **Pancreatic and proteolytic enzymes**: Orally administered pancreatic/proteolytic enzyme combinations are remarkably safe and have applicability for a wide range of clinical problems, including resolution of acute and chronic refractory sinusitis (bromelain)[200], clinical benefit in traumatic contusions, sprains, lacerations, strains (papain-containing preparation)[201], alleviation of hip[202] and knee[203] pain (bromelain), and alleviation of knee pain (bromelain-trypsin-rutosid combination).[204,205] For the concentrations and combinations generally available, orally consumed enzymes might be prescribed as 4-8 tablets thrice daily between meals; doctors will have to customize the doses used based on the products chosen and the details of the patient and condition being treated. At the highest end of the dosage spectrum, Gonzalez[206] reports using as much as "25-40 grams of porcine lyophilized pancreas product daily, taken in capsule form, away from meals, and spread evenly throughout the day. ... The particular formulation for pancreatic enzymes we use tests at 30-80 UPS units of

[197] Ferenci et al. Silibinin is a potent antiviral agent in patients with chronic hepatitis C not responding to pegylated interferon/ribavirin therapy. *Gastroenterology*. 2008 Nov;135(5):1561-7

[198] Min K, Yoon WK, Kim SK, Kim BH. Immunosuppressive effect of silibinin in experimental autoimmune encephalomyelitis. Arch Pharm Res. 2007 Oct;30(10):1265-72

[199] Lee et al. Silibinin polarizes Th1/Th2 immune responses through the inhibition of immunostimulatory function of dendritic cells. *J Cell Physiol*. 2007 Feb;210(2):385-97

[200] Taub SJ. The use of bromelains in sinusitis: a double-blind clinical evaluation. Eye Ear Nose Throat Mon. 1967 Mar;46(3):361-5

[201] Trickett P. Proteolytic enzymes in treatment of athletic injuries. *Appl Ther*. 1964;30:647-52

[202] Klein et al. Efficacy and tolerance of an oral enzyme combination in painful osteoarthritis of the hip. *Clin Exp Rheumatol*. 2006 Jan-Feb;24(1):25-30

[203] Walker et al. Bromelain reduces mild acute knee pain and improves well-being in a dose-dependent fashion in an open study of otherwise healthy adults. *Phytomedicine*. 2002;9:681-6

[204] Akhtar et al. Oral enzyme combination versus diclofenac in the treatment of osteoarthritis of the knee. *Clin Rheumatol*. 2004 Oct;23(5):410-5

[205] Tilwe et al. Efficacy and tolerability of oral enzyme therapy as compared to diclofenac in active osteoarthrosis of knee joint. *J Assoc Physicians India*. 2001 Jun;49:617-21

[206] Gonzalez et al. Evaluation of pancreatic proteolytic enzyme treatment of adenocarcinoma of the pancreas, with nutrition and detoxification support. *Nutr Cancer*. 1999:117-24

proteolytic activity per milligram and 15-40 units of lipolytic activity per milligram." Relevant to this discussion of infectious diseases, we note that oral consumption of pancreatic/proteolytic enzymes has immunostimulatory actions[207] as well as anti-edematous and anti-inflammatory actions.[208]

- o Pilot study in patients with pityriasis lichenoides chronica: Role of bromelain in the treatment of patients with pityriasis lichenoides chronica (PLC) (*J Dermatolog Treat.* 2007[209]): "RESULTS: All patients showed complete clinical recovery after treatment. … CONCLUSIONS: In conclusion bromelain **can** be considered an effective therapeutic option for PLC; its efficacy could be related to its anti-inflammatory, immunomodulatory and/or anti-viral properties."

- o Double-blind, randomized, controlled phase III study at a tertiary care center: Efficacy and safety of phlogenzym—a protease formulation, in sepsis in children (*J Assoc Physicians India.* 2002 Apr;50:527-31[210]): The authors of this study hypothesize that oral administration of proteolytic enzymes may regulate the host's immune system and promote early recovery from sepsis. This study used enteric-coated tablets with bromelain 90 mg, trypsin 48 mg, and rutin 100 mg as adjuvant therapy in treatment of 60 children (aged one month to 12 years) with sepsis; patients were given 1 tablet/10 kg body weight up to maximum six tablets a day in two or three divided doses for 14-21 days along with appropriate antibiotics and supportive treatment. Results are as follows: "Median time taken for fever to subside was three days in the [enzyme] group vs four days in the placebo group; hemodynamic support was needed for two days in the [enzyme] group but three days in the placebo group. The modified Glasgow coma scale score normalized in three days in the [enzyme] group vs 5.5 days in the placebo group. Oral feeds could be started in four days in the [enzyme] group vs five days in the placebo group. Two patients died in the placebo group. CONCLUSION: [Orally administered enzyme therapy] is effective as an adjuvant with antibiotics and supportive treatment for early improvement of pediatric patients with sepsis."

- o Immune stimulation in humans via oral administration of combination enzymes. (*Cancer Biother.* 1995 Summer[211]): A combination of enzymes—pancreatin, papain, bromelain trypsin and chymotrypsin—has been used for decades for the treatment of infections, inflammation, and cancer; this study shows that oral administration of these enzymes increases free-radical production by the immune system, one of the main mechanisms by which the immune system fights infections and possibly cancer cells. Here, the authors summarize the results of administering the polyenzyme preparation (WE): "Depending on dose WE stimulates the cytotoxic capacity of PMN in vitro against tumor cells (50 micrograms/ml). Exposure of PMN to Wobenzym caused a time-dependent significant (p < 0.02) increase in release of ROS. Similarly, oral administration of Wobenzym to healthy volunteers (n = 28) resulted in significant increases (p < 0.01) in ROS production, depending on dose (peak with 20 tablets) and time (peak 4 hours after Wobenzym administration). In contrast, ROS production was not elevated in the PMN of healthy volunteers receiving placebo (n = 8) or no treatment (n = 16). These findings point to an immunomodulatory capacity of WE in adjuvant tumor therapy."
  - ▪ http://www.ncbi.nlm.nih.gov/pubmed/7663574

---

[207] "Similarly, oral administration of Wobenzym to healthy volunteers (n = 28) resulted in significant increases in ROS production, depending on dose (peak with 20 tablets) and time (peak 4 hours after Wobenzym administration). … These findings point to an immunomodulatory capacity of WE in adjuvant tumor therapy." Zavadova et al. Stimulation of reactive oxygen species production and cytotoxicity in human neutrophils in vitro and after oral administration of a polyenzyme preparation. *Cancer Biother.* 1995;10(2):147-52

[208] Taub SJ. The use of bromelains in sinusitis: a double-blind clinical evaluation. Eye Ear Nose Throat Mon. 1967 Mar;46(3):361-5

[209] Massimiliano et al. Role of bromelain in the treatment of patients with pityriasis lichenoides chronica. *J Dermatolog Treat.* 2007;18(4):219-22

[210] Shahid et al. Efficacy and safety of phlogenzym--a protease formulation, in sepsis in children. *J Assoc Physicians India.* 2002 Apr;50:527-31

[211] Zavadova et al. Stimulation of reactive oxygen species production and cytotoxicity in human neutrophils in vitro and after oral administration of a polyenzyme preparation. *Cancer Biother.* 1995 Summer;10(2):147-52

Understanding two types of counterinflammation: how antiinflammatory nutrients (and other treatments) improve immune responsiveness against microbial invasion

I first saw the use of the term "counterinflammation" in the 2004 article by Bistrian wherein the term was used three times to describe active antiinflammatory and proresolution processes that halt inflammation and promote tissue healing yet when carried to excess can have an immunosuppressant effect. I am not fully convinced of this definition of counterinflammation and I think it is largely theoretical; a descriptive quote from Bistrian states, "Although under most circumstances the systemic inflammatory response is beneficial to the host, improving the eventual outcome of injury, infection, or inflammation, excessive proinflammation, leading to cardiac, hepatic, and mitochondrial dysfunction, or excessive **counterinflammation** [which is antiinflammatory and immune depressant, turning off inflammation and promoting wound healing], leading to immune depression, can worsen outcome." With all due respect for Dr Bistrian's work, I found this particular concept weakly supported in his review.

In 2010, I presented a different and perhaps opposing view of counterinflammation, particularly that of "excessive inflammation leading to immune dysregulation and resulting immunoimpairment." My idea was then and remains as follows: excessive nonspecific inflammation causes a discoordination of immune responses leading to impaired immune responsiveness against microbial infections—in this manner, the inflammation is counterproductive, hence my use of the term **counterinflammation**. I think my use of the term explains the commonly-observed phenomena of immunosuppression in diabetic and acutely ill ICU patients, because the immune system should send and receive cytokines in a manner analogous to the precision of tunes played by an expert pianist or guitarist; with excessive systemic inflammation the resulting cytokine cacophony leads to "immune confusion" or "cytokine confusion" that discoordinates/uncoordinates the immune response to microbes. To extend the metaphor and make it more clear: imagine that cytokines are the music, and cells of the immune system must dance to the tune of orchestrated cytokines in order to effectively clear microbial infections while also not damaging host tissues; with excess inflammation—my use of the term counterinflammation—the resultant chaotic cytokine cacophony causes "confusion" and misdirection in the immune system, resulting in impaired antimicrobial responsiveness along with increased tendency toward autoimmunity. This is exactly what we see in clinical care and in the research literature.

Supporting my model and definition of "**counterinflammation: excess inflammation that is counterproductive to immune responsiveness to microbes**" is the recent paper showing that ibuprofen administration leads to enhanced anti-microbial immune responsiveness in an animal model of tuberculosis infection. Research published in 2014 Sep/Oct showed that "both mouse and human lungs develop the same profile of proinflammatory proteins and fatty molecules with age, creating an environment that impairs the immune response to infection" and that in an animal model this inflammation-induced immunoimpairment could be reduced by anti-inflammatory intervention.

1. Bistrian BR. Practical recommendations for immune-enhancing diets. *J Nutr*. 2004 Oct
2. Vasquez A. Immune Module 2010 presented for the Institute for Functional Medicine in Austin Texas and surpassed by later works including especially *Functional Inflammology: Volume 1* (ISBN: 978-0990620402) and *Functional Medicine Rheumatology* (ISBN: 9781502481368) and newer presentations (vimeo.com/DrVasquez).
3. Caldwell E. Making Old Lungs Look New Again: Animal research suggests ibuprofen can reduce lung inflammation in elderly. 2014 Oct news.osu.edu/news/2014/10/02/making-old-lungs-look-new-again/ based on Canan et al. Characterization of lung inflammation and its impact on macrophage function in aging. *J Leukoc Biol*. 2014 Sep;96:473-80

Strategy #4: Support the Cells and Whole System

Antiviral	Antireplication	Immunonutrition	Cell-system support
			Optimization of sleep, modulation of stress, avoidance of sugar, appropriate exercise and physical medicine

<u>**Therapeutic and Interventional Considerations for Use in Patients *with* and *Who Wish to Avoid* Viral Infections**</u>: Clinicians can use any combination of safe noncontraindicated nutrients, botanicals, and dietary modifications to support immune function and the clearance or amelioration of acute or chronic viral infections. These treatments are listed by the current author's preference, with appreciation for naturopathy's hierarchy of therapeutics, and/or by the level of available evidence (i.e., clinical trials over in vitro studies), given the current healthcare trend in favor of evidence-based medicine. General benefits derived from the use of immunonutrition are reductions in severity/frequency/duration of major infections, abbreviated hospitalization (i.e., early discharge due to expedited healing and recovery), reductions in the need for medications, significant improvements in survival, and hospital savings.[212,213,214,215,216,217,218] Doses listed here and throughout this book are for adults unless otherwise specified. Doctors are expected to use these interventions in combination, with individual nutrients and doses customized for each patient.

> **Importance of Whole-Foods Nutrition**
>
> "Given the increased micronutrient requirements, **nutrition counseling with HIV-infected youths should focus on early increase of intake of foods rich in micronutrients** to improve growth, slow disease progression, and increase survival. ... Young patients with HIV are at highest risk of being deficient in vitamins A and E and zinc."
>
> Kruzich et al. US youths in the early stages of HIV disease have low intakes of some micronutrients important for optimal immune function. *J Am Diet Assoc.* 2004 Jul

- **Paleo-Mediterranean Diet**: The health-promoting diet of choice for the majority of people is a diet based on abundant consumption of fruits, vegetables, seeds, nuts, omega-3 and monounsaturated fatty acids, and lean sources of protein such as lean meats, fatty cold-water fish, soy and whey proteins. This diet prohibits and obviates overconsumption of chemical preservatives, artificial sweeteners, and carbohydrate-dominant foods such as candies, pastries, breads, potatoes, grains, and other foods with a high glycemic load and high glycemic index. This "Paleo-Mediterranean Diet" is a combination of the "Paleolithic" or "Paleo diet" and the well-known "Mediterranean diet", both of which are well described in peer-reviewed journals and the lay press. The Mediterranean diet is characterized by increased proportions of legumes, nuts, seeds, whole grain products, fruits, vegetables (including potatoes), fish and lean meats, and monounsaturated and n-3 fatty acids.[219] Consumption of this diet is consistently associated with improvements in insulin sensitivity and

---

[212] "To evaluate the metabolic and immune effects of dietary arginine, glutamine and omega-3 fatty acids (fish oil) supplementation, we performed a prospective study... CONCLUSIONS: The feeding of Neomune in critically injured patients was well tolerated as Traumacal and significant improvement was observed in serum protein. Shorten ICU stay and wean-off respirator day may benefit from using the immunonutrient formula." Chuntrasakul et al. Comparison of a immunonutrition formula enriched arginine, glutamine and omega-3 fatty acid, with a currently high-enriched enteral nutrition for trauma patients. *J Med Assoc Thai.* 2003 Jun;86(6):552-6

[213] "CONCLUSIONS: In conclusion, arginine-enhanced formula improves fistula rates in postoperative head and neck cancer patients and decreases length of stay." de Luis et al. Randomized clinical trial with an enteral arginine-enhanced formula in early postsurgical head and neck cancer patients. *Eur J Clin Nutr.* 2004;58(11):1505-8

[214] "In this prospective, randomised, double-blind, placebo-controlled study, we randomly assigned 50 patients who were scheduled to undergo coronary artery bypass to receive either an oral immune-enhancing nutritional supplement containing L-arginine, omega3 polyunsaturated fatty acids, and yeast RNA (n=25), or a control (n=25) for a minimum of 5 days... Intake of an oral immune-enhancing nutritional supplement for a minimum of 5 days before surgery can improve outlook in high-risk patients who are undergoing elective cardiac surgery." Tepaske et al. Effect of preoperative oral immune-enhancing nutritional supplement on patients at high risk of infection after cardiac surgery: a randomised placebo-controlled trial. *Lancet.* 2001 Sep 1;358(9283):696-701

[215] "The feeding of IMMUNE FORMULA was well tolerated and significant improvement was observed in nutritional and immunologic parameters as in other immunoenhancing diets. Further clinical trials of prospective double-blind randomized design are necessary to address the so that the necessity of using immunonutrition in critically ill patients will be clarified." Chuntrasakul et al. Metabolic and immune effects of dietary arginine, glutamine and omega-3 fatty acids supplementation in immunocompromised patients. *J Med Assoc Thai.* 1998 May;81(5):334-43

[216] "enteral diet supplemented with arginine, dietary nucleotides, and omega-3 fatty acids (IMPACT, Sandoz Nutrition, Bern, Switzerland) " Senkal et al. Early postoperative enteral immunonutrition: clinical outcome and cost-comparison analysis in surgical patients. *Crit Care Med* 1997;25(9):1489-96

[217] "...supplemented diet with glutamine, arginine and omega-3-fatty acids... It was clearly established in this trial that early postoperative enteral feeding is safe in patients who have undergone major operations for gastrointestinal cancer. Supplementation of enteral nutrition with glutamine, arginine, and omega-3-fatty acids positively modulated postsurgical immunosuppressive and inflammatory responses." Wu et al. Modulation of postoperative immune and inflammatory response by immune-enhancing enteral diet in gastrointestinal cancer patients. *World J Gastroenterol.* 2001 Jun;7(3):357-62 wjgnet.com/1007-9327/7/357.pdf

[218] "using a formula supplemented with arginine, mRNA, and omega-3 fatty acids from fish oil (Impact)... CONCLUSIONS: Immune-enhancing enteral nutrition resulted in a significant reduction in the mortality rate and infection rate in septic patients admitted to the ICU. These reductions were greater for patients with less severe illness." Galban et al. An immune-enhancing enteral diet reduces mortality rate and episodes of bacteremia in septic intensive care unit patients. *Crit Care Med.* 2000 Mar;28(3):643-8

[219] Curtis et al. Understanding the Mediterranean diet. Could this be the new "gold standard" for heart disease prevention? *Postgrad Med.* 2002 Aug;112(2):35-8, 41-5

reductions in cardiovascular disease, diabetes, cancer, and all-cause mortality.[220] The Paleolithic diet detailed by collaborators Eaton, O'Keefe, and Cordain[221] is similar to the Mediterranean diet except for stronger emphasis on fruits and vegetables (preferably raw or minimally cooked), omega-3-rich lean meats, and reduced consumption of starchy foods such as potatoes and grains, the latter of which were not staples in the human diet until the last few thousand years. The current author expects that habitual consumption of this Paleo-Mediterranean Diet is immunosupportive/immunoempowering due to both ❶ increased intake of micronutrients, phytonutrients, and the alkalinizing pro-homeostatic benefits in addition to ❷ avoidance of nutrient-poor high-carbohydrate high-fat foods which are immunosuppressive and pro-inflammatory. Given that the pro-inflammatory effect of high-carbohydrate and/or high-fat foods is mediated at least in part via NFkB, and that NFkB stimulation is important for viral replication, we can easily see how a high-carbohydrate high-fat diet can promote viral replication by enhancing activity of NFkB. High-carbohydrate diets deal a double-punch to the human host; first, consumption of a high-carbohydrate load causes immunosuppression, and then secondly the high-carbohydrate load promotes activation of NFkB which then promotes viral replication. Although raw fruits and vegetables have—by definition and virtue of their "rawness"—not been exposed to the potentially near-sterilizing heat of cooking, the bacterial loads of raw fruit and vegetable consumption do not appear to present a risk to immunosuppressed patients[222,223], even though such patients should not take undue culinary risks. The Mediterranean diet has shown unparalleled safety and efficacy in the prevention of cardiovascular disease, cancer, and all-cause mortality; its specific application in reducing the burden of infectious diseases has not been adequately studied in clinical trials, other than by the indirect inference that a reduction in all-cause mortality by the Mediterranean diet implies a reduction in infection-related mortality. Absence of *direct* evidence is not *direct* evidence of absence. We must also appreciate that diet-and-lifestyle studies are much more complicated to implement than are "pill-based" studies; diet and lifestyle interventions reflect the complexity of human physiology and are thus at odds with the medical model of single-intervention double-blind clinical trials.

- o <u>Standard American diet (SAD) meal causes systemic inflammation (*Am J Clin Nutr* 2004 Apr[224])</u>: Consumption of the standard American diet (SAD) causes oxidative stress, systemic inflammation, and activation of NFkB; clinicians must appreciate that each of these three adverse effects leads to a biochemical milieu that supports the development and perpetuation of infections, particularly viral infections. Subjects in this study consumed an egg-muffin and sausage-muffin sandwiches and 2 hash browns, which contained 81 g carbohydrate, 51 g fat, and 32 g protein "RESULTS: ROS generation by mononuclear cells and polymorphonuclear leukocytes and p47(phox) expression increased significantly. The expression of IKKalpha and IKKbeta and DNA-binding activity of NF-kappaB increased significantly, whereas IkappaBalpha expression decreased. Plasma CRP concentrations increased. The intake of 300 mL water did not induce a change in any of the above indexes. CONCLUSIONS: These data show that the ==intake of a mixed [fast-food] meal results in significant inflammatory changes== characterized by a decrease in IkappaBalpha and an increase in NF-kappaB binding, plasma CRP, and the expression of IKKalpha, IKKbeta, and p47(phox) subunit. These proinflammatory changes are probably relevant to the state of chronic hypertension and obesity and to its association with atherosclerosis." Thus, some of the benefit of the Paleo-Mediterranean diet comes not only from the inherent benefits of the diet itself, but also from the avoidance of the negative effects of the SAD eating pattern that is typical in industrialized nations.

- o <u>Glucose ingestion causes sustained inflammation in healthy human subjects (*Metabolism* 2006 Sep[225])</u>: Subjects in this study received glucose ingestion consistent with normal dietary habits: 300 kcal (75 g) glucose in water (300 mL). Results showed that 300 kcal of glucose causes NFkB activation, systemic

[220] Knoops et al. Mediterranean diet, lifestyle factors, and 10-year mortality in elderly European men and women: the HALE project. *JAMA*. 2004 Sep 22;292(12):1433-9

[221] Cordain L, Eaton SB, Sebastian A, Mann N, Lindeberg S, Watkins BA, O'Keefe JH, Brand-Miller J. Origins and evolution of the Western diet: health implications for the 21st century. *Am J Clin Nutr*. 2005 Feb;81(2):341-54

[222] "No clear evidence exists that the neutropenic diet makes a difference in overall rates of infection." DeMille et al. The effect of the neutropenic diet in the outpatient setting: a pilot study. *Oncol Nurs Forum*. 2006 Nov 3;33(2):337-43

[223] "CONCLUSION: In patients treated in a [protected environment], a neutropenic diet did not prevent major infection or death." Gardner et al. Randomized comparison of cooked and noncooked diets in patients undergoing remission induction therapy for acute myeloid leukemia. *J Clin Oncol*. 2008 Dec 10;26(35):5684-8

[224] Aljada et al. Increase in intranuclear nuclear factor kappaB and decrease in inhibitor kappaB in mononuclear cells after a mixed meal. *Am J Clin Nutr*. 2004 Apr;79(4):682-90

[225] Aljada et al. Glucose ingestion induces an increase in intranuclear nuclear factor kappaB, a fall in cellular inhibitor kappaB, and an increase in tumor necrosis factor alpha messenger RNA by mononuclear cells in healthy human subjects. *Metabolism*. 2006 Sep;55(9):1177-85

inflammation, and increased expression of pro-inflammatory TNF-alpha. Clinicians should appreciate that many of the new drugs for rheumatic diseases specifically target TNF-alpha. "We conclude that glucose intake induces an immediate increase in intranuclear NF-kappaB binding, a fall in IkappaBalpha, an increase in IKKalpha, IKKbeta, IKK activity, and messenger RNA expression of TNF-alpha in MNCs (mononuclear cells) in healthy subjects. These data are consistent with profound acute pro-inflammatory changes in MNCs after glucose intake." When patients overconsume simple carbohydrates several times per day, they are inducing a clinically significant oxidative stress and pro-inflammatory state several times per day that lasts for several hours. Thus, by following the SAD eating pattern and lifestyle, patients unwittingly cause in themselves the oxidative stress and pro-inflammatory milieu that predisposes them toward diseases in general and acute and chronic viral infections in particular; additional details to follow.

o   Acute hyperglycemia adversely impacts the innate immune system (*Crit Care Med.* 2005 Jul[226]): "The most obvious findings related to hyperglycemia included reduced neutrophil activity (e.g., chemotaxis, formation of reactive oxygen species, phagocytosis of bacteria), despite accelerated diapedesis of leukocytes into peripheral tissue, as well as specific alterations of cytokine patterns with increased concentrations of the early proinflammatory cytokines tumor necrosis factor-alpha and interleukin-6. Furthermore, a reduction of endothelial nitric oxide formation takes place, thus decreasing microvascular reactivity to dilating agents such as bradykinin, and complement function (e.g., opsonization, chemotaxis) is impaired, despite elevations of certain complement factors. CONCLUSIONS: Acute, short-term hyperglycemia affects all major components of innate immunity and impairs the ability of the host to combat infection."

o   Mediterranean diet reduces mortality (*JAMA.* 2004 Sep[227]): "Among individuals aged 70 to 90 years, adherence to a Mediterranean diet and healthful lifestyle is associated with a more than 50% lower rate of all-causes and cause-specific mortality." The Mediterranean diet has shown safety and efficacy in protection against cardiovascular disease, cancer, and all-cause mortality; its specific application in reducing the burden of infectious diseases has not been adequately studied in clinical trials, other than by the indirect inference that a reduction in all-cause mortality by the Mediterranean diet implies a reduction in infection-related mortality.

o   Infection-induced increased metabolic demands require heightened nutritional density via whole (Paleo) foods (*J Am Diet Assoc.* 2004 Jul[228]): "HIV-infected youths may have increased micronutrient needs related to impaired immune function and metabolic complications of the disease. Dietitians and health care professionals should focus on setting individualized behavioral goals with HIV-infected youths, emphasizing foods rich in micronutrients early in the infection."

o   Food influences systemic inflammation in adolescents (*J Am Diet Assoc.* 2009 Mar[229]): In this study, serologic markers of inflammation and oxidative stress were correlated with dietary intake. Urinary F(2)-isoprostane (a combined marker for inflammation, oxidative stress, and arachidonate intake), interleukin-6 (IL-6), tumor necrosis factor-alpha (TNF), and C-reactive protein (CRP) were inversely correlated with intakes of total fruit and vegetables, legumes, vitamin C, beta carotene, luteolin, folate, and flavonoids; in other words, the lower the intake of fruits and phytonutrients, the higher the level of isoprostane, CRP, TNF, and IL-6.

o   Fruit and vegetable intake reduces incidence of upper respiratory tract infection (URTI) in pregnant women (*Public Health Nutr.* 2009 Jun[230]): Subjects were asked retrospectively about their fruit/vegetable intake during the six months before the pregnancy and their occurrences of URTI during the first half of pregnancy "CONCLUSIONS: Women who consume more fruits and vegetables have a moderate reduction in risk of URTI during pregnancy, and this benefit appears to be derived from both fruits and vegetables instead of either alone."

[226] Turina et al. Acute hyperglycemia and the innate immune system: clinical, cellular, and molecular aspects. *Crit Care Med.* 2005;33(7):1624-33
[227] Knoops et al. Mediterranean diet, lifestyle factors, and 10-year mortality in elderly European men and women: the HALE project. *JAMA.* 2004 Sep 22;292(12):1433-9
[228] Kruzich et al. US youths in the early stages of HIV disease have low intakes of some micronutrients important for optimal immune function. *J Am Diet Assoc.* 2004 Jul;104(7):1095-101
[229] Holt et al. Fruit and vegetable consumption and its relation to markers of inflammation and oxidative stress in adolescents. *J Am Diet Assoc.* 2009 Mar;109(3):414-21
[230] Li L, Werler MM. Fruit and vegetable intake and risk of upper respiratory tract infection in pregnant women. *Public Health Nutr.* 2009 Jun 25:1-7

- o Double-blinded placebo-controlled clinical trial: Regulatory effects of a fermented food concentrate on immune function parameters in healthy volunteers (*Nutrition* 2009 May[231]): This study sought to assess the influence of a "cascade-fermented food consisting of fruits, nuts, and vegetables rich in polyphenols (Regulat)" twice daily for 4 weeks on the immune system in healthy volunteers: 48 healthy men 20-48 y of age with regular low to moderate intake of fruit and vegetables. "The intake of Regulat significantly enhanced intracellular glutathione content in lymphocytes, monocytes, and natural killer cells. Furthermore, activation of natural killer cell cytotoxicity in response to interleukin-2 stimulation...were found in the Regulat but not in the placebo group." Other biochemical benefits included reductions of the following: total lipid peroxidation, soluble vascular cell adhesion molecule-1, soluble intercellular adhesion molecule-1—each of these serve as blood markers for inflammation. Regulat is produced under patent by a "cascade fermentation process" and is made mainly from fruits, vegetables, and nuts (lemons, dates, figs, walnuts, soy beans, coconuts, onions, sprouts, celery, artichokes, millet, peas, spices, saffron). This mixture is fermented over several weeks in various steps with the aid of five different strains of *Lactobacilli* probiotics. In the final product, no viable *Lactobacilli* are present.

- **Multivitamin/multimineral supplementation**: As would be expected, clinical trials of multivitamin supplementation are impressively heterogeneous. In some studies, "multivitamin" is used to describe supplementation with only a handful of vitamins (this should be called *oligo*vitamin supplementation rather than *multi*vitamin supplementation), often in doses so low that they hardly would seem worthwhile to any practitioner of integrative/functional nutrition. In other studies, "multivitamin" does indeed include a broader spectrum of nutrients, but often these are in poor form, for example, cyanocobalamin rather than hydroxy-/methyl-/adenosyl-cobalamin, ergocalciferol rather than cholecalciferol, and pyridoxine HCl rather than pyridoxal-5-phosphate. In essentially 100% of these studies, no consideration is given to nutrients such as magnesium, nor to phytonutrients, nor to the critically important effects of whole-foods nutrition such as urinary/systemic alkalinization to overcome the acidogenic effect of the Western diet which causes mild diet-induced chronic metabolic acidosis.[232] Historically, most nutrients have been considered largely from the perspective of correcting deficiencies or generally supporting the immune system to combat microbes; these days, our understanding is much more sophisticated, emphasizing nutrients to retard viral replication via suppression of inflammatory transcription factors (e.g., selenium and lipoic acid) and viral DNA transcription (folinic acid and methylfolate).

  - o General rationale for routine nutritional supplementation #1—Vitamins for chronic disease prevention in adults (*JAMA* 2002 Jun[233]): "However, suboptimal intake of some vitamins, above levels causing classic vitamin deficiency, is a risk factor for chronic diseases and common in the general population, especially the elderly. ...low levels of the antioxidant vitamins (vitamins A, E, and C) may increase risk for several chronic diseases. Most people do not consume an optimal amount of all vitamins by diet alone. Pending strong evidence of effectiveness from randomized trials, it appears prudent for all adults to take vitamin supplements. ... Physicians should make specific efforts to learn about their patients' use of vitamins to ensure that they are taking vitamins they should...."
    - http://jama.jamanetwork.com/article.aspx?articleid=195039
    - http://www.ncbi.nlm.nih.gov/pubmed/12069676
  - o General rationale for routine nutritional supplementation #2—Prevention of long-latency deficiency disease: insights from calcium and vitamin D (*Am J Clin Nutr* 2003 Nov[234]): "Nutrient intake recommendations and national nutritional policies have focused primarily on prevention of short-latency deficiency diseases. Most nutrient intake recommendations today are based on prevention of the index disease only. However, inadequate intakes of many nutrients are now recognized as contributing to several of the major chronic diseases that affect the populations of the industrialized nations. Often taking many years to manifest themselves, these disease outcomes should be thought of as long-latency deficiency diseases."

---

[231] Schoen et al. Regulatory effects of a fermented food concentrate on immune function parameters in healthy volunteers. *Nutrition*. 2009 May;25(5):499-505
[232] Cordain et al. Origins and evolution of the Western diet: health implications for the 21st century. *Am J Clin Nutr*. 2005 Feb;81(2):341-54
[233] Fletcher RH, Fairfield KM. Vitamins for chronic disease prevention in adults: clinical applications. *JAMA*. 2002 Jun 19;287(23):3127-9
[234] Heaney RP. Long-latency deficiency disease: insights from calcium and vitamin D. *Am J Clin Nutr*. 2003 Nov;78(5):912-9

- o General rationale for routine nutritional supplementation #3—Promotion of optimal metabolism in lieu of the expense and unavailability of extensive laboratory testing for each patient (*Am J Clin Nutr* 2002 Apr[235]): "As many as one-third of mutations in a gene result in the corresponding enzyme having an increased Michaelis constant, or K(m), (decreased binding affinity) for a coenzyme, resulting in a lower rate of reaction. About 50 human genetic dis-eases due to defective enzymes can be remedied or ameliorated by the administration of high doses of the vitamin component of the corresponding coenzyme, which at least partially restores enzymatic activity. Several single-nucleotide polymorphisms, in which the variant amino acid reduces coenzyme binding and thus enzymatic activity, are likely to be remediable by raising cellular concentrations of the cofactor through high-dose vitamin therapy."
  - http://www.ncbi.nlm.nih.gov/pubmed/11916749
  - http://ajcn.nutrition.org/content/75/4/616.long
- o General rationale for routine nutritional supplementation #4—Vitamin D deficiency is the most common and most clinically significant nutrient deficiency seen regularly in the practice of primary care medicine (*Altern Ther Health Med* 2004 Sep[236]): Beyond vitamin and mineral supplementation in general is the clinicians' need to focus on vitamin D3 supplementation, especially given that most multivitamin formulations do not meet the physiologic requirement in adults of approximately 4,000 IU/d; per my 2004 "paradigm shift with implications for all healthcare providers" all readers should know that vitamin D deficiency causes—in large percentages of patients per diagnosis—hypertension, migraine headaches, widespread body pain identical to fibromyalgia, local pain consistent with low-back pain, insulin resistance, systemic inflammation and autoimmunity.
  - http://www.ncbi.nlm.nih.gov/pubmed/15478784
  - http://inflammationmastery.com/D3/vasquez_2004_vitamindmonograph-athm.pdf
  - http://inflammationmastery.com/D3/vasquez_2005_bmj_letter.pdf
  - http://inflammationmastery.com/D3/vasquez_2005_lancet_letter_website.pdf
  - http://inflammationmastery.com/D3/vasquez_2011_five-part_protocol_revisited.pdf
- o Review: Selected vitamins and trace elements support immune function by strengthening epithelial barriers and cellular and humoral immune responses (*Br J Nutr* 2007 Oct[237]): The abstract from the review published in 2007 by Maggini, Wintergerst, Beveridge, and Hornig is so succinct and clear that I feel compelled to quote it here in its entirety for the benefit of clinicians and our worldwide audience of patients in order to give appropriate credit to those authors for their skill in distilling massive amounts of information into a comprehensible summary of the effect of nutrients in immune function. Readers are encouraged to obtain the full text of the article from the publisher's website for free per the links that follow: "Adequate intakes of micronutrients are required for the immune system to function efficiently. Micronutrient deficiency suppresses immunity by affecting innate, T cell mediated and adaptive antibody responses, leading to dysregulation of the balanced host response. This situation increases susceptibility to infections, with increased morbidity and mortality. In turn, infections aggravate micronutrient deficiencies by reducing nutrient intake, increasing losses, and interfering with utilization by altering metabolic pathways. …Micronutrients contribute to the body's natural defenses on three levels by supporting physical barriers (skin/mucosa), cellular immunity and antibody production. Vitamins A, C, E and the trace element zinc assist in enhancing the skin barrier function. The vitamins A, B6, B12, C, D, E and folic acid and the trace elements iron, zinc, copper and selenium **work in synergy to support the protective activities of the immune cells.** …Overall, inadequate intake and status of these vitamins and trace elements may lead to suppressed immunity, which predisposes to infections and aggravates malnutrition. Therefore, supplementation with these selected micronutrients can support the body's natural defense system by enhancing all three levels of immunity."
  - http://www.ncbi.nlm.nih.gov/pubmed/17922955
  - http://journals.cambridge.org/action/displayAbstract?fromPage=online&aid=1364128&fileId=S0007114507832971

---

[235] Ames BN, et al. High-dose vitamin therapy stimulates variant enzymes with decreased coenzyme binding affinity (increased Km). *Am J Clin Nutr* 2002 Apr;75:616-58
[236] Vasquez A, Manso G, Cannell J. The clinical importance of vitamin D (cholecalciferol): a paradigm shift. *Altern Ther Health Med.* 2004 Sep-Oct;10(5):28-36
[237] Maggini et al. Selected vitamins and trace elements support immune function by strengthening epithelial barriers and cellular and humoral immune responses. *Br J Nutr.* 2007 Oct;98 Suppl 1:S29-35

- o Clinical trial: Effect of a multivitamin and mineral supplement on infection and quality of life. A randomized, double-blind, placebo-controlled trial (*Ann Intern Med* 2003 Mar[238]): "A multivitamin and mineral supplement reduced the incidence of participant-reported infection and related absenteeism in a sample of participants with type 2 diabetes mellitus and a high prevalence of subclinical micronutrient deficiency."
- o Review: Contribution of selected vitamins and trace elements to immune function (*Ann Nutr Metab* 2007 Sep[239]): "Adequate intake of vitamins B(6), folate, B(12), C, E, and of selenium, zinc, copper, and iron supports a Th-1 cytokine-mediated immune response with sufficient production of proinflammatory cytokines, which maintains an effective immune response and avoids a shift to an anti-inflammatory Th2 cell-mediated immune response and an increased risk of extracellular infections."
- o Review: Nutritional strategies to boost immunity and prevent infection in elderly individuals (*Clin Infect Dis* 2001 Dec[240]): "Nutritional supplementation strategies can reduce this risk and reverse some of the immune dysfunction associated with advanced age. ... The data support use of a daily multivitamin or trace-mineral supplement that includes zinc (elemental zinc, >20 mg/day) and selenium (100 microg/day), with additional vitamin E, to achieve a daily dosage of 200 mg/day."
- o Clinical trial: Nutritional supplements [cod liver oil and a children's multivitamin-mineral with selenium] as adjunctive therapy for children with chronic/recurrent sinusitis: pilot research (*Int J Pediatr Otorhinolaryngol.* 2004 Jun[241]): "Four, six, and eight weeks after beginning study supplements, the responders had decreased sinus symptoms, fewer episodes of acute sinusitis, and fewer doctor visits for acute illnesses. Their parents reported that they had begun to recover from upper respiratory illnesses without complications, which was unusual for these children..."
- o Clinical trial: Lemon-flavored cod liver oil and a multivitamin-mineral supplement for the secondary prevention of otitis media in young children (*Ann Otol Rhinol Laryngol.* 2002 Jul[242]): "...8 children received 1 teaspoon of lemon-flavored cod liver oil (containing both EPA and vitamin A) and 1 half-tablet of a selenium-containing children's chewable multivitamin-mineral tablet per day. During this OM season, study subjects received antibiotics for OM for 12.3% fewer days during supplementation than before supplementation."
- o Clinical trial: Effect of daily cod liver oil and a multivitamin-mineral supplement with selenium on upper respiratory tract pediatric visits by young, inner-city, Latino children (*Ann Otol Rhinol Laryngol.* 2004 Nov[243]): "The supplementation group had a statistically significant decrease in the mean number of upper respiratory tract [infection] visits over time... Use of these nutritional supplements was acceptable to the inner-city Latino families and their young children, and was associated with a decrease in upper respiratory tract [infection] pediatric visits over time...."
- o Clinical trial: A randomized trial of multivitamin supplements and HIV disease progression and mortality (*N Engl J Med.* 2004 Jul[244]): "Multivitamins also resulted in significantly higher CD4+ and CD8+ cell counts and significantly lower viral loads. ... Multivitamin supplements delay the progression of HIV disease and provide an effective, low-cost means of delaying the initiation of antiretroviral therapy in HIV-infected women."
- o Review: Effects of antioxidant and non-antioxidant vitamin supplementation on immune function (*Nutr Rev.* 2007 May[245]): "There is evidence to support causal effects of supplementation with vitamins E and C and the carotenoids singly and in combination on selected aspects of immunity, including the functional capacity of innate immune cells, lymphocyte proliferation, and the delayed-type hypersensitivity (DTH) response. Controlled intervention trials of B vitamin-containing multivitamin supplements suggest beneficial effects on immune parameters and clinical outcomes in HIV-positive individuals."

[238] Barringer et al. Effect of a multivitamin and mineral supplement on infection and quality of life. *Ann Intern Med.* 2003 Mar 4;138(5):365-71

[239] Wintergerst et al. Contribution of selected vitamins and trace elements to immune function. *Ann Nutr Metab.* 2007;51(4):301-23

[240] High KP. Nutritional strategies to boost immunity and prevent infection in elderly individuals. *Clin Infect Dis.* 2001 Dec 1;33(11):1892-900

[241] Linday et al. Nutritional supplements as adjunctive therapy for children with chronic/recurrent sinusitis: pilot research. *Int J Pediatr Otorhinolaryngol.* 2004 Jun;68(6):785-93

[242] Linday et al. Lemon-flavored cod liver oil and a multivitamin-mineral supplement for secondary prevention of otitis media in young children. *Ann Otol Rhinol Laryngol.* 2002 Jul;111(7 Pt 1):642-52

[243] Linday et al. Effect of daily cod liver oil and a multivitamin-mineral supplement with selenium on upper respiratory tract pediatric visits by young, inner-city, Latino children: randomized pediatric sites. *Ann Otol Rhinol Laryngol.* 2004 Nov;113(11):891-901

[244] Fawzi et al. A randomized trial of multivitamin supplements and HIV disease progression and mortality. *N Engl J Med.* 2004 Jul 1;351(1):23-32

[245] Webb AL, Villamor E. Update: effects of antioxidant and non-antioxidant vitamin supplementation on immune function. *Nutr Rev.* 2007 May;65(5):181-217

o <u>Clinical trial: Effects of maternal vitamin supplements on malaria in children born to HIV-infected women</u> (*Am J Trop Med Hyg.* 2007 Jun[246]): "Compared with placebo, multivitamins excluding VA/BC [vitamin A / beta-carotene] reduced the incidence of clinical malaria by 71% (95% CI = 11-91%; P = 0.02), whereas VA/BC alone resulted in a nonsignificant 63% reduction (95% CI = -4% to 87%; P = 0.06). Multivitamins including VA/BC significantly reduced the incidence of high parasitemia by 43%."

o <u>Clinical trial: Multivitamin supplementation improves hematologic status in HIV-infected women and their children in Tanzania</u> (*Am J Clin Nutr.* 2007 May[247]): "Multivitamin supplementation provided during pregnancy and in the postpartum period resulted in significant improvements in hematologic status among HIV-infected women and their children, which provides further support for the value of multivitamin supplementation in HIV-infected adults."

o <u>Randomized controlled trial: Multivitamin supplementation (vitamins B, C, and E) in HIV-positive pregnant women: impact on depression and quality of life in a resource-poor setting</u> (*HIV Med.* 2007 May[248]): "Multivitamin supplementation (B-complex, C and E) resulted in a reduction in risk of elevated depressive symptoms comparable to MDD [major depressive disorder] and improvement in quality of life in HIV-positive pregnant women in Tanzania." This article reminds us of two important clinical considerations: 1) that the negative effects of any illness extend beyond the illness/infection itself—in this case to include depression, and 2) that nutritional supplementation can help correct the biochemical imbalances that contribute to the psychosocial experience and clinical manifestations of depression. Clinicians would be wise to consider nutritional deficiencies in their depressed patients before jumping to the conclusion that the patient has a Prozac deficiency or insufficiency of electroconvulsive shocks, now again increasingly used in the "medical" management of mental depression, especially among older patients[249]—that is, among patients most likely to have the nutritional deficiencies known to cause depression.[250]

o <u>Review: Effects of vitamins, including vitamin A, on HIV/AIDS patients</u> (*Vitam Horm.* 2007[251]): "Further, multivitamin supplementation reduces the rate of HIV disease progression among patients in early stage of disease, thus delaying the need for ART [antiretroviral treatment] by prolonging the pre-ART stage. In brief, there is no evidence to recommend vitamin A supplementation of HIV-infected pregnant women; however, periodic vitamin A supplementation of HIV-infected infants and children is beneficial in reducing all-cause mortality and morbidity and is recommended. Similarly, multivitamin supplementation of people infected with HIV, particularly pregnant women, is strongly suggested."

o <u>Prospective randomized, placebo-controlled trial of intravenous copper, selenium, and zinc in burn patients: Trace element supplementation after major burns modulates antioxidant status and clinical course by way of increased tissue trace element concentrations</u> (*Am J Clin Nutr.* 2007 May[252]): Due to increased metabolic needs compounded by fluid losses through skin and secondary to hyperhydration, trace element (TE) deficiencies are common in multi-trauma and burn patients. This study used "large, intravenous doses of TE supplements" containing copper, selenium, and zinc. "The number of infections in the first 30 d was significantly lower in the TE group, with a median number of 2 versus 4 infections per patient in the TE and V groups, respectively, as a result of a reduction in pulmonary infections."

- **Probiotics**: Generally speaking, probiotics are beneficial bacteria which colonize the human gastrointestinal tract; related terms are prebiotics (nutritional substrate such as inulin and fructooligosaccharides [FOS]

---

[246] Villamor et al. Effects of maternal vitamin supplements on malaria in children born to HIV-infected women. *Am J Trop Med Hyg.* 2007 Jun;76(6):1066-71

[247] Fawzi et al. Multivitamin supplementation improves hematologic status in HIV-infected women and their children in Tanzania. *Am J Clin Nutr.* 2007 May;85(5):1335-43

[248] Smith Fawzi et al. Multivitamin supplementation in HIV-positive pregnant women: impact on depression and quality of life in a resource-poor setting. *HIV Med.* 2007 May;8(4):203-12

[249] "Electroconvulsive therapy (ECT) is used increasingly in the older adult population for major depression, particularly when depression is not responsive to medications, when antidepressants are not tolerated due to side effects, ..." Kelly et al. Update on electroconvulsive therapy (ECT) in older adults. *J Am Geriatr Soc.* 2000 May;48(5):560-6

[250] "A low serum vitamin B-12 concentration was found in 6% and 5%, low folate in 5% and 19%, and low vitamin B-6 in 9% and 51%, and one or more metabolites were elevated in 63% and 83% of healthy elderly subjects and elderly hospitalized patients, respectively. These results strongly suggest that the prevalence of tissue deficiencies of vitamin B-12, folate, and vitamin B-6 as demonstrated by the elevated metabolite concentrations is substantially higher than that estimated by measuring concentrations of the vitamins." Joosten et al. Metabolic evidence that deficiencies of vitamin B-12 (cobalamin), folate, and vitamin B-6 occur commonly in elderly people. *Am J Clin Nutr.* 1993 Oct;58(4):468-76

[251] Mehta S, Fawzi W. Effects of vitamins, including vitamin A, on HIV/AIDS patients. *Vitam Horm.* 2007;75:355-83

[252] Berger et al. Trace element supplementation after major burns modulates antioxidant status and clinical course by way of increased tissue trace element concentrations. *Am J Clin Nutr.* 2007 May;85(5):1293-300

consumed with the intention of promoting and supporting the intestinal growth of probiotics or endogenous beneficial bacteria) whereas synbiotics are combinations of probiotics and prebiotics.

- o Systematic review: Probiotics for the prevention of respiratory tract infections (*Int J Antimicrob Agents.* 2009 Sep[253]): In this systematic review, Vouloumanou et a evaluated the clinical evidence regarding probiotic use for the prevention of respiratory tract infections (RTIs) which ultimately included fourteen randomized controlled trials (RCTs). These studies used various Lactobacillus strains (7 studies), combinations of *Lactobacillus* and *Bifidobacterium* strains (5 studies), and a *Bifidobacterium* strain and a non-pathogenic *Enterococcus faecalis* strain (1 study). While the incidence of RTIs was often not affected (10 studies showed no difference; 4 studies showed reduced frequency of viral RTIs), the severity of the infections was shown to be reduced in 5 of 6 studies. Regarding duration, 3 studies showed a reduction in sick time, while 6 studies reported no difference. The authors wrote, "In conclusion, probiotics may have a beneficial effect on the severity and duration of symptoms of RTIs but do not appear to reduce the incidence of RTIs."

- o Clinical trial: Dietary supplementation of probiotic *Bacillus polyfermenticus*, Bispan strain, modulates natural killer cell and T cell subset populations and immunoglobulin G levels in human subjects (*J Med Food.* 2006 Fall[254]): This study used the probiotic *Bacillus polyfermenticus* in twenty-five male subjects, 20-35 years of age, randomly assigned to placebo control or *B. polyfermenticus* tablets at a dose of 3.1 x 10(8) colony-forming units/day for 8 weeks. Results: "The concentration of IgG in the experimental group was 12% higher than in the placebo group after 8 weeks of Bispan supplementation. Also, the percentages of CD4+ helper T cells, CD8+ cytotoxic T cells, and CD56+ NK cells in the Bispan strain-supplemented group were 32%, 28%, and 35% higher, respectively, compared with the control group. Because of a higher increment of the CD4+ T cell subset than CD8+ T cells, the ratio of CD4+/CD8+ T cells was greater in the experimental group. This study suggests that the supplementation of *B. polyfermenticus* has a potentially positive effect on immune function by enhancing IgG production as well as by modulating the number of immune cell population such as CD4+ and CD8+ T cells and NK cells."

- o Randomized, double-blind, placebo-controlled clinical trial: Effect of a dietary supplement containing probiotic bacteria plus vitamins and minerals on common cold infections and cellular immune parameters (*Int J Clin Pharmacol Ther.* 2005 Jul[255]): This very large study included 477 healthy men and women (aged 36 +/- 13 years) who had not been vaccinated against influenza; subjects were randomly assigned to daily probiotic/multivitamin/mineral supplement or a placebo, for up to 5.5 months. "RESULTS: The incidence of respiratory tract infections regarded as being virally induced was 13.6% lower in the probiotic/multivitamin/mineral supplement group compared to the placebo group." All symptoms of common cold and influenza-like infection were lower in the probiotic/multivitamin/mineral supplement group. Total symptom score was reduced by 19%, influenza symptoms by 25%, number of days with fever by 54%. Illness duration was not affected. Patients receiving the daily probiotic/multivitamin/mineral supplement showed significantly higher levels of leukocytes, lymphocytes, and in particular T-lymphocytes including CD4+ and CD8+ cells, as well as monocytes during the first 14 days of supplementation compared to placebo.

- o In vitro (cell culture) study: Probiotic *Leuconostoc mesenteroides* ssp. *cremoris* and *Streptococcus thermophilus* induce IL-12 and IFN-γ production (*World J Gastroenterol.* 2008 Feb[256]): The authors of this study observed responses of human immunocytes in culture following response to probiotic bacteria; their results

---

[253] Vouloumanou et al. Probiotics for the prevention of respiratory tract infections: a systematic review. *Int J Antimicrob Agents.* 2009 Sep;34(3):197.e1-10

[254] Kim et al. Dietary supplementation of probiotic Bacillus polyfermenticus, Bispan strain, modulates natural killer cell and T cell subset populations and immunoglobulin G levels in human subjects. *J Med Food.* 2006 Fall;9(3):321-7

[255] Winkler et al. Effect of a dietary supplement containing probiotic bacteria plus vitamins and minerals on common cold infections and cellular immune parameters. *Int J Clin Pharmacol Ther.* 2005 Jul;43(7):318-26

[256] Kekkonen et al. Probiotic Leuconostoc mesenteroides ssp. cremoris and Streptococcus thermophilus induce IL-12 and IFN-gamma production. *World J Gastroenterol.* 2008 Feb 28;14(8):1192-203

showed increased production of anti-inflammatory IL-12 and antiviral IFN-γ (gamma-interferon). The authors note that the increased production of IL-12 and IFN-γ is consistent with the TH1 response, which is important for anti-viral immunity. They write, "...novel probiotic *S. thermophilus* and *Leuconostoc* strains were extremely good inducers of these Th1 type cytokines. ... A strong Th1 type cytokine response is also an important factor in the fight against viral infections such as that caused by influenza A virus."

- o Randomized clinical trial: Synbiotics, prebiotics, glutamine, or peptide in early enteral nutrition: a randomized study in trauma patients (*JPEN*. 2007 Mar[257]): One hundred thirteen multiple injured patients were prospectively randomized into 4 groups: group A, glutamine; B, fermentable fiber; C, peptide diet; and D, standard enteral formula with fibers combined with Synbiotic 2000 (Synbiotic 2000 Forte; Medifarm, Sweden), a formula containing live lactobacilli and specific bioactive fibers. Intestinal permeability was evaluated by measuring lactulose-mannitol excretion ratio on days 2, 4, and 7. Results showed no differences in days of mechanical ventilation, duration of intensive care unit stay, or multiple-organ failure scores. Researchers documented a total of 51 infections with 38 pneumonias; of these, only 5 infections and 4 pneumonias occurred in group D, which was significantly less than the infections and pneumonias in groups A, B, and C. Intestinal permeability decreased only in group D, from 0.148 on day 4 to 0.061 on day 7 whereas in group A, the lactulose-mannitol excretion ratio increased significantly from 0.050 on day 2 to 0.159 on day 7. Clearly and appropriately, the authors of this study concluded, "Patients supplemented with synbiotics did better than the others, with lower intestinal permeability and fewer infections."

- o Clinical trial: Daily ingestion of fermented milk containing *Lactobacillus casei* DN114001 improves innate-defense capacity in healthy middle-aged people (*J Physiol Biochem*. 2004 Jun[258]): "...the probiotic-treated group increased oxidative burst capacity of monocytes, as well as NK cells tumoricidal activity. Results showed that daily intake of fermented milk containing *Lactobacillus casei* DN114001 could have a positive effect in modulating the innate immune defense in healthy-middle-age people."

- **Physical medicine: spinal manipulation, mobilization, massage, exercise:**
  - o Physical exercise: Susceptibility to infections in elite athletes: Generally speaking, the compilation of most research on this subject has shown that lack of exercise increases the risk of infection, while moderate exercise reduces the risk of infection, and extreme athleticism again increases the risk of infection. Moderate exercise reduces the risk of infection by modulating the immune system, reducing superfluous systemic inflammation, and promoting lymphatic flow (animal study[259]), which is critical for immune function. Malm[260] summarized the generally-held view of the relationship between exercise and immunity/infection by writing, "The susceptibility to upper respiratory tract infections (URTIs) after physical exercise has been described with a J-shaped curve, suggesting protection from infections with moderate exercise and increased risk for URTI's in elite athletes." The increase in infections following extreme exercise such as marathon running appears related to the oxidative stress, hormonal activation (e.g., cortisol), and nutrient/antioxidant depletion rather than due to the exercise itself insofar as nutritional supplementation with immunosupportive nutrients such as ascorbate and glutamine can reduce the incidence and severity of such post-exertional infections. In this context, *elite athleticism* describes marathon runners, competitive triathletes, and athletes with extreme training regimens, particularly when combined with dietary restriction, such as bodybuilders under severe caloric limitations before competition; this distinction is necessary because many Westerners have been erroneously convinced that walking around the

> **Musculoskeletal manipulation vs AOM**
>
> "CONCLUSIONS: The results of this study suggest a potential benefit of **osteopathic manipulative treatment as adjuvant therapy in children with recurrent AOM; it may prevent or decrease surgical intervention or antibiotic overuse.**"
>
> Mills et al. The use of osteopathic manipulative treatment as adjuvant therapy in children with recurrent acute otitis media. *Arch Pediatr Adolesc Med*. 2003 Sep;157(9):861-6

[257] Spindler-Vesel et al. Synbiotics, prebiotics, glutamine, or peptide in early enteral nutrition: a randomized study in trauma patients. *JPEN*. 2007 Mar-Apr;31(2):119-26
[258] Parra et al. Daily ingestion of fermented milk containing Lactobacillus casei DN114001 improves innate-defense capacity in healthy middle-aged people. *J Physiol Biochem*. 2004 Jun;60(2):85-91
[259] Knott EM, Tune JD, Stoll ST, Downey HF. Increased lymphatic flow in the thoracic duct during manipulative intervention. *J Am Osteopath Assoc*. 2005 Oct;105(10):447-56
[260] Malm C. Susceptibility to infections in elite athletes: the S-curve. *Scand J Med Sci Sports*. 2006 Feb;16(1):4-6

block after dinner is exercise, and that by extension, "working out" to the point that actually causes perspiration is a rather extreme form of exercise, which is generally to be followed by supplementation with Häagen-Dazs or other confectionery. More accurately, knowledgeable clinicians should re-educate patients to appreciate that walking is a form of *activity*, and that activity does not equate to exercise. *Activity* simply means moving the body, while *exercise* means moving the body either quickly or against resistance for sufficient duration and intensity as to result in diaphoresis and significant physiological adaptations; *athleticism* defines a sufficient frequency-intensity of exercise such that one is approaching optimal fitness, marked by excellent cardiovascular fitness (e.g., at least the ability to run 6 miles within an hour) and low body fat

Osteopathic manipulation vs pneumonia
The seven treatment techniques in the standardized portion of the protocol are:
1. Bilateral paraspinal inhibition
2. Bilateral rib raising
3. Diaphragmatic myofascial release ("redoming the diaphragm")
4. Condylar decompression
5. Soft tissue technique to the cervical muscles
6. Myofascial release to the anterior thoracic inlet
7. The thoracic lymphatic pump.
Noll et al. Benefits of osteopathic manipulative treatment for hospitalized elderly patients with pneumonia. *J Am Osteopath Assoc.* 2000 Dec:776-82

percentage (bf%) (e.g., "optimal fitness" defined as 12-18 bf% for men and 16-25 bf% for women[261]). Per the study by Farrell et al[262], men with body fat percentage <17.5% have the lowest cancer mortality compared to men with higher body fat percentage. Several recent articles support the contention that greater cardiopulmonary/aerobic fitness[263,264,265] and greater muscular strength[266,267] are more important than obesity/adiposity/BMI for reducing all-cause mortality.

o Spinal manipulation and myofascial treatments (chiropractic and/or osteopathic): Studies show clinical benefit for patients treated with spinal/myofascial manipulation on the clinical outcomes in pneumonia and acute otitis media; minor adverse effects are outweighed by the benefits of manual treatments.[268,269]

o Osteopathic manipulative treatment for adult pneumonia—results of a pilot study: "To evaluate the benefit of osteopathic manipulative treatment in the elderly with pneumonia, the authors recruited 21 individuals older than 60 years who were hospitalized with acute pneumonia. ... Osteopathic manipulative treatment may reduce antibiotic use and length of stay; however, a larger study is needed to clarify this outcome."[270]

o Osteopathic manipulative treatment for adult pneumonia—results of a randomized trial: "Elderly patients hospitalized with acute pneumonia were recruited and randomly placed into two groups: 28 in the treatment group and 30 in the control group. The treatment group received a standardized OMT protocol, while the control group received a light touch protocol. There was no statistical difference between groups for age, sex, or simplified acute physiology scores. The treatment group had a significantly shorter duration of intravenous antibiotic treatment and a shorter hospital stay."[271]

---

[261] Data from Kravitz L, Heyward VH. Getting a Grip on Body Composition. http://www.unm.edu/~lkravitz/Article%20folder/underbodycomp.html Accessed July 17, 2009. Attributed to Wilmore JH, Buskirk ER, DiGirolamo M, Lohman TG. Body Composition: A round table. *The Physician and Sportsmedicine* 1986:14(3):144-162

[262] "When grouped into categories of fit and unfit (upper 80% and lower 20% of CRF distribution, respectively), mortality rates (per 10,000 man-years) were significantly lower in fit compared with unfit men within each stratum of BMI, WC, and percent body fat. DISCUSSION: Higher levels of CRF are associated with lower cancer mortality risk in men, independently of several adiposity measures." Farrell SW, Cortese GM, LaMonte MJ, Blair SN. Cardiorespiratory fitness, different measures of adiposity, and cancer mortality in men. *Obesity* (Silver Spring). 2007 Dec;15(12):3140-9

[263] "...our data show that fit men had greater longevity than unfit men regardless of their body composition or risk factor status." Lee CD, Blair SN, Jackson AS. Cardiorespiratory fitness, body composition, and all-cause and cardiovascular disease mortality in men. *Am J Clin Nutr.* 1999 Mar;69(3):373-80

[264] "Although BMI did not prove to be an independent risk factor for mortality from CVD, CHD or from all causes combined, perceived physical fitness and functional capability did. An increase in [leisure time physical activity] seems to have a similar beneficial effect on the mortality risk of obese and nonobese men and women, and the effect also seems to be similar for fit and unfit subjects." Haapanen-Niemi et al. Body mass index, physical inactivity and low level of physical fitness as determinants of all-cause and cardiovascular disease mortality--16 y follow-up of middle-aged and elderly men and women. *Int J Obes Relat Metab Disord.* 2000 Nov;24(11):1465-74

[265] "Accumulating evidence suggests that higher physical activity or fitness attenuates the health risks of obesity." LaMonte MJ, Blair SN. Physical activity, cardiorespiratory fitness, and adiposity: contributions to disease risk. *Curr Opin Clin Nutr Metab Care.* 2006 Sep;9(5):540-6

[266] "CONCLUSIONS: Higher levels of muscular strength are associated with lower cancer mortality risk in men, independent of clinically established measures of overall and central adiposity, and other potential confounders." Ruiz et al. Muscular strength and adiposity as predictors of adulthood cancer mortality in men. *Cancer Epidemiol Biomarkers Prev.* 2009 May;18(5):1468-76

[267] "CONCLUSION: Muscular strength is inversely and independently associated with death from all causes and cancer in men, even after adjusting for cardiorespiratory fitness and other potential confounders." Ruiz et al. Association between muscular strength and mortality in men: prospective cohort study. *BMJ.* 2008 Jul 1;337

[268] "Evidence was promising for potential benefit of manual procedures for children with otitis media and elderly patients with pneumonia." Hawk et al. Chiropractic care for nonmusculoskeletal conditions: a systematic review with implications for whole systems research. *J Altern Complement Med.* 2007 Jun;13(5):491-512

[269] "CONCLUSIONS: The results of this study suggest a potential benefit of osteopathic manipulative treatment as adjuvant therapy in children with recurrent AOM; it may prevent or decrease surgical intervention or antibiotic overuse." Mills et al. The use of osteopathic manipulative treatment as adjuvant therapy in children with recurrent acute otitis media. *Arch Pediatr Adolesc Med.* 2003 Sep;157(9):861-6

[270] Noll et al. Adjunctive osteopathic manipulative treatment in the elderly hospitalized with pneumonia: a pilot study. *J Am Osteopath Assoc.* 1999 Mar;99(3):143-6, 151-2

[271] Noll et al. Benefits of osteopathic manipulative treatment for hospitalized elderly patients with pneumonia. *J Am Osteopath Assoc.* 2000 Dec;100(12):776-82

o <u>Chiropractic spinal manipulation increases phagocytic cell respiratory burst</u>: <mark>"The CL [chemiluminescence] responses of both PMN and monocytes from subjects who received spinal manipulation were significantly higher after than before treatment</mark>, and significantly higher than the response in sham or soft-tissue treated subjects. Measurement of the force applied by sham and spinal manipulation suggested a force threshold for the enhancement of the CL response."[272] <mark>"The response of polymorphonuclear neutrophils isolated from blood collected 15 min after manipulation was significantly higher than the response of cells isolated from blood collected 15 min before and 30 and 45 min after manipulation. Mononuclear cells were also primed for enhanced endotoxin-stimulated tumor necrosis factor production by spinal manipulation."</mark>[273]

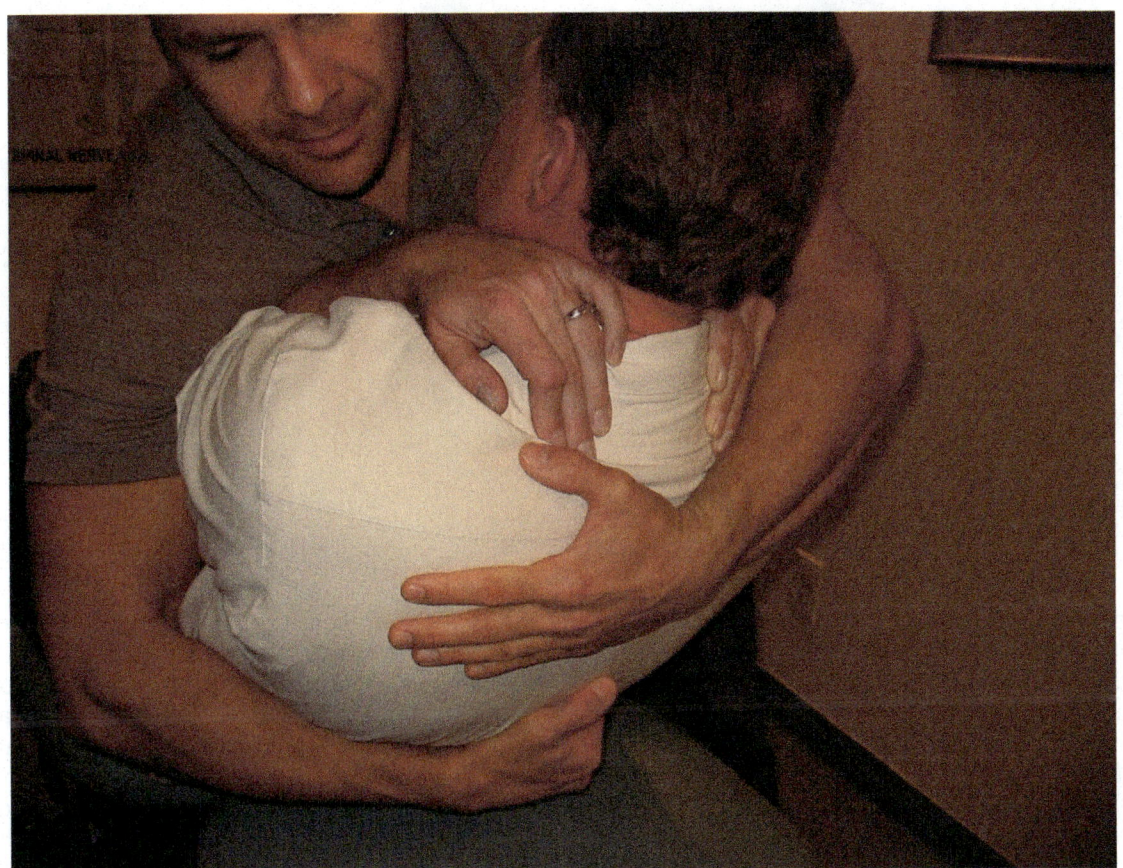

Manual manipulative treatment (inducing flexion) of the thoracic spine—one of many manipulative procedures for this region: In this procedure, the doctor uses body drop thrust technique at 45° toward the ground and toward the head of the table; the trust should simultaneously generate compression and long-axis traction; the contact hand remains tense to provide solid leverage *inferior* to the targeted motion segment; the supporting hand and arm pull toward doctor at time of impulse to accentuate traction and spinal flexion; patient is instructed to breathe deeply then relax and exhale; upon exhalation, the doctor establishes and maintains premanipulative tension to achieve joint flexion, then applies HVLA thrust; the thrust must be fast and shallow; slow and deep impulses can sprain the interspinous ligaments. Image and text originally from *Integrative Orthopedics, Third Edition* and later *Functional Inflammology, Volume 1*.

---

[272] Brennan et al. Enhanced phagocytic cell respiratory burst induced by spinal manipulation: potential role of substance P. *J Manipulative Physiol Ther*. 1991 Sep;14(7):399-408
[273] Brennan et al. Enhanced neutrophil respiratory burst as a biological marker for manipulation forces: duration of the effect and association with substance P and tumor necrosis factor. *J Manipulative Physiol Ther*. 1992 Feb;15(2):83-9

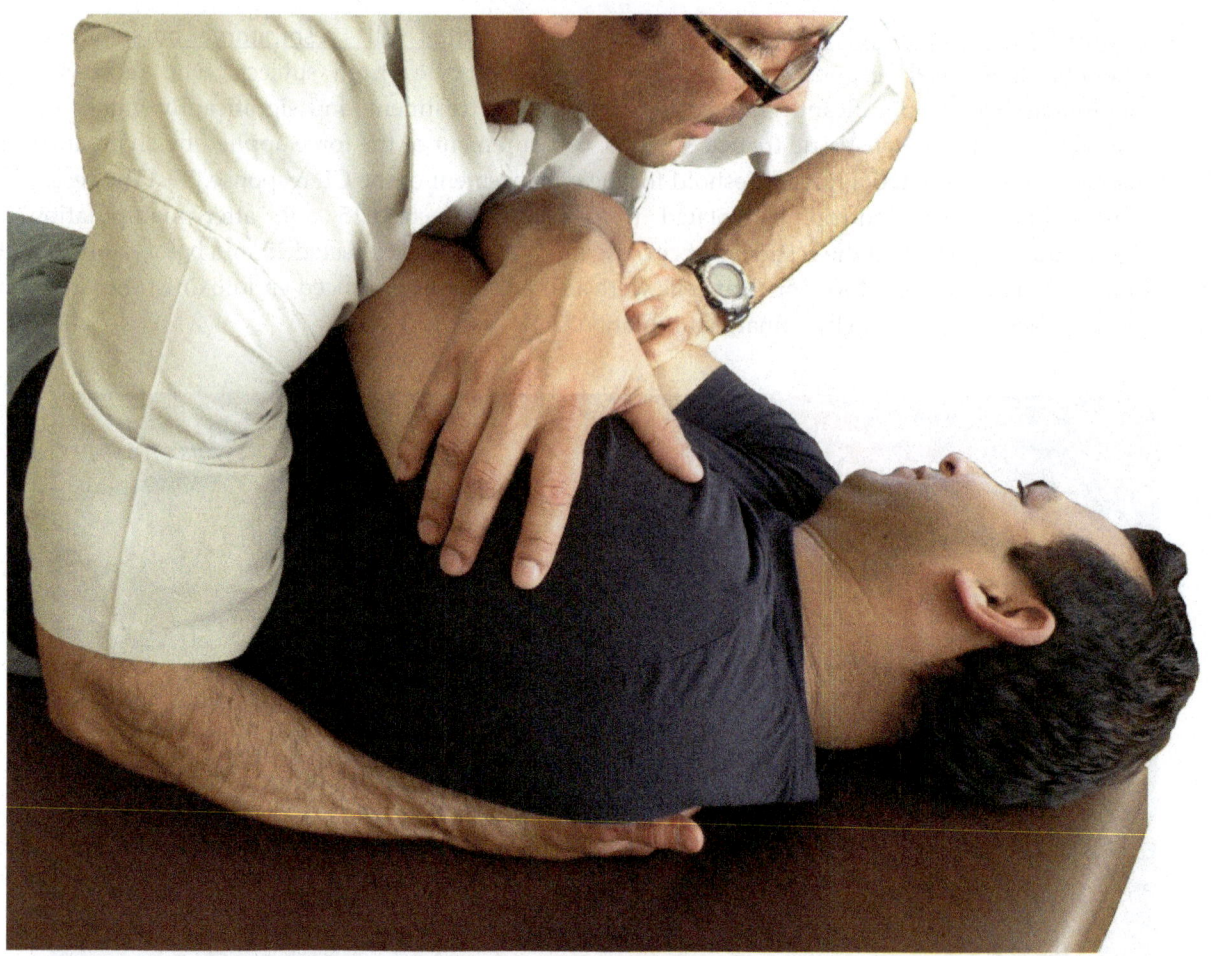

Posterior Ribs: Manipulation of the Costovertebral Junction: *Patient position*: Supine on table; to facilitate positioning, patient's leg opposite doctor may be flexed at hip and knee with foot flat on table. Patient's arms are crossed over the front of their body; my preference is that the arm closest to the doctor (the arm opposite to the side of the thorax being treated) is atop. *Doctor position*: Modified fencer's stance facing cephalad. *Assessment*: *Subjective*: mechanical paraspinal pain; often discomfort with inhalation. *Motion palpation*: stiffness at the affected costotransverse junction. *Static palpation*: prominence in the posterior direction of the rib near the costotransverse junction. *Soft tissue*: local tenderness to palpation is very common. *Treatment contact*: Contact on the specific rib immediately lateral to the costotransverse junction is made with the doctor's thenar eminence with the doctor's hand in a firm, pursed position. Initial contact is made superior and medial to the final location of manipulative contact in order to attain proper premanipulative tissue tension; the contact hand is then pulled against tissue tension in the lateral and inferior direction. *Supporting contact*: The doctor's supporting (noncontact) hand along with the doctor's torso deliver the manipulative thrust through the patient's arm atop the patient's thorax. *Pretreatment positioning*: Patient is supine; after positioning the contact hand posteriorly, the doctor grasps the patient's upper arm, then pulls downward and then applies progressively compressive force (body weight, not muscular force) while raising the supporting contact and rolling the patient over atop the contact hand. *Thrust*: Body-drop thrust generally superiorly and laterally in the direction of the patient's opposite shoulder; the angle of the thrust changes depending on the spinal-costal level being treated, with more superior segments requiring a more superiorly directed thrust, while lower segments require a progressively laterally-yet-sagittally directed thrust. Notably, the manipulative thrust is applied to the anterior thorax via contact with the patient's upper arm, yet the true manipulative force is from posterior to anterior via the doctor's thenar eminence positioned posteriorly. Image and text originally from *Integrative Orthopedics, Third Edition* and later *Functional Inflammology, Volume 1*.

❸ Nutritional Immunomodulation:
Nutritional Interventions to Induce Regulatory T-cells (Treg)

Major Concepts in this Section

"Inflammatory balance" is largely a biochemical endpoint whereas "immune balance" refers more directly to immunophenotypic predominance. In this section, I will outline a nutrition-based clinical protocol for the induction of active cell-mediated anti-inflammation via selective induction of regulatory T-cells ("Treg"). The goal with this component of the functional Inflammology protocol is to utilize the body's own immunomodulating ability by providing the appropriate nutritional climate for epigenetic upregulation of expression of the transcription factor FoxP3, which is the main identifier of the Treg phenotype. Components of this protocol are proven to provide clinical benefit; this nutritional immunomodulation protocol performs best when utilized within an intact functional inflammology protocol, as described throughout this chapter.

Anti-inflammatory/anti-allergy/antirheumatic nutritional immunomodulation: Although the term "nutritional immunomodulation" can be used to include nearly any dietary pattern or nutrient intake that has a meaningful effect on immune function (in which case, the term would encompass the totality of all food and nutrient intake), in this section I will use the term to specifically denote epigenetic induction of regulatory T-cells (Treg) from their precursors—the undifferentiated (indicated by the number zero, or "0") naïve T-helper cells—known as Th0 cells. This is a new, exciting, and remarkably well-documented therapeutic tool that we now have in our food-based armamentarium in the battles against common immune diseases such as metabolic inflammation (e.g.,

> **Treg/Th17 imbalance = autoimmunity**
>
> "Imbalance between effector and regulatory T-cells (Treg) underlies the loss of immune-tolerance to self-antigens in autoimmune disease."
>
> Holder et al. *J Autoimmun.* 2014 Feb

diabetes mellitus and the metabolic syndrome), allergy (e.g., asthma) and autoimmunity (e.g., psoriasis, rheumatoid arthritis, SLE, and multiple sclerosis). For this discussion of nutritional immunomodulation, readers need a practical understanding of the following cell types, their nutritional influences and physiologic/pathologic effects:

- <u>CD3(+)CD4(-)CD8(-) double negative T cells</u>: These cells arrived from the bone marrow to the thymus, but have not yet been fully "programed" for their ultimate functions; however, these cells are not benign and appear to contribute to autoimmune-type inflammation via necrotic-inflammatory cell death via a mechanism that is activated by mitochondrial dysfunction: activation of mTOR.

- <u>Th0—naive T-cells</u>: These cells have been "partially programmed" to become effector cells, particularly Th1, Th2, Th17, or T-regulatory cells.

- <u>Th1 cells</u>: Contribute to cell-mediated "chronic inflammation."

- <u>Th2 cells</u>: Contribute to antibody-mediated inflammation, allergies, and formation of autoreactive antibodies such as ANA.

- <u>Th17 cells</u>: Contribute very significantly to autoimmune-type inflammation as seen in SLE and multiple sclerosis.

- <u>T-regulatory cells (Treg)</u>: Treg are immunomodulatory and generally anti-inflammatory; they dampen the activity of Th1, Th2, Th17 cells, and thereby promote *active* anti-inflammation and immune tolerance to self and environment. Treg surface markers are CD4 and CD25; the transcription factor is FOXp3. Two main subtypes of Treg exist: "natural Tregs" (nTregs) are thymically derived; "induced Tregs" (iTregs) are converted in the periphery in the gastrointestinal associated lymphoid tissue (GALT) from CD4+ CD25- Foxp3- effector T-cells (Teffs). Clinicians need to pay attention to the fact that dietary interventions (or dietary negligence) can affect GALT function and directly and potently promote Treg induction (or Th17 induction); furthermore, iTregs maintain their induced Treg phenotype and function only if the conditions for such are favorable—namely: proper nutritional environment in the absence of microbial pathogens. Again, the fact that the distinction between Treg (immune tolerance) and Th17 (inflammation, autoimmunity) occurs in the GALT makes the importance of diet and gastrointestinal eubiosis/dysbiosis so obvious that refutation of the importance of these environmental determinants for shaping immunologic health is on the verge of being obscene. Further, the facts that nTreg cells produce TGF-beta and iTreg cells produce IL-10 gives prominence to iTreg for active immunosuppression and thus gives prominence to the following nutritional immunomodulation protocol as a key component of any modern treatment plan for inflammatory, allergic, or autoimmune disease.

- γδ T cells, gamma delta T cells: Gamma-delta T-cells are notorious for promoting of autoimmunity and allergic inflammation, in part via their production of IL-17; one animal study (cited previously) showed that the population of gamma-delta T-cells is doubled by consumption of genetically modified food (corn).

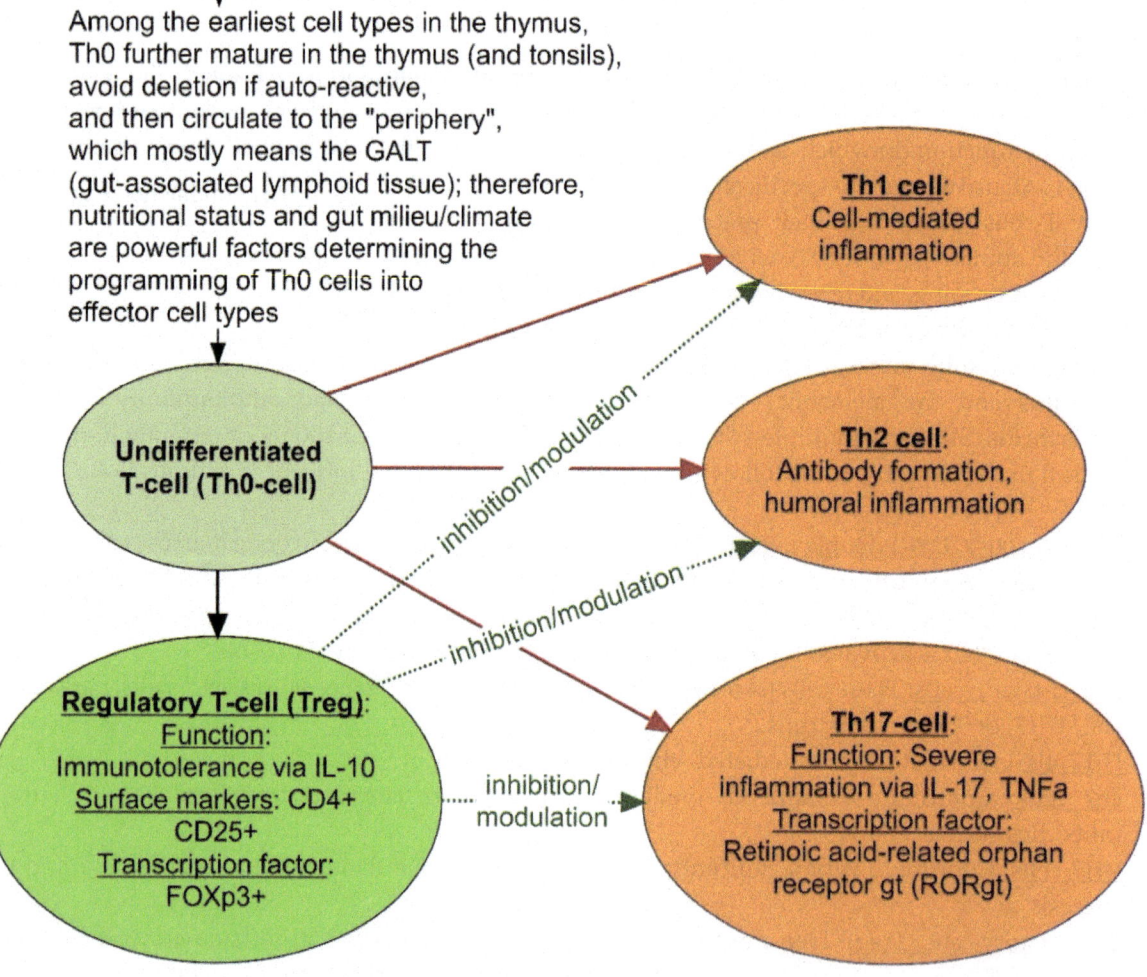

The earliest thymocytes, formed by cells originated in the bone marrow, are CD3(+)CD4(-)CD8(-) **double-negative** T cells. Far from being benign, these double-negative cells contribute to autoimmunity (especially ANA formation, notably in the setting of mitochondrial dysfunction) via inflammatory necrosis and stimulation of DAMP (damage-associated molecular pattern) receptors.

Among the earliest cell types in the thymus, Th0 further mature in the thymus (and tonsils), avoid deletion if auto-reactive, and then circulate to the "periphery", which mostly means the GALT (gut-associated lymphoid tissue); therefore, nutritional status and gut milieu/climate are powerful factors determining the programming of Th0 cells into effector cell types

Undifferentiated T-cell (Th0-cell)

Regulatory T-cell (Treg): Function: Immunotolerance via IL-10 Surface markers: CD4+ CD25+ Transcription factor: FOXp3+

Th1 cell: Cell-mediated inflammation

Th2 cell: Antibody formation, humoral inflammation

Th17-cell: Function: Severe inflammation via IL-17, TNFa Transcription factor: Retinoic acid-related orphan receptor gt (RORgt)

inhibition/modulation

inhibition/modulation

inhibition/modulation

Immunophenotype determination per inflammatory/microbial/nutritional climate: The cytokine climate, nutritional status, and microbial balance determine which immunocyte phenotype will be selected. If the climate is "hostile" then pro-inflammatory immunocytes will be selected; if nutritional needs are met and the internal milieu is relatively un-inflamed and un-infected, then tolerogenic T-regulatory cells will predominate. Thus, when dealing with disorders of sustained inflammation/allergy/autoimmunity, the task of the physician is to create or re-create the conditions for immunotolerance to predominate. Regulatory T-cells (Treg) provide anti-inflammatory immunomodulation and are characterized by the surface markers CD4 CD25 and transcription factor FOXp3 while Th-17 cells promote severe inflammation, autoimmunity, and are marked by the transcription factor RORγt—retinoic acid-related orphan receptor γt, also known as RORC in humans.

<u>DrV's "recipe" for optimized induction of the Treg phenotype is as follows</u>: I first published this protocol in 2012 in *Functional Immunology and Nutritional Immunomodulation*[1], and I am happy to see that clinical trials have now validated the last component of the protocol (vitamin A); now all components of the protocol are supported by clinical trials in humans. Of additional note regarding the induction of Treg versus Th-17 cells, I have chosen to not discuss transforming growth factor-β (TGF-β, TGF-beta) since this cytokine is clearly nondeterministic with regard to Treg/Th-17 induction; TGF-beta can stimulate both/either Treg/Th-17 induction depending on other cytokines and determinants, and thus these deciding factors should be the recipients of our attention.

- <u>Mitochondrial optimization, mTOR inhibition</u>: Recently, mitochondrial dysfunction in general and mTOR activation in particular has been shown to inhibit induction of Treg cells; inhibition of mTOR with NAC 4,800mg/d in divided doses was shown to inhibit mTOR and promote induction of the FoxP3 phenotype Treg cells and result in clinical alleviation of disease in patients with SLE. My basic, foundational, and initial protocol for optimizing mitochondrial function includes: carbohydrate avoidance and/or MTC/caprylate supplementation to enhance endogenous production of BHB, moderate physical exercise/activity 1 h/d, CoQ10 100 mg/d, NAC 1,500 mg TID, lipoic acid 200-400 mg TID, acetyl-carnitine 1 g BID-QID, and biotin 1-10 mg/d.

  - <u>N-acetylcysteine reduces disease activity by blocking mammalian target of rapamycin in T cells from systemic lupus erythematosus patients</u> (*Arthritis Rheum* 2012 Sep[2]): "NAC up to 2.4 gm/day was tolerated by all patients, while 33% of those receiving 4.8 gm/day had reversible nausea. ... Considered together, 2.4 gm and 4.8 gm NAC reduced the SLEDAI score after 1 month, 2 months, 3 months (P = 0.0030), and 4 months; the BILAG score after 1 month and 3 months; and the FAS score after 2 months and 3 months. NAC increased Δψm [mitochondrial inner membrane potential] in all T cells, profoundly reduced mTOR activity, enhanced apoptosis, reversed expansion of CD4-CD8- T cells, stimulated FoxP3 expression in CD4+CD25+ T cells, and reduced anti-DNA production. CONCLUSION: This pilot study suggests that NAC safely improves lupus disease activity by blocking mTOR in T lymphocytes."

- <u>Biotin</u>: Normal dietary intake of biotin is less than 97.5 microg (0.4 micromol); genotropic biotinopathy is treated with pharmacological/supranutritional doses of biotin 5–20 mg/d in children and adults while some patients may require higher doses of 40–200 mg/d.[3] Biotin is necessary for histone biotinylation; the effect is dose-dependent, regional, and repressive[4], notably of TNF-alpha gene transcription—correspondingly, biotin deficiency promotes inflammation while biotin supplementation reduces inflammation.[5]

  - <u>Biotin deficiency up-regulates and biotin supplementation reduces TNF-alpha production in murine macrophages</u> (*J Leukoc Biol* 2008 Apr): Significant decreases in serum biotin levels have been reported in patients with chronic inflammatory diseases. Cell proliferation and biotinylation of intracellular proteins were decreased significantly in biotin-deficient cells compared with biotin-sufficient cells, and this corresponded with significantly higher production and mRNA expression of TNF-alpha. TNF-alpha induction by biotin deficiency was down-regulated by biotin supplementation in vitro and in vivo. These results show that biotin deficiency up-regulates TNF-alpha production and that biotin supplementation down-regulates TNF-alpha production, suggesting that biotin status may influence inflammatory diseases.

  - <u>Biotin supplementation at a pharmacologic dose decreases proliferation rates of human peripheral blood mononuclear cells (PBMC) and decreases cytokine release</u> (*J Nutr* 2001 May[6]): Oral administration of biotin 756.1 microg/d (3.1 micromol/d) for 14 d "caused a significant decrease of PBMC proliferation. At 2 d after mitogen stimulation, [3H]thymidine uptake by postsupplementation PBMC was 66 % of the uptake by presupplementation PBMC. Similarly, concentrations of interleukin-1β (2 d after mitogen) and interleukin-2 (1 d after mitogen) in media

[1] Vasquez A. *Functional Immunology and Nutritional Immunomodulation*. Published June 5, 2012, ISBN-10: 1477603859, ISBN-13: 978-1477603857

[2] Lai ZW et al. N-acetylcysteine reduces disease activity by blocking mammalian target of rapamycin in T cells from systemic lupus erythematosus patients: a randomized, double-blind, placebo-controlled trial. *Arthritis Rheum*. 2012 Sep;64(9):2937-46

[3] Baumgartner MR. Vitamin-responsive disorders: cobalamin, folate, biotin, vitamins B1 and E. *Handb Clin Neurol*. 2013;113:1799-810

[4] Hassan YI, Zempleni J. A novel, enigmatic histone modification: biotinylation of histones by holocarboxylase synthetase. *Nutr Rev*. 2008 Dec;66(12):721-5

[5] Kuroishi T, Endo Y, Muramoto K, Sugawara S. Biotin deficiency up-regulates TNF-alpha production in murine macrophages. *J Leukoc Biol*. 2008 Apr;83(4):912-20

[6] Per the authors 2.46 micromol = 600 microg, and thus 3.1 micromol = 756.1 microg. Zempleni J, Helm RM, Mock DM. In vivo biotin supplementation at a pharmacologic dose decreases proliferation rates of human peripheral blood mononuclear cells and cytokine release. *J Nutr*. 2001 May;131(5):1479-84

from postsupplementation PBMC were 65% and 44%, respectively, of those for presupplementation PBMC. ... Overall, this study provides evidence that administration of pharmacologic doses of biotin [756.1 microg/d] for 14 d decreases PBMC proliferation and synthesis of interleukin-1β and interleukin-2." These impressive results show that low-dose orally administered biotin reduces monocyte proliferation by -34%, IL-1 by -35%, and IL-2 by -56%.

- Vitamin E: The *gamma* form of tocopherol inhibits cyclooxygenase and has anti-inflammatory activity.[7] Alpha-tocopherol has been shown to decrease CRP levels in patients with CVD and in those with risk factors for CVD; alpha-tocopherol inhibits protein kinase C, 5-lipoxygenase, tyrosine-kinase, and cyclooxygenase-2.[8] Clinical trials and case reports have demonstrated benefit of vitamin E supplementation in patients with rheumatoid arthritis[9,10], spondylosis[11] and osteoarthritis[12], and autoimmune diseases including scleroderma, discoid lupus erythematosus, porphyria cutanea tarda, vasculitis, and polymyositis.[13,14,15] In 2013, we as clinicians gained valuable insight into the mechanism of action of vitamin E thanks to the work of Salinthone et al[16] who showed that, rather than functioning simply/solely as an antioxidant, vitamin E significantly raises cyclic adenosine monophosphate (cAMP) levels and thereby has an anti-inflammatory effect; they showed that "vitamin E resulted in a greater than 2-fold increase in cAMP level (29.19 pmol/mg protein) compared to baseline. Lipoic acid was used as a positive control, which generated 45.49 pmol/mg protein of cAMP." Elevation of cAMP—such as by alpha-tocopherol and lipoic acid—results in a dose-dependent inhibition of inflammatory IL-2 and IL-17 cytokine generation and by this mechanism—additive/synergistic with the antioxidant and mitochondrial-supportive effects—reduces inflammation. Most cAMP-elevating agents demonstrate anti-inflammatory actions by increasing production of anti-inflammatory IL-10 and reducing production of pro-inflammatory TNF-alpha.[17]

Vitamin E nutritional immunomodulation
Vitamin E *increases*:
• IL-10
• Antioxidant defenses
• Mitochondrial performance
Vitamin E *decreases*:
• Protein kinase C
• 5-lipoxygenase
• Tyrosine-kinase
• Cyclooxygenase-2
• IL-2
• IL-17
• TNF-alpha
• IgE
• CRP
• Serum AGE
• Oxidative, oxidized, and inflammatory molecules that would otherwise trigger and perpetuate inflammation

  o Vitamin E for atopic dermatitis and effect on immunoglobulin E (*Int J Dermatol.* 2002 Mar[18]): This notable placebo (PL)-controlled study used "natural origin" vitamin E (VE) 400 IU (268 mg) in 96 subjects with atopic dermatitis and for 8 months and found that "23 of the 50 subjects treated with VE showed great improvement, compared to only one in the PL group; and almost complete remission of atopic dermatitis in seven of the 50 subjects in the VE group, but none in the PL group. ... Subjects with great improvement and near remission of atopic dermatitis in the VE group demonstrated a decrease of 62% in serum IgE levels based on initial conditions, while, in subjects taking PL, the difference was approximately 34.4%. ... A remarkable improvement in facial

---

[7] Jiang Q, Christen S, Shigenaga MK, Ames BN. gamma-tocopherol, the major form of vitamin E in the US diet, deserves more attention. *Am J Clin Nutr* 2001;74(6):714-22

[8] Singh et al. Vitamin E, oxidative stress, and inflammation. *Annu Rev Nutr.* 2005;25:151-74

[9] Helmy M, Shohayeb M, Helmy MH, el-Bassiouni EA. Antioxidants as adjuvant therapy in rheumatoid disease. A preliminary study. *Arzneimittelforschung.* 2001;51(4):293-8

[10] Edmonds SE, et al. Putative analgesic activity of repeated oral doses of vitamin E in the treatment of rheumatoid arthritis. *Ann Rheum Dis.* 1997 Nov;56(11):649-55

[11] "Vitamin E administration at a dose of 100 mg daily for three weeks resulted in a significant increase in serum vitamin E level accompanied by complete relief of pain... The results therefore strongly indicate that vitamin E is effective in curing spondylosis and most probably due to its antioxidant activity." Mahmud Z, Ali SM. Role of vitamin A and E in spondylosis. *Bangladesh Med Res Counc Bull.* 1992 Apr;18(1):47-59. See also "The results of this double-blind controlled clinical trial showed that vitamin E was superior to placebo with respect to the relief of pain (pain at rest, pain during movement, pressure-induced pain) and the necessity of additional analgetic treatment. Improvement of mobility was better in the group treated with vitamin E." Blankenhorn G. [Clinical effectiveness of Spondyvit (vitamin E) in activated arthroses. A multicenter placebo-controlled double-blind study] [Article in German—information from abstract] *Z Orthop Ihre Grenzgeb* 1986;124:340-3. See also This is a very interesting study because the clinical response to vitamin E was proportional to the increase in plasma levels of vitamin E, thus confirming the dose-response relationship that implies causality as well as indicating that the failure of such treatment in some patients may be due to malabsorption or unquenchable systemic oxidative stress rather than the inefficacy of vitamin E supplementation, per se. "There were no significant differences in the efficacy of the two drugs, although one patient of the V-group refused further treatment after 8 days because of inefficacy. V reduced or abolished the pain at rest in 77% (D in 85%), the pain on pressure in 67% (D in 50%), and the pain on movement in 62% (D in 63%). Both treatments appeared to be equally effective in reducing the circumference of the knee joints and the walking time and in increasing the joint mobility." Scherak O, et al. [High dosage vitamin E therapy in patients with activated arthrosis] [Article in German—information from abstract] *Z Rheumatol.* 1990 Nov-Dec;49(6):369-73

[12] Machtey I, Ouaknine L. Tocopherol in Osteoarthritis: a controlled pilot study. *J Am Geriatr Soc.* 1978 Jul;26(7):328-30

[13] Killeen RN, Ayres S Jr, Mihan R. Polymyositis: response to vitamin E. *South Med J.* 1976 Oct;69(10):1372-4

[14] Ayres S Jr, Mihan R. Lupus erythematosus and vitamin E: an effective and nontoxic therapy. *Cutis.* 1979 Jan;23(1):49-52, 54

[15] Ayres S Jr, Mihan R. Is vitamin E involved in the autoimmune mechanism? *Cutis.* 1978 Mar;21(3):321-5

[16] Salinthone et al. α-Tocopherol stimulates cyclic AMP production in human peripheral mononuclear cells and alters immune function. *Mol Immunol.* 2013 Mar;53(3):173-8

[17] Eigler et al. Anti-inflammatory activities of cAMP-elevating agents: enhancement of IL-10 synthesis and suppression of TNF production. *J Leukoc Biol.* 1998 Jan;63(1):101-7

[18] Tsoureli-Nikita et al. Evaluation of dietary intake of vitamin E in the treatment of atopic dermatitis: a study of the clinical course and evaluation of the immunoglobulin E serum levels. *Int J Dermatol.* 2002 Mar;41(3):146-50

erythema, lichenification, and the presence of apparently normal skin was reported. Eczematous lesions healed mostly as a result of decreased pruritus."

- o <u>No effect of ineffective nondescript vitamin E supplementation on nasal symptoms and specific IgE levels in patients with perennial allergic rhinitis (*Ann Allergy Asthma Immunol.* 2006 Jan[19]):</u> This clinical trial by Velazquez et al showed no benefit of "vitamin E 400 IU/d" in symptoms nor IgE levels; importantly however, 1) the authors did not specify the type or source of "vitamin E" that was used and therefore we might assume that it was the inexpensive ineffective DL racemic mixture, 2) serum lipid peroxides did not change, thus strongly suggesting inefficacy and lack of potency of the vitamin E supplement used, and 3) the study was conducted in an industrial region of Mexico City, an area internationally notorious for severe airborne pollution. Further differentiating this study and greatly reducing the opportunity to observe efficacy was the assessment of specific (very limited) IgE rather than total IgE.

- **<u>Sodium avoidance</u>:** Sodium—independent from the chloride anion—induces the Th17 phenotype via induction of serum glucocorticoid kinase 1 (SGK1) which stabilizes the IL-23 receptor necessary for maintaining the Th17 phenotype and inflammatory disease.
  - o <u>Sodium drives autoimmune disease by induction of pathogenic TH17 cells (*Nature* 2013 Apr[20]):</u> Changes in environmental factors must ultimately be driving the marked increase in the incidence of autoimmune diseases in the past half-century. "The newly identified population of interleukin (IL)-17-producing CD4(+) helper T cells (TH17 cells) has a pivotal role in autoimmune diseases. ... Here we show that increased salt (sodium chloride, NaCl) concentrations found locally under physiological conditions in vivo markedly boost the induction of murine and human TH17 cells. ... The TH17 cells generated under high-salt conditions display a highly pathogenic and stable phenotype characterized by the upregulation of the pro-inflammatory cytokines GM-CSF, TNF-α and IL-2. ... Thus, increased dietary salt intake might represent an environmental risk factor for the development of autoimmune diseases through the induction of pathogenic TH17 cells."
  - o <u>Induction of pathogenic TH17 cells by sodium (*Nature* 2013 Apr[21]):</u> "TH17 cells (interleukin-17 (IL-17)-producing helper T cells) are highly proinflammatory cells that are critical for clearing extracellular pathogens and for inducing multiple autoimmune diseases. IL-23 has a critical role in stabilizing and reinforcing the TH17 phenotype by increasing expression of IL-23 receptor (IL-23R) and endowing TH17 cells with pathogenic effector functions." Here, the researchers discovered that serum glucocorticoid kinase 1 (SGK1), a serine/threonine kinase, is critical for regulating IL-23R expression and stabilizing the TH17 cell phenotype and that a modest increase in salt concentration induces SGK1 expression, promotes IL-23R expression and enhances TH17 cell differentiation in vitro and in vivo, accelerating the development of autoimmunity. "These data demonstrate that SGK1 has a critical role in the induction of pathogenic TH17 cells and provide a molecular insight into a mechanism by which an environmental factor such as a high salt diet triggers TH17 development and promotes tissue inflammation."

- **<u>Transgenic food avoidance—including avoidance of the associated pesticides</u>:** Per the animal study summarized below, the finding that GMO corn—but not natural corn—lead to increases in IL-6 (which promotes Th-17 cell development, as well as cardiometabolic disease) and gamma-delta T cells (which also produce tissue-damaging IL-17) is sufficient to mechanistically connect GMO foods with inflammatory and dysmetabolic disease in humans. Thus, the implications of this data are that, given that gamma-delta T-cells make IL-17, currently the most notorious cytokine in autoimmune inflammation, humans should avoid GMO foods.
  - o <u>Intestinal and peripheral immune response to MON810 maize ingestion in weaning and old mice (*J Agric Food Chem* 2008 Dec[22]):</u> The authors' abstract understates the importance of their findings, noting immune system abnormalities and an increase in the pro-inflammatory cytokine IL-6

[19] Montaño Velázquez et al. Vitamin E effects on nasal symptoms and serum specific IgE levels in patients with perennial allergic rhinitis. *Ann Allergy Asthma Immunol.* 2006 Jan;96(1):45-50

[20] Kleinewietfeld et al. Sodium chloride drives autoimmune disease by the induction of pathogenic TH17 cells. *Nature.* 2013 Apr 25;496(7446):518-22

[21] Wu et al. Induction of pathogenic TH17 cells by inducible salt-sensing kinase SGK1. *Nature.* 2013 Apr 25;496(7446):513-7

[22] Finamore et al. Intestinal and peripheral immune response to MON810 maize ingestion in weaning and old mice. *J Agric Food Chem.* 2008 Dec 10;56(23):11533-9

following consumption of GMO corn compared with natural corn. The increase in IL-6 is by itself significant, given the role of inflammation in essentially all human diseases and the ability of IL-6 to induce Th-17 phenotype characteristic of more severe allergic and autoimmune diseases. However, per my reading of the full text of the article, I find this article to sound the alarm on GMO foods per the authors' report, "One of the more recurrent alterations in lymphocyte phenotypes observed in this study was an increase in the TCRγδ+ (gamma-delta T-cells) population. A high percentage of these lymphocytes are localized in the gut and ... γδT cells seem to be important regulatory elements of the immune system, being capable of modulating inflammatory response associated with infectious agents and autoantigens. Higher numbers of γδT cells have been observed in humans with asthma, in intraepithelial lymphocytes (IELs) of children with untreated food allergy, and in the duodenum of children with juvenile idiopathic arthritis or connective tissue disease with gastrointestinal symptoms." Further, gamma-delta T-cells are known to secrete IL-17, the cytokine responsible for the massive tissue damage seen in autoimmune diseases such as multiple sclerosis, rheumatoid arthritis, and psoriasis, and which is also elevated in autism.[23]

- Probiotics: Molecular signatures from probiotic bacteria synergize to promote epigenetic induction of Treg cells; probiotic metabolites—particularly butyrate—also promote the histone acetylation which is a common theme in FoxP3 induction.

  o Probiotics induce Treg at the expense of Th-1/2/17 (*Clin Exp Allergy* 2014 Apr[24]): "There is emerging evidence that resident symbionts induce tolerogenic gut-associated Treg cells and dendritic cells that ensure the preferential growth of symbionts; keeping pathogenic strains in check and constraining proinflammatory Th1, Th2 and Th17 clones."

  o Regulatory dendritic cells and CD4+Foxp3+ T cells by probiotics administration suppresses immune disorders (*Proc Natl Acad Sci* 2010 Feb[25]): "Administration of probiotics had therapeutical effects in experimental inflammatory bowel disease, atopic dermatitis, and rheumatoid arthritis. The therapeutical effect of the probiotics is associated with enrichment of CD4(+)Foxp3(+) Tregs in the inflamed regions. Collectively, the administration of probiotics that enhance the generation of rDCs and Tregs represents an applicable treatment of inflammatory immune disorders."

Probiotic immunomodulation
Components:
1. *Lactobacillus acidophilus* (LA),
2. *Lactobacillus casei* (LC),
3. *Lactobacillus reuteri* (LR),
4. *Bifidobacterium bifidium* (BB),
5. *Streptococcus thermophilus* (ST).
Effects:
• Induction of T-cell and B-cell hyporesponsiveness,
• Suppression of Th1, Th2, and Th17 cytokines,
• Induction and maintenance of CD4(+)Foxp3(+) Tregs,
• Alleviation of intestinal hyperpermeability, allergy, inflammation, autoimmunity.
Kwon et al, *Proc Natl Acad Sci* 2010 Feb

  o Cytokine and clinical response to Saccharomyces boulardii therapy in diarrhea-dominant irritable bowel syndrome. (*Eur J Gastroenterol Hepatol.* 2014 Jun[26]): "This was a randomized, double blind, placebo-controlled trial in which S. boulardii, 750 mg/day, or placebo was administered for 6 weeks in IBS-D patients, in addition to ispaghula husk standard treatment. Thirty-seven patients received S. boulardii and 35 patients received the placebo. As compared with placebo, the S. boulardii group showed a significant decrease in blood and tissue levels of proinflammatory cytokines interleukin-8 (IL-8) and tumor necrosis factor-alpha and an increase in anti-inflammatory IL-10 levels, as well as an increase in the tissue IL-10/IL-12 ratio. No significant change in the blood and tissue levels of cytokines was found in the placebo group. Bowel-related IBS-D symptoms reported in the patients' daily diary improved in both groups. However, overall improvement in the quality of life was more marked in the S. boulardii group. Although baseline histological findings were mild, an improvement was observed in the probiotic group in the lymphocyte and neutrophil infiltrates, epithelial mitosis, and intraepithelial lymphocytes. No serious adverse events were found in either group. Conclusion: S. boulardii with ispaghula husk was superior to placebo with ispaghula husk in improving the cytokine profile, histology, and quality of life of patients with IBS-D."

[23] Al-Ayadhi LY, Mostafa GA. Elevated serum levels of interleukin-17A in children with autism. *J Neuroinflammation*. 2012 Jul 2;9:158
[24] West CE et al. The gut microbiota and its role in the development of allergic disease: a wider perspective. *Clin Exp Allergy*. 2014 Apr 29
[25] Kwon et al. Generation of regulatory dendritic cells and CD4+Foxp3+ T cells by probiotics administration suppresses immune disorders. *Proc Natl Acad Sci* 2010 Feb:2159-64
[26] Abbas et al. Cytokine and clinical response to Saccharomyces boulardii therapy in diarrhea-dominant irritable bowel syndrome. *Eur J Gastroenterol Hepatol*. 2014 Jun:630-9

- **Lipoic acid**: LA is an antioxidant and direct inhibitor of NFkB; a clinical trial in humans with multiple sclerosis showed that lipoic acid 400mg PO TID reduced IL-17 levels by 35-50%—the clinical importance of this is massive, given that IL-17 is a major effector of tissue destruction in autoimmune diseases.
  - Lipoic acid attenuates inflammation via cAMP and protein kinase A signaling (*PLoS One* 2010 Sep[27]): "Oral administration of 1200 mg LA to MS subjects resulted in increased cAMP levels in PBMCs four hours after ingestion. Average cAMP levels in 20 subjects were 43% higher than baseline. ... [In vitro] We show that LA reduces IL-6 production in a dose-dependent manner...Pretreatment with 50 and 100 μg/ml LA prior to LPS stimulation resulted in reduced IL-6 levels by 19 and 34%, respectively. ... Stimulation with anti-CD3/CD28 resulted in dramatic and statistically significant increases in IL-17 levels compared to untreated controls. Pretreatment with 50 and 100 μg/ml LA inhibited IL-17 production by 35 and 50%, respectively. Collectively, these data indicate that LA exerts anti-inflammatory functions in part by inhibiting IL-6 and IL-17 synthesis. ... Collectively, the data presented here indicate that LA inhibits T cell proliferation and activation....Collectively, the cytokine data suggest that LA is exerting its anti-inflammatory effects by lowering the concentrations of pro-inflammatory cytokines (IL-6 and IL-17) while possibly having a biphasic effect on IL-10."
- **Vitamin A, retinoic acid, RA**: Retinoic acid is required for Treg induction and for maintenance of Treg phenotype, especially in an inflammatory/IL-6 milieu. Vitamin A enhances histone acetylation at the promoter region of the Foxp3 gene, thereby enhancing FOXp3 transcription and the resultant Treg phenotype. Many patients have insufficient intake of preformed vitamin A and must therefore use oral vitamin A supplementation; relatedly, 27-45% of women (volunteers from UK) are "slow converters" of beta-carotene to vitamin A, and they must likewise supplement with vitamin A in order to meet physiologic needs.[28] Hypothyroidism also impairs conversion of beta-carotene to vitamin A; zinc is also needed for this conversion. Women who are pregnant or might become pregnant are generally advised to keep vitamin A intake below 8,000-9,000 IU/day from all sources. When treating acute viral infections, I have traditionally used a time-limited loading dose of 100,000-300,000 IU/d for 7-10 days followed by a maintenance dose of 10,000-25,000 IU/d for children and adults; I think this is a reasonable approach for the rapid repletion of vitamin A stores for the treatment of acute illness. However, after seeing the success of two clinical trials demonstrating successful FOXp3 and Treg induction in humans with inflammatory diseases following vitamin A 25,000 IU/d, I am inclined to describe the loading dose as optional, particularly for patients wary of the vitamin A headache, which can occur with loading dose without real vitamin A overload or toxicity (i.e., some patients get a headache from high-dose vitamin A supplementation even after the first day, when they are clearly *not* vitamin A toxic). Vitamin A toxicity is monitored clinically with six main findings: "two pains"—bone pain and headache, "two skins"—dry skin and chapped lips, and "two labs"—elevated GGT and triglycerides. The *in vitro* data showing that vitamin A promotes the Treg phenotype is impressively strong; the clinical data that is accumulating is showing that vitamin A supplementation promotes improved Treg/Th-17 balance in humans.
  - Retinoic acid stabilizes antigen-specific regulatory T-cell function in autoimmune hepatitis type 2 (*J Autoimmun* 2014 Feb[29]): This study is not a clinical trial; data are in vitro / ex vivo. The authors introduce their paper with a clear summary, "Imbalance between effector and regulatory T-cells (Treg) underlies the loss of immune-tolerance to self-antigens in autoimmune disease" and they go on to note that "In autoimmune hepatitis type 2 (AIH-2), effector CD4 T-cell immune responses to cytochrome P450IID6 (CYP2D6) are permitted by **numerically** and **functionally** impaired Treg. ... Treg exposure to inflammatory challenge results in decreased suppressive function and up-regulation of Th1/Th2/Th17 transcription factors both in health and AIH-2. ... inflammation-induced decrease in Treg function is also abrogated by retinoic acid (RA) / rapamycin (RP) in health and RA in patients."

---

[27] Salinthone S, et al. Lipoic acid attenuates inflammation via cAMP and protein kinase A signaling. *PLoS One*. 2010 Sep 28;5(9). pii: e13058

[28] "The extent to which β-carotene is converted to vitamin A is highly variable between well-nourished healthy individuals. This variable response to β-carotene has led to the characterization of the poor [slow] converter phenotype in 27–45% of volunteers in double-tracer studies." Leung et al. Two common single nucleotide polymorphisms in the gene encoding beta-carotene 15,15'-monoxygenase alter beta-carotene metabolism in female volunteers. *FASEB J.* 2009 Apr;23(4):1041-53

[29] Holder et al. Retinoic acid stabilizes antigen-specific regulatory T-cell function in autoimmune hepatitis type 2. *J Autoimmun*. 2014 Feb 21. pii: S0896-8411(14)00040-7

- All-trans retinoic acid sustains the stability and function of natural regulatory T cells in an inflammatory milieu (*J Immunol* 2010 Sep[30]): "Recent studies have demonstrated that plasticity of naturally occurring CD4(+)Foxp3(+) regulatory T cells (nTregs) may account for their inability to control chronic inflammation in established autoimmune diseases. All-trans retinoic acid (atRA), the active derivative of vitamin A, has been demonstrated to promote Foxp3(+) Treg differentiation and suppress Th17 development. In this study, we report a vital role of atRA in sustaining the stability and functionality of nTregs in the presence of IL-6. We found that nTregs treated with atRA were resistant to Th17 and other Th cell conversion and maintained Foxp3 expression and suppressive activity in the presence of IL-6 in vitro. atRA decreased IL-6R expression and signaling by nTregs. Of interest, adoptive transfer of nTregs even from arthritic mice treated with atRA suppressed progression of established collagen-induced arthritis. We suggest that nTregs treated with atRA may represent a novel treatment strategy to control established chronic immune-mediated inflammatory diseases."

- Clinical use of vitamin A supplementation on retinoic acid-related orphan receptor γt (RORγt) and interleukin-17 (IL-17) gene expression in Avonex-treated multiple sclerosis patients (*J Mol Neurosci* 2013 Nov[31]): Patients received retinyl palmitate 25,000 IU/d per day for 6 months; results showed that vitamin A downregulates IL-17 gene expression (reported as 1.7-fold reduction) and RORγt gene expression (reported as 50-fold reduction). The authors proudly state, "An attractive feature of our survey is that, for the first time in the world, an assessment of the effect of retinyl palmitate supplementation on IL-17 gene expression in multiple sclerotic patients has been performed. Results of our study show that supplementation with vitamin A decreases IL-17 and RORγt gene expression significantly, while there was no change at the end of the study in the placebo group."

- Clinical use of vitamin A supplementation for Foxp3 induction in atherosclerotic patients (*J Nutrigenet Nutrigenomics* 2013 Jan[32]): Patients with atherosclerosis and healthy controls received retinyl palmitate 25,000 IU/d for 4 months. The levels of Foxp3 expression increased significantly in both groups, more so in the patients with atherosclerosis (10-fold to 14-fold) than in healthy controls (5-fold to 7-fold) as expected. The authors concluded that "...vitamin A has the effect of increasing expression of regulatory T cells, it can be concluded that supplementation with vitamin A in atherosclerotic patients may be effective in slowing disease progression. No adverse effects were reported.

- Inflammation reduction: Reducing inflammation in general and IL-6, IL-17, and TNFa in particular is important for decreasing induction of inflammatory phenotypes—Th1, Th2, Th17—and optimizing

---

Vitamin A: clinical pearls and observations

- Use vitamin A *with* or *following* vitamin D, or start with a low dose of vitamin A: Preformed vitamin A should not be used without concomitant or previous supplementation with physiologic doses of vitamin D3. What may possibly occur in patients with inflammatory/autoimmune diseases who are deficient in both vitamin A and vitamin D is that monotherapy with vitamin A partly restores immune function but does so in a way that is skewed toward Th17 responses due to the lack of vitamin D3; the resulting clinical exacerbation may be a form of (analogous to) what we might call *nutritionally-induced immune reconstitution inflammatory syndrome* (IRIS, or in this case nIRIS). Another clinical approach is to avoid the loading dose of vitamin A unless the patient is already replete with vitamin D. Noted is the fact that studies using vitamin A 25,000 IU/d in the treatment of inflammatory disease for Treg induction have *not* observed disease flares.
- Acute loading dose is not necessary: The vitamin A loading dose commonly used for acute viral infections is not necessary when vitamin A is being used for FOXp3 and Treg induction.
- Early headache with vitamin A loading dose does not indicate "vitamin A toxicity": Some patients are intolerant of high-dose vitamin A, especially if given in an emulsified form (thus with better absorption). Vitamin A loading dose is really only indicated when a rapid response is needed, as with acute viral infections, not with long-term immunomodulation.

---

[30] Zhou X et al. Cutting edge: all-trans retinoic acid sustains stability and function of natural regulatory T cells in inflammatory milieu. *J Immunol.* 2010 Sep;185:2675-9
[31] Mohammadzadeh Honarvar et al. The effect of vitamin A supplementation on retinoic acid-related orphan receptor γt (RORγt) and interleukin-17 (IL-17) gene expression in Avonex-treated multiple sclerotic patients. *J Mol Neurosci.* 2013 Nov;51(3):749-53
[32] Mottaghi et al. Influence of vitamin A supplementation on Foxp3 and TGF-ß gene expression in atherosclerotic patients. *J Nutrigenet Nutrigenomics.* 2012;5(6):314-26

induction of Treg. Of clinical importance are the following facts: summarized as *inflammation becomes a vicious cycle*, and therefore the clinician's task is to break these cycles as effectively and consistently as possible using wide range of modalities:

- o IL-6 vicious cycle: IL-6 promotes Th-17 induction, and the Th-17 phenotype directly/indirectly promotes additional IL-6 production; in my earlier review of NFkB, I noted that IL-6 and TNF-alpha both stimulate NFkB activation, leading to a vicious cycle of inflammation,
- o IL-17 is the main cytokine causing tissue damage: IL-17 is the effector of tissue damage, and tissue damage then causes additional immune response and subsequent cytokine release,
- o IL-21 vicious cycle: IL-21 promotes Th-17 induction; the Th-17 phenotype produces IL-21[33],
- o TNF-alpha vicious cycle: TNFa promotes Th-17 induction; Th-17 phenotype produces TNFa.

Thus, means to reduce IL-6, IL-17, and TNFa help to break the vicious cycles of inflammation, such means include but are not limited to:

- o IL-6 reduction: IL-6 can be reduced by multivitamin/mineral supplementation, CoQ10, vitamin D, low-carbohydrate diets, moderate exercise, weight loss, lipoic acid, antidysbiosis/antimicrobial treatments as needed; vitamin A helps maintain iTreg phenotype and activity in an inflammatory milieu,
- o IL-17 reduction: IL-17 can be reduced by lipoic acid (per in vitro and ex vivo research),
- o IL-21 reduction: Animal studies have shown that vitamin D deficiency increases responsiveness to IL-21 (pro-inflammatory effect), and that vitamin D supplementation reduces responsiveness to IL-21 (anti-inflammatory effect),
- o TNF-alpha reduction: TNFa can be reduced by fish oil and biotin (per in vitro and ex vivo research),

- Vitamin D3: Several clinical trials in humans have shown that vitamin D3 supplementation (detailed previously and throughout in this textbook) induces higher number and function of Treg cells within approximately 1 month in adult humans who are "apparently healthy" and those who have autoimmune diseases such as multiple sclerosis (MS) and systemic lupus erythematosus (SLE, lupus).
  - o Small study shows that vitamin D increases anti-inflammatory IL-10 and reduces frequency of pro-inflammatory Th-17 cells (*Mult Scler* 2012 Dec[34]): Four healthy individuals (n=4) took 5000-10,000 IU/day of vitamin D over 15 weeks, after which serum 25(OH) vitamin D levels rose significantly from baseline, with a corresponding increase in IL-10 production by peripheral blood mononuclear cells and a reduced frequency of Th17 cells.
  - o Vitamin D supplementation increases regulatory T cells in apparently healthy subjects (*Isr Med Assoc J* 2010 Mar[35]): In this study, most "healthy" subjects were vitamin D deficient at the start of this study, then received one dose of vitamin D 140,000 IU (nonphysiologic dosing) and were not corrected to optimal vitamin D status. Nonetheless, participants showed an increase in Tregs.
  - o T-cell modulating effects of high dose vitamin D3 supplementation in multiple sclerosis (*PLoS One* 2010 Dec[36]): N=15 RRMS patients were supplemented with 20,000 IU/d vitamin D3 for 12 weeks. "All patients finished the protocol without side-effects, hypercalcemia, or hypercalciuria. The median vitamin D status increased from 50 nmol/L (31-175) at week 0 to 380 nmol/L (151-535) at week 12 (P<0.001). During the study, 1 patient experienced an exacerbation of MS and was censored from the T cell analysis. The proportions of (naïve and memory) CD4+ Tregs remained unaffected. Although Treg suppressive function improved in several subjects, this effect was not significant in the total cohort. An increased proportion of IL-10+ CD4+ T cells was found after supplementation."
  - o One of the most important studies ever ignored: Intake of vitamin D and risk of type 1 diabetes *Lancet* 2001 Nov[37]): This is one of the most important studies ever published in medicine and nutrition, showing that among more than 10,000 infants, vitamin D supplementation 2,000 IU/d for the first year of life showed complete safety and a dose-dependent reduction in autoimmune type-

---

[33] Korn et al. IL-17 and Th17 Cells. *Annu Rev Immunol*. 2009;27:485-517

[34] Allen AC et al. A pilot study of the immunological effects of high-dose vitamin D in healthy volunteers. *Mult Scler*. 2012 Dec;18(12):1797-800

[35] Prietl et al. Vitamin D supplementation and regulatory T cells in apparently healthy subjects: vitamin D for autoimmune diseases? *Isr Med Assoc J*. 2010;12:136-9

[36] Smolders J et al. Safety and T cell modulating effects of high dose vitamin D3 supplementation in multiple sclerosis. *PLoS One*. 2010 Dec 13;5(12):e15235

[37] Hyppönen et al. Intake of vitamin D and risk of type 1 diabetes: a birth-cohort study. *Lancet*. 2001 Nov 3;358(9292):1500-3

1 diabetes mellitus up to -78% over 30 years of follow-up. If any drug showed this level of safety, affordability, and efficacy, its use would almost certainly be medically and legally mandatory; the continued ignoring of this data by the medical/pediatrician/ObGyn communities is one of many nutritional-medical travesties in medicine and healthcare.

Vitamin D prevention of autoimmune diabetes: lessons learned and ignored

- More than 10,000 human infants were to receive 2,000 IU/d of vitamin D for the first year of life,
- No report of adverse effects.
- Dose-dependent reduction in autoimmune diabetes up to -78% with 30 years of follow-up,
- Published in *The Lancet*
- Virtually completely ignored by the medical and healthcare community

Hyppönen et al. *Lancet.* 2001 Nov

- o Vitamin D restores Treg:Th17 balance in patients with SLE (*Arthritis Res Ther* 2012 Oct[38]): Cholecalciferol 100,000 IU per week for 4 weeks followed by 100,000 IU of cholecalciferol per month for 6 months in 20 SLE patients with hypovitaminosis D resulted in increased serum 25(OH)D levels from 18 ng/mL to 51 ng/mL at 2 months and to 41 ng/mL. "Vitamin D was well tolerated and induced a preferential increase of naïve CD4+ T cells, an increase of regulatory T cells and a decrease of effector Th1 and Th17 cells. Vitamin D also induced a decrease of memory B cells and anti-DNA antibodies."

- Fatty acids—N3 fatty acids and GLA: N3 fatty acids and n6 GLA have shown the ability to reduce the biochemical and clinical manifestations of inflammatory and autoimmune diseases. At first (i.e., in the 1980s-1990s) we thought this was primarily mediated via enzyme and prostaglandin competition, and then later (> years 2000s) we added nutrigenomic and resolvin (et al) effects; by now (> year 2013) we are inclined to include Treg/Th17 modulation as a component of the effectiveness of CFAT—combination fatty acid therapy—via interaction with the human fatty acid receptors, which are all-to-commonly known by the popular and animal-specific (because this is where most basic science research is performed) name of PPAR—peroxisome proliferator-activated receptors. Students and clinicians can easily recall the relative specificity of fatty acids for PPARs by remembering that PPAR-*gamma* is activated by n6 *gamma*-linolenic acid, GLA, while EPA activates PPAR-alpha. Given then that PPAR-*gamma* is activated by *gamma*-linolenic acid, and given that PPAR-gamma activation promotes dendritic cells to produce retinoic acid (vitamin A) to induce Tregs[39], then a logical deduction is that GLA (especially with additional vitamin A, or—at the very least—a diet high in plant material for provision of beta-carotene) should help induce Treg for the control of inflammation/autoimmunity. Increased dietary intake of n3 fatty acids has been shown to reduce the incidence of autoimmune diabetes in humans, suggesting n3FA-mediated immunomodulation, not merely anti-inflammation.

- Infection/dysbiosis clearance: Gastrointestinal dysbiosis prompts formation of pro-inflammatory effector cells: Th1, Th2, Th17. Therefore, eliminating/reducing problematic microbes and promoting systemic eubiosis is important for inducing immunophenotype balance. I am particularly interested in and impressed by the role of segmented filamentous bacteria (SFB) in this regard (detailed in the section on dysbiosis in this book).

- Green tea: Green tea component EGCG induces Treg cells. Patients are recommended to have two cups per day and/or use standardized oral supplementation (caffeinated or decaffeinated).

- o Treg induction by green tea polyphenol EGCG (*Immunol Lett* 2011 Sep[40]): "Regulatory T cells (Treg) are critical in maintaining immune tolerance and suppressing autoimmunity. The transcription factor Foxp3 serves as a master switch that controls the development and function of Treg. Foxp3 expression is epigenetically regulated by DNA methylation, and DNA methyltransferase (DNMT) inhibitors can induce Foxp3 expression in naive CD4(+) T cells. We showed that EGCG, a major green tea polyphenol, could act as a dietary DNMT inhibitor, and induced Foxp3 and IL-10 expression in CD4(+) Jurkat T cells at physiologically relevant concentrations in vitro. We further showed that mice treated with EGCG in vivo had significantly increased Treg frequencies and

[38] Terrier et al. Restoration of regulatory and effector T cell balance and B cell homeostasis in systemic lupus erythematosus patients through vitamin D supplementation. *Arthritis Res Ther.* 2012 Oct 17;14(5):R221
[39] "Overall, our present results suggest that PPARγ ligation may be an important factor in stimulating DCs to produce RA and that the associated ability to enhance generation of iTregs may be one mechanism by which PPARγ ligands can ameliorate autoimmune diseases." Housley et al. PPARgamma regulates retinoic acid-mediated DC induction of Tregs. *J Leukoc Biol.* 2009 Aug;86(2):293-301
[40] Wong et al. Induction of regulatory T cells by green tea polyphenol EGCG. *Immunol Lett.* 2011 Sep 30;139(1-2):7-13

numbers in spleen and lymph nodes and had inhibited T cell response. Induction of Foxp3 expression correlated with a concomitant reduction in DNMT expression and a decrease in global DNA methylation. Our data suggested that EGCG can induce Foxp3 expression and increase Treg frequency via a novel epigenetic mechanism. ...the ability of dietary agents to target similar mechanisms offers opportunities for potentially sustained and longer-term exposures with lower toxicity [compared with drugs]."

o Green tea EGCG ameliorates obesity and autoinflammatory arthritis by altering T-cell balance (*Immunol Lett* 2014 Jan[41]): Paraphrasing the authors: Epigallocatechin-3-gallate (EGCG) is the most biologically active catechin in green tea and has therapeutic effects in autoinflammatory diseases and obesity. Obesity is an inflammatory condition because of the inflammatory cytokines and higher Th1 cell differentiation detected in both obese animals and humans. In this work using animal models of diet-induced obesity and obesity+RA, EGCG reduced the body weight and fat infiltration in liver tissue while improving serum lipid profiles in obese mice and induced a higher Treg/Th17 cell ratio in obese and obese+RA mice. "Thus, EGCG has an anti-inflammatory effect by suppressing STAT3 proteins and Th17-cell differentiation. EGCG thus shows promise for treating autoimmune conditions related to STAT3 or Th17 cells, such as metabolic syndrome, inflammatory arthritis, and some neoplastic diseases."

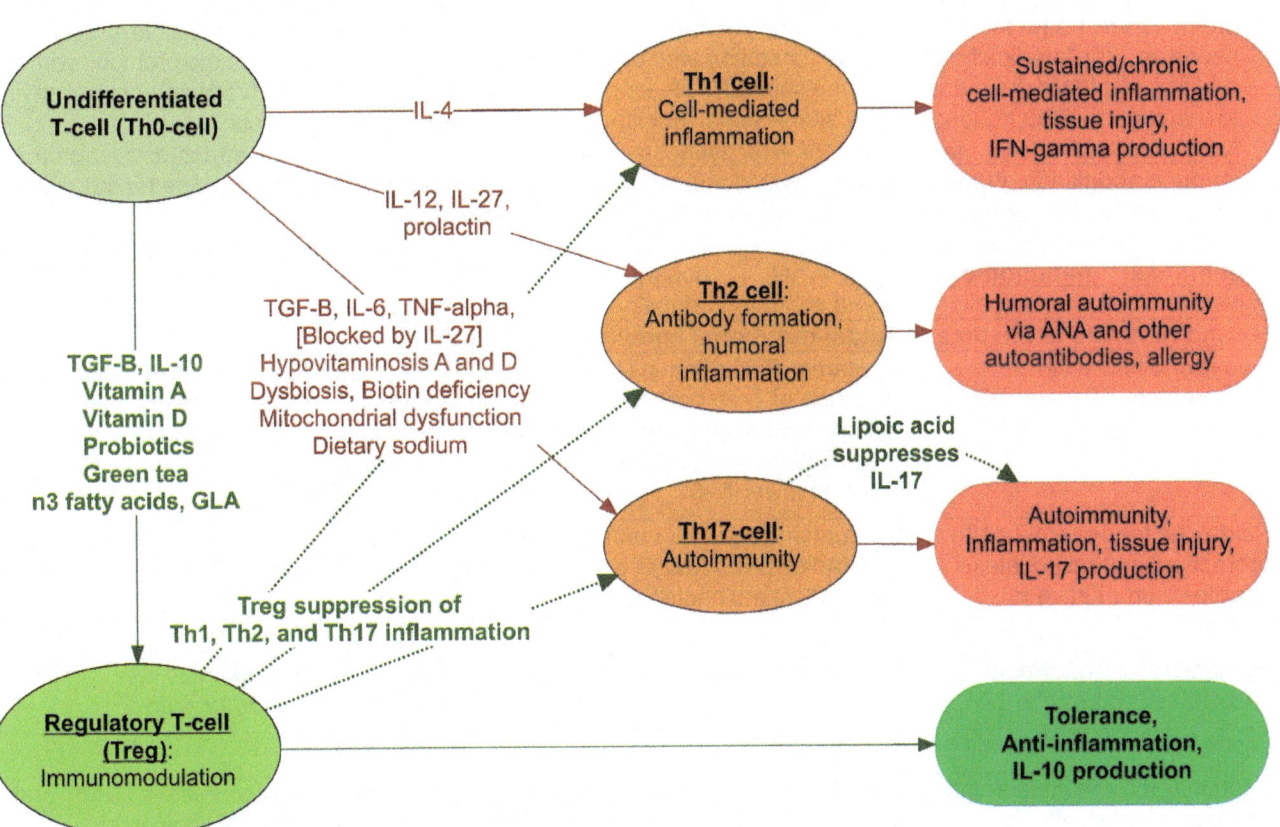

Nutritional immunomodulation of immunophenotype via induction of Treg phenotype: Specific nutrients and an anti-inflammatory milieu promote immune tolerance and avoidance of allergic, inflammatory, and autoimmune diseases by several mechanisms, including induction of Treg phenotype for suppression of Th-1/2/17 hyperactivity.

---

[41] Byun et al. Epigallocatechin-3-gallate ameliorates both obesity and autoinflammatory arthritis aggravated by obesity by altering the balance among CD4+ T-cell subsets. *Immunol Lett.* 2014 Jan-Feb;157(1-2):51-9

Case Report **Remarkable nutritional cure of ~18 years of untreatable psoriasis**: Paradoxically, many of us in the clinical nutrition field have been employing components of nutritional immunomodulation for many years without fully realizing the mechanisms behind the clinical benefits that we consistently observed. I recall the case of a young woman I treated in approximately 2003 for her then 18-year history of treatment-resistant full-body psoriasis; her recovery was so rapid and nearly complete that the case has always stood out in my memory. This case (included below) was published in print and on the internet in 2005 in the professional magazine *Nutritional Wellness*[42] in a discussion of my 5-part nutrition protocol (detailed in the previous section of this chapter); an updated version of the case is provided here:

- Case: This is an 18-year-old woman with head-to-toe psoriasis since childhood. She wears long pants and long-sleeved shirts year-round to conceal her skin lesions, and the psoriasis is a major interference to her social life. Palliative medications have ceased to help. I recall the first time that I saw this patient, I either thought to myself or said aloud, "This psoriasis looks like a second-degree burn" because the inflammation was pervasive, extremely red/erythematous, and had caused thickening of the skin.

- Treatment: The Paleo-Mediterranean diet[43] was implemented, with an emphasis on food allergy identification. We used a multivitamin-mineral supplement with 200 mcg selenium to compensate for the nutritional insufficiencies and selenium deficiency common in patients with psoriasis; likewise, 10 mg of folic acid was added to address the relative vitamin deficiencies and elevated homocysteine common in these patients.[44] Fish oil and GLA from borage oil was used for the anti-inflammatory and skin-healing benefits.[45] Vitamin E (1,200 IU of mixed tocopherols) and lipoic acid (1,000 mg per day) were added for their anti-inflammatory benefits and to combat the oxidative stress that is characteristic of psoriasis.[46] Of course, probiotics were used to modify gut flora, which is commonly deranged in patients with psoriasis.[47]

- Results: Within a few weeks, this patient's "lifelong psoriasis" was essentially gone. Food allergy identification and avoidance played a major role in the success of this case; in her case, the offending food was chicken broth. When I saw the patient again nine months later for her second visit, she had no visible evidence of psoriasis. Her "medically untreatable" condition was essentially cured by the use of my basic protocol, with the addition of a few extra nutrients. At the second visit—approximately 4-5 weeks after the first visit—I recall saying to the patient, "You no longer have skin lesions consistent with the diagnosis of psoriasis."

- New perspective and mechanisms of effectiveness: The success of this case was effected via nutritional immunomodulation. Without knowing I was doing so, I had implemented nearly a perfect recipe for induction of Treg cells for the endogenous suppression of pathogenic Th17-mediated inflammation.

Unintentional immunomodulation: What I thought was anti-inflammatory and antioxidant nutritional supplementation was actually nutritional immunomodulation

Rx and rationale at the time	Actual nutritional immunomodulation
Cod liver oil for anti-inflammatory EPA and DHA	❶ vitamin A, ❷ vitamin D, ❸ EPA and DHA in the cod liver oil stimulated induction of Treg cells to provide endogenous cell-mediated anti-inflammation; retinoic acid and vitamin D both inhibit pathogenic Th17 cells and promote Treg, and the effect is likely additive/synergistic, particularly given vitamin D's ability to lower IL-6.
Paleo diet for general health promotion, increased intake of potassium relative to sodium	Elimination of wheat, common allergens, and increased consumption of vegetables promoted ❹ anti-inflammatory climate and modified gastrointestinal bacteria; ❺ sodium avoidance.
Lipoic acid for antioxidant and anti-NFkB activity	❻ 35-50% reduction in IL-17; ❼ lipoic acid also helps to optimize mitochondrial function an effect which is expected to promote Treg.
Probiotics for global benefit	❽ Probiotics promote Treg.
Vitamin E for antioxidant/anti-inflammatory benefit	New data published in 2014 shows that alpha-tocopherol increases cAMP and thereby reduces IL-6 and IL-17 in a manner similar to that of lipoic acid.

[42] Vasquez A. Implementing the Five-Part Nutritional Wellness Protocol for the Treatment of Various Health Problems. *Nutritional Wellness* 2005 Nov

[43] Vasquez A. Revisiting the Five-Part Nutritional Wellness Protocol: The Supplemented Paleo-Mediterranean Diet. *Nutritional Perspectives* 2011 January

[44] Vanizor Kural B, et al. Plasma homocysteine and its relationships with atherothrombotic markers in psoriatic patients. *Clin Chim Acta* 2003;332(1-2):23-3.

[45] Vasquez A. New insights into fatty acid supplementation and its effect on eicosanoid production and genetic expression. *Nutritional Perspect* 2005: Jan: 5-16

[46] Kokcam I, Naziroglu M. Antioxidants and lipid peroxidation status in the blood of patients with psoriasis. *Clin Chim Acta* 1999;289(1-2):23-31

[47] Waldman A, et al. Incidence of Candida in psoriasis: a study on the fungal flora of psoriatic patients. *Mycoses* 2001;44(3-4):77-81.

Nutritional Immunomodulation: Induction of Treg at the expense/suppression of Th-1/2/17

1. Mitochondrial optimization

2. Biotin

3. E-vitamin

4. Sodium avoidance

5. Transgenic food avoidance

6. Probiotics

7. Lipoic acid

8. A-vitamin

9. Infection/dysbiosis clearance

10. D-vitamin

11. Fatty acids: EPA-DHA and GLA

12. IL-6 reduction: create overall antiinflammatory milieu for Treg induction

13. Green tea

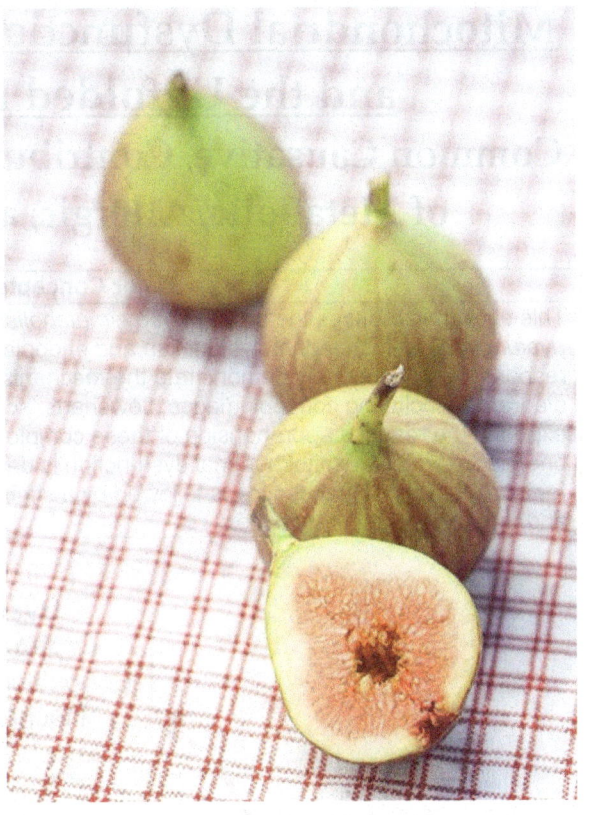

DrV's nutritional immunomodulation protocol: The new (as of Jun 2014) acronym is "My BEST PLAID FIG", as demonstrated above.

In 2015, following my review of the clinical data showing that NAC promotes immunotolerance in large part by inhibiting mTOR (or perhaps more accurately by dissociating mTOR from the underlying mitochondrial hyperpolarization) as shown in the very important study by Lai, Perl, and colleagues[48]—see my video review available online vimeo.com/123342139—I extended the acronym to what can be written as "Mi.B.E.S.T.P.L.A.I.D.F.I.G.iNaC" with the "iNaC" recalled by "in a can", with the latter representing N-acetyl-cysteine. Thus, in early 2015, the complete mnemonic was "My best plaid fig in a can."

In 2016, with increasing appreciation of the anti-inflammatory and immunomodulatory benefits of *Cannabis* generally and cannabidiol (CBD) specifically (along—of course—with the "entourage effect"—of other cannabinoids, especially [endogenous] agonists of cannabinoid receptor CB2[49]) and the noted immunomodulatory effect of increasing Treg and anti-inflammatory cytokines such as IL-10[50,51], I think that we as clinicians and researchers have an obligation to surpass the bias of indoctrination against *Cannabis* as I discussed in Chapter 3 and to appreciate that cannabinoids (whether endogenous, exogenous, or endogenous-potentiated-by-exogenous (see op cit footnote below) indeed show anti-inflammatory and immunomodulatory benefits for the immune system generally but also for the microglia in particular, thereby explaining the anti-seizure and neuroprotective benefits of cannabinoids. As such, "in a can" can represent both NAC along with the "can" representing cannabinoids. Thus, "my best plaid fig in a can" is the mnemonic for the acronym "Mi.B.E.S.T.P.L.A.I.D.F.I.G.NacCan."

---

[48] Lai et al. N-acetylcysteine reduces disease activity by blocking mammalian target of rapamycin in T cells from systemic lupus erythematosus patients: a randomized, double-blind, placebo-controlled trial. *Arthritis Rheum*. 2012 Sep;64(9):2937-46

[49] "CBD has little binding affinity to either the CB1 or CB2 cannabinoid receptors. Instead, CBD indirectly stimulates endogenous cannabinoid signaling by suppressing the enzyme fatty acid amide hydroxylase (FAAH)—the enzyme that breaks down anandamide, the first endocannabinoid discovered in the mammalian brain in 1992. ... CBD also stimulates the release of 2-AG, another endocannabinoid that activates both CB1 and CB2 receptor." projectcbd.org/how-cbd-works Accessed 2016 Mar.

[50] "The increase in IL-10 was confirmed by measuring IL-10 protein levels in MLR culture supernatants. Further, an increase in the percentage of regulatory T-cells (Tregs) was observed in MLR cultures." Robinson et al. A CB2-Selective Cannabinoid Suppresses T-Cell Activities and Increases Tregs and IL-10. *J Neuroimmune Pharmacol*. 2015 Jun;10(2):318-32

[51] Cabral et al. Turning Over a New Leaf: Cannabinoid and Endocannabinoid Modulation of Immune Function. *J Neuroimmune Pharmacol*. 2015 Jun;10(2):193-203

❹ Dysmetabolism & Dysfunctional Organelles: Mitochondrial Dysfunction; Endoplasmic Reticulum Stress and the Unfolded Protein Response; mTOR:

Common Causative, Contributing, and Consequential Components of Metabolic, Allergic, and Autoimmune Inflammation

---

Major Concepts in this Section—Overview

This section introduces the concept of *dysmetabolism* and then uses the best described components of *organelle dysfunction*—mitochondrial dysfunction and endoplasmic reticulum stress (and the consequent unfolded protein response)—to concretely demonstrate the mechanisms of and solutions to subcellular dysfunction. Numerous diagrams—including concept images, flowcharts, scanning electron micrographs—are provided to facilitate and expedite the reader's apprehension of these complex, important and ultimately simple clinical entities. Following the briefest introduction, mitochondrial dysfunction is described in sufficient clinical detail followed by a practical protocol for its remediation; that section is followed by a similar "problem and solution" review of endoplasmic reticulum stress and unfolded protein response.

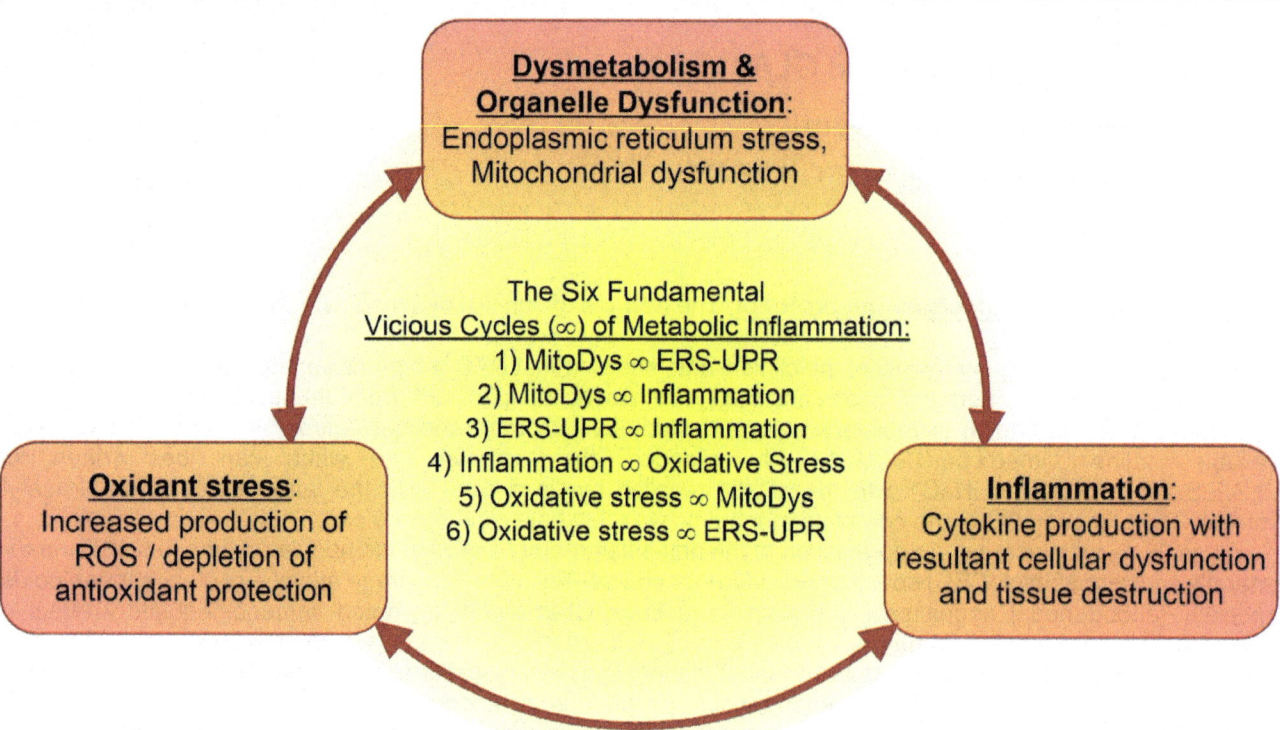

Conceptual diagram demonstrating the major components and vicious cycles of dysmetabolism, organelle dysfunction, and the inflammatory and oxidative consequences: This diagram allows us to appreciate the following vicious cycles, discussed in the text and respective citations:

1. Endoplasmic reticulum stress causes mitochondrial dysfunction, and mitochondrial dysfunction (MitoDys) causes endoplasmic reticulum stress (ERS).
2. MitoDys causes inflammation, and inflammation causes MitoDys.
3. ERS causes inflammation, and inflammation causes ERS.
4. Inflammation causes oxidative stress, and oxidative stress causes inflammation.
5. Oxidative stress causes MitoDys, and MitoDys causes oxidative stress.
6. Oxidative stress causes ERS, and ERS causes oxidative stress.

Major Concepts in this Section on Mitochondrial Dysfunction

Mitochondria do much more than simply produce ATP; they also sense and respond to nutritional status (not simply metabolize available carbon substrates), sense and respond to microbes, are vulnerable to the presence of bacteria and viruses, create reactive oxygen (ROS) and nitrogen species (RNS), are involved in the secretion and reception of insulin, and can promote inflammation and immune imbalance via elaboration of cytokines and Th-17 cells, respectively. Mitochondria are also key players in the determination of the timing and type of cell death, whether by apoptosis or necrosis. When mitochondria are functioning "normally" and "optimally", the various roles of mitochondria can be said to be mostly efficient and beneficent; however, when mitochondria become injured, impaired, or otherwise "dysfunctional" then the ATP-producing and other roles played by mitochondria are adversely affected to the detriment of the human host. The physiologic roles and consequences of dysfunction are outlined in the table below:

Physiologic roles of mitochondria	Consequences of mitochondrial dysfunction
1) Efficiently produce ATP	Inefficient production of ATP with reduced total output.
2) Sense and respond to microbes	Exaggerated response to microbes with inefficient and excessive immune and inflammatory responses.
3) Theoretically, mitochondria perform normal duties especially ATP production without regard for infectious disease status	Mitochondria can be destroyed by infectious agents, such as herpes simplex virus; other microbes and their products (such as bacterial endotoxin) cause mitochondrial dysfunction.
4) Create ROS and RNS as a side-effect of metabolism	Produce excessive ROS and RNS which leads to damage at four levels: 1) mitochondrial—e.g., mitochondrial inner membrane (MIM) and mitochondrial DNA, 2) cellular—e.g., nuclear DNA, 3) tissue—e.g., substantia nigra in Parkinson's disease, 4) systemic—e.g., measureable alterations in oxidative markers, such as TBARS and GSH. Note that oxidative damage to the MIM causes increased oxidant production via dysfunction of the ETC, thereby creating a vicious cycle.
5) Secretion and reception of insulin	Mitochondrial dysfunction contributes to the "diabetic phenotype of hyperglycemia" via impaired pancreatic secretion of insulin and also by impaired peripheral reception of insulin.
6) Normally, mitochondria should not have an appreciable or adverse effect on immune and inflammatory balance	Mitochondrial dysfunction in general and mitochondrial hyperpolariziation in particular promote increased production of inflammatory cytokines, cyclooxygenase, and Th-17 cells while retarding induction of Treg cells.
7) Mitochondrial-triggered apoptosis needs to be appropriately timed per cell.	An excess of apoptosis leads to premature tissue failure, while a failure of cell-killing and relative immortalization of cells contributes to autoimmunity and also cancer. Inflammatory cell death—necrosis—promotes additional inflammation via DAMP-receptor activation; this is noted as a consequence of mitochondrial dysfunction in autoimmune diseases such as SLE.

The three most classic characteristics of mitochondrial dysfunction are ❶ impaired ATP production: reduced efficiency and reduced amount of ATP production, ❷ increased free radical production, and ❸ increased inflammatory tendency, via chemical and enzymatic mediators (such as cytokines and cyclooxygenase, respectively) and cellular effectors (especially Th-17 cells). Given the consequences (introduced above) and high prevalence of mitochondrial disorders in routine outpatient clinical practice, physicians need to appreciate the practical, efficient, and effective, clinical means by which mitochondrial function can be restored, protected, and optimized.

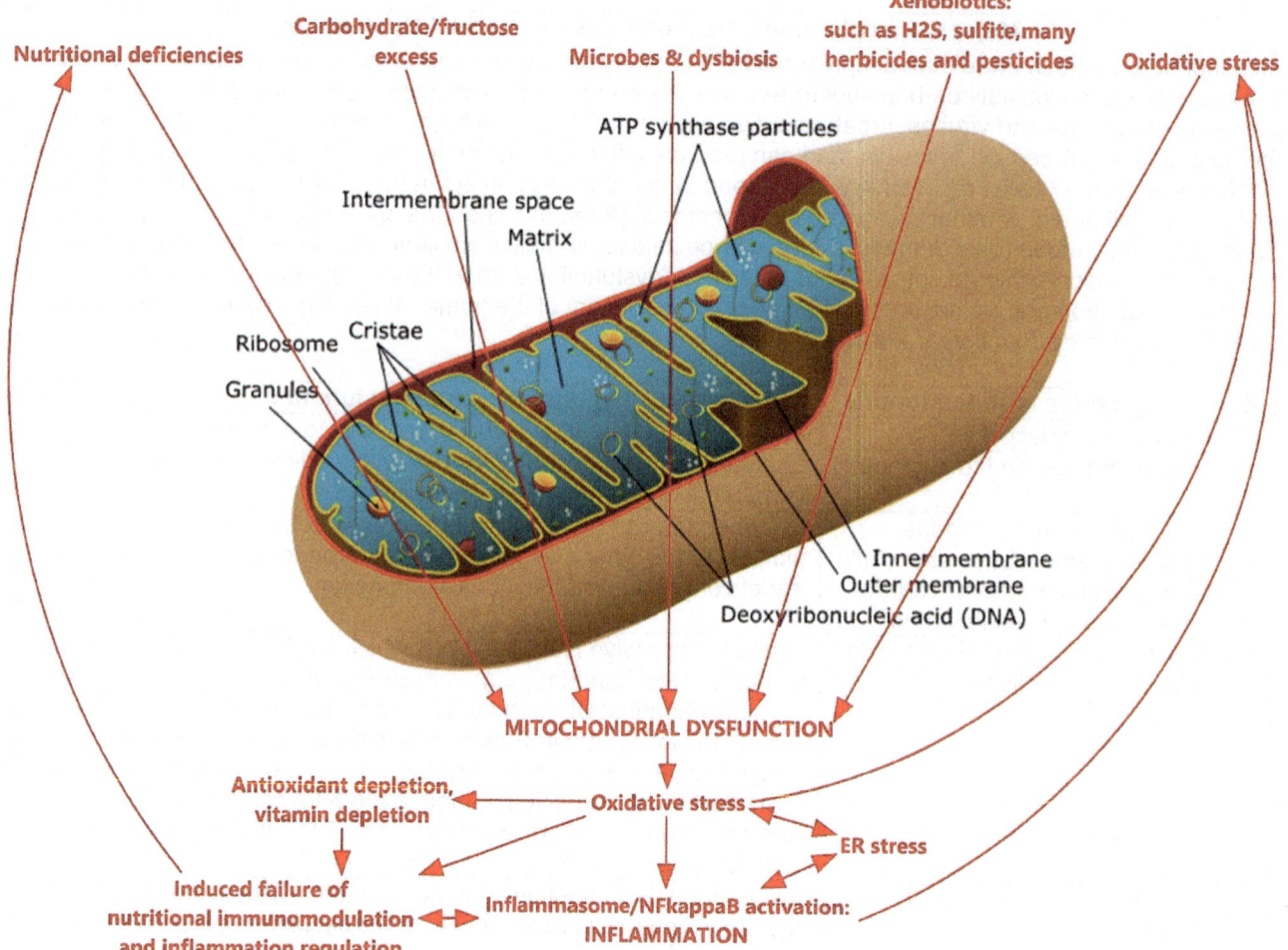

Nutritional deficiencies

Carbohydrate/fructose excess

Microbes & dysbiosis

Xenobiotics: such as H2S, sulfite, many herbicides and pesticides

Oxidative stress

ATP synthase particles

Intermembrane space

Matrix

Ribosome   Cristae

Granules

Inner membrane
Outer membrane
Deoxyribonucleic acid (DNA)

MITOCHONDRIAL DYSFUNCTION

Antioxidant depletion, vitamin depletion

Oxidative stress

ER stress

Induced failure of nutritional immunomodulation and inflammation regulation

Inflammasome/NFkappaB activation: INFLAMMATION

Schematic overview of mitochondrial dysfunction's major causes and consequences: Notice the presence of vicious cycles whereby cause becomes consequence, and then consequence becomes cause. Several dietary, nutritional, botanical, pharmaceutical/microbiologic, and sociopolitical interventions are obvious from the diagram.

Mitochondria—Re-Introduction and New Perspectives:

- Production of cellular energy in the form of ATP: Mitochondria are organelles ("small organs") within each cell that produce the majority of cellular energy for biochemical reactions and cellular processes. The primary fuel used by cells of the body is ATP—adenosine triphosphate. Everyone who has studied mitochondria—ranging from high-school and undergraduate students of Biology all the way to doctorate-level medical/healthcare professionals—is familiar with the fact that mitochondria make ATP; in fact, for most people, whether they are general public or doctors, this is all they know about mitochondria. New research, however, has shown us that mitochondria have many roles in addition to their ability to produce cellular energy. Most importantly, mitochondria are now known to play important roles in perpetuating chronic inflammation, responding to microbial infections, triggering of cell death, and controlling various metabolic processes.[1,2]

- Perpetuation of chronic inflammation: Most relevant to the focus of this work on clinical conditions related to inflammation is the fact that mitochondria have the ability to trigger inflammatory responses via activation of the nuclear transcription factor kappa-B (NFkB). Transcription factors are intracellular molecules that bind to the genetic material (DNA) in the nucleus of the cell to influence the activation or transcription of specific genes; in this case the transcription factor kappaB is most notorious for its activation of genes that promote inflammatory responses—necessary for short-term responses to injury or infection, but harmful when protracted and nonspecific. In this way, certain types of mitochondrial stimulation/activation/dysfunction can

[1] Pieczenik SR, Neustadt J. Mitochondrial dysfunction and molecular pathways of disease. *Exp Mol Pathol*. 2007 Aug;83(1):84-92
[2] Green DR, Galluzzi L, Kroemer G. Mitochondria and the autophagy-inflammation-cell death axis in organismal aging. *Science*. 2011 Aug 26;333(6046):1109-12

contribute to "chronic inflammation"; conversely, interventions that restore/improve proper mitochondrial function have generally been shown to provide anti-inflammatory benefits.

- <u>Responsiveness to microbial infections</u>: Very interestingly, mitochondria have the ability to sense and respond to microbial infections, particularly infections due to viruses and Gram-negative bacteria. This may be related to the evolutionary origin of mitochondria, which is generally perceived to be that of aerobic bacteria that formed a symbiotic intercellular relationship with eukaryotic cells; the primitive bacteria would have needed the ability to respond to stresses in its environment, particularly potential invasion by or competition from infectious agents.

- <u>Triggering of cell death via apoptosis and/or necrosis</u>: Mitochondria are known to play a dual role in relation to a particular form of cell death called "apoptosis" which can be thought of as a peaceful/programmed/noninflammatory death of a cell (in contrast to "necrosis" which is inflammatory cellular death, and "autoschizis" which is cellular self-destruction through progressive fragmentation such as seen in cancer cells, for example, following administration of vitamins C and K3[3]). Mitochondria have a two-part function, either promoting or resisting cell death; stated more simply and clearly: mitochondria play a role in keeping healthy cells alive, while promoting the death/apoptosis of unhealthy/dysfunctional/malignant cells. Mitochondrial dysfunction, as should be expected, impairs normal function and thus leads to the opposite of what we normally expect from mitochondria. In mitochondrial dysfunction, instead of promoting the death of dysfunctional cells, these cells become immortal and resistant to death; examples of this are autoreactive cells and cancer cells, which should have been "killed off" by apoptosis before being allowed to accumulate to such an extent that they cause harm to the host, either by autoimmunity or malignancy, respectively. In mitochondrial dysfunction, instead of keeping healthy cells alive, mitochondria promote the death of otherwise healthy cells; e.g., the loss of neurons that help control movement or which contribute to learning and thinking, thus resulting in Parkinson's disease or Alzheimer's disease, respectively.

- <u>Contribution to control of various metabolic processes</u>: Mitochondria play an integral role in several physiologic processes, including blood pressure control and blood glucose control. The release of insulin from the beta-cells in the pancreas is triggered by a cascade of events beginning with elevated levels of blood glucose and resulting in the entry of calcium into these cells with subsequent release of insulin into the blood; thus, mitochondrial dysfunction results in impaired pancreatic responsiveness to elevated glucose levels, thereby contributing to the complex condition we know as type-2 diabetes mellitus. Mild impairment of muscle contractility in the heart, which can be due to mitochondrial dysfunction and nutrient deficiencies/imbalances, leads to reduced heart function, which causes reflex activation of the sympathetic nervous system—the "panic response" of the nervous system that causes the "fight or flight" phenomenon. Chronic low-level activation of the sympathetic nervous system promotes several adverse effects associated with stress/fight/flight/panic, including elevated blood pressure (hypertension), activation of the renin-aldosterone system (water retention), vasoconstriction (reduced peripheral circulation) and hypercoagulability (promotion of blood clots, thrombosis). Natural treatments that restore or support mitochondrial function generally lower blood pressure in hypertensives, reduce blood glucose levels in diabetics, and reduce markers of inflammation in healthy patients as well as patients with inflammatory diseases; these examples will be further detailed throughout the multivolume textbook of *Inflammation Mastery* starting in 2014.

An accurate contemporary understanding of mitochondria in clinical medicine requires ❶ an updated conceptual appreciation of the roles of mitochondria in normal physiology and the consequences of mitochondrial dysfunction and the implications for various diagnoses and disease states, ❷ a "detailed familiarity" with ATP-producing processes and pathways, of which five are most important: 1) glycolysis, 2) pyruvate dehydrogenase, 3) Krebs cycle, citric acid cycle, 4) electron transport chain, and 5) alternate fuel (e.g., fructose, ketones, fatty acids, amino acids, ethanol) inputs into glycolysis and the citric acid cycle, and ❸ knowledge about how to improve/restore/optimize mitochondrial function—a customizable clinical strategy.

---

[3] Lasalvia-Prisco et al. Serum markers variation consistent with autoschizis induced by ascorbic acid-menadione in patients with prostate cancer. *Med Oncol*. 2003;20(1):45-52

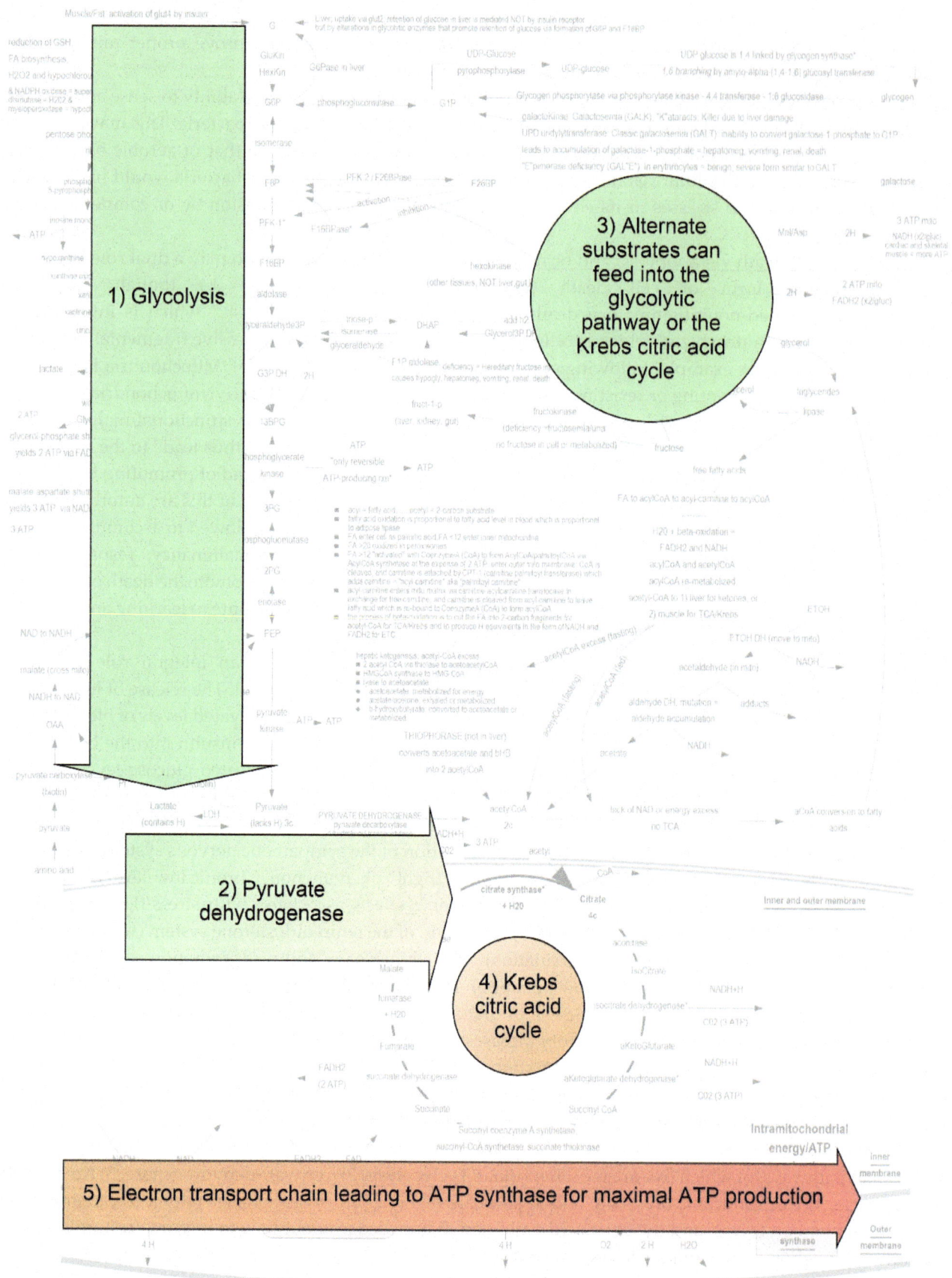

Conceptual overview of 1) glycolysis, 2) PDH complex, 3) the accessory pathways, 4) Krebs' citric acid cycle, and 5) electron transport chain: Clinical implications are discussed in the text.

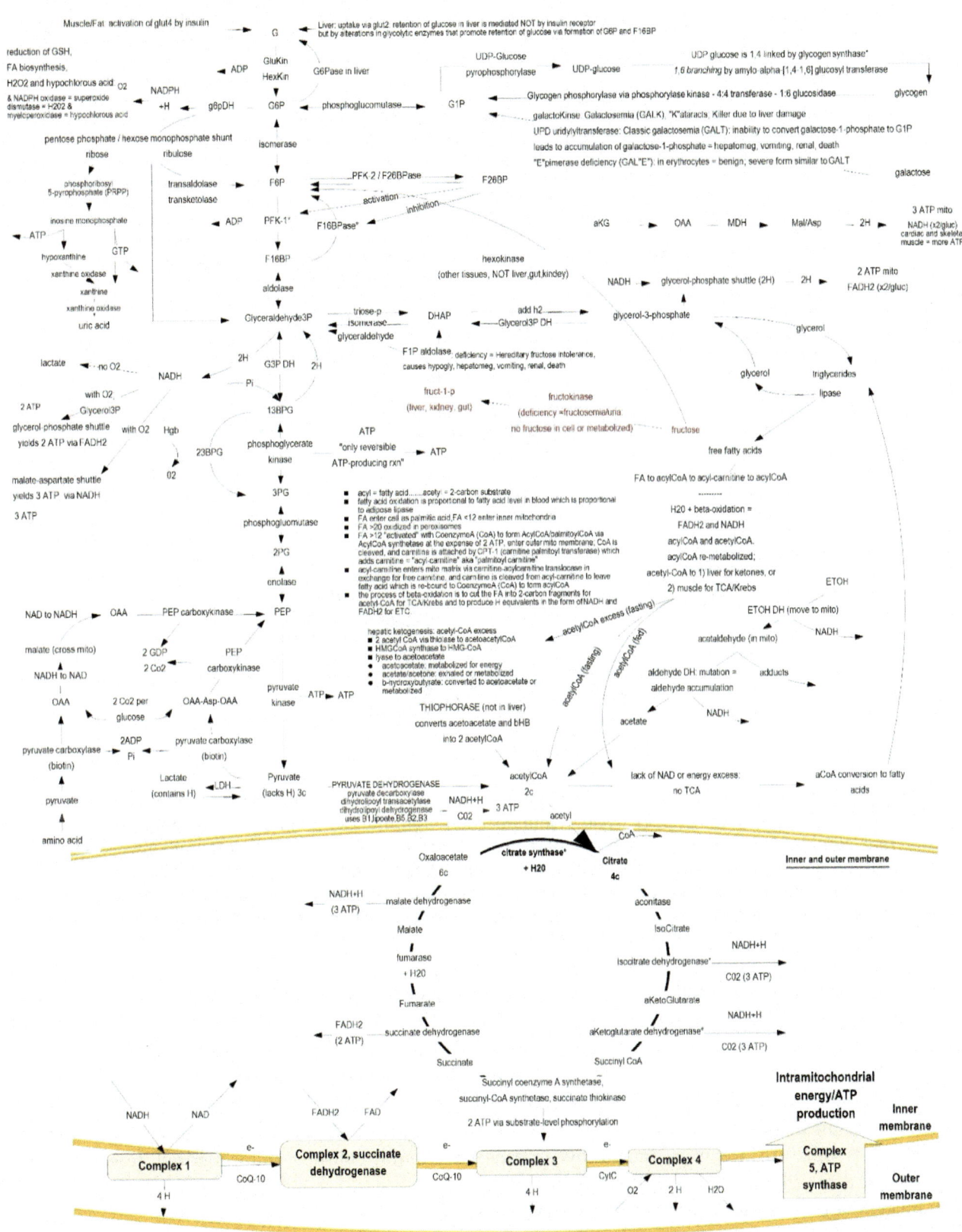

Detailed overview of glycolysis, pyruvate dehydrogenase complex, accessory input pathways, Krebs' cycle, and ETC: Note that the entry of fructose into the pathway via fructokinase to produce fructose-1-phosphate (colored in red) costs ATP, and thereby overconsumption of fructose—most obviously and specifically in the form of high-fructose corn syrup—causes ATP depletion with resultant metabolic and inflammatory consequences which promote insulin resistance and hypertension. These and other clinical implications are discussed in the text.

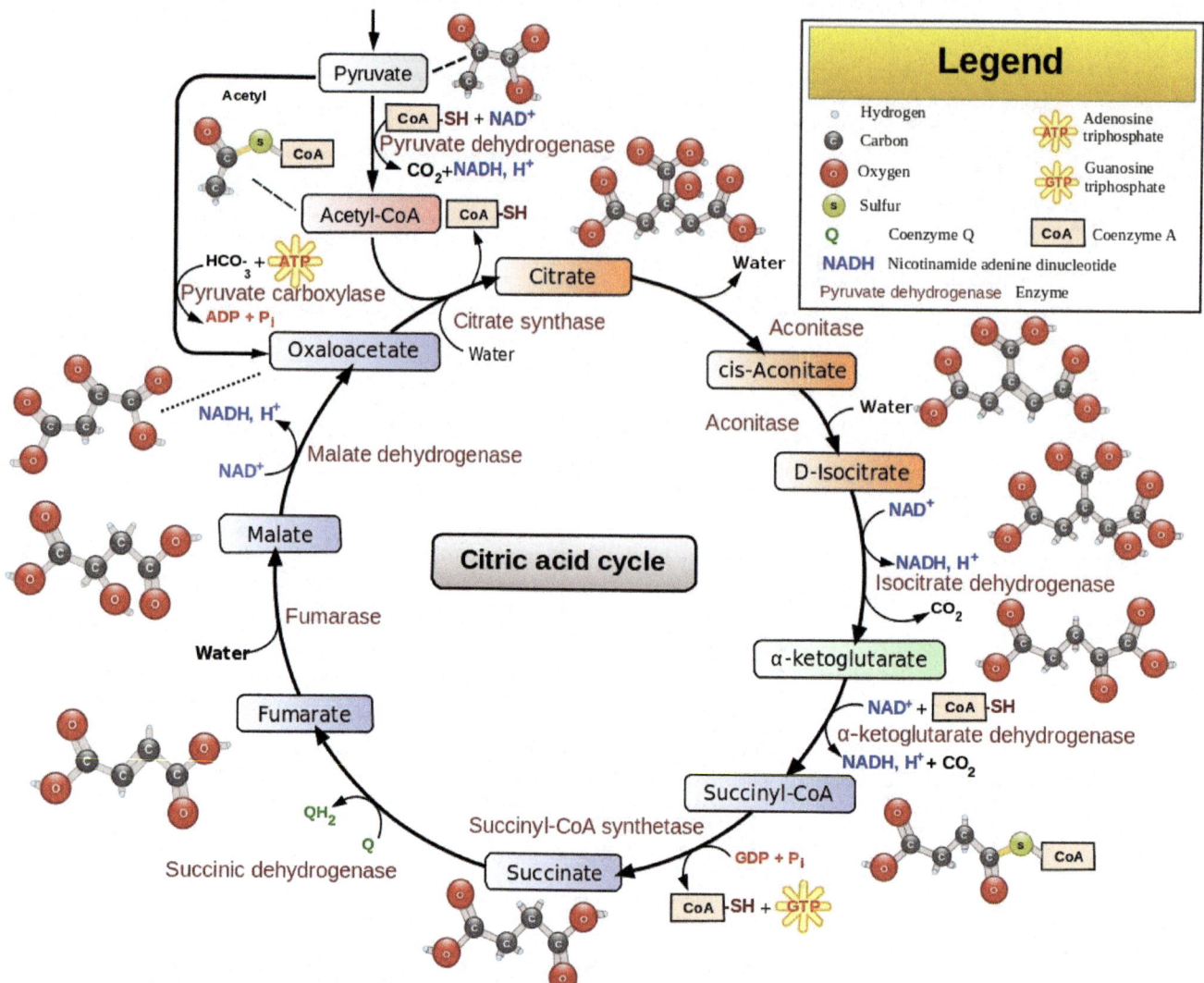

Krebs cycle, citric acid cycle: Excellent review diagram respectfully used from and credited to the open-access resource en.wikipedia.org/wiki/Citric_acid_cycle.[4] Note per the diagram (colored in blue) the importance of vitamin B3—niacin/niacinamide. Not depicted here but of particular importance is the input of glutamate via conversion by glutamate dehydrogenase into alpha-ketoglutarate; of high clinical relevance is the inhibition of glutamate dehydrogenase by (dietary) sulfite, which results in a massive reduction in ATP production and helps explain the migraine-generating and inflammation-exacerbating effect of dietary sulfites in susceptible persons, particularly those with primary and secondary mitochondrial defects.

<u>**Krebs cycle enzymes, with a (partial) listing of cofactors and other comments and considerations**</u>:

- **Pyruvate dehydrogenase (complex)**: This is not a single enzyme but rather an "enzyme complex" with several subunits, each with its own nutritional cofactor. Vitamin B1 (thiamine pyrophosphate): pyruvate dehydrogenase subunit requires B1. Lipoic acid: dihydrolipoyl transacetylase subunit requires lipoic acid. Vitamin B2: dihydrolipoyl dehydrogenase subunit requires B2 and B3; also, B2 is needed for formation of NADH. Vitamin B3: dihydrolipoyl dehydrogenase subunit requires B2 and B3. Vitamin B5 (?): In medical school (class of 2010) we were taught by a respectable/multipublished mitochondrial researcher that pantothenic acid—vitamin B5—was also required for this step.
- **Citrate synthase**: Irreversible reaction. [no coenzyme noted]
- **Aconitase**: Isomeration reaction. [no coenzyme noted]

---

[4] "Citric acid cycle with aconitate 2" by Narayanese, WikiUserPedia, YassineMrabet, TotoBaggins - biocyc.org/META/NEW-IMAGE?type=PATHWAY&object=TCA. Image adapted from :Image:Citric acid cycle noi.svg(uploaded to Commons by wadester16). Licensed under Creative Commons Attribution-Share Alike 3.0 via Wikimedia Commons - commons.wikimedia.org/wiki/File:Citric_acid_cycle_with_aconitate_2.svg#mediaviewer/File:Citric_acid_cycle_with_aconitate_2.svg.

- **Isocitrate dehydrogenase**: Vitamin B3: conversion of isocitrate to oxalosuccinate produces NADH. Magnesium or manganese[5]
- **Alpha-ketoglutarate dehydrogenase (complex), oxoglutarate dehydrogenase (complex)**: Vitamin B3: produces NADH, Vitamin B1 (thiamine pyrophosphate): oxoglutarate dehydrogenase, Lipoic acid: dihydrolipoyl succinyltransferase, Vitamin B2: dihydrolipoyl dehydrogenase subunit requires; also, B2 is needed for formation of NADH. *Comment*: This is not a single enzyme but rather an "enzyme complex" with several subunits, each with its own nutritional cofactor; one of the main end-products is the formation of NADH from B3. Glutamate is converted to alpha-ketoglutarate by glutamate dehydrogenase, which is blocked by sulfite, which is itself derived from certain foods and medications and which can also be chelated by hydroxocobalamin; excess sulfite impairs formation of alpha-ketoglutarate and can reduce ATP production by more than 50%.[6]
- **Succinyl-CoA synthetase**: [no coenzyme noted]
- **Succinate dehydrogenase, succinate-coenzyme Q reductase, Complex 2 of the ETC**: This is a complex enzyme with several subunits. Uses oxidized CoQ-10 in the form of ubiquinone to form the reduced form ubiquinol. This is the only enzyme complex that participates in both the citric acid cycle and the electron transport chain. CoQ-10: enzyme binds directly with CoQ-10, Vitamin B2: a flavoprotein is part of the enzyme's structure, Iron: an iron-sulfur protein is part of the enzyme's structure, Cardiolipin (containing the fatty acid DHA) and phosphatidylethanolamine (which can contain DHA, arachidonic acid, and/or oleic acid) are components of two hydrophobic membrane anchor subunits.
- **Fumarase**: Vitamin B3: produces NADH; however, the enzyme itself appears to function without cofactors or coenzymes.
- **Malate dehydrogenase**: Vitamin B3: produces NADH

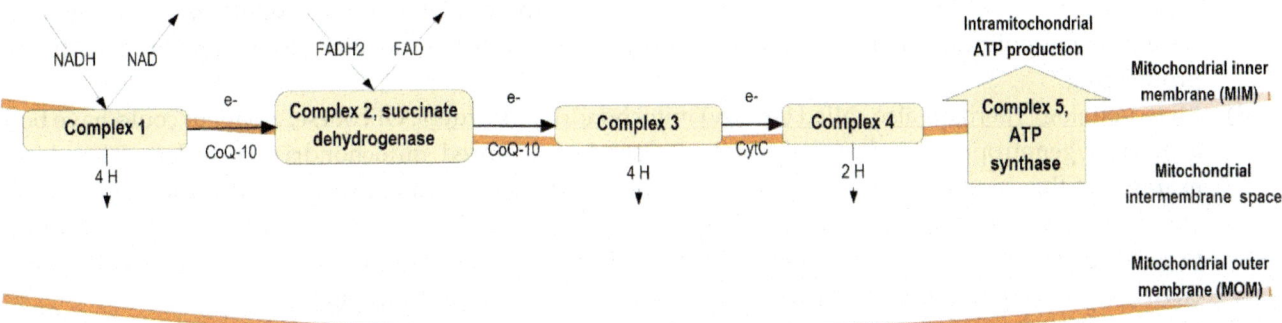

Electron transport chain (ETC) structure, with additional emphasis on the "nonstructure" of the innermembrane space created by the inner and outer mitochondrial membranes, permeability of both of which must be tightly regulated for optimal mitochondrial performance, including but not limited to ATP production: The semi-contained mitochondrial intermembrane space allows the accumulation of protons from the electron transport chain (ETC) to concentrate into a "pressurized" electromechanical gradient that powers ETC Complex #5, also called ATP synthase. ATP synthase is powered via the transmittal of protons from their high concentration gradient in the intermembrane space through the structure of the ATP synthase enzyme, which acts as a "pore" or "pressure valve" allowing protons to move to an area of lesser concentration inside the mitochondria. If the ATP synthase enzyme is bypassed due to a defective or "leaky" inner membrane that allows protons to leak back into the mitochondria, then the production of cellular energy will be reduced, leading to metabolic impairments such as increased free radical production (as the ETC works harder to compensate for reduced efficiency) and clinical manifestations such as fatigue, dyscognition, and muscle (e.g., heart) impairment including body aches and pains consistent with clinical presentations of fibromyalgia and chronic fatigue syndrome. Transmembrane potential of the mitochondrial inner membrane (MIM) is essential for the electromechanical gradient that drives ATP synthase; compromise of this membrane due to dietary faults (e.g., fatty acid deficiency, antioxidant deficiency) or biochemical faults (e.g., overproduction of free radicals which damage the MIM) will lead to hyperpermeability of the MIM ("leaky mitochondria") and reduced ATP synthesis. Clinical implications and interventions are discussed in the text; most of the clinical work with regard to nutritional optimization of the MIM has been led by Professor Garth Nicolson PhD.

---

[5] en.wikipedia.org/wiki/Isocitrate_dehydrogenase#Detailed_mechanism Accessed April 2012
[6] "Intracellular ATP measured 3 h later was significantly depleted by 100 μM sulfite, with about 50–60% decrease in both [neural and hepatic] cell lines." Zhang X, Vincent AS, Halliwell B, Wong KP. A mechanism of sulfite neurotoxicity: direct inhibition of glutamate dehydrogenase. *J Biol Chem.* 2004 Oct 8;279(41):43035-45

A Practical, Cost-Effective, Safe, Ethical Clinical Approach to Improving Mitochondrial Function—DrV's Strategy Suitable for Most Cases of Mitochondrial Dysfunction Seen in General Outpatient Practice

Mitochondrial disorders can be categorized based on the underlying etiology or combination of etiologies:

1) <u>Primary/genotropic mitochondrial disorders</u>: These can range from mild to severe, from occult to life-threatening, and although usually apparent in infancy-childhood, these primary/genotropic disorders can present later in adult life. Manifestations can be generalized affecting multiple organ systems or specific to one system—most commonly either the heart or central nervous system. Due to their rarity, severity, and need for specialist management, these primary/genotropic disorders are not the focus of the following section, although much of the information will be relevant, and conceptually and clinically applicable. For example, the rather common *and notably mild* primary/genotropic mitochondrial disorders associated with migraine headaches are a clear example of a heritable/primary/genotropic mitochondriopathy that responds very well to the interventions described below, especially nutrients that support the electron transport chain (ETC), namely coenzyme Q10 (CoQ-10), riboflavin, magnesium as discussed and cited below. In the main, primary/genotropic mitochondrial disorders are relatively rare.

2) <u>Secondary/acquired mitochondrial disorders</u>: Mitochondrial performance can be severely impaired by secondary/acquired conditions, such as exposure to certain pharmaceutical drugs, toxic industrial chemicals, toxic metals, and bacterial or viral infections; these types of mitochondrial disorders have been previously underappreciated but are progressively gaining a foothold in the consciousness of researchers and clinicians worldwide. These secondary/acquired mitochondrial disorders can affect anyone at any time. The clinical strategy for these conditions should be obvious, focusing on the support of optimal mitochondrial function (outlined below) while eliminating the problematic infection and/or toxic exposure (customized per patient's exposure). Importantly, secondary/acquired mitochondrial disorders are increasingly recognized as common (as more physicians become aware of the clinical frequency and implications of mitochondrial dysfunction) and are becoming more common (as our environment becomes more polluted with herbicides, pesticides, and other persistent organic pollutants as a result of governmental-political failure to regulate industry and protect humanity from unfettered corporate profiteering.

3) <u>Mixed-etiology (perhaps also called tertiary) mitochondrial disorders</u>: Of course, a patient could have both a primary/genotropic disorder along with a secondary/acquired mitochondrial disorder. The classic example of this combination is migranogenic mitochondrial impairment (primary disorder) exacerbated by one or more secondary disorders such as microbial colonization, a pro-inflammatory diet, or nutrient (e.g., magnesium) deficiency; this model helps explain—and place into perspective—the hereditary and environmental contributions to such mixed-etiology mitochondrial disorders.

When possible, the cause of the mitochondrial dysfunction should be treated directly; however, in practical reality of clinical practice, we often have to use an empirical and eclectic approach. Note that eclecticism and empiricism are not the same as random and illogical; even when using an empirical and eclectic approach, we clinicians can choose among the more efficacious and applicable interventions per research and nuances of patient history and assessment. For more complicated or severe cases, we can use laboratory assessments, depending on the problem suspected clinically; however, more skilled and experienced clinicians tend to find that laboratory tests for the assessment of mitochondrial function are not needed on a routine basis. On the contrary, the vast majority of mitochondrial dysfunction observed or suspected in routine outpatient clinical practice can be treated without mitochondria-specific, time-consuming, resource-depleting, and treatment-delaying laboratory assessments.

<u>**Understanding mitochondrial function for clinical intervention**</u>: As a group of intracellular organelles numbering from—for example, and not including the zero per erythrocyte—200 per cell in the biceps to 3,500 per cardiomyocyte, **mitochondria are a heterogeneous group**, populated by those with a theoretical optimal performance ("Olympians") down to those with cell-threatening and body-damaging effects ("misfits"). The mitochondrial population must therefore be occasionally culled for the health of the cell and of the larger organism.[7] Generally, the interconnected eliminative and regenerative processes can be described with the following terminology; additional terms are also listed here for convenience.

1) <u>Fusion</u>: The binding of two mitochondria into one single mitochondria,

2) <u>Reallocation/partitioning</u>: The redistribution of "better" and "worse" mitochondrial components into regions that will eventually split to generate progeny.

3) <u>Fission</u>: The splitting of the large mitochondrion into two daughter mitochondria: 90% of the time, both offspring will be sufficiently healthy and will have benefitted from the reallocation of genetic and structural material, while approximately 10% of the time, one mitochondrion will have received the better components and thus has significantly improved function, and the other ("the runt") will have been allocated a disproportionate share of the damaged/expended/oxidized mitochondrial goods and will therefore have severely impaired function, which targets it for destruction via mitophagy.

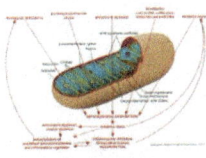
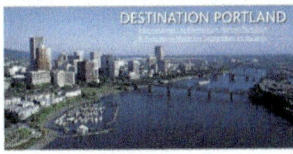
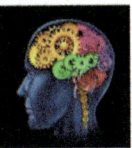

2013 INTERNATIONAL CONFERENCE ON HUMAN NUTRITION AND FUNCTIONAL MEDICINE
PORTLAND OREGON CONVENTION CENTER • SEPTEMBER 25-29, 2013

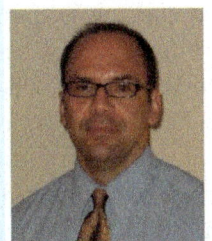

Mitochondrial Nutrition *and Beyond*:
Mitochondrial Optimization for Optimal Health

▸ **Brief introduction and review**

▸ **Mitochondrial interventions**

Alex Vasquez D.C., N.D., D.O., F.A.C.N.

4) <u>Mitophagy/autophagy</u>: Targeted destruction of dysfunctional mitochondria; this can occur following the fusion-fission cycle or likely—in the case of a severely dysfunctional *misfit* mitochondria—directly, i.e., without preceding fusion and fission. Although

2013 presentation and slides:
- Presentation slides: CreateSpace.com/4478800
- Video access: vimeo.com/ichnfm/2013mito-drv
- Password: DrV_mito_protocol2013
- Album access: vimeo.com/album/3033545
- Password: DrV_Mito_and_More

destruction/removal often has a negative connotation (perhaps mostly in Western cultures unconsciously dominated by the Greek-Roman "progressive and additional" Apollonian ideal without the balancing "regressive and subtractive" Dionysian construct), readers should appreciate that mitophagy is necessary for sustaining cellular and organismal health; defects in mitophagy are inconsistent with health and survival. As discussed below, **some significant benefits derived from carbohydrate restriction, fasting, and exercise are mediated by the promotion of mitophagy**, because mild cellular stresses prompt the fusion/fission/mitophagy process, which generally leads to enhanced health and performance of the remaining mitochondrial population, also referred to *en masse* as the "mitochondrial mass." Obviously, if mitophagy proceeds unchecked, then cells will lose the mitochondria's ability to form sufficient ATP and carry out other functions, and cell death will result. In sum: **Insufficient mitophagy promotes oxidative and inflammatory injury, while excess mitophagy leads to insufficient production of ATP and causes cell death and resultant tissue/organism failure**.

5) <u>Biogenesis</u>: Just as mitophagy can occur without a preceding fusion-fission cycle, so can fission; if a mitochondrion is a reasonably robust *Olympian* and if it is stimulated by intracellular signals indicating sufficient nutrients and need are present, it can split, accumulate nutrients, and grow, thus contributing directly to an enhanced mitochondrial population and expanded mitochondrial biomass.

---

[7] Twig G, et al. Mitochondrial fusion, fission and autophagy as a quality control axis: the bioenergetic view. *Biochimica et Biophysica Acta* 2008 May; 1777: 1092–1097

6) Δψm, MIM transmembrane potential (MIMtmp): MIM transmembrane potential (MIMtmp) is a quantification of proton concentration in the intermembrane space. For optimal mitochondrial performance, MIMtmp needs to be conceptually "in the middle"—neither too high nor too low.

- **Excess MIM transmembrane potential—mitochondrial hyperpolarization**—essentially turns off ETC flow and "shuts down" or "hibernates" the mitochondria, which is now resistant to triggering of apoptosis, thus promoting cell immortalization seen in cancer, autoimmunity, and vascular smooth muscle hyperproliferation: Excessive polarization of the transmembrane potential (MIM hyperpolarization, MIMhp) can be caused by LPS activation of TLR, and it can also be caused by immune activation itself, with the latter resulting in a vicious cycle because immune activation causes MIMhp which then triggers activation of mTOR, which promotes additional inflammation and autoimmunity as well as resistance to apoptosis, allowing autoreactive lymphocytes to evade deletion. While mitochondrial hyperpolarization impairs apoptosis, cell death via necrosis is enhanced, and this "inflammatory death" of immunocytes contributes to total inflammatory load since necrotic debris from cells and mitochondria activates damage associated molecular pattern (DAMP) receptors which promote inflammation. Clearly, and documented from different sources, mitochondrial hyperpolarization leads to mTOR activation as well as greatly increased ROS production; mTOR activation suppresses FoxP3 activation and thereby suppresses Treg generation while increased

  > **MIM hyperpolarization is characteristic of cancer and autoimmunity, with the latter secondary to mTOR activation and its inhibition of FoxP3+ Treg generation**
  >
  > - "Maximal hyperpolarization stalls respiration and oxidative phosphorylation, essentially "*shutting off mitochondria*" and shifting energy production to the cytoplasm, with glycolysis becoming the primary source of ATP. A glycolytic phenotype is associated with resistance to apoptosis, in part because the "inactive" hyperpolarized mitochondria cannot induce apoptosis. The majority of human cancers are characterized by hyperpolarized mitochondria, and this metabolic remodeling might be the basis of the Warburg effect in cancer."*
  > - "Mitochondrial hyperpolarization and the resultant ATP depletion sensitize T cells for necrosis, which may significantly contribute to inflammation in patients with SLE."**
  > - Mitochondrial hyperpolarization increases ROS production which activates Signal transducer and activator of transcription 3, also known as STAT3, a transcription factor essential for the differentiation of the TH17 helper T cells, which are implicated in a variety of autoimmune diseases.
  >
  > *Michelakis ED. Mitochondrial medicine: a new era in medicine. *Circulation*. 2008 May **Gergely et al. Mitochondrial hyperpolarization and ATP depletion in patients with SLE. *Arthritis Rheum*. 2002 Jan

  ROS promotes cellular dysfunction, enhanced cytokine elaboration, and necrotic therefore inflammatory death of T cells.[8] Also, ROS → activation of Stat3 transcription factor → activation of Th17 cells → autoimmunity (eg, lupus nephritis). By these mechanisms, mitochondrial hyperpolarization directly promotes autoimmune inflammation; notice that mitochondrial hyperpolarization drives Treg down and Th-17 upward, thereby specifically exacerbating this imbalance in favor of inflammation/allergy/autoimmunity.

- **Insufficient MIM transmembrane potential** "deflates" the proton gradient that is needed to drive ATP synthase; an excessive reduction triggers MTP-mediated apoptosis: A reduction in MIMtmp can be caused by 1) reduced Krebs' and/or ETC performance causing reduced proton generation, or by leakage of protons back through the MIM via 2) unregulated *basal* transmembrane permeability ("leaky mitochondria") due to oxidative damage to the MIM or dietary lack of appropriate fatty acids and phospholipids for MIM structure and maintenance, 3) heightened *augmented physiologic* channel-mediated transmembrane conductance via UPC (uncoupling proteins) or the dreaded MTP (mitochondrial transition pore) which is activated by reduced MIMtmp and leads to further rapid "deflating" of the mitochondria, spewing of apoptotic mediators to the cytoplasm and resultant cell death, 4) artificial *pharmacologic/xenobiotic* ionophore-mediated transmembrane conductance via substances such as salicylate and 2,4-dinitrophenol, and/or possibly 5) leakiness of the MOM, which is generally incompatible with mitochondrial and cell survival. **When MIMtmp is reduced by whatever**

---

[8] Perl A. Systems biology of lupus: mapping the impact of genomic and environmental factors on gene expression signatures, cellular signaling, metabolic pathways, hormonal and cytokine imbalance, and selecting targets for treatment. *Autoimmunity*. 2010 Feb;43(1):32-47

means, then ATP synthase's rotary catalysis of ATP production will be reduced, thus severely compromising the generation of cellular energy.

Conceptually and therefore practically, clinicians benefit from organizing information into categories that can then be subdivided into individual therapeutics; the three main categories of "interventional mitochondrial medicine" as I am defining it are ❶ therapeutic mitophagy—interventions which support therapeutic mitophagy such as carbohydrate/calorie restriction and physical exercise, ❷ mitochondrial support and stimulation—nutritional/phytonutritional support of biochemical processes (e.g., Krebs' cycle and ETC) and physiologic processes (e.g., biogenesis), and ❸ therapeutic disinhibition—removing the obstacles to mitochondrial performance such as xenobiotics and infections. Practically and respectively, these three steps are applied as 1) lifestyle, 2) supplementation, and 3) removal; skilled clinicians should be able to address each of these components simultaneously, prioritizing each particular treatment plan per the needs and responses of the patient. Students/clinicians implementing these protocols should already be familiar with dosing and administration and therefore such information is not included here; further, doses have to be modified per patient not simply based on age, weight, renal function, and (poly)pharmacy, but also per the level of need for and engagement with the overall treatment plan. With regard to the latter two considerations, the dose, duration, and variety of interventions is determined by severity of the illness(es) and the willingness vs resistance of the patient to do the whole program or simply a fewer parts of it. Indeed, doing every aspect of every component of the FINDSEX protocol would be prohibitively expensive and impractically time-consuming for most patients; here, physicians will have to guide patients to the most effective and necessary components of the protocol to customize the plan for the needs, abilities, and nuances of each patient.

❶ **Therapeutic mitophagy *via lifestyle*:** My concept of "therapeutic mitophagy" is this: the intentional induction/promotion of mitophagy—for either/both of the following: reduction in mitochondrial mass for a reduction in inflammatory signaling and oxidant production, and the "culling of the mitochondrial herd" to eliminate the lower-performing mitochondria. Carbohydrate restriction and moderate exercise are two safe and universally available and affordable means to therapeutically/intentionally induce mitophagy and achieve numerous anti-oxidant and anti-inflammatory benefits.

1. **Carbohydrate restriction/avoidance, fasting, ketogenic diet:**
   - Mitochondrial mechanism(s): High dietary loads of carbohydrates overwhelm the nonregulated enzymatic systems involved in substrate conversion, leading to what can be described as a short-term "mitochondrial burnout" due to excess subsequent free radical generation; evidence of this appears quite clear, with an irrefutable collection of data from human trials showing that 100g glucose leads to oxidative stress, antioxidant depletion, a measurable inflammatory response, and immune/phagocytic suppression. Conversely, carbohydrate restriction promotes mitochondrial function generally by allowing mitochondria to adapt to being fueled by a variety of sources (leading to structural reorganization of ETC supercomplex assembly[9]), rather than the "easy currency" and "quick fix" of carbohydrate; specifically, carbohydrate restriction promotes ketogenesis and resultant endogenous production of beta-hydroxy-butyrate (bHB) which stimulates complexes 3 and 4 of the ETC. Whereas consumption/provision of "simple" carbohydrates appears to overwhelm mitochondria and lead to oxidative stress and inflammation; carbohydrate avoidance and promotion of a mildly ketotic state have the opposite effects—anti-inflammatory and antioxidant benefits. The mild stress of caloric/carbohydrate restriction prompts a wide range of physiologic adaptations, one of which is mitophagy, which has the overall effect of reducing oxidant stress and pro-inflammatory signaling.
   - Clinical benefits: Carbohydrate avoidance—and its physiologic converse of ketogenesis promotion—demonstrates an unsurpassed cure rate of hypertension and diabetes mellitus type-2. Carbohydrate avoidance promotes endogenous antioxidant defenses, systemic anti-inflammation, longevity in multiple species, and a rejuvenative phenotype via—among several other means—histone acetylation.

---

[9] Lapuente-Brun et al. Supercomplex assembly determines electron flux in the mitochondrial electron transport chain. *Science.* 2013 Jun 28;340(6140):1567-70

2. **Exercise**:
   - <u>Mitochondrial mechanism(s)</u>: Improves oxygen delivery via vasodilation and increased cardiovascular output (heart rate × stroke volume). Promotes mito-availability of magnesium due to systemic alkalinization secondary to physiologic hyperventilation and resultant respiratory alkalosis; alkalinity promotes renal retention of magnesium and increases intracellular uptake of magnesium thereby increasing magnesium's availability to various enzymes, including the phosphorylating ATP synthase. The stress of exercise prompts a wide range of physiologic adaptations, one of which is mitophagy, which has the overall effect of reducing oxidant stress and pro-inflammatory signaling; exercise also promotes mitochondrial biogenesis and induction/upregulation of ATP-producing substrate-converting enzymes.
   - <u>Clinical benefits</u>: Weight loss, anti-inflammation via elaboration of myokines and via reduction in (visceral) adipose), enhanced insulin responsiveness via muscle uptake of glucose as well as increased elaboration of GLUT-4 receptors, reduced mental depression and psychological dependency, enhanced appearance and self-esteem, likely increased competence and intelligence via skill-building and exercise-induced neurogenesis assuming that one is in [has created for oneself] an environment conducive to intellectual optimization; obviously, this requires more than simply the provision of exercise for neurogenesis and synaptic plasticity; one must give these new neuroconnections something to ponder and perform.

❷ **Mitochondrial support *via supplementation***: Many interventions are available which serve to either support or stimulate mitochondrial function. Simply "stimulating" mitochondrial function would likely be a bad idea if a sizeable portion of the individual's mitochondrial population is dysfunctional; stimulating dysfunctional mitochondria would be expected to promote inflammation and oxidative stress. Clinicians should seek to—as we say in naturopathic medicine—*reestablish the foundation for* (mitochondrial) *health* before employing attempts at mitochondrial stimulation or interventions that promote biogenesis. Thus, in this second category, I will list—in somewhat of a prioritized sequence—those therapeutics which generally support and can later be used to optimize mitochondrial function generally and ATP production specifically. The prioritization of these is somewhat—but not entirely—conceptual; the actual "priority" is the one-many that will best benefit the individual patient.

3. **Five-Part Supplemented Paleo-Mediterranean Diet[10]**: **Plant-based protein-adequate organic diet supplemented with vitamins, minerals, fatty acids, and probiotics.**
   - <u>Mitochondrial mechanism(s)</u>: Vitamins (coenzymes) and minerals (cofactors) must be present in sufficient amounts in order for biochemical reactions to proceed with health-optimizing efficiency; nutritional deficiencies impair biochemical efficiency and initiate the progressive reductions in cellular function that initiates/promotes/mimics and contributes to various disease states. Most people are nutrient deficient and should take a multivitamin and multimineral supplement[11,12], and people with metabolic impairments such as those due to single nucleotide polymorphisms (SNPs) will need to use "high-dose vitamin therapy" for the duration of their lives in order to stimulate their variant enzymes[13] and—speaking casually—push sluggish enzymes to complete their reactions. More specifically, B1 (thiamine), B2 (riboflavin), B3 (niacin), B5 (pantothenate), and lipoic acid are required components for the pyruvate dehydrogenase complex[14] which transfers/converts pyruvate made in the cytoplasm into acetyl-CoA in the mitochondria. B2 is required for the formation of flavin adenine dinucleotide (FAD), and B3 is required for the formation of niacinamide adenine dinucleotide (NAD)—both of these constituents are absolutely required for mitochondrial production of ATP. Further, B2 is a cofactor for glutamate dehydrogenase which converts glutamate to alpha-ketoglutarate for use in the Krebs' cycle. Magnesium is required for phosphorylation reactions, e.g., phosphorylation of ADP to ATP by Complex 5—ATP synthase. Antioxidants, such as tocopherols in general (especially gamma) and tocopherol succinate in particular, help to protect oxidation-vulnerable phospholipids and nuclear and mitochondrial DNA. For general biochemical and antioxidant "support" of mitochondrial function, and for the prevention and

[10] Vasquez A. Revisiting the Five-Part Nutritional Wellness Protocol: The Suppplemented Paleo-Mediterranean Diet. *Nutritional Perspectives* 2011 Jan: 19-25
ichnfm.org/faculty/vasquez/pdf/vasquez_2011_five-part_protocol_revisited.pdf
[11] Fletcher RH, Fairfield KM. Vitamins for chronic disease prevention in adults: clinical applications. *JAMA*. 2002 Jun 19;287(23):3127-9
[12] Heaney RP. Long-latency deficiency disease: insights from calcium and vitamin D. *Am J Clin Nutr*. 2003 Nov;78(5):912-9
[13] Ames et al. High-dose vitamin therapy stimulates variant enzymes with decreased coenzyme binding affinity (increased K(m)). *Am J Clin Nutr*. 2002 Apr;75:616-58
[14] My source of information on this list of coenzymes is my professor in medical school at UNTHSC, Ladislav Dory PhD. I realize some might debate this list of cofactors; but likewise my professor—based on his intimate work with mitochondria—would likely refute those debates. So, I think this list is reasonable for purposes presented here.

treatment of mitochondrial disorders—regardless of cause—routine use of a high-quality broad-spectrum multivitamin and multimineral supplement is reasonable.

- Clinical benefits: B1 improves renal function in DM. B2 improves mood, especially in women, and doses of 400mg daily are remarkably effective for migraine prophylaxis with the most likely effect being mediated via improved function of ETC Complex #2. Vitamin B2 is also necessary conversion of vitamin B6 to its active form of pyridoxal-5-phosphate (P5P); conversion of pyridoxine to pyridoxine phosphate requires magnesium while oxidative conversion to pyridoxal requires riboflavin. B3 is also effective against migraine, perhaps partly via vasodilation, but more likely via stimulation of ETC Complex #1. The vitamin CoQ-10 is necessary for ETC Complexes #1-3. These and other nutrient-specific locations are illustrated in the diagram below of the ETC.

4. **Coenzyme-Q10**: CoQ-10 would have received better public acceptance if Folkers had named it "vitamin Q" instead of "coenzyme Q", per his own admission.

- Mitochondrial mechanism(s): Transfers electrons between complexes 1, 2, and 3. Functions as lipid-soluble antioxidant. Direct anti-inflammatory effect via inhibition of NFkB.
- Clinical benefits: The single most effective "vitamin" treatment for hypertension; alleviates hypertension and insulin resistance probably via improvement of mitochondrial function. Remarkably effective for migraine prophylaxis in adults and children; clinical benefits also shown for Parkinson's disease and Huntington's disease (delayed progression) and asthma (reduced medication dependency). The best nutritional treatment for renal insufficiency is CoQ-10 100-300mg/d and thiamine 100mg TID.

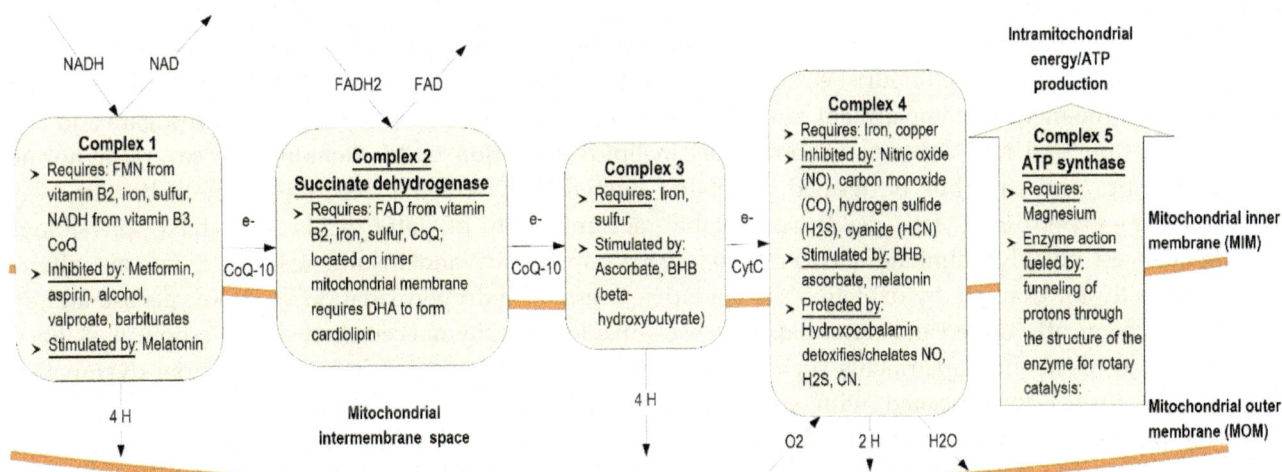

Reduce mitochondrial protein synthesis: Tetracyclines, chloramphenicol
Cause mtDNA depletion: Adriamycin/doxorubicin, zidovudine, herpes simplex virus

Electron transport chain (ETC) with some requirements, inhibitors, stimulators, and protectors: Clinical implications are obvious from the diagram and are additionally discussed in the text.

5. **"Vitamin E"**: What is meant here by "vitamin E" is mixed tocopherols with at least 40% gamma-tocopherol; additionally, alpha-tocopherol succinate has been described as being somewhat "mitochondria specific" and might be used alongside mixed tocopherols. A reasonable *supplemental* dose of tocopherols is 400 IU/d while a more assertive *interventional* dose is 1,200-1,600 IU/d.

- Mitochondrial mechanism(s): Generalized anti-inflammatory and anti-oxidant effects; specifically helps to protect cell membranes in general and mitochondrial membranes in particular.
- Clinical benefits: Anti-inflammatory and immune-modulating effects (e.g., reductions in IgE in patients with eczema, and reductions in ANA in patients with various autoimmune diseases). Alleviates pain in osteoarthritis; can help to restore/normalize mitochondrial function in patients with mitochondrial disease. Important experimental (not clinical) research published in 2013 by Salinthone et al[15] showed for the first time that (alpha) tocopherol raises cAMP and has a potent anti-inflammatory effect, with a notable maximal reduction of PHA-stimulated IL-17 production by 73-79% in human peripheral blood mononuclear cells

---

[15] Salinthone et al. α-Tocopherol stimulates cyclic AMP production in human peripheral mononuclear cells and alters immune function. *Mol Immunol*. 2013 Mar:173-8

(PBMC); of additional note and importance, the authors report their findings using various other nutrients on cAMP production, "cAMP levels were 7.56, 10.57, 14.23 and 5.21 pmol/mg protein for GSE, EGCG, ascorbic acid, and resveratrol, respectively. Conversely, treatment with α-tocopherol resulted in a greater than 2-fold increase in cAMP level (29.19 pmol/mg protein) compared to baseline. Lipoic acid was used as a positive control, which generated 45.49 pmol/mg protein of cAMP."

6. **Lipoic acid**:
   - Mitochondrial mechanism(s): Coenzyme for various enzymatic reactions, including pyruvate dehydrogenase. Water-soluble and lipid-soluble antioxidant. Anti-inflammatory benefits via direct inhibition of NFkB as well as via reductions in IL-17.
   - Clinical benefits: Diabetic neuropathy, hypertension, diabetes mellitus type-2. Per the work of Bruce Ames and based largely on animal studies, we note that lipoic acid and acetyl-L-carnitine function additively/synergistically and should generally be used together. Lipoic acid has a short half-life and should therefore be administered in divided doses throughout the day, e.g., 300-400mg TID-QID.

7. **L-carnitine and Acetyl-L-carnitine (the "carnitines"): 2-4 g/d**
   - Mitochondrial mechanism(s): L-carnitine is required for mitochondrial beta-oxidation of long-chain fatty acids for ATP production; long-chain fatty acids must be in the form of esters of L-carnitine (acylcarnitines) in order to enter the mitochondrial matrix where beta-oxidation occurs.[16] Carnitines also lessen the cellular load of ceramide—inhibition of ceramide-generating sphingomyelinase has been documented, and promotion of ceramide degradation is hypothesized—thereby improving cellular metabolic function and reducing the secondary inflammation.
   - Clinical pearl: One might reasonably wonder how/why supplementation with "carnitines" can be of benefit among patients who are well-nourished via dietary protein intake from animal sources; the answer is found in the fact that the metabolic impairment caused by the Westernized diet (notably high in both sugars and fats, especially saturated fats) leads to abnormalities in lipid deposition which demonstrate several abnormal characteristics and can thus be termed *metabolic dyslipidosis*, which I describe in the following way: *quantitative*—excess total fat, *qualitative*—notable accumulation of fatty acids that have physiologic consequences: notably palmitate and ceramide, *altered*—in obesity and insulin resistance, fats are altered biochemically for example by oxidation via oxidative stress or hydroperoxidation via lipoxygenase and are therefore chemically altered and abnormal, *locational*—inside parenchymal cells (not simply adipocytes) where they lead to metabolic impairments such as endoplasmic reticulum stress and mitochondrial dysfunction. Hence, in disorders associated with endoplasmic reticulum stress, mitochondrial dysfunction, insulin resistance, cardiomyopathy, and biological aging, supplemental carnitines can help rectify abnormal intracellular lipid accumulation/deposition via promotion of mitochondrial metabolism (beyond "fat burning" and more toward "trash burning") thereby alleviating part of the fuel overload problem that triggers metabolic impairment and its inflammatory consequences.
   - Clinical benefits of carnitine supplementation: Alzheimer's disease, hypertension, insulin resistance, Peyrone's disease, erectile dysfunction. Per Bruce Ames and based largely on animal studies, we note that lipoic acid and acetyl-L-carnitine function additively/synergistically and should be used together for optimal benefit.
     - In vitro study: L-carnitine prevents doxorubicin-induced apoptosis of cardiac myocytes via inhibition of ceramide generation (*FASEB J* 1999 Sep[17]): This study showed that L-carnitine blocked ceramide production via sphingomyelinase following metabolic stress induced by doxorubicin/Adriamycin. The authors wrote, "Moreover, in vitro studies conducted on cell extracts or with purified acid sphingomyelinase demonstrated that L-carnitine exerted a dose-dependent, sphingomyelinase inhibitory effect (through V(max) reduction). Taken together, these findings show that by inhibiting a (perhaps novel) drug-activated acid sphingomyelinase and ceramide generation, L-carnitine can prevent doxorubicin-induced apoptosis of cardiac myocytes."

---

[16] Linus Pauling Institute Micronutrient Information Center. L-Carnitine. lpi.oregonstate.edu/infocenter/othernuts/carnitine/
[17] Andrieu-Abadie N, et al. L-carnitine prevents doxorubicin-induced apoptosis of cardiac myocytes: role of inhibition of ceramide. *FASEB J*. 1999 Sep;13(12):1501-10

- o Clinical trial and proof of principle: Carnitines versus testosterone in the treatment of sexual dysfunction, depressed mood, and fatigue associated with male aging (*Urology* 2004 Apr[18]): 120 male ~66yo patients were randomized into three groups: 1) testosterone (undecanoate, oral) 160 mg/day, 2) propionyl-L-carnitine 2 g/day plus acetyl-L-carnitine 2 g/day, 3) placebo for 6 months. "Testosterone and carnitines significantly improved the peak systolic velocity, end-diastolic velocity, resistive index, nocturnal penile tumescence, International Index of Erectile Function score, Depression Melancholia Scale score, and fatigue scale score. Carnitines proved significantly more active than testosterone in improving nocturnal penile tumescence and International Index of Erectile Function score. Testosterone significantly increased the prostate volume and free and total testosterone levels and significantly lowered serum luteinizing hormone; carnitines did not. CONCLUSIONS: Testosterone and, especially, carnitines proved to be active drugs for the therapy of symptoms associated with male aging." Very importantly, all of the men in this study—per inclusion criteria—demonstrated decreased libido and erectile quality, depressed mood and intellectual concentration ability, irritability, fatigue, and free testosterone lower than 6 pg/mL (normal range 8.7 to 54.7 pg/mL); despite the fact that they were all fatigued, depressed, and hypogonadal, carnitines 4g/d proved more effective than testosterone. Of additional note, this article repeatedly and uniquely emphasized that "carnitines" serve, via promotion of acetyl groups into Krebs cycle, to enhance ATP production and reduce ROS production, e.g., "*Carnitines boost the increase and transport of acetyl groups, thereby enhancing Krebs cycle and aerobic metabolism*" and "*Carnitines restore [normalize] the ROS physiologic concentration by acting on the Krebs cycle.*" This study showed that partial restoration of metabolic function using two forms of L-carnitine 4g/d is clinically effective and in fact more effective than testosterone for improving mood and sexual health in elderly hypogonadal men.

> **Multiple benefits of carnitines**
>
> "In humans and experimental models, carnitines have several activities that might influence aging. Fatty acid peroxidation proved depleted, and **carnitines restored the phospholipid composition of mitochondrial membranes and enhanced the cellular energetics in mitochondria**, increasing cytoplasmic acetyl-coenzyme A concentrations through the higher availability of **acetyl** groups. In addition, **carnitines stabilized cell membrane fluidity by regulating phospholipid levels** and **reduced ceramide production and insulin-like growth factor**, preventing cellular death and apoptosis."
>
> Cavallini et al, *Urology* 2004 Apr

8. **Biotin: 2-10 mg/d (rarely up to 200 mg/d)**
   - Mitochondrial mechanism(s): The water-soluble nutrient biotin, generally classified as a B-complex vitamin, is required by all organisms but is synthesized only by "lower" organisms such as bacteria, yeast, molds, algae, and some plants; therefore, it is essential that humans have an adequate external source of the nutrient. Normal dietary intake of biotin is less than 97.5 microg (0.4 micromol); biotin absorption/bioavailability from oral administration is nearly 100% even with pharmacologic dosing[19] thus indicating that parenteral administration is largely unnecessary except in the rarest of cases. Biotin performs its biochemical functions via attachment to proteins (biotinylation) such as enzymes and histones; attachment occurs via holocarboxylase synthetase and release via biotinidase. Biotin is an enzyme cofactor for the following five enzymes: (1 and 2) *Acetyl-CoA carboxylase I and II* for binding bicarbonate to acetyl-CoA to form malonyl-CoA. Malonyl-CoA is required for the synthesis of fatty acids. The former is crucial in cytosolic fatty acid synthesis, and the latter functions in regulating mitochondrial fatty acid oxidation. (3) *Pyruvate carboxylase* for gluconeogenesis, (4) *Methylcrotonyl-CoA carboxylase* for catabolism of leucine, (5) *Propionyl-CoA carboxylase* for the metabolism of certain amino acids, cholesterol, and odd-chain fatty acids.[20] Genotropic defects in either the *attaching* holocarboxylase synthetase or the *releasing* biotinidase leads

> **Benefits of biotin**
>
> Biotin is a nontoxic water-soluble vitamin necessary for several metabolic pathways, mitochondrial fatty acid oxidation, and repression of TNF-alpha gene transcription.

---

[18] Cavallini G, Caracciolo S, Vitali G, Modenini F, Biagiotti G. Carnitine versus androgen administration in the treatment of sexual dysfunction, depressed mood, and fatigue associated with male aging. *Urology*. 2004 Apr;63(4):641-6

[19] "Biotin was administered orally (2.1, 8.2, or 81.9 micromol) or intravenously (18.4 micromol) to 6 healthy adults in a crossover design with > or =2 wk between each biotin administration. Before and after each administration, timed 24-h urine samples were collected. Urinary recoveries of biotin plus metabolites were similar (approximately 50%) after the 2 largest oral doses and the 1 intravenous dose, suggesting 100% bioavailability of the 2 largest oral doses... Our data provide evidence that oral biotin is completely absorbed even when pharmacologic doses are administered. Zempleni et al. Bioavailability of biotin given orally to humans in pharmacologic doses. *Am J Clin Nutr* 1999;69:504-8

[20] lpi.oregonstate.edu/infocenter/vitamins/biotin/ Reviewed 2014 Jun

to –as would be expected– metabolic impairments (metabolic acidosis, neurologic and dermatologic disorders), the severity of which is dependent on the degree of enzyme impairment; biotinidase deficiency leads to biotin depletion due to failure of biotin recycling and failure to detach biotin from dietary proteins. Genotropic biotinopathy is treated with pharmacological/supranutritional doses of biotin 5–20 mg/d in children and adults; some patients may require higher doses of 40–200 mg/d.[21] Secondary/acquired biotin deficiency is caused by insufficient/blocked dietary intake/absorption (e.g., due to raw egg white, malabsorption, long-term parenteral nutrition), increased need during pregnancy (note that biotin deficiency is teratogenic and occurs in humans[22,23]), excess loss with hemodialysis, or drug-induced depletion as with long-term anticonvulsant therapy—note that pharmacologic anticonvulsant therapy commonly causes deficiency of folate and cholecalciferol as well, with the latter two deficiencies contributing to increased seizure activity and therapeutic recalcitrance. Biotinylation of histones affects gene transcription in a manner similar (in concept) to the better known means of methylation and acetylation; in the case of histone biotinylation, the effect is dose-dependent, regional, and repressive[24], notably of TNF-alpha gene transcription.[25] Since biotin is a small molecule that can bind to many proteins without affecting biological activity, the finding of biotin-binding antibodies/immunoglobulins (BBI) is not surprising. A low percentage (3-6%) of the population has biotin-binding IgM antibodies[26] while the incidence of BBI is markedly higher in patients with metabolic/inflammatory/allergic/autoimmune diseases; given the role of biotin in mitochondrial function and suppression of TNF-alpha transcription, this finding warrants clinical consideration. Muratsugu et al[27] quantified biotin-binding IgG, IgA, IgM among healthy and infirmed patients to find that while levels were generally low in the healthy population and within the IgM subclass, both biotin-binding IgA and *especially* biotin-binding IgG were impressively higher (frequency and quantity) among patients with bronchial asthma, atopic dermatitis, epilepsy, and juvenile rheumatoid arthritis (IgG range of positivity: 28-62%) compared with levels among the apparently healthy (7%); biotin-binding IgM was *lower* among infirmed than healthy. Likewise, Nagamine et al (1994)[28] found a higher prevalence of BBI in patients with Grave's thyropathy (47% vs 10% in nonGrave's). The question then becomes whether this finding is an *insignificant epiphenomenon*, a *pathogenic cause or consequence*, or *if a subclass might even be protective*; the former hypothesis—that BBI are a clinically insignificant epiphenomenon—appears to be the victor. Muratsugu M et al (op cit) concluded, "The clinical significance of biotin-binding immunoglobulin is not clear at the present time…" Nagamine et al (op cit 1994) found "no significant relationship between BBI prevalence and thyroid hormone concentrations, anti-thyroglobulin antibody (TGAb) or anti-thyroid microsomal antibody (McAb) titers. In addition, biotin levels in peripheral blood and red blood cells and biotinidase activity did not differ in the BBI detected and non-detected groups"; this data strongly suggests that although BBI are found in patients with thyroid autoimmunity, these BBI are not of pathogenic and clinical significance. Nagamine et al (1996)[29] studied the prevalence of biotin-binding immunoglobulin in patients with allergic and autoimmune diseases and found a higher prevalence of BBI among patients with Crohn's disease, ulcerative colitis, atopic dermatitis, lupus, progressive systemic sclerosis; however, the lack of clinical correlation and the lack of correlation with serum biotin levels and clinical biotin status again appear to indicate that that BBI are a clinically insignificant epiphenomenon and—therefore—that biotin supplementation is not contraindicated in patients with (or without) BBI. Supranutritional biotin supplementation might provide clinical benefits via maintenance of mitochondrial performance and —*of potentially massive importance*—nutraceutical suppression of TNF-alpha transcription; in support of this component of anti-inflammatory/antirheumatic nutritional immunomodulation is the finding

[21] Baumgartner MR. Vitamin-responsive disorders: cobalamin, folate, biotin, vitamins B1 and E. *Handb Clin Neurol.* 2013;113:1799-810

[22] "Biotin deficiency is teratogenic in several mammalian species. ... The conclusion that marginal biotin deficiency occurs frequently in the first trimester further raises concern about potential human teratogenicity." Mock et al. Marginal biotin deficiency during normal pregnancy. *Am J Clin Nutr.* 2002 Feb;75(2):295-9

[23] "Taken together, such studies provide evidence that a substantial proportion of pregnant women are marginally biotin deficient. In mice, degrees of biotin deficiency that are metabolically similar to those seen in pregnant women are very teratogenic. Moreover, in mice, a marginal degree of biotin deficiency in the dam causes a much more severe degree of deficiency in the fetus. These observations further raise concerns that biotin deficiency does occur and does cause human birth defects." Mock DM. Marginal biotin deficiency is common in normal human pregnancy and is highly teratogenic in mice. *J Nutr.* 2009 Jan;139(1):154-7

[24] Hassan YI, Zempleni J. A novel, enigmatic histone modification: biotinylation of histones by holocarboxylase synthetase. *Nutr Rev.* 2008 Dec;66(12):721-5

[25] Kuroishi T, Endo Y, Muramoto K, Sugawara S. Biotin deficiency up-regulates TNF-alpha production in murine macrophages. *J Leukoc Biol.* 2008 Apr;83(4):912-20

[26] "These IgM antibodies were present in 3% adults regardless of age, but were rarely found in children." Chen T et al. Biotin IgM antibodies in human blood: a previously unknown factor eliciting false results in biotinylation-based immunoassays. *PLoS One.* 2012;7(8):e42376

[27] Muratsugu M et al. Quantitation of biotin-binding immunoglobulins G, A, and M in Human Sera Using F(ab')2anti-human immunoglobulin-coated microplates. *Biol Pharm Bull.* 2008 Mar;31(3):507-10

[28] Nagamine et al. Clinical evaluation of biotin-binding immunoglobulin in patients with Graves' disease. *Clin Chim Acta.* 1994 Apr;226(1):47-54

[29] Nagamine T et al. Prevalence of biotin-binding immunoglobulin in patients with allergic and autoimmune diseases. *Clin Chim Acta.* 1996 Feb 28;245(2):209-17

that **orally-administered biotin supplementation can decrease proliferation rates of peripheral blood mononuclear cells and decreases cytokine release in humans.**

- Clinical benefits of biotin supplementation:
  - Biotin supplementation at a pharmacologic dose decreases proliferation rates of human peripheral blood mononuclear cells (PBMC) and decreases cytokine release (*J Nutr* 2001 May[30]): Oral administration of biotin 756.1 microg/d (3.1 micromol/d) for 14 d "caused a significant decrease of PBMC proliferation. At 2 d after mitogen stimulation, [3H]thymidine uptake by postsupplementation PBMC was 66 % of the uptake by presupplementation PBMC. Similarly, concentrations of interleukin-1β (2 d after mitogen) and interleukin-2 (1 d after mitogen) in media from postsupplementation PBMC were 65% and 44%, respectively, of those for presupplementation PBMC. ... Overall, this study provides evidence that administration of pharmacologic doses of biotin [756.1 microg/d] for 14 d decreases PBMC proliferation and synthesis of interleukin-1β and interleukin-2." These are very impressive results, showing that a modest dose of orally administered biotin reduces monocyte proliferation by -34%, IL-1 by -35%, and IL-2 by -56%.
  - Drug-induced biotin deficiency in children with valproic acid (VPA) monotherapy (*Epilepsia.* 2001 Oct[31]): "Strong inverse correlations were observed between liver enzymes and VPA blood levels with the activity of the enzyme. Additionally, no inhibitory effect on biotinidase activity was found, when the enzyme was incubated in vitro with high (1.2 mM) concentrations of the drug. Skin lesions (seborrheic rash, alopecia) were improved in our patients after biotin (10 mg/day) supplementation. It is suggested that VPA impairs the liver mitochondrial function, resulting in a low biotinidase activity and or biotin deficiency." What interested me most about this article was the mention of drug-induced biotin deficiency/dysfunction and the connection with mitochondrial dysfunction; the full text of the article did not provide (likely through no fault of the authors) additional explication but rather a correlative hypothesis that "A possible speculation, as regards the VPA mechanism over biotinidase activity, could be related with an expected impairment of a number of carboxylases involved in the biotin cycle of mitochondrial function. Finally, the absence on an in vitro effect of the drug on biotinidase reinforces the suggestion that an indirect mechanism takes place between VPA and the enzyme." Biotinidase activity was dose-dependently reduced by approximately 20-80% *in vivo* despite the fact that the enzyme was not inhibited by the drug *in vitro*; therefore, VPA "somehow" causes impaired enzyme transcription or production, which the authors related to impaired mitochondrial function.
  - Chromium and biotin improves coronary risk factors in hypercholesterolemic type 2 diabetes mellitus (*J Cardiometab Syndr.* 2007 Spring[32]): "The authors report here a randomized, double-blind placebo-controlled trial (N=348; chromium picolinate and biotin combination [CPB]: 226, placebo: 122; T2DM participants with hemoglobin A1c [HbA1c] >or=7%) evaluating the effects of CPB on lipid and lipoprotein levels. Participants were randomly assigned (2:1 ratio) to receive either CPB (600 microg chromium as chromium picolinate and 2 mg biotin) ... In the primary analysis, CPB lowered HbA1c (P<.05) and glucose (P<.02) significantly compared with the placebo group. No significant changes were observed in other lipid levels. In participants with HC and T2DM, significant changes in total cholesterol and low-density lipoprotein cholesterol (LDL-C) levels and atherogenic index were observed in the CPB group (P<.05). Significant decreases in LDL-C, total cholesterol, HbA1c, and very low-density cholesterol levels (P<.05) were observed in the CPB group taking statins. CPB treatment was well tolerated with no adverse effects, dissimilar from those associated with placebo. These data suggest that intervention with CPB improves cardiometabolic risk factors."
  - Chromium picolinate and biotin combination improves glucose metabolism in treated, uncontrolled overweight/obese patients with type-2 diabetes (*Diabetes Metab Res Rev* 2008 Jan-Feb): N = 447 subjects

[30] Per the authors 2.46 micromol = 600 microg, and thus 3.1 micromol = 756.1 microg. Zempleni J, Helm RM, Mock DM. In vivo biotin supplementation at a pharmacologic dose decreases proliferation rates of human peripheral blood mononuclear cells and cytokine release. *J Nutr.* 2001 May;131(5):1479-84

[31] Schulpis KH et al. Low serum biotinidase activity in children with valproic acid monotherapy. *Epilepsia.* 2001 Oct;42(10):1359-62

[32] Albarracin C et al. Combination of chromium and biotin improves coronary risk factors in hypercholesterolemic type 2 diabetes mellitus. *J Cardiometab Syndr.* 2007;2(2):91-7

with poorly controlled type 2 diabetes (HbA(1c) > or = 7.0%) were enrolled and received either chromium picolinate (600 microg Cr(+3)) with biotin (2 mg), or matching placebo, for 90 days in combination with stable oral anti-diabetic agents (OADs). ... Change in HbA(1c) was significantly different between treatment groups (p = 0.03). HbA(1c) in the chromium picolinate/biotin group decreased 0.54%. The decrease in HbA(1c) was most pronounced in chromium picolinate/biotin subjects whose baseline HbA(1c) > or = 10%, and highly significant when compared with placebo (-1.76% vs - 0.68%; p = 0.005). Fasting glucose levels were reduced in the entire chromium picolinate/biotin group versus placebo (-9.8 mg/dL vs 0.7 mg/dL; p = 0.02). Reductions in fasting glucose were also most marked in those subjects whose baseline HbA(1c) > or = 10.0%, and significant when compared to placebo (-35.8 mg/dL vs. 16.2 mg/dL; p = 0.01). Treatment was well tolerated with no adverse effects dissimilar from placebo.

9. **Magnesium (Mg): 600 mg/d or bowel tolerance; urinary alkalinization is important for cellular uptake**
   - Mitochondrial mechanism(s): Magnesium plays a pivotal role in formation of the transition state of ATP synthase enzyme (complex 5) where ATP is synthesized from ADP and inorganic phosphate.[33]
   - Clinical benefits: Hypertension, seizures/epilepsy, migraine and all types of headaches, insulin resistance, heart failure, depression, anxiety, bruxism and muscle cramps. Mg alleviates neurogenic inflammation in animal models.

10. **Medium-chain triglycerides (MTC): dose varies per source and concentration (e.g., crude food extract versus purified concentrate), but generally 1-2 TBS = 15-30 ml = 14-28 g lipid = 100-200 calories; true toxicity is very low; gastrointestinal intolerance / diarrhea occurs with very large doses; margin of safety is very high**
    - Mitochondrial mechanism(s): MTC and the ketone bodies (KB) into which they are converted are clearly the preferred fuel source for most mitochondria under normal conditions. MTC and KB actually improve mitochondrial function via upregulation/induction of key enzymes and ETC complexes 3 and 4; in contrast to CHO such as fructose which cause mitochondrial damage, MTC and KB improve and restore mitochondrial function while serving as a fuel source. Beta-hydroxybutyrate (bHB) bolsters antioxidant defenses and promotes histone acetylation for induction of a rejuvenative phenotype.
    - Clinical benefits: Administration of MTC (e.g., coconut oil), caprylic acid and relative derivatives, and/or fasting—which promotes endogenous bHB production—leads to clinical improvements in and alleviation of Alzheimer's disease, asthma and various inflammatory disorders. Note that ketogenic therapy is the most safe and effective treatment for both chronic epilepsy and status epilepticus.

11. **Resveratrol: 250 mg/d or more**
    - Mitochondrial mechanism(s): Resveratrol promotes mitochondrial biogenesis, hence its expoited reputation for being the botanical mimic of exercise, as if exercise did not provide other benefits by other means. Resveratrol also stimulates the SIRT enzymes which directly stimulate the proteins/enzymes of the mitochondrial electron transport chain (ETC). Resveratrol has anti-oxidant and anti-inflammatory actions; paradoxically, resveratrol may have an estrogenic effect at the level of the estrogen receptor while also suppressing activity of aromatase.
    - Clinical benefits: Improvement in endothelial function; cardioprotective benefits.

12. **DHA (docosahexaenoic acid) from fish oil or blue-green algae: 500-2,000 mg/d or more**
    - Mitochondrial mechanism(s): DHA becomes integrated into the phospholipid phosphatidylserine, which is the structural anchor for succinate dehydrogenase—a key enzyme in the Krebs' cycle and ETC (complex 2).
    - Clinical benefits: Anti-inflammatory, cardioprotective, neuroprotective, improves cardiovascular health, improves brain function in various neuropsychiatric disorders such as depression, anxiety, bipolar, schizophrenia.

13. **Optimization of iron status—avoiding iron deficiency (both systemic and cerebral) while also avoiding iron overload**: Iron deficiency impairs mitochondrial function because iron is needed for several biochemical reactions in the electron transport chain; conversely, iron overload also impairs mitochondrial function due to free radical damage. The amount of iron in the body can be accurately determined by the blood test "serum ferritin." Per my publications on this topic and review of the literature (more than 300 papers read), optimal iron status correlates with a serum ferritin of 40-70 ng/ml; the only exception to this rule appears to be a subset

---

[33] Ko YH, Hong S, Pedersen PL. Chemical mechanism of ATP synthase. *J Biol Chem.* 1999 Oct 8;274(41):28853-6

of patients with restless leg syndrome (RLS) who have a defect in the transport of iron into the brain, such that they need higher levels of iron correlating with a serum ferritin up to 120 ng/ml. Stated again and differently, some patients with RLS have a defect in the transport of iron into the brain, and this defect can be overcome by allowing the patient to have higher-than-normal levels of iron, up to 120 ng/ml. Iron overload is a common problem, too, either due to lifestyle factors such as overconsumption of alcohol and/or iron-rich foods such as beef and liver, or due to diseases such as type-2 diabetes, metabolic syndrome, or the genetic iron-accumulation disorder hemochromatosis, which is

> **Optimal iron status is necessary for optimal mitochondrial function**
> ---
> - Measure serum ferritin: For most patients, optimal iron status correlates with a serum ferritin of 40-70 ng/ml.
> - Avoid iron deficiency: Iron is a required component of cytochrome C in the electron transport chain (ETC) that produces ATP.
> - Avoid iron overload: Excess iron causes free radical damage that impairs mitochondrial function.

one of the most common genetic diseases seen in humans with a frequency of approximately 1 per 200-250 in the general population. Hereditary iron overload disorders are seen in people of all genetic backgrounds and ethnicities; they appear most common in persons of African descent (perhaps as high as 1 per 80 persons). Serum ferritin levels higher than 200 ng/ml in a woman or 300 ng/ml in a man strongly suggest the probability of excess iron and warrant evaluation and treatment, even in the absence of clinical pathology[34]; overt pathologic damage caused by iron is generally seen with ferritin values greater than 1,000 mcg/L. [Note: when discussing ferritin, the measurement units mcg/L and ng/ml are equivalent.]

- Mitochondrial mechanism(s): Iron is necessary for ETC complexes 3 and 4; iron deficiency causes ETC dysfunction, which generally results in reduced ATP formation and increased oxidant formation. Iron overload promotes lipid oxidation and DNA damage, both of which can contribute to mitochondrial impairment. Iron obviously plays other roles, such as formation of hemoglobin, synthesis of dopamine, function of thyroid hormones, fatty acid metabolism, etc.
- Clinical benefits: Patients feel better when their iron status is optimized so that they are neither iron-deficient nor iron-overloaded. For most patients, optimal iron status correlates with a serum ferritin of 40-70 ng/ml.

14. **N-Acetyl-Cysteine (NAC)**: 500-1,500 mg TID IC
   - Mitochondrial mechanism(s): NAC provides cysteine for GSH production (antioxidant defense, detoxificiation) and also inhibits NFkB (inflammatory pathway). NAC inhibits viral replication (e.g., HIV) more effectively than *and independently from its conversion to* GSH. In 2012, NAC at relatively high doses of 4,800mg/d in divided doses was shown to modulate mitochondrial hyperpolarization (by dissociating the generally resultant mTOR activation) and lead to very important clinical and immunological improvements in patients with SLE; NAC was shown to be safe and well-tolerated by all SLE patients up to 2.4g/d with reversible nausea in 33% of patients receiving 4.8g/d. This study by Lai, Hanczko, Bonilla, et al[35] is truly a landmark

> **Mechanistic and clinical proof that mitochondrial dysfunction directly contributes to autoimmunity**
> ---
> "Similar to the effect of rapamycin, **suppression of mTOR by NAC was accompanied by increased FoxP3 expression in CD4+/CD25+ T cells**. These results suggest that the effect of NAC on the immune system is 1) cell type-specific and 2) it occurs through disconnecting the activation of mTOR from the elevation of Δψm in lupus T cells, similar to the effect of rapamycin."
>
> Lai et al. *Arthritis Rheum* 2012 Sep

contribution and advance in the field of rheumatology and immunology because it proves 1) that mitochondrial dysfunction directly leads to an autoimmune phenotype, and 2) that inhibition of mTOR by NAC is safe and effective in patients with SLE; important insights from this remarkable work are as follows:
   - Safety and effectiveness: NAC 4,800mg/d in divided doses proved safe and clinically beneficial in patients with SLE, leading to reductions in disease activity and ANA levels.
   - Mechanism of action: Mitochondrial hyperpolarization (MHP) causes mTOR activation which in turn suppresses the expression of the FoxP3 transcription factor necessary for induction of T-regulatory cells. Note that the mTOR activation is the cause of the FoxP3 suppression; ironically, NAC actually increases MHP but dissociates it from mTOR by having a greater effect via mTOR suppression. The

---

[34] Barton JC, McDonnell SM, Adams PC,et al. Management of hemochromatosis. *Ann Intern Med.* 1998 Dec 1;129(11):932-9
[35] Lai ZW, Hanczko R, Bonilla E, et al. N-acetylcysteine reduces disease activity by blocking mammalian target of rapamycin in T cells from systemic lupus erythematosus patients: a randomized, double-blind, placebo-controlled trial. *Arthritis Rheum.* 2012 Sep;64(9):2937-46

nutritional supplement NAC works in a similar manner as does the immunosuppressive drug rapamycin, with a mechanism of suppression of mTOR and the effect of enhancing endogenous anti-inflammatory immunomodulation via CD4+ CD25+ FoxP3+ T-regulatory cells. Stated again and differently, NAC paradoxically worsens mitochondrial hyperpolarization in patients with SLE but does so at the same time that it has a more significant impact on mTOR; NAC's rapamycin-like targeting of mTOR dissociates mitochondrial hyperpolarization from mTOR activation. The reduction in mTOR activity (which is of greater consequence than the increase in MIM polarization) allows enhanced expression of FoxP3 for increased elaboration of T-regulatory cells, thereby providing endogenous immunoregulation.

  o Additional details: "MHP of lupus T cells, which most prominently affects DN [double-negative, autoimmunity-promoting] T cells, was associated with resistance to activation-induced apoptosis. In 27 SLE patients receiving daily NAC doses of 1.2 g, 2.4 g, and 4.8 g considered together, both **spontaneous and CD3/CD28-induced apoptosis of DN T cells were markedly increased** and the **expansion of these cells was effectively reversed**. The **elimination of DN T cells, which are known promote anti-DNA autoantibody production by B cells**, is likely to contribute to reduced anti-DNA titers and to the efficacy of NAC.

  o Better effectiveness, less cost, less risk = the new clinical standard: "The therapeutic importance of NAC for SLE is reflected by: 1) achieving clinical improvement in two validated disease activity scores within 3 months; 2) diminishing fatigue (21), which is considered the most disabling symptom in a majority of SLE patients (22); 3) absence of significant side-effects; and 4) affordability of this medication. A monthly supply of 600-mg NAC capsules (120–240 capsules) costs $15–$30 on the retail market. This sharply contrasts with average annual direct medical costs estimated to be ~$22,580 per patient in 2009.Thus, the cost of NAC at $180–$360/year would be negligible in comparison to the overall expenditures to society and the expected benefit in reducing the need for vastly more expensive medications burdened with potentially serious side-effects."

15. **General antioxidant support**: Naturally-derived antioxidants in general tend to have anti-inflammatory, disease-alleviating, and health-promoting benefits; much of the benefit from eating a complex plant-based diet is derived from the additive and synergistic biochemical and physiologic benefits provided by phytonutrients, of which 5,000-8,000 exist.[36] Hence, as I have stated and published for many years, the best approach is a plant-based diet that provides adequate protein, reduces intake of starchy phytonutrient-deficient carbohydrates such as wheat/rye/barley/potatoes, and to which is added a broad-spectrum high-potency multivitamin and multimineral supplementation.[37]

  • Mitochondrial mechanism(s): Speaking generally, broadly, and accurately, we can estimate that anti-inflammatory and antioxidant therapeutics/diets/interventions/supplements will tend to improve mitochondrial function; some might argue against this by stating that oxidative stress induces hormesis to which I'll reply that chronic/sustained/long-term minute-by-minute adaptation is not possible because adaptive mechanisms are not long to be depleted. I think a better approach is to provide sufficient and perhaps supraphysiologic antioxidant support via diet and supplements and to then punctuate that biochemical bliss reasonable bouts of hormetic shock such as fasting, exercise, and ethanol to which defensive/adaptive mechanisms can respond—this is the best of both words, to which a few exceptions are noted, such as blunting of physiologic responsiveness to exercise with antioxidant supplementation in patients with DM-2/MetSyn. Identical arguments are valid or invalid within different clinical contexts, and the argument in favor of high(er) dosing of antioxidants is—as logically anticipated—more easily made when treating *autoimmune/hyperinflammatory/hyperoxidative* patients with more severe oxidant and inflammatory stress.

  • Clinical benefits: Paraphrasing Dr Bruce Ames: Mitochondrial oxidative decay is a major contributor to aging and is accelerated by many common micronutrient deficiencies; an optimum intake of micronutrients can "tune-up mitochondrial metabolism" and give a marked increase in health, particularly for the poor, elderly, and obese, at little cost.[38]

---

[36] Liu RH. Health benefits of fruit and vegetables are from additive and synergistic combinations of phytochemicals. *Am J Clin Nutr.* 2003 Sep;78(3 Suppl):517S-520S
[37] Vasquez A. Revisiting the Five-Part Nutritional Wellness Protocol. *Nutr Perspect* 2011 Jan: 19-25
[38] Ames BN, Atamna H, Killilea DW. Mineral and vitamin deficiencies can accelerate the mitochondrial decay of aging. *Mol Aspects Med.* 2005 Aug-Oct;26(4-5):363-78

16. <u>**General anti-inflammatory support**</u>:
    - <u>Mitochondrial mechanism(s)</u>: Pro-inflammatory cytokines such as interferon (IFN)-gamma, interleukin (IL)-1b, and tumor necrosis factor (TNF)-alpha impair mitochondrial function via cytokine-stimulated iNOS-induced nitric oxide (NO) production[39], and mitochondrial dysfunction increases elaboration of ROS which act as signaling molecules to increase the production of pro-inflammatory cytokines[40]; additively, mitochondrial dysfunction also increases cellular sensitivity to pro-inflammatory cytokines.[41] Obviously, the stage is thus set for a self-perpetuating cycle.
    - <u>Clinical benefits</u>: Vitamin D3 supplementation, low-carbohydrate diets, and multivitamin-multimineral supplementation are excellent examples of anti-inflammatory interventions that are safe and effective. Additional anti-inflammatory benefit can be obtained by eradicating dysbiotic infections, correcting hormone imbalances, reducing obesity, etc. *Refer to my NFkB mini-monograph earlier in Chapter 4.*

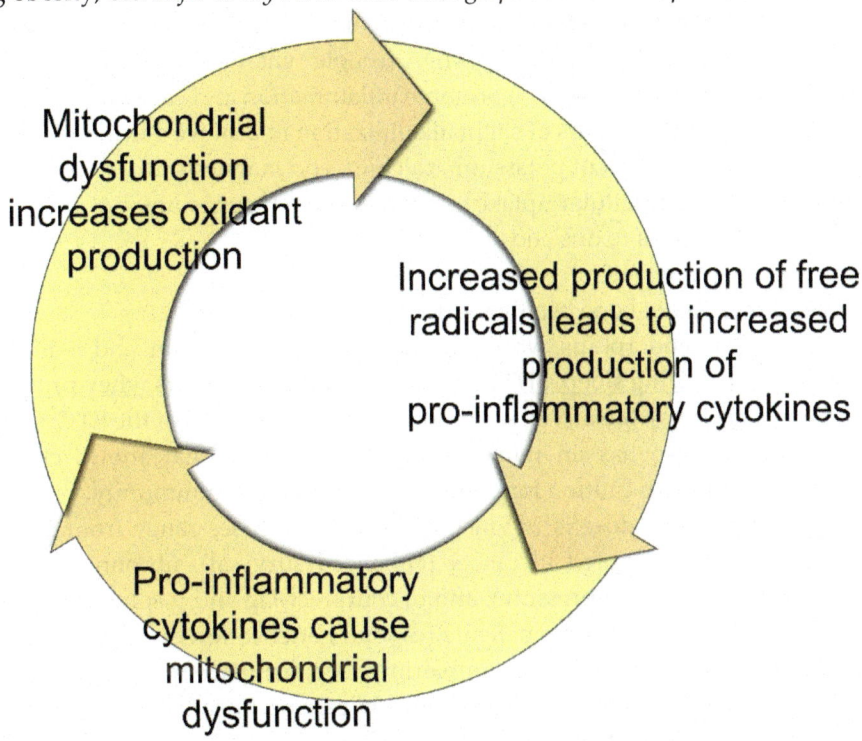

Mitochondrial dysfunction as cause and consequence of oxidative stress and inflammation: Clinical implications are obvious from the diagram and are additionally discussed in the text.

17. <u>**High-salicylate diet and/or low-dose aspirin to provide salicylate for ionophore alleviation of mitochondrial hyperpolarization—hypothesis**</u>:
    - <u>Mitochondrial mechanism(s)</u>: To the best of my knowledge, I am the first to propose that the well-documented benefits of plant-based diets against cancer and autoimmunity may stem in part from the ionophore action of salicylate against mitochondrial hyperpolarization which is common both in cancer and autoimmunity.
    - <u>Clinical benefits</u>: High-plant diets and low-dose aspirin have shown benefit against inflammatory and malignant diseases; what I propose here is that part of the mechanism may be that of alleviation of mitochondrial hyperpolarization by the ionophore action of salicylic acid, a well-absorbed phytochemical that is believed to be significantly responsible for the health-promoting and anticancer benefits of plant-based diets.
18. <u>**Alkalinization, acid-base balance, pH**</u>: Several general statements can be made on this topic that are true and which will serve as an introduction to the topic of acid-base balance in the body. Although I initially approached

---

[39] "These data suggest that IL-1b–induced NO production in cardiac myocytes lowers energy production and myocardial contractility through a direct attack on the mitochondria, rather than through cGMP-mediated pathways." Tatsumi T, Matoba S, Kawahara A, et al. Cytokine-induced nitric oxide production inhibits mitochondrial energy production and impairs contractile function in rat cardiac myocytes. *J Am Coll Cardiol*. 2000 Apr;35(5):1338-46

[40] Naik E, Dixit VM. Mitochondrial reactive oxygen species drive proinflammatory cytokine production. *J Exp Med*. 2011 Mar 14;208(3):417-20

[41] "... mitochondrial dysfunction could amplify the responsiveness to cytokine-induced chondrocyte inflammation through ROS and NF-κB activation." Vaamonde-García et al. Mitochondrial dysfunction increases inflammatory responsiveness to cytokines in human chondrocytes. *Arthritis Rheum* 2012 Sep:2927-36

this topic of acid-base balance with some skepticism and disregard, I have come to have profound and deep respect for this simple concept and intervention that provides numerous very important clinical benefits. Overall, the human body produces and excess of acidic substances that require balancing via internal buffering systems and also via dietary consumption of alkalinizing base-forming substances. The *internal* buffering systems succeed at keeping the acid-base balance within a range compatible for survival; *internal* buffering systems include control of respiratory rate, and the adaptations of the kidneys. The *external* buffering system of dietary consumption of foods that have an alkalinizing effect help to fine-tune the pH of the body in very important ways. My description is: *internal* acid-base buffering via respiration and renal adaptation sustains *life,* while the *external* acid-base buffering of dietarily consumed alkalinizing substances sustains *health.* The Western diet promotes diet-induced metabolic acidosis, while a plant-based Paleolithic diet or vegetarian diet promotes alkalinization.

- Mitochondrial mechanism(s): Alkalinization promotes renal retention and cellular uptake of magnesium, which is an essential nutrient for efficient action of complex 5, ATP synthase. In neurons, magnesium along with zinc also provide partial blockade of NMDA receptor channeling of calcium; high-levels of intracellular calcium ("intracellular hypercalcinosis"[42]) promote inflammation and cause mitochondrial stress.
- Clinical benefits: In sum, the benefits of slight alkalinization to achieve a urine pH of 7.5-8.5 include:
  - Increased renal retention of potassium, calcium, and magnesium
  - Increased (11%) intracellular uptake and retention of magnesium
  - Increased excretion of toxins and xenobiotics[43]
  - Reduction in serum cortisol
  - Improved markers of bone health: reduced bone breakdown
  - Increased serum endorphins, which elevate mood, alleviate pain, and reduce addictiveness.

19. **Melatonin support, including sleep, 5HTP, dietary tryptophan such as whey protein isolate**:
- Mitochondrial mechanism(s): Melatonin stimulates complexes 1 and 4 of the ETC; melatonin is also a powerful antioxidant. Melatonin also has an immune-stimulating action that shows clinical effectiveness against infections but which warrants caution for patients with allergy/autoimmunity.
- Clinical benefits: Physiologic dose is 200 mcg/night; clinical doses range from 200mcg-40mg taken at night before bedtime. Benefits are noted in cancer (enhanced survival), fibromyalgia migraine (reduced pain), hypertension (mild reductions in pressure), and of course jet-lag and insomnia (resynchronization and sleep). With regard to improving sleep, some patients respond better to lower doses <3mg/night while higher doses >6mg/night can have a paradoxical effect of impairing sleep; further, some patients may experience impairment of libido and/or exacerbation of fatigue/depression—in case of the latter, early morning exercise and exposure to bright full-spectrum light are beneficial.

20. **Phospholipid replacement therapy**:
- Mitochondrial mechanism(s): Because the function of the ETC-ATPase is completely dependent on the integrity of the inner mitochondrial membrane, and because oxidative damage and/or biochemical defects in phospholipid composition (e.g., due to poor nutrition and insufficient intake of proper fatty acids) impair function of the ETC and reduce transmembrane potential, phospholipid replacement therapy has conceptual validity, and clinical trials have proven its merit. Professor Dr Garth Nicolson[44] deserves most of the credit for bringing this concept and application to clinical practice, and his research articles and clinical presentation from the 2013 International Conference on Human Nutrition and Functional Medicine (along with presentations from Drs Hirshey, Gonzalez, Vasquez) are online: IntJHumNutrFunctMed.org/events/MitochondrialMedicine/
- Clinical benefits: Phospholipid replacement therapy—whether with soy lecithin or with proprietary phospholipid formulations—has proven in animal studies and human clinical trials to improve health in general and mitochondrial performance in particular.
  - Lipid Replacement Therapy for replacing damaged lipids in cellular membranes and organelles and restoring function (*Biochim Biophys Acta* 2014 Jun[45]): "Various chronic clinical conditions are

[42] Vasquez A. Intracellular Hypercalcinosis. *Naturopathy Digest* 2006 naturopathydigest.com/archives/2006/sep/vasquez.php
[43] Proudfoot AT, Krenzelok EP, Vale JA. Position Paper on urine alkalinization. *J Toxicol Clin Toxicol.* 2004;42(1):1-26
[44] Nicolson GL. Mitochondrial dysfunction and chronic disease: treatment with natural supplements. *Altern Ther Health Med.* 2014 Winter;20 Suppl 1:18-25
[45] Nicolson GL, Ash ME. Lipid Replacement Therapy: a natural medicine approach to replacing damaged lipids in cellular membranes and organelles and restoring function. *Biochim Biophys Acta.* 2014 Jun;1838(6):1657-79

characterized by membrane damage, mainly oxidative but also enzymatic, resulting in loss of cellular function. This is readily apparent in mitochondrial inner membranes where oxidative damage to phospholipids like cardiolipin and other molecules results in loss of trans-membrane potential, electron transport function and generation of high-energy molecules. Recent clinical trials have shown the benefits of Lipid Replacement Therapy in restoring mitochondrial function and reducing fatigue in aged subjects and patients with a variety of clinical diagnoses that are characterized by loss of mitochondrial function and include fatigue as a major symptom."

21. **Oxygen, deep breathing, exercise, hyperbaric oxygen:**
   - Mitochondrial mechanism(s): Oxygen is the molecular "magnet" which pulls protons through the ETC for the formation of water. Without oxygen to receive mitochondrial protons, mammalian cellular respiration ceases. Mild/moderate exercise promotes physiologic hyperventilation and increased cardiac output, increasing blood/nutrient and oxygen delivery to issues while also promoting systemic alkalinization via respiratory alkalosis. Hyperbaric oxygen can be used to "force" oxygen into underperfused tissues and to maximize oxygen-to-cell delivery thereby promoting mitochondrial function; excess oxygen therapy can have a detrimental effect via increased free radical production and also via promotion of vascular hyperproliferation, as noted in the treatment of the retinopathy of prematurity.
   - Clinical benefits: People feel better when they exercise and breathe deeply; doing so regularly improves mitochondrial performance.

22. **Ginkgo, Ginkgo biloba:**
   - Mitochondrial mechanism(s): Antioxidant, vasodilator, specifically improves mitochondria function.
   - Clinical benefits: Alleviation of intermittent claudication, erectile dysfunction, fibromyalgia (combination nutritional intervention with CoQ10), improved cognition and alleviation of dementia and depression.

❸ **Mitochondrial disinhibition *via elimination of infections and xenobiotics*:** If a patient has mitochondrial dysfunction not caused mostly by genetic mutations (e.g., low likelihood of inherited or spontaneous mitochondrial disease) nor by the biochemical impairment caused by coenzyme and cofactor deficiencies (e.g., let's assume the patient is well-nourished and is taking a high-potency broad-spectrum multivitamin and multimineral supplement), then we must ask, "What *exogenous* factors can cause mitochondrial impairment?" Beyond diet-induced impairment of mitochondrial function via consumption of simple carbohydrates (and resultant oxidative stress, fuel overload, ceramide, etc) and nutritional deficiencies (nutritional mitochondriopathy), many patients also demonstrate mitochondrial impairment due to microbes (microbial mitochondriopathy) and xenobiotics (xenobiotic mitochondriopathy).[46]

23. **Detoxification, avoidance of toxins (xenobiotics) that impair mitochondrial function:**
   - Mitochondrial mechanism(s): Many persistent organic pollutants (POPs) such as pesticides (e.g., dieldrin) and dioxin-related compounds cause mitochondrial impairment.
   - Clinical benefits: Xenobiotic mitochondriopathy is noted in Parkinson's disease, as well as insulin resistance and metabolic syndrome. Detoxification is promoted by oral chlorella supplementation, exercise, nutritional supplementation (e.g., NAC for GSH protection and conjugation) as discussed elsewhere in this textbook.
     - Eat organic foods to reduce pesticide/herbicide exposure (*Environ Res* 2014 Jul[47]): "CONCLUSIONS: The consumption of an organic diet for one week significantly reduced organophosphate pesticide exposure in adults."
     - "Effects of the Roundup and glyphosate on mitochondrial oxidative phosphorylation" (*Chemosphere* 2005 Dec[48]): In this study, the researcher used and named a specific brand of chemical formulation. "Roundup stimulates succinate-supported respiration twice, with simultaneous collapse of transmembrane electrical potential, while glyphosate used in the same concentrations does not induce any significant effect. Additionally, Roundup depresses state 3 respiration by about 40%, at 15 mM, whereas uncoupled respiration in the presence of FCCP is depressed by about 50%. Depression of

[46] Vasquez A. Mitochondrial medicine arrives to prime time in clinical care. *Altern Ther Health Med*. 2014 Winter;20 Suppl 1:26-30 ichnfm.org/events/MitochondrialMedicine
[47] Oates et al. Reduction in urinary organophosphate pesticide metabolites in adults after a week-long organic diet. *Environ Res*. 2014 Jul;132:105-11
[48] Peixoto F. Comparative effects of the Roundup and glyphosate on mitochondrial oxidative phosphorylation. *Chemosphere*. 2005 Dec;61(8):1115-22

uncoupled respiratory activity is mediated through partial inhibition of mitochondrial complexes II and III, but not of complex IV. The phosphorylative system was affected by both a direct and an indirect effect on the F0F1 ATPase activity. The addition of uncoupled concentrations of Roundup to Ca2+-loaded mitochondria treated with Ruthenium Red resulted in non-specific membrane permeabilization, as evidenced by mitochondrial swelling... Therefore, the uncoupling of oxidative phosphorylation is also related to the non-specific membrane permeabilization induced by Roundup. Glyphosate alone does not show any relevant effect on the mitochondrial bioenergetics, in opposition to Roundup formulation products. ... these results question the safety of Roundup on animal health."

- Glyphosate is a mitochondrial toxin (*Environ Toxicol Pharmacol* 2012 Sep[49]): This study was performed on the human epidermal cell line HaCaT to examine the cytotoxic effects of glyphosate; researchers "observed an increase in the number of early apoptotic cells at a low cytotoxicity level (15%), and then, a decrease, in favor of late apoptotic and necrotic cell rates for more severe cytotoxicity conditions. At the same time, we showed that the glyphosate-induced mitochondrial membrane potential disruption could be a cause of apoptosis in keratinocyte cultures."

- Glyphosate herbicide is synergistic with common additives to effect mitochondrial toxicity (*Toxicol In Vitro*. 2013 Feb[50]): Glyphosate shows less toxicity alone than when combined with a surfactant, at which point the combination of chemicals is cytotoxic. TN-20 is a common surfactant in glyphosate herbicides. This research shows that the combination of glyphosate with the TN-20 surfactant leads to increased caspase activity (a sign of cell death via apoptosis) and reduced mitochondrial membrane potential. "The results support the possibility that mixtures of glyphosate and TN-20 aggravate mitochondrial damage and induce apoptosis and necrosis. Throughout this process, TN-20 seems to disrupt the integrity of the cellular barrier to glyphosate uptake, promoting glyphosate-mediated toxicity."

- Major pesticides are more toxic to human cells than their declared active principles (*Biomed Res Int* 2014 Feb[51]): Pesticides are used throughout the world as mixtures called formulations. They contain adjuvants, which are often kept confidential and are called "inerts" by the manufacturing companies, plus a declared active principle, which is usually tested alone. In this study, adjuvants were more cytotoxic than the declared active components of the pesticides/herbicides through the disruption of membrane and mitochondrial respiration. "Despite its relatively benign reputation, Roundup was among the most toxic herbicides and insecticides tested." hindawi.com/journals/bmri/2014/179691/

24. **Eradication of gastrointestinal dysbiosis & small intestine bacterial overgrowth (SIBO):**
   - Mitochondrial mechanism(s): Dysbiotic bacteria in the intestines impair systemic mitochondrial function via gut-to-systemic absorption of D-lactic acid, hydrogen sulfide, and endotoxin/LPS.
   - Clinical benefits: Chronic fatigue syndrome, fibromyalgia, migraine headaches; pathophysiology, assessments, and treatments for dysbiosis are detailed elsewhere in this textbook.

25. **Eradication/suppression of any persistent "internal" infections**: Essentially any chronic infection will be associated with immune activation and thus inflammation and elaboration of cytokines; both inflammation as a general process and the elaboration of specific cytokines are known to impair mitochondrial function. Furthermore, some microorganism capable of causing chronic infections such as *Chlamydophila pneumoniae* (*CP*) are called "obligate intracellular bacteria/parasites" because these microbes are incapable of producing their own energy in the form of ATP and thus they must siphon cellular fuel from the host they have infected. Chronic viral infections—particularly those persistent infections caused by members of the herpes family of viruses—should be tested for with blood tests from a standard medical lab; assertive non-drug treatment to suppress viral replication should be implemented for 2-6 months and then serologic (blood) tests can be repeated to determine success of viral suppression. Pathophysiology, assessments, and treatments for dysbiosis are detailed throughout this textbook; note the section on laboratory assessments in Chapter 1. The following table provides examples of pathogens, assessments, and interventions.

---

[49] Heu et al. Glyphosate-induced epidermal cell death: involvement of mitochondrial and oxidative mechanisms. *Environ Toxicol Pharmacol*. 2012 Sep;34(2):144-53
[50] Kim et al. Mixtures of glyphosate and surfactant TN20 accelerate cell death via mitochondrial damage-induced apoptosis and necrosis. *Toxicol In Vitro* 2013 Feb:191-7
[51] Mesnage et al. Major pesticides are more toxic to human cells than their declared active principles. *Biomed Res Int*. 2014;2014:179691

- Mitochondrial mechanism(s): Many microbes—especially those that cause long-term occult/silent infections— impair mitochondrial function; I have referred to this as <mark>microbial mitochondriopathy</mark>[52] and have provided additional details and mechanisms in other sections of this book.
- Clinical benefits: Eradicating mitochondria-impairing microbes with nutritional immunorestoration and/or direct antimicrobial interventions allows restoration and normalization of mitochondrial performance.

Microbial Mitochondriopathy—Introduction to key examples of common clinical relevance

Microbes capable of contributing to fatigue, mitochondrial dysfunction, and energy impairment due to chronic occult/silent infections in humans	Sample interventions
• HSV—herpes simplex viruses types 1 and 2: Although infection with HSV is common, higher antibody titers correlate with higher levels of viral replication; thus [nutritional] treatments should be implemented to reduce viral replication in order to improve energy levels and avoid illness associated with HSV-1 (and to a lesser extent HSV-2) such as Alzheimer's disease, risk of which correlates with IgM antibodies to HSV.[53] Generally, testing IgG antibodies is sufficient. **HSV infection kills mitochondria by destroying mitochondrial DNA.**[54]	**DrV's antiviral protocol**—see digital/print protocol[55] (also Chapter 4, section 2): • Vitamin A: Acute infections are treated with 100,000 international units limited to 7-10 days only followed by daily maintenance dosage
• CMV—cytomegalovirus: Another member of the herpes family of viruses, chronic low-grade CMV infection is very common in humans; IgG antibodies or more direct tests (no perfect test exists) should be performed, nutritional viral suppression implemented, and antibodies are then retested. **CMV infection causes mitochondrial dysfunction.**[56]	• Vitamin D3: 10,000 IU/d for 10 days followed by daily maintenance dosage • Selenium: 600 mcg/d • Lipoic acid: 200 to 400 mg three times per day
• HHV-6—Human herpes virus type-6: Associated with chronic fatigue syndrome, a condition known to be associated with mitochondrial dysfunction. **Proteins of HHV-6 infection alter mitochondrial membrane potential and cause mitochondrial dysfunction.** Generally, testing IgG antibodies is sufficient.	• NAC: 1,500 mg 2 to 3 times per day between meals • Melatonin: 3-20 mg HS • Licorice: tea or capsules; monitor for hypertension and hypokalemia with extended use
• EBV—Epstein Barr virus: EBV is the cause of infectious mononucleosis, a common illness experienced by most people throughout the world. While most patients recover uneventfully from the infection, some patients appear to harbor a chronic ongoing infection with EBV as evidenced by a combination of several laboratory tests available for antibodies and antigens. **Patients who develop chronic fatigue following EBV infection show evidence of alterations in mitochondrial function.**[57]	• CoQ-10: 100-300mg to protect mitochondria and avoid virus-induced fatigue
• CP—*Chlamydophila pneumoniae*: "**Chlamydiae are obligate intracellular gram-negative bacteria and are dependent on the host cell for ATP.** Thus, chlamydial infection may alter the intracellular levels of ATP and affect all energy-dependent processes within the cell."[58] IgG titers of 1/64 to 1/256 suggest of chronic infection and consideration for treatment.[59]	• NAC: 1,000 mg 2 to 3 times per day between meals • Long-term azithromycin: 250-500mg every-other-day for 4-6 months then retest

[52] Vasquez A. Mitochondrial medicine arrives to prime time in clinical care. *Altern Ther Health Med.* 2014 Winter;20 Suppl 1:26-30 ichnfm.org/events/MitochondrialMedicine

[53] Letenneur L, et al. Seropositivity to herpes simplex virus antibodies and risk of Alzheimer's disease: a population-based cohort study. *PLoS One.* 2008;3(11):e3637

[54] "Mitochondria have crucial roles in the life and death of mammalian cells, and help to orchestrate host antiviral defences. Here, we show that the ubiquitous human pathogen herpes simplex virus (HSV) induces rapid and complete degradation of host mitochondrial DNA during productive infection of cultured mammalian cells." Saffran HA, Pare JM, Corcoran JA, Weller SK, Smiley JR. Herpes simplex virus eliminates host mitochondrial DNA. *EMBO Rep.* 2007 Feb;8(2):188-9

[55] Digital format: Vasquez A. *Antiviral Nutrition: Against Colds, Flu, Herpes, AIDS, Hepatitis, Ebola, Dengue, and Autoimmunity.* ICHNFM, 2014. (ASIN: B00OPDQG4W) amazon.com/dp/B00OPDQG4W. Printed in book format: Vasquez A. *Antiviral Strategies and Immune Nutrition,* 2014. (ISBN: 1502894890) AntiviralNutrition.com

[56] McCormick et al. Disruption of mitochondrial networks by human cytomegalovirus UL37 gene product. *J Virol.* 2003 Jan;77(1):631-41

[57] "A comparison of gene expression profiles early and late following EBV infection revealed that those who did not recover had differentially expressed genes implicating mitochondrial perturbations with fatty acid metabolism, mitochondrial function and apoptosis pathways." Vernon SD, Whistler T, Cameron B, et al. Preliminary evidence of mitochondrial dysfunction associated with post-infective fatigue after acute infection with Epstein Barr virus. *BMC Infect Dis.* 2006 Jan 31;6:15

[58] Yaraei K, et al. Effect of Chlamydia pneumoniae on cellular ATP content in mouse macrophages: role of Toll-like receptor 2. *Infect Immun.* 2005 Jul;73(7):4323-6

[59] Ben-Yaakov et al. Prevalence of antibodies to Chlamydia pneumoniae in an Israeli population without clinical evidence of respiratory infection. *J Clin Pathol* 2002 May:355-8

- o **Bacterial** toxins impair mitochondrial function (*IUBMB Life* 2012 May[60]): "Bacterial toxins have been shown to be targeted to the matrix, inner membrane, and outer membrane. The major class of toxins and effectors targeted to mitochondria are predicted to form pores..."
- o **Viral** toxins impair mitochondrial function (*Infect Disord Drug Targets* 2012 Feb[61]): "Viral products alter oxidative balance, mitochondrial permeability transition pore, mitochondrial membrane potential, electron transport and energy production. Moreover, viruses may cause the Warburg Effect, in which metabolism is reprogrammed to aerobic glycolysis as the main source of energy. ... A large number of viral products localize in mitochondria and interact with cellular mitochondrial proteins."
- o Viruses induce mitochondrial dysfunction to promote viral replication (*Int J Biochem Cell Biol* 2013 Jan[62]): "Increase in MMP, disrupts $\Delta\psi$m [MIM transmembrane potential] and affects mitochondrial bioenergetics. Viruses have developed strategies to modulate MMP and to effectively control cell death. In this regard, anti- or pro-apoptotic viral proteins co-opt host mitochondria to modulate MMP, affecting mitochondrial bioenergetics in favor of replication."

26. **Avoidance of dietary sulfite, eradication of H2S-producing dysbiosis, and/or chelation/detoxification of sulfite and H2S with hydroxocobalamin:** Sulfite is a substance found naturally and in significant amounts in some foods such as dried fruit and red wine; it is also added to some foods and drugs as a preservative/antimicrobial/bleaching agent. Sulfite is also produced internally/endogenously from the metabolism of sulfur-containing substances such as amino acids. Sulfite is well-known to trigger asthma and migraine headaches in some patients; of note, both asthma and migraine are complex disorders characterized in part by mitochondrial dysfunction. In 2004 Zhang and coworkers[63] showed that the cellular toxicity of sulfite in brain cells is mediated (at least in part) by inhibition mitochondrial glutamate dehydrogenase, which converts the amino acid and neurotransmitter glutamate into the fuel source alpha-keto-glutarate (AKG); the addition of sulfite increased production of ROS and reduced production of ATP (ATP production was reduced by ~ 50%)—increased ROS and decreased ATP is the classic dyad of mitochondrial impairment. Therefore, sulfite is a mitochondrial toxin; this explains its ability to exacerbate asthma and migraine, two conditions strongly associated with preexisting mitochondrial dysfunction. Vitamin B-12 is available in several different forms—cyanocobalamin, hydroxocobalamin, adenosylcobalamin, methylcobalamin; of these, only the hydroxocobalamin form has been shown to bind to sulfite and neutralize or "detoxify" it in a clinically significant manner with benefits for patients with sulfite-induced asthma as well as migraines. Further, an indirect

> **Hydroxocobalamin can be used clinically to neutralize sulfite and hydrogen sulfide (H2S)**
>
> "Serum concentrations of sulfide before and after administration of hydroxocobalamin were 0.22 and 0.11 µg/mL, respectively; serum concentrations of thiosulfate before and after hydroxocobalamin administration were 0.34 and 0.04 µmol/mL, respectively. **Hydroxocobalamin is believed to form a complex with H2S in detoxification pathways of H2S.** ...The decreased sulfide concentration suggests that hydroxocobalamin therapy may be effective for acute H2S poisoning. The decreased thiosulfate concentration seems to be associated with formation of a thiosulfate/hydroxocobalamin complex, because hydroxocobalamin can form a complex with thiosulfate. ...Therefore, prompt administration of hydroxocobalamin after H2S exposure may be effective for H2S poisoning."
>
> Fujita et al. A fatal case of acute hydrogen sulfide poisoning: hydroxocobalamin therapy. *J Analytical Toxicol* 2011 Mar

mechanism by which sulfur/sulfite-containing foods and drugs may trigger asthma is via the conversion of sulfur/sulfite to sulfur dioxide in the gastrointestinal tract by intestinal bacteria[64]; the sulfur dioxide can then be either absorbed into the intestine and/or released from the gastrointestinal tract via regurgitation (i.e., "burping") to reach the lungs, where it may trigger asthma or be readily absorbed into the systemic circulation. Lastly and very importantly, sulfur-containing substances can be converted by some intestinal bacteria into the potent mitochondrial toxin hydrogen sulfide, which poisons the ETC more powerfully than does cyanide.

- • Mitochondrial mechanism(s): Sulfite is a mitochondrial toxin, especially in brain cells; therefore avoidance or neutralization of sulfite helps avoid interference with normal mitochondrial respiration. Hydrogen sulfide

[60] Jiang et al. Hijacking mitochondria: bacterial toxins that modulate mitochondrial function. *IUBMB Life*. 2012 May;64(5):397-401

[61] Williamson et al. Viral product trafficking to mitochondria, mechanisms and roles in pathogenesis. *Infect Disord Drug Targets*. 2012 Feb;12(1):18-37

[62] El-Bacha T, Da Poian AT. Virus-induced changes in mitochondrial bioenergetics as potential targets for therapy. *Int J Biochem Cell Biol*. 2013 Jan;45(1):41-6

[63] Zhang X, et al. A mechanism of sulfite neurotoxicity: direct inhibition of glutamate dehydrogenase. *J Biol Chem*. 2004 Oct 8;279(41):43035-45

[64] "Inhalation of sulfur dioxide (SO2) generated in the stomach following ingestion of sulfite-containing foods or beverages..." Lester MR. Sulfite sensitivity: significance in human health. *J Am Coll Nutr*. 1995 Jun;14(3):229-32

(H2S) poisons the mitochondrial ETC more powerfully than does cyanide. Sulfite and H2S are both chelated and neutralized by hydroxocobalamin.

- <u>Clinical benefits</u>: Sulfite avoidance helps some patients avoid exacerbations of asthma and migraine. Clinical trials have demonstrated that administration of the sulfite-binding nutrient vitamin B-12 in the form of hydroxocobalamin helps alleviate/prevent migraine and asthma in some patients. Oral administration of hydroxocobalamin 2,000-4,000 mcg per exposure (i.e., taken before exposure to sulfite-containing foods or medications) or daily doses of 4,000-8,000 mcg/day is reasonable; orally administered vitamin B12 at doses of 2,000 mcg/day can achieve higher serum levels than can routine medical protocol of intramuscular vitamin B12.

PERSPECTIVES

Mitochondrial Medicine Arrives to Prime Time in Clinical Care: Nutritional Biochemistry and Mitochondrial Hyperpermeability ("Leaky Mitochondria") Meet Disease Pathogenesis and Clinical Interventions

Alex Vasquez, DC, ND, DO, FACN

Alex Vasquez, DC, ND, DO, FACN, is director of programs at the International College of Human Nutrition and Functional Medicine in Barcelona, Spain and online at ICHNFM.org. (*Altern Ther Health Med.* 2014;20(suppl 1):26-30.)

Corresponding author: Alex Vasquez, DC, ND, DO, FACN
E-mail address: ichnfm@gmail.com

MITOCHONDRIAL MEDICINE ARRIVES TO GENERAL PRACTICE AND ROUTINE PATIENT CARE

Mitochondrial disorders were once relegated to "orphan" status as topics for small paragraphs in pathology textbooks and the hospital-based practices of subspecialists. With the increasing appreciation of the high frequency and ease of treatment of mitochondrial dysfunction, this common cause and consequence of many conditions seen in both primary and specialty care deserves the attention of all practicing clinicians.

We all know that mitochondria are the intracellular organelles responsible for the production of the currency of cellular energy in the form of the molecule adenosine triphosphate (ATP); by this time, contemporary clinicians should be developing an awareness of the other roles that mitochondria play in (patho)physiology and clinical practice. Beyond being simple organelles that make ATP, mitochondria play clinically significant roles in autoimmunity, inflammation, cancer, insulin resistance, cardiometabolic disease such as hypertension and heart failure, and neurologic disorders such as Alzheimer's and Parkinson's diseases. As I stated during the recent International Conference on Human Nutrition and Functional Medicine[1] in Portland, Oregon, in September 2013, we have collectively arrived at a time when mitochondrial therapeutics and the contribution of mitochondrial dysfunction to clinical diseases must be

considered on a routine basis in clinical practice. *Mitochondrial medicine* is no longer an orphan topic, nor is it a superfluous consideration relegated to boutique practices. Mitochondrial medicine is ready for prime time—now—both in the general practice of primary care as well as in specialty and subspecialty medicine. What I describe here as the "new" mitochondrial medicine is the application of assessments and treatments to routine clinical practice primarily for the treatment of secondary/acquired forms of mitochondrial impairment that contribute to common conditions such as fatigue, depression, fibromyalgia, diabetes mellitus, hypertension, neuropsychiatric and neurodegenerative conditions, and other inflammatory and dysmetabolic conditions such as allergy and autoimmunity.

BEYOND BIOCHEMISTRY

Structure and function are of course intimately related and must be appreciated before clinical implications can be understood and interventions thereafter applied with practical precision. The 4 main structures and spaces of the mitochondria are (1) intramitochondrial matrix—the innermost/interior aspect of the mitochondria containing various proteins, enzymes of the Krebs cycle, and mitochondrial DNA; (2) inner membrane—the largely impermeable lipid-rich convoluted/invaginated membrane that envelopes and defines the matrix and which is the structural home of many enzymes, transport systems, and important structures such as cardiolipin and the electron transport chain (ETC); (3) intermembrane space—contains noteworthy molecules: creatine-phosphokinase and cytochrome c; and (4) outer membrane—comparatively more permeable (to molecules <10 000 Dalton) and—like the inner membrane—very lipid-rich and with active and passive transport systems for select molecules that need to enter and exit the mitochondria. Clinicians need to appreciate that mitochondrial membrane integrity is of the highest importance; just as we have come to appreciate the

<u>**2014 Perspective on Mitochondrial Nutrition in Primary Care**</u>: Full-text available online at IntJHumNutrFunctMed.org/events/MitochondrialMedicine.

Food-Induced Activation of Toll-like Receptors, Endoplasmic Reticulum Stress, and the Unfolded Protein Response:
An Integrated Model for Understanding Metabolic Inflammation

> **Metabolic Inflammation: Diet-Induced Metabolic Impairment and Inflammation**
> In this section, I will describe and give structure to a model for understanding what I have previously described—albeit intuitively—as metabolic inflammation.

Introduction: In my model presented starting in 2012,[65] I began differentiating/describing inflammatory conditions as existing along and within an *overlapping continuum* of ❶ metabolic inflammation, ❷ allergic inflammation, and ❸ autoimmune inflammation. The most basic definition/description of metabolic inflammation is simply that it is a pathophysiologic state of nonacute metabolic disruption/dysfunction combined with a state of chronic/sustained mild/nonacute inflammation. What I have also stated is that "chronic inflammation" as most of us were taught in our Pathology coursework does not—for the most part—exist; except for a few rare diseases, the body does not perpetuate clinically significant states of inflammation. So-called ==*chronic* inflammation only occurs via a *sustained inflammatory response*==. Another newer—and perhaps more direct way—of shattering the outdated paradigm of "chronic disease" is to state that such *diseases* do not exist—only *responses* and *accumulated damage* exist. Clinicians should experiment with the possibilities and implications of exchanging their conception of "chronic diseases" in favor of "sustained responses"; I think they will find the experience to be more illuminating/empowering/engaging than resignation to the chronic disease model and its subsequent indefinite noncurative (poly)pharmacotherapy. The illustration below introduces and summarizes several key concepts.

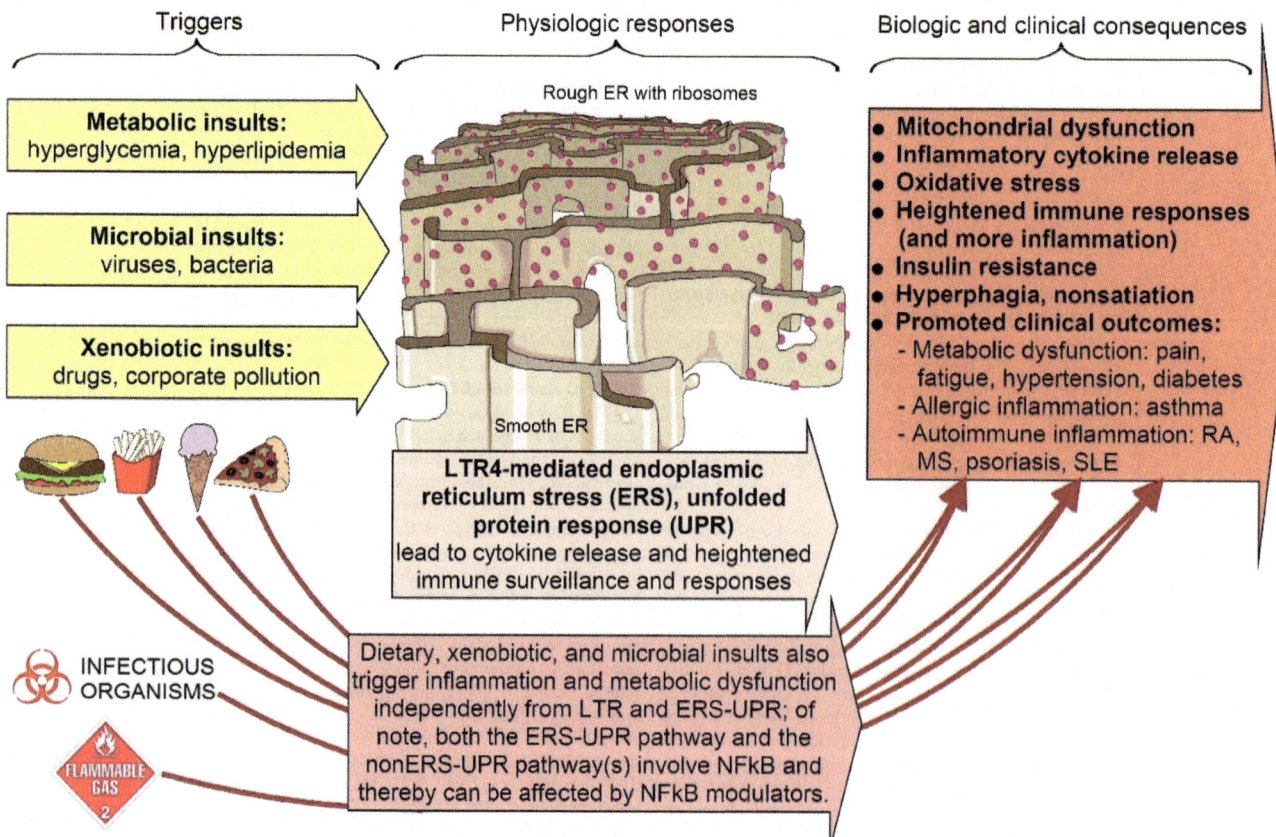

Metabolic, microbial, and xenobiotic insults—often via TLR4—induce endoplasmic reticulum stress (ERS) and the subsequent unfolded protein response (UPR): Consequences include vicious cycles of inflammation, oxidative stress, mitochondrial dysfunction, insulin resistance and hyperphagia—all consistent with sustained sterile nonacute inflammation and metabolic dysfunction/impairment termed here as *metabolic inflammation*.

---

[65] Vasquez A. *Functional Immunology and Nutritional Immunomodulation: Presentation Slides Part 1*. Publication Date: June 5, 2012, ISBN-13: 978-1477603857

Key components of metabolic inflammation: The following points serve to construct an understanding of the major components of metabolic inflammation, starting from the causative metabolic, microbial, and xenobiotic insults and resulting in sustained oxidative stress, inflammation, mitochondrial dysfunction, and insulin resistance.

> **Induction of metabolic inflammation as sequential socioeconomic stress → overeating → cellular fuel overload and intestinal microbial overgrowth → dysmetabolism via LPS, palmitate/ceramide, and xenobiotic accumulation**
>
> **The first manifestation of inflammation is metabolic disturbance.** In my model of sequential and overlapping forms of inflammation—metabolic, allergic, and autoimmune—**metabolic inflammation is generally the primary/first component** and—among most diseases seen in routine practice—is always a component of the other inflammatory states.
>
> "These signs [of inflammation] are typically more prominent in acute inflammation than **in chronic inflammation. A fifth clinical sign, loss of function (functio laesa),** was added by Rudolf Virchow in the 19th century."
>
> Perkins JA. Chapter 2, "Acute and Chronic Inflammation" in *Pathologic Basis of Disease, Eighth Edition* 2010, p43-77

- Fuel overload promotes metabolic stress and inflammation via direct (palmitate, ceramide) and indirect (microbial, xenobiotic) effects—a compilation and review: Stated most simply, overconsumption of simple carbohydrates (e.g., wheat products, sucrose, potatoes) leads to hyperglycemia and hyperinsulinemia, which function synergistically in the formation of palmitate and ceramide, which lead to insulin resistance, inflammation, and metabolic impairment per mitochondrial dysfunction and endoplasmic reticulum stress. The situation is compounded by the fact that these sources of simple carbohydrates (e.g., wheat products, potatoes) also contain indigestible carbohydrates that promote microbial population growth, thereby increasing endotoxin (LPS) load. LPS, glucose, palmitate, and ceramide have additive/synergistic effects in promoting inflammation, mitochondrial dysfunction, and endoplasmic reticulum stress. Gut overgrowth of bacteria secondary to fermentable fuel overload—via LPS—impairs cytochrome p450 "phase 1" detoxification, thereby promoting drug and xenobiotic accumulation; xenobiotic accumulation activates the aryl hydrocarbon receptor to impair GLUT-4 receptor expression and also leads to mitochondrial impairment.[66] In this manner, fuel overload from overconsumption of processed foods can cause inflammation, mitochondrial impairment, and the insulin resistance that causes type-2 diabetes purely by microbial and xenobiotic mechanisms independent from the content of "calories" and resultant adipogenesis. Obviously, the implications of the previous discussion of the AGE/RAGE and the polyol pathway apply here; as a reminder: Processed food + hyperglycemia → AGE → RAGE activation → inflammation

- Toll-like receptors (TLR, e.g., TLR2 and TLR4): Upregulated and activated by microbial motifs such as bacterial endotoxin/LPS as well as by glucose (hyperglycemia), long-chain saturated fatty acids, including palmitate.

- Endoplasmic reticulum (ER) and ER stress (ERS): The ER functions to synthesize and process proteins, whether used intracellularly, within the cell membrane, or secreted from the cell. In certain adverse situations—notably exposure to viruses, bacteria, hyperglycemia and hyper(long-chain saturated)lipidosis, disruption of ER function leads to accumulation of unfolded/misfolded proteins within the ER lumen; this "ER stress" leads to a complex adaptive cellular response termed the "unfolded protein response" (UPR), which increases production and release of proteins and cytokines needed for immune surveillance. Induction of ERS-UPR occurs following activation of the NFkB pathway and/or TLR2 or more potent TRL4 depicted as follows:

  Long-chain saturated fatty acids → TLR4 → NFkB → ERS+UPC → inflammation, orexia, insulin resistance

  ERS is obviously an adaptive mechanism, which most likely developed for sensing microbes, and which becomes maladaptive when chronically stimulated by overconsumption of carbohydrates and saturated fats; the sequel UPR is notably appropriate for response to microbes, and notably harmful when activated by habitual dietary excess. When ERS-UPR activation is sustained, the result is excess inflammation and immune system hypervigilance (e.g., pathophysiologic priming for disorders of metabolic/allergic/autoimmune inflammation); more extreme intensities of ERS-UPR activation may result in cell apoptosis.

- Unfolded protein response (UPR): Endoplasmic reticulum stress is somewhat analogous to a "traffic jam" inside the ER, and the unfolded protein response is a pro-inflammatory "public service announcement" in response. Without the metabolic insults of excess glucose and excess saturated fatty acids—both of which are overpresent

---

[66] "Recently, much evidence has emerged showing that environmental toxins, including POPs, affect mitochondrial function and subsequently induce insulin resistance." Lim et al. Persistent organic pollutants, mitochondrial dysfunction, and metabolic syndrome. *Ann N Y Acad Sci.* 2010 Jul;1201:166-76

in Americanized/Westernized diets but which would have been absent for the vast majority of human history—the main expected stressors for induction of ERS would have been of microbial origin, and thus the resultant "sounding of the alarms" and amplification of immune responses would have clearly been a positive and meaningful response; now that industrialized societies have essentially codified hourly/daily hyperglycemia and higher intakes of saturated fat, this ERS-UPR pathway is maintained in a higher state (quantitatively more) of sustained activation (longer duration).

- <u>NFkB involvement in ERS-UPR inflammatory cytokine release</u>: Saturated long-chain fatty acids activate TLR4 and induce NFkB-mediated inflammation via ERS-UPR and routes that are independent from ERS-UPR. While the ERS-UPR pathway effects elaboration of pro-inflammatory cytokines in an NFkB-dependent manner, the opposite is also true: NFkB activation causes ERS-UPR. Therefore, one would reasonably expect that inhibitors/modulators of the NFkB pathway (detailed elsewhere in this chapter) would be of therapeutic value in conditions of ERS-UPR; however, the clinical focus should always remain on identifying and eliminating the *origin* of the ERS-UPR/NFkB activation.

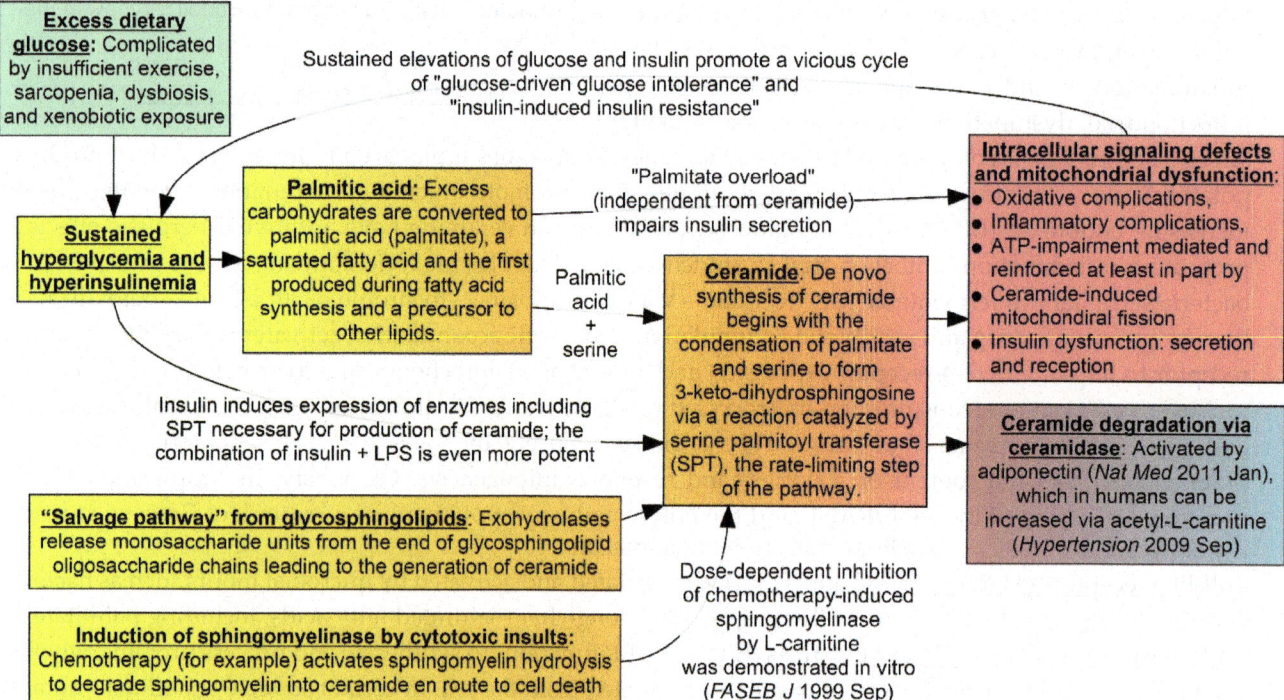

The foundation of metabolic inflammation via confluence of diet, dysbiosis, and xenobiotics: Metabolic inflammation is best understood as a state of inflammation that has a metabolic origin rather than a "normal" origin from infection or injury. The clearest and most concrete examples of metabolic impairment that reciprocate with inflammation are mitochondrial dysfunction and endoplasmic reticulum stress; generally neither of these occur by spontaneous generation, but rather by identifiable and modifiable variables, the three most important of which are dietary excess, dysbiosis, and xenobiotic production/exposure/accumulation and each of which have been independently validated. In the real world—the world in which we live characterized by population-wide economic stress and public promotion and government subsidization of processed food overload, clinically epidemic dysbiosis, and pandemic global pollution—all of these factors converge to promote ==syndemic obesity, inflammation, cardiometabolic syndrome, and brain dysfunction.== Hyperglycemia and hyperinsulinemia upregulate production of palmitate, which is sufficient to promote oxidative and glycemic complications, and which leads to production of ceramide, which furthers the mitochondrial impairment and insulin resistance; these biochemical consequences also lead to brain inflammation which at the level of the hypothalamus reduces satiety and promotes insatiable food cravings while at the level of the cerebral cortex promotes cognitive impairment. Production of ceramide via the other two pathways of exohydrolases and sphingomyelinase appear to be less clinically relevant for most encounters in outpatient practice. Clinically notable is the alleviation of ceramide accumulation via L-carnitine's inhibition of sphingomyelinase[67] and also—more importantly—via induction of ceramidase via adiponectin[68] which is stimulated in humans by supplementation with acetyl-L-carnitine[69], which was reviewed previously.

---

[67] Andrieu-Abadie et al. L-carnitine prevents doxorubicin-induced apoptosis of cardiac myocytes: role of inhibition of ceramide generation. *FASEB J.* 1999 Sep;13(12):1501-10
[68] Holland et al. Receptor-mediated activation of ceramidase activity initiates the pleiotropic actions of adiponectin. *Nat Med.* 2011 Jan;17(1):55-63
[69] Ruggenenti et al. Ameliorating hypertension and insulin resistance in subjects at increased cardiovascular risk: effects of acetyl-L-carnitine. *Hypertension.* 2009 Sep;54:567-74

- **Cytokine-induced and NFkB/inflammation-induced insulin resistance—a vicious cycle**: Milanski et al note, "Cytokines, induced either by TLR activation and/or by ER stress, can play a pathogenetic role in the development of insulin resistance in peripheral tissues." Activation of the NFkB/inflammatory pathway inhibits insulin receptor function via several mechanisms, one of which is the serine phosphorylation of insulin receptor substrates (IRS) 1 and 2[70]; the resultant insulin resistance and hyperinsulinemia obviously promote a sustained state of hyperglycemia and promotion of endogenous saturated fatty acid synthesis thereby creating a vicious cycle of hyperglycemia and hyperlipidosis which further promote inflammatory pathways and insulin resistance, via mechanisms including ERS-UPR, NFkB, mitochondrial dysfunction, and ceramide.

- **ERS-UPR is triggered by xenobiotics and particulate pollution**: Particulate pollution—such as air pollution particles <2.5 micrometers—triggers ERS-UPR in experimental models of lung injury, and these effects—which may become systemic via circulatory distribution of particulate matter—are mediated via oxidative stress.[71] Drugs and nutrients that activate ERS-UPR cytopathology include several HIV-1 protease inhibitors (nelfinavir, atazanavir, ritonavir, lopinavir), the anti-cancer drug sorafenib, the NSAIDs/coxibs indomethacin and celecoxib, and the natural supplement resveratrol (possibly selective for cancer cells); flavonoids baicalein and apigenin and the nutritional supplement N-acetyl cysteine are protective against ERS-UPR.[72]

- **Connecting ERS with mitochondrial dysfunction (MitoDys)**: Given that both ER and mitochondria are nutrient-*sensing* organelles (not simply nutrient *processing* or *metabolizing*), we should reasonably anticipate some coordination between them; indeed per Hotamisligil, "Activation of the nutrient-responsive mTOR signaling pathway stimulates protein synthesis and folding in the ER." ER stress and mitochondrial dysfunction both serve adaptive roles and represent a conceptual point along a continuum spanning function and pathology. An interrelationship between ER stress and mitochondrial dysfunction clearly exists, and the relationship may be most powerful in the direction from mitochondria toward ER; given that mitochondrial mTOR is necessary for ER protein synthesis/folding, then dysfunction in mitochondria/mTOR would be anticipated to promote ER stress and the resultant UPR. ERS adversely impacts mitochondrial function via promotion of inflammation, but this—unlike the effect of mTOR on ER—is indirect and nonspecific. Conversely, correction of mitochondrial dysfunction and optimization of mitochondrial function would be expected to alleviate ER stress via enhanced "ER-Mito coordination"; with regard to the latter, I think this is likely but acknowledge that I am being (reasonably) speculative here. In living systems, and which is already apparent from the previous diagrams, insults against endoplasmic reticulum and mitochondria are often similar/identical, and—also as previously demonstrated—once activated the dysfunctions within ER and mitochondria tend to be self-perpetuating and mutually reinforcing; the cures for these problems are notably similar, namely avoiding the dietary/microbial/xenobiotic (DMX) insults while providing complete nutrition to repeat affected pathways and systems and restore/heal injured molecules/cells/tissues.

- **Fuel overload (excess carbohydrate and saturated long-chain fatty acids) promotes ERS-UPR and mitochondrial dysfunction via oxidative and inflammatory mechanisms (e.g., 12/15-LOX induction) and by inhibition of mitochondrial biogenesis**: The concept of *fuel overload* is highly important; *fuel overload* is the prototype and the major cause of *metabolic stress* to endoplasmic reticulum and mitochondria and which leads to metabolic inflammation.

Overeating → fuel overload → metabolic stress → ER stress & MitoDys → dysmetabolism & inflammation

Of note, when we discuss "fuel overload", we are discussing the biochemical and cellular consequences of overeating; in particular, we are specifying overconsumption of saturated (long-chain) fatty acids and of carbohydrates, which are converted to saturated fatty acids such as palmitate (which leads to induction of pro-inflammatory IL-6, which also promotes induction of TH-17 cells) and ceramide, which causes insulin resistance and mitochondrial dysfunction. Quite obviously, the epidemics of obesity, cardiometabolic disease, and other sustained/chronic diseases/responses are not initiated and maintained by overconsuming lean proteins, whole fruits, vegetables, and seeds. Therefore, overeating (OE) is the psychosocial behavior that leads

---

[70] Hotamisligil GS. Endoplasmic reticulum stress and the inflammatory basis of metabolic disease. *Cell*. 2010 Mar 19;140(6):900-17

[71] Velasco G. Endoplasmic reticulum stressed by pollution. *Am J Physiol Cell Physiol*. 2010 Oct;299(4):C727-8

[72] Lafleur MA, Stevens JL, Lawrence JW. Xenobiotic perturbation of ER stress and the unfolded protein response. *Toxicol Pathol*. 2013 Feb;41(2):235-62

to the cellular and biochemical consequence of fuel overload (FO); since OE precedes and causes FO, the former should be foremost in the discussion. Further, to bring more clarity and specificity to OE, we can specify *acellular/refined/simple* carbohydrates (CHO) and the *harmful-when-overconsumed* fat(ty acid)s—the dietary fatty acids of consequence are saturated, hydrogenated, or the n6 PUFAs linoleic and arachidonic. Given these considerations, then **OverEating Carbohydrates and dangerous Fats** abbreviated as **OECF** is our best phrase for as the proximate cause of *fuel overload* (FO) which causes *metabolic stress* and the resultant *metabolic inflammation*; **OECF-FO** pairs overeating and fuel overload. The specific problem—already noted in the clinical drug protocols and pharmacodevelopment priorities—is the separation of FO from EOCF, so that OECF can be ignored while patients are kept drug-dependent to manage consequences of FO; this is pervasive in current DM2 guidelines.

- Food-induced hypothalamic inflammation: As described in an excellent article by Milanski et al[73], ❶ long-chain saturated fatty acids produce an inflammatory response predominantly through the activation of TLR4 in hypothalamus with resultant local release of cytokines, and ❷ the physiologic consequences of diet-induced hypothalamic inflammation include local endoplasmic reticulum stress, systemic inflammation, adiposity, insulin resistance, and enhanced hunger, the latter via inhibited reception/function of anorexigenic (hunger-suppressing; the roots *orexi-, orex-, -orexia* are Greek with the denotation of hunger, desire, searching) hormones insulin and leptin. Inflammation in the hypothalamic region of the brain, which can occur following TLR activation secondary to glucose, saturated long-chain fatty acids, or exposure to microbial motifs (e.g., bacterial or viral). In the CNS, TLR4 are found in the microglia. Of additional note regarding brain inflammation, "...recent studies in the brain provide in vivo evidence supporting the model that both ER stress and inflammation are able to activate each other and to inhibit normal cellular metabolism."[74] Thus, given that ERS-UPR and inflammation are self-perpetuating, the most logical targets for intervention are 1) blocking initiation of the cycle by reducing triggers, most common of which are dietary, microbial, xenobiotic (DMX), then 2) using safe and effective treatments to address *residual* inflammation and metabolic dysfunction; notice the importance of this sequence and how this approach differs from the "conventional allopathic approach" which usually ignores diet, dysbiosis, detoxification thereby allowing the causative problems to remain, fester, and expand, thereby *creating* the "**need**" for hard-hitting expensive hazardous pharmaceutical interventions.

> **Saturated fatty acids inflame the hypothalamus**
>
> "In animal models of genetic and diet-induced obesity, **the activation of an inflammatory response in the hypothalamus** leads to the molecular and functional resistance to the adipostatic hormones, leptin and insulin, resulting in a defective control of food intake and energy expenditure. ... In conclusion, saturated fatty acids activate TLR2 and TLR4 signaling and ER stress in hypothalamus. ... The presence of a functional TLR4 signaling is required for the development of hyperlipidic dietary obesity."
>
> Milanski et al. *J Neurosci.* 2009 Jan

ER function, ER stress, UPR in a nutshell

- ER functions: Protein folding, maturation, quality control, trafficking; intracellular calcium homeodynamics; "...the ER should be viewed as an essential apparatus in the coordination of metabolic responses through its ability to control the synthetic and catabolic pathways of various nutrients."
- ER stress: Accumulation of newly synthesized unfolded proteins activates the UPR—unfolded protein response
- Three main triggers of ERS-UPR: The main molecular *final common pathways* are TLR4 and NFkB, which are themselves triggered by:
  - ❶ Metabolic stress: Excess glucose, excess saturated long-chain fatty acids, metabolic demands of obesity and hyperglycemia/hyperinsulinemia
  - ❷ Microbial exposure: Viruses and bacteria, especially Gram-negative bacteria
  - ❸ Xenobiotic exposure: Chemical xenobiotics, particulate air pollution
- Five major *fingers* or *branches* of ERS-UPR effects:
  - ❶ Pro-inflammatory: NFkB, JNK-AP1
  - ❷ Oxidative: Pro-oxidant pathways are activated along with Nrf2; despite the latter, ERS-UPR is pro-oxidative
  - ❸ Metabolic: Altered metabolism/reception of glucose, lipids, insulin, leptin, and iron
  - ❹ Catabolism: Reduction in protein synthesis and enhancement of protein degradation to alleviate ER stress
  - ❺ Apoptosis: "All of these signals contribute to the triggering of apoptotic responses when ER stress is excessive, prolonged, or insufficiently neutralized." Hotamisligil, *Cell* 2010 Mar
- Main remedies to ERS-UPR: Avoid triggers, downmodulate TLR activation with fish oil and olive oil, suppress oxidative stress and NFkB as described in this textbook, supplementation with NAC and flavonoids baicalein (*Scutellaria baicalensis*) and apigenin (in many fruits and vegetables, especially parsley, celery and chamomile).

---

[73] Milanski et al. Saturated fatty acids produce inflammatory response predominantly through activation of TLR4 signaling in hypothalamus. *J Neurosci* 2009 Jan;359-70
[74] Hotamisligil GS. Endoplasmic reticulum stress and the inflammatory basis of metabolic disease. *Cell.* 2010 Mar 19;140(6):900-17

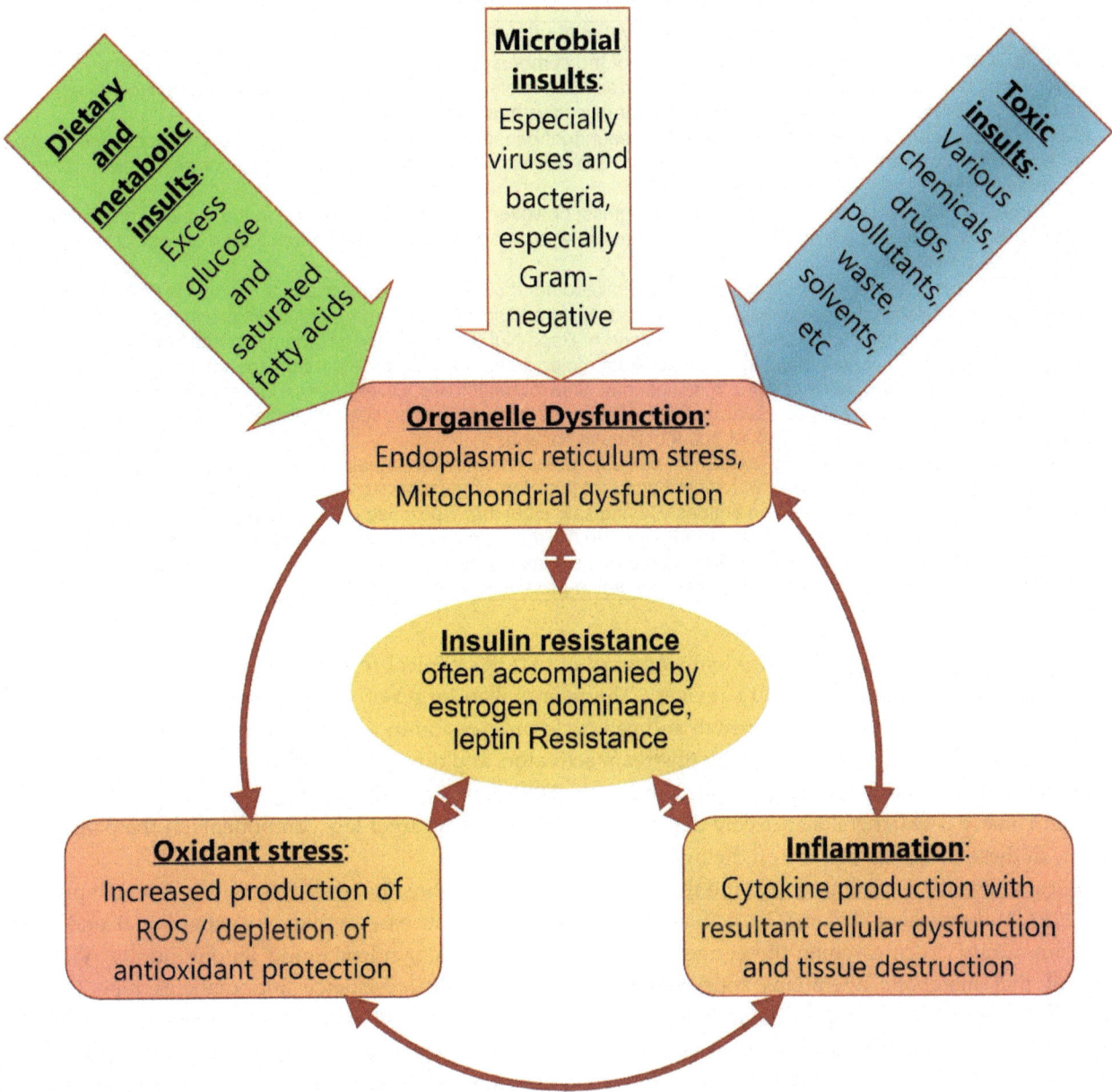

Dietary and metabolic insults: Excess glucose and saturated fatty acids

Microbial insults: Especially viruses and bacteria, especially Gram-negative

Toxic insults: Various chemicals, drugs, pollutants, waste, solvents, etc

Organelle Dysfunction: Endoplasmic reticulum stress, Mitochondrial dysfunction

Insulin resistance often accompanied by estrogen dominance, leptin Resistance

Oxidant stress: Increased production of ROS / depletion of antioxidant protection

Inflammation: Cytokine production with resultant cellular dysfunction and tissue destruction

Genesis and consequences of organelle dysfunction—mitochondrial dysfunction (MitoDys) and endoplasmic reticulum stress (ERS): Common themes in organelle dysfunction include the causes—microbial insults, metabolic insults, xenobiotic insults—and consequences—vicious cycles of organelle dysfunction, inflammation, and oxidative stress. Attentive readers and those who want to master this material at a deeper level should take a few minutes to appreciate the number of vicious cycles represented in the diagram above: hint—ERS reciprocally causes mito-dys and therefore counts as one vicious cycle; each bidirectional arrow represents another vicious cycle, etc. Given that more components can be added to these interactions, these dynamic relationships have an additive tendency to be self-sustaining. The major exogenous triggers to organelle dysfunction (in this conversation: ER and mitochondria) are dietary excess (glucose and saturated fat), microbes (bacteria are quantitatively most important), and corporate-derived toxins such as pollution and pesticides.

mTOR—Mechanistic Target of Rapamycin

mTOR: renaming the so-called Mechanistic Target of Rapamycin

Thankfully, mTOR is a nice short abbreviation in place of the cumbersome common name "Mechanistic Target of Rapamycin" which is cumbersome, grammatically incorrect, and misleading in comparison to a name that would help doctors use mTOR-related information in their clinical practices with greater comfort and ease.

- M—The M can represent "Mechanistic" (which is redundant because all targets are mechanisms; so mechanistic does not add anything meaningful to the conversation) or "Mammalian" (which is unnecessary in a contextualized conversation).
- T—"Target" is nonspecific and biologically meaningless; however, "targets" are common in the world of pharmacology, which is for the most part the science of how to interfere with and generally block the function of biological pathways, enzymes, and receptors.
- O—"Of" is a preposition and should neither be capitalized nor included in an abbreviation; this use is poor grammar.
- R—Rapamycin is an immunosuppressive "drug" that was first discovered as an antibacterial product of the soil bacterium *Streptomyces hygroscopicus* on the island of Rapa Nui (Easter Island). Rapamycin has been officially renamed sirolimus. Of course, naming an intracellular molecule after a drug promotes the idea that this receptor exists to receive this drug, thus reinforcing the medicocentric view of healthcare. Given that mTOR is responsive to antioxidant/Reductive therapies, Resveratrol, and dietary Restriction, we can see that replacing Rapamycin with natural treatments gives us broader conceptual and therapeutic horizons.

For anyone to say that these are simply "semantic" considerations would reveal a painful ignorance of the fact that we as humans *largely but not exclusively* think with words and that therefore linguistic structure is the easiest manner for dictating perceptions and subsequent thoughts and actions. Having said all of that, I propose here a *revisioning* of mTOR via a *renaming* of mTOR, from mammalian target of rapamycin to the more descriptive and clinically applicable Meaningful Therapeutic Opportunity for Reductive/antioxidative therapies, Resveratrol, R-lipoic acid, Restrictive diets and a few Random/Rouge interventions already proven safe and health-promoting.

Clinical relevance, structure and function:

- Clinical relevance—cancer: An excellent summary of mTOR's clinical relevance in cancer was articulated by Tan et al[75] at the start of their 2014 review, "The mammalian target of rapamycin (mTOR) kinase plays an important role in regulating cell growth and cell cycle progression in response to cellular signals. It is a key regulator of cell proliferation and many upstream activators and downstream effectors of mTOR are known to be deregulated in various types of cancers. Since the mTOR signaling pathway is commonly activated in human cancers, many researchers are actively developing inhibitors that target key components in the pathway and some of these drugs are already on the market."

- Clinical relevance—autoimmunity, and the connection with hyperinsulinemia: Fascinating research published in 2012-2014 revealed that mTOR activation precedes clinical disease activity in experiential and human autoimmunity. In researching the connection between metabolic syndrome and autoimmunity, Vilà et al[76] found that metabolic alterations consistent with human insulin resistance and diabetes type-2 such as hyperleptinemia and hyperinsulinemia preceded increased liver mTOR expression, which itself preceded the development of autoimmune disease in a murine model SLE, thereby suggesting the following flow of events— not depicted here but obviously implied are the accompanying and reinforcing mitochondrial dysfunction and oxidative stress, both of which are exacerbated by and supportive of the progressive inflammation and immunometabolic disruption. They also note that leptin, an adipocytokine/adipokine derived from body fat stores, reduces the proliferation of Tregs (and would therefore be expected to exacerbate autoimmunity); leptin resistance (frequently seen with insulin resistance) would therefore be expected to be protective yet is apparently overpowered by the effect of hyperinsulinemia-mTOR.

  Hyperinsulinemia → mTOR activation → immune dysregulation → autoimmune inflammation

  In 2013 Lai et al[77] extended these findings to humans with SLE noting greater mTOR activation in DN (double-negative) T-cells in "preflare" SLE patients relative to those with stable disease or healthy controls, and they concluded [paraphrasing] that "mTOR activation is a trigger of IL-4 production and necrotic death of DN T cells in patients with SLE" thereby allowing us to appreciate the following flow:

  mTOR activation → IL4 production & DN-Tcell necrosis → autoimmune inflammation

[75] Tan HK, et al. The mTOR signalling pathway in cancer and the potential mTOR inhibitory activities of natural phytochemicals. *Asian Pac J Cancer Prev.* 2014;15(16):6463-75
[76] Vilà L et al. Metabolic alterations and increased liver mTOR expression precede development of autoimmune disease in murine lupus erythematosus. *PLoS One.* 2012;7:e51118
[77] Lai et al. mTOR activation triggers IL-4 production and necrotic death of double-negative T cells in patients with systemic lupus erythematosus. *J Immunol* 2013 Sep:2236-46

- <u>Main function: Giving phosphate</u> groups as a serine/threonine kinase: mTOR phosphorylates the OH group of serine or threonine, basically activating/inactivating other pathways and orchestrated responses: proliferation, programmed cell death (apoptosis), differentiation, inflammation via immunophenotype imbalance.

- <u>Structure</u>: Exists as two different multiprotein complexes mTORC1 and mTORC2; rapamycin/sirolimus is specific for mTORC1 while mTORC1 is also activated by bacterial endotoxin (LPS; via TLR4), promoting increased LPS-induced cytokine production and inflammation.

- <u>Downregulation: Receiving phosphate groups from c-Abl protein tyrosine kinase</u> as a means of modulation: While the action of mTOR is to phosphorylate other molecules, mTOR can itself be phosphorylated as thereby inactivated as a means of upstream control, in this case mediated by c-Abl protein tyrosine kinase. Stated planely, "the c-Abl protein tyrosine kinase phosphorylates mTOR and inhibits its action."[78] Additionally, mTOR is inhibited by DEPTOR (DEP domain-containing and mTOR-interactive protein, and the "mTOR pathway" effects are also mitigated by SIRT1; inhibition of the effects of the *mTOR pathway* are promoted by resveratrol via enhanced mTOR-DEPTOR inhibitory interaction and via *mTOR-pathway* modulation/downregulation/neutralization via SIRT1.[79]

> **mTOR controlled (activated/inhibited) by phosphorylation; the effect is dependent on the means (location) of phosphorylation**
>
> "Under normal circumstances, in the presence of growth factor and nutrients, mTOR is constitutively activated. **This activation is achieved**, in part, through the insulin receptor or insulin-like growth factor receptor pathways, via a cascade that involves the activation of phosphatidylinositide-3-kinase (PI3K), then phosphatidyl inositol-3,4,5 phosphate-mediated activation of Akt/PKB-mediated **phosphorylation of mTOR**. Deacetylated tRNA species accumulating as a result of amino acid shortage may act as negative regulators of mTOR... Moreover, the **c-Abl protein tyrosine kinase phosphorylates mTOR and inhibits its action.**"
>
> Castedo et al. *Cell Death & Differentiation* 2002

- <u>Method of activation: Receiving phosphate groups from Akt</u>: Transmembrane phosphatidylinositol-3-3kinase (PI3K), which phosphorylates Akt (also known as protein kinase B or PKB) and which phosphorylates (perhaps at serine residue 2881?[80]) and thereby activates mTOR. Notable and documented from different sources is appreciation that the relationship between Akt and mTOR is bidirectional, self-reinforcing. The flow of sequential activation is as follows (PAM):

  Transmembrane PI3K activation → Akt phosphorylation/activation → mTOR phosphorylation/activation

- <u>mTOR-driven epigenetic changes</u>: In 2014 Oaks and Perl[81] reviewed data showing that mTOR is epigenetically active and conceptually summarized this new data by stating, "mTOR can modify epigenetic pathways including methylation, demethylation, and histone phosphorylation and mediates enhanced T-cell activation in SLE. Beyond their role in metabolism, mitochondria are the main source of reactive oxygen intermediates (ROI), which activate mTOR and regulate the activity of histone and DNA modifying enzymes." While the details and mechanisms are still being explored, the fact that mTOR is epigenetically active clearly broadens its range of influence and clinical implications.

Therefore, per this succinct introduction, we note that mTOR is a major player in cancer and autoimmunity, that it is activated by hyperinsulinemia and oxidative stress, and that its pathogenic mechanisms include alterations in cell growth and proliferation consistent with cancer, as well as the inflammatory/immunologic abnormalities noted in autoimmunity; elucidation of the newly discovered epigenetic changes induced by mTOR may provide additional insight into the mechanisms involved and clinical countermechanisms available. Of additional note is that the mTOR activation complex including but not limited to the direct components of the PAM (PI3K-Akt-mTOR) pathway contain some degree of functional redundancy/feedback such that direct and isolated mTOR targeting (as with drugs) is oft-times met with the development of therapeutic resistance as other pathways (e.g., Akt) are upregulated to compensate for a pharmacologically impaired mTOR; as such, the best clinical approach for downregulating mTOR will utilize an overall *multicomponent* approach rather than targeted *monotherapy*.

---

[78] Castedo M et al. Mammalian Target of Rapamycin (mTOR): Pro- and Anti-Apoptotic. *Cell Death and Differentiation* 2002 Feb;9:99-100

[79] Liu M et al. Resveratrol inhibits mTOR signaling by promoting the interaction between mTOR and DEPTOR. *J Biol Chem.* 2010 Nov 19;285(47):36387-94

[80] Zhong LM et al. Resveratrol inhibits inflammatory responses via the mammalian target of rapamycin signaling pathway in cultured LPS-stimulated microglial cells. *PLoS One.* 2012;7(2):e32195

[81] Oaks Z, Perl A. Metabolic control of the epigenome in systemic Lupus erythematosus. *Autoimmunity.* 2014 Jun;47(4):256-64

Activation leads to:

- Anabolic effects and mechanisms: Cell growth (including muscle), proliferation, promotion of cancer, resistance to anticancer chemotherapy; from this list, obvious is the fact that mTOR is generally anabolic, a trigger for cell growth and proliferation and survival. Mechanisms include enhanced ribosome biogenesis, increased synthesis of lipids and nucleotides, suppression of catabolic processes (especially autophagy).
- Inflammatory disease: Inflammation and immune dysregulation via suppression of FoxP3 activation and thus suppression of Treg generation; mTOR activation is now considered "a key factor in abnormal activation of T and B cells in SLE. ... [mTORC1] is required for transducing T cell activation initiated by cytokines"[82] mTOR suppresses expression of Foxp3 and development of regulatory T cells.
- Promotion of cancer: In their remarkably lucid and clinically relevant review, authors Tan, Moad and Tan[83] wrote, "Hyperactivation of the PI3K/Akt/mTOR signaling pathway is a prominent hallmark of cancer and is frequently implicated in resistance to anticancer therapies such as biologics, tyrosine kinase inhibitors, radiation, and cytotoxics."

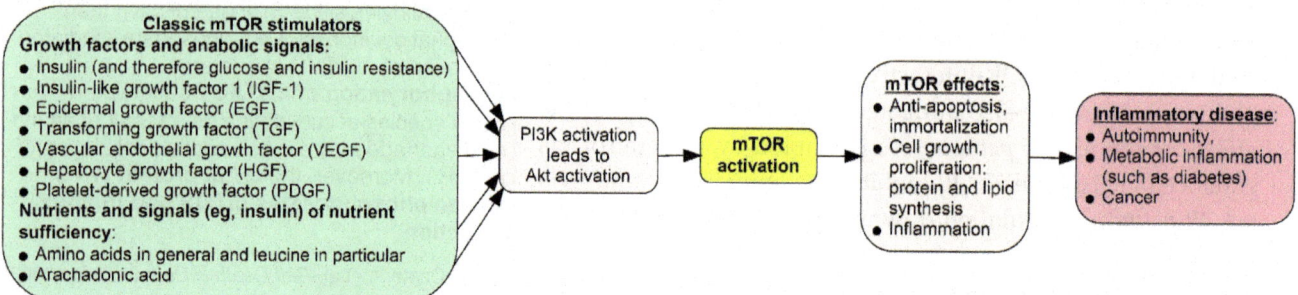

Simplified and "classic" pathway of mTOR activation and its effects: This clear diagram is the basis for understanding the more complex and interconnected pathways represented later in this section.

Means of activation: "Classic" mTOR activation is mostly via activation of the transmembrane PI3K receptor causing Akt phosphorylation/activation causing mTOR phosphorylation/activation. However and importantly, other stimulators, co-stimulators, primers or enhancers can also contribute to mTOR activation and the persistence of that activation. As such, clinicians and researchers need to appreciate both "the classic pathway" as well as "the entire context."

- Growth factors and anabolic hormone-like substances, signals of nutrient abundance/sufficiency:
  - Insulin, and therefore glucose and insulin resistance—see following discussion on mitochondrial hyperpolarization
  - Insulin-like growth factor 1 (IGF-1)
  - Epidermal growth factor (EGF)
  - Transforming growth factor (TGF)
  - Vascular endothelial growth factor (VEGF)
  - Hepatocyte growth factor (HGF)
  - Platelet-derived growth factor (PDGF)
  - Leptin—produced in proportion to adipose load
- Nutrients and signals (e.g., insulin) of nutrient excess:
  - Amino acids: leucine in particular
  - Arachidonic acid
  - Leptin—leptin is both an inflammatory cytokine and a hormone produced in proportion to body adipose load thereby serving as an indicator of nutrient excess; leptin has a hunger-supressing effect in the hypothalamus. Low, basal levels of leptin appear necessary for competent immune responses, while excess leptin contributes to systemic inflammation and autoimmunity via immunocyte activation and enhanced production of pro-inflammatory cytokines such as IL-1, IL-6 and TNF-a. Additionally, leptin activates the mTOR pathway.[84] Leptin's hypothalamic anorexigenic effect is mediated effectively via mTOR and redundantly/directly via leucine. Interestingly, adipogenesis is dependent on mTOR activation, leptin synthesis in adipocytes is dependent on mTOR and leads to additional mTOR activation, thereby forming vicious cycles between adipose, mTOR, leptin and other factors such as

[82] Perl A. Systems biology of lupus. *Autoimmunity*. 2010 Feb;43(1):32-47
[83] Tan et al. The mTOR signalling pathway in cancer and the potential mTOR inhibitory activities of natural phytochemicals. *Asian Pac J Cancer Prev*. 2014;15(16):6463-75
[84] Maya-Monteiro CM, Bozza PT. Leptin and mTOR: partners in metabolism and inflammation. *Cell Cycle*. 2008 Jun 15;7(12):1713-7

mitochondrial dysfunction and hyperglycemia/hyperinsulinemia due to insulin resistance. Obviously, fasting and weight reduction via body fat loss would reduce leptin elaboration and leptin-mediated mTOR activation, as discussed in slightly more detail in the clinical therapeutics section that follows on fasting and restrictive diets.

- **Immunostimulation**: mTORC1 is activated by **bacterial endotoxin (LPS)**[85]; **mTOR is stimulated by inflammation while mTOR also promotes inflammation, thus creating a vicious cycle.** This is to be expected since mTOR induction supports cellular anabolism and activation during immune challenges.

- **Pollution, xenoestrogens:** Including but not limited to **methylparaben** and **bisphenol-A (BPA)**[86]

- **Mitochondrial dysfunction: Mitochondrial hyperpolarization** causes either activation or priming of mTOR; these intracellular characteristics (mitochondrial hyperpolarization and activation of mTOR) are commonly associated together, but the former appears to promote the latter because successful targeting of the latter does not reverse the former. The question therefore becomes, "What causes mitochondrial hyperpolarization?" and answers include: ❶ Physiologic hyperglycemia—Following carbohydrate (CHO) ingestion, glucose uptake by pancreatic beta-cells increases ATP production, and "increased ATP/ADP ratio contributes to inhibition of potassium channel (KATP), which leads to **plasma membrane depolarization**, voltage-gated calcium channel opening, calcium influx, and secretion of insulin."[87] Clearly, in this manner, insulin secretion in response to glucose is dependent upon functional mitochondria that can produce sufficient ATP; defective mitochondria would be expected to cause an impaired secretion of insulin in response to glucose, and this is exactly what is noted in prolonged type-2 diabetes mellitus. Glucose consumption and cellular uptake in excess of what is needed to produce ATP leads to an uncoupling of electron and proton flow with respect to Complex 5 (ATPase) activity; this situation of *more electrons/protons than ATP production* is the hallmark of hyperpolarization of the inner mitochondrial membrane. We can call this *fuel overload induction of mitochondrial hyperpolarization* which is accompanied by *ROS overload induction of mitochondrial hyperpolarization* because the same glucose overload discussed above also triggers excess ROS production. Normally, with a CHO-modest diet and sufficient exercise, this would be a transient experience, and indeed the transient fuel overload and ROS generation is a component of normal insulin secretion. Wikstrom et al[88] summarized, "Beta-cell response to glucose is characterized by mitochondrial membrane potential ($\Delta\Psi$) hyperpolarization and the production of metabolites that serve as insulin secretory signals. We have previously shown that glucose-induced mitochondrial hyperpolarization accompanies the concentration-dependent increase in insulin secretion within a wide range of glucose concentrations." ❷ Pathologic hyperglycemia—With sustained hyperglycemia (whether due for example to carbohydrate excess or sarcopenia), the glucose/ROS induction of mitochondrial hyperpolarization never abates, and ROS-induced oxidative damage persists nonstop (leading to antioxidant depletion, intracellular damage, GSH depletion) and leads to persistent *pathologic* mitochondrial hyperpolarization. Glucose/ROS-induced mitochondrial hyperpolarization has a physiologic role in the secretion of insulin. In an exceptionally excellent and prophetic paper published in 2006, Wiederkehr and Wollheim[89] wrote "In the [pancreatic beta]-cell, glucose has been reported to promote ROS production through its hyperpolarizing effect on mitochondrial membrane potential." From a *common sense* standpoint, nutrient-sensing mTOR would be expected to be activated by carbohydrate overload, because it serves as a growth-stimulating agent; cellular growth is triggered by and dependent upon (over)abundant nutritional reserves. ❸ Oxidized LDL (low density lipoprotein, OxLDL)—Excess dietary CHO drives oxidative stress and LDL production, promoting the formation of oxidized LDL; this is exacerbated in states of insulin resistance and ~~chronic~~ *sustained* hyperglycemia and hyperinsulinemia.[90] OxLDL causes oxidative stress and depletion of GSH, which occur prior to and appear to cause mitochondrial membrane hyperpolarization. Another mechanism of intracellular GSH depletion may be that of active GSH extrusion from cells undergoing apoptosis. Per Giovannini et al[91],

[85] Lee PS et al. mTORC1-S6K activation by endotoxin contributes to cytokine up-regulation and early lethality in animals. *PLoS One.* 2010 Dec 21;5(12):e14399

[86] Goodson WH 3rd1, Luciani MG, Sayeed SA, Jaffee IM, Moore DH 2nd, Dairkee SH. Activation of the mTOR pathway by low levels of xenoestrogens in breast epithelial cells from high-risk women. *Carcinogenesis.* 2011 Nov;32(11):1724-33

[87] Kim JA, Wei Y, Sowers JR. Role of mitochondrial dysfunction in insulin resistance. *Circ Res.* 2008 Feb 29;102(4):401-14

[88] Wikstrom JD et al. beta-Cell mitochondria exhibit membrane potential heterogeneity that can be altered by stimulatory or toxic fuel levels. *Diabetes.* 2007 Oct;56(10):2569-78

[89] Wiederkehr A, Wollheim CB. Minireview: implication of mitochondria in insulin secretion and action. *Endocrinology.* 2006 Jun;147(6):2643-9

[90] Kopprasch S et al. In vivo evidence for increased oxidation of circulating LDL in impaired glucose tolerance. *Diabetes.* 2002 Oct;51(10):3102-6

[91] Giovannini et al. Mitochondria hyperpolarization is early event in oxidized low-density lipoprotein-induced apoptosis in Caco-2 intestinal cells. *FEBS Lett* 2002 Jul;523:200-6

"OxLDL induce mitochondrial membrane hyperpolarization." ❹ Oxidative stress, GSH depletion, mitochondrial hyperpolarization—The interrelationship of ROS stress, GSH depletion, and mitochondrial hyperpolarization has been discussed, or "the last could be the consequence of the first two."[92], and ❺ LPS—"The stimulation of TLR4 by LPS induced a time- and dose-dependent contractile dysfunction, which was associated with a decrease of TLR2 messenger, a rearrangement of microfilament cytoskeleton and an oxidative imbalance, i.e., the formation of reactive oxygen species (ROS) together with the depletion of GSH content. An alteration of mitochondria, namely a hyperpolarization of their membrane potential, was also detected."[93] The means by which LPS induces mitochondrial hyperpolarization includes activation of TLR4, activation of NFkB, and oxidative stress from NADPH oxidase; inhibition of any of these steps leads to resistance to LPS-induced hyperpolarization, ❻ Oligomycin—Oligomycin is a prototypic mitochondrial toxin used experimentally; oligomycin A inhibits ATP synthase by blocking the proton channel (Fo subunit).

Clinical disease associations:

- mTOR and SLE (*Autoimmunity*. 2010 Feb): "Activation of the mammalian target of rapamycin (mTOR) has recently emerged as a key factor in abnormal activation of T and B cells in SLE. In T cells, increased production of nitric oxide and mitochondrial hyperpolarization (MHP) were identified as metabolic checkpoints upstream of mTOR activation. mTOR controls the expression T-cell receptor-associated signaling proteins CD4 and CD3zeta through increased expression of the endosome recycling regulator Rab5 and HRES-1/Rab4 genes, enhances Ca2+ fluxing and skews the expression of tyrosine kinases both in T and B cells, and blocks the expression of Foxp3 and the generation of regulatory T cells. MHP, increased activity of mTOR, Rab GTPases, and Syk kinases, and enhanced Ca2+ flux have emerged as common T and B cell biomarkers and targets for treatment in SLE."

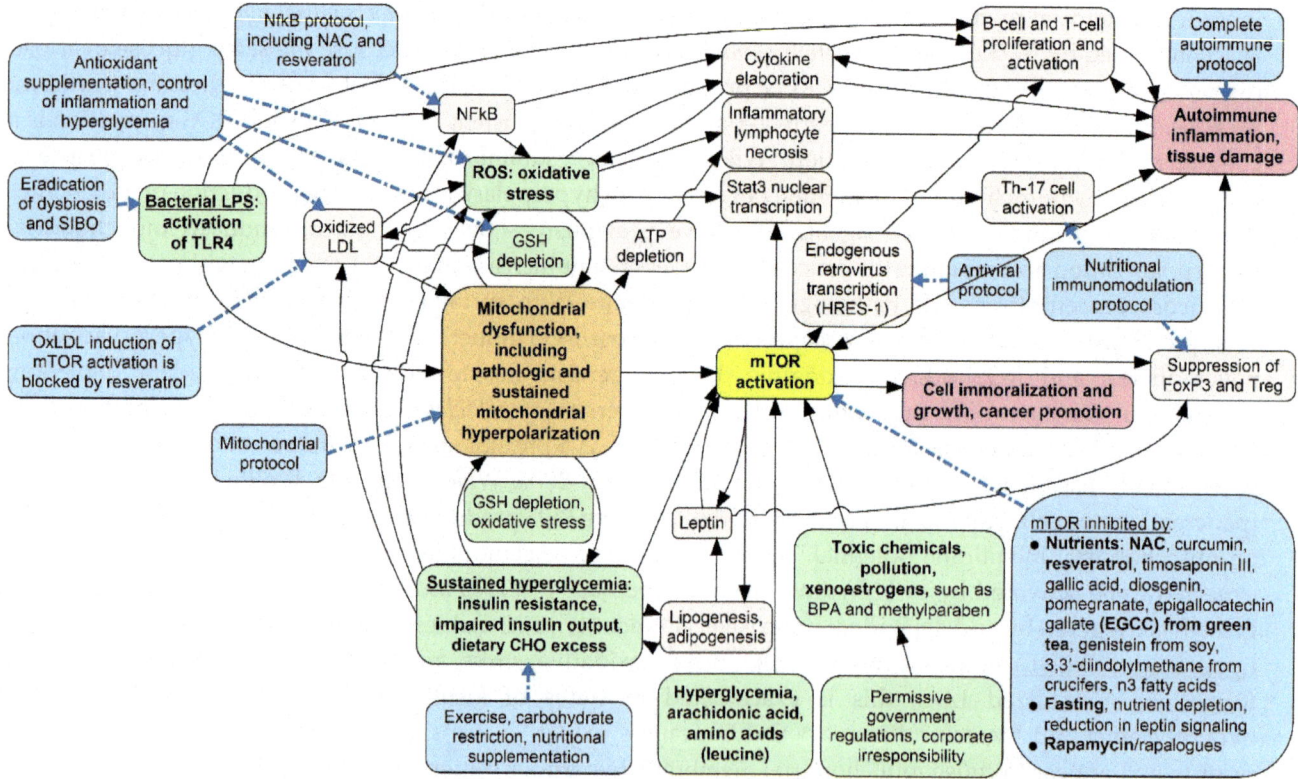

mTOR is best summarized as a cell-survival and growth mechanism that promotes inflammatory disease: Nutrient abundance supports and fuels growth; relatedly but perhaps oppositely and paradoxically, cellular stress also triggers mTOR activation to promote immortalization and proliferation. The worst-case-scenario for mTOR activation would be abundant nutrition (adequate protein with hyperglycemia) with oxidative stress; this is exactly what is noted in diabetes mellitus type-2, which increases the risk for autoimmunity and cancer. In this diagram: green = problems that can be addressed with interventions, blue = clinical interventions, orange, yellow, red = mechanistic steps.

---

[92] Giovannini et al. Mitochondria hyperpolarization is early event in oxidized low-density lipoprotein-induced apoptosis in Caco-2 intestinal cells. *FEBS Lett* 2002 Jul;523:200-6
[93] Scirocco A et al. Exposure of Toll-like receptors 4 to bacterial lipopolysaccharide (LPS) impairs human colonic smooth muscle cell function. *J Cell Physiol.* 2010 May:442-50

Inhibition leads to:

- Normalization of immunophenotype with restored/beneficial balance via increased Treg:Th17 ratios; clinical benefit demonstrated most specifically in autoimmunity and transplant rejection
- Reduced tumor growth, anticancer benefit, notably in lung cancer[94] and also breast cancer cell lines.

The mTOR-inhibition paradox: Lipoic acid and resveratrol block the negative effects of the mTOR signaling pathway as a whole, yet mTOR itself appears responsible for some of this benefit because targeted blockade of mTOR with rapamycin negates some/many benefits from lipoate/resveratrol supplementation, in vitro

An interesting conclusion stated in the mTOR research using lipoic acid as well as reseveratrol is that—depending on the method of study—mTOR appears *necessary* for the induction of the protective response from lipoic acid or resveratrol because administration of rapamycin blocks the beneficial effect of these nutrients; this is potentially of supreme importance in appreciating the differing mechanisms of action of these nutrients from the prototypic drug because this data suggests the possibility that keeping mTOR *at least slightly active* helps the nutrients to work more effectively *either* upstream or downstream but generally **both** upstream *and* downstream as we see with lipoic acid and resveratrol. ❶ Perhaps mTOR activates the pathways or substrates that are more effective targets than mTOR itself, ❷ or perhaps rapamycin-mTOR binding blocks a more powerfully inhibitory effect mediated by the nutrients; of these two possibilities, I suspect that the former is more likely because the impression that I get from the literature is that the mechanism of action of some nutrients—resveratrol and lipoate in particular—is that these nutrients somehow turn mTOR against itself, which would be more consistent with the first of the two possibilities suggested here. ❸ Another possibility is that moderate suppression (without targeted pharmacologic inhibition) of mTOR leads to a better homeodynamic balance which is more moderate and thereby lessens induction of compensatory feedback that might lead to a paradoxical upregulation of mTOR despite administration of a presumed mTOR inhibitor—this would be a paradoxical/hormetic/homeodynamic effect.

I've noticed that the subtlely with regard to mTOR is greater than with other pathways/mechanisms/drugs/nutrients that I have studied; here one must be careful to distinguish in the literature the difference between "inhibition of mTOR" and "inhibition of mTOR signalling" especially because the latter could have its main location of effect either upstream or downstream of mTOR itself. Likewise and per a previous section, "mTOR phosphorylation" as an isolated term is meaningless because it can effect either activation (via Akt) or inhibition (via c-Abl protein tyrosine kinase).

Study	Zhong et al. *PLoS One*. 2012[95]		Xie et al. *Brain Res.* 2012 Oct[96]	
Test	Rat cells: insult (LPS) + resveratrol	Insult + resveratrol + rapamycin	Mouse brain cells: insult (oxygen glucose deprivation [OGD] + lipoate	Insult + lipoate + rapamycin
Findings	"Resveratrol reduced NO, PGE2, inducible nitric oxide synthase (iNOS), cyclooxygenase-2 (COX-2), tumor necrosis factor-α (TNF-α), interleukin-1β (IL-1β) and nuclear factor-κB (NF-κB) in BV-2 cells. "Resveratrol increased PTEN, Akt and mTOR phosphorylation in a dose-dependent manner or a time-dependent manner.	"Rapamycin (10 nM), a specific mTOR inhibitor, blocked the effects of resveratrol on LPS-induced microglial activation. In addition, mTOR inhibition partially abolished the inhibitory effect of resveratrol on the phosphorylation of IκB-α, CREB, extracellular signal-regulated kinase 1/2 (ERK1/2), c-Jun N-terminal protein kinase (JNK), and p38 mitogen-activated protein kinase (p38 MAPK).	"We found that pre-treatment administration of ALA reduced the OGD and simulated reperfusion-induced lactate dehydrogenase (LDH) release in a dose-dependent manner and that 1mM ALA pre- and post-treatments provided protection....	"However, rapamycin, an mTOR inhibitor, was able to thoroughly abolish the protective effects of ALA. Western blotting showed that the ALA pre- and post-treatments up-regulated the phosphorylation of Akt, mTOR, S6K and 4E-BP1 in [cells]. However, after pre-treatment with rapamycin, the level of Akt phosphorylation was decreased in primary cultures of CECs but could still be restored by ALA, whereas the levels of mTOR, S6K and 4E-BP1 phosphorylation were significantly decreased and could not be restored.
Conclusions	"This study indicates that resveratrol inhibited LPS-induced proinflammatory enzymes and proinflammatory cytokines via down-regulation phosphorylation of NF-κB, CREB and MAPKs family in an mTOR-dependent manner."		"These results suggest that ALA pre- and post-treatments provide protective effects against simulated ischemia and reperfusion-induced CEC injury by promoting the Akt/mTOR pathway and that mTOR is required for ALA protection"	
mTOR paradox	Resveratrol blocks the LPS-induced pro-inflammatory effects of the mTOR *pathway*, but does so in a manner that actually activates mTOR and is dependent upon mTOR since the addition of rapamycin reduced the protective effects of resveratrol.		Alpha- blocks the LPS-induced pro-inflammatory effects of the mTOR *pathway*, but does so in a manner that actually activates mTOR and is dependent upon mTOR since the addition of rapamycin reduced the protective effects of resveratrol.	

---

[94] Zarogoulidis P, Lampaki S, Turner JF, et al. mTOR pathway: A current, up-to-date mini-review (Review). *Oncol Lett.* 2014 Dec;8(6):2367-2370
[95] Zhong LM et al. Resveratrol inhibits inflammatory responses via the mammalian target of rapamycin signaling pathway in cultured LPS-stimulated microglial cells. *PLoS One.* 2012;7(2):e32195
[96] Xie et al. Alpha-lipoic acid pre- and post-treatments provide protection against in vitro ischemia-reperfusion injury in cerebral endothelial cells via Akt/mTOR signaling. *Brain Res.* 2012 Oct 30;1482:81-90

The mTOR-inhibition paradox—*continued*

<u>Summary and commentary on studies exemplifying this mTOR paradox:</u>

- <u>Resveratrol inhibits inflammatory responses via mTOR signaling</u> (*PLoS One* 2012 Feb[97]): While resveratrol's antioxidant and NFkB-inhibiting benefits would be expected to reduce downstream effects of mTOR-mediated inflammatory signaling. Paradoxically, in certain in vitro models (freshly isolated monocytes and primary myeloid dendritic cells [DCs]), mTOR activation actually *inhibits* the production of proinflammatory cytokines while enhancing the release of anti-inflammatory cytokines by "blocking NF-kB activation and increasing STAT3 activity"; note that these *micro*antiinflammatory effects are clearly offset clinically and phenotypically when whole-system effects are observed. Apparently noting this paradox, the authors state "Thus, the mTOR pathway might have opposite roles in the immune system." Clearly, increasing Stat3 activity with its resultant promotion of Th-17 cells is pro-inflammatory in whole-systems biology even if it is *micro*antiinflammatory in vitro. Related to this "mTOR-cancer paradox"—which is similar to the pro- and anti-carcinogenic "STAT3 paradox—is that mTOR is both pro- and anti-apoptotic, depending on the overall cellular state and molecular context.[98] By blunting the anti-inflammatory effects of resveratrol with rapamycin, these researchers appear to show that resveratrol's anti-inflammatory effects are mediated at least partly by its interaction with and modulation of mTOR; the authors' conclusion is that "The results of this study indicated that resveratrol activated the mTOR signaling pathway and induced mTOR phosphorylation..." The language of this article is unclear because the authors state that resveratrol "activated the mTOR signaling pathway" when this could be confused with "activated the mTOR signaling" when what is really meant is "activated the signaling pathway upstream of mTOR." What the authors are stating here is that resveratrol's activation of the mTOR *pathway* is what leads to mTOR phosphorylation and inactivation. A (nonexclusively) different/additional and reasonable interpretation from this data is that both resveratrol and rapamycin inhibit mTOR but that rapamycin is weaker in its anti-inflammatory effect but stronger in its binding-site attraction. If this latter model were correct, then both agents would have antiinflammatory effects mediated by (competitive) interaction with mTOR, but each would complete with the other, resveratrol for stronger anti-inflammatory effect, blocked my rapamycin. One impression that I get when reading this article is that part of what occurs with resveratrol and mTOR is that resveratrol interacts with mTOR in such a way as to turn mTOR against itself; the authors note several times that mTOR is necessary for resveratrol's ability to reduce the production of inflammatory cytokines/enzymes/mediators and thus we can summarize from this work that mTOR is necessary for resveratrol-mediated blockade of mTOR-activated inflammation.

- <u>Lipoic acid pre- and post-treatments provide protection against in vitro ischemia-reperfusion injury in cerebral endothelial cells via Akt/mTOR signaling</u> (*Brain Res* 2012 Oct[99]): Authors of this study used a model of simulated ischemia and reperfusion-induced cerebral endothelial cell (CEC) injury by using 6 hours of "oxygen/glucose deprivation (OGD) followed by 4h of simulated reperfusion, either alone or together with aLA administration before (pre-treatment) or immediately after (post-treatment) OGD." Both pre- and post-treatments with aLA provided protection. "However, rapamycin, an mTOR inhibitor, was able to thoroughly abolish the protective effects of aLA. Western blotting showed that the aLA pre- and post-treatments up-regulated the phosphorylation of Akt, mTOR, S6K and 4E-BP1 in both bEnd.3 cells and primary cultures. However, after pre-treatment with rapamycin, the level of Akt phosphorylation was decreased in primary cultures of CECs but could still be restored by aLA, whereas the levels of mTOR, S6K and 4E-BP1 phosphorylation were significantly decreased and could not be restored. These results suggest that aLA pre- and post-treatments provide protective effects against simulated ischemia and reperfusion-induced CEC injury by promoting the Akt/mTOR pathway and that mTOR is required for aLA protection." Again here we see a paradox in that aLA (similar to resveratrol) is able to diminish mTOR pathway singalling and adverse effects yet at the same time mTOR itself appears responsible for part of this benefit, perhaps due to some maintenance of Akt-mTOR feedback, or possibly competition between rapamycin and lipoate/resveratrol.

- <u>Resveratrol inhibits mTOR signaling by promoting the interaction between mTOR and DEPTOR</u> (*J Biol Chem.* 2010 Nov[100]): "We found that RSV inhibits mTOR signaling via a Sirt1-independent mechanism." "How RSV promotes the binding of DEPTOR to mTOR remains unknown. One possibility may be that RSV directly interacts with mTOR or DEPTOR, leading to enhanced interaction between these two proteins. Alternatively, RSV may indirectly promote the interaction between mTOR and DEPTOR by binding to an auxiliary protein. Similar to the latter model, rapamycin has been shown to impair the association between mTOR and Raptor through binding to FKBP12. It is also possible that RSV may activate a signaling pathway that leads to a chemical modification of either mTOR or DEPTOR, thus promoting the interaction between these proteins." "Taken together, our studies reveal that RSV inhibits leucine-stimulated mTORC1 activation by promoting mTOR/DEPTOR interaction and thus uncover a novel mechanism by which RSV negatively regulates mTOR activity." The authors acknowledge the numerous interactions and counteractions and paradoxes, concluding with several possible explanations. The probability for plurality among these mechanism is more certain than this singular "either/or" situation.

<u>Resolution of the paradox:</u> For now, I judge that the best reasonable solution to any cognitive dissonance induced by this mTOR paradox is simply to accept and embrace the complexity and paradox and then to place it (back) into the systems biology context, particularly focusing—as all clinicians must—on the clinical outcomes rather than the isolated molecular biology, the latter of which is highly worthy of consideration and decipherative efforts but not to the extent that it overpowers the larger concern of how to safely and effectively improve patient outcomes. In this regard, we have to keep in mind that, in cells and even more so in whole-body systems, other pathways (eg, NFkB, SIRT1 and SIRT3), whole organelles (eg, mitochondria) and systems (eg, immunologic) are involved and as such any great or small disaster/benefit in an isolated pathway might be offset by effects elsewhere; hence, the ultimate proof is in the clinical outcome. With regard to resveratrol, the three mechanisms that most directly explain the paradox are resveratrol's activation of SIRT1 and SIRT3, promotion of inhibitory DEPTOR binding, inhibition of NFkB, and promotion of mitochondrial biogenesis. Relatedly, lipoate has potent antioxidant effects, supports mitochondrial function, inhibits NFkB, and also promotes immunotolerance via enhancement of IL-10 and reduction of IL-17 and TNF-alpha.

---

[97] Zhong LM et al. Resveratrol inhibits inflammatory responses via the mammalian target of rapamycin signaling pathway in cultured LPS-stimulated microglial cells. *PLoS One.* 2012;7(2):e32195

[98] Castedo M et al. Mammalian Target of Rapamycin (mTOR): Pro- and Anti-Apoptotic. *Cell Death and Differentiation* 2002 Feb;9:99-100

[99] Xie R, Li X, Ling Y, et al. Alpha-lipoic acid pre- and post-treatments provide protection against in vitro ischemia-reperfusion injury in cerebral endothelial cells via Akt/mTOR signaling. *Brain Res.* 2012 Oct 30;1482:81-90

[100] Liu M et al. Resveratrol inhibits mTOR signaling by promoting the interaction between mTOR and DEPTOR. *J Biol Chem.* 2010 Nov 19;285(47):36387-94

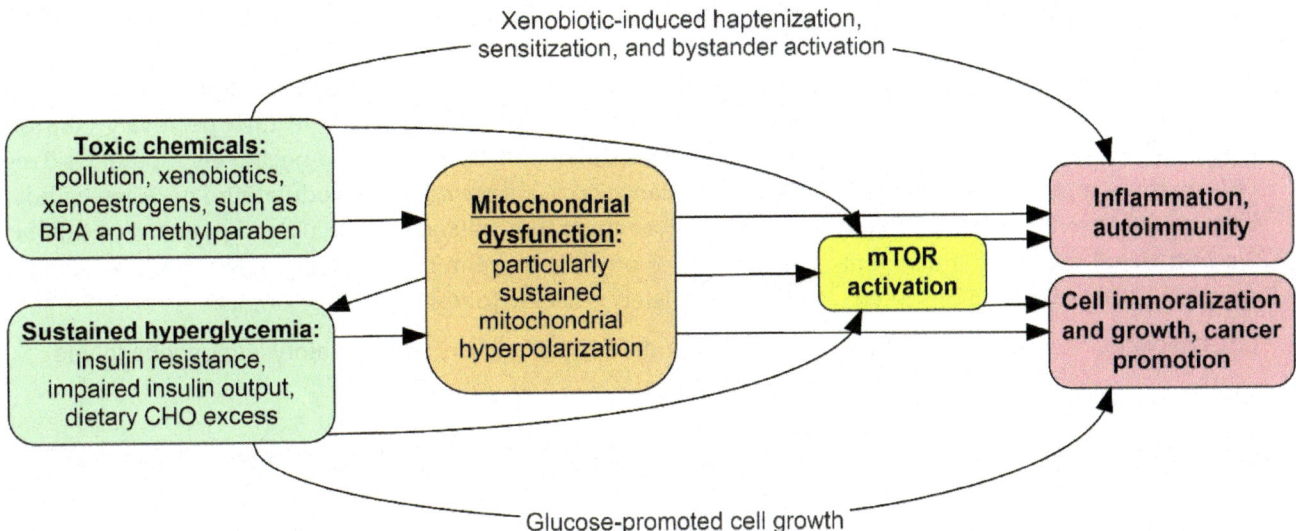

Xenobiotics and hyperglycemia independently and additively/synergistically promote mitochondrial dysfunction (subtype: hyperpolarization) and mTOR activation: Thereafter, hyperglycemia becomes self-reinforcing via induction of and causation by mitochondrial dysfunction and the resulting systemic inflammation. Whether by xenobiotic stimulation or hyperglycemia, both mitochondrial dysfunction and mTOR activation lead to the promotion of inflammation, cell growth and immortizliation leading to promotion of clinical manfestations of autoimmunity and cancer.

Means of inhibition:

- Rapamycin, now renamed for human clinical use as "rapamune" and sirolimus" (*online.epocrates.com* 2015 Mar): "**Black Box Warnings**: **Appropriate Use**—to be aministered only by physicians experienced in immunosuppressive treatment and management of renal transplant patients in adequate medical facility. **Immunosuppressant**—Immunosuppression increases risk of infection, lymphoma, and other malignancy risks. Tablet 2 mg (30 ea): $918; solution 1 mg/mL (1 bottle of oral sol, 60mL): $848. Dose is depenent on weight and "immunologic risk" generally ranges from 2-5 mg/d QD PO with maximum dosage of 40 mg/d. Beyond the FDA-approved use for preventing renal transplant rejection, rapamycin also has utility in the treatment of human autoimmunity; rapamycin 2 mg/d orally reduces disease activity and prednisone dosage in patients (n=9) with SLE—of note, this beneficial suppression of mTOR occurs during and without suppression of mitochondrial hyperpolarization while normalizing very specific aspects of mitochondrial dysfunction (normalization of mitochondrial Ca2+ levels). [101]

- Reductive/antioxidant therapies: Just because a substance can function as an antioxidant and has a consistent physiologic/clinical effect does not imply that the effect is due to the antioxidant property. Nonetheless, a group of therapeutics can be reasonably categorized under reductive/antioxidant therapies; if any sacrifice is made in biomedical accuracy the derived enhancement of clinician memorization and subsequent clinical applicability will more than compensatorily balance the scales of justice. I have grouped most botanicals under this

> Robust redox protection and GSH suppress excess mitochondrial hyperpolarization and the resulting mTOR activation which drive Th17/Treg imbalance; in this manner, GSH and antioxidant/reductive therapies are antiinflammatory via inhibition of mTOR, thereby disinhibiting FoxP3 induction of the Treg phenotype
>
> "**GSH regulates the elevation of mitochondrial transmembrane potential or mitochondrial hyperpolarization**, which in turn **activates the mammalian target of rapamycin (mTOR)** in lupus T cells. The mTOR skews cell death signal processing modulates T cell differentiation, and, in particular, **inhibits the development of CD4 CD25 FoxP3 Treg cells**, which are deficient [and which would be protective if present] in patients with active SLE."
>
> Lai et al. *Arthritis Rheum* 2012 Sep

heading, since most have and function at least in part as reducing/antioxidative agents; resveratrol and R-lipoic acid (lipoate) both take advantage of the fickleness of the universe to gain a separate bulleted header since both

---

[101] Fernandez et al. Rapamycin reduces disease activity and normalizes T cell activation-induced calcium fluxing in patients with systemic lupus erythematosus. *Arthritis Rheum.* 2006 Sep;54(9):2983-8

reasonably deserve their own categories and since both start with the letter *R*. N3 fatty acids block mTOR signaling but don't start with *R* and don't fit into another category; they are thus *Rogue*. *Do we have a "simple truth" that clarifies a large swath of clinical inflammatory chaos into a phrase onto which we can grasp, allowing us to—as we would say in Texas—"take the bull by the horns"?* Yes, because antioxidant balance determines GSH status which is a major inverse modulator of mitochondrial hyperpolarization, which in turn positively controls mTOR activation, which in turn positively modulates induction of Th-17 cells and negatively modulates Treg cells. In this manner, reduction/oxidation (redox) balance is *an important* key to modulating Th17/Treg cellular balance and thereby immunophenotype balance. Given that redox balance is directly and potently modifiable via nutritional intake of antioxidants, the concept of nutritional immunomodulation (detailed in Chapter 4 section 3 [4.3]) can be demonstrated—albeit incompletely—via the following flow of events:

GSH depletion → mitochondrial hyperpolarization → mTOR activation → inflammatory immunophenotype

And therefore conversely, what we expect is:

GSH repletion → mitochondrial eupolarization → mTOR modulation → noninflammatory immunophenotype

Surprisingly, what we see with NAC supplementation is the following, which very similar to the effect of rapamycin—namely, the dissociation from mitochondrial hyperpolarization of mTOR activation:

NAC → mitochondrial hyperpolarization unaffected + mTOR inihibition → noninflammatory immunophenotype

I use the term "noninflammatory phenotype" to represent neutrality, rather than a true anti-inflammatory phenotype; I am basically just being conservative here and not trying to overstate the effect although with a sufficiently robust protocol (Chapter 4 section 3) the immunophenotype might actually become anti-inflammatory (which is generally not the goal, per se, since we are ultimately seeking a homeodynamic state, capable of appropriate responses but not necessarily "preset" toward or against any one direction).

Now, obviously other factors can drive mitochondrial hyperpolarization, such as hyperglycemia and LPS, just as other factors can directly suppress mTOR and/or—more commonly as with resveratrol and lipoate—downwardly modulate mTOR pathway signaling. Further, various other factors can affect immunophenotype balance and subsequent inflammatory pathways, mediators, and effects. However the simple correlation of GSH status, particularly via its upward modulation by the immediate GSH precursor NAC, with immunophenotype balance

> **Mechanistic and clinical proof that mTOR dysfunction directly contributes to autoimmunity**
>
> "Similar to the effect of rapamycin, **suppression of mTOR by NAC was accompanied by increased FoxP3 expression in CD4+/CD25+ T cells**. These results suggest that the effect of NAC on the immune system is 1) cell type-specific and 2) it occurs through disconnecting the activation of mTOR from the elevation of $\Delta\psi m$ in lupus T cells, similar to the effect of rapamycin."
>
> Lai et al. N-acetylcysteine reduces disease activity by blocking mammalian target of rapamycin in T cells from systemic lupus erythematosus patients. *Arthritis Rheum* 2012 Sep

is sufficiently accurate, particularly when contextualized with these aforementioned caveats. Via support of GSH and subsequent suppression of hyperpolarization-induced mTOR activation, antioxidants promote immune and inflammatory tolerance via disinhibition/promotion of Treg generation.

- NAC approximately 4,800 mg/d in divided doses: In a landmark 2012 clinical trial published in the American College of Rheumatology's *Arthritis & Rheumatism*, NAC at relatively high doses of 4,800mg/d in divided doses was shown to modulate mitochondrial hyperpolarization (by dissociating the generally resultant mTOR activation) and lead to very important clinical and immunological improvements in patients with SLE; NAC was shown to be safe and well-tolerated by all SLE patients up to 2.4g/d with reversible nausea in 33% of patients receiving 4.8g/d. This study by Lai, Hanczko, Bonilla, et al[102] is truly a landmark contribution and advance in the field of rheumatology and immunology because it proves 1) that the combination of mitochondrial dysfunction and mTOR activation directly leads to an autoimmune phenotype, and 2) that inhibition of mTOR by NAC is safe and effective in patients with SLE; important insights from this remarkable work are as follows: ❶ safety and effectiveness: NAC 4,800mg/d in divided doses proved safe and clinically beneficial in

---

[102] Lai ZW, Hanczko R, Bonilla E, et al. N-acetylcysteine reduces disease activity by blocking mammalian target of rapamycin in T cells from systemic lupus erythematosus patients: a randomized, double-blind, placebo-controlled trial. *Arthritis Rheum*. 2012 Sep;64(9):2937-46

patients with SLE, leading to reductions in disease activity and ANA levels. ❷ mechanistic understanding: Mitochondrial hyperpolarization (MHP) causes mTOR activation which in turn suppresses the expression of the FoxP3 transcription factor necessary for induction of T-regulatory cells. Note that the mTOR activation is the cause of the FoxP3 suppression; ironically, NAC actually increases MHP but dissociates it from mTOR by having a greater effect on and via mTOR suppression. The nutritional supplement NAC works in a similar manner as does the immunosuppressive drug rapamycin, with a mechanism of suppression of mTOR and the effect of enhancing endogenous anti-inflammatory immunomodulation via CD4+ CD25+ FoxP3+ T-regulatory cells. Stated again and differently, NAC paradoxically worsens mitochondrial hyperpolarization in patients with SLE but does so at the same time that it has a more significant impact on mTOR; NAC's rapamycin-like targeting of mTOR dissociates mitochondrial hyperpolarization from mTOR activation. The reduction in mTOR activity (which is of greater consequence than the increase in MIM polarization) allows enhanced expression of FoxP3 for increased elaboration of T-regulatory cells, thereby providing endogenous immunoregulation. ❸ substantial direct (potential) financial savings: "The therapeutic importance of NAC for SLE is reflected by: 1) achieving clinical improvement in two validated disease activity scores within 3 months; 2) diminishing fatigue (21), which is considered the most disabling symptom in a majority of SLE patients (22); 3) absence of significant side-effects; and 4) affordability of this medication. A monthly supply of 600-mg NAC capsules (120–240 capsules) costs $15–$30 on the retail market. This sharply contrasts with average annual direct medical costs estimated to be ~$22,580 per patient in 2009. Thus, the cost of NAC at $180–$360/year would be negligible in comparison to the overall expenditures to society and the expected benefit in reducing the need for vastly more expensive medications burdened with potentially serious side-effects."

o Curcumin—dose-response relationship with oral doses of curcuma extract 440-2200 mg/day, containing 36-180 mg of curcumin, some short-term cancer studies have used 4-8 grams of curcumin: Downregulation of several components of mTOR pathway; clinical benefit seen in several different types of human cancer per clinical trials using curcuma extract at doses between 440 and 2200 mg/day, containing 36-180 mg of curcumin. Some studies have used higher doses of 4 grams of curcumin for 30 days, results included a five-fold increase in post-treatment plasma curcumin/conjugate levels, thereby suggesting clinically significant bioavailability with high doses. Very obviously, all of the benefits/effects of curcumin—or any other nutrient or intervention which by analogy affects many different pathways—are not mediated solely via mTOR inhibition; curcumin is also an antioxidant, has some antimicrobial effects, and blocks NFkB and lipoxygenase as well.

o Timosaponin AIII (TsA3): TsA3 is a steroidal saponin from *Anemarrhena asphodeloides* Bunge, a traditional Chinese medicine used for its anti-diabetic, antiplatelet aggregation and diuretic effects, and it blocks phosphorylation of Atk and mTOR.[103]

o Gallic acid: This polyphenol from many plants and fruits blocks phosphorylation of Atk and mTOR.

o Diosgenin: This plant steroid blocks phosphorylation of Atk and mTOR and also blocks fatty acid synthase.

o Pomegranate: Studies using 8 ounces (approx. 240 cc) of pomegranate juice daily have shown delayed rise of PSA in men with prostate cancer; obviously the juice should be organic to avoid carcinogenic pesticides/glyphosate/atrazine, and more than 8 ounces can be consumed per day.

o Epigallocatechin gallate (EGCC), the major catechin in green tea: Multiple anti-oxidant and anti-inflammatory effects; antagonizes mTOR by stimulating AMPK (5'AMP-activated protein kinase or 5'adenosine monophosphate-activated protein kinase) and blocking phosphorylation of Akt.

o Genistein 300-600 mg/d from soy: Modest clinical benefit has been shown in some cancer trials; benefits likely enhanced by DIM, vitamin D, and other related nutrients.

---

[103] Tan HK, Moad AI, Tan ML. The mTOR signalling pathway in cancer and the potential mTOR inhibitory activities of natural phytochemicals. *Asian Pac J Cancer Prev.* 2014;15(16):6463-75

- o 3,3'-diindolylmethane (DIM maximum dose 300 mg twice daily) from crucifers: DIM blocks phosphorylation/activation of Akt and mTOR and has demonstrated some modest effectiveness in the treatment/retardation of some human cancers.
- Resveratrol 250-500 mg/d; doses up to 4-5 grams daily have been used in clinical trials (e.g., cancer):
  - o High concentrations of resveratrol inhibit mTOR and suppress cellular senescence (Cell Cycle. 2009 Jun[104]): This is a nice review stating that resveratrol inhibits mTOR directly, via upstream activation of inhibitory phosphorylation, and also likely by activating SIRT pathways; impressively if not provocatively, the authors suggest that mTOR could be an abbreviation for Target of Resveratrol. Also impressively, the authors "speculate that even transient inhibition of mTOR is already sufficient to slightly suppress senescence" and from a clinical pharmacokinetic standpoint, this is important by suggesting that transient peaks in serum levels of resveratrol may be sufficient in this regard. Regarding pharmacokinetics, these authors note, "In humans, 5 g resveratrol as a single oral dose did not cause adverse events. Peak plasma levels of resveratrol was 2.4 microM, which occurred 1.5 h post-dose. Peak levels of two metabolites of resveratrol were 3- to 8-fold higher. These metabolites might be biologically active."
- R-lipoic acid (lipoate, thiotic acid): 100-400 mg TID PO for adults: Lipoic acid (here the term "lipoate" will be used for speed/efficiency) is a dual water-/lipid-soluble stubstance, endogenously formed and also available in foods (kidney, heart, liver, spinach and broccoli) which has been referred to as a vitamin-like substance as well as a "short-chain fatty acid"[105]; as an endogenous substance necessary for life and as a food component and nutritional supplement, lipoate has an impressive history of remarkable tolerability and safety.[106] Lipoate has as been uniquely well-studied in experimental models and in human studies; the latter group includes investigations with large numbers of patients monitored for many years (eg, patients with diabetic neuropathy). This is not at all surprising becaue lipoate has many beneficial properties, mechanisms of effect, and clinical applications that make it an attractive research subject for a wide range of experimental and clinical researchers involved in molecular physiology of mitochondria, cyclic AMP, NFkB, Nrf2, viral inhibition, antioxidant benefits, glutathione recycling, and cytokines such as IL-17 particularly relevant for diabetes mellitus, viral hepatitis, toxicity/poisoning, neurodegeneration, inflammation and autoimmunity. As of early 2015, only 12 studies connect lipoate with mTOR, and these generally show that lipoate does indeed reduce mTOR actiation and/or subsequent signaling. As such a few representative studies showing safety and efficacy in humans will be summarized along with the in vitro/animal studies explicating the mTOR involvement. The mildly positive but otherwise lackluster benefits shown in a 2011 study by Ziegler[107] et al of 450 patients with diabetic neuropathyis likely attributable to the means and timing of lipoate administration—600 mg/d PO QD; this is a ridiculous and inexcusable administration scheme given lipoate's short half-life (following oral administration: peak at 20 minutes, half-life at 40 minutes, almost diasappeared at 60 minutes and completely disappeared at 120 minutes[108]) and suggests stunning ignorance on the part of the researchers or the intention to produce negative/disempowered results. The researchers likely based this dosing scheme one one of their earlier studies which also used inappropriate once-daily dosing; in this earlier study (Ziegler et al. 2006[109]) the authorsed found that once-daily oral dosing with lipoate 600, 1200, or 1800 mg/d produced "dose-dependent increase in nausea, vomiting, and vertigo", and they concluded that "oral dose of 600 mg once daily appears to provide the optimum risk-to-benefit ratio" but this was without considering any divided-dose scheme whatsoever. What the authors should have done is used a divided dosing scheme such as 400 mg TID PO to achieve both fewer adverse effects and potentially/likely better clinical results. One case of lipoic acid-induced

[104] Demidenko ZN, Blagosklonny MV. At concentrations that inhibit mTOR, resveratrol suppresses cellular senescence. *Cell Cycle.* 2009 Jun 15;8(12):1901-4

[105] "Alpha-lipoic acid (ALA) is an endogenous short-chain fatty acid that has beneficial protective effects against various vascular diseases." Xie R, Li X, Ling Y, et al. Alpha-lipoic acid pre- and post-treatments provide protection against in vitro ischemia-reperfusion injury in cerebral endothelial cells via Akt/mTOR signaling. *Brain Res.* 2012 Oct 30;1482:81-90

[106] "Efficacy of lipoic acid is combined with a high safety profile, making this molecule a novel candidate for the management of several diseases. Data reported so far are promising and dietary supplementation with lipoic acid seems a useful tool to contrast neuropathic pain during pregnancy." Costantino et al. Peripheral neuropathy in obstetrics: efficacy and safety of α-lipoic acid supplementation. *Eur Rev Med Pharmacol Sci* 2014; 18 (18): 2766-2771

[107] Ziegler D, Low PA, Litchy WJ, et al. Efficacy and safety of antioxidant treatment with α-lipoic acid over 4 years in diabetic polyneuropathy: the NATHAN 1 trial. *Diabetes Care.* 2011 Sep;34(9):2054-60

[108] Carlson DA, et al. The plasma pharmacokinetics of R-(+)-lipoic acid administered as sodium R-(+)-lipoate to healthy human subjects. *Altern Med Rev.* 2007 Dec;12(4):343-51

[109] Ziegler D, Ametov A, Barinov A, et al. Oral treatment with alpha-lipoic acid improves symptomatic diabetic polyneuropathy: the SYDNEY 2 trial. *Diabetes Care.* 2006 Nov;29(11):2365-70

cholestatic hepatitis (63-yo male with diabetes, hypertension, hypothyroidism, and stage 2 chronic renal failure; thiotic acid 600 mg/day)[110] has been reported.

o Alpha-lipoic acid (aLA) supplementation reduces mTORC1 signaling in skeletal muscle from high-fat fed, obese Zucker rats (*Lipids* 2014 Dec[111]): Following administration of aLA to obese rats, the authors found that, "Phosphorylation of the mTOR substrate, eukaryotic initiation factor (eIF) 4E-binding protein 1 (4E-BP1) and eIF4B were significantly reduced in muscle from aLA supplemented rats. Activation of AMP-activated protein kinase (AMPK), an mTOR inhibitory kinase, was higher in the aLA group. Protein expression of markers of oxidative metabolism, acetyl CoA carboxylase (ACC), cytochrome c oxidase IV (COX IV), peroxisome proliferator-activated receptor (PPAR), and PPAR gamma coactivator 1-alpha (PGC-1a) were significantly higher after aLA supplementation compared to non-supplemented group. Our findings show that aLA supplementation limits the negative ramifications of consuming a high fat diet on skeletal muscle markers of oxidative metabolism and mTORC1 signaling." In summary, these researchers found that aLA exerts inhibitory effects on mTOR signaling affecting both upstream and downstream mechanisms; this multipart benefit via monotherapy appears much more fascinating, much more cliniclially valuable (beneficially impacting multiple pathways) and more clilnically reliable and durable than would be the effect of directly targeting only one molecule—mTOR—directly (e.g., rapamycin).

o Lipoic/thioctic acid for symptomatic diabetic polyneuropathy: a critical review. *Treat Endocrinol.* 2004;3(3):173-89[112]): Meta-analysese of the efficacy of lipoate in the treatment of diabetic neuropathy have encompassed very large numbers of patients, including (in 2004) "the largest sample of diabetic patients (n = 1258) ever to have been treated with a single drug or class of drugs to reduce neuropathic symptoms"; such studies have "confirmed the favorable effects of thioctic acid based on the highest level of evidence (Class Ia: evidence from meta-analyses of randomized, controlled trials)." Many of these large and early studies used lipoate 600 mg/d delivered intravenously; oral treatment has also proven efficacious for diabetic neuropathy (peripheral and autonomic) as well as for improving measures of glycemic control. The safety of lipoic acid is remarkably high.

- Restrictive diets and therapeutic fasting—anti-rheumatic, anti-inflammatory, and mTOR-blocking effects: Given that mTOR's classic means of activation is via stimulation of the PI3K/Akt/mTOR pathway via growth factors and anabolic hormones such as insulin, the obvious and intuitive countermeasure to this flow of events is to block the stream of anabolic signals by promoting *therapeutic catabolism*, specifically via carbohydrate restriction and also via total macronutrient restriction via therapeutic fasting. To be sure, mechanisms besides mTOR inhibition are at work during carbohydrate/macronutrient restriction; these include but are not limited to ❶ allergen avoidance, ❷ reparation of mucosal integrity breached by dietarily-fed microbes or dietary antigens, ❸ stimulation of B-cell mucosal immunity, and beta-hydroxy butyrate's (bHB) ❹ stimulation of histone acetylation for a more rejuvenative phenotype and its ❺ stimulation of antioxidant defenses and ❻ mitochondrial efficiency (via ETC complexes #3 and #4), ❼ the lowering of serum insulin which alleviates sodium retention and thus lowers blood pressure and ❽ the anti-inflammatory effect mediated via blockade of the NLRP3 inflammasome;

> **Fasting: a poem by Jelaluddin Rumi (1207-1276)**
>
> There's hidden sweetness in the stomach's emptiness.
> We are lutes, no more, no less. If the soundbox is stuffed full of anything, no music.
> If the brain and belly are burning clean with fasting, then every moment a new song comes out of the fire.
> The fog clears, and new energy makes you run up the steps in front of you. …
> When you fast, good habits gather like friends who want to help. ...
> If you've lost all will and control, they come back when you fast, like soldiers appearing out of the ground, pennants flying above them...

❾ fasting-induced downregulation of mTOR (mediated via lack of stimulation by insulin, amino acids and growth signals, including leptin) would be expected to provide a buffet of benefits, listed previously and

---

[110] "Because of the presence of symptomatic diabetic neuropathy, he began treatment with thioctic acid 600 mg/day.... Use of the Roussel Uclaf causality assessment scale indicated that the association between thioctic acid treatment and our patient's drug-induced liver injury was highly probable; use of the Maria and Victorino scale indicated that the association was probable." Ridruejo E1, Castiglioni T, Silva MO. Thioctic acid-induced acute cholestatic hepatitis. *Ann Pharmacother.* 2011 Jul;45(7-8):e43

[111] Li Z, Dungan CM, Carrier B, Rideout TC, Williamson DL. Alpha-lipoic acid supplementation reduces mTORC1 signaling in skeletal muscle from high fat fed, obese Zucker rats. *Lipids.* 2014 Dec;49(12):1193-201

[112] Ziegler D. Thioctic acid for patients with symptomatic diabetic polyneuropathy: a critical review. *Treat Endocrinol.* 2004;3(3):173-89

notably including ⑩ enhancement of Treg and suppression of Th-17 effects. Fasting-induced changes in immune parameters—such as antibody titers against dietary or microbial antigens—should not simply be ascribed to reductions in antigen load (reduced antigenic load due to dietary exclusion and microbial elimination/starvation), but also antigen absorption (reduced mucosal permeability) and reduced immune responsiveness due to reductions in Th-17 and increases in Treg. Leptin is a pro-inflammatory cytokine produced in proportion to body fat mass, and leptin inhibits the expansion of CD4+ regulatory T cells (TReg), a subset of T cells with an important role in the maintenance of peripheral immune tolerance to self-antigens; fasting-induced fat loss and fasting-induced reductions in leptin lead to reduction in mTOR signaling and restoration of a noninflammatory/anti-inflammatory immunophenotype.[113] With that understanding of the underlying biochemistry/physiology, we can better appreciate the consistently well-documented benefits of therapeutic fasting contra inflammatory diseases ranging from hypertension and diabetes to asthma and autoimmunity. In case reports and clinical trials, short-term fasting (or protein-sparing fasting) has been documented as safe and effective treatment for SLE, RA[114], and non-rheumatic diseases such as chronic severe hypertension, moderate hypertension, obesity[115,116], type-2 diabetes[117], and epilepsy.[118] The combination of energy restriction and fish oil supplementation was shown highly beneficial in an animal model of SLE.[119] Representative samples are summarized here:

> **Fasting alleviates inflammatory disease via separate mechanisms, particularly including reductions in leptin, an inflammatory mTOR-activating cytokine and hormone that blocks tolerogenic Treg formation**
>
> "Fasting is beneficial in the prevention and amelioration of the clinical manifestations of autoimmune diseases including systemic lupus erythematosus. ... During fasting, there is a dramatic reduction of the levels of circulating leptin, an adipokine with proinflammatory effects. Leptin also inhibits CD4(+)CD25(+)Foxp3(+) regulatory T cells, which are known to contribute significantly to the mechanisms of peripheral immune tolerance. "
>
> Liu et al. Cutting edge: fasting-induced hypoleptinemia expands functional regulatory T cells in systemic lupus erythematosus. *J Immunol.* 2012 Mar

- Brief case reports of medically supervised, water-only fasting associated with remission of autoimmune disease (*Altern Ther Health Med.* 2002 Jul[120]): This is a small case series of six patients—three with RA and one each with SLE (lupus), FM(S) (fibromyalgia), and MCTD (mixed connective tissue disorder). All patinets were transitioned to a vegan diet and discontinued drug treatments before a fasting period of 7-21 days, after which they were all symptomatically and clinically improved and continued thereafter on a nutrient-dense vegan diet. One of the more impressive findings reported is the lack of clinical exacerbation that is so commonly feared and generally expected when "rheumatic" patinets discontinue drug therapy; more accurately in this situation, drug therapy was replaced by therapeutic fasting, the latter of which proved clinically superior. Discontinued medications in this series include the following as reported; dosages were not consistently reported:
    1. **Cyclosporin** 100 mg, **prednisone** 5 mg
    2. **Hydroxychloroquine, tramadol,** cetirizine, **prednisone**
    3. Nefazodone, nortriptyline, propoxyphene, ibuprofen
    4. **Prednisone** 25 mg, **hydroxychloroquine** 5 mg
    5. **Prednisone**
    6. Irbesartan, amlodipine, celecoxib and rofecoxib

  Also of note in terms of practical implementation, all of these patients were fasted in an inpatient facility; chemistry/metabolic panels for blood analysis were performed weekly.

---

[113] Liu Y et al. Cutting edge: fasting-induced hypoleptinemia expands functional regulatory T cells in systemic lupus erythematosus. *J Immunol.* 2012 Mar 1;188(5):2070-3

[114] "An association was found between improvement in inflammatory activity of the joints and enhancement of neutrophil bactericidal capacity. Fasting appears to improve the clinical status of patients with RA." Uden AM, Trang L, Venizelos N, Palmblad J. Neutrophil functions and clinical performance after total fasting in patients with rheumatoid arthritis. *Ann Rheum Dis.* 1983 Feb;42(1):45-51

[115] Vertes V, Genuth SM, Hazelton IM. Supplemented fasting as a large-scale outpatient program. *JAMA.* 1977 Nov 14;238(20):2151-3

[116] Bauman WA, Schwartz E, Rose HG, et al. Early and long-term effects of acute caloric deprivation in obese diabetic patients. *Am J Med.* 1988 Jul;85(1):38-46

[117] Goldhamer AC. Initial cost of care results in medically supervised water-only fasting for treating high blood pressure and diabetes. *J Altern Complement Med.* 2002 Dec;8(6):696-7

[118] "The ketogenic diet should be considered as alternative therapy for children with difficult-to-control seizures. It is more effective than many of the new anticonvulsant medications and is well tolerated by children and families when it is effective." Freeman JM, et al. The efficacy of the ketogenic diet-1998: a prospective evaluation of intervention in 150 children. *Pediatrics.* 1998 Dec;102(6):1358-63 pediatrics.aappublications.org/cgi/reprint/102/6/1358

[119] "In conclusion, our data strongly indicate that ER and FO maintain antioxidant status and GSH:GSSG ratio, thereby protecting against renal deterioration from oxidative insults during ageing." Kelley VE, Ferretti A, Izui S, Strom TB. A fish oil diet rich in eicosapentaenoic acid reduces cyclooxygenase metabolites, and suppresses lupus in MRL-lpr mice. *J Immunol.* 1985 Mar;134(3):1914-9

[120] Fuhrman et al. Brief case reports of medically supervised, water-only fasting associated with remission of autoimmune disease. *Altern Ther Health Med.* 2002 Jul:112, 110-1

○ Clinical performance after total fasting in patients with rheumatoid arthritis (*Ann Rheum Dis* 1983 Feb[121]): Thirteen RA patients were fasted for seven days in a cross-over trial. "During fasting, with a mean weight loss of 5.1 kg, clinical inflammation in the joints and the erythrocyte sedimentation rate (ESR) decreased. …The bactericidal capacity [of neutrophils] improved during fasting, both in comparison with the initial value (p less than 0.005) and with the values from the control period (p less than 0.001). An association was found between improvement in inflammatory activity of the joints and enhancement of neutrophil bactericidal capacity. Fasting appears to improve the clinical status of patients with RA."

○ Open clinical trial: Inpatient water-only fasting in the treatment of hypertension (*Journal of Manipulative Physiological Therapeutics* 2001 Jun[122]): In this open trial, 174 consecutive hypertensive patients were treated in an inpatient setting under clinician supervision. The treatment program began with a short prefasting period (approximately 2 to 3 days on average) during which food consumption was limited to fruits and vegetables, followed by supervised water-only fasting (approximately 10 to 11 days on average) and a refeeding period (approximately 6 to 7 days on average) introducing a low-fat, low-sodium, vegan diet. "RESULTS: Almost 90% of the subjects achieved blood pressure less than 140/90 mm Hg by the end of the treatment program. **The average reduction in blood pressure was 37/13 mm Hg,** with the greatest decrease being observed for subjects with the most severe hypertension. **Patients with stage 3 hypertension (those with systolic blood pressure greater than 180 mg Hg, diastolic blood pressure greater than 110 mg Hg, or both) had an** average reduction of 60/17 mm Hg **at the conclusion of treatment.** All of the subjects who were taking antihypertensive medication at entry (6.3% of the total sample) successfully discontinued the use of medication. CONCLUSION: Medically supervised water-only fasting appears to be a safe and effective means of normalizing blood pressure and may assist in motivating health-promoting diet and lifestyle changes."

○ Water-only fasting in the treatment of borderline hypertension (*Journal of Alternative and Complementary Medicine,* 2002 Oct[123]): 68 consecutive patients with borderline hypertension were treated in an inpatient setting under professional supervision. The treatment program consisted of a short prefasting period (approximately 1-2 days on average) during which food consumption was limited to fruits and vegetables followed by supervised water-only fasting (approximately 13.6 days on average). Fasting was followed by a refeeding period (approximately 6.0 days on average). The refeeding program consisted of a low-fat, low-sodium, plant-based, vegan diet. "RESULTS: Approximately 82% of the subjects achieved BP at or below 120/80 mm Hg by the end of the treatment program. **The mean BP reduction was 20/7 mm Hg,** with the greatest decrease being observed for subjects with the highest baseline BP. A linear regression of BP decrease against baseline BP showed that the estimated BP below which no further decrease would be expected was 96.0/67.0 mm Hg at the end of the fast and 99.2/67.3 mm Hg at the end of refeeding. These levels are in agreement with other estimates of the BP below which stroke events are eliminated, thus suggesting that these levels could be regarded as the "ideal" BP values. CONCLUSION: Medically supervised water-only fasting appears to be a safe and effective means of normalizing BP and may assist in motivating health-promoting diet and lifestyle changes."

○ Retrospective cost-effectiveness and clinical effectiveness analysis for short-term fasting in the treatment of hypertension and diabetes mellitus (*Journal of Alternative and Complementary Medicine* Dec 2002[124]): In this brief report, Dr Goldhamer again reports success with the short-term fasting program in hypertensive patients as well as diabetic patients. Here, Goldhamer reports that the **average reduction in systolic blood pressure was 30/11 mm Hg at the completion of the program and 28/11 mm Hg on follow-up.** "Weight loss averaged 26 pounds after the program and was 28 pounds below

[121] Udén AM, Trang L, Venizelos N, Palmblad J. Neutrophil functions and clinical performance after total fasting in patients with rheumatoid arthritis. *Ann Rheum Dis.* 1983 Feb;42(1):45-51

[122] Goldhamer A, Lisle D, Parpia B, Anderson SV, Campbell TC. Medically supervised water-only fasting in the treatment of hypertension. *J Manipulative Physiol Ther* 2001 Jun;24(5):335-9

[123] Goldhamer AC, Lisle DJ, Sultana P, Anderson SV, Parpia B, Hughes B, Campbell TC. Medically supervised water-only fasting in the treatment of borderline hypertension. *J Altern Complement Med.* 2002 Oct;8(5):643-50

[124] Goldhamer AC. Initial cost of care results in medically supervised water-only fasting for treating high blood pressure and diabetes. *J Altern Complement Med.* 2002 Dec;8(6):696-7

baseline on follow-up. The average cost of medical care and drugs was $5,784.00 per year in the year(s) prior to participation and $3,000.00 in the year after participation for an average reduction of $2,784.00 per subject in the first year alone. This exceeded the cost of the entire program and compound savings are expected in the years to follow."

- ○ Reversal of muscle insulin resistance by weight reduction in young, lean, insulin-resistant *human offspring of parents with type 2 diabetes. (*Proc Natl Acad Sci USA.* 2012 May[125]*): First of all, this is the first study that I've ever read that described human subjects in the title and abstract as "offspring" in a manner that did not clearly state whether these offspring were humans or animals; per the Methods section, the subjects were indeed humans, specifically the authors describe them as " seven (six women: two Black and four Caucasian; one man: Asian), 25 ± 4-y-old, healthy, lean, nonsmoking insulin-resistant individuals with at least one parent with T2DM (IR offspring)." The intervention was a hypocaloric (1,200 Kcal) diet for 9 weeks. Results included: average weight loss of 4.1 kg, 30% reduction of intramyocellular lipid (IMCL) from 1.1 to 0.8 %, and 30% improvement in insulin-stimulated muscle glucose uptake (3.7 to 4.8 ± 0.1 mg/[kg-min]). The author note that these improvements were achieved independently from changes serum levels of TNF-alpha, IL-6, adiponectin, C-reactive protein, acylcarnitines, and branched-chain amino acids. The authors conclude that "these data support the hypothesis that IMCL accumulation plays an important role in causing muscle insulin resistance in young, lean IR offspring, and that both are reversible with modest weight loss." Thus, we are presented here with a nice yet small study exploring the anti-diabetic mechanism of caloric restriction; the authors made no mention of mTOR, despite performing this study within an era of widespread—but not universal—knowledge of mTOR and its significance for diabetes. I won't repeat this latter comment for each article in the "mTOR era" which I subjectively demarcate as having started in 2008 per the open-access publication by Maya-Monteiro and Bozza[126] which was among the first to connect mTOR with adverse metabolic effects and inflammation with particular mention of and relevance to diabetes.

- ○ Reversal of type 2 diabetes: normalization of beta cell function in association with decreased pancreas and liver triacylglycerol. (*Diabetologia.* 2011 Oct[127]): This is one of my favorite studies demonstrating the benefits of caloric restriction in the *reversal*—not *treatment* and not *management*—of diabetes; the authors specifically dismantled the dogma that, "Type 2 diabetes is regarded as inevitably progressive, with irreversible beta cell failure." Eleven people with type 2 diabetes (average age 49.5 years, average BMI 33.6), 9 male and 2 female were treated with a 600 kcal/day diet. Results of this study should have sparked an international change in the so-called "standard of care" for diabetic patients. "After 1 week of restricted energy intake, fasting plasma glucose normalized in the diabetic group (from 9.2 to 5.9 mmol/l). ... The first-phase insulin response increased during the study period (0.19 to 0.46 nmol min[-1] m[-2]) and approached control values (0.62 nmol min(-1) m(-2). Maximal insulin response became supranormal at 8 weeks (1.37 ± 0.27 vs controls 1.15 ± 0.18 nmol min(-1) m(-2)). ... Normalization of both beta cell function and hepatic insulin sensitivity in type 2 diabetes was achieved by dietary energy restriction alone. This was associated with decreased pancreatic and liver triacylglycerol stores. The abnormalities underlying type 2 diabetes are reversible by reducing dietary energy intake." Results were stunning and proved the diet-induced reversibility of diabetes type-2; ironically, these results were published online (2011 Jun) in virtually the same month that a review article by Gavin et al[128] was published in the *JAOA—Journal of the American Osteopathic Association* (a journal that I have publically criticized previously for its weak clinical review articles sponsored by drug companies that ignore dietary and nutritional interventions [Vasquez, 2006[129]]) ignored the value of diet and nutrition and asserted with blatant disrespect for previous research that physicians must "Be absolutely clear that T2DM is a lifelong disease that will require lifelong [drug] treatment." Of

[125] Petersen KF, Dufour S, Morino K, Yoo PS, Cline GW, Shulman GI. Reversal of muscle insulin resistance by weight reduction in young, lean, insulin-resistant *human* offspring of parents with type 2 diabetes. *Proc Natl Acad Sci U S A.* 2012 May 22;109(21):8236-40
[126] Maya-Monteiro CM, Bozza PT.Leptin and mTOR: partners in metabolism and inflammation. *Cell Cycle.* 2008 Jun 15;7(12):1713-7
[127] Lim EL, Hollingsworth KG, Aribisala BS, Chen MJ, Mathers JC, Taylor R. Reversal of type 2 diabetes: normalisation of beta cell function in association with decreased pancreas and liver triacylglycerol. *Diabetologia.* 2011 Oct;54(10):2506-14
[128] Gavin JR 3rd, et al. Type 2 diabetes mellitus: practical approaches for primary care physicians. *J Am Osteopath Assoc.* 2011 May;111(5 Suppl 4):S3-12
[129] Vasquez A. Interventions need to be consistent with osteopathic philosophy [letter]. *J Am Osteopath Assoc.* 2006 Sep;106(9):528-9 InflammationMastery.com/reprints

additional note, *JAOA* published a horrid editorial[130] on the prevention and treatment of viral infections in 2014 by its own Editor, a specialist in Infectious Disease, and then rejected my Letter in response by stating that my "citations were not sufficiently supportive" even though I included more than the Journal's allowance and had cited my own previously published review that contained more than 360 citations[131]; at this point, I replied to the Editor that *JAOA* is an embarrassment to the osteopathic profession—a statement that I still stand by—and basically gave up any additional future hope for that publication given its track-record of ridiculous and drug-promotional babble, occasionally punctuated by quality.

o Serum levels of interleukin-6 and dehydroepiandrosterone sulphate in response to either fasting or a ketogenic diet in rheumatoid arthritis patients. (*Clin Exp Rheumatol.* 2000 May[132]): These researchers investigated the effects of either a 7-day fast or a 7-day ketogenic diet on serum IL-6 and DHEA-sulfate) in 23 patients with active RA; 10 patients followed a 7-day sub-total fast while patients 13 consumed a ketogenic diet (isoenergetic, carbohydrate < 40 g/day) for 7 days. Clinical and laboratory variables were measured at days 0, 7, and 21. The authors found that "Fasting, but not the ketogenic diet, decreased serum IL-6 concentrations by 37% (p < 0.03) and improved disease activity at day 7. Both fasting and the ketogenic diet increased serum DHEAS levels by 34% as compared with baseline (both p < 0.006). Levels of IL-6, but not DHEAS, correlated with several disease activity variables." They concluded, "Both fasting and a ketogenic diet significantly increased serum DHEAS concentrations in RA patients. ==Only fasting significantly decreased serum IL-6 levels and improved disease activity.== As the increases in serum DHEAS were similar in response to both fasting and a ketogenic diet, it is unlikely that the fall in serum IL-6 or clinical improvements after fasting were directly related to increases in serum DHEAS."

- ==Regular exercise—strength training vs endurance exercise==:
  o ==Regular exercise==: Among training-accustomed persons exposed to resistance exericise, endurance exercise, or no exercise, only resistance training—the main purpose of which is to promote anabolism— leads to an expected increase in mTOR activity; "mTORC1 signaling is preferentially activated after hypertrophy-inducing exercise."[133] However, the discussion of the effect of exercise on mTOR opens an important conversation regarding the tissue-specificity of mTOR activation. Anabolism and mTOR activation in muscle tissue, which is generally not susceptible to malignant transformation (e.g., rhabdomyosarcomas are rare), would be considered of lesser concern and consequence than would anabolism/mTOR activation in immunocytes, adipose, hepatic or pancreatic tissue, or potentially premalignant tissues of the prostate or breast. However, to be sure, intracellular compartments are not completely sealed from the surrounding interstitial fluids, and tissue-specific responses frequently have a generalized effect systemically.

- ==Ridding the body of chemical pollutants, detoxification, sauna and the aforementioned exercise==:
  o Xenobiotics/xenoestrogens bisphenol-A (BPA) methylparaben (MP) activate mTOR and promote cellular changes consistent with cancer promotion (*Carcinogenesis.* 2011 Nov[134]): Physiologic (ie, "clinically relevant") low doses of xenoestrogens BPA and methyparaben activate the mTOR pathway in breast epithelial cells from women at high-risk of developing breast cancer. "Breast cancer is an estrogen-driven disease. ... However, increasing male breast cancer rates over the past three decades implicate additional sources of estrogenic exposure including wide spread estrogen-mimicking

---

[130] Orenstein R. Emerging infections: the cauldron of medicine, mobility, and media. *J Am Osteopath Assoc.* 2014 Nov;114(11):e122-3

[131] Vasquez A. *Antiviral Strategies and Immune Nutrition: Against Colds, Flu, Herpes, AIDS, Hepatitis, Ebola, and Autoimmunity.* 2014 Oct. [ISBN 1502894890 / 978-1502894892]. See also: Vasquez A. Unified Antiviral Strategy published by ICHNFM. *Int J Hum Nutr Funct Med* 2014:2(4);1 [ASIN: B00P5AB5RW]

[132] Fraser DA, Thoen J, Djøseland O, Førre O, Kjeldsen-Kragh J.Serum levels of interleukin-6 and dehydroepiandrosterone sulphate in response to either fasting or a ketogenic diet in rheumatoid arthritis patients. *Clin Exp Rheumatol.* 2000 May-Jun;18(3):357-62

[133] "Blood and muscle samples were analyzed for plasma substrates and hormones and for muscle markers of AMPK and Akt-mTORC1 protein signaling. Increases in plasma glucose, insulin, growth hormone (GH), and insulin-like growth factor (IGF)-1, and in phosphorylated muscle phospho-Akt substrate (PAS) of 160 kDa, mTOR, 70 kDa ribosomal protein S6 kinase, eukaryotic initiation factor 4E, and glycogen synthase kinase 3a were observed after strength exercise. ... The results support that in training-accustomed individuals, mTORC1 signaling is preferentially activated after hypertrophy-inducing exercise, while AMPK signaling is less specific for differentiated exercise." Vissing K et al. Differentiated mTOR but not AMPK signaling after strength vs endurance exercise in training-accustomed individuals. *Scand J Med Sci Sports.* 2013 Jun;23(3):355-66

[134] Goodson WH 3rd1, Luciani MG, Sayeed SA, Jaffee IM, Moore DH 2nd, Dairkee SH. Activation of the mTOR pathway by low levels of xenoestrogens in breast epithelial cells from high-risk women. *Carcinogenesis.* 2011 Nov;32(11):1724-33

chemicals or xenoestrogens (XEs), such as bisphenol-A (BPA) [and methylparaben (MP)]." The authors studied human, high-risk donor breast epithelial cells (HRBECs) to "BPA at concentrations that are detectable in human blood, placenta and milk" and found mTOR pathway activation and the expected "prosurvival changes" in human breast cells. In this study, the authors found additional evidence of activation of the PI3K-Akt-mTOR pathway and "marked resistance to rapamycin, the defining mTOR inhibitor. Moreover, HRBECs pretreated with BPA, or the XE, methylparaben (MP), surmounted antiestrogenic effects of tamoxifen showing dose-dependent apoptosis evasion and induction of cell cycling. Overall, XEs, when tested in benign breast cells from multiple human subjects, consistently initiated specific functional changes of the kind that are attributed to malignant onset in breast tissue."

- o Bisphenol-A promotes human preadipocyte differentiation by mTOR pathway activation (*Obesity* 2014 Nov[135]): "The analysis also revealed enrichment of genes following BPA exposure in the thyroid-receptor/retinoic X receptor (TR/RXR) and mammalian target of rapamycin (mTOR) signaling pathways. *CONCLUSIONS*: Our data suggest that potential mechanisms of action of BPA-induced adipogenesis involve SREBF1, the TR/RXR, and the mTOR pathways."

- o Detoxification support (detailed in Chapter 4.7) reduces body-burden of xenobiotics and thereby is expected to reduce mTOR signaling and resultant consequences (inflammation, autoimmunity, malignancy) with an expected benefit of reduction in disease-specific and all-cause mortality: As reviewed in Chapter 4 section 7, the core components of xenobiotic detoxification are ❶ avoidance of ongoing exposure, ❷ detoxification and depuration, ❸ medicial/symptomatic management (ie, "damage control"), and ❹ political action to enforce authentic and meaningful population protection. Of these, the part listed above as "❷ detoxification and depuration" can be further itemized—as initially discussed in Chapter 2—into the following subcomponents" 1) exercise and sauna, 2) bowel cleansing, fiber, probiotics, antibiotics, laxatives, 3) liver and bile stimulators, 4) cofactors for phase 1 oxidation and phase 2 conjugation, 5) chelation for heavy metals, 6) urine alkalinization. Of these, the first—exercise and sauna—both enhance chemical depuration via sweating/diaphoresis; further, the increased heat also likely promotes a nonspecific stress-adaptive hormetic response. Studies have shown that sweating via heat/saunta is an effective means for xenobiotic depuration/cleansing, while others have shown that adsorption of xenobiotics in the gastrointestinal tract interrupts xenobiotic absorption and enterohepatic circulation, thereby reducing the body burden of dioxin-like xenobiotics:

  1. Human Excretion of Bisphenol-A: Blood, Urine, and Sweat (BUS) Study (*Journal of Environmental and Public Health* 2012 Sep[136]): "Bisphenol-A (BPA) is a ubiquitous chemical contaminant that has recently been associated with adverse effects on human health. … Using 20 study participants, this study was designed to assess the relative concentration of BPA in three body fluids—blood, urine, and sweat—and to determine whether induced sweating may be a therapeutic intervention with potential to facilitate elimination of this compound. … In 16 of 20 participants, BPA was identified in sweat, even in some individuals with no BPA detected in their serum or urine samples. *Conclusions*. Biomonitoring of BPA through blood and/or urine testing may underestimate the total body burden of this potential toxicant. Sweat analysis should be considered as an additional method for monitoring bioaccumulation of BPA in humans. Induced sweating appears to be a potential method for elimination of BPA."

  2. Routine sauna bathing reduces fatal cardiovascular and all-cause mortality events (*JAMA Intern Med* 2015 Feb 23[137]): Sauna bathing induces vasodilation and improved hemodynamic function; obviously, sweating promotes excretion of subtances through the skin via sweating. "We performed a prospective cohort study (Finnish Kuopio Ischemic Heart Disease Risk Factor Study) of a population-based sample of 2,315 middle-aged (age range, 42-60 years) men from Eastern Finland. … Increased frequency of sauna bathing [dose-response relationship up to 20 minutes 7 times weekly] is associated with a reduced risk of SCD, CHD, CVD, and all-cause mortality."

[135] Boucher et al. Identification of mechanisms of action of bisphenol a-induced human preadipocyte differentiation by transcriptional profiling. *Obesity*. 2014 Nov;22(11):2333-43
[136] Genuis SJ et al. Human Excretion of Bisphenol A: Blood, Urine, and Sweat (BUS) Study. *Journal of Environmental and Public Health* 2012 Sep, Article ID 185731
[137] Laukkanen et al. Association between Sauna Bathing and Fatal Cardiovascular and All-Cause Mortality Events. *JAMA Intern Med.* 2015 Feb. [Epub ahead of print]

3. Chlorella pyrenoidosa on fecal excretion and liver accumulation of polychlorinated dibenzo-p-dioxin in mice. (*Chemosphere* 2005 Apr[138]): "Among mice fed the 10% *C. pyrenoidosa* diet, cumulative fecal excretion of H6CDD over the first week following administration was significantly greater (9.2-fold) than that observed among mice fed the basal diet. Moreover, excretion during the fifth week following administration of H6CDD was still significantly greater (3.1-fold) among mice fed the 10% C. pyrenoidosa diet than among mice fed the basal diet. Five weeks after administration of H6CDD, liver accumulation of H6CDD in mice fed the 10% C. pyrenoidosa diet was significantly less than that observed among mice fed either the basal diet and the Spinach diet (by 27.9% and 34.8%, respectively). These findings suggest that C. pyrenoidosa may be useful in inhibiting the absorption of dioxins via food and the reabsorption of dioxins stored already in the body in the intestinal tract, thus preventing accumulation of dioxins within the body."

4. Chlorella (Chlorella pyrenoidosa) supplementation decreases dioxin and increases immunoglobulin a concentrations in breast milk (*J Med Food* 2007 Mar[139]): "The present results suggest that Chlorella supplementation not only reduces dioxin levels in breast milk, but may also have beneficial effects on nursing infants by increasing IgA levels in breast milk."

5. Maternal-fetal distribution and transfer of dioxins in pregnant women in Japan, and attempts to reduce maternal transfer with Chlorella (Chlorella pyrenoidosa) supplements (*Chemosphere* 2005 Dec[140]): "Concentrations of 28 dioxin (polychlorinated dibenzo-p-dioxins, polychlorinated dibenzofurans, and co-planar polychlorinated biphenyls) congeners in blood, adipose tissue, breast milk, cord blood and placenta collected from 44 pregnant Japanese women were measured. … Correlations were observed between dioxin total toxic equivalents (total TEQ) in blood and total TEQ in adipose tissue (r=0.913, P<0.0001), breast milk (r=0.695, P=0.0007), and cord blood (r=0.759, P<0.0001). Dioxin levels transferred to fetuses and nursing infants reflect cumulative maternal concentrations of dioxins. … Total TEQ in breast milk were approximately 30% lower in the Chlorella group than in controls (P=0.0113). This finding suggests that maternal transfer of dioxins can be reduced using dietary measures such as Chlorella supplements."

- Rouge/miscellaneous therapeutics including n3 FA:
  - N3 fatty acids 3-6g/d: mTORC1/2 targeted by n-3 polyunsaturated fatty acids in the prevention of mammary tumorigenesis and tumor progression. (*Oncogene*. 2014 Sep[141]): "In breast cancer cell lines, n-3 PUFAs rapidly and efficiently suppress both mTOR complex 1 (mTORC1) and mTORC2 and their downstream signaling, and subsequently inhibit cell proliferation and angiogenesis while promoting apoptosis. … Furthermore, the ability of n-3 PUFAs to block both mTORC1 and mTORC2 could explain why dietary DHA is more effective than the mTORC1 inhibitor rapamycin in the suppression of mammary tumorigenesis. In addition, n-3 PUFAs have been shown to have multiple biological effects on cancers, including alterations in the properties of cancer cells (proliferation, invasion and apoptosis) as well as those of host cells (inflammation, immune response and angiogenesis)."

---

[138] Takekoshi et al. Effect of Chlorella pyrenoidosa on fecal excretion and liver accumulation of polychlorinated dibenzo-p-dioxin in mice. *Chemosphere*. 2005 Apr;59(2):297-304
[139] Nakano et al. Chlorella (Chlorella pyrenoidosa) supplementation decreases dioxin and increases immunoglobulin a concentrations in breast milk. *J Med Food*. 2007 Mar;10(1):134-42
[140] Nakano et al. Maternal-fetal distribution and transfer of dioxins in pregnant women in Japan, and attempts to reduce maternal transfer with Chlorella (Chlorella pyrenoidosa) supplements. *Chemosphere*. 2005 Dec;61(9):1244-55
[141] Chen Z et al. mTORC1/2 targeted by n-3 polyunsaturated fatty acids in the prevention of mammary tumorigenesis and tumor progression. *Oncogene*. 2014 Sep 11;33:4548-57

❺ Stress, Sleep, and Everything Else that starts "S": lifeStyle, Social and pSychological Influences, Self-Esteem, Somatic/Spinal Manipulation, Specialized Supplementation, Surgery,... Stamp Your Passport

Major Concepts in this Section
Initiated with stress modulation/reduction/mastery and sleep deprivation/optimization, this section has since expanded to include additional considerations, as described below, some of which have received additional details and citations, all of which are important.

- **Style of living—lifestyle:** Lifestyle includes many of the considerations below, as well as one's general approach to thinking, problem-solving, and living. Lifestyle is powerfully connected with culture (more accurately: *prevailing cultural morality*) and geography. Many of the relevant concepts and practical applications are included under the naturopathic profession's concept *reestablishing the foundation for health.*

- **Stress management/modulation/optimization:** Eustress is generally considered beneficial; but eventually even eustress can be detrimental if prolonged without respite. Dys-stress or distress impairs would healing, promotes nutrient loss, and promotes microbial pathogenicity via what is generally described as *microbial endocrinology*—the opportunistic enhancement of microbial pathogenicity following microbial reception of the host's elaboration of stress-related hormones/neurotransmitters such as norepinephrine.

  - **Microbial endocrinology—how stress influences susceptibility to infection** (*Trends Microbiol* 2008 Feb[1]): Microbial endocrinology is the transdisciplinary field that represents the intersection of microbiology with mammalian endocrinology and neurophysiology; it is based on the tenet that microorganisms have evolved systems for using neurohormones, which are widely distributed throughout nature, as environmental cues to initiate growth and pathogenic processes.

- **Sleep:** Sleep deprivation/interruption promotes immune dysregulation and a pro-inflammatory response; accordingly, sleep deprivation/interruption is causatively associated with elevations in serum hsCRP and increased risks for obesity, diabetes mellitus and cardiometabolic syndrome.

  - **Sleep disturbance and older adults' inflammatory responses to acute stress** (*Am J Geriatr Psychiatry* 2012 Sep[2]): "RESULTS: Participants categorized as poor sleepers on the basis of Pittsburgh Sleep Quality Index scores had significantly larger IL-6 responses to the cognitive stressors than good sleepers. The association between poor sleep and heightened IL-6 response to acute stress was not explained by other psychosocial factors previously linked to immune dysregulation, including depressive symptoms, perceived stress, and loneliness. CONCLUSIONS: Findings add to the growing evidence for poor sleep as an independent risk factor for poor mental and physical health. Older adults may be particularly vulnerable to effects of sleep disturbance due to significant age-related changes in sleep and inflammatory regulation."

- **pSychology:** One's mental outlook, self-perception, and psychoepistimology, etc. Some of the best contextualized conversations on these topics are by Bradshaw[3], Bly[4], and Branden.[5]

- **Self-esteem:** Brilliantly articulated by Dr Nathaniel Branden to include the following: ❶ Living Consciously, ❷ Self-Acceptance, ❸ Self-Responsibility, ❹ Self-Assertiveness, ❺ Living Purposefully, ❻ Personal Integrity.

---

[1] Freestone PP, Sandrini SM, Haigh RD, Lyte M. Microbial endocrinology: how stress influences susceptibility to infection. *Trends Microbiol*. 2008 Feb;16(2):55-64

[2] Heffner KL et al. Sleep disturbance and older adults' inflammatory responses to acute stress. *Am J Geriatr Psychiatry*. 2012 Sep;20(9):744-52

[3] John Bradshaw's live performance recorded as *Healing the Shame that Binds You* (audio cassette version is different from the digital version and the book by the same name) is a very personal and yet very social and contextual journey and explanation of the personal issues that arise within the context of a fragmented society.

[4] Robert Bly's *Iron John* is famous for having spawned the men's movement in America, but via Bly's knowledge of and sensitivity to historical facts and social trends, the book is also detailed and excellent accounting of the political and social changes that have promoted the degradation of society and which impact our personal self-perceptions and experiences of life; he followed this many years later with lectures titled *Where Have All the Parents Gone?* (audio cassette) related to his masterpiece book *Sibling Society*.

[5] Nathaniel Branden discusses self-esteem and psychoepistimology in *Six Pillars of Self-Esteem* and *Psychology of Self-Esteem*, both in printed books and audiobooks.

- o Branden N. The Six Pillars of Self-Esteem (paper book, audiobook, digital book): "There are realities we cannot avoid. One of them is the importance of self-esteem. Regardless of what we do or do not admit, we cannot be indifferent to our self-evaluation. However, we can run from this knowledge if it makes us uncomfortable. We can shrug it off, evade it, declare that we are only interested in "practical" matters, and escape into baseball or the evening news or the financial pages or a shopping spree or a sexual adventure or a drink. Yet self-esteem is a fundamental human need. ==Its impact requires neither our understanding nor our consent.== It works its way within us with or without our knowledge. We are free to seek to grasp the dynamics of self-esteem or to remain unconscious of them, but in the latter case we remain a mystery to ourselves and endure the consequences." *I personally (DrV) consider this to be one of the most brilliant, practical, and important books/audios ever produced, despite what I perceive as a few imperfections; if the entire world (so to speak) read/understood/applied this book, our collective worldwide and lifetime reality would be improved for the better.*

- • Specialized supplementation: Atop the nutritional considerations discussed in this text, patients often benefit from additional custom-tailored supraphysiologic supplementation; beyond those already mentioned in this book, a few additional examples are provided in the table below. More examples are provided within the context of clinical protocols in *Chiropractic and Naturopathic Mastery of Common Clinical Disorders* (2009) and the 2016 versions of "Volume 2" including *Functional Medicine Clinical Protocols for Inflammatory Disorders*. As always throughout my books, doses listed are for adults unless otherwise specified. Gaby's *Nutritional Medicine* is mentioned here again as an excellent archive and clinical resource.

Examples of "specialized supplementation"	Corresponding applications
Magnesium: 600 mg/d or to bowel tolerance	• Constipation (assuming no bowel obstruction, renal insufficiency) • Headaches of most kinds, including post-traumatic headaches, tension headaches, migraine headaches
Pyridoxine: 250-800mg/d, always administered with magnesium, with food, within a context of dietary sufficiency, multivitamin/mineral supplementation, dietary alkalinization; pyridoxine HCL is generally sufficient while pyridoxal-5-phosphate is appreciated as the active form	• Premenstrual problems, as pyridoxine has an impressive alterative/normalizing/balancing effect via lowering estrogen levels, raising progesterone levels, promoting diuresis[6], and reducing excess glutaminergic neurotransmission which is consistently associated with depression/anxiety/moodiness • Excess glutaminergic neurotransmission, monosodium glutamate (MSG) sensitivity[7]—see discussion in Chapter 5 sections on Migraine and Fibromyalgia
Pyridoxine: 50-250 mg/d Methylfolate or folinic acid: 400 mcg-5 mg/d Cobalamin*: 2,000-6,000 mcg/d PO NAC: 1,500-4,500 mg/d Betaine: 3-6 g/d[8] Soy lecithin: 2-10 tablespoons/d	• Elevated homocysteine—see Chapter 5 • Methylation defects *Cobalamin should always be used in the form of hydroxocobalamin, methylcobalamin, or adenosylcobalamin—not cyanocobalamin, which contains cyanide, a mitochondrial toxin

- • Sweat as metaphor for daily exercise and *exertion*—not simply *activity*.: For many people in industrialized societies, "work" is mostly intellectual/nonphysical/professional and therefore physically inactive; punctuating an inactive lifestyle and daily schedule with occasional spasms of activity (i.e., time-constrained ventures to the gym for "working out") is not the same as having a physically active lifestyle but—for many of us—it is the best

---

[6] Abraham GE. Nutritional factors in the etiology of the premenstrual tension syndromes. *J Reprod Med*. 1983 Jul;28(7):446-64
[7] Mousain-Bosc M, et al. Magnesium VitB6 intake reduces central nervous system hyperexcitability in children. *J Am Coll Nutr*. 2004;23(5):545S-548S
[8] "Ten patients with cystathionine beta-synthase deficiency that was not responsive to pyridoxine and one patient with homocystinuria due to a defect in cobalamin metabolism were treated with 6 g daily of betaine added to conventional therapy, to improve homocysteine remethylation. All patients had a substantial decrease in plasma total homocysteine levels..." Wilcken et al. Homocystinuria—effects of betaine in the treatment of patients not responsive to pyridoxine. *N Engl J Med*. 1983;309:448-53

we can do. We should seek as much physical activity and engagement with the life experience as possible and reasonable per our individual needs and responsibilities. Life and its components have to be customized for an optimal personal experience and self-actualization; we might also appreciate that the vast majority of people in the world (presently and historically) have never had the luxury of time and freedom for such. Current guidelines[9] encourage five 60-minute sessions per week emphasizing aerobic/endurance

exercise and 2 sessions per week of resistance training *engaging all major muscle groups* (legs, hips, back, abdomen, chest, shoulders, arms)—such as calisthenics or weight-lifting; some activities such as hiking and yoga provide endurance and resistance training simultaneously. Exercise promotes "brain health"[10], intellectuality, vitality, social adaptability and relationships, and appropriate assertiveness via neurogenesis, synaptogenesis, improved posture and physical strength, adaptability, and flexibility; avoidance of sarcopenia and adiposity helps liberate/disinhibit mental capacities from the stupifying effects of chronic/sustained inflammation, mitochondrial dysfunction, and rapid/expedited biological aging. Furthermore by analogy: physical exercise preparatory for life in a similar way that work-hardening/conditioning programs are—via physical therapy and occupational rehabilitation—preparatory for work performance; exercise and physicality are synergistic with intellectual development and help to bridge the mind-body gap and thus blur this dichotomy, promoting the development and maintenance generally stronger and more life-appropriate individuals, organizations, and societies by merging the intellectual/ideational with the practical/physical, by promoting individual and societal vitality and robustness.

- o Physicality and intellectuality: Thucydides (460-395 BC), "A society that separates its scholars from its warriors will have its thinking done by cowards and its fighting done by fools."
- o Physicality and intellectuality: Emerson (1803-1882), "Our culture has truckled to the times, - to the senses. It is not manworthy. If the vast and the spiritual are omitted, so are the practical and the moral. It does not make us brave or free. We teach boys to be such men as we are. We do not teach them to aspire to be all they can. We do not give them a training as if we believed in their noble nature. We scarce educate their bodies. We do not train the eye and the hand. We exercise their understandings to the apprehension and comparison of some facts, to a skill in numbers, in words; we aim to make accountants, attorneys, engineers, but not to make able, earnest, great-hearted men. The great object of Education should be commensurate with the object of life. It should be a moral one; to teach self-trust: to inspire the youthful man with an interest in himself; with a curiosity touching his own nature; to acquaint him with the resources of his mind, and to teach him that there is all his strength, and to inflame him with a piety towards the Grand Mind in which he lives. Thus would education conspire with the Divine Providence."
- o Physicality and intellectuality: Nietzsche (1845-1900), "All truly great thoughts are conceived while walking." "To exercise power costs effort and demands courage. That is why so many fail to assert rights to which they are perfectly entitled – because a right is a kind of power but they are too lazy or too cowardly to exercise it. The virtues which cloak these faults are called patience and forbearance." "Error is not blindness, error is cowardice . . . Every achievement, every step forward in knowledge, comes from courage, from harshness towards oneself, from cleanliness with respect to oneself."
- Spinal health and Somatic dysfunction: Spinal manipulative therapy is remarkably effective for certain health problems for which no pharmaceutical/nutritional/botanical treatment is equally effective. Spinal health/function/manipulation/adjustment has obviously been the focus of the chiropractic profession, and "somatic dysfunction"—encompassing spinal health, fascia, ligaments, muscles as well as arterial, lymphatic, and venous flow—has been the focus (within its study of manipulative medicine) of the osteopathic profession.
  - o Clinical trial: Chiropractic atlas vertebra realignment and achievement of arterial pressure goal in hypertensive patients (*J Hum Hypertens* 2007 May[11]): "Using a double blind, placebo-controlled design

---

[9] cdc.gov/physicalactivity/everyone/guidelines/adults.html Accessed 2014 Jun

[10] Cotman et al. Exercise builds brain health: key roles of growth factor cascades and inflammation. *Trends Neurosci.* 2007 Sep;30(9):464-72

[11] Bakris et al. Atlas vertebra realignment and achievement of arterial pressure goal in hypertensive patients. *J Hum Hypertens.* 2007 May;21(5):347-52

at a single center, 50 drug naïve (n=26) or washed out (n=24) patients with Stage 1 hypertension were randomized to receive a National Upper Cervical Chiropractic (NUCCA) procedure or a sham procedure. ... At week 8, there were differences in ==systolic BP (-17 mm Hg==, NUCCA versus -3 mm Hg, placebo; P<0.0001) and ==diastolic BP (-10 mm Hg==, NUCCA versus -2 mm Hg; P=0.002). ... ==No adverse effects were recorded. We conclude that restoration of Atlas alignment is associated with marked and sustained reductions in BP similar to the use of two-drug combination therapy.=="

- T4 syndrome (*J Manipulative Physiol Ther* 1995 Jan[12]): "Upper extremity symptoms of nocturnal or early morning paresthesias, especially in a glove-like distribution, coupled with headaches and a stiff upper thoracic spine without neurological signs of disease may indicate a T4 syndrome. Manipulation of the dysfunctional upper thoracic segments may relieve these symptoms."

- A small example from the author's personal experience: I notice that I get a muscle twitch around my right eye when I carry—even very temporarily—a backpack on my right shoulder; this apparently results in a subluxated/dysfunctional right upper rib (approximately right posterior rib #2 or 3), manipulation/adjustment of which consistently and immediately resolves the eye twitch. *Without chiropractic-type manipulation of this rib, how would this problem be treated medically—muscle relaxant drugs, antianxiety drugs, with some lame excuse about how "it will go away on its own" which never happens?* I think what I experience—which might be described as costovertebral-dysfunction-induced spasm of the orbicularis occuli—is analogous to a mixture of the T4 syndrome described by DeFranca and Levine[13] and the cervico-ocular/spino-ocular phenomenon described by Gorman et al.[14]

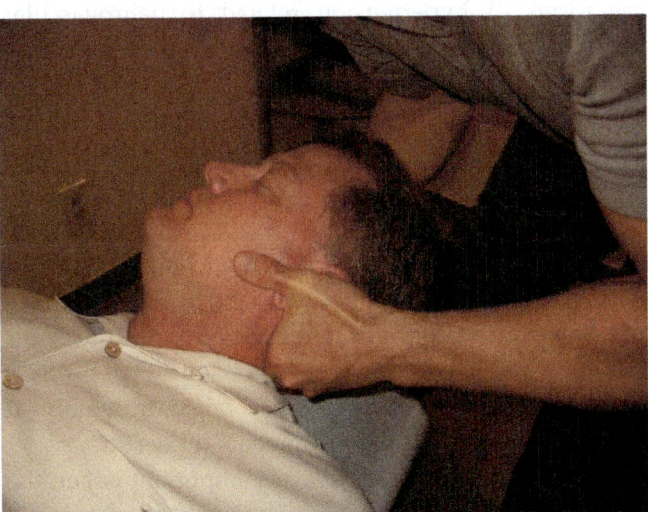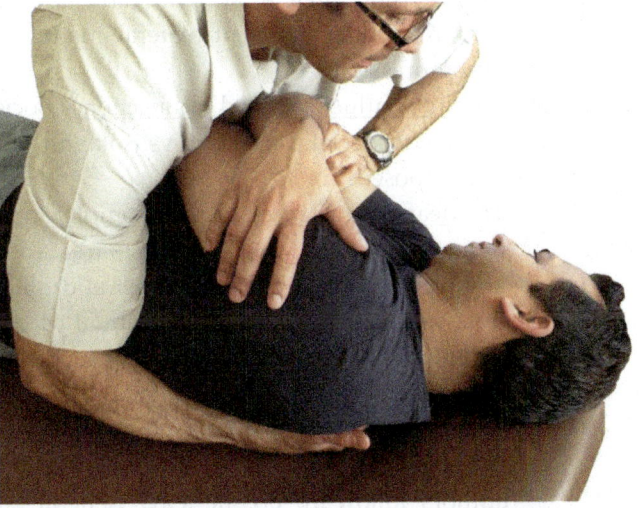

Examples of spinal manipulation and somatic manipulative medicine: *Left*: Cervical spine manipulation has been shown to be several-fold more safe than use of NSAIDs for the treatment of neck pain[15] while being as least as effective or more effective (and likely more cost-effective) than drug treatment for HTN.[16] *Right*: Dr Vasquez demonstrates his favorite manipulative procedure for dysfunctional costovertebral articulations and subluxated posterior ribs (i.e., the posterior aspect of the rib); I (DrV) am consistently impressed at the effectiveness of this maneuver and the scarcity of clinicians who know how to deliver it.

---

[12] DeFranca GG, Levine LJ. The T4 syndrome. *J Manipulative Physiol Ther*. 1995 Jan;18(1):34-7

[13] DeFranca GG, Levine LJ. The T4 syndrome. *J Manipulative Physiol Ther*. 1995 Jan;18(1):34-7

[14] Gorman RF. Automated static perimetry in chiropractic. *J Manipulative Physiol Ther*. 1993 Sep;16(7):481-7. Gorman RF. Monocular visual loss after closed head trauma: immediate resolution associated with spinal manipulation. *J Manipulative Physiol Ther* 1995;18:308-14. Gorman RF. The treatment of presumptive optic nerve ischemia by spinal manipulation. *J Manipulative Physiol Ther*. 1995;18(3):172-7. Gorman RF. Monocular scotomata and spinal manipulation: the step phenomenon. *J Manipulative Physiol Ther*. 1996 Jun;19(5):344-9. Stephens D, Gorman F, Bilton D. The step phenomenon in the recovery of vision with spinal manipulation. *J Manipulative Physiol Ther*. 1997;20(9):628-33. Stephens D, Gorman RF. Does 'normal' vision improve with spinal manipulation? *J Manipulative Physiol Ther*. 1996 Jul-Aug;19(6):415-8. Stephens D, Gorman F. The association between visual incompetence and spinal derangement. *J Manipulative Physiol Ther*. 1997 Jun;20(5):343-50. Stephens D, Pollard H, Bilton D, Thomson P, Gorman F. Bilateral simultaneous optic nerve dysfunction after periorbital trauma: recovery of vision in association with chiropractic spinal manipulation therapy. *J Manipulative Physiol Ther*. 1999 Nov-Dec;22(9):615-21

[15] "The best evidence indicates that cervical manipulation for neck pain is much safer than the use of NSAIDs, by as much as a factor of several hundred times. There is no evidence tha indicates NSAID use is any more effective than cervical manipulation for neck pain." Dabbs V, Lauretti WJ. A risk assessment of cervical manipulation vs. NSAIDs for the treatment of neck pain. *J Manipulative Physiol Ther*. 1995 Oct;18(8):530-6

[16] Bakris et al. Atlas vertebra realignment and achievement of arterial pressure goal in hypertensive patients. *J Hum Hypertens*. 2007 May;21(5):347-52

- **Surgery:** Surgery is an important treatment consideration not simply for trauma and the removal of structural and gross pathologies, but also for more "functional" problems such as migraine headaches associated with patent foramen ovale and hypertension secondary to neurovascular compression of the ventrolateral medulla oblongata.

  - Surgery/procedure—Improving migraine by means of primary transcatheter patent foramen ovale (PFO) closure (*Am J Cardiovasc Dis* 2012 May[17]): Obviously, migraine patients should be treated with the migraine protocol I have outlined in order to correct the primary (often accompanied by secondary contributions) mitochondrial dysfunction that is the fundamental cause of migraine.[18] Following successful implementation of the mitochondrial protocol, for patients who continue to have symptoms, procedural correction of PFO closure can be considered. "RESULTS: 70/80 of patients (87.5%) reported improved migraine symptomatology (mean MIDAS score decreased 33 to 10) whereas 12.5% reported no amelioration... Auras were definitively cured in 61/63 patients with migraine with aura (96.8%). CONCLUSIONS: Transcatheter PFO closure in a selected population of patients with severe migraine at high risk of paradoxical embolism resulted in a significant reduction in migraine over a long-term follow-up."

  - Surgery—Decrease of blood pressure by surgical ventrolateral medullary decompression in essential hypertension (*Lancet* 1998 Aug[19]): "3 months after surgery, blood pressure and antihypertensive regimens had decreased substantially in three patients. ... No complications associated with decompression occurred. One patient experienced a transient vocal-cord paresis after the laryngeal part of the vagus nerve was maneuvered during surgery. We showed a direct causal relation between raised blood pressure and irritation of cranial nerves IX and X. A subgroup of patients with essential hypertension may exist who have secondary forms of hypertension related to neurovascular compression at the ventrolateral medulla and who may be successfully treated with [surgical] decompression."

- **Social cohesion, influences, and connections:** Social influences on inflammatory and immune status are mediated via food, social connection vs isolation, xenobiotic pollution, and the level of sociopolitical chaos to which one is exposed.

  - The deafening silence: the near-complete absence of social perspectives in American medical schools): In medical school, we are taught to treat social problems of depression, anxiety, and isolation without any regard for their social context and political causes. As students and clinicians, we are taught to treat social problems with individual diagnoses and —essentially always— prescriptions for drugs (allopathic/osteopathic), or herbs or meditation (naturopathic), or nutritional supplements or exercise (chiropractic). The dominant allopathic medical profession as a whole has failed miserably at maintaining public health via representation of the human needs and requirements for health.

  - Social isolation in the USA (*American Sociological Review* 2006 Jun[20]): In this very important paper, the authors follow-up on the 1985 General Social Survey (GSS) which collected the first nationally representative data on the confidants with whom Americans discuss important matters; the 2004 GSS replicated those questions to assess social change in core network structures. The findings show that American society is increasingly fragmented and isolationist. "Discussion networks are smaller in 2004 than in 1985. The number of people saying there is no one with whom they discuss important matters nearly tripled. The mean network size decreases by about a third (one confidant), from 2.94 in 1985 to 2.08 in 2004. The modal respondent now reports having no confidant; the modal respondent in 1985 had three confidants. Both kin and non-kin confidants were lost in the past two decades, but the greater decrease of non-kin ties leads to more confidant networks centered on spouses and parents, with fewer contacts through voluntary associations and neighborhoods. Most people have densely interconnected confidants similar to them. Some changes reflect the changing demographics of the U.S. population. Educational heterogeneity of social ties has decreased, racial heterogeneity has increased. The data may

---

[17] Rigatelli et al. Improving migraine by means of primary transcatheter patent foramen ovale closure: long-term follow-up. *Am J Cardiovasc Dis*. 2012;2(2):89-95
[18] My "migraine protocol" is detailed in *Integrative Orthopedics, Third Edition* (2012, text) and *Mitochondrial Nutrition and Endoplasmic Reticulum Stress in Primary Care, Second Edition* (2014, text and presentation slides).
[19] Geiger et al. Decrease of blood pressure by ventrolateral medullary decompression in essential hypertension. *Lancet*. 1998 Aug 8;352(9126):446-9
[20] McPherson et al. Social Isolation in America: Changes in Core Discussion Networks over Two Decades. *Am Sociological Rev* 2006 June: 71;353-375

overestimate the number of social isolates, but these ==shrinking networks reflect an important social change in America=="

- o Relative deprivation—institutionalized inequality—makes people sick and "crazy" (*Soc Sci Med.* 2007 Nov[21]): "==… many problems associated with relative deprivation are more prevalent in more unequal societies.== We summarize previously published evidence suggesting that this may be true of <u>morbidity</u> and <u>mortality</u>, <u>obesity</u>, <u>teenage birth rates</u>, <u>mental illness</u>, <u>homicide</u>, low trust, <u>low social capital</u>, <u>hostility</u>, and <u>racism</u>. To these we add new analyses which suggest that this is also true of <u>poor educational performance</u> among school children, the proportion of the population <u>imprisoned</u>, <u>drug overdose mortality</u> and <u>low social mobility</u>. That ill health and a wide range of other social problems associated with social status within societies are also more common in more unequal societies, may imply that income inequality is central to the creation of the apparently deep-seated social problems associated with poverty, relative deprivation or low social status."

Social inequality increases physical and mental illness, and it cannot exist without government assistance

- <u>Low-quality public education</u>: Reduces opportunities for advancement among low-income persons, while higher-income persons are able to access better quality education through private institutions; increases likelihood that low-income persons will choose military as occupation, thus fragmenting lower-income parts of society (mostly by removing men and fathers), weakening lower-income sections financially, socially, and politically.
- <u>Weak labor protection laws</u>: Reduces fairness in the workplace, creating more of a master-slave relationship; generally increases profitability of the ownership while increasing poverty and hazards among workers.
- <u>No or very low minimum wage</u>: Increases profitability of owners, increases poverty among workers, depletes government coffers via increased demand on government-sponsored social support (health, housing, food) programs; in this way, the government directly subsidizes corporate profitability by compensating for programmatic underpayment of employees while employees are kept at a financial and social level that barely provides for survival.
- <u>Tax policies that protect high-income profitability and burden low-income survivability</u>: The exemplar of government-imposed inequality.
- <u>Institutionalized inequality causes physical and mental health problems (treated with drugs)</u>: These social problems are generally treated with drugs (or [privatized] imprisonment), increasing medical debts, profiting drug companies (and prison companies).
- <u>International trade agreements that allow large-wealthy corporations to "off-shore" labor to countries that pay almost-slave wages to workers in horrid working conditions</u>: This allows a few major corporations to make massive profit while forcing smaller local/domestic companies that pay fair wages to local workers to face bankruptcy; this results in corporate enrichment at the cost of domestic business-owner and worker—and thus lower/middle class—unemployment and disempowerment.
  - o The plain and simple fact is that American corporations such as Nike, McDonalds, WalMart, Target, HomeDepot, Sears, Apple and most electronics companies use the Chinese and "Third world" labor pool as a source almost-slave labor: a situation where the workers are so poor that they have no option other than to work long hours in horrid conditions with innumerable worker and human rights violations, where mistreatment and underpayment are deliberately concealed, and American corporations feign the appearance of concern but not to the extent that productivity and profitability are inconvenienced, nor that child labor is excluded, and where "employees at garment, electronics, and other export factories typically work more than 80 hours a week and make only 42 cents an hour" and are forced to work for consecutive weeks at a time without days off from work, according to the international business magazine *Business Week*. Many experts have claimed that this hurts the American economy by depleting the US of millions of jobs under the title of "free trade agreements" and designated agreements such as "permanent normal trade relations" (PNTR), formerly "most favored nation" (MFN).
  - o "Most of what we buy from developing countries is grown or manufactured by workers whose rights are ignored in important ways. Cell-phone components from China, fruit grown in Mexico, and the Indian cotton in your shirt are commonly processed by workers who were not paid minimum wage, who were exposed to hazardous chemicals or dangerous machinery, who were forced to work overtime, or who were prevented from organizing to negotiate changes in such conditions." Viederman D. Overseas sweatshops are a US responsibility. *BusinessWeek*.com

  businessweek.com/stories/2006-11-26/secrets-lies-and-sweatshops
  businessweek.com/debateroom/archives/2007/06/overseas_sweatshops_are_a_us_responsibility_1.html

---

[21] Wilkinson RG et al. The problems of relative deprivation: why some societies do better than others. *Soc Sci Med.* 2007 Nov;65(9):1965-78

- Social isolation, loneliness, and all-cause mortality in older men and women (*Proc Natl Acad Sci* 2013 Apr[22]): "We found that mortality was higher among more socially isolated and more lonely participants. However, after adjusting statistically for demographic factors and baseline health, social isolation remained significantly associated with mortality (hazard ratio 1.26, 95% confidence interval, 1.08-1.48 for the top quintile of isolation), but loneliness did not (hazard ratio 0.92, 95% confidence interval, 0.78-1.09). ... Both social isolation and loneliness were associated with increased mortality. However, the effect of loneliness was not independent of demographic characteristics or health problems and did not contribute to the risk associated with social isolation. Although both isolation and loneliness impair quality of life and well-being, efforts to reduce isolation are likely to be more relevant to mortality."

- Economic inequality causes social harm (*TEDGlobal* 2011 Jul[23]): Greater economic inequality correlates very strongly with the worst health/social outcomes. Adding more are more drugs to individual patients' treatment plans is not the solution; the solution to socially and politically fostered problems is meaningful social engagement and authentic political representation, both focused on the goal of optimizing education, *health*care, sustainability, working conditions, and the fabric (people, time, resources) of society.

- Social inequality is an underacknowledged source of mental illness/distress (*Br J Psychiatry* 2010 Dec[24]): "Greater income inequality is associated with higher prevalence of mental illness and drug misuse in rich societies. There are threefold differences in the proportion of the population suffering from mental illness between more and less equal countries."

- Social inequality, systematic incarceration, and social-financial consequences (*Frontline* 2014 May[25]): The United States now incarcerates more of its citizens per capita than any other country in the world. "The past 40 years have seen the United States become home to more prisoners than any other country in the world. Yet despite this dramatic boom in incarceration rates, a new report finds that the deterrent effect of tough-on-crime policies remain 'highly uncertain.' The report, published Wednesday by the National Research Council, describes the rise of incarceration in America as "historically unprecedented and internationally unique." It found that from 1973 to 2009, the prison population grew from about 200,000 to approximately 2.2 million. With this spike, the U.S. now holds close to a quarter of the world's prisoners, even though it accounts for just 5 percent of the global population. "We are concerned that the United States is past the point where the number of people in prison can be justified by social benefits," said Jeremy Travis, president of John Jay College of Criminal Justice and the chair of the committee behind the study." America's use of imprisonment does not reflect the rates of crime but rather political policies and campaigns such as "the war on drugs", which itself is impressively focused on the use of *Cannabis* (*sativa* and related variants), a plant with numerous well-documented medical benefits (e.g., alleviation of chronic and neuropathic pain, nausea, glaucoma, spasticity in multiple sclerosis[26]), low cost, ease of cultivation, and many numerous nonmedical uses such as rapid growth of plant fiber for industrial uses such as clothing, rope, and paper manufacturing. NonCaucasians—Hispanics and African Americans specifically—are disproportionately affected by the "war on drugs" and the for-profit incarceration system of privatized prisons in America. According to the new report, the *purported social benefit* of such a system of incarceration does not appear to be offset by its *documented social harms*, most notably the decimation of human potential among those incarcerated and the impressively focal destruction of family systems and social cohesion especially among poor African American communities, wherein minor legal and behavioral issues (e.g., schoolyard fights, truancy) are treated with severe punishment (arrest, prison sentences) in ways that would not be *imposed within* nor *tolerated among* the more affluent and politically/financially advantaged sections of society.

---

[22] Steptoe A, et al. Social isolation, loneliness, and all-cause mortality in older men and women. *Proc Natl Acad Sci U S A.* 2013 Apr 9;110(15):5797-801

[23] https://ted.com/talks/richard_wilkinson/transcript

[24] Pickett KE, Wilkinson RG. Inequality: an underacknowledged source of mental illness and distress. *Br J Psychiatry.* 2010 Dec;197(6):426-8

[25] pbs.org/wgbh/pages/frontline/criminal-justice/locked-up-in-america/new-report-slams-unprecedented-growth-in-us-prisons/

[26] Leung L. Cannabis and its derivatives: review of medical use. *J Am Board Fam Med.* 2011 Jul-Aug;24(4):452-62

Political genesis of the cycles of poverty, crime, imprisonment and blocked access to voting, housing, employment, and education

As a political-governmental creation, social inequality can be imposed directly (e.g., segregation, voting prohibitions) or—much more commonly—indirectly via substandard healthcare, substandard education, reduced opportunity for scholarship and higher education, higher per-percentage-of-income taxation, more frequent use of social-medical "labels" such as behavioral-psychiatric disorders and expedited imprisonment, which results in loss of voting and employment opportunities, and prohibited access to federal funding for education, low-cost housing, and food support. Pulling minorities into the military depletes these communities of men and fathers (and women and mothers to a lesser but growing extent), thus ensuring the fragmentation of families and the modeling of adult behavior and relationships for children. The consequences of **institutionalized social inequality** impact individual people, with outcomes including physical illness, mental illness and drug abuse; medical care is one of the leading causes of personal bankruptcy, and victimless crimes such as *Cannabis* possession are the most common causes of imprisonment.

The American Paradox: "land of the free" has 25% of world's prisoners yet only 5% of world population

"From 1973 to 2009, the [American] prison population grew from about 200,000 to approximately 2.2 million. With this spike, the U.S. now holds close to a quarter of the world's prisoners, even though it accounts for just 5 percent of the global population. ... In 2009, 62 percent of black children age 17 or younger, whose parents had not completed high school, had experienced a parent being sent to prison. Among white children, the rate was 15 percent."

New Report Slams "Unprecedented" Growth in US Prisons. May 1, 2014.
pbs.org/wgbh/pages/frontline/criminal-justice/locked-up-in-america/new-report-slams-unprecedented-growth-in-us-prisons/

---

o **Quantifying imprisonment—interview with Michelle Alexander (*Frontline* 2014 Apr[27]):** "The United States actually has a crime rate that is lower than the international norm, yet our incarceration rate is six to 10 times higher than other countries' around the world… Many people imagine that our explosion in incarceration was simply driven by crime and crime rates, but that's just not true… I think most Americans have no idea of the scale and scope of mass incarceration in the United States… But the reality is that today there are more African Americans under correctional control in prison or jail, on probation or parole, than were enslaved in 1850, a decade before the civil war began."

Institutionalized social fragmentation

"The impact that the system of mass incarceration has on entire communities, virtually decimating them, destroying the economic fabric and the social networks that exist there… The psychological impact, the emotional impact, the level of grief and suffering—it's beyond description."

Alexander M. Edited transcript of an interview conducted on 2013 Sep.
pbs.org/wgbh/pages/frontline/criminal-justice/locked-up-in-america/michelle-alexander-a-system-of-racial-and-social-control

---

o **Xenobiotic pollution is a social phenomenon:** Xenobiotic pollution could have only become a global, massive and inescapable problem if three essential components have likewise existed and persisted: ❶ a culture of corporate greed: Xenobiotic pollution results from failure of large-scale producers/polluters to fully consider and be accountable to the fate and consequences of their toxic products, ❷ failure of government accountability: Governments have failed to be accountable to maintaining the safety of their populations, and governments have failed to hold themselves accountable to the performance of this duty, ❸ failure of social engagement: Populations worldwide have participated in their own marginalization by failing to engage effectively with whatever political structure they have; more often than not, populations are marginalized by their governments in such a way that popular political concern and activity (including "voting") really has no meaningful effect on the pervasive and largely invisible political-industrial infrastructure and core decisions and accountabilities that would promote preservation of our biological and social environments.

---

[27] pbs.org/wgbh/pages/frontline/criminal-justice/locked-up-in-america/michelle-alexander-a-system-of-racial-and-social-control/

> **"The only thing necessary for the triumph of evil is for good men to do nothing."** Ed. Burke (1729-1797)
>
> "Probably the greatest responsibility for the cancer epidemic we're faced with lies with you. Your lack of interest in the past, your lack of involvement, your unwillingness to develop coherent strategies, your unwillingness to challenge authority— **these have created a vacuum in decision-making, that has been filled by professional groups with mindsets, with conflicts of interests, in some instances with close relationships with the chemical industries**—professional groups that are uninterested in [disease] prevention. By your quiescence and your acquiescence, you have allowed these situations to develop. … **It is high time that empowerment and democracy and decision-making on these vital issues should be at least shared by you, if you should not indeed take a more prominent role.**"
>
> Samuel Epstein, M.D. Professor of Occupational and Environmental Medicine at the School of Public Health, University of Illinois Medical Center Chicago. Excerpted from 1993 lecture converge.org.nz/pirm/pestican.htm

- **Spirituality**: Obviously "spirituality" and religion mean different things to different people; people generally feel good if they have some sense of connection with God(s)/god(s) and the Universe/universe and a story that makes sense to them and which assuages feelings of loneliness and existential angst and disorientation. Spirituality and religion are commonly used interchangeably or in connection with each other despite their clear distinctions, for example the former is a decidedly personal and therefore creative experience whereas the latter is culturally codified. Clearly, one can have *spirituality without religion, religion without meaningful spirituality, religion and spirituality together*, or *neither*[28], but some type of "spiritual practice" and/or metaphysical ritual and renewal—even if it is a simple orienting mediation—is good, reasonable, and helpful; the transcultural work of the late Joseph Campbell is noteworthy (e.g., his *Power of Myth* series) and clearly extends beyond the overused soundbite "Follow your bliss" which is more intended to imply *fun and passion* rather than *irresponsibility*.

  > **Hospital-provided "spirituality services" are often a decoy from authentic and effective "CAM"**
  >
  > "We are oft to blame in this—it is too much proved: that with devotion's visage and pious action, we do sugar o'er the devil himself."
  >
  > William Shakespeare, *Hamlet*, Act 3, Scene 1

  - *Spirituality—the emperor's new clothes?* (*J Clin Nurs* 2004 Jan[29]): "The paper concludes that: (i) 'Spirituality' is an elastic term not capable of universal definition as each person's spirituality is an individual matter for them and (ii) tools that are being developed for identifying a person's spirituality run the risk of making wrong presuppositions about what comprises spirituality."

    > **"Spirituality" defined**
    >
    > "Spirituality is defined as: that most human of experiences that seeks to transcend self and find meaning and purpose through connection with others, nature, and/or a Supreme Being, which may or may not involve religious structures or traditions."
    >
    > Buck HG. Spirituality: concept analysis and model development. *Holist Nurs Pract*. 2006 Nov-Dec;20:288-92

  - Use of spirituality for laziness/ease/comfort: "Spirituality" can be used by patients and doctors as a means to circumvent harsh reality, the complexity of biochemistry, and predicted unfavorable outcomes. Spirituality should connect one with reality, not distance one from it; I am not in agreement with "spirituality" being (mis)used for ego-preserving escapism.

  - Use of spirituality for maintenance of institutional and professional power: My observation is that many hospitals provide "spiritual care" under the auspice of *complementary and alternative medicine* (CAM), and that this is done to decoy patients, to satiate them and discourage them from seeking truer and more effective "alternatives" to drugs that are often expensive, hazardous, and inefficacious. Most importantly, decoying/satiating patients with less potent "CAM" therapies reduces the likelihood of use of more highly potent "CAM" treatments such as interventional nutrition which are quite often affordable, safe, and highly efficacious. In this manner, hospitals and insurance companies retain clients (i.e., patients paying for drugs and other medical treatments) via use of "spirituality" and "CAM", and the most clear examples of this are noted in medical cancer treatment centers where "spirituality" is encouraged but effective CAM treatments such as dietary interventions and enzyme therapy are eschewed as *unscientific* despite records of safety and efficacy.

---

[28] "A philosophy can serve either to satisfy those [religious, existential] needs or to set them aside." Nietzsche FW. *Human, all too human*. Section #27. Also contextualized brilliantly in Schacht R. *Giants of Philosophy: Nietzsche*. Knowledge Products, especially the longer audio cassette format
[29] Bash A. Spirituality: the emperor's new clothes? *J Clin Nurs*. 2004 Jan;13(1):11-6

- o Spirituality (S) and religiosity (R) correlate with dietary practices, intake of fruits and vegetables (*Evid Based Complement Alternat Med* 2013[30]): "Overall, the denominational studies showed that religious denomination is significantly related to fruit, vegetable, and fat intake. Specifically, the Adventists consumed more fruit and vegetable and less fat than non-Adventists. However, the relationship between the degree of R/S and dietary intake is mixed."

- **Silliness:** Even the most intellectually robust of us need simple fun now and again; per the famous 1985 essay by Bob Black aptly titled and freely available *The Abolition of Work*, "It does mean creating a new way of life based on play; in other words, a *ludic* conviviality, commensality, and maybe even art. There is more to play than child's play, as worthy as that is. I call for a collective adventure in generalized joy and freely interdependent exuberance. Play isn't passive. Doubtless we all need a lot more time for sheer sloth and slack than we ever enjoy now, regardless of income or occupation, but once recovered from employment-induced exhaustion nearly all of us want to act. ...You may be wondering if I'm joking or serious. I'm joking *and* serious. To be ludic is not to be ludicrous. Play doesn't have to be frivolous, although frivolity isn't triviality: very often we ought to take frivolity seriously. I'd like life to be a game -- but a game with high stakes. ... Such is "work." Play is just the opposite. Play is always voluntary. What might otherwise be play is work if it's forced. This is axiomatic. Bernie de Koven has defined play as the "suspension of consequences." This is unacceptable if it implies that play is inconsequential. The point is not that play is without consequences. This is to demean play. The point is that the consequences, if any, are gratuitous. Playing and giving are closely related, they are the behavioral and transactional facets of the same impulse, the play-instinct. They share an aristocratic disdain for results. The player gets something out of playing; that's why he plays. But the core reward is the experience of the activity itself (whatever it is). ... There are many good games (chess, baseball, Monopoly, bridge) which are rule-governed but there is much more to play than game-playing. Conversation, sex, dancing, travel: these practices aren't rule-governed but they are surely play if anything is. And rules can be *played with* at least as readily as anything else."

- Stamp your passport: Conscious and periodic implementation of *geographic cure* is reasonable and is a great way to renew, recharge, and see amazing things in the world that are inspiring for our lives. Importantly, vacation/travel allows us to get completely out of our ruts and *vicious cycles of thought and behavior* to see ourselves and life anew.

Recreation is Re-creation

"Truth, however, must meet with opposition and be able to fight, and we must be able to rest from it at times in falsehood otherwise truth will grow tiresome, powerless, and insipid, and will render us equally so."

Friedrich Nietzsche, Daybreak, #507

"Take a break from the work before the work breaks you."

Hernando Vasquez

"I should mention that a purposeful, self-disciplined life does not mean a life without time or space for rest, relaxation, recreation, random or even frivolous activity. It merely means that such activities are chosen consciously, with the knowledge that it is safe and appropriate to engage in them. And in any event, the temporary abandonment of purpose also serves a purpose, whether consciously intended or not: that of regeneration."

Nathaniel Branden, Six Pillars of Self-Esteem

When was the last time you had real (healthy [nonescapist, nonselfharmful, nonintoxicated]) fun?

---

[30] Tan et al. Religiosity and Spirituality and the Intake of Fruit, Vegetable, and Fat: A Systematic Review. *Evid Based Complement Alternat Med.* 2013;2013:146214

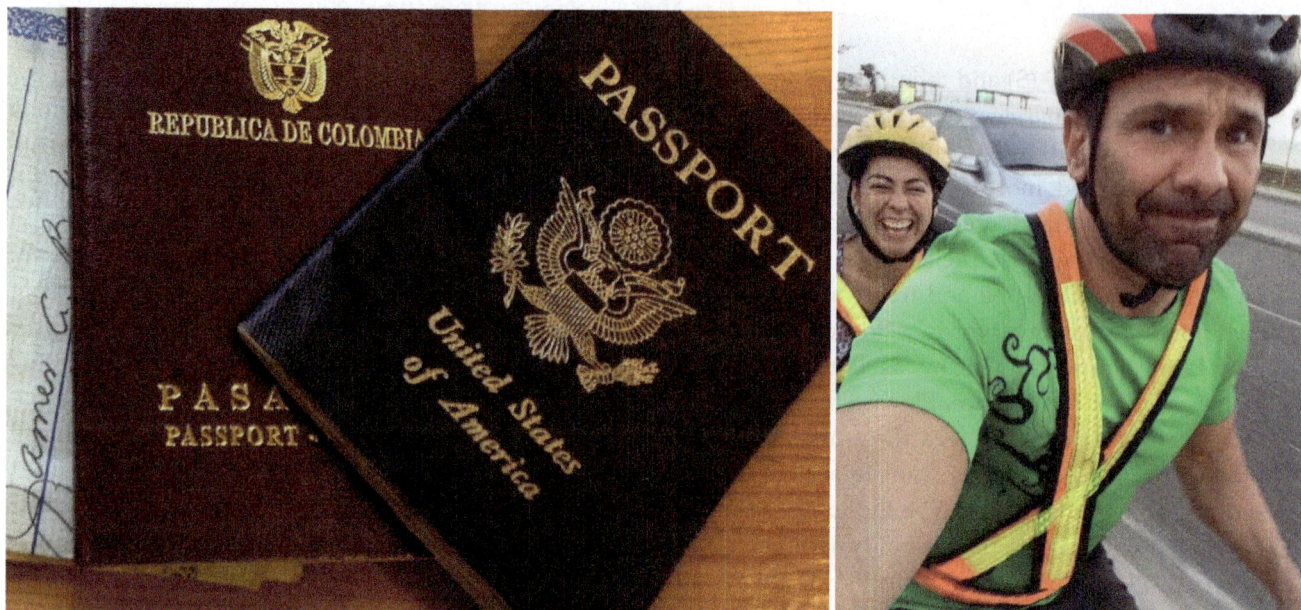

Passports, fun, social cohesion and sustainability: *Above*: Utilize the passport; having fun on a tandem bike in Cartagena Colombia (2014 Apr). *Below*: Notice how cities like Amsterdam have integrated fun with sustainability—massive public parking garages for bicycles are unheard of in the United States, where citizens have been denied access to mass transit and easy pleasurable living while being forced into privately owned, petroleum-dependent and ultimately isolating societal structures dependent on cars—"shiny metal boxes"—per the lyrics aptly describing worklife in America. Contrasted with most countries in North/Central/South America, most European countries have generally achieved and maintained the highest levels of quality of life (ie, enjoyment of daily living for the majority of the population) while also advancing their standard of living (ie, logistics and access to commodities).

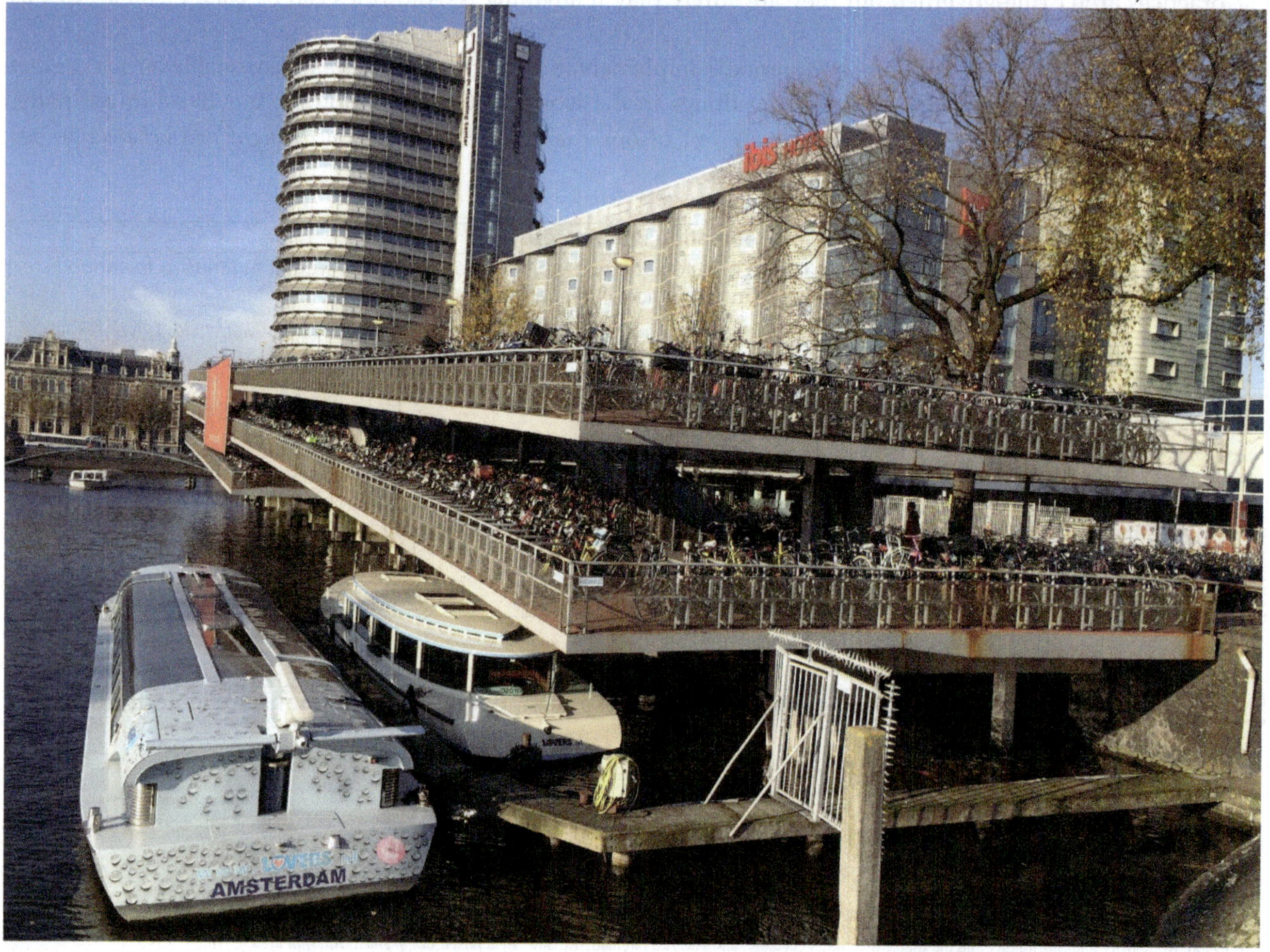

- <u>Sustainability</u>: Any culture or nation—or person—that does not consciously and deliberately provide for its/his/her own sustainability is manifesting either stupidity/naivety/ignorance, self-hatred, political/external manipulation, disdain for future generations or life itself, or some combination of all of these. A culture/nation/person that can only survive by enslaving or exploiting others is at best morally/ethically corrupt, if not in violation of generally accepted modern intercultural standards and international laws. In these modern times, supporting and advancing sustainability measures—ranging from the simple to complex, including recycling, transitioning away from petroleum (by definition: limited and polluting) and toward renewable-sourced electricity and human-power (by definition: practically unlimited and clean[er]), redesigning city infrastructures to support co-ecology and minimal energy and resource investment for their construction, use, and maintenance.

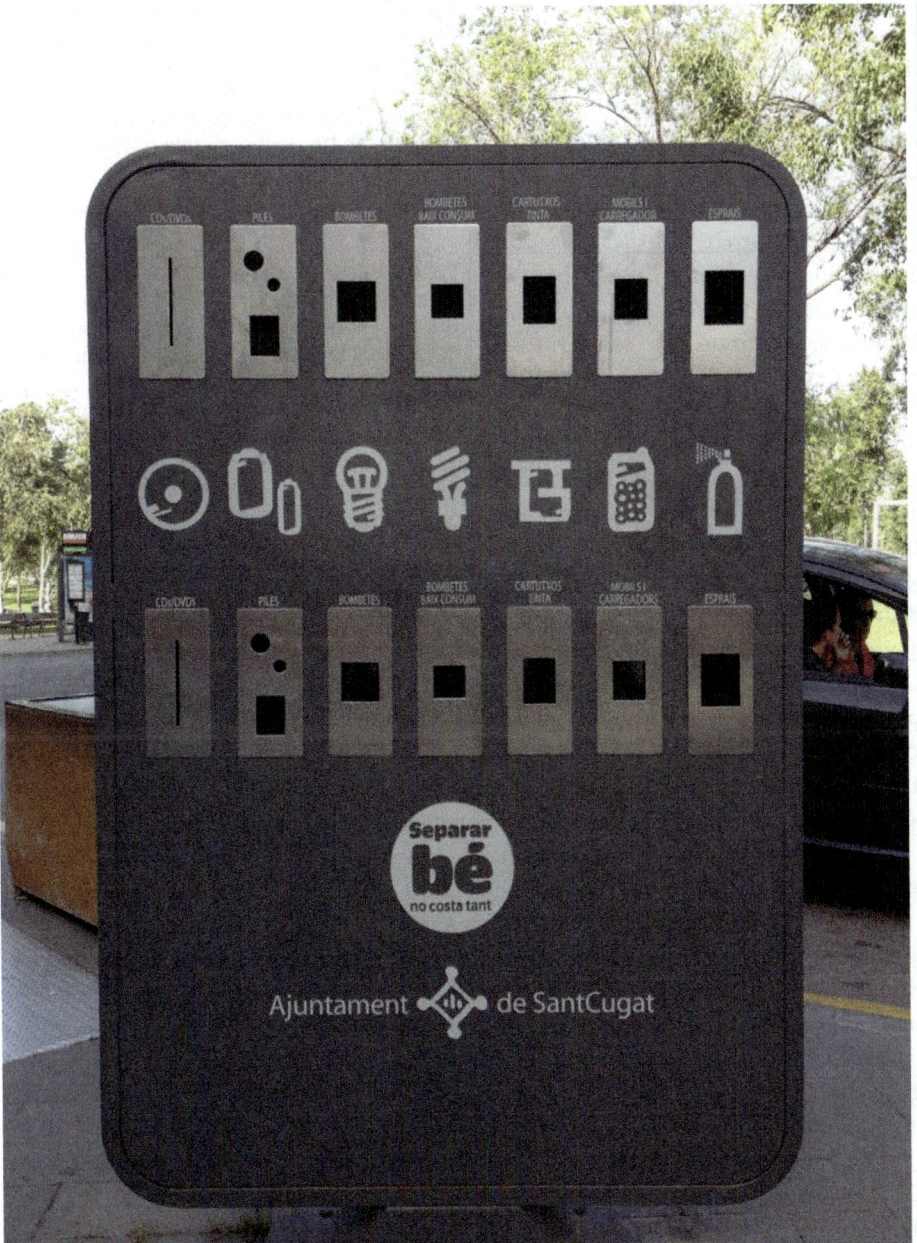

The work of Jacque Fresco —TheVenusProject.org— as an example of intelligent sustainable humanistic social design

"The Venus Project is a veritable blueprint for the genesis of a new world civilization, one that is based on human concern and environmental reclamation. The plans for The Venus Project offer society a broader spectrum of choices based on the scientific possibilities directed toward a new era of peace and sustainability for all. Through the implementation of a resource-based economy, and a multitude of innovative and environmentally friendly technologies directly applied to the social system, The Venus Project proposals will dramatically reduce crime, poverty, hunger, homelessness, and many other pressing problems that are common throughout the world today. One of the cornerstones of the organization's findings is the fact that many of the dysfunctional behaviors of today's society stem directly from the dehumanizing environment of a monetary system. …This is also in perfect accord with the spiritual aspects and ideals found in most religions throughout the world. ..The Venus Project…proposes to translate these ideals into a working reality."

<u>S</u>ustainability: This neighborhood sidewalk recycling station for small items is simple, and yet the implied sophistication of the accompanying forethought and infrastructure dwarfs what is commonly available in most other countries. One could reasonably be baffled at the lack of international progress in sustainability, of which recycling is only one part, because it defies reason and is based on the synergism and interdependence of profiteering, politics, inertia. Many forces within society work directly against peace, progress, and sustainability; their goals are perpetual consumerism, international resource exploitation, and orchestration of public passivity to allow these.

- **Science**: Whether we live in a religious social environment or not and/or whether or not we personally choose by our own independent volition to live in accord with religion/metaphysics, what is very certain is that we are all obligated—via our fundamental need to survive and engage in the concrete world—to live in accord with logic and the physical laws/facts which have been described to govern the majority of our earthly physical experiences. This conversation would be unnecessary except for the major resurgence of anti-science that we now witness in public discourse, notably in critical areas such as international politics, medicine, general science, and society/culture.

  - Antiscientific denial of climate change: Among the grossest examples of anti-science are currently those which deny climate change—the denial is made worse when the very legislators entrusted to manage complexity on behalf of the public make the conversation itself illegal, as happened in North Carolina in the United States.

    - New Law in North Carolina Bans Latest Scientific Predictions of Sea-Level Rise (20/20 ABC news 2012 Aug[31]): "A new law in North Carolina will ban the state from basing coastal policies on the latest scientific predictions of how much the sea level will rise, prompting environmentalists to accuse the state of disrespecting climate science. ... The bill's passage in June triggered nationwide scorn by those who argued that the state was deliberately blinding itself to the effects of climate change." Legally-mandated ignorance sabotages society, endorses/enforces idiocy.

  - Antiscientific denial of the potential dangers of genetically manipulated foods and the heavy chemical and sociopolitical burden resultant from their use: Another example of absurdity is the American Medical Association's (AMA) position against the labeling of foods produced into genetically manipulated

> ### Science and a logical open-eyied and inquisitive approach to life is necessary for happiness/success/survival
>
> "But to think is an act of choice. The key to ... "human nature" ... is the fact that man is a being of volitional consciousness. Reason does not work automatically; thinking is not a mechanical process; the connections of logic are not made by instinct. The function of your stomach, lungs or heart is automatic; the function of your mind is not. In any hour and issue of your life, you are free to think or to evade that effort. But you are not free to escape from your nature, from the fact that reason is your means of survival—so that for you, who are a human being, the question "to be or not to be" is the question "to think or not to think.'"
>
> Rand A. *Atlas Shrugged*. Random House, 1012
>
> "Man's basic means of survival is his mind, his capacity to reason. ...For man, survival is a question—a problem to be solved. The perceptual level of his consciousness—the level of passive sensory awareness, which he shares with animals—is inadequate to solve it. To remain alive, man must think—which means: he must exercise the faculty which he alone, of all living species, possesses: the faculty of abstractions, of conceptualizing. The conceptual level of consciousness is the human level, the level required for man's survival. It is upon his ability to think that man's life depends."
>
> Branden N. *The Psychology of Self-Esteem*. John Wiley and Sons, 231

corporate products—some examples of which are "foods" that are patented as pesticides yet sold to an ignorant public under the guise of "substantial equivalence", promoting the absurd paradox that a patented corporate food-like product can simultaneously be sufficiently *natural* to pass for normal food yet sufficiently *different* to qualify for patents due to genetic manipulations that include insertion of genes from other phylogenetic kingdoms, including genes that produce insecticides and antibiotics. Components of this utter absurdity include but are not limited to these facts: ❶ The organization's members have no training in nutrition: Medical physicians generally and very clearly those in the United States receive absolutely zero training in clinical nutrition[32]; therefore, the AMA's having a position on a topic as nuanced and delicate as that of genetically manipulated nutrition—exacerbated by their defense of nutritional ignorance via publishing a position *against* labeling genetically manipulated (GM) foods—is an example of abuse of cultural authority and biotechnology/multinational corporation favoritism (not unlike the AMA's enabling of the tobacco industry for 25 lethal years after the negative health effects of tobacco were known[33]). ❷ Failure to take a stand for the basic tenets of medical ethics: For the sake of their own integrity/façade, the AMA should have favored GM labeling just as they should uphold two of the basic four tenets of medical ethics, namely those of 1) autonomy—allowing patients/public to decide, and 2) informed consent—providing patients/public the information necessary in order to make reasonable, independent, autonomous decisions. ❸ Failure to implement the precautionary principle: The World Trade Organization (WTO)[34] provides the

---

[31] Harish A. New Law in North Carolina Bans Latest Scientific Predictions of Sea-Level Rise. *ABC news, 20/20* 2012 Aug abcnews.go.com
[32] Vetter et al. What do resident physicians know about nutrition? *J Am Coll Nutr.* 2008;27:287-98. Halsted CH. The relevance of clinical nutrition education and role models to the practice of medicine. *Eur J Clin Nutr.* 1999 May:S29-34. Raman et al. How much do gastroenterology fellows know about nutrition? *J Clin Gastroenterol.* 2009 Jul;43:559-64
[33] Gardner MN, Brandt AM. "The doctors' choice is America's choice": the physician in US cigarette advertisements, 1930-1953. *Am J Public Health.* 2006 Feb;96(2):222-32
[34] World Trade Organization. The "Precautionary Principle" wto.org/english/tratop_e/sps_e/sps_agreement_cbt_e/c8s2p1_e.htm 2014 Dec

following description (see also United Nations Educational Scientific and Cultural Organization[35]), "The "precautionary principle" is a notion which supports taking protective action *before* there is complete scientific proof of a risk; that is, action should not be delayed simply because full scientific information is lacking. The "precautionary principle" or precautionary approach has been incorporated into several international environmental agreements, and some claim that it is now recognized as a general principle of international environmental law. In the fields of food safety, plant and animal health protection, the need for taking precautionary actions in the face of scientific uncertainty has long been widely accepted."

- The AMA's Strange Position on GM Foods: Test but Don't Label (*The Atlantic* 2012 Jun[36]): "Here's what surprises me: in recommending premarket safety testing, which is not now required, the AMA appears to be raising serious questions about the safety of GM foods. If such doubts exist, shouldn't GM foods be labeled so the public has a choice?"

- **Social justice**: What we have begun witnessing in 2014 is a rapid resurgence in social injustice—the police killings of several unarmed African-American men in the United States along with societal eavesdropping and profiteering "asset forfeiture", the government-

> **Social justice is necessary for personal and societal health— gross divergencies from this promote neuroses and addictive/escapist thoughts and behaviours**
> "Injustice anywhere is a threat to justice everywhere."
> Martin Luther King Jr., Letter from Birmingham Jail, 1963

crime collusion that effected the deaths of more than 40 student teachers in Mexico, the ongoing social oppression in countries such as Colombia, Thailand, and China. Social injustice and the previously discussed "inequality" are similar in their cause (oligarchical social oppression) and effect (anguish, impoverishment), with the latter being distress, unrest, that promotes neurotic thoughts and behaviors (e.g., overeating)—neurotic and *pathogenic* existence for those who must witness and endure ongoing social injustice. For personal and societal health, we need justice.

- **Sexuality and sensuality**: Just about everyone has endured some type of familial/societal-induced sexual repression or disorientation, even if that disorientation was "merely" the absence of affirmation. As such, just about everyone should engage in some reflection upon and recovery

> **Sexuality and Sensuality**
> "The degree and kind of a person's sexuality reaches up into the furthermost peaks of their spirit." Nietzsche F. *Beyond Good and Evil*. #75

from this in order to have access to a full, complete, free, and nonneurotic life. Excellent discussions on this have been provided by Robert Bly, John Bradshaw, Alice Miller, Arthur Janov, and David Deida. Health requires integration of our physical needs, wants, desires; denying these leaves us either partly/wholly numb or neurotic.

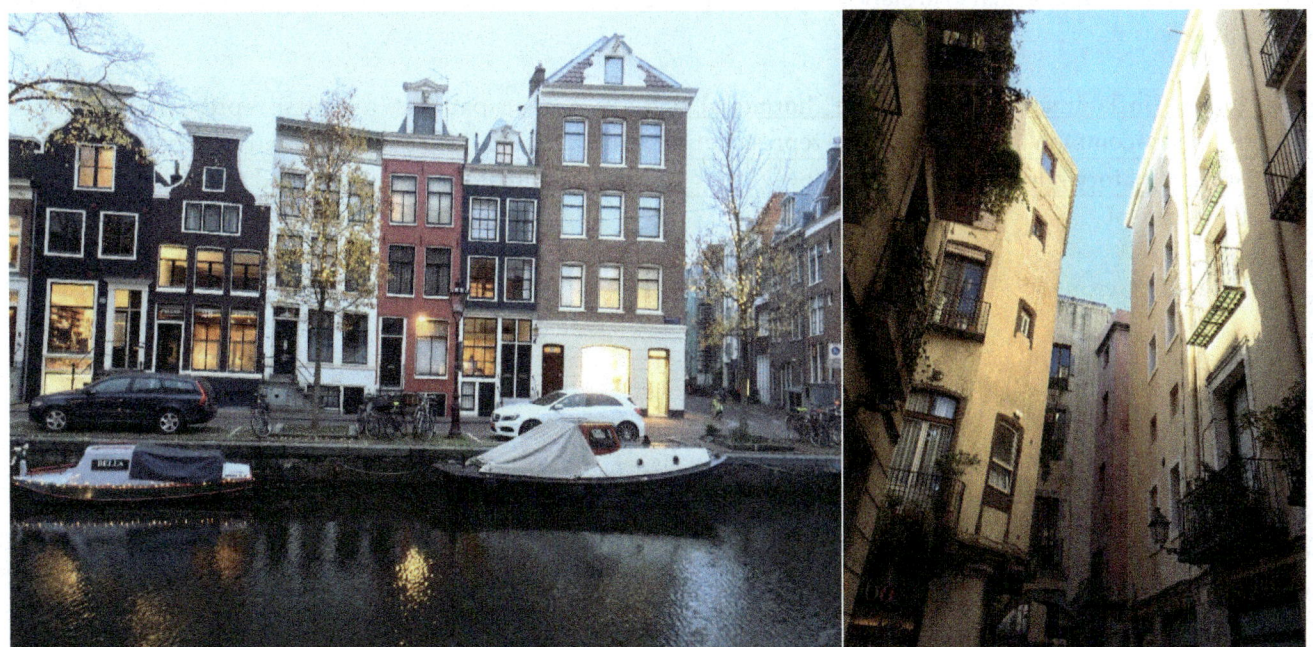

Photos above showing the colorfulness of European life—Amsterdam and Barcelona: Europeans seem to lead the world in quality of life, public works, and work-life balance.

---

[35] United Nations Educational Scientific and Cultural Organization. The Precautionary Principle. 2005 Mar unesdoc.unesco.org/images/0013/001395/139578e.pdf
[36] Nestle M. The AMA's Strange Position on GM Foods: Test but Don't Label. *The Atlantic* 2012 Jun theatlantic.com/

❻ Endocrine Imbalances (Dysendocrinism):
Hormonal Evaluations and Interventions:
Anti-inflammatory Orthoendocrinology

Major Concepts in this Section

Hormones affect and are affected by inflammatory status. In this section, I will focus on the seven hormones of greatest significance to inflammatory homeodynamics. Readers should mentally organize this information in the following way:
❶ Hormones that are commonly **elevated** and **need to be reduced** in inflammatory states: Prolactin, Insulin, Estrogen
❷ Hormones that are commonly **reduced** and **need to be elevated** in inflammatory states: Cortisol, DHEA, Testosterone
❸ Thyroid status is considered separately: See Chapter 1 for discussion of a novel way (contrasted to the standard allopathic viewpoint) of assessing and treating hypothyroidism in general and functional/peripheral/metabolic hypothyroidism in particular. Thyroid status is less potent as an influence on inflammatory balance when compared to the 6 other hormones listed above; however, occasionally a patient will have severe musculoskeletal inflammation (e.g., bilateral adhesive capsulitis, oligoarthritis, proximal myopathy[37]) responsive solely to thyroid hormone monotherapy.

Introduction: Steroidal and peptide hormones have significant immunomodulating properties, and a characteristic pattern of disruption is commonly seen in patients with autoimmunity. Relatively simple natural and/or pharmacologic interventions can be used to safely and effectively correct hormonal disturbances with the dual benefits of improved overall health and the amelioration of autoimmunity. I have coined the term "orthoendocrinology"[38] to describe this technique of

> **Hormones affect inflammation**
>
> "The altered hormonal status could result in relative immunological hyperactivity contributing to enhance tissue damage and disease severity."
>
> Mirone et al. Androgen and prolactin levels in systemic sclerosis: relationship to disease severity. *Ann N Y Acad Sci* 2006

addressing numerous disturbances in endocrine function by using the "right hormones" based on a similar conceptual model to Linus Pauling's suggestion that health might be optimized by the use of the "right molecules" (orthomolecular medicine, orthomolecular nutrition) rather than endless reliance on the cyclical prescriptions of what he called "toximolecular" substances. I will keep this overview and application straightforward, simple, and clinically relevant.

The typical "inflammatory/autoimmune" hormonal pattern: Among patients, a partial representation of this pattern is more common than the complete representation. Clinicians should assess *each* and treat *each* as indicated.

Anti-inflammatory hormones tend to be low	Pro-inflammatory hormones tend to be elevated
• **Low cortisol** • **Low DHEA** • **Low testosterone**	• **High prolactin** • **High estrogen** • **High insulin** (surrogate marker for dietary CHO excess and insulin resistance, the latter of which is a marker of ERS and mitochondrial dysfunction, and thus also of microbial and xenobiotic loads)

Additional considerations:

- Growth hormone: Variable and apparently less important; can be assessed per patient.
- Progesterone: Variable and apparently less important; can be assessed per patient.
- Pregnenolone: Less potent with regard to inflammation than are prolactin, estrogen, cortisol, DHEA, and testosterone; can be measured by laboratory and treated per patient need. Earlier studies showed anti-inflammatory benefit with supplementation.
- Thyroid: Hypothyroidism and/or thyroid autoimmunity; see Chapter 1 for additional discussion, detailed review of assessments, case reports, and treatments.

---

[37] Bowman CA, et al. Bilateral adhesive capsulitis, oligoarthritis and proximal myopathy as presentation of hypothyroidism. *Br J Rheumatol*. 1988 Feb;27(1):62-4
[38] As of November 15, 2005 the word "orthoendocrinology" cannot be found either on Pubmed/Medline or Internet search using Google, Yahoo, or MSN search engines.

<u>**Testing and treatment hormonal status in patients with autoimmunity**</u>: Patients with autoimmune disorders commonly have deficiencies and imbalances in their hormones, particularly steroid and "sex" hormones, which are potent immunomodulators. The classic pattern which may be expressed incompletely in an individual patient, is that of excess prolactin and estrogen, and insufficient cortisol, testosterone, and DHEA. The role of progesterone seems less clear, with some patients showing normal, excess, or insufficient amounts; obviously, this can be tested in an individual patient (random serum test in men or 21st-day/midluteal serum sample from a premenopausal woman). All testing methods—via serum, saliva, or urine—have their individual advantages and disadvantages. Generally however, serum is considered the standard; following this I prefer polyhormonal assessment with 24-hour urine collections, and the last resort is saliva testing, which is the most controversial and least reliable. Thyroid autoimmunity and hypothyroidism are both common in autoimmune/inflammatory patients; comprehensive thyroid assessment with TSH, T4, and anti-TPO antibodies can be justified in nearly any rheumatic patient.

- <u>**Hyperprolactinemia and latent hyperprolactinemia**</u>: Besides its obvious role in lactation, prolactin is a polyfunctional hormone that, at the very least, stimulates the liver to produce excess sex-hormone-binding globulin (SHBG) which adsorbs sex hormones, rendering them less effective due to reduced bioavailability; the resultant *functional hypogonadism* deprives the immune system of the modulation/suppression normally effected by these hormones. Beyond these well-known physiologic roles, **prolactin is now known to be powerfully proinflammatory.**[39] **Patients with RA and SLE have higher basal and stress-induced levels of prolactin compared with**

  > **Prolactin is pro-inflammatory, and anti-prolactin interventions provide an anti-inflammatory benefit**
  >
  > "Multiple lines of evidence support the concept that the anterior pituitary hormone **prolactin has a pathogenic role in rheumatic and autoimmune diseases** including, but not limited to, rheumatoid arthritis (RA), systemic lupus erythematosus (SLE), Reiter's syndrome, psoriatic arthritis, and uveitis."
  >
  > McMurray RW. *Semin Arthritis* Rheum. 2001

  normal controls.[40,41] **Patients with scleroderma have relatively high prolactin**[42] **and low DHEA.**[43] **Patients with polymyalgia rheumatica have elevated prolactin that correlates with increased symptomatology.**[44] Elevated prolactin levels may further exacerbate immune dysfunction by increasing hepatic production of sex-hormone binding globulin and reducing bioavailability of testosterone, thus depriving cells and tissues of testosterone's potent anti-inflammatory and immunoregulatory properties. Prolactin is routinely measured in serum; high values should be reduced with effective treatment, whether nutritional, botanical, or pharmacologic.

  - <u>Thyroid hormone</u>: **Hypothyroidism frequently causes hyperprolactinemia** that is reversible upon effective treatment of hypothyroidism. Conversely, due to its immunodysregulating effects, elevated prolactin appears capable of inducing hypothyroidism and autoimmune thyroiditis.[45] Assessing hyperprolactinemic patients for thyroid disturbances with TSH, T4, T3, and anti-TPO antibodies is strongly advised. Thyroid status should be evaluated in all patients with hyperprolactinemia.

  - <u>High-dose pyridoxine</u>: B6 (250 mg qd-bid with food) is used by some doctors to lower prolactin despite the lack of consistently demonstrated benefit in the research literature.

[39] "Multiple lines of evidence support the concept that the anterior pituitary hormone prolactin has a pathogenic role in rheumatic and autoimmune diseases including, but not limited to, rheumatoid arthritis (RA), systemic lupus erythematosus (SLE), Reiter's syndrome, psoriatic arthritis, and uveitis." McMurray RW. Bromocriptine in rheumatic and autoimmune diseases. *Semin Arthritis Rheum.* 2001 Aug;31(1):21-32

[40] Dostal C, et al. Serum prolactin stress values in patients with systemic lupus erythematosus. *Ann Rheum Dis.* 2003 May;62(5):487-8

[41] "RESULTS: A significantly higher rate of elevated PRL levels was found in SLE patients (40.0%) compared with the healthy controls (14.8%). No proof was found of association with the presence of anti-ds-DNA or with specific organ involvement. Similarly, elevated PRL levels were found in RA patients (39.3%)." Moszkorzova L, et al. Hyperprolactinaemia in patients with systemic lupus erythematosus. *Clin Exp Rheumatol.* 2002 Nov-Dec;20(6):807-12

[42] Straub RH, Zeuner M, Lock G, Scholmerich J, Lang B. High prolactin and low dehydroepiandrosterone sulphate serum levels in patients with severe systemic sclerosis. *Br J Rheumatol.* 1997 Apr;36(4):426-32 rheumatology.oxfordjournals.org/cgi/reprint/36/4/426

[43] "CONCLUSION: Our data show that, as in other autoimmune diseases, low serum DHEAS is a feature of premenopausal SSc patients. More extensive prospective studies are needed to define the exact role of DHEAS dysregulation in SSc." La Montagna G, Baruffo A, Buono G, Valentini G. Dehydroepiandrosterone sulphate serum levels in systemic sclerosis. *Clin Exp Rheumatol.* 2001 Jan-Feb;19(1):21-6

[44] Straub RH, Georgi J, Helmke K, Vaith P, Lang B. In polymyalgia rheumatica serum prolactin is positively correlated with the number of typical symptoms but not with typical inflammatory markers. *Rheumatology* (Oxford). 2002 Apr;41(4):423-9 rheumatology.oxfordjournals.org/cgi/content/full/41/4/423

[45] "...PRL level is higher in SLE patients and that in the presence of hyperPRL there is increased prevalence of antithyroid antibodies, evidencing the association of PRL and autoimmunity and pointing to the appropriateness of assessing and monitoring the progress of these markers in patients affected by these disorders." Kramer CK, Tourinho TF, de Castro WP, da Costa Oliveira M. Association between systemic lupus erythematosus, rheumatoid arthritis, hyperprolactinemia and thyroid autoantibodies. *Arch Med Res.* 2005 Jan-Feb;36(1):54-8

o   *Vitex astus-cagnus* and other supporting botanicals and nutrients: **Vitex lowers serum prolactin in humans**[46,47] **via a dopaminergic effect.**[48] Vitex is considered safe for clinical use; mild and reversible adverse effects possibly associated with Vitex include nausea, headache, gastrointestinal disturbances, menstrual disorders, acne, pruritus and erythematous rash. No drug interactions are known, but given the herb's dopaminergic effect it should probably be used with some caution in patients treated with dopamine antagonists such as the so-called antipsychotic drugs (most of which do not work very well and/or carry intolerable adverse effects[49,50]). In a recent review, Bone[51] stated that daily doses can range from 500 mg to 2,000 mg DHE (dry herb equivalent) and can be tailored to the suppression of prolactin. Due at least in part to its content of L-dopa, *Mucuna pruriens* **shows clinical dopaminergic activity** as evidenced by its effectiveness in Parkinson's disease[52]; up to 15-30 gm/d of mucuna has been used clinically but doses will be dependent on preparation and phytoconcentration. Triptolide and other **extracts from *Tripterygium wilfordii* Hook F** exert clinically significant anti-inflammatory action in patients with rheumatoid arthritis[53,54] and also offer protection to dopaminergic neurons.[55,56] Ironically, even though tyrosine is the nutritional precursor to dopamine with evidence of clinical effectiveness (e.g., narcolepsy[57], enhancement of memory[58] and cognition[59]), **supplementation with tyrosine appears to actually increase rather than decrease prolactin levels**[60]**; therefore tyrosine should be used cautiously if at all in patients with systemic inflammation.** Furthermore, the finding that **high-protein meals stimulate prolactin release**[61] may partly explain the benefits of vegetarian diets in the treatment of systemic inflammation; since vegetarian diets are comparatively low in protein compared to omnivorous diets, they may lead to a relative reduction in prolactin production due to lack of stimulation.

---

[46] "Since AC extracts were shown to have beneficial effects on premenstrual mastodynia serum prolactin levels in such patients were also studied in one double-blind, placebo-controlled clinical study. Serum prolactin levels were indeed reduced in the patients treated with the extract." Wuttke W, Jarry H, Christoffel V, Spengler B, Seidlova-Wuttke D. Chaste tree (Vitex agnus-castus)--pharmacology and clinical indications. *Phytomedicine.* 2003 May;10(4):348-57

[47] German abstract from Medline: "The prolactin release was reduced after 3 months, shortened luteal phases were normalised and deficits in the luteal progesterone synthesis were eliminated." Milewicz A, Gejdel E, Sworen H, Sienkiewicz K, Jedrzejak J, Teucher T, Schmitz H. [Vitex agnus castus extract in the treatment of luteal phase defects due to latent hyperprolactinemia. Results of a randomized placebo-controlled double-blind study] *Arzneimittelforschung.* 1993 Jul;43(7):752-6

[48] "Our results indicate a dopaminergic effect of Vitex agnus-castus extracts and suggest additional pharmacological actions via opioid receptors." Meier B, Berger D, Hoberg E, Sticher O, Schaffner W. Pharmacological activities of Vitex agnus-castus extracts in vitro. *Phytomedicine.* 2000 Oct;7(5):373-81

[49] "The majority of patients in each group discontinued their assigned treatment owing to inefficacy or intolerable side effects or for other reasons." Lieberman JA, Stroup TS, McEvoy JP, Swartz MS, Rosenheck RA, Perkins DO, Keefe RS, Davis SM, Davis CE, Lebowitz BD, Severe J, Hsiao JK; Clinical Antipsychotic Trials of Intervention Effectiveness (CATIE) Investigators. Effectiveness of antipsychotic drugs in patients with chronic schizophrenia. *N Engl J Med.* 2005 Sep 22;353(12):1209-23

[50] Whitaker R. The case against antipsychotic drugs: a 50-year record of doing more harm than good. *Med Hypotheses.* 2004;62(1):5-13

[51] "In conditions such as endometriosis and fibroids, for which a significant estrogen antagonist effect is needed, doses of at least 2 g/day DHE may be required and typically are used by professional herbalists." Bone K. New Insights into Chaste Tree. *Nutritional Wellness* 2005 November nutritionalwellness.com/archives/2005/nov/11_bone.php

[52] "CONCLUSIONS: The rapid onset of action and longer on time without concomitant increase in dyskinesias on mucuna seed powder formulation suggest that this natural source of L-dopa might possess advantages over conventional L-dopa preparations in the long term management of PD." Katzenschlager R, Evans A, Manson A, Patsalos PN, Ratnaraj N, Watt H, Timmermann L, Van der Giessen R, Lees AJ. Mucuna pruriens in Parkinson's disease: a double blind clinical and pharmacological study. *J Neurol Neurosurg Psychiatry.* 2004 Dec;75(12):1672-7

[53] "The ethanol/ethyl acetate extract of TWHF shows therapeutic benefit in patients with treatment-refractory RA. At therapeutic dosages, the TWHF extract was well tolerated by most patients in this study." Tao X, Younger J, Fan FZ, Wang B, Lipsky PE. Benefit of an extract of Tripterygium Wilfordii Hook F in patients with rheumatoid arthritis: a double-blind, placebo-controlled study. *Arthritis Rheum.* 2002 Jul;46(7):1735-43

[54] "CONCLUSION: The EA extract of TWHF at dosages up to 570 mg/day appeared to be safe, and doses > 360 mg/day were associated with clinical benefit in patients with RA." Tao X, Cush JJ, Garret M, Lipsky PE. A phase I study of ethyl acetate extract of the Chinese antirheumatic herb Tripterygium wilfordii hook F in rheumatoid arthritis. *J Rheumatol.* 2001 Oct;28(10):2160-7

[55] "Our data suggests that triptolide may protect dopaminergic neurons from LPS-induced injury and its efficiency in inhibiting microglia activation may underlie the mechanism." Li FQ, Lu XZ, Liang XB, Zhou HF, Xue B, Liu XY, Niu DB, Han JS, Wang XM. Triptolide, a Chinese herbal extract, protects dopaminergic neurons from inflammation-mediated damage through inhibition of microglial activation. *J Neuroimmunol.* 2004 Mar;148(1-2):24-31

[56] "Moreover, tripchlorolide markedly prevented the decrease in amount of dopamine in the striatum of model rats. Taken together, our data provide the first evidence that tripchlorolide acts as a neuroprotective molecule that rescues MPP+ or axotomy-induced degeneration of dopaminergic neurons, which may imply its therapeutic potential for Parkinson's disease." Li FQ, Cheng XX, Liang XB, Wang XH, Xue B, He QH, Wang XM, Han JS. Neurotrophic and neuroprotective effects of tripchlorolide, an extract of Chinese herb Tripterygium wilfordii Hook F, on dopaminergic neurons. *Exp Neurol.* 2003 Jan;179(1):28-37

[57] "Of twenty-eight visual analogue scales rating mood and arousal, the subjects' ratings in the tyrosine treatment (9 g daily) and placebo periods differed significantly for only three (less tired, less drowsy, more alert)." Elwes RD, Crewes H, Chesterman LP, Summers B, Jenner P, Binnie CD, Parkes JD. Treatment of narcolepsy with L-tyrosine: double-blind placebo-controlled trial. *Lancet.* 1989 Nov 4;2(8671):1067-9

[58] "Ten men and 10 women subjects underwent these batteries 1 h after ingesting 150 mg/kg of l-tyrosine or placebo. Administration of tyrosine significantly enhanced accuracy and decreased frequency of list retrieval on the working memory task during the multiple task battery compared with placebo." Thomas JR, Lockwood PA, Singh A, Deuster PA. Tyrosine improves working memory in a multitasking environment. *Pharmacol Biochem Behav.* 1999 Nov;64(3):495-500

[59] "Ten subjects received five daily doses of a protein-rich drink containing 2 g tyrosine, and 11 subjects received a carbohydrate rich drink with the same amount of calories (255 kcal)." Deijen JB, Wientjes CJ, Vullinghs HF, Cloin PA, Langefeld JJ. Tyrosine improves cognitive performance and reduces blood pressure in cadets after one week of a combat training course. *Brain Res Bull.* 1999 Jan 15;48(2):203-9

[60] "Tyrosine (when compared to placebo) had no effect on any sleep related measure, but it did stimulate prolactin release." Waters WF, et al. A comparison of tyrosine against placebo, phentermine, caffeine, and D-amphetamine during sleep deprivation. *Nutr Neurosci.* 2003;6(4):221-35

[61] "Whereas carbohydrate meals had no discernible effects, high protein meals induced a large increase in both PRL and cortisol; high fat meals caused selective release of PRL."Ishizuka, et al. Pituitary hormone release in response to food ingestion. *J Clin Endocrinol Metab* 1983Dec;57:1111-6

o   <u>Bromocriptine</u>: Bromocriptine has long been considered the pharmacologic treatment of choice for elevated prolactin.[62] Typical dose is 2.5 mg per day (effective against lupus[63]); gastrointestinal upset and sedation are common.[64] **Clinical intervention with bromocriptine appears warranted in patients with RA, SLE, Reiter's syndrome, psoriatic arthritis, and probably multiple sclerosis and uveitis.[65]**

o   <u>Cabergoline/Dostinex</u>: Cabergoline/Dostinex is a newer dopamine agonist with few adverse effects; typical dose starts at 0.5 mg per week (0.25 mg twice per week).[66] Several studies have indicated that cabergoline is safer and more effective than bromocriptine for reducing prolactin levels[67] and the dose can often be reduced after successful prolactin reduction, allowing for reductions in cost and adverse effects.[68] Although fewer studies have been published supporting the antirheumatic benefits of cabergoline than bromocriptine, the scientific rationale for its use is derived from the success of bromocriptine in various rheumatic/autoimmune diseases. Furthermore, clinicians need to appreciate that prolactin is an active proinflammatory signal within the immune system (functioning in an autocrine/paracrine manner among immunocytes) and that treatment can be implemented and is often effective regardless of serum prolactin levels; if a high serum prolactin is found then it should be treated, while a normal serum prolactin does not preclude use of antiprolactin treatment.

▪ <u>Case report: Control of unremitting rheumatoid arthritis by the prolactin antagonist cabergoline</u>: Erb et al[69] published a case report of a woman with unremitting rheumatoid arthritis who achieved remarkable clinical improvement and who was able to reduce her need for other antirheumatic drugs with the use of cabergoline 0.5 mg per day. They wrote, "The present case demonstrates a dramatic improvement of previously uncontrollable RA soon after treatment of coincidental hyperprolactinemia [serum prolactin 1623 mU/l (normal range 0–440 mU/l)] with the prolactin antagonist cabergoline. ... Treatment with the prolactin antagonist cabergoline 500 µg daily was commenced. Within 2 months her menstrual cycle and prolactin levels were normal. She had no active synovitis in any of her joints, morning stiffness had declined to less than 30 min, and her ESR and CRP had almost normalized, at 25 mm in the first hour and 6 mg/l respectively. Her RA remains clinically and serologically controlled to the present day, despite gradual but continuous reduction of her anti-rheumatic medication."

▪ <u>Pilot randomized double-blind clinical trial: The effect of cabergoline on clinical and laboratory findings in active rheumatoid arthritis (*Iran Red Crescent Med J* 2011 Oct[70])</u>: "In this study, improvement of tender and swollen joint count, patient assessment of pain and patient global assessment of disease activity were significant when patients were treated by cabergoline [1 mg/week]. Prolactin is secreted not only by anterior pituitary gland, but also by immune cells that may have small effect on total serum prolactin level and a significant effect on immunomedulatory system, so cabergoline suppressed both kinds of

[62] Beers MH, Berkow R (eds). *Merck Manual. 17ᵗʰ Edition*. Whitehouse Station; Merck Research Laboratories 1999 Page 77-78

[63] "A prospective, double-blind, randomized, placebo-controlled study compared BRC at a fixed daily dosage of 2.5 mg with placebo... Long term treatment with a low dose of BRC appears to be a safe and effective means of decreasing SLE flares in SLE patients." Alvarez-Nemegyei J, Cobarrubias-Cobos A, Escalante-Triay F, Sosa-Munoz J, Miranda JM, Jara LJ. Bromocriptine in systemic lupus erythematosus: a double-blind, randomized, placebo-controlled study. *Lupus*. 1998;7(6):414-9

[64] Serri O, Chik CL, Ur E, Ezzat S. Diagnosis and management of hyperprolactinemia. *CMAJ*. 2003 Sep 16;169(6):575-81 cmaj.ca/cgi/content/full/169/6/575

[65] "...clinical observations and trials support the use of bromocriptine as a nonstandard primary or adjunctive therapy in the treatment of recalcitrant RA, SLE, Reiter's syndrome, and psoriatic arthritis and associated conditions unresponsive to traditional approaches." McMurray RW. Bromocriptine in rheumatic and autoimmune diseases. *Semin Arthritis Rheum*. 2001 Aug;31(1):21-32

[66] Serri O, Chik CL, Ur E, Ezzat S. Diagnosis and management of hyperprolactinemia. *CMAJ*. 2003 Sep 16;169(6):575-81 cmaj.ca/cgi/content/full/169/6/575

[67] "CONCLUSION: These data indicate that cabergoline is a very effective agent for lowering the prolactin levels in hyperprolactinemic patients and that it appears to offer considerable advantage over bromocriptine in terms of efficacy and tolerability." Sabuncu T, Arikan E, Tasan E, Hatemi H. Comparison of the effects of cabergoline and bromocriptine on prolactin levels in hyperprolactinemic patients. *Intern Med*. 2001 Sep;40(9):857-61

[68] "Cabergoline also normalized PRL in the majority of patients with known bromocriptine intolerance or -resistance. Once PRL secretion was adequately controlled, the dose of cabergoline could often be significantly decreased, which further reduced costs of therapy." Verhelst J, Abs R, Maiter D, van den Bruel A, Vandeweghe M, Velkeniers B, Mockel J, Lambertigts G, Petrossians P, Coremans P, Mahler C, Stevenaert A, Verlooy J, Raftopoulos C, Beckers A. Cabergoline in the treatment of hyperprolactinemia: a study in 455 patients. *J Clin Endocrinol Metab*. 1999 Jul;84(7):2518-22 jcem.endojournals.org/cgi/content/full/84/7/2518

[69] Erb N, et al. Control of unremitting rheumatoid arthritis by the prolactin antagonist cabergoline. *Rheumatology* (Oxford). 2001 Feb;40(2):237-9

[70] Mobini M, et al. The effect of cabergoline on clinical and laboratory findings in active rheumatoid arthritis. *Iran Red Crescent Med J*. 2011 Oct;13(10):749-50

prolactin. The improvement in RA activity may be due to a significant suppression in secretion of prolactin by immune cells without a significant change in prolactin level."

- **Insulin, hyperinsulinemia:** As a marker for insulin resistance and perhaps xenobiotic exposure, fasting serum insulin is a surrogate marker for an inflammatory state. A challenge exists in determining the accurate pro- or anti-inflammatory effect of insulin itself, because the net effect of the hormone *in vivo* is inflammation-lowering via glucose-lowering. Although major medical labs such as LabCorp (website reviewed January 2014) use a reference range of 2.6-24.9 μIU/mL, such a range is clinically ridiculous except for screening for overt pathology and should be replaced with the following:
  - o **Healthy** fasting serum insulin: <5 μIU/mL
  - o **Mild-moderate insulin resistance** fasting serum insulin: 5-15 μIU/mL
  - o **Marked-severe insulin resistance** fasting serum insulin: 15 μIU/mL

  The goal when considering serum insulin within the context of alleviating inflammation is not to lower serum insulin per se, but rather to alleviate the causative insulin resistance. Stated perhaps more plainly, an elevation in fasting serum insulin is indicative of insulin resistance (except in the exceedingly rare case of insulinoma or exogenous insulin administration which can be distinguished by concomitant measurement of C-peptide) which is itself a proinflammatory state; thus, our goal is to reduce fasting serum insulin not because we are targeting insulin per se but rather because we are measuring serum insulin as a marker for insulin resistance and thus a particular type of *metabolic inflammation*. First-line therapy for insulin resistance is carbohydrate restriction via plant-based low-carbohydrate Paleo diet, exercise and physical activity >60 minutes/day, vitamin and mineral supplementation, especially vitamin D3, chromium, magnesium, CoQ-10, and mixed tocopherols.

- **Estrogen:** Nearly all autoimmune disorders are more common in females than males, and occasionally a menstrual exacerbation is noted, suggesting a possible immunodysregulation by estrogen. Despite the complex and multifaceted nature of the endocrine system, we may safely generalize that the estrogens are immunostimulatory and immunodysregulatory while androgens are immunosuppressive and immunoregulatory[71]; thus, elevated estrogen:androgen ratios promote/exacerbate autoimmunity. Furthermore, many chemical/pollutant xenobiotics have

> **Estrogen is pro-inflammatory, and anti-estrogen interventions provide an anti-inflammatory benefit**
>
> "Using **antiestrogen** medication [tamoxifen or **anastrozole**] in women with dermatomyositis may result in a significant improvement in their rash, possibly via the inhibition of TNF-alpha production by immune or other cells."
>
> Sereda and Werth. *Arch Dermatol.* 2006

estrogen-like effects ("xenoestrogens") and are consistently associated with induction or exacerbation of autoimmunity. So-called **"estrogen-replacement therapy" used in postmenopausal women increases the risk for lupus and scleroderma.**[72] **Men with rheumatoid arthritis show an excess of estradiol** and a decrease in DHEA, and the **excess estrogen is proportional to the degree of inflammation.**[73] Estrogen(s) can be measured in serum and/or 24-hour urine samples. Beyond looking at estrogens from a *quantitative* standpoint, they can also be *qualitatively* analyzed with respect to the ratio of estrone:estradiol:estriol as well as the balance between the "good" 2-hydroxyestrone relative to the purportedly carcinogenic and proinflammatory 16-alpha-hydroxyestrone. Interventions to lower estrogen levels can include the following:

  - o <u>Weight loss and weight optimization</u>: Excess adiposity and obesity raise estrogen levels due to high levels of aromatase (the hormone that makes estrogens from androgens) in adipose tissue; weight optimization and loss of excess fat helps normalize hormone levels and reduce inflammation. In overweight patients, *weight loss* is the means to attaining the goal of *weight optimization*; the task is not complete until the body mass index is normalized/optimized.
  - o <u>Avoidance of ethanol</u>: Ethanol stimulates estrogen production, particularly in men.

---

[71] "In general, androgens seem to inhibit immune activity, while oestrogen seems to have a more powerful effect on immune cells and to stimulate immune activity." Tanriverdi F, Silveira LF, MacColl GS, Bouloux PM. The hypothalamic-pituitary-gonadal axis: immune function and autoimmunity. *J Endocrinol.* 2003 Mar;176(3):293-304 joe.endocrinology-journals.org/cgi/content/abstract/176/3/293

[72] "These studies indicate that estrogen replacement therapy in postmenopausal women increases the risk of developing lupus, scleroderma, and Raynaud disease..." Mayes MD. Epidemiologic studies of environmental agents and systemic autoimmune diseases. *Environ Health Perspect.* 1999 Oct;107 Suppl 5:743-8

[73] "RESULTS: DHEAS and estrone concentrations were lower and estradiol was higher in patients compared with healthy controls. DHEAS differed between RF positive and RF negative patients. Estrone did not correlate with any disease variable, whereas estradiol correlated strongly and positively with all measured indices of inflammation." Tengstrand B, Carlstrom K, Fellander-Tsai L, Hafstrom I. Abnormal levels of serum dehydroepiandrosterone, estrone, and estradiol in men with rheumatoid arthritis: high correlation between serum estradiol and current degree of inflammation. *J Rheumatol.* 2003 Nov;30(11):2338-43

o   Surgical correction of varicocele in affected men: Men with varicocele have higher estrogen levels due to temperature-induced alterations in enzyme function in the testes; surgical correction of the varicocele lowers estrogen levels.

o   "Anti-estrogen diet": Foods and supplements such as green tea, diindolylmethane (DIM), indole-3-carbinol (I3C), licorice, and a high-fiber crucifer-based "anti-estrogenic diet" can also be used; monitoring clinical status and serum estradiol will prove or disprove efficacy. Whereas **16-alpha-hydroxyestrone is pro-inflammatory and immunodysregulatory, 2-hydroxyestrone has anti-inflammatory action**[74] and has been described as "the good estrogen"[75] due to its anticancer and comparatively health-preserving qualities. **In a recent short-term study using I3C in patients with SLE, I3C supplementation at 375 mg per day was well tolerated and resulted in modest treatment-dependent clinical improvement as well as favorable modification of estrogen metabolism away from 16-alpha-hydroxyestrone and toward 2-hydroxyestrone.**[76]

o   Pharmacologic aromatase inhibition: In our office, we commonly measure serum estradiol in men and administer the aromatase inhibitor anastrozole/Arimidex 1 mg (≥2-3 doses per week) to men whose estradiol level is greater than 32 picogram/mL. The Life Extension Foundation[77] advocates that the optimal serum estradiol level for a man is 10-30 picogram/mL. Clinical studies using anastrozole/Arimidex in men have shown that aromatase blockade lowers estradiol and raises testosterone[78]; generally speaking, this is exactly the result that we want in patients with severe systemic autoimmunity. Whether using anastrozole/Arimidex, frequency of dosing is based on serum and clinical response. Letrozole/Femara is a newer pharmacologic aromatase inhibitor which appears to have slight superiority over anastrozole in terms of anti-estrogen efficacy; however, I am quite convinced that Letrozole/Femara is also an androgen receptor agonist and therefore I generally avoid this drug like the plague. Relatedly, the botanical *Rhodiola rosea* can elevate testosterone and estradiol, making the latter particularly difficult to control. On occasion, we have seen some men make so much testosterone→estradiol that they require both anastrozole/Arimidex *and* Letrozole/Femara along with licorice daily in order to control their testosterone and estradiol levels. Licorice lowers testosterone and thus the precursor to estradiol in both men and women within about four days of oral administration, whether by standardized capsules or by tea from the root. Of course, anastrozole/Arimidex can be administered to women in 1 mg doses ranging from once per week to 5-7 times per week depending on clinical and serologic response. **In two recent case reports, administration of anti-estrogen medication— either tamoxifen or anastrozole—resulted in clinical improvements in two women with dermatomyositis.**[79]

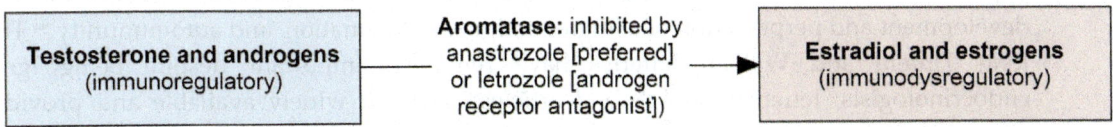

The aromatase enzyme converts androgens to estrogens: If estrogens are high and androgens are low, then estrogens can be lowered and androgens raised via inhibition of aromatase. If androgens are low and estrogens are low, then administration of androgens will raise both the androgens and the estrogens, possibly necessitating coadministration of an aromatase inhibitor.

[74] "Micromolar concentrations of beta-estradiol, estrone, 16-alpha-hydroxyestrone and estriol enhance the oxidative metabolism of activated human PMNL's. The corresponding 2-hydroxylated estrogens 2-OH-estradiol, 2-OH-estrone and 2-OH-estriol act on the contrary as powerful inhibitors of cell activity." Jansson G. Oestrogen-induced enhancement of myeloperoxidase activity in human polymorphonuclear leukocytes--a possible cause of oxidative stress in inflammatory cells. *Free Radic Res Commun.* 1991;14(3):195-208

[75] "Even more dramatically, in the case of laryngeal papillomas induction of 2-hydroxylation with indole-3-carbinol (I3C) has resulted in inhibition of tumor growth during the time that the patients continue to take I3C or vegetables rich in this compound." Bradlow et al. 2-hydroxyestrone: the 'good' estrogen. *J Endocrinol.* 1996 Sep;150 Suppl:S259-65

[76] "Women with SLE can manifest a metabolic response to I3C and might benefit from its antiestrogenic effects." McAlindon TE, Gulin J, Chen T, Klug T, Lahita R, Nuite M. Indole-3-carbinol in women with SLE: effect on estrogen metabolism and disease activity. *Lupus.* 2001;10(11):779-83

[77] Male Hormone Modulation Therapy, Page 4 Of 7: lef.org/protocols/prtcl-130c.shtml Accessed October 30, 2005

[78] "These data demonstrate that aromatase inhibition increases serum bioavailable and total testosterone levels to the youthful normal range in older men with mild hypogonadism." Leder et al. Effects of aromatase inhibition in elderly men with low or borderline-low serum testosterone levels. *J Clin Endocrinol Metab.* 2004 Mar;89:1174-80

[79] "Using antiestrogen medication in women with DM may result in a significant improvement in their rash, possibly via the inhibition of TNF-alpha production by immune or other cells." Sereda D, Werth VP. Improvement in dermatomyositis rash associated with the use of antiestrogen medication. *Arch Dermatol.* 2006 Jan;142(1):70-2

- **Testosterone:** Androgen deficiencies predispose to, are exacerbated by, and contribute to autoimmune/inflammatory disorders. **A large proportion of men with lupus or RA have low testosterone**[80] and suffer the effects of hypogonadism: fatigue, weakness, depression, slow healing, low libido, and difficulties with sexual performance. Particularly in men, blood samples should be drawn for *free* and *total* testosterone (fT and tT, respectively) along with serum estradiol. Since some labs accept ridiculously low levels of testosterone as "within normal limits" clinicians should not necessarily wait until the patient is pathologically hypogonadal before implementing treatment. Clinicians must appreciate the interrelationship of testosterone with estrogen in order to interpret the patient's status appropriately and implement proper treatment. Since testosterone is converted to estradiol by aromatase, a patient with low testosterone and high estradiol is properly treated with aromatase inhibition (e.g., Arimidex/anastrozole) rather than testosterone; administration of Arimidex/anastrozole to men simultaneously lowers estradiol and raises testosterone.[81] Conversely, low testosterone along with low estrogen indicates the appropriateness of testosterone replacement and/or corrective treatment of the cause of the hypogonadism. The need for co-administration of testosterone and Arimidex/anastrozole is not uncommon in order to raise testosterone without leading to an iatrogenic increase in estrogen due to "estrogen shunting" by aromatase. Follow-up testing of testosterone and estradiol 4-8 weeks after the implementation of testosterone replacement is advised to ensure optimal hormone status and that the additional *immunoregulatory* testosterone is not being shunted into *immunodysregulatory* estradiol. For the purpose of gently but effectively modulating/lowering estrogen levels, Arimidex/anastrozole is typically administered as 1 mg administered 1-4 times *per week*; the drug appears to have a wide margin of safety, and doses of 1 mg *per day* (doses up to 10 mg/d have been used) are commonly and appropriately—as one of the safest and most effective treatments against breast cancer—used in women with estrogen-responsive breast cancer. As with any modulation/administration of testosterone and estrogen, follow-up testing of hormones and serum lipids is recommended to ensure the attainment of optimal status and the avoidance of complications, such as suppression of HDL synthesis which would be expected to have adverse cardiovascular consequences. Assessing serum PSA is a prerequisite to testosterone administration in men. **Testosterone therapy improves clinical status and wellbeing in women with rheumatoid arthritis**.[82] Transdermal testosterone creams can be used with dose tailored to serum and clinical response.
- **Cortisol:** In physiologic doses cortisol is immunoregulatory and mildly yet significantly immunosuppressive (*"physiologic immunosuppression"*), while at higher doses *and particularly in its synthetic forms such as prednisone and prednisolone* the hormone becomes immunosuppressive (*"pharmacologic immunosuppression"*) and brings additional adverse effects such as weight gain, truncal obesity, hypertension, glucose intolerance and increased susceptibility to infections—the classic manifestations of hypercortisolemia seen in Cushing's disease.[83] Insufficiencies of cortisol production contribute to the development and perpetuation of allergies, fatigue, inflammation, and autoimmunity.[84] The works of Drs. John Tintera and William Jefferies have remained important despite being ignored by most endocrinologists; Jefferies' books[85] and articles[86] are still widely available and provide concepts and

---

[80] Karagiannis A, Harsoulis F. Gonadal dysfunction in systemic diseases. *Eur J Endocrinol*. 2005 Apr;152(4):501-13 eje-online.org/cgi/content/full/152/4/501

[81] "These data demonstrate that aromatase inhibition increases serum bioavailable and total testosterone levels to the youthful normal range in older men with mild hypogonadism. Serum estradiol levels decrease modestly but remain within the normal male range." Leder BZ, Rohrer JL, Rubin SD, Gallo J, Longcope C. Effects of aromatase inhibition in elderly men with low or borderline-low serum testosterone levels. *J Clin Endocrinol Metab*. 2004 Mar;89(3):1174-80 jcem.endojournals.org/cgi/content/full/89/3/1174

[82] "An improvement in ESR, Dutch health assessment questionnaire, and pain was noted. …Testosterone may improve the general wellbeing of postmenopausal women with active rheumatoid arthritis." Booji A, Biewenga-Booji CM, Huber-Bruning O, Cornelis C, Jacobs JW, Bijlsma JW. Androgens as adjuvant treatment in postmenopausal female patients with rheumatoid arthritis. *Ann Rheum Dis*. 1996 Nov;55(11):811-5

[83] Kirk LF Jr, Hash RB, Katner HP, Jones T. Cushing's disease: clinical manifestations and diagnostic evaluation. *Am Fam Physician*. 2000 Sep 1;62(5):1119-27, 1133-4 aafp.org/afp/20000901/1119.html

[84] "Yet evidence that patients with rheumatoid arthritis improved with small, physiologic dosages of cortisol or cortisone acetate was reported over 25 years ago, and that patients with chronic allergic disorders or unexplained chronic fatigue also improved with administration of such small dosages was reported over 15 years ago…" Jefferies WM. Mild adrenocortical deficiency, chronic allergies, autoimmune disorders and the chronic fatigue syndrome: a continuation of the cortisone story. *Med Hypotheses*. 1994 Mar;42(3):183-9 thebuteykocentre.com/Irish_%20Buteykocenter_files/further_studies/med_hyp2.pdf and members.westnet.com.au/pkolb/med_hyp2.pdf

[85] Jefferies WMcK. Safe Uses of Cortisol. Second Edition. Springfield, CC Thomas, 1996

[86] "Yet evidence that patients with rheumatoid arthritis improved with small, physiologic dosages of cortisol or cortisone acetate was reported over 25 years ago, and that patients with chronic allergic disorders or unexplained chronic fatigue also improved with administration of such small dosages was reported over 15 years ago…" Jefferies WM. Mild adrenocortical deficiency, chronic allergies, autoimmune disorders and the chronic fatigue syndrome: a continuation of the cortisone story. *Med Hypotheses*. 1994 Mar;42(3):183-9 thebuteykocentre.com/Irish_%20Buteykocenter_files/further_studies/med_hyp2.pdf and members.westnet.com.au/pkolb/med_hyp2.pdf

clinically relevant applications. In a 1998 summary by Jefferies[87] on the etiology of rheumatoid arthritis, he reviewed evidence suggesting that subacute hypoadrenalism results in insufficiencies of cortisol and DHEA, both of which are necessary for immunomodulation and immunocompetence; insufficiencies of these hormones leaves the body vulnerable to chronic infections (i.e., multifocal dysbiosis, as detailed previously) and the systemic proinflammatory sequelae that result in so-called "autoimmunity." Differential diagnoses in patients with low adrenal function include congenital adrenal hypoplasia, adrenoleukodystrophy, autoimmune Addison disease, and chronic hypopituarism. A small short-term randomized crossover clinical trial published in *The Lancet* showed benefit of 5-10 mg/day of cortisol in patients with chronic fatigue syndrome.[88] Supplementation with up to 20 mg per day of cortisol/Cortef is physiologic; higher doses in the range of 40 mg per day may benefit patients, especially during times of stress, but are adrenosuppressive. My preference is to dose 10 mg first thing in the morning, then 5 mg in late morning and 5 mg in midafternoon in an attempt to replicate the diurnal variation and normal morning peak of cortisol levels. In patients with hypoadrenalism, administration of pregnenolone in doses of 10-60 mg in the morning may also be beneficial; DHEA supplementation is beneficial for patients with adrenal insufficiency.

Criteria for the diagnosis of adrenal insufficiency in children and adults

- First-morning cortisol less than 8-10 mcg/dL: An 8:00 am serum cortisol concentration less than 8-10 mcg/dL suggests adrenal insufficiency.
- Serum cortisol less than 18 mcg/dL during illness or stress or with elevated ACTH: Serum cortisol concentration less than 18 mcg/dL in a sick and stressed patient, or associated with an elevated ACTH, is highly suggestive of adrenal insufficiency.
- Post-ACTH serum cortisol less than 18 mcg/dL: Serum cortisol less than 18 mcg/dL obtained 30-60 minutes following ACTH injection is diagnostic of adrenal insufficiency.
- Serum cortisol that fails to double within 30-60 minutes after ACTH injection: This test involves three steps: 1) blood sample is taken for serum cortisol, 2) ACTH is injected, 3) blood sample for serum cortisol is taken again at 30-60 minutes. Cortisol production should double following injection of ACTH; this is a demonstration of adrenal reserve and the ability of the adrenal glands to respond to stress.
- Low output of adrenal hormones measured in 24-hour urine samples: This provides sufficient objective data to justify a clinical trial of cortisol replacement in patients with a suggestive clinical picture and lack of contraindications.
- Proper dosing of cosyntropin/ACTH: Injections of "ACTH" are generally performed with the intravenous or intramuscular injection of "Cosyntropin" which is a synthetic peptide fragment of ACTH used for adrenal stimulation. According to the review by Wilson, the **standard dose for adults is 250 mcg**. "For infants, the author suggests 50 mcg of cosyntropin (approximately 250 mg/m2)."

Jefferies WMcK. Safe Uses of Cortisol. Second Edition. Springfield, CC Thomas, 1996 page 39
medicinenet.com/cosyntropin-injectable/article.htm Accessed December 7, 2006
Wilson TA. Adrenal Hypoplasia. *eMedicine* emedicine.com/PED/topic45.htm Accessed November 18, 2005

- **DHEA (insufficiency and supraphysiologic supplementation):** Patients with autoimmunity should be tested for DHEA insufficiency by measurement of serum DHEA-sulfate; insufficiencies should generally be corrected except in cases of concomitant hormone-responsive cancer such as breast cancer or prostate cancer. Physiologic doses are approximately 15-25 mg for women and 25-50 mg for men. However, many patients with autoimmunity will respond favorably to supraphysiologic doses in the range of 200 mg per day. The rationale for using high-dose DHEA in patients with autoimmune diseases is supported by the following:
  1. DHEA is a natural metabolite/hormone of the human body made in the adrenal glands.
  2. Patients with autoimmune diseases are commonly treated with prednisone and other corticosteroids for months or years at a time. Use of prednisone causes adrenal suppression with resultant suppression of DHEA levels.[89]

---

[87] "The etiology of rheumatoid arthritis ...explained by a combination of three factors: (i) a relatively mild deficiency of cortisol, ..., (ii) a deficiency of DHEA, ...and (iii) infection by organisms such as mycoplasma,..." Jefferies WM. The etiology of rheumatoid arthritis. *Med Hypotheses*. 1998 Aug;51(2):111-4

[88] "In some patients with chronic fatigue syndrome, low-dose hydrocortisone reduces fatigue levels in the short term." Cleare AJ, Heap E, Malhi GS, Wessely S, O'Keane V, Miell J. Low-dose hydrocortisone in chronic fatigue syndrome: a randomised crossover trial. *Lancet*. 1999 Feb 6;353(9151):455-8

[89] "Basal serum DHEA and DHEAS concentrations were suppressed to a greater degree than was cortisol during both daily and alternate day prednisone treatments. ...Thus, adrenal androgen secretion was more easily suppressed than was cortisol secretion by this low dose of glucocorticoid, but there was no advantage to alternate day therapy." Rittmaster et al. Effect of daily and alternate day low dose prednisone on serum cortisol and adrenal androgens in hirsute women. *J Clin Endocrinol Metab*. 1988 Aug;67(2):400-3

3. As a consequence of prednisone treatment, many patients lose bone mass and develop osteoporosis. DHEA has been shown to reverse the osteoporosis and loss of bone mass induced by corticosteroid treatment.[90]

4. DHEA shows no acute or subacute toxicity even when used in supraphysiologic doses, even when used in sick patients. For example, in a study of 32 patients with HIV, DHEA doses of 750 mg – 2,250 mg per day were well tolerated and produced no dose-limiting adverse effects.[91] This lack of toxicity compares favorably with any and all so-called "antirheumatic" drugs, nearly all of which show alarming comparable toxicity.

5. DHEA is inexpensive. Even at the relatively high dose of 200 mg per day, the cost is less than $40 per month.

6. When used at doses of 200 mg per day, DHEA safely provides clinical benefit for patients with various autoimmune diseases, including ulcerative colitis, Crohn's disease[92], and SLE.[93]

7. 200 mg per day of DHEA allows SLE patients to reduce their dose of prednisone (thus avoiding its adverse effects) while achieving symptomatic improvement. In other words, it allows for improved health and reduced medication use and therefore fewer side effects.[94]

Thus, based on these financial, safety, and effectiveness considerations, the administration of DHEA is reasonable for patients with moderate or severe autoimmune disease. Furthermore, since optimal clinical response appears to correlate with serum levels that are supraphysiologic[95], treatment may be implemented with little regard for initial DHEA levels, particularly when 1) the dose of DHEA is kept as low as possible, 2) duration is kept as short as possible, 3) other interventions are used to address the underlying cause of the disease, 4) the patient is deriving benefit and the risk-to-benefit ratio is favorable.

- **Thyroid (insufficiency or autoimmunity):** Hypothyroidism is a common concomitant to many of the autoimmune diseases. Overt or imminent hypothyroidism is suggested by TSH greater than 2 mU/L[96] or 3 mU/L[97], low T4 or T3, and/or the presence of anti-thyroid peroxidase antibodies.[98] Specific treatment considerations include the following:
  - Selenium: Supplementation with either selenomethonine[99] or sodium selenite[100,101] can reduce thyroid autoimmunity and improve peripheral conversion of T4 to T3. Selenium may be started at 500-800 mcg per day (for 1-3 months) and tapered to 200-400 mcg per day for maintenance.[102]
  - L-thyroxine/levothyroxine/Synthroid—prescription synthetic T4: 25-50 mcg per day is a common starting dose which can be adjusted based on clinical and laboratory response. Thyroid hormone supplements must be consumed separately from soy products (by at least 1-2 hours) and preferably

[90] "CONCLUSION: Prasterone treatment prevented BMD loss and significantly increased BMD at both the lumbar spine and total hip in female patients with SLE receiving exogenous glucocorticoids." Mease PJ, Ginzler EM, Gluck OS, Schiff M, Goldman A, Greenwald M, Cohen S, Egan R, Quarles BJ, Schwartz KE. Effects of prasterone on bone mineral density in women with systemic lupus erythematosus receiving chronic glucocorticoid therapy. *J Rheumatol.* 2005 Apr;32(4):616-21

[91] "Thirty-one subjects were evaluated and monitored for safety and tolerance. The oral drug was administered three times daily in doses ranging from 750 mg/day to 2,250 mg/day for 16 weeks. ... The drug was well tolerated and no dose-limiting side effects were noted." Dyner TS, Lang W, Geaga J, et al. An open-label dose-escalation trial of oral dehydroepiandrosterone tolerance and pharmacokinetics in patients with HIV disease. *J Acquir Immune Defic Syndr.* 1993 May;6(5):459-65

[92] "CONCLUSIONS: In a pilot study, dehydroepiandrosterone was effective and safe in patients with refractory Crohn's disease or ulcerative colitis." Andus T, et al. Patients with refractory Crohn's disease or ulcerative colitis respond to dehydroepiandrosterone: a pilot study. *Aliment Pharmacol Ther.* 2003 Feb;17(3):409-14

[93] "CONCLUSION: The overall results confirm that DHEA treatment was well-tolerated, significantly reduced the number of SLE flares, and improved patient's global assessment of disease activity." Chang DM, Lan JL, Lin HY, Luo SF. Dehydroepiandrosterone treatment of women with mild-to-moderate systemic lupus erythematosus: a multicenter randomized, double-blind, placebo-controlled trial. *Arthritis Rheum.* 2002 Nov;46(11):2924-9

[94] "CONCLUSION: Among women with lupus disease activity, reducing the dosage of prednisone to < or = 7.5 mg/day for a sustained period of time while maintaining stabilization or a reduction of disease activity was possible in a significantly greater proportion of patients treated with oral prasterone, 200 mg once daily, compared with patients treated with placebo." Petri MA, Lahita RG, Van Vollenhoven RF, et al and GL601 Study Group. Effects of prasterone on corticosteroid requirements of women with systemic lupus erythematosus: a double-blind, randomized, placebo-controlled trial. *Arthritis Rheum.* 2002 Jul;46(7):1820-9

[95] "CONCLUSION: The clinical response to DHEA was not clearly dose dependent. Serum levels of DHEA and DHEAS correlated only weakly with lupus outcomes, but suggested an optimum serum DHEAS of 1000 microg/dl." Barry NN, McGuire JL, van Vollenhoven RF. Dehydroepiandrosterone in systemic lupus erythematosus: relationship between dosage, serum levels, and clinical response. *J Rheumatol.* 1998 Dec;25(12):2352-6

[96] Weetman AP. Hypothyroidism: screening and subclinical disease. *BMJ.* 1997 Apr 19;314(7088):1175-8 bmj.bmjjournals.com/cgi/content/full/314/7088/1175

[97] "Now AACE encourages doctors to consider treatment for patients who test outside the boundaries of a narrower margin based on a target TSH level of 0.3 to 3.0. AACE believes the new range will result in proper diagnosis for millions of Americans who suffer from a mild thyroid disorder, but have gone untreated until now." American Association of Clinical Endocrinologists (AACE). 2003 Campaign Encourages Awareness of Mild Thyroid Failure, Importance of Routine Testing aace.com/pub/tam2003/press.php November 26, 2005

[98] Beers MH, Berkow R (eds). *Merck Manual. 17th Edition.* Whitehouse Station; Merck Research Laboratories 1999 Page 96

[99] Duntas et al. Effects of a six month treatment with selenomethionine in patients with autoimmune thyroiditis. *Eur J Endocrinol.* 2003 Apr;148(4):389-93

[100] Gartner R, Gasnier BC, Dietrich JW, Krebs B, Angstwurm MW. Selenium supplementation in patients with autoimmune thyroiditis decreases thyroid peroxidase antibodies concentrations. *J Clin Endocrinol Metab.* 2002 Apr;87(4):1687-91 jcem.endojournals.org/cgi/content/full/87/4/1687

[101] "We recently conducted a prospective, placebo-controlled clinical study, where we could demonstrate, that a substitution of 200 wg sodium selenite for three months in patients with autoimmune thyroiditis reduced thyroid peroxidase antibody (TPO-Ab) concentrations significantly." Gartner R, Gasnier BC. Selenium in the treatment of autoimmune thyroiditis. *Biofactors.* 2003;19(3-4):165-70

[102] Bruns F, Micke O, Bremer M. Current status of selenium and other treatments for secondary lymphedema. *J Support Oncol.* 2003 Jul-Aug;1(2):121-30 supportiveoncology.net/journal/articles/0102121.pdf

on an empty stomach to avoid absorption interference by food, fiber, and minerals, especially calcium. Doses are generally started at one-half of the daily dose for the first 10 days after which the full dose is used. Caution must be applied in patients with adrenal insufficiency and/or those with cardiovascular disease.

- o Liothyronine, Cytomel®: Cytomel is prescription synthetic T3. Except in patients with myxedema for whom the appropriate starting dose is 5 mcg per day, treatment generally starts with 25 mcg per day and can be increased to 75 mcg per day; dose is adjusted based on clinical and laboratory response. As stated previously, thyroid hormone supplements must be consumed separately from soy products (by at least 1-2 hours) and preferably on an empty stomach to avoid absorption interference by food, fiber, and minerals, especially calcium. Time-released T3 can be obtained from a compounding pharmacy.

- o Armour thyroid—prescription natural T4 and T3 from cow/pig thyroid gland: 60 mg (one grain) is a common starting and maintenance dose. Since administration of Armour thyroid frequently increases serum levels of anti-thyroid antibodies in patients with preexisting thyroid autoimmunity, **many doctors choose to not use Armour thyroid in patients with thyroid autoimmunity**. Some patients prefer to divide their daily dose to maintain constant serum levels of T3.

- o Thyrolar/Liotrix—prescription synthetic T4 with T3: Dosed incrementally as "1", "2", or "3." This product has been difficult to obtain for the past few years due to manufacturing problems (thyrolar.com/); previously it was my treatment of choice due to the combination of T4 and T3 and the lack of antigenicity compared to gland-derived products.

- o Thyroid glandular—nonprescription T3: Producers of nutritional products are able to distribute T3 because it is not listed by the FDA as a prescription item. Nutritional supplement companies may start with Armour thyroid, remove the T4, and sell the thyroid glandular with active T3 thereby providing a nonprescription source of active thyroid hormone. For many patients, one tablet per day is at least as effective as a prescription source of thyroid hormone. Since it is derived from a glandular and therefore potentially antigenic source, thyroid glandular is not used in patients with thyroid autoimmunity due to its ability to induce increased production of anti-thyroid antibodies.

- o L-tyrosine and iodine: Some patients with mild hypothyroidism respond to supplementation with L-tyrosine and iodine. Tyrosine is commonly used in doses of 4-9 grams per day in divided doses. According to Abraham and Wright[103], doses of iodine may be as high as 12.5 milligrams (12,500 micrograms), which is slightly less than the average daily intake in Japan at 13.8 mg per day.

- **Pregnenolone:** Several reviews and clinical trials from the early 1950s showed moderate clinical effectiveness and absence of adverse effects from oral administration of pregnenolone in doses as high as 500-1,000 mg/d in patients with rheumatoid arthritis and other rheumatic conditions.[104,105,106,107] Following oral administration of pregnenolone in doses of approximately 500 mg/d, beneficial results are noted in approximately 50-80% of patients. Responders will show reduced pain, swelling, and objective reductions in inflammation measured by ESR and will have increased strength and mobility. No important adverse effects have been reported, particularly with regard to pulse rate, blood pressure, or glucose homeostasis. In contrast to the adverse withdrawal effects noted with prednisone/prednisolone, discontinuance of pregnenolone does not immediately result in exacerbation of inflammation and has never been reported to incite adrenal insufficiency. Oral administration of pregnenolone produces better clinical response than does intramuscular administration, apparently due to the relative insolubility of parenteral pregnenolone. The low cost and absence of adverse effects makes pregnenolone a reasonable therapeutic intervention in patients with rheumatic disease because the treatment may provide benefit and/or mitigate the need for treatments with greater toxicity and cost. However, this treatment should not be relied upon as

---

[103] Wright JV. Why you need 83 times more of this essential, cancer-fighting nutrient than the "experts" say you do. *Nutrition and Healing* 2005; volume 12, issue 4.
[104] Freeman H, Pincus G, Johnson CW, et al. Therapeutic efficacy of delta-5-pregnenolone in rheumatoid arthritis. *J American Medical Association* 1950; April 15: 1124-8
[105] Stock JP, McClure EC. Pregnenolone in the treatment of rheumatoid arthritis. *Lancet* 1950 Jul 22;2(4):125-8
[106] Dordick JR, Ehrlich ME, Alexander S, Kissin M. Pregnenolone in rheumatoid arthritis. *N Engl J Med*. 1951 Mar 1;244(9):324-6
[107] Freeman H, Pincus G, Bachrach S, et al. Oral steroid medication in rheumatoid arthritis. *J Clin Endocrinol Metab*. 1950 Dec;10(12):1523-32

monotherapy and/or in patients with important inflammatory complications such as iritis, scleritis, or temporal arteritis. In contrast to the much higher doses of 500-1,000 mg/d reported in the studies cited above in this paragraph, I generally limit pregnenolone doses to 10-50 mg/d taken in the morning in patients who may derive benefit; some patients—generally those with hypoadrenalism—notice a marked improvement in energy (to the point of causing insomnia) with doses as low as 5-10 mg/d.

DrV's Summary and Practical Guide to Orthoendocrinology: Read preceding discussions

Assessments	Interventions and Notes
Serum prolactin	• Reduce elevations or treat empirically regardless of serum prolactin level; cabergoline 0.25-0.5 mg twice weekly; also consider using pyridoxine 250-500 mg/d, *Vitex* to effect. • Many studies have now demonstrated that empiric cabergoline is a reasonable, safe, and effective treatment for the more severe inflammatory disorders; cabergoline produces is anti-inflammatory benefit via blocking prolactin signaling within the immune system and not by primarily affecting pituitary output of prolactin.
Serum fasting insulin as a marker of insulin resistance and metabolic inflammation	• Improve insulin sensitivity by reducing carbohydrate intake and improving insulin secretion and reception. Insulin resistance most commonly results from 1) systemic inflammation, 2) xenobiotic down-regulation of GLUT receptors via the aryl-hydrocarbon receptor, 3) micronutrient deficiencies, 4) cortisol excess, 5) physiologic and protective insulin resistance secondary to ceramide accumulation as a result of cellular carbohydrate overload.
Serum estradiol	• Reduce serum estradiol with adipose loss, alcohol and caffeine avoidance, treatment for obesity, surgical correction of varicocele in men, anastrozole 1mg 2-3 times weekly is effective and safe in most cases, especially for men • Consider monitoring osteoporosis risk in cases of prolonged hypoestrogenemia, which should generally be avoided.
Serum DHEA sulfate	• Physiologic doses are 15 mg/d for women and 25 mg/d for men; supraphysiologic dosing up to 200mg/d is effective, safe, and well-represented in the rheumatology literature for the treatment of RA, SLE, and IBD.
Serum cortisol, preferably before and after ACTH	• See interpretive guide provided previously. • Physiologic doses of ≤ 10-20 mg/d orally administered cortisol can be used empirically under appropriate supervision, with the first dose of 10mg administered upon waking in the morning and optional additional doses of 5 mg each administered in the late morning and early afternoon to mimic physiologic secretion.
Serum free and total testosterone	• If total testosterone is low, evaluate for primary or secondary hypogonadism. • If testosterone is low and estrogen is low, consider transdermal testosterone therapy. • If free testosterone is low and total testosterone is normal, likely due to elevated SHBG, generally due to excess estrogen or excess prolactin. • If testosterone is low and estrogen is high, then use aromatase inhibition and/or correct the hypogonadism resulting from obesity/inflammation. • Always assess free and total testosterone in conjunction with serum estradiol.

Always use the lowest dose of hormonal intervention necessary to achieve the desired result based on dual consideration of laboratory results and the patient's response to treatment; lower doses of each intervention can be used when more interventions (e.g., nutritional, mitochondrial, antidysbiotic) are used.

❼ Xenobiotic Immunotoxicity:
Exposure, Accumulation, Detoxification

Major Concepts in this Section
Exposure to "foreign substances" such as toxic chemicals and toxic metals is inescapable in our polluted world and modern lives; exposure invariably results in some level of accumulation. Accumulation of toxic metals and chemicals produces additive and synergistic toxic effects on the entire organism, notably via endocrine disruption, immune imbalance and suppression, oxidative stress, immunogenic modification of endogenous antigens via xenobiotic haptenization, and mitochondrial dysfunction, which then leads to systemic inflammation, reduced cell/tissue performance, and additional oxidative stress. Despite these facts and the obvious clinical implications, most doctorate-level physicians—except for naturopathic clinicians—receive no training in these topics and the clinical remediation via therapeutic detoxification. Thus, the naturopathic profession stands clearly preeminent in its profession-wide training in the appreciation, assessment and treatment of xenobiotic-induced illness.

Xenobiotic Immunotoxicity and Treatment by Therapeutic Detoxification: Ultracondensed Clinical Review

Chemicals such as pesticides, synthetic fertilizers, herbicides, fungicides, industrial pollution, car exhaust, solvents, and innumerable others are bioaccumulative and can alter immune function. The classic manifestation of xenobiotic immunotoxicity is the combination of reduced resistance to infections and increased allergic and autoimmune disorders. The subject of environmental medicine and detoxification is much too broad and complex to review completely in this textbook, and while naturopathic physicians are trained in these topics, other healthcare professionals are not unless they attend post-graduate training and take the time to read articles and textbooks on these topics. Readers for whom these topics are new are encouraged to access the following citations for additional information.[108,109,110,111,112] What follows here will be an ultracondensed clinical review focusing on major concepts and problem-specific solutions.

For the sake of simplicity and with recognition of the various nuances of different xenobiotics, I generalize toxicity into two categories, either *chemicals* or *heavy metals*. Most patients have an overlay of these two problems, so that the clinical manifestations and treatments have several commonalities.

- Chemical toxicity: Accumulation of xenobiotics can cause immune dysfunction and can contribute to the development of "autoimmunity." Examples of xenobiotic-induced autoimmunity include 1) the increased autoimmunity seen in farmers exposed to pesticides[113], 2) the scleroderma-like disease that results from exposure to vinyl chloride[114], 3) the association of mercury and pesticide exposure with lupus[115], and 4) the well-recognized connection between drug and chemical exposure and various autoimmune syndromes such as drug-induced lupus.[116] More than 40 pharmaceutical drugs are known to cause drug-induced lupus.[117] Every one of us is exposed to toxic chemicals every day, and every one of us has chemical

---

[108] "Caffeine enemas cause dilation of bile ducts, which facilitates excretion of toxic cancer breakdown products by the liver and dialysis of toxic products from blood across the colonic wall. The therapy must be used as an integrated whole." Gerson M. The cure of advanced cancer by diet therapy: a summary of 30 years of clinical experimentation. *Physiol Chem Phys.* 1978;10(5):449-64

[109] "The writer has observed numerous cases suffering from such conditions as chronic arthritis, hypertension, coronary disease, chronic abdominal distention, constipation, and colitis, in which the element of constipation, auto-intoxication and possible colon infection seemed to play a prominent part, which responded very satisfactorily to colonic irrigations after failure to improve following the usual forms of medical treatment." Snyder RG. The value of colonic irrigations in countering auto-intoxication of intestinal origin. *Medical Clinics of North America* 1939; May: 781-788

[110] Gonzalez et al. Evaluation of pancreatic proteolytic enzyme treatment of adenocarcinoma of pancreas, with nutrition and detoxification support. *Nutr Cancer* 1999;33:117-24

[111] Crinnion WJ. Results of a decade of naturopathic treatment for environmental illness: a review of clinical records. *J Naturopathic Med* 1997;7:21-27

[112] Sherman JD. *Chemical exposure and disease. Diagnostic and investigative techniques.* Princeton Scientific Publishing; 1994

[113] "IgG levels decreased with increasing p,p'-DDE levels, with a statistically significant decrease of approximately 50% in the highest two categories of exposure. Sixteen (12%) were positive for antinuclear antibodies... These analyses provide evidence that p,p'-DDE modulates immune responses in humans." Cooper GS, et al. Associations between plasma DDE levels and immunologic measures in African-American farmers in North Carolina. *Environ Health Perspect.* 2004 Jul;112(10):1080-4

[114] "Vinyl chloride (VC) monomer can induce a scleroderma-like syndrome in a proportion of workers exposed to it during production of polyvinyl chloride." Black CM, Welsh KI, Walker AE, et al. Genetic susceptibility to scleroderma-like syndrome induced by vinyl chloride. *Lancet.* 1983 Jan 1;1(8314-5):53-5

[115] "...reported occupational exposure to mercury (OR 3.6), mixing pesticides for agricultural work (OR 7.4), and among dental workers (OR 7.1). ...these associations were fairly strong and statistically significant..." Cooper GS, et al. Occupational risk factors for development of systemic lupus erythematosus. *J Rheumatol.* 2004 Oct;31:1928-33

[116] Hess EV. Environmental chemicals and autoimmune disease: cause and effect. *Toxicology.* 2002 Dec 27;181-182:65-70

[117] "Drug-induced lupus has been reported as a side-effect of long-term therapy with over 40 medications... Several mechanisms for induction of autoimmunity will be discussed, including bystander activation of autoreactive lymphocytes due to drug-specific immunity or to non-specific activation of lymphocytes, direct cytotoxicity with release of autoantigens ..." Rubin RL. Drug-induced lupus. *Toxicology.* 2005;209(2):135-47

accumulation and the potential for xenobiotic-induced disease. Except for denial (shown to be clinically ineffective), we cannot escape from the chemical consequences of living in a world with tens of thousands of synthetic chemicals. According to limited analyses, the average American has accumulated at least 18 different chemicals[118], and analyses that are more detailed show that even more chemicals and metals have been accumulated.[119] Common sources of these chemicals include pesticides, synthetic fertilizers, herbicides, fungicides, industrial pollution, car exhaust, solvents, paints, perfumes, plastic food/drink containers, non-stick cookware, Styrofoam, trichloroethylene from dry cleaning, rubber, carpet, plastics, glues, propellants, petroleum fuels such as gasoline, detergents, and other "cleaners." Clinical consequences of chemical toxicity are diverse, can affect nearly every organ system, and may be predicted to some extent by the pattern of chemical exposure since some chemicals have characteristic sequelae. Most chemicals, especially those which are fat-soluble, can readily enter the body via respiratory, gastrointestinal, and transdermal routes. Once in the bloodstream, chemicals are either detoxified (inactivated and/or solubilized) by the liver and then excreted via urine or bile, or to a lesser extent exhaled from the lungs or excreted via sweat. Chemicals which are not excreted from the body are stored in the tissues, particularly lipid-rich organs such as the liver, adipose, and brain. Molecular turnover and recycling (particularly lipolysis) liberates fat-stored xenobiotics for another opportunity for either detoxification or additional toxicity. The main route for detoxification is the liver, which hydrosolubilizes xenobiotics via oxidation ("phase one") and conjugation ("phase two"). Generally speaking, oxidation reactions are dependent on the cytochrome P-450 system, which can be inhibited by various drugs (e.g., ketoconazole, erythromycin, ritonavir, cimetidine, omeprazole, ethanol), foods such as ethanol and grapefruit juice, bacterial endotoxin from bacterial overgrowth of the intestines, and/or by genetic defects known as single nucleotide polymorphisms ("SNiPs") which reduce xenobiotic clearance. Similarly, conjugation reactions can be inhibited by a low-vegetable diet, SNiPs, and insufficiencies of conjugation moieties such as glutathione, glycine, glutamine, taurine, ornithine, sulfur, and methyl groups. If oxidation is too slow, then xenobiotics are insufficiently detoxicated and insufficiently processed for conjugation, leading to xenobiotic accumulation. If oxidation is too fast relative to conjugation, then reactive intermediates are formed which are commonly more toxic than the original xenobiotic, and insufficient conjugation results in accumulation of reactive xenobiotics which are inherently prone to tissue haptenization (which can incite autoimmunity) and DNA intercalation (which promotes damage to DNA and the resultant mutation and oncogenesis). Optimally oxidized and conjugated xenobiotics are excreted in the urine (smaller molecules with molecular weight less than 400-600) or expelled in the bile (larger molecules with molecular weight greater than 400-600). Supranormal hydration and urinary alkalinization enhance renal clearance of weakly acidic xenobiotics and drugs, whereas dehydration and urinary acidity impair toxin excretion, generally speaking. Conjugated toxins expelled in the bile can be deconjugated by bacteria so that the toxin is reabsorbed, a phenomenon commonly referred to as "enterohepatic recycling"[120] or "enterohepatic recirculation."[121] Such recirculation is obviously less likely if gastrointestinal status and diet have been optimized to minimize the presence of deconjugating bacteria and to maximize fiber intake and laxation for the adsorption and expulsion of intraluminal toxins. Therapeutic colonics and enemas can be employed to stimulate bile flow from the liver[122,123] and to remove bile-secreted toxins from the gut before deconjugation and re-absorption occur. Bile formation and expulsion are further stimulated by botanical

[118] Kristin S. Schafer, Margaret Reeves, Skip Spitzer, Susan E. Kegley. Chemical Trespass: Pesticides in Our Bodies and Corporate Accountability. Pesticide Action Network North America. May 2004 panna.org/campaigns/docsTrespass/chemicalTrespass2004.dv.html

[119] Body Burden: The Pollution in People. ewg.org/issues/siteindex/issues.php?issueid=5004

[120] "Enterohepatic recycling occurs by biliary excretion and intestinal reabsorption of a solute, sometimes with hepatic conjugation and intestinal deconjugation. ... Of particular importance is the potential amplifying effect of enterohepatic variability in defining differences in the bioavailability, apparent volume of distribution and clearance of a given compound." Roberts MS, et al. Enterohepatic circulation: physiological, pharmacokinetic and clinical implications. *Clin Pharmacokinet.* 2002;41(10):751-90

[121] Liska DJ. The detoxification enzyme systems. *Altern Med Rev.* 1998 Jun;3(3):187-98

[122] Garbat, AL, Jacobi, HG: Secretion of Bile in Response to Rectal Installations. *Arch Intern Med* 1929; 44: 455-462

[123] "Caffeine enemas cause dilation of bile ducts, which facilitates excretion of toxic cancer breakdown products by the liver and dialysis of toxic products from blood across the colonic wall. The therapy must be used as an integrated whole." Gerson M. The cure of advanced cancer by diet therapy: a summary of 30 years of clinical experimentation. *Physiol Chem Phys.* 1978;10(5):449-64

medicines such as beets, ginger[124], curcumin/turmeric[125], *Picrorhiza*[126], milk thistle[127], *Andrographis paniculata*[128] and *Boerhaavia diffusa*.[129] Respiratory exhalation of toxins is enhanced by deep breathing and exercise, and hyperventilation promotes respiratory alkalosis which elevates urine pH and promotes excretion of weakly acidic drugs and xenobiotics as previously mentioned. Dermal excretion of toxins via sweat and expedited lipolysis are stimulated via low-temperature saunas and regular aerobic exercise. Xenobiotic oxidation can be promoted (cautiously) by reducing endotoxins from the gut and by the use of botanicals such as *Hypericum perforatum* which induce several isoforms of cytochrome P-450 via activation of the pregane X receptor. Xenobiotic conjugation is likewise promoted via nutrigenomic induction stimulated by cruciferous vegetables and their derivatives such as indole-3-carbinol (I3C) and dimethylindolylemethane (DIM). The plant-based diet is employed to provide fiber for bowel cleansing and the urinary alkalinization that is necessary for optimal urinary excretion of toxins, the majority of which are weak acids and are thus excreted more efficiently in alkaline urine. Sodium bicarbonate can also be used to induce urinary alkalinization. The diet must contain high-quality protein and can be supplemented with amino acids to support amino acid and glutathione conjugation. Serum, urine, and adipose samples can be analyzed to determine the intensity and diversity of chemical accumulation; I tend reserve such testing for patients who have been exposed to a specific chemical, particularly in occupational settings. For most patients, their chemical accumulation is so diverse that they may not display abnormally high levels of a specific chemical; their clinical manifestations are rather a manifestation of a wide plethora of different chemicals, which individually may be only modestly increased. Detoxification genotype can be determined by genomic testing for SNPs in oxidation and conjugation enzymes. Phenotype can be assessed by serum and urine measurements of post-challenge detoxification of benzoate, caffeine, acetylsalicylic acid, and acetaminophen. Amino acid status can be quantified and qualified via serum or urine amino acid analysis. Stool testing assesses digestion, absorption, and microflora status. Clinical implementation follows a screening physical examination and basic laboratory assessment (minimally including CBC, metabolic panel, and urinalysis). Stool testing is always reasonable when working with patients with fatigue and/or autoimmunity; however, this and the other detoxification-related tests can often be deferred and/or used selectively. The Paleo-Mediterranean diet provides ample high-quality protein, alkalinization, fiber, and phytonutrients to which may be added supplements of protein, amino acids (especially NAC, glycine, and glutamine), and vitamins and minerals. Antioxidant teas and fresh fruit and vegetable juices are consumed to increase frequency of urination and promote urinary alkalinization, due primarily to the content of potassium citrate. Exercise and low-temperature saunas promote sweating and xenobiotic-mobilizing lipolysis. Colonics and enemas cleanse the bowel and stimulate bile flow.[130,131] Bile flow is further stimulated by consumption of beets, ginger, curcumin/turmeric, *Picrorhiza*, milk thistle, *Andrographis paniculata* and *Boerhaavia diffusa*. These interventions work in concert to enhance xenobiotic depuration ("The act or process of depurating or freeing from foreign or impure matter "[132]) and cleanse the tissues of accumulated toxins. Intervention can be acute or periodic, but must be maintained for the long-term in order to resist the re-accumulation that is destined to result from the chemical onslaught that is inescapable in our polluted world.

---

[124] "Further analyses for the active constituents of the acetone extracts through column chromatography indicated that [6]-gingerol and [10]-gingerol, which are the pungent principles, are mainly responsible for the cholagogic effect of ginger." Yamahara et al. Cholagogic effect of ginger and its active constituents. *J Ethnopharmacol.* 1985;13:217-25

[125] "On the basis of the present findings, it appears that curcumin induces contraction of the human gall-bladder." Rasyid A, Lelo A. The effect of curcumin and placebo on human gall-bladder function: an ultrasound study. *Aliment Pharmacol Ther.* 1999 Feb;13(2):245-9

[126] "Significant anticholestatic activity was also observed against carbon tetrachloride induced cholestasis in conscious rat, anaesthetized guinea pig and cat. Picroliv was more active than the known hepatoprotective drug silymarin." Saraswat B, Visen PK, Patnaik GK, Dhawan BN. Anticholestatic effect of picroliv, active hepatoprotective principle of Picrorhiza kurrooa, against carbon tetrachloride induced cholestasis. *Indian J Exp Biol.* 1993 Apr;31(4):316-8

[127] "We conclude that SIL counteracts TLC-induced cholestasis by preventing the impairment in both the BS-dependent and -independent fractions of the bile flow." Crocenzi FA, et al. Preventive effect of silymarin against taurolithocholate-induced cholestasis in the rat. *Biochem Pharmacol.* 2003 Jul 15;66(2):355-64

[128] "Andrographolide from the herb Andrographis paniculata (whole plant) per se produces a significant dose (1.5-12 mg/kg) dependent choleretic effect (4.8-73%) as evidenced by increase in bile flow, bile salt, and bile acids in conscious rats and anaesthetized guinea pigs." Shukla B, Visen PK, Patnaik GK, Dhawan BN. Choleretic effect of andrographolide in rats and guinea pigs. *Planta Med.* 1992 Apr;58(2):146-9

[129] "The extract also produced an increase in normal bile flow in rats suggesting a strong choleretic activity." Chandan BK, Sharma AK, Anand KK. Boerhaavia diffusa: a study of its hepatoprotective activity. *J Ethnopharmacol.* 1991 Mar;31(3):299-307

[130] Garbat, AL, Jacobi, HG: Secretion of Bile in Response to Rectal Installations. *Arch Intern Med* 1929; 44: 455-462

[131] "Caffeine enemas cause dilation of bile ducts, which facilitates excretion of toxic cancer breakdown products by the liver and dialysis of toxic products from blood across the colonic wall. The therapy must be used as an integrated whole." Gerson M. The cure of advanced cancer by diet therapy. *Physiol Chem Phys.* 1978;10(5):449-64

[132] "The act or process of depurating or freeing from foreign or impure matter." thefreedictionary.com/Depuration Verified March 11, 2007

- <u>Heavy metal toxicity</u>: In contrast to chemical toxicity for which a generalized non-specific cleansing protocol is appropriate, toxic metals more commonly require specific interventions; treatment is determined by the identity of the metal. Metals which are considered toxic or which are linked to the induction of human diseases include aluminum, arsenic, cadmium, lead, and mercury. Other metals and minerals such as manganese, lithium, copper, and iron can be toxic when present in high amounts. In this section I will limit the discussion to mercury since this metal is 1) commonly elevated in chronically toxic patients, and 2) because this metal can contribute to autoimmunity.

  - <u>Mercury</u>: Chronic mercury toxicity is commonly discovered in clinical practice in patients with chronic unwellness, and a recent study published in *JAMA* showed that 8% of American women of childbearing age have sufficient levels of mercury in their bodies to produce neurologic damage in their children.[133] Accumulating evidence implicates mercury in the induction of immune dysfunction and the exacerbation of autoimmunity and allergy, and clinical trials indicate the benefit of mercury removal.

    - Mercury induces autoimmunity, immune complex formation and deposition, and the formation of antinuclear antibodies and antinucleolar antibodies in animal experiments.[134,135,136]

    - In a case-control study of 265 recently diagnosed lupus patients, occupational exposure to mercury increased the risk of developing lupus by 360%, while working in a dental office increased the risk by 710%.[137]

    - Patients with eczema have an increase body burden of mercury[138], suggesting the probability that mercury accumulation induces immune dysfunction and contributes to the clinical picture of immune-induced skin inflammation, to which is affixed the label of "eczema."

    - Leukocytes from autistic patients produce autoantigens when exposed to ethyl mercury (Thimerosal), thus clearly implicating mercury in the incitement and perpetuation of autoimmunity.[139]

    - A slight increase in risk for multiple sclerosis was noted among patients with many long-term mercury amalgam fillings.[140]

    - It is highly probable that chronic mercury exposure, whether from diet or dental amalgams, alters gastrointestinal flora in favor of dysbiosis in general and antibiotic resistance in particular.[141] Thus, mercury may indirectly contribute to autoimmunity by

---

[133] "However, approximately 8% of women had concentrations higher than the US Environmental Protection Agency's recommended reference dose (5.8 microg/L), below which exposures are considered to be without adverse effects. Women who are pregnant or who intend to become pregnant should follow federal and state advisories on consumption of fish." Schober SE, et al. Blood mercury levels in US children and women of childbearing age, 1999-2000. *JAMA*. 2003 Apr 2;289(13):1667-74

[134] "It is well established that in susceptible mouse strains, chronic treatment with subtoxic doses of mercuric chloride (HgCl2) induces a systemic autoimmune disease, which is characterized by increased serum levels of IgG1 and IgE antibodies, by the production of anti-nucleolar antibodies and by the development of immune complex-mediated glomerulonephritis." al-Balaghi S, Moller E, Moller G, Abedi-Valugerdi M. Mercury induces polyclonal B cell activation, autoantibody production and renal immune complex deposits in young (NZB x NZW)F1 hybrids. *Eur J Immunol*. 1996 Jul;26(7):1519-26

[135] "It is well demonstrated that mercury induces a systemic autoimmune disease in susceptible mouse strains... The dominant antibody in the kidney eluate of mercury-injected mice was of IgG1 isotype and found to be directed against double-stranded DNA, collagen, cardiolipin, phosphatidylethanolamine, and the hapten trinitrophenol, but not against nucleolar antigens." Abedi-Valugerdi M, Hu H, Moller G. Mercury-induced renal immune complex deposits in young (NZB x NZW)F1 mice: characterization of antibodies/autoantibodies. *Clin Exp Immunol*. 1997 Oct;110(1):86-91

[136] Abedi-Valugerdi et al. Mercury-induced anti-nucleolar autoantibodies can transgress the membrane of living cells in vivo and in vitro. *Int Immunol*. 1999 Apr;11(4):605-15

[137] "...reported occupational exposure to mercury (OR 3.6), mixing pesticides for agricultural work (OR 7.4), and among dental workers (OR 7.1, 95% CI 2.2, 23.4). ...these associations were fairly strong and statistically significant..." Cooper GS, Parks CG, Treadwell EL, St Clair EW, Gilkeson GS, Dooley MA. Occupational risk factors for the development of systemic lupus erythematosus. *J Rheumatol*. 2004 Oct;31(10):1928-33

[138] Weidinger et al. Body burden of mercury is associated with acute atopic eczema and total IgE in children from southern Germany. *J Allergy Clin Immunol* 2004;114:457-9

[139] Vojdani A, Pangborn JB, Vojdani E, Cooper EL. Infections, toxic chemicals and dietary peptides binding to lymphocyte receptors and tissue enzymes are major instigators of autoimmunity in autism. *Int J Immunopathol Pharmacol*. 2003 Sep-Dec;16(3):189-99

[140] "Although a suggestive elevated risk was found for those individuals with a large number of dental amalgams, and for a long period of time, the difference between cases and controls was not statistically significant." Bangsi D, Ghadirian P, Ducic S, Morisset R, Ciccocioppo S, McMullen E, Krewski D. Dental amalgam and multiple sclerosis: a case-control study in Montreal, Canada. *Int J Epidemiol*. 1998 Aug;27(4):667-71 ije.oxfordjournals.org/cgi/reprint/27/4/667

[141] Pike R, Lucas V, Stapleton P, Gilthorpe MS, Roberts G, Rowbury R, Richards H, Mullany P, Wilson M. Prevalence and antibiotic resistance profile of mercury-resistant oral bacteria from children with and without mercury amalgam fillings. *J Antimicrob Chemother*. 2002 May;49(5):777-83 jac.oxfordjournals.org/cgi/content/full/49/5/777 This seems to be a rather tragic article insofar as the researchers' conclusions are inconsistent with their findings; they state that mercury does not contribute to increased prevalence or numbers of antibiotic resistant bacteria, yet their data in Table 4 clearly demonstrate that patients with dental amalgams have more drug-resistant isolates than do patients without such implants. Note also that the bacteria studied here were from the oral cavity, not the gastrointestinal tract. A much better article on this topic is the following: "Our findings indicate that mercury released from amalgam fillings can cause an enrichment of mercury resistance plasmids in the normal bacterial floras of primates. Many of these plasmids also carry antibiotic resistance, implicating the exposure to mercury from dental amalgams in an increased incidence of multiple antibiotic resistance plasmids in the normal floras of nonmedicated subjects." Summers AO, Wireman J, Vimy MJ, Lorscheider FL, Marshall B, Levy SB, Bennett S, Billard L. Mercury released from dental "silver" fillings provokes an increase in mercury- and antibiotic-resistant bacteria in oral and intestinal floras of primates. *Antimicrob Agents Chemother*. 1993 Apr;37(4):825-34 pubmedcentral.gov/articlerender.fcgi?tool=pubmed&pubmedid=8280208

promoting treatment-resistant dysbiosis, which then directly effects pro-inflammatory immune dysfunction.

- In a clinical trial with 35 patients, 71% experienced improvement in overall health following removal of mercury amalgams; the patients with the most improvement were patients with multiple sclerosis.[142] Whether this was due to reducing autoimmunity or to reducing neurotoxicity is not clear; certainly both mechanisms may explain the improvement. Mercury is directly neurotoxic independently from its almost certain ability to contribute to neuroautoimmunity; this is visually demonstrated in a video of brain neuron degeneration following exposure to mercury, available on-line from the University of Calgary at commons.ucalgary.ca/mercury/.[143]

Very interestingly, the patients most sensitive to mercury compounds appear to be those with a genotypic defect in phase-2 xenobiotic conjugation, specifically glutathione-S-transferase (GST).[144] What makes this even more interesting is the finding that mercury compounds can inhibit GST and produce a GST-deficient phenotype even when the original genotype was GST-normal.[145] Even though this latter finding was documented in *ex vivo* research with human erythrocytes, it correlates with the clinical experience of doctors who specialize in environmental medicine, namely that mercury accumulation appears to inhibit chemical xenobiotic detoxification. Thus mercury and chemical xenobiotics may work synergistically for the induction of immune dysfunction, with the former inhibiting the detoxification/conjugation of the latter. Regardless of the mechanisms involved, which are clearly numerous and synergistic, given that no safe level of mercury has been established, clinicians are justified in treating patients with evidence of mercury accumulation, chronic mercury toxicity. Based on numerous case reports documenting safety and efficacy of dimercaptosuccinic acid (DMSA), when used in children and adults[146,147,148,149,150], it is my chelating agent of choice for most patients with lead and mercury toxicity as I review in the DMSA monograph in the pages that follow. Clinical implementation of metal detoxification can be performed simultaneously with the chemical detoxification program described previously and outlined in the pages that follow. The difference is the addition of DMSA first thing in the morning on an empty stomach at a dose of 10-30 mg per kg. Screening examination for overall health and kidney function should be performed before full-dose administration of DMSA, and sensitivity testing with <100 mg of DMSA is also reasonable to exclude allergy or idiosyncratic reactions to DMSA, which may indeed occur. DMSA is given in an "on and off" schedule, such as four days "on" and 3 days "off." Bile flow stimulation with botanicals and colonics for expulsion of mercury is the same as for xenobiotic detoxification. Two to four hours after consumption of DMSA, metal adsorbents such as phytochelatins and alginate can be used to bind metals in the gut and reduce enterohepatic recirculation. Antioxidants, especially selenium, are supplemented, and the diet is fresh, hypoallergenic, and Paleo-Mediterranean.

---

[142] "Out of 35 patients, 25 patients (71%) showed improvement of health... The highest rate of improvement was observed in patients with multiple sclerosis... Mercury-containing amalgam may be an important risk factor for patients with autoimmune diseases." Prochazkova J, Sterzl I, Kucerova H, Bartova J, Stejskal VD. The beneficial effect of amalgam replacement on health in patients with autoimmunity. *Neuro Endocrinol Lett*. 2004 Jun;25(3):211-8

[143] University of Calgary. How Mercury Causes Brain Neuron Degeneration. commons.ucalgary.ca/mercury/ Accessed November 24, 2005

[144] "The combined deletion (GSTT1-/GSTM1-) was markedly more frequent among thimerosal-sensitized patients than in healthy controls (17.6% vs. 6.5%, P = 0.0093) and in the "para-compound" group (17.6% vs. 6.1%, P =0.014), revealing a synergistic effect of these enzyme deficiencies." Westphal GA, Schnuch A, Schulz TG, Reich K, Aberer W, Brasch J, Koch P, Wessbecher R, Szliska C, Bauer A, Hallier E. Homozygous gene deletions of the glutathione S-transferases M1 and T1 are associated with thimerosal sensitization. *Int Arch Occup Environ Health*. 2000 Aug;73(6):384-8

[145] "Thus, sufficiently high doses of thimerosal may be able to change the phenotypic status of an individual--at least in vitro--by inhibition of the GST T1 enzyme." Muller M, et al. Inhibition of the human erythrocytic glutathione-S-transferase T1 (GST T1) by thimerosal. Int *J Hyg Environ Health*. 2001 Jul;203(5-6):479-81

[146] Bradstreet J, Geier DA, Kartzinel JJ, Adams JB, Geier MR. A case-control study of mercury burden in children with autistic spectrum disorders. *Journal of American Physicians and Surgeons* 2003; 8: 76-79 jpands.org/vol8no3/geier.pdf

[147] Crinnion WJ. Environmental medicine, part three: long-term effects of chronic low-dose mercury exposure. *Altern Med Rev*. 2000 Jun;5(3):209-23

[148] Forman J, Moline J, Cernichiari E, et al. A cluster of pediatric metallic mercury exposure cases treated with meso-2,3-dimercaptosuccinic acid (DMSA). *Environ Health Perspect*. 2000 Jun;108(6):575-7 ehp.niehs.nih.gov/docs/2000/108p575-577forman/abstract.html

[149] Miller AL. Dimercaptosuccinic acid (DMSA), a non-toxic, water-soluble treatment for heavy metal toxicity. *Altern Med Rev*. 1998 Jun;3(3):199-207

[150] DMSA. *Altern Med Rev*. 2000 Jun;5(3):264-7 thorne.com/altmedrev/.fulltext/5/3/264.pdf

Problems and Solutions in Clinical Detoxification

Effects	Cause	Solutions
1) Toxicant exposure and accumulation	• Excess exposure in relation to genotypic/phenotypic detoxification capabilities	• Total load of all xenobiotics must be reduced because of the similar/identical pathways used for the elimination of chemicals. Avoid the following: paint fumes, perfume, varnish, new carpet, formaldehyde, food colors, food additives, artificial sweeteners, pesticides, herbicides, and industrial waste.[151] • Since the vast majority of toxicants originate from irresponsible corporations, social/political action is necessary to effect fundamental change.[152]
2) Phase 1 Oxidation inhibited, too slow	• SNiPs and genotypic variations • Certain drugs • Certain food components: arachidonate and flavonoids such as bergapten (67%), quercetin (55%), naringenin (39%) naringin (6%) • Viral infections • Heavy metals • Nutritional deficiencies • Gut-derived LPS/endotoxin	• Reduce drug need by restoring health and addressing underlying problems • Address viral infections and promote glutathione production, e.g., NAC[153] and lipoic acid[154] • Vitamin/mineral supplements to correct common deficiencies in American diet[155] and to induce activity of detoxifying enzymes[156] • Paleo[157]/Mediterranean diet[158] to provide foundational nutrition and improve health • Avoidance of excess arachidonate and grapefruit • Eliminate unfavorable microflora and reflorestate to reduce LPS/endotoxin load[159] • Chelate metals with chelating agent such as DMSA[160]

[151] Ross GH. Treatment options in multiple chemical sensitivity. *Toxicol Ind Health*. 1992 Jul-Aug;8(4):87-94

[152] Kristin S. Schafer, Margaret Reeves, Skip Spitzer, Susan E. Kegley. Chemical Trespass: Pesticides in Our Bodies and Corporate Accountability. Pesticide Action Network North America. May 2004 Available at panna.org/campaigns/docsTrespass/chemicalTrespass2004.dv.html on August 1, 2004

[153] "NAC treatment was well tolerated and resulted in a significant decrease in the frequency of influenza-like episodes, severity, and length of time confined to bed. Both local and systemic symptoms were sharply and significantly reduced in the NAC group." De Flora S, Grassi C, Carati L. Attenuation of influenza-like symptomatology and improvement of cell-mediated immunity with long-term N-acetylcysteine treatment. *Eur Respir J*. 1997 Jul;10(7):1535-41 Available on-line at erj.ersjournals.com/cgi/reprint/10/7/1535 on October 18, 2004

[154] "These findings confirm the involvement of ROI in NFkB-mediated HIV gene expression as well as the efficacy of LA as a therapeutic regimen for HIV infection and acquired immunodeficiency syndrome (AIDS)." Merin JP, Matsuyama M, Kira T, Baba M, Okamoto T. Alpha-lipoic acid blocks HIV-1 LTR-dependent expression of hygromycin resistance in THP-1 stable transformants. *FEBS Lett*. 1996 Sep 23;394(1):9-13

[155] Fletcher RH, Fairfield KM. Vitamins for chronic disease prevention in adults: clinical applications. *JAMA*. 2002 Jun 19;287(23):3127-9

[156] Ames BN, Elson-Schwab I, Silver EA. High-dose vitamin therapy stimulates variant enzymes with decreased coenzyme binding affinity (increased K(m)): relevance to genetic disease and polymorphisms. *Am J Clin Nutr*. 2002 Apr;75(4):616-58

[157] O'Keefe JH Jr, Cordain L. Cardiovascular disease resulting from a diet and lifestyle at odds with our Paleolithic genome: how to become a 21st-century hunter-gatherer. *Mayo Clin Proc*. 2004 Jan;79(1):101-8

[158] Knoops KT, de Groot LC, Kromhout D, Perrin AE, Moreiras-Varela O, Menotti A, van Staveren WA. Mediterranean diet, lifestyle factors, and 10-year mortality in elderly European men and women: the HALE project. *JAMA*. 2004 Sep 22;292(12):1433-9

[159] Shedlofsky SI, Israel BC, Tosheva R, Blouin RA. Endotoxin depresses hepatic cytochrome P450-mediated drug metabolism in women. *Br J Clin Pharmacol*. 1997 Jun;43(6):627-32

[160] Miller AL. Dimercaptosuccinic Acid (DMSA), A Non-Toxic, Water-Soluble Treatment For Heavy Metal Toxicity. *Altern Med Rev* 1998;3(3):199-207

Problems and Solutions in Clinical Detoxification—*continued*

Effects	Cause	Solutions
3) Phase 1 Oxidation imbalanced, too fast relative to Phase 2	▪ Certain drugs or other toxicant exposure from endogenous or exogenous sources leads to upregulation of Phase 1	▪ Reduce drug need by restoring health and addressing underlying problems ▪ Suspect excess enterohepatic recirculation (via excess fecal β-glucuronidase): assess and optimize gastrointestinal flora by eliminating harmful bacteria and using probiotics[161] ▪ Upregulate phase 2 with diet and botanicals, such as cruciferous vegetables[162,163]
4) Phase 2 Conjugation too slow	▪ SNiPs: single nucleotide polymorphism defects in detoxification enzymes ▪ Fluoridated water: inhibits glucuronidation in some patients with Gilbert's syndrome[164] ▪ Lack of stimulation with diet and botanicals (i.e., insufficient intake of cruciferous vegetables)	▪ Avoid fluoridated water ▪ Upregulate phase 2 with diet and botanicals (citations above) ▪ Create balance by addressing the toxicant exposure that is upregulating phase 1
5) Phase 2 Conjugation Unsupported	▪ Insufficient protein for amino acids and sulfur; insufficient vitamins/minerals ▪ Poor digestion	▪ Paleo-Mediterranean diet with plenty of protein (this is not the time to be a *junkitarian* or *breaditarian*)[165] ▪ Cofactor supplementation: NAC, glutamine, glycine, taurine, sulfur, whey[166,167] ▪ Custom amino acid blend for recalcitrant cases[168]

[161] "Also they inhibited the harmful enzymes (beta-glucosidase, beta-glucuronidase, tryptophanase and urease) and ammonia production of intestinal microflora, and lowered pH of the culture media by increasing lactic acid bacteria of intestinal microflora." Park HY, Bae EA, Han MJ, Choi EC, Kim DH. Inhibitory effects of Bifidobacterium spp. isolated from a healthy Korean on harmful enzymes of human intestinal microflora. *Arch Pharm Res*. 1998 Feb;21(1):54-61

[162] "In conclusion, consumption of glucosinolate-containing Brussels sprouts for 1 week results in increased rectal GST-alpha and -pi isozyme levels. We hypothesize that these enhanced detoxification enzyme levels may partly explain the epidemiological association between a high intake of glucosinolates (cruciferous vegetables) and a decreased risk of colorectal cancer." Nijhoff WA, Grubben MJ, Nagengast FM, Jansen JB, Verhagen H, van Poppel G, Peters WH. Effects of consumption of Brussels sprouts on intestinal and lymphocytic glutathione S-transferases in humans. *Carcinogenesis*. 1995 Sep;16(9):2125-8

[163] "...human CYP1A2 and other CYP enzymes involved in oestrone 2-hydroxylation are induced by dietary broccoli." Kall MA, Vang O, Clausen J. Effects of dietary broccoli on human in vivo drug metabolizing enzymes: evaluation of caffeine, oestrone and chlorzoxazone metabolism. *Carcinogenesis*. 1996 Apr;17(4):793-9

[164] Lee J. Gilbert's disease and fluoride intake. *Fluoride* 1983; 16: 139-45

[165] O'Keefe JH Jr, Cordain L. Cardiovascular disease resulting from a diet and lifestyle at odds with our Paleolithic genome: how to become a 21st-century hunter-gatherer. *Mayo Clin Proc*. 2004 Jan;79(1):101-8 thepaleodiet.com/articles/Hunter-Gatherer%20Mayo.pdf

[166] "CONCLUSION: Supplementation with whey proteins persistently increased plasma glutathione levels in patients with advanced HIV-infection. The treatment was well tolerated." Micke P, Beeh KM, Buhl R. Effects of long-term supplementation with whey proteins on plasma glutathione levels of HIV-infected patients. *Eur J Nutr*. 2002 Feb;41(1):12-8

[167] "A significant increase in mononuclear cell glutathione was also observed in subjects receiving the WPI supplement following the 40 km simulated cycling trial." Middleton N, Jelen P, Bell G. Whole blood and mononuclear cell glutathione response to dietary whey protein supplementation in sedentary and trained male human subjects. *Int J Food Sci Nutr*. 2004 Mar;55(2):131-41

[168] Bralley JA, Lord RS. Treatment of chronic fatigue syndrome with specific amino acid supplementation. *Journal of Applied Nutrition* 1994; 46(3): 74-78

Effects	Cause	Solutions
6) Insufficient bile flow	• "Normal" bile flow appears too slow to keep pace with supraphysiologic toxicant exposure	• Stimulate bile flow with rectal instillations[169,170] and botanical medicines such as *Picrorhiza kurroa*[171] and *Andrographis paniculata*[172]
7) Urinary excretion insufficient due to insufficient hydration	• Subclinical dehydration is common and is exacerbated by diuretics such as ethanol and caffeine	• Drink water and antioxidant-rich teas and juices
8) Renal pH too acidic for optimal toxicant excretion	• Western/American diet promotes an acidic renal pH[173] which is known to reduce toxicant excretion[174]	• Vegetarian or Paleo-Mediterranean diet to alkalinize renal pH • Fruit/vegetable juices provide potassium and citrate for effective alkalinization of urine[175] • Use sodium bicarbonate[176] and/or potassium citrate as needed
9) Enterohepatic recirculation	• Constipation • Excess microflora (quantitative or qualitative) producing β-glucuronidase • Leaky gut	• Promote generous laxation: magnesium, fiber, vegetables, fruit, nuts, seeds • Optimize gastrointestinal microflora • Assess and normalize mucosal integrity • Rectal instillations may be used to cleanse the bowel and to increase bile flow as previously documented radiographically[177]; this appears to improve detoxification clinical results[178,179] presumably due to expedition of toxicant removal[180]

---

[169] Garbat, AL, Jacobi, HG: Secretion of Bile in Response to Rectal Installations. *Arch Intern Med* 1929; 44: 455-462

[170] "Caffeine enemas cause dilation of bile ducts, which facilitates excretion of toxic cancer breakdown products by the liver and dialysis of toxic products from blood across the colonic wall. The therapy must be used as an integrated whole." Gerson M. The cure of advanced cancer by diet therapy: a summary of 30 years of clinical experimentation. *Physiol Chem Phys.* 1978;10(5):449-64

[171] Vaidya AB, Antarkar DS, Doshi JC, Bhatt AD, Ramesh VV, Vora PV, Perissond DD, Baxi AJ, Kale PM. Picrorhiza kurroa (Kutaki) Royle ex Benth as a hepatoprotective agent--experimental & clinical studies. *J Postgrad Med* 1996;42:105-8 Available on October 18, 2004 at jpgmonline.com/article.asp?issn=0022-3859;year=1996;volume=42;issue=4;spage=105;epage=8;aulast=Vaidya

[172] "Andrographolide from the herb Andrographis paniculata (whole plant) per se produces a significant dose (1.5-12 mg/kg) dependent choleretic effect (4.8-73%) as evidenced by increase in bile flow, bile salt, and bile acids in conscious rats and anaesthetized guinea pigs." Shukla B, Visen PK, Patnaik GK, Dhawan BN. Choleretic effect of andrographolide in rats and guinea pigs. *Planta Med* 1992 Apr;58(2):146-9

[173] Cordain L: *The Paleo Diet: Lose weight and get healthy by eating the food you were designed to eat.* John Wiley & Sons Inc., New York 2002

[174] Proudfoot AT, Krenzelok EP, Vale JA. Position Paper on urine alkalinization. *J Toxicol Clin Toxicol.* 2004;42(1):1-26

[175] "New Guinean hunter-gatherer tribal group living in "the primitive feral condition" …urine pH of adults was usually between 7.5 and 9.0." Sebastian A, Frassetto LA, Sellmeyer DE, Merriam RL, Morris RC Jr. Estimation of the net acid load of the diet of ancestral preagricultural Homo sapiens and their hominid ancestors. *Am J Clin Nutr.* 2002 Dec;76(6):1308-16

[176] "Urine alkalinization is a treatment regimen that increases poison elimination by the administration of intravenous sodium bicarbonate to produce urine with a pH > or = 7.5." Proudfoot AT, Krenzelok EP, Vale JA. Position Paper on urine alkalinization. *J Toxicol Clin Toxicol.* 2004;42(1):1-26

[177] "Caffeine enemas cause dilation of bile ducts, which facilitates excretion of toxic cancer breakdown products by the liver and dialysis of toxic products from blood across the colonic wall. The therapy must be used as an integrated whole." Gerson M. The cure of advanced cancer by diet therapy: a summary of 30 years of clinical experimentation. *Physiol Chem Phys.* 1978;10(5):449-64

[178] Snyder RG. The value of colonic irrigations in countering auto-intoxication of intestinal origin. *Medical Clinics of North America* 1939; May: 781-788

[179] Gonzalez NJ, Isaacs LL. Evaluation of pancreatic proteolytic enzyme treatment of adenocarcinoma of the pancreas, with nutrition and detoxification support. *Nutr Cancer.* 1999;33(2):117-24

[180] Crinnion WJ. Results of a decade of naturopathic treatment for environmental illness: a review of clinical records. *J Naturopathic Med* 1997;7:21-27

Problems and Solutions in Clinical Detoxification—*continued*

Effects	Cause	Solutions
10) Deconjugation by microflora	<ul><li>Excess microflora (quantitative or qualitative) producing β-glucuronidase</li><li>Constipation must be eliminated[181]</li></ul>	<ul><li>Botanical and/or pharmaceutical antimicrobials/antifungals to reduce bacterial load in the intestines, similar to the use of antibiotics in the treatment of hepatic encephalopathy</li><li>Prebiotics and probiotics to optimize gut flora</li><li>Dietary fiber may be used to promote laxation and excretion of toxicants before enterohepatic recirculation; cholestyramine may be used in selected cases to augment fecal elimination of toxicants such as pesticides[182]</li></ul>
11) Heavy metal toxicity 12) Metal-induced alteration of detoxification (upregulation or downregulation of specific processes)	<ul><li>Heavy metal exposure appears to inhibit Phase 1 oxidation (*in vitro*[183])</li></ul>	<ul><li>Reduce exposure to toxicants</li><li>Chelation, such as with DMSA which appears effective for mercury[184] and lead[185]</li><li>Promote generous laxation: magnesium, fiber, vegetables, fruit, nuts, seeds</li><li>Optimize gastrointestinal microflora</li><li>Fruit/vegetable juices provide potassium and citrate for effective urinary alkalinization</li></ul>
13) Disease promotion via toxicants stored in body tissues, particularly adipose and brain	<ul><li>Chemical toxicants are inherently biologically persistent</li><li>Defective detoxification</li></ul>	<ul><li>Sauna, hyperthermia, exercise to promote sweating and lipolysis[186,187]</li><li>"Fat exchange" via low-fat diet to effect weight loss followed by supplementation of health-promoting uncontaminated fatty acids[188]</li><li>Weight loss for obese patients only after detoxification program is well established</li></ul>

---

[181] "Enemas and suppositories stimulate colonic contractions and soften stools. Water, saline, soap suds, hypertonic sodium phosphate, and mineral oil are used as enemas. Acute water intoxication can occur with water enemas, especially in infants, children, and the elderly, if they have difficulty evacuating the water." Dosh SA. Evaluation and treatment of constipation. *J Fam Pract*. 2002 Jun;51(6):555-9 Available at jfponline.com/content/2002/06/jfp_0602_00541.asp on October 18, 2004

[182] "Output of chlordecone in bile was 10 to 20 times greater than in stool, suggesting that chlordecone is reabsorbed in the intestine. Cholestyramine, an anion-exchange resin that binds chlordecone, increased its fecal excretion by seven times." Cohn WJ, Boylan JJ, Blanke RV, Fariss MW, Howell JR, Guzelian PS. Treatment of chlordecone (Kepone) toxicity with cholestyramine. Results of a controlled clinical trial. *N Engl J Med*. 1978 Feb 2;298(5):243-8

[183] "All four of the metals investigated decreased the extent of CYP1A1 induction in HepG2 cells by at least one of the five PAHs, in some cases decreases were marked. The same order of effectiveness of metal-mediated decreases in CYP1A1 were cadmium > arsenic > lead > mercury for all the PAHs." Vakharia DD, Liu N, Pause R, Fasco M, Bessette E, Zhang QY, Kaminsky LS. Polycyclic aromatic hydrocarbon/metal mixtures: effect on PAH induction of CYP1A1 in human HEPG2 cells. Drug Metab Dispos. 2001 Jul;29(7):999-1006 Available at dmd.aspetjournals.org/cgi/content/full/29/7/999 on October 18, 2004

[184] "Thus, oral chelation with DMSA produced a significant mercury diuresis in these children. We observed no adverse side effects of treatment. DMSA appears to be an effective and safe chelating agent for treatment of pediatric overexposure to metallic mercury." Forman J, Moline J, Cernichiari E, Sayegh S, Torres JC, Landrigan MM, Hudson J, Adel HN, Landrigan PJ. A cluster of pediatric metallic mercury exposure cases treated with meso-2,3-dimercaptosuccinic acid (DMSA). *Environ Health Perspect*. 2000 Jun;108(6):575-7 Available at ehp.niehs.nih.gov/members/2000/108p575-577forman/108p575.pdf on October 18, 2004

[185] "To conclude, awareness and early diagnosis of lead toxicity is important. Succimer is an effective chelator in patients for lead toxicity. It can be administered orally and hospitalization eliminated. However, chelation therapy should never be used as a substitute for environmental assessment and lead abatement for lead poisoned children." Kalra V, Dua T, Kumar V, Kaul B. Succimer in symptomatic lead poisoning. *Indian Pediatr*. 2002 Jun;39(6):580-5 Available at indianpediatrics.net/june2002/june-580-585.htm on October 18, 2004

[186] Schnare DW, Ben M, Shields MG. Body Burden Reductions of PCBs, PBBs and Chlorinated Pesticide Residues in Human Subjects. *Ambio* 1984; 13 (5-6): 378-380

[187] Krop J. Chemical sensitivity after intoxication at work with solvents: response to sauna therapy. *J Altern Complement Med* 1998 Spring;4(1):77-86

[188] "Repeated fasting and refeeding with fish oil facilitated plasma exchange of n-3 for n-6 PUFA, improved BP, clinical metabolic parameters and lowered platelet reactivity in the vessel wall (primary hemostasis)." Yosefy C, Viskoper JR, Varon D, Ilan Z, Pilpel D, Lugassy G, Schneider R, Savyon N, Adan Y, Raz A. Repeated fasting and refeeding with 20:5, n-3 eicosapentaenoic acid (EPA): a novel approach for rapid fatty acid exchange and its effect on blood pressure, plasma lipids and hemostasis. *J Hum Hypertens* 1996 Sep;10 Suppl 3:S135-9

Toxicant Exposure: solvents, pesticides, herbicides, plastics, fire-proofing, dioxins, exhaust, PCB, mercury, lead, cadmium, and thousands of others; the ultimate causes and therefore solutions are found primarily in addressing corporate environmental policies and influence on government regulations, societal structure/expectations regarding materialism/independence/convenience/passivity

Biological Persistence: lipolysis/redistribution; detoxification/reabsorption

lipophilic chemicals are deposited in cell membranes/adipose

metals circulate and are deposited in tissues where they impair function and thereby contribute to 'disease'

some heavy metals may alter detoxification

Promote lipolysis with diet, exercise, sauna

treatment

DMSA chelation

hydration/urination, bile formation/expulsion, maintenance of conjugation, botanical adsorbents, daily defecation

Phase One: activation / oxidation
Rapidly inducible by toxicant exposure and some drugs; the main clinical problems here are
1) **inhibition** by SNiPs, nutrient deficiencies, drugs, LPS, heavy metals
2) **relative excess activity**: rapid phase one in relation to slow conjugation: the body is not making a mistake here; it is simply responding to exposure; the solutions are to reduce exposure and support conjugation

Clinical Solutions:
1) nutritional supplementation and diet improvement,
2) reduce exposure to drugs and other 'inducers' including enterohepatic recirculation (check increased permeability and fecal b-glucuronidase)
3) clean the gut to restore mucosal integrity and reduce LPS and b-glucuronidase

insufficient oxidation

sufficient oxidation

failure

excretion in urine, excretion via bile flow and defecation

enterohepatic recirculation

chemical toxicant accumulation: increased disease risk: autoimmunity, Parkinson's disease, cancer, multiple chemical sensitivity, adverse drug reactions

a few chemicals are excreted following Phase 1 (without Conjugation)

sufficient oxidation

Phase Two: conjugation
Insufficiently induced by toxicant exposure; failure of conjugation following oxidation is highly problematic; the main clinical problems here are
1) **slow action**: phase 2 is commonly slower than phase 1; slow action can be caused by nutritional deficiencies, insufficient intake of vegetables/crucifers, and SNiPs, which are surprisingly common and are consistently associated with increased risk for disease;
2) **insufficient nutrient intake for conjugation**: recall that most conjugation factors are, of course, derived from foods: amino acids and sulphur

Clinical Solutions:
1) general nutritional supplementation and diet improvement,
2) reduce exposure to all endogenous and exogenous toxicants: drugs, chemicals, enterohepatic recirculation, hyperabsorption due to increased permeability and fecal b-glucuronidase
3) induce conjugation with cruciferous vegetables and specific botanicals
4) stimulate bile flow and bowel cleansing

insufficient conjugation

successful conjugation

excretion in urine

hydration, healthy renal function (and alkalosis)

Toxicant is solublized for excretion in bile or urine

failure of bile formation, blockage in bile flow, dehydration, dysbiosis causing deconjugation constipation promoting reabsorption, insufficient fiber

bile formation, bile expulsion, maintenance of conjugation, daily defecation

excretion via bile flow and defecation

enterohepatic recirculation

Overview of Toxicant Exposure and Detoxification/Depuration: Pathways and therapeutic implications

Outline of the Use of Dimercaptosuccinic acid (DMSA)

Therapeutic:	***Dimercaptosuccinic acid***
Common name:	**DMSA**
Applications and mechanisms of action:	<ul><li>DMSA is a well-documented chelating agent that is FDA-approved for the treatment of lead poisoning.[189] It has been used safely and successfully in children and adults with lead and/or mercury toxicity, whether acute or chronic. The sulfur-containing moiety of the molecule binds to heavy metals, rendering them soluble, and then the metal-DMSA complex is excreted in urine or bile.</li></ul> A few of the better articles on this topic are listed here: <ul><li>**DMSA-mercury testing in autistic children**: Two-hundred-twenty-one children with autism were challenged with 30 mg/kg of DMSA and showed significantly higher urinary mercury excretion compared to control subjects. The specific protocol is described as follows: "The Arizona State University Institutional Review Board approved our retrospective examination of cases and controls in this study. ... Informed consent was obtained from both cases and controls for DMSA chelation treatment. Controls and cases were both challenged with a three-day oral treatment of **DMSA (10 mg/kg per dose given three times daily).** After the ninth dose, the first voided morning urine was collected (when possible), or an overnight urine collection bag was worn. All laboratory analyses were performed by the Doctors Data, Inc., in Chicago, Ill."[190] No adverse effects were reported.</li><li>**Mercury review by Dr. Walter Crinnion**: As one of the most experienced environmental medicine doctors in the US, Dr. Crinnion provides his perspective on the treatment of mercury toxicity, and states, "DMSA can be given to an adult at a dose of 500 mg tid... DMSA (30 mg/kg)... It is generally recommended that these agents be given in several day courses repeatedly, with rest periods in between."[191]</li><li>**Nine cases of pediatric mercury poisoning safely treated with DMSA**: Nine mercury-poisoned children were treated with DMSA 30 mg/kg for 5 days followed by 20 mg/kg for 2 weeks; mercury levels declined in all children, and no adverse effects occurred.[192]</li><li>**DMSA monographs**: monographs on the basic science and clinical applications of DMSA.[193,194]</li><li>**Acute poisoning review**: See also Greene SL, Dargan PI, Jones AL. Acute poisoning: understanding 90% of cases in a nutshell. *Postgrad Med J.* 2005 Apr for a "nutshell" review of the management of acute poisoning.[195]</li></ul>

---

[189] "The Food and Drug Administration has recently licensed the drug DMSA (succimer) for reduction of blood lead levels >/= 45 micrograms/dl. This decision was based on the demonstrated ability of DMSA to reduce blood lead levels. An advantage of this drug is that it can be given orally." Goyer RA, Cherian MG, Jones MM, Reigart JR. Role of chelating agents for prevention, intervention, and treatment of exposures to toxic metals. *Environ Health Perspect.* 1995 Nov;103(11):1048-52 ehp.niehs.nih.gov/docs/1995/103-11/meetingreport.html

[190] Bradstreet J, Geier DA, Kartzinel JJ, Adams JB, Geier MR. A case-control study of mercury burden in children with autistic spectrum disorders. *Journal of American Physicians and Surgeons* 2003; 8: 76-79 jpands.org/vol8no3/geier.pdf

[191] Crinnion WJ. Environmental medicine, part three: long-term effects of chronic low-dose mercury exposure. *Altern Med Rev.* 2000 Jun;5(3):209-23 thorne.com/altmedrev/.fulltext/5/3/209.pdf

[192] Forman J, Moline J, Cernichiari E, Sayegh S, Torres JC, Landrigan MM, Hudson J, Adel HN, Landrigan PJ. A cluster of pediatric metallic mercury exposure cases treated with meso-2,3-dimercaptosuccinic acid (DMSA). *Environ Health Perspect.* 2000 Jun;108(6):575-7 ehp.niehs.nih.gov/docs/2000/108p575-577forman/abstract.html

[193] Miller AL. Dimercaptosuccinic acid (DMSA), a non-toxic, water-soluble treatment for heavy metal toxicity. *Altern Med Rev.* 1998 Jun;3(3):199-207 thorne.com/altmedrev/.fulltext/3/3/199.pdf

[194] DMSA. *Altern Med Rev.* 2000 Jun;5(3):264-7 thorne.com/altmedrev/.fulltext/5/3/264.pdf

[195] Greene SL, Dargan PI, Jones AL. Acute poisoning: understanding 90% of cases in a nutshell. *Postgrad Med J.* 2005 Apr;81(954):204-16 pmj.bmjjournals.com/cgi/content/full/81/954/204

Toxicity:	▪ DMSA has a very favorable risk:benefit ratio when used in patients without renal/hepatic impairment and who are at average or greater-than-average risk for heavy metal accumulation/toxicity. Toxicity is very rare. Some articles make fleeting mention of bone marrow suppression, but this is almost never precipitated clinically and is practically never documented in the case reports and clinical studies using DMSA for the treatment of heavy metal toxicity. Patients should be tested for hematologic and metabolic status prior to DMSA administration; a CBC and metabolic/chemistry panel is sufficient. ▪ Allergic-type reactions to DMSA and/or the mobilization of heavy metals, especially mercury, are infrequent but not rare. To reduce the risk of precipitating such reactions, a trial dose of 100 mg (or less for children) should be used on a single occasion to ensure that IgE-mediated allergy or anaphylaxis does not occur with the higher doses used therapeutically. Like any drug, DMSA may precipitate idiosyncratic reactions, but these are by definition nearly impossible to predict. However, since idiosyncratic drug reactions appear to reflect imbalanced Phase 1 / Phase 2 detoxification, the likelihood of such a reaction can probably be reduced by ensuring that the patient is supplemented with antioxidants, fortified with sufficient protein for supporting Phase 2 conjugation reactions, and abstinent from other drugs which induce Phase 1 upregulation. Patients with adverse reactions to DMSA should either not use DMSA or should do so carefully, such as with a lower dose or after the underlying cause of the sensitivity has been addressed.
Dosage and administration:	▪ <u>Screening laboratory tests</u>: Urinalysis, CBC and chemistry panel with BUN, creatinine, and hepatic markers are sufficient for assessing renal, hepatic, and marrow status. ▪ <u>Empty stomach</u>: DMSA should be taken on an empty stomach, preferably 1-2 hours away from food. In particular, mineral supplements containing zinc and copper (etc) should be avoided for 4 hours before and after DMSA supplementation. Generally, first morning supplementation with a delayed or skipped breakfast is ideal. ▪ <u>The lowest therapeutic dose is generally 10 mg/kg per day, and the highest therapeutic dose is generally 30 mg/kg per day</u>. The 30 mg/kg dose is generally delivered in three divided doses (i.e., 10 mg/kg TID); however, a single-dose 30 mg/kg dose may be used provocatively for diagnostic purposes. Lower dosage schemes are appropriate for children or those with severe sensitivities. The highest scheme may also be appropriate for children but might otherwise be reserved for adult patients who are in otherwise good health. My clinical preference is to use 10mg/kg 3 days "on" and 4 days "off" with periodic monitoring of CBC and chemistry/metabolic parameters. <table><tr><th>Body weight in lbs (kg)</th><th>10 mg/kg dose</th><th>30 mg/kg dose (bolus or divided)</th></tr><tr><td>40 lbs (18 kg)</td><td>180 mg</td><td>540 mg</td></tr><tr><td>80 lbs (36 kg)</td><td>360 mg</td><td>1080 mg</td></tr><tr><td>120 lbs (54 kg)</td><td>540 mg</td><td>1620 mg</td></tr><tr><td>160 lbs (72 kg)</td><td>720 mg</td><td>2,160 mg (limit to 2,000) mg</td></tr><tr><td>200 lbs (90 kg)</td><td>900 mg</td><td>2,700 (limit to 2,000) mg</td></tr><tr><td>240 lbs (108 kg)</td><td>1080 mg</td><td>3,240 (limit to 2,000) mg</td></tr><tr><td>280 lbs (126 kg)</td><td>1260 mg</td><td>3,780 (limit to 2,000) mg</td></tr></table>

Outline of the Use of Dimercaptosuccinic acid (DMSA)—*continued*

Dosage and administration (continued):	▪ <u>Cyclical dosing</u>: DMSA is generally "cycled" which means that it is taken for a few days, the discontinued for a few days, then resumed, etc. This can be customized per patient for ease of compliance and variations in scheduling. For example, the patient might use DMSA for 5 days of the week, taking the weekends "off", or might use DMSA for 4 days on and 3 days off, etc. Every-other-day dosing is also reasonable. Treatment is generally continued for 1-2 months. ▪ <u>Plenty of water</u>: DMSA should be taken with 16 ounces of water. An additional 1-2 liters should be consumed over the next 2-4 hours.

Additional information:	▪ DMSA increases urinary excretion of copper in humans[196]; if treatment were excessively prolonged then theoretically this might lead to copper deficiency. Additionally, DMSA might be useful for people with excess copper. These areas require more research.
	
	▪ Co-supplementation with the following can increase urinary metal excretion and/or reduce enterohepatic recycling of toxic metals. These can be used during DMSA treatment but should not be taken within 2-4 hours of DMSA supplementation so as not to bind with or otherwise interfere with DMSA absorption and utilization.
	
	    • *Fruit and vegetable juices*: Potassium citrate has been shown to significantly increase mercury excretion in humans when used alone and/or with DMSA.[197,198] Fruit and vegetable juices are rich sources of potassium citrate and should be consumed liberally by patients undergoing detoxification. Furthermore, since urinary alkalinization greatly increases the urinary excretion of chemical/xenobiotics toxicants[199], essentially all patients undergoing detoxification programs should increase consumption of fruit and vegetable juices as well as fruits and vegetables.
	
	    • *Phytochelatins*: Phytochelatins are metal-binding moieties from plants and algae.[200] Clinically, doctors use phytochelatin supplementation to bind metals in the gut for enhanced excretion, i.e., to prevent re-absorption of metals that have been detoxified into the gut lumen via the bile. High-fiber plant-based diets are beneficial for the same purpose.
	
	    • *Selenium*: Selenium (Se) has many important actions in the body, one of which is that of an antioxidant. It is generally dosed at 200 mcg per day, but doses up to 800-1,000 mcg per day are generally safe for most adults. The study by Seppanen et al[201] showed 34% reduction in hair mercury following Se 100mcg/d.

[196] "The Food and Drug Administration has recently licensed the drug DMSA (succimer) for reduction of blood lead levels >/= 45 micrograms/dl. This decision was based on the demonstrated ability of DMSA to reduce blood lead levels. An advantage of this drug is that it can be given orally." Goyer RA, Cherian MG, Jones MM, Reigart JR. Role of chelating agents for prevention, intervention, and treatment of exposures to toxic metals. *Environ Health Perspect*. 1995 Nov;103(11):1048-52 ehp.niehs.nih.gov/docs/1995/103-11/meetingreport.html

[197] "Based on the increase in urinary Hg concentrations after single doses, compared with controls, the order of efficacy was: DMPS plus K Cit., NAC plus K Cit. and DMSA (each producing an increase of 163%), then in descending order, DMSA plus K Cit., DMPS, NAC and K Cit." Hibberd AR, Howard MA, Hunnisett AG. Mercury from dental amalgam fillings studies on oral chelating agents for assessing and reducing mercury burdens in humans. *J Nutr Environ Med* 1998;8:219-231

[198] Crinnion WJ. Environmental medicine, part three: long-term effects of chronic low-dose mercury exposure. *Altern Med Rev*. 2000 Jun;5(3):209-23

[199] Proudfoot AT, Krenzelok EP, Vale JA. Position Paper on urine alkalinization. *J Toxicol Clin Toxicol*. 2004;42(1):1-26. This is a very important paper. Posted by the European Association of Poisons Centres and Clinical Toxicologists at eapcct.org/publicfile.php?folder=congress&file=PS_UrineAlkalinization.pdf

[200] Cobbett CS. Phytochelatins and their roles in heavy metal detoxification. *Plant Physiol*. 2000 Jul;123(3):825-32 plantphysiol.org/cgi/content/full/123/3/825 This is a basic science review with relevance for plant biology that discusses the use of phytochelatins to bind metals in the plant's environment. It does not discuss relevance of phytochelatins for the treatment of heavy metal exposure in humans.

[201] "The selenium supplementation group received daily 100 micrograms of selenomethionine. Selenium supplementation reduced pubic hair mercury level by 34% (p = 0.005) and elevated serum selenium by 73% and blood selenium by 59% in the supplemented group (p < 0.001 for both). The study indicates that mercury accumulation in pubic hair can be reduced by dietary supplementation with small daily amounts of organic selenium in a short range of time." Seppanen K, et al. Effect of supplementation with organic selenium on mercury status as measured by mercury in pubic hair. *J Trace Elem Med Biol*. 2000 Jun;14(2):84-7

Outline the functional Inflammology protocol on this page to assess your ability to apply the information clinically:

_____

_____

_____

_____

_____

_____

Chapter 5: Clinical Applications of the Functional Inflammology Protocol

Introduction

- The functional inflammology protocol is a decipherative technology for understanding complex chronic illnesses and for organizing an effective treatment approach: The functional inflammology protocol is a decipherative technology for understanding complex chronic illnesses and for organizing an effective treatment approach; the FINDSEX ® acronym reminds clinicians of the most important lifestyle, nutritional, environmental, and (patho)physiologic contributors and interventions
- History of this Chapter: The bulk of this chapter was updated for *Rheumatology v3.5* (2014); an appendix of less common autoimmune/rheumatic disease has been added at the end of this chapter, imported with minimal revision from *Integrative Rheumatology v2* (2007) and *Integrative Rheumatology and Inflammation Mastery v3* (2014). Sections on migraine, hypertension, diabetes and allergy were imported from previous publications, specifically *Chiropractic and Naturopathic Mastery of Common Clinical Disorders* (2009). The section on fibromyalgia has been completely restructured for this publication and embellished with new diagrams and new information, especially on glial activation and central sensitization which also applies to migraine and other disorders of sustained inflammation and secondary pain sensitization. The detailed information in Chapter 4 and the clinical applications in Chapter 5 are more than sufficient for application to the newly imported conditions from previous publications, even while the FINDSEX ® acronym and structured protocol were developed in 2012.
- Foundational Belief in a Comprehensible and Rational/Orderly Universe: Rheumatologic disorders are multifactorial, not idiopathic. The Functional Inflammology Protocol reviewed in Chapter 4 covers the most important concepts; in this chapter those concepts will encounter opportunities for clinical application in the management/comanagement of rheumatologic diseases, better described as rheumatologic/autoimmune disease *states*, with the latter added to imply their temporal and potentially escapable nature. Stated differently, let us begin with the assumption that we are intelligent and capable, and that while we do not now and never will have "all of the answers", we have enough talent and information within our current grasp to allow us to rationally approach these multifactorial conditions and address the largest components, as outlined by the FINDSEX® acronym. Knowledge is—commonly if not generally—asymptotic; we get closer and closer to the truth without actually touching all components at all times; but this is no rationale for us either as humans generally or clinicians specifically to languish in nihilistic repose. We are obligated to act on what we know and to orchestrate rational treatment.
- Comanagement and Risk Management: A wise clinical strategy when managing any serious or potentially-life threatening condition is for the clinician to arrange for co-management with a specialist, and this is particularly true for conditions that might necessitate hospitalization or acute immunosuppression. Autoimmune diseases such as lupus are notorious for acute flares that can cause permanent damage (e.g., transverse myelitis resulting in paralysis); likewise, giant cell arteritis is notorious for causing rapid-onset visual loss, which is generally permanent and thus debilitating. Reviews of patient management, risk management, and common musculoskeletal emergencies are provided in Chapter 1—this information should be reviewed prior to the reading of this chapter and implementation of the clinical applications herein. Pharmaceuticalization of these patients offers no chance of cure but is useful for "controlling" inflammation with limited efficacy and numerous adverse long-term effects. The best general approach is one that is etiotherapeutic/polyetiotherapeutic—directed at treating the cause(s) of the disorder while accessing pharmacoimmunosuppression on an "as needed" basis.
- Video Presentations and Tutorials: These are provided to help reinforce—*not replace*—the written material in this chapter, and these additional videos should be viewed *following* the videos corresponding to the overall protocol (Chapter 4), mitochondrial dysfunction (Chapter 4), the detailing of dysbiosis (Chapter 4 plus additional presentation slides—see presentation slides for video access). One of the major goals with these videos, in addition to simply providing more information and reinforcing the material in the text, is that these will promote learning of the material in a conversational style, because ultimately the material must be understood in words and communicable in words in order to be understood and applied: vimeo.com/album/3000884, password: DrV_Allergy_Rheum. Updates and sample syllabi: InflammationMastery.com/books/rheum/
- Understanding autoimmunity as "patterns of inflammation": My perspective for years—supported by the phrase "patterns of inflammation" by WG Meggs MD PhD—is that autoimmune disorders as we appreciate them (phenomenonistically and diagnostically) are simply "variations on the theme" of the seven factors I've identified via the FINDSEX® acronym and functional inflammology protocol. As such, readers should note the consistency of the pattern, and also how research "specific" for one disease might well apply to a particular autoimmune/inflamed/autoinflamed patient even if he/she has a different diagnostic label; such is the rule, rather than the exception. As such, the information in this textbook needs to be appreciated and integrated in its entirety, not simply accessed for information on a specific topic without consideration of the provided—and synergistic—context.

❶ Metabolic inflammation, mitochondrial dysfunction
1. Hypertension
2. Diabetes
3. Migraine
4. Fibromyalgia

❷ Allergic inflammation
5. Allergy (general), asthma and reactive airway disease—note that allergy in general and eczema is covered in several locations of the book, particularly Chapter 4, Sections 1 and 3

❸ Autoimmune/rheumatic inflammation
6. Rheumatoid arthritis
7. Psoriasis and psoriatic arthritis
8. Systemic lupus erythematosus
9. Scleroderma, systemic sclerosis Vasculitic diseases
10. Spondyloarthropathies
11. Sjögren syndrome/disease
12. Raynaud's syndrome/phenomenon/disorder
13. Clinical Notes on Additional Conditions: Behçet's Disease, Sarcoidosis, Dermatomyositis and Polymyositis

Layout of each section—listed once here to avoid unnecessary repetition at each section:

- Introduction and Overview
- Clinical Presentation
- Prevalence, Symptoms, and Clinical Findings
- Pathophysiology
- Differential Diagnosis
- Diagnosis
- Standard Medical Treatment
- Therapeutic Interventions—Clinical Application of the Functional Inflammology Protocol via FINDSEX™ acronym

The Functional Inflammology Protocol is a deciperative clinical approach—"a scheme of behavior"—for the understanding and treatment of complex inflammatory-metabolic disorders implemented via the F.I.N.D.S.E.X.® mnemonic acronym
"In order for a particular species to maintain itself and increase its power, its conception of reality **must comprehend enough of the calculable and constant** for it to base a **scheme of behavior** on it."
Nietzsche FW. *Will to Power*, 1901, #480

Factors that are "calculable and constant" in sustained inflammatory diseases: F.I.N.D.S.E.X.®
- Food and nutritional variables
- Infections, dysbiosis
- Nutritional (deficiency) alternations in immune phenotype and function
- Dysmetabolism of mitochondria, ER
- Sleep disturbance, social stressors, sweating deficiency (lack of exercise)
- Endocrine imbalances
- Xenobiotic immunotoxicity

Twilight of the Idiopathic Era and the Dawn of New Possibilities in Health and Healthcare

This article was originally published in *Naturopathy Digest* in 2006; minor edits were made in 2010 and 2014
naturopathydigest.com/archives/2006/mar/idiopathic.php

Among the perplexing paradoxes that exist in healthcare is coexistence of our adoration of allopathy for its "scientific method" along with the description of most chronic diseases as "idiopathic." If the allopathic use of the scientific method were so adroit, then why are so many conditions described as having "no known cause"? Is the scientific method inadequate, or is the allopathic lens incapable of bringing disease causation into focus? Perhaps a third option exists: that some groups—namely the medical profession generally and the pharmaceutical companies specifically—benefit by convincing us that most diseases have "no known cause" and that therefore the best that doctors and patients can hope for is additive and endless pharmaceuticalization of all health problems. When the cause of our health problems is "unknown", we are disempowered, and we must depend on "experts" and those who have "the cure" to help us and save us. When the causes of our problems are known, we are empowered to take effective action. Certainly, some groups have financial and political interests in keeping us *as professionals* and *as patients* confused and disempowered.

The End of the Idiopathic Era: A stark contrast exists between primary research literature and the "facts" that are selectively reported in medical textbooks and which are used to buttress "conventional wisdom" and the resultant status quo. While I have been aware of this contrast for many years, the divergence was impressed upon me with renewed vigor during the preparation of a recent article[1] and the completion of my 2006 textbook *Integrative Rheumatology*.[2] Arthritis in general and autoimmune and rheumatic diseases in particular are frequently described as "idiopathic" and as having "no known cause" by most mainstream medical books like *The Merck Manual* and *Current Medical Diagnosis and Treatment*; these contentions are inconsistent with the abundant and diverse research showing that—rather than being *idiopathic*—most chronic musculoskeletal disorders are *multifactorial*. When a disease is codified as *idiopathic*, doctors lose their incentive to look for and treat the *causes* [plural] of the disease because the codified conventional wisdom has already stated that "The cause [singular] of the disease has not been identified." Similarly, patients are convinced to give up their hope of ever being *cured*; they chose what appears to be the second best option: lifelong medicalization. In these instances, acceptance of the codified conventional wisdom benefits doctors and patients by freeing them of the obligation to think, to mobilize their consciousness; the price paid for this exoneration from consciousness is perpetuated unconsciousness and drug dependence for doctors and patients. Being told by powerful institutions and ensconced authorities that "There's nothing else you can do, and nothing more to think about" lulls us all into apathy and conformity at the price of our individual and collective lives and consciousness.

Multifactorial—not idiopathic: Let's look at psoriasis and rheumatoid arthritis as two shining examples of *idiopathicity*. If one looks into a standard medical textbook, one sees that these conditions have *no known cause* and *therefore* the lifelong prescription of anti-inflammatory medications is presumptively justified. On the contrary, if one spends a few days in any medical library, one can find articles that point to the causes of these diseases and which then illuminate the path (and paths) by which doctors and patients can arrive at authentic improvement or permanent cure. Most patients can be cured of psoriasis, and a large percentage of rheumatoid arthritis patients can avoid the complications and medicalization associated with their disease, particularly if *the causes* of their condition are treated early. We now know that most autoimmune diseases are caused by and/or perpetuated by ~~chronic~~ sustained infections, phenotypic/epigenetic immune imbalances, a proinflammatory lifestyle, hormonal imbalances, and exposure to chemicals and metals that cause immune dysfunction/activation. When the cause(s) of the disease is treated, the disease has the potential to be cured, provided that it is treated comprehensively and hopefully before the onset of irreversible damage. When the disease is cured, lifelong medicalization becomes unnecessary, the patient is free to fully resume his/her life, and doctors are liberated from their roles as drug representatives and can resume their proper positions as healers and creative free-thinking individuals.

Asserting an empowered stance toward disease prevention and treatment carries implications beyond those for the doctor and the patient. These implications also point to new ways of living and stewarding the world. When we look at a disease like Parkinson's disease and then determine that it is *idiopathic*, then nothing happens to change or shape our view of the world, our place in it, and the interconnected components of health and disease. Everyone agrees that that clinical manifestations of Parkinson's disease result from the death (or perhaps impairment?) of dopaminergic neurons. From the allopathic perspective, the disease is *idiopathic*, while from an integrative naturopathic perspective, we see Parkinson's disease as a *multifaceted disorder* associated with defective mitochondrial function, impaired xenobiotic detoxification, and occupational and/or recreational exposure to toxicants, particularly pesticides. These associations align to create a new model for the illness based on exposure to neurotoxicants such as pesticides[3] which are ineffectively detoxified[4] and then accumulate in the brain[5] and induce mitochondrial dysfunction[6] and resultant oxidative stress[7] which leads to impairment/death of dopaminergic neurons. Therefore, from the perspective of both prevention and treatment, the clinical approach to Parkinson's disease should include pesticide avoidance and optimization of detoxification to prevent the cellular accumulation of neurotoxic mitochondrial poisons. The plan must also include optimization of nutritional status, antioxidant capacity, and mitochondrial function.[8] Further, if our goal is to reduce the societal prevalence of

---

[1] Vasquez A. Nutritional and Botanical Treatments against "Silent Infections" and Gastrointestinal Dysbiosis. *Nutritional Perspectives* 2006; January
[2] Vasquez A. *Integrative Rheumatology*. First Edition. 2006
[3] Ritz B, Yu F. Parkinson's disease mortality and pesticide exposure in California 1984-1994. *Int J Epidemiol*. 2000 Apr;29(2):323-9
[4] Menegon A, Board PG, Blackburn AC, et al. Parkinson's disease, pesticides, and glutathione transferase polymorphisms. *Lancet*. 1998;352(9137):1344-6
[5] Kamel F, Hoppin JA. Related Articles, Association of pesticide exposure with neurologic dysfunction and disease. *Environ Health Perspect*. 2004;112(9):950-8
[6] Parker WD Jr, Swerdlow RH. Mitochondrial dysfunction in idiopathic Parkinson disease. *Am J Hum Genet*. 1998;62(4):758-62
[7] Davey GP, Peuchen S, Clark JB. Energy thresholds in brain mitochondria. Potential involvement in neurodegeneration. *J Biol Chem*. 1998;273(21):12753-7
[8] Kidd PM. Parkinson's disease as multifactorial oxidative neurodegeneration: implications for integrative management. *Altern Med Rev*. 2000 Dec;5(6):502-29

Parkinson's disease, then we must begin living in better harmony with nature and thinking of ways to reduce our use of pesticides and herbicides, the chemicals that are consistently shown to cause premature neuronal death and which are increasingly pervasive in our home, work, and outdoor environments.

The Dawn of New Possibilities in Health and Healthcare: The time is now past when credible physicians can assert that most diseases are "of unknown origin." The truth is that we already have access to the information we need to help our patients. The truth is that we can often offer our patients the *probability of cure* rather than *lifelong and endless prescriptions for symptom-modifying drugs*. These truths imply that healthcare and our systems of healthcare delivery must change, because the pharmaceutical and medical icons that stand before us were built upon feet and legs of clay and interspersed lead. We stand at the dawn of a new era in healthcare—one in which patients with chronic diseases in general and autoimmune diseases in particular—have a tangible and authentic opportunity to regain their health.

Higher education

"Our real problem is to determine: *what is the goal of education?*

Are we forming children who are only capable of learning what is already known?

Or should we try to develop creative and innovative minds, capable of discovery from the preschool age onward, throughout life?"

Jean Piaget (1896-1980), Swiss developmental psychologist and philosopher known for his epistemological studies with children

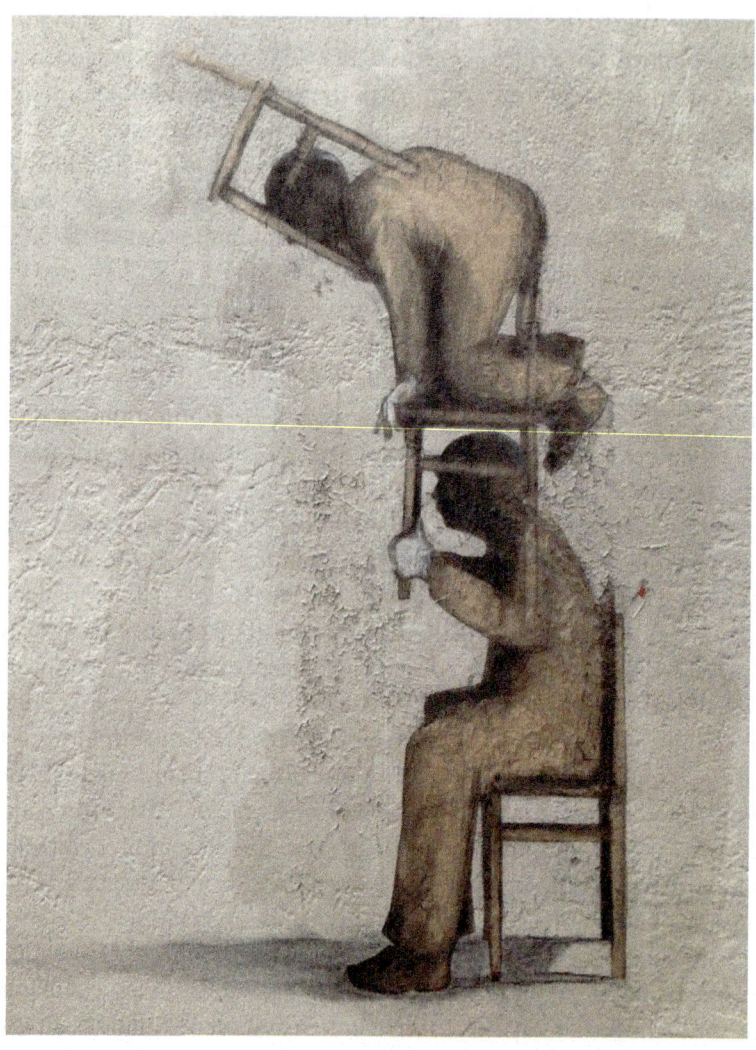

Anonymous art-quality graffiti in Paris, France—photo by Dr Vasquez in 2013: This image reminds me of the (common, American) educational process, which is often stupefying and *stupidifying*. Throughout most of my educational experience—including 12 years of doctorate-level study—I found that most schools have impressively little commitment to *instruction* (Latin: *instruere*: to pack in, to load) and even less to *education* (Latin: *educare*: to lead out); in fact, most "professional" academicians and so-called "administrators" do not appreciate these words or concepts for their meanings nor their implications. In my experience as a Professor and Director at various schools, I frequently found so-called "senior administrators" to be completely incompetent in their roles, and completely corrupt in their willingness to literally sell-out quality faculty for personal gain and financial advantage, even at major cost to students, programs, courses, and the institution—I have seen this in various schools in various professions, including professions and some schools which I previously cherished. The pervasiveness and high level of incompetence and corruption in healthcare professions and institutions is bewildering. What I strive for with my books and courses is to resist the "dumbing down" of students and the dehumanization and eunuchification of academia in general and intellectuality in particular.

Review of the Functional Inflammology Protocol and each of the FINDSEX® Components:
Summarized here to reduce redundancy and repeated citations throughout the clinical application subsections

---

The Functional Inflammology Protocol is reviewed and substantiated in Chapter 4; the protocol is reviewed/outlined here with the most important components cited. In the clinical application sections that follow, the protocol is applied, and its disease-specific implications are emphasized; the abbreviated overview/summary is included in each subsection with nuances noted and citations omitted to enhance safety/efficacy/applicability and space/time efficiency, respectively.

- **FOOD & NUTRITION** The 5-part "supplemented Paleo-Mediterranean diet" (SPMD—reviewed in Chapter 4, Section 1) consists of ❶ foundational plant-based low-carbohydrate diet of fruits, vegetables, nuts, seeds, berries and lean sources of protein: the plant-based diet optimizes antioxidant and phytonutrient intake[9] while promoting favorable modification of gastrointestinal flora for a systemic anti-inflammatory benefit[10]; carbohydrate intake is minimized and tailored per individual need for weight maintenance and exercise recovery/compensation; maintaining mild ketosis via low carbohydrate intake helps maintain optimal body weight, mitochondrial efficiency, bHB's antioxidant function and a rejuvenative phenotype via histone acetylation[11]; plant-based diets promote alkalinization and counteract the Western diet's promotion of diet-induced acidosis[12]; renal insufficiency mandates vigilance for hyperkalemia, especially when considering implementation of a potassium-rich diet ❷ multivitamin and multimineral supplementation: this component serves to correct pandemic nutritional deficiencies[13], prevent long-latency deficiency diseases[14], improve mood[15], reduce systemic inflammation[16], and provide some/partial/complete compensation for genotropic metabolic defects[17], ❸ physiologic doses of vitamin D3 (range 2,000-10,000 IU/d): vitamin D3 supplementation[18] alleviates pain, improves mood, reduces inflammation, enhances immunity, normalizes hypertension, ❹ combination fatty acid therapy (CFAT) with n3-ALA, n6-GLA, n3-EPA, n3-DHA, and phytochemical-rich olive oil which contains n9-oleate: anti-inflammatory, mood-enhancing, and cardioprotective benefits are conclusively documented, ❺ probiotics: probiotics promote immunotolerance via several mechanisms including induction of Treg; probiotic supplementation helps prevent and treat insufficiency dysbiosis, which causes 1) decreased colonization resistance, 2) increased bacterial translocation, and 3) failure of optimal Treg induction. Per "Expert consensus document: The International Scientific Association for Probiotics and Prebiotics consensus statement" published in *Nature Reviews Gastroenterology and Hepatology* 2014 Aug[19], probiotics—by definition—require administration of at least one billion (1,000,000,000 or 1x10^9) colony forming units (CFU); many probiotic nutritional supplements in the form of powders and capsules contain 1-20 billion organisms yet not all organisms are viable at time of consumption and not all viable organisms become CFU. Importantly, some benefits of probiotic supplementation are not dependent on viable microorganisms but rather on the molecular signature of the microbe; other—and obviously more complete—benefits require microbial viability and are mediated via metabolites, which are themselves interdependent on microbes and the host's diet. Bertazzoni et al[20] extensively reviewed the issue of microbial/CFU count number and concluded that the appropriate dose is patient-dependent, disease-dependent, and strain-dependent and thus cannot be generalized; their review included several studies that safely and effectively used varying doses, e.g., 1, 30, 70,

---

[9] Liu RH. Health benefits of fruit and vegetables are from additive and synergistic combinations of phytochemicals. *Am J Clin Nutr.* 2003 Sep;78(3 Suppl):517S-520S

[10] Peltonen R et al. Faecal microbial flora and disease activity in rheumatoid arthritis during a vegan diet. *Br J Rheumatol.* 1997 Jan;36(1):64-8

[11] Shimazu T, Hirschey MD, et al. Suppression of oxidative stress by β-hydroxybutyrate, an endogenous histone deacetylase inhibitor. *Science* 2013 Jan;339:211-4. To access more of Dr Matt Hirschey's work and video presentations, please see ichnfm.org/events/MitochondrialMedicine. For additional information on the rejuvenative effect of histone acetylation, see: Matuoka et al. Rapid reversion of aging phenotypes by nicotinamide through possible modulation of histone acetylation. *Cell Mol Life Sci.* 2001 Dec;58:2108-16

[12] Adeva et al. Diet-induced metabolic acidosis. *Clin Nutr.* 2011 Aug;30:416-21. Cordain et al. Origins and evolution of the Western diet. *Am J Clin Nutr.* 2005 Feb;81(2):341-54

[13] Fletcher RH, Fairfield KM. Vitamins for chronic disease prevention in adults: clinical applications. *JAMA.* 2002 Jun 19;287(23):3127-9

[14] Heaney RP. Long-latency deficiency disease: insights from calcium and vitamin D. *Am J Clin Nutr.* 2003 Nov;78(5):912-9

[15] Benton D, Haller J, Fordy J. Vitamin supplementation for 1 year improves mood. *Neuropsychobiology.* 1995;32(2):98-105

[16] Church TS, Earnest CP, Wood KA, Kampert JB. Reduction of C-reactive protein levels through use of a multivitamin. *Am J Med.* 2003 Dec 15;115(9):702-7

[17] Ames BN, et al. High-dose vitamin therapy stimulates variant enzymes with decreased coenzyme binding affinity (increased K(m)). *Am J Clin Nutr.* 2002 Apr;75(4):616-58

[18] See discussion and citaitons throughout Chapter 4. Vasquez A, Manso G, Cannell J. The clinical importance of vitamin D (cholecalciferol): a paradigm shift with implications for all healthcare providers. *Altern Ther Health Med.* 2004 Sep-Oct;10(5):28-36 ichnfm.academia.edu/AlexVasquez /

[19] Hill et al. Expert consensus document: The International Scientific Association for Probiotics and Prebiotics consensus statement on the scope and appropriate use of the term probiotic. *Nat Rev Gastroenterol Hepatol.* 2014 Aug;11(8):506-14

[20] Bertazzoni et al. Probiotics and clinical effects: is the number what counts? *J Chemother.* 2013 Aug;25(4):193-212

300 billion CFU/d. Per expert clinical opinion, a clinician might use one billion [units = microbes or CFU] for a small or young child, and a starting dose of 10 billion scaling up to 90 billion per day for adults.[21]

- o Additional details—implementation of the "low-carbohydrate (low fermentation) supplemented Paleo-Mediterranean diet" ("low-carb SPMD"): The diet should be plant-based, but not necessarily vegan or vegetarian; I refer to this diet at "plant-based Paleo" since "the Paleo diet" as commonly discussed is simply a diet of whole natural foods which can generally be consumed without cooking or processing. For purposes of meeting physiologic expectations and attaining the highest satiety, weight optimization, and nutrient density with a phytonutrient-dense low-fermentation diet, the diet should primarily consist of fruits, vegetables, nuts, seeds, berries, and lean sources of protein; carbohydrate intake is modulated per caloric and carbohydrate needs while protein intake is tailored to lean body mass, exercise and healing/recuperation needs. Preferred sources of protein are grass-fed land animals as well as wild-caught cold-water fish, both of which are low in total fat and high in the anti-inflammatory and immunomodulatory omega-3 fatty acids, especially EPA and DHA. Whey protein isolate can also be used as it is an inexpensive convenient source of high-quality protein well-tolerated for most patients and as it also contains many functional components such as glutathione precursors, tryptophan, immunoglobulins, and growth factors anti-gastrin effects which help to heal/protect damaged intestinal mucosa. Plant-based diets, which can be further phyto-supplemented with food concentrates and fruit/vegetable smoothies/juices, provide the greatest dietary density and diversity of phytonutrients which generally have antioxidant and anti-inflammatory effects; also very important is the highly important modulation of gastrointestinal flora by plant-based diets which serves as a major mechanism by which such diets exert their clinically significant systemic anti-inflammatory benefits. I have detailed this diet—"the Supplemented Paleo-Mediterranean diet" as a combination of the "Paleolithic" or "Paleo diet" and the well-known "Mediterranean diet", both of which are well described in peer-reviewed journals and the lay press. (See Chapter 2 and my other publications[22,23] for details). This diet is the most nutrient-dense diet available, and its benefits are further enhanced by supplementation with vitamins, minerals, and the health-promoting fatty acids: ALA, GLA, EPA, DHA, and oleic acid. Vitamin and mineral supplementation is warranted in the general population and even more so among patients[24], who are more likely to be nutrient deficient due to their disease processes, mediations, and concomitant problems such as mild metabolic acidosis, malabsorption, and drug-induced nutrient depletions. Beyond routine vitamin-mineral supplementation, additional vitamin D3 supplementation is generally needed to meet the physiologic requirement of approximately 4,000 IU per day and to achieve the physiologic and clinical benefits including prevention/alleviation of depression, chronic pain, diabetes mellitus, hypertension, immunosuppression, immune activation, and cancer.[25] Likewise, absolute or relative deficiencies/insufficiencies of health-promoting anti-inflammatory fatty acids—namely: ALA, GLA, EPA, DHA, and oleic acid—are common and clinically consequential insofar as these deficiencies/insufficiencies promote chronic/sustained inflammation, pain, and neuroemotional impairment; thus, combination fatty acid therapy/replacement/supplementation (CFAT) is indicated based on its physiological effects and clinical benefits. Probiotics, especially when consumed in conjunction with a plant-based diet which promotes an enhanced milieu for their growth and effect, provide clear clinical benefits which are both local to the gut (e.g., reduced incidence of opportunistic infections/colonizations, prevention/amelioration of increased intestinal permeability) and systemic via the anti-inflammatory benefits of enhanced induction of Treg cells at the reciprocal expense of Th-17 cells. This "supplemented Paleo-Mediterranean diet" obviates overconsumption of chemical preservatives, artificial sweeteners, and carbohydrate-dominant foods such as candies, pastries, breads, potatoes,

---

[21] Conversation and personal communication 2014 Aug with my friend and colleague Mike Ash DO ND, an international expert on probiotics and mucosal immunology, "But some studies suggest 1 billion is the number needed to generate an effect (of clinical relevance), and this may suit a small or young child. I tend to start at 10 billion and rarely ever exceed 90 billion in a day [for adults]."

[22] Vasquez A. A Five-Part Nutritional Protocol that Produces Consistently Positive Results. *Nutritional Wellness* 2005 September

[23] Vasquez A. Implementing the Five-Part Nutritional Wellness Protocol for the Treatment of Various Health Problems. *Nutritional Wellness* 2005 November

[24] "However, suboptimal intake of some vitamins, above levels causing classic vitamin deficiency, is a risk factor for chronic diseases and common in the general population, especially the elderly. ... Most people do not consume an optimal amount of all vitamins by diet alone. Pending strong evidence of effectiveness from randomized trials, it appears prudent for all adults to take vitamin supplements. ... Physicians should make specific efforts to learn about their patients' use of vitamins to ensure that they are taking vitamins they should, ..." Fletcher RH, Fairfield KM. Vitamins for chronic disease prevention in adults: clinical applications. *JAMA*. 2002 Jun 19;287(23):3127-9

[25] Vasquez et al. The clinical importance of vitamin D (cholecalciferol): a paradigm shift. *Altern Ther Health Med*. 2004 Sep-Oct;10(5):28-36

grains, and other foods with a high glycemic load and high glycemic index (from a practical and conceptual standpoint: glycemic load x glycemic index = glycemic impact = more oxidative stress, antioxidant depletion, immunosuppression, and mitochondrial impairment).

- **Supplemented Paleo-Mediterranean diet / Specific Carbohydrate Diet**: The specifications of the *specific carbohydrate diet* (SCD) detailed by Gottschall[26] are met with adherence to the Paleo diet by Cordain.[27] The combination of both approaches and books will give patients an excellent combination of informational understanding and culinary versatility.

- The use of a low starch diet in the treatment of patients suffering from ankylosing spondylitis: alleviation of dysbiosis and immune complex formation via nutritional intervention (*Clin Rheumatol* 1996 Jan[28]): "The majority of ankylosing spondylitis (AS) patients not only possess HLA-B27, but during active phases of the disease have elevated levels of total serum IgA, suggesting that a microbe from the bowel flora is acting across the gut mucosa. .... Furthermore AS patients from 10 different countries have been found to have elevated levels of specific antibodies against Klebsiella bacteria. It has been suggested that these Klebsiella microbes, found in the bowel flora, might be the trigger factors in this disease and therefore reduction in the size of the bowel flora could be of benefit in the treatment of AS patients. Microbes from the bowel flora depend on dietary starch for their growth and therefore a reduction in starch intake might be beneficial in AS patients. A "low starch diet" involving a reduced intake of "bread, potatoes, cakes and pasta" has been devised and tested in healthy control subjects and AS patients. The "low starch diet" leads to a reduction of total serum IgA in both healthy controls as well as patients, and furthermore to a decrease in inflammation and symptoms in the AS patients."

  o Celiac disease and autoimmunity (*J Gastroenterol Hepatol* 2013 Jan[29]): 356 patients with CD participated in this study. "Autoimmune thyroiditis (10.6% vs 0.4%), insulin dependent diabetes mellitus (IDDM) (2.2% vs 1.7%), systemic lupus erythematosus (SLE) (1.1% vs 0), and psoriasis (12.9% vs 5.5%) occurred more frequently in CD patients."

  o Refractory immune thrombocytopenia successfully treated with high-dose vitamin D supplementation and hydroxychloroquine: two case reports (*J Med Case Rep.* 2013 Apr[30]): "In our two case reports, we found an association between vitamin D deficiency and immune thrombocytopenia where platelet levels responded to vitamin D treatment and hydroxychloroquine but not to prednisone. We believe there may be synergism between vitamin D supplementation and hydroxychloroquine."

- **INFECTIONS & DYSBIOSIS** Essentially all autoimmune/rheumatic disorders are associated with microbial colonization and intolerance to same; the presence of persistent microbial colonization is *prima facie* evidence of immunosuppression, commonly due to nutritional deficiencies, psychoemotional stress, sleep deprivation, overconsumption of simple carbohydrates, or—most commonly since all of these are common—a combination of all of these. The eight areas of dysbiosis (multifocal)—listed here from head to toe and inside out—are: ❶ sinorespiratory, ❷ orodental, ❸ gastrointestinal, ❹ urogenital/genitourinary, ❺ parenchymal/tissue, ❻ microbial (dysbiosis within microbes, e.g., bacteriophages), ❼ dermal/cutaneous, and ❽ environmental. Patients with low mucosal sIgA levels, recurrent mucosal infections, or autoimmunity are candidates for serum IgA testing to evaluate for genotropic selective secretory IgA deficiency.

  o Interventions and antimicrobial agents for gastrointestinal dysbiosis:

    - *Saccharomyces boulardii*: A non-colonizing, non-pathogenic yeast that increases sIgA production and can aid in the elimination of pathogenic/dysbiotic yeast, bacteria, and parasites. It is particularly useful during antibiotic treatment to help prevent secondary *Candida* and *Clostridium difficile* infections. Common dose is 250 mg thrice daily for adults and twice daily for children.

---

[26] Gotschall E. *Breaking the Vicious Cycle: Intestinal health though diet*. Kirkton Press; Rev edition (August, 1994) scdiet.com/

[27] Cordain L. *The Paleo Diet*. John Wiley & Sons Inc., New York 2002 thepaleodiet.com/

[28] Ebringer A, Wilson C. The use of a low starch diet in the treatment of patients suffering from ankylosing spondylitis. *Clin Rheumatol*. 1996 Jan;15 Suppl 1:62-66

[29] Iqbal et al. Celiac disease arthropathy and autoimmunity study. *J Gastroenterol Hepatol*. 2013 Jan;28(1):99-105

[30] Bockow et al. Refractory immune thrombocytopenia successfully treated with high-dose vitamin D supplementation and hydroxychloroquine. *J Med Case Rep.* 2013 Apr 4;7:91

- Berberine (generally available as generic berberine hydrochloride or as a plant-based standardized extract with synergistic phytochemicals[31]) 1,000-1,500 mg/d in divided doses PO for up to 3 months: Berberine is a botanical alkaloid extracted from plants such as *Berberis vulgaris,* and *Hydrastis canadensis* with millennia of clinical use for various conditions and also specifically for the treatment of infectious diseases, such as those caused by *E coli, Giardia lamblia* (comparable to metronidazole), *Entamoeba histolytica, Streptococcus* and *Chlamydia trachomatis.*[32] Many clinicians use berberine as a standard treatment for gastrointestinal dysbiosis due to bacteria, yeast, and/or other microbes; it is very safe and has a wide range of antimicrobial action. Oral dose of 400 mg per day has been traditionally common for adults[33]; however newer clinical research has shown that berberine 1,000-1,5000 mg/d for three months provides major clinical benefits and is effective treatment for dyslipidemia, insulin resistance, diabetes mellitus type-2 (comparable to metformin), and overweight/obesity.[34,35,36,37] Berberine is available in a "generic" form from many companies.
- Oregano oil (time-released emulsified preparation named "ADP" from Biotics Research Corporation) 600 mg/d generally given as 200 mg/d PO TID for 6 weeks: Oil of Mediterranean oregano *Oreganum vulgare* was orally administered to 14 adult patients whose stools tested positive for enteric parasites, *Blastocystis hominis, Entamoeba hartmanni* and *Endolimax nana.* Six weeks of supplementation with 600 mg emulsified oil of oregano daily resulted in complete disappearance of *Entamoeba hartmanni* (four cases), *Endolimax nana* (one case), and *Blastocystis hominis* in eight cases. *Blastocystis hominis* scores declined in three additional cases.[38] An *in vitro* study[39] and clinical experience support the use of emulsified oregano against *Candida albicans* and various gastrointestinal microbes. Many clinicians use ADP as a standard treatment for gastrointestinal dysbiosis due to bacteria, yeast, and/or other microbes; it is very safe and has a wide range of antimicrobial action.
- Undecylenic acid (also known as 10-undecenoic acid, available as "Formula SF722" from Thorne Research, each gelcap contains 10-undecenoic acid 50 mg) dosed at "450-750 mg undecylenic acid daily in three divided doses"[40] equates to 10-15 capsules per day, or 5 capsules 2-3 times per day: An eleven-carbon monounsaturated fatty acid found naturally in the body (occurring in sweat) and produced commercially by the vacuum distillation of castor bean oil, undecylenate shows laboratory and clinical human-trial effectiveness against *Herpes Simplex, Candida albicans,* and tinea pedis caused by *Trychophyton rubrumor* and *Trychophyton mentagrophytes.*
- Combination botanical antimicrobials ("Tricycline" from Allergy Research Group; "Dysbiocide" and "FC-Cidal" from Biotics Research Corporation): Tricycline contains black walnut, artemesinin, berberine, and citrus seed extract; in the early days of my clinical practice, I used this product routinely with a standard dosing of 2 capsules BID for 2-4 weeks. Two capsules BID each of Dysbiocide and FC-Cidal for 4 weeks is effective—more effective than rifaxamin—against SIBO.[41]
- DrV's (in)famous "vitamin C purge"—the author's perspective and rationale: Generally when I lecture on the topic of dysbiosis to post-graduate audiences, I mention one of my preferred

[31] Stermitz et al. Synergy in a medicinal plant: antimicrobial action of berberine potentiated by 5'-methoxyhydnocarpin. *Proc Natl Acad Sci U S A.* 2000 Feb 15;97(4):1433-7
[32] [No authors listed]. Berberine. *Altern Med Rev.* 2000 Apr;5(2):175-7
[33] Berberine. *Altern Med Rev.* 2000 Apr;5(2):175-7 thorne.com/altmedrev/.fulltext/5/2/175.pdf
[34] Kong et al. Berberine is a novel cholesterol-lowering drug working through a unique mechanism distinct from statins. *Nat Med.* 2004 Dec;10(12):1344-51
[35] "...obese human subjects (Caucasian) were given 500 mg berberine orally 3 times a day for 12 weeks. ... Results demonstrate that berberine treatment produced mild weight loss (average 5 lb/subject) in obese human subjects. But more interestingly, treatment significantly reduced blood lipid levels (23% decrease of triglyceride and 12.2% decrease of cholesterol levels) in human subjects." Hu et al. Lipid-lowering effect of berberine in human subjects and rats. *Phytomedicine* 2012 Jul;19:861-7
[36] "In study A, 36 adults with newly diagnosed type 2 diabetes mellitus were randomly assigned to treatment with berberine or metformin (0.5 g 3 times a day) in a 3-month trial. The hypoglycemic effect of berberine was similar to that of metformin. Significant decreases in hemoglobin A1c (from 9.5% to 7.5%), fasting blood glucose (from 10.6 mmol/L to 6.9 mmol/L), postprandial blood glucose (from 19.8 to 11.1 mmol/L), and plasma triglycerides (from 1.13 to 0.89 mmol/L) were observed in the berberine group. In study B, 48 adults with poorly controlled type 2 diabetes mellitus were treated supplemented with berberine in a 3-month trial. Berberine acted by lowering fasting blood glucose and postprandial blood glucose from 1 week to the end of the trial. Hemoglobin A1c decreased from 8.1% to 7.3%." Yin J, Xing H, Ye J. Efficacy of berberine in patients with type 2 diabetes mellitus. *Metabolism.* 2008 May;57(5):712-7
[37] "One hundred sixteen patients with type 2 diabetes and dyslipidemia were randomly allocated to receive berberine (1.0 g daily) and the placebo for 3 months. ... In the berberine group, fasting and postload plasma glucose decreased from 7.0 +/- 0.8 to 5.6 +/- 0.9 and from 12.0 +/- 2.7 to 8.9 +/- 2.8 mm/liter, HbA1c from 7.5 +/- 1.0% to 6.6 +/- 0.7%, triglyceride from 2.51 +/- 2.04 to 1.61 +/- 1.10 mm/liter, total cholesterol from 5.31 +/- 0.98 to 4.35 +/- 0.96 mm/liter, and low-density lipoprotein-cholesterol from 3.23 +/- 0.81 to 2.55 +/- 0.77 mm/liter,..." Zhang et al. Treatment of type 2 diabetes and dyslipidemia with the natural plant alkaloid berberine. *J Clin Endocrinol Metab.* 2008 Jul;93(7):2559-65
[38] Force M, Sparks WS, Ronzio RA. Inhibition of enteric parasites by emulsified oil of oregano in vivo. *Phytother Res.* 2000 May;14(3):213-4
[39] Stiles JC, Sparks W, Ronzio RA. The inhibition of Candida albicans by oregano. *J Applied Nutr* 1995;47:96–102
[40] [No authors listed] Undecylenic acid. Monograph. *Altern Med Rev.* 2002 Feb;7(1):68-70
[41] Chedid et al. Herbal therapy is equivalent to rifaximin for the treatment of small intestinal bacterial overgrowth. *Glob Adv Health Med.* 2014 May;3(3):16-24

treatments for GI dysbiosis, for which I seem to be either famous or infamous, namely the "vitamin C purge." The application is essentially as straightforward as the underlying logic: the *per os* use of vitamin C (20-60 grams in 1 liter of water, preferably with two cups of coffee) for its osmotic laxative effect to rapidly reduce the quantity of bacteria/microorganisms throughout the gut by introduction of a cleansing water bolus; while the vitamin C and water serve as an osmotic nonstimulant laxative (perhaps with some antimicrobial effect), the coffee/caffeine serves as a bowel stimulant. I have used this treatment empirically with great success in achieving rapid quantitative reductions in gastrointestinal microbes. For many years plain ascorbic acid was used at doses of 20-60 grams 20,000-60,000 mg) to induce therapeutic laxation (occasionally described as "do-it-yourself top-to-bottom gastrointestinal lavage") with onset of action generally within 30-60 minutes following consumption of powered ascorbate in approximately one liter of water, preferably *and often necessarily* with a bowel peristalsis stimulant such as coffee. The goal and purpose are to achieve a cleansing water bolus that purges the bowels of dysbiotic microbes and their pro-inflammatory debris and mitochondria-impairing metabolites. The use of therapeutic laxatives for the treatment of intestinal parasitic disease is well represented in the Infectous Disease and Tropical Medicine literature; in this instance, we are using ascorbic acid as an osmotic laxative and the coffee as a bowel stimulant. In high concentrations, ascorbic acid is directly microbicidal, at least against *E coli* (per Gaby, c 1993). The vitamin C can be administered as ascorbic acid—perfectly fine but very acidic, Ca/Mg/K buffered ascorbate—same laxative effect with the additional nutritive or laxative effect of minerals, or as home-made buffered ascorbate by mixing—per my own use—one heaping teaspoon or tablespoon of ascorbic acid with 1/2-one teaspoon baking soda (sodium bicarbonate). Additional agents can be ingested simultaneously for additional antimicrobial effect (e.g., iodine-iodide 12-48 mg [given that the standard antimicrobial dose for systemic/dermal infections usually starts at 1,000mg/d]) or intraluminal adsorption (e.g., activated charcoal). Patient selection excludes those who are generally frail and those with renal impairment, cardiac arrhythmia, bowel obstruction, electrolyte imbalance, dementia/psychosis, postural instability and/or reduced mobility to attend the toilet promptly, etc; patients with iron overload are reasonably be excluded—thus serum ferritin should be tested as described in Chapter 1—given that oral vitamin C administration may lead to clinical deterioration in patients with hemochromatosis, per a single case report.[42] As a general rule, the vitamin C purge is initiated only in the morning 1-2 hours before the first meal and is followed later in the day—especially when used for several days consecutively—some effective form of electrolyte replacement, whether in supplemental pill/powder form or as salted vegetable juice; patients can use this treatment PRN, at the beginning of antimicrobial therapy especially to break the vicious cycle of SIBO and resultant GI stasis resulting from microbial methane and H2S, or consecutively; when the latter, periodic assessment of serum electrolytes is reasonable, with one standard interval for monitoring dietary intervention being weekly.

Coffee as a gastrointestinal stimulant

"Coffee stimulates gastrin release and gastric acid secretion... Coffee induces cholecystokinin release and gallbladder contraction... Coffee increases rectosigmoid motor activity within 4 min after ingestion in some people. Its effects on the colon are found to be comparable to those of a 1000 kCal meal. ... Coffee promotes gastro-esophageal reflux, but is not associated with dyspepsia. Coffee stimulates gallbladder contraction and colonic motor activity.

        Boekema et al. Coffee and gastrointestinal function: facts and fiction. *Scand J Gastroenterol*. 1999;230:35-9

"Caffeinated coffee, decaffeinated coffee and meal induced more activity in the colon with a greater area under the curve of pressure waves and a greater number of propagated contractions when compared with water. Caffeinated coffee, decaffeinated coffee and meal induced greater motor activity in the transverse/descending colon when compared with the rectosigmoid colon. ... Caffeinated coffee stimulates colonic motor activity. Its magnitude is similar to a meal, 60% stronger than water and 23% stronger than decaffeinated coffee."

        Rao et al. Is coffee a colonic stimulant? *Eur J Gastroenterol Hepatol*. 1998 Feb;10(2):113-8

---

[42] "We describe rapidly fatal cardiomyopathy in a young man. He had for twelve months ingested large amounts of ascorbic acid and was admitted with severe heart failure having been symptomatic for two months. He died after eight days. Idiopathic haemochromatosis was diagnosed at autopsy." McLaran et al. Congestive cardiomyopathy and haemochromatosis--rapid progression possibly accelerated by excessive ingestion of ascorbic acid. *Aust N Z J Med*. 1982 Apr;12(2):187-8

> ### Laxatives promote eradication of intestinal microbes and are especially useful in patients with stasis/constipation
>
> "Our case shows that although the dose of praziquantel is an important issue, supportive care, including the optimal use of an oral laxative and enemas to ensure smooth evacuation of the worm, is also important. This is especially true for young patients who are usually constipated or who cannot evacuate feces intentionally.
>
> Fujita et al. A 2-year-old girl with Diphyllobothrium nihonkaiense infection treated with oral praziquantel and a laxative. J Nippon Med Sch. 2008 Aug
>
> For irritable bowel syndrome with constipation: "Treatment with osmotic laxatives (milk of magnesia or polyethylene glycol) may increase stool frequency, improve stool consistency, and reduce straining."
>
> Papadakis M, McPhee SJ, Rabow MW (eds). Current Medical Diagnosis and Treatment, 2014

- *Artemisia annua*: Artemisinin has been safely used for centuries in Asia for the treatment of malaria, and it also has effectiveness against anaerobic bacteria due to the pro-oxidative sesquiterpene endoperoxide.[43,44] This author has commonly used artemisinin at 200 mg per day in divided doses for adults with dysbiosis. Given its pro-oxidative mechanism, treatment should probably be of limited duration, i.e., 1-2 months; concomitant neuroprotection with CoQ-10 (et al) would be reasonable.

- St. John's Wort (*Hypericum perforatum*): Hyperforin from *Hypericum perforatum* shows impressive antibacterial action *in vitro*, particularly against gram-positive bacteria such as *Staphylococcus aureus*, *Streptococcus pyogenes*, *Streptococcus agalactiae*[45] and perhaps gram-negative *Helicobacter pylori*.[46] Up to 600 mg three times per day of a 3% hyperforin standardized extract is customary in the treatment of depression.

- Bismuth: Bismuth is commonly used in the empiric treatment of diarrhea (e.g., "Pepto-Bismol") and is commonly combined with other antimicrobial agents to reduce drug resistance and increase antibiotic effectiveness.[47]

- Peppermint *(Mentha piperita)*: Peppermint shows antimicrobial and antispasmodic actions and has demonstrated clinical effectiveness in patients with bacterial overgrowth of the small bowel.

- Commonly used antibiotic/antifungal drugs: The most commonly employed drugs for intestinal bacterial overgrowth are described here.[48] Treatment duration is generally at least 2 weeks and up to 8 weeks, depending on clinical response and the severity and diversity of the intestinal overgrowth. With all anti*bacterial* treatments, use empiric anti*fungal* treatment to prevent yeast overgrowth; some patients benefit from antifungal treatment that is continued for *months* and occasionally *years*. Probiotic yeast and bacteria are generally appropriate except in patients with hypersensitivity, severe immunosuppression, or extreme or recalcitrant bacterial overgrowth of the intestines. Drugs can generally be co-administered with natural antibiotics/antifungals for improved efficacy. Treatment can be guided by identification of the dysbiotic microbes, results of culture and sensitivity tests, and response to treatment. Examples of doses are provided below, but clinicians must choose dose and duration per their judgment, experience, and the patient's situation, comorbidity, age, hepatic and renal function, and accompanying polypharmacy; the use of dosing and drug-interaction data (e.g., *Epocrates*) is strongly recommended.

  - Metronidazole: 250-500 mg BID-QID (generally limit to 1.5-2 g/d); metronidazole has systemic bioavailability and effectiveness against a wide range of dysbiotic microbes, including protozoans, amebas/Giardia, *H. pylori*, *Clostridium difficile* and most anaerobic gram-negative bacilli.[49] Adverse effects are generally limited to stomatitis, nausea, diarrhea, and—rarely and/or with long-term use—peripheral neuropathy, dizziness, and metallic taste; the drug must not be consumed with alcohol. Metronidazole resistance by *Blastocystis hominis* and other parasites has been noted.

  - Erythromycin: 250-500 mg TID-QID; this drug is a widely used antibiotic that also has intestinal promotility benefits (thus making it an ideal treatment for intestinal bacterial overgrowth associated

[43] Dien et al. Effect of food intake on pharmacokinetics of oral artemisinin in healthy Vietnamese subjects. *Antimicrob Agents Chemother.* 1997 May;41(5):1069-72

[44] Giao et al. Artemisinin for treatment of uncomplicated falciparum malaria: is there a place for monotherapy? *Am J Trop Med Hyg.* 2001 Dec;65(6):690-5

[45] Schempp et al. Antibacterial activity of hyperforin from St John's wort, against multiresistant Staphylococcus aureus and gram-positive bacteria. *Lancet.* 1999 Jun 19; 2129

[46] "A butanol fraction of St. John's Wort revealed anti-Helicobacter pylori activity with MIC values ranging between 15.6 and 31.2 microg/ml." Reichling J, Weseler A, Saller R. A current review of the antimicrobial activity of Hypericum perforatum L. *Pharmacopsychiatry.* 2001 Jul;34 Suppl 1:S116-8

[47] Veldhuyzen van Zanten SJ, Sherman PM, Hunt RH. Helicobacter pylori: new developments and treatments. *CMAJ.* 1997;156(11):1565-74 cmaj.ca/cgi/reprint/156/11/1565.pdf

[48] Saltzman JR, Russell RM. Nutritional consequences of intestinal bacterial overgrowth. *Compr Ther.* 1994;20(9):523-30

[49] Tierney ML. McPhee SJ, Papadakis MA. *Current Medical Diagnosis and Treatment 2006. 45th edition.* New York; Lange Medical Books: 2006, pages 1578-1577

with or caused by intestinal dysmotility/hypomotility such as seen in scleroderma[50,51]). Do not combine erythromycin with the promotility drug **cisapride** due to risk for serious cardiac arrhythmia.

- Tetracycline: 250-500 mg QID
- Ciprofloxacin: 500 mg BID, Caution: tendonopathy and tendon rupture can occur within 72 hours; new data connects fluoroquinolone with aortic aneurysm.[52]
- Cephalexin/Keflex: 250 mg QID
- Minocycline: Minocycline (200 mg/day)[53] has received the most attention in the treatment of rheumatoid arthritis due to its superior response (65%) over placebo (13%)[54]; in addition to its antibacterial action, the drug is also immunomodulatory and anti-inflammatory. Ironically, minocycline can cause drug-induced autoimmunity, especially lupus.[55,56]
- Nystatin: Nystatin 500,000 units BID-TID with food; duration of treatment begins with a minimum duration of 2-4 weeks and may continue as long as the patient is deriving benefit.

  o Antiviral (phyto)nutrition: Antiviral therapeutics should include those with the greatest safety, efficacy, synergistic/additive/collateral benefits, most obviously—per my antiviral protocol[57]—1) 5pSPMD discussed previously, 2) vitamin D3 2,000-10,000 IU/d for its tolerogenic (via Treg) and antimicrobial (via AMP) benefits, 3) vitamin A 25,000 IU/d with discussion and monitoring for toxicity; particularly important given the high percentage of (female) patients who cannot effectively convert carotene to retinol, 4) selenium 600 mcg/d to retard viral mutagenesis and replication, 5) melatonin 2-20 mg nightly for antioxidant, immunostimulatory, antiinflammatory, and mitochondrial-protective benefits, 6) NAC 1,500 mg TID for antioxidant, GSH-promoting, anti-mTOR, anti-NFkB and antiviral benefits, to be used with 7) lipoic acid 400 mg TID for antioxidant, GSH-preserving, anti-IL-17, anti-NFkB and antiviral benefits, 8) zinc 20-50 mg/d for immunosupportive, pro-thymulin, anti-NFkB, and direct antiviral effects in its ionized form, 9) glycyrrhizin from licorice—doses of glycyrrhizin in the treatment of human viral diseases can be set at 40 mg per day, 5 mg/kg, or dosed reasonably from tea and supplements with periodic monitoring for hypokalemia and hypertension; the generally accepted safe daily dose of glycyrrhizin is 0.2 mg/kg[58], 10) lysine 2-3 g/d is effective and perhaps specific for HSV infections but may be generalizable for all herpes virus infections; generally, the treatment is administered along with a low-arginine diet but arginine itself is necessary for immunocompetence, 11) additional antiviral treatments include injectable adenosine monophosphate, oral/topical lemon balm (*Melissa officinalis*), and oral/topical lithium.

- **NUTRITIONAL IMMUNOMODULATION** Nutrients and therapeutic approaches that promote Treg or IL-10 induction and/or Th-17, IL-17 suppression include 1) mitochondrial optimization and mTOR suppression, 2) biotin, 3) vitamin E, 4) sodium avoidance, 5) transgenic/GMO food avoidance, 6) probiotics, 7) lipoic acid, 8) vitamin A, 9) inflammation reduction, 10) vitamin D, 11) fatty acid supplementation with GLA and n3, 12) infection and dysbiosis remediation, 13) green tea EGCG. Readers should recall the MiBESTPLAIDFIG acronym outlined in Chapter 4.

---

[50] "Prokinetic agents effective in pseudoobstruction include metoclopramide, domperidone, cisapride, octreotide, and erythromycin. ... The combination of octreotide and erythromycin may be particularly effective in systemic sclerosis." Sjogren RW. Gastrointestinal features of scleroderma. *Curr Opin Rheumatol*. 1996 Nov;8(6):569-75

[51] "Erythromycin accelerates gastric and gallbladder emptying in scleroderma patients and might be helpful in the treatment of gastrointestinal motor abnormalities in these patients." Fiorucci et al. Effect of erythromycin administration on upper gastrointestinal motility in scleroderma patients. *Scand J Gastroenterol* 1994 Sep:807-13

[52] Fluoroquinolone use associated with aortic aneurysm. *Pharmaceutical Journal* 2015 Nov pharmaceutical-journal.com/news-and-analysis/research-briefing/fluoroquinolone-use-associated-with-aortic-aneurysm/20200171.article

[53] "...48-week trial of oral minocycline (200 mg/d) or placebo." Tilley et al. Minocycline in rheumatoid arthritis. A 48-week, double-blind, placebo-controlled trial. MIRA Trial Group. *Ann Intern Med*. 1995 Jan 15;122(2):81-9

[54] "In patients with early seropositive RA, therapy with minocycline is superior to placebo." O'Dell et al. Treatment of early rheumatoid arthritis with minocycline or placebo: results of a randomized, double-blind, placebo-controlled trial. *Arthritis Rheum*. 1997 May;40(5):842-8

[55] "...many cases of drug-induced lupus related to minocycline have been reported. Some of those reports included pulmonary lupus..." Christodoulou et al. Respiratory distress due to minocycline-induced pulmonary lupus. *Chest*. 1999 May;115(5):1471-3 chestjournal.org/cgi/content/full/115/5/1471

[56] Lawson TM, Amos N, Bulgen D, Williams BD. Minocycline-induced lupus: clinical features and response to rechallenge. *Rheumatology* (Oxford). 2001 Mar;40(3):329-35

[57] Chapter 4, Section 2b, "Antiviral Protocol" in *Inflammation Mastery, 4th Edition* (2015) and *Antiviral Strategies and Immune Nutrition: Against Colds, Flu, Herpes, AIDS, Hepatitis, Ebola, Dengue, and Autoimmunity* (2014). Digital book ASIN: B00OPJXMTS; Printed book ISBN: 1502894890

[58] Fiore et al. Antiviral effects of Glycyrrhiza species. *Phytother Res*. 2008 Feb;22(2):141-8

- ○ <u>Altered Th17 cells and Th17/regulatory T-cell ratios indicate the subsequent conversion from undifferentiated connective tissue disease [UCTD] to definitive systemic autoimmune disorders</u> (*Hum Immunol.* 2013 Dec[59]): "Th17-cells were increased in UCTD vs. controls, which further increased in those, whom developed SAIDs eventually. The Th17/nTreg ratio gradually increased from controls through UCTD patients, reaching the highest values in SAID-progressed patients. The derailed Th17/Treg balance may contribute to disease progression therefore could function as a prognostic marker."

- **DYSMETABOLISM & DYSFUNCTIONAL MITOCHONDRIA** The major clinical considerations in this section are mitochondrial dysfunction, endoplasmic reticulum stress, unfolded protein response, TLR activation, and the dysmetabolic effects of sustained hyperglycemia and hyperinsulinemia and resultant oxidative stress, inflammation, RAGE activation, and accumulation of AGE, palmitate and ceramide. The review of this information in Chapter 4 covered approximately 30 interventions relevant to dysmetabolism, mitochondrial dysfunction, ERS-UPR, etc; these will not be reviewed here except to mention those most commonly, easily, empirically, synergistically, and effectively used: 1) low-carbohydrate diet with 2) moderate exercise, 3) CoQ-10, 4) acetyl-carnitine with 5) lipoic acid, 6) NAC, 7) resveratrol, and 8) melatonin.

- **STYLE OF LIVING (LIFESTYLE) & SPECIAL CONSIDERATIONS** This is a buffet of mostly lifestyle-based interventions yet also including: sleep optimization, sociopsychology, stress management/avoidance, somatic/spinal treatments, special supplementation, sweat/exercise, sauna/detoxification, surgery, stamp your passport and vacate current reality, and sensory deprivation therapy.

- **ENDOCRINE IMBALANCE & OPTIMIZATION** Common hormonal imbalances seen among autoimmune/inflammatory patients and which contribute to the genesis and perpetuation of these same autoimmune/inflammatory diseases are easily assessed with standard serum laboratory measurements; conveniently, three hormones tend to be elevated, and three tend to be reduced: ❶ *elevated* prolactin, ❷ *elevated* estrogen, ❸ *elevated* insulin—as a surrogate marker (insulin itself actually appears to have an anti-inflammatory effect, counteracting the effect of excess glucose; however the net effect of hyperglycemia-hyperinsulinemia is conclusively pathogenic) for excess carbohydrate intake, insufficient exercise, sarcopenia, mitochondrial dysfunction, nutrient deficiencies, xeobiotic exposure, palmitate and ceramide accumulation, etc, ❹ *reduced* DHEA, ❺ *reduced* cortisol, and ❻ *reduced* testosterone; see Chapter 4 for discussion of these hormones and respective interventions. Thyroid evaluation (history + exam + labs + response to treatment) should be comprehensive, as discussed in Chapter 1, with a low threshold for empiric treatment.

- **XENOBIOTIC ACCUMULATION & DETOXIFICATION** The clinical relevance and pathogenic mechanisms of xenobiotic accumulation are irrefutably well documented and described. Population-wide toxin accumulation results from corporate irresponsibility and government collusion with industry via lax regulations; at times the situation is so grave that one might wonder if corporations and government are intentionally trying to poison the population (e.g., glyphosate application to water supply, rivers, and population-wide food despite consistently documented adverse effects[60]). These persistent organic pollutants (POPs) promote disease primarily via mitochondrial dysfunction and endoplasmic reticulum stress (thus directly promoting ATP production failure, oxidative injury, insulin resistance, antioxidant nutrient depletion, inflammation and promotion of Treg/Th-17 imbalance) and via additional immunogenic effects including bystander activation and haptenization—see discussion and review in Chapter 4. Clinical assessments include history, physical examination, and laboratory assessment (using serum, whole blood, urine or—rarely yet accurately—fat biopsy), and response to treatment. Treatments include nutritional support for Phases 1 and 2 of detoxification (e.g., oxidation and conjugation) and excretion via bile and urine; for the latter, urinary alkalinization is generally recommended. Chemical toxins can be bound in the gut using activated charcoal[61],

---

[59] Szodoray et al. Altered Th17 cells and Th17/regulatory T-cell ratios indicate the subsequent conversion from undifferentiated connective tissue disease to definitive systemic autoimmune disorders. *Hum Immunol.* 2013 Dec;74(12):1510-8

[60] Krüger et al. Detection of glyphosate residues in animals and humans. *J Environ Anal Toxicol* 2014, 4:2 omicsonline.org/open-access/detection-of-glyphosate-residues-in-animals-and-humans-2161-0525.1000210.pdf

[61] Goel et al. Pesticide poisoning. *Nat Med J India* 2007:20;182-191

cholestyramine[62], or Chlorella (6 g/d [2g TID cc] taken after breakfast, lunch, and dinner)[63]—all of these three treatments have documented safety and effectiveness; clinically and empirically, phytochelatin (plant-derived peptides that bind toxic metals[64]) concentrates appear safe and effective despite lack of conclusive published data supporting clinical use.

- o Chlorella pyrenoidosa on fecal excretion and liver accumulation of polychlorinated dibenzo-p-dioxin in mice. (*Chemosphere* 2005 Apr[65]): "Among mice fed the 10% *C. pyrenoidosa* diet, cumulative fecal excretion of H6CDD over the first week following administration was significantly greater (9.2-fold) than that observed among mice fed the basal diet. Moreover, excretion during the fifth week following administration of H6CDD was still significantly greater (3.1-fold) among mice fed the 10% C. pyrenoidosa diet than among mice fed the basal diet. Five weeks after administration of H6CDD, liver accumulation of H6CDD in mice fed the 10% C. pyrenoidosa diet was significantly less than that observed among mice fed either the basal diet and the Spinach diet (by 27.9% and 34.8%, respectively). These findings suggest that C. pyrenoidosa may be useful in inhibiting the absorption of dioxins via food and the reabsorption of dioxins stored already in the body in the intestinal tract, thus preventing accumulation of dioxins within the body."

- o Chlorella (Chlorella pyrenoidosa) supplementation decreases dioxin and increases immunoglobulin a concentrations in breast milk (*J Med Food* 2007 Mar[66]): "The present results suggest that Chlorella supplementation not only reduces dioxin levels in breast milk, but may also have beneficial effects on nursing infants by increasing IgA levels in breast milk."

- o Maternal-fetal distribution and transfer of dioxins in pregnant women in Japan, and attempts to reduce maternal transfer with Chlorella (Chlorella pyrenoidosa) supplements (*Chemosphere* 2005 Dec[67]): "Concentrations of 28 dioxin (polychlorinated dibenzo-p-dioxins, polychlorinated dibenzofurans, and co-planar polychlorinated biphenyls) congeners in blood, adipose tissue, breast milk, cord blood and placenta collected from 44 pregnant Japanese women were measured. ... Correlations were observed between dioxin total toxic equivalents (total TEQ) in blood and total TEQ in adipose tissue (r=0.913, P<0.0001), breast milk (r=0.695, P=0.0007), and cord blood (r=0.759, P<0.0001). Dioxin levels transferred to fetuses and nursing infants reflect cumulative maternal concentrations of dioxins. ... Total TEQ in breast milk were approximately 30% lower in the Chlorella group than in controls. This finding suggests that maternal transfer of dioxins can be reduced using dietary measures such as Chlorella supplements."

> **Corporate-derived government-enabled pollution: Now broadly acknowledged as a major contributor to disease and rising healthcare expenses**
>
> Humans in the general population worldwide have become living repositories for industrial pollutants and environmental contaminants, generally referred to in contemporary literature as POPs—persistent organic pollutants. POP retention/accumulation is causatively associated with induction of insulin resistance and the resulting hyperinsulinemia and hyperglycemia via suppression of GLUT-4 receptor expression via xenobiotic-induced activation of the aryl hydrocarbon receptor. Additively or synergistically, POP-induced mitochondrial dysfunction retards insulin secretion from the pancreas and insulin reception in the periphery, thereby synergizing to create the essential pathophysiology that characterizes type-2 diabetes.
>
> "Health care spending in the U.S. has surged more than eightfold since the 1960s. Skyrocketing in that same time: Rates of chronic disease, use of synthetic chemicals, and evidence that many of these widely used substances may be wreaking havoc on human health. ... The use of bisphenol A, or BPA, in food and beverage containers, according to the study, is responsible for an estimated $3 billion a year in costs associated with childhood obesity and adult heart disease."
>
> Peeples L. BPA among Toxic Chemicals Driving Up Health Care Costs. 2014 Jan huffingtonpost.com/2014/01/22/bpa-health-care-costs_n_4644372.html

---

[62] Cohn WJ et al. Treatment of chlordecone (Kepone) toxicity with cholestyramine. Results of a controlled clinical trial. *N Engl J Med.* 1978 Feb 2;298(5):243-8

[63] Nakano S, Takekoshi H, Nakano M. Chlorella (Chlorella pyrenoidosa) supplementation decreases dioxin and increases immunoglobulin a concentrations in breast milk. *J Med Food.* 2007 Mar;10(1):134-42. Nakano S, Noguchi T, Takekoshi H, Suzuki G, Nakano M. Maternal-fetal distribution and transfer of dioxins in pregnant women in Japan, and attempts to reduce maternal transfer with Chlorella (Chlorella pyrenoidosa) supplements. *Chemosphere.* 2005 Dec;61(9):1244-55

[64] Cobbett CS. Phytochelatin biosynthesis and function in heavy-metal detoxification. *Current Opinion in Plant Biology* 2000, 3:211–216. Cobbett CS. Phytochelatins and their roles in heavy metal detoxification. *Plant Physiology* 2000 Jul; 825–832. Readers should have noticed that these are plant physiology journals—not clinical journals. These articles substantiate that phytochelatins are plant-produced metal-binding peptides; in clinical practice, extracts from certain vegetables rich in phytochelatins are used to bind heavy metals in the gut to reduce absorption and enterohepatic recirculation and promote fecal excretion, in a manner analogous to that of cholestyramine and chlorella.

[65] Takekoshi et al. Effect of Chlorella pyrenoidosa on fecal excretion and liver accumulation of polychlorinated dibenzo-p-dioxin in mice. *Chemosphere.* 2005 Apr;59(2):297-304

[66] Nakano et al. Chlorella pyrenoidosa supplementation decreases dioxin and increases immunoglobulin a concentrations in breast milk. *J Med Food.* 2007 Mar;10(1):134-42

[67] Nakano et al. Maternal-fetal distribution and transfer of dioxins in pregnant women in Japan, and attempts to reduce maternal transfer with Chlorella (Chlorella pyrenoidosa) supplements. *Chemosphere.* 2005 Dec;61(9):1244-55

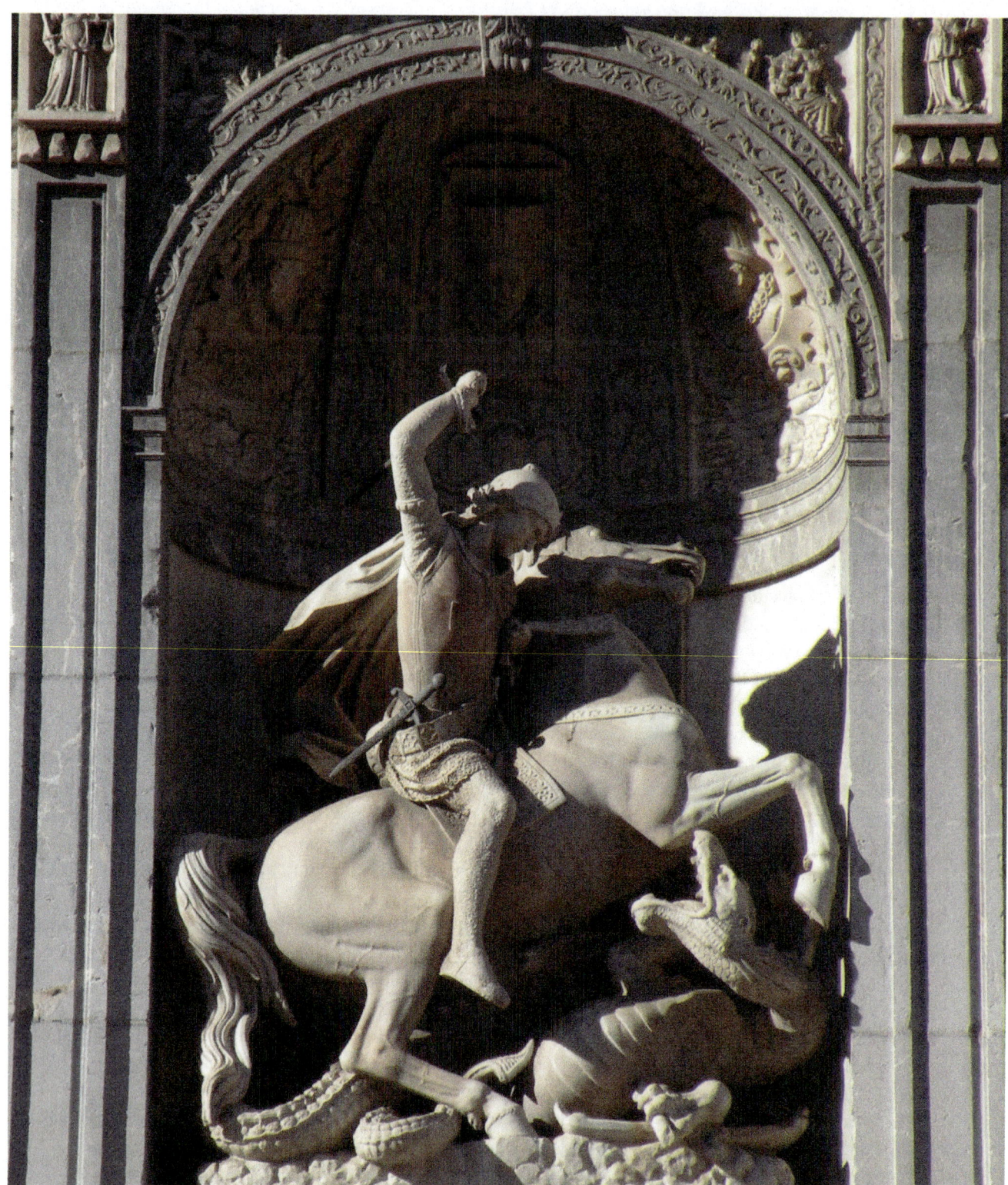

Palau de la Generalitat de Catalunya: In Western societies, one of the dominating paradigms has been that of "man versus nature", which is commonly represented in history, myth, and art as humanity's combat with and attempts at dominance over nature, commonly viewed as hostile or at the very least mysterious, therefore unknown, therefore uncontrollable. As such, nature—despite its beauty and life-giving properties—is often represented as monstrous and demonic, as in the sculpture above. We continue to see this "combat" in science and medicine. Especially in Western/pharmacocentric medicine, the body is depicted as chaotic and in need of outside control and "medical management", and diseases are described as "idiopathic"—from an unknown source. Indeed, Western medicine is full of its own myths, not appreciated as such, which continue to drive thought and action. Wiser approaches to both life and medicine encourage synergy, acceptance, nurturance, and orchestration rather than attempts to outwardly dominate and artificially—and therefore temporarily—control. Photo and caption by DrV, 2016.

High Blood Pressure (HBP) & Hypertension (HTN)

Introduction:

This section reviews clinically relevant information related to chronic hypertension—its cause(s), its social and economic impacts, selected aspects of its pathophysiology and complications, differential diagnosis, assessments, overall management and specific treatments. This chapter is a stand-alone clinical monograph detailing the clinical considerations and etiologic contributors necessary for an accurate multidimensional grasp of this phenomenon and its effective management, both at the level of the individual patient and also at the level of public health and population-wide disease prevention. This chapter also includes the most (or at least one of the most) comprehensive list of differential diagnoses for hypertension that has ever been published. An easy-to-implement clinical approach rooted in the functional inflammology FINDSEX® protocol is detailed, followed by an overview of drug treatments, followed by additional considerations and previously published articles. Throughout, emphasis is placed—not on simply clinical accuracy, therapeutic efficacy, and patient safety—but on the patient-centered rather than disease-centered goal of the best possible outcome for the patient, which is health preservation and optimization, not simply the lowering of arterial pressure.

Treatment options reviewed include drugs, diet, lifestyle, metabolic modifications such as weight loss and improvement in insulin sensitivity, nutritional supplementation, manipulative therapeutics and surgical treatment for the alleviation of medullary neurovascular compression. Recent updates to the clinical approach include the focus on alleviating mitochondrial dysfunction and the restoration of immune and inflammatory balance via nutritional immunomodulation; these newer considerations are clearly relevant for the treatment of hypertension as an isolated finding and are even more relevant for the treatment of cardiometabolic syndrome, of which hypertension is merely one component.

Clearly, most of the non-drug non-surgery treatments reviewed here are natural, non-patentable, and widely available; they work with the body's physiology to improve metabolic function and to thereby improve overall health and cardiovascular, endothelial, endocrine and neuroregulatory homeodynamics. As with most nutritional and natural interventions, side-effects are minimal, and collateral benefits are many; therefore, as overall health improves, various complaints and disorders are alleviated, vitality is enhanced, and patient compliance increases while the need for medical management of other issues decreases.

A quantitative compilation can effect a qualitative transformation in the reader's perception of the nature of the disease and its place in clinical care and healthcare policy; such is the goal of this section on ~~chronic~~ *sustained* hypertension. The strength of the evidence supporting this disease model and the treatment approach is consistent, robust, and much more attractive—both clinically and intellectually—than is the ascribing of hypertension to some "idiopathic" cause which somehow evades biomedical science and the collective human intellect except for the extent to which it allows itself to be appropriately targeted by population-wide polypharmacy. Hypertension is only "chronic" when its causes are ignored and/or not effectively treated; as such, a more accurate descriptor is "sustained." This review of contributors to ~~chronic~~ *sustained* hypertension will provide patients and clinicians a conceptual and factual framework from which to perceive and address the causes of sustained elevations in arterial pressure.

Sustained hypertension is a major risk factor for cardiovascular disease, exacerbated by hyperglycemia and other metabolic factors such as hypercholesterolemia and hyperhomocysteinaemia, all of which are reviewed in the following section on diabetes, obesity, and insulin resistance.

Description, Pathophysiology, and Key Concepts:

- <u>Sustained/chronic high blood pressure—the most common clinical diagnosis</u>: High blood pressure (chronic hypertension) is the most common disease diagnosis encountered in clinical practice worldwide. As such, the diagnosis and successful integrative management of chronic hypertension represents an opportunity for clinicians to achieve higher levels of practice success and for patients to receive the healthcare that they need. In America, 30% of adults have hypertension. For those of us specializing in adult healthcare, these hypertensive adults in the population can be thought of as belonging to two categories: ❶ patients receiving comprehensive integrative functional medicine care (very small minority), and ❷ patients who are either undiagnosed, untreated, or treated only with drugs and therefore in need of comprehensive integrative functional medicine care for optimal hypertension management, disease prevention, and wellness promotion (the vast majority of hypertensive patients).

  Most hypertensive patients have no symptoms of their disorder and are therefore reliant upon a competent clinician to reveal the problem and to provide the appropriate education and the motivation to initiate and maintain compliance with treatment. Clinicians have the responsibility to detect and effectively manage high blood pressure. High blood pressure accelerates the development of cardiovascular disease and additional complications including stroke, heart attack (myocardial infarction), heart failure, renal failure, blindness, peripheral vascular disease and endothelial dysfunction which can contribute to (for example) lower leg amputation and sexual dysfunction[1] in both men and women.

Clinicians have three core responsibilities related to hypertension management. First, the condition must be diagnosed by the clinician; this is a simple physical exam procedure. Second, the patient must be assessed for underlying causes and disease complications. Third, the patient must be enrolled in a treatment program to ensure proper lowering of elevated pressures; this is best accomplished with diet optimization, nutritional supplementation, therapeutic lifestyle changes, spinal manipulation, and—rarely—use of medications.

- Overview and perspective: The emphasis of this section will be the integrative management of so-called "primary" or "essential" hypertension (HTN), which is generally considered "idiopathic" from an outdated medical perspective that has failed to appreciate and integrate the research that has clarified the numerous causes of and contributors to HTN. From the allopathic medical perspective, >90-95% of HTN is considered idiopathic and thus by definition "of no known cause" and therefore appropriate for treatment with drugs. Most (more than 70%) medically managed patients with HTN take two or more antihypertensive drugs from the time of diagnosis until the end of their lives; these drugs commonly cause adverse effects, are relatively devoid of collateral benefits, and do not address the underlying causative physiologic imbalances. Patients managed with nutritional and lifestyle modifications must likewise remain compliant with the prescribed health-promoting treatment-diet-lifestyle, but they generally experience clinically and statistically meaningful collateral benefits; for example, ❶ correction of vitamin D deficiency can alleviate hypertension[2] and musculoskeletal pain[3] while improving mood[4,5]; ❷ fish oil supplementation slightly lowers blood pressure but tremendously and safely lowers cardiovascular mortality and all-cause mortality[6] while also improving mental health[7] and alleviating pain and inflammation[8,9]; ❸ CoQ10 is very effective for the treatment of HTN[10] while also restoring lost renal function[11,12], alleviating migraine headaches[13], and helping to control asthma.[14] The exemplary nutritional interventions listed in the previous sentence are virtually devoid of adverse effects when employed with a modicum of competence, and each of these natural and nonpatentable interventions is widely available. Furthermore, **their clinical benefit (in this case, the reduction of elevated blood pressure) is derived from their ability to restore proper physiologic function** rather than—as with most pharmaceutical drugs—the blockade of normal physiology. If the routine outpatient medical treatment of HTN were to shift away from synthetic chemical drugs that function by interfering with normal physiology (e.g., beta-adrenergic

---

[1] "Available data indicate that essential hypertension is a risk factor for sexual dysfunction, as male and female sexual dysfunction is more prevalent in hypertensive patients than normotensive individuals. Several mechanisms have been implicated in the pathogenesis of sexual dysfunction in hypertensive patients, and major determinants include severity and duration of hypertension, age, and antihypertensive therapy. Female sexual dysfunction, although more frequent than its male counterpart, remains largely under-recognized." Manolis A, Doumas M. Sexual dysfunction: the 'prima ballerina' of hypertension-related quality-of-life complications. *J Hypertens.* 2008 Nov;26(11):2074-84

[2] "A short-term supplementation with vitamin D(3) and calcium is more effective in reducing SBP than calcium alone. Inadequate vitamin D(3) and calcium intake could play a contributory role in the pathogenesis and progression of hypertension and cardiovascular disease in elderly women." Pfeifer et al. Effects of a short-term vitamin D(3) and calcium supplementation on blood pressure and parathyroid hormone levels in elderly women. *J Clin Endocrinol Metab.* 2001 Apr;86(4):1633-7

[3] "Findings showed that 83% of the study patients (n = 299) had an abnormally low level of vitamin D before treatment with vitamin D supplements. After treatment, clinical improvement in symptoms was seen in all the groups that had a low level of vitamin D, and in 95% of all the patients (n = 341). CONCLUSIONS: Vitamin D deficiency is a major contributor to chronic low back pain in areas where vitamin D deficiency is endemic." Al Faraj S, Al Mutairi K. Vitamin D deficiency and chronic low back pain in Saudi Arabia. *Spine.* 2003;28:177-9

[4] Vieth R, Kimball S, Hu A, Walfish PG. Randomized comparison of the effects of the vitamin D3 adequate intake versus 100 mcg (4000 IU) per day on biochemical responses and the wellbeing of patients. *Nutrition Journal* 2004, 3:8 nutritionj.com/content/3/1/8

[5] Lansdowne AT, Provost SC: Vitamin D3 enhances mood in healthy subjects during winter. *Psychopharmacology* (Berl) 1998, 135:319-323

[6] GISSI-Prevenzione Investigators. Dietary supplementation with n-3 polyunsaturated fatty acids and vitamin E after myocardial infarction: results of the GISSI-Prevenzione trial. Gruppo Italiano per lo Studio della Sopravvivenza nell'Infarto miocardico. *Lancet.* 1999 Aug 7;354(9177):447-55

[7] Peet M, Stokes C. Omega-3 fatty acids in the treatment of psychiatric disorders. *Drugs.* 2005;65(8):1051-9

[8] Maroon JC, Bost JW. Omega-3 fatty acids (fish oil) as anti-inflammatory: alternative to nonsteroidal anti-inflammatory drugs for discogenic pain. *Surg Neurol.* 2006 Apr:326-31

[9] "Many of the placebo-controlled trials of fish oil in chronic inflammatory diseases reveal significant benefit, including decreased disease activity and a lowered use of anti-inflammatory drugs." Simopoulos AP. Omega-3 fatty acids in inflammation and autoimmune diseases. *J Am Coll Nutr.* 2002 Dec;21(6):495-505

[10] Singh et al. Hydrosoluble coenzyme Q10 on blood pressures and insulin resistance in hypertensive patients with coronary artery disease. *J Hum Hypertens* 1999 Mar;13:203-8

[11] Singh et al. Randomized, double-blind placebo-controlled trial of coenzyme Q10 in chronic renal failure: discovery of a new role. *J Nutr Environ Med* 2000;10:281-8

[12] Singh et al. Randomized, Double-blind, Placebo-controlled Trial of Coenzyme Q10 in Patients with Endstage Renal Failure. *J Nutr Environ Med* 2003; 13 (1): 13–22

[13] Rozen et al. Open label trial of coenzyme Q10 as a migraine preventive. *Cephalalgia* 2002;22(2):137-41

[14] Gvozdjáková et al. Coenzyme Q10 supplementation reduces corticosteroids dosage in patients with bronchial asthma. *Biofactors.* 2005;25(1-4):235-40

blockers, calcium channel *blockers*, ACE *inhibitors*, angiotensin-2 receptor *blockers*, etc) and toward the favor of natural treatments—diet optimization, body weight reduction/optimization, and evidence-based nutritional supplementation—that promote normalization of blood pressure by helping restore balance to the body's physiology (i.e., by facilitating the restoration of homeostasis), then meaningful and authentic progress in the otherwise never-ending "fight against hypertension" would be made. (For more discussion, see "Thinking Outside the (Pill) Box" at the end of this chapter.)

> **"Prehypertension" is deadly: mortality increases starting at 115/75 mm Hg**
>
> "Hypertension-related diseases are the leading causes of morbidity and mortality in industrially developed societies. Surprisingly, **68% of all mortality attributed to high blood pressure (BP) occurs with systolic BP between 120 and 140 mm Hg and diastolic BP below 90 mm Hg.** Dietary and lifestyle modifications are effective in the treatment of borderline hypertension."
>
> Goldhamer et al. Medically supervised water-only fasting in the treatment of borderline hypertension. *J Altern Complement Med.* 2002 Oct

- <u>Blood pressure and mortality</u>: Increased risk for cardiovascular mortality begins with blood pressures that are still well within the accepted normal range; therefore blood pressure that is consistent with an official diagnosis of hypertension—blood pressure consistently greater than 140 mm Hg systolic and/or greater than 90 mm Hg diastolic—is clearly worthy of treatment if part of the clinical goal is—*as it should be*—to reduce unnecessary morbidity and early mortality. Benowitz[15] wrote, "Starting at 115/75 mm Hg, cardiovascular risk doubles with each increment of 20/10 mm Hg throughout the blood pressure range." Thus, from both *wellness-centered* as well as *disease-prevention* perspectives, pro-active integrative clinicians can define mild HTN as > 115/75 mm Hg. Data from the Framingham study showed that sustained BP > 140/90 induces left ventricular hypertrophy.[16] A reduction of systolic BP (sBP) of -5 mm Hg correlates with a -7% reduction in cardiovascular mortality[17]; thus, patients must be encouraged to take HTN and its effective treatment seriously, since even small numerical decrements in BP can have impressive ameliorating effects on the risk for cardiovascular complications. Except in younger age groups, sBP is more predictive of adverse cardiovascular outcomes than is diastolic BP. Systolic hypertension indicates the presence of vascular abnormalities including reductions in elasticity/compliance of large and medium arteries; thus, the finding of systolic HTN simultaneously indicates *current* vascular abnormalities and *future* cardiovascular disease (CV) risk elevation.

> **Affective interpretations: emotional needs influence intellectual perspectives**
>
> "...to see differently in this way for once, to *want* to see differently, is no small discipline and preparation of the intellect for its future "objectivity"—the latter understood not as "contemplation without interest" (which is a nonsensical absurdity), but as the ability *to control* one's Pro and Con and to dispose of them, so that one knows how to employ a *variety* of perspectives and *affective interpretations* in the service of knowledge."
>
> Nietzsche FW. <u>*Genealogy of Morals*</u>, 1887. Essay #3, section #12.

- <u>Hypertension and vascular disease</u>: Sustained HTN accelerates the development of CVD and end-organ damage by several mechanisms including promotion of endothelial damage resulting in accelerated atherosclerosis (e.g., stroke, myocardial infarction, peripheral vascular disease), direct pressure (e.g., retinal hemorrhages, aortic aneurysm), hyperplastic arteriolosclerosis and occlusive vasculopathy due to smooth muscle proliferation, fibrosis, and hyaline deposition (e.g., hypertensive nephrosclerosis), interstitial edema (e.g., cerebral edema, peripheral edema), and pathologic myocardial adaptation (e.g., hypertrophic cardiomyopathy, hypertensive heart disease, congestive heart failure). Hyperplastic arteriolosclerosis causes hypertensive nephrosclerosis, characterized by renal ischemia which triggers release of renin and increased formation of angiotensin-2 which exacerbates renal ischemia and systemic hypertension.[18]

- <u>Medical physiology-pharmacology of hypertension</u>: Drug treatment of hypertension must have some physiologic basis, even if this basis is simplistic, limited, and outdated by current research and emerging paradigms that might surpass and supplant previous and well entrenched models. In the medical/allopathic paradigm, "physiology" must be tailored to support pharmacology, since the latter is the profession's primary intervention. Thus, the study of physiology must be made to fit pharmacology by limiting the variables

---

[15] Benowitz NL. "Antihypertensive Agents." In Katzung BG (editor). <u>*Basic and Clinical Pharmacology. 10th Edition*</u>. New York: McGraw Hill Medical; 2007, 159

[16] Kumar V, Abbas AK, Fausto N (Editors). <u>*Robbins and Cotran Pathologic Basis of Disease. 7th Edition*</u>. Philadelphia: Elsevier; 2005, 587

[17] Nahas R. Complementary and alternative medicine approaches to blood pressure reduction: An evidence-based review. *Can Fam Physician*. 2008 Nov;54(11):1529-33

[18] Kumar V, Abbas AK, Fausto N (Editors). <u>*Robbins and Cotran Pathologic Basis of Disease. 10th Edition*</u>. Philadelphia: Elsevier; 2005, 1007-8

considered to those which are amenable to drug intervention. Thus, per medical pharmacology textbooks[19], the primary variables considered for the support of antihypertensive pharmacotherapy are ❶ cardiac output ("to be controlled with beta-blockers"), ❷ peripheral resistance ("to be treated with vasodilators such as ACEi and CCB"), and ❸ blood volume ("to be reduced by the first-line use of diuretics"). While this perspective is necessarily limited in the service of the medical paradigm, it is also useful for provisionally grasping a view of some of the key factors involved in blood pressure regulation, including those that are relevant for drug intervention in the acute care setting as well as the long-term nondrug treatment of HTN. Given that this text details the "functional" and "integrative" management of HTN and must therefore provide a variety of perspectives, a concise review of medical physiology is appropriate. The medical paradigm views

> ### Antihypertensive drugs function by blocking *normal* physiology (rather than by *correcting* dysfunctional physiology)
>
> "All antihypertensive [drugs]... produce their effects by interfering with normal mechanisms of blood pressure regulation."
>
> Benowitz NL. "Antihypertensive Agents." In Katzung BG (editor). *Basic and Clinical Pharmacology. Tenth Edition*. New York: McGraw Hill Medical; 2007, p159
>
> "In Western medicine, because of the prevailing mechanistic view, we treat our bodies as dumb machines. We move in with surgery and drugs to make them do what we want [a reflection of the *power-over model*, or the *control paradigm*], bypassing strategies that support the body's capacity to solve its own problems, learn, and regenerate itself."
>
> Breton D, Largent C. *The paradigm conspiracy: why our social systems violate human potential and how we can change them*. Hazelden Publishing; 1998, pages 147-148

most HTN as idiopathic and "somehow" resulting from a complex dysregulation of normal physiology; thereby, the "appropriate" intervention is to interfere with the normal physiologic mechanisms that have gone astray. One interconnecting theme in this paradigm is that of activation of the sympathetic nervous system by some unknown insult or combination thereof. Whether due to "stress", faulty disinhibition of baroreceptors in the aortic arch, carotid sinuses, or renal juxtaglomerular cells, sympathetic activation increases cardiac output via increased rate and contractility, increases peripheral resistance via vasoconstriction, and increases blood volume via aldosterone-enhanced sodium retention. The enzyme renin converts angiotensinogen into angiotensin-1, which is converted via angiotensin converting enzyme (ACE) into angiotensin-2, which is a powerful vasoconstrictor and trigger for the release of aldosterone, which promotes sodium reabsorption and thus sodium-water retention. With this simple and simplistic model, one can grasp the rationale employed for antihypertensive pharmacotherapeutics as well as some of the natural and *eu*physiologic[20] interventions detailed in this text; drug treatments for HTN are detailed toward the end of this chapter.

- Acceleration of atherogenesis and atherosclerosis: HTN is the single most important risk factor for the development of CVD. On a population-wide basis, achieving the target of ≤ 140 mmHg systolic would result in a 28-44% reduction in stroke and a 20-35% reduction in ischemic heart disease (IHD). In describing these benefits for the United Kingdom (population ~60 million in 2005), Tomson and Lip[21] noted in 2005 that control of HTN would prevent approximately 42,800 strokes and 82,800 IHD events per year.
- Basic pathology: Reviewed here are several of the more direct and salient effects of high blood pressure on important organs, the most relevant of which are brain, eye, heart, and kidney.
  - Brain—intracerebral hemorrhage, lacunar infarcts, slit hemorrhages, hypertensive encephalopathy: HTN can cause intracerebral hemorrhage and cerebellar hemorrhage. Arteriolar sclerosis of small vessels can lead to ischemia of the basal ganglia, cerebral white matter, and brainstem. Cavitary lacunar ("lake-like") infarcts classically affect the lenticular nucleus, thalamus, internal capsule, caudate nucleus, and pons. Rupture of small vessels can leave a slit-like cavity of discoloration, cell destruction, and gliosis termed a *slit hemorrhage*. Hypertensive encephalopathy presents with headache, confusion, vomiting, seizure, and/or coma; cerebral edema, petechiae, and transtentorial or tonsillar herniation may be noted at autopsy.[22]
  - Eye—ocular vascular disease and hypertensive retinopathy: Hypertensive sclerosis of arteries and arterioles serving the eye results in the "copper wire" then "silver wire" fundoscopic changes that occur as

---

[19] Harvey RA, Champe PC (eds). *Lippincott's Illustrated Reviews: Pharmacology, 3rd Edition*. Philadelphia, Lippincott Williams and Wilkins; 1997

[20] The prefix "eu" means good or beneficial. The term "euphysiologic" was used more commonly in medical literature of the early 1900's than it is today. Here, euphysiologic means "properly-working physiology" or "beneficial to physiology" in contrast to interventions that are contrary to normal physiology ("antiphysiologic" or—per Greenblatt [*Obstet Gynecol Clin North Am*. 1987;14:251-68]—"contraphysiologic") such as enzyme-blocking drugs which have their therapeutic and adverse effects by working against normal physiology and enzyme function.

[21] Tomson J, Lip GY. Blood pressure demographics: nature or nurture...genes or environment? *BMC Med*. 2005;3:3 biomedcentral.com/1741-7015/3/3

[22] Frosch et al. "Chapter 28: Central nervous system." in Kumar, Abbas, Fausto (eds). *Robins and Cotran Pathologic Basis of Disease. 7th Edition*. Elsevier; 2005, 1368-1369

the arteriole wall thickens and obscures visualization of luminal blood. Within the nerve fiber layer of the retina, "cotton-wool spots" are infarcts, and "flame hemorrhages" are due to vascular rupture. Retinal exudates secondary to vascular leak due to severe hypertension may induce retinal detachment and acute vision loss. Occlusion of retinal arterioles causes retinal infarction.[23]

- **Heart—hypertensive cardiomyopathy and cardiac hypertrophy**: HTN increases the work demands placed on the heart and leads to myocyte hypertrophy followed by altered proportions of cardiac anatomy as well as functional abnormalities: left atrial enlargement leads to conduction defects such as atrial fibrillation; ventricular walls thicken and encroach upon intraventricular volume leading to reduced ejection volume. Adaptations to chronically increased blood pressure lead to alterations in cardiac anatomy, histology, physiology, and gene expression that—if persistent and progressive—eventually culminate in cardiac failure.[24] Acute-onset hypertension can induce oxygen/nutrient delivery-demand mismatch resulting in myocardial infarction.

- **Kidney—malignant hypertension and accelerated nephrosclerosis**: Malignant hypertension—the full syndrome of which includes diastolic pressure > 130 mm Hg, papilledema/retinopathy, encephalopathy, renal failure, and cardiovascular complications—occurs in 1-5% of hypertensive patients; it is more common in patients who are male, young, and of African descent. Risk factors include pre-existing chronic hypertension (whether primary or secondary), scleroderma, and preexisting renal disease such as reflux nephropathy or glomerulonephritis. The main pathophysiologic sequence appears to include intrarenal vascular damage followed by vascular occlusion secondary to intimal smooth muscle hypertrophy and hyperplastic arteriolosclerosis; eventually this leads to renal hypoperfusion and ischemia. Renal hypoperfusion, besides leading to azotemia and oliguria in acute severe hypertension, leads to activation of the renin-angiotensin-aldosterone system (RAAS) which leads to additional vasoconstriction and the cascade of events (including sodium and water retention) which leads to further elevations in blood pressure. Histologic changes in the kidney include fibrinoid necrosis of the arterioles, hyperplastic arteriolitis, intrarenal arterial thrombosis, and glomerular necrosis.[25]

- **Treatment-resistant hypertension**: "Resistant hypertension" was defined in a December 2010 review as "elevated blood pressure despite patient adherence to optimal dosages of three antihypertensive agents, including a diuretic."[26]

- **Obesity, type-2 diabetes mellitus, and hypertension—*unnecessary epidemics*: In the United States (population ~300 million in 2005), 65% of adults are overweight or obese**, generally as a direct result of *overconsumption malnutrition* and physical inactivity). In the US, the number of deaths attributable to obesity is greater than 280,200 yearly. At least 11 million Americans have type-2 diabetes mellitus, while **50 million Americans have hypertension**.[27]

Prevalence of HTN
• 50 million people in the U.S.
• 1 billion worldwide
• European Americans:
o 15% of women,
o 25% of men > age 45 years
• African Americans:
o 35% of women,
o 40% of men > age 45 years
Villela T. Hypertension: Diagnosis and Management. University of California, San Francisco-San Francisco General Hospital. Family and Community Medicine Residency Program. July 2010

- **Hypertension diagnosis and control—an international health priority**: Control of HTN is a worldwide healthcare priority. According to a 2001 editorial by Chobanian[28] in *New England Journal of Medicine*, "…more than one-fourth of the estimated 42 million people with hypertension in the United States remain unaware that they have the disorder, and approximately three-fourths of those with known hypertension have blood pressure that exceeds recommended levels." Dr Chobanian goes on to note that the prevalence and severity of the problem is comparable in the rest of the world, where approximately 20% of the adult population (more than 800 million people) are hypertensive, and rates of control are even worse than in the United States. According to an extensive review of international data published in *The Lancet* in 2005, the global prevalence of HTN was 26.4% (972 million people) in 2000 and is projected to increase to

---

[23] Folberg R. "Chapter 29: The eye." in Kumar V, Abbas AK, Fausto N (eds). *Robins and Cotran Pathologic Basis of Disease. 7th Ed*. Elsevier; 2005, 1436-1437

[24] Schoen FJ. "Chapter 12: The heart" in Kumar V, Abbas AK, Fausto N (eds). *Robins and Cotran Pathologic Basis of Disease. 7th Ed*. Elsevier; 2005, 560-562

[25] Alpers CE. "Chapter 20: The kidney" in Kumar V, Abbas AK, Fausto N (eds). *Robins and Cotran Pathologic Basis of Disease. 7th Ed*. Elsevier: Philadelphia; 2005, 1007-1008

[26] Viera AJ, Neutze DM. Diagnosis of secondary hypertension: an age-based approach. *Am Fam Physician*. 2010 Dec 15;82(12):1471-8

[27] Cordain L, Eaton SB, Sebastian A, Mann N, Lindeberg S, Watkins BA, O'Keefe JH, Brand-Miller J. Origins and evolution of the Western diet: health implications for the 21st century. *Am J Clin Nutr*. 2005 Feb;81(2):341-54 ajcn.org/cgi/content/full/81/2/341 This will forever be an important publication and landmark in nutritional science.

[28] Chobanian AV. Control of hypertension--an important national priority. *N Engl J Med*. 2001 Aug 16;345(7):534-5

29.2% (1.56 billion people) by the year 2025; the authors concluded, "Hypertension is an important public-health challenge worldwide."[29]

- Hypertension—a multifaceted entity with clinical, political, social, and economic components and implications: First, as previously noted, HTN is a treatable and therefore avoidable contributor to CVD and other forms of end-organ damage— stroke, myocardial infarction, congestive heart failure, peripheral vascular disease, renal failure, and hypertensive retinopathy. Second, HTN as a clinical manifestation is *always* a sign of underlying dysfunction or disease; HTN does not cause itself (at least initially) and therefore the "treatment of hypertension" should focus on the identification and "treatment of underlying dysfunction" rather than simply suppressing the visible manifestation of this dysfunction—the elevated blood pressure. **The finding of HTN is a sign to the clinician that one or more underlying physiologic imbalances are present and in need of detection and/or corrective intervention.** The environmental-social factors that predispose toward the development of HTN—including overconsumption malnutrition, lack of exercise, and psychoemotional stress—tend to disproportionately affect people of lower socioeconomic status. Third, HTN is not merely a disease; it is a *business* (leading diagnosis in Family Medicine practices[30]), and an industry (direct costs approach $200 billion per year in the United States). Among allopathic and osteopathic physicians, HTN is the most common clinical diagnosis in Family Medicine practice. For the medical profession and pharmaceutical industry, antihypertensive medications and services are a major source of revenue. Direct annual medical expenses related to HTN exceed $185 billion per year in the United States. Most patients treated exclusively with drugs require *multiple drugs* for adequate BP control[31], and—from the day of diagnosis—they are prescribed to take these drugs for the rest of their lives. **Thus, the term "hypertension" describes much more than one individual patient's elevated blood pressure; the term refers to an entity that spans and interconnects clinical, political, social, and economic phenomena and institutions.** To change the management of hypertension is to change—or at least begin changing in an important way—the practice of medicine as previously known. By perceiving high blood pressure as a barometer of poor health rather than as an isolated clinical entity, clinicians have license to intervene in numerous ways to improve each patient's overall health, thereby reducing suffering and death *beyond that attributable to hypertension-related illness* because most of the natural interventions described in this chapter provide clinically meaningful collateral benefits and reduce blood pressure *en passant*.[32]

- Hypertension—primarily a "disease of Western civilization": The prevalence of HTN among hunter-gatherer societies is virtually zero.[33] Contrasting the absence of CVD noted in *physically active* societies that consume *natural diets* against the pandemics of HTN and CVD seen in Westernized/industrialized nations, O'Keefe and Cordain[34] wrote, "**The lifetime incidence of hypertension [among Americans] is an astounding 90%**, and the metabolic syndrome is present in up to 40% of middle-aged American adults. **Cardiovascular disease remains the number 1 cause of death**, accounting for 41% of all fatalities, and the prevalence of heart disease in the United States is projected to double during the next 50 years." In industrialized nations, the prevalence of HTN in adults is approximately 1 per 4-5 (20-25%) with the vast majority of these considered idiopathic, chronic, and unresponsive to diet and lifestyle improvements from the dominant allopathic medical perspective. Integrative clinicians who appreciate the broad range of causes of and **synergistic contributors to hypertension** do not generally view this disorder as *idiopathic,* nor as necessarily *chronic,* nor as *unresponsive,* but rather find it *understandable* and *highly amenable* to numerous interventions—necessarily specific for each patient (e.g., food allergies and/or hypothyroidism and/or nutrient deficiencies)—supported by publications in peer-reviewed biomedical journals. **The high prevalence of primary hypertension seen in industrial "Westernized" societies does not necessarily imply that the people in these societies are as a group genetically defective and**

---

[29] Kearney PM, Whelton M, Reynolds K, Muntner P, Whelton PK, He J. Global burden of hypertension: analysis of worldwide data. *Lancet*. 2005 Jan 15-21;365(9455):217-23

[30] Sloane PD, Slatt LM, Ebell MH, Jacques LB, Smith MA (Eds). *Essentials of Family Medicine, 5th Edition*. Lippincott Williams & Wilkins, 2007

[31] Domino FJ (editor in chief). *The 5-Minute Clinical Consult. 2010. 18th Edition*. Philadelphia; Wolters Kluwer: 2009, 656-7

[32] French: *in passing* or *in passage*. Capturing "en passant" is a strategy used in the game of chess wherein a player is allowed to capture an opponent's pawn in an adjacent row after the opponent has moved the pawn forward by two spaces. In this context, I use the phrase *en passant* to denote that most of the natural treatments detailed in the following pages do not directly and intentionally target hypertension *per se* but rather reduce hypertension *in passing* as overall health is improved.

[33] Eaton SB, Shostak M, Konner M. *The Paleolithic Prescription*. New York: Harper and Row Publishers; 1988, 49

[34] O'Keefe JH Jr, Cordain L. Cardiovascular disease resulting from a diet and lifestyle at odds with our Paleolithic genome. *Mayo ClinProc* 2004;79:101-8

therefore **"in need of medical intervention"** but perhaps rather that the **industrialized/Westernized lifestyle is inherently adverse to the preservation of human health, well-being, and longevity.**[35] In early biomedical and socioanthropologic literature such as Dr Weston Price's *Nutrition and Physical Degeneration: A Comparison of Primitive and Modern Diets and Their Effects*[36] published in 1945, hypertension—just like diabetes mellitus, dental carries, malocclusion, chronic dermatopathies such as acne, eczema, and psoriasis, and a myriad of clinical and subclinical neuropsychiatric problems—was often described as one of the "diseases of Western civilization", i.e., a disease that did not generally exist within primitive hunter-gatherer societies until such societies were infiltrated with white flour, white sugar, alcohol, salt [sodium chloride], and other aspects of the Western/industrialized way of existing and surviving.

- The clinician's responsibilities: The obligations imposed upon clinicians in the management of hypertension include:
  - Comprehensive clinical assessment: Assess for urgent situations (BP > 210/120 mm Hg) and end-organ damage, particularly of the **eyes** (fundoscopic examination), **kidneys** (measure serum BUN and creatinine; determine GFR; obtain UA, perhaps also look for albumin:creatinine ratio to detect early proteinuria), and **cardiovascular system** (cardiopulmonary auscultation and blood pressure measurement with every visit; consider bruit screening, ECG, echocardiography, ankle-brachial index, and assessment for other cardiovascular risk factors such as hyperglycemia, dyslipidemia, and inflammation with hsCRP. Assessing for other risk factors such as n-3 fatty acid insufficiency (generally dietary history is sufficient for assessment; laboratory analysis is expensive and generally not required), vitamin D3 insufficiency, serum cystatin C, serum ferritin, lipoprotein a (Lp-a), aldosterone, renin, and fibrinogen can also be performed.

"Diseases of Western civilization"

- Primary hypertension
- Diabetes mellitus, type-2
- Metabolic syndrome
- Dental carries and malocclusion
- Common neuropsychiatric problems
- Obesity
- Dermatopathies: eczema, psoriasis, and acne

"Diseases of Western civilization" can be understood by appreciation of the physiologic effects caused by the lifestyle and dietary changes historically imposed upon indigenous hunter-gather societies from incoming Westerners/Europeans. These changes include what was *added* (white flour, grains, table salt, white sugar, alcohol, and other so-called "refined" foods, which were poor in substance and vitality compared to their more "natural" and "primitive" counterparts) and what was *removed* (exercise, whole fruits, vegetables, nuts, seeds, berries, roots [i.e., fiber and phytonutrients], multigenerational community, natural living, full-body exposure to sunshine and therefore ensured adequacy of vitamin D). Important to appreciate is that these diseases were once exceedingly rare but are now commonplace. The fact that most of these conditions are common these days in children dispels the shibboleth espoused by pharmacosurgical proponents that these diseases have become more common simply because people are living longer due to "advances in medicine." Quite to the contrary, medicine as generally practiced has reinforced and abetted the conditions which generate many of these illnesses; thankfully, we are seeing positive changes in medicine, but only recently, and mainly due to outside pressures and the popularity of and market demand for open-mindedness toward healthy living.

The classic text on this subject is Price WA. *Nutrition and Physical Degeneration: A Comparison of Primitive and Modern Diets and Their Effects*. 1945

  - Differential diagnosis: Competently assess for and exclude genuine causes of HTN before ascribing HTN to a "genetic" or familial cause requiring perpetual medicalization; detailed information on assessment (e.g., physical exam, lab tests, and diagnostic/therapeutic interventions) is reviewed later in this chapter.
  - Effective treatment: Effective intervention must be prescribed by the physician and implemented by the patient; results must be documented in the patient's chart. The clinician has the responsibility to effect improved outcome, document patient noncompliance, and/or initiate a *complete referral* to a specialist for recalcitrant cases, for additional testing, advanced treatment, and/or liability defense.
  - Patient education: Because hypertension—like diabetes and hemochromatosis—is generally asymptomatic in its early stages and in milder cases, doctors (derived from the Latin *docere*, which means "to teach"[37]) have the responsibility to instruct patients on the nature of their disorder, its effects and treatment options, and the consequences of nontreatment. Patients have the responsibility to comply with the treatment plan, implement an effective alternate plan, or absorb the consequences of noncompliance and disease progression.

---

[35] O'Keefe JH Jr, Cordain L. Cardiovascular disease resulting from a diet and lifestyle at odds with our Paleolithic genome. *Mayo ClinProc* 2004;79:101-8
[36] Price WA. *Nutrition and Physical Degeneration: A Comparison of Primitive and Modern Diets and Their Effects*. Price-Pottinger Nutrition Foundation, 1945
[37] Prakash R, Misra R, Misra R. Doctors as Teachers. *Psychiatric News* 2002; 37: 37 pn.psychiatryonline.org/content/37/9/37.1.full

- o Implement a follow-up plan: Doctors must (pre)schedule patients for follow-up in-office visits to monitor treatment adherence and therapeutic effectiveness.
- o Complete referral for nonresponsive or noncompliant patients: "Complete referral" includes a professional letter of referral including the patient's history, examination findings, lab results, and any imaging and other assessments that are within the referring clinician's scope of competence/practice. Generally, the referring clinician's office should call the specialist's office to make the appointment for the patient, then provide the appointment time and address to the patient; the components of this complete referral are then documented in the patient's chart. Simply telling a patient, "You need to see a specialist" is often insufficient because doing so places the burden of responsibility onto the patient, and many of our patients lack the sophistication and knowledge to successfully navigate various overlapping healthcare systems. By ensuring that the patient's appointment is made with the specialist, the physician facilitates patient care and protects herself/himself from undue liability.

Consequences of failing to adequately manage hypertension
• Accelerated atherosclerosis, CVD
• Hemorrhagic and ischemic stroke,
• Peripheral arterial disease,
• Mesenteric ischemia,
• Erectile dysfunction in men,
• Myocardial infarction,
• Heart failure,
• Cerebral and aortic aneurysm,
• Nephropathy, dialysis, transplant,
• Retinopathy, intra ocular hemorrhage, vision loss,
• Patient dissatisfaction
• Physician dissatisfaction, malpractice litigation

Clinical Presentations:

- Clearly the vast majority of clinical presentations of HTN are silent, discovered only when the clinician finds elevated blood pressure on routine examination. This underscores the importance of hypertension screening among asymptomatic patients. The second and remaining group of clinical presentations of HTN includes those of end-organ damage: nephropathy, retinopathy, cardiomyopathy, and the consequences of HTN-accelerated CVD including stroke, myocardial infarction, aortic dissection, and rupture of an enlarged (generally >5.5 cm) abdominal aortic aneurysm.
- Typical clinical presentations of the hypertensive patient can range from incidental to catastrophic and include the following:
  - o Asymptomatic: incidental finding during presentation and evaluation for another concern such as routine examination, injury, or infection
  - o Headache, altered mental status
  - o Congestive heart failure presenting with fatigue, lower extremity edema, or dyspnea
  - o Retinopathy, vision impairment
  - o Myocardial infarction or sudden death due to accelerated CVD complicated by cardiac hypertrophy (i.e., supply-demand mismatch)
  - o Hypertensive nephropathy presenting with renal insufficiency: azotemia, edema, malignant hypertension, anuria/oliguria

Major Differential Diagnoses: Characteristics of secondary hypertension include therapeutic recalcitrance (defined as inefficacy or subefficacy of simultaneous use of three or more drugs[38]), onset at an early age (< 30y) or at a more advanced age (>50y), and the typical associated features of the causative disorder, such as hypokalemia with hyperaldosteronism, depression or musculoskeletal pain with hypovitaminosis D, and cold intolerance, bradycardia, and delayed Achilles reflex return with hypothyroidism. Listed below are most of the primary causes of hypertension with a brief sketch of their classic clinical characteristics, including physical examination and laboratory findings. Additionally, the December 2010 review by Vierra and Neutze[39] recommends an age-based approach which will also be included in the following descriptions of differential diagnoses; of note, 70-85% of hypertension in children is secondary to an identifiable primary disorder. While the purpose of this text is to focus on *adult* hypertension, many of the diagnostic and treatment considerations are appropriately applicable to children. Normal and abnormal values for blood pressure in infants and children differ from those of adults and are stratified based on age, gender, and height in a chart from the International Pediatric Hypertension Association available at PediatricHypertension.org.

---

[38] Viera AJ, Neutze DM. Diagnosis of secondary hypertension: an age-based approach. *Am Fam Physician*. 2010 Dec 15;82(12):1471-8
[39] Viera AJ, Neutze DM. Diagnosis of secondary hypertension: an age-based approach. *Am Fam Physician*. 2010 Dec 15;82(12):1471-8

- <u>Aortic coarctation</u>: Coarctation of the aorta is the second most common cause of HTN in children. (Kidney disease is the most common cause of HTN in children, as reviewed later.) Aortic coarctation is 2-5x more common in males, and typical age of diagnosis is 5 years. Classic presentation includes upper extremity hypertension with lower extremity hypotension/hypoperfusion/claudication, with or without discrepancies in bilateral brachial pressure, in a child or young adult; secondary activation of the renin-angiotensin system due to renal hypoperfusion exacerbates the HTN and complicates this *focal* anatomic disorder by adding a *systemic* neurohormonal component. Physical examination findings may include leg blood pressure at least 20 mm Hg less than arm blood pressure, delayed or absent femoral pulses, and an audible murmur or bruit. Imaging modalities of choice are transthoracic ultrasonography for children and MRI for adults; computed tomography (CT), magnetic resonance angiography/aortography (MRA) may also be used. Treatment includes antihypertensive interventions (reviewed in the section on *Therapeutic Considerations*) to manage the hypertension until surgery corrects the coarctation.

- <u>Cocaine use</u>: Cocaine use can cause acute and chronic elevations in blood pressure. Drug cessation is the key to treatment; urine drug testing is appropriate for patients suspected of undisclosed drug use or noncompliance with cessation. In hospital practice, patients presenting with hypertensive disorders, chest pain, and other cardiovascular syndromes are routinely tested for acute (serum drug screen) and chronic (urine drug screen) drug exposure; an impressive number of these tests come back positive even among patients who swear to have never used or not recently used recreational drugs.

- <u>Cushing's disease/syndrome, hypercortisolism</u>: Excess glucocorticoids whether endogenous or exogenous promote sodium retention directly via their mineralocorticoid effect and by causing hyperinsulinemia via induction of peripheral insulin resistance; both of these pathophysiologic processes contribute to HTN. Determination of iatrogenic hypercortisolism can be determined by reviewing the patient's medication intake. Endogenous hypercortisolism (2-5 diagnoses per million patients per year) can be assessed with measurements of serum adrenocorticotropic hormone (ACTH), 24-hour urinary free cortisol, nighttime salivary cortisol, and the low-dose dexamethasone suppression test in addition to looking for the clinical characteristics of moon facies, striae, sarcopenia, and abdominal obesity. Treatment is withdrawal of exogenous steroids (if possible) for iatrogenic Cushing's syndrome, or surgical removal of the ACTH-producing pituitary corticotroph adenoma (classically) in cases of endogenous Cushing's disease. An additional type of Cushing's syndrome can result from ectopic ACTH production from tumors such as small cell carcinoma of the lung or a carcinoid tumor.

- <u>Drug side-effect</u>: Many pharmaceutical drugs can cause an elevation in blood pressure. Reviewing the adverse effects of each drug that a patient is taking may be sufficient to identify the offending agent; a clinical trial of discontinuation may be appropriate to determine if a drug causes or contributes to elevated blood pressure in a particular patient. Many options to the use of pharmaceutical drugs exist, allowing the prevention and alleviation of many diseases and disorders commonly encountered in clinical practice. Several common hypertension-inducing drugs are listed in separate paragraphs within this section on differential diagnosis; drugs worthy of specific mention include amphetamines, buspirone, carbamazapine, clozapine, fluoxetine, lithium, tricyclic antidepressants, prednisone and methylprednisolone, and sympathomimetic decongestants.[40]

- <u>Estrogen, oral contraceptives</u>: As a group of various hormones with divergent effects, estrogens generally tend to promote sodium and water retention, which promotes volume overload and the development of HTN. For women with "estrogen dominance" due to excess endogenous production or exogenous administration of estrogens, supplementation with pyridoxine 50-250 mg/d (nearly always co-administered with magnesium 600-1,200 mg/d or to bowel tolerance; pyridoxal-5-phosphate [p5p] might also be used) and/or natural progesterone (rather than a synthetic progestin, since many of these preparations have inherent glucocorticoid/mineralocorticoid activity) can frequently offset the HTN-inducing effects of estrogens. Clinicians desiring a more comprehensive anti-estrogen protocol within a context of practical hormone optimization ("orthoendocrinology") may find helpful the review in chapter 4.

- <u>Ethanol overconsumption</u>: Excess ethanol consumption raises blood pressure and makes HTN more difficult to treat. Many patients fail to accurately disclose the extent and duration of their alcohol consumption. In acute

---

[40] Viera AJ, Neutze DM. Diagnosis of secondary hypertension: an age-based approach. *Am Fam Physician.* 2010 Dec 15;82(12):1471-8

care and hospital settings, plasma ethanol (blood alcohol concentration, BAC) can be measured, along with either serum toxicology screening for acute/recent intoxication or urinary toxicology screening for chronic/past drug use. Many patients who claim to have not used drugs ever or recently will be found to have positive drug tests with replicable results. Clues to occult alcoholism may include socioeconomic problems and elevations of serum AST (aspartate transaminase) greater than ALT (alanine transaminase), along with elevations of GGT (gamma glutamyl transpeptidase) and triglycerides; hepatic cirrhosis, splenomegaly, and pancytopenia may also be noted among patients with chronic alcoholism, even among patients who deny alcohol use. Differential diagnosis of occult alcoholism includes chronic viral hepatitis B or C, hemochromatosis and other forms of iron overload, overuse of other drugs or medications, and psychiatric disorders.

> **Rapid-onset HTN must be managed early and assertively**
>
> Rapid-onset HTN of 160 mm Hg systolic or 110 mm Hg diastolic requires urgent treatment. *Rapid-onset* HTN can cause stroke at pressures generally tolerated in *chronic* HTN because, in the latter, the vasculature has time to adapt to the higher pressures, while in the former, the cardiovascular system has not had time to adapt, thus leaving the patient particularly vulnerable to hemorrhagic stroke. Acute-onset HTN *from any cause* should be treated urgently when pressures approximate or exceed 160-180 mm Hg systolic or 110 mm Hg diastolic, especially *but not exclusively* if accompanied by complications such as angina (test serum cardiac enzymes), shortness of breath (consider pulmonary edema and auscultate for crackles), vision changes, papilledema, headache/ confusion/ seizures (which suggest cerebral edema or cerebral vasospasm), proteinuria, or edema of the face, peripheral extremities, or of the general body (anasarca, check for sacral edema and weight gain).

- Gestational hypertension and preeclampsia: Pregnancy-induced (after week 20 of gestation) hypertension without proteinuria is termed *gestational hypertension*; gestational hypertension with concomitant proteinuria is termed *preeclampsia*, while the addition of seizures advances the diagnosis to *eclampsia*—all of these pregnancy-related hypertensive syndromes can present with acute HTN. Preeclampsia can accelerate rapidly and cause life-threatening complications for the mother and/or fetus; treatment requires parenteral therapy (intravenous magnesium sulfate for seizure prophylaxis; hydralazine and/or labetolol for HTN control) and/or emergency interventions—namely, delivery.[41] Some evidence suggests that the incidence of preeclampsia can be reduced via increased intake of aspirin, ascorbate, calcium, tocopherol(s), and magnesium[42], and by pre-pregnancy treatment/cure of obesity, diabetes mellitus, and HTN.

- Hypercalcemia: Easily diagnosed by routine laboratory testing, hypercalcemia may be caused by hyperparathyroidism, malignancy, Paget's disease of bone, sarcoidosis, or rarely by nutritional excesses of calcium and/or vitamin D. Most hypercalcemia (80-90%) is due to hyperparathyroidism or malignancy; the most common cause of hypercalcemia in the outpatient setting is hyperparathyroidism, while in the hospital setting the most common cause is malignancy, particularly multiple myeloma, lymphoma, lymphosarcomas, and metastatic disease.[43] While other differential diagnoses also need to be considered, some endocrinologist particularly advocate testing 24-h urinary calcium levels as a test for familial hypocalciuric hypercalcemia. When primary hyperparathyroidism is suspected, the serum level of intact parathyroid hormone (iPTH) is tested. When malignancy is suspected (particularly from the finding of an unexplained serum calcium > 13 mg/dL [> 3.25 mmol/L]), patient-centered evaluation is performed, which often includes initial chest radiograph followed by *pan-scanning* with CT for occult malignancies in the thorax (e.g., lung cancers), abdomen and pelvis (e.g., gastrointestinal tumors).

- Insulin resistance and hyperinsulinemia: Insulin promotes renal retention of sodium which leads to water retention and the subsequent volume overload and systemic hypertension which logically follow in sequence. This explains the well proven and replicable benefit of low-carbohydrate diets in treating "idiopathic" HTN in the general population. Elevated or high-normal serum insulin along with chronic hyperglycemia is most suggestive of insulin resistance; the most effective treatments for insulin resistance are integrative nutritional interventions.[44]

- Licorice (*Glycyrrhiza glabra*) over-consumption: Used medicinally for thousands of years with excellent safety and effectiveness, *Glycyrrhiza glabra* is particularly useful against several common human viral infections. The active constituent glycyrrhizin (also known as glycyrrhizic acid, the hydrolysis product of which is

[41] Wagner LK. Diagnosis and management of preeclampsia. *Am Fam Physician*. 2004 Dec 15;70(12):2317-24
[42] Domino FJ (editor in chief). *The 5-Minute Clinical Consult. 2010. 18th Edition*. Philadelphia; Wolters Kluwer: 2009, 1062
[43] Bent S, Gensler LS, Frances C. *Saint-Frances Guide: Clinical Clerkship in Outpatient Medicine. 2nd Edition*. Philadelphia; Wolters Kluwer: 2008, 490
[44] Vasquez A. *Chiropractic and Naturopathic Mastery of Common Clinical Disorders*. IBMRC 2009. And later versions published in the Inflammation Mastery series.

glycyrrhetinic acid) can cause clinically severe hypertension with hypokalemia via potentiation of endogenous mineralocorticoids leading to clinical syndrome called "pseudo-hyperaldosteronism." More specifically, glycyrrhizin inhibits 11-beta hydroxysteroid dehydrogenase thus preventing cortisol's inactivation to cortisone in the kidney; this potentiates the mineralocorticoid effect of endogenous cortisol leading to sodium retention and potassium excretion. The hypertension resolves following discontinuation of the excess licorice.

- Mercury toxicity: Mercury is an established neurotoxin, immunotoxin, and nephrotoxin. Because pathophysiologic effects are noted even with very small doses of exposure, one could reasonably argue that no safe amount exists and therefore that any detected mercury is an indication for therapeutic intervention to remove this toxicant. According to an article by Schober et al[45] published in *JAMA—Journal of the American Medical Association* in 2003, "Approximately 8% of [1,709 American] women had [blood mercury] concentrations higher than the US Environmental Protection Agency's recommended reference dose (5.8 µg/L), below which exposures are considered to be without adverse effects." Sources of exposure include dental amalgams, vaccinations, airborne pollution, and fish; recently, high-fructose corn syrup was shown to contain mercury.[46] Mercury impairs catecholamine degradation and can thereby cause a clinical syndrome that can include hypertension, tremor, tachycardia, diaphoresis, and neurocognitive changes.[47] Per Shih and Gartner[48], "Mercury combines with the sulfhydryl group of S-adenosylmethionine, which is a cofactor for catecholamine-O-methyltransferase (COMT), and this inhibition of COMT allows accumulation of norepinephrine, epinephrine, and dopamine." The clinical presentation of mercury toxicity can include any of the following: diffuse erythematosus rash, dermatitis (acrodynia), anorexia, malaise, fatigue, muscle pain, proximal and/or distal muscle weakness, tremor, weight loss, insomnia, night sweats, burning peripheral neuropathy (axonal neuropathy), renal insufficiency/failure, inattention, neurocognitive compromise, personality changes, depression, diaphoresis, tachycardia, and hypertension. Differential diagnoses for mercury toxicity are numerous, including pheochromocytoma, hyperthyroidism, conversion disorder, viral infection, toxic shock syndrome, and Kawasaki disease. Laboratory assessment can include 24-hour urinary catecholamines, random urine mercury, and whole blood mercury; these tests are particularly appropriate for acute and subacute intoxications. For distant and chronic mercury intoxications, many clinicians including this author prefer to use dimercaptosuccinic acid (DMSA) dosed orally at 10 mg per kilogram of body weight to enhance the sensitivity of urine toxic metal testing. The use of DMSA for children and adults is supported by peer-reviewed literature[49,50,51,52,53] and has been reviewed in more detail by this author in *Integrative Rheumatology*[54] and to a lesser extent in *Musculoskeletal Pain: Expanded Clinical Strategies*.[55] DMSA chelation is approved by the US Food and Drug Administration (FDA) for the treatment of lead toxicity in children.[56]

- Neurogenic hypertension: In the context of discussing HTN, "neurogenic" was historically interchangeable with "essential", "primary", and "idiopathic." Since *neurogenic* is no longer

> **Physiologic irritation of the nucleus tract solitarius (NTS) and other nearby structures in the brainstem appears to contribute to some cases of hypertension**
>
> "Impaired NTS (CNS) function can produce an amplification of the action of the environmental stresses on blood pressure. Thus environmental stimuli or the expression of behaviors which normally result in trivial elevations of blood pressure will, after the NTS is perturbed, result in marked elevations (of blood pressure)."
>
> Reis DJ. The nucleus tractus solitarius and experimental neurogenic hypertension. *Adv Biochem Psychopharmacol* 1981

[45] Schober et al. Blood mercury levels in US children and women of childbearing age, 1999-2000. *JAMA*. 2003 Apr;289:1667-74 jama.ama-assn.org/content/289/13/1667.long
[46] "Average daily consumption of high fructose corn syrup is about 50 grams per person in the United States. With respect to total mercury exposure, it may be necessary to account for this source of mercury in the diet of children and sensitive populations." Dufault R, LeBlanc B, Schnoll R, Cornett C, Schweitzer L, Wallinga D, Hightower J, Patrick L, Lukiw WJ. Mercury from chlor-alkali plants: measured concentrations in food product sugar. *Environ Health*. 2009 Jan 26;8:2. See also: "High fructose corn syrup has been shown to contain trace amounts of mercury as a result of some manufacturing processes, and its consumption can also lead to zinc loss." Dufault et al. Mercury exposure, nutritional deficiencies and metabolic disruptions may affect learning in children. *Behav Brain Funct*. 2009 Oct 27;5:44.
[47] Wössmann W, Kohl M, Grüning G, Bucsky P. Mercury intoxication presenting with hypertension and tachycardia. *Arch Dis Child*. 1999 Jun;80(6):556-7
[48] Shih H, Gartner JC Jr. Weight loss, hypertension, weakness, and limb pain in an 11-year-old boy. *J Pediatr*. 2001 Apr;138(4):566-9
[49] Bradstreet et al. A case-control study of mercury burden in children with autistic spectrum disorders. *J Am Physicians Surg* 2003; 8: 76-79 jpands.org/vol8no3/geier.pdf
[50] Crinnion WJ. Environmental medicine, part three: long-term effects of chronic low-dose mercury exposure. *Altern Med Rev*. 2000 Jun;5(3):209-23
[51] Forman J, Moline J, Cernichiari E, Sayegh S, Torres JC, Landrigan MM, Hudson J, Adel HN, Landrigan PJ. A cluster of pediatric metallic mercury exposure cases treated with meso-2,3-dimercaptosuccinic acid (DMSA). *Environ Health Perspect*. 2000 Jun;108(6):575-7 ehp.niehs.nih.gov/docs/2000/108p575-577forman/abstract.html
[52] Miller AL. Dimercaptosuccinic acid (DMSA), a non-toxic, water-soluble treatment for heavy metal toxicity. *Altern Med Rev*. 1998 Jun;3(3):199-207
[53] DMSA. *Altern Med Rev*. 2000 Jun;5(3):264-7
[54] Vasquez A. *Integrative Rheumatology*. IBMRC 2006, 2007 and all future editions, most recently updated as *Inflammation Mastery, 4th Edition* (2016).
[55] Vasquez A. *Musculoskeletal Pain: Expanded Clinical Strategies*. Institute for Functional Medicine (2008), most recently updated as *Inflammation Mastery, 4th Edition* (2016).
[56] "The Food and Drug Administration has recently licensed the drug DMSA (succimer) for reduction of blood lead levels >/= 45 micrograms/dl. This decision was based on the demonstrated ability of DMSA to reduce blood lead levels. An advantage of this drug is that it can be given orally." Goyer et al. Role of chelating agents for prevention, intervention, and treatment of exposures to toxic metals. *Environ Health Perspect*. 1995 Nov;103(11):1048-52 ehp.niehs.nih.gov/docs/1995/103-11/meetingreport.html

generally used for this purpose, and because new research advocates the term's reinstitution, *neurogenic hypertension* should be exonerated from its previous identification with *idiopathicity* and given revised meaning. For the purposes of this discussion and as detailed later in this chapter, **the term "neurogenic hypertension" will mean what its name implies,** namely **chronic HTN induced principally by the nervous system due to**

> ### Facilitation: chronic low-threshold nerve discharge
>
> "Previous studies have indicated the existence, in man, of pools of spinal extensor motoneurons which are in a state of enduring excitation, as reflected in low reflex thresholds. ... The data indicate that differences in pressure thresholds reflect differences in central facilitation, and that the facilitation is due to a bombardment of the motoneurons by impulses originating, in part at least, from points other than the spinous process which was the site of stimulation."
>
> Denslow, Korr, et al. Quantitative studies of chronic facilitation in human motoneuron pools. *Am J Physiology* 1947

irritation or *functional disturbance* **rather than overt pathology**. Given its basis in physiology rather than pathology per se, the term "functional neurogenic hypertension" would serve to further emphasize the functional and therefore largely reversible mechanism of the disorder. Foci of neurogenic hypertension can reside in the central nervous system (CNS) or peripheral nervous system (PNS). In this text, **"central neurogenic hypertension"** describes hypertensive states induced by irritation of the central nervous system, in particular at the level of the brainstem (i.e., medulla oblongata in general and the root entry zones [REZ] of cranial nerves 9 and 10 as well as the nucleus tract solitarius [NTS] in particular) as will be reviewed in a following section on surgical interventions for the treatment of medullary neurovascular compression. The first use of the term "central neurogenic hypertension" of which this author is aware was published by Reis[57] in a 1981 review, mostly of animal research. In this review, Reis included the hypothesis that irritation of the CNS by either mechanical or neurochemical means could serve as a predisposition or antecedent to the manifest development of clinical HTN. The diagnosis of central neurogenic hypertension is generally based upon ❶ MRI/MRA or CT findings of neurovascular compression of the left medulla oblongata in conjunction with ❷ reduction in blood pressure following decompressive intervention.

"**Peripheral neurogenic hypertension**" as an entity is more theoretical, less studied, and might be exemplified by irritation of spinal nerve roots and sympathetic ganglia as discussed primarily in the chiropractic[58,59,60,61,62] and osteopathic literature.[63,64] Functional compromise in general and **facilitation**[65] in particular of the nerve roots and sympathetic ganglia as a potential *cause of* or *contributor to* chronic HTN supports the rationale for the use of spinal manipulation and manual medicine for the treatment of HTN and other nonmusculoskeletal disorders. Peripheral neurogenic hypertension may be diagnosed based on clinical/electrographic/vasodynamic evidence of functional PNS compromise/ facilitation/ irritation and alleviation of HTN following appropriate regional intervention such as manual manipulative treatment of the spine and adjacent neuromusculoskeletal structures applied to effect restoration of proper nervous system function and balance. Central and peripheral types of neurogenic HTN will be discussed in more detail later in this chapter within the context of their surgical and manipulative treatments, respectively.

- <u>Nonsteroidal anti-inflammatory drugs (NSAIDs):</u> NSAIDs in general such as ibuprofen and naproxen and COX-2 inhibitors (coxibs) in particular reduce endogenous production of vasodilating prostacyclin and thus cause pharmacologic/iatrogenic renal artery constriction, which leads to varying degrees of HTN via activation of the renin-angiotensin system. This explains, in part, the increased cardiovascular mortality due to overutilization of coxibs such as rofecoxib/Vioxx, withdrawn from the US market in 2005 by the US FDA due to its causal role in increasing cardiovascular deaths.[66] Evidence of increased cardiovascular morbidity and mortality secondary to coxib use was widely publicized for several years before rofecoxib/Vioxx and a similar

---

[57] "The abnormalities of pressure control resulting from abnormal transmission in NTS met most of the criteria of an animal model of central neurogenic hypertension. ... Impaired NTS function can produce an amplification of the action of the environmental stresses on blood pressure." Reis DJ. The nucleus tractus solitarius and experimental neurogenic hypertension: evidence for a central neural imbalance hypothesis of hypertensive disease. *Adv Biochem Psychopharmacol.* 1981;28:409-20

[58] Bakris et al. Atlas vertebra realignment and achievement of arterial pressure goal in hypertensive patients: a pilot study. *J Hum Hypertens.* 2007 May;21(5):347-52

[59] Plaugher G, Bachman TR. Chiropractic management of a hypertensive patient. *J Manipulative Physiol Ther.* 1993 Oct;16(8):544-9

[60] Yates et al. Effects of chiropractic treatment on blood pressure and anxiety: a randomized, controlled trial. *J Manipulative Physiol Ther.* 1988 Dec;11(6):484-8

[61] Plaugher et al. Practice-based randomized controlled-comparison clinical trial of chiropractic adjustments and brief massage treatment at sites of subluxation in subjects with essential hypertension: pilot study. *J Manipulative Physiol Ther.* 2002 May;25:221-39

[62] Crawford et al. Management of hypertensive disease: review of spinal manipulation and the efficacy of conservative therapeusis. *J Manipulative Physiol Ther* 1986 Mar ;:27-32

[63] Celander E, Koenig AJ, Celander DR. Effect of osteopathic manipulative therapy on autonomic tone as evidenced by blood pressure changes and activity of the fibrinolytic system. *J Am Osteopath Assoc.* 1968 May;67(9):1037-8

[64] Fichera AP, Celander DR. Effect of osteopathic manipulative therapy on autonomic tone as evidenced by blood pressure changes and activity of the fibrinolytic system. *J Am Osteopath Assoc.* 1969 Jun;68(10):1036-8

[65] Denslow JS, Korr IM, Krems AD. Quantitative studies of chronic facilitation in human motoneuron pools. *Am J Physiol.* 1947 Aug;150(2):229-38

[66] Topol EJ. Failing the public health—rofecoxib, Merck, and the FDA. *N Engl J Med.* 2004 Oct 21;351(17):1707-9

drug valdecoxib/Bextra were belatedly withdrawn from the consumer market.[67,68] The multiple failures involved in this politicopharmaceutical phenomenon include ❶ failure of Merck to act on data showing that its popular and profitable new drug was harming and killing an unacceptable proportion of patients who took it, ❷ failure of the US FDA to regulate the pharmaceutical industry, ❸ failure of the medical profession as a whole to police itself and call for a ban on the use of this drug before either Merck or the FDA took action. See Topol's "Failing the public health—rofecoxib, Merck, and the FDA" published in the October 21, 2004 issue of *New England Journal of Medicine* for authoritative discussion.

> **Fraudulent marketing of valdecoxib/Bextra contributed to the largest healthcare fraud settlement in the history of the US Department of Justice—US $2.3 billion**
>
> Pharmacia and Upjohn Company, a subsidiary of Pfizer Inc, pled guilty to a felony violation of the Food, Drug & Cosmetic Act for misbranding the drug Bextra with the intent to defraud or mislead. Pharmacia and Upjohn Company admitted to its criminal conduct in the promotion of Bextra and agreed to pay a criminal fine of $1.195 billion, the largest criminal fine ever imposed in the United States for any matter. Pharmacia and Upjohn Company also agreed to forfeit $105 million, for a total criminal resolution of $1.3 billion. In addition Pfizer agreed to pay an additional $1 billion plus interest to settle civil allegations that it fraudulently promoted and marketed Bextra, as well as three other drugs in its portfolio, Geodon, an anti-psychotic drug, Zyvox, an antibiotic, and Lyrica, an anti-epileptic drug, as well as claims that it paid kickbacks for these, as well as other drugs, to induce physician prescribing.
>
> justice.gov/usao/ma/Press Office Press Release Files/Sept2009/PharmaciaPlea.html. Posted September 15, 2009. Accessed November 23, 2010. See also news.bbc.co.uk/2/hi/business/8234533.stm

- Pheochromocytoma: An exceedingly rare cause of secondary HTN (0.5%) in contrast to the high frequency with which it is covered in textbooks and licensing board exams, pheochromocytoma's classic presentation includes episodic HTN, headache, tremor, and diaphoresis. Pheochromocytoma is diagnosed with increased 24-hour urinary catecholamines, metanephrines, and vanillylmandelic acid with or without plasma free metanephrines followed by CT/MRI to localize the secreting neuroendocrine tumor. Mercury intoxication whether acute or chronic must be considered in the differential diagnosis of pheochromocytoma and similar clinical presentations.[69,70] Treatment is surgical excision of the adrenal/extra-adrenal catecholamine-producing tumor.

- Primary hyperaldosteronism (Conn's syndrome): Primary hyperaldosteronism is caused by a unilateral adrenal adenoma or bilateral adrenal hyperplasia; this condition accounts for approximately 6% of adult HTN and 10-20% of cases of treatment-resistant HTN.[71] The classic finding is HTN with hypokalemia (30%), occasionally with slight hypernatremia, and the diagnosis is established by documentation of an elevated serum aldosterone:renin ratio. Importantly, aldosterone must be tested with renin (i.e., plasma renin activity) since measurement of serum aldosterone alone is insensitive; 25% of patients with hyperaldosteronism will have a normal serum aldosterone level.[72] Per *The Merck Manual*:

  > "Initial laboratory testing consists of plasma aldosterone levels and plasma renin activity (PRA). Ideally, tests are done with the patient off of drugs that affect the renin-angiotensin system (e.g., thiazide diuretics, ACE inhibitors, angiotensin antagonists, β-blockers) for 4 to 6 wk. PRA is usually measured in the morning with the patient recumbent [or upright[73]]. Patients with primary aldosteronism typically have plasma aldosterone > 15 ng/dL (> 0.42 nmol/L, [or > 416.10 pmol/L[74]]) and low levels of PRA, with a ratio of plasma aldosterone (in nanograms/dL) to PRA (in nanograms/mL/h) > 20."[75]

Diagnosis is confirmed by an endocrinologist performing a salt-suppression test. CT imaging is insensitive for detecting microadenomas and milder degrees of glandular hyperplasia. Curative treatment is laparoscopic removal/resection of the hypersecreting adrenal tumor; for patients who are not surgical candidates, drug treatment with an aldosterone-blocking drug (e.g., spironolactone or eplerenone) is used.

---

[67] "The results from VIGOR showed that the relative risk of developing a confirmed adjudicated thrombotic cardiovascular event (myocardial infarction, unstable angina, cardiac thrombus, resuscitated cardiac arrest, sudden or unexplained death, ischemic stroke, and transient ischemic attacks) with rofecoxib treatment compared with naproxen was 2.38 (95% confidence interval, 1.39-4.00; P =.002)." Mukherjee et al. Risk of cardiovascular events associated with selective COX-2 inhibitors. *JAMA* 2001 Aug 22-29;286(8):954-9

[68] "Systolic blood pressure increased significantly in 17% of rofecoxib- compared with 11% of celecoxib-treated patients (P = 0.032) at any study time point. Diastolic blood pressure increased in 2.3% of rofecoxib- compared with 1.5% of celecoxib-treated patients (P = 0.44)." Whelton et al; SUCCESS VI Study Group. Cyclooxygenase-2--specific inhibitors and cardiorenal function: a randomized, controlled trial of celecoxib and rofecoxib in older hypertensive osteoarthritis patients. *Am J Ther* 2001 Mar-Apr;8(2):85-95

[69] Wössmann W, Kohl M, Grüning G, Bucsky P. Mercury intoxication presenting with hypertension and tachycardia. *Arch Dis Child.* 1999 Jun;80(6):556-7

[70] Shih H, Gartner JC Jr. Weight loss, hypertension, weakness, and limb pain in an 11-year-old boy. *J Pediatr.* 2001 Apr;138(4):566-9

[71] Viera AJ, Neutze DM. Diagnosis of secondary hypertension: an age-based approach. *Am Fam Physician.* 2010 Dec 15;82(12):1471-8

[72] Viera AJ, Neutze DM. Diagnosis of secondary hypertension: an age-based approach. *Am Fam Physician.* 2010 Dec 15;82(12):1471-8

[73] Viera AJ, Neutze DM. Diagnosis of secondary hypertension: an age-based approach. *Am Fam Physician.* 2010 Dec 15;82(12):1471-8

[74] Viera AJ, Neutze DM. Diagnosis of secondary hypertension: an age-based approach. *Am Fam Physician.* 2010 Dec 15;82(12):1471-8

[75] unboundmedicine.com/merckmanual/ub/view/Merck-Manual-Pro/503850/all/Primary_Aldosteronism Accessed October 2, 2010

Pseudohyperaldosteronism can be caused by overconsumption of *Glycyrrhiza glabra* (licorice) and by Liddle's syndrome, a genotropic disorder causing increased sodium reabsorption, characterized by early onset (<35y) HTN with hypokalemia, low urinary sodium levels, and normal serum aldosterone levels.

- Renal artery (renovascular) stenosis: Partial obstruction of the renal arteries whether by thrombus (rare), atherosclerosis, or fibromuscular dysplasia causes renal hypoperfusion and activation of the renin-angiotensin system. Accounting for approximately 10% of renal artery stenosis (RAS), fibromuscular dysplasia is the most common cause of renovascular stenosis in young adults (19-39 years of age); women are affected much more commonly than are men. The other 90% of renovascular

> **Clinical pearl: Increase in serum K, BUN, or creatinine following ACEi or ARB treatment suggests RAS**
>
> An increase in serum creatinine (0.5-1.0 mg/dL [44.2-88.4 micromol/L]) following initiation of ACEi or ARB treatment suggests renal artery stenosis (RAS). Additional considerations include heart failure, renal insufficiency, dehydration, and drug intolerance with secondary acute renal injury. The drug does not necessarily have to be stopped until the creatinine has increased >30% over baseline or unless another compelling reason exists; monitor serum K and recheck GFR within 10 days.

stenosis is caused by atherosclerosis and is therefore mostly seen in older adults (>50y), particularly those with clinically significant CVD risk factors such as smoking and dyslipidemia and/or already established vascular disease. Renovascular stenosis is suggested by elevation of serum potassium, BUN, and/or creatinine following administration of an ACEi or an ARB; a high-pitched holosystolic renal artery bruit may be heard upon careful physical examination. The diagnosis of renal artery stenosis, per review by Zhang et al[76] in December 2009, can be made via imaging or invasive procedures, each with distinct advantages, disadvantages, safety profiles and costs. Catheter angiography with pressure gradient measurements is the definitive gold standard but is invasive, expensive, and thus reserved for surgical revascularization candidates. Ultrasonography is safe and inexpensive but the least accurate. Contrast-enhanced computed tomographic angiography and magnetic resonance angiography are intermediate in safety and accuracy. Magnetic resonance angiography *without any contrast* has become progressively more accurate and can rival contrast-enhanced techniques in its clinical utility, thereby making it the preferred imaging assessment for patients with renal insufficiency. Captopril-augmented renography lacks sensitivity and specificity and is no longer recommended. Treatment options are generally surgical (e.g., stent placement, angioplasty, or other revascularization technique) and/or pharmaceutical, with surgical approaches generally preferred for fibromuscular dysplasia and pharmaceutical treatment preferred for atherosclerotic renovascular stenosis.

- Renal parenchymal disease (nephrogenic hypertension): Renal disease can both lead to and result from HTN. Kidney diseases are the most common cause of hypertension in childhood; the leading primary etiologies are glomerulonephritis, congenital abnormalities, and reflux nephropathy. Over time and especially in adults, chronic HTN causes renal parenchymal damage, and parenchymal damage (whether due to HTN or another cause such as glomerulonephritis, pyelonephritis, polycystic kidneys, etc) leads to water retention and activation of the renin-angiotensin-aldosterone system, thus promoting a vicious cycle of progressive HTN and renal failure. The clinical picture commonly includes edema, elevated BUN and creatinine, proteinuria, anemia due to insufficient production of erythropoietin, and osteomalacia and osteodystrophy due to hyperphosphatemia, hypocalcemia, and insufficient renal formation of 1,25-dihydroxyvitamin D3. The diagnosis of renal disease is suggested by the finding of elevated BUN and creatinine on routine chemistry/metabolic panel blood tests; the diagnosis is further verified and refined by the use of CT, MRI, or US imaging, followed if necessary by renal biopsy. The Cockcroft-Gault formula has commonly been used for bedside estimation of renal function based on the patient's age, weight, gender, and serum creatinine (sCr); the formula is provided below in two versions, one using American-favored mg/dL as the unit for sCr, and the other using the international units of micromol/L—note that the latter formula employs a different constant value per gender in the numerator of the equation. The Cockcroft-Gault formula estimates creatinine clearance, which in turn is an estimate of the glomerular filtration rate (GFR), a measure of kidney function; thus creatinine clearance and GFR are somewhat interchangeable from a practical clinical perspective. Clinicians should appreciate the importance of the patient's age in determining GFR; sCr in the upper end of the normal range may indicate renal insufficiency in a patient of advanced age. Variants can be used per units in mg/dL or micromol/L, as shown in the following formulas:

---

[76] Zhang HL, Sos TA, Winchester PA, Gao J, Prince MR. Renal artery stenosis: imaging options, pitfalls, and concerns. *Prog Cardiovasc Dis*. 2009 Nov-Dec;52(3):209-19

Estimated Creatinine Clearance =	$\dfrac{(140 - \text{age in years}) \times \text{Weight in kilograms} \times (0.85 \text{ if female})}{72 \times \text{serum \textbf{creatinine in mg/dL}}}$
Estimated Creatinine Clearance =	$\dfrac{(140 - \text{age in years}) \times \text{Weight in kilograms} \times (1.23 \text{ for men or } 1.04 \text{ for women})}{72 \times \text{serum \textbf{creatinine in micromol/L}}}$

Although the Cockcroft-Gault formula is the *best-known* and *longest-used* formula for the estimation of GFR, currently the *best* equation for *more accurately* estimating GFR from serum creatinine is the Modification of Diet in Renal Disease (MDRD) Study equation, available on-line: nkdep.nih.gov/professionals/gfr_calculators/.[77]

Finally on this topic of renal disease, clinicians should be aware of measuring serum cystatin C to assess renal function. Cystatin C is a cysteine protease inhibitor produced by all nucleated cells, and its serum level is not affected by diet or muscle mass (unlike serum creatinine). The normal range for cystatin C when measured by particle-enhanced nephelometric immunoassay (PENIA) is <0.28 mg/L or <0.95 mg/L when measured by other immunologic methods. Cystatin C is a more sensitive indicator of declining renal function than is serum creatinine, and—like elevating serum creatinine or declining GFR (or elevated CRP for that matter)—cystatin C predicts risk and severity of CVD, CHF, and CKD; furthermore, cystatin C is directly involved in the pathogenesis of atherosclerosis.[78]

> **Clinical pearls for managing the patient with declining renal function**
> - When the GFR < 60 (CKD stage 3), modify dosages or withdraw certain drugs. Treat the causative problem and/or begin specialist co-management. Avoid intravenous contrast agents and other nephrotoxic drugs when feasible. Blood pressure and glucose control are important; initiation of ACEi or ARB should be considered.
> - When the GFR < 30 (CKD stage 4), the patient needs to consult a nephrologist.
> - When the GFR < 15 (CKD stage 5), the patient needs transplant or dialysis.

- Sleep apnea: Obstructive sleep apnea (OSA) is a risk factor for HTN, and treatment for OSA with continuous positive airway pressure (C-PAP) can produce modest reductions in BP that are proportionate to the severity of the HTN and compliance with treatment. Diagnosis is suggested by history of unrestful sleep, fatigue, depression, and/or a spouse's report of interrupted nighttime breathing. Physical exam may show obesity and impairment of upper airway airflow. An overnight sleep study (polysomnography) provides data on sleep, respiratory effort, and blood oxygenation and has been considered the standard for the diagnosis of sleep apnea; however, nocturnal pulse oximetry may be sufficient for the diagnosis in selected high-index patients and is less cumbersome and less expensive.

- Systemic sclerosis: HTN in general and treatment-resistant HTN in particular are seen in systemic sclerosis, a disease in which cardiopulmonary disease (e.g., pulmonary hypertension, congestive heart failure) and renal compromise (e.g., acute renal crisis heralded by nephrogenic hypertension) are the most common causes of death. Abnormalities disclosed on history and physical exam may include Raynaud's phenomenon, sclerodactyly, mask-like face, telangiectasia, and esophageal dysfunction. Laboratory findings typically include some combination of positive antinuclear antibodies (ANA), anticentromere antibodies, anti-SCL-70 antibodies, and (more rarely) anti-fibrillarin antibodies. Treatment for scleroderma and other common autoimmune disorders is reviewed in *Integrative Rheumatology*.[79]

- Thyroid disease, including both hyperthyroidism and hypothyroidism: Hypothyroidism generally causes diastolic HTN, whereas hyperthyroidism generally causes systolic HTN and widened pulse pressure. Assess clinically (e.g., pulse rate, physical exam, weight loss/gain, Achilles reflex return speed, body temperature), and with laboratory testing. A low TSH and elevated free T4 is sufficient to diagnose hyperthyroidism. The diagnosis of hypothyroidism is indicated by any one or more of the following: elevated TSH, low free T4, low free T3 and/or total T3. Elevated titers of antithyroid antibodies (e.g., either anti-thyroid peroxidase or anti-thyroglobulin) can provide sufficient indication for treatment with thyroid hormone to prevent overt hypothyroidism from developing. Elevated reverse T3 and/or a ratio of total T3 to reverse T3 less than 10:1 indicates impaired peripheral metabolism of thyroid hormones; many integrative clinicians—including this

---

[77] National Kidney Disease Education Program, National Institutes of Health (NIH). nkdep.nih.gov/professionals/gfr_calculators/

[78] "Prospective studies have shown in various clinical scenarios that patients with increased cystatin C are at a higher risk of developing both CVD and CKD. Importantly, cystatin C appears to be a useful marker for identifying individuals at a higher risk for cardiovascular events among patients belonging to a relatively low-risk category as assessed by both creatinine and estimated glomerular filtration rate values." Taglieri N, Koenig W, Kaski JC. Cystatin C and cardiovascular risk. *Clin Chem.* 2009 Nov;55(11):1932-43

[79] Vasquez A. *Integrative Rheumatology.* IBMRC 2006, 2007 and all future editions, most recently updated as *Inflammation Mastery, 4th Edition* (2016).

author—hold that the ratio of total T3 to reverse T3 should be > 10:1 to ensure proper peripheral thyroid metabolism.[80]

- **Tobacco use**: Tobacco smoke constituents cause arterioconstriction which promotes HTN. Constituents and free radicals in tobacco smoke are more pathogenic than nicotine, while the latter in isolation indeed causes adverse cardiovascular effects via vasoconstriction. Conversely, nicotine (*sin* tobacco smoke) provides synaptogenic and anti-inflammatory benefits.
- **Upper cervical spine dysfunction/subluxation**: A remarkable clinical trial published in *Journal of Human Hypertension* in 2007 by Bakris et al[81] showed that **correction of upper cervical spine subluxation/dysfunction by chiropractic spinal manipulation causes "marked and sustained reductions in BP [blood pressure] similar to the use of two-drug combination therapy."** These results suggest and perhaps indicate that subtle biomechanical dysfunction of the upper cervical spine can cause hypertension, perhaps via neuronal reflex mechanisms or possibly—as suggested by Bakris et al—by alleviating neurovascular compression and/or by alleviating circulatory compromise of the vertebral artery.
- **Vitamin D deficiency**: Vitamin D deficiency is common in the general population—often up to 90-100% of subjects in large population-based studies—and causes intracellular hypercalcinosis[82] via elevated PTH levels and contributes to chronic HTN[83] via endothelial dysfunction, systemic inflammation, insulin resistance, and activation of the renin-angiotensin-aldosterone system.[84] **Correction of vitamin D deficiency can cause a reduction in elevated blood pressure comparable to that which can be achieved by single-drug oral antihypertensive medication[85] while also providing numerous collateral benefits (including reductions in depression, pain, and risks for autoimmune and malignant diseases) at lower cost and greater safety than can be achieved with pharmaceutical drugs.**[86,87]

Clinical Assessments:

- **History/subjective**: As stated previously, **most patients with HTN are asymptomatic** and only become symptomatic as a result of severe HTN which results in end-organ compromise, such as renal insufficiency, cerebral edema, or transient myocardial ischemia. The clinical history should include inquiry about chest pain, shortness of breath, family history of CVD or diabetes mellitus (DM), morning occipital headaches, new stressors, tobacco/caffeine use, and current medications/drugs including antihypertensives, nonsteroidal anti-inflammatory drugs (NSAIDs), estrogens, ethanol, cocaine, sympathomimetics and decongestants. During this standard *history of the present illness* (HPI) which all clinicians are taught to master before graduation from their respective colleges, astute clinicians have already begun the psychographic assessment (described hereafter as "BVG-LOC profiling") which will enable them to couch the treatment objectives and details in a manner tailored for that particular patient. In this context, the patient's BVG-LOC profile (i.e., personal profile of beliefs, values, goals, and locus of control) must be appreciated by the clinician since each aspect is essential to the understanding needed by the clinician in order to address or "speak to" the patient in such a way as to improve treatment compliance—these concepts are discussed more under the section *Clinical Management* below.
- **Physical Examination/Objective**: A screening physical examination is necessary (with details emphasized below) along with documentation of findings and vital signs, including blood pressure, pulse rate, breathing rate, temperature, pain level; weight and body mass index should be noted. Auscultation of the heart, lungs, carotid and renal arteries is performed, and cranial nerves are screened.
  - Blood pressure measurement: Screening for HTN should be performed at least once every two years starting at 18 years of age. The blood pressure cuff must be at heart level and properly fitted to the patient; the patient should be seated and relaxed for 5-10 minutes prior to blood pressure measurement. At initial

[80] McDaniel AB. Thyroid Assessment: Controversies and Conundrums. Institute for Functional Medicine 14th International Symposium. Tuscon, Arizona, 2007. Detailed in: Vasquez A. *Musculoskeletal Pain: Expanded Clinical Strategies*. Institute for Functional Medicine (2008), most recently updated as *Inflammation Mastery, 4th Edition* (2016).
[81] Bakris et al. Atlas vertebra realignment and achievement of arterial pressure goal in hypertensive patients: a pilot study. *J Hum Hypertens*. 2007 May;21(5):347-52
[82] Vasquez A. Intracellular Hypercalcinosis: A Functional Nutritional Disorder with Implications Ranging from Myofascial Trigger Points to Affective Disorders, Hypertension, and Cancer. *Naturopathy Digest* 2006 Previously published in-print and on-line at naturopathydigest.com/archives/2006/sep/vasquez.php and included in this book.
[83] Vasquez A. Nutritional Treatments for Hypertension. *Naturopathy Digest* 2006. Previously published in-print and on-line at naturopathydigest.com and included herein.
[84] Pilz S, Tomaschitz A, Ritz E, Pieber TR; Medscape. Vitamin D status and arterial hypertension: a systematic review. *Nat Rev Cardiol*. 2009 Oct;6(10):621-30
[85] "Inadequate vitamin D(3) and calcium intake could play a contributory role in the pathogenesis and progression of hypertension and cardiovascular disease in elderly women." Pfeifer M, Begerow B, Minne HW, Nachtigall D, Hansen C. Effects of a short-term vitamin D(3) and calcium supplementation on blood pressure and parathyroid hormone levels in elderly women. *J Clin Endocrinol Metab*. 2001 Apr;86(4):1633-7
[86] Vasquez et al. The clinical importance of vitamin D: a paradigm shift with implications for all healthcare providers. *Altern Ther Health Med*. 2004 Sep-Oct;10(5):28-36
[87] Faloon B. Millions of Needless Deaths. *Life Extension Magazine*. 2009 January lef.org/magazine/mag2009/jan2009_Millions-of-Needless-Deaths_01.htm

evaluation and periodically thereafter, blood pressure should be assessed in both the right and left arms; a significant side-to-side discrepancy > 20/10 mm Hg suggests a partial unilateral occlusion and is worthy of further evaluation. The two measurements upon which the diagnosis of HTN is being considered should occur on different visits at least 3 days apart; alternatively, if the blood pressure is >160/100 mm Hg on any one visit, then a presumptive diagnosis of HTN can be made and treatment initiated—in the pharmaceutical paradigm, treatment for BP >160/100 mm Hg is often initiated with two drugs. Blood pressure 120/80-139/89 mm Hg is considered "prehypertension" and is observed for progression without drug treatment in standard allopathic medicine[88] but is obviously a prime opportunity to intervene with nutritional and lifestyle improvements for those clinicians more progressively inclined. Blood pressure ≥140/90-160/100 is considered "stage 1 hypertension" and in the medical model is initially treated with one drug—generally a thiazide—while blood pressure ≥160/100-210/120 ("stage 2 hypertension") is often treated initially with a two-drug combination, with one of those drugs generally being a thiazide and the other drug selected based on patient characteristics. (Antihypertensive drug treatments are summarized at the end of this chapter). Blood pressures ≥210/120 are worthy of urgent or emergency treatment, based on the absence or presence of symptoms or organ damage, respectively, in an emergency hospital setting—additional details are provided in a following section on *Clinical Management*.

- <u>Cardiopulmonary examination</u>: Auscultation for rate, rhythm, rales/crackles; localize the cardiac point of maximal impulse (PMI) for evidence of lateral displacement or increased intensity which could indicate cardiomegaly or left ventricular hypertrophy.

- <u>Eye and fundoscopic examination</u>: Look for cotton-wool spots, retinal/flame hemorrhages, arteriovenous nicking, and papilledema; manifestations of diabetic retinopathy may also be seen if DM is concomitant. Patients with DM are referred for ophthalmologic evaluation at the time of diagnosis and annually/biannually thereafter depending on severity and compliance with and effectiveness of treatment.

- <u>Inspection for diagonal ear lobe crease</u>: Numerous studies have shown that the diagonal ear lobe crease is one of the easiest and most sensitive (~75%) and specific (~80%) physical examination findings to correlate with advanced atherosclerosis and cardiovascular disease.[89,90]

- <u>Examination of the extremities</u>: Assess pulse strength, arm:leg blood pressure differences[91] (ankle:brachial index should be > 1), lower extremity edema, capillary refill/perfusion and trophic changes consistent with peripheral vascular disease.

- <u>Renal disease survey</u>: Renal diseases are the most common causes of secondary hypertension. No physical examination finding correlates specifically with renal disease; peripheral edema is correlative but not indicative. Laboratory assessments include serum BUN, serum creatinine, serum cystatin C, and urine albumin:creatinine ratio (microalbuminuria) and/or urine albumin (proteinuria).

- <u>Auscultation for bruits</u>: Use the stethoscope bell over the carotid arteries (atherosclerosis) and renal arteries (renovascular hypertension due to atherosclerosis or fibromuscular dysplasia). Occasionally, an aortic bruit may be heard, particularly in cases of malformation or dissection. Higher degrees of arterial occlusion may reduce blood flow to such an extent that no bruit is heard.

- <u>Neurologic examination</u>: Observation for facial symmetry, inquiry about headache and mental status, and quick screening for symmetric and normal extremity muscle strength and reflexes may be sufficient for "low index" cases of mild hypertension in middle-aged patients without concomitant disease, such dyslipidemia or diabetes mellitus. However, as the number and severity of risk factors accumulate, the case becomes progressively worthy of a "high index" examination to establish a comprehensive assessment of baseline status and to screen for underlying causes or contributors to the HTN, as well as for other risk factors for CVD and complications from HTN. Situations indicating the appropriateness of a more thorough examination include younger or older patients in whom the HTN is more likely to be secondary to an underlying cause, patients with comorbidities or increased risk for complications, patients with more severe hypertension, and in patients with possible or impending complications from chronic HTN. Deep

[88] Le T, Dehlendorf C, Mendoza M, Ohata C. *First Aid for the Family Medicine Boards*. New York: McGraw-Hill Medical; 2008, 50
[89] Edston E. The earlobe crease, coronary artery disease, and sudden cardiac death: an autopsy study of 520 individuals. *Am J Forensic Med Pathol*. 2006 Jun;27(2):129-33
[90] Motamed M, Pelekoudas N. The predictive value of diagonal ear-lobe crease sign. *Int J Clin Pract*. 1998 Jul-Aug;52(5):305-6
[91] Ankle-brachial index test. webmd.com/heart-disease/ankle-brachial-index-test Referenced January 2010

tendon reflexes are checked for hyperreflexia (particularly with preeclampsia), and the Achilles reflex return is assessed for noteworthy delay that can indicate hypothyroidism[92], a well-documented cause of HTN and dyslipidemia. All patients deserve a thorough exam, whether for the assessment of baseline status, complications, contributions, or for the reassurance (for both doctor and patient) that is attained after a competent professional evaluation reveals no abnormalities.

- Body mass index (BMI) for assessing current BMI and predicting amount and duration of weight loss: Given that the average citizen of industrialized nations is overweight, nearly all patients can benefit from developing a specific goal-oriented and time-oriented plan for the achievement of weight optimization. **Contrasting current BMI with optimal BMI** clarifies the **amount of weight** that needs to be lost and provides an estimate of the **duration of the weight loss program**, given that adherent patients can lose an average of 4-8 lbs (~9-15 kg) per month. Although some patients can achieve highly significant improvements in various parameters such as glycemic control and blood pressure *without* significant weight loss, the fact remains that obesity (more specifically, abdominal obesity) is a **risk**

> **Clinical wisdom**
>
> Patients with lifestyle-generated diseases should be coached in the reversal of the patterns that have caused their disease rather than being enabled to pursue their disease-promoting lifestyles while surrogate markers of metabolic-physiologic dysfunction (e.g., hypertension) are pharmacologically suppressed.

factor and often the **primary determinant** for CVD-HTN-dyslipidemia-hyperglycemia-inflammation as well as osteoarthritis, many types of cancer, and significant but immeasurable (and generally unspoken) suffering associated with diminished self-esteem, inefficacy, social isolation, and depression. Patients have a myriad of reasons and rationalizations for maintaining their overweight status quo—every excuse from being "big boned" to "big framed" to "I've always been big" to "Everyone in my family is big" to "I don't have time to take care of myself" to "I don't know how to cook" to "I simply cannot [eat right, exercise, say 'no' to candy, give up wheat, give up ice cream, drink coffee without sugar and cream, etc]." Clinicians need to anticipate this resistance and have a diverse array of techniques—ranging from patient to insistent, from gentle to confrontational, from emotional to intellectual—to use *as appropriate to the individual patient's needs* to coax, inspire, lead, or push the patient who will benefit from weight loss. Elevated BMI correlates with numerous biochemical risk factors for CVD—progressively elevated levels of blood glucose, insulin, triglycerides, increasing

> **How to measure waist circumference**
>
> "To measure your waist circumference, place a tape measure around your bare abdomen just above your hip bone. [Waist circumference is the distance around your natural waist (just above the navel).*] Be sure that the tape is snug (but does not compress your skin) and that it is parallel to the floor. Relax, exhale, and measure your waist."
>
> Weight and Waist Measurement: Tools for Adults. win.niddk.nih.gov/Publications/tools.htm
> * Body Composition Tests. americanheart.org/presenter.jhtml?identifier=4489
> Accessed February 2009

severity of insulin resistance, and progressively lower levels of beneficial high-density lipoprotein (HDL) cholesterol—and an increased risk for cardiovascular death, various cancers, psychosocial problems including low self-esteem, reduced academic performance, and impaired interpersonal relationships, e.g., being a target for prejudice.[93] Elevated BMI is a preventable and treatable condition; physicians should not ignore this problem simply because it is common or difficult for some patients to acknowledge and effectively address. Relatedly, BMI should be viewed in context, especially with that of cardiovascular fitness, patient's symptoms (or lack thereof) of pain (joint pain and inflammatory diseases such as asthma and psoriasis are more common among the obese) and shortness of breath (dyspnea on exertion); also and importantly, several studies have shown that xenobiotic load is a more powerful predictor of insulin resistance than is obesity/BMI. Not surprisingly, the combination of obesity with either/both 1) lack of cardiovascular fitness and/or 2) elevated xenobiotic load is more problematic than obesity by itself. Obesity and elevated BMI are the easiest to detect and most obvious to discuss; patients and doctors alike need to be aware of the importance of enhancing both cardiovascular fitness (e.g., increasing the level of activity and exercise) and reducing the total xenobiotic load (e.g., avoiding exposure, promoting detoxification/depuration, and supporting governmental regulations to protect the public) rather than focusing solely on the obvious and easy: obesity and BMI.

---

[92] Degowin RL. *DeGowin and DeGowin's Diagnostic Evaluation. 6th Edition*. New York: McGraw Hill: 1994, 900. See also Khurana AK, Sinha RS, Ghorai BK, Bihari N. Ankle reflex photomotogram in thyroid dysfunctions. *J Assoc Physicians India*. 1990 Mar;38(3):201-3
[93] Costa et al. Body mass index has a good correlation with proatherosclerotic profile in children and adolescents. *Arq Bras Cardiol*. 2009 Sep;93(3):261-7

Laboratory Assessments:

- <u>Chemistry/metabolic panel</u>: Heightened attention is given to glucose, BUN, creatinine, calcium, and potassium. To screen for a renal cause of HTN, test serum BUN and creatinine and check urine albumin:creatinine ratio on a random urine sample; these tests are generally sufficient to confirm or refute a renal etiology of HTN. Renal US or CT imaging can be used for further renal evaluation. Glomerular filtration rate (GFR) can be estimated by the Cockcroft-Gault equation (DrV's tutorial: <u>vimeo.com/152296851</u>) and should be used by clinicians to monitor renal function in patients at risk for renal insufficiency, namely patients with HTN, diabetes mellitus, advanced age, and known renal disease. **Estimated GFR = (140 - age) x weight (kg) / (72 x serum creatinine); in women, multiply this result by .85.** GFR values consistently less than 60 for 3 months are consistent with chronic kidney disease and approximately 50% loss of renal function; at this level of impaired renal function, drug doses need to be modified. Hypercalcemia is a rare cause of HTN and requires evaluation for underlying cause, such as hyperparathyroidism, hyperthyroidism, malignancy (especially multiple myeloma, lymphoma, or cancer of the breast, lung, or kidney), granulomatous diseases such as sarcoidosis, vitamin D or vitamin A excess, adverse drug effect (especially lithium or thiazide diuretics), Paget disease of bone, adrenal insufficiency, or genotropic metabolic disorder such as familial hypocalciuric hypercalcemia.

- <u>Renal assessment, urinalysis (UA)</u>: Test for hematuria, proteinuria, and glucosuria; random albumin:creatinine ratio to assess for microalbuminuria. See Chapter 1 (lab interpretation), video archive <u>vimeo.com/152293616</u>.

- <u>Thyroid assessment—glandular function, peripheral metabolism, and autoimmunity</u>: The purpose of thyroid assessment is to determine the overall functionality of the pituitary-thyroid-metabolic axis, and therefore thyroid testing should be comprehensive and include TSH, free T4, free or total T3, and reverse T3, and the antibodies directed against thyroid peroxidase (anti-TPO) and thyroglobulin (anti-thyroglobulin). Overt or imminent hypothyroidism is suggested by TSH greater than 2 mU/L[94] or 3 mU/L[95], low T4 or T3, and/or the presence of anti-thyroid peroxidase antibodies.[96] Objective laboratory abnormality suggesting hypothyroidism in a patient with compatible clinical symptomatology or objective findings is sufficient justification to warrant a clinical trial of thyroid hormone supplementation provided that no contraindications are present and that the apparent hypothyroidism is not due to another cause such as hyperestrogenemia, which reduces thyroid hormone cellular bioavailability due to increased production of thyroxine binding globulin (TBG). Common clinical manifestations of hypothyroidism include fatigue, depression, cold hands and feet, dry skin, constipation, bradycardia, adult acne, hypertension, head hair loss, hypercholesterolemia, dysthymia/anhedonia, menstrual irregularities in women, and hypogonadism and subfertility in both men and women. Several approaches to the treatment of hypothyroidism are described in the section of *Therapeutic Considerations*.

- <u>Serum 25-hydroxy-vitamin D</u>: In 2004, Vasquez, Manso, and Cannell[97] proposed a "paradigm shift" for clinicians' appreciation of vitamin D that summarized new applications for the clinical use of this nutrient beyond its application in patients with osteoporosis or malabsorption. A novel concept at its time, our article admonished clinicians to use empiric supplementation and/or laboratory assessment of all patients seen in clinical practice. The goal with vitamin D supplementation is to get serum 25-hydroxy-vitamin D (25-OH-D) levels into the optimal range, as currently defined in the illustration. As the cardioprotective role of vitamin D becomes more clear, the peer-reviewed

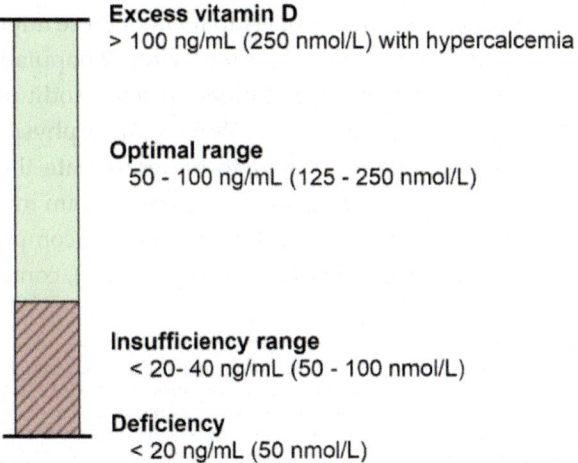

Excess vitamin D
> 100 ng/mL (250 nmol/L) with hypercalcemia

Optimal range
50 - 100 ng/mL (125 - 250 nmol/L)

Insufficiency range
< 20- 40 ng/mL (50 - 100 nmol/L)

Deficiency
< 20 ng/mL (50 nmol/L)

---

[94] Weetman AP. Hypothyroidism: screening and subclinical disease. *BMJ*. 1997 Apr 19;314(7088):1175-8 bmj.bmjjournals.com/cgi/content/full/314/7088/1175

[95] "Now AACE encourages doctors to consider treatment for patients who test outside the boundaries of a narrower margin based on a target TSH level of 0.3 to 3.0. AACE believes the new range will result in proper diagnosis for millions of Americans who suffer from a mild thyroid disorder, but have gone untreated until now." American Association of Clinical Endocrinologists (AACE). 2003 Campaign Encourages Awareness of Mild Thyroid Failure, Importance of Routine Testing aace.com/pub/tam2003/press.php November 26, 2005

[96] Beers MH, Berkow R (eds). *Merck Manual. 17th Edition*. Whitehouse Station: Merck Research Laboratories; 1999, Page 96

[97] Vasquez et al. The clinical importance of vitamin D: a paradigm shift with implications for all healthcare providers. *Altern Ther Health Med*. 2004 Sep-Oct;10(5):28-36

medical research increasingly advocates that **"vitamin D supplementation should be prescribed to patients with hypertension and 25-hydroxyvitamin D levels below target values."**[98]

- Uric acid: Many years ago uric acid was generally included in the standard chemistry/metabolic panel; these days it has to be ordered as a separate test. For at least a decade, "a strong, specific, stepwise, independent association of increasing serum uric acid and cardiac morbidity and mortality" has been noted[99], and recent research has shown that inhibition of uric acid production with allopurinol prevents fructose-induced urate-mediated metabolic disturbances that contribute to CVD, HTN, and the metabolic syndrome.[100] The roles of fructose and uric acid are discussed in greater detail in a following section.

- Urine pH: Urine pH can easily be monitored in-office or at home with the use of simple pH strips. Urine pH fluctuates throughout the day and therefore the most reliable evaluations are made with multiple daily assessments (easy and practical) and/or 24-h urine collections (cumbersome, inconvenient, and relatively impractical); an additional and important advantage to using multiple daily assessments of urine pH is that it allows the patient and doctor to observe how dietary and lifestyle fluctuations alter the whole-body biochemical-physiologic milieu. A urine pH of 7.0-8 is desirable as an indicator of dietary compliance and avoidance of the acidogenic Western diet, which is generally HTN-inducing due to its content of sodium, chloride, simple sugars and insufficiency of magnesium, potassium, calcium, and phytonutrients. Mild urinary alkalosis is the natural and optimal state of human physiology[101,102,103], and its induction is therefore simply a restoration of normalcy rather than an intervention or treatment per se. Caution might be employed when using this (or any other) treatment in patients with severe hepatorenal disease (who have lost the ability to buffer efficiently) and in patients with pre-existing electrolyte disturbances. Patients susceptible to urinary tract infections (UTIs) might experience an increased frequency of UTIs due to urinary alkalinization and may need to improve hygiene, supplement with additional ascorbic acid to prevent urine from becoming excessively alkaline, and/or correct gastrointestinal dysbiosis—this latter point is particularly important for women who experience recurrent UTIs, since urovaginal flora is strongly influenced by intestinal flora.[104]

- Urine sodium and potassium: Urine sodium (Na) and potassium (K) can be measured as markers for dietary intake and therefore as direct markers for compliance with dietary optimization. Urinary Na excretion ranges widely (thousand-fold) between human populations and individuals based mostly on dietary intake; among Yanomamo Indians in Brazil uNa is 0.2 mmol/24 h while among the northern Chinese the uNa is 242 mmol/24 h.[105] Very obviously, the general therapeutic goal in the treatment of HTN is to increase intake of potassium and reduce intake of sodium; the inverse ratio of these two cations positively correlates with blood pressure and other metabolic markers such as insulin sensitivity and endothelial function; thus measurement of urine sodium/potassium is more than a marker for nutritional compliance since is reflective and predictive of key aspects of cardiovascular health. Excepting sodium and potassium losses through perspiration, emesis, and diarrhea the urinary measurement of these minerals is clinically meaningful and correlates with dietary intake; the large Intersalt Study[106] involving 52 population samples in 32 countries for a total of 10,074 men and women aged 20-59 showed that higher urinary sodium excretion correlated positively and directly with systolic and diastolic blood pressures. While patient/physician-estimated potassium intake correlates with 24-h urinary K excretion, "patients tend to underestimate their sodium intake by 30% to 50%; therefore, urinary sodium excretion is more accurate to assess sodium intake."[107] Per the clinical trial by McCullough et al[108], patients on a low-Na diet (10 mEq/d) with excellent compliance have 24-hr Na excretion of approximately 4.6 - 13.4 mEq (outpatients and inpatients, respectively), compared with 24-hr Na excretion of 184.5 - 195.3 mEq for patients

[98] Pilz S, Tomaschitz A, Ritz E, Pieber TR; Medscape. Vitamin D status and arterial hypertension: a systematic review. *Nat Rev Cardiol*. 2009 Oct;6(10):621-30

[99] Alderman M. Uric acid in hypertension and cardiovascular disease. *Can J Cardiol* 1999 Nov;15 Suppl F:20F-2F

[100] News release from American Heart Association's 63rd High Blood Pressure Research Conference. High-sugar diet increases men's blood pressure; gout drug protective. Abstract P127. Sept. 23, 2009. americanheart.mediaroom.com/index.php?s=43&item=829 Accessed December 19, 2009

[101] Sebastian et al. Estimation of the net acid load of the diet of ancestral preagricultural Homo sapiens and their hominid ancestors. *Am J Clin Nutr*. 2002 Dec;76(6):1308-16

[102] Maurer et al. Neutralization of Western diet inhibits bone resorption independently of K intake and reduces cortisol secretion in humans. *Am J Physiol Renal Physiol*. 2003 Jan;284(1):F32-40

[103] Frassetto L, Morris RC Jr, Sellmeyer DE, Todd K, Sebastian A. Diet, evolution and aging--the pathophysiologic effects of the post-agricultural inversion of the potassium-to-sodium and base-to-chloride ratios in the human diet. *Eur J Nutr*. 2001 Oct;40(5):200-13

[104] Miles MR, Olsen L, Rogers A. Recurrent vaginal candidiasis. Importance of an intestinal reservoir. *JAMA*. 1977 Oct 24;238(17):1836-7

[105] Intersalt Cooperative Research Group. Intersalt: an international study of electrolyte excretion and blood pressure. Results for 24 hour urinary sodium and potassium excretion. Intersalt Cooperative Research Group. *BMJ*. 1988 Jul 30;297(6644):319-28

[106] Elliott et al. Intersalt revisited: further analyses of 24 hour sodium excretion and blood pressure within and across populations. *BMJ*. 1996 May 18;312(7041):1249-53

[107] Leiba et al. Does dietary recall adequately assess sodium, potassium, and calcium intake in hypertensive patients? *Nutrition*. 2005 Apr;21(4):462-6

[108] McCullough ML, Swain JF, Malarick C, Moore TJ. Feasibility of outpatient electrolyte balance studies. *J Am Coll Nutr*. 1991 Apr;10(2):140-8

on a higher Na diet (200 - 250 mEq/d); the differences seen here in 24-hr Na excretion of approximately 9 mEq in low-Na groups compared to approximately 190 mEq in high-Na groups is plain to see, even for the mathematically impaired and those stalwart skeptics who continue to resist appreciating the ability of dietary modification to have measurable and meaningful effects. The urinary sodium:creatinine (uNa/uCr) ratio can be assessed; for example, in the study by Kwok et al[109] among 111 ambulatory vegetarians, hypertensives had uNa/uCr ratio of 32.6 compared with a ratio of 12.4 among normotensives. In this same study, the urinary sodium:potassium (uNa/uK) ratio was 4.7 for hypertensives and 3.4 for normotensives; blood pressure also correlated with calcium intake, and the review by Ruilope et al[110] showed that calcium increases renal excretion of sodium (in a prostaglandin-dependent mechanism). With this latter data in mind, a clinician might speculate that part of vitamin D3's HTN-ameliorating effect may be derived *in part* from its ability to increase intestinal absorption of calcium and thereby promote renal loss of sodium.

- Fasting serum insulin: A direct relationship exists between elevated serum insulin, peripheral insulin resistance, and cardiovascular mortality.[111,112] Insulin promotes renal retention of sodium which leads to water retention and the subsequent volume overload and systemic hypertension. Clinicians can consider testing fasting serum insulin in patients likely to have hyperinsulinemia and insulin resistance; this can be used to tailor treatment, monitor benefit and compliance, and as a teaching aid for patients requiring or requesting additional details and insight. One of the largest medical laboratories in the US uses a reference range of "0.0-24.9 µIU/mL" (micro-IU [international units] per milliliter) for insulin.[113] Elevated fasting insulin concentration is generally defined as > 100 pmol/L (16.6 mU/L); however, leaning toward 60 pmol/L (10 mU/L)—or more conservatively 90 pmol/L (15 mU/L)—as the upper acceptable limits would provide for more sensitive detection of insulin resistance *as a marker for metabolic dysfunction* in appropriate clinical settings.[114] Per Vølund[115], the correct conversion factor for human insulin is 1 mU/L = 6 pmol/L.

- Hemoglobin A1c (Hgb-A1c): Hgb-A1c is also known as glycosylated hemoglobin, levels of which increase in direct proportion to average blood glucose levels. Thus, Hgb-A1c can be used on random blood samples to estimate blood glucose levels to establish or exclude a diagnosis of prediabetes or diabetes mellitus. Interpretation of Hgb-A1c levels is as follows:

A1c Percentage	Description
<5.7	<u>Normal:</u>
5.7 - 6.4	<u>Prediabetic:</u> Interestingly, the phrase "prediabetic" reflects the allopathic medical paradigm of the unidirectionality and unavoidability of diabetes. A more proper term could be "borderline diabetes" indicating that the patient is *not* diabetic but showing a tendency toward *insulin resistance* or *glucose intolerance*—note that either of the two latter phrases are better and more "actionable" than the pseudoprophetic phrase *prediabetic*. Unlike *"insulin resistance"*, the phrase *"glucose intolerance"* is actionable because the common-sense implication is that if a patient has a metabolic impairment to the efficient utilization and metabolism of glucose then this substance should be avoided. By popularizing the phrases insulin resistance and—even worse—*metabolic syndrome*, physicians and patients alike are distracted from the importance of reducing carbohydrate intake in the treatment of these conditions.
>6.5	<u>Diabetes mellitus:</u> Diabetes mellitus and insulin resistance are reviewed elsewhere.

---

[109] Kwok TC, Chan TY, Woo J. Relationship of urinary sodium/potassium excretion and calcium intake to blood pressure and prevalence of hypertension among older Chinese vegetarians. *Eur J Clin Nutr.* 2003 Feb;57(2):299-304

[110] "...calcium influences renal function and enhances renal sodium excretion. The intrarenal effects of low doses of calcium are dependent on the renal production of prostaglandins." Ruilope LM, Lahera V, AraqueA,SuarezC,RodicioJL,RomeroJC. Electrolyte excretion and sodium intake. *Am J Med Sci.* 1994;307 Suppl 1:S107-11

[111] "The magnitude and direction of the relationship between insulin concentration and incident CVD were similar. CONCLUSIONS: We found a significant association between HOMA-IR and risk of CVD after adjustment for multiple covariates." Hanley AJ, Williams K, Stern MP, Haffner SM. Homeostasis model assessment of insulin resistance in relation to the incidence of cardiovascular disease: the San Antonio Heart Study. *Diabetes Care.* 2002 Jul;25(7):1177-84

[112] "Hyperinsulinemia was associated with increased all-cause and cardiovascular mortality in Helsinki policemen independent of other risk factors,..." Pyörälä et al. Plasma insulin and all-cause, cardiovascular, and noncardiovascular mortality: the 22-year follow-up results of the Helsinki Policemen Study. *Diabetes Care.* 2000;23(8):1097-102

[113] Insulin. Test Number: 004333 CPT Code: 83525. https://labcorp.com Accessed November 24, 2010

[114] Personal communications, November 2010. I am grateful to Bill Beakey of Professional Laboratory Co-Op, James Bogash DC, Kara Fitzgerald ND, Dan Lukaczer, and Todd Lepine MD for their conversations with me about serum insulin.

[115] Vølund A. Conversion of insulin units to SI units. *Am J Clin Nutr.* 1993 Nov;58(5):714-5

- Tests for lead accumulation: In the United States, a consistent correlation has been found between body burden of lead and HTN, even when blood lead levels are well below the current US occupational exposure limit guidelines (40 microg/dl).[116] Harlan et al[117] analyzed data from the second National Health and Nutrition Examination Survey (1976-1980) and thereby found a direct relationship between blood lead levels and systolic and diastolic pressures for men and women and for white and black persons aged 12 to 74 years; they concluded, "Blood lead levels were significantly higher in younger men and women (aged 21 to 55 years) with high blood pressure, but not in older men or women (aged 56 to 74 years). In multiple regression analyses, the relationship of blood lead to blood pressure was independent of other variables for men, but not for women. Dietary calcium and serum zinc levels were inversely related to blood pressure." Schwartz and Stewart[118] contrasted blood lead, dimercaptosuccinic acid (DMSA)-chelatable lead, and tibial lead to find that blood lead was the assessment that most strongly correlated with HTN; they concluded, "**Systolic blood pressure was elevated by blood lead levels as low as 5 microg/dl**." Thus, clinicians might first measure blood lead levels, which do not measure total body burden but rather the lead that is mobile or *in transit* within the body and which appears to have the best correlation with HTN; the finding of normal blood lead results could then be followed with the more sensitive DMSA-provoked heavy metal testing before concluding that heavy metals are noncontributory to that particular patient's HTN. For heavy metal testing in various clinical scenarios, this author's preference is to use DMSA-provoked measurement of urine toxic metals. After a minimal test dose of DMSA (e.g., in the range of 50-100 mg) to screen for hypersensitivity, patients take oral DMSA 10 mg/kg as a single oral dose in the morning on an empty stomach after emptying the bladder and send a sample from the next urination for laboratory analysis; follow laboratory protocol if different from these instructions. Use of DMSA for lead and mercury chelation/detoxification and for diagnostic purposes is generally safe and effective[119,120,121,122,123]; see Chapter 4 of _Functional Inflammology_ / _Inflammation Mastery_ (2014 and later).
- Plasma aldosterone-to-renin ratio: As the screening blood test for primary hyperaldosteronism, this test is indicated in any hypertensive patient with unexplained hypokalemia. When the plasma aldosterone measured in ng per dL is > 20 times the level of plasma renin activity in ng *per* mL *per* hour, hyperaldosteronism is suspected, confirmatory testing can be performed by an endocrinologist using an available salt-suppression test.[124]
- Plasma and urine levels of epinephrine and norepinephrine: Plasma and urine levels of epinephrine and norepinephrine can be measured while the patient is on a stable low-sodium diet. In a review and exemplary case report summarized in a following section, Morimoto et al[125] describe the use of plasma and urine epinephrine and norepinephrine as markers of sympathetic nervous system activity in a patient treated with neurovascular decompression (detailed later in this chapter); their strategy employed a sodium intake of 120 mmol/d with fasting blood samples taken via indwelling catheter at 7:30am after the patient had rested for 30 minutes in the supine position. Over the course of four months following surgical neurovascular decompression of the left ventrolateral medulla oblongata, Morimoto et al report the following postsurgical changes:
  - Plasma epinephrine: Reduced from 0.22 to <0.05 (reference range <0.93 nmol/L).
  - Plasma norepinephrine: Reduced from 0.95 to 0.30 (range 0.89 - 3.37 nmol/L).
  - Urine epinephrine: Reduced from 83.5 to 26.2 (range 5.5 – 76.4 nmol/d).
  - Urine norepinephrine: Reduced from 0.52 to 0.39 (range 0.06 – 0.024 mmol/d).

The importance of their case report is, among other considerations, that it shows that a post-intervention reduction in sympathetic nerve activity can be documented objectively, and that antihypertensive benefits can

[116] Nash et al. Blood lead, blood pressure, and hypertension in perimenopausal and postmenopausal women. *JAMA.* 2003 Mar 26;289(12):1523-32 jama.ama-assn.org

[117] Harlan et al. Blood lead and blood pressure. Relationship in the adolescent and adult US population. *JAMA.* 1985 Jan 25;253(4):530-4

[118] "Systolic blood pressure was elevated by blood lead levels as low as 5 microg/dl." Schwartz BS, Stewart WF. Different associations of blood lead, meso 2,3-dimercaptosuccinic acid (DMSA)-chelatable lead, and tibial lead levels with blood pressure in 543 former organolead manufacturing workers. *Arch Environ Health.* 2000 Mar-Apr;55(2):85-92

[119] Bradstreet J, Geier DA, Kartzinel JJ, Adams JB, Geier MR. A case-control study of mercury burden in children with autistic spectrum disorders. *Journal of American Physicians and Surgeons* 2003; 8: 76-79 jpands.org/vol8no3/geier.pdf

[120] Crinnion WJ. Environmental medicine, part three: long-term effects of chronic low-dose mercury exposure. *Altern Med Rev.* 2000 Jun;5(3):209-23

[121] Forman J, Moline J, Cernichiari E, Sayegh S, Torres JC, Landrigan MM, Hudson J, Adel HN, Landrigan PJ. A cluster of pediatric metallic mercury exposure cases treated with meso-2,3-dimercaptosuccinic acid (DMSA). *Environ Health Perspect.* 2000 Jun;108(6):575-7 ehp.niehs.nih.gov/docs/2000/108p575-577forman/abstract.html

[122] Miller AL. Dimercaptosuccinic acid (DMSA), a non-toxic, water-soluble treatment for heavy metal toxicity. *Altern Med Rev.* 1998 Jun;3(3):199-207

[123] DMSA. *Altern Med Rev.* 2000 Jun;5(3):264-7

[124] Viera AJ, Neutze DM. Diagnosis of secondary hypertension: an age-based approach. *Am Fam Physician.* 2010 Dec 15;82(12):1471-8

[125] Morimoto S, Sasaki S, Takeda K, Furuya S, Naruse S, Matsumoto K, Higuchi T, Saito M, Nakagawa M. Decreases in blood pressure and sympathetic nerve activity by microvascular decompression of the rostral ventrolateral medulla in essential hypertension. *Stroke.* 1999 Aug;30(8):1707-10

be significant and associated with *relative* reductions in catecholamine levels that may be *within* or *outside of* the normal reference range. With the awareness that reference ranges for plasma and urine levels of epinephrine and norepinephrine were established exclusively for the detection of *overt pathology* (i.e., autonomic failure at the bottom of the range and pheochromocytoma at the top of the range) rather than for *functional disorders* such as neurogenic hypertension, clinicians may judiciously utilize measurements of plasma and urine

> **Applied physiology**
>
> Epinephrine levels reflect activity of the adrenal medulla, while norepinephrine levels are a more general indicator of overall sympathetic nervous system activity. Post-intervention reductions in epinephrine and norepinephrine indicate reduced sympathetic activity, generally an important benefit in patients with hypertensive and cardiovascular diseases.

epinephrine and norepinephrine to assess for hypersympathotonia and to monitor patient's response to treatment by documenting reductions in catecholamine production after intervention.

- Other cardiovascular risk factors: Lipids (and an increasing number of lipid fractions), homocysteine, high-sensitivity C-reactive protein (hsCRP) can also be assessed to evaluate overall long-term cardiovascular risk.

Imaging:

- Electrocardiography (ECG, EKG): To assess for injury or pathophysiologic adaptation, ECG is appropriate for patients with HTN[126] and those at high risk for or with evidence of CVD, MI, PVD, CHF, chest pain (CP, including angina), or shortness of breath (SOB).
- Upper cervical radiographs: Clinicians highly skilled in manual manipulative therapeutics might choose to radiograph the upper cervical spine as a means to determine the appropriateness and application of spinal manipulative therapy to effect "marked and sustained reductions in BP similar to the use of two-drug combination therapy."[127] Generally however, radiographs prior to spinal manipulative therapy are not advised unless indicated by specific clinical characteristics such as recent trauma, neurologic deficit, or increased possibility for congenital anomaly (e.g., Sprengel's deformity), atlantoaxial instability (e.g., Down syndrome, rheumatoid arthritis, ankylosing spondylitis), or underlying disease (e.g., suspicion of malignant disease).
- Other imaging: CT, US, and angiographic techniques are commonly used to assess for HTN-related tumors, vascular anomalies/occlusion, and renal abnormalities. More specifically, US or IV contrast CT assessment for abdominal aortic aneurysm is indicated for hypertensive patients with any history of smoking aged >65yo and patients with documented CAD/CVD.[128]
- Biopsy/Procedure: Tissue biopsy is generally not required except when investigating a specific pathoetiologic consideration. Angioplasty and stent placement for the treatment of renal artery stenosis, and aldosterone measurement in the adrenal vein to lateralize the side of an aldosterone-secreting tumor are examples of procedures used in some cases of HTN. Renal biopsy specifies type and severity of intrinsic renal disease when history, labs, and imaging are inconclusive.

Establishing the Diagnosis of Hypertension in Adults: The diagnosis of adult hypertension is established after at least two measurements of blood pressure with either component greater than 140/90 mm Hg. Patients with systolic blood pressure 120-139 mm Hg or diastolic blood pressure 80-89 mm Hg are considered "prehypertensive"[129] and should be differentially diagnosed then treated with lifestyle and non-pharmacologic measures unless a *true primary cause* of the hypertension is discovered. Patients with diabetes mellitus, renal disease, or CVD should have their blood pressure controlled to ≤ 130/80 mm Hg. Patients with elevated systolic and normal diastolic pressures have **isolated systolic hypertension**, which in adults indicates an increased risk for stroke, heart failure, myocardial infarction, and overall mortality that can be ameliorated by effective intervention.[130] Given that mortality increases with chronic blood pressures greater than 115/75 mm Hg[131], progressive clinicians should appreciate 115/75 mm

---

[126] Bent S, Gensler LS, Frances C. *Saint-Frances Guide: Clinical Clerkship in Outpatient Medicine. 2nd Edition*. Philadelphia; Wolters Kluwer: 2008, 90
[127] Bakris et al. Atlas vertebra realignment and achievement of arterial pressure goal in hypertensive patients: a pilot study. *J Hum Hypertens*. 2007 May;21(5):347-52
[128] "In-hospital screening of AAA is very efficient among patients with coronary artery disease. Therefore, patients with CAD may be considered for routine AAA screening." Monney et al. High prevalence of unsuspected abdominal aortic aneurysms in patients hospitalised for surgical coronary revascularisation. *Eur J Cardiothorac Surg* 2004 Jan:65-8
[129] Bent S, Gensler LS, Frances C. *Saint-Frances Guide: Clinical Clerkship in Outpatient Medicine. 2nd Edition*. Philadelphia; Wolters Kluwer: 2008, 87
[130] Chobanian AV. Control of hypertension—an important national priority. *N Engl J Med*. 2001 Aug 16;345(7):534-5
[131] Benowitz NL. "Antihypertensive Agents." In Katzung BG (editor). *Basic and Clinical Pharmacology. 10th Edition*. New York: McGraw Hill Medical; 2007, 159

Hg as the upper end of the ideal range; from this perspective, the diagnostic threshold of 140/90 mm Hg for hypertension is appropriately seen as a great deviation from normal.

- **Hypertension in infants, children, and adolescents**: As previously mentioned, normal and abnormal values for blood pressure in infants and children are different from those of adults and are stratified based on age, gender, and height in a chart from the International Pediatric Hypertension Association. Please see their website at PediatricHypertension.org for downloadable charts and additional information helpful when dealing with childhood hypertension.

Blood pressure description and clinical considerations

BP in mm Hg	Description and clinical considerations
115/75 or slightly lower	Optimal blood pressure: "Starting at 115/75 mm Hg, cardiovascular risk doubles with each increment of 20/10 mm Hg throughout the blood pressure range."[132]
120/80 to 139/89	Prehypertension: Elevated risk for adverse cardiovascular outcomes; begin assessment and assertive lifestyle and nutritional interventions.
≤ 130/80	Blood pressure goal for patients with diabetes mellitus, renal disease, or CVD: Patients with multiple risk factors for adverse cardiovascular outcomes must have each variable treated to more assertively than if only one risk factor was present.
140/90 to 159/99	Stage 1 hypertension: Implement effective treatment and management strategies and reviewed here and elsewhere. Drug-treated patients are generally started with **one** medication, most commonly hydrochlorothiazide. See the concise pharmacotherapy review at the end of this chapter for more information on drug therapy.
160/100 or greater	Stage 2 hypertension: Implement effective treatment and management strategies and reviewed here and elsewhere. Drug-treated patients are generally started with **two** medications, most commonly hydrochlorothiazide plus another medication prescribed based on the patient's comorbidities and tolerance. See the concise pharmacotherapy review at the end of this chapter for more information on drug therapy. The *acute onset* of blood pressures greater than 160/100 – 160/110 must be treated as a potentially life-threatening emergency, because *acute onset* hypertension by definition of its acute onset poses a higher risk of complications because physiologic adaptations have not had time to accommodate the higher pressures. In inpatient hospital settings, sBP > 160 is commonly used as a threshold for use of hydralazine, generally administered as 10 mg IV PRN each 1-2 hours.
200/120 or greater *without* complications	Hypertensive urgency: Severe HTN *without* symptoms or evidence of end-organ damage. These patients are appropriately treated in the emergency department with *orally administered* medications—see details that follow.
200/120 or greater *with* complications	Hypertensive emergency: Severe HTN with symptoms or evidence of end-organ damage such as headache, blurred vision, chest pain, shortness of breath, or renal insufficiency. Must be treated in an intensive/critical care setting with *intravenous* antihypertensive medications—see details that follow.

Disease Complications:

- The increased morbidity and mortality of HTN can manifest as any of the following:
    - Congestive heart failure presenting with fatigue, lower extremity edema, rales, dyspnea or orthopnea
    - Retinopathy and visual impairment
    - Hypertensive nephropathy presenting as azotemia, edema, recalcitrant HTN
    - Stroke—hemorrhagic or ischemic
    - Atrial fibrillation due to atrial enlargement
    - Myocardial infarction or sudden death due to accelerated CVD complicated by cardiac hypertrophy (i.e., supply-demand mismatch)
    - Abdominal aortic aneurysm, especially with HTN plus tobacco smoking

---

[132] Benowitz NL. "Antihypertensive Agents." In Katzung BG (editor). *Basic and Clinical Pharmacology. 10th Edition*. New York: McGraw Hill Medical; 2007, 159

Clinical Management: For routine outpatients, the obvious goal is to get the blood pressure down below 140/90 mm Hg as quickly, safely, and cost-effectively as possible while treating any primary underlying disorders; treatments that provide *collateral benefits* are preferred over those which cause *side effects*. Attention to naturopathic medicine's "hierarchy of therapeutics"[133] is important here in order to prioritize the implementation of therapeutic interventions. Correction of nutritional deficiencies (e.g., vitamin D, magnesium, potassium, calcium,

> **The physician's judgment remains paramount**
>
> "Positive experiences, trust in the clinician, and empathy improve patient motivation and satisfaction. This report serves as a guide, and the committee continues to recognize that the responsible physician's judgment remains paramount."
>
> Seventh Report of the Joint National Committee on Prevention, Detection, Evaluation and Treatment of High Blood Pressure [JNC 7]

phytonutrients), nutritional imbalances (e.g., insulin resistance and hyperglycemia, diet-induced metabolic acidosis), and hormonal imbalances (e.g., thyroid deficiency/excess, estrogen excess, aldosterone excess) should take precedence over the simple utilization of **antihypertensive drugs which suppress the manifestation of underlying dysfunction and thus allow it to perpetuate**; because of the latter, pharmacotherapy often abets rather than abates chronic disease. Following the exclusion of pathologic causes of HTN, the diagnosis of HTN should be explained to the patient as a sign of internal (e.g., nutritional, hormonal, metabolic, or structural) imbalance or otherwise as an opportunity to use this marker (blood pressure) as a barometer of overall health and compliance with a health-promoting lifestyle, including optimization of diet, exercise, relationships, and nutritional intake.

- <u>Stratification of HTN management</u>: Factors that direct the management of HTN include severity, manifestations of associated organ damage, and the patient's general condition and comorbidities.
  - <u>Hypertensive emergency</u> = >200/120 mm Hg *with evidence of end-organ damage or symptoms possibly attributable to the hypertension such as headache, blurred vision, chest pain, or shortness of breath*: Accompanying clinical manifestations may include renal failure, hematuria, proteinuria, altered mental status, papilledema, retinal vascular changes, MI, angina, stroke, aortic dissection, and pulmonary edema. Treat in intensive/critical care setting with *intravenous* antihypertensive medications such as nitroprusside, nitroglycerine, esmolol, hydralazine, labetolol, nicardipine then transition to oral beta-blockers and ACEi (angiotensin converting enzyme inhibitor) drugs. Add diuretics such as furosemide/Lasix as needed to alleviate volume overload, pulmonary edema, HTN, and heart failure. The initial drop in blood pressure should not exceed 25% in order to prevent precipitation of organ ischemia due to reflexive arteriospasm.
  - <u>Hypertensive urgency</u> = blood pressure >220/120 mm Hg[134] or >220/125 mm Hg[135] *without end-organ damage and without symptoms*: These patients are appropriately treated in the emergency department with *orally administered* medications such as nifedipine (oral, not sublingual), clonidine, and/or captopril. Patients can be discharged following normalization of blood pressure, but these patients require timely follow-up with a primary care provider. Complicating factors and concomitant disease may necessitate hospital admission.
  - <u>Acute-onset HTN</u>: Acute HTN in a previously normotensive patient can lead to stroke and other complications at pressures of 160 mm Hg systolic or 110 mm Hg diastolic. Acute-onset HTN can cause stroke at pressures generally tolerated in chronic cases because in the latter vascular adaptations accommodate higher pressures. **Acute-onset HTN *from any cause* should be treated emergently/urgently when pressures approximate or exceed 160-180 mm Hg systolic or 110 mm Hg diastolic**, especially but not exclusively if accompanied by complications such as angina, shortness of breath, vision changes, papilledema, headache/confusion/seizures (which suggest cerebral edema or cerebral vasospasm), proteinuria, or edema of the face, peripheral extremities, or of the general body (anasarca, check for sacral edema and weight gain).
  - <u>Malignant HTN</u>: Severe, intractable, and generally progressive HTN characterized by diastolic HTN > 130 mm Hg with clinical complications including renal failure, encephalopathy, or papilledema. Treat in hospital setting with intravenous antihypertensive medications (reviewed above for hypertensive emergency).

---

[133] The "hierarchy of therapeutics" is a guiding principle of naturopathic medicine providing a conceptual framework for prioritizing and sequencing of therapeutic interventions, reviewed in the section on "Naturopathic Medicine" in Chapter 1 and—in concepts and applications—throughout Chapter 2.
[134] Bent S, Gensler LS, Frances C. *Saint-Frances Guide: Clinical Clerkship in Outpatient Medicine. 2nd Edition*. Philadelphia; Wolters Kluwer: 2008, 89
[135] McPhee SJ, Papadakis MA (editors). *Current Medical Diagnosis and Treatment. 2009. 48th Edition*. New York; McGraw Hill Medical: 401

- Routine recommendations that should be communicated then documented in the patient's chart: These include ❶ encouragement of smoking cessation, ❷ a minimum of 30 minutes of exercise per day (for patients healthy enough to exercise), ❸ weight loss/optimization, ❹ limit alcohol intake to no more than 1-2 drinks per day, ❺ restrict sodium to ≤ 2,400 mg/d (i.e., ≤ 6 grams/d of sodium chloride), ❻ increase intake of fruits and vegetables, and ❼ reduce intake of total and saturated fat in order to promote weight loss and optimize serum lipids.[136] In the allopathic model, these lifestyle recommendations are used for three months before initiating drug treatment of HTN.

- Drug management and comanagement of HTN may be required. Drug management is appropriate in urgent situations, recalcitrant cases, patients with initial BP > 160/100 mm Hg, and for patients who are noncompliant with treatment. Patients and clinicians can facilitate progression through the "stages of change"[137] by appreciating the barriers and requirements that characterize the overcoming of each stage until the final stage of termination/integration is achieved. In common medical practice, lifestyle interventions, the processes of change, nutritional supplementation, and spinal manipulation are almost never given their full due consideration; thus, by default, drug treatment of hypertension is the allopathic standard of care because it is the only treatment given priority. Failure to discuss nondrug treatments with hypertensive patients is unethical because many nondrug treatments are superior in safety, affordability, and effectiveness when compared with drug treatments; failure to discuss nondrug treatments is also a violation of medical ethics' principles of beneficence, autonomy and informed consent.

> **Clinical insight**
>
> Patients with lifestyle-generated diseases should be coached in the reversal of the patterns that have caused their disease rather than being enabled to pursue their disease-promoting lifestyles while surrogate markers of metabolic-physiologic dysfunction (e.g., hypertension) are pharmacologically suppressed.

- Tailor treatment recommendations and goals to the patient's specific psychographics and BVG-LOC profile. More than 90-95% of HTN patients will be found to have no pathologic/medical cause of their HTN, thus implicating diet and lifestyle as the most responsible factors. In some situations, the resolution of the patient's HTN comes expeditiously through the simple and imperfect implementation of weight loss, diet modification, correction of nutritional deficiencies, and avoidance or reduced intake of infamous triggers such as tobacco, alcohol, and excess caffeine. **For many patients with HTN— especially when the HTN is part of a larger cluster of clinical findings such as type-2 diabetes mellitus or the metabolic syndrome—the successful management of their HTN will rely on the implementation of numerous changes in various aspects of "lifestyle" including diet, preparation/procurement of food, social interactions, core relationships, exercise involvement, time and money allocation, and—most importantly— changes in self-image, and the establishment and "affirmation-through-action" of core values.** These issues can appear complex to the point of being "too complicated" for doctors and patients who are not personally accustomed to living consciously and for whom dispensing and consuming pills, respectively, are easier than the consciousness-raising and the self-disciplined and self-directed living required to advocate and manifest a health-centered life. Complexity and convenience should not be the determinants of care. Patients with lifestyle-generated diseases should be coached in the reversal of the patterns that have caused their disease rather than being enabled to pursue these disease-promoting lifestyles while surrogate markers of metabolic-physiologic dysfunction are pharmacologically suppressed. Therapeutic lifestyle changes must be merged with the patient's **beliefs** (important but changeable paradigms), **values** (subjective-objective rules), and **goals** (conscious and subconscious aspirations and trajectory). In order to facilitate this merger, the clinician must— first—understand the patient's position on these variables, then—second—deliver the treatment plan in such a way as to "speak to" the patient's beliefs, values, and goals. Most people do not have consciously-chosen and declarable beliefs, values, and goals for their lives; thus, this process of the physician's gaining an understanding of the patient's unconscious psychographic details is generally not completed on the first visit and may not be completed until the patient has done the requisite "homework" (perhaps facilitated by a professional therapist or lay counselor/coach) and has thereafter returned with a perceptible level of self-awareness. Clinicians who **seek first to understand, then to be understood**[138] will have advantages over clinicians who steamroll patients with lifestyle impositions and a "to do" list that is foreign to the patient's

[136] Bent S, Gensler LS, Frances C. _Saint-Frances Guide: Clinical Clerkship in Outpatient Medicine. 2nd Edition_. Philadelphia; Wolters Kluwer: 2008, 90
[137] Prochaska, JO, Norcross, JC, and DiClemente, CC. _Changing for Good_. NY, William Morrow and Company; 1994
[138] Covey SR. _The Seven Habits of Highly Effective People_ (1989); see also _The 8th Habit: From Effectiveness to Greatness_ (2004).

inner and previous experiences. With regard to psychographic information, clinicians are wise to remember the three tenets of evidence-based medicine, one of which rests upon this psychographic information: ❶ published research, ❷ the clinician's experience and expertise, and ❸ the patient's preferences and goals.

Psychographic profiling: Understanding patients to help them connect personal goals with health goals
• <u>Beliefs</u>: What are the fundamental beliefs and expectations that the patient has for his/her future? Is life merely "suffering and toil" or is it meant to be "a well of delight"? Patients who expect misery are generally successful in its attainment unless they are guided and provoked toward a more positive life expectancy. The clinician can correct errors in thought and information. • <u>Values</u>: What does the patient value? "*Autonomy and independence*"—will this manifest as resistance to the clinician's advice or as a willingness to comply with treatment so as to avoid future disability? "*Strength*"—will this be resistance to the plan or disciplined adherence to the plan? "*Love*"—is this self-sacrificing 'love' for other people or is it a wholesome and healthy love that includes the self? "*My family*"—does this include avoiding disability, being alive to support and encourage family members and upcoming generations? "*Nothing really*"—what are the mental barriers and painful experiences that have resulted in this emotional numbness; what would his/her life be like if he/she were to engage in life consciously and with purpose? The clinician assigns homework for the patient to clarify—and later manifest in action—a list of personal values. Patients need to understand how their *personal* goals are connected to their *health* status and goals. • <u>Goals</u>: What are the patient's social, physical, professional, personal, and spiritual goals? Is the current lifestyle and health/disease trajectory consistent with the attainment and extended enjoyment of these goals? Are the goals too limited, and has the patient accommodated small goals with small effort and the resulting lackluster results that reinforce self-depreciation and low self-esteem, thus perpetuating a vicious cycle? Goals are a reflection of core values and one's intimate belief about what is possible and what levels of success, love, and happiness are appropriate for one's life. • <u>Locus of Control</u>: Does the patient view the world as chaotic and menacing (external locus of control), or as understandable and thus worthy of meaningful engagement (internal locus of control)? If the patient views him/herself as a victim, then compliance will be low because every and any excuse will serve as a rationalization for why he/she "couldn't" exercise, eat right, and take medications or nutrients as prescribed. Patients who experience their health problems as incomprehensible and "idiopathic" are less likely to engage in purposeful health activities and are more likely to be noncompliant with treatment(s) and more passive in their willingness to rely on "doctor's orders" and drug treatments. Physicians should encourage the best self-image in and self-efficacy from patients by reminding them by either Socratic-dialectic education or direct verbalization that the patient has the power and thus the "response-ability" to strongly influence his/her health outcomes via positive health expectations and behaviors.

• <u>Patients must receive instruction on at-home blood pressure monitoring and/or follow-up in-office assessments</u>: At the time of diagnosis, patients are instructed of the importance of proper treatment and follow-up visits (ranging from weekly to biweekly to monthly) to facilitate compliance and monitor treatment effectiveness. HTN must never be taken lightly by the clinician or the patient as it represents and indicates a significant departure from optimal health and the failure of internal homeostatic mechanisms; more concretely, HTN is generally a silent and progressive disorder which prematurely undercuts health and vitality and which tends to culminate in unnecessary morbidity (e.g., pain, suffering, loss of function, renal dialysis, and stroke) and early death. Patients can use office-calibrated home blood pressure monitoring equipment to self-monitor compliance, lifestyle effects, and effectiveness of treatment; patients are advised that at-home monitoring does not substitute for in-office visits and that in-office blood pressure measurements are the standard by which treatment decisions are made. "White coat hypertension" (WCH) is explained as an exaggerated stress response to innocuous stimuli that has parallels in other areas of the patient's life and is therefore not an excuse for normal at-home readings; accordingly, studies have shown that patients with WCH show increased risk for cardiovascular complications.[139,140] Depending on HTN severity and the protocol being followed, patients might be seen in the office for a quick follow-up assessment once every 2-7 days, or less frequently if BP checks are occurring reliably at home. Patients with metabolic syndrome, obesity, or who are likely to be noncompliant are followed-up more frequently than medically indicated in order to promote compliance and patient-physician alliance. Generally, after the normalization of blood pressure with treatment, patients are reevaluated every 3-6 months in the office. Laboratory tests are performed at least annually and can be performed on an as needed basis with any evidence or suspicion of problems such as nephropathy, dyslipidemia, DM, or drug side effects.

---

[139] "Coronary disease may be more severe among patients with WCH than among those without." Kostandonis et al. Topography and severity of coronary artery disease in white-coat hypertension. *Eur J Intern Med*. 2008 Jun;19(4):280-4

[140] "Our findings also further stress the interest of assessing the presence of a white-coat effect as a means to further identify patients at increased cardiovascular risk and guide treatment accordingly." Bochud et al. Association between White-Coat Effect and Blunted Dipping of Nocturnal Blood Pressure. *Am J Hypertens*. 2009 Oct;22(10):1054-61

- Patients already taking antihypertensive medications are likely to require a dosage adjustment or medication discontinuation after using diet, lifestyle, and nutritional interventions. Clinicians should anticipate this benefit and inform the patient and prescribing doctor appropriately. Failure to anticipate the normalization of blood pressure and to adjust medications appropriately may result in hypotension, most commonly manifested by fatigue and/or (pre)syncope.
- Document everything: Document all relevant clinical findings, laboratory/imaging results, treatments with rationale, patient education, plan of scheduled follow-up, and referal/comanagment. Ensure that chart notes document education, consent to treatment, and that "patient verbalizes understanding; all questions are answered and concerns addressed."

Clinical management of HTN

1. Assessment for urgency and end-organ damage
2. Differential diagnosis and comprehensive assessment
3. Effective treatment or appropriate referral
4. Patient education—legitimate, effective education, not simply drug indoctrination buttressed by ineffective diet and lifestyle advice
5. Scheduled follow-up
6. Monitor for compliance, treatment effectiveness, adverse effects, and new complications; clinicians have the responsibility to implement effective treatment or refer for effective treatment. Non-treatment is not an appropriate option. Nonresponsive and noncompliant patients need in-office and/or written information regarding risk; referrals need to include written letter to the other physician plus scheduling of the patient's appointment, with the patient clearly informed of the date, time, and location of the appointment.
7. Document all of the above in the patient chart, signed and dated.

Treatment Considerations for "Primary" Hypertension—An Evidence-based Article-by-Article Review with Commentary: Reviewed here are the most successful and/or most common treatments for HTN; these treatments can generally be categorized as **dietary** (i.e., foods consumed), **nutritional** (i.e., foods consumed plus the use of nutritional supplements), **hormonal** (e.g., correction of hypothyroidism, hyperaldosteronism, hyperparathyroidism), **surgical** (reviewed here: microvascular decompression of the left ventrolateral medulla oblongata), **manipulative** (reviewed here: spinal and paraspinal soft tissue manipulation), and **lifestyle intervention**, with the latter being a large general category that includes but is not limited to exercise, weight optimization (generally weight *loss* for the treatment of HTN), Qigong, controlled breathing, meditation, and acupuncture. Readers will be better able to appreciate the clinical significance of the blood pressure reductions achieved if they are aware that ❶ most blood-pressure-lowering drugs used chronically on an outpatient basis achieve reductions in the magnitude of approximately 12/6 mm Hg while reductions of 20/10 mm Hg generally require combination (i.e., at least two drugs) therapy[141], ❷ the vast majority (more than 70%) of medically-treated HTN patients take at least two blood-pressure-lowering drugs to achieve or approach their BP goal, and ❸ the criteria to establish efficacy of an antihypertensive effect as defined by the US Food and Drug Administration for approval of a new antihypertensive drug requires proof of both efficacy and safety in a blinded-design study; proof of efficacy is defined as a placebo-subtracted reduction in diastolic BP of 4-5 mm Hg or more, and "…most single agent antihypertensive [drugs] yield an 8 mm Hg drop in pressure in people with Stage 1 hypertension…"[142] Upon close reading of the following sections, readers will note that most of the nonpharmacologic therapeutics reviewed can achieve reductions greater than 5 mm Hg in BP.

FOOD & NUTRITION The first component of "DrV's functional inflammology protocol" recalled by the FINDSEX® acronym is the (re)establishment of nutritional sufficiency and nutrition-related biochemical balance via implementation of a healthy foundational diet and basic nutritional supplementation. Paleolithic diets—defined as those which emphasize fruits, vegetables, nuts, seeds, berries and sufficient intake of lean protein—are the most nutrient-dense, satiating, and neuro-enhancing diets available; the diet can be customized to meet the needs of all patients. Atop this foundational diet, supplementation of vitamins, minerals, fatty acids—specifically ALA, GLA,

---

[141] Magill MK, Gunning K, Saffel-Shrier S, Gay C. New developments in the management of hypertension. *Am Fam Physician*. 2003 Sep 1;68(5):853-8

[142] "The criteria used in this study to establish efficacy of an antihypertensive effect are those defined by the Food and Drug Administration for approval of a new antihypertensive drug. Specifically, it would require a blinded design with a placebo-subtracted reduction in diastolic BP of 5 mm Hg or more and be free of serious side effects to be approvable." Bakris et al. Atlas vertebra realignment and achievement of arterial pressure goal in hypertensive patients: a pilot study. *J Hum Hypertens*. 2007 May;21(5):347-52. See also information from the US FDA website (fda.gov/RegulatoryInformation/Guidances/ucm129461.htm, accessed June 12, 2010) which states, "…because the effect of active drugs is often small (diastolic blood pressure change of 4-5 mm Hg more than placebo), studies conducted in a blinded fashion and with placebo controls are essential."

EPA, DHA, and oleic acid, and probiotics provides the optimal base from which metabolic/physiologic balance and function can be restored/maintained, and from which balance and function can be further optimized by the skilled addition of other components of the protocol.

- **The supplemented Paleo-Mediterranean Diet**: The health-promoting diet of choice for the majority of people is a diet based on abundant consumption of fruits, vegetables, seeds, nuts, omega-3 and monounsaturated fatty acids, and lean sources of protein such as lean meats, fatty cold-water fish, soy and whey proteins. This diet prohibits and obviates overconsumption of chemical preservatives, artificial sweeteners, and carbohydrate-dominant foods such as candies, pastries, breads, potatoes, grains, and other foods with a high glycemic load and high glycemic index. This "Paleo-Mediterranean Diet"—first detailed by Vasquez[143] in 2005—is a combination of the "Paleolithic" or "Paleo diet" and the well-known "Mediterranean diet", both of which are well described in peer-reviewed journals and the lay press. The Paleo-Mediterranean Diet is wholly consistent with the "polymeal"—a multicomponent cardioprotective diet plan characterized by emphasis on phytonutrient-rich foods including fish, red wine, garlic, almonds, dark chocolate, and most (low-carbohydrate) fruits and vegetables—which is estimated to have the potential to lower the incidence of CVD by 76%.[144]

  In the subsections that follow, various studies related to dietary intervention for hypertension will be summarized; these dietary patterns can be viewed in a continuum ranging from the ❶ SAD diet to ❷ the DASH diet to ❸ the Paleo-Mediterranean diet. Also included is the fourth most common dietary pattern, that of ❹ the vegetarian diet and its related variants of veganism, pescovegetarianism, and lacto-ovo-vegetarianism.

> **Cardiovascular and metabolic benefits of the Paleolithic hunter-gatherer diet pattern**
>
> ☑ **Significant reductions in blood pressure**,
> ☑ Improved arterial distensibility,
> ☑ **Significant reduction in plasma insulin**,
> ☑ Large significant reductions in total cholesterol, low-density lipoproteins (LDL) and triglycerides,
> ☑ Consistently improved status of circulatory, carbohydrate and lipid metabolism/physiology.
>
> "Conclusions: Even **short-term consumption of a Paleolithic type diet improves BP and glucose tolerance, decreases insulin secretion, increases insulin sensitivity and improves lipid profiles without weight loss in healthy sedentary humans**."
>
> Frassetto et al. Metabolic and physiologic improvements from consuming a Paleolithic, hunter-gatherer type diet. *Eur J Clin Nutr*. 2009 Feb

Combining the Paleo-Mediterranean diet with multivitamin/multimineral supplementation (including physiologic doses of vitamin D3 to optimize serum levels), with balanced combination fatty acid (ALA, GLA, EPA, DHA) supplementation and probiotics forms the "supplemented Paleo-Mediterranean diet" (sPMD)[145], the five basic components of which are outlined below:

1. Paleo-Mediterranean Diet: The most nutrient-dense diet available; more amenable to social integration and greater nutrient content compared to vegetarianism; provides sufficient protein to promote satiety and therefore reduced caloric intake. The importance of carbohydrate restriction is commonly underappreciated, and it provides an anti-hypertensive benefit regardless of weight change/loss; carbohydrate restriction provides numerous eumetabolic benefits such as promoting depletion of ceramide and promoting mitochondrial autophagy/biogenesis—ie, mitochondrial recycling. Importantly and very easy to understand mechanistically, low-carbohydrate diets lower blood glucose and thereby lower insulin levels; because (elevated) insulin serves to promote sodium and water retention, reducing insulin (in this case by reducing the carbohydrate load) reduces hypertension by reducing sodium and water retention, thereby functioning in a *poly*beneficial manner, one that is partly analogous to diuretic therapy.

2. Multivitamin and multimineral supplementation: Routine vitamin and mineral supplementation is warranted because dietary intake (based on SAD) is generally insufficient to provide sufficient vitamins and minerals[146]; supranutritional doses of vitamins and minerals stimulates variant/defective enzymes with decreased coenzyme binding affinity (increased K[m]).[147]

---

[143] Vasquez A. A Five-Part Nutritional Protocol that Produces Consistently Positive Results. *Nutritional Wellness* 2005 Sept. Vasquez A. Importance of Integrative Chiropractic Health Care in Treating Musculoskeletal Pain and Reducing the Nationwide Burden of Medical Expenses and Iatrogenic Injury and Death. *Original Internist* 2005; 12(4): 159-182

[144] Franco OH, Bonneux L, de Laet C, Peeters A, Steyerberg EW, Mackenbach JP. The Polymeal: a more natural, safer, and probably tastier (than the Polypill) strategy to reduce cardiovascular disease by more than 75%. *BMJ*. 2004 Dec 18;329(7480):1447-50

[145] Vasquez A. The Importance of Integrative Chiropractic Health Care in Treating Musculoskeletal Pain and Reducing the Nationwide Burden of Medical Expenses and Iatrogenic Injury and Death. *Original Internist* 2005; 12(4): 159-182

[146] Fletcher RH, Fairfield KM. Vitamins for chronic disease prevention in adults: clinical applications. *JAMA*. 2002 Jun 19;287(23):3127-9

[147] Ames BN, Elson-Schwab I, Silver EA. High-dose vitamin therapy stimulates variant enzymes with decreased coenzyme binding affinity (increased K(m)): relevance to genetic disease and polymorphisms. *Am J Clin Nutr*. 2002 Apr;75(4):616-58

3. <u>Vitamin D3 in physiologic doses to optimize serum 25-OH-D levels</u>: Vitamin D3 deficiency and insufficiency are common in the general population and are causatively and/or epidemiologically associated with HTN, CVD, CHF, type-1 and type-2 diabetes mellitus, mental depression and schizophrenia, systemic inflammation, and various cancers and autoimmune disorders. The physiologic requirement for vitamin D3 is approximately 4,000 IU per day for adult men. Dosages should be sufficient to effect serum 25-OH-D levels within the optimal range of 50-100 ng/ml.

4. <u>Balanced combination fatty acid supplementation with ALA, GLA, EPA, DHA, with dietary oleic acid</u>: Patients consuming the SAD may be presumed to have numerous fatty acid imbalances (e.g., excess arachidonate and *trans*-fatty acids) along with insufficiencies of ALA, GLA, EPA, DHA, and oleic acid. Hunter-gather intake of omega-3 fatty acids is approximately 7 grams per day contrasted to 1 gram per day provided by Westernized/industrialized diets. Fatty acid imbalances/deficiencies commonly seen in patients consuming Westernized/industrialized/SAD diets—similar to and probably additive to if not synergistic with vitamin D deficiency/insufficiency—contributes to HTN, CVD, CHF, type-1 and type-2 diabetes mellitus, mental depression and schizophrenia, systemic inflammation, and various cancers and autoimmune disorders.

5. <u>Probiotics</u>: Probiotics are safe and effective anti-inflammatory, immunoenhancing, and immunomodulating agents[148,149] and are—based on published research and clinical experience—suitable for routine use, ideally as a rotating combination of yogurts, kefir, other fermented foods, and—particularly for dairy-intolerant patients—supplements.

The Four Main Food-Consumption Patterns

Diet pattern	Characteristics
❶ SAD: Standard American Diet	<ul><li>Food choices in this diet are based on convenience, recent advertisements, coupons and cost, popular trends, social pressure, and instant gratification at the expense of the feeling of health or its authentic attainment.</li><li>This diet tends to be high in sucrose, fructose, sodium, chloride, and chemical colorants, preservatives, and artificial flavors. It is generally low in essential fatty acids, minerals, vitamins in their natural form, fiber and phytonutrients.</li><li>This diet is largely responsible for the modern epidemics of *overconsumption malnutrition* which causes obesity, hypertension, cardiovascular disease, and increased risk for various cancers and other chronic diseases.</li><li>Because the foods tend to be mass-produced, of low quality, and of durable shelf life due to lack of nutritional value, chemical preservatives, and packaging, the economics of these products is that of low cost for consumers and high profit for producers and sellers. Tertiary profitability is enjoyed by drug companies, so-called "health insurance" corporations, and hospital and clinic systems that have to implement the damage control and rescue remedies necessary to sustain life following long-term consumption of this diet.</li><li>If not for the SAD dietary pattern and the physical inactivity that generally accompanies it, hypertension would not exist as the epidemic that it currently is, and antihypertensive medications would be *orphan drugs*.</li><li>Because of the characteristic incorporation of "flavor enhancers" such as monosodium glutamate and carrageenan, and because of the high content of sodium and sugars, the *supranormal* stimulation provided to taste receptors downregulates the subtle perception of taste so that consumers become accustomed to (i.e., *addicted to*) the supranormal stimulation and are thereby disinclined to consume a normal natural diet due to its comparatively "bland" taste. ***Clinical pearl***: Generally, 1-2 weeks are required following discontinuation of the SAD diet before gustatory sensitivity is restored so that foods in their natural state can be appreciated. Patients need to lean toward going "cold turkey" (pun intended) and thereby avoiding excess sugar, sodium, flavor-enhancers and other supranormal stimulation for 1-2 weeks so that they can thereafter consume and enjoy a *natural* whole foods diet.</li></ul>

---

[148] Neish AS. Microbes in gastrointestinal health and disease. *Gastroenterology*. 2009 Jan;136(1):65-80

[149] Galdeano et al. Proposed model: mechanisms of immunomodulation induced by probiotic bacteria. *Clin Vaccine Immunol*. 2007 May;14(5):485-92

The Four Main Food-Consumption Patterns—*continued*

Diet pattern	Characteristics
❷ DASH: Dietary Approaches to Stop Hypertension	• *Better* food choices than the SAD diet, with emphasis placed on: • *Reduced* consumption of saturated fat, cholesterol, and total fat, red meat, sweets, added sugars, and sugar-containing beverages compared to the SAD. • *Increased* consumption of fruits, vegetables, and fat-free or low-fat milk and milk products, whole grain products, fish, poultry, and nuts. • Compared to the SAD, DASH provides more potassium, magnesium, calcium, protein, and fiber and less sodium and sugars such as sucrose and fructose. • In sum, the DASH diet a *better* diet pattern compared to the random and nonlogical convenience- and pleasure-based eating habits followed by most Americans and others seduced by the convenience, low cost, and supranormal stimulation of the SAD or "Westernized" diet. However, the inclusion of grains and excess carbohydrates makes it suboptimal, particularly when compared to diets based on vegetables, nuts, berries, seeds.
❸ Paleo-Mediterranean Diet	• The Paleo-Mediterranean diet consists almost exclusively of unprocessed and as-fresh-as-possible and as-raw-as-possible fruits, vegetables, nuts, seeds, berries and lean sources of protein, especially fish, poultry, and lean grass-fed meats and game meats. A modern modification allows the inclusion of whey and soy protein isolates for their functional benefits beyond the mere provision of protein to include functionally active proteins, peptides, amino acid profiles, whey immunoglobulins and lactoferrin, and the soy phytonutrients genistein, daidzein, and beta-sitosterol. Dark chocolate, olive oil, and red wine are also accepted staples of this dietary pattern. • The Mediterranean diet as commonly described also includes "whole grains" such as wheat and starchy vegetables such as potatoes; these are best avoided. Knowledgeable clinicians will appreciate that the modern notion of "whole grains" is a farce because of mechanical processing which pulverizes the husk and bran of the grain into oblivion, rendering its natural-state physiochemical properties powerless. • In its highest form (i.e., excluding grains and other mechanically processed and overcooked food items), the Paleo-Mediterranean diet is the most nutrient-dense and physiologically appropriate diet for human beings with the greatest promise of health optimization and disease prevention.[150]
❹ Vegetarian diet, and related variants	• Plant-based diets *should* consist of fruits, vegetables, nuts, seeds, berries consumed as raw and as fresh as possible; this might seem obvious except that many (pseudo)vegetarians rely on grains and processed foods and are thus only vegetarians to the extent that they avoid meat (perhaps "acarneists") and not to the extent that they rely on vegetables, as the term *vegeta*rianism implies. Consumption of legumes for their relatively higher protein content is common. Avoidance of grains due to their allergenicity and low phytonutrient and micronutrient content is advised. • The lack of sufficient vitamin B-12 along with the relatively higher content of anti-nutrients such as phytic acid makes a purely vegetarian diet of tenuous durability for the unskilled, unknowledgeable, and undisciplined consumer. Many people adopt a so-called vegetarian diet for sociopolitical reasons without becoming aware of its proper implementation; such persons can consume a protein-deficient diet consistent with "breaditarianism"[151]—which is basically equal to or worse than the SAD diet due to its lack of adequate protein and overreliance on simple carbohydrates • <u>Vegan</u> = exclusive consumption of plant foods only. • <u>Vegetarian</u> = reliance upon plant foods, with the occasional inclusion of diary, eggs, and fish. • <u>Pescovegetarian</u> = consumption of plants and fish. • <u>Lacto-ovo-vegetarian</u> = consumption of plants, milk, eggs (i.e., animal protein without the killing of animals).

---

[150] Cordain et al. Origins and evolution of the Western diet: health implications for the 21st century. *Am J Clin Nutr.* 2005 Feb;81(2):341-5 ajcn.org/cgi/content/full/81/2/341
[151] O'Keefe JH Jr, Cordain L.Cardiovascular disease resulting from a diet and lifestyle at odds with our Paleolithic genome. *Mayo Clin Proc* 2004;79:101-8

Most of the studies reviewed in the following section pertain to the Paleo-Mediterranean diet (PMD) and its optimized expression in the supplemented Paleo-Mediterranean diet (sPMD). Studies on the DASH diet generally showed benefit when contrasted to the SAD eating pattern which is the norm for most Americans and increasingly among other nationalities. In this text, the DASH diet is advocated only insofar as it is an improvement over the SAD eating pattern; it is secondary to the PMD and tertiary to the sPMD in its effectiveness for disease treatment and prevention.

- Small clinical trial: Metabolic and physiologic improvements from consuming a Paleolithic, hunter-gatherer type diet (*European Journal of Clinical Nutrition* 2009 Feb): Despite the small subject size (n = 9), this study demonstrates safety and beneficial effectiveness of the Paleolithic diet in addressing several of the perturbations that characterize the metabolic syndrome and lifestyle-induced predisposition to CVD. "Results: Compared with the baseline (usual) diet, we observed (a) **significant reductions in BP** associated with improved arterial distensibility; (b) **significant reduction in plasma insulin** vs time AUC [area under the curve], during the OGTT [oral glucose tolerance testing]; and (c) large significant reductions in total cholesterol, low-density lipoproteins (LDL) and triglycerides (-0.8, -0.7 and -0.3 mmol/l respectively). In all these measured variables, either **eight or all nine participants had identical directional responses when switched to Paleolithic type diet, that is, near consistently improved status of circulatory, carbohydrate and lipid metabolism/physiology.**"[152]

- Randomized 3-month cross-over pilot study: Beneficial effects of a Paleolithic diet on cardiovascular risk factors in type 2 diabetes (*Cardiovascular Diabetology* 2009 Jul): Although small (n=13), this study is impressive because it shows not only the benefits of the Paleolithic diet but also its superiority over the commonly recommended "diabetic diet" which is advocated by so-called conventional-standard-mainstream-government and medical groups that claim to advocate health and victory in the so-called war against obesity and diabetes mellitus. "Compared to the diabetes diet, the Paleolithic diet resulted in lower mean values of HbA1c (-0.4% units), triacylglycerol (-0.4 mmol/L), **diastolic blood pressure (-4 mmHg)**, weight (-3 kg), BMI (-1 kg/m2) and waist circumference (-4 cm), and higher mean values of high density lipoprotein cholesterol (+0.08 mmol/L)."[153]

- Randomized controlled trial: Effects of the DASH diet alone and in combination with exercise and weight loss on blood pressure and cardiovascular biomarkers in men and women with high blood pressure (*Archives of Internal Medicine* 2010 Jan): This publication reports results of a randomized controlled clinical trial among 144 overweight/obese hypertensive patients for 4 months; intervention was either DASH diet alone, DASH diet with a weight management program, or usual control diet.

Intervention	Results
DASH diet alone	☺ BP was reduced by -11.2/-7.5 mm Hg
DASH diet *with* aerobic exercise *and* caloric restriction	☺ BP was reduced by **-16.1/-9.9** mm Hg ☺ Greater improvement was noted in this group than with DASH alone for pulse wave velocity, baroreflex sensitivity, and left ventricular mass
Usual control (UC) diet	☺ Nonsignificant BP reduction of -3.4/-3.8 mm Hg

The authors reported the results and conclusion as follows: "Clinic-measured BP was reduced by 16.1/9.9 mm Hg (DASH plus weight management); 11.2/7.5 mm (DASH alone); and 3.4/3.8 mm (usual diet controls). … Greater improvement was noted for DASH plus weight management compared with DASH alone for pulse wave velocity, baroreflex sensitivity, and left ventricular mass. CONCLUSION: For overweight or obese persons with above-normal BP, the addition of exercise and weight loss to the DASH diet resulted in even larger BP reductions, greater improvements in vascular and autonomic function, and reduced left ventricular mass."[154]

---

[152] Frassetto et al. Metabolic and physiologic improvements from consuming a paleolithic, hunter-gatherer type diet. *Eur J Clin Nutr*. 2009 Feb 11.

[153] Jonsson et al. Beneficial effects of a Paleolithic diet on cardiovascular risk factors in type 2 diabetes: a randomized cross-over pilot study. *Cardiovasc Diabetol*. 2009;8:35.

[154] Blumenthal JA, Babyak MA, Hinderliter A, et al. Effects of the DASH diet alone and in combination with exercise and weight loss on blood pressure and cardiovascular biomarkers in men and women with high blood pressure: the ENCORE study. *Arch Intern Med*. 2010 Jan 25;170(2):126-35

- <u>Randomized controlled trial with n=144: Effects of the Dietary Approaches to Stop Hypertension (DASH) diet alone and in combination with exercise and caloric restriction on insulin sensitivity and lipids</u> (<u>*Hypertension*</u> 2010 May[155]): In this study lead by Blumenthal published in 2010, the authors examined the effects of the DASH diet on insulin sensitivity and lipids in a randomized controlled trial with 144 overweight (BMI: 25 to 40) men (n=47) and women (n=97) with BP up to 159/99 mm Hg. Study subjects were randomly assigned for 4 months to one of three groups with the following results (table below), respectively. Of important note is the worsening of glucose control and insulin sensitivity on the DASH diet; this suggests that the DASH diet may ultimately promote development of metabolic syndrome despite appearing to be cardioprotective based on short-term reductions in blood pressure. Note that the weight loss induced by *caloric restriction + exercise* of 19 lbs over 4 months equates to 4.75 lbs per month; this is consistent with what clinicians should expect in clinical practice, namely patients' weight loss of 4-8 lbs per month with dietary optimization plus increased physical activity.

Intervention	Results
DASH diet alone	☺ <u>Weight loss</u>: Imperceptible, only -0.3 kg ☺ <u>Exercise capacity</u>: No improvement ☹ <u>Glucose control</u>: Slight worsening of glucose levels after the oral glucose load; fasting serum insulin actually increased from 16.6 to 17.6 mcu/ml ☹ <u>Lipids</u>: No change; slight worsening of triglycerides ☺ <u>Blood pressure</u>: Clinically significant reductions in blood pressure
DASH diet *with* aerobic exercise *and* caloric restriction	☺ <u>Weight loss</u>: Clinically and statistically significant at -8.7 kg (-19.2 lbs) ☺ <u>Exercise capacity</u>: Significant increase in aerobic capacity ☺ <u>Glucose control</u>: Lower fasting glucose; lower glucose levels after the oral glucose load; improved insulin sensitivity; fasting serum insulin reduced from 18.1 to 12.5 mcu/ml ☺ <u>Lipids</u>: Meaningful reductions in total cholesterol, triglycerides, and low-density lipoprotein cholesterol (LDL) ☺ <u>Blood pressure</u>: Clinically significant reductions in blood pressure
Usual control (UC) diet	☹ <u>Weight *gain*</u>: +0.9 kg ☺ <u>Exercise capacity</u>: No improvement ☺ <u>Glucose control</u>: No improvement ☺ <u>Lipids</u>: No improvement ☺ <u>Blood pressure</u>: No improvement

- <u>Randomized clinical trial: Effects of the dietary approaches to stop hypertension diet, exercise, and caloric restriction on neurocognition in overweight adults with high blood pressure</u> (<u>*Hypertension*</u> 2010 Jun[156]): In this clinical trial, 124 subjects with either prehypertension or stage 1 hypertension (sBP 130 to 159 mm Hg or dBP 85 to 99 mm Hg) who were sedentary and overweight or obese (BMI: 25 to 40) were randomized to the DASH diet alone, DASH with exercise and caloric restriction, or a usual control (UC) diet group. Subjects completed tests of executive function, memory, and learning and psychomotor speed at baseline and at the end of the 4-month trial. Results showed the following: "Participants on the DASH diet combined with a behavioral weight management program exhibited greater improvements in executive function-memory-learning and psychomotor speed, and DASH diet alone participants exhibited better psychomotor speed compared with the usual diet control. Neurocognitive improvements appeared to be mediated by increased aerobic fitness and weight loss. … In conclusion, combining aerobic exercise with the DASH diet and caloric restriction improves neurocognitive function among sedentary and overweight/obese individuals with prehypertension and hypertension." Specific to changes in blood pressure, the following results were noted (per Table 2 of the original article):

---

[155] Blumenthal et al. Effects of dietary approaches to stop hypertension diet alone and in combination with exercise and caloric restriction on insulin sensitivity and lipids. *Hypertension*. 2010 May;55(5):1199-205
[156] Smith et al. Effects of dietary approaches to stop hypertension diet, exercise, and caloric restriction on neurocognition in overweight adults with high blood pressure. *Hypertension*. 2010 Jun;55(6):1331-8

Intervention	Initial BP	Final BP	BP change
DASH diet alone	137.5/87.2	127.8/79.5	-9.7/-7.7
DASH diet *with* aerobic exercise *and* caloric restriction	138.6/85.4	125.1/77.2	**-13.5/-8.2**
Usual control (UC) diet	138.6/85.7	136.2/82.7	-2.2/-3

Thus, as we should expect, dietary improvement plus caloric restriction and exercise resulted in greater reductions in BP than diet improvement alone, which was better than no change at all. The neurocognitive improvements associated with improved diet and increased exercise are consistent with the previously documented neurogenic/neuroprotective/synaptogenic effects of exercise[157], as well as improved neuronal function seen with increased phytonutrient intake.[158] *Consider the implications: the "standard American diet" along with the standard American lifestyle of inactivity basically dumbs people down.* As discussed in Chapter 4.4, Kihn's 2013 essay "Political Roots of American Obesity" is an impressive alignment of compelling ideas.[159]

What might be the cumulative additive/synergistic neuro-intellectual results—on a personal, interpersonal, social, and national level—of dietary optimization, frequent exercise, decided application of one's efforts and abilities, and habitual exposure to complex neurointellectual phenomena—for example, the combination of humanistic psychology, authentic (not "pop") philosophy, and highly structured music?[160,161] Synergism of these events would likely elevate humanity toward its positive potential.

- Review: Effects of exercise, diet and weight loss on high blood pressure (*Sports Medicine* 2004[162]): The authors of this review note that HTN "is a major health problem in the US, affecting more than 50 million people" and that "anti-hypertensive medications are not effective for everyone, and may be costly and result in adverse effects that impair quality of life and reduce adherence. Moreover, abnormalities associated with high BP, such as insulin resistance and hyperlipidemia, may persist or may even be exacerbated by some anti-hypertensive medications." Thereafter, their expert review of the literature may be summarized in the table below. The benefits of exercise and weight loss extend beyond BP reduction to include reductions in left ventricular mass and wall thickness (i.e., reductions in left ventricular hypertrophy), reduced arterial stiffness and improved endothelial function.

Intervention	Blood pressure reduction
Exercise alone: without intentional weight loss or diet intervention	-3.5/-2.0 mm Hg
DASH diet	-5.5/-3.0 mm Hg
Weight loss of 17.6 lbs (8 kg)	-8.5/-6.5 mm Hg
Combined exercise & weight loss	**-12.5/-7.9 mm Hg**

- The 2009 Canadian Hypertension Education Program recommendations for the management of hypertension: Part 2—therapy (*Canadian Journal of Cardiology* 2009 May[163]): These are very conventional and standard recommendations from the medical community which are included here for the sake of completeness so that doctors have a recent reference guideline from which they can move beyond in the delivery of superior clinical care. "RECOMMENDATIONS: For lifestyle modifications to prevent and treat hypertension, restrict dietary sodium to less than 2300 mg (100 mmol)/day (and 1500 mg to 2300 mg [65 mmol to 100 mmol]/day in hypertensive patients); perform 30 min to 60 min of aerobic exercise four to seven days per week; maintain a healthy body weight (body mass index 18.5 kg/m(2) to 24.9 kg/m(2)) and waist circumference (smaller than 102 cm for men and smaller than 88 cm for women); limit alcohol consumption to no more than 14 units [drinks] per week in men or nine units per week in women; follow

[157] Cotman CW, Berchtold NC, Christie LA. Exercise builds brain health: key roles of growth factor cascades and inflammation. *Trends Neurosci.* 2007 Sep;30(9):464-72
[158] Spencer JP. The impact of fruit flavonoids on memory and cognition. *Br J Nutr.* 2010 Oct;104 Suppl 3:S40-7 and Spencer JP. Flavonoids and brain health: multiple effects underpinned by common mechanisms. *Genes Nutr.* 2009 Dec;4(4):243-50
[159] Kihn ED. The Political Roots of American Obesity. 2013 May truth-out.org/opinion/item/16149-the-political-roots-of-american-obesity
[160] Suda M, Morimoto K, Obata A,Koizumi H, Maki A.Cortical responses to Mozart's sonata enhance spatial-reasoning ability.*Neurol Res* 2008;30:885-8
[161] Jausovec N, Jausovec K, Gerlic I. The influence of Mozart's music on brain activity in the process of learning. *Clin Neurophysiol.* 2006;117:2703-14
[162] Bacon SL, Sherwood A, Hinderliter A, Blumenthal JA. Effects of exercise, diet and weight loss on high blood pressure. *Sports Med.* 2004;34:307-16
[163] Khan et al. 2009 Canadian Hypertension Education Program recommendations for the management of hypertension: Part 2—therapy. *Can J Cardiol.* 2009 May;25(5):287-98

a diet that is reduced in saturated fat and cholesterol, and that emphasizes fruits, vegetables and low-fat dairy products, dietary and soluble fiber, whole grains and protein from plant sources; and consider stress management in selected individuals with hypertension." These guidelines would have been better if they had advised complete avoidance of grains (sources of generally acidogenic phytonutrient-poor carbohydrates) and other sources of simple carbohydrate including candies and soft drinks in general and those pseudofoods laden with high-fructose corn syrup in particular.

- Meta-analysis: Adherence to Mediterranean diet and health status (*British Medical Journal* 2008 Sep[164]): "Greater adherence to a Mediterranean diet is associated with a significant improvement in health status, as seen by a **significant reduction in overall mortality** (-9%), mortality from **cardiovascular diseases** (-9%), incidence of or mortality from **cancer** (-6%), and incidence of **Parkinson's disease and**

> **Lifestyle recommendations from the Canadian Hypertension Education Program**
> - Restrict dietary sodium to less than 2300 mg (100 mmol)/day (and 1500 mg to 2300 mg [65 mmol to 100 mmol]/day in hypertensive patients).
> - Perform 30 min to 60 min of aerobic exercise four to seven days per week.
> - Maintain a healthy body weight (body mass index 18.5 kg/m(2) to 24.9 kg/m(2)) and waist circumference (< 102 cm for men and < 88 cm for women).
> - Limit alcohol consumption to no more than 14 units per week in men or nine units per week in women.
> - Follow a diet that is reduced in saturated fat and cholesterol.
> - Follow a diet that emphasizes fruits, vegetables and low-fat dairy products, dietary and soluble fiber, ~~whole grains~~ and protein from plant sources.
> - Consider stress management in selected individuals with hypertension.
>
> Khan NA, Hemmelgarn B, Herman RJ, et al. The 2009 Canadian Hypertension Education Program recommendations for the management of hypertension: Part 2—therapy. *Can J Cardiol*. 2009 May;25(5):287-98

Alzheimer's disease (-13%). These results seem to be clinically relevant for public health, in particular for **encouraging a Mediterranean-like dietary pattern for primary prevention of major chronic diseases.**" The results of this meta-analysis have major implications for clinical practice and public health policy.

- **Short-term water-only fasting**: The anti-hypertensive and anti-diabetic benefits of low-carbohydrate diets and short-term fasting have been substantiated in the research literature for several decades. However, the chiropractic physician Alan Goldhamer deserves credit for the most recent revival of short-term fasting as a therapeutic tool for chronic hypertension and diabetes mellitus.

  - Open clinical trial: Chiropractic-supervised water-only fasting in the treatment of hypertension (*Journal of Manipulative Physiological Therapeutics* 2001 Jun[165]): In this open trial, 174 consecutive hypertensive patients were treated in an inpatient setting under clinician supervision. The treatment program began with a short prefasting period (approximately 2 to 3 days on average) during which food consumption was limited to fruits and vegetables, followed by supervised water-only fasting (approximately 10 to 11 days on average) and a refeeding period (approximately 6 to 7 days on average) introducing a low-fat, low-sodium, vegan

> **Clinical Pearl: lowering plasma glucose → lower insulin levels → less sodium-water retention → alleviation of hypertension**
> Treatments that lower plasma glucose levels, either via reduced intake of carbohydrates or by increasing glucose disposal (i.e., increasing insulin sensitivity) have an anti-hypertensive effect via lowering insulin levels. **Because insulin promotes sodium-water retention, any treatment that lowers glucose-insulin levels will help correct the contribution of hyperinsulinemia to hypertension.** Likewise, avoidance of dietary fructose is now known to avoid the fructose-induced elevations in serum uric acid which contribute to endothelial dysfunction, hypertension, and the metabolic syndrome.

diet. "RESULTS: Almost 90% of the subjects achieved blood pressure less than 140/90 mm Hg by the end of the treatment program. **The average reduction in blood pressure was 37/13 mm Hg**, with the greatest decrease being observed for subjects with the most severe hypertension. **Patients with stage 3 hypertension (those with systolic blood pressure greater than 180 mg Hg, diastolic blood pressure greater than 110 mg Hg, or both) had an average reduction of 60/17 mm Hg at the conclusion of treatment.** All of the subjects who were taking antihypertensive medication at entry (6.3% of the total sample) successfully discontinued the use of medication. CONCLUSION: Medically supervised water-only fasting appears to be a safe and effective means of normalizing blood pressure and may assist in motivating health-promoting diet and lifestyle changes."

[164] Sofi F, Cesari F, Abbate R, Gensini GF, Casini A. Adherence to Mediterranean diet and health status: meta-analysis. *BMJ*. 2008 Sep 11;337:a1344
[165] Goldhamer et al. Medically supervised water-only fasting in the treatment of hypertension. *J Manipulative Physiol Ther* 2001 Jun;24(5):335-9

- Open clinical trial: Chiropractic-supervised water-only fasting in the treatment of borderline hypertension (*Journal of Alternative and Complementary Medicine* 2002 Oct[166]): 68 consecutive patients with borderline hypertension were treated in an inpatient setting under professional supervision. The treatment program consisted of a short prefasting period (approximately 1-2 days on average) during which food consumption was limited to fruits and vegetables followed by supervised water-only fasting (approximately 13.6 days on average). Fasting was followed by a refeeding period (approximately 6.0 days on average). The refeeding program consisted of a low-fat, low-sodium, plant-based, vegan diet. "RESULTS: Approximately 82% of the subjects achieved BP at or below 120/80 mm Hg by the end of the treatment program. **The mean BP reduction was 20/7 mm Hg,** with the greatest decrease being observed for subjects with the highest baseline BP. A linear regression of BP decrease against baseline BP showed that the estimated BP below which no further decrease would be expected was 96.0/67.0 mm Hg at the end of the fast and 99.2/67.3 mm Hg at the end of refeeding. These levels are in agreement with other estimates of the BP below which stroke events are eliminated, thus suggesting that these levels could be regarded as the "ideal" BP values. CONCLUSION: Medically supervised water-only fasting appears to be a safe and effective means of normalizing BP and may assist in motivating health-promoting diet and lifestyle changes."

- Retrospective analysis of the cost-effectiveness and clinical effectiveness of short-term fasting: Initial cost of supervised water-only fasting for treating high blood pressure and diabetes (*Journal of Alternative and Complementary Medicine* 2002 Dec[167]): In this brief report, Dr Goldhamer again reports success with the short-term fasting program in hypertensive patients as well as diabetic patients. Here, Goldhamer reports that the **average reduction in systolic blood pressure was 30/11 mm Hg at the completion of the program and 28/11 mm Hg on follow-up.** "Weight loss averaged 26 pounds after the program and was 28 pounds below baseline on follow-up. The average cost of medical care and drugs was $5,784.00 per year in the year(s) prior to participation and $3,000.00 in the year after participation for an average reduction of $2,784.00 per subject in the first year alone. This exceeded the cost of the entire program and compound savings are expected in the years to follow."

- **Specific food items to be avoided or reasonably minimized**: Clinicians and patients should be aware that dietary intake of food allergens, fructose, sodium chloride, and arachidonic acid can contribute to the development, perpetuation, and therapeutic recalcitrance of chronic HTN.

  - Food allergen avoidance, customized per patient (*The Lancet* 1979 May[168]): According to a clinical study of migraineurs (n = 60) published in *The Lancet*, identification and avoidance of food allergens can generally normalize blood pressure in migraine patients who have concomitant hypertension; findings of this study included, "The commonest foods causing reactions were wheat (78%), orange (65%), eggs (45%), tea and coffee (40% each), chocolate and milk (37%) each), beef (35%), and corn, cane sugar, and yeast (33% each). When an average of ten common foods was avoided there was a dramatic fall in the number of headaches per month, 85% of patients becoming headache-free. The 25% of patients with hypertension became normotensive."

  - Minimization of dietary sodium chloride: Excess sodium (Na) promotes water retention and subsequent volume expansion, while also contributing to vasoconstriction and arterial stiffness via enhanced adrenergic reactivity and via promotion of "intracellular hypercalcinosis" (per Vasquez[169]) possibly due to enhanced sodium-calcium exchange.[170] When consumed in common table salt, the chloride (Cl) anion promotes acidosis which results in the progression of CAD/CVD morbidity and mortality and the exacerbation of HTN with increased renal losses of magnesium, potassium, and calcium. These effects justify the advice for HTN patients to avoid dietary NaCl and also justify the use of drug diuretics that enhance Na excretion by the kidney. Clinical responsiveness to low-sodium diets ranges from clinically insignificant to a maximum reduction in the range of -22/-14 to -16/-9.[171] Contraindications to low-sodium

---

[166] Goldhamer et al. Medically supervised water-only fasting in the treatment of borderline hypertension. *J Altern Complement Med*. 2002 Oct;8(5):643-50

[167] Goldhamer AC. Initial cost of care results in medically supervised water-only fasting for treating high blood pressure and diabetes. *J Altern Complement Med*. 2002 Dec;8(6):696-7

[168] Grant EC. Food allergies and migraine. *Lancet*. 1979 May 5;1(8123):966-9

[169] Vasquez A. Intracellular Hypercalcinosis: A Functional Nutritional Disorder with Implications Ranging from Myofascial Trigger Points to Affective Disorders, Hypertension, and Cancer. *Naturopathy Digest* 2006 Previously published in-print and on-line at naturopathydigest.com/archives/2006/sep/vasquez.php and included in this book.

[170] Benowitz NL. "Antihypertensive Agents." In Katzung BG (editor). *Basic and Clinical Pharmacology. 10th Edition*. New York: McGraw Hill Medical; 2007, 163

[171] "The average fall in blood pressure from the highest to the lowest sodium intake was 16/9 mm Hg." MacGregor et al. Double-blind study of three sodium intakes and long-term effects of sodium restriction in essential hypertension. *Lancet*. 1989 Nov 25;2(8674):1244-7

diet are uncommon (e.g., hyponatremia, adrenal failure); low-sodium/NaCl diets should generally be a component of all anti-hypertensive treatment plans. Approximately 20% of patients will show antihypertensive benefit from sodium restriction.[172] As previously noted, Canadian guidelines published in 2009 support the restriction of dietary sodium to less than 2300 mg (100 mmol)/day and to less than 1500-2300 mg [65 mmol to 100 mmol]/day in hypertensive patients.[173] One might hope that readers would appreciate that human physiology developed over millennia wherein the addition of manufactured table salt was a logistical impossibility; in an excellent paradigm-shifting compilation and integration of research, Cordain and his pioneering expert co-authors[174] noted, "the addition of manufactured salt to the food supply and the displacement of traditional potassium-rich foods by foods introduced during the Neolithic and Industrial periods caused a 400% decline in the potassium intake while simultaneously initiating a 400% increase in sodium ingestion. The inversion of potassium and sodium concentrations [dietary sodium-potassium ratio] in hominin diets had no evolutionary precedent and now plays an integral role in eliciting and contributing to numerous diseases of civilization." Adverse effects of NaCl can be at least partly offset by administration of calcium, vitamin D, magnesium, potassium, bicarbonate and citrate.

> **The importance of potassium**
>
> "Adults should consume at least 4.7 grams of potassium per day to lower blood pressure, blunt the effects of salt, and reduce the risk of kidney stones and bone loss. However, most American women 31 to 50 years old consume no more than half of the recommended amount of potassium, and men's intake is only moderately higher. There was no evidence of chronic excess intakes of potassium in apparently healthy individuals and thus no UL [upper limit of intake] was established."
>
> Food and Nutrition Board of the Institute of Medicine of the National Academies. "Dietary Reference Intakes: Water, Potassium, Sodium, Chloride, and Sulfate." Released: February 11, 2004 iom.edu/Reports/2004/Dietary-Reference-Intakes-Water-Potassium-Sodium-Chloride-and-Sulfate.aspx

- Potassium supplementation, preferably via fruits, vegetables, and their juices: Antihypertensive mechanisms of potassium include vasodilator activity, diuretic and naturietic effects, and suppression of renin, angiotensin, and adrenergic tone.[175] In February 2004, the Institute of Medicine (IOM) set the Adequate Intake of potassium for adults at 4.7 grams a day—more than double previous recommendations; more than 90% of American adults do not meet these recommendations. If 90% of the population is not meeting recommended intakes of potassium, and these recommendations from the IOM come after an extensive review of the scientific literature, then potassium assessment and supplementation should be routine components of patient care; furthermore, this shows to the inadequacy of current laboratory assessments for evaluating potassium status and potassium balance. The commonly used "serum potassium" test detects only the most extreme potassium deficiency and is wholly and obviously insensitive for detection of subtle long-term potassium *insufficiency*.

An irony exists in the observations that 1) metabolic syndrome is a very common lethal condition with a hypertensive component, and 2) thiazide diuretics are first-line treatment for most cases of hypertension, and 3) thiazide diuretics exacerbate many CVD-inducing aspects of the metabolic syndrome, such as insulin resistance and dyslipidemia. A 2007 experimental [animal] study published in *Journal of the American Society of Nephrology* showed that potassium supplementation—alone or in combination with treatment to reduce fructose-induced hyperuricemia—can ameliorate exacerbation of metabolic syndrome caused by thiazide diuretics.[176] This is yet another example of nutritional intervention being used to treat the primary disease as well as alleviate the secondary metabolic disturbances caused by the current drug-of-choice.

True to what is to be expected from studies conducted by researchers with little or no previous training in clinical nutrition, most studies of potassium supplementation for the treatment of HTN have been methodologically flawed due to ❶ utilization of potassium in the form of potassium chloride (KCl), ❷ failure to simultaneously reduce intake of dietary NaCl so as to normalize the K:Na ratio and ❸ also reduce total Cl intake; furthermore, ❹ the notion that "potassium intake from foods is associated with reduced blood pressure and that potassium supplementation (e.g., KCl) could be equivalent to potassium intake from food" is a *colossal failure* to appreciate the manifold cardioprotective benefits of the phytonutrients *consumed along with potassium*

[172] Domino FJ (editor in chief). *The 5-Minute Clinical Consult. 2010. 18th Edition*. Philadelphia; Wolters Kluwer: 2009, 656-7

[173] Khan et al. 2009 Canadian Hypertension Education Program recommendations for the management of hypertension: Part 2—therapy. *Can J Cardiol*. 2009 May;25(5):287-98

[174] Cordain et al. Origins and evolution of the Western diet: health implications for the 21st century. *Am J Clin Nutr*. 2005 Feb;81(2):341-5 ajcn.org/cgi/content/full/81/2/341

[175] Patki et al. Efficacy of potassium and magnesium in essential hypertension: a double-blind, placebo controlled, crossover study. *BMJ*. 1990 Sep 15;301(6751):521-3

[176] Reungjui et al. Thiazide diuretics exacerbate fructose-induced metabolic syndrome. *J Am Soc Nephrol*. 2007 Oct;18(10):2724-31

when obtained from its richest natural food sources—fruits, vegetables, nuts, seeds, berries. Furthermore, reverence for KCl reveals ignorance of the cardiovasculotoxic and acidogenic effects of chloride. Respective amounts of potassium per serving of food or juice (1 cup = 8 fluid ounces =240 milliliters) are provided in the table below.

Potassium content of common foods

Food serving	Potassium in mg (sodium as available)
One papaya	780
One cup of mixed vegetable juice	740 (35 mg sodium, up to 630 mg sodium)
One cup of prune juice	700
One cup of carrot juice	520 (160 mg sodium)
One cup plain low-fat yogurt	510 (150 mg sodium)
One cup of cantaloupe	490
One cup of orange juice	470
One small banana	465
One cup of honeydew melon	460
One-third cup of raisins	365
One cup of carrot-orange juice	360 (35 mg sodium)
One medium mango	320
One medium kiwi	250
One small orange	240
One medium pear	210

Note again that the physiologic effect of potassium is influenced by the potassium:sodium ratio (sodium reduces effectiveness and retention of potassium), potassium:chloride ratio (chloride reduces effectiveness and retention of potassium), and the overall pH acid-base balance of the human host (i.e., metabolic acidosis reduces effectiveness and retention of potassium, while an alkaline state improves retention and effectiveness of potassium). Importantly, magnesium status is an important positive-direct determinant of potassium status, particularly in patients with recalcitrant hypokalemia and/or hyperaldosteronism.[177]

- Double-blind, placebo controlled, crossover study: Efficacy of potassium and magnesium in essential hypertension (*British Medical Journal* 1990 Sep[178]): The authors conducted a double-blind randomized placebo-controlled crossover trial of 32 weeks' duration among 37 adults with mild hypertension (diastolic blood pressure less than 110 mm Hg); patients received either placebo or potassium 60 mmol/day (approximately 2,250 mg/d) alone or in combination with magnesium 20 mmol/day (approximately 480 mg/d) in a crossover design without other intervention. More specifically, patients were treated with either placebo, K alone, or K+Mg for 8 weeks each with a 2-week washout period between treatments. While blood pressure in the placebo group did not change after 8 weeks of treatment, BP in the K group dropped from 157/101 to 143/85 (drop of **-14/-16 mm Hg**) and from 154/99 to 146/88 (drop of -8/-11) in the K+Mg group. The reduction in serum cholesterol was from the initial value of 7.5 mmol/l (290 mg/dL) to 6.0 mmol/l (232 mg/dL) and 6.1 mmol/l (235 mg/dL) in the K and K+Mg groups, respectively. The authors wrote, "RESULTS: **Potassium alone or in combination with magnesium produced a significant reduction in systolic and diastolic blood pressures** (p less than 0.001) and a **significant reduction in serum cholesterol concentration** (p less than 0.05); other biochemical variables did not change. Magnesium did not have an additional effect. ... The drug was well tolerated and compliance was satisfactory. CONCLUSION: Potassium 60 mmol/day lowers arterial blood pressure in patients with mild hypertension. Giving magnesium as well has no added advantage." While the reduction in blood pressure by potassium is to be expected, two surprising findings in this study are 1) the reduction in serum cholesterol and 2) the

---

[177] "Magnesium deficiency is frequently associated with hypokalemia. Concomitant magnesium deficiency aggravates hypokalemia and renders it refractory to treatment by potassium. Herein is reviewed literature suggesting that magnesium deficiency exacerbates potassium wasting by increasing distal potassium secretion. A decrease in intracellular magnesium, caused by magnesium deficiency, releases the magnesium-mediated inhibition of ROMK channels and increases potassium secretion. Magnesium deficiency alone, however, does not necessarily cause hypokalemia. An increase in distal sodium delivery or elevated aldosterone levels may be required for exacerbating potassium wasting in magnesium deficiency." Huang CL, Kuo E. Mechanism of hypokalemia in magnesium deficiency. *J Am Soc Nephrol*. 2007 Oct;18(10):2649-52
[178] Patki et al. Efficacy of potassium and magnesium in essential hypertension: a double-blind, placebo controlled, crossover study. *BMJ*. 1990 Sep 15;301(6751):521-3

lack of additive benefit by the magnesium supplementation, particularly when other studies have shown antihypertensive benefit of magnesium when used alone. In this study, both the potassium and the magnesium were provided in a liquid form as KCl and MgCl, respectively; better sources would have been the citrate or malate chelates for alkalinization and enhanced bioavailability. Attentive readers might have also noted one additional curious finding from this study: none of the 37 patients were reported to have developed diarrhea or loose stools from the magnesium 480 mg/d; this may or may not be significant to the credibility of the study; in clinical practice, some patients will report loose stools with magnesium doses as low as 200 mg per day.

- Meta-analysis: Potassium supplementation for the management of primary hypertension in adults (*Cochrane Database of Systematic Reviews* 2006 Jul[179]): Using reasonable inclusion/exclusion criteria, the authors of this meta-analysis found that "Six RCT's (n=483), with eight to 16 weeks follow-up, met our inclusion criteria. Meta-analysis of five trials (n=425) with adequate data indicated that potassium supplementation compared to control resulted in a large but statistically non-significant reductions in **SBP** (mean difference: **-11.2**, 95% CI: -25.2 to 2.7) and **DBP** (mean difference: **-5.0**, 95% CI: -12.5 to 2.4)." The conclusion that potassium supplementation resulted in "large but statistically non-significant reductions" would appear to be an example of *statistical methodology* trumping *clinical practicality* insofar as a reduction of -11/-5 mm Hg is indeed clinically significant and also meets criteria for drug efficacy/approval per the US FDA (assuming that the difference is placebo subtracted). The authors reviewed "two high quality trials (n=138)" showing blood pressure reductions of **-7.1/-5.5** mm Hg but again concluded that these findings represented "non-significant reductions in blood pressure." Given the safety and *essentiality* of potassium, its inadequate consumption from Westernized diets, its facilitated urinary excretion due to consumption of salt/sugar/caffeine/alcohol and many diuretic drugs, and its demonstrated efficacy, clinicians are justified in utilizing potassium in the treatment of HTN especially when sourced from *natural whole foods* and fruit/vegetable juices; indeed, a recent clinical trial[180] utilizing the DASH diet (described previously) in all subjects showed that blood pressure reductions were enhanced among the subset of subjects consuming 8-16 ounces of vegetable juice daily, even when the sodium:potassium ratio was nonphysiologic at >1 since 8 ounces of the juice contained 480 mg of sodium and 470 mg of potassium.

- Randomized trial with 1-year follow-up and a title that says it all: Increasing the dietary potassium intake reduces the need for antihypertensive medication (*Annals of Internal Medicine* 1991 Nov[181]): The stated purpose of this study was "To determine whether an increase in dietary potassium intake from natural foods reduces the need for antihypertensive medication in patients with essential hypertension." Forty-seven patients with medication-controlled hypertension completed one year of dietary treatment (or control nonintervention) and follow-up; the dietary intervention focused on increasing intake of potassium-rich foods, with compliance monitored by 3-day food records and by measuring 24-hour urinary potassium excretion. Results showed the following: "After 1 year, the average drug consumption (number of pills per day) relative to that at baseline was 24% in group 1 (potassium-rich diet) and 60% in group 2 (control diet) (P less than 0.001). By the end of the study, blood pressure could be controlled using less than 50% of the initial therapy in 81% of the patients in group 1 compared with 29% of the patients in group 2 (P = 0.001). Patients in group 1 ended the study with a lower number of reported symptoms compared with patients in the control group (P less than 0.001). CONCLUSION: Increasing the dietary potassium intake from natural foods is a feasible and effective measure to reduce antihypertensive drug treatment." With powerful results such as these, world-wise clinicians will not be surprised that US National Heart, Lung, and Blood Institute (NHLBI)'s endorsed dietary program "Stay Young at Heart: Cooking the Heart-Healthy Way"[182] is notably low in potassium; this will be reviewed in a section toward the end of this chapter.

---

[179] Dickinson et al. Potassium supplementation for the management of primary hypertension in adults. *Cochrane Database Syst Rev*. 2006 Jul 19;3:CD004641

[180] Shenoy et al. The use of a commercial vegetable juice as a practical means to increase vegetable intake: a randomized controlled trial. *Nutr J*. 2010 Sep 17;9:38

[181] Siani et al. Increasing the dietary potassium intake reduces the need for antihypertensive medication. *Ann Intern Med*. 1991 Nov 15;115(10):753-9

[182] US National Heart, Lung, and Blood Institute (NHLBI). Stay Young at Heart: Cooking the Heart-Healthy Way. nhlbi.nih.gov/health/public/heart/other/syah/index.htm Accessed December 2009 and re-reviewed in November 2010.

- Magnesium (Mg) dosed at 600 mg per day or to bowel tolerance: Given the safety and low cost of magnesium, along with the high prevalence of magnesium deficiency in the general population, routine oral magnesium supplementation is warranted. The standard replacement dose for oral magnesium supplementation is 600 mg per day; some patients may tolerate less or need more, with a typical range of 200-1,800 mg/d being used in clinical practice. Insufficient doses are inefficacious, while excess doses are generally benign (causing only transient loose stools). Renal insufficiency and/or treatment with the magnesium-retaining diuretic spironolactone indicate the need for cautious dosing and more frequent clinical and laboratory monitoring. Measurement of *intracellular* Mg levels in erythrocytes or leukocytes is more accurate than is measurement of *serum* Mg levels.

> **Key concept: Subphysiologic doses of nutrients are generally subtherapeutic**
>
> In order to obtain a physiologic effect and an optimal clinical benefit from nutritional supplementation, the supplementation must be of adequate *duration, dose*, and *bioavailability* to optimally supply cellular processes. *Cofactors, co-nutrients*, and the *proper biochemical milieu* (pH in particular) are also required for optimal effectiveness of the nutritional intervention.
>
> Vasquez A. **Subphysiologic doses of vitamin D are subtherapeutic**: comment on study by The Record Trial Group. *TheLancet.com*. Published online May 6, 2005

  - Oral magnesium supplementation reduces ambulatory blood pressure in patients with mild hypertension (*American Journal of Hypertension* 2009 Oct[183]): For a 12-week period, 48 patients with mild uncomplicated hypertension were assigned either to treatment with 600 mg (25 mmol) of magnesium pidolate orally twice a day for 12 weeks + lifestyle recommendations (n=24) or to treatment with lifestyle recommendations only. "RESULTS: In the Mg(2+) supplementation group, **small but significant reductions in mean 24-h systolic and diastolic BP levels were observed**, in contrast to control group (**-5.6** vs. -1.3 mm Hg, and **-2.8** vs. -1 mm Hg, respectively). These effects of Mg(2+) supplementation were consistent in both daytime and night-time periods. Serum Mg(2+) levels and urinary Mg(2+) excretion were significantly increased in the intervention group. Intracellular Mg(2+) and K(+) levels were also increased, while intracellular Ca(2+) and Na(+) levels were decreased in the intervention group. None of the intracellular ions were significantly changed in the control group. CONCLUSION: This study suggests that oral Mg(2+) supplementation is associated with small but consistent ambulatory BP reduction in patients with mild hypertension." Readers should note that magnesium supplementation in this study was shown to reduce intracellular calcium and to increase intracellular potassium simultaneously with the reduction in BP. These findings are consistent with my proposal for treatment of intracellular hypercalcinosis[184] published in 2006 and with the fact that magnesium sufficiency is mandatory for the intracellular uptake of potassium; **any patient with chronic hypokalemia should be tested and/or treated for magnesium insufficiency**. *How do we translate "600 mg (25 mmol) of magnesium pidolate orally twice a day" into an understanding of the clinical dosage which is generally expressed in milligrams of elemental Mg?* The physiologic action of magnesium supplements depends upon their content of magnesium ion. Magnesium pidolate is the magnesium salt of pidolic acid (pyroglutamic acid), which is only 8.7% Mg by weight. Thus, "600 mg (25 mmol) of magnesium pidolate orally twice a day" provides 1,200 mg of magnesium pidolate which provides 8.7% of 600 mg of elemental magnesium, which is only 104 mg of elemental Mg per day. Given that the standard replacement dose for Mg is 600 mg per day of elemental Mg, we see that the dose used in this study was suboptimally therapeutic (only 17% of the standard dose of Mg) and that therefore the clinical results are less impressive than those which would have likely been obtained if the study subjects had used a more substantial amount of Mg.

- Fructose avoidance for caloric moderation and uric acid reduction (American Heart Association, news release 2009 Sep[185]): Production of uric acid is stimulated by ingestion of fructose (most notoriously in the form of high-fructose corn syrup, common in many processed foods and cola drinks), and uric acid directly contributes to the development of insulin resistance and HTN and other classic features of the metabolic syndrome. In a clinical trial published in 2009, 74 adult men added fructose 200 g/d to their regular diet (typical American diet averages 50-70 g/d of fructose) for 2 weeks and experienced a 6/3 elevation in BP, elevations in serum triglycerides and LDL cholesterol, and a more than doubling of the incidence of metabolic syndrome from

---

[183] Hatzistavri et al. Oral magnesium supplementation reduces ambulatory blood pressure in patients with mild hypertension. *Am J Hypertens*. 2009 Oct;22(10):1070-5

[184] Vasquez A. Intracellular Hypercalcinosis: A Functional Nutritional Disorder with Implications Ranging from Myofascial Trigger Points to Affective Disorders, Hypertension, and Cancer. *Naturopathy Digest* 2006 Previously published in-print and on-line at naturopathydigest.com/archives/2006/sep/vasquez.php and included at the end of this chapter.

[185] News release from American Heart Association's 63rd High Blood Pressure Research Conference. High-sugar diet increases men's blood pressure; gout drug protective. Abstract P127. Sept. 23, 2009. americanheart.mediaroom.com/index.php?s=43&item=829 Accessed December 19, 2009

approximately 20% to 50% as determined by two sets of international criteria. The authors logically concluded, "These results suggest that fructose may be a cause of metabolic syndrome. They also suggest that excessive fructose intake may have a role in the worldwide epidemic of obesity and diabetes." Men in this trial who were randomized to receive the xanthine oxidase inhibitor allopurinol (dose not reported; common adult amount is 200-600 mg/d in divided doses, preferably with food) did not develop adverse effects from the increased fructose ingestion, thus clearly implicating fructose-induced hyperuricemia as the biochemical pathway involved. Clinicians should appreciate that the rapid (within 2 weeks) development of HTN and a doubling of the incidence of metabolic syndrome by the addition of fructose to the diet is of undeniably major importance as it clearly implicates high-fructose corn syrup as a major culprit in the burgeoning epidemics of HTN, type-2 diabetes mellitus, and the metabolic syndrome. In a study[186] involving adolescents with elevated uric acid levels (serum uric acid levels > or = 6 mg/dL), allopurinol 200 mg twice daily resulted in a reduction in blood pressure of approximately -7/-5 mm Hg (compared to approximately -2/-2 for placebo); this was a proof-of-concept study (i.e., that uric acid contributes to HTN) and not necessarily an endorsement to use allopurinol for the treatment of HTN. Adverse effects due to allopurinol can include skin rash that may be followed by more severe hypersensitivity reactions such as "exfoliative, urticarial and purpuric lesions as well as Stevens-Johnson syndrome (erythema multiforme exudativum) and/or generalized vasculitis, irreversible hepatotoxicity and on rare occasions, death."[187] Adherence to the Paleo-Mediterranean Diet in general and a low-fructose diet in particular can help reduce elevated serum uric acid levels without the use of drugs because this dietary profile is low in fructose and promotes urinary alkalinization; alkalinizing the urine via avoidance of acidogenic foodstuffs such as dairy and sodium chloride and by increased intake of fruits and vegetables (or supplemental forms of citrate and bicarbonate[188]) promotes renal excretion of uric acid, thus lessening the adverse metabolic effects of uric acid on insulin resistance and endothelial dysfunction. Clinicians should note that, as a result of the manufacturing process, high-fructose corn syrup contains mercury[189], a toxic metal for which no known "safe" and free-from-harm dose exists; adverse effects of mercury exposure include renal damage and clinical hypertension, the latter is promoted by the former while also being generated independently by increased catecholamine release (according to case reports[190]). Per the 2009 review by Houston[191], "The clinical consequences of mercury toxicity include hypertension, CHD, MI, increased carotid IMT [intima media thickness] and obstruction, CVA, generalized atherosclerosis, and renal dysfunction with proteinuria." Mercury contamination of corn syrup ranks among the better examples of how industrialization of the food supply causes untoward [i.e., unexpected and negative] effects; it also exemplifies how one problem (overconsumption of processed "junk" food which contains pro-hypertensive fructose in nonphysiologic/unnatural concentrations) can lead/contribute to other types of problems (adverse effects of mercury, neurotoxicity, nephrotoxicity, and chronic overstimulation of the sympathetic nervous system). Rapid induction of hypertension and the metabolic syndrome in humans by fructose consumption is almost certainly *not* mediated by the mercury content; the extent to which mercury from corn syrup contributes to hypertension is not known, but facts that are already established include the following: ❶ mercury is a known immunotoxin, nephrotoxin, and neurotoxin, ❷ mercury can cause hypertension in humans, ❸ mercury causes hypertension in humans via at least two mechanisms—inhibition of catecholamine breakdown, and induction of renal damage, ❹ corn syrup contains two agents known to cause hypertension in humans: mercury and fructose.

---

[186] "Allopurinol, 200 mg twice daily for 4 weeks,... For casual BP, the mean change in systolic BP for allopurinol was -6.9 mm Hg vs -2.0 mm Hg for placebo, and the mean change in diastolic BP for allopurinol was -5.1 mm Hg vs -2.4 for placebo. CONCLUSIONS: In this short-term, crossover study of adolescents with newly diagnosed hypertension, treatment with allopurinol resulted in reduction of BP." Feig et al. Effect of allopurinol on blood pressure of adolescents with newly diagnosed essential hypertension: a randomized trial. *JAMA.* 2008 Aug 27;300(8):924-32

[187] Brinker AD. Allopurinol and the role of uric acid in hypertension. [letter] *JAMA.* 2009 Jan 21;301(3):270

[188] "The treatment of uric acid stones should focus on alkalinization of the urine with citrate or bicarbonate salts." Liebman SE, Taylor JG, Bushinsky DA. Uric acid nephrolithiasis. *Curr Rheumatol Rep.* 2007 Jun;9(3):251-7

[189] "Average daily consumption of high fructose corn syrup is about 50 grams per person in the United States. With respect to total mercury exposure, it may be necessary to account for this source of mercury in the diet of children and sensitive populations." Dufault et al. Mercury from chlor-alkali plants: measured concentrations in food product sugar. *Environ Health.* 2009 Jan 26;8:2. See also: "High fructose corn syrup has been shown to contain trace amounts of mercury as a result of some manufacturing processes, and its consumption can also lead to zinc loss." Dufault et al. Mercury exposure, nutritional deficiencies and metabolic disruptions may affect learning in children. *Behav Brain Funct.* 2009 Oct 27;5:44.

[190] "Because of the clinical presentation [severe hypertension in children] and the finding of elevated catecholamines, most of the patients were first studied for possible pheochromocytoma. Subsequently, elevated levels of mercury were found." Torres AD, Rai AN, Hardiek ML. Mercury intoxication and arterial hypertension: report of two patients and review of the literature. *Pediatrics.* 2000 Mar;105(3):E34

[191] Houston MC. The role of mercury and cadmium heavy metals in vascular disease, hypertension, coronary heart disease, and myocardial infarction. *Altern Ther Health Med.* 2007 Mar-Apr;13(2):S128-33

- Arachidonate avoidance: Arachidonate promotes intracellular calcium accumulation which promotes the development of HTN. Avoidance of arachidonic acid helps restore intracellular ion homeostasis and results in reduction of elevated BP. Restoration of fatty acid balance via simultaneous reduced intake of arachidonate and increased intake of oleic acid (found in olive oil), gamma-linolenic acid (found in borage seed oil, hemp seed oil, black currant seed oil, and evening primrose oil), and eicosapentaenoic acid (EPA) and docosahexaenoic acid (DHA) (both from cold-water fish oil) helps reduce intracellular hypercalcinosis that promotes chronic HTN in addition to effecting beneficial changes in inflammatory, hemorrheologic, and coagulation indices.

- Fish oil or combination fatty acid supplementation: The cardioprotective benefits of fish oil are insufficiently represented by the minimal numerical reduction in blood pressure that is achieved with this intervention. Despite only lowering blood pressure by a few points (if at all), n-3 fatty acids are safer, less expensive, and more effective than statin and fibrate antihypercholesterolemic drug treatment for reducing total and cardiovascular mortality.[192] Thus, combination fatty acid supplementation should be used for its pronounced cardioprotective benefits regardless of its modest ability to reduce elevated blood pressure. The combination of EPA+DHA from fish oil and GLA from borage oil (or other source) in a ratio of approximately 2:1 (e.g., daily intake of 4 grams EPA+DHA along with 2 grams GLA) appears to provide the best cardioprotective benefit based on favorable changes in serum lipids, according to a speculative prospective clinical trial by Laidlaw and Holub.[193]

- Correction of vitamin D deficiency: Vitamin D3 (cholecalciferol)—with or without calcium supplementation—can reduce blood pressure in cholecalciferol-deficient hypertensive patients as effectively as the use of antihypertensive medication. As I have discussed in extensive detail elsewhere, a reasonable dose of vitamin D3 for adults is in the range of 4,000-10,000 IU per day, and doctors new to vitamin D therapy should read our clinical monograph published in 2004 and available on-line.[194] The most important drug interaction with vitamin D3 is seen with hydrochlorothiazide (HCTZ), a commonly-used antihypertensive diuretic that promotes hypercalcemia. Vitamin D supplementation in patients taking HCTZ must be implemented slowly, with professional supervision, and with laboratory monitoring of serum calcium at days 10, 30, and 60 following the use of combined cholecalciferol-HCTZ treatment. The goal of vitamin D3 supplementation is for serum 25-OH-vitamin D3 levels to reach the optimal range of 50-100 ng/ml, as shown in the diagram.

  - Controlled clinical trial: Effects of short-term calcium supplementation with or without vitamin D3 supplementation on blood pressure and parathyroid hormone levels in elderly women. (*Journal of Clinical Endocrinology and Metabolism* 2001 Apr[195]): In an 8-week study of 148 elderly women (average age 74 years) with a 25-hydroxycholecalciferol (25OHD(3)) level <20 ng/ml (<50 nmol/l), daily administration of 1200 mg calcium plus 800 IU vitamin D3 (note: very low dose of vitamin D) was superior to 1200 mg calcium without vitamin D. Vitamin D plus calcium resulted in an increase in serum 25OHD(3) of 72%, a decrease in serum PTH of 17%, a decrease in heart rate of 5.4%, and a decrease in blood pressure of approximately -13/-7 mm Hg. These results are clinically important because of the significant alleviation of hypertension that is noted, even despite the low dose of vitamin D3 that was used. Collateral benefits in muscle strength, mood, cognition, balance (and reduced falling), and enhanced resistance to infection are commonly noted with vitamin D3 supplementation; such benefits are not seen with antihypertensive drug use.

  - Placebo-controlled clinical trial: Vitamin D improves endothelial function and reduces blood pressure in patients with Type 2 diabetes mellitus and low vitamin D levels (*Diabetic Medicine* 2008 Mar[196]): In a double-blind, parallel group, placebo-controlled randomized trial, a single dose of 100,000 IU vitamin D2 (note the use of ergocalciferol, the less effective form of vitamin D compared with cholecalciferol, vitamin D3) or placebo was administered to patients with Type-2 diabetes mellitus (DM-2) who were vitamin D deficient

---

[192] "Compared with control groups, risk ratios for overall mortality were 0.87 for statins, 1.00 for fibrates, 0.84 for resins, 0.96 for niacin, 0.77 for n-3 fatty acids, and 0.97 for diet. Compared with control groups, risk ratios for cardiac mortality indicated benefit from statins (0.78), resins (0.70) and n-3 fatty acids (0.68)." Studer M, Briel M, Leimenstoll B, Glass TR, Bucher HC. Effect of different antilipidemic agents and diets on mortality: a systematic review. *Arch Intern Med*. 2005 Apr 11;165(7):725-30

[193] "A mixture of 4 g EPA+DHA and 2 g GLA favorably altered blood lipid and fatty acid profiles in healthy women. On the basis of calculated PROCAM values, the 4:2 group was estimated to have a 43% reduction in the 10-y risk of myocardial infarction." Laidlaw M, Holub BJ. Effects of supplementation with fish oil-derived n-3 fatty acids and gamma-linolenic acid on circulating plasma lipids and fatty acid profiles in women. *Am J Clin Nutr*. 2003 Jan;77(1):37-42

[194] Vasquez A, Manso G, Cannell J. The clinical importance of vitamin D (cholecalciferol). *Altern Ther Health Med*. 2004 Sep-Oct;10(5):28-36

[195] "A short-term supplementation with vitamin D(3) and calcium is more effective in reducing SBP than calcium alone. Inadequate vitamin D(3) and calcium intake could play a contributory role in the pathogenesis and progression of hypertension and cardiovascular disease in elderly women." Pfeifer et al. Effects of a short-term vitamin D(3) and calcium supplementation on blood pressure and parathyroid hormone levels in elderly women. *J Clin Endocrinol Metab*. 2001 Apr;86(4):1633-7

[196] Sugden et al. Vitamin D improves endothelial function in patients with Type 2 diabetes mellitus and low vitamin D levels. *Diabet Med*. 2008 Mar;25(3):320-5

with an average baseline 25-hydroxyvitamin D level <20 ng/ml (<50 nmol/l). Benefits of vitamin D supplementation included significantly improved flow mediated vasodilatation (FMD) of the brachial artery by 2.3% and significantly decreased systolic blood pressure by -14 mmHg compared with placebo. Total reduction in blood pressure for vitamin D compared to placebo (per Table 2 of the original article) was -13.9/-4.5 mm Hg.

- <u>Vitamin C (ascorbic acid) 3 g/d or bowel tolerance</u>: Since ascorbic acid is biochemically synthesized from glucose, these molecules remain structurally similar; not surprisingly therefore, an excess of glucose (i.e., as in hyperglycemia) reduces cellular uptake of ascorbic acid, leading to a relative "cellular scurvy" even in the absence of the classic presentation of scurvy. "In neutrophils from different volunteers, glucose inhibited uptake and accumulation of ascorbic acid by both transport activities 3-9-fold. ... Glucose-induced inhibition of both ascorbic acid transport activities occurred in neutrophils of all donors tested and was fully reversible."[197]

  - <u>Clinical trial: Vitamin C for refractory hypertension in elderly patients</u> (*Arzneimittelforschung* 2006[198]): Treatment with ascorbic acid 600 mg/d for 6 months was evaluated for effects on blood pressure and levels of C-reactive protein, 8-isoprostane, and malondialdehyde-modified low-density lipoproteins among 12 elderly patients (average age 78.3y) and 12 adult patients (average age 54.6y) with refractory hypertension. Treatment with ascorbic acid markedly reduced systolic blood pressure in the elderly group from 154.9 to 134.8 mmHg (p < 0.001); pulse pressure reduced from 79.1 to 63.4. These benefits of vitamin C supplementation were accompanied by an increase in the serum levels of ascorbic acid and decreases in the levels of C-reactive protein, 8-isoprostane, and malondialdehyde-modified low-density lipoproteins. In contrast, ascorbic acid did not affect blood pressure in the adult nonelderly group. These results suggest that ascorbic acid is useful for controlling blood pressure in elderly patients with refractory hypertension." Clinicians should appreciate that elevated systolic blood pressure is an important predictor of cardiovascular mortality in elderly patients, and that its ascorbate-induced reduction by -20 mmHg is highly clinically significant.

- <u>Urinary alkalinization</u>: In non-pathologic states, the pattern of dietary intake is the single most important determinant of systemic/urine acid-base balance.[199] The two main classes of acids of physiologic importance are 1) carbonic acid—formed when carbon dioxide (CO_2) from metabolism of carbohydrates and fatty acids combines with water (H_2O) to form carbonic acid (H_2CO_3), and 2) noncarbonic acids—these are primarily generated from the oxidation of sulfur-containing amino acids which results in the formation of sulfuric acid (H_2SO_4); avoidance of the former is mostly achieved via respiration (i.e., removal of CO_2) while elimination of the latter requires bicarbonate and renal excretion.[200] Average urine pH among societies consuming a Paleo-Mediterranean diet and obtaining daily physical exercise is 7.5-9; clearly this very alkaline state reflects a diet high in fruits and vegetables, and provides physiologic benefits including increased excretion of xenobiotics[201] and renal retention of potassium, magnesium, and calcium. For example, among New Guinean hunter-gatherer tribal groups living in the *primitive feral condition*, "urine pH of adults was usually between 7.5 and 9.0 because of potassium bicarbonate and carbonate excretion."[202] Excess urine alkalinity can predispose to urinary tract infections; thus some clinicians may be more comfortable with a urine pH goal of approximately 7.5-8.0.

  - <u>Clinical trial: Neutralization of Western diet inhibits bone resorption independently of K intake and reduces cortisol secretion in humans</u> (*American Journal of Physiology - Renal Physiology* 2003 Jan[203]): Acid-base neutralization by substituting equimolar amounts of sodium bicarbonate and potassium bicarbonate for NaCl and KCl "induced a significant cumulative calcium retention (10.7 +/- 0.4 mmol) and significantly reduced the urinary excretion of deoxypyridinoline, pyridinoline, and n-telopeptide. Mean daily plasma cortisol decreased from 264 to 232 nmol/l (P = 0.032), ... An acidogenic Western diet results in mild

---

[197] Washko P, Levine M. Inhibition of ascorbic acid transport in human neutrophils by glucose. *J Biol Chem.* 1992 Nov 25;267(33):23568-74

[198] Sato et al. Effects of ascorbic acid on ambulatory blood pressure in elderly patients with refractory hypertension. *Arzneimittelforschung.* 2006;56(7):535-40

[199] "Nutrition has long been known to strongly influence acid-base balance. Recently, we have shown that it is possible to appropriately estimate the renal net acid excretion (NAE) of healthy subjects from the composition of their diets." Remer T. Influence of nutrition on acid-base balance--metabolic aspects. *Eur J Nutr.* 2001 Oct;40(5):214-20

[200] Rennke HG, Denker BM. *Renal Physiology: The Essentials. 2nd Edition.* Philadelphia: Lippincott Williams and Wilkins; 2007, p129

[201] "Urine alkalinization is a treatment regimen that increases poison elimination by the administration of intravenous sodium bicarbonate to produce urine with a pH > or = 7.5." Proudfoot AT, Krenzelok EP, Vale JA. Position Paper on urine alkalinization. *J Toxicol Clin Toxicol.* 2004;42(1):1-26

[202] Sebastian et al. Estimation of the net acid load of the diet of ancestral preagricultural Homo sapiens and their hominid ancestors. *Am J Clin Nutr.* 2002 Dec;76(6):1308-16

[203] Maurer M, Riesen W, Muser J, Hulter HN, Krapf R. Neutralization of Western diet inhibits bone resorption independently of K intake and reduces cortisol secretion in humans. *Am J Physiol Renal Physiol.* 2003 Jan;284(1):F32-40

metabolic acidosis in association with a state of cortisol excess, altered divalent ion metabolism, and increased bone resorptive indices. Acidosis-induced increases in cortisol secretion and plasma concentration may play a role in mild acidosis-induced alterations in bone metabolism and possibly in osteoporosis associated with an acidogenic Western diet." Clinicians should appreciate that long-term reductions in cortisol along with renal retention of calcium would be expected to have a favorable effect on blood pressure.

- Review: Diet, evolution and aging—the pathophysiologic effects of the post-agricultural inversion of the potassium-to-sodium and base-to-chloride ratios in the human diet (*European Journal of Nutrition* 2001 Oct[204]): This excellent review article discusses the changes in mineral intake (i.e., less potassium complicated by more sodium) and the shift from a plant-based alkalinizing diet to a pseudo-food acidifying diet and the physiological ramifications of these dietary changes. Note their conclusion in the following quote which states that any level of acidosis may be unacceptable and that (conversely) a state of alkalinization is the normal and ideal human condition: "We argue that any level of acidosis may be unacceptable from an evolutionarily perspective, and indeed, that **a low-grade metabolic alkalosis may be the optimal acid-base state for humans.**"

- Clinical trial: Urine alkalization facilitates uric acid excretion (*Nutrition Journal* 2010 Oct[205]): Highly consistent with and positively affirming of the protocol and paradigm advocated in this text, this clinical trial published in *Nutrition Journal* in 2010, authors of this study note that "Increase in the incidence of hyperuricemia associated with gout as well as hypertension, renal diseases and cardiovascular diseases has been a public health concern." Their clinical trial therefore sought to increase renal excretion of uric acid by altering urine pH via dietary improvement, moving in the direction of a more plant-based and more Paleo-Mediterranean diet. The authors made recipes consisting of "protein-rich and less vegetable-fruit food materials" (acid diet) and of "less protein but vegetable-fruit rich food materials" (alkali diet). Urine pH reached a steady state 3 days after switching from ordinary daily diets to specified regimens. Results showed that H+ (acidity) in urine is directly affected by the metabolic degradation of food materials, and that uric acid and excreted urine pH retained a linear relationship; the higher

> **Diet optimization is the "safest and most economical" intervention to lower the total body load of uric acid**
>
> "This study has clarified that alkalization of urine by the manipulation of food materials promotes the removal of uric acid. When one pays enough attention to the construction of a nutritionally balanced menu, dietary intervention becomes the safest and the most economical way for the prevention of hyperuricemia."
>
> Kanbara et al. Urine alkalization facilitates uric acid excretion. *Nutrition Journal* 2010, 9:45 nutritionj.com/content/9/1/45

the pH (more alkaline), the greater the uric acid excretion. The authors concluded, "We conclude that alkalization of urine by eating nutritionally well-designed food is effective for removing uric acid from the body." Given the increasing evidence that intracellular urate directly contributes to microvascular disease and the anticipated pathological complications in the brain, kidneys, and cardiovascular system[206], reducing the total body load of uric acid (i.e., the composite load in intracellular and extracellular/plasma compartments) is justified and warranted.

- Cocoa & Dark Chocolate (*Theobroma cacao*): Cacao has been cultivated for thousands of years in South and Central America; currently most production comes from Africa as well as various other countries such as Belize. The word chocolate came into English from Spanish and entered Spanish either from the Aztecs ("chocolatl" or "chicolatl") or the Maya ("chokol"). Among its numerous constituents, alkaloids such as theobromine and phenethylamine and various antioxidants such as epicatechin and procyanidins have received the most attention. Dark chocolate *without added sugar* and *without the addition of excess fat or cow's milk* provides antioxidant, cardioprotective, neuroprotective, and anticancer benefits. People who regularly consume higher levels of cocoa (suggested range 10-30 grams up to 100 grams daily) have lower BP and a -50% relative reduction in cardiovascular and all-cause mortality; regarding the mechanism of action for the BP-lowering

[204] Frassetto L, Morris RC Jr, Sellmeyer DE, Todd K, Sebastian A. Diet, evolution and aging—the pathophysiologic effects of the post-agricultural inversion of the potassium-to-sodium and base-to-chloride ratios in the human diet. *Eur J Nutr.* 2001 Oct;40(5):200-13

[205] "We conclude that alkalization of urine by eating nutritionally well-designed food is effective for removing uric acid from the body." Kanbara A, Hakoda M, Seyama I. Urine alkalization facilitates uric acid excretion. *Nutrition Journal* 2010, 9:45 nutritionj.com/content/9/1/45

[206] "...dietary intake of sugars rich in fructose may be driving the development of microvascular disease as a consequence of raising intracellular uric acid." Kanbay M, Sánchez-Lozada LG, Franco M, Madero M, Solak Y, Rodriguez-Iturbe B, Covic A, Johnson RJ. Microvascular disease and its role in the brain and cardiovascular system: a potential role for uric acid as a cardiorenal toxin. *Nephrol Dial Transplant.* 2010 Oct 8. [Epub ahead of print]

effect of chocolate: flavonoids in cacao upregulate nitric oxide synthase in endothelial cells, and thus chocolate improves endothelial function.[207] The cocoa content should be at least 65% and preferably 85%-90%. In December 2009, MD Anderson Cancer Center endorsed dark chocolate for its probable cancer-preventive benefits.[208] Because of its stimulating effects, cocoa should be consumed in the earlier part of the day in order to avoid sleep disturbance.

- **Systematic review and meta-analysis: Benefits of cocoa products on blood pressure** (*American Journal of Hypertension* 2010 Jan[209]): For this systematic review, the authors performed a meta-analysis of randomized controlled trials assessing the antihypertensive effects of flavanol-rich cocoa products. They found that among 10 randomized controlled trials with a total of 297 individuals (either healthy normotensive adults or patients with prehypertension/stage 1 hypertension), systolic BP dropped -4.5 mm Hg while diastolic BP dropped -2.5 mm Hg following cocoa consumption for durations of 2-18 weeks. The authors concluded that "The meta-analysis confirms the BP-lowering capacity of flavanol-rich cocoa products...." Rather than rendering the typical cautionary note ("...questions such as the most appropriate dose and the long-term side effect profile warrant further investigation before cocoa products can be recommended as a treatment option in hypertension."), the authors might have been more wise to suggest increased consumption of chocolate for its antihypertensive and cardioprotective benefits and its greater safety profile compared to pharmaceutical drugs.

- **Randomized controlled trial: Effects of habitual cocoa intake on blood pressure and bioactive nitric oxide** (*JAMA—Journal of the American Medical Association* 2007 Jul[210]): The authors of this clinical trial review previously published research and note that regular intake of cocoa-containing foods is linked to lower cardiovascular mortality and that short-term interventions show that **high doses of cocoa can improve endothelial function and reduce BP due to the action of the cocoa polyphenols**. Their clinical trial design was a randomized, controlled, investigator-blinded, parallel-group trial involving 44 adults aged 56 through 73 years (24 women, 20 men) with untreated upper-range prehypertension or stage 1 hypertension without comorbidity; the treatment was 6.3 g (30 kcal) per day of dark chocolate containing 30 mg of polyphenols or a placebo of polyphenol-free white chocolate. Main outcome measures were ❶ BP, ❷ plasma markers of vasodilative nitric oxide (S-nitrosoglutathione), ❸ oxidative stress (8-isoprostane), and ❹ bioavailability of cocoa polyphenols. "RESULTS: From baseline to 18 weeks, **dark chocolate reduced mean systolic BP by -2.9 mm Hg and diastolic BP by -1.9 mm Hg** without changes in body weight, plasma levels of lipids, glucose, and 8-isoprostane. **Hypertension prevalence declined from 86% to 68%.** The BP decrease was accompanied by a sustained increase of S-nitrosoglutathione by 0.23 nmol/L, and a dark chocolate dose resulted in the appearance of cocoa phenols in plasma. White chocolate intake caused no changes in BP or plasma biomarkers. CONCLUSIONS: Data in this relatively small sample of otherwise healthy individuals with above-optimal BP indicate that **inclusion of small amounts of polyphenol-rich dark chocolate as part of a usual diet efficiently reduced BP and improved formation of vasodilative nitric oxide.**"

- **Randomized controlled single-blind crossover trial: Benefits of acute dark chocolate and cocoa ingestion on endothelial function** (*American Journal of Clinical Nutrition* 2008 Jul[211]): The purpose of this clinical trial (n = 45, BMI = 30, age = 53y) was to assess the acute effects of solid dark chocolate and liquid cocoa intake on endothelial function and blood pressure in overweight adults. First, subjects were randomly assigned to consume a solid dark chocolate bar (containing 22 g cocoa powder) or a cocoa-free placebo bar (containing 0 g cocoa powder). In the second part of the trial, subjects were randomly assigned to consume sugar-free cocoa (containing 22 g cocoa powder), sugared cocoa (containing 22 g cocoa powder), or a placebo (containing 0 g cocoa powder). "RESULTS: Solid dark chocolate and liquid cocoa ingestion improved endothelial function (measured as [ultrasound-visualized] flow-mediated dilatation) compared

---

[207] Nahas R. Complementary and alternative medicine approaches to blood pressure reduction: An evidence-based review. *Can Fam Physician*. 2008 Nov;54(11):1529-33

[208] "In addition to being delicious, moderate amounts of dark chocolate may play a role in cancer prevention. ... To get those cancer prevention benefits, the chocolate should contain at least 65% cocoa. Winters R. Focused on Health - December 2009. mdanderson.org/publications/focused-on-health/issues/2009-december/share-the-health.html Accessed January 15, 2010

[209] Desch et al. Effect of cocoa products on blood pressure: systematic review and meta-analysis. *Am J Hypertens*. 2010 Jan;23(1):97-103

[210] Taubert et al. Effects of low habitual cocoa intake on blood pressure and bioactive nitric oxide: a randomized controlled trial. *JAMA*. 2007 Jul 4;298(1):49-60

[211] Faridi et al. Acute dark chocolate and cocoa ingestion and endothelial function: a randomized controlled crossover trial. *Am J Clin Nutr*. 2008 Jul;88(1):58-63

with placebo (dark chocolate: 4.3% compared with -1.8% [for placebo]; sugar-free and sugared cocoa: 5.7% and 2.0% compared with -1.5%). Blood pressure decreased after the ingestion of dark chocolate and sugar-free cocoa compared with *placebo* (dark chocolate: systolic, -3.2 mm Hg compared with 2.7 mm Hg; and diastolic -1.4 mm Hg compared with 2.7 mm Hg; sugar-free cocoa: systolic, -2.1 mm Hg compared with 3.2 mm Hg; and diastolic: -1.2 mm Hg compared with 2.8 mm Hg. Endothelial function improved significantly more with sugar-free than with regular cocoa (5.7 % compared with 2.0%). CONCLUSIONS: The acute ingestion of both solid dark chocolate and liquid cocoa improved endothelial function and lowered blood pressure in overweight adults. Sugar content may attenuate these effects, and sugar-free preparations may augment them." The practical application of this research is important to communicate to patients: to obtain the cardioprotective benefits of chocolate, the chocolate must be consumed without added sugar, i.e., it must be **dark chocolate**, *not* sugar-sweetened milk chocolate.

- Population-based inception cohort study with 8-year follow-up: Chocolate consumption and mortality following a first acute myocardial infarction: the Stockholm Heart Epidemiology Program (*Journal of Internal Medicine* 2009 Sep[212]): Authors of this study followed 1,169 non-diabetic patients hospitalized with a confirmed first acute myocardial infarction (AMI) between 1992 and 1994. Participants self-reported usual chocolate consumption over the preceding 12 months with a standardized questionnaire distributed during hospitalization. Participants were followed for 8 years. "RESULTS: Chocolate consumption had a strong inverse association with cardiac mortality. When compared with those never eating chocolate, the multivariable-adjusted hazard ratios were 0.73 (95% confidence interval, 0.41-1.31) for those consuming chocolate less than once per month, 0.56 (0.32-0.99) for up to once per week, and 0.34 (0.17-0.70) and twice or more per week respectively. [Note: dose-response relationships suggest causality.] Chocolate consumption generally had an inverse but weak association with total mortality and nonfatal outcomes. In contrast, intake of other sweets was not associated with cardiac or total mortality. CONCLUSIONS: Chocolate consumption was associated with lower cardiac mortality in a dose dependent manner in patients free of diabetes surviving their first AMI. Although our findings support increasing evidence that chocolate is a rich source of beneficial bioactive compounds, confirmation of this strong inverse relationship from other observational studies or large-scale, long-term, controlled randomized trials is needed." The importance of this study is that it suggests that the cardioprotective benefits of cocoa are not limited to short-term alleviation of hypertension but extend to a more generalized cardioprotective benefit; beyond this, the reduction in all-cause mortality is what we would expect from a functional food rich in bioactive health-promoting constituents. Limitations to this study include the self-selected nature of the intervention and lack of randomization; however, the large number of subjects (n = 1,169) serves to mitigate these methodological limitations.

- **Whey peptides, casokinins, and lactokinins**: Yet another benefit of whey protein consumption is the salutary effect on blood pressure, probably mediated by whey protein's anti-stress, anti-oxidant/pro-glutathione, and ACE-inhibiting properties. Very interestingly, the anti-hypertensive effects of milk peptides may depend on their specific hydrolysation by lactic acid producing bacteria in the intestines; thus, clinical anti-hypertensive benefit of milk/whey peptides may require establishment of eubiosis, eradication of intestinal dysbiosis, and/or co-supplementation with probiotics. (For extensive reviews on the clinical consequences of dysbiosis and the [re]establishment of eubiosis, see monographs[213] and book chapters[214] by Vasquez). Whey protein is commonly consumed in doses that provide 20-80 grams of protein per day; individual antihypertensive responses will, of course, vary.

  - Clinical trial: The long-term effects of whey protein isolate on blood pressure, vascular function, and inflammatory markers in overweight individuals. (*Obesity* 2010 Jul[215]): This study evaluated the effects of whey protein isolate (27 grams twice daily) on blood pressure, vascular function and inflammatory markers compared to the effects of casein and glucose (control) supplementation in overweight/obese individuals. Seventy men and women with average BMI of 31.3 completed this 12-week study. Blood pressure

---

[212] Janszky et al. Chocolate consumption and mortality following a first acute myocardial infarction. *J Intern Med*. 2009 Sep;266(3):248-57

[213] Vasquez A. Reducing Pain and Inflammation Naturally - Part 6: Nutritional and Botanical Treatments against "Silent Infections" and Gastrointestinal Dysbiosis, Commonly Overlooked Causes of Neuromusculoskeletal Inflammation and Chronic Health Problems. *Nutritional Perspectives* 2006; 29 (January): 5-21

[214] Chapter Four in: Vasquez A. *Integrative Rheumatology*. IBMRC 2006, 2007 and all later versions.

[215] Pal S, Ellis V. The chronic effects of whey proteins on blood pressure, vascular function, and inflammatory markers in overweight individuals. *Obesity*. 2010 Jul;18(7):1354-9

reductions due to whey protein isolate were noted at 6 weeks and were significant for systolic and diastolic pressures at 12 weeks of supplementation. No significant changes in inflammatory markers were noted. This study demonstrated that supplementation with whey protein improves blood pressure and vascular function (assessed by the augmentation index) in overweight and obese individuals. Systolic blood pressure (SBP) decreased significantly by 3% at week 6 (115.5 mm Hg) and by 4% at week 12 (114.5 mm Hg) compared to baseline (119.3 mm Hg) in the whey protein group. A significant decrease of 3.3% in diastolic blood pressure (DBP) at week 12 (62.0 mm Hg) compared with baseline (64.1 mm Hg) in the whey protein group was noted. Thus, the total BP reduction by whey protein isolate in this study is approximately -4.8/-2.1 mm Hg.

- Clinical trial: Effects of whey protein isolate on body composition, lipids, insulin and glucose in overweight and obese individuals. (*British Journal of Nutrition* 2010 Sep[216]): Whey protein isolate supplementation in 70 men and women with a mean age of 48.4 years and a mean BMI of 31.3 for 12 weeks in a parallel study design resulted in no significant change in body composition or serum glucose at 12 weeks compared with the control (glucose) or casein group. A significant decrease in total cholesterol and LDL cholesterol at week 12 in the whey protein isolate group compared with the casein and control groups was noted. Fasting insulin levels and homeostasis model assessment of insulin resistance scores were also significantly decreased in the whey protein isolate group compared with the control group. The present study demonstrated that supplementation with whey protein isolate improves fasting lipids and insulin levels in overweight and obese individuals.

- Randomized cross-over clinical trial: The acute effects of four protein meals on insulin, glucose, appetite, and energy intake in lean men. (*British Journal of Nutrition* 2010 Oct[217]): The authors note that different dietary proteins vary in their ability to influence satiety and reduce food intake. The present study compared the effects of four protein meals—whey, tuna, turkey, and egg albumin—on postprandial glucose and insulin concentrations as well as on appetite measures and energy intake in 22 lean healthy men. Results showed that blood glucose response after the consumption of the test meal measured as area under the curve (AUC) was significantly lower with the whey meal and tuna meal than with the turkey and egg meals. The AUC blood insulin was significantly higher with the whey meal than with the tuna, turkey and egg meals; however, the AUC rating of hunger was significantly lower with the whey meal than with the tuna, turkey, and egg meals. Mean energy intake at the ad libitum meal following the protein meal was significantly lower with the whey meal than with the tuna, egg, and turkey meals. Results showed that whey protein meal produced a greater acute insulin response, reduced appetite and decreased ad libitum energy intake at a subsequent meal compared with the other protein meals, indicating a potential for appetite suppression and weight loss in overweight or obese individuals. This is a very interesting study showing that even though whey protein acutely elevates insulin levels postprandially, the reduced appetite and calorie intake induced by whey protein consumption may actually help patients lose weight.

- Review: Lactokinins are whey protein-derived ACE inhibitory peptides (*Nahrung* 1999 Jun[218]): Whey protein contains lactokinins, peptides that function as ACE-inhibitors. "Peptides derived from the major whey proteins, i.e. alpha-lactalbumin (alpha-la) and beta-lactoglobulin (beta-lg) in addition to bovine serum albumin (BSA), inhibit ACE. ... While they do not have the inhibitory potency of synthetic drugs commonly used in the treatment of hypertension, these naturally occurring peptides may represent nutraceutical/functional food ingredients for the prevention/treatment of high blood pressure."

- Review: Milk protein-derived peptide inhibitors of angiotensin-I-converting enzyme (*British Journal of Nutrition* 2000 Nov[219]): "Numerous casein and whey protein-derived angiotensin-I-converting enzyme (ACE) inhibitory peptides/hydrolysates have been identified. Clinical trials in hypertensive animals and humans show that these peptides/hydrolysates can bring about a significant reduction in hypertension. These peptides/hydrolysates may be classified as functional food ingredients and nutraceuticals due to

[216] Pal et al. Effects of whey protein isolate on body composition, lipids, insulin and glucose in overweight and obese individuals. *Br J Nutr*. 2010 Sep;104(5):716-23

[217] Pal S, Ellis V. The acute effects of four protein meals on insulin, glucose, appetite and energy intake in lean men. *Br J Nutr*. 2010 Oct;104(8):1241-8

[218] FitzGerald RJ, Meisel H. Lactokinins: whey protein-derived ACE inhibitory peptides. *Nahrung*. 1999 Jun;43(3):165-7

[219] FitzGerald RJ, Meisel H. Milk protein-derived peptide inhibitors of angiotensin-I-converting enzyme. *Br J Nutr*. 2000 Nov;84 Suppl 1:S33-

their ability to provide health benefits i.e. as functional food ingredients in reducing the risk of developing a disease and as nutraceuticals in the prevention/treatment of disease."

- ▪ Review: Hypotensive peptides from milk proteins (*Journal of Nutrition* 2004 Apr[220]): "Milk proteins, both caseins and whey proteins, are a rich source of ACE inhibitory peptides. Several studies in spontaneously hypertensive rats show that these casokinins and lactokinins can significantly reduce blood pressure. Furthermore, a limited number of human studies have associated milk protein-derived peptides with statistically significant hypotensive effects (i.e., lower systolic and diastolic pressures)."

- **L-Arginine**: L-arginine (Arg) is the amino acid precursor for the formation of vasodilating nitric oxide (NO) produced via the action of endothelial nitric oxide synthase. A significant number of hypertensive patients have impaired conversion of Arg into NO, and a subset of these patients benefit from oral Arg supplementation. As usual, amino acid supplementation is delivered between meals (empty stomach) to facilitate absorption, and coadministration of simple carbohydrate can facilitate insulin-mediated cellular amino acid uptake. Recently, asymmetric dimethylarginine (ADMA) has been identified as an independent cardiovascular risk factor; per the excellent review by Böger[221], clinicians should appreciate that ADMA—formed from degradation of methylated proteins and an endogenous competitive inhibitor of NO synthase (NOS)—is a vasoconstrictor found in elevated levels among patients with hypercholesterolemia, atherosclerosis, hypertension, chronic renal failure, chronic heart failure, hyperthyroidism, hyperhomocysteinemia and folate deficiency. As expected, administration of Arg has demonstrated antihypertensive benefit, particularly among patients with high ADMA levels; indeed, elevated ADMA may identify which patients are likely to respond to Arg supplementation via a more favorable Arg:ADMA ratio. Laboratory testing for ADMA is available now from some research centers (such as Baylor[222]) and will surely become more widely available in the future. The predictable clinical take-home messages are that ❶ intravenous Arg administration generally produces a greater response than does oral administration, ❷ the hypotensive benefits of Arg supplementation are short-lived, ❸ the hypotensive benefits of Arg are more consistently seen in the groups expected to have high ADMA levels as previous listed, and ❹ younger patients (with less atherosclerosis and arterial calcification) are more likely to respond. Clinicians should appreciate that the cardioprotective benefits of Arg extend beyond and are not entirely dependent upon its antihypertensive benefit; other benefits include decreased platelet aggregation and adhesion, decreased monocyte adhesion, antiproliferative effects on vascular smooth muscle, and improved endothelium-dependent vasodilation which can occur locally and systemically without an accompanying hypotensive effect. Very importantly, concomitant administration of the amino acid N-acetyl-cysteine (NAC) appears to enhance the cardioprotective efficacy of Arg according to recent research.[223] Aside from the possibility of promoting reactivation of herpes simplex outbreaks, Arg is remarkably safe and is commonly used in immunonutrition formulas as a life-saving treatment in critically ill patients; Zhou and Martindale[224] recently noted, "The numerous potential beneficial effects of arginine in the critically ill patient include: 1) stimulation of immune function via its influence on lymphocyte, macrophage, and dendritic cells; 2) improved wound healing; 3) increased net nitrogen balance; 4) increased blood flow to key vascular beds; and 5) decreased clinical infections and length of hospital stay." The doses employed have ranged widely from 1,200 mg/d to 30,000 mg/d, (i.e., 1.2-30 g/d) and have included both oral and intravenous administration. Of course, Arg can be used with other dietary and nutritional interventions and with drug treatments with the caveat that common sense is employed to minimize the risk of hypotension by not initiating too many new treatments simultaneously in a given patient. While oral administration of L-arginine is generally considered beneficial at best and benign at worst, a report published in 2009 by Jahangir et al[225] showed that L-arginine supplementation at 9 grams per day for 4 days did not alter vascular reactivity but did increase methylation demand (shown by increased homocysteine to methionine ratio); this study and its implications (namely that

[220] FitzGerald RJ, Murray BA, Walsh DJ. Hypotensive peptides from milk proteins. *J Nutr*. 2004 Apr;134(4):980S-8S

[221] Böger RH. Asymmetric dimethylarginine, an endogenous inhibitor of nitric oxide synthase, explains the "L-arginine paradox" and acts as a novel cardiovascular risk factor. *J Nutr*. 2004 Oct;134(10 Suppl):2842S-2847S jn.nutrition.org/cgi/content/full/134/10/2842S

[222] Institute of Metabolic Disease at Baylor Research Institute. Asymmetric dimethylarginine (ADMA). baylorhealth.edu/imd/researchtests/asymmetric.htm Accessed Dec 2009

[223] Martina V, Masha A, Gigliardi VR, et al. Long-term N-acetylcysteine and L-arginine administration reduces endothelial activation and systolic blood pressure in hypertensive patients with type 2 diabetes. *Diabetes Care*. 2008 May;31(5):940-4 care.diabetesjournals.org/content/31/5/940.long

[224] "The numerous potential beneficial effects of arginine in the critically ill patient include: 1) stimulation of immune function via its influence on lymphocyte, macrophage, and dendritic cells; 2) improved wound healing; 3) increased net nitrogen balance; 4) increased blood flow to key vascular beds; and 5) decreased clinical infections and length of hospital stay." Zhou M, Martindale RG. Arginine in the critical care setting. *J Nutr*. 2007 Jun;137(6 Suppl 2):1687S-1692S jn.nutrition.org/cgi/content/full/137/6/1687S

[225] Jahangir et al. The effect of L-arginine and creatine on vascular function and homocysteine metabolism. *Vasc Med*. 2009 Aug;14(3):239-48

methylation factors such as folate, betaine, pyridoxine, and cobalamin might be coadministered with L-arginine to optimize vascular health and endothelial function) are reviewed at the end of this section on L-arginine.

- Open clinical trial: The effects of sustained-release L-arginine on blood pressure and vascular compliance in 29 healthy individuals (normotensives and hypertensives) treated for one week (*Alternative Medicine Review* 2006 Mar[226]): Miller used 2.1 g/d Arg administered in two divided doses in a sustained release preparation to find that approximately 65% of hypertensive patients responded favorably with an average reduction of -4/-3.7 mm Hg for the group as a whole that included normotensives and hypertensives. Among patients who were "borderline or hypertensive" the average BP reduction was -11/-4.9 mm Hg. Vascular elasticity assessed by digital pulse wave analysis showed a significant increase in large artery compliance (mean 23% improvement). Given the low dose, the short duration, and the low cost and absence of adverse effects, these results are worthy of clinical consideration and additional study. Consistent with many studies in clinical nutrition, the intervention provided an *alterative*, homeostatic effect in that—in contrast to the effects of pharmaceutical drugs—the effects are benign and rather minimal in healthy-normotensive persons and are clinically significant and therapeutic in patients with the index disease.

- Randomized placebo-controlled trial with 123 patients: Effect of L-arginine on blood pressure in pregnancy-induced hypertension (*Journal of Maternal-Fetal and Neonatal Medicine* 2006 May[227]): Inclusion criteria for this trial included maternal age range 16-45 years, diagnosis of gestational hypertension without proteinuria (patients normotensive until the 20th week), and gestational age ranging between 24 and 36 weeks. Subjects were allocated to receive either Arg 20 g/500 mL intravenously or placebo treatment through an i.v. line. Treatment or placebo was administered in the morning from 8-10 a.m. and was repeated for four consecutive days. The final analysis was performed on 62 women in the Arg group and 61 in the placebo group. "RESULTS: Maternal clinical features such as age, height, weight, and gestational age at inclusion were similar between groups. Both systolic and diastolic blood pressures were reduced by treatment, the effect of L-arginine being significantly higher than that of the placebo (systolic values F = 8.59, p < 0.005; diastolic values F = 3.36; p < 0.001). … CONCLUSIONS: In conclusion, these data support the use of L-Arg as an antihypertensive agent for gestational hypertension especially in view of the other beneficial effects nitric oxide donors display in pregnancy. Further, L-Arg seems well tolerated since in this sample none of the patients reported adverse effects requiring study interruption." According to Figure 4 of the article, BP reductions due to arginine supplementation were approximately -5/-8 mm Hg.

- Double-blind placebo-controlled clinical trial: Long-term N-acetylcysteine and L-arginine administration reduces endothelial activation and systolic blood pressure in hypertensive patients with type 2 diabetes (*Diabetes Care* 2008 May[228]): This double-blind trial included 24 male patients with type-2 DM and HTN divided into two groups of 12 patients that randomly received either placebo or NAC 1,200 mg/d and ARG 1,200 mg/d orally for 6 months. "RESULTS—The NAC + ARG treatment caused a reduction of both systolic and diastolic mean arterial blood pressure, total cholesterol, LDL cholesterol, oxidized LDL, high-sensitive C-reactive protein, intracellular adhesion molecule, vascular cell adhesion molecule, nitrotyrosine, fibrinogen, and plasminogen activator inhibitor-1, and an improvement of the intima-media thickness during endothelial postischemic vasodilation. HDL cholesterol increased. No changes in other parameters studied were observed. CONCLUSIONS—NAC + ARG administration seems to be a potential well-tolerated antiatherogenic therapy because it improves endothelial function in hypertensive patients with type 2 diabetes by improving NO bioavailability via reduction of oxidative stress and increase of NO production. Our study's results give prominence to its potential use in primary and secondary cardiovascular prevention in these patients." The **BP change in the treatment group was -5/-5 mm Hg**; the results of this study are remarkable considering the low dose of Arg employed and the manifold biochemical benefits attained.

---

[226] Miller AL. The effects of sustained-release-L-arginine formulation on blood pressure and vascular compliance in 29 healthy individuals. *Altern Med Rev.* 2006 Mar;11(1):23-9
[227] Neri et al. Effect of L-arginine on blood pressure in pregnancy-induced hypertension: a randomized placebo-controlled trial. *J Matern Fetal Neonatal Med.* 2006 May:277-81
[228] Martina V, Masha A, Gigliardi VR, et al. Long-term N-acetylcysteine and L-arginine administration reduces endothelial activation and systolic blood pressure in hypertensive patients with type 2 diabetes. *Diabetes Care.* 2008 May;31(5):940-4 care.diabetesjournals.org/content/31/5/940.long

- Review: L-arginine and cardiovascular system (*Pharmacological Reports* 2005 Jan-Feb[229]): "The majority of experimental and clinical studies clearly show a beneficial effect of L-arginine on endothelium in conditions associated with its hypofunction and thus with reduced NO synthesis. Some clinical studies involving healthy volunteers or patients suffering from hypertension and diabetes indicate that it may also regulate vascular hemostasis." The full text of this article goes on to itemize several clinical trials (at variable level of detail), the majority of these synopses related to HTN are summarized here:

Adverse effects of elevated homocysteine
• Activation of coagulation
• Stimulation of monocyte adhesion
• Enhanced oxidation of low density lipoprotein (LDL),
• Impairment of NO-mediated vascular responses (vasodilation)
• Adverse effects on bone health and increased risk for osteoporosis
• Neuroinflammation, activation of glutamate receptors
• Mitochondrial impairment
• Endothelial dysfunction, relative or absolute vasoconstriction

  - Placebo controlled trial of 30 g (thirty grams) Arg infused intravenously over 30 minutes to healthy volunteers: Diastolic BP was "markedly reduced" more than was systolic BP; another study conducted in women found similar results.
  - Consumption of an Arg-enriched diet by healthy volunteers: BP reduction.
  - Oral administration of 21g daily to healthy young men for 3 days: No correlation of Arg with blood pressure.
  - Oral administration of 20g daily to healthy men for 28 days: No reduction in BP.
  - Oral administration of 9g daily to healthy subjects for 6 months: No reduction in BP; however, "long-term administration of this amino acid had a favorable effect on endothelium, improving its function and reducing concentration of endothelin." (Endothelins are peptides that constrict blood vessels and contribute to HTN.)
  - Intravenous Arg given at a dose of 500 mg/kg in patients with primary and secondary hypertension: "Considerable reduction both in systolic and diastolic pressure in all the cases."
  - Intravenous Arg given at a dose of 30g over 60 minutes in patients with treated/untreated HTN: Previously untreated HTN patients had the best clinical response, followed by ACEi-treated patients, and a slight BP reduction in normal volunteers.
  - Oral Arg 5.6 or 12.6 g/day for 6 weeks in patients with heart failure: Reduction in arterial blood pressure.
  - Oral Arg 21 g for 3 days to young men with coronary artery disease: No changes in blood pressure despite improvement in brachial artery dilation.
  - Intravenous bolus of 3g Arg to healthy subjects and patients with insulin-independent diabetes, hypercholesterolemia and primary hypertension: Best response was seen in young healthy patients (response inverse to age), then hypertensives, and lastly in patients with hypercholesterolemia and DM.
  - Oral Arg 21 g/d for 4 weeks in young patients with hypercholesterolemia: Improved endothelium-dependent dilatation.
  - Intravenous infusion of Arg 30 g for 60 minutes in patients with limb ischemia: "Marked reduction in diastolic and systolic pressure and an increased blood flow in the femoral artery."
- Randomized placebo-controlled clinical trial: The effect of L-arginine and creatine on vascular function and homocysteine metabolism (*Vascular Medicine* 2009 Aug[230]): The authors introduce their study by noting that studies with L-arginine supplementation have shown inconsistent effects on endothelial function (readers will have noted this from the studies reviewed above). The authors point out that, while L-arginine is a nitric oxide precursor, it is also the precursor to guanidinoacetate (GAA), which leads to the formation of creatine and the consumption of methionine to produce homocysteine, thereby utilizing methyl groups and increasing methylation demand. The purpose of this study was to investigate the effect of supplementation with L-arginine and creatine (alone or in combination) on vascular function and methylation/homocysteine metabolism. Patients with documented CAD (n=109) were randomized to

---

[229] Cylwik D, Mogielnicki A, Buczko W. L-arginine and cardiovascular system. *Pharmacol Rep.* 2005 Jan-Feb;57(1):14-22 if-pan.krakow.pl/pjp/pdf/2005/1_14.pdf
[230] Jahangir et al. The effect of L-arginine and creatine on vascular function and homocysteine metabolism. *Vasc Med.* 2009 Aug;14(3):239-48

receive L-arginine (9gm/d), creatine (21gm/day), L-arginine plus creatine, or placebo for 4 days (n=26–29 per group); brachial artery flow-mediated dilation and plasma levels of L-arginine, creatine, homocysteine, methionine, and GAA were measured at baseline and follow up. Results of this study showed that L-arginine and creatine supplementation had no effects on vascular function; we could argue that 4 days is insufficient duration to produce changes in physiologic function. L-arginine increased GAA (P<0.01) and the ratio of homocysteine to methionine (from 0.7 to 0.9; P<0.01) suggesting increased methylation demand. Supplementation with L-arginine increased plasma homocysteine from 11.1 micromol/L to 11.2 micromol/L (P=0.006); one could easily argue that such a minute change is clinically insignificant, while one could also argue that a negative change within the span of 4 days of supplementation portends a potentially hazardous trend if carried out for months and years, especially in the large number of patients with defective or deficient methylation pathways.

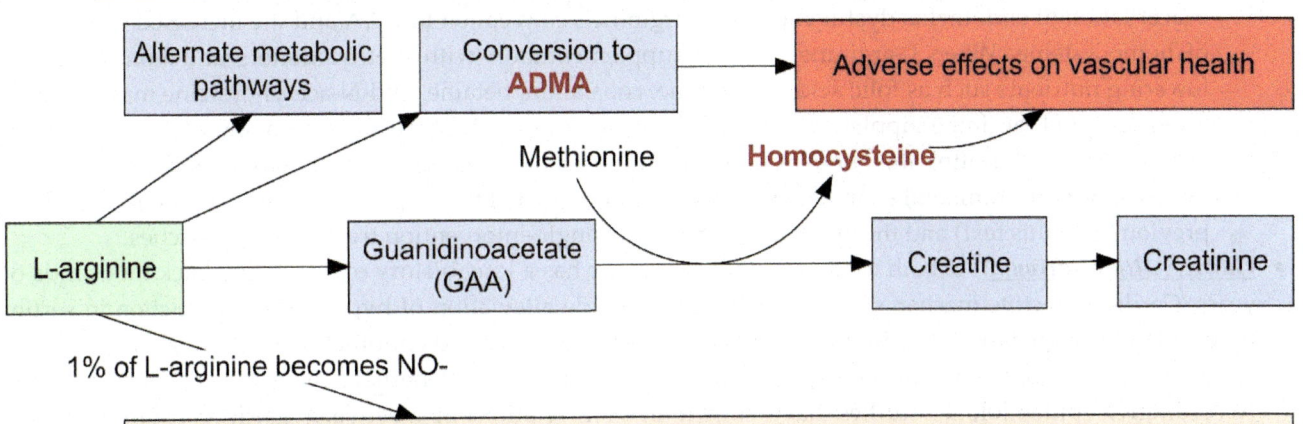

L-arginine conversion to nitric oxide and ADMA, effect on methionine-homocysteine metabolism: Beyond the lure and lore of biochemistry, this pathway shows that administration of arginine might promote depletion of methyl groups in patients deficient (nutritionally) or impaired (genetically, hormonally) in this pathway. Utilization of methyl groups via S-adenosyl methionine (SAMe) results in elevated homocysteine and depletion of methyl groups if methylation factors such as folate are in short supply. L-arginine (whether as an isolated supplement or as contained within dietary proteins) can be converted into asymmetric dimethylarginine (ADMA)—notably by Gram-negative and dysbiotic bacteria (or possibly via the inflammatory response thereto) such as *Helicobacter pylori*, but also endogenously (e.g., in adipocytes), especially in patients at heightened cardiometabolic risk—which, despite some antiinflammatory actions, appears mostly vasculotoxic. Thus, administration of arginine for the sake of vascular health for enhancement of endothelial function and nitric oxide production, can—depending on host factors of nutritional (in)sufficiency and/or dysbiosis—actually have vasculotoxic effects via homocysteine and ADMA, respectively. Administration of L-arginine can clearly lead to elevations of ADMA in humans.[231] Böger[232] summarized the "arginine paradox" as follows: "Asymmetric dimethylarginine (ADMA) is an endogenous competitive inhibitor of NO synthase. ADMA inhibits vascular NO production in concentrations found in pathophysiological conditions; ADMA also causes local vasoconstriction when it is infused intraarterially. Thus, elevated ADMA levels may explain the "L-arginine paradox," i.e., the observation that supplementation with exogenous L-arginine improves NO-mediated vascular functions in vivo, although its baseline plasma concentration is about 25-fold higher than the Michaelis-Menten constant K(m) of the isolated, purified endothelial NO synthase in vitro. ... Thus, ADMA may explain the discrepant results of clinical trials in which L-arginine sometimes improves endothelial function and sometimes does not—a discrepancy that has so far remained unexplained." Administration of L-citrulline as an L-arginine precursor might be preferred to use of L-arginine itself.

More important than the change in homocysteine levels is the more sensitive increase in the ratio of homocysteine to methionine, indicating increased methylation demand which is likely to have adverse effects in various metabolic pathways; the authors note, "Thus, it remains possible that L-arginine

---

[231] "Patients were later randomized to either L-arginine (2 g tid or 4 g tid) or placebo. ... Additionally plasma ADMA concentrations after 28 days of L-arginine supplementation significantly exceeded initial concentrations. CONCLUSIONS: L-arginine supplementation increases plasma arginine, citrulline and TAS in patients with mild arterial hypertension. It confirms the thesis that augmented concentrations of L-arginine stimulate NO biosynthesis which leads to reduction of oxidative stress. Increase of ADMA plasma level after L-arginine supplementation confirms correlation between ADMA and L-arginine." Jabecka et al. Oral L-arginine supplementation in patients with mild arterial hypertension and its effect on plasma level of asymmetric dimethylarginine, L-citruline, L-arginine and antioxidant status. *Eur Rev Med Pharmacol Sci.* 2012 Nov;16(12):1665-74
[232] Böger RH. Asymmetric dimethylarginine, an endogenous inhibitor of nitric oxide synthase, explains the "L-arginine paradox" and acts as a novel cardiovascular risk factor. *J Nutr.* 2004 Oct;134(10 Suppl):2842S-2847S

metabolism imposes a methylation demand that counterbalances the effects of NO generated despite the absence of a change in measured plasma homocysteine." The average GFR of patients in this study was 68 ml/min by the Cockcroft–Gault formula (consistent with stage 2—almost stage 3—kidney disease), and previous studies have shown that patients with kidney disease are less likely to respond to treatments that improve endovascular health, including L-arginine, due in part to higher levels of circulating ADMA and homocysteine. The combination of creatinine and L-arginine did not suppress GAA production or prevent the increase in homocysteine-to-methionine ratio. Unexpectedly, the authors found that creatine supplementation (alone or in combination with L-arginine) was associated with an 11 to 20% increase in plasma homocysteine; other studies *of longer duration* using *lower doses of creatine* (<5.5 gm/d for 4 weeks) have shown the opposite effect—namely that creatine supplementation lowers plasma homocysteine. Altogether, these findings raise the possibility that L-arginine's effects on vascular function may be dependent on the patient's methylation ability; patients with poor methylation ability may experience exacerbation of endothelial dysfunction via L-arginine's conversion to GAA and the increased production of homocysteine. When L-arginine is used, supplementation with methyl donors and homocysteine-lowering nutrients such as folic acid, pyridoxine, cobalamin, betaine, and N-acetyl-cysteine may improve the efficacy of L-arginine supplementation while additively or synergistically improving vascular reactivity and endothelial health; this underscores the importance of dietary optimization and foundational multivitamin/multimineral supplementation (as a component of the "5-part nutritional protocol" described previously in this text) and the general need to avoid single-intervention treatment approaches.

- **Garlic, *Allium sativum*:** As both food and medicine, garlic has a long history of use dating back thousands of years. Cardioprotective mechanisms are reported to include alleviation of hypertension, reduction in serum lipids, platelet aggregation, and improvements in insulin sensitivity and endothelial function; obviously these vasculoprotective effects would be expected to produce additive and perhaps synergistic clinical benefits. Accordingly, epidemiologic studies have shown inverse relationships between garlic consumption and cardiovascular disease prevalence; while various mechanisms are in effect, a recent *in vitro* study showed that human RBCs convert garlic-derived organic polysulfides (allyl-substituted sulfur compounds) into hydrogen sulfide (H_2S), an endogenous cell signaling molecule that exerts vasculoprotective effects in endothelial cells.[233] Per *in vitro* studies, extracts from garlic leaf and bulbs have shown ability to inhibit 5-lipoxygenase, cyclooxygenase, thrombocyte aggregation, and angiotensin-converting enzyme (ACE).[234] Garlic's antimicrobial properties and its numerous immune-enhancing effects might also be included in its spectrum of cardioprotective properties, since occult infections in general (i.e., multifocal polydysbiosis, particularly the orodental and gastrointestinal subtypes[235]) and bacterial lipopolysaccharide (LPS) in particular are correlated in humans with HTN, diabetes mellitus, and cardiovascular disease; additionally, garlic's ability to modulate cytokine expression and inhibit activation of NFkB could further mitigate the cardiovasculotoxic effects of inflammation and dysbiosis.

  - Critical review: Garlic and cardiovascular disease (*Journal of Nutrition* 2006 Mar[236]): The authors note that epidemiologic studies show an inverse correlation between garlic consumption and progression of cardiovascular disease and that garlic has many cardioprotective properties:
    - Garlic inhibits enzymes involved in lipid synthesis, most notably beta-hydroxy-beta-methylglutaryl-CoA (HMG-CoA) reductase, the rate limiting enzyme in cholesterol biosynthesis,
    - Garlic decreases platelet aggregation,
    - Garlic prevents lipid peroxidation of erythrocytes and LDL,
    - Garlic improves antioxidant status,
    - Garlic inhibits angiotensin-converting enzyme (ACE).

Garlic's inconsistent results on BP, the authors suggest, is due ❶ to a combination of usage of different garlic preparations, ❷ uncertainty about which active constituents should be provided, and their respective

---

[233] Benavides et al. Hydrogen sulfide mediates the vasoactivity of garlic. *Proc Natl Acad Sci* U S A. 2007 Nov 13;104(46):17977-82

[234] "The inhibition rates as IC50 values of both extracts for 5-LO, CO, and TA showed a good correlation with %-content of the major S-containing compounds (thiosulfinates and ajoenes) of the various extracts. ... In ACE test, water extract of the leaves of wild garlic containing glutamyl-peptides showed the highest inhibitory activity followed by that of the garlic leaf and the bulbs of both drugs." Sendl et al. Comparative pharmacological investigations of Allium ursinum and Allium sativum. *Planta Med.* 1992 Feb;58(1):1-7

[235] Vasquez A. *Integrative Rheumatology*. IBMRC 2006, 2007 and all future editions. Vasquez A. Nutritional and Botanical Treatments Against "Silent Infections" and Gastrointestinal Dysbiosis, Commonly Overlooked Causes of Neuromusculoskeletal Inflammation and Chronic Health Problems. *Nutritional Perspectives* 2006; January

[236] Rahman K, Lowe GM. Garlic and cardiovascular disease: a critical review. *J Nutr.* 2006 Mar;136(3 Suppl):736S-740S

bioavailability, ❸ inadequate randomization, ❹ selection of inappropriate subjects, and ❺ insufficient duration of trials. However, the gestalt of garlic's cardioprotective benefits strongly suggest its value in dietary utilization for patients with elevated cardiovascular risk, which obviously includes patients with hypertension.

- Double-blind, placebo-controlled trial: Time-released garlic powder tablets lower systolic and diastolic blood pressure in men with mild and moderate arterial hypertension (*Hypertension Research* 2009 Jun[237]): This double-blind placebo-controlled trial with 84 hypertensive men employed either ❶ time-released garlic powder tablets (600-2400 mg Allicor) or ❷ "regular garlic pills" (900 mg Kwai). Allicor (600 mg daily) resulted in a reduction of both systolic and diastolic blood pressures by 7.0 mm Hg and 3.8 mm, respectively, with no advantage noted at the higher 2400 mg/d dose. Use of Kwai resulted in a similar decrease in systolic blood pressure (-5.4 mm Hg), but no decrease in diastolic blood pressure was observed with Kwai. Noting that both garlic preparations provided an antihypertensive benefit, the authors concluded, "The results of this study show that time-released garlic powder tablets are more effective for the treatment of mild and moderate arterial hypertension than are regular garlic supplements."[238] Of note, a different study by the same primary author (Igor Sobenin) also demonstrated lipid-modifying effects of time-released garlic powder tablets, (Allicor 600 mg daily) in a double-blinded placebo-controlled randomized study among 42 men: total cholesterol reduced by >7%, LDL cholesterol reduced by approximately 12%, and HDL cholesterol increased by 11.5%.
- Systematic review and meta-analysis: Effect of garlic on blood pressure (*BioMed Central - Cardiovascular Disorders* 2008 Jun[239]): The authors reviewed eleven criteria-selected studies published between 1955 and October 2007 identified from Medline and Embase databases. Results showed, "…the mean decrease in the hypertensive subgroup was 8.4 mm Hg for SBP (n = 4; p < 0.001), and 7.3 mm Hg for DBP (n = 3; p < 0.001). Regression analysis revealed a significant association between blood pressure at the start of the intervention and the level of blood pressure reduction (SBP: R = 0.057; p = 0.03; DBP: R = -0.315; p = 0.02). CONCLUSION: Our meta-analysis suggests that garlic preparations are superior to placebo in reducing blood pressure in individuals with hypertension."
- Meta-analysis: Effects of garlic on blood pressure in patients with and without systolic hypertension (*Annals of Pharmacotherapy* 2008 Dec[240]): For this meta-analysis, the authors performed a systematic search of MEDLINE, CINAHL, and the Cochrane Central Register of Controlled Trials to identify randomized controlled trials in humans evaluating garlic's effect on blood pressure; to this was added a manual search of published literature, and the complete search yielded 10 trials for review. The authors write, "Garlic reduced SBP by **16.3 mm Hg** (95% CI 6.2 to 26.5) and DBP by **9.3 mm Hg** (95% CI 5.3 to 13.3) compared with placebo in patients with elevated SBP. … This meta-analysis suggests that garlic is associated with blood pressure reductions in patients with an elevated SBP although not in those without elevated SBP. Future research should focus on the impact of garlic on clinical events and the assessment of the long-term risk of harm." While the authors' cautionary note is reasonable given the potential for adverse effects from nearly any agent, the risk-benefit scales appear to tip in favor of garlic's overall cardioprotective, antihypertensive, eulipidemic benefits in addition to its wide availability and low cost; indeed, given these results, an argument could be made that withholding garlic—like CoQ10 and fish oil and vitamin D3— could be unethical in patients at elevated CVD risk.
- Garlic (*Allium sativum* L.) modulates cytokine expression in lipopolysaccharide-activated human blood thereby inhibiting NF-kappaB activity (*Journal of Nutrition* 2003 Jul[241]): Given the well-established role of inflammation in CVD initiation and progression, and the potential role of occult infections (i.e., various types and locations of dysbiosis), an anti-inflammatory mechanism to garlic's cardioprotective benefits is intriguing. The authors write, "This paper shows that garlic powder extracts (GPE) and single garlic metabolites modulate lipopolysaccharide (LPS)-induced cytokine levels in human whole blood" and that

[237] Sobenin et al. Lipid-lowering effects of time-released garlic powder tablets in double-blinded placebo-controlled randomized study. *J Atheroscler Thromb*. 2008 Dec;15:334-8
[238] Sobenin et al. Time-released garlic powder tablets lower systolic and diastolic blood pressure in men with mild/moderate arterial hypertension. *Hypertens Res*. 2009 Jun:433-7
[239] Ried et al. Effect of garlic on blood pressure: a systematic review and meta-analysis. *BMC Cardiovasc Disord*. 2008 Jun 16;8:13
[240] Reinhart et al. Effects of garlic on blood pressure in patients with and without systolic hypertension: a meta-analysis. *Ann Pharmacother*. 2008 Dec;42(12):1766-71
[241] Keiss et al. Garlic modulates cytokine expression in lipopolysaccharide-activated human blood thereby inhibiting NF-kappaB activity. *J Nutr*. 2003 Jul;133(7):2171-5

these favorable modifications in GPE-altered cytokine levels "reduced nuclear factor (NF)-kappaB [NFkB] activity in human cells exposed to these samples." Pretreatment with garlic extracts reduced LPS-induced production of proinflammatory cytokines interleukin (IL)-1beta from 15.7 to 6.2 micro g/L (greater than 50% reduction) and tumor necrosis factor (TNF)-alpha from 8.8 to 3.9 micro g/L (greater than 50% reduction). In an additional experiment, exposure of human embryonic kidney cell line (HEK293) cells to GPE-treated blood sample supernatants reduced NFkB activity by 25% (unfertilized garlic) and 41% (sulfur-fertilized garlic). The authors conclude, "In summary, garlic may indeed promote an anti-inflammatory environment by cytokine modulation in human blood that leads to an overall inhibition of NFkB activity in the surrounding tissue." Beyond demonstrating an anti-inflammatory effect of garlic, this study also serves as a reminder that suppression of proinflammatory cytokines can favorably downregulate NFkB activity in a "retroactive" manner, since NFkB activation generally precedes elaboration of proinflammatory cytokines; thus, garlic extracts appear capable of breaking the proinflammatory vicious cycle.

- **Nattokinase**: Nattokinase is an enzyme extracted and purified from a Japanese food called Natto, a cheese-like food made from fermented soybeans.
  - Randomized, controlled trial: Effects of nattokinase on blood pressure (*Hypertension Research* 2008 Aug[242]): 86 participants with pre-hypertension or stage-1 hypertension received nattokinase (2,000 FU/capsule) or a placebo capsule for 8 weeks. **Net changes in systolic and diastolic blood pressure were -5.55 mmHg and -2.84 mmHg, respectively, after the 8-week intervention**. Renin activity levels dropped by -1.17 ng/mL/h for the nattokinase group compared with the control group. The authors concluded, "…nattokinase supplementation resulted in a reduction in SBP and DBP. These findings suggest that increased intake of nattokinase may play an important role in preventing and treating hypertension."

INFECTIONS/DYSBIOSIS Over the past many years—and perhaps due to changes in the environment such as the overuse of the antibiotic glyphosate and the superabundance of other metabolism-inhibiting corporate chemicals, all of which have culminated in increased metabolic fragility and pro-inflammatory tendencies—we have become increasingly aware of the role of the gut microbiome in mitochondrial dysfunction and the resulting insulin resistance, obesity, and hypertension.

- **Berberine**: Used for its health-promoting properties for thousands of years, berberine is a naturally-occurring plant alkaloid present in *Hydrastis canadensis* (goldenseal), *Coptis chinensis* (goldenthread), *Berberis aquifolium* (Oregon grape), *Berberis vulgaris* (barberry), and *Berberis aristata* (tree turmeric). Naturopathic physicians have commonly employed berberine-containing treatments for anti-infective benefits, particularly against gastrointestinal dysbiosis and respiratory tract infections. Within the past few years, numerous experimental studies in animals and clinical trials in humans have clearly demonstrated that berberine possesses many cardioprotective benefits, only one of which is its ability to promote normalization of elevated blood pressure. Given its well-documented antimicrobial effects, berberine quite likely improves overall health by reducing microbe-induced total inflammatory load (TIL) in addition to its direct benefits on metabolic and genomic processes. The current author appreciates berberine's numerous benefits demonstrated in clinical practice and in recent research, but prefers to limit its high-dose (1,000 mg/d) use to 3-6 months.
  - Clinical trial: Treatment of type 2 diabetes and dyslipidemia with the natural plant alkaloid berberine (*Journal of Clinical Endocrinology and Metabolism* 2008 Jul[243]): In this randomized placebo-controlled trial, 116 patients with diabetes mellitus type-2 and dyslipidemia were randomly allocated to receive berberine (1,000 mg/d) or placebo for 3 months. Significant benefits were shown by berberine in insulin sensitivity, glucose homeostasis, and plasma lipids; except for mild to moderate constipation in five subjects in the berberine group, no major adverse effects were observed. With regard to blood pressure, results showed that systolic blood pressure decreased from 124 to 117 mm Hg and diastolic blood pressure decreased from 81 to 77 mm Hg in subjects treated with berberine (i.e., total reduction of -7/-4 mm Hg); this effect was superior to that shown in patients treated with placebo, who showed reduction of -3/-3 mm Hg. Note that these patients—even though they were diabetic—were not hypertensive. The authors concluded the text of their article by stating, "Given the benefits of berberine in lowering blood glucose, lipids, body weight,

---

[242] Kim et al. Effects of nattokinase on blood pressure: a randomized, controlled trial. *Hypertens Res.* 2008 Aug;31(8):1583-8
[243] Zhang et al. Treatment of type 2 diabetes and dyslipidemia with the natural plant alkaloid berberine. *J Clin Endocrinol Metab.* 2008 Jul;93(7):2559-65

and blood pressures, we speculate that berberine may be used for patients with type-2 diabetes and metabolic syndrome."

- **Probiotics**: The term "probiotics" generally refers to beneficial microorganisms—most commonly bacteria but also including the probiotic yeast *Saccharomyces boulardii*—that are consumed either in the supplement/nutraceutical form of tablets, capsules, powders or as fermented foods such as yogurt, kefir, kombucha, miso, tempeh, cottage cheese (some types), and sauerkraut. Due to their numerous benefits, probiotics have been included as the fifth component of the 5-part nutritional protocol published by Vasquez[244] in 2005. As science has continued to progress (both qualitatively and quantitatively), so has our knowledge of the diversity and mechanisms of the health-promoting benefits of probiotic supplementation. This section reviews several of the mechanisms behind the antihypertensive (and also cardioprotective, antidiabetic, antidyslipidemic, and anti-inflammatory) benefits of probiotic supplementation. Starting with and strongly relying upon a review article by Lye et al[245] named "The improvement of hypertension by probiotics: effects on cholesterol, diabetes, renin, and phytoestrogens", this section will concisely review the more prominent antihypertensive benefits and mechanisms of probiotic supplementation. Lye et al emphasize the role of dyslipidemia in the genesis of HTN by stating, "...lipid metabolism disorders are often the causes of hypertension." Relevant to this paradigm, they review data from controlled studies in humans, rats, and/or pigs showing that antidyslipidemic benefits (reduction in total serum cholesterol, very low density lipoprotein, intermediate density lipoprotein, and LDL cholesterol and increase in HDL cholesterol) have been documented due to the use of *Lactobacillus acidophilus*, *Lactobacillus casei*, *Bifidobacterium longum*, and *Saccharomyces boulardii* (when used with bacterial probiotics). The antidyslipidemic benefit of supplementation with *L. acidophilus*, *B. breve*, *Lactococcus lactis* and other probiotics is mediated in part or in whole part via ❶ cholesterol assimilation during growth (i.e., the bacteria actively take up cholesterol for their own use), ❷ binding of cholesterol to the cellular surface, in part via exopolysaccharides (EPS) which adhere to the cell surface and absorb cholesterol, and ❸ probiotic elaboration of the enzyme bile salt hydrolase (BSH; cholyglycine hydrolase) which catalyzes the hydrolysis of glycine- and/or taurine-conjugated bile salts into amino acid residues and free bile acids, the latter of which contain cholesterol and are preferentially excreted in the feces rather than being reabsorbed in the intestines. Thus, probiotics function in part (mechanisms 1 and 2) similarly to the anticholesterolemic drug cholestyramine, which exerts its cholesterol-lowering effect via enhanced fecal excretion of cholesterol. Also, the authors note the correlation between diabetes mellitus, insulin resistance, and HTN, and that probiotics may also mediate an antihypertensive benefit by ❹ ameliorating diabetes and insulin resistance; in their words, "The consumption of probiotics is a new therapeutic strategy in preventing or delaying the onset of diabetes and subsequently reducing the incident of hypertension." With regard to this fourth mechanism, the postulated mechanism of the antihypertensive and antidiabetic benefit is worthy of appreciation both as a mechanism and as an independent benefit. The authors state that the antidiabetic benefit of probiotics is due to the reduction in systemic inflammation mediated via improvements in intestinal microecology which effect a reduction in systemic absorption of intestinally-derived bacterial lipopolysaccharides [LPS], which are inherently proinflammatory; the authors write, "...the composition of natural intestinal gut microflora often determine the degree of inflammation contributing to the onset of diabetes and obesity. The concentration of plasma lipopolysaccharides, the proinflammatory factor, is inversely correlated with the population of *Bifidobacterium* spp. ... Several studies have also shown that bifidobacteria can reduce the intestinal endotoxin levels and improve mucosal barrier thus reducing systemic inflammation and subsequently reduced the incidence of diabetes." This **systemic anti-inflammatory benefit derived from the (re)establishment of eubiosis** is wholly consistent with the model of dysbiosis-induced systemic inflammation and autoimmunity detailed in both the 2006 and 2007 editions of *Integrative Rheumatology*.[246] In summarizing this mechanism, we must (again) conclude that probiotics are antidysbiotic and anti-inflammatory (dependent on and independent from LPS reduction) and that ❺ the antihypertensive benefit of probiotic supplementation is mediated at least in part via reducing systemic LPS-induced inflammation and thus subsequent insulin resistance and endothelial dysfunction, which independently and synergistically promote HTN. In either *in vitro*, animal, or human studies, the

---

[244] Vasquez A. A Five-Part Nutritional Protocol that Produces Consistently Positive Results. *Nutritional Wellness* 2005 September

[245] Lye et al. The improvement of hypertension by probiotics: effects on cholesterol, diabetes, renin, and phytoestrogens. *Int J Mol Sci.* 2009 Aug 27;10(9):3755-75

[246] Vasquez A. *Integrative Rheumatology*. IBMRC 2006, 2007 and all future editions

beneficial effects of probiotic supplementation have been demonstrated (in descending order of efficacy) from the use of living and growing probiotic populations, non-growing probiotics, and dead cells. Finally but not exhaustively, we should appreciate as mentioned previously that ❻ probiotic bacteria interact with dietary components—especially proteins from cow's milk—to produce antihypertensive peptides which, in particular, have ACE-inhibiting functions. As summed by Lye et al, "Probiotics are able to grow in milk products because they possess a proteolytic system that degrades casein along with lactose hydrolyzing enzymes. Upon fermentation, the proteinases of various probiotics are capable of releasing ACE inhibitory peptides and thus a blood-pressure lowering effect can be derived from the milk proteins. Several studies have demonstrated that *Lactobacillus helveticus* are capable of releasing antihypertensive peptides which are ACE inhibitory tripeptides Val-Pro-Pro (VPP) and Ile-Pro-Pro (IPP) from milk protein casein."

- Randomized, placebo-controlled, double-blind study: Effect of powdered fermented milk with *Lactobacillus helveticus* on subjects with high-normal blood pressure or mild hypertension (*Journal of the American College of Nutrition* 2005 Aug[247]): This study used a randomized, placebo-controlled, double-blind design in 40 subjects with high-normal blood pressure (HN group: SBP 130–139 mm Hg and DBP 85–89 mm Hg) and 40 subjects with mild hypertension (MH group: SBP 140–159 mm Hg and DBP 90–99 mm Hg). Each subject ingested 12 g of powdered fermented milk (in tablet form) with *L. helveticus* CM4 daily for 4 weeks (test group) or the same amount of placebo tablets for 4 weeks (placebo group). The authors noted that **among the patients with high-normal blood pressure, the change in SBP in the test group was 3.2 mm Hg lower than that in the placebo group, and DBP decreased more in the test group than in the placebo group during treatment, by 5.0 mm Hg** at the end of week 4. Further, they write, "**In the [Mild Hypertension] group, SBP decreased by 11.2 mm Hg and there was a statistically non-significant decrease in DBP of 6.5 mm Hg** compared with the placebo group." Their conclusions read, "Daily ingestion of the tablets containing powdered fermented milk with *L. helveticus* CM4 in subjects with high-normal blood pressure or mild hypertension reduces elevated blood pressure without any adverse effects." Readers should appreciate that this group with mild hypertension (SBP 140–159 mm Hg and DBP 90–99 mm Hg) represents the largest group of HTN patients and that this benefit of peptides from fermented milk—a reduction in blood pressure of -11.2/-6.5—is on par with the antihypertensive effect derived from many commonly used FDA-approved pharmaceutical drugs.

NUTRITIONAL IMMUNOMODULATION Evidence is accumulating that proinflammatory immune imbalances contribute to sustained hypertension.[248] What is becoming more and more clear—to the amazement of many of us—is the interrelationship between mitochondrial dysfunction and immunophenotype imbalance: **clearly at this time we must acknowledge that a bidirectional relationship exists between mitochondria and the immune system**—a fact that is not commonly within the curriculum of most medical schools nor the intellectual armamentarium of most clinicians. Per the illustration that follows, this section will discuss the role of immunophenotype imbalance in the genesis and perpetuation of sustained hypertension; therapeutic correction of immunophenotype imbalance—simplified as "excess Th17 and insufficient Treg"—is discussed in Chapter 4. I call this the "mito-immunologic model of hypertension."

- Evidence for immunophenotype imbalance—functional usurpation by Th1, Th2, and Th17 with functional abdication of Treg—in sustained hypertension: See section on Nutritional Immunomodulation in Chapter 4 for important pathophysiologic details and therapeutic interventions; this section serves solely to describe and substantiate the causal connection between immunophenotype imbalance and sustained hypertension. In sum, mitochondrial ROS (mtROS) directly contribute to the pro-hypertensive response of immune cells[249], mediated significantly by Th17 cells and their signature cytokine IL-17. [250]
  - The immune system in in hypertension (*Can J Cardiol* 2013 May[251]): The author of this article provides an efficient review and summary by reminding us that various lymphocyte subsets and their respective cytokines are involved in vascular remodeling, hypertensive renal disease, and cardiovascular disease.

[247] Aihara K, Kajimoto O, Hirata H, Takahashi R, Nakamura Y. Effect of powdered fermented milk with Lactobacillus helveticus on subjects with high-normal blood pressure or mild hypertension. *J Am Coll Nutr.* 2005 Aug;24(4):257-65

[248] Schiffrin EL. The immune system: role in hypertension. *Can J Cardiol.* 2013 May;29(5):543-8

[249] Nazarewicz RR, Dikalov SI. Mitochondrial ROS in the prohypertensive immune response. *Am J Physiol Regul Integr Comp Physiol.* 2013 Jul 15;305(2):R98-100

[250] Wang J et al. Elevated Th17 and IL-23 in hypertensive patients with acutely increased blood pressure. *American Journal of Immunology* 2012: 8: 27-32

[251] Schiffrin EL. The immune system: role in hypertension. *Can J Cardiol.* 2013 May;29(5):543-8

Among the effector lymphocytes, Th1 produce interferon-γ, Th2 produce IL-4, Th17 produce IL17), and Tregs are anti-inflammatory and express the FoxP3 transcription factor. **These immune cells mediate the cardiovascular effects of angiotensin-2 and mineralocorticoids.** Further, "....neoantigens could be generated by elevated blood pressure through damage-associated molecular pattern [DAMP] receptors [rDAMP] or other mechanisms. When activated, Th1 may contribute to blood pressure elevation by affecting the kidney, vascular remodeling of blood vessels directly via effects of the cytokines produced, or through their effects on perivascular fat. **T regulatory cells protect from blood pressure elevation** acting on similar targets. These novel findings may open the way for new therapeutic approaches to improve outcomes in hypertension and cardiovascular disease in humans."

> **Immune activation and pro-inflammatory cytokines are "essential" for the sustenance of "essential HTN"**
>
> **"T-cells are critical for hypertension;** however, the exact mechanism of T-cell activation in hypertension has not been fully understand. Once activated, T-cells intensively proliferate, produce cytokines that further stimulate immune system, **alter vascular function** and stimulate ROS production. **MtROS regulates cellular signaling, cell functions, and metabolism.**" Inhibition of NOX2 prevents production of **TNFα, a cytokine that is critical for the development of hyp**ertension. Inhibition of TNFα mutes hypertension; thus, scavenging ROS in immune cells may attenuate their pro-hypertensive effect.
>
> Nazarewicz RR, Dikalov SI. Mitochondrial ROS in the prohypertensive immune response. *Am J Physiol Regul Integr Comp Physiol* 2013 Jul

- Elevated Th17 and IL-23 in hypertensive patients with acutely increased blood pressure (*American Journal of Immunology* 2012[252]): "The involvement of **immune activation in hypertension has been well demonstrated** by many research groups... **Th17**, a recently discovered subset of CD4+T cells, is believed to play a role in the **pathogenesis of vascular dysfunction and hypertension.** In the current study, demonstrated an increased level of Th17 and IL-17 in hypertensive patients with acute increases of blood pressure..."

- Mitochondrial ROS in the prohypertensive immune response (*Am J Physiol Regul Integr Comp Physiol* 2013 Jul[253]): This nice article provides insight into the connection between mitochondrial dysfunction and the immune system's role in sustaining hypertension. In a nutshell, evidence supports circular and bidirectional connections between mitochondrial dysfunction and proinflammatory and immunodysfunctional contributions to sustaining the hypertensive phenotype. Mechanistically, intramitochondrial and intracellular ROS function as intracellular signals independent from systemic oxidative stress to induce additional mitochondrial dysfunction, dependence on glycolysis, inhibition of mitochondrial electron transport chain (ETC) function, additional mtROS formation, enhanced elaboration of pro-inflammatory cytokines, and increased hypertensive sensitivity to angiotensin. Cutting to the clinical chase, these authors state that "… angiotensin II-induced hypertension leads to endothelial dysfunction dependent on mtROS and NADPH oxidases. These pathological conditions can be reversed by preventing mitochondrial superoxide production. … It is conceivable that mitochondria-targeted antioxidants interfere with signal transduction in vascular cells; resulting in protection against the development of hypertension." Inhibition of NOX2 prevents production of TNFα, a cytokine that is critical for the development of hypertension. Inhibition of TNFα mutes hypertension; thus, scavenging ROS in immune cells may attenuate their pro-hypertensive effect. I think this likely explains the extraordinary effectiveness of CoQ10 in the treatment *and reliable clinical cure* of HTN, the mechanism being the mitochondria-specific sequestration of ROS with the simultaneous enhancement/support of ETC complexes 1, 2, and 3.

- T-cells in the genesis of angiotensin-2-induced hypertension and vascular dysfunction (*J Exp Med* 2007 Oct[254]): Experimental studies show that hypertension is blunted in animals lacking T-cells and/or the oxidant-producing enzyme nicotinamide adenosine dinucleotide phosphate (NADPH) oxidase discussed previously (see diagram). In fact, the pro-hypertensive effect of the prototypic prohypertensive hormone angiotensin-2 appear to be mediated via activity of nicotinamide adenosine dinucleotide phosphate (NADPH) oxidase via the resultant oxidant stress which mediates changes in (pro)inflammatory immune function resulting in the hypertensive clinical phenotype. Angiotensin-2 causes immune activation which

---

[252] Wang J et al. Elevated Th17 and IL-23 in hypertensive patients with acutely increased blood pressure. *American Journal of Immunology* 2012: 8: 27-32

[253] Nazarewicz RR, Dikalov SI. Mitochondrial ROS in the prohypertensive immune response. *Am J Physiol Regul Integr Comp Physiol*. 2013 Jul 15;305(2):R98-100

[254] Guzik TJ et al. Role of the T cell in the genesis of angiotensin II induced hypertension and vascular dysfunction. *J Exp Med*. 2007 Oct 1;204(10):2449-60

is dependent upon ROS produced via nicotinamide adenosine dinucleotide phosphate (NADPH) oxidase. Thus, we see a tripartite overlapping and vicious cycle via which ❶ angiotensin-2 activates NADPH oxidase to produce ROS which then leads to immune activation (i.e., angiotensin-2 is proinflammatory, and its hypertensive effects are ROS-dependent and immunocytes-dependent), and ❷ heightened immune activation leads to increased secretion of IL-17 and TNFa, both of which promote hypertension, and ❸ hypertension itself leads to immune activation. These authors articulated part of the vicious cycle as follows, "Hypertension also increased T lymphocyte production of tumor necrosis factor (TNF) alpha, and treatment with the TNFalpha antagonist etanercept prevented the hypertension and increase in vascular superoxide caused by angiotensin II. These studies identify a previously undefined role for T cells in the genesis of hypertension and support a role of inflammation in the basis of this prevalent disease. T cells might represent a novel therapeutic target for the treatment of high blood pressure."

Hypertensive immune imbalance via deficient Treg and excess Th17, IL-17, TNFa

Material/physical (not simply biochemical) predisposition toward inflammation, allergy, and autoimmunity; overproduction of pro-inflammatory and tissue-damaging cytokines which lead to synergistic production of ROS as well as alteration of native molecules and the activation of DAMP receptors (rDAMP), thereby promoting a vicious cycle of tissue damage, metabolic dysfunction, and "inflammation dysfunction."

Immunophenotype imbalance promotes hypertension

Mechanisms include inflammation-driven 1) insulin resistance, 2) endothelial dysfunction, 3) phagocytic production of NADPH oxidase (Nox2) augments mtROS pro-hypertensive cell signaling. Prohypertensive actions of angiotensin-2 are largely dependent on Nox2-mediated ROS production, which augments prohypertensive cytokine (TNFa) production. Hypertensive HTN patients show elevations in Th17 cells and the proinflammatory cytokines IL-6, IL-17, and TNFa.

Vicious cycles: mtROS is produced by immune activation and also leads to immune activation; immunocyte involvement is significant for the induction of the hypertensive response promoted by angiotensin-2 and mineralocorticoids

1) mtROS-induced mtROS production
2) Immune-driven immunoactivation
3) mtROS-induced immune-mediated mitochondrial dysfunction and immunoimbalance which promotes dysmetabolism, dysinsulinism, hypertension, autoimmunity, etc.
4) Hypertension is itself pro-inflammatory, and the resulting inflammation and ROS sustain the HTN.

Mitochondrial dysfunction promotes HTN

Mitochondrial dysfunction promotes HTN via dysinsulinism, endothelial dysfunction, altered intracellular signaling mediated by mtROS, and via enhanced elaboration of prohypertensive cytokines, especially IL-17 and TNFa. Mitochondrial dysfunction promotes prohypertensive "priming" of the immune system toward an exaggerated hypertensive response to glucocorticoids and angiotensin-2. Excessive mtROS from the ETC in the form of superoxide leads directly to neutralization of vasodilating nitric oxide and formation of peroxinitrite

Mitochondrial dysfunction

Mitochondrial hyperpolarization, activation of mTOR, and increased mitochondrial ROS production function *independently* and *synergistically* to inhibit Treg maturation, to promote Th17 maturation, and to promote molecular damage which provokes additional unnecessary/nonproductive immune responsiveness and inflammation. Superoxide radical combines with and therefore neutralizes what would otherwise be vasodilating nitric oxide, resulting in the production of the aggressive free radical peroxinitrite.

The mitoimmunology and mitoinflammology model: Immune phenotype imbalance and mitochondrial dysfunction can exist independently (at least initially) but eventually become interconnected and pathosynergistic

Proinflammatory cytokines are—in many experimental models—either necessary or sufficient for the establishment of sustained hypertension, and recent evidence shows elevated Th17 cells and serum IL-17 in acutely hypertensive patients. Elaboration of prohypertensive cytokines is increased by mitochondrial dysfunction; simultaneously, immune-mediated damage and resultant release of DAMP and activation of rDAMP likely perpetuates the cycle. rDAMP = receptor for damaged associated molecular pattern (DAMP), mtROS = mitochondrial reactive oxygen species. Nox2 = nicotinamide adenosine dinucleotide phosphate (NADPH) oxidase or NADPH oxidase, a ROS-generating enzyme in phagocytes and also in nonphagocytic tissues such as renal parenchyma and vascular endothelium

- <u>Therapeutic nutritional immunomodulation and immunophenotype (im/re)balance in hypertension</u>: Briefly, we can surmise that the "immune system" and inflammatory responses are necessary for the maintenance of the hypertensive clinical phenotype. Prohypertensive hormones such as glucocorticoids and angiotensin-2 effect elevated blood pressure through various means, some of which are completely dependent on induction of mitochondrial oxidative stress and the resultant pro-inflammatory immune response; I have termed this interdependency "**mitoimmunology**" and "**mitoinflammology.**"

   Correction of **mitochondrial dysfunction** and **immunophenotype imbalance** are both now-appreciated means by which clinicians can modulate dysfunctional pro-hypertensive pathophysiologic tendencies; furthermore, we must now appreciate the intimate connection between mitochondrial dysfunction (especially the role played by intramitochondrial ROS as cell signaling molecules that promote inflammation, hypertension, and autoimmunity) and the immune system, which can now be seen as the effector of the mitochondria's direction. Stated more plainly: Mitochondrial signals (e.g., mtROS) direct the proinflammatory and hypertensive response of the immune system (which will "over-react" if already in a state of pro-inflammatory imbalance) to promote harmful inflammation, which I categorize as ❶ metabolic (e.g., hypertension), ❷ allergic, and ❸ autoimmune. These insights provide access to "new" and nonpharmaodependent means by which clinicians can address hypertension via correction and optimization of physiologic function rather than dependence on pharmacomonkeywrenching—using drugs to interfere with a system that is already dysfunctional.

   Clinicians have generally considered oxidative stress to be "bad" and antioxidants to be "good" and while this is generally true in a quantitative sense, we as intellectually competent clinicians should discern more than such broad categories of "good and bad" given that the information is now available to us thanks to the efforts of innumerable named/unnamed researchers, their students, and assistants. Further to this deepening understanding, we need to discern the names and characteristics, roles and functions, location and compartmentalization of ROS to better appreciate their participation in health and disease; with this knowledge we will be better able to help our patients and strengthen the science of our healthcare and art.

MITOCHONDRIA/METABOLIC IMPAIRMENT CoQ10 is the most safe, effective, and reliable nutritional/physiological treatment for hypertension; its nearest competitors (and biochemical synergists) are potassium, magnesium, and vitamin D3). Not too many years ago, we were not perfectly clear on the mechanism of action, and indeed many different antihypertensive actions exist, including antioxidant, antiinflammatory, and mitochondrial. However, at this time, the mitochondrial mechanism clearly prevails: CoQ10 facilitates electron transfer in the electron transport chain, reducing free radical elaboration: notably reducing superoxide production and thereby reducing the binding of nitric oxide with superoxide which thereby leads to inhibited vasodilation, endothelial dysfunction, and the relative/absolute vasoconstriction that promotes vascular resistance and the resultant hypertension.

   In a personal communication by email in which the current author corresponded with world-renowned CoQ10 researcher Peter Langsjoen MD FACC (citations[255,256]) about CoQ10's mechanism of action in the treatment of hypertension, the following reply was received, as quoted in the textbox, with permission:

Personal communication from Peter H. Langsjoen, MD, FACC
January 25, 2011

Dear Alex,
   In regards to the antihypertensive effect of coenzyme Q10, I do have a couple of thoughts.
   The first theory is that coenzyme Q10 (CoQ10) has some influence on endothelial function, which may thereby have some benefit in hypertension. There is one thing that is quite clear, and that is that CoQ10 cannot have any direct vasodilator function because we never see a decrease in blood pressure in patients who already have low-normal blood pressures.
   My own theory on this subject is that the decrease in blood pressure from CoQ10 supplementation is a secondary phenomenon. We have observed that patients with established hypertension quite frequently have underlying diastolic dysfunction and it is clear that CoQ10 supplementation improves diastolic function because this is in large part an active process requiring a large amount of ATP to re-establish calcium gradients such that the actin and myosin fibrils can uncouple. When diastolic function improves, there is a secondary gradual decrease in hypertension. The theory is that the

---

[255] Langsjoen PH, Langsjoen AM. Supplemental ubiquinol in patients with advanced congestive heart failure. *Biofactors.* 2008;32(1-4):119-28
[256] Langsjoen P, Langsjoen P, Willis R, Folkers K. Treatment of essential hypertension with coenzyme Q10. *Mol Aspects Med.* 1994;15 Suppl:S265-72

CoQ10's safety and efficacy in the treatment of hypertension are very well established, and the mechanism(s) of action are manifold rather than singular. CoQ10 has been shown to improve glycemic control, reduce serum insulin levels, promote beneficial redistribution of adipose, provide anti-inflammatory and anti-allergy benefits, and to improve mitochondrial bioenergetics. Peer-reviewed articles on the use of CoQ10 for cardiovascular health are reviewed and summarized in the sections that follow.

- **Coenzyme Q-10 (CoQ10) with doses ranging from 100-300 mg per day**: Average dietary intake of CoQ10 is 2-5 mg/d. CoQ10 is made endogenously; however, some patients—particularly those with migraines, asthma, hypertension, allergies, heart failure and idiopathic dilated cardiomyopathy—may have an inborn or acquired error of metabolism that prevents them from making sufficient amounts of this vitally important substance. Hypertensive patients generally have lower serum CoQ10 levels than normotensive persons. **Typical blood levels of CoQ10 range from 0.7-1 mcg/ml; however clinical benefit in CVD may require serum levels of 2-3 and up to 4 mcg/ml to attain maximal clinical benefit.**[257] Testing of serum CoQ10 levels is not necessary before starting treatment; however, patients who do not benefit as expected should have their CoQ10 levels measured and supplementation increased to attain optimal serum levels before deciding that treatment is inefficacious. While clinical benefit may occur within the first week of supplementation, maximal improvement generally takes 4-8 weeks in order to obtain tissue saturation and beneficial changes in cell physiology. CoQ10 is clearly one of the most powerful and broadly-beneficial nutritional supplements on the nutrition-healthcare market; research literature shows clinically meaningful benefit of CoQ10 supplementation in patients with myocardial infarction, HTN, heart failure, renal failure, allergies, asthma, migraine, Parkinson's disease, and chronic viral infections such as HIV. CoQ10 has generally been produced and studied in its oxidized form as "ubiquinone" however more current research and clinical trends suggest that the reduced form "ubiquinol" is better absorbed (perhaps 3x); a small clinical trial (n=7) showed impressive improvements in serum CoQ10 and clinical status followed by ubiquinol treatment compared to ubiquinone treatment in CHF patients with malabsorption-inducing bowel wall edema.[258] Whether ubiquinol has clinical advantage over ubiquinone to such an extent that the higher cost is justified in other clinical scenarios—especially those which are not associated with malabsorption and/or the bowel wall edema seen in severe heart failure—remains to be determined. **In hypertensive patients, CoQ10 doses of 60-120 mg/d can typically lower BP by about -15/-9 mm Hg.** CoQ10 can be safely used with antihypertensive medications and is generally safer than all antihypertensive medications. CoQ10 may rarely interfere with coumadin/warfarin action in some patients; a cross-over study of 24 patients on chronic warfarin showed that neither CoQ10 nor *Ginkgo biloba* affected coagulation indices nor warfarin dosage.[259] More frequent monitoring of INR is routinely advised following any change in diet or medication. CoQ10 supplementation provides numerous collateral benefits; research literature shows clinically meaningful benefit of CoQ10 supplementation in patients with myocardial infarction, HTN, heart failure, renal

[257] Kumar A, Kaur H, Devi P, Mohan V. Role of coenzyme Q10 (CoQ10) in cardiac disease, hypertension and Meniere-like syndrome. *Pharmacol Ther.* 2009 Dec;124(3):259-68

[258] "Patients with CHF, NYHA class IV, often fail to achieve adequate plasma CoQ10 levels on supplemental ubiquinone at dosages up to 900 mg/day. These patients often have plasma total CoQ10 levels of less than 2.5 microg/ml and have limited clinical improvement. It is postulated that the intestinal edema in these critically ill patients may impair CoQ10 absorption. ... Ubiquinol has dramatically improved absorption in patients with severe heart failure and the improvement in plasma CoQ10 levels is correlated with both clinical improvement and improvement in measurement of left ventricular function." Langsjoen PH, Langsjoen AM. Supplemental ubiquinol in patients with advanced congestive heart failure. *Biofactors.* 2008;32(1-4):119-28

[259] "The study indicated that Coenzyme Q10 and Ginkgo biloba do not influence the clinical effect of warfarin." Engelsen J, Nielsen JD, Hansen KF. [Effect of Coenzyme Q10 and Ginkgo biloba on warfarin dosage in patients on long-term warfarin treatment. A randomized, double-blind, placebo-controlled cross-over trial]. [Article in Danish] *Ugeskr Laeger.* 2003 Apr 28;165(18):1868-71. See also Engelsen et al. The healthcare products coenzyme Q10 and ginko biloba do not interact with warfarin. Abstracdt P796. *Thrombosis and Haemostasis.* 2001: July Presented at Eighteenth Congress of the International Society on Thrombosis and Haemostasis, July 6-12, 2001 in Paris, France.

failure, allergies, asthma, migraine, fibromyalgia, gingivitis, male infertility/subfertility, Parkinson's disease, and chronic viral infections.

> **NYHA Stages of Heart Failure**
>
> 1. **Class 1**: Comfortable at all times. No limitation of physical activity. Ordinary activity does not cause undue fatigue, palpitation, dyspnea or anginal pain.
> 2. **Class 2**: Comfortable at rest. Slight limitation of physical activity. Ordinary activity causes fatigue, palpitation, dyspnea, or anginal pain.
> 3. **Class 3**: Comfortable at rest. Marked limitation of physical activity. Less than ordinary activity causes fatigue, palpitation, dyspnea or anginal pain.
> 4. **Class 4**: Symptomatic at rest. Cannot perform any physical activity without progressive discomfort.
>
> American Heart Association. 1994 Revisions to Classification of Functional Capacity and Objective Assessment of Patients with Diseases of the Heart. http://americanheart.org Accessed Nov 2010.

- Correlational study: CoQ10 is an independent predictor of mortality in chronic heart failure (*Journal of the American College of Cardiology* 2008 Oct[260]): Plasma samples from 236 patients admitted to the hospital with heart failure were assayed for LDL and total cholesterol, and total CoQ10. "CONCLUSIONS: Plasma CoQ10 concentration was an independent predictor of mortality in this cohort. The **CoQ10 deficiency might be detrimental to the long-term prognosis of CHF [chronic heart failure]**, and there is a rationale for controlled intervention studies with CoQ10."

- Review: Role of coenzyme Q10 (CoQ10) in cardiac disease, hypertension and Meniere-like syndrome (*Pharmacology and Therapeutics* 2009 Dec[261]): In this excellent review that covers the role of CoQ10 in the treatment of cardiovascular diseases—heart failure, HTN, myocardial infarction, arrhythmia—and Meniere syndrome and hearing loss, Kumar et al review the literature to conclude that CoQ10 provides major clinical benefit in all of these conditions and without adverse effects. Cardioprotective properties of CoQ10 include its role as an antioxidant, vasodilator, and membrane stabilizer in addition to its ability to decrease blood viscosity, proinflammatory cytokines, endothelial dysfunction, insulin resistance, and to promote proper diastolic and systolic function of the myocardium. Additional functions of CoQ10 specific to its benefit in HTN appear related to the ability of CoQ10 to antagonize aldosterone and/or angiotensin; if confirmed, these functions would support the concept that CoQ10 functions in part like an aldosterone antagonist (such as spironolactone) and/or an angiotensin 2 receptor blocker (such as losartan). **Typical blood pressure reduction with use of CoQ10 can be as high as -18/-11 mm Hg,** depending on dose, attained serum levels; other common nutritional deficiencies such as magnesium, potassium, and vitamin D can also be addressed to improve efficacy. Maximal improvement might take 4–8 weeks; however, some patients will respond more quickly—within the first week—and this observation underscores the importance of frequent BP monitoring and the need to adjust doses of antihypertensive drugs as needed to avoid hypotension and its complications such as syncope.

- Randomized, double-blind, placebo-controlled trial of coenzyme Q10 in isolated systolic hypertension (*Southern Medical Journal* 2001 Nov[262]): Twice daily administration of 60 mg of oral CoQ10 was given to 46 men and 37 women with isolated systolic hypertension in a 12-week randomized, double-blind, placebo-controlled trial. "**RESULTS: The mean reduction in systolic blood pressure of the CoQ-treated group was 17.8 mm Hg.** None of the patients exhibited orthostatic blood pressure changes. CONCLUSIONS: Our results suggest CoQ may be safely offered to hypertensive patients as an alternative treatment option."

- Open clinical trial: Coenzyme Q-10 in essential hypertension (*Molecular Aspects of Medicine* 1994[263]): In this open trial with no comparative placebo group, 26 patients with essential hypertension received oral CoQ10 50 mg twice daily for 10 weeks. Results of this study showed the following:
    - Systolic BP decreased from 164.5 to 146.7 mmHg (reduction of -17.8 mmHg).
    - Diastolic BP decreased from 98.1 to 86.1 mmHg (reduction of -12 mmHg).
    - Plasma CoQ10 values increased from 0.64 mcg/ml to 1.61 mcg/ml. Of particular note is that eight of 26 patients (30%) had baseline values of plasma CoQ10 that were subnormal before treatment and which normalized with supplementation.
    - Serum total cholesterol decreased from 222.9 mg/dl to 213.3 mg/dl.
    - Serum HDL cholesterol increased slightly from 41.1 mg/dl to 43.1 mg/dl.

---

[260] Molyneux et al. Coenzyme Q10: an independent predictor of mortality in chronic heart failure. *J Am Coll Cardiol*. 2008 Oct 28;52(18):1435-41

[261] Kumar A, Kaur H, Devi P, Mohan V. Role of coenzyme Q10 (CoQ10) in cardiac disease, hypertension and Meniere-like syndrome. *Pharmacol Ther*. 2009 Dec;124(3):259-68

[262] Burke et al. Randomized, double-blind, placebo-controlled trial of coenzyme Q10 in isolated systolic hypertension. *South Med J*. 2001 Nov;94(11):1112-7

[263] Digiesi et al. Coenzyme Q10 in essential hypertension. *Mol Aspects Med*. 1994;15 Suppl:s257-63

- Plasma renin activity, urinary aldosterone, serum and urinary sodium and potassium, plasma endothelin, electrocardiographic and echocardiographic findings and did not change.
  - In a subgroup of 5 patients tested, peripheral vascular resistances were 2,283 dyne·s·cm−5 before treatment and 1,627 dyne·s·cm−5 after treatment, thus indicating a clear reduction in peripheral resistance by CoQ10. The authors concluded that the antihypertensive effect of CoQ10 is probably mediated by reduction in peripheral resistance.

==These anti-hypertensive results, the collateral benefits, and the absence of adverse effects make CoQ10 superior to drug treatment for the treatment of chronic/persistent/sustained HTN.==

- Clinical trial with water-soluble CoQ10: Effect of hydrosoluble coenzyme Q10 on blood pressures and insulin resistance in hypertensive patients with coronary artery disease (*J Hum Hyperten* 1999 Mar[264]): In this randomized double-blind placebo-controlled trial among patients receiving antihypertensive medication and with coronary artery disease (n=59: 30 in treatment group, 29 in placebo group), patients received oral coenzyme Q10 (60 mg twice daily) for 8 weeks. **In the coenzyme Q10 group, beneficial reductions were noted in systolic and diastolic blood pressures (average 168/106 reduced to 152/97 [-16/-9] mm Hg),** heart rate, **waist–hip ratio**, fasting and 2-h plasma insulin and glucose levels, triglyceride levels and angina; CoQ10 supplementation raised HDL-cholesterol. The authors concluded, "These findings indicate that treatment with coenzyme Q10 decreases blood pressure possibly by decreasing oxidative stress and insulin response in patients with known hypertension receiving conventional antihypertensive drugs."

- Open trial using average dose of CoQ10 225 mg/d for the treatment of essential hypertension (*Molecular Aspects of Medicine* 1994[265]): This study was one of the first to use dosage adjustments to ==attain serum CoQ10 levels of at least 2 mcg/ml==. "A total of 109 patients with symptomatic essential hypertension presenting to a private cardiology practice were observed after the addition of CoQ10 (average dose, 225 mg/day by mouth) to their existing antihypertensive drug regimen. … A definite and gradual improvement in functional status was observed with the ==concomitant need to gradually decrease antihypertensive drug therapy within the first one to six months==. Thereafter, clinical status and cardiovascular drug requirements stabilized with a ==significantly improved systolic and diastolic blood pressure==. Overall New York Heart Association (NYHA) functional class improved from a mean of 2.40 to 1.36 (P < 0.001) and 51% of patients came completely off of between one and three antihypertensive drugs at an average of 4.4 months after starting CoQ10. … In the 9.4% of patients with echocardiograms both before and during treatment, we observed a highly significant improvement in left ventricular wall thickness and diastolic function."

- **Acetyl-L-carnitine and L-carnitine**: Acetyl-L-carnitine (ALC) first made its impression on clinicians when it was found to be effective treatment for Alzheimer's disease; later research found application for this nutrient in the treatment of hepatic coma, Peyronie's disease, male sexual dysfunction, various types of peripheral neuropathy, dysthymia, fibromyalgia, and various types of physical and mental fatigue. The primary mechanism of action is most likely the support/enhancement of mitochondrial function, while other mechanisms clearly exist and are additive/synergistic. Common therapeutic doses are 1,500-3,000 mg per day of either or both of ALC and/or L-carnitine, taken orally, between meals; clinicians should appreciate that amino acid therapy is generally administered between meals to avoid problems arising from competitive blockade among amino acids as they are absorbed/utilized. L-carnitine and ALC can be administered together; use of one does not necessarily preclude use of the other. For example in the study by Cavallini et al[266] among aging men, L-carnitine 2 g/day plus acetyl-L-carnitine 2 g/day proved significantly more effective than testosterone in improving nocturnal penile tumescence and International Index of Erectile Function score.
  - Review: Carnitine insufficiency caused by aging and overnutrition compromises mitochondrial performance and metabolic control (*Journal of Biological Chemistry* 2009 Jun[267]): The authors wrote, "…we hypothesized that **carnitine insufficiency might contribute to mitochondrial dysfunction and obesity-related impairments in glucose tolerance.** Consistent with this prediction, whole body carnitine diminution was identified as a common feature of insulin resistant states such as advanced age, genetic

[264] Singh et al. Hydrosoluble coenzyme Q10 on blood pressures and insulin resistance in hypertensive patients with coronary artery disease. *J Hum Hypertens.* 1999 Mar;13:203-8
[265] Langsjoen P, Langsjoen P, Willis R, Folkers K. Treatment of essential hypertension with coenzyme Q10. *Mol Aspects Med.* 1994;15 Suppl:S265-72
[266] Cavallini et al. Carnitine versus androgen administration in the treatment of sexual dysfunction, depressed mood, fatigue associated with male aging. *Urology.* 2004 Apr:641-6
[267] Noland et al. Carnitine Insufficiency Caused by Aging and Overnutrition Compromises Mitochondrial Performance and Metabolic Control. *J Biol Chem.* 2009 Jun 24

diabetes and diet-induced obesity." This impressive study documented that carnitine deficiency is noted in patients with obesity and insulin resistance; thus, carnitine supplementation—either as L-carnitine or acetyl-L-carnitine, or a combination of the two—appears warranted in such groups simply from the standpoint of correcting this nutrient deficiency/insufficiency.

- <u>Clinical trial: Ameliorating hypertension and insulin resistance in subjects at increased cardiovascular risk. Effects of acetyl-L-carnitine therapy</u> (*Hypertension* 2009 Sep[268]): In a previous trial, acetyl-L-carnitine infusion acutely ameliorated insulin resistance in type-2 diabetics. In this sequential off-on-off pilot study, the authors prospectively evaluated the effects of 24-week oral acetyl-L-carnitine (1 g twice daily) therapy on the glucose disposal rate (GDR), assessed by hyperinsulinemic euglycemic clamps, and components of the metabolic syndrome in nondiabetic subjects at increased cardiovascular risk. "Acetyl-L-carnitine increased GDR from 4.89+/-1.47 to 6.72+/-3.12 mg/kg per minute (P=0.003, Bonferroni-adjusted) and improved glucose tolerance in patients with GDR </=7.9 mg/kg per minute, whereas it had no effects in those with higher GDRs. ... Systolic blood pressure decreased from 144.0 to 135.1 mm Hg and from 130.8 to 123.8 mm Hg in the lower and higher GDR groups, respectively... Acetyl-L-carnitine safely ameliorated arterial hypertension, insulin resistance, impaired glucose tolerance, and hypoadiponectinemia in subjects at increased cardiovascular risk. Whether these effects may translate into long-term cardioprotection is worth investigating." Total adiponectin increased from 4.7 to 6.0 meq/L, while HMW adiponectin increased from 2.2 to 3.0 meq/L (p<0.05 for both changes). The finding of relative carnitine deficiency in patients with HTN and DM along with the finding that acetyl-L-carnitine supplementation raises adiponectin in these patient groups suggests that the hypoadiponectinemia in HTN and DM may be a direct result from hypocarnitinemia.

- <u>Randomized placebo-controlled double-blind crossover study: Effect of combined treatment with alpha-lipoic acid (400 mg/d) and acetyl-L-carnitine (1,000 mg/d) on vascular function and blood pressure in patients with documented coronary artery disease</u> (*Journal of Clinical Hypertension* 2007 Apr[269]): The authors note that mitochondria produce reactive oxygen species that may contribute to vascular dysfunction, and that both oxidative stress and mitochondrial dysfunction can be ameliorated by alpha-lipoic acid and acetyl-L-carnitine. Among 36 subjects with coronary artery disease, active treatment for 8 weeks increased brachial artery diameter by 2.3%, consistent with reduced arterial tone. "Active treatment **decreased systolic blood pressure** for the whole group and had a significant effect in the subgroup with blood pressure above the median (151 to 142 mm Hg) and in the subgroup with the metabolic syndrome (139 to 130 mm Hg)." Although this study used low-modest doses of acetyl-carnitine and lipoic acid, it showed that antihypertensive benefits were greatest in patients with systolic blood pressure >135 mm Hg—blood pressure was reduced by approximately -9/-5 mm Hg—and in patients with metabolic syndrome—blood pressure was reduced by approximately -7/-3 mm Hg. More significant results probably would have been obtained with higher doses, but these results are still statistically and clinically significant.

Acetyl-L-carnitine increases adiponectin: clinical significance and mechanism of action against hypertension

Discovered in 1996, adiponectin is a beneficial protein hormone secreted from adipose tissue, and as such it is an adipokine (adipocyte-derived hormone). Adiponectin is secreted in two forms: a low molecular weight form and a more metabolically active high molecular weight (HMW) multimer. Adiponectin is unique among adipokines in that its effects are largely beneficial; it has anti-diabetic, anti-atherogenic, and anti-inflammatory properties. Another unique feature of adiponectin is that—even though it is made in adipose tissue—its production is inversely proportional to the total load of visceral fat. Per Matsuzawa: "Hypoadiponectinemia induced by visceral fat accumulation is closely associated with type 2 diabetes, lipid disorders, **hypertension** and also certain inflammatory diseases."

Metabolic effects of adiponectin include:
- Decreases gluconeogenesis and reduces serum glucose,
- Increases peripheral glucose uptake, indicating improved insulin sensitivity,
- Enhances β-oxidation of fatty acids, promotes triglyceride clearance,
- Protects from endothelial dysfunction and atherosclerosis,
- Promotes weight loss.

Matsuzawa Y. Adiponectin. *Curr Pharm Des.* 2010 Jun

---

[268] Ruggenenti et al. Ameliorating Hypertension and Insulin Resistance in Increased Cardiovascular Risk. Effects of Acetyl-L-Carnitine Therapy. *Hypertension.* 2009 Sep:567-74
[269] McMackin et al. Combined treatment alpha-Lipoic acid and acetyl-L-carnitine on vascular function and blood pressure in coronary disease. *J Clin Hypertens* 2007 Apr:249-55

and other considerations are listed here, notably including surgery (for reduction of neurovascular compression) and spinal manipulation.

- **Exercise**: Current guidelines indicate that everyone should obtain 30-60 minutes of exercise 4-7 times per week unless specific contraindications exist. Patients with or at risk for CAD should receive baseline and stress/exercise ECG before commencing vigorous exercise; if ECG abnormalities are detected or if angina is reported, then stress echocardiography and/or perfusion scan should be considered.

- **Weight optimization**: All patients *and doctors* should maintain a healthy body weight. Canadian guidelines published in 2009 specify a body mass index 18.5-24.9 and waist circumference (<102 cm [40.2 inches] for men and <88 cm [34.6 inches] for women).[270] In most patients and clinical situations, body weight and body mass can be used as an indicator of compliance with a health-promoting diet and plan of regular *sufficiently intense* exercise. Exercise sufficiency can be assessed by the ability of the activity to produce mild breathlessness, diaphoresis, and changes in or favorable maintenance of body composition and optimal weight.

> **Weight loss for overweight patients provides numerous psychosocial and physical benefits**
>
> "With a substantial weight loss of 35 kg and 42% loss of excessive weight, and correction of disturbed metabolic parameters, they significantly improved in general well-being, health distress, and perceived attractiveness, approaching halfway the values of a normal-weight reference group. ... In physical activity, they bypassed the reference group. Days of sick leave decreased to the level of the reference group. **Improvements in HRQL [health-related quality-of-life] paralleled the rate of weight loss.**"
>
> Mathus-Vliegen et al. Health-related quality-of-life in patients with morbid obesity after gastric banding for surgically induced weight loss. *Surgery*. 2004 May

- **Mind-Body Approaches including Qigong, controlled breathing, transcendental meditation, and acupuncture**: Traditional therapeutics and lifestyle activities such as Qigong, controlled breathing, meditation, and acupuncture can effect statistically and clinically significant reductions in BP among hypertensive patients. Mechanisms of action include induction of beneficial neurohormonal responses (e.g., increased dehydroepiandrosterone and melatonin levels following meditation) as well as induction of a relaxed state. Avoidance of physiological stressors can play a role in blood pressure control and should be implemented on an as-appropriate basis. Sympathetic neural activity via beta-adrenergic receptors in the kidney stimulates release of renin, which is a peptidase enzyme that converts angiotensinogen to angiotensin-1 and thereby expedites the formation of angiotensin-2 in the lungs; angiotensin-2 is a vasoconstrictor and stimulates aldosterone production which increases sodium resorption and thus water retention.[271]; Thus, the net effect of sympathetic nervous activation is increased volume within a constricted vasculature, thus causing HTN. Data on therapeutic interventions in the following four subsections are derived from the review by Nahas[272] (*Canadian Family Physician* 2008 Nov) unless otherwise noted.

  - Qigong: A Chinese medicine form of movement, breathing, and meditation: As a part of traditional Chinese medicine (TCM), Qigong incorporates movement, breathing, and meditation. Two systematic reviews involving hundreds of patients (n = > 900 to > 1,200 subjects) have examined the role of Qigong in the treatment of hypertension. Despite some methodological shortcomings, evidence shows that Qigong can reduce BP among hypertensives by -12 to -17 mm Hg systolic and -8.5 to -10 mm Hg diastolic. Thus, the BP-lowering results obtained by Qigong are comparable to drug treatment of HTN.

  - Controlled breathing: Most studies (4 of 5) using slow controlled breathing have shown an antihypertensive benefit presumably mediated through increased parasympathetic and reduced sympathetic activity; as expected, diabetics with autonomic dysfunction tend to receive less benefit.

  - Transcendental meditation: Twice-daily sessions of sitting quietly while repeating a specific mantra can effect a BP-lowering effect of approximately -4.7/-3.2 mm Hg.

  - Acupuncture: Acupuncture is difficult to study in a placebo-controlled manner due to the physical, individualized, and experiential nature of the treatment. Antihypertensive benefits of acupuncture have ranged from no different from the so-called placebo to reductions of -6 to -14 mm Hg for systolic BP and -3 to -7 mm Hg for diastolic BP.

---

[270] Khan et al. 2009 Canadian Hypertension Education Program recommendations for the management of hypertension: Part 2—therapy. *Can J Cardiol*. 2009 May;25(5):287-98

[271] Benowitz NL. "Antihypertensive Agents." In Katzung BG (editor). *Basic and Clinical Pharmacology. 10th Edition*. New York: McGraw Hill Medical; 2007, 161

[272] Nahas R. Complementary and alternative medicine approaches to blood pressure reduction: An evidence-based review. *Can Fam Physician*. 2008 Nov;54(11):1529-33

- **<u>Treatment of "central neurogenic hypertension" with surgical techniques—focus on neurovascular (de)compression at the level of the left ventrolateral medulla oblongata</u>**: Physical compression or mechanical irritation of neuronal structures can result in systemic hypertension through a variety of mechanisms; these mechanisms have been most thoroughly described in the biomedical research literature under the disciplines of Surgery as well as of Manipulative Medicine and Spinal Manipulation. Readers should appreciate the basic commonality between surgical intervention and physical manipulation: both interventions have the potential to change physiological relationships experienced between two or more anatomical components via either direct means (i.e., physical alteration) or indirect mechanisms (e.g., reflexive or adaptive changes). Several studies describing surgical alleviation of neurogenic hypertension will be reviewed and summarized here, while those focusing on manipulative treatments will be discussed in the subsection immediately following. Dr Peter Jannetta (MD) is generally attributed with the origination of the concept of medulla oblongata vascular compression by the vertebral artery as one of the causes of hypertension; he has demonstrated that neurovascular compression can be surgically treated by microvascular decompression (MVD) with resultant antihypertensive benefits.[273] Initially, patients selected for surgery (generally either left retromastoid craniectomy or lateral suboccipital craniectomy) were chosen for their cranial nerve deficits such as trigeminal neuralgia, hemifacial spasm, glossopharyngeal neuralgia, Bell's palsy, and spasmodic torticollis, and alleviation of HTN was a "side benefit" of the surgery. Later, severe recalcitrant HTN alone without overt CN deficits has become sufficient basis for surgery in carefully selected patients in appropriate treatment centers, perhaps within a prospective research protocol (per Geiger *et al* in 1998, reviewed below). Also, as stated in a previous section, the perspectives offered by Reis[274] is worthy of recall because of the two truths contained therein, namely that neurogenic contributors to HTN can be ❶ *omnipotent* (Reis: "A neural or neurochemical imbalance in brain **can produce** hypertension"), or ❷ *contributory/amplificatory* (Reis: "Impaired NTS [nucleus tract solitarius] function can produce an **amplification** of the action of the environmental stresses on blood pressure. Thus environmental stimuli or the expression of behaviors which normally result in trivial elevations of blood pressure will, after the NTS is perturbed, result in marked elevations [of blood pressure]).'" Per descriptions in the literature, central neurogenic hypertension is typically difficult to control, chronic, and progressive.
  - <u>Review and case series: Neurogenic hypertension etiology and surgical treatment: observations in 53 patients (*Annals of Surgery* 1985 Mar[275])</u>: Among 53 patients with simultaneous cranial nerve (CN) dysfunctions and systemic hypertension, 51 of these 53 patients were noted to have arterial compression of the **left lateral medulla oblongata** by looping arteries at the base of the brain (note: neurovascular compression was *not* noted in *normotensive* patients); all 53 patients underwent left retromastoid craniectomy and microvascular decompression (MVD) for treatment of the cranial nerve dysfunctions. More specifically, treatment by vascular decompression of the medulla was performed in 42 of the 53 patients. Relief in the hypertension was seen in 32 of 42 (76% of total) patients and improvement in four; "improvement" was defined in this article as "more than a 20-mm drop in both systolic and diastolic pressures", and thus the total number of patients with a highly meaningful antihypertensive response was 36 of 42 (85% of total). Generally, the problem appears localized to the left vagal nerve and the left lateral medulla oblongata (more specifically between the inferior olive anteriorly and the root entry zone (REZ) or CN 9 and CN 10 posteriorly) and is most commonly caused by arteriosclerosis and arterial ectasia which contribute to arterial elongation and looping, which can eventually lead to pulsatile compression of the left lateral medulla; hypertension can then develop from compromise of the balance in the neural control systems that regulate blood pressure. Because systemic HTN can further contribute to arterial elongation, a vicious cycle of HTN followed by progressive arterial ectasia followed by additional neuronal compromise which results in additional HTN may be established. Specific arteries that can contribute to medulla and/or cranial nerve neurocompression include the left vertebral artery (due to normal anatomy, ectasia, or severe atherosclerosis), posterior inferior cerebellar artery, superior cerebellar artery, basilar

273 See "Discussion": ncbi.nlm.nih.gov/pmc/articles/PMC1346999/pdf/annsurg00224-0102.pdf
274 Reis DJ. Nucleus tractus solitarius and experimental neurogenic hypertension: central neural imbalance hypothesis of hypertensive disease. *Adv Biochem Psychopharmacol.* 1981;28:409-20
275 Jannetta PJ, Segal R, Wolfson SK Jr. Neurogenic hypertension: etiology and surgical treatment. I. Observations in 53 patients. *Ann Surg.* 1985 Mar;201(3):391-8

artery, and anterior inferior cerebellar artery. Neural pathways involved in BP control relevant to this discussion as reviewed by Jannetta *et al* include ❶ carotid baroreceptors with afferents traveling in CN 9 to the nucleus tractus solitarius, ❷ aortic baroreceptors with afferents traveling in CN 10 (i.e., aortic vagal afferents), ❸ cardiac vagal afferents, ❹ descending sympathetic output to vascular smooth muscle; of these, *vasodepressive* cardiac vagal afferent fibers are unmyelinated and are thus most susceptible to compression (per Jannetta *et al*, 1985) thus neurovascular compressive compromise at the REZ of the medulla likely causes HTN (at least in large part) by disinhibition, i.e., impairment of vasodepressive cardiac vagal afferent input. Furthermore, the pulsatile nature of arterial compression may cause greater damage than constant pressure and may desynchronize neural cardiac-pressor control centers. Following surgical displacement of the offending artery away from the brainstem by use of an implant of plastic sponge, muscle, or synthetic felt, many of these patients with chronic systemic HTN who had been taking "large doses of strong medications" were able to reduce or altogether discontinue their drug dependency over the course of days to months following the surgical microvascular decompression. Thus, neurovascular decompression of the left medulla oblongata is a treatment option worth considering in affected and appropriately selected patients with chronic hypertension.

- Exemplary case report: Decreases in blood pressure and sympathetic nerve activity by microvascular decompression of the rostral ventrolateral medulla in essential hypertension (*Stroke* 1999 Aug[276]): The authors of this report begin by noting that neurovascular compression of the rostral ventrolateral medulla, a major center regulating sympathetic nerve activity, may be causally related to essential hypertension, and that microvascular decompression of the rostral ventrolateral medulla decreases elevated blood pressure in some patients. A 47-year-old male with "essential hypertension" and hemifacial nerve spasms was found to have neurovascular compression of the rostral ventrolateral medulla and facial nerve; **microvascular decompression of the rostral ventrolateral medulla successfully reduced blood pressure from 152/110 mm/Hg** while on amlodipine, quinapril, and doxazosin **to 108/74** with only low-dose quinapril (the authors note that quinapril was being tapered to discontinuation at time of publication). Microvascular decompression of the rostral ventrolateral medulla also reduced plasma and urine norepinephrine levels, and reduced other markers of excessive sympathetic nerve activity. Reductions in plasma and urine epinephrine and norepinephrine following MVD in their case report were listed previously in this chapter and are included here again in context to show that post-intervention reduction in sympathetic nerve activity can be documented objectively, and that clinical antihypertensive benefits (BP reductions of 10–30% at 48h postsurgery) can be associated with *relative* reductions in catecholamine levels that may be *within* or *outside of* the normal reference range:
  - Plasma epinephrine: Reduced from 0.22 to <0.05 (reference range <0.93 nmol/L).
  - Plasma norepinephrine: Reduced from 0.95 to 0.30 (range 0.89 - 3.37 nmol/L).
  - Urine epinephrine: Reduced from 83.5 to 26.2 (range 5.5 – 76.4 nmol/d).
  - Urine norepinephrine: Reduced from 0.52 to 0.39 (range 0.06 – 0.024 mmol/d).
- Prospective study (n=14) with long-term follow-up: Temporary reduction of blood pressure and sympathetic nerve activity in hypertensive patients after microvascular decompression (*Stroke* 2009 Jan[277]): Fourteen patients with essential hypertension underwent microvascular decompression of the brain stem. Vasoconstrictor muscle sympathetic nerve activity (recorded by microneurography: burst frequency, bursts/min) and blood pressure (24-hour profiles) were measured before surgery and 7 days, 3 months, and every 6 months postoperatively. **Muscle sympathetic nerve activity** decreased from preoperative levels (35 bursts/min) a nadir of 19 bursts/min before spontaneously rising again to 34 bursts/min; in more detail, the sympatholytic benefits were noted as follows: a reduction from preoperative levels of 35 bursts/min to 19 bursts/min (at 3 months postoperatively), 19 bursts/min (at 6 months), and 23 bursts/min (at 12 months) but were minimized to statistical and clinical insignificance to 28 bursts/min (at 18 months) and 34 bursts/min (at 24 months). **Systolic and diastolic blood pressure** decreased from 162/98 mm Hg preoperatively to 133/85 mm Hg (at 7 days postoperatively), 136/86 mm Hg (at 3 months), 132/85 mm Hg

[276] Morimoto S, Sasaki S, Takeda K, Furuya S, Naruse S, Matsumoto K, Higuchi T, Saito M, Nakagawa M. Decreases in blood pressure and sympathetic nerve activity by microvascular decompression of the rostral ventrolateral medulla in essential hypertension. *Stroke*. 1999 Aug;30(8):1707-10

[277] Frank H, Heusser K, Geiger H, Fahlbusch R, Naraghi R, Schobel HP. Temporary reduction of blood pressure and sympathetic nerve activity in hypertensive patients after microvascular decompression. *Stroke*. 2009 Jan;40(1):47-51 stroke.ahajournals.org/cgi/content/full/40/1/47

(at 6 months), 132/85 mm Hg (at 12 months), and then increased to 158/96 mm Hg at 24 months; thus both blood pressure and hypersympathotonia were reduced by MVD surgery but both returned many months thereafter. The fact that hypersympathotonia returned before HTN would appear to indicate that the former caused the latter despite the fact that the latter can cause the former as discussed in a preceding section. (For review: hypersympathotonia causes HTN via vasoconstriction and activation of the renin-angiotensin system, while HTN causes activation of the sympathetic nervous system when chronic HTN induces elongation and tortuosity of the arteries [left vertebral artery, posterior inferior cerebellar artery, superior cerebellar artery, basilar artery, and anterior inferior cerebellar artery] that are in close proximity to the nucleus tract solitarius and related pressure-controlling neurologic structures.) The authors of the study conclude that, "The data are a hint for sympathetic overactivity as a pathomechanism in this subgroup of patients" while also noting that in the patients selected for this study, the life-threatening severity of their hypertension was probably of such an extent that end-organ damage and various neurohormonal vicious cycles had probably already been established so as to make long-term suppression of HTN particularly challenging. The authors of this paper, published in 2009 in the American Heart Association's journal *Stroke*, close with the following four main conclusions:

- Neurovascular compression of the RVLM causes neurogenic hypertension mediated by a central sympathetic hyperactivity.
- Surgical microvascular decompression reduces central sympathetic outflow and reduces blood pressure, at least temporarily.
- In this study, neither blood pressure improvement nor sympathetic deactivation was sustained effectively for the long-term.
- Until more conclusions are established regarding appropriate imaging and patient selection, MVD is not recommended as cure for HTN and should be performed only in prospective study protocols.

○ Case series (n=8) using microvascular decompression as therapy for severe chronic HTN: Decrease of blood pressure by ventrolateral medullary decompression in essential hypertension (*The Lancet* 1998 Aug[278]): Previously, this group of authors showed that 83% of patients with primary HTN, 24% of patients with secondary HTN, and 7% of normotensive controls showed evidence of looping vessels at the left ventrolateral medulla consistent with neurovascular compression as seen on magnetic resonance imaging. In this study, the authors investigated whether neurosurgical microvascular decompression substantially decreases blood pressure long-term in patients with severe essential hypertension. Eight patients—all of whom had experienced one or more life-threatening hypertensive crises—who had received *three or more* antihypertensive drugs without adequate control of blood pressure, intolerable side-effects, or both, underwent microvascular decompression at the root-entry zone (REZ) of cranial nerves 9 and 10 after neurovascular compression of the ventrolateral medulla oblongata was seen with magnetic resonance angiography (MRA). Three months after surgery, blood pressure and antihypertensive drug regimens had decreased substantially in 7 of 8 patients. Four patients who were followed up for more than 1 year became normotensive. No complications associated with decompression occurred except that one patient experienced a transient vocal-cord paresis after the laryngeal part of the vagus nerve was maneuvered during surgery. The authors concluded, "We showed a direct causal relation between raised blood pressure and irritation of cranial nerves 9 and 10. A subgroup of patients with essential hypertension may exist who have secondary forms of hypertension related to neurovascular compression at the ventrolateral medulla and who may be successfully treated with decompression."

- **Treatment of "central and peripheral neurogenic hypertension" with chiropractic and osteopathic manipulative techniques**: Spinal manipulative therapy has proven safe and effective for musculoskeletal spinal pain as well as some extra-spinal disorders, notably asthma.[279] Chiropractic manipulation differs from the types of manipulation provided by other professions (e.g., osteopathic, naturopathic) and thus research substantiating the effectiveness of chiropractic manipulation may not be applicable to different manipulative approaches. Based on the material reviewed in the previous section, readers should already have some

---

[278] Geiger et al. Decrease of blood pressure by ventrolateral medullary decompression in essential hypertension. *Lancet*. 1998 Aug 8;352(9126):446-9
[279] Mein et al. Manual medicine diversity: research pitfalls and the emerging medical paradigm. *J Am Osteopath Assoc*. 2001 Aug;101(8):441-4

appreciation of the rationale, potential benefits, and potential limitations of upper cervical spinal manipulation for the treatment of HTN via reduction of **central neurogenic hypertension** (i.e., potentially via reduction in medullary compression and NTS irritation) as well as via reduction of **peripheral neurogenic hypertension** insofar as upper cervical and cranial/occipital manipulation has been suggested—mainly by theory, extrapolation of anatomy, and less so by strong clinical trials—to potentially decompress, de-facilitate, or otherwise generally relieve from mechanical (and thus physiologic) irritation CN 9, CN 10, and the cervical sympathetic ganglia, all of which are involved in regulation of blood pressure, heart rate, and/or peripheral resistance.

- <u>Double-blind, placebo-controlled pilot study of chiropractic upper cervical manipulation for treatment of hypertension: Atlas vertebra realignment and achievement of arterial pressure goal in 50 *pain-free* hypertensive patients (*Journal of Human Hypertension* 2007 May[280]):</u> The authors introduce this study by writing, "Anatomical abnormalities of the cervical spine at the level of the Atlas vertebra are associated with relative ischemia of the brainstem circulation and increased blood pressure (BP). Manual correction of this mal-alignment has been associated with reduced arterial pressure." The authors used a double-blind, placebo-controlled design at a single center among 50 *pain-free* drug-naïve (n=26) or washed-out (n=24) patients with Stage 1 hypertension; patients were randomized (n=25 in each treatment or placebo group) to receive a National Upper Cervical Chiropractic (NUCCA) procedure or a sham

> ### Cervical spine manipulation for chronic hypertension
>
> "At week 8, there were differences in **systolic BP (-17 mm Hg, NUCCA [chiropractic]** versus -3 mm Hg, placebo) and **diastolic BP (-10 mm Hg, NUCCA [chiropractic]** versus -2 mm Hg). … No adverse effects were recorded. We conclude that restoration of Atlas alignment is associated with marked and sustained reductions in BP similar to the use of two-drug combination therapy.
>
> … most single agent antihypertensive [drugs] yield an 8 mm Hg drop in pressure in people with Stage 1 hypertension…"
>
> Bakris et al. Atlas vertebra realignment and achievement of arterial pressure goal in hypertensive patients: a pilot study. *J Hum Hypertens.* 2007 May.

procedure. Significant findings included the following, "At week 8, there were differences in **systolic BP (-17 mm Hg, NUCCA** versus -3 mm Hg, placebo) and **diastolic BP (-10 mm Hg, NUCCA** versus -2 mm Hg [placebo]). … No adverse effects were recorded. We conclude that restoration of Atlas alignment is associated with marked and sustained reductions in BP similar to the use of two-drug combination therapy." Because the patients were pain-free at the start of the study, relief of neck pain due to treatment with chiropractic manipulation does not explain antihypertensive benefit. Pretreatment patient assessment for NUCCA-specific chiropractic treatment (rather than all forms of chiropractic treatment, of which exist many different techniques) includes ❶ assessment for dynamic functional leg-length discrepancy in the supine position while the patient actively rotates the neck left and right in the transverse/horizontal plane, ❷ paracervical skin temperature measurement, ❸ postural analysis with a proprietary device named Anatometer[281] for precise static biomechanical measurements, and ❹ craniocervical radiographs which are then assessed with NUCCA-specific roentgenometric techniques. As with any procedure involving exposure to ionizing radiation, long-term risk-to-benefit ratios need to be determined and compared to the risk-to-benefit ratios of other treatments; if radiographic evaluation could be eliminated from the assessment protocol without compromising treatment safety efficacy then both costs and risks would be reduced. Impressively, **85% of patients in the chiropractic-treated group required only one treatment to maintain the antihypertensive benefit during the study's duration of two months.** NUCCA treatment of the atlas vertebra resulted in significant measurable changes in atlas lateral and rotational positioning (measured by the pre- and post-treatment radiographs), lateral displacement of C-7 vertebra, frontal-plane pelvic distortion, and lateral-plane pelvic distortion which correlated with the reductions in blood pressure. Lastly for this discussion, readers should appreciate that the NUCCA chiropractic technique uses a gentle direct technique of spinal manipulation which is not the typical, more forceful, high-velocity low-amplitude (HVLA) type which is more commonly used by the majority of chiropractic and (to a lesser extent) osteopathic clinicians; in the current article, NUCCA treatment was described as "A series of precise, subtle, external nudges causes Atlas to recoil into normalized alignment, reseating occipital

---

[280] Bakris et al. Atlas vertebra realignment and achievement of arterial pressure goal in hypertensive patients: a pilot study. *J Hum Hypertens.* 2007 May;21(5):347-52
[281] Anatometer is manufactured by Benesh Corporation: anatometer.com

condyles into Atlas' lateral masses", and the technique's delivery can be observed in the video hyperlinks provided and specifically at nucca.org. Readers of this section may have—hopefully—seen beyond the "data" of this study to appreciate the paradigm shifts implied, which are built upon and/or include but are not limited to the following: ❶ a single gentle musculoskeletal manipulation delivered to the atlas vertebra can lower blood pressure just as effectively as the use of two-drug antihypertensive treatment; ❷ a single gentle musculoskeletal manipulation delivered to the atlas vertebra can affect the positioning of the C-7 vertebra as well as pelvic positioning in the frontal and lateral planes; ❸ subtle changes (invisible to the naked eye) in the positioning of the atlas vertebra, the C-7 vertebra, and pelvis correspond to clinically and statistically significant changes in arterial pressure that can be sustained for at least two months; ❹ individually and collectively, these findings present us with paradigm shifts regarding the local effects of spinal manipulation, body-wide musculoskeletal effects of spinal manipulation, and the systemic nonmusculoskeletal effects of spinal manipulation.

- Case report: Chiropractic management of a hypertensive patient (*Journal of Manipulative and Physiological Therapeutics* 1993 Oct[282]): In this single illustrative case report, the clinician authors describe their experience with a 38-year-old male previously diagnosed with and medicated for chronic essential HTN; the patient's presenting complaints were HTN, drug-related side effects, and low back pain. Chiropractic treatment emphasized specific contact, short lever arm spinal adjustments as the primary mode of chiropractic care. The authors noted, "**During the course of chiropractic treatment, the patient's need for hypertensive medication was reduced.** The patient's medical physician gradually withdrew the medication over 2 months." Appreciating the BP-normalizing benefits of chiropractic manipulation and how these benefits may—paradoxically—lead to iatrogenic complications in patients whose physiologic homeostasis is restored, the authors caution that "specific contact short lever arm spinal adjustments may cause a hypotensive effect in a medicated hypertensive patient that may lead to complications (e.g., hypotension). Since a medicated hypertensive patient's blood pressure may fall below normal while he or she is undergoing chiropractic care, it is advised that the blood pressure be closely monitored and medications adjusted, if necessary, by the patient's medical physician." This point about the very real potential of drug-induced iatrogenic hypotension is analogous to the drug-induced iatrogenic hypoglycemia that can occur when patients' utilization of non-drug integrative treatments overlaps with their previously prescribed drug treatments. When working with medicated and particularly *polymedicated* HTN patients, clinicians have the responsibility to implement treatment in such a way as to minimize the risk for hypotension (and other complications, such as hypoglycemia, respectively)—for example, by starting with lower doses of nutritional supplements, implementing treatment in a step-wise manner, coordinating modifications/reductions in drug doses, and having the patient use more frequent self-monitoring (of blood pressure, blood glucose [etc], respectively); patient education and documentation of informed consent are standards of care for all interventions.

- Randomized, controlled trial (active treatment, placebo treatment, or no treatment): Effects of chiropractic treatment on blood pressure and anxiety (*Journal of Manipulative and Physiological Therapeutics* 1988 Dec[283]): This study (n=21) differs from the previously cited article "Atlas vertebra realignment and achievement of arterial pressure goal in hypertensive patients" in that ❶ the thoracic spine (T1-T5) rather than the upper cervical spine was the area of treatment, ❷ the treatment used a mechanical chiropractic adjusting device rather than manual manipulation, and ❸ the study included assessment for anxiety as well as for changes in BP, rather than BP alone. The mechanical chiropractic adjusting device used in this study is the Activator Adjusting Instrument[284], which delivers a highly-localized 28-pound thrust within 1/300 of a second. The authors concluded, "Results indicated that systolic and diastolic blood pressure decreased significantly in the active treatment condition, whereas no significant changes occurred in the placebo and control conditions. State anxiety significantly decreased in the active and control conditions. Results provide support for the hypothesis that blood pressure is reduced following chiropractic treatment."[285]

---

[282] Plaugher G, Bachman TR. Chiropractic management of a hypertensive patient. *J Manipulative Physiol Ther*. 1993 Oct;16(8):544-9

[283] Bakris et al. Atlas vertebra realignment and achievement of arterial pressure goal in hypertensive patients: a pilot study. *J Hum Hypertens*. 2007 May;21(5):347-52

[284] Activator Methods International, Ltd. (AMI) produces the Activator Adjusting Instrument. See also activatoronline.com

[285] Yates et al. Effects of chiropractic treatment on blood pressure and anxiety: a randomized, controlled trial. *J Manipulative Physiol Ther*. 1988 Dec;11(6):484-8

Cervical Spine: Rotation Emphasis

Patient:	• Supine, neck slightly flexed
Doctor position:	• At 45° angle from head of table; may also be in a more lateral position aside the patient's head and neck; while it is acceptable to assess and set-up with straight legs, at the time of impulse, doctor's legs should be bent to provide the doctor with greater power, stability, and biomechanical safety
Assessment:	• <u>Subjective</u>: neck pain, headaches
	• <u>Motion palpation</u>: rotation restriction; primary or compensatory hypermobile segments may be detected above or below the restricted segment
	• <u>Static palpation</u>: vertebra may feel relatively posterior on the side opposite the rotational restriction, e.g., a right rotational restriction may present with a relative left rotational malposition that brings the vertebral lamina and articular pillars posterior on the left
	• <u>Soft tissue</u>: tenderness, may also have muscle spasm
Treatment contact:	• Doctor uses either an index or proximal phalange contact on the posterior aspect of the transverse process and/or articular pillar
	• The doctor's vector and hence the positioning of the forearm of the contact hand must change depending on the level of the cervical spine that is being treated
	• Notice in this photograph that the thumb of the doctor's contact hand is placed on the angle of the mandible, this is more to help anchor the contact and stabilize the doctor's wrist than to assist with the manipulation; very little pressure and zero thrust are applied to the mandible
Supporting contact:	• Head is held into rotation and slight flexion; as with all techniques, nuanced adjustments in flexion-extension, rotation, and side-bending are made until the premanipulative tension is localized to the specific direction/tissue of restriction
Pretreatment positioning:	• Slight flexion and extension may be used below and above the treatment contact to create motion restriction at the adjacent motion segments; this helps to focus the motion and therapeutic force at the specific; importantly the support hand is largely responsible for proper positioning with the correct amount of nuanced flexion-extension and side-bending so that the rotational force is accurately delivered
Thrust:	• Rotational thrust with contact hand; support hand keeps head off table allowing rotation
Image:	

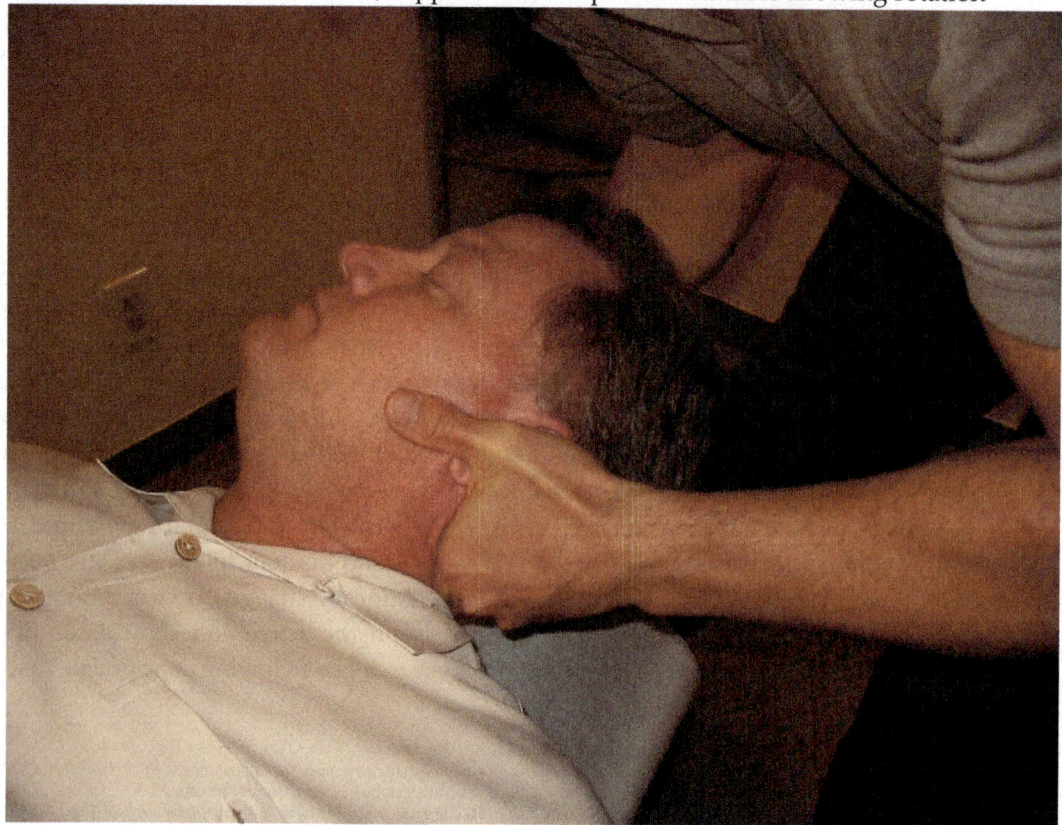

	Cervical Spine: Lateral Flexion (Side-Bending) Emphasis; Treatment of Lateral Malposition
Patient position:	• Supine, head is neutrally placed—neither flexed nor extended; slight flexion is allowed; this technique can also be adapted for use in a seated position
Doctor position:	• At 45° angle from head of table; may also be in a more lateral position aside the patient's head and neck
Assessment:	• <u>Subjective</u>: neck pain, headaches • <u>Motion palpation</u>: lateral flexion restriction • <u>Static palpation</u>: vertebra may *feel* laterally displaced • <u>Soft tissue</u>: tenderness, may also have muscle spasm
Treatment contact:	• Using an index (metacarpal-phalangeal) contact at the tip of the transverse process or slightly posterior to the transverse process; an index phalangeal contact can also be used on the articular pillars as long as doctor is careful not to thrust in a rotational direction; notice in this picture how Dr Harris has the forearm of his contact hand perfectly aligned in the treatment vector, which is almost purely in the patient's transverse/horizontal plane; notice also that Dr Harris has his knees bent and is forward flexed to bring his torso closer to his contact and thereby minimize stress and strain on his own shoulders; with slight modifications in vector direction, this technique can be applied throughout the cervical spine from C0-C7
Supporting contact:	• Lateral aspect of head, opposite contact; generally the supporting hand is neutral, however it can supply some traction and can help induce lateral flexion at impulse; with more aggressive adjustments, the supporting hand can supply a counterforce to minimize motion following the application of a faster and more powerful thrust
Pretreatment positioning:	• Lateral flexion at the targeted segment; the slightest amount of contralateral rotation is applied
Therapeutic action:	• Establish minimal premanipulative tension once the end range of motion has been reached, then use quick and very shallow trust to induce lateral flexion
Image:	

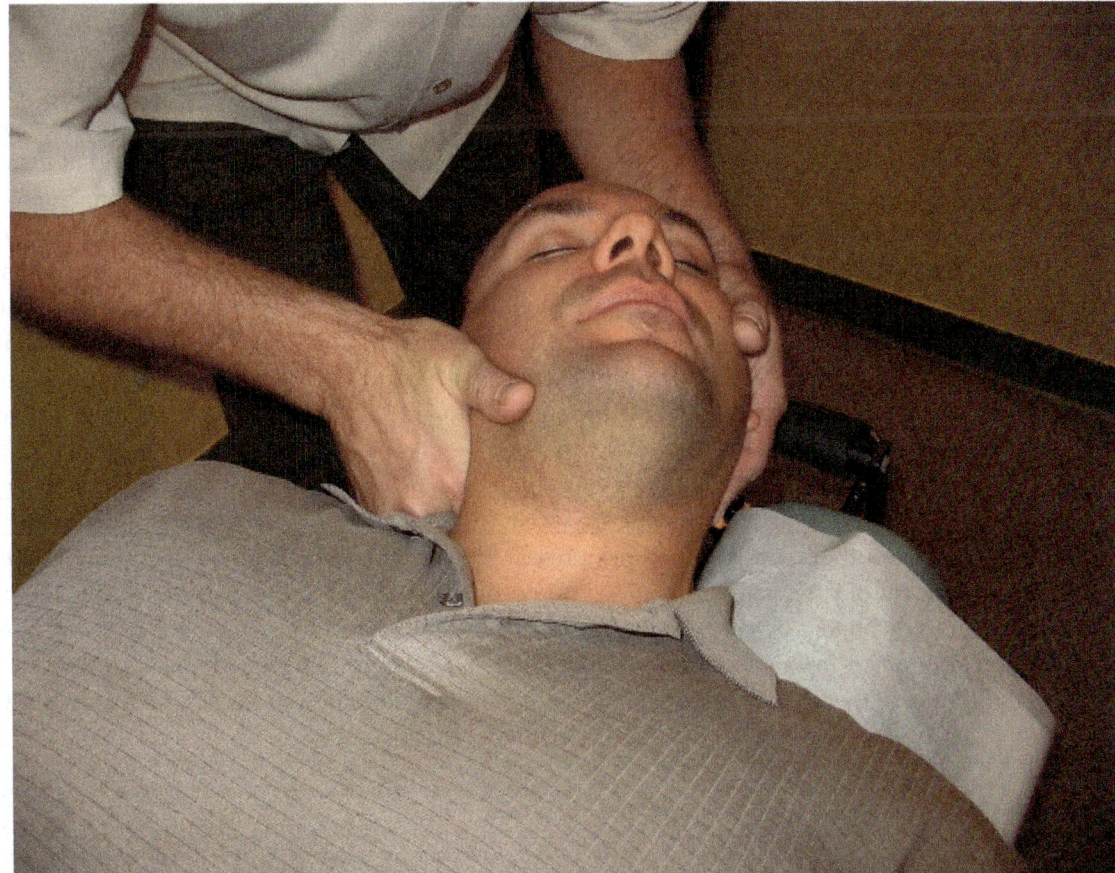

- Pilot study to determine the feasibility of a practice-based randomized controlled clinical trial with three parallel groups: Chiropractic adjustments and brief massage treatment at sites of subluxation in subjects with essential hypertension (*Journal of Manipulative and Physiological Therapeutics* 2002 May[286]): Treatment groups in this study consisted of ❶ chiropractic manipulation, ❷ brief soft tissue massage, or ❸ nontreatment control group. The patient group consisted of 23 subjects, 24-50 years of age, with systolic or diastolic primary HTN. In the active chiropractic treatment group, the intervention consisted of 2 months of full-spine chiropractic care using Gonstead technique, described as specific-contact, short-lever-arm adjustments delivered at motion segments exhibiting signs of subluxation. The massage group received brief effleurage at localized regions of the spine believed to be exhibiting signs of subluxation. The nontreatment control group rested alone for a period of approximately 5 minutes in a treatment room. In both the chiropractic and massage therapy groups, all subjects were classified as either overweight or obese; in the control group, only 2 subjects were overweight—these baseline differences in the study groups are important as they suggest that more patients in the chiropractic treatment group probably had HTN as a component of the metabolic syndrome rather than HTN due specifically and solely to a musculoskeletal lesion. The authors report that at the end of the study period, the BP change was -6.3 mm Hg in the chiropractic group, -1.0 mm Hg in the massage group, and -7.2 mm Hg in the relaxation "control" group. The authors of this pilot feasibility study noted several methodological shortcomings and logistical complications of their study, most notably the limited subject pool of patients who have hypertensive disease but who are not taking medications for its control. A larger study group would have allowed improved randomization and thus equilibration of baseline patient characteristics such as body mass index, which shows a strong correlation with severity of HTN.
- Review: Spinal manipulation and the efficacy of conservative therapeusis for the treatment of hypertension (*Journal of Manipulative and Physiological Therapeutics* 1986 Mar[287]): These authors review relevant chiropractic and osteopathic literature of the day (published in 1986) and conclude that manipulative therapy has a rational basis in the treatment of HTN based on the potential for spinal manipulation to promote restoration of homeostasis via reducing excess sympathetic tone and effecting a relative increase in parasympathetic tone. Spinal regions that are emphasized are ❶ the upper cervical spine (occiput-atlas) which correlates anatomically with the superior cervical sympathetic ganglia, ❷ the upper thoracic spine (T1-T6, especially T2-T3) which correlates with the thoracic sympathetic ganglia, and ❸ the lower thoracic spine (T11-T12) which correlates with sympathetic innervation via the renal ganglia/plexus that services the kidney. Clinicians should recall that sympathetic activation of the kidney increases production of renin (the enzyme), angiotensin-2 (the product of renin acting upon angiotensin-1), and aldosterone (produced by the adrenal cortex in response to stimulation by angiotensin-2) to effect systemic vasoconstriction and retention of sodium and water to increase blood volume and blood pressure. Comprehensive chiropractic treatment should include (but not be limited to) manipulation of spinal segments, massage and manipulation of regional soft tissues, mobilization of the ribs, and the implementation of dietary, nutritional, exercise/lifestyle, sleep pattern, and psychoemotional interventions. The authors conclude that alleviating HTN via resolution of musculoskeletal dysfunction and restoration of homeostasis is a more logical and ethical approach than is the suppression of HTN with the use of drugs that commonly have iatrogenic consequences.
- Review: Effect of osteopathic manipulative therapy on autonomic tone as evidenced by blood pressure changes and activity of the fibrinolytic system (*JAOA—Journal of the American Osteopathic Association* 1968 May[288]): The authors describe their prior research experience with humans and animals in the investigation of the effects of osteopathic manipulation on blood pressure and activation of the sympathetic nervous system as evaluated by changes in the fibrinogen/fibrinolytic system; they wrote, "In research which has been conducted in this laboratory to date, the relationship between changes in blood pressure and the manipulative therapeutic approach not only has been validated in human beings with hypertension, but

---

[286] Plaugher et al. Practice-based randomized controlled-comparison clinical trial of chiropractic adjustments and brief massage treatment at sites of subluxation in subjects with essential hypertension: pilot study. *J Manipulative Physiol Ther*. 2002 May;25(4):221-39

[287] Crawford et al. Management of hypertensive disease: spinal manipulation and the efficacy of conservative therapeusis. *J Manipulative Physiol Ther* 1986 Mar ;9(1):27-32

[288] Celander E, Koenig AJ, Celander DR. Effect of osteopathic manipulative therapy on autonomic tone as evidenced by blood pressure changes and activity of the fibrinolytic system. *J Am Osteopath Assoc*. 1968 May;67(9):1037-8

has also been demonstrated in normal persons as well as in experimental dogs. **Soft tissue manipulation of the upper thoracic and cervical vertebrae leads in almost every case to a decrease in blood pressure.**" These authors go on to note that "…a cumulative effect does occur, four or five treatments accomplishing a greater effect than a single treatment…" and that a reduction in pro-coagulative tendency occurs as evidenced by reductions in fibrinogen and other serum levels of coagulation factors.

- <u>Clinical trial: Effect of osteopathic manipulative therapy on autonomic tone as evidenced by blood pressure changes and activity of the fibrinolytic system</u> (*JAOA—Journal of the American Osteopathic Association* 1969 Jun[289]): The authors describe the use of an interventional protocol consisting of ❶ 15 minutes of rest in the supine position during measurement of blood pressure and laboratory indices, ❷ 5 minutes of soft tissue manipulation in the prone position ("The patient then assumes the prone position for 5 minutes. During this time soft tissue manipulation is applied equally to the left and right posterior cervical and thoracic areas. In the control experiment, no soft tissue manipulation is performed during this time interval.", and ❸ 15 minutes of rest in the supine position during measurement of blood pressure and laboratory indices. The authors wrote, "In our study after an initial rest period followed by manipulation there was a significant decrease (p<0.01) in both diastolic and systolic pressure in the hypertensive group." Furthermore, they noted laboratory evidence of reduced hemoconcentration, erythrocyte sedimentation rate, and a reduction in fibrinogen levels in 96% of patients with hypertension; among normotensive patients, fibrinogen levels decreased in 32% and increased in 51%.

- <u>Blinded randomized clinical trial using chiropractic and diet to treat hypertension: Treatment of Hypertension with Alternative Therapies (THAT) Study</u> (*Journal of Hypertension* 2002 Oct[290]): Given the potential implications of the use of "chiropractic spinal manipulation and diet" for the treatment of HTN, this study is potentially important and therefore worthy of detailed analysis; this is even more true when we appreciate that the authors titled this study "Treatment of Hypertension with Alternative Therapies" and thus broadened the implications of this article to all modes, genres, professions, and interventions that might fall under the rubric of "alternative medicine." The authors begin their abstract by stating that the objective of the study is to "To examine the effect of spinal manipulation on blood pressure" and then go on to describe the design of the study to be "This randomized clinical trial compared the effects of chiropractic spinal manipulation and diet with diet alone for lowering blood pressure in participants with high-normal blood pressure or stage I hypertension."; thus, from the outset, the study was not designed to truly investigate "alternative therapies" *per se* as the term should be applied (if it is to be used at all[291]) but rather only "chiropractic spinal manipulation" (within which many techniques exist) and "diet" (which can mean different things to different clinicians and can be variously applied to and implemented by diverse groups of patients). Per the study description, "One hundred and forty men and women, aged 25-60 years, with high-normal blood pressure or stage I hypertension, were enrolled. One hundred and twenty-eight participants completed the study. INTERVENTIONS: (i) A dietary intervention program administered by a dietitian [Diet] or (ii) a dietary intervention program administered by a doctor of chiropractic in conjunction with chiropractic spinal manipulation [DC+diet]. The frequency of treatment for both groups was three times per week for 4 weeks, for a total of 12 visits"; this might appear to be a reasonable study design insofar as it distinguishes the effectiveness of Diet from the effectiveness of DC+diet however the comparison is not balanced insofar as the Diet group was seen by a full-time dietician (who focuses only on nutrition) versus the diet advice administered by a full-time clinician with a broader range of responsibilities and daily actions who then by definition has less time to dedicate to dietary advice. Results of the study showed that "Average decreases in systolic/diastolic blood pressure were -4.9/5.6 mmHg for diet group and -3.5/4.0 mmHg for the chiropractic group. Between group changes were not statistically significant. CONCLUSIONS: For patients with high normal blood pressure or stage I hypertension, chiropractic spinal manipulation in conjunction with a dietary modification program offered

---

[289] Fichera AP, Celander DR. Effect of osteopathic manipulative therapy on autonomic tone as evidenced by blood pressure changes and activity of the fibrinolytic system. *J Am Osteopath Assoc.* 1969 Jun;68(10):1036-8

[290] Goertz et al. Treatment of Hypertension with Alternative Therapies (THAT) Study: a randomized clinical trial. *J Hypertens.* 2002 Oct;20(10):2063-8

[291] MacIntosh A. "Understanding the Differences between Conventional, Alternative, Complementary, Integrative and Natural Medicine" *Townsend Letter* 1999 July tldp.com/medicine.htm This is a brilliant -- if not obvious -- explanation that was powerful for the time it was written, and beyond. This article should be required reading for politicians, clinicians, and policy-makers and others with a stake in so-called "CAM."

no advantage in lowering either diastolic or systolic blood pressure compared to diet alone." This conclusion could easily be interpreted to imply that chiropractic manipulation is inefficacious and/or that the dietary advice given by the chiropractic doctors in this study was of poor quality or that it even negated the potential benefits of spinal manipulation (or vice versa). For many clinicians and policy-makers, this is probably as far as they might go with this study, with the take-away message being that both diet and spinal manipulation are essentially inefficacious for the treatment of hypertension. However, detailed reading of the article reveals several study

characteristics that may have contributed to the report of inefficacy, which is suspiciously noteworthy for its severity in both groups treated with diet therapy. Critique of the article follows:

❶ <u>Participants in this study did not have hypertension to begin with</u>. Participants for this study were relatively healthy with systolic pressures below 160 mmHg and diastolic pressures of 85–99 mmHg. Since patients with less severe degrees of hypertension would be expected to show less numerical improvement, this study's use of subjects with average blood pressure of 135/88 mm Hg—a level which is considered nonhypertensive—slanted the scales toward a conclusion of inefficacy because the subjects had no disease. In a very real sense therefore, the title of this article "Treatment of Hypertension with Alternative Therapies" is doubly misleading; first, the subjects did not have hypertension to begin with, and second, among the hundreds of "alternative therapies" available, only two were chosen for this study. A more accurate title of this article (as will become more clear in the following discussion) would have been "Treatment of nonhypertensive patients with weak dietary advice and nonspecific chiropractic manipulation lowers blood pressure by approximately 4/5 mm Hg."

❷ <u>The diet advice given was standardized rather than customized</u>. The study reads "DC/Diet patients received all of the written diet information received by the Diet group, but from the chiropractor. In addition, DC/Diet participants received chiropractic spinal manipulation." Regardless of whether the information was delivered by a chiropractic doctor or an experienced registered dietitian, the information was "prefabricated" rather than customized per patient. Better results are obtained when treatments are customized per patient; thus, this study failed to offer optimal diet therapy and not surprisingly found lackluster results.

❸ <u>The study prohibited the use of several of the most effective "alternative therapies" for hypertension despite being titled "Treatment of Hypertension with Alternative Therapies"</u>. The requirement that "All treating clinicians agreed not to offer dietary advice other than that included in the standard diet instructions (e.g. supplements), aerobic exercise advice, acupuncture or activator treatment to participants" was good for the standardization of the study but it eliminates the possibility of implementing some of the most valuable "alternative therapies" that exist for the treatment of HTN, such as vitamin D3, CoQ10, exercise, and weight loss. Again, the study was given a misleading title.

❹ <u>The "specific diet intervention instructions" used in this study were suspiciously inefficacious and were not disclosed in the materials and methods</u>. The authors fail to disclose the details of their diet intervention, thus ensuring that their study can never be subjected to scientific scrutiny by replication. Further, the only details provided are that subjects were given "written instructions on how to modify their current diet and were also given diet sheets, which included low-fat, low-salt recipes. The nutritionist explained the diet and covered a pre-set list of topics." The low-fat aspect of the diet strongly suggests that the diet was low in the health-promoting cardioprotective fatty acids previously reviewed, namely ALA, GLA, EPA, DHA, and oleic acid; the diet pattern suggested was probably neither Paleo nor Mediterranean. Diets that are relatively lower in fat tend to be by default relatively higher in carbohydrates, which leads to insulin release, retention of sodium and water, systemic inflammation, endothelial dysfunction, and the perpetuation of hypertension. That the diet was highly inefficacious is made obvious by the results provided in Table @ of their study, which shows that participants in both groups lost essentially zero weight (-0.8 lbs) during the 4-week study duration; this proves the inappropriate design of the intervention diet provided to both groups because clinical experience and clinical trials have repeatedly demonstrated that patients on effective optimized diets generally lose 4-8 lbs per month. Failure of the diet intervention to effect weight loss in both therapeutic groups

having an average BMI of 30.5 *which clearly shows that most patients in this study met objective criteria for obesity* provides objective proof that the interventional diet was of faulty design; again, these patients should have lost 4-8 lbs during the study period had the diet been appropriately designed, delivered, and implemented.

❺ The subjects in the chiropractic group were healthier than those in the diet group. "The diet group overall weighed more than the chiropractic group at 200 versus 187 lbs, and this difference was borderline significant (P = 0.06)." Regardless of statistical significance, the clinical significance of a 13-pound weight difference is noteworthy. Because the DC+diet group was healthier from the start of the study, less improvement would have been expected. The DC+diet group also had fewer smokers and fewer patients taking medications; these differences between groups were not mathematically significant, but they may have been additively or synergistically clinically significant.

❻ Exclusion of patients with pain negates the recognition of chiropractic's probable antihypertension-via-analgesia benefit from spinal manipulation. The authors acknowledge, "Because spinal manipulation has been reported to lower pain levels for individuals with back pain, and there is a correlation between pain levels and blood pressure, participants reporting average pain levels of five or above on a 0–10 point visual analog type scale were also excluded." In the real world, if a patient with pain and hypertension has both conditions relieved via spinal manipulation's antinociceptive benefits, then this would be documented as a dual benefit from a single therapy. This study's design eliminated the possibility of detecting and documenting this benefit.

❼ Positive selection of subjects likely confused the findings of the study. Recruitment methods quite likely selected patients already using "alternative therapies" and who may have already been "maximally improved" from their former baseline of hypertension severity. "All methods [of subject recruitment] incorporated the same message and highlighted the alternative therapy aspect of the study."; this would have resulted in positive selection of patients interested in and perhaps already using CAM treatments including nutritional supplements and exercise. Since the authors did not include use of nutritional supplements, exercise, acupuncture, diet therapy (etc) in their exclusion criteria, some of the test

subjects may have already been maximally treated with self-selected or professionally-directed treatments. The exclusion criteria failed to control for this important variable.

❽ With all of these problems invalidating the design, implementation, and conclusions of the study, its publication calls into question the intent and/or the wakefulness of the journal's editorial board. Supposedly, the purpose of having an Editor and an Editorial Board is to create what is called the "peer-review" process by which an article undergoes at least some modicum of scientific *or perhaps even intellectual* scrutiny prior to publication so that drivel is not incorporated into our collective body of knowledge that we use to direct patient care. Bad research is bad enough, but when it becomes codified by publication in a journal such as *Journal of Hypertension* and then indexed into Medline by the US National Library of Medicine, then it has the power to influence the healthcare received by thousands of patients, nationally and internationally. The publication of articles such as this calls into question the value and reliability of the peer-review process, the quality and intent of journal editors and editorial boards, and the value of doctorate-level training *prima facie* if its results are such as these. In sum, this study had numerous flaws—the three most important are ❶ the patients were nonhypertensive from the start, ❷ the dietary intervention was standardized (rather than individualized) and was clearly inefficacious as demonstrated by its inability to effect weight loss in a group of obese patients, and ❸ the interventional diet was prefabricated rather than reflecting the type of dietary intervention that a chiropractic doctor might actually use in real clinical practice. Thus, this study completely failed to offer any legitimate insight into the "treatment of hypertension with alternative therapies" and it unscientifically and inaccurately slanders both chiropractic manipulation and dietary intervention for the treatment of hypertension.

Clinical pearls: Ways to objectively assess treatment involvement (compliance)
1. **Vitamin D levels**: Serum 25-OH-cholecalciferol can be tested as a surrogate marker for compliance with nutritional supplementation (detailed later); levels should rise within one month and plateau at the optimal range within 2-3 months if dose and compliance are appropriate. Since most patients will have low levels of 25-OH-D at initial assessment, retesting serum levels after 1-2 months of supplementation is an easy way to assess compliance with and effectiveness of this aspect of the treatment plan.
2. **Recall**: Patients should be able to recite their daily regimen of nutritional supplementation, pharmaceutical drugs, dietary prescriptions/proscriptions, and exercise-lifestyle habits. *If the patient cannot recall their daily health-promoting activities, then compliance is likely either low or nonexistent.*
3. **Consciousness**: Ideally, patients should be able to recite their personal values and goals, as these are the driving forces that either *support* or *subvert* their daily health-related behaviors. Conscious physicians should encourage consciousness-raising in their patients.
4. **Weight optimization**: Often, the "scale of truth" can be used for objective determination of compliance with the Paleo-Mediterranean Diet and particularly its low-carbohydrate and ketogenic variants. Overweight patients who comply with dietary optimization and lifestyle modification can generally achieve weight loss of 4-8 lbs (13-18 kg) per month. Certainly not all benefits of diet optimization are mediated through weight loss; however, the fact remains that weight loss is an important goal for the majority of hypertensive patients. Failure of weight loss can also be used to assess compliance and effectiveness of clinical trials involving dietary intervention; obviously, those trials that fail to effect weight loss were affected by inadequate compliance on behalf of the group of subjects (unlikely) or failure to design an appropriate dietary intervention on behalf of the researchers (more likely).
5. **Urinary sodium and potassium**: With a decided and consistent shift away from the Standard American-type diet (SAD) and toward the health-promoting Paleo-Mediterranean Diet (PMD) and particularly with its supplemented version (sPMD), the urinary sodium:creatinine ratio will decrease, as will the urinary sodium:potassium ratio.

ENDOCRINE Generally speaking: estrogen promotes water retention and thus hypertension; an excess or deficiency of thyroid hormone/function can lead to systolic or diastolic hypertension, respectively. Melatonin is an antioxidant (among its many functions) and can help reduce elevated blood pressure; obviously, melatonin is take only at night.

- **Treatment of hypothyroidism**: Obviously, HTN caused by primary, secondary, or peripheral/metabolic hypothyroidism is not primary/essential HTN because it is due to the thyroid hormone disorder/dysfunction. Clinicians can choose any of several—or a combination thereof—methods to correct thyroid dysfunction, not the least of which are gluten avoidance in gluten-intolerant patients[292], zinc[293] and selenium supplementation[294,295,296,297], administration of *inactive* T4 (levothyroxine) and/or T3 (liothyronine, the most active thyroid hormone[298,299]), or the use of bovine/porcine-sourced glandular thyroid products—the latter should be avoided in patients with antibody-positive thyroid autoimmunity.

- **Melatonin**: Melatonin is an endogenously produced hormone from the pineal gland that plays numerous physiologic roles beyond its sedative effect for sleep promotion. Trace amounts of melatonin are found in food;

---

[292] "In most patients who strictly followed a 1-yr gluten withdrawal (as confirmed by intestinal mucosa recovery), there was a normalization of subclinical hypothyroidism. ... CONCLUSIONS: The greater frequency of thyroid disease among celiac disease patients justifies a thyroid functional assessment. In distinct cases, gluten withdrawal may single-handedly reverse the abnormality." Sategna-Guidetti et al. Prevalence of thyroid disorders in untreated adult celiac disease patients and effect of gluten withdrawal: an Italian multicenter study. *Am J Gastroenterol*. 2001 Mar;96(3):751-7

[293] "RESULTS: Thirteen had low levels of serum free T3 and normal T4. ... After oral supplementation of Zn sulphate (4-10 mg/kg body weight) for 12 months, levels of serum free T3 and T3 normalized, serum rT3 decreased, and the TRH-induced TSH reaction normalized. ... CONCLUSION: Zn may play a role in thyroid hormone metabolism in low T3 patients and may in part contribute to conversion of T4 to T3 in humans." Nishiyama et al. Zinc supplementation alters thyroid hormone metabolism in disabled patients with zinc deficiency. *J Am Coll Nutr*. 1994 Feb;13(1):62-7

[294] Duntas et al. Effects of a six month treatment with selenomethionine in patients with autoimmune thyroiditis. *Eur J Endocrinol*. 2003 Apr;148(4):389-93

[295] Gartner R, Gasnier BC, Dietrich JW, Krebs B, Angstwurm MW. Selenium supplementation in patients with autoimmune thyroiditis decreases thyroid peroxidase antibodies concentrations. *J Clin Endocrinol Metab*. 2002 Apr;87(4):1687-91 jcem.endojournals.org/cgi/content/full/87/4/1687

[296] "We recently conducted a prospective, placebo-controlled clinical study, where we could demonstrate, that a substitution of 200 wg sodium selenite for three months in patients with autoimmune thyroiditis reduced thyroid peroxidase antibody (TPO-Ab) concentrations significantly." Gartner R, Gasnier BC. Selenium in the treatment of autoimmune thyroiditis. *Biofactors*. 2003;19(3-4):165-70

[297] "A highly significant linear correlation between the T3/T4 ratio and indices of Se status was observed in the older group of subjects. Indices of Zn status did not correlate with thyroid hormones, ... We concluded that reduced peripheral T4 conversion is related to impaired Se status in the elderly." Olivieri et al. Selenium, zinc, and thyroid hormones in healthy subjects: low T3/T4 ratio in the elderly is related to impaired selenium status. *Biol Trace Elem Res*. 1996 Jan;51(1):31-41

[298] McDaniel AB. Thyroid Assessment: Controversies and Conundrums. Institute for Functional Medicine Fourteenth International Symposium. Tuscon, Arizona. May 23-26, 2007. Reviewed in more detail in: Vasquez A. *Integrative Rheumatology*. IBMRC 2006, 2007 and all future editions and Vasquez A. *Musculoskeletal Pain: Expanded Clinical Strategies*. Institute for Functional Medicine. May 2008

[299] Friedman et al. Supraphysiological cyclic dosing of sustained release T3 in order to reset low basal body temperature. *P R Health Sci J*. 2006 Mar;25(1):23-9

when taken as a dietary supplement, melatonin demonstrates chronobiologic, sedative, antioxidant, antitumor, and immunomodulatory benefits.

- Double-blind placebo-controlled clinical trial: Melatonin reduces night blood pressure in patients with nocturnal hypertension (*American Journal of Medicine* 2006 Oct[300]): The authors begin by noting that "Nocturnal hypertension is associated with a high risk of morbidity and mortality." In this study, 38 adult patients medicated for HTN were randomized to receive melatonin 2 mg or placebo for 4 weeks. The results read as follows, "Melatonin treatment reduced nocturnal systolic BP significantly from 136 to 130 mm Hg (P=.011), and diastolic BP from 72 to 69 mm Hg (P=.002), whereas placebo had no effect on nocturnal BP." Thus, the authors concluded, "**Thus, an addition of melatonin 2 mg at night to stable antihypertensive treatment may improve nocturnal BP control in treated patients with nocturnal hypertension.**" This study showed that the addition of melatonin to standard drug treatment for HTN resulted in a **decrease in nighttime blood pressure of -6/-3 mm Hg** among patients with nocturnal HTN.

- Randomized placebo-controlled double-blind crossover study: Blood pressure response to melatonin in type 1 diabetes (*Pediatric Diabetes* 2004 Mar[301]): Eleven normotensive adolescent patients with type 1 diabetes of average 7-year duration and 10 healthy controls aged 14-18y participated in a randomized placebo-controlled double-blind crossover study of 5 mg melatonin for 1 week followed by a 1-week washout. Results showed that, "In the patients with type 1 diabetes, the decline in **diastolic blood pressure** during sleep was significantly greater on melatonin (17.8 mmHg) than on placebo (16.0 mmHg, p < 0.01)." This study showed use of melatonin 5 mg resulted in a **decrease in nighttime diastolic pressure of -1.6 mm Hg** among type-1 diabetic patients.

- Randomized, double-blind, placebo-controlled, crossover trial: Daily nighttime melatonin reduces blood pressure in male patients with essential hypertension (*Hypertension* 2004 Feb[302]): The authors of this study show uncommon insight in their introduction which partly reads: "Our objective was to determine whether enhancement of the functioning of the biological clock by repeated nighttime melatonin intake might reduce ambulatory blood pressure in patients with essential hypertension." Sixteen men with untreated essential HTN were given oral melatonin 2.5 mg at 1 hour before sleep, while 24-hour ambulatory blood pressure and actigraphic estimates of sleep quality were measured. Results showed that **repeated melatonin intake reduced systolic and diastolic blood pressure during sleep by -6 and -4 mm Hg, respectively**, with no effect on heart rate.

XENOBIOTICS Xenobiotics and "toxins" such as lead, mercury, and the wide range of POPs—persistent organic pollutants—such as dioxin have a long record of causing or contributing to hypertension and many other health problems; these facts are so well established that citation to research is not necessary for this section—see details in Chapter 2 and Chapter 4, Section 7. As such, all patients need to live a "detoxification lifestyle" including the following:	**Xenobiotic-induced HTN** Pesticides and other pollutants commonly induce mitochondrial dysfunction, thereby contributing to insulin resistance and vasoconstriction, both of which promote HTN.

1. Organic diet
2. Political activism—the only way to stop the daily chemical assault is to get governments to *write* and *enforce* pollution-control and to deter corporate irresponsibility. Failure to effect political and social change will lead to continued poisoning of the population, while partially salvaging only the more affluent and educated portions of the population able to afford and knowledgeable about detoxification; we are witnessing negative selection of the entire population, with only the more educated and affluent able to avoid or detoxify chemicals that are poisoning everyone. In the United States for example, large portions of the population are exposed to glyphosate in air and water; clearly eating "an organic diet" is only of partial help if the air is contaminated.
   - **America's air and (rain) water are contaminated with pesticides** (*Environ Toxicol Chem* 2014 Jun[303]): "Seven compounds in 1995 and 5 in 2007 were detected in ≥50% of both air and rain samples. Atrazine, metolachlor,

[300] Grossman et al. Melatonin reduces night blood pressure in patients with nocturnal hypertension. *Am J Med.* 2006 Oct;119(10):898-902
[301] Cavallo A, Daniels SR, Dolan LM, Khoury JC, Bean JA. Blood pressure response to melatonin in type 1 diabetes. *Pediatr Diabetes.* 2004 Mar;5(1):26-31
[302] Scheer et al. Daily nighttime melatonin reduces blood pressure in male patients with essential hypertension. *Hypertension.* 2004 Feb;43(2):192-7
[303] Majewski et al. Pesticides in Mississippi air and rain: a comparison between 1995 and 2007. *Environ Toxicol Chem.* 2014 Jun;33(6):1283-93

and propanil were detected in ≥50% of the air and rain samples in both years. Glyphosate and its degradation product, aminomethyl-phosphonic acid (AMPA), were detected in ≥75% of air and rain samples in 2007... The 1995 seasonal wet depositional flux was dominated by methyl parathion (88%) and was >4.5 times the 2007 flux. Total herbicide flux in 2007 was slightly greater than in 1995 and was dominated by glyphosate."

3. Avoid exposure, e.g., plastics and consumption of foods from cans lined with BPA—bisphenol A.
4. Establish and maintain urine pH of ~7.5-8 to promote reductions in cortisol, retention of magnesium and potassium, and urinary excretion of toxins/xenobiotics.
5. Optimization of gut flora to avoid LPS inhibition of detoxification.
6. Exercise to promote lipolysis, circulation of toxins (for hepatic and renal clearance), and sweating/diaphoresis for dermal clearance of toxins.
7. Basic mitochondrial and detoxification support with NAC and CoQ10 at the very least.

The connection between xenobiotic exposure and mitochondrial dysfunction is so strong and consistent that the former term is becoming synonymous with the latter. Xenobiotic-induced mitochondrial dysfunction promotes ROS production, persistent systemic inflammation, pro-inflammatory phenotype, insulin resistance, and vasoconstriction—any one of which independently and all of which additively/synergistically promote HTN.

| Using models of interconnection to understand chronic hypertension | Among variations on this theme, this diagram provides a reasonable representation of several of the key factors that generate and perpetuate the common clinical syndromes of overweight-obesity, hypertension, insulin resistance and diabetes type-2.

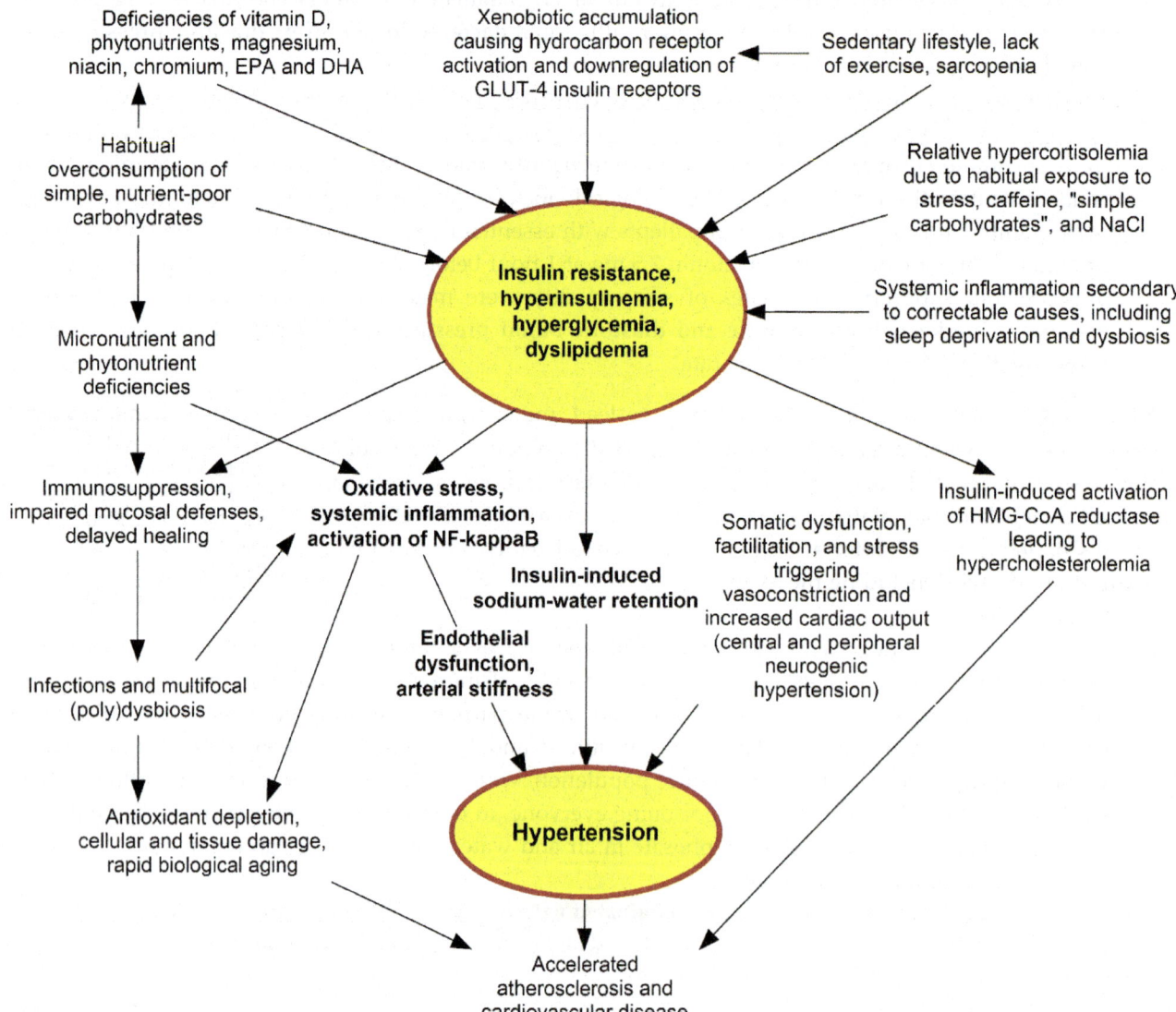

Simple Integrated Model of "Primary Hypertension": Interconnected lifestyle-physiologic mechanisms contribute to the hyperinsulinemia-inflammation-hypertension syndrome commonly known as "idiopathic hypertension" and metabolic syndrome.

- <u>Decipherative contextualization</u>: The social (and therefore political and economic) context in which "hypertension" exists is of supreme and generally neglected importance. Hypertension as a common disease does not exist in cultures that follow healthy lifestyles, particularly characterized by sufficient physical activity, Paleo-Mediterranean diets, and low to moderate societal stress; in sharp contrast, hypertension is an epidemic in countries like the United States where the social scene is littered with physical inactivity, unhealthy processed-food diets including overconsumption of high-fructose corn syrup and underconsumption of micronutrients (including vitamins [e.g., vitamin D], minerals [e.g., magnesium and potassium], and phytonutrients), and high levels of psychosocial and political stress coupled with epidemic individual isolation and pervasive social fragmentation.[304] I consider this fact self-evident: "hypertension" as we generally "know"/perceive it in the industrialized world would not exist in its epidemic form were it not for the social context and corporate-political climate which synergistically nurture it. This does not imply the need necessarily for political change to precede the treatment of hypertension, nor is such necessary in order to quantitatively reduce the number of affected individuals; what it does imply is that we as healthcare providers will be more successful in the achievement of our goals—if those goals are the beneficent alleviation of individual and societal disease burden and the optimization of individual and societal health—if we attend to the social-political-paradigmatic environment that contributes to patterns of disease pathogenesis. The goal here is to contextualize hypertension so thoroughly that the "disease" itself—as it exists in industrialized societies (pandemic) and we have been taught to see it (idiopathic, and therefore drug-dependent)—vanishes into comprehensibility and manageability and therefore loses its enigmatic power. I call this approach "decipherative contextualization" from the perspective that describing the disease as an extension of the social context from which it arises allows us to conceptually and intellectually apprehend the condition and thus decipher/decode/deflate its illusory enigmacity; of course, this model and each component therein has to be based on verified facts, as are readily abundant. My "decipherative contextualization" seeks to explain—to a sufficiently thorough degree—these enigmatic diseases so that they lose their phenomenalistic luster and can thereafter be managed dexterously, hopefully with ease, eventually with pleasure.

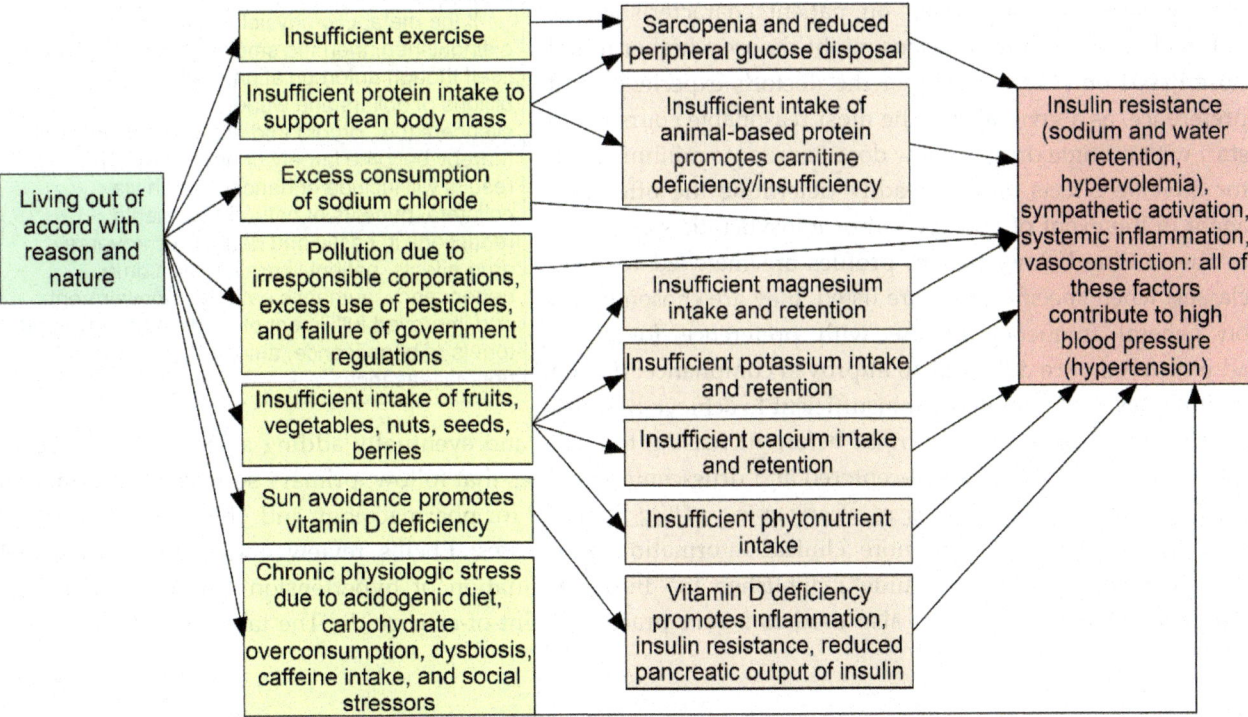

HTN—a singular etiology, multiple etiologies, or both?: Failure to meet nature-based physiologic expectations is a major cause of different secondary causes of hypertension: The above diagram shows how the simple act of what is referred to here as "living out of accord with nature" sets the stage for numerous biochemical and physiologic factors which contribute to HTN. Thus, this singular etiology or cause leads to numerous secondary etiologies or causes which all culminate in volume

---

304 Kihn, E Douglas. The Political Roots of American Obesity. truth-out.org/opinion/item/16149-the-political-roots-of-american-obesity. 2013 May. Excellent article.

overload, sympathetic activation, systemic inflammation, and vasoconstriction. "Living out of accord with nature" has been a theme of so-called modernized/ Westernized/ industrialized societies since their subtle and progressive development. Dr Price's *Nutrition and Physical Degeneration: A Comparison of Primitive and Modern Diets and Their Effects*[305] documented in 1945 the effects that this "progress" was having on the health of societies that became "modernized"—their health status and social structures fell into decline, often complete ruin. More recently, O'Keefe and Cordain[306] wrote in their review article entitled *Cardiovascular disease resulting from a diet and lifestyle at odds with our Paleolithic genome: how to become a 21st-century hunter-gatherer* that, "Accumulating evidence suggests that this mismatch between our modern diet and lifestyle and our Paleolithic genome is playing a substantial role in the ongoing epidemics of obesity, hypertension, diabetes, and atherosclerotic cardiovascular disease. ... Although the human genome has remained largely unchanged (DNA evidence documents relatively little change in the genome during the past 10,000 years), our diet and lifestyle have become progressively more divergent from those of our ancient ancestors." Whether we call the problem "living out of accord with nature" or "the mismatch between our modern diet and lifestyle and our Paleolithic genome" the concept is the same, and the biophysiologic and social results are obviously negative. America's social fabric has deteriorated to the point that most Americans have only 2-3 friends and no confidants[307], and the progressively larger epidemics of obesity, depression, cancer, diabetes mellitus, and cardiovascular disease are well publicized and known to all.

- **Drug treatments for chronic HTN**: From a practical standpoint, the many drugs used for the suppression of HTN can be placed in one of five categories; the mnemonic offered in the *Saint-Frances Guide*[308] is "A.B.C.D.E." which stands for ❶ ACEis (angiotensin converting enzyme inhibitors) and ARBs (angiotensin II Receptor Blockers), ❷ BBs (beta-blockers), ❸ CCBs (calcium channel blockers), ❹ diuretics, and ❺ everything else (e.g., central alpha-agonists, alpha-blockers, vasodilators). For uncomplicated HTN, the initial treatment is a diuretic, generally hydrochlorothiazide (HCTZ), since the thiazide diuretics have the best cost-effectiveness of various drug classes; as noted by Howland and Mycek[309], "Current treatment recommendations are to **initiate therapy with a thiazide diuretic unless there are compelling reasons to employ other drug classes**. ... Recent data suggest that diuretics are superior to beta-blockers in older adults." For complicated HTN (resistant to treatment or with concomitant illness), a different first-line or additive second drug is chosen from a different class based on patient characteristics, as outlined below. While clinicians might choose a higher initial dose based on HTN severity or the doctor's experience and preference, as a general rule the most reasonable course is to start with a single drug at a low dose in order to minimize risk for adverse effects and to readily determine the offending agent in the event of an expected or idiosyncratic side effect. In the outline below, patient profiles are matched to drug classes; when specific drugs are listed, they are chosen based on general frequency of use with preference for those administered once daily due to improved compliance. If drug treatment is well tolerated but insufficient to achieve BP goal,

> **Analogy: "Treating hypertension" simply by using drugs to lower blood pressure is like turning off a smoke alarm and then letting the fire continue to blaze.**
>
> High blood pressure is a manifestation of dysfunction. Rather than directing treatment toward the manifestation (i.e., the blood pressure elevation), clinicians would be more wise to address the nature and cause of the imbalance that is causing the elevation in blood pressure.
>
> If the metabolic-physiologic fire is extinguished, then the smoke alarm will silence itself though autoregulation, and spending billions of dollars and work-hours on alarm silencers (i.e., drugs) and alarm specialists will thereby become largely unnecessary. The results will include enhanced health via collateral benefits of natural treatments, reductions in costly and dangerous adverse drug effects, patient liberation from drug dependency, authentic patient empowerment, and improved fulfillment of medicine's purported tenets of beneficence, autonomy, and nonmalfeasance.

then *treatment compliance is verified* before increasing the dose and eventually adding a second drug from a different class. For the patient-centered and drug-centered tables that follow, primary sources of information are *Lippincott's Illustrated Reviews: Pharmacology, Third Edition*[310] for pharmacology and The 5-Minute Clinical Consult, 18th Edition[311] for more clinical information and doses; Ebell's review and clinical worksheet ("Hypertension Encounter Guide") published in "Initial evaluation of hypertension" in *American Family Physician* (March 2004)[312] was also used as a very practical point-of-care guide. The tables that follow were

[305] Price WA. *Nutrition and Physical Degeneration: A Comparison of Primitive and Modern Diets and Their Effects*. Price-Pottinger Nutr Foundtn: 1945

[306] O'Keefe JH Jr, Cordain L. Cardiovascular disease resulting from a diet and lifestyle at odds with our Paleolithic genome. *Mayo Clin Proc*. 2004 Jan;79(1):101-8

[307] McPherson et al. Social Isolation in America: Changes in Core Discussion Networks over Two Decades. *American Sociological Review* 2006; 71: 353-75 asanet.org

[308] Bent S, Gensler LS, Frances C. *Saint-Frances Guide: Clinical Clerkship in Outpatient Medicine. 2nd Edition*. Philadelphia; Wolters Kluwer: 2008, 90

[309] Howland RD, Mycek MJ. *Lippincott's Illustrated Reviews: Pharmacology, 3rd Edition*. Baltimore: Lippincott Williams and Wilkins; 2006, 213-226

[310] Howland RD, Mycek MJ. *Lippincott's Illustrated Reviews: Pharmacology, 3rd Edition*. Baltimore: Lippincott Williams and Wilkins; 2006, 213-226

[311] Domino FJ (editor in chief). *The 5-Minute Clinical Consult, 2010. 18th Edition*. Philadelphia; Wolters Kluwer: 2009, 656-7

[312] Ebell MH. Initial evaluation of hypertension. *Am Fam Physician*. 2004 Mar 15;69(6):1485-7 aafp.org/afp/2004/0315/p1485.html

originally written by Alex Vasquez and reviewed by Robert Richard DO[313] in January 2010 for the publication of *Chiropractic Management of Chronic Hypertension* (from which this more current text is derived); later editions of this publication have undergone additional professional and peer review.

- The medical profession's near-exclusive reliance upon drug treatments for HTN is fraught with problems, particularly including adverse drug effects, failure to address the underling primary cause(s) of the metabolic disturbance(s), of which, HTN is only the tip of the proverbial iceberg, and patient noncompliance. According to a 2001 editorial published in the *New England Journal of Medicine*, "Approximately one-half of patients who are prescribed antihypertensive medications discontinue therapy by the end of the first year."[314]

- In representative medical pharmacology textbooks[315] the primary variables considered for the support of antihypertensive pharmacotherapy are ❶ cardiac output (controlled with beta-blockers), ❷ peripheral resistance (treated with vasodilators such as ACEi and CCB), and ❸ blood volume (reduced by the first-line use of diuretics). One interconnecting theme in this paradigm is that of activation

> **Sequential HTN Drug Protocol**
>
> 1. **Thiazide diuretic: Hydrochlorothiazide 12.5-25 mg/d po** initially for most patients, not with renal insufficiency. For patients with DM or proteinuria, start with ACEi. Add **spironolactone 25-50 mg/d** if hypokalemia develops.
> 2. **ACEi: Lisinopril 10-40 mg/d po**, give the first dose in the office to monitor for hypotensive syncope or angioedema. If cough or angioedema develop, switch to ARB, particularly **losartan 25-100 mg/d** due to modest uricosuric effect. ACEi and ARB are contraindicated in pregnancy.
> 3. **CCB: Amlodipine 2.5-10 mg/d po**, particularly for patients with migraine, COPD, asthma.
> 4. **BB: Metoprolol 50-100 mg/d po** (up to bid), especially with angina or MI; not with bradycardia, insulin-requiring DM, depression, or sexual dysfunction.
> 5. **Loop diuretic: Furosemide 20-320 mg/d po** if patient has severe volume overload; effective with renal insufficiency.
>
> Ebell MH. Initial evaluation of hypertension. *Am Fam Physician*. 2004 Mar 15;69:1485-7 aafp.org/afp/2004/0315/p1485.html Domino FJ (editor-in-chief). *The 5-Minute Clinical Consult. 2010. 18th Edition*: 2009, 656-7

of the sympathetic nervous system by some unknown insult or combination thereof. Whether due to "stress", faulty disinhibition of baroreceptors in the aortic arch, carotid sinuses, or renal juxtaglomerular cells, sympathetic activation increases cardiac output via increased rate and contractility, increases peripheral resistance via vasoconstriction, and increases blood volume via aldosterone-enhanced sodium (and thus water) retention. The enzyme renin converts angiotensinogen into angiotensin-1, which is converted via angiotensin converting enzyme (ACE) into the vasoconstrictor and trigger for aldosterone release angiotensin-2.

- Suggested doses of course need to be tailored to individual patient needs; doses suggested are for adults of average adult size and are administered by mouth (per os, p.o.) unless otherwise indicated. Note that IV and IM doses are generally much smaller than oral doses.

Comorbidity profile suggesting specific first- or second-line treatment of hypertension

- **Tailoring drug selection per comorbidities:** Although the first choice for an antihypertensive drug is generally hydrochlorothiazide, the second drug and occasionally the first-line drug are selected based on patient tolerance and co-morbidities. The following quote by Chobanian[316] summarizes the general approach: "…for those who have had a heart attack, beta blockers and ACE inhibitors are preferred; for those at high risk for coronary heart disease, ACE inhibitors, beta blockers, calcium channel blockers, as well as diuretics are recommended; and for chronic kidney disease, ACE inhibitors and angiotensin receptor blockers are drugs of first choice." Additional details are provided below:
  - o **Uncomplicated**: Thiazide diuretics (especially **HCTZ**) are first choice (can worsen gout and dyslipidemia); BB have historically been a common second choice, but recently atenolol has fallen out of favor[317] and with the increasing prevalence of DM which indicates ACEi and ARB treatment, these

---

[313] Robert Richard DO is Medical Director of the John Peter Smith Polytechnic Clinic and Chair of Community Medicine at Texas College of Osteopathic Medicine. Dr Richard's review of these tables does not imply his endorsement of their content nor of the content of this document as a whole. Furthermore, Dr Richard's review does not imply endorsement by JPS Health Network or Texas College of Osteopathic Medicine.
[314] Chobanian AV. Control of hypertension—an important national priority. *N Engl J Med*. 2001 Aug 16;345(7):534-5
[315] Harvey RA, Champe PC (eds). *Lippincott's Illustrated Reviews: Pharmacology, 3rd Edition*. Philadelphia, Lippincott Williams and Wilkins; 1997
[316] Chobanian AV. Press Conference Remarks: The Seventh Report of the Joint National Committee on Prevention, Detection, Evaluation, and Treatment of High Blood Pressure (JNC 7). May 14, 2003. nhlbi.nih.gov/guidelines/hypertension/speaker2.htm Accessed November 2010
[317] Domino FJ (editor in chief). *The 5-Minute Clinical Consult. 2010. 18th Edition*. Philadelphia; Wolters Kluwer: 2009, 656-7

medications may become the preferred second line; the ARB **losartan** would seem particularly favorable in patients with metabolic syndrome and type-2 DM due to its uricosuric effect.

- o **Diabetes mellitus**: ACEis are renoprotective (but not used with renovascular disease), ARB's are second choice due to cost and less historical use; beta-blockers are generally avoided in insulin-requiring DM due to blunting of protective responses to hypoglycemia.
- o **Renal disease**: ACEis are renoprotective (but not used with renovascular disease), ARBs are second choice. Nondihydropyridine CCBs reduce intrarenal filtration pressure thus reducing proteinuria. Thiazides require renal function and are generally not useful if creatinine is >2 mg/dl.
- o **African American**: African-Americans tend to respond better to diuretics and CCB than to BB or ACEi.[318]
- o **Asthma and COPD**: Use a CCB. Generally avoid beta-blockers with any airway disease, B1-selective metoprolol might be considered
- o **Angina**: BB and CCB improve outcomes independent of BP-lowering; when BB and CCB are combined, the CCB should be a dihydropyridine (i.e., from the class of "-pyridines" or "-pines"). Do not combine a BB with a negative inotropic non-dihydropyridine CCB so as to avoid inducing heart block.
- o **Erectile dysfunction**: Avoid beta-blockers; thiazides may exacerbate. Consider concomitant administration of arginine and/or a phosphodiesterase-5 inhibitor; also consider treatment for excess estrogen in men with a serum estradiol greater than 30 picogram/mL (for details see the anti-estrogen protocol outlined in chapter 4 of *Integrative Rheumatology/ Inflammation Mastery*[319]). Implement diet and lifestyle modification for weight optimization; optimize endothelial health.
- o **Systolic HTN**: Dihydropyridine CCB ("-pyridines" or "-*pines*") are preferred because of their relative selectivity for the peripheral vasculature—the vascular *tree*.
- o **CAD or prior MI**: BB are top choice if not contraindicated by problematic asthma, COPD, or DM.
- o **Pregnancy**: Use methyldopa, hydralazine, magnesium; pregnancy contraindicates ACEi and ARB due to teratogenic effects.
- o **CHF**: BB are particularly useful for diastolic CHF to slow heart rate and allow greater filling time: Carvedilol is BB of choice in this situation. Monitor for signs of excessive cardiosupresion such as edema, SOB, rales, bradycardia. Carvedilol is a non-selective beta blocker/alpha-1 blocker indicated in the treatment of mild to moderate CHF. Do not use BB or CCB with bradycardia; generally do not use verapamil (negative inotrope CCB) with CHF. Diuretics such as Lasix are mainstays of CHF treatment, particularly for exacerbations. ACEi and ARB drugs are also routinely used in CHF.
- o **Bradycardia**: Do not use BB or CCB with bradycardia.
- o **Edema**: Sodium and water restriction along with use of loop diuretics (e.g., furosemide/Lasix) is common treatment. Lasix is generally dosed "to effect."

The next several pages provide a review of each drug class. Preferred/representative drugs are listed based on the author's experience, training (especially observed prescribing patterns by attending physicians) and research; following the so-called preferred drug is optional at the discretion of the clinician.

ACEi: angiotensin-2 converting enzyme inhibitors

- • Pharmacology and introduction: Blocking formation of angiotensin-2 reduces peripheral vascular resistance and aldosterone secretion; vasodilation is effected by reduced breakdown of bradykinin; sympathetic tone may be reduced. For best safety, the initial dose of an ACEi can be given in the office under supervision due to risks for first-dose syncope and life-threatening angioedema; this advised practice is rarely followed.
- • Unique benefits of class: ACE inhibitors provide renoprotection, hence their routine use in patients with DM, with or without HTN. Thiazide, BB, and ACEi can be safely used together. As summarized by Domino (editor, *5-Minute Clinical Consult*), "ACE inhibitors should be used in patients with diabetes, proteinuria, atrial fibrillation, or CHF but not in pregnancy."
- • Unique adverse effects and contraindications: Not used with **renal artery stenosis** (can cause acute renal failure) or **pregnancy** (teratogenic); may cause **cough (10%) and angioedema** due to reduced breakdown of bradykinin. Reduced aldosterone secretion promotes hypotension and **hyperkalemia—potassium levels should be monitored**

---

[318] Howland RD, Mycek MJ. *Lippincott's Illustrated Reviews: Pharmacology, 3rd Edition*. Baltimore: Lippincott Williams and Wilkins; 2006, 213-226
[319] Vasquez A. *Integrative Rheumatology*. IBMRC 2006, 2007 and all future editions.

especially in diabetic patients and those with **renal insufficiency and/or renal vascular stenosis; coadministration of ACEi and spironolactone is generally contraindicated** due to risk of hyperkalemia.
- Representative drug of class (dose range): Lisinopril 10 mg/d — see table

---

ARB: angiotensin-2 receptor blocker/antagonist

- Pharmacology and introduction: ARBs block reception of angiotensin-2 and thus reduce vasoconstriction and aldosterone secretion; risk-benefit profile is similar to ACEi except that bradykinin-mediated benefits (vasodilation) and risks (cough, angioedema) are not seen. ARBs improve endothelial dysfunction in patients with HTN and/or CAD, reduce cardiovascular mortality and morbidity, and have anti-inflammatory benefits.
- Unique benefits of class: Hypotensive and renoprotective benefits without the risks of cough and angioedema compared with ACEi.
- Unique adverse effects and contraindications: Fetotoxicity contraindicates ARB use in pregnancy — this is a black box warning.
- Representative drug of class (dose range): Losartan 50 mg/d — see table

---

BB: beta-adrenergic receptor blockers, "beta blockers"

- Pharmacology and introduction: Primary mechanism of drug action is via blockade of B1 receptors; this reduces cardiac output, sympathetic tone, and renin secretion. Major adverse effects include bradycardia, fatigue, depression, sexual dysfunction, exacerbation of asthma and COPD, and **rebound hypertension with rapid discontinuation of drug**.
- Unique benefits of class: Thiazide, BB, and ACEi can be safely used together. BB considered more effective in Caucasians than Africans, more effective in young than elderly. BB are particularly used in HTN patients who also have **supraventricular tachyarrhythmia, previous MI, angina, migraine, and anxiety**.
- Unique adverse effects and contraindications: Do not use BB or CCB with **bradycardia** due to potential for inducing **heart block or hypotension**. Nonselective BB such as propranolol which target B1 (heart) and B2 (lungs) have potential to **exacerbate asthma and COPD**; however, **propranolol's B1 blockade helps reduce renin levels**. Patients with PVD may have a worsening of limb ischemia secondary to reduced perfusion. **Hypotension, fatigue, depression, sexual dysfunction,** and **rebound hypertension** are common adverse BB effects; lowering of HDL and elevation of TRIGs has also been noted. Sudden discontinuation of BB can result in **rebound hypertension** (presumably due to upregulation of beta-adrenergic receptors under prolonged suppression). Of note, **atenolol** is no longer considered first-line treatment due to recent evidence of **inefficacy** in preventing HTN complications.[320]
- Representative drug of class (dose range): Metoprolol in extended release (Toprol-XL) 25 mg/d — see table

---

CCB: calcium channel blockers (dihydropyridine class)

- Pharmacology and introduction: The "-pyridines" block calcium entry into vascular smooth muscle and thus cause relative arterial dilation and thus a reduction in peripheral resistance. *Memory tool*: Remember that *pyridines* sounds like *pines* and that these drugs work on the *vascular tree* to lower blood pressure via systemic arterial dilation.
  - Not detailed here are the non-dihydropyridine class of CCB (i.e., including diltiazem/Cardizem and Verapamil) which are not used for HTN but rather are used for their cardioselective effects. *Memory tool*: Remember that the *non*-dihydropyridine CCBs are cardiosuppressive via a *negative* inotropic effect.
- Unique benefits of class: Generally safe in HTN patients with asthma, DM, angina, and PVD.
- Unique adverse effects and contraindications: Do not use BB or non-dihydropyridine CCB with bradycardia. Adverse effects include constipation (10%, especially with nifedipine), headache, and fatigue.
- Representative drug of class (dose range): Amlodipine 5 mg/d, or start with 2.5 mg/d — see table

---

Diuretic — loop class: furosemide /Lasix

- Pharmacology and introduction: A key mechanism of action of most diuretics is enhanced excretion of sodium. Sodium (Na) retention promotes water retention and subsequent volume expansion, while also contributing to vasoconstriction

> **Loop diuretics infamously cause electrolyte and thiamine loss**
>
> Loop diuretics such as furosemide/Lasix are commonly used in the treatment of heart failure and other edematous states in elderly patients, but the depletion of thiamine, magnesium, potassium, and calcium can exacerbate heart failure and contribute to co-morbidity such as depression, delirium, and dementia.
>
> Felípez et al. Drug-induced nutrient deficiencies. *Pediatr Clin North Am.* 2009

---

[320] Domino FJ (editor in chief). *The 5-Minute Clinical Consult. 2010. 18th Edition*. Philadelphia; Wolters Kluwer: 2009, 656-7

and arterial stiffness via enhanced adrenergic reactivity and via promotion of intracellular hypercalcinosis (possibly due to enhanced sodium-calcium exchange).[321]

- Unique benefits of class: Fast action even in patients with renal insufficiency; efficacy of Lasix is via diuresis and venodilation.
- Unique adverse effects and contraindications: Chronic use promotes depletion of potassium, magnesium, and thiamine. Diuretic effect is potent and acute.
- Representative drug of class (dose range): Furosemide 20 mg/d po is reasonable starting dose—see table

Diuretic—thiazide class: hydrochlorothiazide (HCTZ)

- Pharmacology and introduction: Drug of choice for initial treatment of HTN. Sulfa sensitivity does not necessarily contraindicate thiazide use, even though thiazides are sulfa derivatives; use with caution. Thiazide diuretics are ineffective in patients with renal insufficiency; the loop diuretic furosemide is effective in patients with renal insufficiency.
- Unique benefits of class: Thiazide, BB, and ACEi can be safely used together. Particularly beneficial in elderly (as long as renal function is intact) and Africans. Promotion of calcium retention may benefit osteoporosis and reduce calcium nephrolithiasis. Thiazide diuretics reduce peripheral vascular resistance, perhaps via sodium elimination.
- **Unique adverse effects and contraindications**: Not useful in patients with renal insufficiency (creatinine clearance < 50 mL/min).
  - Thiazide diuretics can worsen **hyperuricemia** (70% of patients) and **gout** due to competition for renal excretion (organic acids).
  - **Hypokalemia** (70%)—potassium levels should be monitored in patients predisposed to cardiac arrhythmia and those treated with digitalis. Coadministration with ACEi/lisinopril helps negate the tendency toward hypokalemia.
  - **Hyperglycemia (10%), dyslipidemia, hypomagnesemia**
  - Promotion of calcium retention can promote **hypercalcemia** when HCTZ is combined with vitamin D3, even with the use of modest doses of vitamin D (e.g., 2,000 IU/d).[322]
  - Exacerbation of (fructose-induced) metabolic syndrome was recently proven experimentally [animal study] and published in a peer-reviewed journal[323]; this effect is mediated at least in part due to potassium depletion.
- Representative drug of class (dose range): Hydrochlorothiazide, started at 12.5-25 mg/d—see table

Diuretic—potassium-sparing: spironolactone

- Pharmacology and introduction: Potassium-sparing diuretics are weak diuretics; **spironolactone** is the prototype and also has anti-androgen action and is therefore used in hirsutism.
- Unique benefits of class: Spironolactone is commonly used with HCTZ; it beneficially diminishes cardiac remodeling seen in CHF. Spironolactone reduces incidence of spontaneous bacterial peritonitis (SBP) in patients with cirrhosis.
- Unique adverse effects and contraindications: Spironolactone has antiandrogen effects, can promote sexual dysfunction in men and gynecomastia; can precipitate hyperkalemia and hypermagnesemia.
- Representative drug of class (dose range): Spironolactone, start HTN dose at 12.5 mg/d—see table

Alpha-1-blocker: alpha-adrenergic receptor type-1 antagonist

- Pharmacology and introduction: Reduce BP via relaxation of venous and arterial smooth muscle. These drugs are certainly not used as first-line treatments for HTN, generally speaking.
- Unique benefits of class: Can be used when other drugs have not been effective; can benefit men with prostatic hyperplasia.
- Unique adverse effects and contraindications: Sodium-water retention, hypotension, syncope, and reflex tachycardia are common; reflex tachycardia can be prevented with BB.
- Representative drug of class: Prazosin, start with 1 mg/d—see table

Alpha-2 agonists: alpha-adrenergic receptor class-2 agonist

- Pharmacology and introduction: Centrally acting drugs reduce sympathetic output via central feedback inhibition. Rebound hypertension with clonidine withdrawal mandates tapering discontinuation.
- Unique benefits of class: Safe for use in renal disease; generally used with diuretic.

---

[321] Benowitz NL. "Antihypertensive Agents." In Katzung BG (editor). *Basic and Clinical Pharmacology. 10th Edition*. New York: McGraw Hill Medical; 2007, 16
[322] Vasquez et al. The clinical importance of vitamin D: a paradigm shift with implications for all healthcare providers. *Altern Ther Health Med*. 2004 Sep-Oct;10(5):28-36
[323] Reungjui et al. Thiazide diuretics exacerbate fructose-induced metabolic syndrome. *J Am Soc Nephrol*. 2007 Oct;18(10):2724-31

- Unique adverse effects and contraindications: Generally used with a diuretic to counteract the sodium-water retention. Sedation and dry nose may occur. Rebound hypertension mandates *tapering* discontinuation. **Alpha-2 agonists are best avoided due to high risk of rebound HTN following noncompliance or missed/skipped dose.**
- Representative drug of class: Clonidine, start at 0.1 mg bid—see table

---

Vasodilators: Direct-acting smooth muscle relaxants: hydralazine

- Pharmacology and introduction: Vasodilators are used for treatment-resistant HTN, acute severe HTN, and pregnancy-related HTN. During my hospital training, we used these drugs commonly in emergency settings and in obstetrics; generally these drugs were administered intravenously at 10 mg per dose repeated as needed for HTN control. Hydralazine's mechanism of action includes limiting calcium release from the sarcoplasmic reticulum of smooth muscle thereby resulting in relaxation of arterioles and veins; hydralazine recently has been identified as a nitric oxide donor.
- Unique benefits of class: Rapid onset of action; safe for use during pregnancy.
- Unique adverse effects and contraindications: Sodium-water retention can be avoided with BB and diuretic. BB can be used to avoid vasodilator-induced tachycardia.
- Representative drug of class: Hydralazine—see table

Common anti-hypertensive drugs listed in alphabetical order per class: ACE-inhibitor, ARB, Beta-blocker, Calcium channel blocker, Diuretics, Extra (less commonly used) drugs: alpha1-blocker, alpha2-agonist, Vasodilators (ie, direct-acting vasodilators)

Drug, starting dose, comments	Benefits	Risks
Lisinopril: 10 mg/d (up to 80 mg/d; max dose in renal failure is 40 mg/d) po; available as 2.5 mg, 5 mg, 10 mg, 20 mg, 30 mg and 40 mg tablets. Lisinopril is an orally administered long-acting angiotensin converting enzyme inhibitor. This is a very commonly used medication in medical practice and hospitals. Half-life is approximately 12 hours; absorption of Lisinopril is approximately 25%, with large intersubject variability (6% to 60%) at all doses tested (5 mg to 80 mg).	☑ Antihypertensive, vasodilatory, anti-aldosterone effect, ☑ Beneficial in CHF, ☑ Beneficial after MI, ☑ Benefits within 1 hour, peak at 6 hours, duration 24 hours; full benefit takes weeks, ☑ Concomitant administration of Lisinopril and hydrochlorothiazide further reduces blood pressure in Black and non-Black patients.	☒ Contraindicated in **pregnancy**—black box warning. Do not use during lactation. ☒ Not to be used in patients with ACEi hypersensitivity, higher risk for **life-threatening angioedema** in African-American patients, ☒ Benefit blunted by NSAIDs, ☒ Can reduce renal filtration of potassium, **lithium**—especially use caution in patients with sCr >2mg/dL. ☒ Removal of angiotensin II negative feedback on renin secretion leads to increased plasma renin activity.
Losartan: 50 mg/d (up to 100 mg/d), available as 25 mg, 50 mg and 100 mg; among the ARBs, this drug provides the additional benefit of reducing uric acid levels, which is relevant for fructose-induced urate-mediated metabolic syndrome; however, a recent clinical trial showed no differences between ramipril and losartan in lowering BP and both drugs showed a trend to improve metabolic parameters such as serum glucose, serum triglycerides, and uric acid equally.[324]	☑ Half-life is 6-9 hours with no plasma accumulation after repeated daily dosing. ☑ Food slows and reduces absorption but this is not clinically significant.	☒ Contraindicated in **pregnancy**—black box warning. Do not use during lactation. ☒ Less effective in African-American patients. ☒ Most of the anti-HTN benefits of Losartan are due to its active carboxylic acid metabolite formed via the action of cytochrome P450 2C9 and 3A4. Generally, 14% of Losartan is converted into the active metabolite; in 1% of patients, they only convert 1% of Losartan to the active metabolite and therefore the drug is inefficacious for them. ☒ Consider caution and lower doses in patients with renal disease: plasma concentrations are increased by 50 to 90% in patients with mild (creatinine clearance of 50 to 74 mL/min) or moderate (creatinine clearance 30 to 49 mL/min) renal insufficiency.

---

[324] Spinar et al; CORD Invesigators. CORD: COmparsion of Recommended Doses of ACE inhibitors and angiotensin II eceptor blockers. *Vnitr Lek*. 2009 May;55(5):481-8

Drug, starting dose, comments	Benefits	Risks
Metoprolol in extended release (Toprol-XL): 25 mg/d; available as 25 mg, 50 mg, 100 mg, 200 mg: This drug is preferred in patients with angina or MI.	☑ Benefits HTN, supraventricular tachyarrhythmia, previous MI, angina, migraine, and anxiety.	☒ Patients must not discontinue drug without tapering dose; sudden discontinuation can cause severe rebound HTN, angina, and MI. ☒ Do not use in patients with bradycardia or heart block. Fatigue, depression, sexual dysfunction, and weight gain can be caused by beta-blockers. ☒ Beta-blockers blunt the physiologic responses to hypoglycemia and are thus associated with hypoglycemic risk in diabetic patients taking glucose-lowering drugs such as insulin.
Amlodipine: 5 mg/d, or start with 2.5 mg/d if being used as a secondary drug or if patient has liver disease; available as 2.5 mg, 5 mg, 10 mg	☑ Amlodipine is indicated for HTN, chronic stable angina, vasospastic angina, and CAD if the ejection fraction is >40%. ☑ Generally safe in HTN patients with asthma, DM, angina, and PVD.	☒ Generally do not use this drug if patient has aortic stenosis, hypersensitivity, severe CAD or severe CHF. ☒ CCB are generally fourth-line drugs after thiazide diuretics, followed by either ACI/ARB and then BB. ☒ Numerous drug interactions, including barbiturates, phenytoin, rifampin, antipsychotics, amiodarone, erythromycin, fluconazole, and the related drugs sildenafil (Viagra) and tadalafil (Cialis).
Furosemide: 20 mg/d po is reasonable starting dose; may increase up to 600 mg/d as needed; available as 20 mg, 40 mg, 80 mg: Dose must be step-wise increased to find patient-specific threshold dose and frequency for individual patient, works for 6 hours (hence the name Lasix); higher doses not better than threshold dose.	☑ This is a very commonly used drug; commonly used PRN for outpatients with edema, including idiopathic edema. ☑ Used for systemic edema, pulmonary edema, CHF, hypercalcemia. ☑ This drug can be used in patients with renal insufficiency, but not with anuria or urethral obstruction	☒ This is a potent diuretic that can cause volume depletion and secondary syncope and hypoperfusion. This is a potent diuretic that can cause electrolyte depletion, including hyponatremia. Scheduled follow-up and laboratory tests for electrolytes are required. ☒ Avoid nighttime use to avoid nocturia.
Hydrochlorothiazide: Started at 12.5-25 mg/d; may use up to 50 mg/d for HTN. When used for the treatment of peripheral edema (rare), the dose is as high as 200 mg/d po qd.	☑ HCTZ is the first-line drug of choice for the routine outpatient management of chronic hypertension. Other drugs such as ACEi/ARB and BB are commonly added as second line agents after the initiation of HCTZ.	☒ HCTZ exacerbates many of the pathophysiologic components of the metabolic syndrome, such as hyperuricemia, potassium insufficiency, hyperglycemia, dyslipidemia, hypomagnesemia and magnesium insufficiency.
Spironolactone: Start HTN dose at 12.5 mg/d; available as 25 mg, 50 mg, 100 mg; dosed as high as 200 mg/d for edema and 400 mg po qd x21-28 days for the diagnosis of hyperaldosteronism.	☑ Useful as a second line or third line drug in the treatment of HTN following the use of HCTZ; also used as second line agent with Lasix. ☑ Used in the treatment of hypokalemia, hyperaldosteronism, ascities, hirsutism, CHF, and edema due to CHF, renal failure, and cirrhosis.	☒ Tumorigenic effect noted in animals suggests that spironolactone may exacerbate cancer and should therefore be used sparingly. ☒ Hyperkalemia is a real clinical concern associated with potassium-sparing diuretics such as spironolactone.

<u>**Common anti-hypertensive drugs listed in alphabetical order per class**</u>—*continued*

Drug, starting dose, comments	Benefits	Risks
<u>**Prazosin**</u>: start with 1 mg/d for the treatment of HTN; available as 1 mg, 2 mg, 5 mg; highest recommended dose for HTN is 15 mg/d.	☑ Used in the treatment of HTN, prostate enlargement (1 mg po bid).	☒ First-dose syncope and hypotension are common with prazosin.
<u>**Clonidine**</u>: start at 0.1 mg bid for HTN; max dose is 2.4 mg; available as 0.1 mg, 0.2 mg, and 0.3 mg for oral administration, also available for injection.	☑ **Useful for acute and severe HTN; not routinely used for routine chronic HTN.** Can be administered orally or intravenously for the rapid reduction of severe hypertension. ☑ Epidural administration is used in the treatment of severe pain.	☒ **High risk of rebound HTN following noncompliance or missed/skipped dose.** Taper dose over 4 days to reduce risk of rebound HTN.
<u>**Hydralazine**</u>: oral dose for moderate-severe HTN is 10-50 mg po starting with 10 mg po qid for 2-4 days then 25 mg po qid for 1 week; max dose is 300 mg po qd25-150 mg twice daily; available for oral administration 10 mg, 25 mg, 50 mg, 100 mg. For acute HTN, the parenteral dose is 10-20 mg IM or IV each 2-4 hours; switch to oral dosing as soon as possible.	☑ Monotherapy is generally only used in the treatment of pregnancy-induced HTN and moderate-severe treatment-resistant HTN. This drug is commonly used in hospitals for the treatment of pregnancy-induced HTN and pre-eclampsia.	☒ Side effects include headache due to vasodilation and drug-induced systemic lupus erythematosus (SLE). May also cause neutropenia and other blood disorders. ☒ **Warning**: Vasodilators cause reflex tachycardia that can precipitate MI and CHF.

Nutritional Treatments for Hypertension

This article was originally published in *Naturopathy Digest* in 2006
naturopathydigest.com/archives/2006/nov/vasquez.php

<u>**Introduction**</u>: Clinical problems associated with hypertension can be divided into two categories dependent upon the severity and duration of the elevated blood pressure. Mild elevations in blood pressure that are sustained over a period of many years and decades increases the risk of atherosclerosis, stroke, myocardial infarction, heart failure, and renal failure. Acute elevations in blood pressure, even if sustained for a relatively short time, can cause hypertensive encephalopathy, stroke, retinal hemorrhage, acute myocardial infarction, and acute left ventricular failure with pulmonary edema. Many different etiologies exist for hypertension, including but not limited to metabolic syndrome, hypothyroidism, renal failure, and adverse drug effects; the scope of this article is limited to uncomplicated prehypertension and Stage One Hypertension. Obviously, the goals of therapy are to bring the blood pressure down into the normal range and to prevent end-organ damage, especially to heart, brain, eyes, and kidneys.

<u>**Diagnosis**</u>: Blood pressure is assessed with a sphygmomanometer. Elevated blood pressure is a clinical finding that—if confirmed by at least two readings—leads to the diagnosis of hypertension.

<u>**Management**</u>: Guidelines for the assessment and therefore management of hypertension change periodically based on new consensus and new research data. "Prehypertension" or early hypertension begins at 120 systolic over 80 diastolic, while "Stage One hypertension" is in the range of 140/90 - 160/100. Patients beyond Stage One

Hypertension or those with a complex clinical presentation should generally be co-managed pharmaceutically (at least initially); a table describing hypertensive categories is provided below (Table 1). Doctors who choose to manage hypertension for their patients must include proper history, physical examination, laboratory assessment (e.g., chemistry/metabolic panel, urinalysis, thyroid and cardiovascular panels), and the treatment plan must include frequent follow-up (e.g., every 2-4 weeks) until the problem is resolved. If effectiveness cannot be obtained, sustained, or documented then the patient should receive both verbal and written referral to another physician, particularly an internist or cardiologist.

Table 1: Hypertension categorization and management*	
Prehypertension: >120/80	These patients are essentially normal but might take steps to lower blood pressure to a safer level.
Stage One: 140/90 - 160/100	These are perfect candidates for diet/lifestyle/integrative treatments. As with any condition: high-risk, noncompliant, and nonresponsive patients are referred for medical management.
Stage Two: 160/100 - 210/120 without symptoms and without end-organ damage (i.e., no renal damage, headache, or edema).	All integrative treatments can be used; drugs might also be used initially to reduce hypertension. Nonmedical/nonprescribing clinicians should generally refer or co-manage these patients.
Urgent: SBP ≥ 220 or DBP 125 - 129, or Stage 2 with symptoms or end-organ damage.	Immediate referral for drug treatment is appropriate.
Emergency: >220/130 is an emergency	Emergency: Intravenous medications in a hospital or urgent care clinic
* Additional considerations that affect treatment and management: Insulin resistance / pre-diabetes / metabolic syndrome: dyslipidemia / high cholesterol, obesity, inactivity, tobacco use, concomitant diseases, personal and family medical history, other chief complaints and clinical and laboratory findings.	

Nutritional treatments for hypertension: Nutritional treatments for hypertension include the following considerations, which can generally be used in combination (rather than in isolation, as studied in the research). These will be listed and discussed in order of general effectiveness (see Table 2).

1. Short-term supervised fasting: Short-term inpatient supervised fasting appears to be the most effective treatment for chronic hypertension that has ever been documented. Working closely with his multidisciplinary team, pioneering chiropractic physician Alan Goldhamer DC documented reductions in hypertension of 60/17 in patients with severe hypertension and reductions of 37/13 in patients with moderate hypertension.[325,326,327] Generally the program begins with 4-7 days of a raw vegetarian diet followed by 1-2 weeks of fasting and concluded with reintroduction of a vegetarian and health-promoting diet. Laboratory tests and professional supervision help ensure patient safety.

2. Healthy diet and exercise: Health-promoting diets such as either Paleo- and Mediterranean-style diets can lower blood pressure by as much as 17/13 according to some reports. Please see my previous articles in this magazine for description of the "supplemented Paleo-Mediterranean Diet."[328]

3. CoQ10: CoQ-10 in doses of 100-225 mg/day can lower blood pressure quite effectively, as documented in several clinical studies, some of which showed that CoQ10 is more effective and safer than the use of antihypertensive drugs.[329,330,331] Reductions in blood pressure are generally in the range of 17/12 and are dose-

[325] Goldhamer A, et al. Medically supervised water-only fasting in the treatment of hypertension. *J Manipulative Physiol Ther* 2001 Jun;24(5):335-9
[326] Goldhamer AC, et al. Medically supervised water-only fasting in the treatment of borderline hypertension. *J Altern Complement Med.* 2002 Oct;8(5):643-50
[327] Goldhamer AC. Initial cost of care results in medically supervised water-only fasting for treating high blood pressure and diabetes. *J Altern Complement Med.* 2002 Dec;8(6):696-7
[328] Vasquez A. Five-Part Nutritional Protocol that Produces Consistently Positive Results.*NutrWellness*2005 Sep
[329] "RESULTS: The mean reduction in systolic blood pressure of the CoQ-treated group was 17.8 +/- 7.3 mm Hg (mean +/- SEM). None of the patients exhibited orthostatic blood pressure changes. CONCLUSIONS: Our results suggest CoQ may be safely offered to hypertensive patients as an alternative treatment option." Burke BE, Neuenschwander R, Olson RD. Randomized, double-blind, placebo-controlled trial of coenzyme Q10 in isolated systolic hypertension. *South Med J.* 2001 Nov;94(11):1112-7
[330] "These findings indicate that treatment with coenzyme Q10 decreases blood pressure possibly by decreasing oxidative stress and insulin response in patients with known hypertension receiving conventional antihypertensive drugs." Singh RB, Niaz MA, Rastogi SS, Shukla PK, Thakur AS. Effect of hydrosoluble coenzyme Q10 on blood pressures and insulin resistance in hypertensive patients with coronary artery disease. *J Hum Hypertens.* 1999 Mar;13(3):203-8
[331] "...51% of patients came completely off of between one and three antihypertensive drugs at an average of 4.4 months after starting CoQ10." Langsjoen P, Langsjoen P, Willis R, Folkers K. Treatment of essential hypertension with coenzyme Q10. *Mol Aspects Med.* 1994;15 Suppl:S265-72

dependent. A patient who does not respond to 100 mg per day may respond very well to 200 mg per day. Since it is a fat-soluble nutrient, CoQ10 should be administered with dietary fat and/or consumed in a "pre-emulsified" form to enhance absorption which is a prerequisite for clinical effectiveness. Several trials have been reported showing enhanced absorption of CoQ10 when administered in pre-emulsified form. CoQ10 is very safe, and drug interactions are rare; caution should be used in patients taking coumadin.

4. <u>Sodium restriction</u>: Clinical responsiveness to low-sodium diets ranges from minimal to a maximal reduction in the range of 22/14 - 16/9.[332] Contraindications to low-sodium diet are uncommon (e.g., hyponatremia); low-sodium diets should generally be a component of all anti-hypertensive treatment plans.

5. <u>Vitamin D and calcium</u>: Vitamin D3 (cholecalciferol) and calcium supplementation can reduce blood pressure in hypertensive patients by approximately 13/7.[333] As I have discussed in extensive detail elsewhere, a reasonable dose of vitamin D3 for adults is in the range of 2,000 - 4,000 IU per day, and doctors new to vitamin D therapy should read my clinical monograph published in 2004 and available on-line.[334] The most important drug interaction with vitamin D is seen with hydrochlorothiazide, a commonly-used antihypertensive diuretic that promotes hypercalcemia; vitamin D therapy in patients taking hydrochlorothiazide must be implemented slowly, with professional supervision, and with weekly laboratory monitoring of serum calcium. Vitamin D probably corrects hypertension via several mechanisms, including but not limited to increased absorption of magnesium and reduction in intracellular calcium, as I described previously in this magazine.[335] Since vitamin D absorption decreases with age and in patients with intestinal disease (including dysbiosis[336]), absorption of fat-soluble vitamin D3 is enhanced when administered in pre-emulsified form.[337]

6. <u>Prescription drugs</u>: Use of the nutritional treatments described in this article can complement or replace antihypertensive drug therapy in many patients. When used singly, prescription antihypertensive drugs average a reduction in blood pressure of approximately 12/6. Initial reductions of 20/10 require combination therapy, according to a review article published in *American Family Physician* in 2003.[338]

7. <u>Exercise</u>: Moderate exercise can reduce blood pressure by approximately 7/7 in the short term. Longer-term exercise, particularly along with diet improvements and weight loss, can result in synergistic and curative benefits. Patients who have been sedentary for years and those with probable or documented cardiovascular disease should be evaluated by a physician and ECG before beginning an exercise program.

8. <u>Fish oil</u>: Fish oil supplementation had been shown to reduce blood pressure by approximately 3/2. For reasons that I have detailed elsewhere[339], fish oil should be co-administered with a source of GLA such as borage oil in order to maximize effectiveness and minimize subtle biochemical adverse effects. Importantly, fish oil is safer, less expensive, and more effective than "statin" antihypercholesterolemic drug treatment for reducing total and cardiovascular mortality.

9. <u>Food allergy elimination</u>: According to a clinical study of migraineurs published in *The Lancet*, identification and avoidance of food allergens can normalize blood pressure in hypertensive migraine patients.[340] The anti-hypertensive response to food allergy avoidance can be seen clinically even in patients who do not have migraine or other manifestations of allergy, but the more allergic symptoms that are seen and the more complete the response to allergy elimination, the more likely is a reduction in blood pressure.

---

[332] "The average fall in blood pressure from the highest to the lowest sodium intake was 16/9 mm Hg." MacGregor GA, Markandu ND, Sagnella GA, Singer DR, Cappuccio FP. Double-blind study of three sodium intakes and long-term effects of sodium restriction in essential hypertension. *Lancet*. 1989 Nov 25;2(8674):1244-7

[333] "A short-term supplementation with vitamin D(3) and calcium is more effective in reducing SBP than calcium alone. Inadequate vitamin D(3) and calcium intake could play a contributory role in the pathogenesis and progression of hypertension and cardiovascular disease in elderly women." Pfeifer et al. Effects of a short-term vitamin D(3) and calcium supplementation on blood pressure and parathyroid hormone levels in elderly women. *J Clin Endocrinol Metab*. 2001 Apr;86(4):1633-7

[334] Vasquez A, Manso G, Cannell J. The clinical importance of vitamin D (cholecalciferol). *Altern Ther Health Med*. 2004 Sep-Oct;10(5):28-36

[335] Vasquez A. Intracellular Hypercalcinosis. *Naturopathy Digest* 2006, September

[336] Vasquez A. Nutritional and Botanical Treatments against "Silent Infections" and Gastrointestinal Dysbiosis. *Nutritional Perspectives* 2006; January

[337] Vasquez A. Subphysiologic Doses of Vitamin D are Subtherapeutic: Comment on the Study by The Record Trial Group. *Lancet* 2005 published online May 6

[338] Magill MK, Gunning K, Saffel-Shrier S, Gay C. New developments in the management of hypertension. *Am Fam Physician*. 2003 Sep 1;68(5):853-8

[339] Vasquez A. New Insights into Fatty Acid Supplementation and Its Effect on Eicosanoid Production and Genetic Expression. *Nutritional Perspectives* 2005; January: 5-16

[340] Grant EC. Food allergies and migraine. *Lancet*. 1979 May 5;1(8123):966-9

Table 2: Anti-hypertensive effectiveness relative to standard drug treatment for outpatient chronic HTN	
1. **Short-term supervised fasting**	-60/17 for severe HTN and -37/13 for moderate HTN
2. **Healthy diet and exercise**	-17/13
3. **CoQ10 100-225 mg/day**	-17/12
4. **Sodium restriction**	Reduction ranges from -16/9 up to -22/14
5. **Vitamin D and calcium**	Reductions up to -13/7 in vitamin D-deficient hypertensive patients
6. <u>Prescription drugs</u>	-12/6 Reductions of -20/10 require two-drug therapy
	"Initial combination therapy is suggested by JNC 7 for patients whose blood pressure is more than 20/10 mm Hg above their goal blood pressure." *Am Fam Physician* 2003 Sep
7. Exercise	-7/7
8. Fish oil	-3/2
9. Food allergy elimination	Variable response ranging from insignificant to curative

Conclusions: Many nutritional treatments for hypertension are documented in the research literature, and several of these treatments appear safer and more cost-effective than pharmaceutical antihypertensive drugs. Furthermore, the synergistic use of the nutritional and lifestyle interventions described above—e.g., supplemented Paleo-Mediterranean diet along with exercise, fish oil, vitamin D, CoQ10, and sodium restriction-results in clinical benefits that far exceed the results published in the single-intervention clinical trials that have documented the effectiveness of the individual components. The major drug interaction that one must look out for is the combination of vitamin D with hydrochlorothiazide. Switching from pharmaceutical drugs to nutrients for the management of hypertension requires diligent follow-up, informed consent, and documentation of beneficial clinical response and should be undertaken only by skilled and experienced clinicians.

Promoting Unhealthy Eating: Proatherosclerotic Recipes Endorsed by the US National Heart, Lung, and Blood Institute (NHLBI)

The following is a partial list of atherosclerosis-promoting recipes listed under the title "Stay Young at Heart: Cooking the Heart-Healthy Way"[341] advocated on the website of the NHLBI in December 2009; *horror of horrors— these recipes are still posted and advocated in 2015*. Notice the lack of nutrient density, the emphasis on simple carbohydrates, the lack of raw foods, paucity of phytonutrients, and the frequent use of baking with oil to create the effect of frying:

- <u>Stir-fried beef</u> with boiled potatoes and white rice
- <u>Beef stroganoff</u> with 6 cups of cooked macaroni pasta
- <u>Crispy oven-fried chicken</u> cooked in cornflakes and buttermilk
- <u>Classic macaroni and cheese</u>
- <u>Candied yams</u> with brown sugar, margarine, white flour, and orange juice
- <u>Oven French fries</u> (white potatoes oven-fried in vegetable oil)
- <u>White rice</u> cooked with vegetable oil and salt
- <u>Sunshine (white) rice</u> cooked with vegetable oil, orange juice, and lemon juice
- <u>Homestyle biscuits</u> made from white flour, salt, and sugar
- <u>Banana-nut bread</u> made from mashed ripe bananas, low-fat buttermilk, packed brown sugar, margarine, all-purpose white flour, egg and salt
- <u>Apricot-orange bread</u> made from dried apricots, margarine, white sugar, egg, white flour, dry milk powder, salt and orange juice
- <u>Apple coffee cake</u> made with peeled apples (please note that >90% of the antioxidants contained in apples are in the peel—thus when the peel is removed, virtually all that remains is antioxidant-poor carbohydrate), one cup of sugar, one cup of dark raisins, one-quarter cup vegetable oil, 1 egg, and two-and-a-half cups of sifted all-purpose white flour

---

[341] US National Heart, Lung, and Blood Institute (NHLBI). Stay Young at Heart: Cooking the Heart-Healthy Way. nhlbi.nih.gov/health/public/heart/other/syah/index.htm Accessed December 23, 2009. This index of recipes has been relocated to nhlbi.nih.gov/health/resources/heart/syah-html/; reviewed 2015 Nov.

- <u>Frosted cake</u> with 2 1/4 cups cake flour, 4 tablespoons margarine, 1 1/4 cups sugar, 4 eggs, low fat cream cheese, and 2 cups sifted confectioners' sugar!
- <u>Tropical fruit compote</u> with sugar
- <u>Peach cobbler</u> with sugar, white flour, margarine, canned peaches "packed in juice", peach nectar, and cornstarch
- <u>Rice pudding</u> with white rice, 3 cups of skim milk, and 2/3 cup sugar

> **The war is not meant to be won**
>
> "Their lives are dedicated to world conquest, but they also know that it is necessary that the war should continue everlastingly and without victory."
>
> George Orwell in *Nineteen Eighty-four (1984)*.
> Chapter 3, *War is Peace*, approximately page 249

The list goes on to include many other proatherosclerotic and prodiabetic meals. Any reasonable person—*the general public has the option but healthcare professionals have the obligation*—might ask why **the US National Heart, Lung, and Blood Institute has been promoting a diet plan that is ensured to contribute to the pandemics of hypertension, obesity, and diabetes mellitus.** Actually, asking the question simply delays and allows for additional delay of the obvious solution.

Thinking Outside the (Pill) Box: Is the "Battle Against Hypertension and Diabetes" Truly Meant to be "Won" for Patients...or for the Drug Companies?

<u>**The Most Profitable "Wars" are the ones that are Fought Indefinitely and which Require Reliance on Private Industry**</u>: As with most modern sociopolitical fights, wars, and missions, a keen observer (or any high-school student who read George Orwell's classic novel *1984*) might question whether the current "**Mission: To Combat High Blood Pressure in America**"[342] is actually meant to ever be won. The US National Heart, Lung, and Blood Institute (NHLBI) invokes the language of battle, e.g., "to **mobilize** all Americans in the **fight against high blood pressure** and reduce the more than 1 million heart attacks, strokes, and kidney failure cases that it causes each year. The CDC and the NHLBI have **joined forces** to **disseminate** these materials…"[343] Ironically, the NHLBI's document entitled "Physician Fact Sheet: What Every Physician Should Know" hp2010.nhlbihin.net/mission/partner/physcian_factsheet.pdf **contains zero practical information on diet, exercise, or nutritional supplementation.** Likewise, the document under the heading "Real Possibilities for America's Health Care Providers"[344] provides nothing that a clinician or patient could use to authentically correct the common causes of HTN; it provides near-meaningless mention of "diet and exercise" accompanied by a photo of people sitting at a table with food and encourages that doctors "Support Adherence to Treatment" accompanied by a photo of a woman taking pills.

<u>**"Common Objectives" …with Drug Companies**</u>: For more than a decade, the American Heart Association has been "advised" by their "Pharmaceutical Roundtable" (PRT) comprised of **monolithic drug companies each of which must pay a least $1 million per year for each 3-year term of membership.**[345] According to the American Heart Association's website in a document last reviewed in August 2009[346], "The American Heart Association Pharmaceutical Roundtable (PRT) is a strategic coalition of 10 leading pharmaceutical companies and association volunteers and staff. It allows our association and members of the **pharmaceutical industry** to identify and pursue **common objectives** to improve cardiovascular health in the United States through research, patient education, and public and professional programs." Current (or recent) members of the American Heart Association Pharmaceutical Roundtable include:

1. AstraZeneca L.P.
2. Eli Lilly and Company
3. Bristol-Myers Squibb Company
4. GlaxoSmithKline
5. Merck/Schering-Plough Pharmaceuticals
6. Merck Pharmaceuticals
7. Novartis Pharmaceuticals Corporation
8. Pfizer, Inc.
9. Sanofi-Aventis
10. Takeda Pharmaceuticals

---

[342] National Heart, Lung, and Blood Institute (NHLBI). The Mission: To Combat High Blood Pressure in America hp2010.nhlbihin.net/mission/ Accessed December 22, 2009
[343] State Heart Disease and Stroke Prevention Program Addresses High Blood Pressure. cdc.gov/dhdsp/library/fs_state_hbp.htm Accessed December 22, 2009
[344] National Heart, Lung, and Blood Institute (NHLBI). nhlbi.nih.gov/health/prof/heart/hbp/mp/mp_health.htm Accessed December 22, 2009
[345] "Each industry participant of the PRT will sign a separate agreement with AHA that will be binding only between the AHA and that individual industry member. The agreements will commit each industry member to contribute $1,000,000 per year for three years." Letter dated March 20, 1998 from Joel I. Klein (Assistant Attorney General), US Department of Justice Antitrust Division. justice.gov/atr/public/busreview/1608.htm Accessed December 23, 2009
[346] americanheart.org/presenter.jhtml?identifier=2366 Accessed December 23, 2009

Diabetes Mellitus Type-2 & Metabolic Syndrome

<table>
<tr><td>

Introduction:

Long ago and far away are the epochs and perspectives holding that "adult onset diabetes" resulted simply from overeating and underexcercising; we now appreciate powerful contributions from dysbiosis, mitochondrial impairment, systemic inflammation, and persistent organic pollutants (POPs) such as pesticides and plastics. The clinical phenotype of diabetes is likely changing as pollutant-induced mitochondrial dysfunction, exacerbated by gastrointestinal dysbiosis from consumption of artificial foods/sweeteners and hidden consumption of glyphosate, leads to massive preclinical and prediabetic metabolic impairment, later manifesting as insulin resistance and overt diabetes. As such, pharmacocentric treatments—ie, the drug model of treating diabetes—that focus simply and solely on reducing glucose levels are intellectually absurd and scientifically ridiculous; hyperglycemia is simply the outward manifestation—the signal, the alarm—of underlying metabolic impairment and defective cellular signaling. Outside of urgent and emergency situations, treatment of insulin resistance should be founded upon dietary improvement (e.g., carbohydrate restriction, which is clinically superior to insulin therapy), microbiome modification (e.g., especially gut flora modification, such as with berberine, which is superior to drug treatment with metformin), mitochondrial support (e.g., CoQ10 is a superior intervention for long-term management of hypertension), and pesticide/pollution avoidance and depuration. Metabolic syndrome is a clinical cluster of several components—always including hyperglycemia, dyslipidemia, abdominal obesity, and hypertension, and per more broad/inclusive criteria also encompassing inflammation and hypercoagulability—which sum to effect accelerated atherosclerosis, hence the related term cardiometabolic syndrome. Because of this, a wide range of cardiovascular risk factors are discussed in this section, with treatments for each.

</td></tr>
</table>

Description & Pathophysiology:

- Origins of terms: The term "diabetes mellitus" is from ancient Greek, *diabetes* means "to pass through" while *mellit* refers to "honey" or "sugar." Obviously, these are references to the voluminous output of urine seen passing through untreated diabetic patients who are experiencing hyperglycemic diuresis due to the osmotic effect of excess glucose in renal filtrate.

- Introduction: Diabetes mellitus (DM) can refer to any pathological states characterized by chronic hyperglycemia. Generally, DM is divided into type-1 (DM-1), which typically begins in childhood following autoimmune destruction of pancreatic beta cells leading to insulinopenia and the resulting hyperglycemia, and type-2 (DM-2), which typically begins in adulthood as a result of an interplay of genes, poor diet, insufficient exercise, numerous vitamin and mineral deficiencies, and a myriad of metabolic malfunctions including most prominently the phenomenon of peripheral tissue insulin resistance. Thus, we could oversimplify these disorders by saying that DM-1 is a pancreatic failure of insulin output while DM-2 is a tissue failure of insulin receptivity; in both instances, hyperglycemia is the most obvious physiologic result, and hyperglycemia-induced pathophysiologic disorders are the result. Clinicians should appreciate that the insulinopenic clinical picture of DM-1 can be produced by any condition that causes destruction of pancreatic beta-cells (e.g., chronic or acute pancreatitis, iron overload and hemochromatosis [see chapter from this textbook on iron overload]) and that the clinical picture of peripheral insulin resistance can occur secondary to acromegaly, severe acute illness and excess internal production or exogenous administration of corticosteroids.

- Clinical picture of DM-2: Insulin levels are always low in DM-1, whereas in DM-2 the insulin levels typically start high (fasting hyperinsulinemia) as the pancreas produces more insulin in an appropriate physiologic response to hyperglycemia; later as DM-2 progresses, pancreatic output of insulin progressively fails, thus exacerbating the hyperglycemia. DM-2 and "the metabolic syndrome" (MetSyn, also "syndrome X") have practically become synonymous over the last few years, due to the high concordance of these two clinical entities. DM-2 can, however, exist without the full picture of the two-part (up to six-part) definition of the metabolic syndrome. Various definitions of the metabolic syndrome include at least the first 4 of the following, with increasing appreciation of the additional last two characteristics: ❶ central adiposity, abdominal obesity, ❷ hyperglycemia, ❸ dyslipidemia, ❹ hypertension, ❺ systemic inflammation, and ❻ hypercoagulability. Metabolic syndrome is more aggressive and malignant than simple diabetes mellitus because of the former's inclusion of greater degrees of dyslipidemia, oxidative stress, and systemic inflammation; thus, these patients need to be managed assertively. Because the abbreviation "MS" is synonymous with multiple sclerosis, the contraction MetSyn will be used here for expediency when discussing metabolic syndrome.

- Pathoetiology of DM-2/MetSyn: Regarding DM-2/MetSyn, a more detailed pathoetiologic list of phenomena that contribute to peripheral insulin resistance includes ❶ genetic predisposition, ❷ sedentary lifestyle, ❸ caloric excess, ❹ sarcopenia, ❺ micronutrient deficiencies (especially magnesium, cholecalciferol, chromium), ❻ metabolic perturbations due to consumption of artificial "junk foods" (e.g., fructose excess, overconsumption of *trans* fatty acids), ❼ xenobiotic exposure and accumulation with resultant activation of the aryl hydrocarbon receptor which downregulates expression of peripheral GLUT-4 glucose-insulin receptors thus leading directly to peripheral insulin resistance, and ❽ systemic inflammation, which contributes directly to insulin resistance. Chronic hyperglycemia places constant demand and therefore physiologic strain on pancreatic beta cells, leading to what has been referred to in earlier literature as "high output failure." Hyperglycemia itself is toxic to pancreatic beta-cells such that regardless of the original cause of the hyperglycemia, the final common pathway of disease progression includes impaired production of insulin, thus exacerbating the hyperglycemia. The link between diabetes and obesity is so strong that the two are increasingly merged into the single term "diabesity."[347]

Cardiovascular risk:
Inflammation, hyperglycemia, oxidant stress, dyslipidemia, hypertension, peripheral and central atherosclerosis

Infection risk:
Counterinflammation, immunocompromise, predisposition to gingival infections and skin lesions, poor tissue healing

Diabetes Mellitus type-2 & Metabolic Syndrome

Organ damage / tissue injury:
Renal failure, diabetic neuropathy, eye damage (cataracts, retinopathy), vasculopathy

Nutritional deficiencies and excesses:
Excess carbohydrate and arachidonate; deficiencies of vitamin D3, zinc, ascorbate, chromium, selenium, magnesium and numerous other vitamins, minerals, and phytonutrients; consequences include depression and infection

Venn Diagram Showing 4 Important Clinical Considerations for the Management of DM-2/MetSyn: Clinicians should consider these 4 priorities when planning a risk-management strategy for patients with DM-2/MetSyn: 1) cardiovascular risk, 2) infection risk, 3) organ damage including blindness, renal failure, and neuropathy, and 4) the underlying nutritional imbalances and dietary carbohydrate excess that underlie these pathophysiologic processes. What underlies the nutritional imbalances and carbohydrate excess?—The answer to this question will vary somewhat per patient, but clinicians should assess the psychoemotional environment that has enabled a patient to adopt the unhealthy lifestyle and mindset that allowed this situation to develop in the first place. To get to the core of these issues, integrative clinicians should appreciate concepts such as the reciprocal causality between self-esteem and self-efficacy, as well as the importance of values, self-assertiveness, self-responsibility, living purposefully and consciously (reviewed by Branden[348]) and how these core psychoemotional issues can be integrated into a program for behavior change (reviewed by Prochaska[349]).

---

[347] "Lifestyle is an expression of individual choices and their interaction with the environment and is closely associated with risks for obesity, diabetes, and cardiovascular disorders. If taken cumulatively this syndrome may be referred to as "diabesity." Mobley CC. Lifestyle interventions for diabesity. *Compend Contin Educ Dent*. 2004 Mar:207-18
[348] Branden N. *The Six Pillars of Self-Esteem*. Bantam Books, 1994
[349] Prochaska JO, Norcross JC, and DiClemente CC. *Changing for Good*. William Morrow and Company; 1994

- <u>Prevalence</u>: In the US, approximately 21 million Americans have DM with about 15 million cases diagnosed and another 6 million undiagnosed. DM-1 accounts for about 5%, with the remaining 95% due to DM-2 including MetSyn and less commonly DM secondary to drugs (e.g., exogenous corticosteroids) and diseases such as acromegaly. Costs attributed to DM are approximately $132 billion per year in direct and indirect costs.

Clinical Presentation:

- The clinical presentation is extremely variable, which is why diabetes mellitus (like hemochromatosis and syphilis) is known as a "great imitator."
- DM/MetSyn patients may be asymptomatic and "apparently healthy" or may have the following:
  - Cataracts, retinopathy, macular edema
  - Recurrent infections (most commonly presenting as gingivitis, yeast vaginitis, and skin infections)
  - Underweight with DM-1
  - Obesity (especially abdominal/visceral)
  - Peripheral neuropathy (paresthesias, burning, tingling, insensate injuries and ulcerations)
  - Slow-healing wounds
  - Dyslipidemia
  - Hypertension
  - CVD (MI, stroke)
  - PVD (peripheral vascular disease)
  - Erectile dysfunction in men
  - Menstrual disorders in women: PCOS, infertility, menstrual irregularity
  - <u>Hyperglycemic crises</u>: These require emergency management in a hospital/ambulance setting.
  - <u>Diabetic ketoacidosis (DKA)</u>: Classic presentation for DM-1 characterized by the triad of ❶ **hyperglycemia, ❷ ketosis, ❸ acidosis**; 20% of DKA presentations represent new DM-1 cases. 80% of DKA presentations occur in previously diagnosed diabetics who had an acute failure of glucose control and resultant hyperglycemia due to insulin noncompliance, infection such as UTI or pneumonia, alcohol abuse, trauma or cardiopulmonary insult. The onset of DKA is typically rapid (<24h) and presents with nausea, vomiting, and abdominal pain; thus the presentation of DM DKA resembles other presentations of acute abdomen, such as pancreatitis, food poisoning, or infectious gastroenteritis. Clinical signs in addition to the triad of hyperglycemia, ketosis, and acidosis include **Kussmaul breathing** (deep labored respirations as a sign of respiratory compensation for metabolic acidosis), **fruity acetone breath, dehydration, and mental status changes**. "Paradoxical hyperkalemia" in response to acidosis may be present; acidotic patients are generally depleted of potassium, and the hyperkalemia (shift of potassium from *intra*cellular to *extra*cellular) is a buffering response to the acidosis. A "normal" potassium level in a setting of acidosis potentially portends severe hypokalemia, especially upon correction of the acidosis.
  - <u>Hyperosmolar hyperglycemic state (HHS) or hyperosmolar hyperglycemic nonketotic coma (HHNK)</u>: Occurs with severe uncontrolled DM-2; plasma glucose exceeds 800-1,000 mg/dL but ketosis and acidosis are not present with hyperosmolar hyperglycemia. Massive glucosuria leads to osmotic diuresis and resultant severe dehydration and hyperosmolarity; the clinical presentation primarily includes severe dehydration and complications from hypovolemia as well as mental status changes including disorientation, obtundation, seizures, visual loss, paralysis and focal neurologic deficits, and coma.

Major Differential Diagnoses:

- **Corticosteroid iatrogenesis**: Assess medication history and intake.
- **Post-pancreatitis insulinopenia**: Assess for history of pancreatitis or its classic precursors (e.g., alcoholism, hypertriglyceridemia, common bile duct obstruction). Measure serum insulin and use CT imaging of pancreas as indicated.
- **Iron overload and hemochromatosis**: Assess serum ferritin and transferrin saturation in all patients with DM and MetSyn. These patients have a greater-than-average incidence of iron overload, both primary and secondary forms.
- **Acromegaly**: Clinical evaluation for classic physical manifestations; measure serum insulin-like growth factor-1 (IGF-1) as a marker for growth hormone overproduction.
- **Diabetes insipidus**: Polyuria without the hyperglycemia due to failure of secretion or reception of antidiuretic hormone (ADH, same as arginine vasopressin). Inquire about lithium use, previous head injury or other intracranial lesion. Hypernatremia may be present; careful rehydration is warranted.

Clinical Assessments:

- **History/subjective**: The classic history associated with untreated DM is either ❶ asymptomatic, ❷ the presentation of a complicating manifestation such as infection, renal failure, or tissue ischemia (e.g., stroke or MI), ❸ or the textbook presentation of polyuria, polydipsia, and hyperphagia which are all complications hyperglycemia/hyperglucosuria. Any history of recurrent yeast infections in females and balantitis in men warrants testing for DM.

- **Physical Examination/Objective**: The physical examination focuses on assessment for the presence and severity of the expected complications from the disease.

  - Body mass index, assessment of body habitus: To calculate the "Body Mass Index" simply chart height and weight to determine the BMI number. Numbers greater than 25 correlate with being "overweight" while numbers greater than 30 meet the criteria for "obesity." BMI determinations may not be reflective of disease risk for people who are pregnant, highly muscular, or for young children or the frail elderly. Waist-hip ratios can also be determined. Overweight patients need to be made acutely aware of their body weight and the use of body weight as an indicator of compliance and progress toward disease regression and health restoration. Excess weight of only a few pounds/kilograms significantly increases the risk for diabetes, so patients should be reminded that *"Every pound/kilogram counts."* Mobley wrote, "An increase in body weight of approximately 2.2 pounds (1 kg) has been shown to increase risk for diabetes by 4.5%."[350]

    Adipose tissue is biologically active, promoting systemic inflammation and "estrogen dominance", thereby promoting the development of inflammatory and malignant diseases such as psoriasis and cancers of the breast, prostate, and colon. The previous view that fat (adipose) tissue was merely serving as an inert and inactive depot for lipid/energy storage is now replaced with the view that adipose tissue is biologically-active, influencing overall health via complex mechanisms that are biochemical-inflammatory-endocrinologic and not merely mechanical (i.e., excess weight, excess mass).[351] **Excess fat tissue— especially visceral/abdominal adipose—creates a systemic proinflammatory state** evidenced most readily by the elevations in hsCRP commonly seen in patients with obesity and the metabolic syndrome.[352] Adipokines are cytokines secreted by adipose tissue and include tumor necrosis factor-alpha, interleukin-6, and leptin—a cytokine derived from fat cells that promotes inflammation and immune activation; levels are higher in obese patients and decrease after weight loss. Obese patients also appear to have "leptin resistance" with regard to the suppression of appetite by leptin. **Adipose creates excess estrogens;** concomitant hyperglycemia increases androgen production[353], and these androgens are subsequently converted to estrogens by aromatase in the adipose tissue. For example, the adrenal gland makes androstenedione, which can be converted by aromatase in adipose tissue into estrone.[354] These proinflammatory and hormonal perturbations manifest clinically as an increased risk for breast, prostate, endometrial, colon and gallbladder cancers, insulin resistance and cardiovascular disease. The combination of inflammation, reduced testosterone, and elevated estrogen is also predisposes toward the development of autoimmune/inflammatory diseases.

  - **Obesity**: Obesity is a major risk factor for cardiovascular disease, cancer, diabetes mellitus, depression, joint degeneration and pain. Obese people also commonly report difficulties with performing daily activities, and they also report higher rates of depression and social isolation than do people of normal weight. "Body Mass Index" is a clinically valuable measure of height-weight proportionality and therefore adiposity, since an excess of height-proportionate weight is more commonly due to excess adipose than to excess muscle. To calculate BMI simply chart height and weight in the table below. Numbers greater than 25 correlate with being "overweight" while numbers greater than 30 meet the criteria for "obesity." BMI

---

[350] Mobley CC. Lifestyle interventions for "diabesity": the state of the science. *Compend Contin Educ Dent.* 2004 Mar;25(3):207-8, 211-2, 214-8

[351] "The fat cell is a true endocrine cell that secretes a variety of factors, including metabolites such as lactate, fatty acids, prostaglandin derivatives and a variety of peptides, including cytokines (leptin, tumor necrosis factor, interleukin-1 and -6, adiponectin), angiotensinogen, complement D (adipsin), plasminogen activator inhibitor-1 and undoubtedly many others." Bray GA. The underlying basis for obesity: relationship to cancer. *J Nutr.* 2002 Nov;132(11 Suppl):3451S-3455S

[352] "Our results indicate a strong relationship between adipocytokines and inflammatory markers, and suggest that cytokines secreted by adipose tissue could play a role in increased inflammatory proteins secretion by the liver." Maachi M, et al. Systemic low-grade inflammation is related to both circulating and adipose tissue TNFalpha, leptin and IL-6 levels in obese women. *Int J Obes Relat Metab Disord.* 2004;28:993-7

[353] Christensen et al. Elevated levels of sex hormones and sex hormone binding globulin in male patients with insulin dependent diabetes mellitus. *Dan Med Bull.* 1997;44:547-50

[354] "Conversion of androstenedione secreted by adrenal gland into estrone by aromatase in adipose tissue stroma provides an important source of estrogen for the postmenopausal woman. This estrogen may play an important role in development of endometrial and breast cancer." Bray GA. Underlying basis for obesity. *J Nutr* 2002;3451S-3455S

determinations may not be reflective of disease risk for people who are pregnant, highly muscular, or for young children or the frail elderly. Several articles have subjugated BMI (the greatest variable of which is adiposity), under the greater importance of cardiorespiratory fitness; regardless, obesity directly encourages/causes many physical and psychosocial health problems and directly impairs cardiorespiratory fitness. Several studies have also shown that xenobiotic load is a more powerful predictor of insulin resistance than is higher adiposity/BMI. For optimal health in all dimensions, the goals remain optimization of total physical fitness, acquiring a (near-)optimal BMI, and reducing xenobiotic burden.

- ❑ Severely underweight: < 16.5
- ❑ Underweight: 16.5 - 18.4
- ❑ **Normal: 18.5 - 24.9**
- ❑ Overweight: 25 - 29.9

- ❑ Obese Class 1: 30 - 34.9
- ❑ Obese Class 2 (severe obesity): 35 - 39.9
- ❑ Obese Class 3 (morbid obesity): 40 - 47.9
- ❑ Obese Class 4 (supermorbid obesity): ≥ 48

Weight in kilograms (*derived from pounds and inches from original table below; BMI is approximate)

Height cm*	45	50	55	59	63	68	73	77	82	86	90	95	100	104	109	114
152	20	21	23	25	27	29	31	33	35	37	39	41	43	45	47	49
155	19	21	23	25	26	28	30	32	34	36	38	40	42	43	45	47
157	18	20	22	24	26	27	29	31	33	35	37	38	40	42	44	46
160	18	19	21	23	25	27	28	30	32	34	35	37	39	41	43	44
162	17	19	21	22	24	26	27	29	31	33	34	36	38	39	41	43
165	17	18	20	22	23	25	27	28	30	32	33	35	37	38	40	42
167	16	18	19	21	23	24	26	27	29	31	32	34	36	37	39	40
170	16	17	19	20	22	23	25	27	28	30	31	33	34	36	38	39
173	15	17	18	20	21	23	24	26	27	29	30	32	33	35	36	38
175	15	16	18	19	21	22	24	25	27	28	30	31	32	34	35	37
177	14	16	17	19	20	22	23	24	26	27	29	30	32	33	34	36
180	14	15	17	18	20	21	22	24	25	26	27	28	30	32	33	35
182	14	15	16	18	19	20	22	23	24	26	27	28	30	31	33	34
185	13	15	16	17	18	20	21	22	24	25	26	28	29	30	32	33
188	13	14	15	17	18	19	21	22	23	24	26	27	28	30	31	32
190	12	14	15	16	17	19	20	21	22	24	25	26	27	29	30	31
193	12	13	15	16	17	18	19	21	22	23	24	26	27	28	29	30

Weight in pounds

Height: (Ft'inch")	100	110	120	130	140	150	160	170	180	190	200	210	220	230	240	250
5'0"	20	21	23	25	27	29	31	33	35	37	39	41	43	45	47	49
5'1"	19	21	23	25	26	28	30	32	34	36	38	40	42	43	45	47
5'2"	18	20	22	24	26	27	29	31	33	35	37	38	40	42	44	46
5'3"	18	19	21	23	25	27	28	30	32	34	35	37	39	41	43	44
5'4"	17	19	21	22	24	26	27	29	31	33	34	36	38	39	41	43
5'5"	17	18	20	22	23	25	27	28	30	32	33	35	37	38	40	42
5'6"	16	18	19	21	23	24	26	27	29	31	32	34	36	37	39	40
5'7"	16	17	19	20	22	23	25	27	28	30	31	33	34	36	38	39
5'8"	15	17	18	20	21	23	24	26	27	29	30	32	33	35	36	38
5'9"	15	16	18	19	21	22	24	25	27	28	30	31	32	34	35	37
5'10"	14	16	17	19	20	22	23	24	26	27	29	30	32	33	34	36
5'11"	14	15	17	18	20	21	22	24	25	26	27	28	30	32	33	35
6'0"	14	15	16	18	19	20	22	23	24	26	27	28	30	31	33	34
6'1"	13	15	16	17	18	20	21	22	24	25	26	28	29	30	32	33
6'2"	13	14	15	17	18	19	21	22	23	24	26	27	28	30	31	32
6'3"	12	14	15	16	17	19	20	21	22	24	25	26	27	29	30	31
6'4"	12	13	15	16	17	18	19	21	22	23	24	26	27	28	29	30

- ▪ Neurologic exam: Assess baseline central and peripheral neurological status to determine history of stroke or neuropathy; assessment should include monofilament and/or vibration testing.

- **Fundoscopic eye exam**: All DM/MetSyn patients should be evaluated by an ophthalmologist. Because MetSyn is a more aggressive multisystem disorder than DM, these patients with the former should receive appropriate referral within the first year of diagnosis unless treatment is rapidly curative and compliance is high and maintained. Patients must be educated about the risks of vision loss.
- **Cardiovascular exam**: Cardiac auscultation, peripheral vascular exam, and blood pressure assessment are components of a competent clinical examination. As of August 2009, "U.S. Preventive Services Task Force (USPSTF) found insufficient evidence to recommend for or against routine screening with ECG, exercise treadmill test (ETT), or electron-beam computerized tomography (EBCT) scanning for coronary calcium for either the presence of severe coronary artery stenosis (CAS) or the prediction of CHD events in adults at increased risk for CHD events." Doppler evaluation and ankle:brachial index can be evaluated in patients with suspected PVD.
- **Foot examination**: DM patients often lose sensation in their feet; this lack of sensation can predispose them to injury, and when injury occurs it may be painless due to the anesthesia caused by the peripheral neuropathy. Add to this increased risk of infection and poor circulation and clinicians should understand why a visual and manual examination of the feet should be performed on a frequent basis. Podiatric referral and the acquisition of orthoses/orthotics and particularly well-made and properly fitting footwear should be strongly considered, especially in patients with the common combination of PDV, neuropathy, and obesity—these patients are particularly prone to foot injuries that can lead to serious complications.

- **Laboratory Assessments**: Laboratory assessments—prior to the initiation of treatment and periodically to assess the efficacy of treatment and the patient's compliance—are absolutely essential in the proper management of diabetes mellitus and the related syndromes of insulin resistance and metabolic syndrome. Renal function should be checked before the initiation of nutritional or pharmacologic treatment.
  - **Chemistry/metabolic panel**: Serum glucose, electrolytes, blood urea nitrogen, creatinine levels, and liver markers are all assessed by this battery of tests. Renal function must be assessed from "both sides" of the kidney—serum (BUN and creatinine) and urine (albumin:creatinine ratio). Keep in mind that advanced renal failure can become a contraindication to certain treatments, such as a high-potassium diet and supplementation with vitamin D, calcium, and/or magnesium.
  - **Serum glucose**: Generally this is assessed with the chemistry/metabolic panel but can be ordered separately, particularly via finger-stick blood sample. The following serum glucose levels in mg/dL are described:
    - ☺ **< 85 mg/dL**: Optimal fasting glucose; obviously symptomatic hypoglycemia would not be optimal
    - ☺ **> 85-125 mg/dL**: Impaired fasting glucose (functional), candidate for lifestyle/nutritional intervention
    - ☺ **100-125 mg/dL**: Impaired fasting glucose (medical), "prediabetes"
    - ☹ **≥ 126 mg/dL on two separate occasions**: Fasting hyperglycemia, diagnostic of diabetes mellitus
    - ☹ **≥ 200 mg/dL with nonfasting blood sample or 2 hours after of 75 g oral glucose tolerance test (GGT)**: Non-fasting severe hyperglycemia, diagnostic of DM
  - **Serum insulin (fasting)**: In patients with DM-1, insulin and C-peptide are low. In patients with DM-2, insulin levels tend to be *elevated* early in the disease due to insulin resistance and increased pancreatic output, *normal* as pancreatic function declines, and then *low(er)* after the pancreas is sufficiently "burnt out" from years of overwork in a milieu of chronic glucose toxicity. Measuring fasting serum insulin can be helpful in determining if a patient's recalcitrant hyperglycemia is due to failure to comply with treatment or failure to produce endogenous insulin—obviously these two different scenarios would need to be managed with increased compliance or exogenous insulin (or pancreatic restoration), respectively. Although the laboratory reference range can be > 24 uIU/mL as shown in the example below, clinicians should view this upper reference limit as ridiculous except when searching for insulinoma; insulin >15 uIU/mL indicates severe insulin resistance, > 10 uIU/mL is problematic, and <5 uIU/mL is optimal.

Lab results showing optimal fasting serum insulin in a 39yo physician: <5 uIU/mL (shown) is optimal

Account Number	Patient ID	Control Number	Date and Time Collected	Date Reported	Sex	Age(Y/M/D)	Date of Birth
		53023	12/18/10 11:43	12/23/10	M	39	

TESTS	RESULT	FLAG	UNITS	REFERENCE INTERVAL
Insulin	2.3		uIU/mL	0.0 - 24.9

- Glycosylated hemoglobin (Hgb-A1c): As a marker for long-term (120 days) glucose levels, Hgb-A1c is an excellent marker for assessing glucose levels and thus treatment compliance for the past month. "Healthy" Hgb-A1c is less than 6%; "at risk" Hgb-A1c is 6 to <6.5%, and an Hgb-A1c level equal to or greater than 6.5% is now considered diagnostic of DM according to criteria published in June 2009. For the treatment of DM, the goal "target" Hgb-A1c is <7%; however, pushing for this level of strict control in a population of diabetics is likely to produce a significant number of hypoglycemic events, some of which could be serious and/or result in hospitalization, and thus some clinician experts will accept 7.5% as a sufficient level of compliance and efficacy. A correlation can be found between Hgb-A1c levels and average glucose levels:

Percentage	Description	Estimated serum glucose
< 5.7	Normal:	
5.7 - 6.4	Prediabetic: Interestingly, the phrase "prediabetic" reflects the allopathic medical paradigm of the unidirectionality and unavoidability of diabetes. A more proper term could be "borderline diabetes" indicating that the patient is *not* diabetic but showing a tendency toward *insulin resistance* or *glucose intolerance*—note that either of the two latter phrases are better and more "actionable" than the pseudoprophetic phrase *prediabetic*. Unlike *insulin resistance*, the phrase *glucose intolerance* is actionable because the common-sense implication is that if a patient has a metabolic impairment to the efficient utilization and metabolism of glucose then this substance should be avoided. By popularizing the phrases insulin resistance and—even worse—*metabolic syndrome*, physicians and patients alike are distracted from the importance of reducing carbohydrate intake in the treatment of these conditions.	A1c 6% correlates with average glucose of 126 mg/dL or 7 mmol/L
> 6.5	Diabetes mellitus: Diabetes mellitus and insulin resistance are reviewed elsewhere.	A1c 6.5% correlates with average glucose of 140 mg/dL or 7.8 mmol/L
7	Goal for DM treatment: Tighter control tends to result in more hypoglycemic complications in the context of drug management	154 mg/dL or 8.6 mmol/L
7.5	Higher Hgb-A1c values (listed progressively below) indicate poor control:	169 mg/dL or 9.4 mmol/L
8		183 mg/dL or 10.1 mmol/L
8.5		197 mg/dL or 10.9 mmol/L
9		212 mg/dL or 11.8 mmol/L
9.5		226 mg/dL or 12.6 mmol/L
10		240 mg/dL or 13.4 mmol/L

- High-sensitivity C-reactive protein (hsCRP): HsCRP predicts the onset of and correlates with the severity of the systemic inflammation seen in patients with DM and MetSyn. This is an excellent objective marker (along with Hgb-A1c and body weight) to determine the effectiveness of and compliance with treatment. In a 51-year-old male patient with MetSyn and concomitant rheumatoid arthritis, the current author was able to achieve a lowering of hsCRP from 124 mg/L (normal: 1-3 mg/L) to 7.8 mg/L within about one month of multifaceted interventions as described in *Inflammation Mastery*[355]; the details of this case and the

---

[355] Vasquez A. *Integrative Rheumatology, Second Edition*. IBMRC; 2008

interventions utilized were first published in *Musculoskeletal Pain: Expanded Clinical Strategies*[356] for CME credits.

- **Fasting lipid profile**: Elevations of total Cholesterol, LDL, and triglycerides with depression of HDL is the classic pattern of dyslipidemia. Total cholesterol should be reduced to <200 mg/dl and LDL cholesterol should generally be brought to less than 100 mg/dl and is physiologically optimized—and consistent with a Paleo-Mediterranean diet and appropriate exercise at 50-70 mg/dl.[357]

> **LDL levels should be <100 mg/dl and ideally <70 mg/dl**
>
> "The normal low-density lipoprotein (LDL) cholesterol range is 50 to 70 mg/dl for native hunter-gatherers, healthy human neonates, free-living primates, and other wild mammals (all of whom do not develop atherosclerosis). Randomized trial data suggest atherosclerosis progression and coronary heart disease events are minimized when LDL is lowered to <70 mg/dl."
>
> O'Keefe JH Jr, Cordain L, et al. Optimal low-density lipoprotein is 50 to 70 mg/dl: lower is better and physiologically normal. *J Am Coll Cardiol*. 2004 Jun

- **Serum homocysteine and other cardiovascular risk factors**: Other cardiovascular risk factors such as homocysteine and—more controversially—lipoprotein-A might also be tested in any patient with a high risk of cardiovascular disease.

- **Serum ferritin (with or without transferrin saturation)**: DM is one of the classic presentations for hemochromatosis, which is generally considered to be one of the most common hereditary disorders in all human populations. Routine use of serum ferritin is the most reasonable and cost-effective means for diagnosing iron overload condition in symptomatic and asymptomatic patients. Elevations of ferritin (i.e., >200 mcg/L in women and >300 mcg/L in men) need to be retested along with CRP (to rule out false elevation due to excessive inflammation) before making the presumptive diagnosis of iron overload. In the absence of significant inflammation, ferritin values >200 mcg/L in women and >300 mcg/L in men indicate iron overload and the need for treatment/phlebotomy regardless of the absence of symptoms or end-stage complications.[358] Another benefit to the use of serum ferritin is the frequent detection of iron deficiency. Transferrin saturation is a good test for detecting *genetic* hemochromatosis before iron overload has occurred; values greater than 40% should be repeated *in conjunction with a measurement of serum ferritin*. As a general rule, lab tests should be performed under fasting conditions.

- **Thyroid assessment**: Among the numerous metabolic perturbations that characterize DM-2 and MetSyn, clinical and functional hypothyroidism are both quite common. Detailed thyroid assessment should include measurements of TSH, free T4, free T3, total T3, reverse T3, and anti-thyroid antibodies (anti-thyroid peroxidase and anti-thyroglobulin). TSH levels above 2 uIU/mL[359] (uIU/mL = mU/L) or 3.0 uIU/mL[360] warrant consideration for intervention as these indicate subtle thyroid dysfunction and increased risk for future thyroid disease. Progressive clinicians note the importance of the ratio of total T3 to reverse T3 (tT3:rT3 ratio) and consider the optimal range to be 10-14 with lower ratios indicating impaired formation of T3 and/or excess production of rT3.[361] Contrary to the previous view which held that rT3 was simply inactive, we now appreciate that rT3 actually impairs normal thyroid hormone metabolism thus functioning as an thyrometabolic monkeywrench or "brake" on normal metabolism. Elevated rT3 levels predict mortality among critically ill patients.[362] Aberrancies in thyroid hormone levels may reflect organic disease, psychoemotional stress, or nutritional deficiency[363], and therefore such serologic abnormalities warrant consideration of underlying problems and direct treatment when possible. If no underlying cause is apparent, then a trial of thyroid hormone(s) is reasonable in appropriately selected

---

[356] Vasquez A. *Musculoskeletal Pain: Expanded Clinical Strategies*. Institute for Functional Medicine, 2008

[357] "Randomized trial data suggest atherosclerosis progression and coronary heart disease events are minimized when LDL is lowered to <70 mg/dl. No major safety concerns have surfaced in studies that lowered LDL to this range of 50 to 70 mg/dl." O'Keefe JH Jr, Cordain L, Harris WH, Moe RM, Vogel R. Optimal low-density lipoprotein is 50 to 70 mg/dl: lower is better and physiologically normal. *J Am Coll Cardiol*. 2004 Jun 2;43(11):2142-6

[358] Barton et al. Management of hemochromatosis. Hemochromatosis Management Working Group. *Ann Intern Med*. 1998 Dec 1;129(11):932-9

[359] Weetman AP. Fortnightly review: Hypothyroidism: screening and subclinical disease. *BMJ* 1997;314: 1175

[360] American Association of Clinical Endocrinologists: "Until November 2002, doctors had relied on a normal TSH level ranging from 0.5 to 5.0 to diagnose and treat patients with a thyroid disorder who tested outside the boundaries of that range. Now AACE encourages doctors to consider treatment for patients who test outside the boundaries of a narrower margin based on a target TSH level of 0.3 to 3.04. AACE believes the new range will result in proper diagnosis for millions of Americans who suffer from a mild thyroid disorder, but have gone untreated until now." Available at aace.com/pub/tam2003/press.php on January 2004. For more current information, see "The target TSH level should be between 0.3 and 3.0 μIU/mL." American Association of Clinical Endocrinologists Medical Guidelines for Clinical Practice for the Evaluation and Treatment of Hyperthyroidism and Hypothyroidism. aace.com/pub/pdf/guidelines/hypo_hyper.pdf December 20,2005

[361] McDaniel AB. Thyroid Assessment: Controversies and Conundrums. Institute for Functional Medicine 14th International Symposium. Tucson, Arizona. May 23-26, 2007

[362] Peeters et al. Serum 3,3',5'-triiodothyronine (rT3) and 3,5,3'-triiodothyronine/rT3 are prognostic markers in critically ill patients and are associated with postmortem tissue deiodinase activities. *J Clin Endocrinol Metab*. 2005 Aug;90(8):4559-65

[363] Kelly GS. Peripheral metabolism of thyroid hormones: a review. *Altern Med Rev*. 2000 Aug;5(4):306-33

patients. Beyond stress reduction and nutritional supplementation with iodine, selenium, and zinc (as indicated per patient), correction of overt, subclinical, and functional hypothyroidism generally centers on the administration of natural or synthetic thyroid hormones in the form of T4 and T3. Correction of functional hypothyroidism (relatively reduced total T3 and increased rT3) is accomplished with either time-released or twice-daily dosing of T3 without T4 to suppress endogenous T4 conversion to T3. This allows temporary downregulation of transforming enzymes so that rT3 production is reduced and thyroid metabolism is normalized following withdrawal of T3 treatment.[364]

- Serum 25-hydroxy-vitamin D: Per our review by Vasquez, Manso, and Cannell[365] in 2004, we fulfilled our promise of creating a "paradigm shift" that summarized new applications for the clinical use of vitamin D beyond its application in patients with osteoporosis or malabsorption to include the mandate of empiric treatment or laboratory assessment of all patients seen in clinical practice. Daily doses generally average between 4,000-10,000 IU/d for adults, with an acceptable one-time loading dose of 100,000-300,000 IU in patients for whom it is advantageous and safe to raise serum 25-hydroxy-vitamin D levels quickly and without

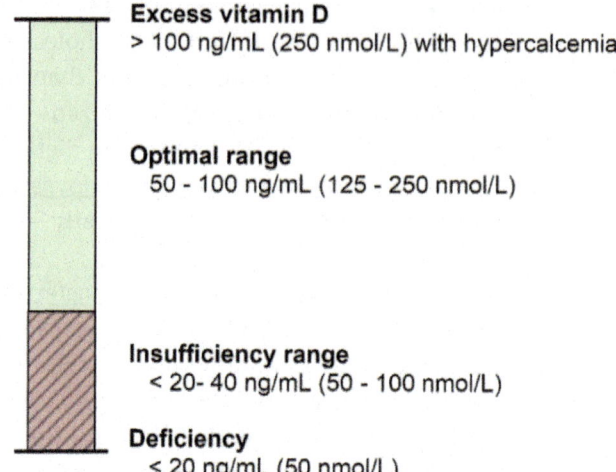

Excess vitamin D
> 100 ng/mL (250 nmol/L) with hypercalcemia

Optimal range
50 - 100 ng/mL (125 - 250 nmol/L)

Insufficiency range
< 20- 40 ng/mL (50 - 100 nmol/L)

Deficiency
< 20 ng/mL (50 nmol/L)

concern for compliance failure. The goal with vitamin D supplementation is to get serum 25-hydroxy-vitamin D levels into the optimal range, as illustrated.

- Androgens and estrogens: For a myriad of reasons, obese patients have adverse alterations in their sex hormones; typically "estrogens" are high in both genders, while androgens are low, particularly in males. Indeed, "Cross-sectional studies have found that between 20 and 64% of men with diabetes have hypogonadism, with higher prevalence rates found in the elderly."[366] In diabetic men, the low testosterone and high estrogens have a pathogenic role in insulin resistance; a review in 2008 by Cohen[367] concluded, "In males with increasing obesity there is increased aromatase activity, which irreversibly converts testosterone to estradiol resulting in decreased testosterone and elevated estrogen levels. Since androgens reduce the expression of ER [estrogen receptor] beta activity, **decreased testosterone levels** release the normally suppressed ER beta expression and **results in the down regulation of GLUT4 with resultant insulin resistance.**" In DM/MetSyn men with low testosterone, the exogenous/transdermal administration of testosterone is often the *wrong* solution to the problem because for many of these men the problem is not that they are not *making* enough testosterone *per se* but rather that their adipose tissue which contains the aromatase enzyme is *converting* their testosterone into estradiol. Giving these men more testosterone simply gives their adipose more substrate for converting into estrogens.

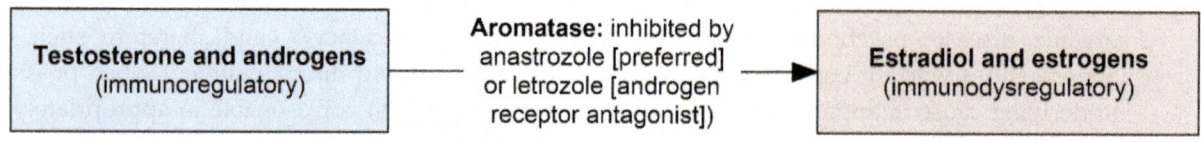

The aromatase enzyme converts androgens to estrogens: If estrogens are high and androgens are low, then estrogens can be lowered and androgens raised via inhibition of aromatase. If androgens are low and estrogens are low, then administration of androgen will raise both the androgens and the estrogens, possibly necessitating the coadministration of an aromatase inhibitor.

---

[364] "The WT3 protocol involves the use of SR-T3 taken orally by the patient every 12 hours according to a cyclic dose schedule determined by patient response. The patient is then weaned once a body temperature of 98.6 degrees F has been maintained for 3 consecutive weeks." Friedman M, Miranda-Massari JR, Gonzalez MJ. Supraphysiological cyclic dosing of sustained release T3 in order to reset low basal body temperature. *P R Health Sci J*. 2006 Mar;25(1):23-9

[365] Vasquez A, Manso G, Cannell J. The clinical importance of vitamin D (cholecalciferol). *Altern Ther Health Med*. 2004 Sep-Oct;10(5):28-36

[366] Kalyani RR, Dobs AS. Androgen deficiency, diabetes, and the metabolic syndrome in men. *Curr Opin Endocrinol Diabetes Obes*. 2007 Jun;14(3):226-34

[367] "Since androgens reduce the expression of ER beta activity, decreased testosterone levels release the normally suppressed ER beta expression and results in the down regulation of GLUT4 with resultant insulin resistance." Cohen PG. Obesity in men: the hypogonadal-estrogen receptor relationship. *Med Hypotheses*. 2008;70(2):358-60

Giving a "hypogonadal" man testosterone *without first measuring his serum estradiol level* should, in this author's opinion, be considered *mal-practice* because ❶ many of these men make sufficient testosterone but they are "rapid converters" to estradiol, ❷ giving them more testosterone raises their testosterone but can easily lead to high enough levels of estradiol to compromise sexual function, ❸ high estradiol in men appears to cause depression and fatigue, ❹ high estradiol in men appears to be a risk factor for prostate cancer. In our office, we commonly measure serum estradiol in men and administer the aromatase inhibitor anastrozole/Arimidex 1 mg (≥2-3 doses per week) to men whose estradiol level is greater than 32 picogram/mL. The Life Extension Foundation[368] advocates that the optimal serum estradiol level for a man is 10-30 picogram/mL. Clinical studies using anastrozole/Arimidex in men have shown that aromatase blockade lowers estradiol and raises testosterone[369]; generally speaking, this is exactly the result that we want. When using anastrozole/Arimidex, frequency of dosing is based on serum and clinical response. On occasion, we have seen some men who make so much endogenous testosterone→estradiol that they require both anastrozole/Arimidex *and* licorice daily in order to control their testosterone and estradiol levels. Licorice lowers testosterone[370] and thus reduces the precursor to estradiol in both men and women within about four days of oral administration. Licorice is effective for this purpose whether by standardized capsules or by tea from the cut and sifted root.

- Dipstick urinalysis: Begin with a urine dipstick test for overt proteinuria; results may be falsely elevated due to urinary tract infection or hematuria. Confirm positive result with repeat dipstick test within one month. Urine pH should be 7.5 to avoid chronic (diet-induced) metabolic acidosis.

- Sensitive tests for occult proteinuria: Urine dipstick testing is insufficiently sensitive to accurately detect minor renal damage that almost invariably affects all patients with DM and MetSyn. Urine tests for microalbuminuria include the random microalbumin-to-creatinine ratio or the timed 24-hour urine collection; these are both valid and the trend in clinical practice is away from the 24-hour urine collection toward the more convenient random microalbumin-to-creatinine ratio, with values >30 mg albumin per gram of creatinine considered positive.

- Xenobiotic accumulation and toxicity; functional detoxification profiles, body burden of persistent organic pollutants (POPs): Patients with DM-2 and MetSyn have much higher-than-average levels of and diversity of toxins and xenobiotics; this literature was reviewed by Vasquez[371] in 2007 and the original article is provided at the end of this chapter. The "take home" message is that DM-2/MetSyn patients have consistent evidence of supranormal xenobiotic accumulation. Several xenobiotics stimulate the aryl hydrocarbon receptor which leads to downregulation of GLUT-4 receptors; therefore the physiologic mechanisms are clearly in place by which xenobiotic accumulation can lead directly to peripheral insulin resistance. Recent reviews have highlighted the importance of xenobiotic accumulation over obesity as an important risk factor for diabetes.[372,373] Tests of serum, whole blood, and adipose tissue can be used to test for levels of specific xenobiotics; the current author has not found that approach particularly useful because most patients with xenobiotic accumulation and the often resultant multiple chemical sensitivity syndrome (MCS) have low-level elevations of *innumerable* xenobiotics rather than isolated elevations of

> **Toxic chemical burden correlates strongly with DM-2/MetSyn**
>
> "...the expected association between obesity and diabetes was absent in people with low concentrations of persistent organic pollutants in their blood. ...the association between obesity and diabetes became stronger as the concentrations of such pollutants in the blood increased."
>
> Jones et al. Environmental pollution and diabetes. *Lancet.* 2008 Jan

---

[368] Male Hormone Modulation Therapy, Page 4 Of 7: lef.org/protocols/prtcl-130c.shtml Accessed October 30, 2005

[369] "These data demonstrate that aromatase inhibition increases serum bioavailable and total testosterone levels to the youthful normal range in older men with mild hypogonadism." Leder et al. Effects of aromatase inhibition in elderly men with low or borderline-low serum testosterone levels. *J Clin Endocrinol Metab.* 2004 Mar;89:1174-80

[370] "The mean testosterone values decreased by 26 % after one week of treatment." Armanini D, Bonanni G, Mattarello MJ, Fiore C, Sartorato P, Palermo M. Licorice consumption and serum testosterone in healthy man. *Exp Clin Endocrinol Diabetes.* 2003 Sep;111(6):341-3

[371] Vasquez A. Chemical Exposure as a Major Contributor to the Epidemic of Diabetes Mellitus and Disorders of Insulin Resistance: From Molecular Mechanisms to Clinical Implications. *Naturopathy Digest* 2006; April.

[372] "Recent studies in populations exposed to polychlorinated biphenyls (PCBs) and chlorinated pesticides found a dose-dependent elevated risk of diabetes. An elevation in risk of diabetes in relation to levels of several POPs [persistent organic pollutants] has been demonstrated by two different groups using the National Health and Nutrition Examination Survey (NHANES), a random sampling of US citizens. The strong associations seen in quite different studies suggest the possibility that exposure to POPs could cause diabetes. One striking observation is that obese persons that do not have elevated POPs are not at elevated risk of diabetes, suggesting that the POPs rather than the obesity per se is responsible for the association." Carpenter DO. Environmental contaminants as risk factors for developing diabetes. *Rev Environ Health.* 2008 Jan-Mar;23(1):59-74

[373] "...the expected association between obesity and diabetes was absent in people with low concentrations of persistent organic pollutants in their blood. ...the association between obesity and diabetes became stronger as the concentrations of such pollutants in the blood increased." Jones et al. Environmental pollution and diabetes. *Lancet.* 2008 Jan:287-8

individual xenobiotics (unless the patient had a specific overdosing exposure). Functional assessments of hepatic detoxification ability are available commercially through specialty laboratories that cater to progressive integrative clinicians; these tests can be useful either for documenting baseline, assessing response to treatment, or demonstrating to patients, colleagues, or insurers the validity of detoxification interventions. However, much of this information can be determined empirically via a thorough patient history, which specifically asks about drug intolerances, caffeine sensitivity, multiple chemical sensitivity, and to a much lesser extent known xenobiotic exposures.

- **Imaging**: From a practical clinical standpoint, clinicians may choose to provide resting/stress ECG for asymptomatic patients at high risk of CAD/CVD, especially before implementing an exercise program; the level of evidence for this recommendation is neutral.[374] Some clinicians choose to practice more defensively than others, especially if the patient's condition or demeanor indicate the need for increased caution. Patients with any CAD/CVD symptoms should receive cardiovascular evaluation. Resting and stress ECG is appropriate for screening patients at high risk for cardiovascular disease and before low-moderate risk patients begin exercise. Patients with long-standing DM/MetSyn are at high risk for cardiovascular disease, especially if they also have hypertension, dyslipidemia, any evidence of PVD, or any history of smoking. Echocardiography may be added with evidence of impaired cardiac output or ventricular hypertrophy.

- **Biopsy/Procedure**: These are generally not indicated except in special circumstances. Liver biopsies show that DM and MetSyn patients have higher-than-average rates of hepatic iron accumulation and iron overload[375,376] but iron overload can generally be determined by serologic testing with ferritin and transferrin saturation as discussed previously thus making liver biopsy unnecessary.

- **Establishing the Diagnosis**: The diagnosis of MetSyn is made by connecting the clinical constellation previously listed: ❶ central adiposity, abdominal obesity, ❷ hyperglycemia, ❸dyslipidemia, ❹ hypertension, ❺ systemic inflammation, and ❻ hypercoagulability. The diagnosis of DM-2 is made by finding a compelling clinical picture, elevated glucose levels (discussed previously and repeated in abbreviated format below) and by excluding the differential diagnoses.

  - Serum glucose: The interpretive guide below describes fasting/nonfasting glucose in units of mg/dl.
    - Fasting; diagnostic of DM: ≥126 on two separate occasions.
    - Non-fasting, diagnostic of DM: ≥ 200 with nonfasting blood sample or 2 hours after oral consumption of 75 g glucose (glucose tolerance test, GGT).

Hgb-A1c for DM diagnosis

"The diagnosis of diabetes is made if the A1C level is ≥6.5%. Diagnosis should be confirmed with a repeat A1C test unless clinical symptoms and glucose levels >200 mg/dl (>11.1 mmol/l) are present."

International Expert Committee report on the role of the A1C assay in the diagnosis of diabetes. *Diabetes Care*. 2009 Jul

Disease Complications: Major complications of DM and MetSyn are listed below and displayed graphically in the previous Venn diagram.

- Cardiovascular disease (CVD): MI, peripheral/visceral/cerebral/ocular vascular disease. More than 60% of nontraumatic limb amputations are due to complications from DM. Impaired circulation contributes to impaired wound healing. Hypercoagulability promotes atherosclerosis and thrombosis and resultant arterial occlusion, particularly in the coronary arteries of the heart (myocardial infarction, MI), cerebral circulation of the brain (stroke), retinal arteries of the eyes (retinal ischemia), peripheral limbs (digital necrosis), and internal organs (e.g., mesenteric ischemia, renal artery occlusion). Hypertension is highly prevalent in DM-2/MetSyn patients. Control of hypertension reduces disease-related complications by 24% while tight glucose control lowers these complications by 12%.

---

[374] "U.S. Preventive Services Task Force (USPSTF) found insufficient evidence to recommend for or against routine screening with ECG, exercise treadmill test (ETT), or electron-beam computerized tomography (EBCT) scanning for coronary calcium for either the presence of severe coronary artery stenosis (CAS) or the prediction of CHD events in adults at increased risk for CHD events." Screening for Coronary Heart Disease. Release Date: February 2004. ahrq.gov/clinic/uspstf/uspsacad.htm Accessed August 12, 2009

[375] Phelps G, Chapman I, Hall P, Braund W, Mackinnon M. Prevalence of genetic haemochromatosis among diabetic patients. *Lancet*. 1989 Jul 29;2(8657):233-4

[376] "Most of the patients (95%) had one or more of the following conditions; obesity, hyperlipidaemia, abnormal glucose metabolism, or hypertension. INTERPRETATION: We have found a new non-HLA-linked iron-overload syndrome which suggests a link between iron excess and metabolic disorders." Moirand R, Mortaji AM, Loréal O, Paillard F, Brissot P, Deugnier Y. A new syndrome of liver iron overload with normal transferrin saturation. *Lancet*. 1997 Jan 11;349(9045):95-7

- <u>Ocular diseases</u>: DM is the leading cause of blindness in adults; blindness results from cataracts (due to sorbitol accumulation and ROS production), vascular and neuropathic eye diseases. Due to the speed and severity of ocular complications of DM-2, all patients with DM-2 must be referred for ophthalmologist's evaluation upon diagnosis; follow-up exams are generally every 1-2 years.
- <u>Kidney failure, renal insufficiency</u>: Hyperglycemia is toxic to nephrons; chronic hyperglycemia eventually causes renal damage and chronic renal failure (CRF). The hypertension that is often part of the clinical picture in patients with DM/MetSyn further accelerates and exacerbates the renal disease; renal disease then becomes an additional cause of hypertension. Pharmacologic renoprotection is provided by early use of angiotensin converting enzyme (ACE) inhibitors and angiotensin receptor blockers (ARBs). Nutritional renoprotection is provided by treating the underlying cause of the syndrome and promoting its clinical resolution, as well as by CoQ10, which separately lowers blood pressure and rejuvenates nephrons, as discussed later in this chapter and in more detail in the chapter on hypertension. Assessment of renal function (detailed in Chapter 1) is mandatory in hypertensive and diabetic patients for many reasons, one of which is to screen for predisposition to hyperkalemia—which may be induced by a high-potassium diet—as discussed in a video tutorial by DrV available online: https://vimeo.com/152293616
- <u>Neuropathy</u>: Peripheral neuropathy is primarily *sensory*, predisposing to unattended injuries and proprioceptive defects that classically result in neuropathic osteoarthropathy (previously called Charcot joints). Autonomic neuropathy results in orthostatic hypotension, gastroparesis (with secondary small intestine bacterial overgrowth and tertiary malabsorption), erectile dysfunction and retrograde ejaculation.
- <u>Gingival disease</u>: DM patients have an increased incidence of gum and dental disease. The relationship is bidirectional: gum disease causes systemic inflammation which exacerbates peripheral insulin resistance; hyperglycemia causes immune suppression and nutrient/antioxidant depletion which predisposes DM patients to gum disease.
- <u>Immunosuppression</u>: Most commonly presenting as gingivitis, yeast vaginitis/balantitis, and skin infections; each of these may be the presenting manifestation of DM. Clinicians must attend to each of the above clinical manifestations of DM as potential signs of DM when a new patient presents.
- <u>Hyperosmolar hyperglycemic nonketotic coma</u>: Uncontrolled DM-2 leads to extreme hyperglycemia (glucose >800-1,000 mg/dL) with resultant hyperosmolar diuresis and profound dehydration, which can result in altered mental status, stroke, or seizures.
- <u>Pregnant mothers with DM deliver babies with increased prevalence and severity of birth defects</u>: Some women may choose to delay conception until DM is resolved; risks, contraceptive options, and *most importantly* safe and effective treatments for alleviation of diabetes should be discussed with women of child-bearing potential.

Initial Checklist for managing DM-2/MetSyn

☑ <u>Implement "the supplemented (low-carb) Paleo-Mediterranean diet"</u> with multivitamin/multimineral, combination fatty acids, physiologic vitamin D dosage, magnesium and other nutrients as indicated

☑ <u>Blood pressure</u>: <130/85

☑ <u>Hgb-A1c</u>: <7%

☑ <u>Check renal function with serum BUN and creatinine and urine albumin:creatinine ratio</u>: Renal failure may contraindicate certain nutritional interventions and may necessitate referral to a specialist

☑ <u>LDL cholesterol</u>: <70-100 mg/dl

☑ <u>Triglycerides</u>: <100-150 mg/dl

☑ <u>HDL</u>: >40 mg/dl in men; >50 mg/dl in women

☑ <u>Serum ferritin</u>: 40-70 mcg/l

☑ <u>hsCRP</u>: 1-3 mg/L, ideal is <1

☑ <u>25(OH)vitamin D</u>: 50-100 ng/ml

☑ <u>Estradiol</u>: <30 picogram/mL in men

☑ <u>Assessments</u>: Foot exam, ophthalmology referral, ECG for patients with cardiac symptoms

☑ <u>Smoking cessation</u>

☑ <u>Low-dose aspirin for most patients >40y</u>: This recommendation has become increasingly questioned in the past few years, but is still a reasonable recommendation, especially in patients at low/normal risk for gastrointestinal bleeding and hemorrhagic stroke. "Diabetics are at high risk for atherosclerotic cardiovascular disease (ASCVD) and are considered a coronary heart disease risk equivalent. The utility of aspirin in primary prevention of ASCVD in diabetic patients has been widely studied and is still debated. Overall, the current evidence suggests a modest benefit for reduction in ASCVD events with the greatest benefit among those with higher baseline risk, but at the cost of increased risk of gastrointestinal bleeding. Diabetic patients at higher risk (with 10-year ASCVD risk >10 %) are generally recommended for aspirin therapy if bleeding risk is felt to be low. A patient-provider discussion is recommended before prescribing aspirin therapy." Desai et al. Preventing cardiovascular disease in patients with diabetes: use of aspirin for primary prevention. *Curr Cardiol Rep.* 2015 Mar

---

Clinical Management:

- <u>Goals</u>: The goals are ❶ to address any urgent problems such as imminent MI, impending CRF, infection, electrolyte imbalance, or dehydration, ❷ assess and address anticipated complications such as CRF, CVD, dyslipidemia, retinopathy; also screen for primary causes of the clinical picture as appropriate, including iron overload, iatrogenesis (e.g., corticosteroid overdose), Cushing's disease, acromegaly, acute/chronic pancreatitis, ❸ ensure proper patient education about the nuances and curative potential of dietary and lifestyle management of uncomplicated DM-2 and the utmost importance of dietary control and overall treatment compliance—remind them that DM/MetSyn is a kidney-, heart-, limb-, vision-, and life-threatening condition, ❹ use drugs as needed to complement lifestyle and nutritional interventions, particularly for patients with complications or noncompliance; typical drugs include oral hypoglycemics, injectable insulin, aspirin, statins, antihypertensive drugs, and renoprotective drugs such as ACE-inhibitors and angiotensin receptor blockers (ARBs), ❺ practice defensively with appropriate documentation, education, co-management, and timely referral. Noncompliant patients must receive documented education, access to appropriate treatments and resources, encouragement, and co-management/referral. Clinicians should appreciate that transitioning from an unhealthy lifestyle to one compatible with health is a major challenge for many DM-2 patients; clinicians should be compassionate, patient, and diligent about documenting clinical encounters and education. Noncompliant patients put themselves at risk for devastating adverse health outcomes including blindness, death, injury, and limb amputation; likewise, noncompliant nonresponsive patients place the clinician at risk for medicolegal complications. In certain situations, clinicians may choose to provide a complete referral (i.e., call and make a confirmed appointment for the patient) to a specialist; more rarely, dangerously noncompliant patients should be appropriately referred to a specialist and then discharged from the practice by certified mail.

- <u>Patient referral, co-management and education</u>: DM and MetSyn are serious disorders that mandate thorough patient education about the disease and its treatments, and the procedures/alternatives/risks/benefits (PAR-B) for each treatment. Guidelines from the American College of Physicians[377] include the following (with slight modifications):

  1. Refer all patients for diabetes self-management education, to cover diet, glycemic management, exercise programs, and strategies to prevent complications. Review and support self-management topics at every visit.
  2. Consider referral to an endocrinologist for help in managing complex patients.
  3. Refer all patients with DM-2 to an ophthalmologist. Obtain consult to screen for diabetic eye disease at diagnosis and every 1 to 3 years, depending on risk, to reduce the risk of visual loss from diabetic retinopathy and macular edema.
  4. Consult for cardiology to perform a cardiac stress test in patients with typical/atypical cardiac symptoms and an abnormal resting ECG; consider a screening/stress cardiac stress test for those with a history of peripheral or carotid artery occlusive disease and those over age 35 with a sedentary lifestyle who plan to begin a vigorous exercise program. Exercise can induce hypoglycemia; patients are justified in starting their exercise regimen slowly so that they can adapt to the experience physiologically as well as psychologically. Patients who smoke are expediting the development of cardiovascular complications atop a condition characterized by accelerated atherosclerosis. All patients who smoke must be advised to stop smoking and this must be documented in the chart, preferably at each visit.
  5. For DM/MetSyn patients over age 40y, the benefits of a daily aspirin (75-162 mg/d) outweigh the risks for medically managed patients (common practice, yet consistently debated).

<u>Food & Nutrition</u> Food intake and nutritional status/supplementation always has and always will be foundational in the treatment of various forms of diabetes; carbohydrate restriction and nutritional density are the everlasting keystones of the dietary management of diabetes.

- **Low-carbohydrate Paleo-Mediterranean Diet**: The health-promoting diet of choice for the majority of people is a diet based on abundant consumption of fruits, vegetables, seeds, nuts, omega-3 and monounsaturated fatty acids, and lean sources of protein such as lean meats, fatty cold-water fish, soy and whey proteins. This diet prohibits and obviates overconsumption of chemical preservatives, artificial sweeteners, and carbohydrate-

---

[377] pier.acponline.org/physicians/public/d296/mgt.consult/d296-s9.html Accessed July 17, 2009

dominant foods such as candies, pastries, breads, potatoes, grains, and other foods with a high glycemic load and high glycemic index. This "Paleo-Mediterranean Diet" is a combination of the "Paleolithic" or "Paleo diet" and the well-known "Mediterranean diet", both of which are well described in peer-reviewed journals and the lay press. The Mediterranean diet is characterized by increased proportions of legumes, nuts, seeds, whole grain products, fruits, vegetables (including potatoes), fish and lean meats, and monounsaturated and n-3 fatty acids.[378] Consumption of this diet is consistently associated with improvements in

> **Clinical Pearl**
>
> Because inflammation is a key component of DM and MetSyn, clinicians are wise to treat DM/MetSyn as if it were an inflammatory disorder. Inflammation promotes insulin resistance, and insulin resistance promotes inflammation; both cause oxidative stress and nutritional depletion. Essentially all nutrients and dietary plans that have shown benefit in the treatment of DM/MetSyn are simultaneously inhibitors of inflammation in general and NFkB in particular, while they sensitize peripheral insulin receptors to improve glucose and serum lipid control.

insulin sensitivity and reductions in cardiovascular disease, diabetes, cancer, and all-cause mortality.[379] The Paleolithic diet detailed by collaborators Eaton[380], O'Keefe[381], and Cordain[382] is similar to the Mediterranean diet except for stronger emphasis on fruits and vegetables (preferably raw or minimally cooked), omega-3-rich lean meats, and reduced consumption of starchy foods such as potatoes and grains, the latter of which were not staples in the human diet until the last few thousand years. The current author expects that habitual consumption of this Paleo-Mediterranean Diet is immunosupportive/immunoempowering due to both ❶ increased intake of micronutrients, phytonutrients, and the alkalinizing pro-homeostatic benefits in addition to ❷ avoidance of nutrient-poor high-carbohydrate high-fat foods which are immunosuppressive and pro-inflammatory. High-carbohydrate diets deal a double-punch to the human host; first, consumption of a high-carbohydrate load causes immunosuppression, and then secondly the high-carbohydrate load promotes activation of NFkB which then promotes systemic inflammation. The Mediterranean diet has shown unparalleled safety and efficacy in the prevention of cardiovascular disease, cancer, and all-cause mortality.

- Review: Mediterranean diet and the metabolic syndrome (*Mol Nutr Food Res* 2007 Oct[383]): "Some recent studies dealing specifically with the effect of interventions on the resolution of the metabolic syndrome have demonstrated a 25% net reduction in the prevalence of the syndrome following lifestyle changes mainly based on nutritional recommendations. ... The favorable benefit/hazard ratio makes Mediterranean-style diets particularly promising to reduce the cardiovascular burden associated with the metabolic syndrome."

- Cross-sectional study: Swedish pre-school children eat too much junk food and sucrose (*Acta Paediatr* 2007 Feb[384]): An interesting finding in this study, which proved a point that integrative clinicians have been proclaiming for decades, is that obesity and nutritional deficiency can certainly co-exist. Excess caloric intake coupled with physical inactivity does not ensure against nutritional deficiencies, despite the appearance of being "overnourished." "Eighteen percent of children were overweight/obese. ... Junk food supplied 24% of energy. Ninety-two percent had low vitamin D intake, 70% low iron and 21% low calcium intake." Astute clinicians will note that the 92% prevalence of insufficient vitamin D intake would virtually guarantee that these children will have pandemic vitamin D deficiency, since year-round sunbathing is unlikely, particularly among this group of pre-school children in Sweden.

> **Clinical Insight**
>
> Question: Why do low-carbohydrate diets cause a rapid reduction/normalization in blood pressure among hypertensive patients even before significant weight loss has taken place?
>
> Answer: Because carbohydrate ingestion triggers insulin release, and insulin promotes renal retention of sodium, and therefore promotes retention of water and the development of the volume overload that is characteristic of hypertension. Low-carbohydrate diets cause a rapid reduction in serum insulin levels, and thus the endogenous trigger for sodium-water retention is abated; blood pressure then has the opportunity to normalize rapidly.

[378] Curtis et al. Understanding the Mediterranean diet. Could this be the new "gold standard" for heart disease prevention? *Postgrad Med.* 2002 Aug;112(2):35-8, 41-5
[379] Knoops et al. Mediterranean diet, lifestyle factors, and 10-year mortality in elderly European men and women: the HALE project. *JAMA.* 2004 Sep 22;292(12):1433-9
[380] Eaton SB, Shostak M, Konner M. *The Paleolithic Prescription: A program of diet & exercise and a design for living.* New York: Harper & Row, 1988
[381] O'Keefe JH Jr, Cordain L. Cardiovascular disease resulting from a diet and lifestyle at odds with our Paleolithic genome. *Mayo Clin Proc.* 2004 Jan;79(1):101-8
[382] Cordain L. *The Paleo Diet: Lose Weight and Get Healthy by Eating the Food You Were Designed to Eat.* Indianapolis; John Wiley and Sons, 2002
[383] Esposito K, Ciotola M, Giugliano D. Mediterranean diet and the metabolic syndrome. *Mol Nutr Food Res.* 2007 Oct;51(10):1268-74
[384] Garemo M, Lenner RA, Strandvik B. Swedish pre-school children eat too much junk food and sucrose. *Acta Paediatr.* 2007 Feb;96(2):266-72

- Cross-sectional study: Micronutrient deficiency and the prevalence of mothers' overweight/obesity in Egypt (_Econ Hum Biol_ 2007 Dec [385]): This study showed that micronutrient deficiency greatly increases the risk for overweight/obesity. "The ordered logit results show an overlap between micronutrient deficiency and the prevalence of mothers' overweight/obesity in Egypt. The odds of being overweight/obese are 80.8% higher for micronutrient deficient mothers than for non-deficient mothers, keeping all other variables constant." Given the firmly-established role of vitamins and minerals in basic cellular metabolism, a simple model could hold that patients with multiple micronutrient deficiencies simply do not have the enzyme cofactors to metabolize energy substrates such as lipids/adipose, and that they therefore have a biochemical predisposition toward overweight/obesity by shear virtue of not being able to metabolize energy. A second theory holds that nutritional deficiencies cause a form of _junk food pica_ (note that **pica**—defined as an abnormal appetite for nonnutritive substances—is well

established in relation to iron deficiency) in which nutrient-depleted patients eat more as a result of either a biochemical disturbance in the brain or a starvation-prevention instinct which is attempting to compensate for the malnutrition, or both.

- Negative effects of the standard American diet (SAD): Increase in intranuclear nuclear factor kappaB and decrease in inhibitor kappaB in mononuclear cells after a mixed meal (_Am J Clin Nutr_ 2004 Apr[386]): Consumption of the standard American diet (SAD) causes oxidative stress, systemic inflammation, and activation of NFkB; clinicians must appreciate that each of these three adverse effects leads to a biochemical milieu that supports the development and perpetuation of infections, particularly viral infections. Subjects in this study consumed an egg-muffin and sausage-muffin sandwiches and 2 hash browns, which contained 81 g carbohydrate, 51 g fat, and 32 g protein "RESULTS: ROS generation by mononuclear cells and polymorphonuclear leukocytes and p47(phox) expression increased significantly. The expression of IKKalpha and IKKbeta and DNA-binding activity of NF-kappaB increased significantly, whereas IkappaBalpha expression decreased. Plasma CRP concentrations increased. The intake of 300 mL water did not induce a change in any of the above indexes. CONCLUSIONS: These data show that the intake of a mixed meal results in significant inflammatory changes characterized by a decrease in IkappaBalpha and an increase in NF-kappaB binding, plasma CRP, and the expression of IKKalpha, IKKbeta, and p47(phox) subunit. These proinflammatory changes are probably relevant to the state of chronic hypertension and obesity and to its association with atherosclerosis." Thus, some of the benefit of the Paleo-Mediterranean diet comes not only from the inherent benefits of the diet itself, but also from the avoidance of the negative effects of the SAD eating pattern that is typical in industrialized nations.

- Prospective diet-disease correlation among more than 21,000 subjects: Plasma vitamin C level, fruit and vegetable consumption, and the risk of new-onset type-2 diabetes mellitus (_Arch Intern Med_ 2008 Jul[387]): This study aimed to determine whether fruit and vegetable intake and plasma vitamin C level are associated with the risk of incident type 2 diabetes by correlating fruit-vegetable intake with plasma vitamin C levels and then monitoring for development of DM-2 over the next 12 years. "RESULTS: A strong inverse association was found between plasma vitamin C level and diabetes risk. The odds ratio of diabetes in the top quintile of plasma vitamin C was 0.38 (95% confidence interval, 0.28-0.52) in a model adjusted for demographic, lifestyle, and anthropometric variables. In a similarly adjusted model, the odds ratio of diabetes in the top quintile of fruit and vegetable consumption was 0.78 (95% confidence interval, 0.60-1.00). CONCLUSIONS: **Higher plasma vitamin C level and, to a lesser degree, fruit and vegetable intake** were associated with a substantially **decreased risk of diabetes.**"

---

[385] Asfaw A. Micronutrient deficiency and the prevalence of mothers' overweight/obesity in Egypt. _Econ Hum Biol_. 2007 Dec;5(3):471-83

[386] Aljada A, Mohanty P, Ghanim H, Abdo T, Tripathy D, Chaudhuri A, Dandona P. Increase in intranuclear nuclear factor kappaB and decrease in inhibitor kappaB in mononuclear cells after a mixed meal: evidence for a proinflammatory effect. _Am J Clin Nutr_. 2004 Apr;79(4):682-90

[387] Harding et al. Plasma vitamin C level, fruit and vegetable consumption, and the risk of new-onset type 2 diabetes mellitus. _Arch Intern Med_. 2008 Jul 28;168(14):1493-9

- Adherence to a Mediterranean-type diet reduces the prevalence of clustered cardiovascular risk factors among 3,204 high-risk patients (*Eur J Cardiovasc Prev Rehabil* 2008 Oct[388]): "Adherence to **MeDiet [Mediterranean diet]** was inversely associated with individual risk factors and, above all, with the clustering of them. ... CONCLUSION: Following a **MeDiet** was inversely associated with the clustering of hypertension, diabetes, obesity, and hypercholesterolemia among high-risk patients."

- Pro-inflammatory effects of glucose ingestion: Glucose induces an increase in intranuclear nuclear factor kappaB, a fall in cellular inhibitor kappaB, and an increase in tumor necrosis factor alpha messenger RNA by mononuclear cells in healthy human subjects (*Metabolism* 2006 Sep[389]): Subjects in this study received glucose ingestion consistent with normal dietary habits: 300 kcal (75 g) glucose in water (300 mL). Results showed that 300 kcal of glucose causes NFkB activation, systemic inflammation, and increased expression of pro-inflammatory TNF-alpha. Clinicians should appreciate that many of the new drugs for rheumatic diseases specifically target TNF-alpha. "We conclude that glucose intake induces an immediate increase in intranuclear NF-kappaB binding, a fall in IkappaBalpha, an increase in IKKalpha, IKKbeta, IKK activity, and messenger RNA expression of TNF-alpha in MNCs (mononuclear cells) in healthy subjects. These data are consistent with **profound acute pro-inflammatory changes in MNCs after glucose intake.**"

When patients overconsume simple carbohydrates several times per day, they are inducing a clinically significant oxidative stress and pro-inflammatory state several times per day that lasts for several hours.

- Cohort study of the Mediterranean diet in elderly humans (*JAMA* 2004 Sep[390]): "Among individuals aged 70 to 90 years, **adherence to a Mediterranean diet and healthful lifestyle is associated with a more than 50% lower rate of all-causes and cause-specific mortality.**" The Mediterranean diet has shown unparalleled safety and efficacy in the prevention of cardiovascular disease, cancer, and all-cause mortality.

- Twelve-month randomized clinical trial shows that the low-carb Atkins diet is superior to other diets for weight loss (*JAMA* 2007 Mar[391]): In this 12-month randomized trial, 311 free-living, overweight/obese (body mass index, 27-40) nondiabetic, premenopausal women were randomly assigned to follow the Atkins (n = 77), Zone (n = 79), LEARN (n = 79), or Ornish (n = 76) diets. Subjects received weekly instruction for 2 months with 10-month follow-up. Body weight and laboratory parameters were measured. "RESULTS: **Weight loss was greater for women in the Atkins diet group compared with the other diet groups at 12 months**, and mean 12-month weight loss was significantly different between the Atkins and Zone diets (P<.05). Mean 12-month weight loss was

> **Diets that emphasize more protein and less carbohydrate clearly provide more metabolic and weight-loss benefits than other eating patterns, especially when combined with exercise**
>
> "Thus, a high-protein diet combined with a moderate-intensity combination aerobic and resistance training protocol **seems the ideal program** for short-term weight loss in this subject population."
>
> Meckling KA, Sherfey R. A randomized trial of a hypocaloric high-protein diet, with and without exercise, on weight loss, fitness, and markers of the Metabolic Syndrome in overweight and obese women. *Appl Physiol Nutr Metab.* 2007 Aug

> **Clinical Insight**
>
> Error: Diabetes mellitus type-2 and the metabolic syndrome are "chronic diseases" from which the patient cannot recover.
>
> Correction: Diabetes mellitus type-2 and the metabolic syndrome are conditions reflected by acute and subacute maladaptations (to nutritional deficiencies, nutrient imbalances, carbohydrate excess and possibly xenobiotic accumulation) that persist because the conditions for their perpetuation continue to exist. When these primary problems are addressed, the condition either partially abates or completely resolves, depending on the comprehensiveness of the plan, the level of compliance, and the duration/damage of the previous state. Thus, diabetes mellitus type-2 and the metabolic syndrome are not so much "chronic diseases" as they are "acute/subacute diseases that are repeated hourly and daily for many years", perhaps the rest of the patient's life, until and unless a skilled clinician and compliant patient address and correct the causes of the repetitive maladaptations.

---

[388] Sánchez-Taínta et al; PREDIMED group. Adherence to a Mediterranean-type diet and reduced prevalence of clustered cardiovascular risk factors in a cohort of 3,204 high-risk patients. *Eur J Cardiovasc Prev Rehabil.* 2008 Oct;15(5):589-93

[389] Aljada A, Friedman J, Ghanim H, Mohanty P, Hofmeyer D, Chaudhuri A, Dandona P. Glucose ingestion induces an increase in intranuclear nuclear factor kappaB, a fall in cellular inhibitor kappaB, and an increase in tumor necrosis factor alpha messenger RNA by mononuclear cells in healthy human subjects. *Metabolism.* 2006 Sep;55(9):1177-85

[390] Knoops et al. Mediterranean diet, lifestyle factors, and 10-year mortality in elderly European men and women: the HALE project. *JAMA.* 2004 Sep 22;292(12):1433-9

[391] Gardner CD, Kiazand A, Alhassan S, Kim S, Stafford RS, Balise RR, Kraemer HC, King AC. Comparison of the Atkins, Zone, Ornish, and LEARN diets for change in weight and related risk factors among overweight premenopausal women: the A TO Z Weight Loss Study: a randomized trial. *JAMA.* 2007 Mar 7;297(9):969-77

as follows: **Atkins, -4.7 kg**, Zone, -1.6 kg, LEARN, -2.6 kg, and Ornish, -2.2 kg. ... While questions remain about long-term effects and mechanisms, a low-carbohydrate, high-protein, high-fat diet may be considered a feasible alternative recommendation for weight loss." Clinicians should appreciate not only the exoneration of Dr Atkins, who was ostracized and harassed by groups in "conventional medicine" for his advocation of a health-promoting diet, but also that the negative associations with the *ad libitum* fat consumption are not necessarily a requirement for the success of this diet. Patients can still achieve success on a low-carb diet even if they do not overindulge in dietary lipids; what the study proves is that carbohydrate avoidance is the key to weight loss, and that avoidance of dietary fat is of lesser importance. The diet should focus on ❶ adequate consumption of high-quality protein to avoid decrements in muscle mass and immune function that are reported when patients follow a "normal" diet that is low in protein, ❷ *ad libitum* consumption of **low-carbohydrate** fruits, **vegetables, nuts, seeds**, and berries, ❸ avoidance of all dietary carbohydrate (from starchy foods such as potatoes and wheat and other grains, including rice and

> ### Carbohydrate restriction shows therapeutic equivalence to—and therefore clinical superiority over—insulin therapy in severe diabetics
>
> Avoidance of the following foods:
> 1. <u>Staple foods</u>: rice, bread, corn, spaghetti, noodle made of wheat or buckwheat, potato, sweet potato, taro and yam
> 2. <u>Fruits</u>: pear, apple, persimmon, mikan, orange, grapefruit, peach, grape, melon, water melon, banana, pineapple.
> 3. <u>Vegetables</u>: carrot, pumpkin, and autumn squash
> 4. <u>Confectioneries</u>: all
> 5. <u>Drink</u>: beverages containing sugar, glucose and fructose, and milk
> 6. <u>Alcohol</u>: sake, beer and wine (Distilled liquor was not restricted)
>
> The main principle of the carbohydrate-restricted diet was to eliminate carbohydrate-rich food twice a day at breakfast and dinner, or eliminate it three times a day at breakfast, lunch and dinner. There were no other restrictions. Patients on the carbohydrate-restricted diet were permitted to eat as much protein and fat as they wanted, including saturated fat.
>
> Haimoto et al. Effects of a low-carbohydrate diet on glycemic control in outpatients with severe type 2 diabetes. *Nutr Metab* 2009:6;21

corn) except what is found from whole-foods sources, and from the inevitable "cheating", ❹ broad-spectrum supplementation with the fatty acids ALA, GLA, EPA, and DHA along with oleic acid and the requisite polyphenolics found in olive oil, ❺ supplemental vitamin D in physiologic doses targeted to attain and maintain optimal serum levels of 25-OH-vitamin D3, and ❻ regular consumption of probiotics, either in pills or as yogurt/kefir.

- Randomized clinical trial with 100 women: Comparison of high-protein vs high-carbohydrate diet on markers of cardiovascular health in obese women (*Am J Clin Nutr* 2005 Jun[392]): Subjects were randomly assigned to 1 of 2 isocaloric 5600-kJ dietary interventions for 12 wk: either 1) a high-protein (HP) or 2) a high-carbohydrate (HC) diet. "RESULTS: ... Weight loss was 7.3 +/- 0.3 kg with both diets. Subjects with high serum triacylglycerol (>1.5 mmol/L) lost more fat mass with the HP than with the HC diet and had a greater decrease in triacylglycerol concentrations with the HP than with the HC diet. ... Fasting LDL-cholesterol, HDL-cholesterol, glucose, insulin, free fatty acid, and C-reactive protein concentrations decreased with weight loss. Serum vitamin B-12 increased 9% with the HP diet and decreased 13% with the HC diet. Folate and vitamin B-6 increased with both diets; homocysteine did not change significantly. ... CONCLUSION: An energy-restricted, high-protein, low-fat diet provides nutritional and metabolic benefits that are equal to and sometimes greater than those observed with a high-carbohydrate diet."

- Review: Metabolic effects of low glycemic index diets (*Nutr J* 2009 Jan[393]): "The currently available scientific literature shows that low glycemic-index diets acutely induce a number of favorable effects, such as a rapid weight loss, decrease of fasting glucose and insulin levels, reduction of circulating triglyceride levels and improvement of blood pressure."

- Two-year clinical trial: Weight loss with a low-carbohydrate, Mediterranean, or low-fat diet (*N Engl J Med.* 2008 Jul[394]): 322 moderately obese subjects were randomized to one of three diets: ❶ low-fat, restricted-calorie; ❷ Mediterranean, restricted-calorie; or ❸ low-carbohydrate, non–restricted-calorie. "The mean weight loss was 2.9 kg for the low-fat group, 4.4 kg for the Mediterranean-diet group, and 4.7 kg for the

[392] Noakes M, Keogh JB, Foster PR, Clifton PM. Effect of an energy-restricted, high-protein, low-fat diet relative to a conventional high-carbohydrate, low-fat diet on weight loss, body composition, nutritional status, and markers of cardiovascular health in obese women. *Am J Clin Nutr*. 2005 Jun;81(6):1298-306
[393] Radulian G, Rusu E, Dragomir A, Posea M. Metabolic effects of low glycaemic index diets. *Nutr J*. 2009 Jan 29;8:5
[394] Shai I, Schwarzfuchs D, Henkin Y, et al. Weight loss with a low-carbohydrate, Mediterranean, or low-fat diet. *N Engl J Med*. 2008 Jul 17;359(3):229-41

low-carbohydrate group; among the 272 participants who completed the intervention, the mean weight losses were 3.3 kg, 4.6 kg, and 5.5 kg, respectively. Among the 36 subjects with diabetes, changes in fasting plasma glucose and insulin levels were more favorable among those assigned to the Mediterranean diet than among those assigned to the low-fat diet. Mediterranean and low-carbohydrate diets may be effective alternatives to low-fat diets. The more favorable effects on lipids (with the low-carbohydrate diet) and on glycemic control (with the Mediterranean diet) suggest that personal preferences and metabolic considerations might inform individualized tailoring of dietary interventions." I suggest that a *low-carb Mediterranean diet is the diet of choice because it provides the "best of both worlds"* for lipid control, weight loss, cancer prevention, mortality reduction, and the numerous other health benefits already well-established to result from habituation to the Mediterranean diet.

- Moderately low-carb diet is comparable to insulin therapy for diabetics: Effects of a low-carbohydrate diet on glycemic control in outpatients with severe type 2 diabetes (*Nutr Metab* 2009 May[395]): A 30%-carbohydrate diet was used in 33 outpatients with severe type-2 diabetes (Hgb-A1c levels of 9.0% or above). "HbA1c levels decreased sharply from a baseline of 10.9 to 7.8 at 3 months and to 7.4 at 6 months. Body mass index decreased slightly from baseline (23.8 +/- 3.3) to 6 months (23.5 +/- 3.4). ... No adverse effects were observed except for mild constipation. The number of patients on sulfonylureas decreased from 7 at baseline to 2 at 6 months. No patient required inpatient care or insulin therapy. **In summary, the 30%-carbohydrate diet over 6 months led to a remarkable reduction in HbA1c levels, even among outpatients with severe type 2 diabetes, without any insulin therapy, hospital care or increase in sulfonylureas. The effectiveness of the diet may be comparable to that of insulin therapy.**"

- Randomized clinical trial: A randomized trial of a hypocaloric high-protein diet, with and without exercise, on markers of the Metabolic Syndrome in overweight and obese women (*Appl Physiol Nutr Metab* 2007 Aug[396]): This study evaluated the effects of hypocaloric diets with 3:1 and 1:1 carbohydrate-to-protein ratios, with/without exercise on physical and serologic parameters. Four groups were designated: ❶ control diet (CON), ❷ control diet with exercise (CONEx), ❸ high-protein (HP), and ❹ high-protein with exercise (HPEx)—exercise for the purpose of this study meant only three times per week (and is thus not truly representative of *exercise*, but merely of *activity*). Weight loss was as follows, with results favoring the group randomized to high-protein+exercise: -2.1 kg for the CON group, -4.0 kg in the CONEx group, -4.6 kg in the HP group, and **-7.0 kg in the HPEx**. Benefits seen in all groups were weight loss, improved body composition, decreased blood pressure, and decreased waist and hip circumference. **"A high-protein diet was superior to a low-fat, high-carbohydrate diet either alone or when combined with an aerobic/resistance-training program in promoting weight loss and nitrogen balance**, while similarly improving body composition and risk factors for the Metabolic Syndrome in overweight and obese Canadian women."

> **Nutrition-drug coordination**
>
> Clinicians must appreciate that a low-carbohydrate diet may make antihyperglycemic and antihypertensive drugs less necessary or completely unnecessary; patients need to be educated appropriately and warned of potential hypoglycemic or hypotensive complications that could occur if drug doses are not adjusted appropriately. Nutritional interventions need to be coordinated with adjustments in drug dosage so that hypoglycemic or hypotensive complications are avoided.

- Inpatient fasting as treatment for diabetes type-2 and obesity (*Am J Med* 1988 Jul[397]): "Sixty-four poorly controlled obese diabetic patients were hospitalized and placed on a precisely defined, hypocaloric diet. ... **Average weight loss was 13 pounds in a mean of 23 days.** During hospitalization, the mean fasting **plasma glucose value for the group fell from 221 +/- 10 to 122 +/- 5 mg/dl.** In 45 patients (73 percent), the final fasting plasma glucose level was less than 125 mg/dl (mean: 102 +/- 2 mg/dl). Oral glucose tolerance even in those patients in whom fasting plasma glucose levels normalized was still grossly diabetic at the end of the hospital stay, deteriorating further after three days of liberalized caloric intake. In part this may have been due to decreased insulin secretory reserve as reflected by blunted plasma C-peptide response. **Forty of 42 patients who entered the study taking insulin were able to discontinue the drug within one to**

[395] Haimoto et al. Low-carbohydrate diet on glycemic control in outpatients with severe type-2 diabetes. *Nutr Metab* 2009 May:21 nutritionandmetabolism.com/content/6/1/21
[396] Meckling KA, Sherfey R. A randomized trial of a hypocaloric high-protein diet, with and without exercise, on weight loss, fitness, and markers of the Metabolic Syndrome in overweight and obese women. *Appl Physiol Nutr Metab*. 2007 Aug;32(4):743-52
[397] Bauman et al. Early and long-term effects of acute caloric deprivation in obese diabetic patients. *Am J Med*. 1988 Jul;85(1):38-46

seven days of hospitalization. After a mean follow-up period of 19 months, only 10 of 50 patients continued to maintain fasting euglycemia; five were on diet alone, and five were receiving oral hypoglycemic agents. Thirteen patients [down from 42 patients who were originally taking insulin] were receiving insulin therapy. **CONCLUSION: Diet therapy in these patients resulted in short-term improvement of glycemic control and, in the majority, normalization of fasting plasma glucose levels.** However, long-term outpatient follow-up revealed that relapse occurred in most patients." Part of the significance of this study is that it again shows the remarkable effectiveness of low-carbohydrate diet therapy for the treatment of DM-2; notice that most patients had normalization of their glucose levels, were able to discontinue insulin, and they succeeded in significant weight loss. The fact that these accomplishments were short-lived does not reflect a failure of the treatment but rather of compliance; this underscores the importance of patient support during the initiation of a low-carbohydrate diet and lifestyle.

- Clinical trial: Supplemented fasting as a large-scale outpatient program (*JAMA* 1977 Nov[398]): "Although supplemented fasting is now established as an efficient means of achieving substantial weight reduction in massively obese persons, widespread application of this treatment is contingent on its successful adaptation to a large-scale outpatient regimen. Of 519 patients treated as outpatients, 78% lost a minimum of 18.2 kg during the course of treatment. The overall rate of weight loss was 1.5 kg/wk, with females averaging 1.3 kg/wk and males, 2.1 kg/wk. The majority of patients tolerated the regimen well and were able to continue normal daily activities without experiencing any serious side effects." The importance of this study is that it showed that fasting programs can be administered safely and effectively on an outpatient basis; this does not mean that all patients will tolerate or are candidates for this treatment. Clinicians have the responsibility to select patients carefully, to screen them appropriately (e.g., ensure normal kidney function, electrolytes, and cardiac function), and to monitor them during the supervised fast with weekly or twice weekly in-office clinical assessments including blood pressure, mental status, serum electrolytes, and cardiac status assessed with auscultation and ECG.

- Outpatient diet and exercise treatment of 106 patients with massive obesity (*Arch Intern Med* 1975 Dec[399]): "This study demonstrates that massively obese persons can achieve marked weight reduction, even normalization of weight, without hospitalization, surgery, or pharmacologic intervention. Accompanying cardiovascular risk factors show great decrements concomitant with weight loss."

- **Multivitamin/multimineral supplementation**: DM/MetSyn patients generally achieved their clinical status via a lifetime of "overconsumption malnutrition." DM/MetSyn patients are at risk of nutritional deficiency because of poor dietary habits, oxidative destruction of vitamins, increased urinary losses of minerals, and—in patients with diabetes-induced autonomic neuropathy—nutrient malabsorption due to bacterial overgrowth of the small bowel due to gastroparesis or delayed intestinal transit (functional/overt hypothyroidism also contributes to the latter).

  - Review: Vitamins for chronic disease prevention in adults: clinical applications (*JAMA* 2002 Jun[400]): "Most people do not consume an optimal amount of all vitamins by diet alone. ...it appears prudent for all adults to take vitamin supplements. ... Physicians should...ensure that [patients] are taking vitamins they should..."

  - Clinical trial: Effect of a multivitamin and mineral supplement on infection and quality of life. A randomized, double-blind, placebo-controlled trial (*Ann Intern Med* 2003 Mar[401]): "A multivitamin and mineral supplement reduced the incidence of participant-reported infection and related absenteeism in a sample of participants with type 2 diabetes mellitus and a high prevalence of subclinical micronutrient deficiency."

  - Review: Contribution of selected vitamins and trace elements to immune function (*Ann Nutr Metab* 2007 Sep[402]): "Adequate intake of vitamins B(6), folate, B(12), C, E, and of selenium, zinc, copper, and iron supports a Th-1 cytokine-mediated immune response with sufficient production of proinflammatory

[398] Vertes V, Genuth SM, Hazelton IM. Supplemented fasting as a large-scale outpatient program. *JAMA*. 1977 Nov 14;238(20):2151-3

[399] Kempner et al. Treatment of massive obesity with rice/reduction diet program. Analysis of 106 patients with at least a 45-kg weight loss. *Arch Intern Med*. 1975 Dec:1575-84

[400] Fletcher RH, Fairfield KM. Vitamins for chronic disease prevention in adults: clinical applications. *JAMA*. 2002 Jun 19;287(23):3127-9

[401] Barringer et al. Effect of a multivitamin and mineral supplement on infection and quality of life. *Ann Intern Med*. 2003 Mar 4;138(5):365-71

[402] Wintergerst ES, Maggini S, Hornig DH. Contribution of selected vitamins and trace elements to immune function. *Ann Nutr Metab*. 2007;51(4):301-23

cytokines, which **maintains an effective immune response** and avoids a shift to an anti-inflammatory Th2 cell-mediated immune response and an increased risk of extracellular infections."

- Review: Nutritional strategies to boost immunity and prevent infection in elderly individuals (*Clin Infect Dis* 2001 Dec[403]): **"Nutritional supplementation strategies can reduce this risk and reverse some of the immune dysfunction associated with advanced age.** ... The data support use of a daily multivitamin or trace-mineral supplement that includes zinc (elemental zinc, >20 mg/day) and selenium (100 microg/day), with additional vitamin E, to achieve a daily dosage of 200 mg/day."

> **Clinical Perspective**
>
> Remember that DM/MetSyn is a form of immunosuppression insofar as patients with these conditions have an increased risk for infection, poor circulation, and delayed wound healing and tissue repair. Thus, a comprehensive plan should address not only the obvious hyperglycemic, hypertensive, and pro-inflammatory issues, but also the immunocompromise that can be addressed at least partly through comprehensive nutritional supplementation.

- Clinical trial: Effect of vitamin C on blood glucose, serum lipids & serum insulin in type 2 diabetes patients (*Indian J Med Res* 2007 Nov[404]): These authors evaluated the effect of different doses of vitamin C on blood glucose, serum lipids and serum insulin in individuals with DM-2; 84 patients with DM-2 referred to a specialty diabetic clinic in Iran were included in the study. "They received randomly either 500 mg or 1000 mg daily of vitamin C for six weeks. ... RESULTS: A significant decrease in FBS [fasting blood sugar], TG, LDL, HbA1c and serum insulin was seen in the group supplemented with 1000 mg vitamin C. The dose of 500 mg vitamin C, however, did not produce any significant change in any of the parameters studied. INTERPRETATION & CONCLUSION: Our results indicate that **daily consumption of 1000 mg supplementary vitamin C may be beneficial in decreasing blood glucose and lipids in patients with type 2 diabetes and thus reducing the risk of complications**." To their credit, the authors of this study used a high enough dose to produce benefit. The results of 500 mg vitamin C per day are obvious—in this case, they were insignificant, and the "inefficacy of nutritional supplementation in patients with diabetes" would have made headlines in every newspaper in America, as is common when poorly conducted and underpowered trials of nutritional therapy fail.

- Randomized double-blind placebo-controlled pilot study: High-dose thiamine therapy for patients with type 2 diabetes and microalbuminuria (*Diabetologia* 2009 Feb[405]): The authors review data showing that high-dose supplements of thiamine prevent the development of microalbuminuria in experimental diabetes. "METHODS: Type 2 diabetic patients (21 male, 19 female) with microalbuminuria were recruited at a diabetic clinic and randomized to placebo and treatment arms. Patients were given 3 x 100 mg capsules of thiamine or placebo per day for 3 months with a 2 month follow-up washout period. The primary endpoint was change in **urinary albumin excretion (UAE).** "RESULTS: UAE was **decreased in patients receiving thiamine therapy for 3 months with respect to baseline (median -17.7 mg/24 h**; p < 0.001, n = 20). There was no significant decrease in UAE in patients receiving placebo after 3 months of therapy (n = 20). UAE was significantly lower in patients who had received thiamine therapy compared with those who had received placebo (30.1 vs 35.5 mg/24 h, p < 0.01) but not at baseline. UAE continued to decrease in the 2 month washout period in both groups, but not significantly. There was no effect of thiamine treatment on glycemic control, dyslipidemia or BP. There were no adverse effects of therapy. CONCLUSIONS/INTERPRETATION: **In this pilot study, high-dose thiamine therapy produced a regression of UAE in type 2 diabetic patients with microalbuminuria. Thiamine supplements at high dose may provide improved therapy for early-stage diabetic nephropathy.**" This remarkable study disproves the medically purported "dangers" of using nutritional supplementation in patients with DM in general and DM-related renal insufficiency in particular. The mechanism of action is probably related to improved mitochondrial bioenergetics; based on this proposed mechanism of action, clinicians should readily hypothesize which other nutrient(s) would be expected to have similar clinical application—answer(s) will be provided later in this text.

[403] High KP. Nutritional strategies to boost immunity and prevent infection in elderly individuals. *Clin Infect Dis.* 2001 Dec 1;33(11):1892-900

[404] Afkhami-Ardekani et al. Effect of vitamin C on blood glucose, serum lipids & serum insulin in type 2 diabetes patients. *Indian J Med Res.* 2007 Nov;126(5):471-4

[405] Rabbani et al. High-dose thiamine therapy for patients with type 2 diabetes and microalbuminuria. *Diabetologia.* 2009 Feb;52(2):208-12

- Review: The potential role of thiamine (vitamin B1) in diabetic complications (*Curr Diabetes Rev* 2005 Aug[406]): Hyperglycemia causes accumulation of triose-phosphates, which are believed to contribute to the development of diabetic complications. The disposal of excess triose-phosphates via the reductive pentose-phosphate pathway relies upon the thiamine-dependent enzyme, transketolase. Correction of thiamine deficiency or supplemental thiamine has prevented diabetic complications in experimental diabetes. Given the potential clinical benefits and the paucity of adverse effects, the author concludes, "even mild thiamine deficiency in diabetes should be avoided and thiamine supplementation to high dose should be considered as adjunct nutritional therapy to prevent dyslipidemia and the development of vascular complications in clinical diabetes."

- Randomized, double-blind, controlled study: Antioxidant supplementation improves insulin sensitivity, endothelial adhesion molecules, and oxidative stress in normal-weight and overweight young adults (*Metabolism* 2009 Feb[407]): Participants (n=48) received "antioxidants" (AOX) as vitamin E 800 IU, vitamin C 500 mg, beta-carotene 10 mg or placebo for 8 weeks. The HOMA [homeostasis model assessment: a test of insulin sensitivity] values were initially higher in the overweight subjects and were lowered with AOX by week 8 (15% reduction, P = .02). Adiponectin increased in both AOX groups. (Adiponectin is a protein hormone that modulates glucose regulation and fatty acid catabolism. Adiponectin is exclusively secreted from adipose tissue, and levels of the hormone are inversely correlated with body fat percentage in adults. Adiponectin plays a protective role in the suppression of the metabolic derangements that may result in type 2 diabetes, obesity, atherosclerosis, non-alcoholic fatty liver disease (NAFLD) and the metabolic syndrome.) Furthermore, "Soluble intercellular adhesion molecule-1 and endothelial-leukocyte adhesion molecule-1 decreased in overweight AOX-treated groups by 6% and 13%, respectively (P < .05). Plasma lipid hydroperoxides were reduced by 0.31 and 0.70 nmol/mL in the normal-weight and overweight AOX-treated groups, respectively, by week 8 (P < .05)." In summary, this study showed that overweight patients have several positive and important biochemical responses to multivitamin supplementation with vitamin E 800 IU, vitamin C 500 mg, beta-carotene 10 mg for 8 weeks; integrative clinicians should appreciate the application of this protocol within a larger context that includes other nutrients as well as diet and exercise optimization.

- **Vitamin D3 (cholecalciferol, not ergocalciferol): 4,000-10,000 IU per day; for acute infections in deficient patients consider a one-time loading dose of 50,000-100,000 (up to 300,000) IU followed by a more conservative maintenance dose**: In our 2004 monograph by Vasquez, Manso, and Cannell[408], we fulfilled our promise of creating a "paradigm shift" that summarized new applications for the clinical use of vitamin D beyond its application in patients with osteoporosis or malabsorption to include the mandate of empiric treatment or laboratory assessment of all patients seen in clinical practice. Daily doses generally average between 4,000-10,000 IU/d for adults, with an acceptable one-time loading dose of 100,000-300,000 IU in patients for whom it is advantageous and safe to raise serum 25-hydroxy-vitamin D levels quickly and without concern for compliance failure; the logistical goal with vitamin D supplementation is to get serum 25-hydroxy-vitamin D levels into the optimal range, as defined in the illustration. The particular importance for using vitamin D in all diabetic patients is established by the following: ❶ DM/MetSyn patients tend to be more sedentary than the average American (who is also too sedentary), and "being sedentary" generally equates to "being indoors" where no sun exposure can occur; thus the prevalence of vitamin D deficiency is increased above the pandemic levels seen in the rest of the population. ❷ DM/MetSyn patients tend to be overweight or grossly obese, and the risk of vitamin D deficiency increases with increasing obesity/adiposity/BMI. ❸ Vitamin D levels correlate inversely with risk for heart disease, insulin resistance, renal failure, infection, cancer, and heart failure—all of these are increased in patients with DM/MetSyn. ❹ Lack of exercise that characterizes the lifestyle (or more accurately: *deathstyle*) of many patients with DM/MetSyn may also predispose a good number of these patients to osteopenia/osteoporosis; obviously vitamin D has a role in preventing this complication. ❺ Vitamin D levels correlate directly and positively with pancreatic insulin output and peripheral insulin sensitivity. ❻ DM/MetSyn patients have an increased incidence of depression, and by this time at least three separate clinical trials have shown that vitamin D has a mood-elevating and antidepressant benefit. ❼ Vitamin D can be safely

[406] Thornalley PJ. The potential role of thiamine (vitamin B1) in diabetic complications. *Curr Diabetes Rev.* 2005 Aug;1(3):287-98
[407] Vincent et al. Antioxidant supplementation on insulin sensitivity, endothelial adhesion molecules, oxidative stress in normal/overweight adults. *Metabolism* 2009 Feb:254-62
[408] Vasquez A, Manso G, Cannell J. The clinical importance of vitamin D (cholecalciferol). *Altern Ther Health Med.* 2004 Sep-Oct;10(5):28-36

administered to DM/MetSyn patients; patients who require more frequent monitoring of serum calcium are those with end-stage renal insufficiency and those taking hydrochlorothiazide, both of which can predispose to hypercalcemia.

- Chart review: Very high prevalence of vitamin D insufficiency in obese children and adolescents (*J Pediatr Endocrinol Metab* 2007 Jul[409]): Charts of 217 obese children were reviewed and correlated with laboratory results. **Severe vitamin D deficiency was found in 55% of obese children**, and this single nutritional **deficiency correlated with increased overweight/obesity, systolic blood pressure, and lower levels of cardioprotective HDL**. "CONCLUSION: **More than half of the obese children had vitamin D levels <20 ng/ml** with equal gender distribution. Vitamin D insufficiency was associated with increased age, BMI, and SBP, and decreased HDL-C."

Improvements in Hgb-A1c per various non-insulin treatments: ranked per safety and effectiveness, and cost-effectiveness
1. **Low-carbohydrate diet: -3.1 %***
2. **Oral magnesium supplementation: -2 %****
3. **Berberine: -1.2-2 %*****
4. Metformin: -1.5-2 %******
5. Sulfonylurea drugs: -1.5-2 %******
6. Thiazolidinedione drugs: -1.5-2 %******
*Haimoto et al. Effects of a low-carbohydrate diet on glycemic control in outpatients with severe type 2 diabetes. *Nutr Metab* 2009
** Rodríguez-Morán et al. Oral magnesium supplementation improves insulin sensitivity and metabolic control in type 2 diabetic subjects. *Diabetes Care* 2003 Apr
***Yin et al. Efficacy of berberine in patients with type 2 diabetes mellitus. *Metabolism*. 2008 May
****Sloan PD et al [eds]. *Essentials of Family Medicine, Fifth Edition*. Lippincott Williams & Wilkins: 2008, pages 233-235

- Double-blind, parallel group, placebo-controlled randomized trial: Vitamin D improves endothelial function in patients with DM-2 and low vitamin D levels (*Diabet Med* 2008 Mar[410]): Unfortunately, this is an example of a trial that started with the wrong intervention, but was able to produce meaningful results nonetheless. The investigators used a single dose 100,000 IU vitamin D2 (they should have used vitamin D3, because it is much more effective) to see if this would improve endothelial function in patients with DM-2 and low serum 25-hydroxyvitamin D level (baseline 25-hydroxyvitamin D level was < 50 nmol/l). Significant results of this study are as follows: ❶ 49% of screened patients were vitamin D deficient. ❷ Vitamin D supplementation increased 25-hydroxyvitamin D levels by 15.3 nmol/l relative to placebo from a baseline 25-OH-vitamin D level of 38.3 nmol/l; thus the average increased to about 54 nmol/l—this is only slightly higher than the minimum of the optimal range defined and discussed previously (and again below). ❸ Vitamin D supplementation significantly improved flow mediated vasodilatation (FMD) of the brachial artery by 2.3%. ❹ **Vitamin D supplementation significantly decreased systolic blood pressure by 14 mmHg** compared with placebo; readers should note that this reduction in blood pressure is clinically meaningful and that it supports the earlier findings by Pfeifer et al[411] who found a reduction in blood pressure of approximately -13/-7 following the administration of low-dose vitamin D and calcium to elderly women.

- **Magnesium—600-1,200 mg per day or to bowel tolerance; use caution in patients predisposed to hypermagnesemia (renal failure, spironolactone):**
  - Randomized double-blind controlled trial: Oral magnesium supplementation improves insulin sensitivity and metabolic control in type 2 diabetic subjects (*Diabetes Care* 2003 Apr[412]): Oral supplementation with placebo or magnesium chloride (50 ml MgCl(2) solution containing 50 g MgCl(2) per 1,000 ml solution) was given to 63 subjects with DM-2 and hypomagnesaemia (serum magnesium levels </=0.74 mmol/l) for 16 weeks. "RESULTS: At the end of the study, **subjects who received magnesium supplementation showed significant higher serum magnesium concentration** (0.74 +/- 0.10 vs. 0.65 +/- 0.07 mmol/l, P = 0.02) and **lower HOMA-IR index** (3.8 +/- 1.1 vs. 5.0 +/- 1.3, P = 0.005), **fasting glucose levels** (8.0 +/- 2.4 vs. 10.3 +/- 2.1 mmol/l, P = 0.01), and **HbA(1c) (8.0** +/- 2.4 vs. **10.1** +/- 3.3%, P = 0.04) than control subjects. CONCLUSIONS: Oral supplementation with MgCl(2) solution restores serum magnesium levels, improving insulin sensitivity and metabolic control in type-2 diabetic patients with decreased serum magnesium levels." These results are truly remarkable considering the dramatic clinical response that these

[409] Smotkin-Tangorra et al. Prevalence of vitamin D insufficiency in obese children and adolescents. *J Pediatr Endocrinol Metab*. 2007 Jul;20(7):817-23

[410] Sugden et al. Vitamin D improves endothelial function in patients with Type 2 diabetes mellitus and low vitamin D levels. *Diabet Med*. 2008 Mar;25(3):320-5

[411] Pfeifer et al. Short-term vitamin D(3) calcium supplementation on blood pressure and parathyroid hormone levels in elderly women. *J Clin Endocrinol Metab* 2001 Apr:1633-7

[412] Rodríguez-Morán M, Guerrero-Romero F. Oral magnesium supplementation improves insulin sensitivity and metabolic control in type 2 diabetic subjects: a randomized double-blind controlled trial. *Diabetes Care*. 2003 Apr;26(4):1147-52

DM-2 patients showed to simple intervention with oral magnesium. Magnesium chloride is one of the least desirable forms of magnesium supplementation, with the citrate and malate forms being generally preferred by clinicians. The remarkable drop in Hgb-A1c levels from 10% (very poor control) to 8% (markedly improved control nearing the target of 7%) is sufficient to justify Mg supplementation in all diabetic patients (assuming result replicability).

- Randomized clinical trial: Efficacy and safety of oral magnesium supplementation in the treatment of depression in the elderly with type 2 diabetes (*Magnes Res* 2008 Dec[413]): Unfortunately, these researchers used what is generally considered to be an inferior form of magnesium supplementation—magnesium chloride—to evaluate the efficacy and safety of oral magnesium supplementation in the treatment of newly diagnosed depression in elderly hypomagnesemic patients with DM-2. Twenty-three subjects were enrolled and randomly allocated to receive either 50 mL of MgCl2 5% solution (equivalent to **450 mg of elemental magnesium**) or Imipramine 50 mg daily during 12 weeks. For inclusion criteria, hypomagnesemia was defined as serum magnesium levels < 1.8 mg/dL and depression by Yasavage and Brink score > or = 11 points; astute readers should appreciate that serum magnesium is reasonably specific but is not sensitive for magnesium deficiency. Results included the following, "At end of follow-up, there were no significant differences in the Yasavage and Brink score (11.4 +/- 3.8 and 10.9 +/- 4.3, p = 0.27) between the groups in study; whereas serum magnesium levels were significantly higher in the group with MgCl2 (2.1 +/- 0.08 mg/dL) than in the subjects with imipramine (1.5 +/- 0.07 mg/dL), p < 0.0005. **In conclusion, MgCl2 is as effective in the treatment of depressed elderly type 2 diabetics with hypomagnesemia as imipramine 50 mg daily.**" In the end, this turned out to be a remarkable study showing not only safety of oral magnesium 450 mg per day, but more importantly that magnesium is as effective as a commonly used but somewhat dangerous tricyclic antidepressant; given that the probably of *magnesium deficiency* in elderly DM-2 patients is higher than the probability of *imipramine deficiency* in these patients, correcting the underlying nutritional deficiency by the use of oral magnesium supplementation is more logical than using a tricyclic antidepressant with its numerous and serious adverse effects. Further, Mg benefits insulin sensitivity, blood pressure and other aspects of DM-2 which are not beneficially impacted by the more expensive and dangerous imipramine.

- 3-month randomized double-blind placebo-controlled trial: Oral magnesium supplementation improves insulin sensitivity in non-diabetic subjects with insulin resistance (*Diabetes Metab* 2004 Jun[414]): In this study, the researchers used oral magnesium chloride (MgCl2) 2.5 g daily in "apparently healthy" non-diabetic subjects with insulin resistance (HOMA-IR index equal or greater than 3.0) and hypomagnesemia (serum magnesium levels equal or lower than 0.74 mmol/l). Subjects were randomized to receive either, MgCl2 2.5 g daily or placebo by 3-months. "RESULTS: At baseline there were not significant anthropometric or laboratory differences between both groups. At ending of the study, magnesium-supplemented subjects significantly increased their serum magnesium levels (0.61 +/- 0.08 to 0.81 +/- 0.08 mmol/l, p<0.0001) and reduced HOMA-IR index (4.6 +/- 2.8 to 2.6 +/- 1.1, p<0.0001), whereas control subjects did not (0.62 +/- 0.08 to 0.61 +/- 0.08 mmol/l, p=0.063 and 5.2 +/- 1.9 to 5.3 +/- 2.9, p=0.087). **CONCLUSIONS: Oral magnesium supplementation improves insulin sensitivity in hypomagnesemic non-diabetic subjects.**"

• **Fatty acid supplementation with ALA (from flaxseed oil), GLA (from borage oil), EPA and DHA (from fish oil)—alone or in combination**: Fish oil supplementation is the single most effective intervention for the prevention of cardiovascular disease that has ever been consistently documented. Fish oil supplementation beneficially affects many of the physiologic phenomena that are involved in cardiovascular health and disease, including platelet adhesion, endothelial function, inflammation, serum lipids, insulin sensitivity, and mental depression; furthermore, natural-source fish oil such as cod liver oil is a notable source of cardioprotective vitamin D3, which is pandemically deficient in nearly all populations. For healthcare providers of all disciplines and pedigrees, the evidence is so strong in favor of the routine use of fish oil that—if the standards of care in healthcare truly included beneficence and nonmalfecense—failure to utilize fish oil in all patients and particularly in patients at increased risk for cardiovascular disease should be considered negligent malpractice. No other single treatment—nutritional or pharmacologic—offers the numerous benefits that fish oil

[413] Barragán-Rodríguez et al. Efficacy and safety of oral magnesium supplementation in treatment of depression in the elderly with type 2 diabetes. *Magnes Res.* 2008 Dec:218-23
[414] Guerrero-Romero et al. Oral magnesium supplementation improves insulin sensitivity in non-diabetic subjects with insulin resistance. *Diabetes Metab.* 2004 Jun;30(3):253-8

supplementation provides. Because fatty acids work in combination and synergy with other fatty acids, and because most patients have numerous fatty acid imbalances and deficiencies, fatty acid supplementation should be administered as combination fatty acid therapy that provides—at minimum—the EPA and DHA of fish oil in combination with the GLA sourced from either borage oil (most concentrated source), evening primrose oil (perhaps the best biochemical form of GLA), black currant seed oil, or hemp oil. In an earlier review[415] of this topic, I summarized the benefits of fatty acid supplementation as follows:

☑ N-3 alpha-linolenic acid (ALA): Increased intake of ALA appears to provide cardioprotective[416] and anti-inflammatory benefits[417,418], and ALA can help reduce the frequency and severity of migraine headaches when used as part of a comprehensive natural treatment plan that includes GLA, multivitamins, and dietary modification.[419]

☑ Eicosapentaenoic acid (EPA): EPA used in isolation shows benefit in lupus,[420] cancer[421], borderline personality disorder[422], mental depression[423,424,425], schizophrenia[426], and osteoporosis (when used with GLA).[427]

☑ Docosahexaenoic acid (DHA): Supplementation with DHA (often in the form of fish oil, which includes EPA) has been shown to benefit patients with bipolar disorder[428], Crohn's disease[429], rheumatoid arthritis[430,431,432], lupus[433], cardiovascular disease[434], psoriasis[435], and cancer.[436] DHA appears to have an "anti-stress" benefit manifested by 30% reductions in norepinephrine and improved resilience to psychoemotional stress.[437,438]

☑ Supplementation with EPA+DHA: This combination, naturally found in fish oil, is extremely safe and reduces all-cause mortality.[439]

☑ Gamma-linolenic acid (GLA): Clinical benefit associated with GLA supplementation is seen in patients with, eczema[440], breast cancer (when used with tamoxifen[441]), premenstrual syndrome[442], rheumatoid arthritis[443,444], diabetic neuropathy[445], migraine headaches (when used with ALA[446]), and respiratory distress

[415] Vasquez A. New Insights into Fatty Acid Supplementation and Its Effect on Eicosanoid Production and Genetic Expression. *Nutritional Perspectives* 2005; January: 5-16

[416] Hu et al. Dietary intake of alpha-linolenic acid and risk of fatal ischemic heart disease among women. *Am J Clin Nutr.* 1999 May;69(5):890-7

[417] "CONCLUSIONS: Dietary supplementation with ALA for 3 months decreases significantly CRP, SAA and IL-6 levels in dyslipidaemic patients. This anti-inflammatory effect may provide a possible additional mechanism for the beneficial effect of plant n-3 polyunsaturated fatty acids in primary and secondary prevention of coronary artery disease." Rallidis et al. Dietary alpha-linolenic acid decreases C-reactive protein, serum amyloid A and interleukin-6 in dyslipidaemic patients. *Atherosclerosis.* 2003 Apr;167(2):237-42

[418] Adam O, Wolfram G, Zollner N. Effect of alpha-linolenic acid in the human diet on linoleic acid metabolism and prostaglandin biosynthesis. *J Lipid Res.* 1986 Apr;27(4):421-6

[419] Wagner W, Nootbaar-Wagner U. Prophylactic treatment of migraine with gamma-linolenic and alpha-linolenic acids. *Cephalalgia.* 1997 Apr;17(2):127-30

[420] Duffy et al. The clinical effect of dietary supplementation with omega-3 fish oils and/or copper in systemic lupus erythematosus. *J Rheumatol.* 2004 Aug;31(8):1551-6

[421] Wigmore SJ, Barber MD, Ross JA, Tisdale MJ, Fearon KC. Effect of oral eicosapentaenoic acid on weight loss in patients with pancreatic cancer. *Nutr Cancer.* 2000;36:177-84

[422] Zanarini MC, Frankenburg FR. omega-3 Fatty acid treatment of women with borderline personality disorder. *Am J Psychiatry.* 2003 Jan;160(1):167-9

[423] Nemets et al. Addition of omega-3 fatty acid to maintenance medication treatment for recurrent unipolar depressive disorder. *Am J Psychiatry.* 2002 Mar;159(3):477-9

[424] Puri BK, Counsell SJ, Hamilton G, Richardson AJ, Horrobin DF. Eicosapentaenoic acid in treatment-resistant depression associated with symptom remission, structural brain changes and reduced neuronal phospholipid turnover. *Int J Clin Pract.* 2001 Oct;55(8):560-3

[425] Peet M, Horrobin DF. A dose-ranging study of the effects of ethyl-eicosapentaenoate in patients with ongoing depression despite apparently adequate treatment with standard drugs. *Arch Gen Psychiatry.* 2002 Oct;59(10):913-9

[426] Emsley et al. Randomized, placebo-controlled study of ethyl-eicosapentaenoic acid as supplemental treatment in schizophrenia. *Am J Psychiatry.* 2002 Sep;159(9):1596-8

[427] Kruger et al. Calcium, gamma-linolenic acid and eicosapentaenoic acid supplementation in senile osteoporosis. *Aging* (Milano). 1998 Oct;10(5):385-94

[428] Stoll et al. Omega 3 fatty acids in bipolar disorder: a preliminary double-blind, placebo-controlled trial. *Arch Gen Psychiatry.* 1999 May;56(5):407-12

[429] Belluzzi et al. Effect of an enteric-coated fish-oil preparation on relapses in Crohn's disease. *N Engl J Med.* 1996 Jun 13;334(24):1557-60

[430] Adam et al. Anti-inflammatory effects of a low arachidonic acid diet and fish oil in patients with rheumatoid arthritis. *Rheumatol Int.* 2003 Jan;23(1):27-36

[431] Lau et al. Effects of fish oil supplementation on non-steroidal anti-inflammatory drug requirement in patients with mild rheumatoid arthritis. *Br J Rheumatol.* 1993 Nov:982-9

[432] Kremer et al. Fish-oil fatty acid supplementation in active rheumatoid arthritis. A double-blinded, controlled, crossover study. *Ann Intern Med.* 1987 Apr;106(4):497-503

[433] Walton et al. Dietary fish oil and the severity of symptoms in patients with systemic lupus erythematosus. *Ann Rheum Dis.* 1991 Jul;50(7):463-6

[434] "The recent GISSI (Gruppo Italiano per lo Studio della Sopravvivenza nell'Infarto miocardico)-Prevention study of 11,324 patients showed a 45% decrease in risk of sudden cardiac death and a 20% reduction in all-cause mortality in the group taking 850 mg/d of omega-3 fatty acids." O'Keefe JH Jr, Harris WS. From Inuit to implementation: omega-3 fatty acids come of age. *Mayo Clin Proc.* 2000 Jun;75(6):607-14

[435] Bittiner SB, Tucker WF, Cartwright I, Bleehen SS. A double-blind, randomised, placebo-controlled trial of fish oil in psoriasis. *Lancet.* 1988 Feb 20;1(8582):378-80

[436] Gogos et al. Dietary omega-3 polyunsaturated fatty acids plus vitamin E restore immunodeficiency and prolong survival for severely ill patients with generalized malignancy. *Cancer.* 1998 Jan 15;82(2):395-402

[437] Hamazaki T, Itomura M, Sawazaki S, Nagao Y. Anti-stress effects of DHA. *Biofactors.* 2000;13(1-4):41-5

[438] Sawazaki S, Hamazaki T, Yazawa K, Kobayashi M. The effect of docosahexaenoic acid on plasma catecholamine concentrations and glucose tolerance during long-lasting psychological stress: a double-blind placebo-controlled study. *J Nutr Sci Vitaminol* (Tokyo). 1999 Oct;45(5):655-65

[439] "The recent GISSI (Gruppo Italiano per lo Studio della Sopravvivenza nell'Infarto miocardico)-Prevention study of 11,324 patients showed a 45% decrease in risk of sudden cardiac death and a 20% reduction in all-cause mortality in the group taking 850 mg/d of omega-3 fatty acids." O'Keefe JH Jr, Harris WS. From Inuit to implementation: omega-3 fatty acids come of age. *Mayo Clin Proc.* 2000 Jun;75(6):607-14

[440] Fiocchi et al. The efficacy and safety of gamma-linolenic acid in the treatment of infantile atopic dermatitis. *J Int Med Res.* 1994 Jan-Feb;22(1):24-32

[441] Kenny et al. Gamma linolenic acid with tamoxifen as primary therapy in breast cancer. *Int J Cancer.* 2000 Mar 1;85(5):643-8

[442] Puolakka et al. Biochemical and clinical effects of treating the premenstrual syndrome with prostaglandin synthesis precursors. *J Reprod Med.* 1985 Mar;30(3):149-53

[443] Brzeski et al. Evening primrose oil in patients with rheumatoid arthritis and side-effects of non-steroidal anti-inflammatory drugs. *Br J Rheumatol.* 1991 Oct;30(5):370-2

[444] Rothman D, DeLuca P, Zurier RB. Botanical lipids: effects on inflammation, immune responses, and rheumatoid arthritis. *Semin Arthritis Rheum.* 1995 Oct;25(2):87-96

[445] Jamal GA, Carmichael H. The effect of gamma-linolenic acid on human diabetic peripheral neuropathy. *Diabet Med.* 1990 May;7(4):319-23

[446] Wagner W, Nootbaar-Wagner U. Prophylactic treatment of migraine with gamma-linolenic and alpha-linolenic acids. *Cephalalgia.* 1997 Apr;17(2):127-30

syndrome (when used with EPA).[447] As discussed and detailed in Chapter 4, the major "biochemical risk" from using GLA is that of raising arachidonic acid levels if delta-5-desaturase is not inhibited by concomitant administration of EPA; the major "clinical risk" associated with GLA administration is that of inducing or exacerbating temporal lobe epilepsy, as noted in a few case reports and case series.

Insofar as research and statistical analyses are concerned, we have to appreciate that many of these fatty acid supplementation studies were performed by researchers who thought that olive oil was an inert placebo; no clinician or researcher in his/her right mind would make such a blunder these days—or so we might hope. The olive oil "placebo" is one of the most potent anti-inflammatory and cardioprotective interventions available; olive oil contains numerous substances with anti-cancer, cardioprotective, and anti-inflammatory benefits, including n-9 oleic acid, squalene, and the numerous polyphenolic phytonutrients. Because many of the earlier "fish oil studies" used olive oil as their control group, important benefits of fish oil were underestimated and underappreciated and thus underutilized because the "control group" (i.e., olive oil supplementation) and "treatment group" (i.e., fish oil supplementation) were both being treated with a potent anti-cancer, cardioprotective, and anti-inflammatory intervention.

- Clinical trial with very-low-dose fish oil: Effect of omega-3 fatty acids on cardiovascular risk factors in patients with type 2 diabetes mellitus and hypertriglyceridemia: an open study (*Eur Rev Med Pharmacol Sci* 2009 Jan[448]): In this group of **30 patients** with type-2 diabetes mellitus and hypertriglyceridemia, patients received two capsules of **eicosapentaenoic 465 mg and docosahexaenoic 375 mg daily** for 12 weeks. "RESULTS: Triglycerides levels and non HDL-cholesterol decreased (326 vs. 216.4 mg/dl) and (103.87 vs. 89.6 mg/dl), respectively. HDL-cholesterol levels increased (39.6 vs. 46.4 mg/dl). C-reactive protein decreased (5.98 vs. 3.9 mg/dl) and TNF-alpha levels decreased (16.24 vs. 13.3 pg/dl), without significant changes in IL-6 levels. **In conclusion, an n-3 polyunsaturated intervention improved lipid profile and inflammatory markers in patients with diabetes mellitus type 2 and hypertriglyceridemia.**" The results of this study are remarkable insofar as the dose of fish oil used was very low; generally in clinical practice we use at least 1,000 and often up to 3,000 mg per day of combined EPA and DHA; this study used only 840 mg.

- 8-week, randomized, double-blind, placebo-controlled study: Efficacy and tolerability of adding prescription omega-3 fatty acids 4 g/d to simvastatin 40 mg/d in hypertriglyceridemic patients (*Clin Ther* 2007 Jul[449]): "This study evaluated the effects on non-HDL-C and other variables of adding prescription omega-3-acid **ethyl esters** (P-OM3; Lovaza, formerly Omacor [Reliant Pharmaceuticals, Inc., Liberty Corner, New Jersey]) to stable statin therapy in patients with persistent hypertriglyceridemia. METHODS: This was a multicenter, randomized, double-blind, placebo-controlled, parallel-group study in adults who had received > or = 8 weeks of stable statin therapy and had mean fasting TG levels > or = 200 and < 500 mg/dL and mean low-density lipoprotein cholesterol levels < or = 10% above their NCEP ATP III goal. The study regimen consisted of an initial 8 weeks of open-label simvastatin 40 mg/d and dietary counseling, followed by 8 weeks of randomized treatment with double-blind P-OM3 4 g/d plus simvastatin 40 mg/d or placebo plus simvastatin 40 mg/d. The main outcome measure was the percent change in non-HDL-C from baseline to the end of treatment. RESULTS: The evaluable population included 254 patients, of whom 57.5% (146) were male and 95.7% (243) were white. The mean (SD) age of the population was 59.8 (10.4) years, and the mean weight was 92.0 (19.6) kg. At the end of treatment, the median percent change in non-HDL-C was significantly greater with P-OM3 plus simvastatin compared with placebo plus simvastatin (-9.0% vs -2.2%, respectively; P < 0.001). P-OM3 plus simvastatin was associated with **significant reductions in TG** (29.5% vs 6.3%) **and very-low-density lipoprotein cholesterol** (27.5% vs 7.2%), **a significant increase in high-density lipoprotein cholesterol (HDL-C) (3.4%** vs -1.2%), and a significant reduction in the total cholesterol:HDL-C ratio (9.6% vs 0.7%) (all, P < 0.001 vs placebo). Adverse events (AEs) reported by > or= 1% of patients in the P-OM3 group that occurred with a higher frequency than in the group that received simvastatin alone were nasopharyngitis (4 [3.3%]), upper respiratory tract infection (4 [3.3%]), diarrhea (3 [2.5%]), and dyspepsia (3 [2.5%]). There was no significant difference in the frequency of AEs [adverse

---

[447] Pacht ER, DeMichele SJ, Nelson JL, Hart J, Wennberg AK, Gadek JE. Enteral nutrition with eicosapentaenoic acid, gamma-linolenic acid, and antioxidants reduces alveolar inflammatory mediators and protein influx in patients with acute respiratory distress syndrome. *Crit Care Med.* 2003 Feb;31(2):491-500

[448] De Luis et al. Omega-3 fatty acids on cardiovascular risk factors in patients with type 2 diabetes mellitus and hypertriglyceridemia. *Eur Rev Med Pharmacol Sci.* 2009 Jan:51-5

[449] Davidson et al. Efficacy and tolerability of adding prescription omega-3 fatty acids 4 g/d to simvastatin 40 mg/d in hypertriglyceridemic patients. *Clin Ther.* 2007 Jul:1354-67

events] between groups. No serious AEs were considered treatment related. CONCLUSION: In these adult, mainly white patients with persistent hypertriglyceridemia, P-OM3 plus simvastatin and dietary counseling improved non-HDL-C and other lipid and lipoprotein parameters to a greater extent than simvastatin alone." Although this study was of short duration, the sample size is reasonably large (n=254) and the results are consistent with what we would have expected, namely that adding EPA+DHA supplementation would provide laboratory evidence of cardioprotection. Each 1-gram LOVAZA capsule contains 465 mg of eicosapentaenoic acid (EPA) and 375 mg of docosahexaenoic acid (DHA). Ethyl esters are the synthetic distillation product made by processing fish oil with ethanol; controversy exists about the bioavailability and biological nuances between natural fish oils with a glycerol backbone versus these semi-synthetic fish oils with an ethanol backbone.

- Meta-analysis of n-3 fatty acid supplementation in patients with DM-2: Meta-analysis of the effects of n-3 polyunsaturated fatty acids on lipoproteins and other emerging lipid cardiovascular risk markers in patients with type 2 diabetes (*Diabetologia* 2007 Aug[450]): "RESULTS: There were 23 trials on non-dietary supplementation, involving 1,075 subjects with a mean treatment duration of 8.9 weeks, with sufficient data to permit pooling. Compared with placebo, n-3 PUFA had a statistically significant effect on four outcomes, **reducing levels of (1) triacylglycerol** (18 trials, 969 subjects) by **25%**; (2) **VLDL-cholesterol** (7 trials, 238 subjects) **by 36%**; and (3) VLDL-triacylglycerol (6 trials, 178 subjects) by 39.7%; while *slightly increasing LDL* (16 trials, 565 subjects) *by 5.7%*. There were no significant effects on total cholesterol, apolipoproteins, lipid subfractions or ratios. CONCLUSIONS/INTERPRETATION: In addition to recognized triacylglycerol-lowering effects, n-3 PUFA supplementation decreases VLDL-cholesterol and VLDL-triacylglycerol, but may have an adverse effect on LDL-cholesterol. Larger and longer term clinical trials are required to conclusively establish the effect of n-3 PUFA on cardiovascular risk markers and outcomes in type 2 diabetic patients." Basically, this information reviewed the biochemical effects (rather than the clinical outcomes) of n-3 fatty acid supplementation. The fact that, per this meta-analysis, n-3 fatty acid supplementation increased LDL by 5.7% is a trend in the wrong direction, since LDL is the major target of serum lipid optimization. However, the fact that all meta-analyses that have focused on *clinical outcomes* have concluded that n-3 fatty acid supplementation reduces overall mortality (even to a greater degree than do to the highly touted and heavily advertised statin drugs) implies that clinicians should use n-3 fatty acids even at the biochemical expense of slightly elevated LDL. Furthermore, the trial by Laidlaw and Holub[451] showed that by combining n-3 fatty acids with GLA, the LDL level could be lowered by more than 11%; thus the findings from these two studies suggests that while n-3 fatty acid supplementation shows overall cardiovascular benefits at the expense of a slight increase in LDL, this biochemical adverse effect is offset by more powerful reductions in overall and cardiovascular mortality, and that even the biochemical adverse effect of raising LDL by 5% can be mitigated by combining with GLA for a total reduction in LDL of 11%. The addition of GLA would do more than lower LDL levels; it would cause additive or synergistic improvements in overall health status, given that GLA helps in a variety of clinical scenarios, such as psoriasis, eczema, and inflammatory joint pain such as rheumatoid arthritis.

- Systematic review: Effect of different antilipidemic agents and diets on mortality (*Arch Intern Med* 2005 Apr[452]): "RESULTS: A total of 97 studies met eligibility criteria, with 137,140 individuals in intervention and 138,976 individuals in control groups. Compared with control groups, **risk ratios for overall mortality** were **0.87 for statins** (95% confidence interval [CI], 0.81-0.94), **1.00 for fibrates** (95% CI, 0.91-1.11), **0.84 for resins** (95% CI, 0.66-1.08), **0.96 for niacin** (95% CI, 0.86-1.08), **0.77 for n-3 fatty acids** (95% CI, 0.63-0.94), and 0.97 for diet (95% CI, 0.91-1.04). Compared with control groups, **risk ratios for cardiac mortality** indicated **benefit from statins (0.78**; 95% CI, 0.72-0.84), **resins (0.70**; 95% CI, 0.50-0.99) **and n-3 fatty acids (0.68**; 95% CI, 0.52-0.90). Risk ratios for noncardiovascular mortality of any intervention indicated no association when compared with control groups, with the exception of fibrates (risk ratio, 1.13; 95% CI, 1.01-1.27).

---

[450] Hartweg et al. Meta-analysis of the effects of n-3 polyunsaturated fatty acids on lipoproteins and other emerging lipid cardiovascular risk markers in patients with type 2 diabetes. *Diabetologia*. 2007 Aug;50(8):1593-602

[451] Laidlaw M, Holub BJ. Effects of supplementation with fish oil-derived n-3 fatty acids and gamma-linolenic acid on circulating plasma lipids and fatty acid profiles in women. *Am J Clin Nutr*. 2003 Jan;77(1):37-42

[452] Studer et al. Effect of different antilipidemic agents and diets on mortality: a systematic review. *Arch Intern Med*. 2005 Apr 11;165(7):725-30

CONCLUSIONS: Statins and n-3 fatty acids are the most favorable lipid-lowering interventions with reduced risks of overall and cardiac mortality. Any potential reduction in cardiac mortality from fibrates is offset by an increased risk of death from noncardiovascular causes." This systematic review found that n-3 fatty acids are superior to statin drugs (and all other cholesterol-lowering cardiovascular drugs) for reducing total mortality and cardiac mortality. Clinically significant side-effects of statin drugs commonly include muscle pain and chemical hepatitis, while side effects of n-3 fatty acids such as fish oil commonly include improved mood and alleviation of depression, schizophrenia, bipolar disorder, borderline personality disorder, eczema, psoriasis, and back pain and joint pain. Even at internet prices, generic atorvastatin (same as Lipitor) at 20 mg per day for one month costs about $34 (plus fees for the office visit and follow-up laboratory and clinical monitoring), whereas one teaspoon of cod liver oil (to provide approximately 1 gram of EPA+DHA) per day for one month costs about $8 (without additional medical expenses, plus cost savings from alleviation from other conditions).

- Extrapolation of short-term effect of various fatty acid ratios on long-term cardiovascular risk: Effects of supplementation with fish oil-derived n-3 fatty acids and gamma-linolenic acid on circulating plasma lipids and fatty acid profiles in women (*Am J Clin Nutr* 2003 Jan[453]): This important study used computerized models to determine long-term cardiovascular risk based on alterations in serum lipids effected by combination fatty acid supplementation with various ratios of EPA+DHA to GLA. "DESIGN: Thirty-one women were assigned to 1 of 4 groups, equalized on the basis of their fasting triacylglycerol concentrations. They received supplements providing 4 g EPA+DHA (4:0, EPA+DHA:GLA; control group), 4 g EPA+DHA plus 1 g GLA (4:1), 2 g GLA (4:2), or 4 g GLA (4:4) daily for 28 d. Plasma lipids and fatty acids of serum phospholipids were measured on days 0 and 28. RESULTS: Plasma triacylglycerol concentrations were significantly lower on day 28 than on day 0 in the 4:0, 4:1, and 4:2 groups. **LDL cholesterol decreased significantly (by 11.3%) in the 4:2 group.** Dihomo-gamma-linolenic acid increased significantly in serum phospholipids only in the 4:2 and 4:4 groups; however, total n-3 fatty acids increased in all 4 groups. CONCLUSIONS: A mixture of **4 g EPA+DHA and 2 g GLA** favorably altered blood lipid and fatty acid profiles in healthy women. On the basis of calculated PROCAM values, the **4:2 group was estimated to have a 43% reduction in the 10-y risk of myocardial infarction**." This research shows that combination fatty acid therapy with EPA+DHA+GLA is better than EPA+DHA alone and that a 4g:2g ratio-amount is optimal. Obviously, this is an extrapolated computer model and not a long-term prospective trial, but the acute reduction in LDL of 11% is very promising; the collateral health benefits of combined EPA+DHA+GLA would be enormous if applied as widely as are the statin drugs.

- **Chromium**: Chromium has long been used in disorders of glucose metabolism: both hypoglycemia and hyperglycemia. The problem with the *medical research* in this regard is that it has generally been consistent with the *medical model* of disease, namely: the constant search for the silver bullet that can alleviate disease, without proper consideration to the use of several nutrients together, along with dietary change, and exercise and physical medicine to more accurately reflect the interventions used by integrative chiropractic and naturopathic clinicians. While we must appreciate the earlier single-intervention studies for their preliminary attempts at determining safety and efficacy of nutritional interventions, we must also appreciate what the culmination of this research has consistently shown, namely that nutrients work together synergistically and that a moderate dose of several nutrients is generally safer and more efficacious than a single dose of one nutrient, and that key metabolic pathways must be affected if clinical benefit is to be shown. Nutrients with numerous overlapping functions (especially fish oil and vitamin D) are massively more effective than single nutrients that work on only a fraction of an isolated pathway (such as chromium in the treatment of DM); simultaneously and perhaps conversely, each nutrient is necessary for optimal metabolic and immunologic function.

  - Short-term (4 weeks) placebo-controlled, double-blinded, randomized trial of chromium+biotin: The effect of chromium picolinate and biotin supplementation on glycemic control in poorly controlled patients with type 2 diabetes mellitus (*Diabetes Technol Ther* 2006 Dec[454]): Experimental studies have shown that

---

[453] Laidlaw M, Holub BJ. Effects of supplementation with fish oil-derived n-3 fatty acids and gamma-linolenic acid on circulating plasma lipids and fatty acid profiles in women. *Am J Clin Nutr*. 2003 Jan;77(1):37-42

[454] Singer et al. Effect of chromium picolinate and biotin supplementation on glycemic control in poorly controlled patients with type 2 diabetes mellitus. *Diabetes Technol Ther*. 2006 Dec;8(6):636-43

chromium picolinate together with biotin significantly enhances glucose uptake in skeletal muscle cells. This pilot study was conducted among 43 patients with DM-2 with poor glycemic control (Hgb-A1c > 7%) despite use of oral antihyperglycemic drugs. Study subjects were administered chromium 600 mcg/d (as chromium picolinate) and biotin 2 mg per day; antihyperglycemic drugs were continued during the study. "RESULTS: After 4 weeks, there was a **significantly greater reduction in the total area under the curve for glucose during the 2-h oral glucose tolerance test for the treatment group** (mean change -9.7%) compared with the placebo group (mean change +5.1%). **Significantly greater reductions were also seen in fructosamine** (P < 0.03), **triglycerides** (P < 0.02), and **triglycerides/ high-density lipoprotein cholesterol ratio** (P < 0.05) **in the treatment group**. No significant adverse events were attributed to chromium picolinate and biotin supplementation. CONCLUSIONS: … Chromium picolinate/ biotin supplementation may represent an effective adjunctive nutritional therapy to people with poorly controlled diabetes with the potential for improving lipid metabolism."

- Pilot study (n=8) of chromium in medicated HIV patients with insulin resistance: Chromium picolinate for insulin resistance in subjects with HIV disease: a pilot study (*Diabetes Obes Metab* 2008 Feb[455]): Because multidrug regimens for HIV treatment are associated with an increased incidence of insulin resistance (as much as 50%), the authors of this study used chromium picolinate (1000 mcg/day) to improve insulin sensitivity, determined with a hyperinsulinaemic-euglycaemic insulin clamp, was determined in eight HIV-positive subjects on highly active antiretroviral therapy (HAART). "RESULTS: The mean **rate of glucose disposal** during the clamp was 4.41 mg glucose/kg lean body mass (LBM)/min (range 2.67-5.50), which increased to 6.51 mg/kg LBM/min (range 3.19-12.78, p = .03), an **increase of 25% after 8 weeks of treatment with chromium picolinate**. There were no significant changes in blood parameters, HIV viral burden or CD4+ lymphocytes with

> **Chromium (picolinate) can modulate appetite in depressed overweight patients who crave carbohydrates**
>
> "While these findings require replication in a prospective trial, they suggest that CrPic may be beneficial for patients with atypical depression who are also high carbohydrate cravers."
>
> Docherty et al. A double-blind, placebo-controlled, exploratory trial of chromium picolinate in atypical depression: effect on carbohydrate craving. *J Psychiatr Pract*. 2005 Sep

chromium picolinate treatment. Two subjects experienced abnormalities of liver function during the study. Another subject experienced an elevation in blood urea nitrogen. CONCLUSIONS: The study shows that **chromium picolinate therapy improves insulin resistance in some HIV-positive subjects, but with some concerns about safety in this population**." These findings are of interest for several reasons: ❶ While the dose used in this study is higher than what has been used in most studies (generally 200 mcg), the 1,000 mcg dose is consistent with what clinicians might use in clinical practice. ❷ These results, even though based on a very small number of patients, suggests that clinicians should use a smaller dose or use careful patient selection or frequent laboratory surveillance when using high-dose chromium in patients with HIV who are taking HAART. ❸ The lack of placebo/control group makes impossible the attribution of adverse effects to chromium, but nonetheless, clinicians should use caution when using high-dose chromium in this patient population based on these results.

- Double-blind, placebo-controlled, multicenter, 8-week replication study: Chromium picolinate in overweight patients with atypical depression: effect on carbohydrate craving (*J Psychiatr Pract* 2005 Sep[456]): The authors report that in a pre-publication small pilot trial, patients with atypical depression demonstrated significant positive therapeutic response to chromium picolinate. These 113 overweight (average BMI = 29.7) adult outpatients with atypical depression were randomized 2:1 to receive chromium 600 mcg/d (as chromium picolinate (CrPic)) or placebo. Patients were assessed with the 29-item Hamilton Depression Rating Scale (HAM-D-29) and the Clinical Global Impressions Improvement Scale (CGI-I). "RESULTS: … There was no significant difference between the CrPic and placebo groups in both the ITT [intention to treat] and evaluable populations on the primary efficacy measures, with both groups showing significant improvement from baseline on total HAM-D-29 scores during the course of treatment (p < 0.0001). However, in the evaluable population, **the CrPic group showed significant improvements from**

[455] Feiner et al. Chromium picolinate for insulin resistance in subjects with HIV disease: a pilot study. *Diabetes Obes Metab*. 2008 Feb;10(2):151-8
[456] Docherty et al. A trial of chromium picolinate in atypical depression: effect on carbohydrate craving. *J Psychiatr Pract*. 2005 Sep;11(5):302-14

baseline compared with the placebo group on 4 HAM-D-29 items: appetite increase, increased eating, carbohydrate craving, and diurnal variation of feelings. A supplemental analysis of data from the subset of 41 patients in the ITT population with high carbohydrate craving (26 CrPic, 15 placebo; mean BMI = 31.1) showed that **the CrPic patients had significantly greater response on total HAM-D-29 scores** than the placebo group (65% vs. 33%; p < 0.05) as well as **significantly greater improvements on the following HAM-D-29 items: appetite increase, increased eating, carbohydrate craving, and genital symptoms (e.g., level of libido)**. Chromium treatment was well-tolerated. CONCLUSIONS: In a population of adults with atypical depression, most of whom were overweight or obese, CrPic produced improvement on the following HAM-D-29 items: appetite increase, increased eating, carbohydrate craving, and diurnal variation of feelings. In a subpopulation of patients with high carbohydrate craving, overall HAM-D-29 scores improved significantly in patients treated with CrPic compared with placebo. **The results of this study suggest that the main effect of chromium was on carbohydrate craving and appetite regulation in depressed patients and that 600 mcg of elemental chromium may be beneficial for patients with atypical depression who also have severe carbohydrate craving.** Further studies are needed to evaluate chromium in depressed patients specifically selected for symptoms of increased appetite and carbohydrate craving as well as to determine whether a higher dose of chromium would have an effect on mood." Interpretation of this study may be a little confusing to clinicians unfamiliar with the clinical spectrum of depression, especially when combined with an overweight BMI. On the one hand, we would like to see overweight depressed patients eat less if we are more focused on their weight; on the other hand, since lack of appetite is one of the defining characteristics of depression, the fact that some of these patients actually began to eat more can be interpreted as a reflection of an antidepressant effect. Further the observation that patients with severe carbohydrate craving actually began to eat less shows that, overall, chromium supplementation in depressed+overweight patients might be expected to have a homeostatic effect: following chromium supplementation, patients with anorexia begin to eat more, while patients with food cravings begin to eat less.

- Review: Chromium and polyphenols from cinnamon improve insulin sensitivity (*Proc Nutr Soc* 2008 Feb[457]): "The signs of Cr deficiency are similar to those for the metabolic syndrome and supplemental Cr has been shown to improve all these signs in human subjects. In a double-blind placebo-controlled study it has been demonstrated that glucose, insulin, cholesterol and HbA1c are all improved in patients with type 2 diabetes following Cr supplementation."

- **Cinnamon**: Cinnamon supplementation/consumption has shown benefit in the treatment of DM.
  - Small placebo-controlled study of the impact of cinnamon on glycemic control in healthy patients: Changes in glucose tolerance and insulin sensitivity following 2 weeks of daily cinnamon ingestion in healthy humans (*Eur J Appl Physiol* 2009 Apr[458]): Eight male volunteers underwent two 14-day interventions involving cinnamon 3g/d or placebo supplementation. "Oral glucose tolerance tests (OGTT) were performed on days 0, 1, 14, 16, 18, and 20. Cinnamon ingestion reduced the glucose response to OGTT on day 1 (-13.1 +/- 6.3% vs. day 0; P < 0.05) and day 14 (-5.5 +/- 8.1% vs. day 0; P = 0.09). Cinnamon ingestion also reduced insulin responses to OGTT on day 14 (-27.1 +/- 6.2% vs. day 0; P < 0.05), as well as improving insulin sensitivity on day 14 (vs. day 0; P < 0.05)." This small study shows that orally administered cinnamon 3g/d improves the response of OGTT in healthy humans.
  - Review: Chromium and polyphenols from cinnamon improve insulin sensitivity (*Proc Nutr Soc* 2008 Feb[459]): "It has also been shown that cinnamon polyphenols improve insulin sensitivity in in vitro, animal and human studies. Cinnamon reduces mean fasting serum glucose (18-29%), TAG (23-30%), total cholesterol (12-26%) and LDL-cholesterol (7-27%) in subjects with type 2 diabetes after 40 d of daily consumption of 1-6 g cinnamon. Subjects with the metabolic syndrome who consume an aqueous extract of cinnamon have been shown to have improved fasting blood glucose, systolic blood pressure, percentage body fat and increased lean body mass compared with the placebo group. Studies utilizing an aqueous extract of cinnamon, high in type A polyphenols, have also demonstrated improvements in fasting glucose, glucose

---

[457] Anderson RA. Chromium and polyphenols from cinnamon improve insulin sensitivity. *Proc Nutr Soc.* 2008 Feb;67(1):48-53
[458] Solomon et al. Glucose tolerance and insulin sensitivity following 2 weeks of daily cinnamon ingestion in healthy humans. *Eur J Appl Physiol.* 2009 Apr;105(6):969-76
[459] Anderson RA. Chromium and polyphenols from cinnamon improve insulin sensitivity. *Proc Nutr Soc.* 2008 Feb;67(1):48-53

tolerance and insulin sensitivity in women with insulin resistance associated with the polycystic ovary syndrome."

- Systematic review of the safety and efficacy of common and cassia cinnamon bark: From type 2 diabetes to antioxidant activity (*Can J Physiol Pharmacol* 2007 Sep[460]): Common cinnamon (*Cinnamomum verum, C. zeylanicum*) and cassia cinnamon (*C. aromaticum*) are well known for their centuries-old use as spices and flavoring agents. Regarding cinnamon's applications in DM-2, "Two of 3 randomized clinical trials on type 2 diabetes provided strong scientific evidence that cassia cinnamon demonstrates a therapeutic effect in reducing fasting blood glucose by 10.3%-29%; the third clinical trial did not observe this effect. Cassia cinnamon, however, did not have an effect at lowering glycosylated hemoglobin (HbA1c). One randomized clinical trial reported that cassia cinnamon lowered total cholesterol, low-density lipoprotein cholesterol, and triglycerides; the other 2 trials, however, did not observe this effect."

- **Vanadium**: Vanadium is probably the most controversial nutrient purported to have benefit in the treatment of DM. At current, the lack of documented benefit and the narrow therapeutic window precludes its routine clinical utilization.

  - Systematic review: Vanadium oral supplements for glycemic control in type 2 diabetes mellitus (*QJM* 2008 May[461]): Using reasonable criteria for study inclusion (controlled human trials of vanadium vs. placebo in adults with type 2 diabetes of minimum 2 months duration, and a minimum of 10 subjects per arm) the authors found 151 studies, but none met the inclusion criteria. Using weaker criteria, the authors found five studies: "These demonstrated significant treatment-effects, but due to poor study quality, must be interpreted with caution. Treatment with vanadium often results in gastrointestinal side-effects." Appropriately, the authors concluded, "There is no rigorous evidence that oral vanadium supplementation improves glycemic control in type 2 diabetes. The routine use of vanadium for this purpose cannot be recommended. A large-scale randomized controlled trial is needed to address this clinical question."

Infections, Microbiome Diabetes patients are at increased risk for various types of overt infections and are thus candidates for supportive immunonutrition, such as with glutamine, zinc, and vitamin D3. Beyond the obvious, we now appreciate that diabetes patients have dysbiosis of the mouth, gut, and skin; see overall protocol in Chapter 4, Section 2—a few highlights will be provided here. Berberine has emerged as a superior intervention in DM2, with euglycemic benefits safely mediated via several mechanisms, including that of modulating the gut microbiome; the clinical efficacy of berberine is similar to that of metformin, thus giving berberine clinical superiority due to its low cost, wide availability, collateral benefits, and excellent safety.

- **Berberine: 200-500 mg twice-thrice daily for dyslipidemia**: Most naturopathic physicians would probably and appropriately first think of its antimicrobial benefits when first asked about the clinical benefits of berberine; indeed berberine has been used for thousands of years to help the body's immune system clear infections, particularly gastrointestinal infections such as due to *Giardia lamblia*. More recently, clinical trials have allowed us to expand the clinical applications of this popular botanical extract to the treatment of dyslipidemia. Berberine appears to have a beneficial impact on negative serum lipid profiles by promoting increased production of LDL cholesterol receptors.

  - Review and trials: Berberine is a novel cholesterol-lowering drug working through a unique mechanism distinct from statins (*Nat Med* 2004 Dec[462]): Oral administration of berberine 500 mg orally twice daily for 3 months in 32 hypercholesterolemic patients reduced serum cholesterol by 29%, triglycerides by 35% and LDL-cholesterol by 25%. In an animal study, treatment with berberine in hyperlipidemic hamsters reduced serum cholesterol by 40% and LDL-cholesterol by 42%, with a 3.5-fold increase in hepatic LDL-receptor mRNA and a 2.6-fold increase in hepatic LDL-receptor protein. In vitro studies showed that berberine upregulates LDLR expression through a post-transcriptional mechanism that stabilizes the mRNA. The authors concluded, "These findings show [berberine] as a new hypolipidemic drug with a mechanism of action different from that of statin drugs."

---

[460] Dugoua et al. From type 2 diabetes to antioxidant activity: a systematic review of the safety and efficacy of cinnamon bark. *Can J Physiol Pharmacol.* 2007 Sep;85(9):837-47

[461] Smith DM, Pickering RM, Lewith GT. A systematic review of vanadium oral supplements for glycaemic control in type 2 diabetes mellitus. *QJM.* 2008 May;101(5):351-8

[462] Kong et al. Berberine is a novel cholesterol-lowering drug working through a unique mechanism distinct from statins. *Nat Med.* 2004 Dec;10(12):1344-51

- Randomized clinical trial: Treatment of type 2 diabetes and dyslipidemia with the natural plant alkaloid berberine (*J Clin Endocrinol Metab* 2008 Jul[463]): 116 patients with DM-2 and dyslipidemia were randomly allocated to receive berberine (1.0 g daily) and the placebo for 3 months. Results showed that berberine reduced fasting and postload plasma glucose from 7.0 to 5.6 and from 12.0 to 8.9 mm/liter, HbA1c from 7.5% to 6.6%, triglyceride from 2.51 to 1.61 mm/liter, total cholesterol from 5.31 to 4.35 mm/liter, and low-density lipoprotein-cholesterol from 3.23 to 2.55 mm/liter, with all parameters differing from placebo significantly. Only 5 patients had mild to moderate constipation as the adverse effect in the berberine group. "CONCLUSIONS: Berberine is effective and safe in the treatment of type 2 diabetes and dyslipidemia."
- Animal study and human clinical trial: Combination of simvastatin with berberine improves the lipid-lowering efficacy (*Metabolism* 2008 Aug[464]): Animal studies confirmed that berberine alone was nearly as effective as simvastatin in normalizing lipids, but that the combination of berberine+simvastatin was significantly more effective than either treatment alone. The mechanism of action appears to be stabilization of the low-density lipoprotein receptor (LDLR) messenger RNA. In a human clinical trial, the therapeutic efficacy of the berberine+simvastatin was then evaluated in 63 hypercholesterolemic patients; the combination showed an improved lipid-lowering effect with 31.8% reduction of serum LDL cholesterol with similar efficacies observed in the reduction of total cholesterol as and triglyceride levels. The authors concluded, "Our results display the rationale, effectiveness, and safety of the combination therapy for hyperlipidemia using BBR and SIMVA. It could be a new regimen for hypercholesterolemia."

Nutritional Immunomodulation Obese and diabetic patients tend to demonstrate an excess of inflammation generally and Th-17 dominance in particular. Given such, these patients are candidates for the nutritional immunomodulation protocol detailed in Chapter 4, Section 3.

Dysmetabolism & Dysfunctional Mitochondria Clearly, the vast majority of diabetic patients—like their euglycemic counterparts—show overwhelming evidence of increased body burden of pesticides and other persistent organic pollutants. High levels of chemical accumulation correlate more strongly with hyperglycemia than does obesity, per many studies; likewise, population-wide trends in diabetes incidence are wisely attributed to population-wide exposure to pollutants, rather than simple "lack of willpower" with regard to individual choices in diet and exercise. Indeed, reducing the global burden/prevalence of diabetes will require individual nations and the global community as a whole to implement effective controls against polluting their inhabitants; governments must implement stronger controls against reckless and rampant corporate polluting. As stated plainly by the article and specific example provided by Lee[465], "I do not believe the diabetes epidemic in China occurred because Chinese people were lazy when they were achieving huge economic growth during the period of 2000–2010. They did not live a luxurious life either. They were not even obese when they became diabetic. The mean body mass index of Chinese diabetic patients reported in the 2010 survey was 23.7, and waist circumference was 80.2 cm. ... My Chinese friends should read the very compelling review by Lee et al. showing that various persistent organic pollutants (POPs) are associated with obesity and diabetes. My fellow diabetologists would agree that, rather than a few individual POPs, background exposure to POP mixtures, including organochlorine pesticides and polychlorinated biphenyls, might increase diabetes. All those POPs might enter our body through foods, water and air." Readers are encouraged to review the two interviews by Drs Lee and Vasquez in *International Journal of Human Nutrition and Functional Medicine* (2015, Spring Edition), available freely online: IntJHumNutrFunctMed.org.[466]

- **Carbohydrate avoidance/reduction, fasting**: The major causes of secondary dysmetabolism are 1) carbohydrate excess, 2) nutritional deficiencies, 3) microbial effects, and 4) xenobiotic effects. As such, each must be addressed as noted in the respective sections of Chapter 4. In the case of diabesity, fasting, low-carbohydrate diets, and exercise all serve to "burn" excess saturated fats and ceramide which otherwise

---

[463] Zhang et al. Treatment of type 2 diabetes and dyslipidemia with the natural plant alkaloid berberine. *J Clin Endocrinol Metab*. 2008 Jul;93(7):2559-65

[464] Kong et al. Combination of simvastatin with berberine improves the lipid-lowering efficacy. *Metabolism*. 2008 Aug;57(8):1029-37

[465] Lee HK. Success of 2013-2020 World Health Organization action plan to control non-communicable diseases would require pollutants control. *J Diabetes Investig*. 2014 Nov;5(6):621-2

[466] Vasquez A. "Dr Hong Lee's Personal and Educational Path: The New Field of Mitochondrial Toxicology and Its Clinical Relevance to Endocrine Disruption and Meaningful Control of the Diabetes Epidemic" and "Dr Vasquez's Personal and Educational Path, the 2015 CAM Summit, and Mitochondrial Medicine as the Conversational and Conceptual Hub for Interconnecting Nutrition, Lifestyle, Microbes, and Political Pollution—Beyond Nutritional Myopia into Social Contextualization." *International Journal of Human Nutrition and Functional Medicine* 2015 Spring http://intjhumnutrfunctmed.org/

promote inflammation and mitochondrial impairment. Again, sugar-induced production of dysmetabolic and proinflammatory fatty acids leads to metabolic impairment (e.g., mitochondrial dysfunction via ceramide accumulation[467]) and inflammation, including hypothalamic inflammation that drives nonsatiation and overconsumption.[468] Rather than seeking to always "add something good", clinicians should emphasize "taking away the harmful substances that are causing disease", especially toxins—microbial, xenobiotic, metabolic.

- **Coenzyme Q-10 (CoQ10)**: CoQ10 is an endogenous antioxidant, NFkB inhibitor, favorable immune modulator, and essential component of several steps in the electron transport chain. CoQ10 has shown benefit in hypertensive patients, patients with dyslipidemia, and in patients with renal failure, but as of 2009 the current author is not aware of any studies showing positive benefit of CoQ10 on indexes of glycemic control in patients with DM/MetSyn; CoQ10 may still be used in these patients for cardioprotective, renoprotective, and anti-dyslipidemic benefits.

    - Double-blind crossover study: Coenzyme Q10 improves endothelial dysfunction in statin-treated type 2 diabetic patients (*Diabetes Care* 2009 May[469]): The authors investigated whether oral CoQ10 supplementation (200 mg/d) improves endothelial dysfunction in statin-treated type-2 diabetic patients (n=23). "RESULTS: Compared with placebo, CoQ(10) supplementation increased brachial artery FMD [flow-mediated dilatation] by 1.0%, but did not alter NMD [nitrate-mediated dilatation]. CoQ10 supplementation also did not alter plasma F(2)-isoprostane or urinary 20-HETE levels. CONCLUSIONS: **CoQ10 supplementation improved endothelial dysfunction in statin-treated type 2 diabetic patients**, possibly by altering local vascular oxidative stress."

    - Letter to the editor: Lackluster effect of coenzyme Q10 on microcirculatory endothelial function of subjects with type-2 diabetes mellitus (*Atherosclerosis* 2008 Feb[470]): This trial used 200 mg per day of CoQ10 for 12 weeks in medicated patients with DM-2 and found a serologic response to supplementation (increased CoQ10 levels by 3x over baseline) but no significant benefit to CoQ10 supplementation in this group (treatment n=40; placebo n=40). Furthermore, although CoQ10 levels increased, the metabolism of CoQ10 was impaired in these DM-2 patients in the absence of dietary modification; in this regard the authors write, "CoQ10 supplementation without reducing the burden of other metabolic derangements (e.g. hyperglycemia) could not alter the distribution of ubiquinol/ubiquinone favorably." The authors suggest that a higher dose such as 300 mg per day might have shown benefit, as documented in other trials, and surmise, "In conclusion, oral CoQ10 supplementation can replete the plasma concentration without altering its ubiquinol/ubiquinone composition. This intervention was, however, ineffective in improving microcirculatory endothelial function in subjects with T2DM."

    - Clinical trial with water-soluble CoQ10: Effect of hydrosoluble coenzyme Q10 on blood pressures and insulin resistance in hypertensive patients with coronary artery disease (*J Hum Hypertens* 1999 Mar[471]): In this randomized, double-blind trial, placebo-controlled trial among patients receiving antihypertensive medication and with coronary artery disease (n=59: 30 in treatment group, 29 in placebo group), patients received oral coenzyme Q10 (60 mg twice daily) for 8 weeks. In the coenzyme Q10 group, **beneficial reductions were noted in systolic and diastolic blood pressures (average 168/106 reduced to 152/97 [-16/-9]), heart rate, waist–hip ratio, fasting and 2-h plasma insulin and glucose levels, triglyceride levels and angina; CoQ10 supplementation also effected a net increase in HDL-cholesterol.** The authors concluded, "These findings indicate that treatment with coenzyme Q10 decreases blood pressure possibly by decreasing oxidative stress and insulin response in patients with known hypertension receiving conventional antihypertensive drugs."

- **Lipoic acid (thioctic acid)—oral doses range from 600 mg to 1,800 mg per day in divided doses**: Lipoic acid is produced endogenously as well as consumed in foods; it has been referred to as "the universal antioxidant"

---

[467] Chavez JA, Summers SA. A ceramide-centric view of insulin resistance. *Cell Metab.* 2012 May 2;15(5):585-94

[468] Milanski et al. Saturated fatty acids produce an inflammatory response predominantly through the activation of TLR4 signaling in hypothalamus: implications for the pathogenesis of obesity. *J Neurosci.* 2009 Jan 14;29(2):359-70

[469] Hamilton SJ, Chew GT, Watts GF. Coenzyme Q10 improves endothelial dysfunction in statin-treated type 2 diabetic patients. *Diabetes Care.* 2009 May;32(5):810-2

[470] Lim et al. The effect of coenzyme Q10 on microcirculatory endothelial function of subjects with type 2 diabetes mellitus. *Atherosclerosis.* 2008 Feb;196(2):966-9

[471] Singh RB, Niaz MA, Rastogi SS, Shukla PK, Thakur AS. Effect of hydrosoluble coenzyme Q10 on blood pressures and insulin resistance in hypertensive patients with coronary artery disease. *J Hum Hypertens.* 1999 Mar;13(3):203-8

because it is both water-soluble and fat-soluble. In addition to its antioxidant roles, lipoic acid is also a potent inhibitor of NFkB, and as such has broad applications, including the treatment of viral infections. Lipoic acid is an essential component of the pyruvate dehydrogenase complex, which is the intermediate pathway between glycolysis and the Kreb's cycle. When used in supplemental doses, lipoate should always be used in a comprehensive plan that includes a high-potency broad-spectrum multivitamin and multimineral. With regard to DM-2, lipoate has been mostly studied in the treatment of diabetic polyneuropathy; however, clinicians should not lose sight of its broad anti-oxidant benefits that extend beyond this single application. Nor should diabetic neuropathy be taken lightly as it represents a major health problem; it is responsible for increased mortality as well as substantial morbidity and impaired quality of life. The most important treatment for DM-neuropathy is control of blood glucose levels; specific treatments such as lipoate play a secondary but very important role.

- Literature review: Alpha-lipoic acid in the treatment of diabetic polyneuropathy in Germany: current evidence from clinical trials (*Exp Clin Endocrinol Diabetes* 1999[472]): The authors review at least 15 clinical trials, which, as a group, have shown beneficial effects of lipoic/thioctic acid on either "neuropathic symptoms and deficits due to polyneuropathy or reduced heart rate variability resulting from cardiac autonomic neuropathy." Studies reporting positive results have used at least 600 mg per day. The authors enumerate the following findings:
  1. "Short-term treatment for 3 weeks using 600 mg of thioctic acid i.v. per day appears to reduce the chief symptoms of diabetic polyneuropathy. A 3-week pilot study of 1800 mg per day given orally indicates that the therapeutic effect may be independent of the route of administration, but this needs to be confirmed in a larger sample size.
  2. The effect on symptoms is accompanied by an improvement of neuropathic deficits.
  3. **Oral treatment for 4-7 months tends to reduce neuropathic deficits and improves cardiac autonomic neuropathy**.
  4. Preliminary data over 2 years indicate possible long-term improvement in motor and sensory nerve conduction in the lower limbs.
  5. Clinical and postmarketing surveillance studies have revealed a highly favorable safety profile of the drug."

- Critical review: Thioctic acid for patients with symptomatic diabetic polyneuropathy (*Treat Endocrinol* 2004[473]): The author reviews evidence that oxidative stress resulting from enhanced free-radical formation and/or defects in antioxidant defense is implicated in the pathogenesis of diabetic neuropathy; if this is true, then control of endogenous oxidant production such as through improved glycemic control as well as the administration of supplemental/exogenous antioxidants would appear to be the obvious and reasonable therapeutic interventions. Supporting this oxidative-neuropathic link is the observation that superoxide anion and peroxynitrite production are increased in diabetic patients in relation to the severity of polyneuropathy. **The author also discusses a meta-analysis that included the largest sample of diabetic patients (n = 1258) ever to have been treated with a single drug or class of drugs to reduce neuropathic symptoms, and confirmed the favorable effects of thioctic acid based on the highest level of evidence (Class Ia: evidence from meta-analyses of randomized, controlled trials).** The author enumerates the following conclusions:
  1. Short-term treatment for 3 weeks using intravenous thioctic acid 600 mg/day reduces the chief symptoms of diabetic polyneuropathy to a clinically meaningful degree;
  2. This effect on neuropathic symptoms is accompanied by an improvement of neuropathic deficits, suggesting potential for the drug to favorably influence underlying neuropathy;
  3. Oral treatment for 4-7 months tends to reduce neuropathic deficits and improve cardiac autonomic neuropathy;
  4. Clinical and postmarketing surveillance studies have revealed a highly favorable safety profile of the drug."

---

[472] Ziegler et al. Alpha-lipoic acid in the treatment of diabetic polyneuropathy in Germany: current evidence from clinical trials. *Exp Clin Endocrinol Diabetes*. 1999;107:421-30
[473] Ziegler D. Thioctic acid for patients with symptomatic diabetic polyneuropathy: a critical review. *Treat Endocrinol*. 2004;3(3):173-89

- ▪ <u>Controlled, randomized, open-label study: Alpha-lipoic acid in the treatment of autonomic diabetic neuropathy</u> (*Rom J Intern Med* 2004[474]): In this study, 46 patients with type-1 diabetes and different forms of autonomic neuropathy (mean duration of diabetes 16.8 years) were treated with alpha-lipoic acid 600 mg/d intravenously (IV or iv) for 10 days; thereafter they received 600 mg/d orally for 50 days. The control group consisted of 29 type-1 diabetic patients with autonomic diabetic neuropathy. "RESULTS: **There was a significant improvement** after treatment in the score for severity of cardiovascular autonomic neuropathy--from 6.43 +/- 0.9 to 4.24 +/- 1.8 (p<0.001), while in the control group it worsened from 6.18 +/- 1.3 to 6.52 +/- 0.9 (p>0.1). We found improvement in the Valsalva maneuver after treatment - from 1.05 +/- 0.04 to 1.13 +/- 0.08 (p<0.001); in the deep-breathing test -from 3.4 +/- 2.8 to 10.4 +/- 5.7 (p<0.001); and in the lying-to-standing test--from 0.99 +/- 0.01 to 1.01 +/- 0.02 (p>0.1), while **in the control group there was no improvement**. ... We found improvement in diabetic enteropathy in six patients; in the complaints of dizziness, instability upon standing in six patients; in neuropathic edema of the lower extremities in four patients and in erectile dysfunction in four patients after treatment, while in the control group no change was reported in the symptoms and signs of autonomic neuropathy by the end of the follow-up period. There were changes in the laboratory parameters of oxidative stress after therapy--**total serum antioxidant capacity increased** from 20.42 +/- 1.8 to 22.96 +/- 2.3 microgH2O2/ml/min (p<0.05), **serum SOD activity** - from 269.8 +/- 31.1 to 319.8 +/- 29.IU/l (p=0.02) and **erythrocyte SOD**--from 0.89 +/- 0.10 to 1.11 +/- 0.09 U/gHb (p=0.04). CONCLUSION: Our results demonstrate that alpha-lipoic acid (Thiogamma) appears to be an effective drug in the treatment of the different forms of autonomic diabetic neuropathy."

- ▪ <u>Multicenter clinical trial: The role of alpha-lipoic acid in diabetic polyneuropathy treatment</u> (*Bosn J Basic Med Sci.* 2008 Nov[475]): These researchers investigated the effect of alpha-lipoic acid on the symptoms of diabetic neuropathy by administering lipoate 600 mg intravenously for 3 weeks, followed by 3 months of oral lipoate 300-600 mg/d. The 100 patients in this study had either DM-1 (n=16) or DM-2 (n=80) with 4 patients not classified; average age was 61y, and average duration of disease was 11y. 69 patients were taking insulin and 31 were treated with oral hypoglycemics; average duration of polyneuropathic symptoms was 3y. The authors reported the following results, "**Significant statistic differences in improvement** were recorded (P>0,05) according to Fridman's test for repeated measurements compared to initial findings in assessments: **sensory symptoms of polyneuropathy, pain sensations as polyneuropathy symptoms, total score of polyneuropathy symptoms, subjective assessment of patients, subjective findings of physicians**, and significant differences were not found (P>0,05) in autonomous and motoric neuropathy. Based on the conducted study, we have concluded that the application of **alpha-lipoic acid during 3 months has helped to decrease the symptoms of diabetic neuropathy** and in only one case out of 100 included patients there was no subjective improvement after drug application." Thus, in summary, these authors loaded patients with intravenous administration of lipoate for 3 weeks, then followed with oral administration for 3 months; **they report that 99 out of 100 patients had a positive response** in the reduction of the severity of diabetic polyneuropathy.

- • **Acetyl-L-carnitine 500-1,000 mg three times daily between meals for diabetic neuropathy**:
  - ▪ <u>Review: Acetyl-L-carnitine in the treatment of diabetic peripheral neuropathy</u> (*Ann Pharmacother* 2008 Nov[476]): These authors review data from two large clinical trials (n=1679) using acetyl-L-carnitine (ALC) in the treatment of diabetic peripheral neuropathy (DPN). Results showed, "Subjects who received at least 2 g daily of ALC showed decreases in pain scores. One study showed improvements in electrophysiologic factors such as nerve conduction velocities, while the other did not. Patients who had neuropathic pain reported reductions in pain using a visual analog scale. Nerve regeneration was documented in one trial. The supplement was well tolerated. A proprietary form of ALC was used in both studies. CONCLUSIONS: Data on treatment of DPN with ALC support its use. It should be recommended to patients early in the disease process to provide maximal benefit."

---

[474] Tankova et al. Alpha-lipoic acid in the treatment of autonomic diabetic neuropathy (controlled, randomized, open-label study). *Rom J Intern Med.* 2004;42(2):457-64

[475] Bureković A, Terzić M, Alajbegović S, Vukojević Z, Hadzić N. The role of alpha-lipoic acid in diabetic polyneuropathy treatment. *Bosn J Basic Med Sci.* 2008 Nov;8:341-5

[476] Evans JD, Jacobs TF, Evans EW. Role of acetyl-L-carnitine in the treatment of diabetic peripheral neuropathy. *Ann Pharmacother.* 2008 Nov;42(11):1686-91

- **Acetyl-L-carnitine improves pain, nerve regeneration, and vibratory perception in patients with chronic diabetic neuropathy: an analysis of two randomized placebo-controlled trials** (*Diabetes Care* 2005 Jan[477]): "CONCLUSIONS: These studies demonstrate that ALC treatment is efficacious in alleviating symptoms, particularly pain, and improves nerve fiber regeneration and vibration perception in patients with established diabetic neuropathy."

Style of Living Diabetes must be approached in its totality—socially, politically, emotionally, physically, nutritionally, etc.

- **Sleep**: Sleep deprivation causes systemic inflammation that promotes insulin resistance and the development of DM-2. Patients should be encouraged to practice good "sleep hygiene" by allowing sufficient time for quality sleep; some patients will need to reduce caffeine intake appropriately. Assessment for sleep apnea by history or polysomnography should be employed.

- **Psychological support, group support, and individual counseling**: The development of obesity requires years of under-exercising, overeating, allowing/denying progressive decrements in physical and (generally) social and psychological functioning. These cannot be reversed by a purely nutritional or medical approach. Patients must be willing to receive counseling, feedback, support, and to actively participate in psychological counseling *with a competent therapist* who holds the patient accountable to homework, behavioral change, the achievement of goals, and the integration (or more often *creation*) of important life goals which can pull the patient forward into a positive future via a health-promoting lifestyle. A healthy lifestyle is the means by which patients attain, maintain, and protect an optimized health status which helps them achieve their overall life goals; patients with no goals and without high standards for the expectations of their life experience will readily fall into the pattern of noncompliance and failure that have made obese, DM-2, and MetSyn patients notoriously hard to help and deal with clinically.
  - Review: A comprehensive psychological approach to obesity (*Psychiatr Med* 1983 Sep[478]): "The management of obesity must be a joint venture between psychiatry and medicine. ... Many obese patients lack a fundamental knowledge of nutrition, exercise, and health. In addition, most are poorly socialized and require assistance in learning assertiveness and other interpersonal skills. A behaviorally oriented component is very effective in providing these skills."

- **Specific therapeutic and management considerations for specific aspects of the DM/MetSyn interconnected matrix**: The previous sections have reviewed therapeutics considered by this author to be most poignant in the routine management of DM, particularly DM-2 and MetSyn. The single most important treatment is the low-carbohydrate supplemented Paleo-Mediterranean diet; this is simply a low-carbohydrate version of "the supplemented Paleo-Mediterranean diet" which I described in *Integrative Orthopedics* (2004), *Integrative Rheumatology* (2006), *Musculoskeletal Pain: Expanded Clinical Strategies* (2008) and originally in *Nutritional Wellness* in 2005.[479] In the section that follows, I provide a problem-based itemization of various therapeutics worthy of consideration when specific problems need to be targeted within a context of overall diabetes management. These are "reasonable" considerations based on clinical experience generally with but sometimes without high-quality peer-reviewed trials.
  - **Cardiovascular risk**: Hypertension and hyperglycemia both lead to accelerated atherosclerosis; the combination of hypertension with hyperglycemia is additive/synergistic, hence the term "accelerated atherosclerosis" to describe the cardiometabolic syndrome. Clinicians must address whole-body physiology while also addressing various individualized facets and nuances per patient.
    - Clinical patient assessment with resting/stress ECG, consider adding echocardiography: These are considerations per patient; guidelines do not recommend these for all patients as benefit has not been demonstrated unless clinically indicated.
    - Hyperglycemia, oxidative stress, hypercoagulability: Assess and address with tests and interventions detailed above, especially low-carb supplemented Paleo-Mediterranean diet; add low-dose aspirin for most DM patients over age 40y.

---

[477] Sima et al. Acetyl-L-carnitine improves pain, nerve regeneration, and vibratory perception in patients with chronic diabetic neuropathy. *Diabetes Care*. 2005 Jan;28(1):89-94
[478] Fawzy FI, Pasnau RO, Wellisch DK, Ellsworth RG, Dornfeld L, Maxwell M. A comprehensive psychological approach to obesity. *Psychiatr Med*. 1983 Sep;1(3):257-73
[479] Vasquez A. A Five-Part Nutritional Protocol that Produces Consistently Positive Results. *Nutritional Wellness* 2005 Sept

- o <u>Optimize glycemic control</u>: Use additional chromium, biotin, grapeseed extract, cinnamon, and *Gymnema* as necessary.
- o <u>Co-manage or refer unresponsive or noncompliant patients</u>: The clinician's technical goal is the objective documentation of a positive serologic (e.g., glucose, Hgb-A1c, lipids, CRP) and clinical (e.g., blood pressure, weight loss) response to treatment within not more than 2-3 months' time from the initiation of treatment. If such documentation cannot be made due to treatment failure or patient noncompliance, or if documentable positive responses are not occurring quickly enough and the patient remains at an unacceptable level of risk, the patient should be co-managed with pharmaceutical drugs (especially statins) until the diet and lifestyle interventions have taken effect. Clinicians must be aware of the politics and medicolegal consequences, especially if a state medical board is involved: A patient who dies while taking statins and antihypertensive polypharmacy will be considered "well managed" while a patient who dies despite the prescription of an evidence-based nutritional protocol will likely be considered "mismanaged." The topic being debated is not research or patient care; rather, the issue is "standard of care" which is defined by what doctors and specialists are doing in the community (and nationally). Standard-of-care issues are decided by majority rule; when most cardiologists and internists rely solely on drugs for the treatment of diet-induced disease, the drug treatment is the standard of care, regardless of research showing that nutritional interventions are superior or equivalent. When in doubt, refer or co-manage.

- **Hypercholesterolemia and dyslipidemia**: Assess with serum testing; strongly consider the following interventions.
  - o <u>Low-carb supplemented Paleo-Mediterranean diet</u>: Best single intervention for reducing cardiovascular and total mortality; fish oil, vitamin D, and Mg supplementation make the intervention particularly more powerful.
  - o <u>Berberine 500 mg once or twice or thrice daily</u>: Most studies have been short-term in the range of about 3 months when using the 1,000 mg per day dose; long-term safety of berberine 1,000 mg/d has not been established.
  - o <u>Policosanol 10-20 mg/d</u>: Policosanol appears efficacious for some patients, despite some controversy in the research literature, with some studies showing statin-like results and others showing no benefit. The most effective policosanol comes from sugar cane (not bee's wax) and is standardized for the octacosanol content Early in my (DrV) clinical practice, I recall witnessing the reduction of 100 mg/dL (from 280 mg/dL to 180 mg/dL) within one month simply by use of dietary carbohydrate restriction plus policosanol.
  - o <u>Niacin 500 mg 2-4 times per day</u>: Very effective for raising HDL, but the uncomfortable skin flushing sensation limits its tolerability; pretreatment with aspirin can help mitigate this benign adverse effect. Plain niacin is the product of choice for serum lipid modification; other forms such as niacinamide and inositol hexaniacinate are much less effective in this regard. Niacin, like EFAs when given in excessive doses, may worsen glycemic control.

- **Diabetic neuropathy**:
  - o <u>Biotin 10-20 mg/d</u>: Clinicians should recall from their training in basic/clinical nutrition that biotin is essentially nontoxic; toxicity of biotin has not been reported in patients receiving daily doses of up to 200 mg orally and up to 20 mg intravenously for the treatment of biotin-responsive inborn errors of metabolism and acquired biotin deficiency.[480]
  - o <u>Gamma linolenic acid</u>: 500-1,000 mg/d: Preferably administered with food
  - o <u>Lipoic acid 400 mg 2-4 times daily</u>.
  - o <u>Acetyl-L-carnitine 500 mg 2-6 times daily</u>.
  - o <u>B vitamins especially vitamin B12 and thiamine</u>: Oral B-12 given 2,000-4,000 mcg daily as hydroxocobalamin (or the methyl- or adenosyl- forms); about half that dose if given intramuscularly. Thiamine is available in water-soluble and fat-soluble forms and can be given orally 50-300 mg per day.

---

[480] Ames BN, et al. High-dose vitamin therapy stimulates variant enzymes with decreased coenzyme binding affinity (increased K(m)). *Am J Clin Nutr*. 2002 Apr;75(4):616-58

- o Capsaicin cream: Applied topically for pain relief only, 2-4 times per day. The burning sensation abates with continued use. Avoid contact with eyes and mucus membranes.
- **Diabetic retinopathy**: Emphasize blood pressure control, glycemic control, lipid control, and antioxidants especially zinc, selenium, and phytonutrients from bilberry (e.g., standardized to >25% anthocyanosides given 240-600 mg/day) and other flavonoids (e.g., quercetin) and proanthocyanidins. **Referral to an ophthalmologist is absolutely mandatory for all DM and MetSyn patients**.
- **Nephropathy and renal failure**: These patients are best co-managed by an internist, nephrologist, or excellent family medicine doctor; the legal ramifications and consent and compliance issues, along with preparation for hemodialysis or transplant need to be addressed quickly in preparation for the expenses and procedures likely to come.
  - o Adjust the diet to avoid excess potassium, magnesium, or protein: Adjust the diet and use serum testing as indicated.
  - o High-dose (300 mg per day) thiamine therapy for patients with type-2 diabetes and microalbuminuria: "METHODS: Type 2 diabetic patients (21 male, 19 female) with microalbuminuria were recruited at a diabetic clinic and randomized to placebo and treatment arms. Patients were given 3 x 100 mg capsules of thiamine or placebo per day for 3 months with a 2 month follow-up washout period. The primary endpoint was change in urinary albumin excretion (UAE). "RESULTS: UAE was decreased in patients receiving thiamine therapy for 3 months with respect to baseline (median -17.7 mg/24 h; $p < 0.001$, n = 20). There was no significant decrease in UAE in patients receiving placebo after 3 months of therapy (n = 20). UAE was significantly lower in patients who had received thiamine therapy compared with those who had received placebo (30.1 vs 35.5 mg/24 h, $p < 0.01$) but not at baseline. UAE continued to decrease in the 2 month washout period in both groups, but not significantly. There was no effect of thiamine treatment on glycemic control, dyslipidemia or BP. There were no adverse effects of therapy. CONCLUSIONS/INTERPRETATION: In this pilot study, high-dose thiamine therapy produced a regression of UAE in type 2 diabetic patients with microalbuminuria. Thiamine supplements at high dose may provide improved therapy for early-stage diabetic nephropathy."[481]
  - o CoQ10 200-300 mg/day with food: CoQ10 is one of the most effective treatments for reversing renal failure according to Singh et al.[482,483]
  - o Other nephroprotective nutrients: Selenium and silymarin have also shown nephroprotective benefits in humans treated with nephrotoxic anti-cancer chemotherapy.
- **Hypertension**: See Hypertension section for details and interventions beyond those mentioned in this chapter.
- **Infection risk**: See chapter on Viral Infections, revisit treatments and management strategies throughout this chapter while focusing on:
  - o Foot care: Examine the feet at nearly every visit.
  - o Dental/mouth care: DM and MetSyn patients should receive dental care at least annually. Encourage use of antimicrobial mouthwashes, regular brushing, and frequent sterilization/replacement of toothbrushes.
  - o Treat all infections aggressively: From pneumonia to sinus and ear infections to boils, treat all infected DM patients aggressively and with in-office follow-up within 48-72 hours.
- **Impaired pancreatic function**: Beta-cell failure is the hallmark of DM-1 and—as previously mentioned—it also occurs in DM-2 after the disease has progressed for many years (previously termed "high output failure"). In patients with pancreatic failure due to acute/chronic pancreatitis—such as seen due to hypertriglyceridemia, alcoholism, or (rarely) major abdominal trauma—a clinician might aspire to promote regeneration/protection of remaining pancreatic beta-cells. The following therapeutics might be considered; although they have more experimental/animal research support than support from clinical trials in humans.

[481] Rabbani et al. High-dose thiamine therapy for patients with type 2 diabetes and microalbuminuria. *Diabetologia*. 2009 Feb;52(2):208-12
[482] Singh et al. Randomized, double-blind placebo-controlled trial of coenzyme Q10 in chronic renal failure: discovery of a new role. *J Nutr Environ Med* 2000;10:281-8
[483] Singh et al. Randomized, Double-blind, Placebo-controlled Trial of Coenzyme Q10 in Patients with Endstage Renal Failure. *J Nutr Environ Med* 2003; 13 (1): 13–22

o <u>Niacinamide 2-3 g/d in divided doses</u>: Niacinamide has shown the ability to protect pancreatic beta-cells in several studies in animal models of DM-1. A reasonable daily dose of 2,000 mg should be divided into several smaller doses, such as 500 mg 4 times daily, or 250 mg 8 times daily. As with plain niacin, hepatitis from niacinamide can occur, but this is exceedingly rare; clinicians should monitor liver enzymes before starting treatment, at about 2-4 weeks after starting treatment, again at 3-6 months. Nausea or abdominal pain should prompt appropriate follow-up and testing of serum AST and ALT; patients should be educated appropriately.

o <u>Gymnema (*Gymnema sylvestre*)</u>: Gymnema appears to have some benefit in selected patients. Clinicians might have to try more than one brand/manufacturer in order to find a product that works for a particular patient; in my own clinical experience with difficult-to-control DM-2, I found that some products were inefficacious, while another provided clear benefit by reducing glucose levels. Admittedly, some of the research on Gymnema is not entirely clear; hence my reservation of this intervention as a last resort. The typical therapeutic dose of a standardized extract, standardized to contain 24% gymnemic acids, is 400-600 mg/d, with some preference for dosing with meals.[484]

  ▫ <u>Systematic review: Use of Gymnema sylvestre for diabetes mellitus (*J Altern Complement Med* 2007 Nov[485])</u>: "Given that *G. sylvestre* targets several of the etiological factors connected with diabetes, including chronic inflammation, obesity, enzymatic defects, and pancreatic beta-cell function, and no single oral hypoglycemic drug presently exerts such a diverse range of effects, suggests that *gymnema* may be useful in the management of diabetes and the prevention of associated pathological changes. However, as this systematic review shows, the clinical efficacy of *gymnema* has only been supported by a small number of nonrandomized, open-label trials."

  ▫ <u>Clinical trial: Antidiabetic effect of a leaf extract from Gymnema sylvestre in non-insulin-dependent diabetes mellitus patients (*J Ethnopharmacol* 1990 Oct [486])</u>: "The effectiveness of GS4, an extract from the leaves of Gymnema sylvestre, in controlling hyperglycemia was investigated in 22 Type 2 diabetic patients on conventional oral anti-hyperglycemic agents. GS4 (400 mg/day) was administered for 18-20 months as a supplement to the conventional oral drugs. During GS4 supplementation, the **patients showed a significant reduction in blood glucose, glycosylated hemoglobin and glycosylated plasma proteins, and conventional drug dosage could be decreased.** Five of the 22 diabetic patients were able to discontinue their conventional drug and maintain their blood glucose homeostasis with GS4 alone. These data suggest that the beta cells may be regenerated/repaired in Type 2 diabetic patients on GS4 supplementation. This is supported by the appearance of raised insulin levels in the serum of patients after GS4 supplementation."

▪ **Elevated homocysteine (hyperhomocysteinaemia, hyperhomocysteinuria)**: Reasonable doses are listed; clinicians will have to combine and "dose to effect" per patient. All of these treatments are well-accepted as safe and generally effective.

  o <u>Folinic acid or methylfolate 5 mg/d</u>: Use in combination with other vitamins, especially vitamin B12, in the form of hydroxocobalamin, adenosylcobalamin, or methylcobalamin—cyanocobalamin is obviously to be avoided because of its clinically relevant content of cyanide.

  o <u>Vitamin B12 >2,000 mcg per day</u>: Use in the form of hydroxocobalamin, adenosylcobalamin, or methylcobalamin—cyanocobalamin is to be avoided because of its clinically relevant content of cyanide.

  o <u>Vitamin B6, pyridoxine 50-250 mg/d</u>: The phosphorylated form (P5P) can also be used; when the HCL form is used, additional attention must be given to magnesium status/supplementation and urinary alkalinization.

  o <u>Riboflavin 20-400 mg/d</u>: Small doses of 2 mg/d have been shown to significantly reduce homocysteine levels, and doses of 400 mg/d are common and well-tolerated in the treatment of migraine.

---

[484] [No authors listed] Gymnema sylvestre. *Altern Med Rev.* 1999 Feb;4(1):46-7
[485] Leach MJ. Gymnema sylvestre for diabetes mellitus: a systematic review. *J Altern Complement Med.* 2007 Nov;13(9):977-83
[486] Baskaran et al. Antidiabetic effect of a leaf extract from Gymnema sylvestre in non-insulin-dependent diabetes mellitus patients. *J Ethnopharmacol.* 1990 Oct;30(3):295-300

- NAC 600 mg per day and upward to 500-1,500 mg thrice daily: Doses of NAC 4,800 mg/d have been used with success and safety in the treatment of SLE. NAC binds directly to homocysteine to form a NAC-homocysteine conjugate that is excreted in the urine.
- Thyroid optimization: Hypothyroidism causes elevated homocysteine and promotes insulin resistance[487] and should be treated appropriately per Chapter 1.
- Avoidance of homocysteine-elevating factors: High coffee intake (>5 cups per day), ethanol, tobacco smoking, and medications/treatments (such as methotrexate, metformin, niacin and fibrate drugs); fish oil can raise homocysteine levels in some patients. Metformin is well-known to cause malabsorption of vitamin B12 and to thereby exacerbate "diabetic neuropathy" and promote depression and dementia/psychosis.
- Choline, phosphatidylcholine, lecithin (approximately 2.6 g choline/d): Each TBS (tablespoon, approximately 15 mL) of lecithin contains 275 mg of choline; thus, if the goal is to get to 2.6 g choline, one would need to use 10 TBS (150 mL) per day of granulated lecithin.
- Betaine, trimethylglycine 6–12 g/day: Effects are weak/modest; likely more relevant for patients taking drugs such as metformin and fibrates that promote loss of betaine in urine.

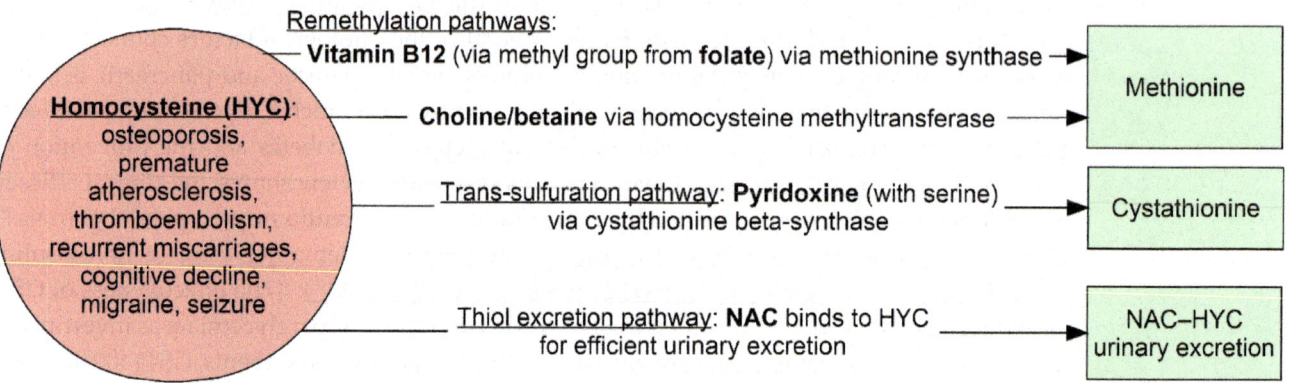

Lowering homocysteine (HYC) via nutritional supplementation: Folate gives methyl group to cobalamin (vitamin B12) to convert HYC via methionine synthase to methionine; choline/betaine can remethylate homocysteine via homocysteine methyltransferase to form methionine. Pyridoxine promotes conversion of HYC via cystathionine beta-synthase to cystathionine. The amino acid N-acetyl-cysteine (NAC) binds to HYC for efficient renal excretion of NAC-HYC.[488]

Endocrine Imbalances Obese/diabetic patients generally have hyperinsulinemia (previously reviewed in this chapter); excesses of estrogen and cortisol with deficiencies of DHEA, testosterone, and thyroid are expected—see Chapter 4, Section 6 for review of assessments and interventions.

Xenobiotic Exposure and Detoxification Detoxification must be optimized, as reviewed in Chapter 4, Section 7.

Drug Treatments The three classes of oral drugs and the injectable insulin can be remembered by the mnemonic "MIST" for metformin, insulin, sulfonylureas, and thiazolidinediones. The sequence of medicalization is generally as follows: ❶ provide cursory and nonspecific diet and lifestyle advice, ❷ start with metformin, increase dose as necessary until maximized at 2,500 mg/d, ❸ add sulfonylurea, ❹ add thiazolidinedione, ❺ discontinue sulfonylurea and add injectable insulin when the previous measures have "failed."

> **Xenobiotic-induced mitochondrial dysfunction is what leads to xenobiotic-induced HTN and diabetes**
>
> Pesticides and other pollutants commonly induce mitochondrial dysfunction, thereby contributing to insulin resistance and vasoconstriction, both of which promote HTN and DM.

---

[487] Yang N et al. Novel Clinical Evidence of an Association between Homocysteine and Insulin Resistance in Patients with Hypothyroidism or Subclinical Hypothyroidism. *PLoS One.* 2015 May 4;10(5):e0125922

[488] "NAC intravenous administration induces an efficient and rapid reduction of plasma thiols, particularly of Hcy; our data support the hypothesis that NAC displaces thiols from their binding protein sites and forms, in excess of plasma NAC, mixed disulphides (NAC-Hcy) with a high renal clearance." Ventura et al. N-Acetyl-cysteine reduces homocysteine plasma levels after single intravenous administration by increasing thiols urinary excretion. *Pharmacol Res.* 1999 Oct;40(4):345-50

Drug treatment of diabetes mellitus

Drugs	Clinical considerations
- Metformin: Promoted as initial pharmacologic management due to benefits (reduction of HgbA1c by 2% max; reduction in mortality) and safety (less hypoglycemia); reduces hepatic gluconeogenesis and increases peripheral insulin sensitivity with additional benefits for lipids, blood pressure, and (hyper)coagulation. Berberine is safer and more effective than metformin per a 3-month equivalent-dose 500mg TID study (Yin et al, *Metabolism* 2008 May)	- Renal excretion of metformin prohibits use in patients with renal insufficiency; relative contraindications are serum creatinine >1.5 in men or >1.4 in women (per what we learned in medical school/training) - Adverse GI effects: anorexia, N/V/D; may be transient. - Hypoglycemia is more likely with fasting exercise, alcohol, and concomitant use of other hypoglycemic treatments. - Lactic acidosis: Occurs 3-5 cases per 100,000 patient-years. Increased risk with hepatic or renal insufficiency/compromise, also older age, diuretics, radiographic contrast, dehydration, diarrhea, vomiting, hepatic insufficiency, alcoholism. Metformin should be avoided 48 hours before and after radiographic contrast. - Contraindicated with pregnancy & lactation - Start at 500 mg with dinner, titrating upward weekly as needed with a max dose of 2,500 mg/d in divided doses with food. Extended-release preparations are conveniently administered once daily.
- Sulfonylurea drugs—glyburide, glipizide, glimepiride: Stimulate pancreatic insulin production and improve peripheral insulin sensitivity.	- Start with low dose with breakfast, titrate upward weekly PRN - **Hypoglycemia is the biggest risk** occurring in 1% of patients per year; reduce dose when fasting. Sulfonylurea "gli-ide" drugs should be discontinued when rapid-acting insulins are added, ie, when moving from "basal only" to "basal-bolus." - Glipizide: Shortest half-life and thus the least hypoglycemia
- Thiazolidinedione drugs— pioglitazone and rosiglitazone: Improve peripheral insulin sensitivity; reduction of HgbA1c by 1.5% max; with reductions in Trigs, increases in LDL and HDL.	- "-glitazones" are extensively metabolized in the liver and are thus contraindicated with liver disease - Liver monitoring by measurement of ALT and AST should occur before treatment and every 2 months for the first year of treatment - Exacerbation of heart failure: Contraindicated in Class 3-4 CHF
- Insulin: Pancreatic beta-cells constantly produce insulin (basal) accentuated by increased production postprandially (bolus). Pharmacologic insulins function as endogenous insulin but vary in their cellular bioavailability and thus onset and duration of action. Patients with type-1 DM require frequent insulin injections with each meal or must use a continuous infusion pump.	- Initial starting dose of insulin: 0.1 units/kg, or divide the fasting glucose level in mg/dL by 18. - Basal insulin is given at bedtime, with the dose adjusted every 3 days; the nighttime basal insulin dose is increased by 2 units every 3 days for as long as the mean fasting glucose level is greater than 100 mg/dl. The long-acting insulins NPH and Glargine (insulin analog) are equally efficacious but Glargine produces less hypoglycemia. "Basal" insulin is given as one nighttime injection of NPH or Glargine. - Basal-bolus therapy is introduced when oral+basal treatments are insufficient: Generally this is a 70/30 combination of rapid and intermediate acting insulins administered twice daily before meals; the original nighttime basal dose of a long-acting insulin is replaced by two doses of 70/30 rapid/intermediate doses administered before breakfast and dinner.
- Inhibitors of dipeptidyl peptidase 4: DPP-4 inhibitors, such as sitagliptin/Januvia	- This relatively new class of drugs provide an antidiabetic effect by increasing pancreatic output of insulin and reducing hepatic gluconeogenesis. In contrast to other agents, sitagliptin/Januvia is reported to cause less weight gain (a side-effect of insulin) and less hypoglycemia (a problem with insulin and the sulfonylurea drugs). - The botanical medicine berberine inhibits DPP-4, which at least partly explains its anti-hyperglycemic activities.[489]

---

[489] "Our findings suggest that DPP IV inhibition is, at least, one of the mechanisms that explain the anti-hyperglycemic activity of berberine." Al-Masri et al. Inhibition of dipeptidyl peptidase IV (DPP IV) is one of the mechanisms explaining the hypoglycemic effect of berberine. *J Enzyme Inhib Med Chem.* 2009 Oct;24(5):1061-6

Chemical Exposure as a Major Contributor to the Epidemic of Diabetes Mellitus and Disorders of Insulin Resistance: From Molecular Mechanisms to Clinical Implications

This article was originally published in *Naturopathy Digest* in 2007
naturopathydigest.com/archives/2007/apr/diabetes.php

Introduction: Evidence has been consistently accumulating over the past few years implicating chemical exposure as a plausible and important cause of insulin resistance and diabetes mellitus. In this article, I will survey current literature and explain the causes, mechanisms, and clinical implications of the toxin-diabetes link, and I will expand some of my previous work on chemical exposure and clinical detoxification methods[490] as specifically related to the genesis and treatment of diabetes. By the time they finish reading this article, chiropractic and naturopathic doctors should appreciate the role of chemical exposure in the genesis and perpetuation of insulin resistance, understand the mechanisms of chemical accumulation and detoxification, and have an awareness of some of the methods used to alleviate and prevent chemical-induced disease.

Chemical Exposure and Type-2 Diabetes in Humans: Numerous animal models have irrefutably established the ability of specific chemicals and toxic metals to destroy pancreatic beta-cells and thus reduce insulin production to such an extent that hyperglycemia and diabetes result; these models establish that toxin exposure can result in a form of type-1 "low insulin" diabetes. However, the largest burden of hyperglycemic diabetes (distinguished from diabetes insipidus) in industrialized nations is associated not with insufficiency of insulin as in type-1 diabetes but rather with the hallmark findings of excess insulin, peripheral insulin resistance, and associated clinical presentations that include overweight/obesity, hypertension, hyperglycemia and dyslipidemia. The current dominant paradigm of type-2 diabetes and its synonyms and closely related conditions including insulin resistance, adult-onset diabetes, metabolic syndrome, and syndrome X is that the condition results from excess caloric intake and an insufficiency of exercise in patients with one or more genetic predispositions. Medical treatment generally consists of inadequate dietary-lifestyle advice and the use of one or more prescription drugs. However, the diet-exercise-gene-drug model of diabetes is clearly incomplete; other factors, including micronutrient status (particularly vitamin D, cholecalciferol[491]) and hormonal milieu also clearly influence adiposity and insulin receptor sensitivity. Exposure to and accumulation of toxic chemicals, either from occupational exposure or chronic background exposure to these chemicals which pervade our environment appears to be a hitherto underappreciated factor influencing insulin receptor sensitivity and the risk and prevalence of diabetes mellitus; a sampling of primary research is provided in the following section.

In 1997, Henriksen et al[492] showed that military veterans exposed to dioxin showed increased prevalence of glucose abnormalities, insulin abnormalities, and diabetes prevalence and faster development of diabetes compared to veterans of the same era who had lower levels of dioxin in their blood. In 1999, Calvert et al[493] showed that among workers occupationally exposed to a highly toxic form of dioxin, those with the highest blood levels of dioxin showed higher average levels of blood glucose. In 2000, Longnecker and Michalek[494] showed that among 1,197 veterans Air Force Veterans with no history of chemical exposure and normal serum levels of dioxins, patients with higher levels of dioxins showed an increased prevalence of diabetes. In 2003, Fierens et al[495] reported that diabetic patients showed significantly increased serum levels of dioxins, coplanar PCBs, and 12 PCB markers compared to unaffected control patients, and the level of chemical accumulation in diabetics was very significant; diabetic patients showed a 62% higher level of PCB toxins than healthy patients, and higher levels of toxins were associated with a higher risk of diabetes in a dose-dependent manner. In 2006, Fujiyoshi et al[496] showed that higher levels of dioxin correlated with higher levels of systemic inflammation (as measured by NFkB activity, which I have reviewed elsewhere[497]) and higher levels of blood glucose and increased risk of clinical diabetes; the results of this

---

[490] Vasquez A. "Detoxification: Clinical Relevance and Interventional Strategies for Adjunctive Treatment and Preventive Healthcare" in AFMCP: Applying Functional Medicine in Clinical Practice hosted by the Institute for Functional Medicine. Tampa, Florida November 2004 and Seattle, Washington March 2005. See Chapter 4.7 for review.

[491] Vasquez A, et al. The clinical importance of vitamin D (cholecalciferol). *Altern Ther Health Med.* 2004 Sep-Oct;10(5):28-36

[492] Henriksen GL, Ketchum NS, Michalek JE, Swaby JA. Serum dioxin and diabetes mellitus in veterans of Operation Ranch Hand. *Epidemiology.* 1997 May;8(3):252-8

[493] Calvert GM, Sweeney MH, Deddens J, Wall DK. Evaluation of diabetes mellitus, serum glucose, and thyroid function among United States workers exposed to 2,3,7,8-tetrachlorodibenzo-p-dioxin. *Occup Environ Med.* 1999 Apr;56(4):270-6. While the findings of this study are significant, the strength of the relationship between chemical exposure and insulin resistance was probably underestimated due to the researchers' focus on the specific dioxin subfraction 2,3,7,8-tetrachlorodibenzo-p-dioxin.

[494] Longnecker et al. Serum dioxin level in relation to diabetes mellitus among Air Force veterans with background levels of exposure. *Epidemiology.* 2000 Jan;11(1):44-8

[495] Fierens et al. Dioxin/polychlorinated biphenyl body burden, diabetes and endometriosis. *Biomarkers.* 2003 Nov-Dec;8(6):529-34

[496] Fujiyoshi et al. Molecular epidemiologic evidence for diabetogenic effects of dioxin exposure in US Air force veterans. *Environ Health Perspect.* 2006 Nov;114(11):1677-83

[497] Vasquez A. Nutritional and Botanical Inhibition of NF-kappaB, the Major Intracellular Amplifier of the Inflammatory Cascade. *Nutritional Perspectives* 2005;July: 5-12

study are particularly alarming because serum levels of toxins that correlated with increased risk of insulin resistance were comparable to levels found in the general population and which are generally considered "normal", assuming that chemical exposure and accumulation could ever be considered normal. **This research shows that background "every day" environmental exposure to dioxins and other chemical increases the risk of diabetes and insulin resistance even among patients with no occupational or accidental acute exposure to these chemicals.** Also in 2006, Vasiliu et al[498] showed that women with higher levels of polychlorinated biphenyls showed increased risk of diabetes. Further in 2006, Lee et al[499] showed a "striking dose-response relations between serum concentrations of six selected POPs [persistent organic pollutants] and the prevalence of diabetes" among a sample of more than 2,000 American citizens; note that this study is unique in that it analyzed a group of chemicals rather than a single or a small number of chemicals as performed in most of the previous studies. In 2007, Lee et al[500] published a follow-up study which again showed a clinically significant correlation between body burden of toxic chemicals and the incidence of insulin resistance and risk of diabetes.

Given the strong and consistent link between diabetes and the accumulation of toxic chemicals, two causal possibilities exist: either chemical accumulation causes diabetes, or diabetes causes chemical accumulation. While the former is more likely, the latter would not exclude clinicians and patients from the need to take action on this data because of the inherent risks associated with chemical accumulation. Toxic chemicals such as the ones associated with diabetes in the aforementioned studies are the same chemicals associated with induction of Parkinson's disease, and current evidence does indeed show increased risk of Parkinson's disease among diabetic patients.

Molecular Mechanisms of Xenobiotic Diabetogenesis: Toxic chemicals (xenobiotics) can cause insulin resistance and clinical diabetes mellitus by several different mechanisms. The aryl hydrocarbon receptor (hereafter: hydrocarbon receptor) is generally viewed as the molecular mechanism by which dioxin-like chemicals exert their adverse biological actions.[501] Stated simply, a leading hypothesis suggests that dioxin-like chemicals stimulate the hydrocarbon receptor to suppress glucohomeostatic activity of PPAR-gamma (peroxisome proliferator activated receptor gamma). PPAR-gamma is an intranuclear receptor that powerfully modulates insulin sensitivity and glucose utilization; indeed PPAR-gamma is the main target of the drug class of thiazolidinediones (TZDs) which are used in diabetes mellitus and other disorders of insulin resistance.[502] PPAR-gamma activation promotes insulin sensitivity and thus has a clear anti-diabetic effect by increasing the number of GLUT-4 receptors on the surface of muscle and adipose cells. Conversely, inhibition of PPAR-gamma (by toxin activation of the hydrocarbon receptor) causes a reduction in the number of GLUT-4 transporters which are required to move glucose from the serum into the intracellular space of muscle and adipose tissue. **Thus, the molecular mechanism and biologic plausibility by which toxic chemicals can lead to insulin resistance is clearly and firmly established based on in vitro studies, animal experiments, and the consistent data reported in humans.** Furthermore, secondary effects such as the estrogen-like action of many toxic chemicals may further complicate and exacerbate the diabetogenic effect of these toxins via upregulation of adipose accumulation. Increased adiposity from whatever cause correlates with increased serum levels of estrogens because adipose tissue expresses the aromatase enzyme which converts androgens into estrogens. Furthermore, adipose tissue is pro-inflammatory via the elaboration of cytokines (adipokines) which induce systemic inflammation and downregulate insulin sensitivity by decreasing the number of insulin receptors in adipose and muscle cell membranes. Many of the toxic chemicals that correlate with increased risk for diabetes have been shown in other studies to adversely affect thyroid function, directly leading to clinical and subclinical hypothyroidism and the resultant reduction in metabolic rate and propensity for weight gain and increased adiposity. Once established, the hyperglycemia of diabetes results in increase urinary excretion of nutrients such as magnesium, which is essential for peripheral insulin sensitivity and hepatic detoxification of xenobiotics; thus diabetes-induced magnesium deficiency can impair xenobiotic detoxification and thus contribute

[498] Vasiliu et al. Polybrominated biphenyls, polychlorinated biphenyls, body weight, and incidence of adult-onset diabetes mellitus. *Epidemiology*. 2006;17(4):352-9.

[499] Lee DH, Lee IK, Song K, Steffes M, Toscano W, Baker BA, Jacobs DR Jr. A strong dose-response relation between serum concentrations of persistent organic pollutants and diabetes: results from the National Health and Examination Survey 1999-2002. *Diabetes Care*. 2006 Jul;29(7):1638-44

[500] Lee et al. Association between serum concentrations of persistent organic pollutants and insulin resistance among nondiabetic adults. *Diabetes Care*. 2007 Mar;30(3):622-8

[501] Remillard RB, Bunce NJ. Linking dioxins to diabetes: epidemiology and biologic plausibility. *Environ Health Perspect*. 2002 Sep;110(9):853-8

[502] "PPAR-gamma is the main target of the drug class of thiazolidinediones (TZDs), used in diabetes mellitus and other diseases that feature insulin resistance." en.wikipedia.org/wiki/PPAR Accessed March 11, 2007

to an exacerbation of chemical accumulation. Lastly, some clinicians have proposed that increased adiposity may be a defensive means by which the body attempts to protect itself from chemical exposure, since increased fat stores will serve to dissipate and dilute absorbed chemicals and thus lessen their toxic effects. Anecdotal reports of rapid and effective weight loss have been observed in some patients following the implementation of clinical detoxification procedures, such as those outlined by the current author (Chapter 4, *Inflammation Mastery*) and detailed by others, notably Walter Crinnion ND as cited below.

Diabetes Treatment by Routine Methods—Unintentional Detoxification: I propose here that some of the commonly used methods for treating diabetes actually derive their benefits at least in part from their ability to enhance excretion of toxic chemicals. Exercise increases lipolysis which liberates fat-stored xenobiotics from adipose tissue, resulting in higher serum levels of toxins which thus increases urinary excretion of these toxins. Furthermore, the hyperventilation induced by exercise promotes respiratory alkalosis and the resultant alkalinization of the urine increases excretion of weakly acidic poisons. Relatedly, increased intake of fruits and vegetables promotes systemic and urinary alkalinization and thereby facilitates urinary excretion of poisons. Given evidence that systemic inflammation (in human studies of endotoxinemia) suppresses hepatic detoxification of xenobiotics, then the glucohomeostatic benefits of exercise, phytonutrient-rich diets, vitamin D3, fatty acid supplementation, and lipoic acid may be derived in part from the ability of these interventions to reduce systemic inflammation and thus facilitate (via derepression) xenobiotic biotransformation. The fiber of fruits and vegetables binds to chemicals which have undergone detoxification/biotransformation and which have been excreted in the bile; high-fiber diets reduce the recycling of toxins excreted into the gut. Magnesium supplementation improves insulin sensitivity, enables hepatic detoxification, and promotes urinary alkalinization. Fruits, vegetables, fiber, exercise, and magnesium supplementation all promote increased frequency of bowel movements to reduce enterohepatic recycling of (de)conjugated toxins. "Statin" cholesterol-lowering drugs (designed to inhibit the HMG-CoA reductase enzyme) activate the pregnane X receptor which upregulates xenobiotic detoxification and results enhanced toxin excretion. Cholestyramine, a drug that binds cholesterol in the gut and that is used in the treatment of diabetic hypercholesterolemia, also binds toxic chemicals excreted in the gut and can be used as effective therapy in patients with chronic chemical poisoning.[503] Therefore, the anti-diabetic, hypocholesterolemic, and insulin-sensitizing clinical effects of many commonly employed therapeutics may result directly and in part from the enhanced elimination of xenobiotics; this is a hitherto unappreciated mechanism of action for these treatments.

Diabetes Treatment by Detoxification—Proposal for Large-Scale Clinical Trials: Given the strength and direction of the research (sampled above) indicating that xenobiotic exposure and chemical accumulation is a major contributor to the epidemic of type-2 diabetes mellitus and other disorders of insulin resistance, all of us as researchers, clinicians, and healthcare consumers are potentially on the verge of a major paradigm shift in regard to our view of these disorders and their clinical management. If chemical exposure and accumulation contributes to insulin resistance, then healthcare professionals will have ethical and professional obligations to address these underlying problems in their patients who present with insulin resistance. Detoxification protocols, rather than endless and additive drug prescriptions to suppress the symptoms of the problem, could become the standard of care if such protocols are shown safe and effective for restoring glucohomeostasis. However, given the ubiquitous nature of xenobiotic exposure and the numeric infinity and methodological complexity of measuring levels of xenobiotics in individual patients, doctors and patients alike will be fighting an uphill battle against the constant onslaught of toxins, and both groups will have to start with an understanding of the body's inherent detoxification processes and the means by which these defense mechanisms can be supported in their respective roles. Given that we already have molecular mechanisms, animal research, and human data linking xenobiotic exposure to the genesis and perpetuation of insulin resistance, the only piece of the diabetes-xenobiotic puzzle that is missing is a large-scale clinical trial of effective therapeutic detoxification in patients with diabetes. If such a trial were to be skillfully designed and successfully implemented and was able to demonstrate amelioration of insulin resistance by interventions that are—to the extent possible—specific to the detoxification process (rather than directed toward

---

[503] "Cholestyramine offers a practical means for detoxification of persons exposed to chlordecone and possibly to other lipophilic toxins." Cohn WJ, Boylan JJ, Blanke RV, Fariss MW, Howell JR, Guzelian PS. Treatment of chlordecone (Kepone) toxicity with cholestyramine. Results of a controlled clinical trial. *N Engl J Med.* 1978 Feb 2;298(5):243-8

enhancement of insulin sensitivity), then an authentic breakthrough in the management of the rising pandemic of diabetes mellitus would have been achieved. Further, such a breakthrough would open the door to other trials in xenobiotic-associated diseases, particularly Parkinson's disease, autism[504], and many of the systemic autoimmune diseases such as systemic lupus erythematosus. In order to design and implement such trials, clinician researchers must start from an understanding of the biochemical and physiologic means by which detoxification occurs and the means by which such process can be supported and expedited to effect rapid elimination of toxins, and an overview of important concepts will be provided in the following section. Citations to research will be limited here due to space restrictions; excellent reviews of this subject include the works of Liska[505] and Crinnion.[506] What follows here is an excerpt from my previous work in the role of therapeutic detoxification in the treatment of musculoskeletal inflammation; see Chapter 4 of *Inflammation Mastery 4th Edition* for the complete list of references to the following paragraph.

Biochemistry and Physiology of Detoxification—Rationale for Clinical Therapeutics: Studies using blood tests and tissue samples from Americans across the nation have consistently shown that **all** Americans have toxic chemical **accumulation** whether or not they work in chemical factories or are exposed at home or work.[507,508] We cannot escape from the chemical consequences of living in a world with tens of thousands of synthetic chemicals. According to limited analyses, the average American has accumulated at least 18 different chemicals[509], and analyses that are more detailed show that even more chemicals and metals have been accumulated.[510] Common sources of these chemicals include pesticides, synthetic fertilizers, herbicides, fungicides, industrial pollution, car exhaust, solvents, paints, perfumes, plastic food/drink containers, non-stick cookware, Styrofoam, trichloroethylene from dry cleaning, rubber, carpet, plastics, glues, propellants, petroleum fuels such as gasoline, detergents, and other "cleaners." Clinical consequences of chemical toxicity are diverse, can affect nearly every organ system, and may be predicted to some extent by the pattern of chemical exposure since some chemicals have characteristic sequelae. Most of these chemicals are fat-soluble and can readily enter the body via respiratory, gastrointestinal, and transdermal routes. Once in the bloodstream, chemicals are either detoxified (inactivated and/or solubilized) by the liver and then excreted via urine or bile, or to a lesser extent exhaled from the lungs or excreted via sweat. Chemicals which are not excreted from the body are stored in the tissues, particularly lipid-rich organs such as the liver, adipose, and brain. Molecular turnover and recycling (particularly lipolysis) liberates fat-stored xenobiotics for another opportunity for either detoxification or additional toxicity. The main route for detoxification is the liver, which hydrosolublizes xenobiotics via oxidation ("phase one") and conjugation ("phase two"). Generally speaking, oxidation reactions are dependent on the cytochrome P-450 system, which can be inhibited by various drugs (e.g., ketoconazole, erythromycin, ritonavir, cimetidine, omeprazole, ethanol), foods such as ethanol and grapefruit juice, bacterial endotoxin from bacterial overgrowth of the bowel, and/or by genetic defects known as single nucleotide polymorphisms ("SNiPs") which reduce xenobiotic clearance. Similarly, conjugation reactions can be inhibited by a low-vegetable diet, SNiPs, and insufficiencies of conjugation moieties such as glutathione, glycine, glutamine, taurine, ornithine, sulfur, and methyl groups. If oxidation is too slow, then xenobiotics are insufficiently detoxicated and insufficiently processed for conjugation, leading to xenobiotic accumulation. If oxidation is too fast *relative to conjugation*, then reactive intermediates are formed which are commonly more toxic than the original xenobiotic. Optimally oxidized and conjugated xenobiotics are excreted in the urine or expelled in the bile. Supranormal hydration and urinary alkalinization enhance renal clearance of weakly acidic xenobiotics and drugs, whereas dehydration and urinary acidity impair toxin excretion, generally speaking. Conjugated toxins expelled in the bile can be deconjugated by bacteria so that the toxin is reabsorbed, a

---

[504] Vasquez A. "Chapter 10: Organ System Function and Underlying Mechanisms: The Interconnected Web." In Jones DS (Editor-in-Chief). *Textbook of Functional Medicine*. Institute for Functional Medicine, 2005. Vasquez A. Web-like Interconnections of Physiological Factors. *Integrative Med* 2006 April: 32-37 ichnfm.academia.edu/AlexVasquez
[505] Liska DJ. The detoxification enzyme systems. *Altern Med Rev*. 1998 Jun;3(3):187-98
[506] Crinnion WJ. Results of a decade of naturopathic treatment for environmental illnesses. *J Naturopathic Med* 1994;17:21-27. Crinnion WJ. Human burden of environmental toxins and their common health effects. *Altern Med Rev*. 2000 Feb:52-63; Crinnion WJ. Health effects of ubiquitous airborne solvent exposure. *Altern Med Rev* 2000 Apr:133-43
[507] "The average concentration of 2,3,7,8-tetrachlorodibenzo-p-dioxin in the adipose tissue of the US population was 5.38 pg/g, increasing from 1.98 pg/g in children under 14 years of age to 9.40 pg/g in adults over 45." Orban JE, Stanley JS, Schwemberger JG, Remmers JC. Dioxins and dibenzofurans in adipose tissue of the general US population and selected subpopulations. *Am J Public Health* 1994;84(3):439-45
[508] "Although the use of HCB as a fungicide has virtually been eliminated, detectable levels of HCB are still found in nearly all people in the USA." Robinson PE, Leczynski BA, Kutz FW, Remmers JC. An evaluation of hexachlorobenzene body-burden levels in the general population of the USA. *IARC Sci Publ* 1986;(77):183-92
[509] Schafer et al. Chemical Trespass: Pesticides in Our Bodies and Corporate Accountability. Pesticide Action Network North America. May 2004 panna.org/ on August 1, 2004
[510] Body Burden: The Pollution in People. ewg.org/issues/siteindex/issues.php?issueid=5004 Accessed February 6, 2006

phenomenon commonly referred to as "enterohepatic recycling" or "enterohepatic recirculation." Such recirculation is obviously less likely if gastrointestinal status and diet have been optimized to minimize the presence of deconjugating bacteria and to maximize fiber intake and laxation for the adsorption and expulsion of intraluminal toxins. Therapeutic colonics and enemas can be employed to stimulate bile flow from the liver[511,512] and to remove bile-secreted toxins from the gut before deconjugation and re-absorption occur. Bile formation and expulsion are further stimulated by botanical medicines such as beets, ginger, curcumin/turmeric[513], *Picrorhiza*, milk thistle, *Andrographis paniculata,* and *Boerhaavia diffusa*. Respiratory exhalation of toxins is enhanced by deep breathing and exercise, and hyperventilation promotes respiratory alkalosis which elevates urine pH and promotes excretion of weakly acidic drugs and xenobiotics as previously mentioned. Dermal excretion of toxins via sweat and expedited lipolysis are stimulated via low-temperature saunas and regular aerobic exercise. Xenobiotic oxidation can be promoted (cautiously) by reducing endotoxins from the gut and by the use of botanicals such as *Hypericum perforatum* which induce several isoforms of cytochrome P-450 via activation of the pregane X receptor. Xenobiotic conjugation is likewise promoted via nutrigenomic induction stimulated by cruciferous vegetables and their derivatives such as indole-3-carbinol (I3C) and dimethylindolylemethane (DIM). The plant-based diet is employed to provide fiber for bowel cleansing and the urinary alkalinization that is necessary for optimal urinary excretion of toxins, the majority of which are weak acids and are thus excreted more efficiently in alkaline urine. Sodium bicarbonate can also be used to induce urinary alkalinization. The diet must contain high-quality protein and can be supplemented with amino acids to support amino acid and glutathione conjugation. Serum, urine, and adipose samples can be analyzed to determine the intensity and diversity of chemical accumulation. For most patients, their chemical accumulation is so diverse that they may not display abnormally high levels of a specific chemical; their clinical manifestations are rather a manifestation of a wide plethora of different chemicals, which individually may be only modestly increased. Detoxification characteristics can be assessed from genotypic and phenotypic perspectives using appropriate laboratory tests. Phenotype can be assessed by serum and urine measurements of post-challenge detoxification of benzoate, caffeine, acetylsalicylic acid, and acetaminophen. Amino acid status can be

> **Xenobiotic-induced HTN and DM**
> Pesticides and other pollutants commonly induce mitochondrial dysfunction, thereby contributing to insulin resistance (impaired insulin secretion and reception) and vasoconstriction (via ROS-induced endothelial dysfunction), which promote HTN and DM.

quantified and qualified via serum or urine amino acid analysis. Stool testing assesses digestion, absorption, and microflora status. Clinical implementation of therapeutic detoxification follows a screening physical examination and basic laboratory assessment (minimally including CBC, metabolic panel, and urinalysis). Stool testing for dysbiosis is always reasonable when working with patients with fatigue and/or autoimmunity[514]; however, this and the other detoxification-related tests can often be deferred and/or used selectively. The Paleo-Mediterranean diet provides ample high-quality protein, alkalinization, fiber, and phytonutrients to which may be added supplements of protein, amino acids (especially NAC, glycine, and glutamine), and vitamins and minerals. Antioxidant teas and fresh fruit and vegetable juices are consumed to increase frequency of urination and promote urinary alkalinization due primarily to the content of potassium citrate. Exercise and low-temperature saunas promote sweating and xenobiotic-mobilizing lipolysis. Bile flow is further stimulated by consumption of beets, ginger, curcumin/turmeric, *Picrorhiza*, milk thistle, *Andrographis paniculata* and *Boerhaavia diffusa*. These interventions work in concert to enhance xenobiotic removal and cleanse the tissues of accumulated toxins. Intervention can be acute or periodic, but must be maintained for the long-term in order to resist the re-accumulation that is destined to result from the chemical onslaught that is inescapable in our polluted world.

Conclusion: Clinicians should now have an appreciation of the emerging research that links chemical accumulation to the development of diabetes. The molecular mechanisms have been explained, and the basic science and clinical research has been reviewed. Lastly, major considerations for the design and implementation of therapeutic detoxification programs have been presented. Formal clinical trials must be pursued, while individual clinicians explore the use of detoxification in their diabetic patients.

---

[511] Garbat, AL, Jacobi, HG. Secretion of bile in response to rectal installations. *Arch Intern Med* 1929; 44: 455-462

[512] "Caffeine enemas cause dilation of bile ducts, which facilitates excretion of toxic cancer breakdown products by the liver and dialysis of toxic products from blood across the colonic wall. The therapy must be used as an integrated whole." Gerson M. The cure of advanced cancer by diet therapy. *Physiol Chem Phys*. 1978;10(5):449-64

[513] "On the basis of the present findings, it appears that curcumin induces contraction of the human gall-bladder." Rasyid A, Lelo A. The effect of curcumin and placebo on human gall-bladder function: an ultrasound study. *Aliment Pharmacol Ther*. 1999 Feb;13(2):245-9

[514] Vasquez A. Nutritional and Botanical Treatments against "Silent Infections" and Gastrointestinal Dysbiosis. *Nutr Perspect* 2006; Jan. ichnfm.academia.edu/AlexVasquez

Migraine, Cluster and Other Headaches

Introduction:

This section focuses on migraine headaches in their classic and prototypic manifestations, originating primarily from the additive/synergistic combination of glial activation (and the related neurogenic inflammation and neuroinflammation) and mitochondrial dysfunction; understood as such, migraine and its closely related variant cluster headache can reasonably and very accurately be categorized within my model of metabolic inflammation— the manifestation of inflammation strongly associated with or caused by metabolic impairment, most generally noted in causal/contributory association with mitochondrial dysfunction. Per the origination of this work in my clinical textbooks (*Integrative Orthopedics*, 2004, 2007, 2012) and clinical monographs (*Musculoskeletal Pain*, 2008), this section includes clinical evaluation and differential diagnosis.

Description/pathophysiology:

- Introduction: Headaches are a common symptom-based diagnosis with a wide variety of underlying causes ranging from commonplace and benign (e.g., muscle tension headache) to catastrophic (e.g., meningitis or stroke). This section deals only with the pathophysiology and amelioration of routine benign headaches (migraine, cluster, allergic, tension, and cervicogenic); emphasis is placed on migraine headaches as the prototype for these disorders. Once serious pathological causes of headache have been excluded, the headache can be treated with symptom-suppressing drugs (which have associated risks and expenses without collateral benefits) or by biological/nutritional/natural interventions that address the underlying causative mechanisms and thereby improve overall health.

- Social and medical significance: Headaches and migraine—while seemingly insignificant compared to life-threatening diseases such as cancer and autoimmune diseases—account for huge losses in quality of life and productivity. Headache is a diagnosis based on the patient's subjective report of pain *in* (deep) or *on* (superficial) the head. The potential causes are numerous, ranging from benign muscle tension to life-threatening intracranial hemorrhage or meningitis. Of important note: migraine headache patients have increased risk for neurologic and cardiovascular diseases[1,2]; simply treating the *pain* of migraine does not address the underlying biochemical, physiologic, and inflammatory disturbances whereas nutritional and anti-inflammatory interventions hold great potential for both *alleviation of pain* and *improvement of overall health* via correction of the underlying pathophysiology.

- Mechanism of pain sensation in headache: The final common pathway for "primary" headaches (e.g., migraine and cluster headaches) is currently reported to be neurogenic/brain inflammation: inflammatory mediators from the brain generally and nerves specifically activate trigeminal (cranial nerve V) neurons to produce both vasoconstriction and the sensation of pain.[3]

- A contemporary integrated model of migraine: The task of

> ### Dysfunction precedes disease; understanding precedes efficacy
>
> The best model of any disease is one that incorporates all of the major known facts into a cohesive and sequential understanding, predicting and being supported by efficacious treatments that are known to address the abnormal physiology—the dysfunction that precedes and causes the disease. The intellectual error of previous models of migraine is that they had no specific starting point, other than to attribute the genesis to "genetic traits and environmental triggers." As such, these earlier descriptions "started from the middle" and simply explained ongoing pathophysiology. By failing to start at the beginning, these earlier models likewise based their treatment on the downstream effects rather than on the treatment of the original cause of the disease. As such, the medical treatments based on this faulty model were necessarily ineffective. Here, I present a complete model, facilitating both understanding and treatment of various headache types.

intellectuals is the creation of cohesion, integration, and understanding; as such, one of the first tasks in the conversation on migraine is to define and characterize the disorder. Effective treatment, excepting blind luck, must be based on a comprehensive and cohesive understanding of the disorder in its *essential* totality. The major

---

[1] "Depression [adjusted OR = 2.12] and migraine [adjusted OR = 3.65] were more commonly recorded before the diagnosis of dementia in the DLB group." Fereshtehnejad et al. Comorbidity profile in dementia with Lewy bodies versus Alzheimer's disease. *Alzheimers Res Ther.* 2014 Oct 6;6(5-8):65

[2] "The migraine cohort had a higher prevalence of diabetes, hypertension, coronary artery disease, head injury and depression at baseline (p < 0.0001). After adjusting the covariates, migraine patients had a 1.33-fold higher risk of developing dementia [hazard ratio (HR) 1.33]. The sex-specific incidence rate of dementia was higher in men than in women in both cohorts, with an HR of 1.09 for men compared to women. Kaplan-Meier analysis shows that the cumulative incidence of dementia was 1.48% greater in the migraine cohort than in the nonmigraine cohort. This study shows that migraines are associated with a future higher risk of dementia after adjusting for comorbidities. Specifically, the association between migraine and dementia is greater in young adults than in older adults." Chuang et al. Migraine and risk of dementia. *Neuroepidemiology.* 2013;41:139-45

[3] Tierney ML. McPhee SJ, Papadakis MA (eds). *Current Medical Diagnosis and Treatment 2006, 45th Edition*. New York: Lange Medical Books; 2006, pages 31-33

themes from experimental studies and clinical trials have to be integrated and reconciled so that the best model of the disorder emerges triumphantly above the trivia of anecdote and the dogma of pharmaceutical profiteering. Beyond, in addition to, and in support of clinical efficacy, we need a grand unified theory (GUT) that helps us perceive the disease and prioritize the treatments; otherwise, a disarticulated understanding will perpetuate the disarrayed medical management and dependency that we currently observe in migraine and headache management. Each of the following components are sequentially ordered, starting with the first most important primary cause: mitochondrial dysfunction. Importantly, given that—as Thoreau noted in *Civil Disobedience* (1849, p. 26)—"We love eloquence for its own sake, and not for any truth which it may utter", we cannot be satisfied with a clear explanation; the explanation has to have high merit in the real world, being proven by the safety and efficacy of the treatments that it advocates. This standard reveals the falsity of the medical model of both migraine and fibromyalgia, since both the models are selectively incomplete in order to justify drug treatment, and the interventions are unnecessarily hazardous and inadequately efficacious.

1. Mitochondrial impairment is the origin of migraine and cluster headache: Patients with migraine (and cluster headache) have very clear and consistent defects in mitochondrial performance, leading to cellular energy/ATP deficiency, excess production of free radicals (reactive oxygen species—ROS, which promote cellular damage and inflammation). Patients with migraine are often deficient in coenzyme Q-10 (CoQ10), and this causes mitochondrial dysfunction and reduced antioxidant protection against the harmful and pro-inflammatory effects of ROS. Nutritional treatments, such as riboflavin and CoQ10, which support mitochondrial function are consistently the safest and most effective anti-migraine treatments available, thereby proving the mitochondrial origin of migraine. Defects in cellular energy/ATP production cause neurons to be more unstable, resulting in excessive activation, resulting in pain sensation and sensitization. Mitochondrial dysfunction always promotes inflammation, at the very least by increasing formation of free radicals and the liberation of free ATP via leaky mitochondrial membranes; these molecules are perceived by cellular receptors as danger signals, thereby triggering the nonspecific alarm response of inflammation. The metabolic impairment likely contributes to vasodilation, as arteries dilate to bring more oxygen to support metabolic demand (in physiology, this is termed "reactive hyperemia").

    Increasingly over the past several years, the model of microglial activation along with mitochondrial dysfunction is gaining strength and due popularity; this model helps explain many divergent aspects of migraine and provides unification of previously fragmented models and disconnected facts. One of the strongest primary drivers of migraine is mitochondrial dysfunction, which shows a severity-response relationship and is maternally inheritable. Mitochondrial dysfunction is sufficient to promote (micro)glial activation, and the two then form a vicious cycle, ultimately promoting neocortical excitation and the resultant pain sensitization, thereby again promoting continuance and reinforcement of this vicious cycle. By analogy, the brains of these patients are "physiologically fragile" with a constant smoldering sterile inflammation; the brain is either constantly smoldering (e.g., chronic neuroinflammation) or actively "on fire" (e.g., migraine attack).

2. Sustained glial activation results from mitochondrial dysfunction and causes brain inflammation and hyperexcitation: Glial cells are the "glue"—the interconnecting cells—of the brain comprised chiefly of microglia and astrocytes. Microglia (the immune cells of the brain) are sensitive to ROS and inflammatory signals, and become "activated" (microglial activation) in response to peripheral inflammation (including obesity, trauma, infection and vaccination) and central "within the nervous system" events such as trauma and stress. When microglia become activated, they signal the astrocytes (cells that physically and chemically support neurons) to change behavior by providing *less protective support* to brain neurons and *causing more stimulation* of these same neurons; more stimulation with less protection causes the neurons to become "sensitized" and hyperresponsive and eventually promotes the "burn-out" of these neurons. The combinations of more excitation, more inflammation, less energy/ATP and less protection is called "excitotoxicity" (neuronal injury by overstimulation) and eventually leads to neurodegeneration, damage to neurons, brain structures, and the brain as a whole. Stated again and differently: microglia cells in the brain receive inflammatory stimuli and then trigger astrocytes to increase stimulation of neurons via the excitatory neurotransmitter glutamate, which activates a receptor called the NMDA receptor (NMDAr, detailed later); in this manner, inflammatory signals are converted into altered levels of neurotransmitters

(especially glutamate, also quinolinic acid [QUIN], a metabolite of tryptophan produced during conditions of inflammation, discussed later) which stimulate neurons to perceive more pain. Excessive stimulation of neurons feeds-back into causing more microglial activation, resulting in a vicious cycle.

3. <mark>Brain inflammation, neuroinflammation, neurogenic inflammation all result from glial activation and promote additional brain inflammation</mark>: Nerve cells become inflamed in response to any insult; this is called **neuroinflammation**, and it promotes various neurologic and psychiatric disorders, such as pain and depression (e.g., the components of **sickness behavior**), respectively. The neurons themselves can also release inflammatory mediators; this is called **neurogenic inflammation** because the inflammation is coming from the nerve cells while also affecting those same nerve cells. When **brain inflammation** is triggered, it affects all of the major cells types of the brain and becomes a self-reinforcing cycle, sometimes called "**brain on fire**."[4] Inflammation in the brain has many consequences; for example, ❶ inflamed neurons release neuropeptides and inflammatory mediators that activate endothelial cells (thereby causing vasoconstriction) and promote additional inflammation, and ❷ activation of mast cells and platelets causes these cells to secrete inflammatory/vasoactive amines, arachidonate metabolites (such as prostaglandins, leukotrienes, isoprostanes); these substances promote additional inflammation and also promote constriction of blood vessels. Remarkably, the brain inflammation and metabolic impairment seen in migraine known as **cortical spreading depression** triggers release of the inflammation-associated and tissue-destructive enzyme matrix metalloproteinase (MMP), which causes leakiness of the blood-brain barrier (BBB), leading to brain edema and enhanced uptake of inflammatory molecules from the blood.[5]

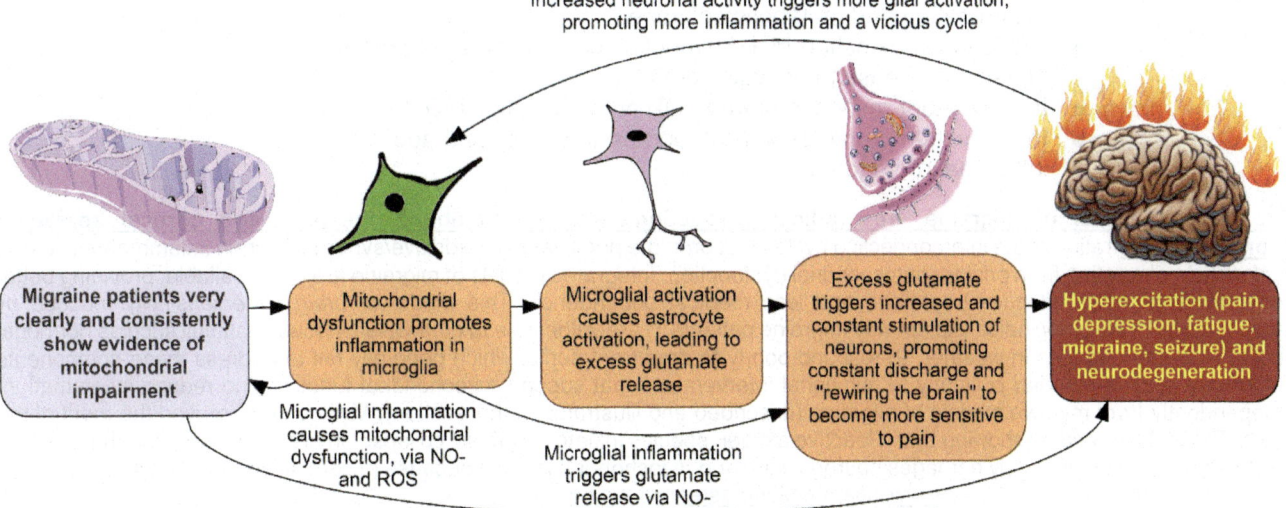

Increased neuronal activity triggers more glial activation, promoting more inflammation and a vicious cycle

| Migraine patients very clearly and consistently show evidence of mitochondrial impairment | Mitochondrial dysfunction promotes inflammation in microglia | Microglial activation causes astrocyte activation, leading to excess glutamate release | Excess glutamate triggers increased and constant stimulation of neurons, promoting constant discharge and "rewiring the brain" to become more sensitive to pain | Hyperexcitation (pain, depression, fatigue, migraine, seizure) and neurodegeneration |

Microglial inflammation causes mitochondrial dysfunction, via NO- and ROS

Microglial inflammation triggers glutamate release via NO-

Mitochondrial impairment causes neurons to be more vulnerable to normal activity and makes these neurons more sensitive to minor insults and stressors such as sound/light stimulation, hormonal fluctuations, emotional stress.
The combination of mitochondrial dysfunction with excess excitation is particularly devastating to neurons, leading to neuron death: neurodegeneration.

Foundational model of migraine: ❶ Migraine patients very clearly and consistently show evidence of mitochondrial impairment: This genotropic mitochondrial dysfunction can be due to different factors, including 1) defects in CoQ10 synthesis, 2) defects in the citric acid cycle, and 3) defects in the function of the electron transport chain (ETC). The majority of these problems can be partly/largely circumvented by use of nutritional interventions. ❷ Mitochondrial dysfunction promotes inflammation in microglia: Sterile inflammation promoted by excess free radicals produced by dysfunctional mitochondria promote microglial activation. Microglial inflammation causes mitochondrial dysfunction via NO- (nitric oxide, causes impairment of Complex #4 in the electron transport chain[ETC], leading to reduced cellular energy/ATP production), ROS (reactive oxygen species, free radicals), and perhaps directly via inflammatory cytokines thereby creating a vicious cycle. ❸ Microglial activation causes astrocyte activation, leading to excess glutamate release. ❹ Excess glutamate triggers increased and constant stimulation of neurons, promoting constant discharge and "rewiring the brain" to become more sensitive to pain. ❺ Hyperexcitation promotes pain, depression, fatigue, seizure, migraine and neurodegeneration. The combination of mitochondrial dysfunction with excess excitation is particularly devastating to neurons, leading to neuron death: neurodegeneration. Image of brain by IsaacMao per Flickr.com via creativecommons.org/licenses/by/2.0. See educational videos and updates at www.inflammationmastery.com/pain

---

[4] Cohen G. The brain on fire? *Ann Neurol.* 1994 Sep;36(3):333-4
[5] Moskowitz MA. Genes, proteases, cortical spreading depression and migraine: impact on pathophysiology and treatment. *Funct Neurol.* 2007 Jul-Sep;22(3):133-6

Brain neuron excitation

- Glutamate/NMDA receptors are activated by glutamate, QUIN and homocysteine
- Reduced mitochondrial performance impairs homeodynamics in response to excessive NMDAr stimulation
- Free radicals from mitochondria, neurons, and glia promote molecular and cellular damage, thereby triggering inflammation and metabolic collapse of neurons
- Excess intracellular calcium triggers inflammation
- Hyperexcitation promotes pain, pain sensitization, and neurodegeneration

Mitochondrial dysfunction

- Increases in oxidant production promote progressive inflammation and metabolic collapse
- Promotes inflammation in all affected cells
- Depletes antioxidant nutrients such as CoQ10, thereby leading to additional vulnerability, inflammation, and mitochondrial dysfunction
- Makes neurons vulnerable/fragile to excessive activation (eg, lowered depolarization threshold) due to oxidant damage and increased intracellular calcium
- Mitochondrial ROS cause mitochondrial damage, which increases ROS production in a vicious cycle

Central sensitization, cortical spreading depression, metabolic collapse
Image © by Dr Alex Vasquez, ICHNFM.ORG

Microglial activation, astrocyte activation

- Increased oxidant production promotes progressive inflammation and metabolic collapse
- NO- causes mitochondrial dysfunction at ETC #4 and triggers glutamate release to activate NMDAr
- Inflammatory response creates QUIN to activate NMDAr
- Inflammation promotes leaky blood-brain barrier and additional inflammation, edema

The vicious cycles of migraine, free radical production/damage, "metabolic collapse" and cortical spreading depression: Illustration of the interconnecting cycles that promote persistent and additive/synergistic brain inflammation, neuron dysfunction, stemming from primary mitochondrial dysfunction. Integrated models of migraine are now available, providing better understanding, more effective treatment, and less medical dependency. This model of *brain hypersensitivity induced by mitochondrial dysfunction* helps explain why migraine patients 1) are vulnerable to otherwise innocuous stimuli such as hormonal fluctuations and changes in weather, 2) respond poorly to drug treatments, which generally fail to address these components sufficiently, and 3) respond brilliantly to nutritional interventions that support mitochondrial function and reduce inflammation. Independently from my own models of migraine (described and illustrated in this section), Malkov et al[6] proved the merit of the model I have illustrated by showing that "Reactive oxygen species initiate metabolic collapse" in brain neurons, and that this free radical damage that tripartitely damages neurons, glia, and mitochondria is a major cause of cortical spreading depression. See educational videos and updates at www.inflammationmastery.com/pain

4. Mitochondrial dysfunction and glial activation combine to cause altered brain neuron function—brain destabilization, metabolic fragility; in its entirety, this three-part combination of mitochondrial dysfunction, glial inflammation, and neuronal dysfunction is called cortical spreading depression (CSD): Neurons are simultaneously hyperactive due to (NMDA) neurotransmitter receptor activation and also hyporesponsive due to the mitochondrial impairment; this "physiologic confusion" contributes to the altered brain function seen in migraine, especially migraine with aura. In migraine, the brain is "destabilized" (per Moskowitz[7]), leading to what I call "metabolic fragility" or "brain fragility" that makes migraine patients more sensitive to changes in diet, climate, hormones, stress and sleep. These combinations of ❶ metabolic/mitochondrial impairment with ❷ increased/altered brain activity (e.g., specifically mediated by glutamate at the NMDA

> **Mitochondrial dysfunction is a key component of migraine**
>
> "In migraine, the degree of the mitochondrial impairment ... is related to the severity of the clinical phenotype."
>
> Lodi et al. *J Neurol Sci*. 1997 Feb

---

[6] Malkov et al. Reactive oxygen species initiate a metabolic collapse in hippocampal slices: potential trigger of cortical spreading depression. *J Cereb Blood Flow Metab*. 2014 Sep;34(9):1540-9

[7] Moskowitz MA. Genes, proteases, cortical spreading depression and migraine: impact on pathophysiology and treatment. *Funct Neurol*. 2007 Jul-Sep;22(3):133-6

receptor) and ❸ glial/neuronal/brain inflammation is what creates the wave of abnormal brain function—cortical spreading depression—that typifies migraine and which promotes its exacerbation; cortical spreading depression (CSD) leads to elaboration of the inflammatory and destructive enzyme MMP9 which causes leakiness of the BBB and subsequent brain edema (secondary to protein and water entry into the brain) and increased brain entry of substances from the blood, such as peripherally derived proinflammatory cytokines.[8,9] Brain edema in migraine is associated with and likely contributes to reduced brain perfusion (ie, reduced blood flow).[10] Very importantly, enhanced glutaminergic neurotransmission is itself sufficient to induce cortical spreading depression in experimental models. In an insightful article published in 2014 that supports the model that I have proposed, Malkov et al[11] showed that cortical spreading depression is caused by elaboration of reactive oxygen species (ROS, free radicals) and that these initiate "metabolic collapse" in brain cells.

> **All of these components are interconnected and thus the terms and components become (ultimately/practically) conceptually synonymous**
>
> Since microglial activation causes astrocyte activation, these terms can be summarized as glial activation. Microglial activation triggers formation of QUIN, which along with glutamate from astrocyte activation, causes stimulation of the NMDA receptor, promoting excitation of neurons. Since glial activation causes neuronal excitation, we can generally state that glial activation is synonymous with hyperexcitation of neurons, which segues into excitotoxic death of neurons and neurodegeneration. Persistent and prolonged hyperexcitation of neurons causes these neurons to strengthen their connections with each other, leading to facilitated pain perception, called central sensitization, as noted in **migraine, fibromyalgia**, and **complex regional pain syndrome**. Microglial activation—via release of nitric oxide (NO-) —causes mitochondrial dysfunction and additional glutamate release, causing the combination of metabolic impairment (e.g., reduced ATP formation) and increased metabolic demand, because activation of the NMDA receptor by glutamate and QUIN imposes increased metabolic demand on the neuron cells as they must control the resulting influx of calcium, which if not controlled will promote additional inflammation, impairment, and neuronal cell death.

5. Pain route—the covering of the brain is sensitive to metabolic and inflammatory changes within the brain, and interprets the inflammatory substances as pain signals: The trigeminal nerve (cranial nerve V, #5) receives transmissions from nerve endings surrounding the blood vessels of the membrane surrounding the brain (pia mater) and inside of the skull (dura mater). Recall as previously discussed and cited that the blood-brain barrier becomes more permeable when the brain is inflamed, thereby promoting passage/diffusion of inflammatory mediators from the brain to nearby neurons that receive noxious stimuli and convert the reception of those substances into nerve impulses received and interpreted as pain signals (nociception). While sensory innervation of the supratentorial dura mater membrane is via small meningeal branches of the trigeminal nerve, the innervation for the infratentorial dura mater is via upper cervical nerves, thereby establishing a bidirectional relationship between neck pain (and other subconscious neurologic inputs) and intracranial stimuli and structures.

6. Pain sensitization: As more pain signals are received, the brain facilitates the reception of these messages and thereby becomes more sensitive to the reception of pain; this is called central sensitization, and is greatly facilitated by brain inflammation and mitochondrial impairment.

7. Blood vessel dilation and constriction, and the role of serotonin-1D receptors: Metabolic impairment can trigger vasodilation, while inflammatory mediators promote vasoconstriction; both vasodilation and vasoconstriction have been noted in migraine.

8. Nuances in the contribution of various factors leads to different clinical presentations (e.g., migraine headaches vs cluster headaches); however, in the main primary headache conditions—migraine and cluster—the main themes of mitochondrial dysfunction and brain inflammation dominate the causal pathophysiology and therefore guide treatment: The model presented and used here is that cluster headache is simply a variant of migraine headache, with secondary rather than primary causes of the

[8] Moskowitz MA. Genes, proteases, cortical spreading depression and migraine: impact on pathophysiology and treatment. *Funct Neurol.* 2007 Jul-Sep;22(3):133-6

[9] Wilson CJ, Finch CE, Cohen HJ. Cytokines and cognition--the case for a head-to-toe inflammatory paradigm. *J Am Geriatr Soc.* 2002 Dec;50(12):2041-56

[10] For evidence of brain edema (with associated hypoperfusion) in patients with migraine: Kim et al. Recurrent steroid-responsive cerebral vasogenic edema in status migrainosus and persistent aura. *Cephalalgia.* 2015 Jul;35:728-34. See also: Bereczki et al. Cortical spreading edema in persistent visual migraine aura. *Headache.* 2008 Sep;48:1226-9

[11] Malkov et al. Reactive oxygen species initiate a metabolic collapse in hippocampal slices: cortical spreading depression. *J Cereb Blood Flow Metab.* 2014 Sep;34(9):1540-9

underlying mitochondrial dysfunction, and with a greater contribution by psychoemotional stress, muscle tension, and nutritional deficiencies. Mitochondrial dysfunction is seen in both migraine and cluster headache.[12] Nutritional deficiencies (e.g., folic acid) and excesses of systemic inflammation and serum homocysteine are noted in various types of headache, in both adult and pediatric populations.[13]

- Pathophysiology—from past to current models: The sensation of headache pain results from activation and sensitization of sensory trigeminal pain neurons that service intracranial blood vessels and meninges. For many years, the debate focused on whether *vasculogenic* or *neurogenic* influences predominated; most if not all headaches appear to involve *both* of these main components, thus allowing for the consensus that headaches have a *neurovascular* component. That said, the weight of evidence increasingly shifted to support the *neurological* origin—from within the brain and neurons (rather than the blood vessels)—of headaches in general and migraines in particular. "Brain-initiated events" such as cortical spreading depression—a wave of electrical and metabolic disturbance that sweeps across the brain surface, making the brain tissue physiologically unstable, and thus more fragile and vulnerable to various insults—culminate in the release of pain-inducing nociceptive substances including hydrogen ions and arachidonate metabolites, which irritate trigeminovascular sensory neurons surrounding pial vessels.[14,15]

Both dilation and constriction of arteries has been noted in migraine. Dilation of arteries may be an early compensatory response to impaired cellular energy/ATP production as mitochondrial dysfunction progresses from mild to more severe as vicious cycles exacerbate an ever-present primary defect; vasodilation in response to impaired energy/ATP production is well known in physiology as "reactive hyperemia." As mitochondrial

Brain sensitization to pain: 4 main components
1. <u>Pain signals</u>: Defects in cellular energy/ATP production cause neurons to be more unstable, resulting in excessive activation, resulting in pain sensation and sensitization. Mitochondrial dysfunction always promotes inflammation, at the very least by increasing formation of free radicals, which are perceived by cellular receptors as danger signals. The metabolic impairment likely contributes to vasodilation, as arteries dilate to bring more oxygen to support metabolic demand (in physiology, this is termed "reactive hyperemia").
2. <u>Brain inflammation</u>: Microglia and astrocytes in the brain transform inflammatory signals into altered levels of neurotransmitters which further activate neurons.
3. <u>Mitochondrial dysfunction</u>: Nerve cells become inflamed in response to any insult; this is called **neuroinflammation**, and it promotes various neurologic and psychiatric disorders. The neurons themselves can also release inflammatory mediators; this is called **neurogenic inflammation** because the inflammation is coming from the nerve cells. When **brain inflammation** is triggered, it affects all of the major cell types of the brain and becomes a self-reinforcing cycle that has been called **brain on fire**. Released neuropeptides activate endothelial cells, mast cells, and platelets to then increase extracellular levels of amines, arachidonate metabolites, peptides, and ions; these substances promote additional inflammation and also promote constriction of blood vessels.
4. <u>Free radicals, reactive oxygen species (ROS)</u>: "We show that ROS accumulation...is capable of triggering an abrupt metabolic collapse (MC) that reproduces most features of cortical spreading depression (CSD). This suggests that oxidative stress may be the primary cause of CSD and not just its consequence. In pathological conditions, the failure to neutralize ROS during the excessive ROS surge and/or deficiency of the neuronal antioxidant system may result in the MC and subsequent ignition of CSD. Indeed, our in vivo results show that when the oxidative stress-induced ROS accumulation is suppressed by an exogenous antioxidant, CSD occurrence is strongly reduced."*
*Malkov et al. Reactive oxygen species initiate a metabolic collapse: potential trigger of cortical spreading depression. *J Cereb Blood Flow Metab.* 2014 Sep

function deteriorates before and during a migraine attack, it segues from a metabolic problem to an inflammatory problem, and the consequences of mitochondrial dysfunction (e.g., ROS, inflammation, failure of calcium homeostasis) plus brain neuron dysfunction due to excessive excitation (e.g., ROS, inflammation, failure of calcium homeostasis) lead to vasoconstriction specifically via increased intracellular calcium in

---

[12] "The maximum rate of mitochondrial ATP production (Qmax), calculated from the rate of post-exercise PCr recovery and the end-exercise [ADP], was low in cluster headache patients as well as in migraine patients except MwoA. In migraine the degree of the mitochondrial impairment, that apparently is associated with a reduced glycolytic flux, is related to the severity of the clinical phenotype." Lodi et al. Quantitative analysis of skeletal muscle bioenergetics and proton efflux in migraine and cluster headache. *J Neurol Sci.* 1997 Feb 27;146(1):73-80

[13] "Mean values for body mass index, C-reactive protein, and homocysteine were higher in children with than without headaches, and more children with headaches were in the highest quintile of risk for these factors. Serum and red blood cell folate levels were lower in children with headache. More children with headache were in the highest quintile of risk for 3 or more of these factors. Several important risk factors for long-term vascular morbidity cluster in children and adolescents with severe or recurrent headache or migraine. Further study and screening of children with headaches may permit improved preventive management." Nelson et al. Headache and biomarkers predictive of vascular disease in a representative sample of US children. *Arch Pediatr Adolesc Med.* 2010 Apr;164(4):358-62

[14] Moskowitz MA. Pathophysiology of headache—past and present. *Headache.* 2007 Apr;47 Suppl 1:S58-63

[15] Moskowitz MA. Genes, proteases, cortical spreading depression and migraine: impact on pathophysiology and treatment. *Funct Neurol.* 2007 Jul-Sep;22(3):133-6

astrocytes and inflammation-triggered phospholipase-A2-catalized formation of vasoconstrictive prostaglandins, specifically prostaglandin E2 (PGE2) and F2-alpha (PGF2), which are also elaborated from endometrial tissue, thereby supporting the biochemical basis of menstrual migraine.[16]

Neurogenic inflammation (in this conversation, the release of neuropeptides from trigeminal nerve [cranial nerve V] neurons to local blood vessels and meninges) is also important and contributes to a vicious cycle of pain and inflammation.[17] Elevated intracellular calcium levels that trigger inflammatory pathways can be promoted by arachidonate, secondary hyperparathyroidism due to vitamin D deficiency, a relative insufficiency of magnesium, and also by mitochondrial impairment. Mast cell degranulation releases inflammatory mediators such as serotonin, prostaglandin I-2, and histamine, which induce local inflammation and activation of meningeal nociceptors[18,19] and might serve as a pathophysiological link between emotional stress or allergen exposure and headache (i.e., the link between environmental stressors and headache pain). Mast cells can also be activated by neuropeptides that originate from neurons in the brain parenchyma/tissue. Further substantiating the role of local inflammation in migraine is the finding of increased activity of nuclear transcription factor-kappa B (NFkB) in jugular blood of migraine patients during migraine episode[20]; NFkB is an important mediator of inflammation through its ability to enhance transcription of genes that encode for inflammatory mediators.[21] This model provides for the often observed continuum between external and biopsychosocial factors such as exposure to bright lights, hypoglycemia, stress, anxiety, allergen exposure, and hormonal fluctuations with the triggering of new or recurrent headaches. An appreciation for the intraneuronal genesis of headaches such as migraines sharpens our focus on events occurring *within the neuronal cell*, particularly impaired mitochondrial bioenergetics, increased intraneuronal calcium, and the elaboration of inflammatory mediators derived from omega-6 (n6) polyunsaturated fatty acids. With the realization of mitochondrial and eicosanoid contributions to headache, clinicians can intervene with nutritional intervention and fatty acid supplementation to enhance mitochondrial function and modulate eicosanoid production, respectively. Failure to appreciate these underlying pathophysiological mechanisms forces clinicians and patients to rely on pharmacological symptom suppression while the underlying processes remain unaddressed.

The historically documented failure of migraine treatments has arisen largely from the incomplete model of the disease upon which those treatments are founded. Without raw luck, a treatment based on an erroneous or incomplete model has no chance of providing *major*—let alone *optimal*—benefit. Any listing of medical treatments for migraine reveals a catalog of chaos: bits and pieces of incomplete and inconsistent models and the resulting therapy—ie, drugs—which address a small fraction of the problem and therefore have to be overpowered in effect to compensate for their minor significance; hence the low efficacy and high risk of adverse effects.

Important for the perpetuation of any ongoing disease are the vicious cycles that are initiated and maintained; skilled clinicians focus on breaking these vicious cycles because failure to do so allows the disease condition to re-initiate and perpetuate, even after limited therapeutic efficacy of incomplete treatment. I might introduce the concept of "double-stranded" or "triple-stranded" (etc) therapies that simultaneously break multiple vicious cycles, in contrast to treatments such as with drugs which focus only on a single molecule or a single pathway, ie, single-stranded therapy. In this metaphor, the "strands" are biochemical and physiologic pathways; the more that we can optimize the maximum number of pathways, the greater our opportunities for restoring and enjoying optimal health.

A 2015 review discussing fibromyalgia (FM) and complex regional pain syndrome (CRPS) focused on "neurogenic neuroinflammation", the essential definition/concept of which is that that neuronal activity in general and its inflammatory effects in particular can become autonomous and self-perpetuating; neuroinflammation could be initiated externally so-to-speak by stress or trauma and then become a vicious

[16] Shaik MM, Gan SH. Vitamin supplementation as possible prophylactic treatment against migraine with aura and menstrual migraine. *Biomed Res Int.* 2015;2015:469529
[17] Tierney ML. McPhee SJ, Papadakis MA (eds). *Current Medical Diagnosis and Treatment 2006, 45th Edition.* New York: Lange Medical Books; 2006, pages 31-33
[18] Levy D, Burstein R, Kainz V, Jakubowski M, Strassman AM. Mast cell degranulation activates a pain pathway underlying migraine headache. *Pain.* 2007 Jul;130(1-2):166-76
[19] Zhang XC, et al. Sensitization and activation of intracranial meningeal nociceptors by mast cell mediators. *J Pharmacol Exp Ther.* 2007 Aug;322(2):806-12
[20] Sarchielli et al. NF-kappaB activity and iNOS expression in monocytes from internal jugular blood of migraine without aura during attacks. *Cephalalgia.* 2006 Sep; 1071-9
[21] Tak PP, Firestein GS. NF-kappaB: a key role in inflammatory diseases. *J Clin Invest.* 2001 Jan;107(1):7-11

cycle within the nervous system promoting chronic pain and neurodegeneration.[22] The existence of neurogenic neuroinflammation is physiologically *likely* and becomes *probable* within dysfunctional and predisposed (i.e., "primed") metabolic and physiologic systems; such "priming factors" clearly include a pro-inflammatory diet, nutrient deficiencies (especially of vitamin B6, magnesium, vitamin D, and CoQ10), mitochondrial dysfunction, and dysbiosis. Hence, the treatment of persistently painful and inflammatory disorders—including but not limited to migraine, recurrent headaches, fibromyalgia and CRPS—needs to focus on the treatment of factors which continue to sustain these disease processes.

- The importance of glutamate and the NMDA receptor in headache, migraine, and chronic pain syndromes: The excitatory neurotransmitter glutamate stimulates neurons by binding to the NMDA (N-methyl-D-aspartate) receptor (NMDAr). As shown in the diagram, excitatory glutamate (which promotes pain, seizure, migraine, anxiety and depression) can be converted into inhibitory GABA (gamma-amino butyric acid, which has an inhibitory, relaxing effect on neurons and the brain as a whole) via the enzyme glutamic acid decarboxylase, which is dependent upon and also dose-dependently stimulated by the vitamin pyridoxine (vitamin B6). Stimulation of the NMDA receptor by glutamate and other receptor activators such as QUIN (quinolinic acid, a "dysfunctional metabolite" of the amino acid L-tryptophan which is formed in response to inflammation and which causes additional inflammation, oxidative damage, and neurotoxicity) causes calcium to enter into the stimulated neuron cells to trigger activation or "firing" of the neuron. A moderate amount of NMDAr stimulation is a normal part of learning and the formation of memories—normal and healthy neurologic function; however, too much NMDAr stimulation causes overstimulation (excitotoxicity) of neurons thereby promoting pain, depression, anxiety, migraine, seizure/epilepsy, and neurodegeneration. Magnesium and zinc partly block the NMDAr calcium channel to reduce/modulate calcium entry into neurons; in this way, magnesium and zinc might be thought of as "softening the effect" of NMDAr activation. The safety and efficacy of supplemental pyridoxine (vitamin B6) in reducing glutamate levels—and thus reducing excessive stimulation of the NMDAr by glutamate—necessitates its inclusion in the treatment of any and all chronic pain disorders, especially migraine and fibromyalgia. Pyridoxine does more than simply lower glutamate levels, as pyridoxine also helps to lower homocysteine (HYC) levels. Glutamate and HYC are both amino acids that activate the NMDAr and mGluR[23]—the metabotropic glutamate receptor (detailed shortly). Generally, higher homocysteine levels correlate with fatigue and pain in patients with fibromyalgia and chronic fatigue syndrome, and with headache pain and increased cardiovascular disease risk in patients with migraine.[24]

- In the treatment of pain—including headaches and fibromyalgia—reducing the effects of glutamate-mediated neurotransmission and cellular effects is of very high importance: Glutamate is an amino acid with many functions, including serving as a precursor to the antioxidant glutathione (GSH), serving as a precursor to alpha-keto-glutarate (a substrate for energy production in the Krebs/citrate cycle in mitochondria) and serving as an excitatory neurotransmitter. Our concern in this conversation is with glutamate's role as a stimulator of neurotransmission in the peripheral and central nervous system; while some minimal glutaminergic stimulation is normal and necessary, excess glutaminergic neurotransmission very clearly promotes anxiety, depression, fibromyalgia pain, myofascial pain and myofascial trigger points, migraine and headaches, seizures and epilepsy; in the extreme, excess glutamate in the brain causes over-excitation of neurons leading to cell death—neurodegeneration—and either mild or massive, acute or chronic, brain damage. In the following image and subsequent descriptors, I provide an accurate and yet simplified overview of important concepts, but I will state plainly here what everyone needs to know about this section: Because glutaminergic neurotransmission promotes pain/anxiety/depression/neurodegeneration, our therapeutic goals are to 1) reduce glutamate levels with vitamin B6 and by avoiding/treating microglial activation (ie, "brain inflammation"), 2) reduce glutamate-triggered influx of calcium with zinc and magnesium, also vitamin D, alkalinization (increased consumption of base-forming foods, such as fruits and vegetables which contain citrate which is converted to bicarbonate to promote alkalinization, one effect of which is to promote magnesium retention, thereby alleviating pain[25]), omega-3 fatty acids such as from fish oil, 3) reduce the effects

[22] Littlejohn G. Neurogenic neuroinflammation in fibromyalgia and complex regional pain syndrome. *Nat Rev Rheumatol.* 2015 Nov;11(11):639-48

[23] Abushik et al. NMDA and mGluR5 in calcium mobilization and neurotoxicity of homocysteine in trigeminal/cortical neurons and glial cells. *J Neurochem.* 2014 Apr; 264-74

[24] "Mean homocysteine plasma levels - as well as the proportion of subjects with hyperhomocysteinaemia - were significantly higher in patients with MA than in healthy controls." Moschiano et al. Homocysteine plasma levels in patients with migraine with aura. *Neurol Sci.* 2008 May;29 Suppl 1:S173-5

[25] Vormann et al. Supplementation with alkaline minerals reduces symptoms in patients with chronic low back pain. *J Trace Elem Med Biol.* 2001;15(2-3):179-83

of glutamate/NMDA receptor activation by counterbalancing with benzodiazepine/GABA receptor activation by promoting conversion of glutamate to GABA and perhaps also by using niacinamide and botanicals that act as ligands for the GABA receptor. Because much of this information is both important and a bit complicated, I will create some teaching videos on this material and make them available per the following internet link/redirect: www.inflammationmastery.com/pain

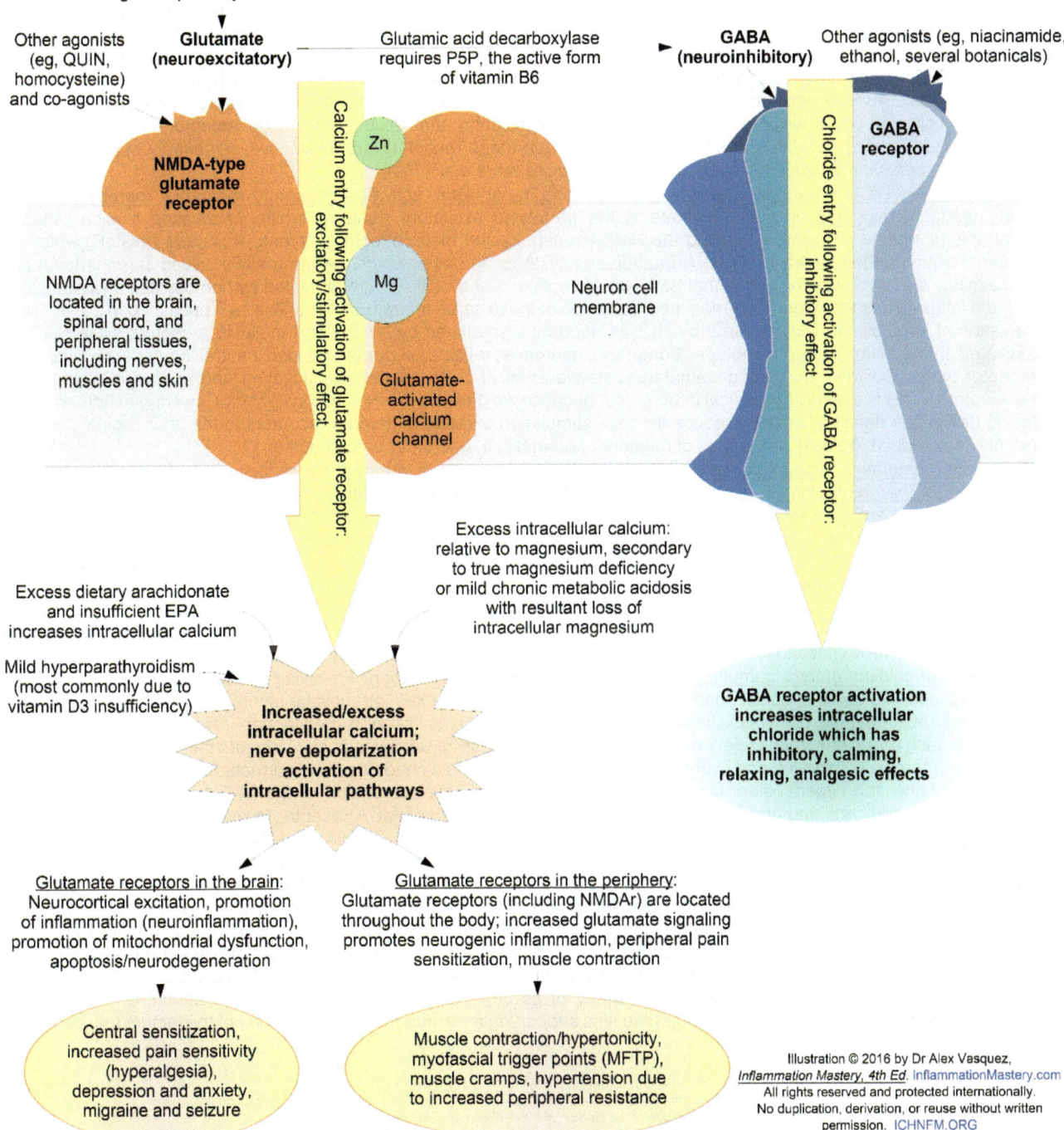

Glutamate is increased by dietary MSG, deficiencies of B6 and Mg, glial activation, genotropic enzyme defects

Other agonists (eg, QUIN, homocysteine) and co-agonists

Glutamate (neuroexcitatory)

Glutamic acid decarboxylase requires P5P, the active form of vitamin B6

GABA (neuroinhibitory)

Other agonists (eg, niacinamide, ethanol, several botanicals)

Calcium entry following activation of glutamate receptor: excitatory/stimulatory effect

GABA receptor

Zn

NMDA-type glutamate receptor

Mg

Chloride entry following activation of GABA receptor: inhibitory effect

NMDA receptors are located in the brain, spinal cord, and peripheral tissues, including nerves, muscles and skin

Neuron cell membrane

Glutamate-activated calcium channel

Excess intracellular calcium: relative to magnesium, secondary to true magnesium deficiency or mild chronic metabolic acidosis with resultant loss of intracellular magnesium

Excess dietary arachidonate and insufficient EPA increases intracellular calcium

Mild hyperparathyroidism (most commonly due to vitamin D3 insufficiency)

Increased/excess intracellular calcium; nerve depolarization activation of intracellular pathways

GABA receptor activation increases intracellular chloride which has inhibitory, calming, relaxing, analgesic effects

Glutamate receptors in the brain: Neurocortical excitation, promotion of inflammation (neuroinflammation), promotion of mitochondrial dysfunction, apoptosis/neurodegeneration

Glutamate receptors in the periphery: Glutamate receptors (including NMDAr) are located throughout the body; increased glutamate signaling promotes neurogenic inflammation, peripheral pain sensitization, muscle contraction

Central sensitization, increased pain sensitivity (hyperalgesia), depression and anxiety, migraine and seizure

Muscle contraction/hypertonicity, myofascial trigger points (MFTP), muscle cramps, hypertension due to increased peripheral resistance

Clinically relevant conceptual illustration of the NMDA-type glutamate receptor (NMDAr), its activation, effects, and nutritional modulation: The image above provides a conceptually accurate and clinically applicable model of glutamate reception and the effects thereof; categorized details are provided below, listed from top to bottom of the image and also prioritized to clinical relevance (top) and additional details and context (bottom). See instructional videos at ICHNFM.ORG.

Image caption—continued from previous page:

- Various types of glutamate receptors in the central nervous system and periphery share the common themes of promoting pain and inflammation: Glutamate receptors are described in two broad categories; **ionotropic glutamate receptors—iGluR**—(divided into three groups: AMPA, NMDA and kainate receptors) transpose ions such as sodium and calcium upon activation and thus can be considered mostly involved with propagation of nerve impulses, while **metabotropic glutamate receptors—mGluR**—(also with several subtypes, such as mGluR5) lead more to activation of intracellular pathways with results dependent on the cell type but generally consistent with some type of cellular activation and/or inflammation.

- Glutamate reception, with the NMDA receptor (NMDAr) as the prototype receptor: Many types and subtypes of glutamate receptors exist, and the specific subtype NMDA is very clearly the most discussed for its relevance in both chronic pain disorders and neurodegenerative diseases. The NMDA receptor is activated by glutamate, QUIN (quinolinic acid, a metabolite of tryptophan made in inflammatory conditions, discussed in more detail in the section on fibromyalgia), aspartate, homocysteine and other substances which act as agonists/activators or required co-activators/co-agonists (e.g., D-serine, glycine). Different forms of the NMDA receptor exist in the central and peripheral nervous systems, each with slightly different characteristics and sensitivity to agonists and requirement for co-agonists; thus, the image presented here is a generalized version that is conceptually accurate (rather than all-inclusive; for more details see reviews[26]) and clinically relevant. Although we have traditionally thought of glutamate/NMDA receptors as existing separately (ie, on different cell types) from the GABA/benzodiazepine receptors, that fact remains true (ie, some cells are clearly dominated by one receptor type over others) while we are also increasingly appreciating that glutamate/NMDA receptors can coexist with GABA/benzodiazepine receptors on the same cell and that these receptors are interactive, not simply oppositional, and occasionally behave/interact in paradoxical and age-specific manners.[27,28]

- Homocysteine (HYC), a toxic intermediate of amino acid metabolism, activates glutamate receptors, thereby promoting pain, headache/migraine/seizure: Glutamate is the prototypic excitatory neurotransmitter, activating a wide range of ionotropic glutamate receptors (including the NMDA receptor) and metabotropic glutamate receptors (mGluR) which are present throughout the central and peripheral nervous systems and all of which are generally involved in (enhanced) pain processing. We have exacting clarity that both NMDA receptors and mGluR5 are activated by homocysteine with resultant calcium influx just as with glutamate-mediated activation of these same receptors; Abushik et al[29] published in 2014, "Thus, elevation of intracellular calcium (Ca2) by HCY in neurons is mediated by NMDA and mGluR5 receptors while SGC are activated through the mGluR5 subtype. Long-term neurotoxic effects in peripheral and central neurons involved both receptor types. Our data suggest glutamatergic mechanisms of HCY-induced sensitization and apoptosis of trigeminal nociceptors." This is of very high clinical importance, because we gain the mechanistic insight that lowering of homocysteine levels (technique detailed later) will reduce the total stimulation of these glutamate receptors in the brain, spinal cord, and periphery to reduce the pain and fatigue of migraine, fibromyalgia, and other pain conditions.

- Glutamate promotes pain and inflammation; therefore, reducing levels of glutamate or reducing the effects of its reception are important therapeutic goals, especially in the treatment of pain, anxiety/depression, migraine, and seizure/epilepsy: Glutamate levels are increased by microglial inflammation and the subsequent astrocyte activation[30]; therefore, reducing inflammation generally and "brain inflammation" specifically is an important therapeutic goal. Reducing inflammation must always focus on the trigger of the inflammation, most commonly microbial (e.g., gastrointestinal dysbiosis[31]) and/or metabolic (e.g., excess sugar and "junk/fast food" in the diet[32], vitamin D deficiency, lack of phytonutrients due to insufficient intake of fruits and vegetables, insufficient omega-3 fatty acids from fish oil, etc). Glutamate is excitatory to neurons, promoting pain, depression, migraine, seizure and neurodegeneration; glutamate is readily converted by the enzyme glutamic acid decarboxylase to GABA—gamma-amino-butyric acid—which has opposing effects to those of glutamate.

- Modulation of calcium entry/accumulation following NMDA receptor activation: Following NMDAr activation, sodium (Na) enters to propagate nerve impulses, and calcium (Ca) enters and promotes intracellular signaling, including the promotion of pain and inflammatory pathways. Intracellular calcium is a famous "second messenger" responsible for physiologic processes such as the pancreatic release of insulin; however, excess intracellular calcium triggers the activation of pathways that can promote pain, migraine and hypertension, hence the well-established use of calcium-channel blocking (CCB) drugs to treat migraine and hypertension. Calcium entry following glutamate stimulation of the NMDA receptor is reduced or "modulated" by both zinc and magnesium, both of which "adhere" to the NMDA receptor to reduce calcium influx; in fact, magnesium is often described as a "cork" or "plug" of the NMDA receptor. Magnesium (Mg) can also be thought of as competing for space with calcium or otherwise blocking some of the effects of intracellular calcium; as such, Mg reduces the effect of glutamate receptor stimulation. Excess intracellular calcium also challenges or stresses the capacity of mitochondria, while magnesium supports mitochondrial function. Intracellular calcium promotes muscle contraction, important in hypertension (due to systemic constriction of arteries/arterioles) and myofascial trigger points (MFTP, an important cause of and contributor to pain in migraine and fibromyalgia), while magnesium promotes muscle relaxation, arterial dilation, and pain relief. Thus, we would expect—and indeed we see clinically—that magnesium supplementation (typically 600 mg per day for adults) provides many of its benefits by offsetting the adverse effects of glutaminergic stimulation and excess intracellular calcium, while also supporting mitochondrial function. Many of the factors that contribute

[26] Vyklicky et al. Structure, function, and pharmacology of NMDA receptor channels. *Physiol Res.* 2014;63 Suppl 1:S191-203

[27] Ben-Ari et al. GABAA, NMDA and AMPA receptors: a developmentally regulated 'ménage à trois'. *Trends Neurosci.* 1997 Nov;20(11):523-9

[28] Ben-Ari Y. Excitatory actions of gaba during development: the nature of the nurture. *Nat Rev Neurosci.* 2002 Sep;3(9):728-39

[29] Abushik et al. The role of NMDA and mGluR5 receptors in calcium mobilization and neurotoxicity of homocysteine in trigeminal and cortical neurons and glial cells. *J Neurochem.* 2014 Apr;129(2):264-74

[30] Béchade C, Cantaut-Belarif Y, Bessis A. Microglial control of neuronal activity. *Front Cell Neurosci.* 2013 Mar 28;7:32

[31] Vasquez A. Nutritional and Botanical Treatments against "Silent Infections" and Gastrointestinal Dysbiosis. *Nutr Perspectives* 2006. Translating Microbiome (Microbiota) and Dysbiosis Research into Clinical Practice. *Int J Hum Nutr Funct Med* 2015 https://ichnfm.academia.edu/AlexVasquez

[32] Aljada et al. Increase in intranuclear nuclear factor kappaB and decrease in inhibitor kappaB in mononuclear cells after a mixed meal: proinflammatory effect. *Am J Clin Nutr.* 2004 Apr;79(4):682-90. Mohanty et al. Glucose challenge stimulates reactive oxygen species (ROS) generation by leucocytes. *J Clin Endocrinol Metab.* 2000 Aug;85(8):2970-3

to excess intracellular calcium—vitamin D deficiency, magnesium deficiency, an acidic acid-base balance, excess omega-6 arachidonic acid relative to omega-3 fatty acids—are easily treated with vitamin D supplementation, magnesium supplementation, promotion of systemic alkalinization, and omega-3 fatty acid supplementation, respectively; proof-of-principle is demonstrated by the observation that each of these interventions provides analgesic, antihypertensive, and other clinical benefits.[33]

- <u>Stimulation of the GABA/benzodiazepine receptor</u>: GABA reception at the GABA receptor—a large multicomponent receptor that also receives benzodiazepine and barbiturate drugs—promotes analgesia, euphoria, relaxation and antiseizure benefits. GABA receptors are also activated by the niacinamide form of vitamin B3 as well as by alcohol/ethanol in beer, wine, and liquors. Botanical medicines that have proven clinical benefit via—at least in large part—their activation of the GABA/benzodiazepine receptor include *Matricaria recutita* (Chamomile), *Melissa officinalis* (lemon balm), *Passiflora incarnata* (passionflower), *Piper methysticum* (kava), *Scutellaria lateriflora* (skullcap), *Valeriana species* (valerian), *Withania somnifera* (ashwagandha).[34]

- <u>Conversion of glutamate to GABA, the importance of vitamin B6 in neuroprotection and pain alleviation</u>: Conversion of glutamate to GABA via glutamic acid decarboxylase requires vitamin B6 (pyridoxine), and the speed/efficiency of this conversion is generally proportionate to the provision of B6. Giving more vitamin B6 results in lower glutamate levels and therefore less activation of the glutamate receptor, thereby providing anti-pain, anti-depression, and anti-seizure benefits. As such, what is obvious is that supplementation with vitamin B6 clearly has an essential role in the treatment of pain, depression, migraine, and seizure; all patients affected by such disorders should receive high-potency vitamin B6 supplementation, at least as a therapeutic trial if not as a default component of therapy. Very importantly, vitamin B6 alleviates pain and the excess brain activity seen with migraine and seizure by means other than serving as a cofactor for glutamic acid decarboxylase; vitamin B6 also provides analgesic and antiinflammatory benefits in peripheral tissues/nerves, in the spinal cord, in the deep brain structures of the brain such as the pain-relaying thalamus, as well as in the neurocortex.

- <u>Activation of the glutamate receptor, especially the NMDA receptor, in the nervous system results in stimulation/depolarization of neurons and the promotion of new connections, promoting memory/learning as well as pain</u>: Activation of the NMDA receptor allows sodium (Na) and calcium (Ca) to enter the cell; entry of Na promotes depolarization of the nerve membrane to allow propagation of the nerve impulse, sometimes called nerve "firing." Entry of Ca following glutamate receptor activation triggers intracellular events, some of which are beneficial for processes such as learning and memory, while others—especially if intracellular calcium levels are too high for too long—are harmful and promote inflammatory responses and mitochondrial stress. While we have typically thought of glutamate receptors and the classic NMDA receptor as existing in the brain and neocortex, we now share the clarity that NMDA receptors exist throughout the nervous system including the spinal cord and peripheral nerves. Activation of NMDAr is important for learning and memory and is also important for the generation of excessive neuronal/brain activity that is seen in seizure/epilepsy, chronic pain, and overactivation of neurons that leads to neuron/brain damage—neuroexcitation, neurodegeneration, and neuroexcitatory neuronal death.

- <u>Activation of the glutamate receptor in peripheral tissues (outside of the nervous system) is not well understood, but again mostly correlates with pain and inflammation</u>: Beyond the NMDA receptor and beyond the nervous system, other types of glutamate receptors are active throughout the body. Given that most tissues and cells are innervated by the nervous system, the distinction between glutaminergic effect via the nervous system and the direct effect on the cells is a bit challenging; however, one of the most important themes observed in the research and science literature is that elevated levels of glutamate in the periphery are clearly and causatively associated with increased pain sensation and to a lesser extent with adverse physiologic changes. For example, activation of mGluR5 in skin is seen with inflammatory and irritating/itchy/pruritic skin disorders, and blockade of the receptor is therapeutic; this same subtype mGluR5 also participates in hypersensitivity to pain in inflammatory diseases.[35] Elevated levels of glutamate are seen in malignant diseases (ie, cancer) and appear to suppress immune function; blockade of iGluR reduces cancer invasiveness. Overall, the associations with excessive glutamate signaling are pain and inflammation; when glutamate is injected into muscles, the result is increased intensity of pain and enlargement of the receptive field (ie, spreading of pain, increased area of heightened sensitivity).[36] Therefore, treatments to reduce glutamate levels (especially vitamin B6) and to reduce the effect of glutamate-triggered increases in intracellular calcium (e.g., magnesium and vitamin D) are expected to reduce glutamate-triggered pain and inflammation.

- <u>Conclusion of this image caption with a few more details and bit of redundancy</u>: Conversion of glutamate to GABA requires vitamin B6 and provides analgesic and "calming" benefits to brain and muscles. Neuroexcitatory glutamate is converted to neuroinhibitory GABA by the enzyme glutamic acid decarboxylase, which—as firmly established in the disease pyridoxine-dependent/responsive epilepsy—shows very clear dose-responsiveness in its ability to reduce glutamate levels in response to high-dose vitamin B6 supplementation. Magnesium and zinc (and perhaps copper) retard the passage of calcium through this channel, thereby mitigating some of the effects of NMDAr activation. Quenching NO- (for example with the hydroxocobalamin form of vitamin B12), which would otherwise trigger glutamate release, and dousing glial activation (for example, with anti-inflammatory nutrients such as vitamin D3 and EPA and DHA from fish oil) which otherwise promotes elaboration of glutamate and QUIN are important considerations not included in this illustration. Glycine is generally considered a necessary co-activator of the NMDAr; but given that glycine is ubiquitous and mostly invariable, it is not immediately malleable and therefore not considered of high relevance as a clinical therapeutic target.

---

[33] Vasquez A. Intracellular Hypercalcinosis. *Naturopathy Digest* 2006 naturopathydigest.com/archives/2006/sep/vasquez.php. Included at the end of this section/chapter.
[34] Sarris et al. Plant-based medicines for anxiety disorders, part 2: a review of clinical studies with supporting preclinical evidence. *CNS Drugs*. 2013 Apr;27(4):301-19
[35] Julio-Pieper et al. Exciting times beyond the brain: metabotropic glutamate receptors in peripheral and non-neural tissues. *Pharmacol Rev*. 2011 Mar;63(1):35-58
[36] Wang et al. Spatial pain propagation over time following painful glutamate activation of latent myofascial trigger points in humans. *J Pain*. 2012 Jun;13(6):537-45

Clinical presentations:

- Headache—general considerations: Head pain, with a wide range of differential diagnoses and possible causes and contributions, ranging from simple "stress" and so-called "reactive hypoglycemia" to life-threatening causes such as stroke, aneurysm, tumor, meningitis. Especially for new headaches or acute-onset headaches, concomitant subjective complaints (e.g., lethargy, sleepiness, mood/cognitive changes, changed vision) and/or objective presentations (e.g., fever, skin rash, galactorrhea, or neurologic deficits) indicate the need for additional evaluation to exclude important intracranial lesions such as pituitary adenoma, meningitis, tumor, or subdural hematoma. Since the trigeminal sensory pathway is activated in any condition associated with brain inflammation, relief of headache with analgesic medications does not exclude serious underlying disease such as hemorrhage or meningitis.

- Migraine: Periodic headache characterized by unilateral distribution, commonly with a pulsatile sensation; severity ranges from moderate to severe and disabling; commonly begin in adolescence; commonly with a maternal inheritance, consistent with inheritance of mitochondrial DNA from the mother; twice as common in women (5-25%) as in men (2-10%); typical duration of migraine "attack" is 4-72 hours. 80% of migraine is "common migraine" or "migraine without aura." Photophobia and phonophobia (excessive sensitivity to light and sound, respectively) are common, as is nausea, sometimes leading to vomiting. Patients with migraine show a consistent pattern of different—additive and synergistic—mitochondrial defects affecting various locations in the pathway of substrate conversion to cellular energy/ATP: ❶ enzymatic impairment of citrate synthase—the first enzyme in the Krebs cycle, ❷ impaired function of complexes #1-4 of the electron transport chain, ❸ deficiency of coenzyme Q-10 due to insufficient endogenous production, thereby promoting failure of performance of the electron transport chain as well as reduced antioxidant and antiinflammatory defense, and ❹ magnesium deficiency—noted in all headache types—which leads to impairment of complex #5 (ATP synthase) of the electron transport chain, and also leading to increased intracellular calcium influx following activation of the NMDA receptor, leading to increased metabolic demand in neurons.

- Migraine with aura: Migraine with aura is characterized by focal neurologic symptoms/deficits; the localization of the neurologic involvement has traditionally been attributed to regional brain vasospasm, leading to reduced blood flow and compromised neuron/brain function in the affected areas. Migraine with aura may present with any combination of the following: blurred/altered vision including scotoma (the perception of "flashing lights"), vertigo/dizziness, hallucinations such as hearing nonreal sounds or seeing nonreal images. Some patients experience the aura as hyper/hypo-activity, depression, food cravings, yawning, mood changes. More than 50% of migraine patients report significant impairment in life tasks and personal relationships as a result.

- Cluster headache: Cluster headache (CH) affects predominantly middle-aged men. Although the "pathophysiology is unclear" according to *Current Medical Diagnosis and Treatment 2014*, triggering of trigeminal pain sensation and vasoconstriction are clearly involved, identically to migraine. CH patients generally lack a family history of headache or migraine. CH manifests with episodes of severe unilateral periorbital pain, generally with one or more of the following: ipsilateral nasal congestion, rhinorrhea (runny nose), lacrimation (tearing), redness of the eye, and Horner syndrome (ptosis/drooping of the eyelid, meiosis/constriction of the pupil, and anhidrosis—reduced sweating on the affected side). CH attacks may occur daily (especially nightly) for several weeks, and patients often feel restless and agitated. CH attacks typically last 15 minutes - 3 hours and occur in clusters for weeks or months, then remit. Triggers include alcohol, stress, glare, or specific foods. The prototypic CH patient is a stressed male entrepreneur who smokes, with varying levels of alcohol intake. Mechanistically, stress promotes muscle tension especially in the neck; ethanol/alcohol and tobacco smoke's cyanide are both mitochondrial toxins, and the prototypical stressed male entrepreneur is not eating sufficient fruits and vegetables to maintain urinary alkalinization and sufficient magnesium intake/retention. The facts that CH patients generally ❶ have no family history of the disorder, ❷ have a characteristic lifestyle pattern known to promote mitochondrial impairment, and ❸ respond acutely to oxygen therapy (obviously a form of mitochondrial support, since the primary function of oxygen in the human body is to drain hydrogen protons from the intramembrane space via the formation of ATP and water), support the contention that these patients have a *secondary* lifestyle-generated mitochondrial impairment leading to their headaches, via the aforementioned glial activation and resultant brain inflammation and the remainder of the pain-inducing cascade of events.

Major differential diagnoses: The differential diagnosis of headache by history, examination, and laboratory and imaging assessments should be familiar to clinicians. In particular, the neurological examination should include psychoemotional assessment, as well as cranial nerve and fundoscopic examination, and any new headache symptoms, even in a patient with a history of headaches, must receive due diligence on the part of the clinician.

- Cervical spondylosis: Cervical spine dysfunction and arthropathy can cause and contribute to head pain and headaches; confer with history and examination.
- Cluster headache: Presents with intense unilateral periorbital pain often associated with ipsilateral nasal congestion, rhinorrhea, lacrimation, eye redness, and transient/chronic Horner's syndrome; more common in men, especially in smokers; exacerbated by alcohol; tend to recur at the same time each day/night.
- Cough headache: Severe transient headache triggered by coughing, straining, sneezing, or laughing; patients with recurrent complaints need to be evaluated with a complete neurologic examination and are candidates for CT/MRI since 10% of patients with persistent cough headache have an intracranial lesion.[37]
- Dental or occlusive disorders: Mouth examination, history, oral/dental exam.
- Depression: Check for history consistent with depression: apathy, recent stressful life events.
- Drug side-effect: Check each drug to see if side-effects correlate with clinical complaints.
- Food allergy: Evaluate with elimination/challenge, history; consider blood tests for recalcitrant cases.
- Head injury: Evaluate with history and examination.
- Hyperparathyroidism: Begin by assessing serum calcium.
- Hypertension: Assess blood pressure; although most patients with hypertension do not have headaches, and most patients with headaches do not have hypertension, acute exacerbations of hypertension commonly precipitate headache. Assess for papilledema and hyperreflexia.
- Hyperthyroidism: Weight loss, tremor; assess TSH (generally low) and free T4 (always high).
- Hypothyroidism: Assess TSH (typically elevated), free T4 (generally low), free T3 (may be low or normal), anti-TPO antibodies (seen with autoimmune hypothyroidism: Hashimoto's disease); effective treatment with thyroid hormone alleviates most headaches in hypothyroid-headache patients.[38]
- HIV infection: Patients with HIV are at increased risk for infections, including intracranial infections, particularly toxoplasmosis; intracranial lymphoma is also more common in HIV-positive patients.
- Intracranial aneurysm: May present with throbbing pain; assessed with contrast angiography. In one large international study with 1449 patients[39], the risk of rupture was less than 1% per year, whereas complications from surgery were seen in approximately 14%. A Japanese study[40] found that 95% of patients had a favorable outcome with surgery, implying that 5% had an unfavorable outcome, which is still greater than the risk of rupture, being less than 1% per year for untreated aneurysms reported previously.[41] A more recent study also suggested that the risks of treatment might exceed the risk of spontaneous rupture.[42] Thus the clinical management of intracranial aneurysms must be determined per patient, neuroanatomic location, available techniques/technology, current research, and experience of the neurosurgeon.
- Iron deficiency: Iron is necessary for function of the mitochondrial electron transport chain as well as for formation of the neurotransmitters dopamine and serotonin, both of which can be said to have an analgesic effect. As such, iron deficiency can promote headaches in general and migraine in particular; iron deficiency might also contribute to the clinical presentation of fibromyalgia.[43] Optimal iron status correlates with serum ferritin values of 40-70 ng/ml; rarely, a person with what can be described as a defect in the blood-brain barrier transport of iron into the brain will need to have a serum ferritin value of 120 ng/ml in order to promote entry of iron into the brain.

[37] Tierney ML. McPhee SJ, Papadakis MA (eds). *Current Medical Diagnosis and Treatment 2002, 41st Edition*. New York: Lange; 2002. Page 999-1005

[38] "Thirty-one patients with hypothyroidism of 102 (30%) presented with headache 1-2 months after the first symptoms of hypothyroidism. The headache was slight, nonpulsatile, continuous, bilateral, and salicylate responsive and disappeared with thyroid hormone therapy." Moreau et al. Headache in hypothyroidism. *Cephalalgia* 1998 Dec:687-9

[39] International UIA Investigators. Unruptured intracranial aneurysms—risk of rupture and risks of surgical intervention. *N Engl J Med* 1998 Dec 10;339(24):1725-33

[40] Orz et al. Risks of surgery for patients with unruptured intracranial aneurysms. *Surg Neurol* 2000 Jan;53(1):21-7; discussion 27-9

[41] International UIA Investigators. Unruptured intracranial aneurysms—risk of rupture and risks of surgical intervention. *N Engl J Med* 1998 Dec 10;339(24):1725-33

[42] Risks associated with spontaneous rupture "were often equaled or exceeded by the risks associated with surgical or endovascular repair of comparable lesions." Wiebers DO, et al. Unruptured intracranial aneurysms: natural history, clinical outcome, and risks of surgical and endovascular treatment. *Lancet*. 2003 Jul 12; 362(9378): 103-10

[43] "The mean serum ferritin levels in the fibromyalgia and control groups were 27.3 and 43.8 ng/ml, respectively, and the difference was statistically significant. Binary multiple logistic regression analysis with age, body mass index, smoking status and vitamin B12, as well as folic acid and ferritin levels showed that having a serum ferritin level <50 ng/ml caused a 6.5-fold increased risk for FMS." Ortancil et al. Association between serum ferritin level and fibromyalgia syndrome. *Eur J Clin Nutr*. 2010 Mar;64(3):308-12

- <u>Iron overload, with or without genetic hemochromatosis</u>: For reasons reviewed in Chapter 1 and per my previous reviews[44], all patients must be tested for iron overload. Iron overload causes headaches; iron depletion can relieve headaches.[45,46] Optimal iron status correlates with serum ferritin values of 40-70 ng/ml.
- <u>Magnesium deficiency</u>: Magnesium deficiency is common in industrialized nations[47,48,49,50] and can be assessed clinically (e.g., response to supplementation) or with laboratory tests (e.g., intracellular magnesium). Associated findings common with magnesium deficiency are muscle cramps, bruxism, constipation, and cravings of sweets/candies and especially chocolate.
- <u>Meningitis</u>: Evaluate fundoscopic examination, skin rash, fever, CBC, CRP; immediate transport to emergency department if meningitis is suspected.
- <u>Migraine</u>: Classic presentation includes periodicity, unilaterality, with prodrome, photophobia, nausea, vomiting, visual changes, and positive family history and onset in early teens or adulthood; a large percentage of migraine patients do not have the classic presentation. Migraine can be associated with transient neurologic deficits: numbness, aphasia, clumsiness, and weakness.
- <u>Muscle tension and tension headaches</u>: Assessed with palpation/provocation of cervical/cranial musculature; worse with stress and generally worse at the end of the workday; generally responsive to manual therapies, stress reduction, stretching of affected musculature, and magnesium supplementation.
- <u>Myofascial trigger points</u>: Palpation/provocation of cervical/cranial musculature; treat with post-isometric stretching, ergonomic improvements, and the supplemented Paleo-Mediterranean diet[51]with an emphasis on supplementation with vitamin D, calcium, and magnesium.
- <u>Ocular disorders</u>: Assess with history (e.g., recent change in prescription, new glasses or contacts), and neurologic, eye, and fundoscopic examination; consider diabetes mellitus, multiple sclerosis, and glaucoma and test or refer appropriately.
- <u>Preeclampsia</u>: Headache in a pregnant woman may indicate preeclampsia; assess for hypertension, edema, and proteinuria; emergency or urgent obstetrical referral will be indicated in most cases.
- <u>Pheochromocytoma</u>: Common presentation is periodic headache concurrent with exacerbations of hypertension, sweats, and tachycardia/palpitations.
- <u>Sinusitis or sinus infection</u>: History, fever, pain with palpation of sinuses, nasal discharge; test CBC and CRP; consider radiographic or CT imaging.
- <u>Temporal arteritis (TA), giant cell arteritis (GCA), polymyalgia rheumatica (PMR)</u>: History of diffuse head/shoulder pain and jaw claudication generally with systemic complaints of myalgia and fatigue in a patient over 50 years of age; if suspected, must assess CRP/ESR and palpation of artery. **Remember that temporal arteritis can result in blindness; any visual change in a patient with TA/PMR should be considered a medical emergency.** "Loss of vision is the most feared manifestation and occurs quite commonly."[52]
- <u>Temporomandibular joint (TMJ) dysfunction</u>: Assess with examination, history, oral/dental exam, pain worse with chewing (DDX temporal arteritis); notably associated with excess interstitial glutamate.
- <u>Tumor other intracranial lesion</u>: One-third of brain tumor patients present with headache[53], typically worse upon waking and worse with exertion. Assess with neurologic exam/imaging as indicated.

---

[44] See Chapter 1 of either <u>Inflammation Mastery</u> / <u>Functional Inflammology</u> (2014 or later) for the most complete reviews, including assessment, management, and radiographic presentations. See also: Vasquez A. Musculoskeletal disorders and iron overload disease: comment on the American College of Rheumatology guidelines for the initial evaluation of the adult patient with acute musculoskeletal symptoms. [Letter] *Arthritis & Rheumatism* 1996; 39:1767-8. Vasquez A. High body iron stores. *Nutr Perspect* 1994 October

[45] In a study involving more than 51,000 patients: "Phenotypic hemochromatosis and the C282Y/C282Y genotype were both associated with an 80% increase in headache prevalence evident only among women. The reason for this association is unclear, but one may speculate that iron overload alters the threshold for triggering a headache by disturbing neuronal function." Hagen K, et al. High headache prevalence among women with hemochromatosis. *Ann Neurol* 2002;51(6):786-9

[46] "...the temporary improvement of headache from depletion of iron stores may indicate a causal relation, possibly mediated by iron deposits in pain-modulating centres in the brainstem." Stovner et al. Hereditary haemochromatosis in two cousins with cluster headache. *Cephalalgia* 2002 May;22(4):317-9

[47] "The American diet is low in magnesium, and with modern water systems, very little is ingested in the drinking water." Innerarity S. Hypomagnesemia in acute and chronic illness. *Crit Care Nurs Q.* 2000 Aug;23(2):1-19

[48] "Altogether 43% of 113 trauma patients had low magnesium levels compared to 30% of noninjured cohorts." Frankel et al. Hypomagnesemia in trauma patients. *World J Surg.* 1999 Sep;23(9):966-9

[49] "There was a 20% overall prevalence of hypomagnesemia among this predominantly female, African American population." Fox et al. An investigation of hypomagnesemia among ambulatory urban African Americans. *J Fam Pract.* 1999 Aug;48(8):636-9

[50] "Suboptimal levels were detected in 33.7 per cent of the population under study. These data clearly demonstrate that the Mg supply of the German population needs increased attention." Schimatschek HF, Rempis R. Prevalence of hypomagnesemia in an unselected German population of 16,000 individuals. *Magnes Res.* 2001 Dec;14(4):283-90

[51] Vasquez A. A Five-Part Nutritional Protocol that Produces Consistently Positive Results. *Nutritional Wellness* 2005Sept.

[52] Tierney ML. McPhee SJ, Papadakis MA (eds). <u>Current Medical Diagnosis and Treatment 2002, 41st Edition</u>. New York: Lange; 2002, page 999-1005

[53] Tierney ML. McPhee SJ, Papadakis MA (eds). <u>Current Medical Diagnosis and Treatment 2002, 41st Edition</u>. New York: Lange; 2002, page 999-1005

Clinical assessment:

- History/subjective:
  - o Subacute or chronic/periodic head pain: Most likely benign if course is not progressive and if no neurologic deficits and other findings are present.
  - o Acute headache: Recent onset of severe headache in a previously healthy patient suggests intracranial lesion or meningitis.[54] Approximately 1% of patients with acute headache who present to emergency departments will have a life-threatening disorder.[55]
- Physical examination/objective:
  - o Neurologic examination should be performed on all patients with a recent onset of new headaches or a change from their previous headache. The finding of any mental abnormality or neurologic deficit indicates immediate need for further evaluation: brain CT/MRI and/or emergency department referral.[56]
  - o Muscle strength and reflexes
  - o Fundoscopic examination for papilledema
  - o Cranial nerve examination
  - o Blood pressure
  - o Spinal and cervical musculature assessment for joint dysfunction and myofascial trigger points[57]
  - o Signs for meningeal irritation:

> **Spinal and myofascial assessment**
> "Because treating myofascial problems may be the only way to offer complete relief from certain types of headache, clinicians must learn to diagnose and manage trigger points in neck, shoulder, and head muscles."
>
> Davidoff RA. *Cephalalgia*. 1998 Sep

  - ▪ Nuchal rigidity (previously referred to as Soto-Hall maneuver): Patient supine on examining table; doctor gently-yet-assertively forces patient's neck into flexion: positive sign for meningeal irritation is undue pain or resistance. This test must not be performed in patients who may have atlantoaxial instability or cervical spine fracture.
  - ▪ Kernig sign: Patient supine with hip flexed, slowly extend knee; positive sign: pain in posterior thigh with or without flexion of opposite knee.
  - ▪ Brudzinski sign: Bilateral hip flexion following forced cervical flexion when the patient is supine.
- Imaging & laboratory assessments:
  - o Imaging: Rarely required except to assess for or exclude intracranial pathology or cervical spondylosis. Importantly, **new onset of headache in an elderly patient or a patient with HIV warrants neuroimaging** *even if the neurologic examination is normal*.[58]
  - o Lumbar puncture for CSF analysis: This procedure assesses for infection and subarachnoid hemorrhage and must not be performed unwittingly in patients with increased intracranial hypertension/papilledema.
  - o Laboratory evaluation is generally routine and includes the following:
    - ▪ 25-OH-vitamin D (serum): Should be between 50-100 ng/mL. All patients with pain need to be assessed for vitamin D deficiency and/or supplemented with 2,000 IU/d (children) or at least 4,000 IU/d (adults).[59]
    - ▪ CBC: Assess for anemia and evidence of infection.
    - ▪ Chemistry panel: Screening for diabetes, hypercalcemia/electrolytes, liver and kidney function.
    - ▪ CRP: Helps to exclude an infectious or inflammatory etiology.
    - ▪ Ferritin: Should be 40-70 and certainly less than 120 mcg/L for most people. Assessment for iron overload is indicated in African Americans[60,61], white men over age 30 years[62], patients with peripheral

---

[54] "The onset of severe headache in a previously well patient is more likely than chronic headache to relate to an intracranial disorder such as subarachnoid hemorrhage or meningitis." Tierney ML. McPhee SJ, Papadakis MA (eds). *Current Medical Diagnosis and Treatment 2002, 41ˢᵗ Edition*. New York: Lange Medical Books; 2002, page 999

[55] Tierney ML. McPhee SJ, Papadakis MA (eds). *Current Medical Diagnosis and Treatment 2006, 45ᵗʰ Edition*. New York: Lange Medical Books; 2006, pages 31-33

[56] Tierney ML. McPhee SJ, Papadakis MA (eds). *Current Medical Diagnosis and Treatment 2006, 45ᵗʰ Edition*. New York: Lange Medical Books; 2006, pages 31-33

[57] Davidoff RA. Trigger points and myofascial pain: toward understanding how they affect headaches. *Cephalalgia*. 1998 Sep;18(7):436-48

[58] Tierney ML. McPhee SJ, Papadakis MA (eds). *Current Medical Diagnosis and Treatment 2006, 45ᵗʰ Edition*. New York: Lange Medical Books; 2006, pages 31-33

[59] Vasquez et al. Clinical Importance of Vitamin D: Paradigm Shift for All Healthcare Providers. *Altern Ther Health Med* 2004; 10: 28-37 ichnfm.academia.edu/

[60] Barton JC, Edwards CQ, Bertoli LF, Shroyer TW, Hudson SL. Iron overload in African Americans. *Am J Med*. 1995 Dec;99(6):616-23

[61] Wurapa RK, Gordeuk VR, Brittenham GM, Khiyami A, Schechter GP, Edwards CQ. Primary iron overload in African Americans. *Am J Med*. 1996;101(1):9-18

[62] Baer DM, et al. Hemochromatosis screening in asymptomatic ambulatory men 30 years of age and older. *Am J Med*. 1995 May;98(5):464-8

arthropathy[63], diabetics[64] and is advisable in children[65], women[66], young adults[67] and the general population.[68] Iron overload causes headaches.[69,70]

- **Homocysteine (serum)**: Optimal level is below 7 micromoles/liter in blood/serum; all patients with pain disorders—including but not limited to migraine/headaches, fibromyalgia and CRPS—should be tested for elevated homocysteine. Importantly, we need to appreciate that the most "pathologic" increases in homocysteine occur in the fluid around the brain—the cerebrospinal fluid (CSF) which is typically not subject to laboratory assessment due to the pain, risk, technical needs and skill involved in the procedure.[71]
- **Thyroid assessment**: Especially in patients with classic manifestations of hypothyroidism: fatigue, depression, cold hands and feet, dry skin, constipation, and delayed Achilles return.[72] See Chapter 1.
- **Food allergy testing**: May be helpful when elimination-and-challenge procedures are nonproductive and when other therapeutic measures have failed. I personally (DrV) think food allergy testing is overused and that addressing mucosal barrier defects and phenotype immunomodulation (Chapter 4, Section 3) is more important than laboratory testing for food allergies.
- **Establishing the diagnosis**:
  - Headache is considered a diagnosis based on the patient's subjective report of head pain. However, the headache is always secondary to some other cause of pain, which is the true diagnosis. A clinical or empirical process of elimination must consider common and dangerous causes of head pain, including meningitis, temporal arteritis, sinus infections, cervicogenic pain, intracranial lesions such as brain tumors, hypertension, drug side-effects, and food intolerances.
  - **Serious causes of head pain must be considered with each recurrence, as a patient with a long-term history of benign headaches may contract meningitis or develop hypertension as a new or additive cause of his/her headaches.**

Complications:

- Pain, nausea/vomiting/diarrhea, secondary inability to engage in work, play, and other daily activities.
- Cost and adverse effects of drugs.
- Complications may arise if an underlying cause (e.g., tumor, meningitis, hemorrhage) is undiagnosed.

Clinical management:

- A complete patient history and the above-mentioned lab tests and a physical examination with neurologic assessment will exclude most of the lethal differential diagnoses, allowing the provisional assessment of "benign headache" or "migraine headache" to be established. New onset of headaches or a progressive headache disorder always requires investigation. Refer to neurologist if clinical outcome is unsatisfactory or if complications become evident. For benign headaches including migraine, standard medical treatment is targeted at the alleviation of symptoms. To this end, analgesics and anti-inflammatory drugs such as acetaminophen, aspirin, ibuprofen, naproxen, and ketoprofen are the medical mainstays. Antidepressant drugs ranging from amitriptyline to fluoxetine also might be used for both migraine and tension headaches. Other drugs used for migraine include beta-adrenergic blockers such as propanolol, calcium-channel antagonists such as verapamil, anticonvulsants such as gabapentin and topiramate, and serotonin-modulating drugs such as methysergide and sumatriptan, as well as monoamine oxidase inhibitors and angiotensin-2 receptor blockers. Treatments unique to cluster headaches include inhaled oxygen, lithium carbonate, and prednisone.

[63] Olynyk J, Hall P, Ahern M, KwiatekR, MackinnonM. Screening for hemochromatosis in a rheumatology clinic. *Aust NZ J Med* 1994; 24: 22-5

[64] Phelps G, Chapman I, Hall P, Braund W, Mackinnon M. Prevalence of genetic haemochromatosis among diabetic patients. *Lancet* 1989; 2: 233-4

[65] Kaikov Y, et al. Primary hemochromatosis in children: report of three newly diagnosed cases and review of the pediatric literature. *Pediatrics* 1992; 90: 37-42

[66] Edwards CQ, Kushner JP. Screening for hemochromatosis. *N Engl J Med* 1993; 328: 1616-20

[67] Gushusrt TP, Triest WE. Diagnosis and management of precirrhotic hemochromatosis. *W Virginia Med J* 1990; 86: 91-5

[68] Balan V, Baldus W, Fairbanks V, et al. Screening for hemochromatosis: a cost-effectiveness study based on 12, 258 patients. *Gastroenterology* 1994; 107: 453-9

[69] Hagen K, Stovner LJ, Asberg A, et al. High headache prevalence among women with hemochromatosis: the Nord-Trondelag health study. *Ann Neurol* 2002 Jun;51(6):786-9

[70] Stovner LJ, Hagen K, Waage A, Bjerve KS. Hereditary haemochromatosis in two cousins with cluster headache. *Cephalalgia* 2002 May;22(4):317-9

[71] "The concentration of free HC did not differ significantly from normal controls, but the total HC concentration was significantly higher in MOA and MWA patients (41% increase in MOA and 376% increase in MWA). These findings suggest that an increase of total HC concentration in the brain is commonly seen in migraine patient and is particularly pronounced in MWA sufferers." Isobe C, Terayama Y. A remarkable increase in total homocysteine concentrations in the CSF of migraine patients with aura. *Headache*. 2010 Nov;50(10):1561-9

[72] DeQowin RL. *DeQowin and DeQowin's Diagnostic Examination. Sixth Edition*. New York, McGraw-Hill; 1994, page 900

Migraine patients may become dependent on prescription narcotic drugs, which carry inherent risks of dependence and abuse. Topiramate (Topomax®) is one of the most commonly used pharmaceutical drugs for the treatment of migraine, and a brief description of its efficacy and expense is warranted in order to provide clinical perspective. A recent clinical trial in a leading headache journal concluded that topiramate "resulted in statistically significant improvements" and that the drug is "safe and generally well tolerated"[73]; these statements would appear to support clinical use of the drug. However, more than 10% of patients stopped using the drug due to adverse

> **Patients with migraine headaches—noted in 50% of patients with fibromyalgia and some patients with hypertension—often have food allergies/sensitivities/intolerances**
>
> "The commonest foods causing reactions were wheat (78%), orange (65%), eggs (45%), tea and coffee (40% each), chocolate and milk (37%) each), beef (35%), and corn, cane sugar, and yeast (33% each). When an average of ten common foods were avoided there was a dramatic fall in the number of headaches per month, 85% of patients becoming headache-free."
>
> Grant EC. Food allergies and migraine. *Lancet.* 1979 May

effects, and the statistically significant benefit largely consisted of a reduction in headache days by 1.5 days per 91 days of treatment compared to placebo. The out-of-pocket cost for 3 months of this drug treatment (not including physician fees, recommended laboratory monitoring, and management of adverse effects) is in the range of $400 to $600. Thus, for a yearly cost of approximately $2000, the total reduction in headache days over placebo would be approximately 6 days per year. This study was funded by the company that makes the drug, and 11 of the 13 authors received funding, employment, or direct payment from Ortho-McNeil Neurologics, Inc. Therapeutic trials are implemented to address the underlying problem(s); natural treatments may be superior to drug treatments especially when used in combination.[74]

- Medical standard for migraine—symptomatic relief: "Management of migraine consists of avoidance of any precipitating factors, together with prophylactic or symptomatic pharmacologic treatment if necessary."[75] The goals of medical management are to reduce pain and other manifestations of migraine such as nausea and aura; this symptom-based approach ignores—conceptually and therapeutically—nearly all of the underlying biochemical and nutritional components of the illness, thereby providing minimal/modest benefit while fostering drug-dependency; additional medical goals are to reduce use of high-cost higher-risk emergency "rescue" drugs as well as the utilization of urgent/emergency medical services.

- Treatments (all benign headaches): Standard medical treatment for headaches is expensive and fraught with adverse effects, drug dependence, and suboptimal efficacy. Further, such symptom-suppressive treatment fails to address the causative food intolerances, nutritional deficiencies, and mitochondrial defects that are common in headache patients and migraineurs. Following the exclusion of serious underlying disease, headache patients should be counseled on allergen identification (free and highly efficacious) and should receive nutritional supplementation with combination fatty acids (e.g., ALA, GLA, EPA, DHA) and therapeutic doses of vitamins and minerals, particularly riboflavin, vitamin D3, and magnesium. CoQ10, 5-HTP, melatonin, spinal manipulation, post-isometric stretching, and the other treatments listed above can be used in combination as appropriate per patient to optimize the therapeutic response.

Food & Nutrition The foundational diet is the 5pSPMD as described previously; this "Paleo template"—a diet of fruits, vegetables, nuts, seeds, berries, and lean sources of protein (thereby excluding grains in general and gluten-containing grains in particular)—immediately helps patients increase potassium and magnesium intake specifically and increase nutritional density and systemic alkalinization generally while reducing intake of sodium chloride, common allergens and triggers such as wheat/gluten and milk/dairy, and chemicals such as MSG and aspartame. Patients should—generally speaking—base the diet on "fruits, vegetables, nuts, seeds, and berries with adequate protein intake." Grains that contain the most inflammatory and allergenic form of gluten are rye, barley, and wheat; these foods should be avoided due to their pro-inflammatory properties, their ability to promote gastrointestinal

[73] Silberstein SD, et al. Efficacy and safety of topiramate for the treatment of chronic migraine. *Headache.* 2007 Feb;47(2):170-80
[74] Vasquez A. Interventions need to be consistent with osteopathic philosophy. *J Am Osteopath Assoc.* 2006 Sep;106(9):528-9 jaoa.org/cgi/content/full/106/9/528
[75] Tierney ML. McPhee SJ, Papadakis MA (eds). *Current Medical Diagnosis and Treatment 2002, 41ˢᵗ Edition.* New York: Lange; 2002. Page 999-1005

dysbiosis generally and small intestine bacterial overgrowth (SIBO) in particular, and their promotion of gastrointestinal damage, release of zonulin and—in some patients—promotion of systemic inflammation and brain inflammation, both leading to pain while also likely promoting neurodegeneration.[76] The ability of gluten-containing grains to trigger brain inflammation (triggering migraine and other headaches) and autoimmune brain conditions (mimicking multiple sclerosis [MS] and amyotrophic lateral sclerosis [ALS]) has been well proven for decades and is irrefutable; a gluten-free diet is curative.[77,78,79] Beyond custom, convenience, and the government subsidies that make "junk foods"—many of

> **Dr Vasquez's Five-part Nutrition Protocol: The "Supplemented Paleo-Mediterranean Diet" (SPMD)**
>
> 1. **Diet: Emphasize fruits, vegetables, nuts, seeds, berries, and lean sources of protein** (fish, grass-fed lamb/beef). Make modifications for patient-specific food allergies and sensitivities; this is especially important for patients with known allergy-related conditions such as migraine headaches. Patients with kidney disease should use caution when consuming a potassium-rich diet. Vasquez A. Revisiting the Five-Part Nutritional Wellness Protocol: The Supplemented Paleo-Mediterranean Diet. *Nutritional Perspectives* 2011 Jan
> 2. **Multivitamin and multimineral supplement**: Nutrient deficiencies are common and are easily treated with nutritional supplementation. Fletcher and Fairfield. Vitamins for chronic disease prevention in adults. *JAMA* 2002 Jun
> 3. **Vitamin D dosed at 2,000-10,000 IU per day**: The adult requirement for vitamin D3 is approximately 4,000 IU per day; some patients may achieve optimal blood levels with lower doses, but generally daily doses of 4,000-10,000 IU are necessary. Vasquez A et al. The Clinical Importance of Vitamin D. *Alternative Therapies in Health and Medicine* 2004 Sep
> 4. **Combination fatty acid supplementation**: A combination of flax oil, borage oil, and fish oil provides the health-promoting fatty acids (ALA, GLA, EPA, DHA). Patients should consume organic virgin olive oil liberally with foods. Vasquez A. New Insights into Fatty Acid Supplementation and Its Effect on Eicosanoid Production and Genetic Expression. *Nutritional Perspectives* 2005; Jan
> 5. **Probiotics**: Health-promoting bacteria can be consumed in the form of powders, pills, and fermented foods such as yogurt and kefir.
>
> For a video review of this foundational diet and introduction to the functional inflammology protocol, see Dr Vasquez "Functional Inflammology Protocol, part 1" from the 2013 International Conference on Human Nutrition and Functional Medicine (ICHNFM.ORG): https://vimeo.com/100089988 Password: "DrVprotocol_volume1"

which contain gluten and other inflammatory dietary components—inexpensive and widely available, no legitimate medical or nutritional reason exists for the consumption of gluten-containing foods; the myth that "whole grain foods promote health" is a lie foisted on an ignorant public and an equally uninformed population of nutritionally ignorant medical professionals.[80]

- Food allergy elimination (*Lancet* 1979 May): Mitochondrial dysfunction promotes inflammation, including allergic inflammation; as a result of mitochondrial dysfunction, elevated glutamate levels, and microglial activation, headache patients in general and migraine patients in particular are more sensitive to triggers (e.g., emotional, environmental, hormonal, nutritional) that might otherwise not cause problems. Food allergy is among the most common causes/triggers of headaches[81,82], particularly migraine headaches, particularly those that do not respond to drug treatments.[83,84] In the important study by Grant[85], the following foods were identified as the most common headache triggers: wheat (78%), orange (65%), eggs (45%), tea and coffee (40% each), chocolate and milk (37% each), beef (35%), corn, cane sugar, and yeast (33% each); when an average of 10 triggering foods were avoided, patients experienced a "dramatic fall in the number of headaches per month, 85% of patients becoming headache-free." Food allergen identification via the *elimination and challenge technique*[86] is accurate and inexpensive, and problem-causing foods are then eliminated from the diet.

---

[76] Daulatzai MA. Non-celiac gluten sensitivity triggers gut dysbiosis, neuroinflammation, gut-brain axis dysfunction, and vulnerability for dementia. *CNS Neurol Disord Drug Targets*. 2015;14(1):110-31

[77] Finsterer J, Leutmezer F. Celiac disease with cerebral and peripheral nerve involvement mimicking multiple sclerosis. *J Med Life*. 2014 Sep 15;7(3):440-4

[78] "The authors describe 10 patients with gluten sensitivity and abnormal MRI. All experienced episodic headache, six had unsteadiness, and four had gait ataxia. MRI abnormalities varied from confluent areas of high signal throughout the white matter to foci of high signal scattered in both hemispheres. Symptomatic response to gluten-free diet was seen in nine patients." Hadjivassiliou et al. Headache and CNS white matter abnormalities associated with gluten sensitivity. *Neurology*. 2001 Feb 13;56(3):385-8

[79] "CD is an autoimmune-mediated disorder of the gastrointestinal tract. Initial symptom presentation is variable and can include neurologic manifestations that may comprise ataxia, neuropathy, dizziness, epilepsy, and cortical calcifications rather than gastrointestinal-hindering diagnosis and management. We present a case of a young man with progressive neurologic symptoms and brain MR imaging findings worrisome for ALS. During the diagnostic work-up, endomysium antibodies were discovered, and CD was confirmed by upper gastrointestinal endoscopy with duodenal biopsies. MR imaging findings suggestive of ALS improved after gluten-free diet institution." Brown et al. White matter lesions suggestive of amyotrophic lateral sclerosis attributed to celiac disease. *AJNR Am J Neuroradiol*. 2010 May;31(5):880-1

[80] Adams et al. Nutrition education in U.S. medical schools: latest update of a national survey. *Acad Med*. 2010 Sep;85(9):1537-42

[81] Egger J, Carter CM, Wilson J, Turner MW, Soothill JF. Is migraine food allergy? A double-blind controlled trial of oligoantigenic diet treatment. *Lancet* 1983 Oct ;2:865-9

[82] Monro J, Brostoff J, Carini C, Zilkha K. Food allergy in migraine. Study of dietary exclusion and RAST. *Lancet* 1980 Jul 5;2(8184):1-4

[83] Monro J, Carini C, Brostoff J. Migraine is a food-allergic disease. *Lancet* 1984 Sep 29;2(8405):719-21

[84] Finn R, Cohen HN. "Food allergy": Fact or Fiction? *Lancet* 1978 Feb 25;1(8061):426-8

[85] Grant EC. Food allergies and migraine. *Lancet* 1979 May 5;1(8123):966-9

[86] "Elimination diets can be both a diagnostic tool and a therapeutic intervention for people with a suspected food sensitivity or allergy." Denton C. The elimination/challenge diet. *Minn Med*. 2012 Dec;95(12):43-4. The classic book on the topic of the elimination and challenge technique is William G. Crook MD's *Detecting Your Hidden Allergies* or *Tracking Down Hidden Food Allergy*. Professional Books; 2 edition (June 1980).

- Gluten-free diet alleviates migraine and fibromyalgia in a significant proportion of affected patients (*Rheumatol Int.* 2014): "The level of widespread chronic pain improved dramatically for all patients; for 15 patients, chronic widespread pain was no longer present, indicating remission of FM. Fifteen patients returned to work or normal life. In three patients who had been previously treated in pain units with opioids, these drugs were discontinued. Fatigue, gastrointestinal symptoms, migraine, and depression also improved together with pain. ... For some patients, the clinical improvement after starting the gluten-free diet was striking and observed after only a few months; for other patients, improvement was very slow and was gradually observed over many months of follow-up."

- Avoidance of food additives: Red wine, aged cheeses, sardines, sausage, bacon, and monosodium glutamate (MSG)-containing foods are common triggers for headache and migraine in susceptible patients and should therefore be avoided or at least trialed, ie, avoided and reintroduced to observe for any reduction and recurrence, respectively, of headache or other inflammatory manifestations. Most of these foods contain tyramine, nitrites, or other neuroexcitatory or vasoactive substances, in addition to components (allergens) to which migraine patients tend to be immunologically sensitized. MSG consumption can trigger headache, nausea, and increased blood pressure in apparently normal healthy people.[87] Sulfites in red wine are also noted to trigger migraine and headache in some patients; many wines are available on the market now which contain no detectable sulfites. Sulfites trigger migraine by directly triggering the release of inflammatory mediators and by impairing mitochondrial function; sulfite inhibits the enzyme glutamate dehydrogenase in its conversion of glutamate into alpha-keto-glutarate thereby blocking substrate/fuel entry into the Krebs/citrate cycle (leading to a 50% reduction in cellular energy/ATP production in an experimental study using rat brain cells[88]) while perhaps also leaving excess glutamate present for NMDAr activation—note here again, as previously mentioned, that the combination of mitochondrial dysfunction with glutamate-mediated NMDAr activation is particularly lethal for neurons because the mitochondrial dysfunction starves the neurons of energy/ATP and mitochondria-mediated calcium homeostasis at the exact moment when these same neurons are overstimulated.

- Fish oil supplying 3,000 mg of eicosapentaenoic acid (n3 EPA) and docosahexaenoic acid (n3 DHA) per day, with additional 400 IU mixed tocopherols: Fish oil has been shown to reduce the frequency, duration, and intensity of migraine headaches[89] and the effectiveness of fish oil may be mediated via alterations in cytokine production.[90] More specifically per current research, we appreciate that EPA and especially DHA alleviate glial activation, thereby reducing excessive glutamate-driven pain-inducing excitatory neurotransmission.

- Gamma-linolenic acid (n6 GLA, from plants such as borage and hemp) and alpha-linolenic acid (n3 ALA, notably from flaxseed oil): Supplementation with GLA and ALA—along with the use of a multivitamin and multimineral supplement and avoidance of dietary arachidonic acid—has been shown to significantly reduce the intensity, frequency, and duration of migraine headaches.[91] Exacerbation of temporal lobe epilepsy (TLE) with GLA combined with n6 linoleic acid has been reported; this exacerbation can be problematic or diagnostically useful (e.g., temporary exacerbation of TLE aids in the differential from schizophrenia).[92] Relatedly and importantly, Al-Khamees et al[93] reported a case of previously well 41-year-old female (i.e., 41yoF) who developed temporal lobe status epilepticus following one week of 1.5-3 g/d borage oil; the amount of GLA and LA and any contaminants in the product were not determined but serum fatty acid analysis showed elevations of GLA 345 microg/g of blood (control 191 microg/g), and LA 259 microg/g of blood (control 165 microg/g). Migraine patients could reasonably limit GLA intake to not more than 500 mg/d; other treatments within this protocol such as vitamin D, pyridoxine, and magnesium have established anti-seizure benefits.

---

[87] "A statistically significant increase in systolic and diastolic blood pressures after MSG administration was observed, as well as a significantly higher frequency of reports of nausea and headache in the MSG group. No robust effect of MSG on muscle sensitivity was found." Shimada et al. Differential effects of repetitive oral administration of monosodium glutamate on interstitial glutamate concentration and muscle pain sensitivity. *Nutrition.* 2015 Feb;31(2):315-23

[88] Zhang et al. A mechanism of sulfite neurotoxicity: direct inhibition of glutamate dehydrogenase. *J Biol Chem.* 2004 Oct 8;279(41):43035-45

[89] "In fact, results of this preliminary study suggest that both fish oil and olive oil may be beneficial in the treatment of recurrent migraines in adolescents." Harel et al. Supplementation with omega-3 polyunsaturated fatty acids in the management of recurrent migraines in adolescents. *J Adolesc Health* 2002 Aug;31(2):154-61

[90] Smith RS. The cytokine theory of headache. *Med Hypotheses* 1992 Oct;39(2):168-74

[91] "In 129 patients available for study, 86% experienced reduction in severity, frequency and duration of migraine attacks, 22% became free of migraine and more than 90% had reduced nausea and vomiting." Wagner et al. Prophylactic treatment of migraine with gamma-linolenic and alpha-linolenic acids. *Cephalalgia.* 1997 Apr;17(2):127-30

[92] Vaddadi KS. The use of gamma-linolenic acid and linoleic acid to differentiate between temporal lobe epilepsy and schizophrenia. *Prostaglandins Med.* 1981 Apr;6(4):375-9

[93] Al-Khamees et al. Status epilepticus associated with borage oil ingestion. *J Med Toxicol.* 2011 Jun;7(2):154-7

Generally, the minimal dose of GLA for systemic anti-inflammatory effect is 500 mg/d; doses up to 2-4 grams per day have been used with safety and efficacy in other inflammatory/metabolic disorders such as cancer, asthma, psoriasis, and rheumatoid arthritis.

- <u>Magnesium supplementation to bowel tolerance (generally with additional pyridoxine)</u>: Magnesium deficiency is common, affecting approximately 30% of different populations in various industrialized nations.[94,95,96,97] Regardless of headache etiology or classification, magnesium deficiency is more common in headache patients than in headache-free controls. Magnesium deficiency directly contributes to headache by at least 4 mechanisms: (1) facilitating brain cortex hyperexcitability and hypesthesia due to a reduction in the partial blockade of N-methyl-D-aspartate (NMDA) neurotransmitter receptor sites by magnesium[98], (2) impairing cellular energy production, specifically at the level of mitochondrial electron chain complex #5, the ATP synthase enzyme, (3) promoting vasoconstriction, and (4) promoting increased muscle tension, with the latter 2 mechanisms caused in part by impaired energy production, as well as altered intracellular calcium-to-magnesium ratios. Conversely, adequate magnesium nutriture and use of magnesium supplementation help prevent headaches by modulation of NMDA receptor sensitivity and support of energy production, vasorelaxation, and myorelaxation. Not only is magnesium deficiency common in female patients with menstrual migraine[99] and in patients with post-traumatic headaches[100], but magnesium supplementation is justified in headache patients based on the findings of "disturbances in magnesium ion homeostasis" which appear to contribute to brain cortex hyperexcitability.[101] **Except when contraindicated due to renal failure or drug interaction, magnesium supplementation is safe, effective, and reasonable for essentially all patients with headache.**[102,103,104,105,106] Intravenous magnesium (sulfate) is more effective than drug therapy with dexamethasone/metoclopramide for the treatment of acute migraine headaches.[107] A reasonable clinical approach is to 1) evaluate patient with history, physical examination, and screening laboratory tests to exclude contraindications such as renal insufficiency (assess with BUN, creatinine, and urinalysis), 2) assess for possible drug interactions, and then 3) begin the patient with 200 mg

> **Clinical Pearl**
>
> The importance of alkalinization for the renal retention and intracellular uptake of magnesium can hardly be overemphasized; so-called failure of magnesium therapy is generally due to failure to attain systemic alkalinization, without which magnesium is both hyperexcreted in the urine and "underabsorbed" into the intracellular space. As discussed in this context, systemic pH can be assessed by measuring urine pH, which should range from 7.5 up to approximately 8.5.

elemental magnesium (citrate or malate) with the dose increased by 200 mg every 1-2 days until bowel tolerance is reached. Reduce dose if excessively loose stools or diarrhea occur. When high-dose magnesium supplementation is used in patients with renal insufficiency or drugs that predispose to hypermagnesemia, cautious professional supervision is warranted, with periodic measurement of serum or ionized magnesium. Efficacy of magnesium supplementation is enhanced with concomitant pyridoxine supplementation (e.g., 100-250 mg per day with food) and with an alkalinizing Paleo-Mediterranean Diet as described in Chapter 2. The Paleo-Mediterranean Diet can promote alkalinization[108] which facilitates systemic mineral and magnesium

[94] Innerarity S. Hypomagnesemia in acute and chronic illness. *Crit Care Nurs Q*. 2000 Aug;23(2):1-19

[95] Frankel H, Haskell R, Lee SY, Miller D, Rotondo M, Schwab CW. Hypomagnesemia in trauma patients. *World J Surg*. 1999 Sep;23(9):966-9

[96] Fox CH, Ramsoomair D, Mahoney MC, et al. An investigation of hypomagnesemia among ambulatory urban African Americans. *J Fam Pract*. 1999 Aug;48(8):636-9

[97] Schimatschek HF, Rempis R. Prevalence of hypomagnesemia in an unselected German population of 16,000 individuals. *Magnes Res*. 2001 Dec;14(4):283-90

[98] Boska et al. Contrasts in cortical magnesium, phospholipid and energy metabolism between migraine syndromes. *Neurology* 2002 Apr 23;58(8):1227-33

[99] "CONCLUSIONS: The high incidence of IMg2+ deficiency and the elevated ICa2+/IMg2+ ratio during menstrual migraine confirm previous suggestions of a possible role for magnesium deficiency in the development of menstrual migraine." Mauskop A, Altura BT, Altura BM. Serum ionized magnesium levels and serum ionized calcium/ionized magnesium ratios in women with menstrual migraine. *Headache* 2002 Apr;42(4):242-8

[100] "Abnormalities in serum IMg(2+) concentrations and ICa(2+)/IMg(2+) ratios were found in children with post-traumatic headaches, but total magnesium levels were normal." Marcus JC, Altura BT, Altura BM. Serum ionized magnesium in post-traumatic headaches. *J Pediatr* 2001 Sep;139(3):459-62

[101] "...disturbances in magnesium ion homeostasis may contribute to brain cortex hyperexcitability and the pathogenesis of migraine syndromes associated with neurologic symptoms." Boska et al. Contrasts in cortical magnesium, phospholipid and energy metabolism between migraine syndromes. *Neurology* 2002 Apr 23;58(8):1227-33

[102] Mazzotta G, Sarchielli P, Alberti A, Gallai V. Intracellular Mg++ concentration and electromyographical ischemic test in juvenile headache. *Cephalalgia* 1999 Nov;19(9):802-9

[103] Mishima K, et al. Platelet ionized magnesium, cyclic AMP, and cyclic GMP levels in migraine and tension-type headache. *Headache* 1997 Oct;37(9):561-4

[104] "After a prospective baseline period of 4 weeks they received oral 600 mg (24 mmol) magnesium (trimagnesium dicitrate) daily for 12 weeks or placebo... High-dose oral magnesium appears to be effective in migraine prophylaxis." Peikert et al. Prophylaxis of migraine with oral magnesium. *Cephalalgia* 1996 Jun;16(4):257-63

[105] Mauskop A, Altura BT, Cracco RQ, Altura BM. Intravenous magnesium sulfate rapidly alleviates headaches of various types. *Headache* 1996 Mar;36(3):154-60

[106] Wang et al. Oral magnesium oxide prophylaxis of frequent migrainous headache in children: a randomized, double-blind, placebo-controlled trial. *Headache*. 2003;43:601-610

[107] "We gave dexamethasone/metoclopramide to one group and magnesium sulfate to the other group, and evaluated pain severity at 20 min and at 1- and 2-h intervals after infusion. ... According to the results, magnesium sulfate was a more effective and fast-acting medication compared to a combination of dexamethasone/metoclopramide for the treatment of acute migraine headaches." Shahrami et al. Comparison of therapeutic effects of magnesium sulfate vs. dexamethasone/metoclopramide on alleviating acute migraine headache. *J Emerg Med*. 2015 Jan;48(1):69-76

[108] Sebastian et al. Estimation of the net acid load of the diet of ancestral preagricultural Homo sapiens and their hominid ancestors. *Am J Clin Nutr* 2002;76:1308-16

retention[109,110] and increases intracellular magnesium levels; alkalinization and increased intracellular magnesium levels are associated with reductions in low-back pain according to a clinical trial.[111] **Magnesium may decrease the absorption or effectiveness of several drugs**, including: Azithromycin (Zithromax), Cimetidine (Tagamet), Ciprofloxacin (Ciloxan, Cipro), Doxycycline (Atridox, Doryx, Doxy, Monodox, Periostat, Vibramycin), Famotidine (Mylanta-AR, Pepcid, Pepcid AC), Hydroxychloroquine (Plaquenil), Levofloxacin (Levaquin), Nitrofurantoin (Furadantin, Macrobid, Macrodantin), Nizatidine (Axid, Axid AR), Ofloxacin (Floxin, Ocuflox), Tetracycline (Achromycin, Sumycin, Helidac), and Warfarin (Coumadin). Misoprostol (Cytotec, Arthrotec) with magnesium may result in diarrhea. **Spironolactone (Aldactone, Aldactazide) or Amiloride (Midamor, Moduretic) may cause hypermagnesemia.**

- Oral magnesium for migraine prophylaxis. (*J Pak Med Assoc.* 2013 Feb[112]): "In this clinical trial study, effects of 500 mg/day oral magnesium oxide for migraine prophylaxis and serum magnesium concentration in 77 migrainous adults (case=33, control=44) aged 34.10±9.61 years, were assessed. Significant reduction in migraines, migraine days, headache severity and migraine index in both the groups compared with baseline, were observed. In magnesium oxide group compared with control group, 50% or greater reduction in migraines (P<0.01) and headache severity (P<0.05) were significant. ... Magnesium supplementation increased significantly (P<0.001) serum magnesium concentration while in control group no difference was seen. Considering that oral oxide magnesium supplementation resulted in positive outcomes in decreasing frequency and severity of migraine seizures without leaving any serious side effects, it seems that magnesium oxide supplementation associated with the routine treatments may be effective especially in patients with low level of serum magnesium."

- Vitamin C, ascorbate: Ascorbate promotes mitochondrial function at cytochrome c, between complexes 3 and 4. My personal hypothesis is that ascorbate provides analgesic benefits via enhancement of central dopaminergic mechanisms and via its ability to lower histamine levels[113] thereby potentially alleviating neurogenic inflammation.[114] Appreciating its safety and efficacy in treating CRPS, migraine, neuropathic and postsurgical pain[115,116], I think all patients with pain should receive ascorbate 2-6 grams daily in divided doses.

- Hydroxocobalamin (hydroxo-vitamin-B12, OH-B12): Hydroxocobalamin is a nitric oxide (NO-) scavenger and appears to benefit the majority of patients with migraine headaches; this study used OH-B12 1 mg/d via aqueous intranasal administration to obviate the need for parenteral administration.[117] If the route of administration is unimportant, then high-dose oral supplementation with 2,000-6,000 mcg/d may prove to be just as effective, according to comparable research using cyanocobalamin.[118] NO- promotes migraine by two mechanisms—induction of mitochondrial dysfunction and promotion of glutamate release—which function synergistically to promote pain amplification, central sensitization as discussed in great detail in the following section on fibromyalgia. Therefore, hydroxocobalamin's effectiveness in migraine is mediated by NO- scavenging is simultaneously mitoprotective (protective of mitochondria) and neuroprotective (protective of neurons).

> **NO- scavenging with hydroxocobalamin**
>
> "Drugs which directly counteract nitric oxide (NO), such as endothelial receptor blockers, NO-synthase inhibitors, and NO-scavengers, may be effective in the acute treatment of migraine, but are also likely to be effective in migraine prophylaxis. ...This is the first prospective, open study indicating that intranasal hydroxocobalamin may have a prophylactic effect in migraine."
>
> van der Kuy et al. Hydroxocobalamin, a nitric oxide scavenger, in the prophylaxis of migraine. *Cephalalgia.* 2002 Sep

[109] Sebastian et al. Improved mineral balance and skeletal metabolism in postmenopausal women treated with potassium bicarbonate. *N Engl J Med.* 1994;330(25):1776-81

[110] Tucker et al. Potassium, magnesium, and fruit and vegetable intakes are associated with greater bone mineral density in elderly men and women. *Am J Clin Nutr.* 1999;69(4):727-36

[111] "The results show that a disturbed acid-base balance may contribute to the symptoms of low back pain. The simple and safe addition of an alkaline multimineral preparate was able to reduce the pain symptoms in these patients with chronic low back pain." Vormann J, Worlitschek M,Goedecke T,Silver B. Supplementation with alkaline minerals reduces symptoms in patients with chronic low back pain. *J Trace Elem Med Biol.* 2001;15(2-3):179-83

[112] Talebi M, Goldust M. Oral magnesium; migraine prophylaxis. *J Pak Med Assoc.* 2013 Feb;63(2):286

[113] Johnston CS, Martin LJ, Cai X. Antihistamine effect of supplemental ascorbic acid and neutrophil chemotaxis. *J Am Coll Nutr.* 1992 Apr;11(2):172-6

[114] Rosa AC, Fantozzi R. The role of histamine in neurogenic inflammation. *Br J Pharmacol.* 2013 Sep;170(1):38-45

[115] Hasanzadeh Kiabi et al. Can vitamin C be used as an adjuvant for managing postoperative pain? A short literature review. *Korean J Pain.* 2013 Apr;26(2):209-10

[116] Mohseni M. Use of vitamin C as placebo in anesthesiology. *Anesth Pain Med.* 2013 Winter;2(3):141

[117] van der Kuy PH, et al. Hydroxocobalamin, a nitric oxide scavenger, in the prophylaxis of migraine: an open, pilot study. *Cephalalgia.*2002; 22:513 –519

[118] "In cobalamin deficiency, 2 mg of cyanocobalamin administered orally on a daily basis was as effective as 1 mg administered intramuscularly on a monthly basis and may be superior." Kuzminski et al. Effective treatment of cobalamin deficiency with oral cobalamin. *Blood* 1998 Aug 15;92(4):1191-8 bloodjournal.org/cgi/content/full/92/4/1191

- Folic acid in the form of folinic acid or methylfolate ("5-methyltetrahydrofolate" or "5-MTHF"): Most nutrition-knowledgeable doctors do not use "folic acid" in the form of folic acid due to concerns about increased free radical generation and possible increased risk of cellular damage and malignant disease; we still use the term "folic acid" but nowadays this is—in practice—meant to imply the use of either folinic acid or methylfolate, two forms of folic acid that are considered safer, if not also more effective. Strictly speaking, "folic acid" refers to the synthetic form of the vitamin, whereas "folate" refers to derivatives of tetrahydrofolate that are found in food, especially leafy green vegetables, of which most people do not consume a sufficient amount. Some people develop antibodies against the folic acid transporter (cerebral folate receptor autoantibodies) that facilitates entry of folate into the brain, and they must receive either folinic acid or methylfolate to avoid neurologic devastation due to cerebral folate deficiency, wherein blood/serum levels of folate are normal but the brain (on the other side of the "wall" formed by the blood-brain barrier) is starved for this nutrient.[119] Folic acid from diet and/or supplementation serves many roles and thereby provides numerous benefits, largely centered on the provision of single-carbon methyl groups for metabolic processes (e.g., homocysteine metabolism) and DNA methylation, which regulates/suppresses gene transcription and thereby reduces risk of cancer and viral activation (e.g., cervical cancer following exposure to the human papilloma virus [HPV][120]). In this conversation, we are primarily concerned with optimizing folate intake to optimize "neurologic function" (i.e., generally speaking: normalization of homocysteine-mediated NMDAr activation in the brain, spinal cord and periphery) by reducing homocysteine levels because elevated homocysteine levels will cause excessive pain/fatigue/depression due to activation of the NMDA-receptor, mostly in the brain but also in the periphery. The most important nutrients for reducing homocysteine are folate (vitamin B9), pyridoxine (vitamin B6), cobalamin (vitamin B12) and the amino acid N-acetyl-cysteine (NAC); some people have a defect in their ability to convert folate into its active form via the enzyme methylenetetrahydrofolate reductase (MTHFR) and therefore need more nutritional supplementation to push this sluggish pathway to metabolic completion and reduce/normalize homocysteine levels. Diagrams illustrating these pathways tend to be repulsively complex, immemorably curvaceous, and/or incomplete and thereby clinically valueless; the illustration below is perhaps the most simple for efficient understanding of the means by which nutritional supplementation lowers homocysteine levels.

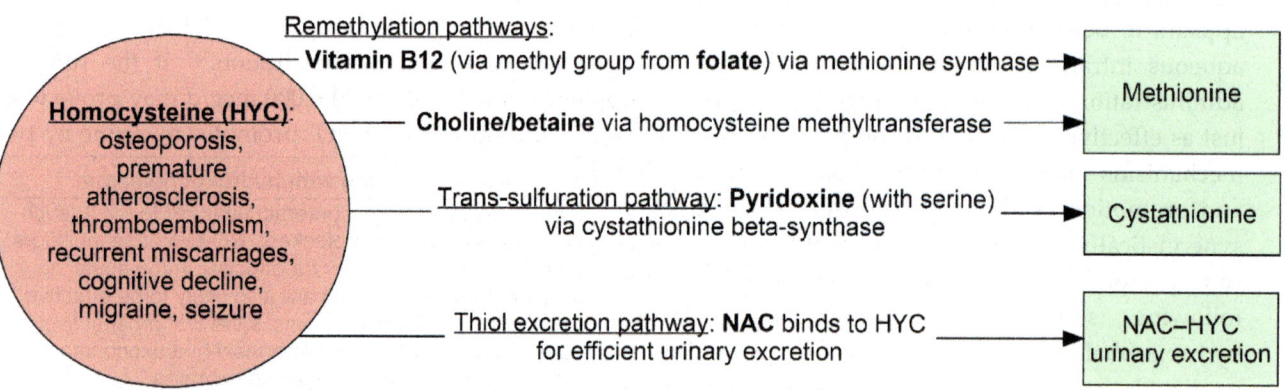

Lowering homocysteine (HYC) via nutritional supplementation: Folate gives methyl group to cobalamin (vitamin B12) to convert HYC via methionine synthase to methionine; choline/betaine can remethylate homocysteine via homocysteine methyltransferase to form methionine. Pyridoxine promotes conversion of HYC via cystathionine beta-synthase to cystathionine. The amino acid N-acetyl-cysteine (NAC) binds to HYC for efficient renal excretion of NAC-HYC.[121]

Increased consumption of folate from diet and/or supplements can alleviate depression, fatigue, and pain and is therefore recommended for all "pain patients", including those with migraine, fibromyalgia, and chronic fatigue syndrome. Adult doses of folate 1-5 mg (1,000-5,000 mcg) per day are reasonable and should be

[119] Gordon N. Cerebral folate deficiency. *Dev Med Child Neurol.* 2009 Mar;51(3):180-2

[120] Piyathilake et al. Indian women with higher serum concentrations of folate and vitamin B12 are significantly less likely to be infected with carcinogenic or high-risk (HR) types of human papillomaviruses (HPVs). *Int J Womens Health.* 2010 Aug 9;2:7-12

[121] "NAC intravenous administration induces an efficient and rapid reduction of plasma thiols, particularly of Hcy; our data support the hypothesis that NAC displaces thiols from their binding protein sites and forms, in excess of plasma NAC, mixed disulphides (NAC-Hcy) with a high renal clearance." Ventura et al. N-Acetyl-cysteine reduces homocysteine plasma levels after single intravenous administration by increasing thiols urinary excretion. *Pharmacol Res.* 1999 Oct;40(4):345-50

coadministered with a roughly equal amount of vitamin B12. Anti-seizure drugs (especially phenytoin, carbamazepine, barbiturates[122]), some of which are used in the treatment of migraine and chronic pain, are notorious for causing folate deficiency and homocysteine elevation[123]; obviously, the drugs would paradoxically promote pain and seizure if folate deficiency develops—coadministration of folate with anti-seizure drugs should be supervised by the prescribing physician.

- Vitamin supplementation to lower homocysteine levels alleviates migraine. (*Pharmacogenet Genomics*. 2009 Jun[124]): "This was a randomized, double-blind placebo, controlled trial of 6 months of daily vitamin supplementation (i.e. 2 mg of folic acid, 25 mg vitamin B6, and 400 microg of vitamin B12) in 52 patients diagnosed with migraine with aura. Vitamin supplementation reduced homocysteine by 39% (approximately 4 mumol/l) compared with baseline, a reduction that was greater than placebo (P=0.001). Vitamin supplementation also reduced the prevalence of migraine disability from 60% at baseline to 30% after 6 months, whereas no reduction was observed for the placebo group. Headache frequency and pain severity were also reduced, whereas there was no reduction in the placebo group. In this patient group the treatment effect on both homocysteine levels and migraine disability was associated with MTHFRC677T genotype whereby carriers of the C allele experienced a greater response compared with TT genotypes."

- Higher levels of dietary folate intake reduce migraine disability and frequency. (*Headache*. 2015 Feb[125]): "A significant inverse relation was observed between dietary folate equivalent and (folic acid) FA consumption and migraine frequency. It was also observed that in individuals with the CC genotype for the methylenetetrahydrofolate reductase (MTHFR) C677T variant, migraine frequency was significantly linked to FA consumption. The results from this study indicate that folate intake in the form of FA may influence migraine frequency in female MA sufferers."

- Pyridoxine (vitamin B6) 50-250 mg/d taken with food and aided by concomitant supplementation with magnesium and riboflavin: Pyridoxine promotes the conversion, via glutamic acid decarboxylase, of neuroexcitatory glutamate into neuroinhibitory GABA, as previously discussed and diagrammed. Pyridoxine also lowers levels of homocysteine, which functions as does glutamate in excitation of the NMDA receptor; thus, pyridoxine protects brain neuron cells from excess stimulation by lowering both glutamate and homocysteine. Experimental and clinical data are both very clear that B6 has analgesic and anti-seizure benefits that are independent from its support of glutamic acid decarboxylase's conversion of glutamate to GABA; pyridoxine functions both peripherally and centrally, with those central locations including the spinal cord, deep brain structures such as the thalamus (where it inhibits neuron firing), and cortex.[126] The conversion of pyridoxine to its intermediate form pyridoxine-5-phosphate requires magnesium (Mg), as expected with phosphorylation reactions; further, magnesium modulates/reduces calcium entry following NMDAr activation, and thus magnesium has a dual effect in reducing excess NMDAr activation. Conversion of pyridoxine-5-phosphate to the fully activated form pyridoxal-5-phosphate (P5P or PLP) requires an oxidase enzyme which requires riboflavin (vitamin B2); thus, as expected, some patients respond to B6 supplementation optimally/only when B2 is coadministered.[127] Not surprisingly, some patients respond better—or exclusively— to administration of the active P5P when pyridoxine previously failed to provide efficacy[128]; thus, what should be obvious by now is that pyridoxine therapy cannot be considered inefficacious until B2, and Mg have been used concomitantly with it and/or until P5P has been used. Furthermore, pyridoxine doses for adults should be in the range of 50-250 (up to 500) mg/d while determining the proper dosage (ie, response to treatment); multiyear use of extremely high doses, e.g., 2,000 mg/d, can cause sensory nerve damage (dorsal root

[122] Morrell MJ. Folic Acid and Epilepsy. *Epilepsy Curr*. 2002 Mar;2(2):31-34
[123] "Patients who consume antiepileptic drugs are susceptible to high levels of homocysteine and low levels of folate in the blood." Paknahad et al. Effects of Common Anti-epileptic Drugs on the Serum Levels of Homocysteine and Folic Acid. *Int J Prev Med*. 2012 Mar;3(Suppl 1):S186-90
[124] Lea et al. Effects of vitamin supplementation and MTHFR (C677T) genotype on homocysteine-lowering and migraine disability. *Pharmacogenet Genomics*. 2009 Jun:422-8
[125] Menon et al. Effects of dietary folate intake on migraine disability and frequency. *Headache*. 2015 Feb;55(2):301-9
[126] Zimmerman M, Bartoszyk GD, Bonke D, et al. Antinociceptive properties of pyridoxine. Neurophysiological and behavioral findings. *Ann N Y Acad Sci*. 1990;585:219-30
[127] Folkers et al. Enzymology of the response of the carpal tunnel syndrome to riboflavin and to combined riboflavin and pyridoxine. *Proc Natl Acad Sci*. 1984 Nov;81(22):7076-8
[128] "We present a female infant with seizures responsive to pyridoxal phosphate but that are resistant to pyridoxine. ... It is suggested that in addition to glutamic acid decarboxylase abnormality, the path from the absorption, transportation, phosphorylation, and oxidation of pyridoxine to pyridoxal phosphate in this patient might be defective. It should be considered whether pyridoxal phosphate can be the drug of choice instead of pyridoxine in treating patients suspected of pyridoxine-dependent epilepsy to reduce failure rate and further delay in seizure control." Kuo MF, Wang HS. Pyridoxal phosphate-responsive epilepsy with resistance to pyridoxine. *Pediatr Neurol*. 2002 Feb;26(2):146-7

ganglionopathy[129]) but this is not a concern when P5P is used (because P5P is considered nontoxic relative to pyridoxine[130]) lower doses are used for shorter periods of time, especially with professional supervision and a modicum of awareness and common sense. Studies using B6 in the treatment of premenstrual syndrome have used doses of 50-500 mg/d; however, regarding dosing, we all need to appreciate the differences between clinical trials (short-term studies with close supervision), use of B6 in epilepsy (high doses are warranted to prevent death and brain damage), and long-term unsupervised use (more likely—although still generally unlikely—to result in adverse effects). Of additional note regarding dosing is the observation that pyridoxine is commonly administered in doses 5-10 mg/kg/d for infants (up to 50 mg/kg/d of P5P[131]) and of 100-500 mg/d for children and adults with the seizure disorder "pyridoxine-dependent epilepsy" (of note: to correct the unfortunate error in the naming of this condition, the name should have been "pyridoxine-responsive epilepsy" or "epilepsy of pyridoxine dependency"). Patients with B6-dependent epilepsy have a gene defect that causes accumulation of a natural substance that blocks the function of P5P; this coenzyme inhibition is overpowered via daily megadosing of B6.[132]

- **Effects of pyridoxine supplementation on severity, frequency and duration of migraine attacks in migraine patients with aura.** (*Iran J Neurol.* 2015 Apr[133]): "This double-blind randomized clinical trial study was conducted on 66 patients with migraine with aura (MA)... Patients were randomly allocated to receive either pyridoxine supplements (80 mg pyridoxine per day) or placebo.... Pyridoxine supplementation led to a significant decrease in headache severity, attacks duration, and HDR (headache diary results) compared with placebo, but was not effective on the frequency of migraine attacks. CONCLUSION: Pyridoxine supplementation in patients with MA was effective on headache severity, attacks duration and HDR, but did not affect the frequency of migraine attacks."

- **Antiseizure benefit of pyridoxine administration in an infant with normal blood levels of pyridoxine and deficient brain levels of GABA** (*Neuropediatrics.* 1992 Oct[134]): "In an infant with typical pyridoxine-dependent seizures, CSF GABA level, was determined before treatment with pyridoxine. Before onset of treatment, level of GABA in CSF was highly lowered (16 pmol/ml), pyridoxine level in serum was within normal range. Immediately after application of 80 mg pyridoxine fits stopped and the EEG was without seizure activity. The data substantiate previous findings in brain tissue from a patient with pyridoxine-dependent seizures. They are proof of a disturbed GABA metabolism in pyridoxine dependent seizures."

- **Pyridoxine deficiency is extremely common in adult patients with severe epilepsy.** (*Epilepsy Behav.* 2015 Nov[135]): "An 8-year-old girl treated at our facility for superrefractory status epilepticus was found to have a low pyridoxine level at 5microg/L. After starting pyridoxine supplementation, improvement in the EEG for a 24-hour period was seen. ... All but six [of 81] patients admitted for status epilepticus [SE] had low normal or undetectable pyridoxine levels. A selective pyridoxine deficiency was seen in 94% of patients with status epilepticus (compared to 39.4% in the outpatients) which leads us to believe that there is a relationship between status epilepticus and pyridoxine levels." Very clearly, all seizure/epilepsy patients must be tested for vitamin B6 deficiency and/or treated empirically with pyridoxine; relatedly and very importantly, several anti-seizure medications cause deficiency of folic acid and/or vitamin D—deficiency of either can promote seizure. Thus, testing for serum pyridoxine, homocysteine, and 25-OH-vitamin D should be mandatory in all seizure/epilepsy patients; empiric nutritional treatment is safe and provides collateral benefits.

- **Pyridoxine lowers serum/blood glutamate levels** (*Am J Clin Nutr* 1992 Apr[136]): "Initially, the plasma PLP concentration of the subjects was 45 ± 2 nmol/L ... and after 7 d of oral supplementation with 27 mg PN-HC1 it reached 377 nmol/L. This represented an 8.5-fold increase from the initial concentration (P < 0.0001).

[129] Baxter P. Pyridoxine-dependent seizures: a clinical and biochemical conundrum. *Biochim Biophys Acta.* 2003 Apr 11;1647(1-2):36-41

[130] Lewis PJ. Pain in the hand and wrist. Pyridoxine supplements may help patients with carpal tunnel syndrome. *BMJ.* 1995 Jun 10;310(6993):1534

[131] Wang HS et al. Pyridoxal phosphate is better than pyridoxine for controlling idiopathic intractable epilepsy. Arch Dis Child. 2005 May;90(5):512-5

[132] The gene defect leads to reduced activity of antiquitin which would leads to accumulation of L-alpha-aminoadipic semialdehyde (L-AASA) and its reciprocal L-alpha-piperideine 6-carboxylate (P6C), the latter of which inhibits P5P. Mills et al. Genotypic and phenotypic spectrum of pyridoxine-dependent epilepsy (ALDH7A1 deficiency). *Brain.* 2010 Jul;133(Pt 7):2148-59

[133] Sadeghi et al. Effects of pyridoxine supplementation on severity, frequency and duration of migraine attacks in migraine patients with aura. *Iran J Neurol.* 2015 Apr 4;14:74-80

[134] Kurlemann et al. Disturbance of GABA metabolism in pyridoxine-dependent seizures. *Neuropediatrics.* 1992 Oct;23(5):257-9

[135] Dave et al. Pyridoxine deficiency in adult patients with status epilepticus. Epilepsy Behav. 2015 Nov;52(Pt A):154-8

[136] Kang-Yoon SA, Kirksey A. Relation of short-term pyridoxine-HCl supplementation to plasma vitamin B-6 vitamers and amino acid concentrations in young women. *Am J Clin Nutr.* 1992 Apr;55(4):865-72

PLP concentration remained essentially unchanged as long as PN supplementation was continued; after 14 d of vitamin supplementation the plasma PLP concentration was 429 ± 16 nmol/L. The increase in plasma PLP concentrations of individuals ranged from 400% to 1400% after supplementation. The concentration of plasma glutamic acid decreased 31% in the supplemented group after 7d of supplementation and 47% after 14 d of supplementation compared with the unsupplemented group." This very important study shows that supplementation with 27mg per day of synthetic pyridoxine hydrochloride raised blood levels of the pyridoxine and the active phosphorylated form P5P—pyridoxal-5-phosphate. Important for patients with migraine, chronic pain and seizures is the fact that serum glutamate levels were reduced by 31%. The authors somewhat erroneously describe 27 mg as a "large oral dose"; most nutritional doctors comfortably and frequently use doses of 50 to 250 to 500 mg per day of pyridoxine. Also noteworthy is that 2 of 10 of the patients showed moderate elevations—not reductions—in serum glutamate. Magnesium (typical adult dose is 600 mg/d) should always be supplemented when vitamin B6 is used. Also of high importance is the fact that—although this study showed clear safety and effectiveness for lowering blood levels of glutamate—levels of glutamate that surround the brain in the CSF were not measured.

- Vitamin administration improves the analgesic efficacy of pharmacotherapy with diclofenac following knee surgery (*Drug Res* 2013 Jun[137]): "Forty eight patients programmed to total knee arthroplasty with a pain level =7 in a 1-10 cm visual analogue scale were allocated to receive a single intramuscular injection of sodium diclofenac (75 mg) alone or combined with thiamine (100 mg), pyridoxine (100 mg) and cyanocobalamin (5 mg), and the pain level was evaluated during 12 h post-injection. Diclofenac+B vitamins mixture showed a superior analgesic effect during the assessed period and also a better assessment of the pain relief perception by patients than diclofenac alone."

- Pyridoxine (vitamin B6) alleviates neuropsychiatric aspects of premenstrual syndrome (*J R Coll Gen Pract.* 1989 Sep[138]): "A randomized double-blind crossover trial was conducted to study the effects of pyridoxine (vitamin B6) at a dose of 50 mg per day on symptoms characteristic of the premenstrual syndrome. ...In these women a significant beneficial effect (P less than 0.05) of pyridoxine was observed on emotional type symptoms (depression, irritability and tiredness)."

- Vitamin D3 (cholecalciferol): All patients with persistent pain must be tested for non-optimal vitamin D status and empirically treated with vitamin D3 to optimize serum vitamin D.[139,140] Failure to assess and correct vitamin D deficiency and implement effective correction in patients with persistent pain is medical-professional negligence; the data is very clear on the induction of chronic and often debilitating pain by vitamin D deficiency and the merits of vitamin D supplementation in alleviating pain. Several case reports have documented the effectiveness of vitamin D supplementation in the treatment and prevention of migraine.[141,142] Vitamin D is

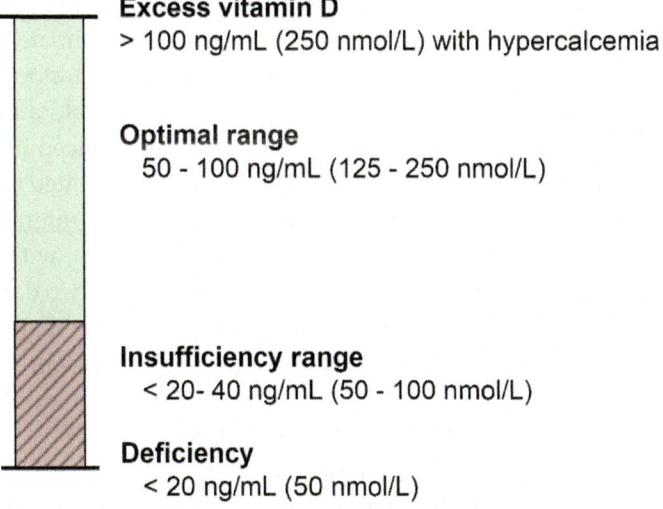

Excess vitamin D
> 100 ng/mL (250 nmol/L) with hypercalcemia

Optimal range
50 - 100 ng/mL (125 - 250 nmol/L)

Insufficiency range
< 20- 40 ng/mL (50 - 100 nmol/L)

Deficiency
< 20 ng/mL (50 nmol/L)

Image © 2004-2015 by Vasquez A in "**Functional Inflammology, volume 1**" published 2014 and "**Inflammation Mastery, 4th Edition**" published 2015. See InflammationMastery.com/reprints for Dr Vasquez's original paper Vasquez et al. The clinical importance of vitamin D (cholecalciferol): a paradigm shift with implications for all healthcare providers. *Altern Ther.Health Med.* 2004 Sep-Oct

---

[137] Magaña-Villa et al. B-vitamin mixture improves the analgesic effect of diclofenac in patients with osteoarthritis: a double blind study. *Drug Res.* 2013 Jun;63(6):289-92

[138] Doll H, Brown S, Thurston A, Vessey M. Pyridoxine (vitamin B6) and the premenstrual syndrome: a randomized crossover trial. *J R Coll Gen Pract.* 1989 Sep;39(326):364-8

[139] Moore D, Wahl R, Levy P. Hypovitaminosis D presenting as diffuse myalgia in a 22-year-old woman: a case report. *J Emerg Med.* 2014 Jun;46(6):e155-8

[140] "The findings suggest a role of low vitamin D levels for heightened central sensitivity, particularly augmented pain processing upon mechanical stimulation in chronic pain patients." von Känel et al. Vitamin D and central hypersensitivity in patients with chronic pain. *Pain Med.* 2014 Sep;15(9):1609-18

[141] "Therapeutic replacement with vitamin D and calcium resulted in a dramatic reduction in the frequency and duration of their migraine headaches." Thys-Jacobs S. Alleviation of migraines with therapeutic vitamin D and calcium. *Headache.* 1994 Nov-Dec;34(10):590-2

[142] "These observations suggest that vitamin D and calcium therapy should be considered in the treatment of migraine headaches." Thys-Jacobs S. Vitamin D and calcium in menstrual migraine. *Headache.* 1994 Oct;34(9):544-6

anti-inflammatory (including reductions in glial activation) and immunomodulatory[143] and also modulates vascular tone by reducing intracellular hypercalcinosis.[144] Reasonable replacement doses are 2,000 IU per day for children and 4,000 IU per day for adults; monitoring serum calcium ensures safety. Optimal vitamin D status correlates with serum 25(OH)D levels of 50-100 ng/mL, or 125-250 nmol/L—see our review article for more details[145]; levels greater than 100 ng/mL are unnecessary and increase the risk of hypercalcemia.

- 5-Hydroxytryptophan (5-HTP)—typical dose is 50-300 mg per day in divided doses: 5-Hydroxytryptophan (5-HTP) is a natural constituent of the human body and is also found in some plants and is thus available as a nutritional supplement. Altered serotonin metabolism has been observed in headache patients, and this observation serves to support the use of selective serotonin reuptake inhibitors (SSRIs) in headache patients, while supplementation with 5-HTP increases serotonin levels naturally. Among various types of headache, migraine would be expected to show the best response to 5-HTP because the conversion of serotonin to melatonin would extend the benefits of serotonin-mediated analgesia to include the protection of mitochondrial function, an important benefit of melatonin.

> **Tryptophan/serotonin insufficiency & glial activation: common in migraine, chronic pain, and fibromyalgia**
>
> "The recently shown **high prevalence of migraine in the population of fibromyalgia sufferers**, suggests a common ground shared by fibromyalgia and migraine. Migraine has been demonstrated to be characterized by a defect in the serotonergic and adrenergic systems. A parallel dramatic failure of serotonergic systems and a defect of adrenergic transmission have been evidenced to affect fibromyalgia sufferers, too."
>
> Nicolodi M, Sicuteri F. Fibromyalgia and migraine, two faces of the same mechanism. Serotonin as the common clue. *Adv Exp Med Biol.* 1996;398:373-9

Conversion of serotonin to melatonin occurs in non-migraine headaches but is of lesser therapeutic importance since these disorders (cluster headaches excepted) are not associated directly with mitochondrial dysfunction. 5-HTP has a better safety and efficacy profile than does the drug methysergide in the treatment of migraine according to a study of 124 adults and children with migraine.[146]

- Vitamin E supplementation with mixed tocopherols 400-1,200 IU/d: As noted previously, free radicals and prostaglandins contribute to migraine pathophysiology; both are reduced by administration of supplemental doses of vitamin E.[147] Vitamin E—known chemically as tocopherol—is present in several forms, arguably the most important of which is the gamma form; most nutritionally competent clinicians generally recommend that vitamin E supplementation contain approximately 40% gamma tocopherol. Another form of vitamin E with more specificity for enhancing/protecting mitochondrial function is known as tocopherol succinate; a combination of various tocopherols is reasonable and is likely to produce enhanced therapeutic efficacy. Isoprostanes are lipid-derrived mediators produced in direct proportion to free radical burden; isoprostanes directly trigger pain and their production is inhibited by antioxidant protection, especially with vitamin E.

  - Vitamin E for the treatment of menstrual migraine. (*Med Sci Monit.* 2009 Jan[148]): "During a placebo-controlled double-blinded trial, 72 women with menstrual migraine received placebo (identical in appearance to vitamin E) daily for five days, two days before to three days after menstruation for two cycles followed by a one-month wash-out and one vitamin E softgel (400 IU) daily for five days in the next two cycles. ... There were statistically significant differences in the pain severity and functional disability scales between the placebo and the vitamin E treatments. Vitamin E effect was also superior to placebo regarding photophobia, phonophobia, and nausea. CONCLUSIONS: Vitamin E is effective in relieving symptoms due to menstrual migraine."

- Combination nutritional supplementation: Patients with migraine show multiple abnormalities in metabolism, inflammation, and oxidative stress; as expected therefore, multi-nutrient supplementation shows benefits via numerous mechanisms.

---

[143] Timms et al. Circulating MMP9, vitamin D and variation in the TIMP-1 response with VDR genotype. *QJM.* 2002 Dec;95(12):787-96
[144] Vasquez A. Intracellular Hypercalcinosis. *Naturopathy Digest* 2006 September naturopathydigest.com/archives/2006/sep/vasquez.php
[145] Vasquez et al. The Clinical Importance of Vitamin D (Cholecalciferol). *Alternative Therapies in Health Med* 2004; 10: 28-37. ichnfm.academia.edu/AlexVasquez
[146] "The most beneficial effect of 5-HTP appears to be felt with regard to the intensity and duration rather than the frequency of the attacks... These results suggest that 5-HTP could be a treatment of choice in the prophylaxis of migraine." Titus et al. 5-Hydroxytryptophan versus methysergide in prophylaxis of migraine. *Eur Neurol.*1986; 25:327-329
[147] Shaik MM, Gan SH. Vitamin supplementation as possible prophylactic treatment against migraine with aura and menstrual migraine. *Biomed Res Int.* 2015;2015:469529
[148] Ziaei S, Kazemnejad A, Sedighi A. The effect of vitamin E on the treatment of menstrual migraine. *Med Sci Monit.* 2009 Jan;15(1):CR16-9

- <u>Alleviation of migraine symptoms with a supplement containing riboflavin, magnesium, Q10, and other nutrients.</u> (*J Headache Pain.* 2015 Dec[149]): "130 adult migraineurs (age 18 - 65 years) with ≥ three migraine attacks per month were randomized into two treatment groups: dietary supplementation or placebo in a double-blind fashion." The product contained "400 mg riboflavin (vitamin B2), 600 mg magnesium, 150 mg coenzyme Q10 along with a multivitamin/trace elements combination per 4 capsules. The amount of additional multivitamin/trace elements per 4 capsules is as follows: 750 mcg vitamin A, 200 mg vitamin C, 134 mg, vitamin E, 5 mg thiamin, 20 mg niacin, 5 mg vitamin B6, 6 mcg vitamin B12, 400 mcg folic acid, 5 mcg vitamin D, 10 mg pantothenic acid, 165 mcg biotin, 0.8 mg iron, 5 mg zinc, 2 mg manganese, 0.5 mg copper, 30 mcg chromium, 60 mcg molybdenum, 50 mcg selenium, 5 mg bioflavonoids." "Migraine days per month declined from 6.2 days during the baseline period to 4.4 days at the end of the treatment with the supplement and from 6.2.days to 5.2 days in the placebo group. The intensity of migraine pain was significantly reduced in the supplement group compared to placebo. The sum score of the HIT-6 questionnaire was reduced by 4.8 points from 61.9 to 57.1 compared to 2 points in the placebo-group. The evaluation of efficacy by the patient was better in the supplementation group compared to placebo."

- <u>Use of a pine bark extract and antioxidant vitamin combination product as therapy for migraine refractory to pharmacologic medication.</u> (*Headache.* 2006 May[150]): "Twelve patients with a long-term history of migraine with and without aura who had failed to respond to multiple treatments with beta-blockers, antidepressants, anticonvulsants, and 5-hydroxytryptamine receptor agonists were selected for the study. They were treated with 10 capsules of an antioxidant formulation of 120 mg pine bark extract, 60 mg vitamin C, and 30 IU vitamin E in each capsule daily for 3 months. ... There was a significant mean improvement in migraine disability assessment (MIDAS) score of 50.6% for the 3-month treatment period compared with the 3 months prior to baseline. The treatment was also associated with significant reductions in number of headache days and headache severity score. Mean number of headache days was reduced from 44.4 days at baseline to 26.0 days after 3 months' therapy and mean headache severity was reduced from 7.5 of 10 to 5.5. CONCLUSION: These data suggest that the antioxidant therapy used in this study may be beneficial in the treatment of migraine possibly reducing headache frequency and severity."

Infections & Dysbiosis Patients with migraine have a higher-than-average prevalence of gastric infection with *H. pylori*, and significant symptomatic improvement is obtained following eradication of *H pylori* in these patients, according to two studies[151,152] and refuted by two others.[153,154] As usual, gastrointestinal dysbiosis should be assessed and corrected on a *per patient* (rather than *per disease*) basis—see Chapter 4 of *Integrative Rheumatology / Functional Inflammology* for details and interventions. For patients with recalcitrant headaches (and for those seeking comprehensive whole-patient health care), assessment of digestion, absorption, and gastrointestinal microecology is a reasonable component of evaluation that can help guide treatment. Although *Helicobacter pylori* is a common inhabitant of the human gastrointestinal tract (found in more than 50% of Americans over age 50), immunologic responses to the organism can range from nonreactive on one end of the spectrum to diverse diseases like chronic gastritis, chronic urticaria, autoimmune thrombocytopenia, or reactive arthritis on the more severe and systemic end of the spectrum. Thus, the host-microbe relationship is of greater significance than the identity and microbiological characteristics of the microbe. As a Gram-negative bacterium that produces endotoxin (LPS), the obvious means by which *H pylori* can contribute to migraine is via LTR-4 mediated systemic inflammation and microglial activation.

---

[149] Gaul et al. Improvement of migraine symptoms with a proprietary supplement containing riboflavin, magnesium and Q10: a randomized, placebo-controlled, double-blind, multicenter trial. *J Headache Pain.* 2015 Dec;16:516

[150] Chayasirisobhon S. Use of a pine bark extract and antioxidant vitamin combination product as therapy for migraine in patients refractory to pharmacologic medication. *Headache.* 2006 May;46(5):788-93

[151] "H. pylori is common in subjects with migraine. Bacterium eradication causes a significant decrease in attacks of migraine. The reduction of vasoactive substances produced during infection may be the pathogenetic mechanism underlying the phenomenon." Gasbarrini et al. Beneficial effects of Helicobacter pylori eradication on migraine. *Hepatogastroenterology.* 1998 May-Jun;45(21):765-70

[152] "Helicobacter pylori should be examined in migranous patients and eradication of the infection may be helpful for the treatment of the disease." Tunca et al. Is Helicobacter pylori infection a risk factor for migraine? A case-control study. *Acta Neurol Belg.* 2004 Dec;104(4):161-4

[153] "Our study suggests that chronic Helicobacter pylori infection is not more frequent in patients with migraine than in controls and that infection does not modify clinical features of the disease." Pinessi et al. Chronic Helicobacter pylori infection and migraine: a case-control study. *Headache.* 2000 Nov-Dec;40(10):836-9

[154] "In conclusion, our results do not support any specific correlation between Hp infection and migraine." Ciancarelli et al. Helicobacter pylori infection and migraine. *Cephalalgia.* 2002 Apr;22(3):222-5

Nutritional Immunomodulation Migraine is most essentially viewed as a combination of mitochondrial dysfunction and glial activation—those two primary components are fundamental, consistent, and explanatory of nearly all other permutations— resulting in physiologic fragility and sensitivity toward (intolerance of) otherwise minor "subclinical" or "subsymptomatic" stressors such as dietary, hormonal, and environmental stressors. With regard to immunohyperresponsiveness—specifically in this case the glial activation, treatments to reduce neuroinflammation should be implemented, such as vitamin D, anti-inflammatory polyphenolics, resveratrol, the n3 fatty acids EPA and DHA, etc. For patients with overt systemic inflammation, allergy, and/or autoimmunity, a more comprehensive antiinflammatory protocol can and should be implemented, especially 1) identifying and removing the inflammatory triggers, and 2) promoting immunotolerance with the complete nutritional immunomodulation protocol outlined in Chapter 4, Section 3. Elevated homocysteine can promote microglial activation, and reducing homocysteine levels with nutritional supplementation is indicated for hyperhomocysteinemic migraineurs as described in protocol component #5: *Style of Living and Special Considerations*.

Dysmetabolism & Mitochondrial Dysfunction We must appreciate that migraine is a multifaceted phenomenon with neuroemotional, structural, allergic-immunologic-inflammatory, and mitochondrial components. With regard to the latter, we can understand migraine from the perspective of defects in the mitochondrial electron transport chain (ETC), namely **NADH-dehydrogenase**, **citrate synthase** and **cytochrome-c-oxidase**; defects in **NADH-cytochrome-c-reductase** appear to be specific to migraine with aura.[155] Thus, not surprisingly, nutrients which are intimately involved with these steps of the ETC have shown impressive efficacy in the treatment and prevention of migraine via the Le Chatelier principle which states—from the perspective of orthomolecular nutrition—that metabolic defects can be compensated for by the administration of supraphysiologic quantities of nutrients to push defective pathways toward completion; this is a main component of Linus Pauling's orthomolecular concept[156] (ie, that using the right molecules in the right amounts can optimize health by optimizing biochemistry and metabolism, as most recently and authoritatively reviewed by his colleague Bruce Ames in a masterful review.[157] In the case of migraine, we are bypassing or compensating for defects in mitochondrial function by supplying supraphysiologic doses of the nutrients involved in those pathways with the end result being enhancement/restoration/normalization/optimization of

> **The evidence of mitochondrial dysfunction in migraine is strong, consistent and irrefutable**
>
> 1. Biochemical evidence: High intracellular calcium, excessive production of free radicals, low activity of superoxide dismutase, activation of cytochrome-c oxidase and nitric oxide, high levels of lactate and pyruvate, and low ratios of phosphocreatine-inorganic phosphate and "deficient oxidative phosphorylation, which ultimately causes energy failure in neurons and astrocytes, thus triggering migraine mechanisms, including spreading depression."
> 2. Cellular, histologic evidence: Muscle biopsy shows ragged red fibers, accumulation of giant mitochondria with paracrystalline inclusions
> 3. Genetic evidence: Various mitochondrial DNA polymorphisms/mutations have been demonstrated
> 4. Therapeutic evidence: "Several agents that have a positive effect on mitochondrial metabolism have shown to be effective in the treatment of migraines. The agents include riboflavin (B2), coenzyme Q10, magnesium, niacin, carnitine, topiramate, and lipoic acid."
>
> Yorns WR Jr, Hardison HH. Mitochondrial dysfunction in migraine. *Semin Pediatr Neurol.* 2013 Sep;20:188-93

mitochondrial function. In the world of nutritional medicine, we would probably not be familiar with these concepts were it not for the independent and synergistic works of Roger Williams, Linus Pauling, Jeff Bland, and Bruce Ames; to these men do we owe gratitude for our understanding of this phenomenon and its clinical application. Furthermore however, we must also appreciate that nutrients have numerous functions and *affect* and *effect* numerous (not singular) pathways and processes, such that a "mitochondrial nutrient" may exert its action via a *non-mitochondrial* effect, as mentioned per nutrient in the itemized section that follows:

- CoQ10—100-400 mg per day: CoQ10 supplementation significantly reduces migraine headache frequency, duration, and intensity.[158] As shown in the diagram below, CoQ10 shuttles electrons from Complex 1 to Complex 2, and from "Complex 2" to Complex 3. Thus, CoQ10 supplementation helps to bypass defects in the electron transport chain (ETC) of mitochondria to promote, preserve, and protect optimal cellular energy/ATP

---

[155] "NADH-dehydrogenase, citrate synthase and cytochrome-c-oxidase activities in both patient groups were significantly lower than in controls, while NADH-cytochrome-c-reductase activity was reduced in migraine with aura." Sangiorgi et al. Abnormal platelet mitochondrial function in migraine with and without aura. *Cephalalgia* 1994 Feb; 21-3
[156] Pauling L. Orthomolecular psychiatry. Varying concentrations of substances normally present in human body may control mental disease. *Science.* 1968 Apr 19;160:265-71
[157] Ames et al. High-dose vitamin therapy stimulates variant enzymes with decreased coenzyme binding affinity (increased K(m)). *Am J Clin Nutr.* 2002 Apr;75(4):616-58
[158] Rozen et al. Open label trial of coenzyme Q10 as a migraine preventive. *Cephalalgia* 2002;22(2):137-41

production. Furthermore, research by Folkers et al[159] strongly suggests that CoQ10 has an anti-allergy and immunomodulatory role; thus the anti-migraine benefits of CoQ10 may be mediated via immunomodulation in addition to enhancement of mitochondrial function.

- <u>Riboflavin (vitamin B2)—50-400 mg per day</u>: Flavin adenine dinucleotide (FAD) is required at Complex 2 of the ETC. High-dose vitamin B2 shows "high efficacy, excellent tolerability, and low cost" in the prevention of migraine headaches.[160] The standard dose for riboflavin in the treatment of migraine is 400 mg taken orally each morning; identical or lower doses can be used in children and/or when riboflavin is used with other nutrients such as CoQ10, magnesium, etc. Riboflavin is safe and effective for long-term use in children and adults[161]; riboflavin is also effective in the long-term treatment of the migraine variant condition known as cyclic vomiting syndrome (CVS) in children.[162] So-called "B vitamins" such as riboflavin—as with zinc and iron— should always be taken with food to avoid the nausea that commonly occurs when vitamins are taken on an empty stomach; other vitamins such as vitamins A, D, and E are generally well tolerated on an empty stomach.
  - <u>Riboflavin prophylaxis in pediatric and adolescent migraine. (*J Headache Pain*. 2009 Oct[163])</u>: "This retrospective study reports on our experience of using riboflavin for migraine prophylaxis in 41 pediatric and adolescent patients, who received 200 or 400 mg/day single oral dose of riboflavin for 3, 4 or 6 months. ... In conclusion, riboflavin seems to be a well-tolerated, effective, and low-cost prophylactic treatment in children and adolescents suffering from migraine."
- <u>Acetyl-L-Carnitine—1,000-2,000 mg taken twice daily between meals</u>: The amino acid L-carnitine is necessary for fatty acid transport into the mitochondria for oxidative metabolism and energy production. Deficiency of or metabolic inability to use carnitine can precipitate or perpetuate migraine headaches, which can be alleviated by carnitine supplementation.[164] As a natural component of the human diet, carnitine has a wide safety margin, and supplemental doses of 2-4 g/d are commonly used; acetyl-L-carnitine is generally the preferred form. Carnitine and acetyl-carnitine provide best benefit when combined with other nutrients, especially CoQ10, magnesium, and lipoic acid. A study in 2015 using 3 grams per day of acetyl-carnitine as monotherapy showed no benefit in the treatment of migraine[165]; one possibility is that 3 grams per day of acetyl-carnitine as monotherapy is an excessive dose. A study using magnesium 500 mg/d and/or carnitine 500 mg/d showed benefit in all groups.[166]
- <u>Lipoic acid—300 mg twice-thrice daily</u>: Lipoic (thiotic) acid is an essential component of the pyruvate dehydrogenase complex, is a potent antioxidant, and it also inhibits NFkB-mediated inflammation. A placebo-controlled clinical trial showed benefit of lipoic acid (600 mg/d) supplementation in migraine patients.[167]
- <u>Melatonin—5-20 mg at night</u>: As mentioned previously, melatonin is a potent protector of mitochondrial function, which has been demonstrated in experimental models of mitochondrial inhibition by bacterial endotoxin. As a powerful antioxidant, melatonin scavenges oxygen and nitrogen-based reactants generated in mitochondria and thereby limits the loss of the intramitochondrial glutathione; this prevents mitochondrial protein and DNA damage. Melatonin increases the activity of Complexes 1 and 4 of the ETC, promoting mitochondrial ATP synthesis under various physiological/experimental conditions.[168]
- <u>Niacin, including inositol hexaniacinate and niacinamide—dose varies per type used</u>: High-dose niacin alleviates migraine headaches and headaches of various etiologies, whether administered orally,

---

[159] Ye CQ, Folkers K, et al. A modified determination of coenzyme Q10 in human blood and CoQ10 blood levels in diverse patients with allergies. *Biofactors*. 1988 Dec;1:303-6

[160] Schoenen J, Jacquy J, Lenaerts M. Effectiveness of high-dose riboflavin in migraine prophylaxis. A randomized controlled trial. *Neurology* 1998;50(2):466-70

[161] Sherwood M, Goldman RD. Effectiveness of riboflavin in pediatric migraine prevention. *Can Fam Physician*. 2014 Mar;60(3):244-6

[162] "They received prophylactic monotherapy with riboflavin for at least 12 months. Excellent response and tolerability was observed." Martinez-Esteve Melnikova et al. Riboflavin in cyclic vomiting syndrome: efficacy in three children. *Eur J Pediatr*. 2015 Jul 31. [Epub ahead of print]

[163] Condò et al. Riboflavin prophylaxis in pediatric and adolescent migraine. *J Headache Pain*. 2009 Oct;10(5):361-5

[164] Kabbouche et al. Carnitine palmityltransferase II (CPT2) deficiency and migraine headache: two case reports. *Headache*. 2003 May;43(5):490-5

[165] "After a four-week run-in-phase, 72 participants were randomized to receive either placebo or 3 g acetyl-l-carnitine for 12 weeks. ...In this triple-blind crossover study no differences were found in headache outcomes between acetyl-l-carnitine and placebo. Our results do not provide evidence of benefit for efficacy of acetyl-l-carnitine as prophylactic treatment for migraine." Hagen et al. Acetyl-l-carnitine versus placebo for migraine prophylaxis: A randomized, triple-blind, crossover study. *Cephalalgia*. 2015 Oct;35(11):987-95

[166] "In this clinical trial, 133 migrainous patients were randomly assigned into three intervention groups: magnesium oxide (500 mg/day), L-carnitine (500 mg/day), and Mg-L-carnitine (500 mg/day magnesium and 500 mg/day L-carnitine), and a control group. .. Oral supplementation with magnesium oxide and L-carnitine and concurrent supplementation of Mg-L-carnitine besides routine treatments could be effective in migraine prophylaxis; however, larger trials are needed to confirm these preliminary findings." Tarighat Esfanjani et al. The effects of magnesium, L-carnitine, and concurrent magnesium-L-carnitine supplementation in migraine prophylaxis. *Biol Trace Elem Res*. 2012 Dec;150(1-3):42-8

[167] Magis D, Ambrosini A, et al. A randomized double-blind placebo-controlled trial of thioctic acid in migraine prophylaxis. *Headache*. 2007 Jan;47(1):52-7

[168] León J, Acuña-Castroviejo D, Escames G, Tan DX, Reiter RJ. Melatonin mitigates mitochondrial malfunction. *J Pineal Res*. 2005 Jan;38(1):1-9

intramuscularly, or intravenously; niacin can also be used to halt acute migraine attacks.[169,170] Niacinamide adenine dinucleotide (NADH) is an essential component of the first stage (Complex 1) of the ETC, a step that is commonly defective in migraine patients. High-dose niacin facilitates this step and thus enhances energy production. Another anti-migraine benefit of high-dose niacin is its sparing effect on tryptophan, allowing its conversion to serotonin. Niacin also has a vasodilating action and may thereby address the vasculogenic component of headache. Efficacious oral doses of niacin can range from 300 to 1500 mg/d; lower doses are used for children. High-dose niacin, particularly in time-released tablets, presents some risk for hepatic damage, and thus safer forms of niacin such as plain niacin, slow-release niacin (e.g., Niaspan®), and inositol hexaniacinate are preferred; niacinamide and NADH might also be efficacious but neither has vasodilating actions provided by the other forms of niacin. Doses of niacin exceeding 500 to 1000 mg/d are probably unnecessary in headache patients if other treatments such as coenzyme Q10 (CoQ10), vitamin D, and fatty acids are being used; before implementing high-dose niacin, patients should be selected, informed, and monitored appropriately.

- Oxygen: One-hundred percent oxygen delivered by facial mask at 8 L/min for 10 minutes can help abort an attack of cluster headache. Oxygen is the required electron and proton acceptor of the mitochondrial electron transport chain (ETC) for ATP production; thus, supraphysiologic oxygen, like supraphysiologic doses of mitochondria-specific nutrients, generally improves mitochondrial energy (ATP) production. The model of pain sensitization in so-called "chronic pain syndromes"—specifically migraine, cluster headache, fibromyalgia, myofascial pain syndrome and complex regional pain syndrome (CRPS)—that I have developed includes a tripartite vicious cycle of mitochondrial dysfunction, glial activation, and neuronal hyperexcitation, all of which promote brain inflammation, central sensitization, and perpetuation and amplification of pain. Strong support for this model comes from both its biochemical and physiologic rationale as well as the efficacy of corresponding treatments that address each of the main components: mitochondrial dysfunction, glial activation, neuronal hyperexcitation, brain inflammation.

  Appreciation of the efficacy of oxygen therapy—whether as normobaric (more available and affordable) or hyperbaric (more effective and more expensive; hyperbaric oxygen therapy [HBOT])—in various pain states invites us to revisit the naturopathic profession's hierarchy of therapeutics. Symptomatic therapy clearly has a role in patient care but, in order to avoid repeated use of urgent/emergency care and the creation of unnecessary medical dependency, repeated acute care or even "maintenance therapy" should never replace treatment of the underlying cause(s). Patients need to receive treatment aimed at the underlying pathophysiology so that health is optimized and patients are moved toward better general well-being and disease-specific health. Oxygen therapy is abortive of pain and shows some contribution to breaking the vicious cycles of mitochondrial impairment (immediate treatment of headaches, current-prospective treatment of fibromyalgia and CRPS) but this therapy does not address the other aspects of mitochondrial dysfunction (e.g., CoQ10 deficiency) and does not address the cause (e.g., small intestine bacterial overgrowth [SIBO] in fibromyalgia) and therefore should remain as supplemental, abortive/acute, and adjunctive therapy not as the foundation of therapy. Obviously, hyperbaric therapy makes more money for doctors/clinics and—(except/including) when patients buy their own home hyperbaric units—will therefore receive more press and more endorsement than therapies that are curative and empowering (ie, autonomous, without medical dependence). Given that most patients with persistent inflammation and pain are antioxidant deficient and therefore at increased risk for oxygen toxicity (including subclinical damage), antioxidant repletion should occur prior to oxygen therapy; the idea of administering supraphysiologic doses of oxygen to pull more protons and electrons through an *already damaged* and *pro-inflammatory* and *ROS-generating* electron transport chain is not meritorious, although some will defend it—weakly—on the theoretic basis of hormesis.

  - High-flow oxygen therapy for all types of headache (*Am J Emerg Med* 2012 Nov[171]): "We performed a prospective, randomized, double-blinded, placebo-controlled trial of patients presenting to the ED with a chief complaint of headache. The patients were randomized to receive either 100% oxygen via nonrebreather mask at 15 L/min or the placebo treatment of room air via nonrebreather mask for 15 minutes in total. ... A total of 204 patients agreed to participate in the study and were randomized to the oxygen

[169] Velling DA, Dodick DW, Muir JJ. Sustained-release niacin for prevention of migraine headache. *Mayo Clin Proc.* 2003 Jun;78(6):770-1
[170] Prousky J, Seely D. The treatment of migraines and tension-type headaches with intravenous and oral niacin (nicotinic acid). *Nutr J.* 2005 Jan 26;4:3
[171] Ozkurt et al. Efficacy of high-flow oxygen therapy in all types of headache: a prospective, randomized, placebo-controlled trial. *Am J Emerg Med.* 2012 Nov;30(9):1760-4

(102 patients) and placebo (102 patients) groups. Patient headache types included tension (47%), migraine (27%), undifferentiated (25%), and cluster (1%). Patients who received oxygen therapy reported significant improvement in visual analog scale scores at all points when compared with placebo: 22 mm vs 11 mm at 15 minutes, 29 mm vs 13 mm at 30 minutes, and 55 mm vs 45 mm at 60 minutes. ... In addition to its role in the treatment of cluster headache, high-flow oxygen therapy may provide an effective treatment of all types of headaches in the ED setting.

- Oxygen (normobaric/hyperbaric) for migraine (*Headache* 1995 Apr[172]): "The purpose of this study was to compare the effects of hyperbaric oxygen and normobaric oxygen in migraine. Twenty migraineurs were divided randomly into two groups and studied in a hyperbaric chamber during a typical headache attack. ... One group received 100% oxygen at 1 atmosphere of pressure (normobaric) while the other received 100% oxygen at 2 atmospheres of pressure (hyperbaric). One of the 10 patients in the normobaric group achieved significant relief of headache symptoms, while 9 of 10 in the hyperbaric group found relief. Based on a chi-square test, this difference is significant at the P < .005 level. Those patients who did not find significant relief from normobaric oxygen were given hyperbaric oxygen as above. All nine found significant relief. The results suggest that hyperbaric (but not normobaric) oxygen may be useful in the abortive management of migraine headache. Possibilities for the mechanism of this effect, in addition to vasoconstriction, include an increase in the rate of energy-producing and neurotransmitter-related metabolic reactions in the brain which require molecular oxygen."

- Hyperbaric oxygen in the treatment of migraine with aura. (*Headache* 1998 Feb[173]): "Female subjects with confirmed migraine were randomly assigned to begin with either the control (100% oxygen, no pressure) or hyperbaric treatment (100% oxygen, pressure). ... Results suggest that hyperbaric oxygen treatment reduces migraine headache pain..."

- Minimal prophylactic/preventive effect of hyperbaric oxygen therapy on migraine. (*Cephalalgia* 2004 Aug[174]): Not surprisingly, this study found that prophylactic administration of oxygen was generally inefficacious in reducing future migraine attacks; while patients with migraine always have a basal level of mitochondrial dysfunction, oxygen administration does not prevent future attacks. Oxygen is of main value in the treatment of active migraine (and other headache) attacks.

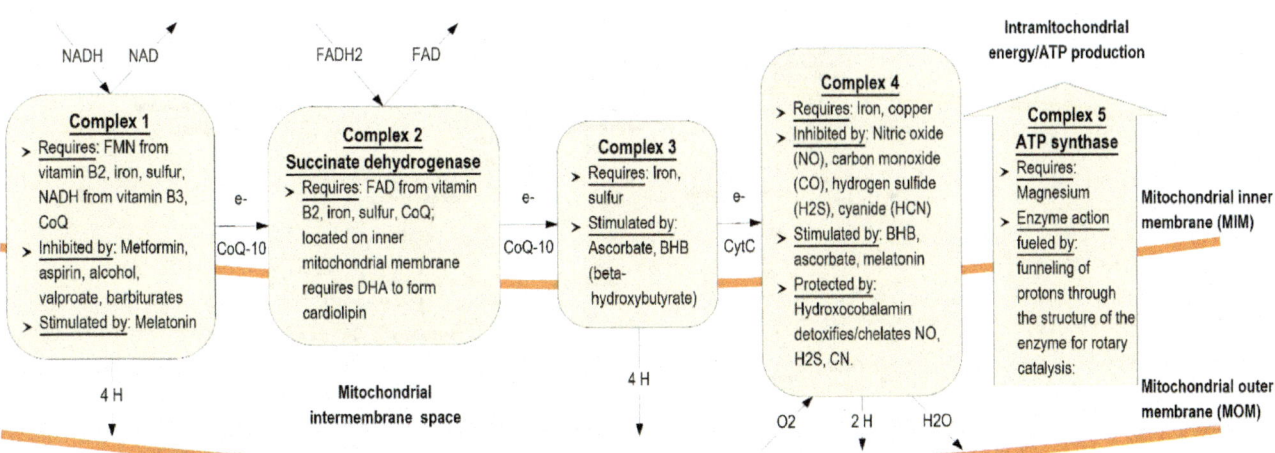

Mitochondrial ETC: Schematic diagram of the electron transport chain, function of which is wholly dependent upon niacin, riboflavin, CoQ10, iron, copper, and—to a lesser extent—vitamin C. Beyond showing where nutrients function in the ETC, this diagram also shows where drugs inhibit ETC function while endogenous substances such as melatonin and beta-hydroxybutyrate stimulate the ETC at complexes 1 and 4 (melatonin) and 3 and 4 (BHB), respectively. For thorough reviews of mitochondrial nutrition and mitochondrial medicine, see vimeo.com/ondemand/mitochondrialmedicine.

[172] Myers DE, Myers RA. A preliminary report on hyperbaric oxygen in the relief of migraine headache. *Headache*. 1995 Apr;35(4):197-9
[173] Wilson et al. Hyperbaric oxygen in the treatment of migraine with aura. *Headache*. 1998 Feb;38(2):112-5
[174] Eftedal et al. A randomized, double blind study of the prophylactic effect of hyperbaric oxygen therapy on migraine. *Cephalalgia*. 2004 Aug:639-44

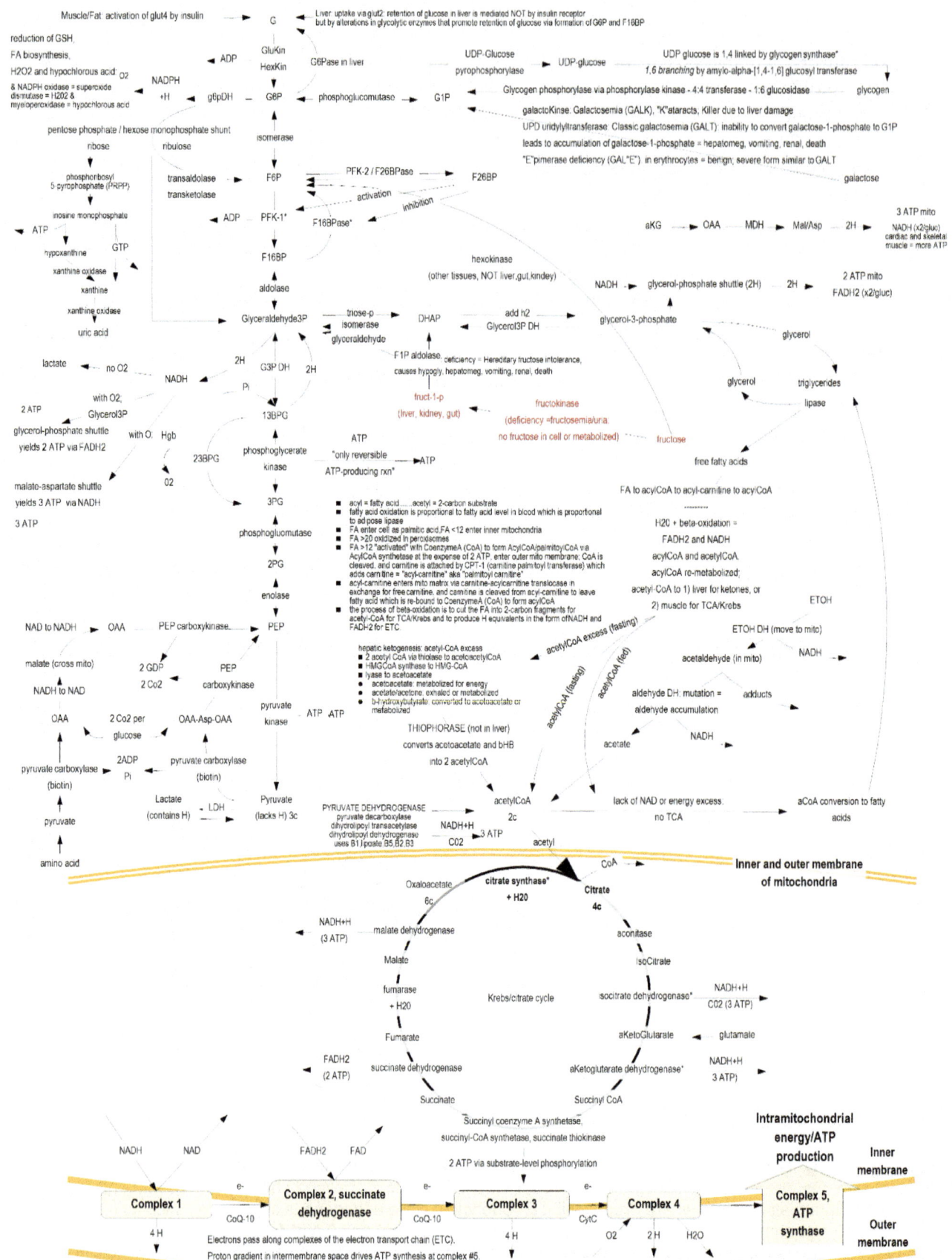

Schematic overview of glycolytic pathways, pyruvate dehydrogenase complex, the Krebs/citrate cycle, and the electron transport chain: Items in bold/red are those which are commonly defective in patients with migraine headaches (and fibromyalgia)—consult your biochemistry text as needed for details and definitions. Note from DrV: The origin of this diagram is from my first year of medical school, during which I created this diagram for my study notes and could recite it from memory.

Style of Living, Special Considerations, Surgical & Somatic/Spinal Treatments

- Style of living—lifestyle optimization: Patients with cluster headaches show a greater percentage of increased work-related stress, self-employment, tobacco smoking, and alcohol use or abuse. These concerns should be addressed per patient as indicated. Lifestyle factors such the standard American diet, overconsumption of caffeine and alcohol, and use of tobacco can result in mitochondrial impairment through various mechanisms, not the least of which are nutrient (especially magnesium) deficiency and accumulation of cyanide (from tobacco smoke), a known mitochondrial poison.

- Self-knowledge—psychological exploration of emotional tension: If someone has chronic "tension headaches" then the question becomes *"Why does this person have chronic tension?"* Generally, the answer is a combination of magnesium deficiency along with some underlying emotional issue(s). If someone feels compelled to maintain a static posture all day without taking a necessary and healthful break to stretch and relax, this suggests that they are over-focusing on their work at the expense of taking care of their body and health—this is not a sign of health, and it suggests an underlying compulsion or dissociation. Patients with cluster headaches show a greater percentage of increased work-related stress, self-employment, tobacco smoking and alcohol use and abuse.[175] Address as indicated.

> **Osteopathic treatment should include manual musculoskeletal medicine and nutritional interventions**
>
> "In contrast to the description of the osteopathic medical profession by the American Osteopathic Association, namely, "doctors of osteopathic medicine, or D.O.s, apply the philosophy of treating the whole person to the prevention, diagnosis and treatment of illness, disease and injury," [the authors of the article in question] essentially reviewed only pharmacologic treatment. ... It is hoped that future reviews in this journal can include a more balanced survey of the literature, inclusive of non-pharmacologic and "holistic" interventions that are consistent with osteopathic philosophy."
>
> **Vasquez A.** Interventions Need to be Consistent with Osteopathic Philosophy. [Letter] *JAOA: Journal of the American Osteopathic Association* 2006 Sep
> http://jaoa.org/cgi/content/full/106/9/528

- Stress reduction, relaxation and biofeedback: Biofeedback is proven effective in the prevention of chronic headaches, including pediatric migraine.[176,177] Relaxation and stress management are more effective than drug treatment with metoprolol for pediatric migraine.[178]

- Somatic treatments—cervical myofascial trigger points: Check the upper cervical spine musculature (especially suboccipital muscles and sternocleidomastoid) for the characteristic manifestations of myofascial trigger points (MFTP, see Chapter 3): palpable nodule, twitch response, and elicitation of referred pain with deep palpation/provocation. Myofascial trigger points are much more common in patients with migraine[179] than in non-headache controls, and they are an important cervicogenic contribution to chronic headaches.[180,181] If located, the MFTP can be effectively treated with in-office/at-home post-isometric stretching and exercises.[182]

> **Post-isometric stretching is of high value in the treatment of cervical MFTP that contribute to headache**
>
> If deep palpation of the upper cervical musculature produces referred pain to the head or face, then you know the patient has MFTP, and you can then treat them with at-home and in-office stretching and exercises. Generally their "chronic pain" will be greatly reduced within 3-10 days. Better results will be obtained with alkalinization and concomitant supplementation with magnesium, vitamin D, and fish oil.

- Somatic treatments—spinal manipulation: Myofascial, arthrogenic, and dyskinetic contributions to headache are significant, and these cervicogenic problems can be addressed with manual spinal and myofascial manipulation. Spinal manipulation can help alleviate headaches with efficacy comparable to commonly used

---

[175] Manzoni GC. Cluster headache and lifestyle: remarks on a population of 374 male patients. *Cephalalgia* 1999 Mar;19(2):88-94

[176] Scharff L, Marcus DA, Masek BJ. A controlled study of minimal-contact thermal biofeedback treatment in children with migraine. *J Pediatr Psychol.*2002; 27:109 –119

[177] "Feedback training was accompanied by significant reduction of cortical excitability. This was probably responsible for the clinical efficacy of the training; a significant reduction of days with migraine and other headache parameters was observed." Siniatchkin et al. Self-regulation of slow cortical potentials in children with migraine: an exploratory study. *Appl Psychophysiol Biofeedback.*2000; 25:13 –32

[178] "The overall results of the study showed that relaxation training combined with stress management training was significantly more effective in reducing the headache index than treatment with the betablocker metoprolol." Sartory et al. A comparison of psychological and pharmacological treatment of pediatric migraine. *BehavResTher*1998;36:1155-1170

[179] "Trigger points were found in 92 (93.9%) migraineurs and in nine (29%) controls (P < 0.0001). The number of individual migraine trigger points varied from zero to 14, and was found to be related to both the frequency of migraine attacks, and the duration of the disease." Calandre et al. Trigger point evaluation in migraine patients: an indication of peripheral sensitization linked to migraine predisposition? *Eur J Neurol.* 2006 Mar;13(3):244-9

[180] "Myofascial trigger points can refer pain to the head and face in the cervical region, thus contributing to cervicogenic headache." Borg-Stein J. Cervical myofascial pain and headache. *Curr Pain Headache Rep.* 2002 Aug;6(4):324-30

[181] "Because treating myofascial problems may be the only way to offer complete relief from certain types of headache, clinicians must learn to diagnose and manage trigger points in neck, shoulder, and head muscles." Davidoff RA. Trigger points and myofascial pain: toward understanding how they affect headaches. *Cephalalgia.* 1998 Sep;18(7):436-48

[182] Lewit K, Simons DG. Myofascial pain: relief by post-isometric relaxation. *Arch Phys Med Rehabil* 1984 Aug;65(8):452-6. This is a classic "must read" article.

first-line prophylactic prescription medications. [183,184,185,186] Spinal manipulation should be performed only by professionals with graduate and postgraduate training in relevant spinal biomechanics, patient assessment, and manipulative technique.[187,188,189,190]

- Somatic treatments—acupuncture: Acupuncture is effective symptomatic treatment for migraine and tension headaches, with cost-effectiveness comparable to standard medical treatment.[191,192,193] Acupuncture is known to affect regional blood flow, and the neurophysiological mechanisms involved include increased release of endogenous analgesics such as endomorphin-1, beta-endorphin, enkephalin, and serotonin.[194] In a head-to-head study of acupuncture versus drug treatment with metoprolol, "2 of 59 patients randomized to acupuncture withdrew prematurely from the study compared to 18 of 55 randomized to metoprolol … The proportion of responders was 61% for acupuncture and 49% for metoprolol. Both physicians and patients reported fewer adverse effects in the acupuncture group."[195] While pain relief is an important benefit, it should not be the primary goal in treatment if an underlying physiological or biochemical disturbance (including nutritional deficiencies or imbalances) can be corrected.

- Somatic treatment—exercise: When people have pain, they are disinclined to move and exercise; however, lack of movement and exercise promotes the continuation of pain via several mechanisms including allowing the formation of myofascial adhesions and contractions, "untraining" of vestibulocerebellar circuits that are necessary for neuromuscular coordination, which is important for reducing musculoskeletal microtrauma that results from uncoordinated/dyscoordinated movements. Exercise and movement are necessary for maintaining myofascial elasticity; all three of these (exercise, movement/stretching, elasticity) support flow of blood, nutrients, oxygen, interstitial fluid, lymph throughout tissues to maintain cellular metabolism and remove wastes and inflammatory mediators. Movement also reduces pain directly via proprioceptive/sensory inhibition of nociception; stated simply: *movement sensation blocks pain reception.*
  - Intensive dynamic training for females with chronic neck/shoulder pain. (*Clin Rehabil.* 1998 Jun[196]): In a clinical research study with 77 women who suffered from chronic neck and shoulder pain, women who performed their exercises **three times per week for 5 sets of 20 repetitions** had better results than those who performed their exercises three times per week for 1 set of 20 repetitions. *More exercise gives better results—faster and more complete relief of pain.*

- Special supplementation for hyperhomocysteinaemia/hyperhomocysteinuria: Reasonable doses are listed; clinicians will have to combine and "dose to effect" per patient. All of these treatments are well-accepted as safe and generally effective. Homocysteine contributes to the increased cardiovascular and stroke risk seen in patients with migraine, while also contributing directly to neuroinflammation and NMDA receptor activation resulting in—identically as with glutamate—increased intracellular calcium and neurotoxicity.[197]
  - Folinic acid or methylfolate 2-5 mg/d: Use in combination with other vitamins, especially vitamin B12, in the form of hydroxocobalamin, adenosylcobalamin, or methylcobalamin—cyanocobalamin is obviously to be avoided because of its clinically relevant content of cyanide.
  - Vitamin B12 >2,000 mcg per day orally, or 1-2 mg per week by injection: Use in the form of hydroxocobalamin, adenosylcobalamin, or methylcobalamin—cyanocobalamin is obviously to be avoided because of its clinically relevant content of cyanide.

[183] Bronfort et al. Efficacy of spinal manipulation for chronic headache: a systematic review. *J Manipulative Physiol Ther* 2001 Sep;24(7):457-66
[184] Tuchin PJ, Pollard H, Bonello R. A randomized controlled trial of chiropractic spinal manipulative therapy for migraine. *J Manipulative Physiol Ther.* 2000 Feb;23(2):91-5
[185] "SMT appears to have a better effect than massage for cervicogenic headache. It also appears that SMT has an effect comparable to commonly used first-line prophylactic prescription medications for tension-type headache and migraine headache." Bronfort et al. Efficacy of spinal manipulation for chronic headache: a systematic review. *J Manipulative Physiol Ther* 2001 Sep;24(7):457-66
[186] "The average response of the treatment group (n = 83) showed statistically significant improvement in migraine frequency (P < .005), duration (P < .01), disability, and medication use..." Tuchin et al. A randomized controlled trial of chiropractic spinal manipulative therapy for migraine. *J Manipulative Physiol Ther.* 2000 Feb;23(2):91-5
[187] Kirk CR, Lawrence DJ, Valvo NL. *States Manual of Spinal, Pelvic, and Extravertebral Technics. Second Edition.* Lombard, Illinois: National College of Chiropractic; 1985
[188] Kimberly PE. *Outline of Osteopathic Manipulative Procedures. The Kimberly Manual 2006.* Kirksville College of Osteopathic Medicine. Walsworth Publishing
[189] Bergmann TF, Peterson DH, Lawrence DJ. *Chiropractic Technique.* New York; Churchill Livingstone: 1993
[190] Gatterman MI. *Chiropractic Management of Spine Related Disorders.* Baltimore; Williams and Wilkins: 1990
[191] Endres et al. Acupuncture for tension-type headache. *J Headache Pain.* 2007 Oct; 8(5): 306–314
[192] Vickers et al. Acupuncture of chronic headache disorders in primary care: randomised controlled trial and economic analysis. *Health Technol Assess.* 2004 Nov;8(48):iii, 1-35
[193] Wonderling D, et al. Cost effectiveness analysis of a randomised trial of acupuncture for chronic headache in primary care. *BMJ.* 2004 Mar 27;328(7442):747
[194] Cabyoglu MT, Ergene N, Tan U. The mechanism of acupuncture and clinical applications. *Int J Neurosci.* 2006 Feb;116(2):115-25
[195] Streng et al. Effectiveness and tolerability of acupuncture compared with metoprolol in migraine prophylaxis. *Headache.* 2006 Nov-Dec;46(10):1492-502
[196] "... pain scores were only significantly improved in the intensive group at 12 months follow-up." Randlov et al. Intensive dynamic training for females with chronic neck/shoulder pain. *Clin Rehabil.* 1998 Jun:200-10
[197] Abushik et al. The role of NMDA and mGluR5 receptors in calcium mobilization and neurotoxicity of homocysteine in trigeminal and cortical neurons and glial cells. *J Neurochem.* 2014 Apr;129(2):264-74

- Vitamin B6, pyridoxine 50-250 mg/d: The phosphorylated form (P5P) can also be used; when the HCL form is used, additional attention must be given to magnesium status/supplementation and urinary alkalinization.
- Riboflavin 20-400 mg/d: Small doses of 2 mg/d have been shown to significantly reduce homocysteine levels, and doses of 400 mg/d are common and well-tolerated in the treatment of migraine.
- Thyroid optimization: Hypothyroidism causes elevated homocysteine and promotes insulin resistance[198] and should be treated appropriately per Chapter 1.
- NAC 600 mg per day and upward to 500-1,500 mg thrice daily: Doses of NAC 4,800 mg/d have been used with success and safety in the treatment of SLE.
- Avoidance of homocysteine-elevating factors: High coffee intake (>5 cups per day), ethanol, tobacco smoking, and medications/treatments (such as methotrexate, metformin, niacin and fibrate drugs); fish oil can raise homocysteine levels in some patients. Metformin is well-known to cause malabsorption of vitamin B12 and to thereby exacerbate "diabetic neuropathy" and promote depression and dementia/psychosis.
- Choline, phosphatidylcholine, lecithin (approximately 2.6 g choline/d): Each TBS (tablespoon, approximately 15 mL) of lecithin contains 275 mg of choline; thus, if the goal is to get to 2.6 g choline, one would need to use 10 TBS (150 mL) per day of granulated lecithin.
- Betaine, trimethylglycine 6–12 g/day: Effects are weak/modest; likely more relevant for patients taking drugs such as metformin and fibrates that promote loss of betaine in urine.

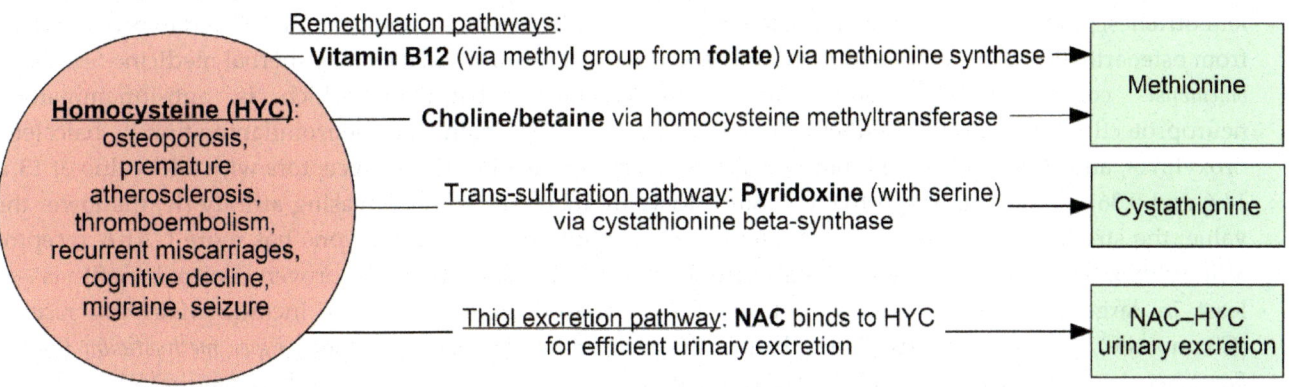

Lowering homocysteine (HYC) via nutritional supplementation: Folate gives methyl group to cobalamin (vitamin B12) to convert HYC via methionine synthase to methionine; choline/betaine can remethylate homocysteine via homocysteine methyltransferase to form methionine. Pyridoxine promotes conversion of HYC via cystathionine beta-synthase to cystathionine. The amino acid N-acetyl-cysteine (NAC) binds to HYC for efficient renal excretion of NAC-HYC.[199]

- Special supplementation—Feverfew (*Tanacetum parthenium*) as monotherapy or with ginger, willow: Results of numerous studies support the use of feverfew for the safe and cost-effective treatment and prevention of migraine headaches. Feverfew has several mechanisms of action including antithrombosis and inhibition of NFkB. Feverfew products are generally concentrated to 0.2% to 0.7% parthenolide, and a reasonable starting dose is 250 mcg/d of parthenolide; lower doses can be used within a context of multicomponent treatment. Feverfew can be used alone, with other nutrients, or with other botanical medicines. The combination of ginger and feverfew has shown efficacy for halting incipient migraine attacks when started within 2 hours of pain onset.[200] Similarly, the combination of feverfew and willow extract was shown to be remarkably safe and effective in preventing and reducing migraine.[201]

[198] Yang N et al. Novel Clinical Evidence of an Association between Homocysteine and Insulin Resistance in Patients with Hypothyroidism or Subclinical Hypothyroidism. *PLoS One*. 2015 May 4;10(5):e0125922
[199] "NAC intravenous administration induces an efficient and rapid reduction of plasma thiols, particularly of Hcy; our data support the hypothesis that NAC displaces thiols from their binding protein sites and forms, in excess of plasma NAC, mixed disulphides (NAC-Hcy) with an high renal clearance." Ventura et al. N-Acetyl-cysteine reduces homocysteine plasma levels after single intravenous administration by increasing thiols urinary excretion. *Pharmacol Res*. 1999 Oct;40(4):345-50
[200] Cady RK, Schreiber CP, Beach ME, Hart CC. Gelstat Migraine (sublingually administered feverfew and ginger compound) for acute treatment of migraine when administered during the mild pain phase. *Med Sci Monit*. 2005 Sep;11(9):PI65-9
[201] Shrivastava R, Pechadre JC, John GW. Tanacetum parthenium and Salix alba (Mig-RL) combination in migraine prophylaxis. *Clin Drug Investig*. 2006;26(5):287-96

- Special supplementation—Butterbur (*Petasites hybridus*): Butterbur/*Petasites* has consistently shown excellent efficacy in the prophylaxis of migraine, with frequency reductions of ~60%.[202,203] Adult doses used in clinical trials have been variantly described per product as "two capsules 25 mg BID" for a total of 100 mg and "Petasites extract 75 mg bid, Petasites extract 50 mg bid" with the higher doses showing greater efficacy. Anderson et al[204] noted that antimigraine and anti-allergy benefits are mediated via sesquiterpene esters of petasin and furanopetasin which reduce leukotriene biosynthesis, inhibit cyclooxygenase (COX-1 and COX-2), ameliorate activation of p38 mitogen–activated protein kinase stress signaling, and reduce NFkB activation in rat microglial cells; partial blockade of calcium channels has also been noted. Rare (< 0.01%) cases of liver damage (acute hepatitis) and liver failure have been reported; Anderson et al (op cit) per their comparative *in vitro* studies recommend limiting the petasin content (<17%) to improve the hepatobiliary safety profile. Differently, Utterback et al[205] attributed the hepatotoxicity to pyrrolizidine alkaloids (PAs) and stated that products should be virtually PA-free, with less than 0.08 ppm PA; their review concluded that butterbur is safe for antimigraine treatment in children (>6yo) and adults. Contraindications include hypersensitivity/allergy to butterbur or any of the related Asteraceae plants: ragweed, marigolds, daisies, and chrysanthemums.
- Special supplementation—botanical medicines with anti-inflammatory and/or GABA agonist effects: Numerous botanical medicines have proven anti-inflammatory and analgesic benefits. *Zingiber officinale* (ginger) demonstrates multiple antiinflammatory mechanisms and is commonly consumed as food, juice and as a nutritional supplement in the form of pills/powder. Components of ginger reduce production of the leukotriene LTB4 by inhibiting 5-lipoxygenase and reduce production of the prostaglandin PG-E2 by inhibiting cyclooxygenase.[206,207] With its dual reduction in the formation of inflammation-promoting prostaglandins and leukotrienes, ginger has been shown to safely reduce musculoskeletal pain in general[208,209] and to provide relief from osteoarthritis of the knees and migraine headaches.[210] The traditional Chinese herbal medicine *Scutellaria baicalensis* contains, among other active phytochemicals, baicalein, which is anti-inflammatory, neuroprotective, and protective/therapeutic against persistent pain and neuroinflammation[211]; baicalein, oroxylin A, and skullcapflavone II bind the benzodiazepine site of GABA-A receptors with a Ki value of 13.1, 14.6 and 0.36 micromol/L, respectively.[212] Since Ki value increases with decreasing affinity (ie, the lower the value, the stronger the ligand-receptor interaction), we note that skullcapflavone has more GABA receptor affinity than does the more "famous" baicalein. Botanical medicines that have proven clinical benefit via—at least in large part—their activation of the GABA/benzodiazepine receptor include *Matricaria recutita* (Chamomile), *Melissa officinalis* (lemon balm), *Passiflora incarnata* (passionflower), *Piper methysticum* (kava), *Scutellaria lateriflora* (skullcap), *Valeriana species* (valerian), and *Withania somnifera* (ashwagandha).[213]
- Special supplementation—intranasal capsaicin: Capsaicin is the "hot" spicy component of hot chili peppers; when applied to the skin or mucus membranes, it damages pain-sensing nerves and thereby reduces the sensation of pain after an initial exacerbation of pain. Intranasal capsaicin (300 mcg/100 microliters) is remarkably well studied in the treatment and prevention of cluster headaches, beginning with the first report published by Sicuteri et al[214] in 1989. Treatment of active cluster headache with intranasal capsaicin (compared

[202] Grossmann M, Schmidramsl H. An extract of Petasites hybridus is effective in the prophylaxis of migraine. *Int J Clin Pharmacol Ther*. 2000 Sep;38(9):430-5. See also Grossman W, Schmidramsl H. An extract of Petasites hybridus is effective in the prophylaxis of migraine. *Altern Med Rev*. 2001 Jun;6(3):303-10

[203] Lipton et al. Petasites hybridus root (butterbur) is an effective preventive treatment for migraine. *Neurology*. 2004 Dec 28;63(12):2240-4

[204] Anderson et al. Toxicogenomics applied to cultures of human hepatocytes enabled an identification of novel petasites hybridus extracts for the treatment of migraine with improved hepatobiliary safety. *Toxicol Sci*. 2009 Dec;112(2):507-20

[205] Utterback et al. Butterbur extract: prophylactic treatment for childhood migraines. *Complement Ther Clin Pract*. 2014 Feb;20(1):61-4

[206] Kiuchi et al. Inhibition of prostaglandin and leukotriene biosynthesis by gingerols and diarylheptanoids. *Chem Pharm Bull* (Tokyo) 1992 Feb;40(2):387-91

[207] Tjendraputra et al. Effect of ginger constituents and synthetic analogues on cyclooxygenase-2 enzyme in intact cells. *Bioorg Chem* 2001 Jun;29(3):156-63

[208] Srivastava KC, Mustafa T. Ginger (Zingiber officinale) in rheumatism and musculoskeletal disorders. *Med Hypotheses*. 1992 Dec;39(4):342-8

[209] Srivastava KC, Mustafa T. Ginger (Zingiber officinale) and rheumatic disorders. *Med Hypotheses*. 1989 May;29(1):25-8

[210] "It is proposed that administration of ginger may exert abortive and prophylactic effects in migraine headache without any side-effects." Mustafa T, Srivastava KC. Ginger (Zingiber officinale) in migraine headache. *J Ethnopharmacol*. 1990 Jul;29(3):267-73

[211] "Baicalein (BE), isolated from the traditional Chinese herbal medicine Scutellaria baicalensis Georgi (or Huang Qin), has been demonstrated to have anti-inflammatory and neuroprotective effects. ...Intrathecal and oral administration of BE at different doses could alleviate the mechanical allodynia in CIBP rats. Intrathecal 100 μg BE could inhibit the production of IL-6 and TNF-α in the spinal cord of CIBP rats. ...The analgesic effect of BE may be associated with the inhibition of the expression of the inflammatory cytokines IL-6 and TNF-α and through the activation of p-p38 and p-JNK MAPK signals in the spinal cord." Hu et al. The Analgesic and Antineuroinflammatory Effect of Baicalein in Cancer-Induced Bone Pain. *Evid Based Complement Alternat Med*. 2015;2015:973524

[212] "A benzodiazepine binding assay directed separation led to the identification of 3 flavones baicalein (1), oroxylin A (2), and skullcapflavone II (3) from the water extract of Scutellaria baicalensis root. Compounds 1, 2, and 3 interacted with the benzodiazepine binding site of GABAA receptors with a Ki value of 13.1, 14.6 and 0.36 micromol/L, respectively." Liao et al. Benzodiazepine binding site-interactive flavones from Scutellaria baicalensis root. *Planta Med*. 1998 Aug;64(6):571-2

[213] Sarris et al. Plant-based medicines for anxiety disorders, part 2: a review of clinical studies with supporting preclinical evidence. *CNS Drugs*. 2013 Apr;27(4):301-19

[214] Sicuteri et al. Beneficial effect of capsaicin application to the nasal mucosa in cluster headache. *Clin J Pain*. 1989;5(1):49-53

with placebo) reduced severity after 7 days of treatment.[215] In a small controlled clinical trial, patients stated that intranasal capsaicin alleviated chronic migraine suffering by 50% to 80%.[216] Burning pain, sneezing, and increased nasal secretions induced by topical capsaicin application are intense for the first few applications but decrease over time, generally within a week or so; clinical benefits generally begin on the eighth day of consecutive treatment. Episodic cluster headache patients appear to benefit more than do chronic cluster headache patients. Cluster headaches are typically unilateral, and capsaicin should be applied to the nostril on the same side as the head pain.[217]

- Surgical closure of patent foramen ovale: While the prevalence of patent foramen ovale in the general adult population is approximately 20% to 30%, patients with migraine—especially migraine with aura—show a higher prevalence (55–65%) of this physiological cardiopulmonary shunt. Surgical closure of a patent foramen ovale can provide relief from headache in many migraine patients.[218,219] If the cardiopulmonary shunt is severe enough to result in reduced blood oxygenation, it can exacerbate the already reduced energy production caused by the aforementioned mitochondrial dysfunction. More likely, bypassing the lungs results in failure of pulmonary degradation of proinflammatory mediators. The lungs inactivate proinflammatory mediators such as prostaglandins E1, E2, and F2-alpha, all of the leukotrienes, and norepinephrine (30% reduction). Thus, surgical closure of the patent foramen ovale stops inflammatory mediators from bypassing the lungs and may provide a systemic anti-inflammatory benefit that reduces migraine severity.

Endocrine Imbalances All hormones have either pro-inflammatory or anti-inflammatory effects. As such, patients with pain and inflammation are candidates for complete hormonal evaluation, as reviewed in Chapter 4, Section 5. Melatonin's utility in migraine—as in fibromyalgia—is more likely related to its antioxidant and mitochondrial-supportive effects than to a true "hormonal" effect. Thyroid status must be optimized in all migraine patients.

- Melatonin—3-20 mg at night: Melatonin is a hormone made in the pineal gland from the neurotransmitter serotonin which is derived from the amino acid tryptophan and 5-hydroxytryptophan. Melatonin levels are low in patients with migraine and cluster headache. According to case reports and studies with small numbers of patients, 10 mg of melatonin taken at night relieves cluster headaches in approximately 50% of patients, with results beginning 3 to 5 days after the start of treatment and continuing for the duration of treatment.[220,221] Clinical trials using melatonin in migraine patients have shown consistently positive results, with a significant number of patients becoming completely migraine-free.[222] Melatonin is generally administered at night in doses ranging from 3 to 10 mg, although studies in cancer patients have safely used doses as high as 20 to 40 mg and have shown antitumor and pro-survival benefits. Melatonin has antioxidant and immunomodulatory actions in addition to its ability to preserve mitochondrial function, which is particularly relevant to migraine and cluster headaches. According to small studies and case reports with small numbers of patients, 10 mg of melatonin taken at night relieves cluster headaches in approximately 50% of patients.[223,224]

- Testosterone: Testosterone has antiinflammatory/immunomodulatory actions, and as such has clinical utility in migraine, cluster headache, rheumatoid arthritis, and fibromyalgia via reduction/modulation of peripheral inflammation and the brain inflammation and microglial activation that promote central sensitization to pain. In this study[225], following subcutaneous testosterone implant, "Improvement in headache severity was noted by 92% of patients and the mean level of improvement was statistically significant (3.3 on a 5 point scale). ... Seventy-four percent of patients reported a headache severity score of '0' (none) on testosterone implant therapy

[215] Marks et al. A double-blind placebo-controlled trial of intranasal capsaicin for cluster headache. *Cephalalgia*. 1993 Apr;13(2):114-6

[216] Fusco et al. Repeated intranasal capsaicin applications to treat chronic migraine. *Br J Anaesth*. 2003 Jun;90(6):812

[217] Fusco et al. Preventative effect of repeated nasal applications of capsaicin in cluster headache. *Pain*. 1994 Dec;59(3):321-5

[218] Rigatelli et al. Primary patent foramen ovale closure to relieve severe migraine. *Ann Intern Med*. 2006 Mar 21;144(6):458-60

[219] Dubiel et al. Migraine Headache Relief after Percutaneous Transcatheter Closure of Interatrial Communications. *J Interv Cardiol*. 2007 Dec 18; [Epub ahead of print]

[220] Leone et al. Melatonin versus placebo in the prophylaxis of cluster headache: a double-blind pilot study with parallel groups. *Cephalalgia* 1996 Nov;16(7):494-6

[221] "Melatonin levels have been found to be decreased in cluster headache patients. ... We report two chronic cluster headache patients who had both daytime and nocturnal attacks that were alleviated with melatonin." Peres MF, Rozen TD. Melatonin in the preventive treatment of chronic cluster headache. *Cephalalgia*. 2001 Dec;21(10):993-5

[222] Vogler et al. Role of melatonin in the pathophysiology of migraine: implications for treatment. *CNS Drugs*. 2006;20(5):343-50

[223] "Five of the 10 treated patients were responders whose attack frequency declined 3-5 days after treatment, and they experienced no further attacks until melatonin was discontinued." Leone et al. Melatonin versus placebo in the prophylaxis of cluster headache: a double-blind pilot study with parallel groups. *Cephalalgia* 1996 Nov;16(7):494-6

[224] "Melatonin levels have been found to be decreased in cluster headache patients. ... We report two chronic cluster headache patients who had both daytime and nocturnal attacks that were alleviated with melatonin." Peres MF, Rozen TD. Melatonin in the preventive treatment of chronic cluster headache. *Cephalalgia*. 2001 Dec;21(10):993-5

[225] Glaser et al. Testosterone pellet implants and migraine headaches: a pilot study. *Maturitas*. 2012 Apr;71(4):385-8

for the 3-month treatment period. Continuous testosterone was effective therapy in reducing the severity of migraine headaches in both pre- and post-menopausal women." In another study, "Seven male and 2 female patients, seen between July 2004 and February 2005, and between the ages of 32 and 56, are reported with histories of treatment resistant cluster headaches accompanied by borderline low or low serum testosterone levels. The patients failed to respond to individually tailored medical regimens, including melatonin doses of 12 mg a day or higher, high flow oxygen, maximally tolerated verapamil, antiepileptic agents, and parenteral serotonin agonists. Seven of the 9 patients met 2004 International Classification for the Diagnosis of Headache criteria for chronic cluster headaches; the other 2 patients had episodic cluster headaches of several months duration. After neurological and physical examination all patients had laboratory investigations including fasting lipid panel, PSA (where indicated), LH, FSH, and testosterone levels (both free and total). All 9 patients demonstrated either abnormally low or low, normal testosterone levels. After supplementation with either pure testosterone in 5 of 7 male patients or combination testosterone/estrogen therapy in both female patients, the patients achieved cluster headache freedom for the first 24 hours. Four male chronic cluster patients, all with abnormally low testosterone levels, achieved remission."[226]

Xenobiotic Accumulation/Detoxification Persistent organic pollutants promote inflammation generally and mitochondrial dysfunction specifically. Treat as described throughout this text and as reviewed in Chapter 2 and also in Chapter 4, Section 7.

---

[226] Stillman MJ. Testosterone replacement therapy for treatment refractory cluster headache. *Headache*. 2006 Jun;46(6):925-33

Fibromyalgia (FM, FMS, FMD) &
Complex Regional Pain Syndrome (CRPS)

Introduction:

Fibromyalgia (FM)—also referred to as fibromyalgia syndrome (FMS) but more properly referred to as fibromyalgia disease (FMD)—is an organic clinical entity that has remained enigmatic to the medical profession despite the consistent publication of research that delineates its cause and its effective treatments. This chapter summarizes clinical assessments, treatments, and essential background information that—when properly applied—should provide empowering knowledge for clinicians and for the patients suffering with this condition. For any disease, we as scientists and clinicians must establish a model of the disease so that we can start with *some shared idea about the disease itself* and have some common language and understanding so that we can engage in meaningful conversations and valuable research. The model of FM that I have been the first and only clinician researcher to construct (starting in 2008) is that FM starts from small intestine bacterial overgrowth, and that the absorbed microbial molecules lead to the pain-amplifying central sensitization and fatigue-inducing mitochondrial dysfunction that clearly characterize this condition; variations of and deviations from the classic model of any disease will undoubtedly be encountered, but they can always be traced back to this classic model.

Fibromyalgia is uniquely exemplary in its clouded diagnostic criteria and etiology; I argue in this review and the associated videos and related articles that the diagnostic criteria for FM have been intentionally clouded and deconstructed via influence of drug companies that want the FM label to be applied to as many patients as possible for the longest duration possible and that the etiology and very nature of the disorder has been clouded and hijacked by medical/science writers who are heavily paid by drug companies that sell the FDA-approved drugs for fibromyalgia and which directly profit from a population of confused doctors and helpless patients which create a multi-billion dollar international drug/medical market.

After considerable literature review and personal deliberation, I have decided to include information about complex regional pain syndrome (CRPS) in this section that is otherwise exclusive to fibromyalgia. At the time of this writing, I am impressed that these are two variants of essentially the same pathophysiology, just as migraine and cluster headaches are variants on the same theme. With all due respect for the differences and distinctions between these conditions, I appreciate that their pathophysiologic similarities are of greater importance for understanding and treating both disorders. Both FM and CRPS share 1) central sensitization, 2) peripheral sensitization, 3) neuroinflammation, 4) neurogenic inflammation, 5) increased glutaminergic/NMDA-mediated central and peripheral neurotransmission, 6) mitochondrial dysfunction, 7) increased intestinal permeability, and 8) gastrointestinal dysbiosis. Relative to my study of migraine and fibromyalgia which has a history of publications over many years, I have only recently begun to study CRPS, but my impression is that it is a spinal cord (SC)-specific regional activation of glia and neurons and failure of regional neuroinhibition; somewhat analogous to a spinal cord migraine/seizure or at least the spinal cord variant of fibromyalgia. I agree with Littlejohn[227] that both FM and CRPS have a component of neurogenic inflammation; I think the role of neurogenic inflammation in CRPS is stronger than it is in FM, also—perhaps obviously—more focal, limited to a region of spinal cord segments. While the pathophysiologic similarities among FM and CRPS suggest that effective nutritional therapeutics for FM will be at least partly efficacious for CRPS, we generally do not have such proof due to lack of studies in CRPS; however, the risk:benefit ratio of these highly safe and frequently efficacious interventions clearly favors empiric implementation followed by monitoring of therapeutic response in a condition notorious for its debilitating severity and therapeutic recalcitrance.

Introduction and Clinical Presentation

- Overview: Fibromyalgia (FM) is commonly described as an "idiopathic" (of unknown origin) syndrome principally characterized by widespread body pain and numerous myofascial tender points at specific locations. FM is most common in women 20-50 years of age, and the condition often presents with associated complaints of fatigue, headaches, subjective numbness, altered sleep patterns, and gastrointestinal disturbances. FM in children and adolescents presents similarly to FM in adults except for the comparatively higher prevalence of sleep disturbance and the finding of fewer tender points in children.[228] Until recently,

---

[227] Littlejohn G. Neurogenic neuroinflammation in fibromyalgia and complex regional pain syndrome. *Nat Rev Rheumatol*. 2015 Nov;11(11):639-48. At the time this citation is added in 2015 Dec, I (DrV) had recently submitted a reply to *Nat Rev Rheumatol*; my reply will be posted at ichnfm.academia.edu/AlexVasquez as soon as possible.
[228] Siegel DM, Janeway D, Baum J. Fibromyalgia syndrome in children and adolescents: clinical features at presentation and status at follow-up. *Pediatrics* 1998;101:377-82

fibromyalgia was considered a *diagnosis of exclusion* after infection, autoimmunity, or other primary causes of widespread pain were excluded by clinical and laboratory assessment. However, current criteria base the diagnosis on positive findings of chronic, widespread musculoskeletal pain in characteristic locations; these criteria will be described below. Fibromyalgia shares several clinical, demographic, and pathologic features with chronic fatigue syndrome (CFS) and irritable bowel syndrome (IBS); the reason for these overlaps is not generally understood by most clinicians and researchers but will be made plain in this writing.

- The common medical view—scientifically inaccurate, financially leveraged: The prevailing medical view, expressed by most medical doctors and the authors of widely cited articles, is that fibromyalgia is idiopathic—*of unknown origin*—with strong neuropsychogenic (*neuro*=nerves and brain, *psyche*=mind, *genic*=origin) influences (in other words, "It's all in your head.") and that, since the underlying causes of the condition have not been identified, the best therapeutic approach is symptom suppression via perpetual pharmacotherapy with adjunctive use of psychotherapy and limited exercise.[229,230,231] This prevailing medical view is unscientific (not based on science) and counterscientific (ignores and contradicts published and validated research), unethical (fails to provide effective treatment when such treatment is available; condemns patients to medicalization and suffering), and commercially leveraged (diagnostic criteria revision and many review articles discussing treatment are sponsored by drug companies; medical profession benefits financially by having many long-term drug-dependent patients).

- <mark>Fibromyalgia—in its original "1990-based" description—is a disease, not a syndrome</mark>: The term *syndrome* connotes that a cluster of symptoms is of a nonorganic, psychogenic, or idiopathic nature, whereas *disease* validates the organic and pathophysiological nature of an illness. This author advocates the use of *disease* rather than *syndrome* when describing fibromyalgia in appreciation of the real, organic, biochemical, and histopathological (*histo*=cells and tissues, *pathological*=disease) findings which clearly indicate that fibromyalgia is a specific disease entity and not simply a psychogenic or enigmatic cluster of symptoms. If fibromyalgia is a real, organic clinical entity (as will be documented here), then the appropriate designation is *fibromyalgia disease* (FMD) rather than *fibromyalgia syndrome* (FMS). For consistency and clarity within this section, the general term "fibromyalgia" will be used. Relatedly, the term "irritable bowel syndrome" (IBS) is also a misnomer that confuses professionals as well as the general public into thinking that the condition does not have identified causes and (nonpharmaceutical) treatments; despite promulgations to the contrary, the cause of IBS is well-known[232], and effective treatment is readily available. When in 2010 the American College of Rheumatology (ACR) mistakenly allowed the diagnostic criteria for FM to be hijacked to leverage more drug sales—facilitate the making of the diagnosis, broaden the number of people affected, and impair the "cure" of and escape from the disease—the legitimate meaning of the diagnosis of course became less specific and much broader and therefore less meaningful. Per the original diagnostic criteria published in 1990, fibromyalgia is a legitimate functional disease and should be described and labeled as such; per the ridiculous diagnostic criteria published in 2010, fibromyalgia is a symptom cluster of aches, pains, and other signs and symptoms that can accompany virtually any other disease. Classic legitimate "FM" or "FMD" is what is described in this section (per the 1990 criteria), not simply the pain and symptom cluster (FMS) per the 2010 criteria. The idea that any and all patients with widespread pain should qualify for a diagnosis of fibromyalgia is ludicrous, and the 2010 ACR criteria for fibromyalgia are an obfuscating disservice to patients, doctors, and researchers while only benefiting the drug companies that can now sell their expensive and ineffective drugs *more quickly* to a *larger audience* for a *longer duration*. Patients develop true *primary* FM/FMD per the description that follows; patients can develop "fibromyalgia-like syndrome" or "fibromyalgia syndrome"—ie, FMS—by many means, including head injury or major trauma—these cases are more legitimately titled *secondary* hyperalgesic/allodynic central sensitization and/or myofascial pain syndromes.

- Prevalence, symptoms, and clinical findings: Fibromyalgia is one of the most common chronic pain conditions, affecting an estimated 10 million people in the U.S. and an estimated 3-6% of people world-wide.[233]

[229] Chakrabarty S, Zoorob R. Fibromyalgia. *Am Fam Physician*. 2007 Jul 15;76(2):247-54

[230] Tierney ML. McPhee SJ, Papadakis MA (eds). *Current Medical Diagnosis and Treatment 2006, 45th Edition*. New York: Lange Medical Books, pages 820-821

[231] Simms RW. Nonarticular soft tissue disorders. In Andreoli TE, Carpenter CCJ, Griggs RC, Benjamin IJ (eds). *Cecil Essentials of Medicine. 7th Edition*. Elsevier 2007:851-2

[232] Lin HC. Small intestinal bacterial overgrowth: a framework for understanding irritable bowel syndrome. *JAMA*. 2004 Aug 18;292(7):852-8

[233] "Fibromyalgia is one of the most common chronic pain conditions. The disorder affects an estimated 10 million people in the U.S. and an estimated 3-6% of the world population." National Fibromyalgia Association. fmaware.org/PageServera6cc.html?pagename=fibromyalgia_affected Accessed Sept 2012.

Approximately 10% of affected patients have severe symptoms resulting in partial or total disability. Affected patients report chronic aches, pains, and stiffness with a proclivity for localization near the neck, shoulders, low back, and hips. Pain and fatigue are typically exacerbated following physical exertion or psychological stress. Associated manifestations include fatigue, sleep disorders (including insomnia, unrefreshing sleep, and objective abnormalities such as an increase in stage 1 sleep, a reduction in delta sleep, and alpha-delta sleep anomaly), subjective numbness, headaches, and gastrointestinal disturbances consistent with a clinical diagnosis of irritable bowel syndrome (IBS). Clinical findings shared between FM and IBS include abdominal pain and discomfort, changed frequency of stool, diarrhea and/or constipation, abdominal bloating/distention/gas and flatulence, dyspepsia/heartburn, headaches especially migraine-type headaches), fatigue, myalgias, restless leg syndrome, anxiety, and depression. The **high prevalence (>50%) of migraine-type headaches in FM patients** suggests an underlying pathogenesis shared between cephalgia (*ceph*=head, *algia*=pain) and widespread myalgia (*myo*=muscle, *algia*=pain); one of the established and most likely causative abnormalities shared between migraine and FM is impaired mitochondrial function, which will be explained in greater detail later in this publication. Cognitive symptoms such as "brain fog" ("fibro-fog") and difficulty with memory and word retrieval, as well as **environmental intolerance (EI) and multiple chemical sensitivity (MCS)**, are seen in both FM and CFS[234]; again, this overlap of shared symptoms suggests a common etiopathogenesis (*etio*=cause, *patho*=disease, *genesis*=initiation). Routine physical examination and laboratory findings are generally normal, with the exception the physical examination finding of fibromyalgia tender points (described and diagrammed below in the section on Diagnosis per the 1990 diagnostic criteria).

Objective "organic" (ie, real) abnormalities in fibromyalgia dispel the myth that the condition is psychogenic
1. Histologic and functional abnormalities in muscle tissue: Disorganization of actin filaments, accumulation of lipofuscin bodies consistent with premature muscle aging, increased DNA fragmentation, and focal areas of chronic muscle contraction, reduced perfusion of muscle tissue during exercise (i.e., reduced blood flow to muscles).
2. Mitochondrial defects: Accumulation of glycogen (muscle sugar) and lipid (fat) indicate that intracellular energy production is impaired and that the cells are unable to efficiently convert fuel sources into energy in the form of ATP, adenosine triphosphate, which is the basic fuel source for cellular metabolism. Also noted are significant reductions in the number of mitochondria, reduced activity of important enzymes such as 3-hydroxy-CoA dehydrogenase, citrate synthase, and cytochrome oxidase. Nutritional deficiencies, such as CoQ-10 deficiency, promote mitochondrial dysfunction, thus leading to mitochondrial destruction (mitophagy) which ultimately results in reduced numbers of mitochondria and perpetuates and aggravates muscle fatigue, pain, and neurocognitive dysfunction (i.e., brain fog, difficulty thinking, depression).
3. Oxidative stress: Increased oxidative stress results from mitochondrial dysfunction and nutrient depletion.
4. Neuroendocrine abnormalities: Hypothalamic-pituitary-adrenal (HPA) disturbance indicates impaired function of the brain and endocrine system.
5. Elevated brain glutamate, homocysteine, and interlukin-8: See in FM, also CFS and CRPS.
6. Low-grade immune activation: Increased cytokine production indicates a pro-inflammatory state.
7. Bacterial overgrowth in the intestines: FM patients have excess/overgrowth of bacteria in their intestines, referred to as SIBO (small intestine bacterial overgrowth); CRPS patients have an abnormal pattern of microbial growth.
8. Increased intestinal permeability, "leaky gut": Generally this indicates a gastrointestinal disorder, including but not limited to microbial imbalance (dysbiosis) or overt infection. Leaky gut is seen in both FM and CRPS.
9. High prevalence of vitamin D deficiency: Common in the general population but more common in patients with chronic pain; vitamin D deficiency causes chronic pain, depression/anxiety, and low-grade inflammation—all of these problems are seen in patients with fibromyalgia.
10. Low blood levels of L-tryptophan: FM patients have low levels of the amino acid tryptophan in their blood, despite adequate dietary intake. The most likely explanation for the deficiency of tryptophan is destruction of tryptophan by bacterial enzyme action. Several intestinal bacteria produce the enzyme tryptophanase, which destroys the amino acid tryptophan. Bacterial overgrowth results in more tryptophanase, resulting in tryptophan deficiency. Deficiency of tryptophan results in deficiencies of the hormones serotonin and melatonin, which result in anxiety, depression, food/sugar cravings, unrestful sleep, and mitochondrial dysfunction, since deficiency of melatonin causes reduced mitochondrial energy-production efficiency.

---

[234] Brown MM, Jason LA. Functioning in individuals with chronic fatigue syndrome: increased impairment with co-occurring multiple chemical sensitivity and fibromyalgia. *Dyn Med.* 2007 May 31;6:6 dynamic-med.com/content/6/1/6

Pathophysiology of Pain and Mitochondrial Dysfunction in Fibromyalgia

- Patients with FM demonstrate multiple biochemical abnormalities, centering on mitochondrial dysfunction, oxidative stress, and increased pain perception: Ultrastructural and biochemical abnormalities appear to be more pathologically significant and clinically relevant than the noted histological changes in skeletal muscle biopsy samples. Importantly, **the biochemical abnormalities *are the cause* of the histologic/tissue abnormalities.** Numerous **mitochondrial enzyme defects are seen**, including reduced activity of 3-hydroxy-CoA dehydrogenase, citrate synthase, and cytochrome oxidase. Levels of free magnesium are reduced by 31%, and levels of complexed ATP-magnesium are reduced by 12% in muscle from FM patients compared with levels seen in healthy controls; these biochemical and bioenergetic defects contribute to rapid-onset fatigue and muscle pain. From a neurophysiological perspective, *magnesium deficiency* can promote hypersensitivity to pain due to a reduction in the partial blockade of N-methyl-D-aspartate (NMDA) neurotransmitter receptor sites.[235] Reduced perfusion of muscle tissue during exercise results in relative tissue hypoxia, reduced muscle healing after the microtrauma of exercise, and promotion of muscle soreness due to accumulation of L-lactate (lactic acid).[236] **Increased oxidative stress** is also seen in FM patients,[237] providing additional objective evidence of the systemic, organic, and non-psychogenic nature of the illness. Evidence of hypothalamic-pituitary-adrenal disturbance and **increased cytokine production (particularly interleukin-8, which promotes sympathetic pain, and interleukin-6, which induces hyperalgesia [increased perception of pain], fatigue, and depression**[238]) further characterize the systemic and organic nature of this condition and are well documented in the research literature. **The majority of fibromyalgia patients demonstrate laboratory evidence of bacterial overgrowth in the small bowel**[239], and the details and important implications of this will be discussed below. **Vitamin D deficiency**—a recognized cause of chronic widespread pain as well as depression, muscle fatigue, and chronic low-grade inflammation—is also common in fibromyalgia patients.[240,241] FM patients have **significantly elevated blood levels of pentosidine**, which is an advanced glycation end-product (AGE) and marker of oxidative stress and glycosylation (sugar-protein binding); AGEs promote chronic inflammation and nociceptive sensitization leading to chronic pain.[242] Another AGE very similar to pentosidine, **carboxy-methyl-lysine (CML) is found in higher levels in the blood and muscle of FM patients**[243]; both pentosidine and CML cause expedited "muscle aging" and promote chronic pain and inflammation. These objective abnormalities of biochemical, histological, nutritional, and microbiological/gastrointestinal status force clinicians to appreciate the valid and organic nature of fibromyalgia. As previously stated, this evidence refutes promulgations espoused within standard allopathic/pharmaceutical medicine that fibromyalgia is an idiopathic condition warranting lifelong medicalization with expensive and potentially hazardous analgesic and antidepressant drugs; the focus on drug treatment to mask/suppress the pain of fibromyalgia detours doctors and patients away from focusing on the legitimate and validated causes of fibromyalgia and physiology-based (rather than pharmacology-based) means for alleviating the suffering and pain that these patients experience. CRPS patients also show evidence of biochemical and metabolic abnormalities, including increased oxidative stress and impaired mitochondrial function.[244]

  - Chronic widespread pain: increased glutamate and lactate concentrations in the trapezius muscle and plasma. (*Clin J Pain.* 2014 May[245]): "Chronic widespread pain (CWP), including fibromyalgia syndrome (FM), is associated with prominent negative consequences. CWP has been associated with alterations in

[235] Park JH, Niermann KJ, Olsen N. Evidence for metabolic abnormalities in the muscles of patients with fibromyalgia. *Curr Rheumatol Rep.* 2000 Apr;2(2):131-40

[236] Elvin et al. Decreased muscle blood flow in fibromyalgia patients during standardised muscle exercise. *Eur J Pain.* 2006 Feb;10(2):137-44

[237] Altindag O, Celik H. Total antioxidant capacity and the severity of the pain in patients with fibromyalgia. *Redox Rep.* 2006;11(3):131-5

[238] Wallace DJ, Linker-Israeli M, Hallegua D, et al. Cytokines play an aetiopathogenetic role in fibromyalgia. *Rheumatology* (Oxford). 2001 Jul;40(7):743-9

[239] Pimentel et al. A link between irritable bowel syndrome and fibromyalgia may be related to findings on lactulose breath testing. *Ann Rheum Dis.* 2004 Apr;63(4):450-2

[240] Huisman AM, White KP, Algra A, et al. Vitamin D levels in women with systemic lupus erythematosus and fibromyalgia. *J Rheumatol.* 2001 Nov;28(11):2535-9

[241] Armstrong DJ, Meenagh GK, Bickle I, et al. Vitamin D deficiency is associated with anxiety and depression in fibromyalgia. *Clin Rheumatol.* 2007 Apr;26(4):551-4

[242] Hein G, Franke S. Are advanced glycation end-product-modified proteins of pathogenetic importance in fibromyalgia? *Rheumatology* (Oxford). 2002 Oct;41(10):1163-7

[243] "In the interstitial connective tissue of fibromyalgic muscles we found a more intensive staining of the AGE CML, activated NF-kappaB, and also higher CML levels in the serum of these patients compared to the controls. RAGE was only present in FM muscle." Rüster M, Franke S, Späth M, Pongratz DE, Stein G, Hein GE. Detection of elevated N epsilon-carboxymethyllysine levels in muscular tissue and in serum of patients with fibromyalgia. *Scand J Rheumatol.* 2005 Nov-Dec;34(6):460-3

[244] "Recent evidence demonstrates that oxidative stress is associated with clinical symptoms in patients with CRPS-I. ... This review summarises the effect of oxidative stress and mitochondrial dysfunction in the pathogenesis of CRPS." Taha R, Blaise GA. Update on the pathogenesis of complex regional pain syndrome: role of oxidative stress. *Can J Anaesth.* 2012 Sep;59(9):875-81

[245] Gerdle et al. Chronic widespread pain: increased glutamate and lactate concentrations in the trapezius muscle and plasma. *Clin J Pain.* 2014 May;30(5):409-20. See also "Significantly higher interstitial concentrations of pyruvate and lactate were found in patients with fibromyalgia- syndrome. The multivariate regression analyses of group membership and pressure pain thresholds of the trapezius confirmed the importance of pyruvate and lactate." Gerdle et al. Increased interstitial concentrations of pyruvate and lactate in the trapezius muscle of patients with fibromyalgia: a microdialysis study. *J Rehabil Med.* 2010 Jul;42(7):679-87

the central processing of nociception. ...CWP patients had significantly increased interstitial muscle and plasma concentrations of lactate and glutamate. No significant differences existed in blood flow between CWP and CON [controls]. The interstitial concentrations-but not the plasma levels-of glutamate and lactate correlated significantly with aspects of pain such as pressure pain thresholds of the trapezius and tibialis anterior and the mean pain intensity in CWP but not in CON." Elevated lactate correlates with and suggests the presence of impaired energy/ATP production, consistent with mitochondrial dysfunction, while elevated glutamate levels is expected to promote enhanced pain reception, given that glutamate is the classic excitatory neurotransmitter (activator of glutamate receptors in general and the NMDA receptor in particular). The combination of elevated lactate (e.g., muscle impairment leading to muscle pain) and elevated glutamate (e.g., enhanced sensitivity to pain) is the perfect recipe and explanation for muscle-generated pain with enhanced sensitivity to pain that might otherwise be well tolerated. In addition to lactate and glutamate, patients with chronic muscle pain also show tissue-specific elevations of pyruvate (again indicating impaired energy/ATP production in muscles, leading to easy fatigability and increased achiness/pain) and elevated serotonin[246]; although we generally think of serotonin as having a relaxing and analgesic effect in the *central* nervous system, serotonin in the *periphery* appears to promote pain perception and sensitization while also promoting inflammation.[247]

- Patients with FM demonstrate abnormalities in muscle tissue and mitochondrial function: Muscle biopsies from patients with fibromyalgia show numerous histological, ultrastructural, and biochemical abnormalities, including defects in mitochondrial structure and function, reduced numbers of capillaries in skeletal muscle (leading to reduced blood supply to muscles), thickened capillary endothelium (thicker vessel walls), and ragged red fibers consistent with the development of **mitochondrial myopathy** (*myo*=muscle, *pathos*=disease). The histological finding of "rubber-band morphology" with reticular threads connecting neighboring cells in muscle biopsies of FM patients is associated with prolonged contractions in adjacent/neighboring muscle fibers; these abnormalities result in and perpetuate a low-energy state within myocytes (*myo*=muscle, *cytes*=cells).[248] Other studies have shown disorganization of actin filaments, accumulation of lipofuscin (cellular debris) consistent with premature muscle aging, accumulation of glycogen and lipid accumulation consistent with **mitochondrial impairment**, increased DNA fragmentation, **significant reductions in the number of mitochondria**, and focal areas of chronic muscle contraction.[249] These histological abnormalities are important and establish the fact that **fibromyalgia is a *disease of metabolic dysfunction*** rather than an *emotional disorder of psychogenic origin*; therefore, attributing the pain and fatigue of fibromyalgia to a mental-psychological cause or a central nervous system disorder such as central sensitization is unscientific and illogical. Patients with CRPS also show evidence of impaired oxygen diffusion and mitochondrial impairment[250], and Tan et al[251] specifically noted that mitochondrial ETC "complex II activity in the CRPS I patients was significantly lower."

[246] "Several studies clearly showed elevated levels of serotonin, glutamate, lactate, and pyruvate in localized chronic myalgias and may be potential biomarkers." Gerdle et al. Chronic musculoskeletal pain: review of mechanisms and biochemical biomarkers as assessed by the microdialysis technique. *J Pain Res.* 2014 Jun 12;7:313-26

[247] "5-HT, acting in combination with other inflammatory mediators, may ectopically excite and sensitize afferent nerve fibers, thus contributing to peripheral sensitization and hyperalgesia in inflammation and nerve injury." Sommer C. Serotonin in pain and analgesia in the periphery. *Mol Neurobiol.* 2004 Oct:117-25. See also: "5-HT sensitizes afferent nerve fibers, thus contributing to hyperalgesia in inflammation and nerve injury." Sommer C. Is serotonin hyperalgesic or analgesic? *Curr Pain Headache Rep.* 2006 Apr; 101-6

[248] Olsen NJ, Park JH. Skeletal muscle abnormalities in patients with fibromyalgia. *Am J Med Sci.* 1998 Jun;315(6):351-8

[249] Sprott H, Salemi S, Gay RE, et al. Increased DNA fragmentation and ultrastructural changes in fibromyalgic muscle fibres. *Ann Rheum Dis.* 2004 Mar;63(3):245-51

[250] "The mean venous oxygen saturation (S(v)O(2)) value (94.3% ± 4.0%) of the affected limb was significantly higher than S(v)O(2) values found in healthy subjects (77.5% ± 9.8%) pointing to a severely decreased oxygen diffusion or utilization within the affected limb. ... Ultrastructural investigations of soleus skeletal muscle capillaries revealed thickened endothelial cells and thickened basement membranes. Muscle capillary densities were decreased in comparison with literature data. High venous oxygen saturation levels were partially explained by impaired diffusion of oxygen due to thickened basement membrane and decreased capillary density. ...The abnormal skeletal muscle findings points to severe disuse but only partially explain the impaired diffusion of oxygen; mitochondrial dysfunction seems a likely explanation in addition." Tan et al. Impaired oxygen utilization in skeletal muscle of CRPS I patients. *J Surg Res.* 2012 Mar;173(1):145-52

[251] "We observed that mitochondria obtained from CRPS I muscle tissue displayed reduced mitochondrial ATP production and substrate oxidation rates in comparison to control muscle tissue. Moreover, we observed reactive oxygen species evoked damage to mitochondrial proteins and reduced MnSOD levels." Tan et al. Mitochondrial dysfunction in muscle tissue of complex regional pain syndrome type I patients. *Eur J Pain.* 2011 Aug;15(7):708-15

<table>
<tr><td style="text-align:center">**CONTROL**</td><td style="text-align:center">**PATIENT**</td></tr>
</table>

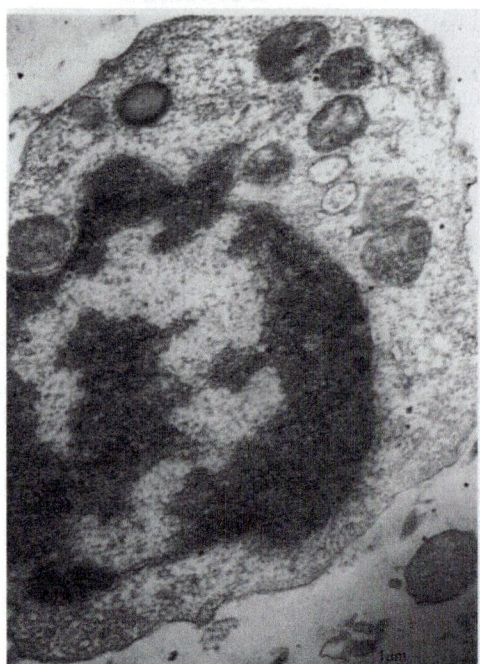 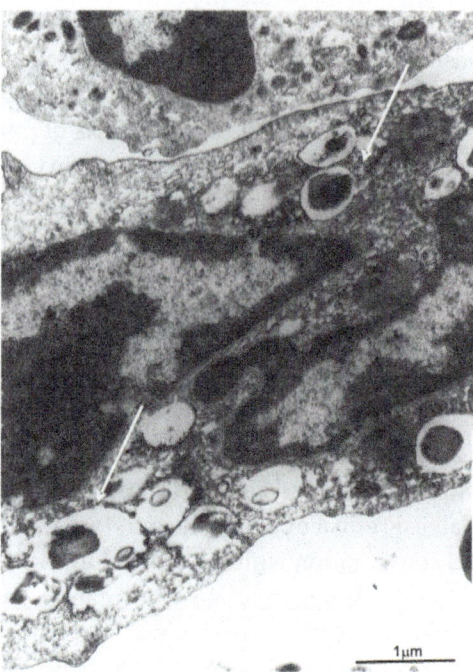

Blood cells in FM patients show mitochondrial destruction (mitophagy), smaller size and lower number of mitochondria: Structure of blood mononuclear cells (BMCs, cells of the immune system) from FM patients. The healthy/control BMCs show mitochondria with a normal structure. Autophagosomes (indicated by arrows), where mitochondria are destroyed (the process of mitophagy [*mito*=mitochondria, *phagy*=consumption], are noted in the BMCs of patients with FM. [Bar = 1 micrometer]. This open-access image is respectfully attributed to the brilliant research published by these researchers Cordero MD, De Miguel M, Moreno Fernández AM, Carmona López IM, Garrido Maraver J, Cotán D, Gómez Izquierdo L, Bonal P, Campa F, Bullon P, Navas P, Sánchez Alcázar JA. Mitochondrial dysfunction and mitophagy activation in blood mononuclear cells of fibromyalgia patients. *Arthritis Res Ther.* 2010;12(1):R17 arthritis-research.com/content/12/1/R17

Mitophagy: The body's inherent mechanism for the destruction of dysfunctional mitochondria

Concept: Autophagic destruction of mitochondria is termed "mitophagy" and is the body's inherent mechanism for eliminating superfluous or dysfunctional mitochondria; this generally has a protective and life-sustaining effect. However, in the case of fibromyalgia wherein the mitochondrial dysfunction is persistent, prolonged mitophagy contributes to failure of adequate energy production and thereby contributes to clinical manifestations of fatigue, dyscognition, and impaired exercise/activity performance. Further, the consistent documentation of significant mitophagy in patients with fibromyalgia proves the biological/organic/real/pathophysiologic character of the illness and refutes the pharmacocentric paradigm which holds that the condition is of psychogenic or neurologic origin and thus to be treated with so-called "antidepressants" and/or analgesic drugs, respectively.

- "The removal of damaged mitochondria that could contribute to cellular dysfunction or death is achieved through process of mitochondrial autophagy, i.e. mitophagy." Novak I. *Antioxid Redox Signal.* 2011
- "Mitochondrial number and health are regulated by mitophagy, a process by which excessive or damaged mitochondria are subjected to autophagic degradation." Rambold. *Cell Cycle.* 2011
- **"Autophagy can be beneficial for the cells by eliminating dysfunctional mitochondria, but massive autophagy can promote cell injury and may contribute to the pathophysiology of FM."** Cordero. *Arthritis Res Ther.* 2010

- **Pain in fibromyalgia originates peripherally and is amplified centrally**: The pain of fibromyalgia originates from the muscles[252] secondary to stimulation by oxidative and inflammatory mediators and is excessively amplified in the brain and spinal cord; another possible peripheral contribution to pain inputs is degeneration of nerve fibers in the skin.[253] To risk redundancy for clarity: **FM pain originates *peripherally* in the muscles**

---

[252] "Results of these studies suggest that FM pain is associated with widespread primary and secondary cutaneous hyperalgesia, which are dynamically maintained by tonic impulse input from deep tissues and likely by brain-to-spinal cord facilitation. Enhanced somatic pains are accompanied by mechanical hyperalgesia and allodynia in FM patients as compared with healthy controls. FM pain is likely to be at least partially maintained by peripheral impulse input from deep tissues. This conclusion is supported by results of several studies showing that injection of local anesthetics into painful muscles normalizes somatic hyperalgesia in FM patients." Staud R. Is it all central sensitization? Role of peripheral tissue nociception in chronic musculoskeletal pain. *Curr Rheumatol Rep.* 2010 Dec;12(6):448-54

[253] "The study's instruments comprised the Michigan Neuropathy Screening Instrument (MNSI), the Utah Early Neuropathy Scale (UENS), distal-leg neurodiagnostic skin biopsies, plus autonomic-function testing (AFT). We found that 41% of skin biopsies from subjects with fibromyalgia vs 3% of biopsies from control subjects were diagnostic for small-fiber polyneuropathy (SFPN), and MNSI and UENS scores were higher in patients with fibromyalgia than in control subjects (all P ≤ 0.001). Abnormal AFTs were equally prevalent, suggesting that fibromyalgia-associated SFPN is primarily somatic. Blood tests from subjects with fibromyalgia and SFPN-diagnostic skin biopsies provided insights into causes. All glucose tolerance tests were normal, but 8 subjects had dysimmune markers, 2 had hepatitis C serologies, and 1 family had apparent genetic causality. These

(and likely in the skin as well, at least in some patients) and is amplified *centrally* **in the spinal cord and brain.** Following reception and amplification of the original muscular pain, the peripheral "receptive field" grows both in size and intensity/hypersensitivity to include the skin, so that various skin inputs are perceived as pain; the two main types of dysfunctional pain sensitivity/sensations are allodynia (reception of nonpainful stimuli as pain) and hyperalgesia (extended duration and increased intensity of pain).

- Enhanced central pain processing of fibromyalgia patients is maintained by muscle afferent input (*Pain.* 2009 Sep[254]): "Lidocaine injections increased local pain thresholds and decreased remote secondary heat hyperalgesia in FM patients, emphasizing the important role of peripheral impulse input in maintaining central sensitization in this chronic pain syndrome; similar to other persistent pain conditions such as irritable bowel syndrome and complex regional pain syndrome."

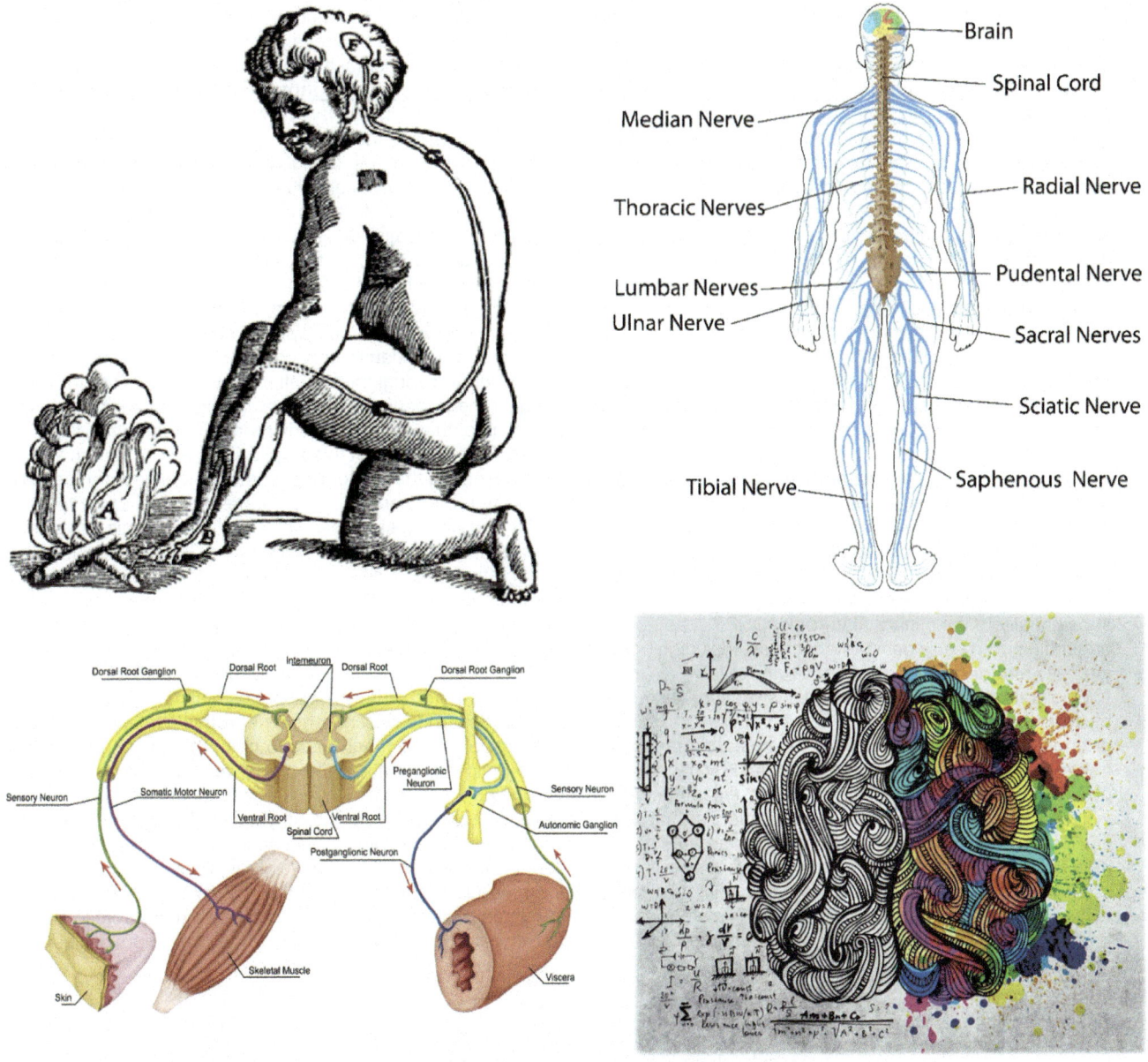

More than 400 years of the history and development of neuroanatomy and neurophysiology represented in four images: These four images in sequence represent the history and development of the fields of neuroanatomy and neurophysiology, ❶ starting with the drawing by Descartes in the 1600s, ❷ the tracing of nerves throughout the body, ❸ what might be called the

findings suggest that some patients with chronic pain labeled as fibromyalgia have unrecognized SFPN, a distinct disease that can be tested for objectively and sometimes treated definitively." Oaklander et al. Objective evidence that small-fiber polyneuropathy underlies some illnesses currently labeled as fibromyalgia. *Pain.* 2013 Nov;154(11):2310-6
[254] Staud et al. Enhanced central pain processing of fibromyalgia patients is maintained by muscle afferent input. *Pain.* 2009 Sep;145(1-2):96-104

start of the "functional neurology revolution" with the work of Melzack and Wall in 1965, and ❹ culminating with today's understanding of neurophysiology and neuropathophysiology as highly dynamic and interactive processes, far advanced from the simple models of sequential reception, perception, and interpretation.

1. ***Image upper left*—Peripheral reception and central perception of pain as simple linear connectivity**: The famous historical image from Rene Descartes (French polymath, 1596-1650) was an important beginning in society's understanding that pain had a neurophysiologic basis; in this model, pain sensations were received peripherally, transmitted by nerves to the brain where they were perceived and acted upon (e.g., reflexive withdrawal from painful stimuli).

2. ***Image upper right*—Nervous system as simple anatomic connectivity**: Advances in anatomy and neuroanatomy later provided more details about neurologic pathways and synapses (connections between nerves), but the overall model remained very mechanical, resembling electric circuitry (e.g., wiring) transmitting signals which were simply received in the brain for interpretation. Important within this obvious, simple, and overly simplistic model of neuroanatomy is the facile assumption of "stimulus-response specificity"—the idea that specific sensory receptors receive only one type of sensory input such as temperature or light touch or vibration; what we appreciate instead is that receptors, nerves, and their connections within the spinal cord, brainstem, and brain can communicate a wide range of sensory inputs in ways that commonly defy anatomic expectations. As stated by Wall[255], "Obviously anatomy does not predict physiology." Wall goes on to dismantle "the specificity theory" with the observations that "nociceptors become sensitized by prolonged or repeated noxious stimulation so that their threshold drops and they are excited by normally innocuous stimuli" and "one should be cautious in attributing one and only one function to a particular cell ...the degree of convergence is under control of other afferents and descending systems and is also dependent on the activity of segmental interneurons."

3. ***Image lower left*—Interconnections of nerves allows for "spill over" of sensory inputs and dynamic changes in perception, including amplification and misinterpretation**: Research published by Melzack and Wall[256] in 1965 is commonly credited with revolutionizing our view of pain processing by changing the paradigm from a static model of linear connectivity (e.g., sensory receptors to peripheral nerve to spinal cord to the brain) to one of dynamic interconnectivity, with interactive interconnections and opportunities for inhibition, amplification and misinterpretation at nearly every level. The perception of pain is neither simple, nor solely anatomy-based, nor static; it is a dynamic process reflecting the sum total interplay of peripheral reception (e.g., modifiable by inflammation), nerve transmission (e.g., modifiable by nutritional status and glutamate levels), reception and "intermixing" (e.g., pre-synaptic inhibition/facilitation, post-synaptic inhibition/facilitation) in the spinal cord, brain stem, subcortical structures such as the thalamus, and the "conscious" brain cortex. Furthermore and very importantly, we know that sensory nerves and sensory nerve endings do much more than simply receive information; in addition to sensing various types of stimuli through various types of sensors in nerve endings, sensory nerves directly influence the peripheral environment by releasing inflammatory mediators via a process called "neurogenic inflammation." Neurogenic (*neuro*—nerve, *genic*—generated, originating) inflammation again forces us to expand our perception of the nervous system and its components; in neurogenic inflammation, stimulated sensory nerves respond to painful stimuli by releasing inflammatory mediators into the self-same environment, thereby adding an inflammatory component to whatever is perceived as pain-inducing. One can think of this as providing a survival advantage in the short-term, as the inflammatory response generated by the release of these pro-inflammatory mediators released by nerves will serve to prepare the area for infiltration by immune cells to remove and repair damage and repel any infectious agents that might have entered with the injury. However, when chronically sustained in so-called "chronic diseases", neurogenic inflammation contributes to tissue injury, as we see in complex regional pain syndrome (CRPS). Indeed, CRPS might be considered a prototype of the effects of neurogenic inflammation. In a review published in 2015, Littlejohn[257] writes, "Neurogenic inflammation—comprising tissue swelling, vasomotor changes and marked allodynia—also contributes substantially to the clinical features of CRPS."; he goes on to mention the clinical sequelae that have a strong or dominant origination from neurogenic inflammation, including bone marrow edema, osteopenia, visceral pain, hyperalgesia (increased intensity and duration of pain sensitivity), allodynia (misperception of sensory input as pain), abnormal hair and nail growth (including absence of same), rashes, sweating, vasodilation (causing heat and redness), vasoconstriction (causing cold and blueness), skin ulceration and fibrosis of skin and joints. Littlejohn goes on to describe how neurogenic inflammation can promote itself, as nerve-released inflammatory mediators cause tissue damage that leads to pain, the self-same sensory nerves respond to the self-generated pain by causing more neurogenic inflammation; the proper term for this concept and phenomenon is "*neurogenic* neurogenic inflammation" or "neurogenic inflammation-induced neurogenic inflammation", a vicious cycle. I (DrV[258]) disagree with Littlejohn that this vicious cycle is at the core of fibromyalgia, although I agree that it could and likely does play a contributing part. Lastly and also included in the review by Littlejohn, the idea of "neurogenic neuroinflammation" likely has merit based on our current understanding of neuropathophysiology; especially in the spinal cord and brain, neuronal activity triggers microglial inflammation, which thereby inflames the nearby nerves for a vicious cycle of neurogenic neuroinflammation. This neurogenic neuroinflammation is almost certain to play a major role in CRPS, importantly but to a lesser degree in FM (chronic) and migraine (periodic). In the context of the brain and spinal cord,

[255] Wall PD. The gate control theory of pain mechanisms. A re-examination and re-statement. *Brain*. 1978 Mar;101(1):1-18

[256] Melzack R, Wall PD. Pain mechanisms: a new theory. *Science*. 1965 Nov 19;150(3699):971–979

[257] Littlejohn G. Neurogenic neuroinflammation in fibromyalgia and complex regional pain syndrome. *Nat Rev Rheumatol*. 2015 Nov;11(11):639-48

[258] At the time this citation is added in 2015 Dec, I (DrV) had recently submitted a reply to the article by Littlejohn (Neurogenic neuroinflammation in fibromyalgia and complex regional pain syndrome. *Nat Rev Rheumatol*. 2015 Nov) pointing out some of the bitemporal hemianopsia of the aforecited article; my reply will be published either by *Nat Rev Rheumatol* or elsewhere and will be posted at ichnfm.academia.edu/AlexVasquez as soon as possible. In reply to the previously cited article, Cordeo —a preeminent researcher in the field of fibromyalgia's mitochondrial dysfunction and its remediation by the vitamin-like substance coenzyme Q10 (CoQ10)—noted that neurogenic neuroinflammation includes activation of the NLRP3 inflammasome, which he suggests could be a therapeutic target (e.g., by CoQ10). "Interestingly, inflammasome activation in the CNS primarily occurs in microglia and macrophages. Microglia have been highly studied as key contributors to pathological and chronic pain mechanisms, and are involved in hyperalgesia and allodynia in both fibromyalgia and chronic fatigue syndrome, as well as pain in CRPS. Microglial inflammasome activation promotes the recruitment of peripheral innate immune cells (macrophages) and adaptive immune cells (T cells and B cells), as well as further activating nearby glial cells." Cordero MD. The inflammasome in fibromyalgia and CRPS: a microglial hypothesis? *Nat Rev Rheumatol*. 2015 Nov;11(11):630. See also Cordero MD et al. NLRP3 inflammasome is activated in fibromyalgia: the effect of coenzyme Q10. *Antioxid Redox Signal*. 2014 Mar 10;20(8):1169-80

neurogenic neuroinflammation contains an important pro-inflammatory contributor that is phenotypically ready to perceive, amplify, and exacerbate neuroinflammation caused by increased neuroactivity—the microglial cells; thus, neurogenic (in this context, including the microglia and astrocytes as components of the brain and spinal cord) neuroinflammation would be expected to participate in seizure disorders and vaccine-induced encephalomyelitis.

4. ***Image lower right*—The nervous system (represented by artistic brain image) is now appreciated as dynamic and interactive receiver and processor of sensory information**: In modern times, pain processing is appreciated as a dynamic, complex, and interactive process at every level, from ❶ peripheral reception of stimuli (e.g., in the skin or muscles), to the ❷ spinal cord, to the ❸ brainstem, to the ❹ subcortical structures especially the thalamus, to the ❺ cortex. Generally appreciated is that much "spill-over", "misinterpretation", inhibition and amplification" can occur in the spinal cord, brainstem, and structures of the brain, so that the initial perception of pain—in the muscles for example in the case of FM—is amplified at multiple levels and "spills over" to be perceived as skin pain, resulting in allodynia (misinterpretation of light touch as pain) and hyperalgesia (pain perception is amplified in intensity and duration). The brain is constantly adapting to input; for example the brain forms neuron-neuron connections in various patterns to produce memory. When the brain is constantly receiving messages of pain, the brain "rewires" the neuron-neuron interconnections to increase pain processing—what might be called a "pain memory"—in a way that facilitates the perception of pain, leading to enhanced pain perception, e.g., more pain felt by the patient.

Diagnosis

- <u>Clinical criteria—description and contrast of the 1990 criteria and the 2010 criteria</u>: Per guidelines published in 1990 by the American College of Rheumatology (ACR), a diagnosis of fibromyalgia can be made in a patient with inexplicable, widespread myofascial pain of at least 3 months' duration; *inexplicable* denotes normalcy of routine laboratory and physical examination findings and failure to find an alternate explanation or diagnosis, while *widespread* denotes bilateral pain above and below the waist not attributable to trauma or rheumatic disease and with pain at 11 of 18 classic tender point locations (see illustration below).

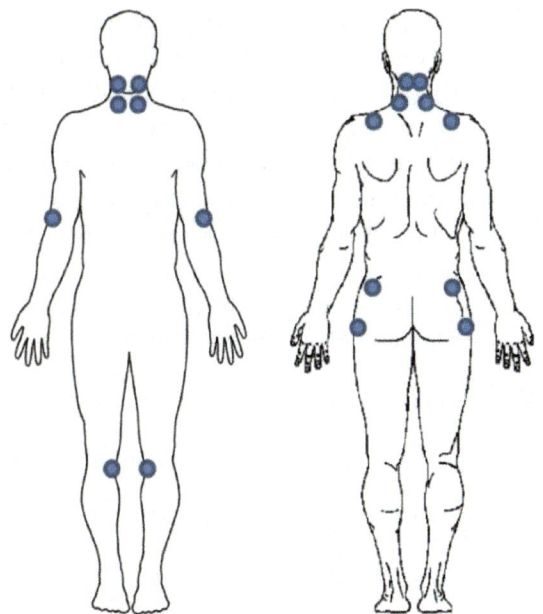

Illustration of the 9 paired locations of FM tender points:
Pain, on digital palpation, must be present in at least 11 of the following 18 tender point sites:
1. <u>Occiput</u>: at the suboccipital muscle insertions.
2. <u>Low cervical</u>: at the anterior aspects of the intertransverse spaces at C5-C7.
3. <u>Trapezius</u>: at the midpoint of the upper border.
4. <u>Supraspinatus</u>: at origins, above the scapula spine near the medial border.
5. <u>Second rib</u>: upper lateral to the second costochondral junction.
6. <u>Lateral epicondyle</u>: 2 cm distal to the epicondyles.
7. <u>Gluteal</u>: in upper outer quadrants of buttocks in anterior fold of muscle.
8. <u>Greater trochanter</u>: posterior to the trochanteric prominence.
9. <u>Knee</u>: at the medial fat pad proximal to the joint line.

Per 1990 ACR guidelines, the diagnosis of FM is supported when at least 11 out of 18 of these locations are painful. Digital palpation should be performed with an approximate force of 4 kg (9 lbs). A tender point has to be painful at palpation, not just "tender."[259]

FM tender points are assessed bilaterally at 9 paired sites: (sub)occiput (below the head at the neckline), low cervical spine (lower neck), trapezius and supraspinatus (two of the shoulder muscles), second rib (anterior, near costosternal [rib-breastbone] junction), lateral epicondyle, gluteal region, greater trochanter, and medial fat pad of the knees. Tender points are provoked by the clinician's application of approximately 9 pounds of fingertip pressure, which is sufficient to cause blanching of the clinician's nail bed. The tender points of fibromyalgia are distinguished from myofascial trigger points (MFTP, described by Travell[260]) and strain-counterstrain tender points (described in the osteopathic literature by Jones[261]). Pain must have been consistent

---

[259] The American College of Rheumatology 1990 Criteria for the Classification of Fibromyalgia. nfra.net/Diagnost.htm Accessed Nov 2011

[260] Simons DG, Travell JG, Simons LS. *Travell & Simons' Myofascial Pain and Dysfunction. The Trigger Point Manual*. Baltimore: Lippincott Williams & Wilkins; 1999

[261] Jones L, Kusunose R, Goering E. *Jones Strain-Counterstrain*. Carlsbad, Jones Strain Counterstrain Incorporated, 1995. [ISBN 0964513544]

for at least three months and must not be attributable to another (obvious) cause. In contrast to MFTP, which are located toward the center of the muscle fiber and which refer pain and show spontaneous electrocontractile activity[262], tender points of fibromyalgia are located near the tendinous insertions of muscle to bone and cause local pain only, without pain referral or contractile activity.

The new 2010 ACR guidelines for the diagnosis and assessment of FM[263] are significantly different from the 1990 guidelines. These new guidelines are mostly illogical and appear to have been structured to broaden the definition of fibromyalgia, to allow patients and nonphysicians to make the diagnosis, and generally to increase the patient population available for a diagnosis of fibromyalgia, thereby increasing the sales of drugs. Very curiously, the authors state that one of their objectives was to create criteria that "do not require a tender point examination"; at first, this seems odd and clinically inconsistent considering that the tender point examination ❶ takes only about 60 seconds to perform, ❷ is noninvasive, ❸ was previously the standard by which the diagnosis was made, and ❹ is reasonable and responsible—physical examination of patients with pain is a reasonable standard of care. Oddly, the authors of the new guidelines note several "important problems" with the 1990 ACR criteria, such as "Patients who improved or whose symptoms and tender points decreased could fail to satisfy the ACR 1990 classification definition" and "there was little variation in symptoms among fibromyalgia patients." Clinicians should note that these so-called "problems" *are not problems at all* because patients who improve and thus no longer meet diagnostic criteria should not be considered to have an active disease/diagnosis, and that high-quality clinical criteria should indeed result in the specific definition of clinical disorder and thus in a well-defined cohort of patients; correcting these "problems" results in patients being diagnosed for longer periods of time (more *long-term* patients) and also results in more patients being diagnosed with fibromyalgia (more *total* patients). Perhaps even more curious is the fact that development of these new guidelines was sponsored by Lilly Research Laboratories—the front page of the article states "these criteria were developed with support from the study sponsor, Lilly Research Laboratories", which is the "research" section of Eli Lilly and Company, one of the world's largest drug companies and the manufacturer of duloxetine/Cymbalta® which is one of the only drugs approved by the US Food and Drug Administration (FDA) for the treatment of fibromyalgia.[264] Among patients labeled with fibromyalgia, the new criteria increase the percentage of patients diagnosable by criteria from 75% to 88%; whether the motivation to expand the patient population diagnosed with fibromyalgia is altruistic or financially motivated is subject to debate. The new criteria rely on a summation of two tallies—"widespread pain index" (WPI) and "symptom severity" (SS, parts 1 and 2)—with the diagnosis being supported by either **"WPI >7 and SS >5"** or **"WPI 3–6 and SS >9"**.

A descriptive video of the distinctions between the 1990 and 2010 diagnostic criteria is available for free from www.InflammationMastery.com/pain.

---

[262] Hubbard DR, Berkoff GM. Myofascial trigger points show spontaneous needle EMG activity. *Spine*. 1993 Oct 1;18(13):1803-7
[263] Wolfe F, et al. The ACR preliminary diagnostic criteria for fibromyalgia and measurement of symptom severity. *Arthritis Care Res*. 2010;62(5):600-10
[264] lilly.com/research/Pages/research.aspx and newsroom.lilly.com/ReleaseDetail.cfm?releaseid=316740 Accessed January 2012

Widespread pain index (WPI): Each positive location receives one point (max = 19)

1. Shoulder girdle, left	7. Hip (buttock/trochanter), left	13. Jaw, left
2. Shoulder girdle, right	8. Hip (buttock/trochanter), right	14. Jaw, right
3. Upper arm, left	9. Upper leg, left	15. Chest (sternum area)
4. Upper arm, right	10. Upper leg, right	16. Abdomen
5. Lower arm, left	11. Lower leg, left	17. Neck
6. Lower arm, right	12. Lower leg, right	18. Upper back
		19. Lower back

Symptom severity (SS)—part 1: Each of these three problems is quantified with the following scale (max = 9):
0 none: no problem **1 mild**: intermittent or mild problems
2 moderate: often present, considerable problems **3 severe**: continuous, life-disturbing problems

0 1 2 3 Fatigue	0 1 2 3 Waking unrefreshed	0 1 2 3 Cognitive symptoms

Symptom severity (SS)—part 2: The clinician considers the patient's "somatic symptoms in general" (listed below) and applies the following scale (max = 3):
0 no symptoms 1 few symptoms
2 a moderate number of symptoms 3 a great deal of symptoms

0 1 2 3 muscle pain	0 1 2 3 itching
0 1 2 3 irritable bowel syndrome	0 1 2 3 wheezing
0 1 2 3 fatigue/tiredness	0 1 2 3 Raynaud's phenomenon
0 1 2 3 thinking or remembering problems	0 1 2 3 hives/welts
0 1 2 3 muscle weakness	0 1 2 3 ringing in ears
0 1 2 3 headache	0 1 2 3 vomiting
0 1 2 3 pain/cramps in the abdomen	0 1 2 3 heartburn
0 1 2 3 numbness/tingling	0 1 2 3 oral ulcers
0 1 2 3 dizziness	0 1 2 3 loss of/change in taste
0 1 2 3 insomnia	0 1 2 3 seizures
0 1 2 3 depression	0 1 2 3 dry eyes
0 1 2 3 constipation	0 1 2 3 shortness of breath
0 1 2 3 pain in the upper abdomen	0 1 2 3 loss of appetite
0 1 2 3 nausea	0 1 2 3 skin rash
0 1 2 3 nervousness	0 1 2 3 sun sensitivity
0 1 2 3 chest pain	0 1 2 3 hearing difficulties
0 1 2 3 blurred vision	0 1 2 3 easy bruising
0 1 2 3 fever	0 1 2 3 hair loss
0 1 2 3 diarrhea	0 1 2 3 frequent urination
0 1 2 3 dry mouth	0 1 2 3 painful urination
	0 1 2 3 bladder spasms

Tally points from above; patients may be diagnosed with FM if **"WPI >7 and SS >5"** or **"WPI 3-6 and SS >9"**.
WPI = ____
SS1 + SS2 = ____

2010 Fibromyalgia diagnostic criteria—summary, chart for clinical use, discussion: Per the 2010 diagnostic criteria[265], patients may be diagnosed with fibromyalgia if "WPI >7 and SS >5" or "WPI 3–6 and SS >9". Of note, these new criteria reflect a major departure from the former criteria published and codified in 1990; of additional note, publication of these new criteria received sponsorship from a drug company which has an FDA-approved drug for this condition—this represents a massive conflict of interest, full manifestation of which would have the same for-profit entity influencing the criteria used by doctors for the diagnosis and then providing (i.e., selling for profit) one of the only approved drug treatment options. I have discussed these conundrums in video format at Vimeo.com/ICHNFM and Vimeo.com/DrVasquez.

- Clinical profile and findings on common laboratory tests: New-onset fibromyalgia is unlikely over age 50, and the condition never causes fever, significant weight loss, or other objective signs of acute or subacute illness. Hypothyroidism is common and can produce widespread myofascial pain along with depression and other complaints, resulting in a clinical picture that closely resembles FM; thus, a complete thyroid evaluation (detailed later) is essential during the initial evaluation of any fibromyalgia-like condition. Common rheumatic

---

[265] Wolfe F, et al. The ACR preliminary diagnostic criteria for fibromyalgia and measurement of symptom severity. *Arthritis Care Res.* 2010;62(5):600-10

conditions such as rheumatoid arthritis (RA) and systemic lupus erythematosus (SLE) are excluded by the lack of other clinical manifestations (e.g., joint pain and swelling) and the lack of positive laboratory findings such as anti-cyclic citrullinated protein (CCP) antibodies and antinuclear antibodies (ANA), respectively. C-reactive protein (CRP) and erythrocyte sedimentation rate (ESR) are normal in FM patients; abnormalities with these or other common laboratory assessments suggest inflammatory disease, infection, or other concomitant illness. Hypophosphatemia (a low level of the electrolyte phosphate in the blood) can cause bone pain and muscle weakness; this condition is easily excluded by demonstration of normal serum phosphate level.

Standard Medical Treatment for Fibromyalgia

- Overview: Mild exercise, "patient education", and the use of pain-relieving drugs are mainstays of standard medical treatment delivered by most allopathic medical doctors (MDs), and osteopathic medical doctors (DOs) may add manual musculoskeletal treatments to enhance the benefits of drugs.[266] These interventions are only partially effective and offer no hope of actually curing the disease; thus, medical treatment relegates patients to a future of drug dependency, potential adverse effects (some of which can be fatal), and therapeutic inefficacy insofar as none of these treatments addresses the underlying cause of the disorder.

  - Amitriptyline: For many years, the most widely used drug for symptomatic treatment of fibromyalgia was amitriptyline (a tricyclic antidepressant), which has been used "off label"—without approval from the FDA—for this application. In the treatment of FM, the drug has low efficacy and high potential for adverse effects; up to 20% of patients suffer from weight gain, constipation, orthostatic hypotension, and/or agitation as a side-effect of the drug. Only 25% to 30% of fibromyalgia patients experience clinically significant improvement with amitriptyline.[267] According to recent research in rats, administration of amitriptyline causes deficiency of CoQ10, impaired mitochondrial function, reduced ATP/energy production, and increased oxidative stress and free radical damage[268]; all of these drug-induced problems (discussed in detail later in this paper) are expected to worsen the pain and suffering experienced by FM patients. Thus, the use of amitriptyline cannot be considered to be consistent with the practice of good medicine due to its low efficacy and unacceptable risks for adverse effects.

  - Pregabalin: In 2007, the United States Food and Drug Administration (US FDA) approved pregabalin (Lyrica® sold/marketed by Pfizer) for symptomatic treatment of fibromyalgia[269]; however, because the drug does not address the primary cause(s) of the disease, patients must continue treatment indefinitely. Adverse effects of pregabalin include

Suicide and depression risk warning for pregabalin/Lyrica from the US FDA
"Antiepileptic drugs (AEDs), including Lyrica, increase the risk of suicidal thoughts or behavior in patients taking these drugs for any indication. Patients treated with any AED for any indication should be monitored for the emergence or worsening of depression, suicidal thoughts or behavior, and/or any unusual changes in mood or behavior." fda.gov/Safety/MedWatch/SafetyInformation/Safety-RelatedDrugLabelingChanges/ucm154524.htm

dizziness, sleepiness, blurred vision, weight gain, dry mouth, swelling of hands and feet, impairment of motor function, and problems with concentration and attention. Pregabalin when given at the recommended dose of 150-225 mg twice per day for fibromyalgia costs $94-190 per month (pricing in 2013).

  - Duloxetine: In 2008, the FDA announced duloxetine (Cymbalta® sold/marketed by Lilly) as the second approved drug for the treatment of fibromyalgia. Ironically, many physicians consider any "approved" drug to have scientific substantiation; however, in the case of duloxetine (as well as pregabalin) the exact mechanism of action is unknown[270] although duloxetine appears to inhibit reuptake of norepinephrine and serotonin, thereby increasing the action of these neurotransmitters in the synaptic cleft. Adverse effects from duloxetine include nausea, dry mouth, sleepiness, constipation, decreased appetite, and increased

[266] Gamber RG, Shores JH, Russo DP, Jimenez C, Rubin BR. Osteopathic manipulative treatment in conjunction with medication relieves pain associated with fibromyalgia syndrome: results of a randomized clinical pilot project. *J Am Osteopath Assoc.* 2002 Jun;102(6):321-5 jaoa.org/content/102/6/321.full.pdf

[267] Leventhal LJ. Management of fibromyalgia. *Ann Intern Med.* 1999 Dec 7;131(11):850-8

[268] "Amitriptyline is a tricyclic antidepressant commonly prescribed for the treatment of several neuropathic and inflammatory illnesses. We have already reported that amitriptyline has cytotoxic effect in human cell cultures, increasing oxidative stress, and decreasing growth rate and mitochondrial activity." Bautista-Ferrufino MR, Cordero MD, Sánchez-Alcázar JA, et al. Amitriptyline induces coenzyme Q deficiency and oxidative damage in mouse lung and liver. *Toxicol Lett.* 2011 Jul 4;204(1):32-7

[269] FDA Approves First Drug for Treating Fibromyalgia. fda.gov/bbs/topics/NEWS/2007/NEW01656.html

[270] "exact mechanism of action unknown; inhibits norepinephrine and serotonin reuptake" https://online.epocrates.com; "Both Lyrica and Cymbalta reduce pain and improve function in people with fibromyalgia. While those with fibromyalgia have been shown to experience pain differently from other people, the mechanism by which these drugs produce their effects is unknown. fda.gov/ForConsumers/ConsumerUpdates/ucm107802.htm. Accessed January 2012

sweating; **duloxetine can also increase the risk of suicidal thinking and behavior and for this reason the drug carries a black box warning on the container.** Duloxetine can cause serious and fatal adverse effects including the following: worsening depression and suicidality, serotonin syndrome, neuroleptic malignant syndrome, seizures, and Stevens-Johnson syndrome. Duloxetine given at the recommended dose of 60 mg per day for FM costs $170 per month (pricing in 2013).

Suicide and depression risk warning for duloxetine/Cymbalta
"WARNING: Suicidality and Antidepressant Drugs: Antidepressants increased the risk compared to placebo of suicidal thinking and behavior (suicidality) in children, adolescents, and young adults in short-term studies of major depressive disorder (MDD) and other psychiatric disorders. Anyone considering the use of Cymbalta or any other antidepressant in a child, adolescent, or young adult must balance this risk with the clinical need. Short-term studies did not show an increase in the risk of suicidality with antidepressants compared to placebo in adults beyond age 24; there was a reduction in risk with antidepressants compared to placebo in adults aged 65 and older. Depression and certain other psychiatric disorders are themselves associated with increases in the risk of suicide. Patients of all ages who are started on antidepressant therapy should be monitored appropriately and observed closely for clinical worsening, suicidality, or unusual changes in behavior. Families and caregivers should be advised of the need for close observation and communication with the prescriber. Cymbalta is not approved for use in pediatric patients."
pi.lilly.com/us/cymbalta-pi.pdf

- Milnacipran: Approved for the treatment of FM by the US FDA in 2009, milnacipran (Savella® sold/marketed by Forest Pharmaceuticals) inhibits norepinephrine and serotonin reuptake, i.e., it potentiates (increases the effect of) the neurotransmitters norepinephrine and serotonin, both of which decrease the experience of pain and elevate mood. Of course, other non-drug treatments (such as nutrients and dietary optimization) can have the same effect, but most medical doctors have no training in nondrug

Suicide and depression risk warning for milnacipran/Savella
"Savella is a selective serotonin and norepinephrine reuptake inhibitor (SNRI), similar to some drugs used for the treatment of depression and other psychiatric disorders. Antidepressants increased the risk compared to placebo of suicidal thinking and behavior (suicidality) in children, adolescents, and young adults in short-term studies of major depressive disorder (MDD) and other psychiatric disorders."
frx.com/pi/Savella_pi.pdf, linked as "Full Prescribing Information" from savella.com/important-risk-information.aspx

treatments[271,272,273,274] and thus habitually turn to drugs as the one-and-only answer to the patients' problems[275], especially when these are sanctified by FDA/government approval. Nondrug treatments that enhance serotonergic and noradrenergic neurotransmission include exercise, relaxation, massage, and nutritional supplementation with omega-3 fatty acids (as found in fish oil), nutritional supplementation in general and vitamin D supplementation in particular. Adverse effects associated with use of milnacipran include seizures, suicidality, depression, worsening hypomania/mania, Stevens-Johnson syndrome (which is a medical emergency that can be fatal), serotonin syndrome, neuroleptic malignant syndrome, hypertensive (elevated blood pressure) crisis, tachycardia (rapid heart rate), hyponatremia (low sodium in the blood, which can occasionally result in permanent brain damage), abnormal bleeding (due to abnormal platelet function), glaucoma, and liver toxicity.[276] Treatment of fibromyalgia is the only FDA-approved use of this medication, which when used at the recommended dose of 50 mg twice daily costs $144 per month (pricing in April 2013).

- Cyclobenzaprine, Tramadol, and acetaminophen: Cyclobenzaprine (a muscle-relaxing drug), Tramadol (a non-typical opioid, centrally-acting narcotic analgesic) and acetaminophen (centrally acting analgesic),

---

[271] "Internal medicine interns' perceive nutrition counseling as a priority, but lack the confidence and knowledge to effectively provide adequate nutrition education." Vetter ML, Herring SJ, Sood M, Shah NR, Kalet AL. What do resident physicians know about nutrition? An evaluation of attitudes, self-perceived proficiency and knowledge. *J Am Coll Nutr.* 2008 Apr;27(2):287-98 ncbi.nlm.nih.gov/pmc/articles/PMC2779722/

[272] "The amount of nutrition education that medical students receive continues to be inadequate." Adams KM, Kohlmeier M, Zeisel SH. Nutrition education in U.S. medical schools: latest update of a national survey. *Acad Med.* 2010 Sep;85(9):1537-42

[273] "Scientific advances on the relationship of dietary substances to the cellular mechanisms of disease occur with regularity and frequency. Yet, despite the prevalence of nutritional disorders in clinical medicine and increasing scientific evidence on the significance of dietary modification to disease prevention, present day practitioners of medicine are typically untrained in the relationship of diet to health and disease." Halsted CH. The relevance of clinical nutrition education and role models to the practice of medicine. *Eur J Clin Nutr.* 1999 May;53 Suppl 2:S29-34

[274] Vasquez A. Interventions need to be consistent with osteopathic philosophy. *J Am Osteopath Assoc.* 2006 Sep;106(9):528-9 jaoa.org/content/106/9/528.full.pdf

[275] Ely et al. Analysis of questions asked by family doctors regarding patient care. *BMJ.* 1999 Aug 7;319(7206):358-61 ncbi.nlm.nih.gov/pmc/articles/PMC28191/

[276] https://online.epocrates.com/noFrame/showPage.do?method=drugs&MonographId=4950 Accessed April 2012.

show low efficacy and have little research supporting their use in the treatment of FM; these drugs also carry important risks for adverse effects, and they do not favorably alter the course of the disease over the long-term.[277] Per recent information from the American College of Rheumatology (ACR), treatment of FM with opioid drugs "may cause greater pain sensitivity or make pain persist."[278]

- Exercise: Low-intensity aerobic exercise may initially exacerbate symptoms but can result in very modest mental and physical improvement. Exercise alone cannot cure FM.
- Cognitive-behavioral therapy (CBT): Cognitive-behavioral therapy helps patients deal with and adapt to the impact of the illness. Therapy alone cannot cure FM.
- Patient (mis)education in standard medicine: "Patient education" from a *medical* perspective generally means telling patients that ❶ they will probably have the condition forever, ❷ they will not immediately die from it, ❸ they need to take it seriously (i.e., comply with medical treatment), and ❹ they need to rely on drugs for alleviation of symptoms since no cause of the condition is known and therefore no direct treatment is available. From the medical perspective, these communications are considered "helpful" and "reassuring"; however, part of the effect that is created is **dependency** ("You need these drugs from me."), **passivity** ("There's nothing you can do about this, so don't even try to think for yourself or seek 'alternative' treatments."), and **co-victimization** ("We are both victims of our ignorance; I am in this with you in that we are both blind and dependent on drug management."). In the examples that follow, I will review and summarize patient educational materials from major medical groups; for efficiency, I will use quotes followed by my comments in *italics*:
- Press release from the American Pain Society "Fibromyalgia Has Central Nervous System Origins", written by an author heavily funded by drug companies[279]:
  - "Fibromyalgia is the second most common rheumatic disorder behind osteoarthritis and, though still widely misunderstood, is now considered to be a lifelong central nervous system disorder, which is responsible for amplified pain that shoots through the body in those who suffer from it." — *This lunacy does not require additional refutation: the American Pain Society clearly affiliates with drug companies and wants to promote drug sales and use of their specialty organization; for this, they need to foster the illusion that FM begins in the brain, has no cure, and needs to be treated with drugs for the duration of patients' lives.*
- "Patient Education" from the American College of Rheumatology, Rheumatology.org[280]:
  - "Though there is no cure, medications can relieve symptoms." — *This is a commonly used statement within the medical community from doctors to patients to create passivity and drug/medical dependency.*
  - "There likely are certain genes that can make people more prone to getting fibromyalgia and the other health problems that can occur with it. Genes alone, though, do not cause fibromyalgia." — *These are common statements in the medical community, basically summed as "We don't know what we are doing but your only hope is to depend on us."*
  - "For the person with fibromyalgia, it is as though the "volume control" is turned up too high in the brain's pain processing centers." — *This promotes the concept of "primary central sensitization" (i.e., the brain has defied normal physiology and has somehow [without known cause, by itself] become too sensitive to pain); this "blame the brain" concept is used to leverage drug sales for pain-relieving and anti-depressant drugs as I have recently reviewed in video: youtube.com/watch?v=41opevN87qs*
  - "There is no cure for fibromyalgia. However, symptoms can be treated with both medication and non-drug treatments." — *This is the standard "party line" for the medical profession, whose chief goal is not to cure diseases but rather to drug them indefinitely, thereby creating a perpetual audience for their services and prescriptions. Honorable mention (more accurately: dishonorable mention) is generally given to "lifestyle modification" but is generally done so in a way that provides vague advice for ineffective interventions, thereby* **creating the illusion of options** *while undercutting any potential for these "options" to actually work.*
  - Non-drug treatments reviewed: relaxation, deep breathing, meditation, sleep, avoidance of nicotine and caffeine, exercise including such miniscule revelations as "take the stairs instead of the elevator, or park further [sic] away from the store", and "education" from other medical and special interest groups. — *These*

[277] Goldenberg DL, Burckhardt C, Crofford L. Management of fibromyalgia syndrome. *JAMA*. 2004 Nov 17;292(19):2388-95
[278] rheumatology.org/practice/clinical/patients/diseases_and_conditions/fibromyalgia.asp Accessed April 2012
[279] Fibromyalgia Has Central Nervous System Origins. americanpainsociety.org/about-us/press-room/fibromyalgia-clauw May 16, 2015
[280] rheumatology.org/practice/clinical/patients/diseases_and_conditions/fibromyalgia.asp Accessed March 31, 2012

are all essentially worthless suggestions, but they are effective distractions for patients and doctors so that effective treatments are marginalized and drug/medical dependency is fostered.

- Prescription drugs are given the primary emphasis in the treatment section.—*Whether drugs are effective or not, the medical profession relies on drugs for its societal position and will therefore reflexively advocate them.*

- Patient education from American Academy of Family Physicians, FamilyDoctor.org[281]:
  - "…your muscles and organs are not being damaged."—*This is false/inaccurate information. Several primary research studies have demonstrated consistently pathologic and biochemical abnormalities in muscle tissue from patients with fibromyalgia; this research has been published in widely available peer-reviewed medical journals. While the muscle damage in FM is not gross or overt myopathy, stating that no damage is occurring is not histologically accurate and supports the drug-friendly model that FM is idiopathic and (neuro)psychiatric.*
  - "This condition is not life-threatening, but it is chronic (ongoing). Although there is no cure,…"—*This is false information because obviously the condition is curable; the statement as it reads produces patient passivity and drug-dependency, which is exactly what the medical profession and the drug industry want.*
  - "There isn't currently a cure for fibromyalgia. Your care will focus on helping you minimize the impact of fibromyalgia on your life and treating your symptoms. Your doctor can prescribe medicine to help with your pain,… The treatment recommendations your doctor makes won't do any good unless you follow them."—*Again, false information promoting passivity and drug-dependency. This is basically drug propaganda, encouraging passivity and compliance on the parts of doctors and patients alike.*
  - Weak recommendations under the guise of "taking an active role in your healthcare" include 1) maintaining a healthy outlook, 2) support groups, 3) **"take medicines exactly as prescribed"**, 4) moderate exercise, 5) stress management, 6) "establish healthy sleep habits", 7) make a routine daily schedule, 8) "make healthy lifestyle choices." —*Most of these recommendations are blatantly passive, vague, and ineffective while fostering drug-dependency.*

The most common pattern in medical books and articles: components of the medical paradigm

1. Diseases are describable yet incomprehensible: The condition generally is described as a complex interplay of genetic factors with numerous environmental factors; generally little or no intellectually worthwhile effort is made to understand these environmental factors, so the ultimate view that medical physicians are taught is the disease is not understood and that drug therapy is the best available treatment.
2. Nearly always the disease is described as chronic and incurable: Even if a cure is known and published in available peer-reviewed research, most medical books and articles conclude that the causes are unknown and that palliative drug treatment is therefore warranted.
3. Characteristics and diagnostic criteria are reviewed: The medical profession is very good at defining and diagnosing problems, but the reliance on drugs often detours from the more effective nondrug treatments. The idea that every disease needs a drug is absurd, but this very same idea is embraced as the axiom of medicine and indeed as proof of its insight and resourcefulness.
4. Drug treatments are emphasized: Drug benefits are inflated and adverse effects are minimized if mentioned at all. Many review articles published in clinical journals are authored by consultants to the drug industry who profit from the sale of the drugs used to treat the condition about which they write; the general conclusion of these articles is that "Medical research is making considerable advances in our understanding of Disease X, which results from a complex interplay of genetic and environmental factors. The appropriate treatment for Disease X is Drug X, then Drug X2…along with generally meaningless lifestyle advice.
5. Nondrug treatments are marginalized: Brief mention is made of diet and lifestyle and other non-drug treatments, but the information is nonspecific, very general, and almost always diluted to the point of inefficacy.
6. Authentic integrative/functional medicine approaches are essentially never mentioned: Generally, the only nondrug treatments that are mentioned are weak or are mentioned so casually that no effective action can be implemented.
7. Hope for the future is always placed back in the hands of "more research" and "drug development": Often some mention of "hope for the future" is made, generally in the guise of "medical research" and "drug development"; all the while, safe and effective non-drug treatment approaches that go far beyond diet and lifestyle are virtually never mentioned.

Most medical students start medical school in their early 20s, when they are notably young and impressionable, with practically zero life experience other than creating the perfect medical school application (ie, high scores plus some foray into volunteer work to appear socially concerned), and eager to "be a doctor." Medical training is typically 7 years—4 years of school followed by 3 years of hospital-based residency training—during which students and residents are stressed, sleep-deprived, hazed, and fearful of expulsion for any minor infraction. Medical training induces a trance-like state, with several features of Stockholm syndrome, wherein doctors become accustomed in their early training to memorize, pathologize, and conform to expectations. They are eager to do the things that define a doctor's authority and privilege—write prescriptions or recommend procedures/surgery; nutrition—a "nonmedical" treatment that is considered "alternative"—is for "quacks" (nonscientists, nonrationalists, especially those who could not enter a "real" medical school) and dieticians (hierarchically inferior to doctors). With the time pressure (2-7 minutes per patient) and formulary restrictions (zero outpatient nutritional options) of hospital/clinic-based training/practice, practically no *conscientious* medical student/clinician would consider deviation from well ingrained (and intellectually inbred) *expectations*.

---

[281] American Academy of Family Physicians. familydoctor.org/familydoctor/en/diseases-conditions/fibromyalgia.html Accessed March 31, 2012

Functional/Naturopathic Considerations, Assessments, and Interventions

- **Foundational perspectives:** Two fundamental premises of are: (1) ~~chronic~~ sustained *diseases* are manifestations of ~~chronic~~ sustained *dysfunctions*, and (2) dysfunction can result from a wide range of interconnected genotropic (gene-influenced), metabolic, nutritional, microbial, inflammatory, toxic, environmental, and psychological and social influences. **Many of these dysfunctions lie outside the narrow, pathology-based, pharmacocentric (drug-centered) view of standard allopathic medicine.** The functional/naturopathic medicine approach to each individual fibromyalgia patient is based firstly on the presumption that the condition has an underlying primary cause (or several interconnected causes) and that the cause(s) can be identified and addressed—in this manner, the clinical approach is one of positive psychoepistimology (ie, affirmative that we can understand this situation), rather than pathodefetism (ie, "we can't understand this disease") resulting pharmacodependency. The cause(s) may be manifold and multifaceted and may differ among patients with the same diagnostic label. This approach includes the diagnostic and therapeutic considerations of standard medicine but extends far beyond these in assessment, treatment, and understanding. Clinicians should appreciate that as a diagnostic label, fibromyalgia is commonly applied to any patient with chronic, widespread pain and that the current trend to limit diagnostic evaluation in such patients will clearly result in failure to identify and address readily diagnosable and treatable problems that can result in a clinical picture that resembles FM. Clinicians must consider chronic infections (such as with hepatitis C virus, *Borrelia burgdorferi* [the bacteria strongly associated with Lyme disease], *Chlamydia/Chlamydophila pneumoniae*, and the protozoan parasite *Babesia*, which is also associated with Lyme disease and co-infection with *Borrelia burgdorferi*), cancerous conditions such as multiple myeloma and lymphoma, and autoimmune/rheumatic diseases such as polymyositis and polymyalgia rheumatica. A few of the other more exemplary conditions to consider in patients with widespread pain are vitamin D deficiency, hypothyroidism, iron overload, and chronic exposure to and accumulation of xenobiotics—perhaps most importantly mercury and lead.

Common differential diagnoses—conditions that can mimic (or contribute to) fibromyalgia

- **Vitamin D deficiency:** A clinical picture nearly identical to fibromyalgia—chronic widespread pain, mental depression/anxiety, headaches, low-grade systemic inflammation—can result from vitamin D deficiency.[282] Fibromyalgia patients are commonly deficient in vitamin D, and indeed, **vitamin D deficiency—with its attendant pain, anxiety/depression, and normal lab values on routine laboratory testing—is often misdiagnosed as fibromyalgia**, as reported by Holick.[283] Increased severity of the deficiency correlates with worsening depression and anxiety in these patients.[284] Correction of vitamin D deficiency by administration of vitamin D3 (cholecalciferol) in doses of 5,000-10,000 IU (international units) per day for several months has resulted in a dramatic alleviation of pain; such intervention among patients with low back pain has resulted in cure rates greater than 95%.[285] Other studies with vitamin D3 using doses 400-4,000 IU/day have shown that vitamin D3 supplementation for the correction of vitamin D deficiency alleviates depression and enhances sense of well-being. Vitamin D3 supplementation—or adequate endogenous production from ultraviolet light exposure (approximately 10-30 minutes per day of full-body exposure at midday, near the equator)—to meet physiological requirements of approximately 4,000 IU/day is safe and results in numerous major health benefits.[286,287,288] The only risk associated with vitamin D supplementation is hypercalcemia—too much calcium in the blood, mostly as a result of increased gastrointestinal absorption of calcium; hypercalcemia can cause abdominal pain, bone pain, fatigue, constipation, abnormal heart rhythm (arrhythmia), kidney stones, increased thirst and urination [additional details[289]]. Hypercalcemia caused solely by vitamin D3 supplementation is extremely rare; vitamin D supplementation in the range of 2,000 – 10,000 IU per day for

---

[282] Plotnikoff GA, Quigley JM. Prevalence of severe hypovitaminosis D in patients with persistent, nonspecific musculoskeletal pain. *Mayo Clin Proc*. 2003;78(12):1463-70

[283] Holick MF. Vitamin D: importance in the prevention of cancers, type 1 diabetes, heart disease, and osteoporosis. *Am J Clin Nutr*. 2004 Mar;79(3):362-71

[284] Armstrong DJ, et al. Vitamin D deficiency is associated with anxiety and depression in fibromyalgia. *Clin Rheumatol*. 2007 Apr;26(4):551-4

[285] Al Faraj S, Al Mutairi K. Vitamin D deficiency and chronic low back pain in Saudi Arabia. *Spine*. 2003;28:177-9

[286] Holick MF. Vitamin D: importance in the prevention of cancers, type 1 diabetes, heart disease, and osteoporosis. *Am J Clin Nutr*. 2004 Mar;79(3):362-71

[287] Vieth R. Vitamin D supplementation, 25-hydroxyvitamin D concentrations, and safety. *Am J Clin Nutr*. 1999 May;69(5):842-56

[288] Zittermann A. Vitamin D in preventive medicine: are we ignoring the evidence? *Br J Nutr*. 2003 May;89(5):552-72

[289] Mild hypercalcemia is not necessarily a problem by itself and must be evaluated within the patient's clinical context. When blood levels of calcium (normal range: 8.7-10.4 mg/dL) reach approximately 12.0 mg/dL, patients will start to develop symptoms; with levels of 14 mg/dL or higher, the patient is generally experiencing symptoms and complications and is in need of treatment (initially with administration of intravenous fluids and a loop diuretic such as furosemide).

adults is remarkably safe.[290,291] The main drug-nutrient interaction of relevance to vitamin D supplementation is with the drug hydrochlorothiazide, which is a diuretic drug used for the treatment of high blood pressure; this drug causes calcium retention by the kidney and when combined with vitamin D supplementation may lead to high levels of calcium in the blood (hypercalcemia). *Note from Dr Vasquez: I have only seen this occur one time in my clinical practice in a hypertensive patient taking hydrochlorothiazide who was vitamin D deficient; vitamin D supplementation at 2,000 IU/d caused a mild hypercalcemia within 10 days which was treated simply by discontinuing the vitamin D supplementation (also note that discontinuation of appropriate nutritional supplementation in favor of continuing a symptom-suppressing drug is generally not my preference but in this particular situation it was the best choice).* A group of conditions called granulomatous diseases—which can include lymphoma, sarcoidosis, and Crohn's disease—increase the risk for hypercalcemia; caution and more frequent laboratory monitoring must be employed when using physiological doses of vitamin D3 in patients with these conditions. Diagnosis of vitamin D3 deficiency is simple and is based upon measurement of serum 25-hydroxy vitamin D3 (25[OH]D) levels. Supplementation effectiveness and safety are monitored by measuring 25(OH)D levels and serum calcium, respectively. The two goals with supplementation of vitamin D3 are ❶ safety—avoidance of hypercalcemia or any calcium-related complications, and ❷ efficacy—serum 25[OH]D levels should enter into the optimal range of 50 – 100 ng/mL (125 - 250 nmol/L).

- Functional/metabolic hypothyroidism: Insufficient levels of thyroid hormone lead to an associated clinical condition called hypothyroidism (*hypo*=low, *thyroidism*=thyroid condition). Both mild and overt hypothyroidism are well known in the rheumatology literature as causes of diffuse body pain. As a cause of diffuse muscle pain, mild-moderate hypothyroidism can mimic fibromyalgia; more severe cases of hypothyroidism cause "hypothyroid myopathy" which typically manifests as polymyositis-like disease with proximal muscle weakness and an increased serum level of the enzyme creatine kinase, indicating muscle damage. In its most extreme, hypothyroid myopathy presents as muscle enlargement (pseudohypertrophy); in adults, this condition is called Hoffmann syndrome while in children it is known as Kocher-Debré-Sémélaigne syndrome.[292] Hypothyroidism is well known to cause depression and low-grade systemic inflammation; these are two findings

> ## Thyroid hormone production and metabolism
> - <u>TSH—thyroid stimulating hormone</u>: Hormone secreted from the anterior pituitary gland to stimulate T4 and T3 production from the thyroid gland.
> - <u>T4</u>: The inactive form of thyroid hormone, accounting for about 80% of thyroid gland output. Oddly and contrary to physiology, doctors have been trained to use this inactive form of the hormone despite known problems in conversion to the active T3 form described immediately below.
> - <u>T3</u>: The active form of thyroid hormone produced from conversion of T4, accounts for about 20% of thyroid gland output. This is the form of thyroid hormone that is most important, because it is active and ready to stimulate metabolic processes; of note, the brain is unable to convert T4 to T3 and thus when patients are deficient in thyroid hormone and substituted with T4 only, they commonly have suboptimal improvement, especially for brain-specific issues of depression and fatigue.
> - <u>rT3—reverse T3</u>: During times of stress and also as a result of some drugs, T4 is preferentially converted to rT3, which is inactive and may actually impair the utilization of active T3. In some people, especially after a period of severe emotional stress, their thyroid hormone metabolism becomes skewed toward rT3 production, perhaps as an adaptive mechanism to conserve energy. However, increased rT3 production results in impaired thyroid hormone function and thereby promotes a clinical picture of hypothyroidism even when gland function is adequate; the problem is the hormone's peripheral metabolism, not its production from the gland.

common in FM. Another related problem commonly seen with both FM and hypothyroidism is IBS and small intestinal bacterial overgrowth (SIBO); hypothyroidism causes a slowing of intestinal motility, promoting stasis in the gastrointestinal tract which leads to an overgrowth of bacteria.[293] Detailed thyroid assessment should include measurements of thyroid stimulating hormone (TSH), free T4, free T3, total T3, reverse T3 (rT3), and antithyroid peroxidase (anti-TPO) and antithyroglobulin antibodies. Management of hypothyroidism is detailed in Chapter 1 of *Inflammation Mastery* / *Functional Inflammology* (2014 and later editions).

---

[290] Vieth R. Vitamin D supplementation, 25-hydroxyvitamin D concentrations, and safety. *Am J Clin Nutr*. 1999 May;69(5):842-56
[291] Vasquez et al. Clinical Importance of Vitamin D: Paradigm Shift for All Healthcare Providers. *Altern Ther Health Med* 2004; 10: 28-37 ichnfm.academia.edu/AlexVasquez
[292] Kedlaya D. Hypothyroid Myopathy. emedicine.medscape.com/article/313915-overview Accessed April 2012
[293] Lauritano EC, Bilotta AL, Gabrielli M, et al. Association between hypothyroidism and small intestinal bacterial overgrowth. *J Clin Endocrinol Metab*. 2007 Nov;92(11):4180-4

- Occult infections, especially with _Mycoplasma_ species and _Chlamydia/Chlamydophila pneumoniae_: Clinicians are increasingly appreciating the role of occult intracellular infections in the genesis and/or perpetuation of chronic health problems, including some previously perplexing problems such as chronic fatigue syndrome (CFS), inflammatory arthritis, and multiple sclerosis (MS). For chronic _Chlamydophila_ (previously _Chlamydia_) _pneumoniae_ infection, testing for serum levels of antibodies is useful followed by treatment with antibacterial drugs such as azithromycin and nutritional supplements such as N-acetyl-cysteine (NAC) in appropriately selected patients; for chronic _Mycoplasma_ infections, because of the various subspecies involved, polymerase chain reaction (PCR) testing appears to be preferred followed by treatment with doxycycline in adults.

  - Review: _Mycoplasma_ blood infection in chronic fatigue and **fibromyalgia** syndromes (_Rheum Int_ 2003 Sep[294]): The author notes that "**Chronic fatigue syndrome (CFS) and fibromyalgia syndrome (FMS)** are characterized by a lack of consistent laboratory and clinical abnormalities. Although they are distinguishable as separate syndromes based on established criteria, a great number of patients are diagnosed with both." He goes on to say, "In studies using **polymerase chain reaction [PCR] methods, mycoplasma blood infection has been detected in about 50% of patients with CFS and/or FMS**, including patients with Gulf War illnesses and symptoms that overlap with one or both syndromes. **Such infection is detected in only about 10% of healthy individuals**, significantly less than in patients. Most patients with CFS/FMS who have mycoplasma infection appear to recover and reach their pre-illness state after **long-term antibiotic therapy with doxycycline**, and the infection cannot be detected after recovery. ... It is not clear whether mycoplasmas are associated with CFS/FMS as causal agents, cofactors, or opportunistic infections in patients with immune disturbances."

  - Clinical investigation: High prevalence of Mycoplasmal infections in symptomatic (chronic fatigue syndrome) family members of _Mycoplasma_-positive Gulf War illness patients (_Journal of Chronic Fatigue Syndrome_ 2003[295]): The authors state, "...a relatively common finding in Gulf War Illness patients is a bacterial infection due to _Mycoplasma_ species, we examined military families (149 patients: 42 veterans, 40 spouses, 32 other relatives and 35 children with at least one family complaint of illness) selected from a **group of 110 veterans with Gulf War Illness who tested positive (~41%) for at least one of four _Mycoplasma_ species**: M. fermentans, M. hominis, M. pneumoniae or M. genitalium. Consistent with previous results, over 80% of Gulf War Illness patients who were positive for blood mycoplasmal infections had **only one _Mycoplasma_ species, in particular M. fermentans** (Odds ratio = 17.9, P <0.001). In healthy control subjects the incidence of mycoplasmal infection was ~8.5% and none were found to have multiple mycoplasmal species."

  - Clinical investigation: Prevalence of antibodies to _Chlamydophila pneumoniae_ in persons without clinical evidence of respiratory infection (_Journal of Clinical Pathology_ 2002 May[296]): The authors note that "Because there is as yet no standardization of serological criteria for persistent infection, we considered antibody titers of > 1/20 in the IgA fraction, together with **IgG titers of 1/64 to 1/256, to be indicative of persistent infection.**" This article supports clinical experience and post-graduate presentations[297] showing that in persons with fatigue and various other chronic health disorders characterized by pain and inflammation (such as chronic inflammatory arthritis[298] or spine[299] inflammation), the finding of IgG antibody levels >1:64 suggests that the patient has a persistent _Chlamydophila pneumoniae_ infection which may be alleviated by the administration of—for example—the antibiotic **azithromycin** (adult dose 250 mg every other day due to the drug's long half-life, given for several weeks or months until symptoms are resolved and/or antibody

---

[294] Endresen GK. Mycoplasma blood infection in chronic fatigue and fibromyalgia syndromes. _Rheumatol Int._ 2003 Sep;23(5):211-5

[295] Nicolson GL, Nasralla MY, Nicolson NL. High prevalence of Mycoplasmal infections in symptomatic (chronic fatigue syndrome) family members of _Mycoplasma_-positive Gulf War illness patients. _Journal of Chronic Fatigue Syndrome_ 2003; 11(2): 21-36 immed.org/GulfWarIllness/10.01.11update/GWIfamilyJCFS_.pdf

[296] Ben-Yaakov et al. Prevalence of antibodies to Chlamydia pneumoniae in an Israeli population without clinical evidence of respiratory infection. _J Clin Pathol._ 2002 May;55(5):355-8 jcp.bmj.com/content/55/5/355.long

[297] Stratton C. The Role of Chlamydophila in Autoimmune Disease. 2011 International Symposium. "The Challenge of Emerging Infections in the 21st Century: Terrain, Tolerance, and Susceptibility" hosted by Institute for Functional Medicine in Seattle, Washington in May 2011

[298] "This study was a 9-month, prospective, double-blind, triple-placebo trial assessing a 6-month course of combination antibiotics as a treatment for Chlamydia-induced ReA. Groups received 1) doxycycline and rifampin plus placebo instead of azithromycin; 2) azithromycin and rifampin plus placebo instead of doxycycline; or 3) placebos instead of azithromycin, doxycycline, and rifampin. ... These data suggest that a 6-month course of combination antibiotics is an effective treatment for chronic Chlamydia-induced ReA." Carter JD, Espinoza LR, Inman RD, et al. Combination antibiotics as a treatment for chronic Chlamydia-induced reactive arthritis: a double-blind, placebo-controlled, prospective trial. _Arthritis Rheum._ 2010 May;62(5):1298-307

[299] "The frequency of Chlamydia-positive ST samples, as determined by PCR, was found to be significantly higher in patients with uSpA than in patients with OA. Our results suggest that in many patients with uSpA, chlamydial infection, which is often occult, may be the cause." Carter et al. Chlamydiae as etiologic agents in chronic undifferentiated spondylarthritis. _Arthritis Rheum._ 2009 May;60(5):1311-6

titers are normalized) and **N-acetyl-cysteine** (NAC: 500-1,200 mg 1-3 times per day by mouth between meals). Positive antibody titers (levels) are common because the infection itself is common *as a transient condition*; the issue here is the determination of which patients have a *chronic* and *persistent* low-grade infection. The finding of an elevated antibody titer—that is a level greater than 1:64—indicates the need to consider long-term antimicrobial intervention.

Chlamydia pneumoniae IgG	**>1:256**	**High**	Neg:<1:16
Chlamydia pneumoniae IgM	<1:10		Neg:<1:10

Elevated titers to *Chlamydia/Chlamydophila pneumoniae* suggesting chronic persistent infection in a 40yo male physician *without pulmonary symptoms* but with a positive history of chronic sinus congestion and low-grade fatigue—improvement with azithromycin and NAC: This patient experienced years of severe psychologic and physiologic stress during a doctorate program and then had an acute upper respiratory illness onset in September 2010 while working in hospital emergency rooms and urgent care clinics; recurrent bouts of upper respiratory illness—attributed to viral infections—persisted for five months until February 2011. By the summer of 2011, the patient was relatively asymptomatic except for persistent sinus congestion and low-grade fatigue. No pulmonary symptoms such as shortness of breath were ever present. Following detection of the elevated antibody titer, the patient started on azithromycin and NAC, which resulted in a short-term (12-hour) exacerbation of symptoms followed by complete and sustained resolution of sinus congestion and improved energy levels and exercise endurance.

- Hemochromatosis and iron overload: Genetic hemochromatosis is a common iron-accumulation disease that causes chronic persistent musculoskeletal pain, even while most routine laboratory tests are normal; thus, the clinical presentation of iron overload may be confused with that of fibromyalgia—both are common conditions commonly presenting with inexplicable (i.e., normal values of routine laboratory tests) nontraumatic musculoskeletal pain. Hemochromatosis is one of the most common hereditary disorders among Caucasians, with a homozygote (two of the same genes, results in more severe disease) frequency of approximately 1 in 200 to 250 persons and a heterozygote (only one affected gene, less severe disease) frequency of approximately 1 in 7 persons. Various other hereditary iron overload disorders affect all races, with the highest prevalence in persons of African descent (as high as 1 in 80 according to some small studies among hospitalized African-American patients).[300,301] Eighty percent of hemochromatosis patients have chronic musculoskeletal pain, which is commonly the earliest or only presenting complaint.[302] In contrast to the clinical presentation of FM, the musculoskeletal manifestations of iron overload are classically arthritic (i.e., in the joints) rather than muscular, with the joints of the hands, wrists, hips, and knees most commonly affected. However, due to the widespread distribution of pain and the normalcy of routine laboratory results, iron overload can mimic fibromyalgia. Given the high population prevalence of iron overload and the high frequency with which it presents with musculoskeletal manifestations, all patients with chronic, nontraumatic musculoskeletal pain must be tested for iron overload. Serum ferritin, which can be used alone or with transferrin saturation, is the best single laboratory test; confirmed results greater than 200 mcg/L in women and 300 mcg/L in men necessitate treatment with diagnostic and therapeutic phlebotomy (frequent "blood donation" is the most effective treatment for chronic iron overload).[303]

- Iron deficiency: Iron is necessary for function of the mitochondrial electron transport chain as well as for formation of the neurotransmitters dopamine and serotonin, both of which can be said to have an analgesic effect. As such, iron deficiency can promote headaches in general and migraine in particular; iron deficiency might also contribute to the clinical presentation of fibromyalgia.[304] Per my previous extensive reviews of the

---

[300] Wurapa RK, Gordeuk VR, Brittenham GM, Khiyami A, Schechter GP, Edwards CQ. Primary iron overload in African Americans. *Am J Med.* 1996 Jul;101(1):9-18

[301] Barton JC, Edwards CQ, Bertoli LF, Shroyer TW, Hudson SL. Iron overload in African Americans. *Am J Med.* 1995 Dec;99(6):616-23

[302] Vasquez A. Musculoskeletal disorders and iron overload disease: comment on the American College of Rheumatology guidelines for the initial evaluation of the adult patient with acute musculoskeletal symptoms. *Arthritis Rheum.* 1996 Oct;39(10):1767-8 Ichnfm.academia.edu/AlexVasquez

[303] Barton JC, McDonnell SM, Adams PC, et al. Management of hemochromatosis. Hemochromatosis Management Working Group. *Ann Intern Med.* 1998 Dec 1;129(11):932-9

[304] "The mean serum ferritin levels in the fibromyalgia and control groups were 27.3 and 43.8 ng/ml, respectively, and the difference was statistically significant. Binary multiple logistic regression analysis with age, body mass index, smoking status and vitamin B12, as well as folic acid and ferritin levels showed that having a serum ferritin level <50 ng/ml caused a 6.5-fold increased risk for FMS." Ortancil et al. Association between serum ferritin level and fibromyalgia syndrome. *Eur J Clin Nutr.* 2010 Mar;64(3):308-12

literature on the topics of iron overload and iron deficiency[305], optimal iron status correlates with serum ferritin values of 40-70 ng/ml. Rarely, a person with what can be described as a defect in the blood-brain barrier transport of iron into the brain will need to have a serum ferritin value of 120 ng/ml in order to promote entry of iron into the brain.

- Accumulation of xenobiotics (including mercury and lead): Xenobiotic (foreign chemical) accumulation may occasionally cause widespread pain resembling fibromyalgia, and xenobiotic detoxification (depuration) can alleviate pain in affected patients. Toxic chemical and toxic metal accumulation is common in humans worldwide and has been well-documented in Americans. Eight percent (8%) of American women of childbearing age have sufficiently high levels of mercury in their blood to increase the risk of health problems such as neurological damage in their

> **Potential benefits of reducing the body burden of mercury in patients with chronic pain and fatigue**
>
> "We suggest that **metal-driven inflammation** may affect the hypothalamic-pituitary-adrenal axis (HPA axis) and indirectly trigger psychosomatic multisymptoms characterizing **chronic fatigue syndrome, fibromyalgia**, and other diseases of unknown etiology."
>
> Sterzl et al. Mercury and nickel allergy: risk factors in fatigue and autoimmunity. *Neuro Endocrinol Lett.* 1999

children.[306] Americans in general show alarmingly high concentrations and combinations of neurotoxic (nerve-damaging), carcinogenic (cancer-causing), diabetogenic (diabetes-causing), and immunotoxic (immune-poisoning) xenobiotics/toxins.[307] Adverse effects of toxic chemicals (e.g., pesticides, herbicides, solvents, plastics, formaldehyde, petroleum byproducts) and heavy metals (especially lead and mercury) are well described throughout the biomedical literature and have been clinically reviewed by Crinnion.[308,309,310,311] Among toxins with the ability to produce chronic muscle pain, mercury may deserve special recognition given its ubiquitous distribution in the human population and the scientific evidence detailing its numerous adverse effects.[312,313] Whether by metabolic, neurological, or endocrinologic means, occult mercury toxicity may manifest as a syndrome of widespread muscle pain that resembles fibromyalgia.[314] Acrodynia is a subacute peripheral pain syndrome due to mercury toxicity classically seen in children.[315] Acute mercury intoxication can result in severe skeletal muscle damage (rhabdomyolysis).[316] Mercury in organic and inorganic forms interferes with acetylcholine reception and several crucial aspects of the sarcoplasmic reticulum, including calcium-magnesium-ATPase and calcium transport; these adverse effects establish a molecular basis for a *mercurial myopathy* (mercury-induced muscle disease).[317,318] The toxicity of mercury is greatly increased by simultaneous accumulation of lead, elevated levels of which are also common in the U.S. population. Demonstration of high mercury and lead levels in urine following administration of a chelating agent such as dimercaptosuccinic acid (DMSA) can be used to diagnose chronic mercury or lead overload, and orally administered DMSA is also used for treatment.[319,320,321,322] Failure to preadminister a chelating agent prior to measurement of urine mercury renders the test insensitive for chronic accumulation and can thus give the false impression that mercury is not contributory to fibromyalgia, as concluded by Kotter et al.[323] Orally administered selenium, phytochelatins (metal-binding peptides from plants[324]), a high-fiber diet, and potassium citrate can be used to augment mercury excretion.

---

[305] See Chapter 1 of either *Inflammation Mastery* / *Functional Inflammology* (2014 or later) for the most complete reviews, including assessment, management, and radiographic presentations. See also: Vasquez A. Musculoskeletal disorders and iron overload disease. [Letter] *Arthritis & Rheumatism* 1996; 39:1767-8. Vasquez A. High body iron stores: causes, effects, diagnosis, and treatment. *Nutritional Perspectives* 1994 October

[306] "However, approximately 8% of women had concentrations higher than US Environmental Protection Agency's recommended reference dose (5.8 µg/L), below which exposures are considered to be without adverse effects." Schober et al. Blood mercury levels in US children and women of childbearing age,1999-2000. *JAMA* 2003;289:1667-74

[307] Kristin et al. Chemical Trespass. Pesticide Action Network North America. Available at panna.org. See also: Body Burden: The Pollution in People. ewg.org/ 2006 Feb

[308] Crinnion WJ. Environmental medicine, part 1: the human burden of environmental toxins and their common health effects. *Altern Med Rev.* 2000 Feb;5(1):52-63

[309] Crinnion WJ. Environmental medicine, part 2: health effects of and protection from ubiquitous airborne solvent exposure. *Altern Med Rev.* 2000 Apr;5(2):133-43

[310] Crinnion WJ. Environmental medicine, part 3: long-term effects of chronic low-dose mercury exposure. *Altern Med Rev.* 2000 Jun;5(3):209-23

[311] Crinnion WJ. Environmental medicine, part 4: pesticides - biologically persistent and ubiquitous toxins. *Altern Med Rev.* 2000 Oct;5(5):432-47

[312] Elemental Mercury Vapor Poisoning -- North Carolina, 1988. cdc.gov/mmwr/preview/mmwrhtml/00001499.htm

[313] Shih H, Gartner JC Jr. Weight loss, hypertension, weakness, and limb pain in an 11-year-old boy. *J Pediatr.* 2001 Apr;138(4):566-9

[314] Sterzl I, Prochazkova J, Hrda P, et al. Mercury and nickel allergy: risk factors in fatigue and autoimmunity. *Neuro Endocrinol Lett.* 1999;20:221-8

[315] Padlewska KK. Acrodynia. Last Updated: February 15, 2007 eMedicine emedicine.com/derm/topic592.htm Accessed October 25, 2007

[316] Chugh KS, Singhal PC, Uberoi HS. Rhabdomyolysis and renal failure in acute mercuric chloride poisoning. *Med J Aust.* 1978 Jul 29;2(3):125-6

[317] Chiu VC, Mouring D, Haynes DH. Action of mercurials on the active and passive transport properties of sarcoplasmic reticulum. *J Bioenerg Biomembr.* 1983 Feb;15(1):13-25

[318] Shamoo AE, Maclennan DH, Elderfrawi ME. Differential effects of mercurial compounds on excitable tissues. *Chem Biol Interact.* 1976 Jan;12(1):41-52

[319] Kalra V, et al. Succimer in Symptomatic Lead Poisoning. *Indian Pediatrics* 2002; 39:580-585 indianpediatrics.net/june2002/june-580-585.htm

[320] Bradstreet et al. Case-control study of mercury burden in children with autistic spectrum disorders. *J Am Physicians Surgeons* 2003; 8: 76-79 jpands.org/vol8no3/geier.pdf

[321] Forman et al. A cluster of pediatric metallic mercury exposure cases treated with meso-2,3-dimercaptosuccinic acid (DMSA). *Environ Health Perspect.* 2000 Jun;108(6):575-7

[322] Miller AL. Dimercaptosuccinic acid (DMSA), a non-toxic, water-soluble treatment for heavy metal toxicity. *Altern Med Rev.* 1998 Jun;3(3):199-207

[323] Kotter I, Durk H, Saal JG, et al. Mercury exposure from dental amalgam fillings in the etiology of primary fibromyalgia. *J Rheumatol.* 1995;22:2194-5

[324] Cobbett CS. Phytochelatins and their roles in heavy metal detoxification. *Plant Physiol.* 2000;123:825-32 plantphysiol.org/content/123/3/825

- **Case report: Therapeutic detoxification to reduce the body burden of lead and mercury in a woman diagnosed with FM leads to complete relief of FM symptoms**: This 54-year-old athletic female with healthy diet, lifestyle, and supportive relationship presented with chronic diffuse musculoskeletal pain. Health history was significant for decades of environmental illness/intolerance (EI) and multiple chemical sensitivity (MCS). Family history was positive for maternal temporal (giant cell) arteritis. Physical examination revealed numerous tender points consistent with FM. Stool analysis was unremarkable and unsupportive of either identifiable infection or nonspecific bacterial overgrowth. Laboratory investigations revealed normal results for hsCRP (high-sensitivity c-reactive protein), CK (creatine kinase, a marker of muscle damage), ANA (anti-nuclear antibodies, elevated in many autoimmune diseases such as lupus/SLE), vitamin D, calcium, phosphorus, and comprehensive thyroid evaluation. The patient was then (defensively) referred to an excellent osteopathic medical internist who diagnosed the patient with fibromyalgia. The patient was unsatisfied with the diagnosis of FM and returned to the current author, who then performed urine heavy metal testing provoked with 10 mg per kilogram of dimercaptosuccinic acid (DMSA). Results revealed the highest levels of lead and mercury encountered in the author's practice at that time. As in the accompanying lab results, lead levels were 6x above the reference range and mercury levels were 7x above the reference range. The patient was commenced on DMSA 10 mg/kg/d three days "on" and 4 days "off" (cyclic dosing is used to avoid toxicity in general and bone marrow toxicity [neutropenia] in particular), selenium 800 mcg/d to promote excretion of toxic metals and to support renal and antioxidant protection, vegetable juices to provide potassium and citrate for urinary alkalinization and enhanced excretion of xenobiotics[325], and a proprietary phytochelatin (metal-binding peptides from plants) concentrate to bind toxic metals in the gut and thereby promote their fecal excretion by blocking enterohepatic recycling/recirculation. DMSA chelation is approved by the US Food and Drug Administration (FDA) for the treatment of lead toxicity in children.[326] The use of DMSA for children and adults is supported by peer-reviewed literature.[327,328,329,330,331] After approximately 8 months of treatment, the patient was completely free of pain, and the clinical improvement was associated with a reduction in both lead and mercury of approximately 50% as demonstrated by follow-up laboratory testing. This case was published in peer-reviewed literature for continuing medical education (CME) for physicians.[332]

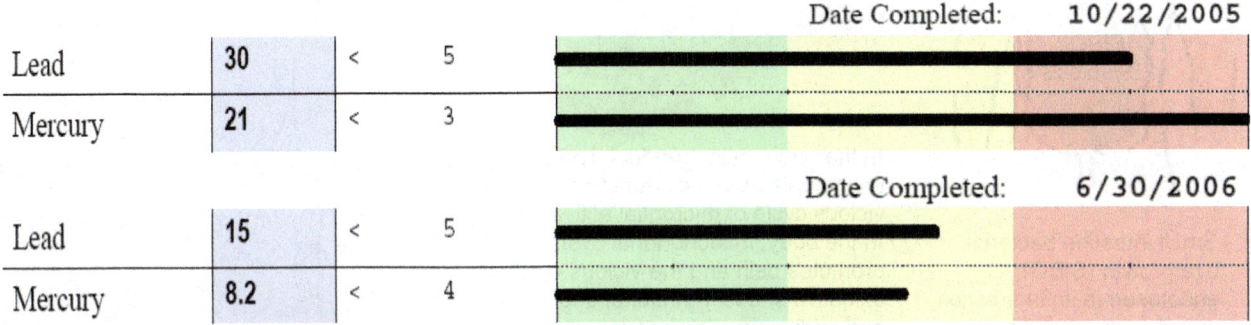

Marked accumulation of lead and mercury in a patient diagnosed with FM—complete elimination of pain and stiffness following identification and reduction in the body burden of lead and mercury: 54yo woman presents with nontraumatic widespread pain consistent with a diagnosis of fibromyalgia; the diagnosis of FM is confirmed by two clinicians. All laboratory test results were normal except for urine toxic metal testing which showed 6x elevations of lead and 7x elevations of mercury. Treatment (DMSA, citrate, selenium, and phytochelatins per above) for 8 months effected safe reductions in body burden of lead and mercury and alleviation of all pain.

---

[325] Crinnion WJ. Environmental medicine, part3:long-term effects of chronic low-dose mercury exposure. *Altern Med Rev* 2000 Jun;5:209-23

[326] "The Food and Drug Administration has recently licensed the drug DMSA (succimer) for reduction of blood lead levels >/= 45 micrograms/dl. This decision was based on the demonstrated ability of DMSA to reduce blood lead levels. An advantage of this drug is that it can be given orally." Goyer RA, Cherian MG, Jones MM, Reigart JR. Role of chelating agents for prevention, intervention, and treatment of exposures to toxic metals. *Environ Health Perspect*. 1995 Nov;103(11):1048-52

[327] Bradstreet et al. A case-control study of mercury burden in children with autistic spectrum disorders. *Journal of American Physicians and Surgeons* 2003; 8: 76-79

[328] Crinnion WJ. Environmental medicine, part three: long-term effects of chronic low-dose mercury exposure. *Altern Med Rev*. 2000 Jun;5(3):209-23

[329] Forman et al. A cluster of pediatric metallic mercury exposure cases treated with meso-2,3-dimercaptosuccinic acid (DMSA). *Environ Health Perspect*. 2000 Jun;108(6):575-7

[330] Miller AL. Dimercaptosuccinic acid (DMSA), a non-toxic, water-soluble treatment for heavy metal toxicity. *Altern Med Rev*. 1998 Jun;3(3):199-207

[331] DMSA. *Altern Med Rev*. 2000 Jun;5(3):264-7 thorne.com/altmedrev/.fulltext/5/3/264.pdf

[332] Vasquez A. *Musculoskeletal Pain: Expanded Clinical Strategies*. Institute for Functional Medicine. 2008

In the restructuring of this work in 2015 from its previous versions, I am—based on a more confident description of FM that moves from hypothesis to assertion—choosing to organize the pathophysiologic descriptions, upon which are based the therapeutic interventions, in the following four categories, each with their respective evidence:

1. The primary cause of fibromyalgia is SIBO—small intestinal bacterial overgrowth.
2. As a result of SIBO, fibromyalgia patients suffer somatic/body fatigue from mitochondrial dysfunction.
3. As a result of SIBO, fibromyalgia patients suffer increased sensitivity to pain due to heightened sensitivity of the brain and spinal cord—central sensitization—as well as from peripheral sensitization and impaired muscle function due to the previously established mitochondrial dysfunction.
4. All other biochemical and pathophysiologic abnormalities seen in fibromyalgia are explained from SIBO.

The primary focus of this section—establishing that SIBO is the cause of FM—is the provision of a cohesive and coherent explanation of FM; examples of treatments will be provided in this section on pathophysiology because the efficacy of treatments substantiates and helps prove the model that I have developed. Following these proofs substantiating this pathophysiologic model, a separate section detailing treatments will be provided. Allowing some repetition of citations used in the establishment of the pathophysiologic model, in the section on therapeutics I will review treatments using the format of my FINDSEX ® acronym to maintain consistency with my treatment protocols. Several diagrams will be provided, each providing novelty, emphasis, and repetition.

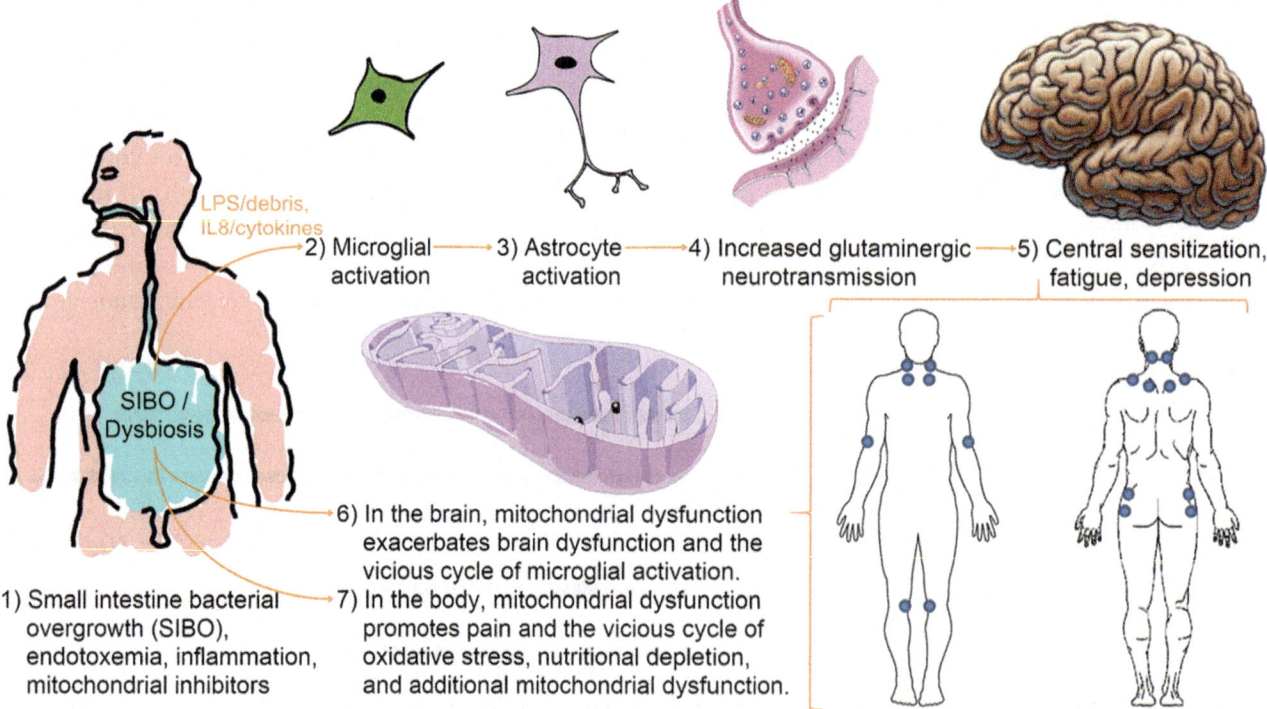

LPS/debris, IL8/cytokines

2) Microglial activation → 3) Astrocyte activation → 4) Increased glutaminergic neurotransmission → 5) Central sensitization, fatigue, depression

SIBO / Dysbiosis

1) Small intestine bacterial overgrowth (SIBO), endotoxemia, inflammation, mitochondrial inhibitors

6) In the brain, mitochondrial dysfunction exacerbates brain dysfunction and the vicious cycle of microglial activation.

7) In the body, mitochondrial dysfunction promotes pain and the vicious cycle of oxidative stress, nutritional depletion, and additional mitochondrial dysfunction.

A simple integrated model of fibromyalgia, emphasizing dysbiosis-induced glial activation and mitochondrial dysfunction—first published in *Nutritional Perspectives* 2015 Oct: Small intestine bacterial overgrowth (SIBO) elaborates endotoxin/lipopolysaccharide (LPS) with other inflammogens and mitochondrial inhibitors (including D-lactate and hydrogen sulfide [H2S]). Microglial activation can be triggered directly by LPS or indirectly by peripheral and central cytokines (especially IL-8), and it then triggers astrocyte activation and results in increased glutaminergic neurotransmission, which promotes central sensitization and the resulting depression, central fatigue, and pain sensitivity. In the brain, mitochondrial dysfunction exacerbates brain dysfunction and the vicious cycle of microglial activation. In the body, mitochondrial dysfunction promotes pain and the vicious cycles of oxidative stress, nutritional depletion, and additional mitochondrial dysfunction. Vitamin D deficiency, common in many conditions of persistent pain, exacerbates central pain by allowing increased microglial activation while also contributing to peripherally-sourced pain from muscle (myalgia) and bone (osteomalacia). Illustration by Vasquez; image of brain by IsaacMao per Flickr.com via creativecommons.org/licenses/by/2.0. See educational videos and updates at www.inflammationmastery.com/pain

❶ Primary Cause of FM—SIBO: The primary cause of fibromyalgia is small intestinal bacterial overgrowth.
Small intestine bacterial overgrowth (SIBO)—also referred to as "intestinal bacterial overgrowth" or simply "bacterial overgrowth"—provides the single best model for explaining the clinical and pathophysiological manifestations of fibromyalgia. Although commonly underappreciated by many clinicians, SIBO is common in clinical practice, affecting for example approximately 40% of patients with rheumatoid arthritis, 84% of patients with IBS, and 90% to 100% of patients with fibromyalgia. **In a study of 42 fibromyalgia patients, all 42 FM patients showed laboratory evidence of SIBO, and the severity of the intestinal bacterial overgrowth correlated positively with the severity of the fibromyalgia**, thus indicating the plausibility of a causal relationship.[333] The links between fibromyalgia and IBS are also strong; **most IBS patients meet strict diagnostic criteria for fibromyalgia, and most fibromyalgia patients meet strict criteria for IBS**. Lubrano et al[334] showed that fibromyalgia severity correlated with IBS severity among patients who met strict diagnostic criteria for both conditions. The high degree of overlap between these two diagnostic labels suggests that these conditions are two variations of a common pathophysiological process—SIBO.[335] SIBO causes altered bowel function, immune activation, and visceral hypersensitivity, and it is the best causative explanation for the clinical and pathophysiological manifestations of IBS; for more details and citations, see the excellent review by Lin published in *Journal of the American Medical Association* in 2004.[336] IBS is characterized by *visceral* hyperalgesia (hypersensitivity to pain), just as fibromyalgia is characterized by *skeletal muscle* hyperalgesia. Given that strong evidence indicates that IBS is caused by SIBO and that IBS and fibromyalgia are variations of the same pathophysiological process, then fibromyalgia may therefore be caused by SIBO. However, these links and interconnections require substantiation, as provided throughout this section.

Bacterial LPS and other antigens absorbed from the intestine during SIBO contribute to a subclinical inflammatory state that results in pain hypersensitivity and increased cytokine release, both of which are characteristics of fibromyalgia. In animal models and in human research studies, exposure to bacterial endotoxin/LPS has been shown to increase the brain's sensitivity to and perception of pain. Immune-mediated and inflammation-mediated pathways that promote pain sensitivity and pain perception include ❶ increased production of nitric oxide with ❷ increased production of prostaglandins and cytokines, resulting in ❸ the sensitization of peripheral and/or central neurons to pain perception/transmission. In support of this concept, Lin[337] wrote in 2004, **"The immune response to bacterial antigen in SIBO provides a framework for understanding the hypersensitivity in both fibromyalgia and IBS."** A later paper by Othmanm, Agüero, and Lin[338] in 2008 stated, "…a recent animal study demonstrated that exposure to endotoxin increased the production of prostaglandins and simultaneously decreased nitrous oxide production, resulting in inflammatory hyperalgesia" and "These observations suggest that SIBO is a common feature in both [IBS and FM] disorders and that altered gut microbiota in SIBO may play a role in the induction of somatic or visceral hypersensitivity, with affected patients meeting the diagnostic criteria for IBS, fibromyalgia or both disorders."

Gut bacteria also affect CNS/brain neurotransmission via vagal stimulation. According to a 2014 review by Galland, "Intrinsic primary afferent neurons (IPANs) are cellular targets of neuroactive bacteria and transmit microbial messages to the brain via the vagus nerve. Live bacteria may not be needed for these effects; in the case of *B. fragilis*, a lipid-free polysaccharide is both necessary and sufficient for IPAN activation. … Gut bacteria influence reactivity of the HPA axis and the induction and maintenance of nREM sleep. They may influence mood, pain sensitivity and normal brain development."[339]

- Fibromyalgia is tightly correlated with irritable bowel syndrome, a condition caused by small intestine bacterial overgrowth: Fibromyalgia and IBS are strongly convergent, and the evidence indicates that IBS is caused largely or completely by SIBO; again, for more details and citations, see the brilliant article by Lin, cited previously. Small intestine bacterial overgrowth is highly prevalent in fibromyalgia. Several studies have

[333] Pimentel et al. A link between irritable bowel syndrome and fibromyalgia may be related to findings on lactulose breath testing. *Ann Rheum Dis.* 2004 Apr;63(4):450-2

[334] Lubrano E, et al. Fibromyalgia in patients with irritable bowel syndrome. An association with the severity of the intestinal disorder. *Int J Colorectal Dis.* 2001 Aug;16(4):211-5

[335] Veale et al. Primary fibromyalgia and the irritable bowel syndrome: different expressions of a common pathogenetic process. *Br J Rheumatol.* 1991 Jun;30(3):220-2

[336] Lin HC. Small intestinal bacterial overgrowth: a framework for understanding irritable bowel syndrome. *JAMA.* 2004 Aug 18;292(7):852-8

[337] Lin HC. Small intestinal bacterial overgrowth: a framework for understanding irritable bowel syndrome. *JAMA.* 2004 Aug 18;292(7):852-8

[338] Othman M, Agüero R, Lin HC. Alterations in intestinal microbial flora and human disease. *Curr Opin Gastroenterol.* 2008 Jan;24(1):11-6

[339] Galland L. The gut microbiome and the brain. *J Med Food.* 2014 Dec;17(12):1261-72

shown that 90% to 100% of fibromyalgia patients have evidence of SIBO; such a strong correlation and the dose-response relationship imply causality and must be integrated into any science-based model of fibromyalgia.

- ▫ Clinical study: Patients with FM have evidence of frequent and severe bacterial overgrowth in the intestines (*Annals of the Rheumatic Diseases* 2004 Apr[340]): The **breath hydrogen test** is used for the detection of SIBO and involves orally administering a carbohydrate (such as lactulose, a source of sugar for bacteria) which is converted to hydrogen through bacterial fermentation; the exhaled hydrogen in the breath is measured as an indirect quantification of the amount of bacteria in the intestines. In this study, 20% of "healthy" control patients were found to have intestinal bacterial overgrowth via an abnormal hydrogen breath test compared with 93/111 (84%) subjects with IBS and **42/42 (100%) with fibromyalgia**. Subjects with fibromyalgia had higher hydrogen production (indicating more severe SIBO), peak hydrogen, and area under the curve than subjects with IBS. **The degree of somatic pain in fibromyalgia correlates significantly with the hydrogen level seen on the breath test.**

- • Small intestine bacterial overgrowth leads to systemic absorption of toxins that impair brain/nerve and muscle/mitochondrial function: SIBO is associated with overproduction and absorption of bacterial cellular debris (e.g., lipopolysaccharide [LPS], bacterial DNA, peptidoglycans, teichoic acid, exotoxins) and antimetabolites—substances which are directly toxic to cellular energy/ATP production and muscle and nerve function—such as D-lactic acid, tyramine, tartaric acid, hydrogen sulfide. Intestinal gram-negative bacteria produce endotoxin (also known as lipopolysaccharide, LPS), which impairs skeletal muscle energy/ATP production (by stimulating skeletal muscle sodium-potassium-ATPase). Endotoxin also raises blood lactate (indicating impaired cellular energy production) under aerobic conditions in humans.[341] **Thus, via direct and indirect effects on cellular metabolism, chronic low-dose bacterial LPS/endotoxin exposure can result in impaired muscle metabolism and reduced ATP synthesis via impairment of mitochondrial function.** Intestinal bacteria also produce D-lactate, a well-known metabolic toxin in humans; SIBO often results in variable levels of D-lactate acidosis, severe cases of which can progress from fatigue and malaise to encephalopathy (e.g., confusion, ataxia, slurred speech, altered mental status) and death.[342] Supporting the proposal that bacterial overgrowth with D-lactate-producing bacteria is a contributor to the chronic fatigue syndromes including fibromyalgia is an excellent study published in 2009 showing that **patients with chronic fatigue syndrome have intestinal overgrowth of bacteria that produce the cellular toxin D-lactate**; specifically the research showed that these chronic fatigue patients have **a 7-fold increase in D-lactate producing *Enterococcus* and 1,100-fold increase in D-lactate producing *Streptococcus*.** Energy/ATP underproduction and lactate overproduction cause muscle fatigue and muscle pain. An additional cellular toxin produced by intestinal bacteria is hydrogen sulfide (H2S), which causes DNA damage[343] (noted previously to be increased in fibromyalgia patients) and which impairs cellular energy production, a finding relevant to *but not necessarily limited to* the pathogenesis of ulcerative colitis.[344,345] Bacteria and yeast in the intestines produce H2S, which can bind to the mitochondrial enzyme cytochrome c oxidase (part of Complex IV of the electron transport chain), thereby impairing oxidative phosphorylation and ATP production; this may partly explain the association of gastrointestinal dysbiosis and small intestine bacterial overgrowth (SIBO) with conditions such as chronic fatigue syndrome (CFS) and fibromyalgia.[346] Given that sulfur-containing molecules such as sulfite and hydrogen sulfide bind to vitamin B12[347,348], we should reasonably expect that patients with excess exposure to H2S from the gastrointestinal tract would have an increased prevalence of vitamin B12 deficiency, and indeed this has been documented; vitamin B12 deficiency in CFS and FM patients promotes fatigue and brain dysfunction via the effects of vitamin B12 deficiency directly (ie, vitamin B12 deficiency is well known to cause

---

[340] Pimentel et al. A link between irritable bowel syndrome and fibromyalgia may be related to findings on lactulose breath testing. *Ann Rheum Dis.* 2004 Apr;63(4):450-2

[341] Bundgaard et al. Endotoxemia stimulates skeletal muscle Na+-K+-ATPase and raises blood lactate under aerobic conditions in humans. *Am J Physiol Heart Circ Physiol.* 2003 Mar;284(3):H1028-34

[342] Vella A, Farrugia G. D-lactic acidosis: pathologic consequence of saprophytism. *Mayo Clin Proc.* 1998 May;73(5):451-6

[343] Attene-Ramos MS, Wagner ED, Gaskins HR, Plewa MJ. Hydrogen sulfide induces direct radical-associated DNA damage. *Mol Cancer Res.* 2007 May;5(5):455-9

[344] Magee et al. Contribution of dietary protein to sulfide production in large intestine: in vitro and controlled feeding study in humans. *Am J Clin Nutr.* 2000 Dec;72(6):1488-94

[345] Babidge W, Millard S, Roediger W. Sulfides impair short chain fatty acid beta-oxidation at acyl-CoA dehydrogenase level in colonocytes. *Mol Cell Biochem.* 1998 Apr:117-24

[346] Lemle MD. Hypothesis: chronic fatigue syndrome is caused by dysregulation of hydrogen sulfide metabolism. *Med Hypotheses.* 2009 Jan;72(1):108-9

[347] Añíbarro et al. Asthma with sulfite intolerance in children: a blocking study with cyanocobalamin. *J Allergy Clin Immunol.* 1992 Jul;90(1):103-9

[348] Fujita et al. A fatal case of acute hydrogen sulfide poisoning caused by hydrogen sulfide: hydroxocobalamin therapy for acute hydrogen sulfide poisoning. *J Anal Toxicol.* 2011 Mar;35(2):119-23

nerve damage and brain damage) and indirectly via impaired metabolism of homocysteine, which then triggers pain sensitivity and accelerated neurodegeneration via activation of NMDA receptors in the brain.[349]

▫ Experimental study: Effect of *E. coli* endotoxin on mitochondrial form and function (*Annals of Surgery* 1971 Dec[350]): Authors of this paper show that treatment of normal rat liver mitochondria with *E. coli* endotoxin results in mitochondrial impairment. They note previous research showing that animal exposure to *E. coli* endotoxin causes inhibition of mitochondrial respiration and uncoupling of oxidative phosphorylation. Near their conclusion, the authors write, "Thus we have evidence to show that topical **E. coli endotoxin has pathologic effects on both membrane integrity and internal mechanochemical systems of isolated mitochondria.**" Readers should appreciate that *E. coli* is a common inhabitant of the gastrointestinal tract of humans and that its population is quantitatively increased during states of bacterial overgrowth of the small bowel, as is commonly seen in most patients with fibromyalgia. More recently, research has shown that impairment of mitochondrial function (noted in patients with fibromyalgia) can lead to destruction of mitochondria by a process termed "mitophagy" (noted in patients with fibromyalgia); over time, loss of mitochondria via mitophagy leads to reduced numbers of mitochondria in muscle and other tissues (noted in patients with fibromyalgia) and contributes to the fatigue and other symptoms which characterize FM.

▫ Clinical study: Increased D-lactic acid intestinal bacteria in patients with chronic fatigue syndrome (*In Vivo* 2009 Jul-Aug[351]): The authors of this 2009 study state in the summary of their research, "Patients with chronic fatigue syndrome (CFS) are affected by symptoms of cognitive dysfunction and neurological impairment, the cause of which has yet to be elucidated. However, these symptoms are strikingly similar to those of patients presented with D-lactic acidosis. A significant increase of Gram-positive facultative anaerobic fecal microorganisms in 108 CFS patients as compared to 177 control subjects is presented in this report. The viable count of D-lactic acid producing *Enterococcus* and *Streptococcus* spp. in the fecal samples from the CFS group (3.5 x 10(7) cfu [colony forming units]/L and 9.8 x 10(7) cfu/L respectively) were significantly higher than those for the control group (5.0 x 10(6) cfu/L and 8.9 x 10(4) cfu/L respectively). [**Note: This is approximately a 7x increase in D-lactate producing *Enterococcus* and 1,100x increase in D-lactate producing *Streptococcus*.**] Analysis of exometabolic profiles of *Enterococcus faecalis* and *Streptococcus sanguinis*, representatives of *Enterococcus* and *Streptococcus* spp. respectively, by NMR and HPLC showed that these organisms produced significantly more lactic acid from (13)C-labeled glucose, than the Gram negative *Escherichia coli*. Further, **both E. faecalis and S. sanguinis secrete more**

> **Patients with "chronic fatigue syndrome" and the associated neurologic dysfunction and muscle dysfunction have intestinal overgrowth of bacteria that produce D-lactic acid, a known neurotoxin and metabolic poison**
>
> In 2007 and 2008, the current author (AV) wrote and published *Musculoskeletal Pain: Expanded Clinical Strategies** with the Institute for Functional Medicine; this chapter on fibromyalgia is derived and updated from that work. In that publication, I reviewed evidence that fibromyalgia—at that time considered mysterious, idiopathic, chronic, relentless, and treatable only by pain-relieving drugs—was most likely caused by small intestine bacterial overgrowth (SIBO) and the resultant absorption of metabolic toxins and immunogenic debris. This perspective has been supported by numerous publications, particularly the article published by Sheedy et al** in 2009, which showed for the first time that patients with chronic fatigue syndrome—a condition tightly correlated with and which often overlaps with fibromyalgia—have SIBO with various bacteria that are high-output producers of D-lactic acid, a known neurotoxin and metabolic poison which potentially contributes to many of the main clinical, biochemical, and histologic manifestations of FM, namely mental fatigue and dyscognition (difficulty thinking), muscle fatigue and pain, biochemical evidence of mitochondrial impairment, and histologic evidence of mitochondrial myopathy.
>
> *Vasquez A. *Musculoskeletal Pain*. Institute for Functional Medicine, 2008. **Sheedy, et al. Increased d-lactic acid intestinal bacteria in patients with chronic fatigue syndrome. *In Vivo*. 2009 Jul

D-lactic acid than E. coli. This study suggests a probable link between intestinal colonization of Gram-positive facultative anaerobic D-lactic acid bacteria and symptom expressions in a subgroup of patients with CFS. Given the fact that **this might explain not only neurocognitive dysfunction in CFS patients but**

---

[349] Regland et al. Increased concentrations of homocysteine in the cerebrospinal fluid in patients with fibromyalgia and chronic fatigue syndrome. *Scand J Rheumatol.* 1997;26(4):301-7

[350] White et al. Effect of E. coli endotoxin on mitochondrial form and function. *Ann Surg.* 1971 Dec;174(6):983-90

[351] Sheedy JR, Wettenhall RE, Scanlon D, et al. Increased d-lactic acid intestinal bacteria in patients with chronic fatigue syndrome. *In Vivo.* 2009 Jul-Aug;23(4):621-8

also mitochondrial dysfunction, these findings may have important clinical implications." A note of personal experience: the current author (Dr Vasquez) had one event of severe headache and dyscognition following consumption of a prebiotic (FOS) supplement during my 6-year bout with a CFS-related condition; from this experience, I furthered my understanding of dysbiosis and continued to do so *via personal experience* for the following 10 years. Of further note, based on my personal experience and review of the biomedical literature, I proposed in the CME monograph *Musculoskeletal Pain: Expanded Clinical Strategies* (Institute for Functional Medicine, 2008) that D-lactic acidosis was one of the pathophysiologic mechanisms by which microbial overgrowth of the intestines causes fibromyalgia; I was therefore gratified to see this article—published in 2009, nearly 2 years after I had proposed this mechanism—verifying my hypothesis.

- <u>Commensal microbiota are necessary for the development of inflammatory pain</u> (*Proc Natl Acad Sci.* 2008 Feb[352]): In this remarkably insightful article, the authors introduce their work by stating, "The sensation of pain can be enhanced by acute or chronic inflammation", and that in their experimental model using germ-free and "conventional" (colonized) mice, they "show that inflammatory hypernociception induced by carrageenan, lipopolysaccharide, TNF-alpha, IL-1beta, and the chemokine CXCL1 was reduced in germ-free mice" while hypernociception induced by prostaglandins and dopamine was not altered by the presence/absence of bacteria. However, "reposition of the microbiota" or systemic administration of LPS essentially restored the pain and inflammation that was absent in germ-free mice, which also produced more IL-10, which—via experiments using anti-IL-10 antibody—proved to mediate both anti-inflammation and anti-nociception. The authors concluded that, "Therefore, these results show that contact with commensal microbiota is necessary for mice to develop inflammatory hypernociception. ... Therefore, these results show that contact with commensal microbiota [or LPS] is necessary for mice to develop inflammatory hypernociception possibly in a TLR-dependent manner."

- <u>Low-dose LPS 'priming' of muscle provides an animal model of persistent elevated mechanical sensitivity for the study of chronic pain</u> (*Eur J Pain* 2011 Aug[353]): In this experiment using intramuscular hypertonic saline with either high or low doses of LPS, the authors found that low-dose LPS exacerbated long-term pain, while high-dose LPS caused the expected acute inflammatory response but did not promote development of chronic pain; the authors speculate that the low dose of LPS "primed" inflammatory and neurologic pathways for the persistence of pain perception while the higher dose may have invoked counter-inflammatory mechanisms ("larger-dose of LPS in this experiment may have provoked a protective effect such as invoking negative feedback loops") that failed to promote the development of central sensitization. By showing that low-level locally-administered systemically-circulated LPS could promote the development of chronic pain, these authors have supported a model consistent with an integrated model of fibromyalgia, in which SIBO/LPS can explain the entirety of this common condition.

---

[352] Amaral et al. Commensal microbiota is fundamental for the development of inflammatory pain. *Proc Natl Acad Sci U S A.* 2008 Feb 12;105(6):2193-7
[353] Yamaguchi et al. Low rather than high dose lipopolysaccharide 'priming' of muscle provides an animal model of persistent elevated mechanical sensitivity for the study of chronic pain. *Eur J Pain.* 2011 Aug;15(7):724-31

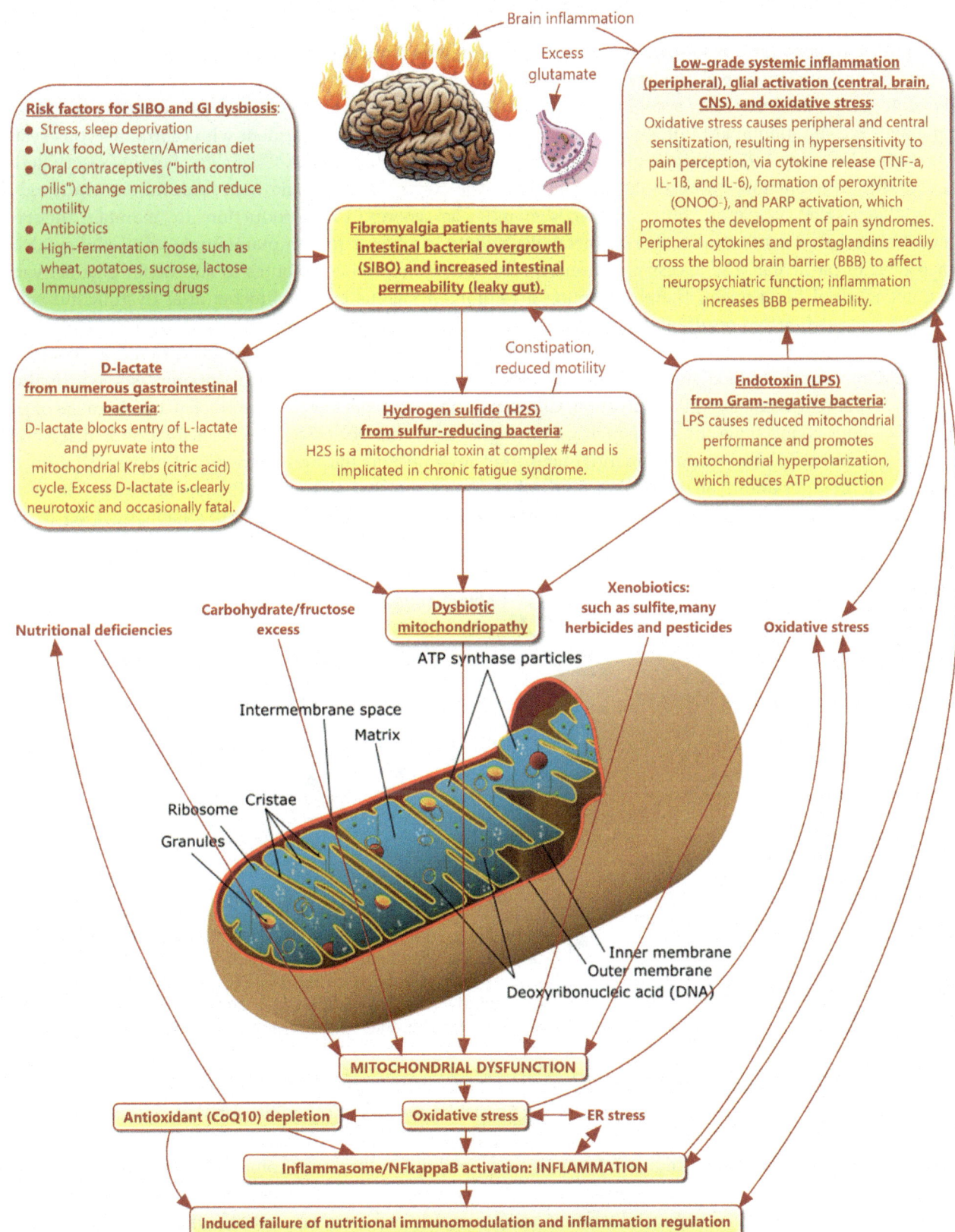

Brain inflammation

Excess glutamate

Risk factors for SIBO and GI dysbiosis:
- Stress, sleep deprivation
- Junk food, Western/American diet
- Oral contraceptives ("birth control pills") change microbes and reduce motility
- Antibiotics
- High-fermentation foods such as wheat, potatoes, sucrose, lactose
- Immunosuppressing drugs

Fibromyalgia patients have small intestinal bacterial overgrowth (SIBO) and increased intestinal permeability (leaky gut).

Low-grade systemic inflammation (peripheral), glial activation (central, brain, CNS), and oxidative stress:
Oxidative stress causes peripheral and central sensitization, resulting in hypersensitivity to pain perception, via cytokine release (TNF-a, IL-1ß, and IL-6), formation of peroxynitrite (ONOO-), and PARP activation, which promotes the development of pain syndromes. Peripheral cytokines and prostaglandins readily cross the blood brain barrier (BBB) to affect neuropsychiatric function; inflammation increases BBB permeability.

D-lactate from numerous gastrointestinal bacteria:
D-lactate blocks entry of L-lactate and pyruvate into the mitochondrial Krebs (citric acid) cycle. Excess D-lactate is clearly neurotoxic and occasionally fatal.

Constipation, reduced motility

Hydrogen sulfide (H2S) from sulfur-reducing bacteria:
H2S is a mitochondrial toxin at complex #4 and is implicated in chronic fatigue syndrome.

Endotoxin (LPS) from Gram-negative bacteria:
LPS causes reduced mitochondrial performance and promotes mitochondrial hyperpolarization, which reduces ATP production

Nutritional deficiencies

Carbohydrate/fructose excess

Dysbiotic mitochondriopathy

Xenobiotics: such as sulfite, many herbicides and pesticides

Oxidative stress

ATP synthase particles

Intermembrane space

Matrix

Ribosome

Cristae

Granules

Inner membrane

Outer membrane

Deoxyribonucleic acid (DNA)

MITOCHONDRIAL DYSFUNCTION

Antioxidant (CoQ10) depletion

Oxidative stress

ER stress

Inflammasome/NFkappaB activation: INFLAMMATION

Induced failure of nutritional immunomodulation and inflammation regulation

Fibromyalgia is a unique combination of SIBO-induced mitochondrial impairment with SIBO-induced glial activation: The synergistic combination of mitochondrial impairment (clearly evidenced in FM) with glial activation and the resulting central sensitization (clearly evidenced in FM) produces the clinical pattern of fibromyalgia. Image copyright © 2016 by Dr Alex Vasquez, all rights reserved and enforced. Image of brain by IsaacMao per Flickr.com via creativecommons.org/licenses/by/2.0.

❷ Secondary Cause of FM (part 1)—Mitochondrial Dysfunction: Fibromyalgia patients suffer somatic/body and central/brain fatigue from mitochondrial dysfunction as a result of SIBO.

The evidence is clear to the point of being irrefutable that FM patients have mitochondrial impairment; given the critical role of mitochondria in somatic and cerebral function, this mitochondrial impairment (dysmitochondriosis) alone would be sufficient to explain virtually all manifestations of FM. Dysmitochondriosis is evident biochemically and histologically, thus obviously accounting for—or at least contributing to—the muscle/somatic pain and fatigue; what makes the situation in FM unique is the coupling of mitochondrial impairment with central nervous system inflammation, ie, brain inflammation, glial activation, and central sensitization. Glial activation is exacerbated by mitochondrial dysfunction, because—at least in part—the hyperglutaminergic neurotransmission induced by microglial-astrocyte activation puts heavier demands on energy/ATP production to maintain neuronal homeostasis, for maintaining the increased metabolic activity in general and for maintaining intracellular calcium homeostasis in particular. The excess glutaminergic neurotransmission contributes to additional glial activation and mitochondrial impairment, thereby forming a reinforced vicious cycle. Mitochondrial dysfunction causes excess ROS production and resultant depletion of multifunctional nutrients/chemicals such as CoQ10, which again feeds back to promote additional mitochondrial impairment and reduction in antioxidant defenses, leading to altered and consequential ROS signaling and the perpetuation of inflammation (e.g., inflammasome activation), mitochondrial impairment, and glial activation. Clinicians and researchers need to appreciate that because of their pathophysiologic connections and consequences, microglial activation leads to astrocyte activation which leads to excessive glutaminergic (hyperglutaminergic) neurotransmission and the brain/neocortical hyperexcitation that promotes the manifestations of depression (and other components of sickness behavior) and pain via central sensitization; as such these terms become interconnected and largely interchangeable when discussed in their totality of effect.

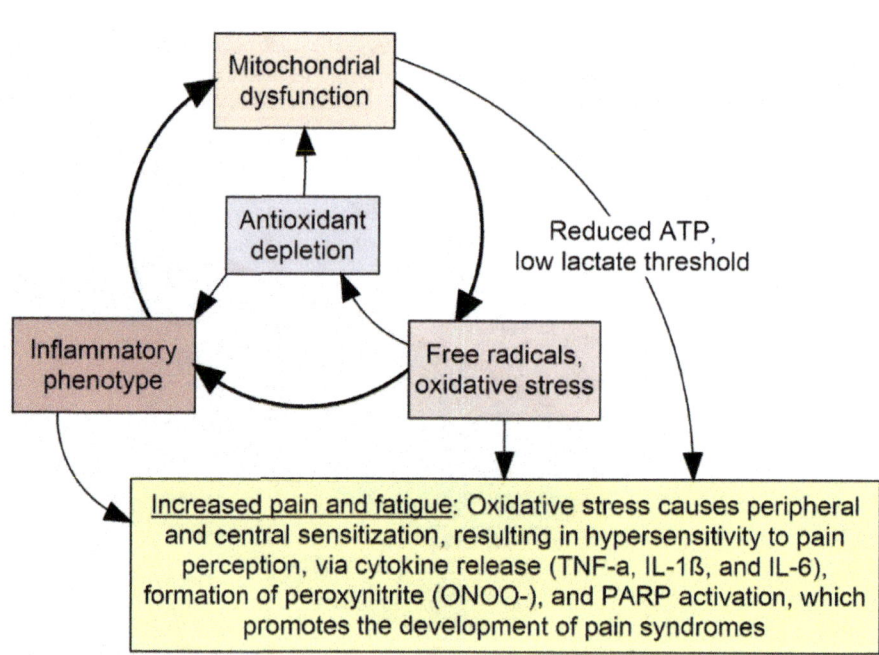

Mitochondrial dysfunction promotes central sensitization via oxidative stress and cytokine release: Mitochondrial dysfunction increases free radical production, which promotes "neurologic hypersensitivity" to pain, i.e., the pain in fibromyalgia is not simply due to muscle fatigue due to mitochondrial dysfunction although that is clearly a major component. The mitochondrial dysfunction also promotes central sensitization, which should be treated directly via alleviating the mitochondrial dysfunction and the causative dysbiosis, in addition to patient-specific factors.

Mitochondrial dysfunction → Antioxidant depletion → Reduced ATP, low lactate threshold → Free radicals, oxidative stress → Inflammatory phenotype

Increased pain and fatigue: Oxidative stress causes peripheral and central sensitization, resulting in hypersensitivity to pain perception, via cytokine release (TNF-a, IL-1ß, and IL-6), formation of peroxynitrite (ONOO-), and PARP activation, which promotes the development of pain syndromes

- Antimetabolites—microbial products that directly and indirectly impair mitochondrial performance: Yeast and bacteria can produce certain molecules which *jam up, monkey wrench,* or otherwise interfere with normal human cellular metabolism. The best example is **D-lactic acid**, which impairs human metabolic pathways that are designed to work with the "human" form of this metabolite—the levo isomer—L-lactic acid. Commonly resulting in headache, fatigue, depression, and sometimes death, D-lactic acidosis is extensively well documented in the medical research literature and commonly occurs in association with bacterial overgrowth of the intestine, particularly following intestinal bypass surgery.[354] Other antimetabolites produced from

---

[354] "D-Lactic acidosis is a potentially fatal clinical condition seen in patients with a short small intestine and an intact colon. Excessive production of D-lactate by abnormal bowel flora overwhelms normal metabolism of D-lactate and leads to an accumulation of this enantiomer in the blood." Vella A, Farrugia G. D-lactic acidosis: pathologic consequence of saprophytism. *Mayo Clin Proc.* 1998 May;73(5):451-6

(intestinal) microbes which are associated with human disease and dysfunction include **ammonia, tryptamine, tyramine, octopamine, mercaptates, aldehydes, alcohol (ethanol), tartaric acid, indolepropionic acid, indoleacetic acid, skatole, indole, putrescine,** and **cadaverine**. Many of these metabolites are seen in higher amounts in patients with migraine, depression, weakness, confusion, schizophrenia, agitation, hepatic encephalopathy, chronic arthritis and rheumatoid arthritis. **Gut-derived neurotoxins** from bacteria and yeast may contribute to autistic symptomatology[355,356], and case reports have consistently demonstrated that excess absorption of bacterial metabolites can alter behavior in humans and result in acute neurocognitive decline and behavioral abnormalities in children.[357] **Hydrogen sulfide (H2S)**, produced by intestinal bacteria such as *Citrobacter freundii*[358], is a mitochondrial poison[359] and is strongly associated with disease activity in ulcerative colitis.[360] Degradation of tryptophan by bacterial tryptophanase predisposes the host to a "functional tryptophan deficiency" and may result in insufficiency of serotonin which would contribute to hyperalgesia, depression, impaired adrenal responsiveness[361] ("hypoadrenalism"), and insomnia; **indole** and **skatole**, which are gut-derived bacterial degradation products of tryptophan, produce an inflammatory arthritis identical to rheumatoid arthritis in animal models.[362,363]

> **D-lactate triad: SIBO, CHO, and IP—bacterial overgrowth, carbohydrate, and increased permeability; the solutions are to reduce SIBO, reduce/modify CHO, heal gut, promote motility**
>
> "D-lactate is usually produced in excess when small bowel resection allows delivery of a high carbohydrate load to the colon. Elevation of D-lactate in plasma may also occur after other types of abdominal surgery, as a result of increased intestinal permeability and bacterial translocation across the intestinal mucosal barrier. Nonsurgical causes of intestinal hyperpermeability also increase absorption of D-lactate from the intestinal lumen."
>
> Galland L. *J Med Food.* 2014 Dec

- **Increased D-lactic acid intestinal bacteria in chronic fatigue syndrome** (*In Vivo* 2009 Jul[364]): The authors report finding a **significant increase of Gram-positive facultative anaerobic fecal microorganisms** in 108 CFS patients as compared to 177 control subjects. Specifically, they report, "The viable count of D-lactic acid producing *Enterococcus* and *Streptococcus* spp. in the fecal samples from the CFS group (3.5 x 10(7) cfu/L and 9.8 x 10(7) cfu/L respectively) were significantly higher than those for the control group (5.0 x 10(6) cfu/L and 8.9 x 10(4) cfu/L respectively). **Readers should note that this is approximately a 10-fold increase in *Enterococcus* and a >1,000-fold increase in *Streptococcus* in the CFS group compared with the control group. These Gram-positive bacteria produced not only more lactic acid in general but specifically they produced more of the dextro isomer D-lactic acid** than the Gram negative *Escherichia coli*. The authors correctly conclude that these findings "might explain not only neurocognitive dysfunction in CFS patients but also mitochondrial dysfunction, these findings may have important clinical implications."

- **Short bowel syndrome and D-lactic acidosis** (*Arch Dis Child* 1980 Oct[365]): The three-sentence abstract of this case report reads, "Metabolic acidosis in a 3-year-old child with short bowel syndrome led to the discovery of massive D-lactic aciduria. After normalization of the intestinal bacterial flora, D-lactate disappeared together with the acidosis. Dysbacteriosis with excessive production of D-lactate by intestinal bacteria (unidentified) and subsequent absorption explains this unusual cause of metabolic acidosis." Note the use

---

[355] Sandler RH, Finegold SM, Bolte ER, et al. Short-term benefit from oral vancomycin treatment of regressive-onset autism. *J Child Neurol.* 2000 Jul;15(7):429-35

[356] Shaw et al. Increased urinary excretion of analogs of Krebs cycle metabolites and arabinose in two brothers with autistic features. *Clin Chem* 1995;41(8Pt1):1094-104

[357] "The neurological features consisted of a depressed conscious state, confusion, aggressive behaviour, slurred speech and ataxia. The organic acid profile of urine demonstrated increased amounts of lactic, 3-hydroxypropionic, 3-hydroxyisobutyric, 2-hydroxyisocaproic, phenyllactic, 4-hydroxyphenylacetic and 4-hydroxyphenyllactic acids. Of the lactic acid 99% was D-lactic acid." Haan et al. Severe illness caused by products of bacterial metabolism in child with short gut. *Eur J Pediatr.* 1985;144:63-5

[358] Lennette EH (editor in chief). *Manual of Clinical Microbiology, Fourth Edition.* Washington DC; American Society for Microbiology: 1985, page 269. See also web.indstate.edu/thcme/micro/GI/general/sld038.htm Accessed 10/27/2005

[359] "Treatment of H2S poisoning may benefit from interventions aimed at minimizing ROS-induced damage and reducing mitochondrial damage." Eghbal MA, Pennefather PS, O'Brien PJ. H2S cytotoxicity mechanism involves reactive oxygen species formation and mitochondrial depolarisation. *Toxicology.* 2004 Oct 15;203(1-3):69-76

[360] "CONCLUSIONS: Metabolic effects of sodium hydrogen sulfide on butyrate oxidation along the length of the colon closely mirror metabolic abnormalities observed in active ulcerative colitis, and increased production of sulfide in ulcerative colitis suggests that the action of mercaptides may be involved in the genesis of ulcerative colitis." Roediger WE, et al. Reducing sulfur compounds of the colon impair colonocyte nutrition: implications for ulcerative colitis. *Gastroenterology* 1993 Mar;104:802-9

[361] "This hypothesis is supported by the findings in chronic MS patients of a significantly diminished adrenal cortisol reactivity to insulin-induced hypoglycemia which is considered a stress response mediated through the 5-HT system. Consequently, since patients with MS exhibit an abnormal response to stress it follows that increased tryptophan availability through dietary supplementation would diminish their vulnerability to psychological stress." Sandyk R. Tryptophan availability and the susceptibility to stress in multiple sclerosis: a hypothesis. *Int J Neurosci.* 1996 Jul;86(1-2):47-53

[362] Nakoneczna I, Forbes JC, Rogers KS. The arthritogenic effect of indole, skatole and other tryptophan metabolites in rabbits. *Am J Pathol.* 1969 Dec;57(3):523-38

[363] Rogers KS, Forbes JC, Nakoneczna I. Arthritogenic properties of lipophilic, aryl molecules. *Proc Soc Exp Biol Med.* 1969 Jun;131(2):670-2

[364] Sheedy JR, et al. Increased d-lactic acid intestinal bacteria in patients with chronic fatigue syndrome. *In Vivo.* 2009 Jul-Aug;23(4):621-8

[365] Schoorel EP, Giesberts MA, Blom W, van Gelderen HH. D-Lactic acidosis in a boy with short bowel syndrome. *Arch Dis Child.* 1980 Oct;55(10):810-2

of "dysbacteriosis" which is more commonly abbreviated to "dysbiosis", with the latter being more accurate in its nonspecificity since the disease-producing microbes may be from several different kingdoms and thus not exclusive to bacteria. The young boy in this case report underwent bowel resection secondary to multiple congenital malformations and complications from infection, i.e., mesenteric thrombosis tertiary to dehydration secondary to infectious diarrhea. After several episodes of neurocognitive dysfunction including weakness and dyspnea, the child was eventually diagnosed with multiple nutritional deficiencies, malabsorption, and lactic acidosis secondary to intestinal overgrowth of Gram-positive D-lactate-producing bacteria and an insufficiency of Gram-negative bacteria. The child was treated only with probiotic supplementation—no antibiotics were given—and D-lactate levels fell quickly within 4 days and were virtually undetectable by day 11. Thus, probiotic therapy alone may be sufficient treatment for some cases of D-lactic acidosis, particularly when an "insufficiency dysbiosis" of beneficial bacteria and a relative or absolute "overgrowth dysbiosis" of harmful bacteria coexist.

❸ Secondary Cause of FM (part 2)—Central Sensitization: As a result of SIBO, fibromyalgia patients suffer increased sensitivity to pain due to heightened sensitivity of the brain and spinal cord—as well as from peripheral sensitization and impaired muscle function due to the previously established mitochondrial dysfunction. In other words, inflammation induced by microbial debris promotes sensitization to pain.

- The *existence* of central sensitization in fibromyalgia—real and generally accepted: Central sensitization—the increased perception of "pain" from otherwise nonpainful stimuli—is a well-accepted component of fibromyalgia; in fact, some authors and medical societies have claimed that sensitization of the brain and spinal cord is indeed the sole cause of fibromyalgia. The emphasis on *central* is to specify that the sensitization is localized in the *central* nervous system (comprised only of the brain and spinal cord) and not in the *peripheral* nervous system—the peripheral nerves (e.g., in the arms and legs) nor in their receptors (e.g., in skin, muscles, and other tissues). Again, the consensus is that central sensitization is present in fibromyalgia, that these patients have heightened sensitivity to pain and the perception of pain from stimuli that would not otherwise be painful to "normal" persons whom do not have fibromyalgia.

- The *origin* of central sensitization—an issue of the highest importance in the treatment of fibromyalgia: What is needed in the conversation on central sensitization is not debating is *presence* but rather an understanding of its *cause*, or purported lack of cause. In medicine, when we say that a condition is "primary" we are saying that conceptually the condition has *no known cause*, that it is *idiopathic*, that the primary origin is *inherent* within the disease condition itself; to say that something is *primary* is to say that it itself is the origin of the disease process. In contrast, when we describe a

> **Dysbiosis—SIBO and LPS—alter brain function, neurotransmission, to promote pain, fatigue, depression**
>
> "Structural bacterial components such as **lipopolysaccharides** provide low-grade tonic stimulation of the innate immune system. Excessive stimulation due to bacterial **dysbiosis**, **small intestinal bacterial overgrowth**, or increased intestinal permeability may produce systemic and/or central nervous system inflammation."
>
> Galland L. *J Med Food*. 2014 Dec

condition or aspect of disease as *secondary*, we are saying that it is due to a preceding primary problem, that it follows some other event, that it is second in line in the disease process. Likewise, we can say that a problem that occurs *causally* (not simply *chronologically*) after a secondary problem is a tertiary problem, and so on. If two events happen at the same time but one event does not cause the other, then the events are *associated* (somehow related) or *concomitant* (occurring at the same time).

- Example—distinguishing *primary*, from *secondary*, from *tertiary*, from *associated*: If a person has an automobile or sporting accident (the *primary* event) and suffers a painful injury, we would say that the injury is *secondary* to trauma, and that any resulting psychological distress would be *secondary* to the pain and impairment from the injury, or *tertiary* to the primary trauma. If the psychological distress were due to the accident itself (e.g., distressing memories of what occurred), then the psychological distress would be *secondary* to experiencing the event of the accident itself, independent from or complicated by any pain or impairment. If the patient also had a skin disease that existed previously, we would say that the patient has a *concomitant* skin disease but that it is unrelated to the accident or the injury, unless perhaps the patient intentionally injured himself/herself as a result of the skin disease (for example in a suicide attempt or some other form of self-harm secondary to the primary illness).

In the conversation on central sensitization in fibromyalgia, the distinction between *primary* and *secondary* is of the highest importance. If we say that central sensitization in fibromyalgia is *primary*, we are saying that the problem originates in the brain and spinal cord, and that the appropriate treatments are therefore those that target the brain and spinal cord, such as pain-relieving drugs; other treatments might be useful, but they are of secondary importance to directly influencing the *primary* problem in the brain and spinal cord. For ethical and professional reasons, doctorate-level physicians are obligated to address the primary cause of disease whenever possible; this is a matter of acumen and beneficence because failing to address the primary cause of the problem when possible firstly allows the primary disease to fester and develop and progress while secondly leaving the patient dependent upon—enslaved to—symptom alleviation.

- o <u>Example—distinguishing *professional* and *ethical* behavior (e.g., treating the primary problem) from *unprofessional/irresponsible/unethical* behavior (e.g., failing to treat the primary problem, promoting dependency and exposing the patient to excess risk and expense, etc) among physicians</u>: If a patient sits on a nail but cannot see the nail and then reports to the physician's office with a complaint of pain, the physician is professionally obligated to assess the situation by providing treatment of the primary problem—in this case, by removing the nail. The cause of the pain is the embedded nail, removing the nail will shortly alleviate the pain (assuming no infection or other complication). But let's say that an unethical physician is paid by a drug company to sell analgesic drugs, and the physician neglects his/her professional responsibility and his/her ethical responsibility to the patient; this physician fails to address the primary problem (the painful nail) and instead prescribes a dangerous drug to partly alleviate the pain at a cost of $200 and the doctor also receives a cash "gift" of $50 from the drug company for having promoted the sale of the drug. Because the doctor failed to address the *primary* problem (the painful nail) and only addressed the *secondary* problem (the pain), the doctor has failed to provide professional and ethical care, and this is further complicated by the physician's nondisclosed conflict of interest and receipt of a cash reward for having ordered the patient to spend $200 on a drug that he/she did not need. What is worse, the patient might be injured from the drug, or might eventually develop and infection because of the ongoing nature of the embedded nail. The doctor has created dependency (e.g., return visits and fees for more prescriptions) and income (e.g., from office fees and from payments by the drug company) while failing to treat the primary cause of the patient's problem.

If we say that pain and central sensitization in fibromyalgia are *primary*—without identifiable cause—then we have to treat symptomatically by suppressing/targeting the pain itself; this is reasonable, but increasingly unlikely as science advances and we better understand the nature and causes of diseases. If we say that pain and central sensitization in fibromyalgia are *secondary*—caused by a primary problem—then we are professionally and ethically obligated to address the primary cause of the pain. If physicians and medical groups say that pain and central sensitization in fibromyalgia are *primary* when in fact the research has made clear the cause of and treatment for the pain, then these physicians and medical groups—possibly to advance their own importance in society and income from drug companies—are behaving unprofessionally and unethically and unscientifically by cheating their patients of the opportunity for cure and putting these patients at risk for complications from the primary disease, at risk for adverse drug effects including injury and death, and burdening patients and the healthcare system with the costs of thousands of dollars individually and billions of dollars collectively/systematically by frauding the nature of the illness and its treatment. There it is; that is the defining line between *ethical* and *professional* behavior and *unethical* and *unprofessional* behavior, whether by individual physicians affecting the lives of hundreds of patients or by medical organizations affecting millions of patients for billions of dollars. If fibromyalgia has a legitimate cause, then doctors have an obligation to treat the cause of the problem rather than profit by unnecessary clinical patronage (coerced by pain, made necessary by the "necessary" need for repeated assessments and prescription refills). Relatedly, medical organizations that fraud the practice of medicine by distributing false information and promoting inefficacious treatment protocols that culminate in nontreatment of the primary disorder, the unnecessary use of dangerous treatments that harm patients, and unnecessary expenses to healthcare systems in the billions of dollars would be culpable for same.

- <u>Describing central sensitization in fibromyalgia as "primary" is unscientific, magical thinking that promotes drug dependency, drug sales, and physician dependency</u>: This promulgation, based on the selective ignoring of a vast and readily integrated body of scientific body of information, harms patients and costs healthcare systems billions of dollars.
- <u>Describing central sensitization in fibromyalgia as "secondary" is scientific, logical thinking</u>: This affirmation, based on the integration of a large body of scientific information, benefits patients, empowers doctors, and saves healthcare systems billions of dollars.

Given that the existence of central sensitization in animal and human models of pain, and that its presence is reasonably well established in human patients with fibromyalgia, the main question(s) to address are ❶ What is the cause of the central sensitization?, ❷ How can the cause be effectively treated?, ❸ Only if no cause can be found are we then allowed to ask, "What treatments—natural or pharmaceutical—are appropriate for the direct treatment of central sensitization?" Anytime that doctors and policymakers are discussing treatments, we have to consider 1) cost, availability, distributive justice, 2) effectiveness, 3) cost-effectiveness ratio, 4) safety, contraindications, adverse effects, and 5) drug-drug and drug-nutrient interactions; in shorthand, we can think of the risk:benefit ratio as a summation of these considerations, wherein "risk" is everything negative and "benefit" is everything positive. Except perhaps in Emergency Medicine and Urgent Care, doctors for the most part are trained to ignore the cause of problems and to just prescribe the "appropriate" drug for each diagnosis[366]; this is why medical care for nonacute/chronic/persistent diseases is so abysmal—because doctors have been trained to turn off their investigative brains, to recite the *idiopathic dogma*[367] that "chronic diseases are a complex interplay genes and environment, and while we don't yet know the exact cause, we can give you medicines that will help", to focus on molecules rather than context and cause, and to basically just practice as MDs—medicine dispensers. Exacerbating the problem are the medical/science writers and the medical organizations (e.g., specialists organizations in pain, rheumatology, and general medicine) that are paid hundreds of thousands and millions of dollars, respectively, to selectively ignore *causal* data and emphasize the *drug-selling* data.

In the following sections, I will establish that ❶ central sensitization in fibromyalgia is caused by microbial debris and secondary metabolic and inflammatory effects, that ❷ rational treatment of microbe-induced pain and inflammation must focus on 1) the eradication/modulation of the inflammatory microbial load, 2) the restoration of barrier defenses (e.g., the defensive lining of the skin and the gut wall) to reduce absorption of and exposure to microbial molecules (enhancing elimination of already-absorbed microbial toxins is a possibility, but is of lesser importance and is mentioned in some of my other writings), and ❸ treatments to directly address the inflammatory pain and central sensitization.

[366] Ely JW, Osheroff JA, Ebell MH, et al. Analysis of questions asked by family doctors regarding patient care. *BMJ*. 1999 Aug 7;319(7206):358-61
[367] Vasquez A. Twilight of the Idiopathic Era and the Dawn of New Possibilities in Health and Healthcare. *Naturopathy Digest* 2006 Mar naturopathydigest.com/archives/2006/mar/idiopathic.php. See also: Ely et al. Analysis of questions asked by family doctors regarding patient care. *BMJ*. 1999 Aug:358-61

Central sensitization in fibromyalgia is caused by microbial debris and secondary metabolic and inflammatory effects: My main thesis is stated immediately above, that central sensitization in fibromyalgia is caused by microbial debris and the secondary metabolic and inflammatory effects. I think this is easily demonstrated in graphic form, and so I will use the following image and its caption do most of the explaining, then I will follow the caption with a bit more discussion before concluding this section with a few notes and comments on research.

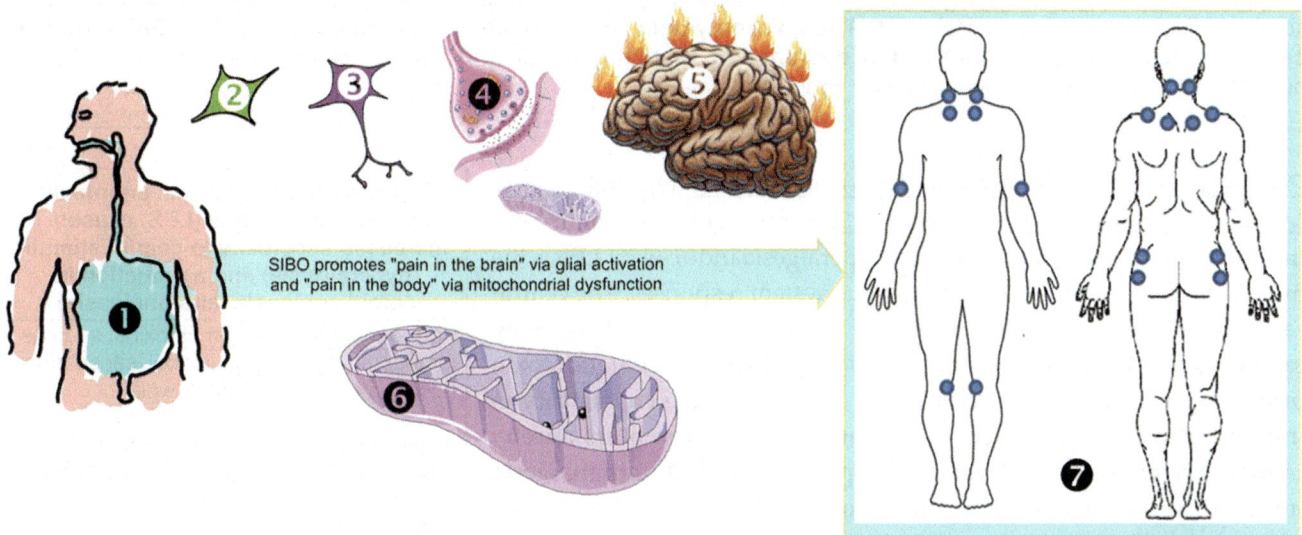

SIBO promotes glial activation and mitochondrial impairment which are the major causes of fibromyalgia syndrome: *From gut to "brain pain"*: ❶ Small intestine bacterial overgrowth (SIBO) leads to intestinal absorption and systemic distribution of low levels of bacterial endotoxin (endotoxemia) and other ***inflamm**ation-**gen**erating molecules* (inflammogens); this results in low-grade inflammation (including release of cytokines, prostaglandins and other inflammatory mediators and oxidants).[368] Microbial inflammogens cause systemic inflammation, and cytokines and prostaglandins produced peripherally (ie, outside of the central nervous system [CNS], which is the brain and spinal cord) can readily traverse the blood-brain barrier (BBB) and enter the CNS to promote glial activation—brain inflammation.[369] Some of these microbial inflammogens may be able to bypass the BBB directly, when the BBB becomes permeable/leaky following induction of systemic inflammation. SIBO can also elaborate mitochondrial inhibitors such as endotoxin (lipopolysaccharide, LPS)[370], hydrogen sulfide (H2S)[371], and D-lactate.[372] In the brain, mitochondrial dysfunction exacerbates brain dysfunction and the vicious cycle of microglial activation.[373] ❷ Microglia are immune cells in the brain that respond to cytokines, prostaglandins, and microbial inflammogens; when microglia become stimulated or "activated" by inflammatory triggers/signals, the microglia signal/activate/irritate the nearby ❸ astrocytes, which are cells in the brain that respond by causing an increase in neuron-to-neuron communication (neurotransmission) via the neurotransmitter glutamate, which is stimulatory to neurons.[374] ❹ While glutamate is necessary in small and regulated amounts, higher levels of glutamate promote central sensitization, pain amplification, "brain fatigue", depression and anxiety; when very elevated, glutamate can promote migraine headaches, seizures and epilepsy.[375] ❺ High levels of glutamate cause excitation of brain neurons, and this increased activity leads to increased production of free radicals, which cause additional local inflammation and mitochondrial dysfunction within the brain, leading back to microglial activation for a vicious cycle. The brain is now in a "positive feedback loop" which promotes additional pain/fatigue/depression independently from ongoing stimulation from the original trigger. As you can see from this description, microglial activation causes astrocyte activation in a close relationship; since microglia—the brain's immune cells—and astrocytes—the brain's supportive or helper or "nurse" cells—are both categorized as glial cells (glia = glue = the mass of cells that creates the supporting structure for the neurons of the brain), you can see that *microglial activation* and *astrocyte activation* and *glial activation* are extensions of each other and can be used somewhat interchangeably. Excess or prolonged microglial activation promotes neurodegeneration via hyperexcitation of neurons, basically causing them to "burn out" in a process

[368] Patel et al. Human experimental endotoxemia in modeling pathophysiology, genomics, and therapeutics of innate immunity in complex cardiometabolic diseases. *Arterioscler Thromb Vasc Biol* 2015 Mar:525-34. Ferguson et al. Omega-3 PUFA supplementation response to endotoxemia in healthy volunteers. *Mol Nutr Food Res* 2014 Mar;601-13

[369] Wilson CJ, Finch CE, Cohen HJ. Cytokines and cognition--the case for a head-to-toe inflammatory paradigm. *J Am Geriatr Soc.* 2002 Dec;50(12):2041-56

[370] Scirocco et al. Exposure of Toll-like receptors 4 to bacterial lipopolysaccharide (LPS) impairs human colonic smooth muscle cell function. *J Cell Physiol.* 2010 May; 442-50

[371] Lemle MD. Hypothesis: chronic fatigue syndrome is caused by dysregulation of hydrogen sulfide metabolism. *Med Hypotheses.* 2009 Jan;72(1):108-9

[372] Sheedy et al. Increased d-lactic Acid intestinal bacteria in patients with chronic fatigue syndrome. *In Vivo.* 2009 Jul-Aug;23(4):621-8

[373] Nguyen et al. A new vicious cycle involving glutamate excitotoxicity, oxidative stress and mitochondrial dynamics. *Cell Death Dis.* 2011 Dec 8;2:e240

[374] Béchade C, Cantaut-Belarif Y, Bessis A. Microglial control of neuronal activity. *Front Cell Neurosci.* 2013 Mar 28;7:32

[375] Devinsky O, Vezzani A, Najjar S, De Lanerolle NC, Rogawski MA. Glia and epilepsy: excitability and inflammation. *Trends Neurosci.* 2013 Mar;36(3):174-84

that has been described as "brain on fire."[376] The exception to this occurs after a period of particularly protracted microglial activation, which can cause damage or "burn out" of the astrocytes, too; this "astrocyte degeneration" leads to neurodegeneration when the astrocytes become impaired and cannot perform their supportive and "nursing" functions to the neurons. ❻ *From gut to "body pain and fatigue"*: SIBO can also elaborate mitochondrial inhibitors such as endotoxin (lipopolysaccharide, LPS), hydrogen sulfide (H2S), and D-lactate, as previously stated and cited. In the body, mitochondrial dysfunction promotes pain and the vicious cycle of oxidative stress, nutritional depletion, and additional mitochondrial dysfunction. Mitochondrial dysfunction in muscle leads to the cellular/cytologic and histologic/tissue changes that are typical and well-documented in cell and muscle samples of patients with fibromyalgia.[377] These peripheral (e.g., non-brain) changes in muscle also prove beyond any doubt that fibromyalgia is not a "brain disease" or solely a "disorder of pain processing." ❼ **Thus, fibromyalgia can be easily explained/understood as SIBO-induced central sensitization and mitochondrial dysfunction, resulting in pain and fatigue**; all other abnormalities in FM can be traced back to these key problems. Image of brain by IsaacMao per Flickr.com via creativecommons.org/licenses/by/2.0. See educational videos and updates at www.inflammationmastery.com/pain

---

Central sensitization (enhanced and autonomous pain hypersensitivity) seen in FM can be caused by bacterial LPS: Somewhat independent from the immune/inflammation-mediated hyperalgesia induced by LPS is the hyperalgesia mediated by central nervous system responses. The central sensitization seen with fibromyalgia[378] might be explained as being caused by intestinally-derived bacterial toxins. **Bacterial LPS/endotoxin promotes central sensitization via (microglia-driven astrocyte-induced glutamate-mediated) activation of NMDA receptors and by inducing hyperalgesia (elevated pain perception) and anti-analgesia (reduced response to pain inhibition).**[379] Accumulated evidence suggests that fibromyalgia may be a disorder of somatic hypersensitivity induced by bacterial toxins derived from quantitative excess or qualitative abnormalities in gut bacteria.[380]

> **Exposure to the bacterial endotoxin lipopolysaccharide (LPS) causes increased sensitivity to painful stimuli (hyperalgesia) and a reduction in opioid analgesia (anti-analgesia)**
>
> "Intraperitoneal injection of toxins, such as the bacterial endotoxin lipopolysaccharide (LPS), is associated with a well-characterized increase in sensitivity to painful stimuli (hyperalgesia) and a longer-lasting reduction in opioid analgesia (anti-analgesia) when pain sensitivity returns to basal levels."
>
> Johnston et al. Inhibition of morphine analgesia by LPS. *Behav Brain Res* 2005 Jan

Gut dysbiosis—generally speaking—can promote syndromes of pain, fatigue and depression via systemic inflammation (triggered directly by microbial molecules), immune activation via increased intestinal permeability, and increased glutaminergic neurotransmission via glial activation—microglial activation followed by astrocyte activation. As the name implies, central sensitization describes a condition of heightened perception of / responsiveness to sensory stimuli, particularly pain. In an authoritative review by Woolf[381] in 2011, the following introduction provides both definition and description, "Nociceptor inputs can trigger a prolonged but reversible increase in the excitability and synaptic efficacy of neurons in central nociceptive pathways, the phenomenon of central sensitization. Central sensitization manifests as pain hypersensitivity, particularly dynamic tactile allodynia, secondary punctate or pressure hyperalgesia, aftersensations, and enhanced temporal summation." Woolf goes on to note that central sensitization (CS) can be elicited in humans by diverse experimental noxious stimuli to skin, muscles or viscera, and that CS "results in secondary changes in brain activity that can be detected by electrophysiological or imaging techniques." Clinical conditions in which CS plays a role include fibromyalgia, osteoarthritis, headache, temporomandibular joint disorders, chronic musculoskeletal pain, dental pain, neuropathic pain, visceral pain hypersensitivity disorders (such as irritable bowel syndrome, IBS), and post-surgical/traumatic pain. In essence, anything that causes pain (e.g., injury) or contributes to increased pain perception (e.g., sleep deprivation, magnesium deficiency, vitamin D deficiency) can contribute to central sensitization simply by virtue of neuronal plasticity, which makes repeatedly activated pathways—in this case the perception of and response to pain—become more permanent via synaptogenesis, e.g., pain chronification via activity/repetition-dependent synaptic plasticity. In experimental models, bacterial LPS has been shown to promote central sensitization via activation of microglial release of extracellular ATP which in turn triggers astrocytes to

---

[376] Cohen G. The brain on fire? *Ann Neurol.* 1994 Sep;36(3):333-4

[377] Cordero et al. Mitochondrial dysfunction and mitophagy activation in blood mononuclear cells of fibromyalgia patients: implications in the pathogenesis of the disease. *Arthritis Res Ther.* 2010;12(1):R17. Olsen NJ, Park JH. Skeletal muscle abnormalities in patients with fibromyalgia. *Am J Med Sci.* 1998 Jun;315(6):351-8

[378] Meeus et al. Central sensitization: biopsychosocial explanation for chronic widespread pain in patients with fibromyalgia and chronic fatigue syndrome. *Clin Rheumatol.* 2007 Apr;26(4):465-73

[379] Johnston IN, Westbrook RF. Inhibition of morphine analgesia by LPS: role of opioid and NMDA receptors and spinal glia. *Behav Brain Res.* 2005;156(1):75-83

[380] Othman M, Agüero R, Lin HC. Alterations in intestinal microbial flora and human disease. *Curr Opin Gastroenterol.* 2008 Jan;24(1):11-6

[381] Woolf CJ. Central sensitization: implications for the diagnosis and treatment of pain. *Pain.* 2011 Mar;152(3 Suppl):S2-15

promote glutaminergic neurotransmission, thereby increasing neurocortical hyperexcitability and promoting pain, depression, central fatigue, and migraine/seizure. As paraphrased here and noted in the diagram from Béchade et al[382], LPS stimulates microglia to externalize the DAMP extracellular ATP, recruiting astrocytes to release glutamate leading to increased excitatory transmission via a glutamate, the major excitatory neurotransmitter. Clinicians should appreciate that LPS is a prototype agonist but certainly not the only "environmental factor" capable of triggering hyperglutaminergic neurotransmission (excess glutamate activating the glutamate-sensitive NMDA receptors) or what might be called glutamate-mediated hypertransmission (normal levels of glutamate triggering a hypersensitive receptor, or a hypersensitive or "loaded" or "primed" intracellular cascade). The clinical correlates of this model are relevant for chronic pain, depression, central fatigue, neurodegeneration, post-traumatic pain, post-traumatic stress disorder (PTSD), epilepsy and migraine. LPS is one of many "noxious stimuli" that can trigger microglia activation for eventual hyperglutaminergic neurocortical hyperexcitability and excitotoxicity; other factors include trauma and inflammatory cytokines and prostaglandins. LPS, other microbial immunogens, and other inflammatory triggers need not originate in the gut, as many long-term/chronic "dysbiotic-like" infections are localized within the brain and central nervous system, such as HSV[383], *Chlamydia pneumoniae*[384], and "algal" chlorovirus ATCV-1[385]; neuropathologic infections, antigens and neurotoxins such as the aluminum used in vaccines/immunizations as an adjuvant can be trafficked from the periphery into the brain by the immune system.[386] This author's perspective is that gut-derived microbial signals do indeed evoke central sensitization, most likely via direct CNS entry (via a "leaky" blood-brain barrier; perhaps trafficked by immunocytes), but at the very least indirectly by peripheral immune activation and the systemic proinflammatory state characterized by increased production of cytokines and prostaglandins which readily cross the blood-brain barrier to produce microglial activation and the subsequent hyperexcitation, excitotoxicity, and sickness behavior—including fatigue, depression, sensitivity. Microglial activation promotes neuronal hyperexcitation/excitotoxicity, and the reverse is also true: neuronal (hyper)activity promotes microglial activation; thereby forming a vicious cycle. Additionally, factors such as heightened glutamate/NMDA receptor sensitivity, depleted antioxidant defenses and specific nutrient deficiencies (e.g., pyridoxine, magnesium, zinc, vitamin D, n3 fatty acids), mitochondrial impairment, and an pro-inflammatory microenvironment combine additively/synergistically to promote the progressively accelerated pace of reciprocal microglial activation and neuronal hyperexcitation/excitotoxicity noted in several neurodegenerative states. This could be complicated by gut *Clostridia* production of 3-3-hydroxyphenyl-3-hydroxypropionic acid (HPHPA) and p-cresol causing neurotransmitter imbalance—elevated dopamine and reduced norepinephrine.

Defining and describing what is meant by "brain inflammation" relative to central sensitization in pain syndromes: Encephalitis (*enceph*—brain, *itis*—inflammation) classically refers to acute brain inflammation resultant from brain infection, such as a viral infection, e.g., herpes encephalitis. However, we now appreciate more subtle forms of chronic/persistent brain inflammation—metabolic-immunologic inflammation—in neurologic and psychiatric conditions such as chronic pain, autism, Parkinson's and Alzheimer's DZs, as well as chronic depression and schizophrenia. As such, we can reasonably expand the use of the term *encephalitis* beyond the acute and infectious to include the chronic and metabolic, ie

---

> **Glial activation = brain inflammation = promotion of central sensitization = pain hypersensitivity and other manifestations of sickness behavior**
>
> Typical manifestations of brain inflammation and sickness behavior include:
> - Reduced physical activity, inertia
> - Reduced food intake
> - Reduced social interaction
> - Reduced sexual behavior
> - Reduced mood, depression
> - Impaired memory
> - Heightened sensitivity to pain
>
> Maier SF, Watkins LR. Consequences of the Inflamed Brain. *Report on Progress 2012, University of Colorado at Boulder. Dana Alliance* 2012 Aug

---

[382] Béchade C, Cantaut-Belarif Y, Bessis A. Microglial control of neuronal activity. *Front Cell Neurosci.* 2013 Mar 28;7:32
[383] Ball et al. Intracerebral propagation of Alzheimer's disease: strengthening evidence of a herpes simplex virus etiology. *Alzheimers Dement.* 2013 Mar;9(2):169-75
[384] Hammond et al. Immunohistological detection of Chlamydia pneumoniae in the Alzheimer's disease brain. *BMC Neurosci.* 2010 Sep 23;11:121
[385] Yolken et al. Chlorovirus ATCV-1 is part human oropharyngeal virome associated changes in cognitive functions in humans and mice. *Proc Natl Acad Sci* 2014 Nov:16106-11
[386] "We previously showed that poorly biodegradable aluminum-coated particles injected into muscle are promptly phagocytosed in muscle and the draining lymph nodes, and can disseminate within phagocytic cells throughout the body and slowly accumulate in brain." Gherardi et al. Biopersistence and brain translocation of aluminum adjuvants of vaccines. *Front Neurol* 2015 Feb;6:4. See also: "Detection of Al(III) in tissues indicated presence of aluminum in the nervous tissue of experimental animals." Luján et al. Autoimmune/autoinflammatory syndrome induced by adjuvants (ASIA syndrome) in commercial sheep. *Immunol Res* 2013 Jul:317-24

chronic/persistent metabolic-immunologic brain inflammation. Not all brain inflammation leads to central sensitization, but all central sensitization has a (neuro)inflammatory component. If we say "central sensitization", then we are a bit lost, because we are describing too many things at once (e.g., pain, emotions, MRI changes, early experiences, neurotransmitters...); as such, overuse of the term central sensitization can lead us astray or leave us unclear and therefore easily manipulated. If we say "brain inflammation" then we can reasonably appreciate a process that is: 1) causal—only so many things cause brain inflammation, so we can organize a plan of discovery and treatment, and 2) limited—we appreciate that most inflammatory disorders and responses should resolve. Any inflammatory trigger will be expected to trigger brain inflammation; while insults to the brain are obvious, peripheral cytokines and immunocytes can cross the blood brain barrier (BBB) to trigger inflammation in the brain, even when the problem started in the periphery. If you know that "the brain has an immune system", and that when the brain's immune system triggers inflammation—whether via central/brain insult or peripheral/body inflammation—that the result is neuroinflammation, pain, depression, and expedited neurodegeneration, then you can appreciate the intermixing of systemic inflammation with brain inflammation, with microglial activation and the resultant changes in neurotransmission that lead to pain sensitivity and changes in mood/affect called "sickness behavior." In this work, I show that fibromyalgia is a unique combination of dysbiosis-induced glial activation and mitochondrial impairment; both of these components need to be treated effectively and at the same time in order to alleviate the brain inflammation—unique—in fibromyalgia. "Glial activation with mitochondrial impairment" is different from and worse than glial activation or mitochondrial impairment by itself; the combination of the two together exacerbates both while also causing a vicious cycle that promotes ongoing pain, fatigue, and emotional/psychiatric changes.

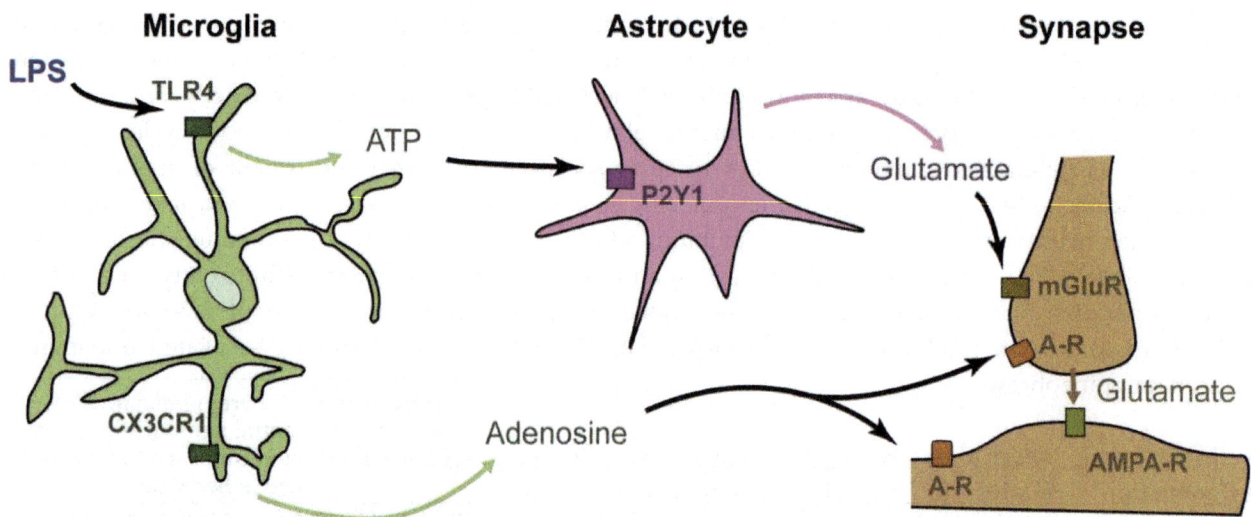

Microglial LPS reception leads to (extracellular) ATP elaboration, which stimulates astrocytes to produce glutamate, which increases glutaminergic neurotransmission: "Upon LPS stimulation, microglia rapidly produce ATP, which recruits astrocytes. Astrocytes subsequently release glutamate, and this leads to increased excitatory transmission via a metabotropic glutamate receptor-dependent mechanism." Illustration and quote from: Béchade C, Cantaut-Belarif Y, Bessis A. Microglial control of neuronal activity. *Front Cell Neurosci*. 2013 Mar 28;7:32[387]

Verified in animal models and likely contributory to clinical pain syndromes such as fibromyalgia is the observation that bacterial endotoxin/LPS can also contribute to central sensitization. This concept is introduced here and will be further substantiated in a following section on clinical pain syndromes and more so in separate writings, whether specific to fibromyalgia[388] or general to rheumatology.[389] The basic pathophysiology is quite simple and linear, as depicted below and itemized with citations thereafter.

Bacterial LPS ➜ microglial activation ➜ astrocyte hyperglutaminogenesis ➜ neurocortical hyperexcitation ➜ pain

[387] Béchade C, Cantaut-Belarif Y, Bessis A. Microglial control of neuronal activity. *Front Cell Neurosci*. 2013 Mar 28;7:32 doi: 10.3389/fncel.2013.00032 journal.frontiersin.org/article/10.3389/fncel.2013.00032/abstract. Copyright © 2013 Béchade, Cantaut-Belarif and Bessis. *Front Cell Neurosci* is an open-access journal distributed under terms of Creative Commons Attribution License, which permits use/distribution/reproduction in other forums, provided original authors/source are credited.
[388] Vasquez A. *Fibromyalgia in a Nutshell: A Safe and Effective Functional Medicine Strategy*. 2012, and later versions.
[389] Vasquez A. *Functional Medicine Rheumatology v3.5*. 2014, and later versions.

However, the correlation of serum LPS (or its indirect marker, anti-LPS antibodies) with increased intestinal permeability provides another interpretation, wherein serum LPS activity is simply a correlate with increased IP which promotes pain via nonspecific and non-LPS mechanisms, as shown in the following sequence:

SIBO/LPS-induced mucosal damage ➔ absorption of gut-derived immunogens and toxins ➔ microglial activation ➔ astrocyte-mediated hyperglutaminogenesis ➔
neurocortical hyperexcitation ➔ pain/depression/fatigue and associated low-grade immune activation

- <u>Endotoxemia induces visceral hypersensitivity and altered pain evaluation in healthy humans</u> (*Pain.* 2012 Apr[390]): "…transient systemic immune activation results in decreased visceral sensory and pain thresholds and altered subjective pain ratings."
- <u>LPS-induced hyperalgesia in healthy humans</u> (*Brain Behav Immun* 2014 Oct[391]): "Our results revealed widespread increases in musculoskeletal pain sensitivity in response to a moderate dose of LPS (0.8 ng/kg), which correlate both with changes in IL-6 and negative mood."
- <u>Widespread hyperalgesia in adolescents with symptoms of irritable bowel syndrome</u> (*J Pain.* 2014 Sep[392]): "We examined pain sensitivity in 961 adolescents from the general population (mean age 16.1 years), including pain threshold and tolerance measurements of heat (forearm) and pressure pain (fingernail and shoulder) and cold pressor tolerance (hand). … Our results indicate that adolescents in the general population with IBS symptoms, like adults, have widespread hyperalgesia. … Our results suggest that central pain sensitization mechanisms in IBS may contribute to triggering and maintaining chronic pain symptoms."

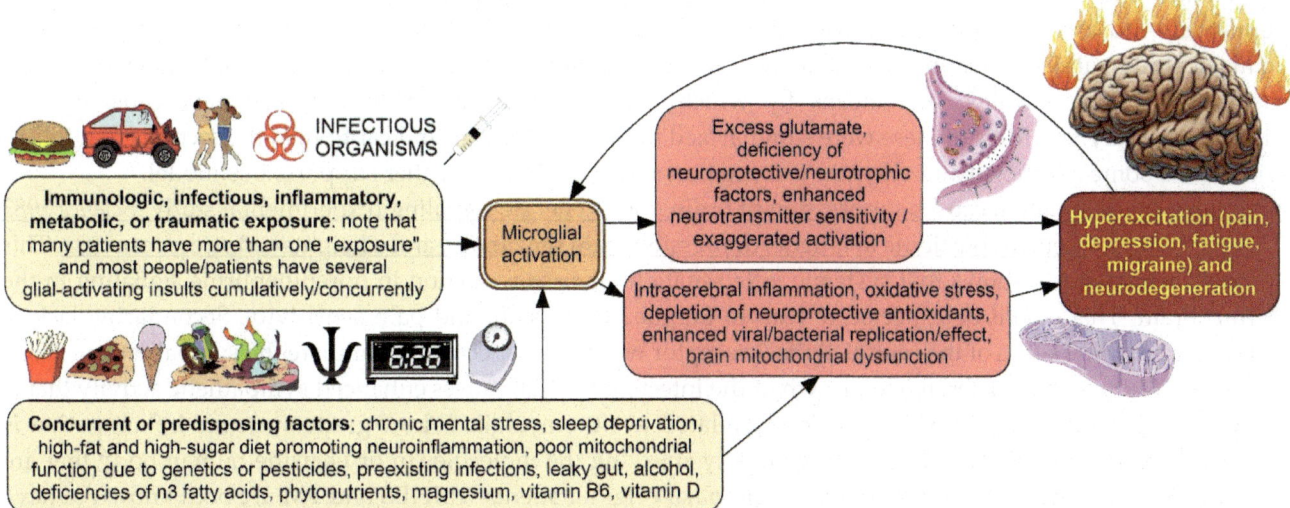

Numerous insults—immunologic, inflammatory, infectious, metabolic, traumatic, toxins—can "team up" or act individually to incite glial activation: Very importantly, glial activation can remain in an activated state promoting neurotransmitter imbalance, hyperexcitation, and neurodegeneration for several years after a single biochemical, infectious, or physical assault. High-fat foods, physical trauma from sports and accidents, psychological and mental stress, sleep deprivation, and the metabolic stress of hyperglycemia, insulin resistance, and obesity all contribute to brain inflammation—also called "the brain on fire" per Cohen, *Annals of Neurology* 1994—to promote pain, depression, migraine/seizure, and neurodegeneration. Images and descriptions above © 2015-2015 by Dr Vasquez except for image of brain by IsaacMao per Flickr.com via creativecommons.org/licenses/by/2.0. See educational videos and updates at www.inflammationmastery.com/pain

<u>Proof of accelerated neurodegeneration in fibromyalgia</u>: The model I have presented—dysbiosis-induced glial activation and mitochondrial dysfunction leading to both pain sensitivity and accelerated neurodegeneration—is supported by research showing accelerated brain aging and loss of gray matter (neuron cell bodies) in patients with fibromyalgia. As such, I consider my model of fibromyalgia to be very complete and consistent.

[390] Benson et al. Acute experimental endotoxemia induces visceral hypersensitivity and altered pain evaluation in healthy humans. *Pain.* 2012 Apr;153(4):794-9
[391] Wegner et al. Inflammation-induced hyperalgesia: timing, dosage, and negative affect on somatic pain in human endotoxemia. *Brain Behav Immun.* 2014 Oct;41:46-54
[392] Stabell et al. Widespread hyperalgesia in adolescents with symptoms of irritable bowel syndrome: results from a large population-based study. *J Pain.* 2014 Sep;15(9):898-906

- Accelerated brain gray matter loss and premature aging of the brain in fibromyalgia patients (*J Neurosci* 2007 Apr[393]): "In this study, we investigate anatomical changes in the brain associated with fibromyalgia. Using voxel-based morphometric analysis of magnetic resonance brain images, we examined the brains of 10 female fibromyalgia patients and 10 healthy controls. We found that fibromyalgia patients had significantly less total gray matter volume and showed a 3.3 times greater age-associated decrease in gray matter than healthy controls. The longer the individuals had had fibromyalgia, the greater the gray matter loss, with each year of fibromyalgia being equivalent to 9.5 times the loss in normal aging. In addition, fibromyalgia patients demonstrated significantly less gray matter density than healthy controls in several brain regions, including the cingulate, insular and medial frontal cortices, and parahippocampal gyri. The neuroanatomical changes that we see in fibromyalgia patients contribute additional evidence of CNS involvement in fibromyalgia. In particular, fibromyalgia appears to be associated with an acceleration of age-related changes in the very substance of the brain."

Additional comments and perspectives on central sensitization—integrating the model of SIBO-induced central sensitization via glial activation and other mechanisms

We appreciate that FM contains the aspect of central sensitization and the associated pain amplification; our intellectual task is to understand the most likely origin or—alternatively—to ascribe the central sensitization

> **Follow the pathophysiologic trail from bacterial exposures to IL-8 to brain inflammation and central sensitization**
>
> Various microbial exposures are known to cause elevations in IL-8, elevated CSF levels of which are characteristic of and perhaps unique to fibromyalgia, a condition causatively associated with intestinal bacterial overgrowth. The best summation of data at this point reads that the brain inflammation of fibromyalgia pain is triggered by microbial exposure. The alternate hypothesis that all of these pathophysiologic characteristics are unrelated is illogical and subintellectually immeritous.

to a magical/idiopathic origination. My contention is that microbial exposure leads to pain amplification via central sensitization in fibromyalgia; the means by which this can occur are both direct/primary causality and indirect/secondary, etc. Most of these were summarized in the above image and caption; in the sections that follow I will review some additional and also new information and show how it further supports this model.

- Systemic inflammation causes suppression of brain noradrenergic signaling (experimental study; *Science* 1983 Aug[394]) and is likely to contribute to fatigue, depression, pain sensitivity, and a heightened stress response: This experimental study shows that systemic inflammation leads to reduction in norepinephrine signaling in the (rat) brain. This would be expected to lead to fatigue, depression, and pain sensitivity. Secondarily, lack of adrenergic stimulation of the central alpha-2 receptor would be expected to stimulate the sympathetic nervous system; we note that bacterial overgrowth of the intestines (SIBO) causes enhanced sympathetic activity that is noted in patients with IBS which is closely related to fibromyalgia.[395] Low-grade systemic inflammation is known to be a component of FM, and generally speaking the molecules in or near the human body that are most likely to trigger inflammation are of microbial origin. Patients with IBS and FM are both known to have small intestine bacterial overgrowth. **In sum, we can reasonably opine that SIBO in FM and IBS leads to low-grade inflammation which leads to suppression of brain noradrenergic signaling, leading directly to fatigue and depression while likely also contributing to a heightened stress/sympathetic response; all of these components are noted in patients with IBS/FM.**
- FM patients have elevated CSF levels of IL-8 (*J Neuroimmunol* 2012 Jan[396] and *J Neuroimmunol* 2015 Mar[397]): Kadetoff et al did good work in 2012 when they were the first to find that patients with FM showed elevated levels of the inflammatory cytokine IL-8 in the cerebrospinal fluid (CSF) of patients with FM; research suggests that IL-8 promotes central sensitization via brain inflammation, and again this is consistent with FM. Although these authors note that "The release of pro-inflammatory cytokines/chemokines (including IL-8), by glia cells

---

[393] Kuchinad et a. Accelerated brain gray matter loss in fibromyalgia patients: premature aging of the brain? *J Neurosci.* (2007 Apr 11;27(15):4004-7

[394] "We report here that the immune response elicits a decrease in NA synthesis in the hypothalamus and that soluble products of activated immunological cells induce a decrease in NA content in the hypothalamus." Besedovsky et al. The immune response evokes changes in brain noradrenergic neurons. *Science.* 1983 Aug 5;221(4610):564-6

[395] Lin HC. Small intestinal bacterial overgrowth: a framework for understanding irritable bowel syndrome. *JAMA.* 2004 Aug 18;292(7):852-8

[396] "To our knowledge, this is the first study assessing intrathecal concentrations of pro-inflammatory substances in fibromyalgia. We report elevated cerebrospinal fluid and serum concentrations of interleukin-8, but not interleukin-1beta, in FM patients." Kadetoff D, Lampa J, Westman M, Andersson M, Kosek E. Evidence of central inflammation in fibromyalgia-increased cerebrospinal fluid interleukin-8 levels. *J Neuroimmunol.* 2012 Jan;242:33-8

[397] Kosek E, Altawil R, Kadetoff D, et al. Evidence of different mediators of central inflammation in dysfunctional and inflammatory pain--interleukin-8 in fibromyalgia and interleukin-1 β in rheumatoid arthritis. *J Neuroimmunol.* 2015 Mar 15;280:49-55

can be triggered by stress, immune activation and afferent nociceptive input [pain]", they ultimately pin the blame on pain by concluding in their abstract that their findings are "in accordance with FM symptoms being mediated by sympathetic activity...and supports the hypothesis of glia cell activation in response to pain mechanisms." The error these authors make is when they prematurely and without citation ascribe the elevation of IL-8 to pain and sympathetic activation in FM. The authors are thereby stating in essence that pain causes stress which causes more pain; they completely failed to both 1) substantiate this claim, and/or to 2) consider alternate hypotheses. Their attribution of the sympathetic activation to pain appears premature at best; they provide no substantiation for this claim, and it appears to have been promulgated and accepted simply because it is convenient and in accord with the prevailing drug-funded model of fibromyalgia which states that, in fibromyalgia, pain/stress causes pain/stress via a vicious cycle of glial activation (central sensitization, brain inflammation). In 2015, this same team of researchers replicated their 2012 finding of elevated IL-8 in FM; however they exacerbated their error of attribution by stating that their findings are—citing the work of Clauw—"in line with the proposal to regard FM as a sympathetically mediated pain syndrome." I believe that these authors are inappropriately connecting their finding of elevated IL-8 in FM with elevated sympathetic activity and pain in FM, and then concluding conveniently and hastily that these are the only variables worth considering and that therefore these must cause each other; they give zero consideration to the fact that these FM patients have SIBO[398] and that microbial molecules and intestinal inflammation can cause elevations in IL-8. So while we can reasonably accept that IL-8 is elevated in FM and may contribute to pain sensitization via brain inflammation and central sensitization, ascribing the elevation of IL-8 to the same pain that it promotes is circular thinking which in this case is also faulty thinking without consideration and exclusion of the obvious microbial overload noted in these patients with FM. Their citation to Clauw is particularly questionable since Clauw has been heavily funded by drug companies and consistently cheerleads the idea that FM is a primary disorder of the brain that needs—in accord with his sources of funding—perpetual drug treatment.[399] While stress and pain may lead to elevations in IL-8, an inflammatory cytokine that appears to promote central pain sensitization, stress and pain alone are less likely to be the primary contributors to the central sensitization in FM than are microbial and mitochondrial contributors, especially in combination. If stress and pain were sufficient to cause central sensitization, then virtually all medical students/residents (and working single mothers, persons living in war zones, persons living in prison and in conditions of gross social inequality, etc) and all competitive athletes would have central sensitization and FM; thus the general lack of population-wide correlation argues against the stress/pain model of *IL-8 induced central sensitization* in FM. Furthermore and even more clearly, the stress/pain model of pain sensitization in FM absolutely fails to account for the mitochondrial and other molecular abnormalities. In contrast, SIBO and microbial exposure is the perfect explanation of/for central sensitization in FM.

- <u>Elevations in IL-8 can be triggered by various bacterial exposures</u>: In an experimental cell culture model, exposure to the Gram-negative bacterium *Pseudomonas aeruginosa* was shown to increase production of IL-8.[400] Similarly, exposure to protein from the Gram-negative bacterium *Streptococcus pyogenes* also triggered expression of IL-8.[401]

- <u>Elevations in IL-8 correlate with gastrointestinal infection with *Blastocystis* in patients with IBS</u>, known to be correlated with FM (*PLoS One* 2015 Sep[402]): "Among 109 (IBS n = 35 and non-IBS n = 74) adults, direct stool

---

[398] Pimentel et al. A link between irritable bowel syndrome and fibromyalgia may be related to findings on lactulose breath testing. *Ann Rheum Dis.* 2004 Apr;63(4):450-2

[399] American Pain Society. Fibromyalgia Has Central Nervous System Origins. May 16, 2015. americanpainsociety.org/about-us/press-room/fibromyalgia-clauw and "Dr Clauw has received grants/research support from Pfizer and Forest Laboratories. He is a consultant and a member of the advisory boards for Pfizer, Eli Lilly and Company, Forest Laboratories, Cypress Biosciences, Pierre Fabre Pharmaceuticals, UCB, and AstraZeneca. Dr Arnold has received grants/research support from Eli Lilly and Company, Pfizer, Cypress Biosciences, Wyeth Pharmaceuticals, Boehringer Ingelheim, Allergan, and Forest Laboratories. She is a consultant for Eli Lilly and Company, Pfizer, Cypress Biosciences, Wyeth Pharmaceuticals, Boehringer Ingelheim, Forest Laboratories, Allergan, Takeda, UCB, Theravance, AstraZeneca, and sanofi-aventis. Dr McCarberg has received honoraria from Cephalon, Eli Lilly and Company, Endo Pharmaceuticals, Forest Laboratories, Merck & Co, Pfizer, and Purdue Pharma. The FibroCollaborative group was sponsored by Pfizer." "Editorial support was provided by Gayle Scott, PharmD, of UBC Scientific Solutions and funded by Pfizer." Clauw DJ, Arnold LM, McCarberg BH; FibroCollaborative. The science of fibromyalgia. *Mayo Clin Proc.* 2011 Sep;86(9):907-11

[400] "Thus, IL-8 mRNA expression was prolonged after P. aeruginosa stimulation in CF epithelial cells, and this sustained IL-8 expression may contribute to the excessive inflammatory response in CF." Joseph T, Look D, Ferkol T. NF-kappaB activation and sustained IL-8 gene expression in primary cultures of cystic fibrosis airway epithelial cells stimulated with Pseudomonas aeruginosa. *Am J Physiol Lung Cell Mol Physiol.* 2005 Mar;288(3):L471-9

[401] "Our results showed that following exposure to SPE B or G308S, the levels of IL-8 protein and mRNA were increased and the increase was inhibited by the addition of anti-Fas antibody, suggesting that the increased production of IL-8 by SPE B is mediated through Fas receptor." Chang CW, Wu SY, Chuang WJ, Lin YS, Wu JJ, Liu CC, Tsai PJ, Lin MT. The IL-8 production by Streptococcal pyrogenic exotoxin B. *Exp Biol Med* (Maywood). 2009 Nov;234(11):1316-26

[402] Ragavan et al. Blastocystis sp. in Irritable Bowel Syndrome (IBS) - Detection in Stool Aspirates during Colonoscopy. *PLoS One.* 2015 Sep 16;10(9):e0121173

examination and culture of colonic aspirates were initially negative for *Blastocystis*. However, PCR analysis detected *Blastocystis* in 6 (17%) IBS and 4 (5.5%) non-IBS patients. In the six positive IBS patients by PCR method, subtype 3 was shown to be the most predominant (3/6: 50%) followed by subtype 4 (2/6; 33.3%) and subtype 5 (1/6; 16.6%). ==IL-8 levels were significantly elevated in the IBS Blasto group and IBS group (p<0.05) compared to non-IBS and non-IBS Blasto group.== … Meanwhile, the IL-5 levels were significantly higher in IBS Blasto group (p<0.05) compared to non-IBS and non-IBS Blasto group. This study implicates that detecting Blastocystis by PCR method using colonic aspirate samples during colonoscopy, suggests that this may be a better method for sample collection due to the parasite's irregular shedding in Blastocystis-infected stools. Patients with IBS infected with parasite showed an increase in the interleukin levels demonstrate that *Blastocystis* does have an effect in the immune system." Additionally, *Blastocystis* is known to cause intestinal damage and to thereby increase intestinal permeability[403], and fibromyalgia patients are also noted to have increased intestinal permeability[404]; the possibility exists that *Blastocystis* induces increased IL-8 via intestinal mucosal damage which leads to increased absorption of microbial debris/inflammogens rather than directly, although an additive and synergistic mechanism/effect is more likely.

- Elevations in IL-8 are seen in patients with IBS, known to be triggered by SIBO and causatively dose-dependently correlated with FM (*Am J Gastroenterol.* 2010 Oct[405]): If my model is correct that the elevated IL-8 in FM is caused by the SIBO and not by the FM itself, then we should see elevated in IL-8 in patients with IBS, which is caused by SIBO. In a study with more than 120 human subjects, results showed that ==patients with IBS/SIBO have increased plasma levels of IL-6 and IL-8.== Note that this study used blood/plasma/serum testing rather than cerebrospinal fluid (CSF) as in the previously reviewed studies; IL-8 levels in blood and CSF tend to correlate, as demonstrated in FM patients who typically have elevations in both locations (ie, peripherally and centrally).

- Bacterial overgrowth in ulcerative colitis patients correlates with increased inflammatory mediator production, including IL-8 (*J Crohns Colitis.* 2014 Aug[406]): Among patients with ulcerative colitis, SIBO is common and correlates with reduced intestinal motility and increased production of inflammatory mediators: "observed that there was a ==significant correlation between SIBO with IL-6, IL-8, TNF-α, and IL-10, LPO and GSH.=="

- Small intestinal bacterial overgrowth association with TLR4 expression and IL-8 (*Dig Dis Sci.* 2011 May[407]): SIBO was more common in nonalcoholic steatohepatitis (NASH) patients than control subjects (77% v 31.25%) and only IL-8 levels were significantly higher in patients than control and correlated positively with TLR-4 expression. "NASH patients have a higher prevalence of small intestinal bacterial overgrowth which is associated with enhanced expression of TLR-4 and release of IL-8. SIBO may have an important role in NASH through interactions with TLR-4 and induction of the pro-inflammatory cytokine, IL-8."

Microbe-induced brain inflammation without brain infection and without high fever, vasculitis or autoimmunity

Viral infections
- Measles
- Mumps
- Rubella
- Influenza A and B
- Herpes simplex
- Epstein-Barr virus
- Varicella
- Vaccinia

Bacterial infections
- Mycoplasma pneumoniae
- Chlamydia
- Legionella
- Streptococcus
- Campylobacter
- Shigella

Immunizations*
- Rabies
- DPT—Diphtheria, pertussis tetanus
- Smallpox
- Measles
- Japanese B encephalitis
- Influenza

*Of important note, vaccinations commonly contain numerous adjuvants, toxic metals such as mercury and aluminum, highly allergenic antibiotics and cell culture components including egg, aborted human cells, and monkey kidney cells; as such, the inflammatory encephalitis that results cannot be ascribed solely to the microbial component of the vaccination.

cdc.gov/vaccines/pubs/pinkbook/downloads/appendices/B/excipient-table-2.pdf
Accessed 2015 Nov

---

[403] "The IP was found to have increased in patients with protozoan infections compared with control patients (7.20+/-5.52 vs. 4.47+/-0.65%, P=0.0017). The IP values were 9.91+/-10.05% in Giardia intestinalis group, 6.81+/-2.25% in Blastocystis hominis group, 5.78+/-2.84% in Entamoeba coli group. In comparison with the control group, the IP was significantly higher in G. intestinalis and B. hominis patients (P=0.0025, P=0.00037, respectively), but not in E. coli patients. In conclusion, the IP increases in patients with G. intestinalis and B. hominis but not with E. coli infection. This finding supports the view that IP increases during the course of protozoan infections which cause damage to the intestinal wall while non-pathogenic protozoan infections have no effect on IP. The increase in IP in patients with B. hominis brings forth the idea that B. hominis can be a pathogenic protozoan." Dagci H, Ustun S, Taner MS, Ersoz G, Karacasu F, Budak S. Protozoon infections and intestinal permeability. *Acta Trop.* 2002 Jan;81(1):1-5
[404] Goebel et al. Altered intestinal permeability in patients with primary fibromyalgia and in patients with complex regional pain syndrome. *Rheumatology* 2008 Aug;47(8):1223-7
[405] Scully et al. Plasma cytokine profiles in females with irritable bowel syndrome and extra-intestinal co-morbidity. *Am J Gastroenterol.* 2010 Oct;105(10):2235-43
[406] Rana et al. Relationship of cytokines, oxidative stress and GI motility with bacterial overgrowth in ulcerative colitis patients. *J Crohns Colitis.* 2014 Aug;8(8):859-65
[407] Shanab et al. Small intestinal bacterial overgrowth in nonalcoholic steatohepatitis: toll-like receptor 4 and plasma levels of interleukin 8. *Dig Dis Sci.* 2011 May;1524-34

Stress/pain is an insufficient explanation for the origination of FM: While stress and pain may lead to elevations in IL-8, an inflammatory cytokine that appears to promote central pain sensitization, stress and pain alone are less likely to be the primary contributors to the central sensitization in FM than are microbial and mitochondrial contributors, especially in combination. If stress and pain were sufficient to cause central sensitization, then virtually all medical students/residents (and working single mothers, persons living in war zones, etc) and all competitive athletes would have central sensitization and FM; thus the general lack of population-wide correlation argues against the stress/pain model of IL8-induction of central sensitization in FM. Furthermore and even more clearly, the stress/pain model of pain sensitization in FM absolutely fails to account for the mitochondrial and other molecular abnormalities. In contrast, **SIBO and microbial exposure is the perfect explanation of/for FM.**

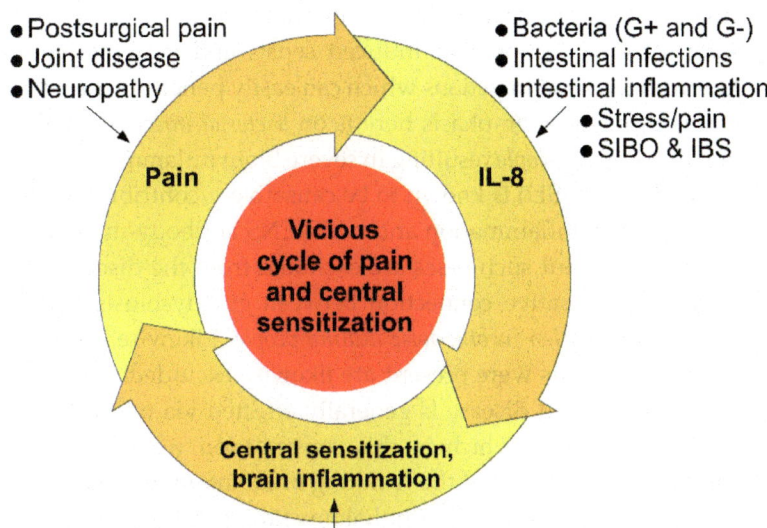

- Postsurgical pain
- Joint disease
- Neuropathy

- Bacteria (G+ and G-)
- Intestinal infections
- Intestinal inflammation
- Stress/pain
- SIBO & IBS

Pain

IL-8

Vicious cycle of pain and central sensitization

Central sensitization, brain inflammation

- Microbial inflammogens and systemic inflammation
- Deficiencies of anti-inflammatory nutrients, such as vitamin D, n3FA and phytochemicals
- Mitochondrial dysfunction, per migraine (primary) and fibromyalgia (secondary)

In sum, the data clearly show that microbial exposure in general and bacterial overgrowth of the small intestine in particular trigger increased IL-8 production. While elevated IL-8 is not specific to a particular disease per se, it is consistently elevated in patients with small intestine bacterial overgrowth, regardless of disease association. Many conditions causatively related to SIBO are noted to have elevated IL-8 levels, and we should reasonably attribute the elevated IL-8 levels in fibromyalgia to bacterial exposure, especially given the exceptionally high and dose-dependent correlation of SIBO with FM. IL-8 promotes pain sensitization, and the hyperalgesic effects of IL-8 are mediated in part by activation of beta-adrenergic receptors[408], chronic/sustained activation of which would be expected to promote depression, anxiety, and fatigue in addition to pain. IL-8 promotes activation of the sympathetic nervous system via beta-adrenergic receptors, and activation of the sympathetic nervous system via beta-adrenergic receptors feeds back to cause additional IL-8 production, thereby promoting a vicious cycle; my contention is that microbial debris is the initiating factor in this cycle, and that exposure to microbial inflammogens from SIBO is both more powerful (microbial debris is clearly pro-inflammatory, and LPS in particular is the most potent inflammogen known to science) and more durable (24/7 for months and years) than any "stress response." As such, the microbial inflammatory load is the more reasonable recipient of the burden of physiologic guilt than is the "stress level" of these patients. Stress is transient, and highly stressed people (e.g., medical students and residents, air traffic controllers, etc) do not show an undue burden of pain and mitochondrial impairment as do patients with an excessive total microbial load, specifically—as previously shown per literature review—SIBO. Thus having established that SIBO is sufficient to induce brain inflammation, I will now review more severe cases of what might be considered true gastrointestinal infection as a cause of severe brain inflammation; I am moving from the *mild and functional* to the truly *infectious and pathologic* to further exemplify this model.

- Gastrointestinal infection/dysbiosis as a cause of severe brain inflammation: criteria and review: We might reasonably expect that if *comparatively/relatively mild* cases of dysbiosis and SIBO can cause *mild* brain inflammation, then cases may have been reported wherein *more severe* gastrointestinal infections have led to *more severe* brain inflammation (ie, encephalitis and encephalomyelitis), and indeed such cases are impressively

---

[408] Kosek E, Altawil R, Kadetoff D, et al. Evidence of different mediators of central inflammation in dysfunctional and inflammatory pain--interleukin-8 in fibromyalgia and interleukin-1 β in rheumatoid arthritis. *J Neuroimmunol.* 2015 Mar 15;280:49-55. Kadetoff D, Lampa J, Westman M, Andersson M, Kosek E. Evidence of central inflammation in fibromyalgia-increased cerebrospinal fluid interleukin-8 levels. *J Neuroimmunol.* 2012 Jan;242:33-8

abundant. The most important distinction is that of what is being discussed here, specifically brain inflammation induced by gastrointestinal-specific microbes, their inflammatory debris, and the resulting inflammatory response within the brain, *versus* an infection that originated in the gut and then spread to the brain, or an infection that induced sepsis and systemic complications that resulted in altered cognition. Accordingly, viral infections which can easily penetrate the brain are selected against (e.g., essentially omitted) in this discussion; emphasis here is on *bacterial infections* with *no evidence of direct brain/meningeal infection* in *otherwise healthy people* resulting in severe brain inflammation via "indirect" inflammatory effects. Inflammatory bowel disease (IBD) is known to be causatively/contributively associated with gut dysbiosis; IBD patients can develop brain inflammation and brain/CNS antibody-mediated autoimmunity[409], apparently triggered by the gut dysbiosis, but such cases are excluded from the discussion below for the sake of clarity in establishing a more pure causative connection between gut dysbiosis and brain inflammation *mediated via cytokines and microglial activation* in *otherwise healthy people.* Likewise, cases of infection-induced encephalitis wherein high fever or vasculitis were present are likewise excluded. As I have discussed and presented recently in 2015[410], dysbiosis-induced disease is generally effected via multiple mechanisms, one of which is the inflammatory-cytokine response, which in this conversation would "spill from the periphery into the brain" to cause microglial activation and the resulting brain inflammation—encephalitis.

- Acute disseminated encephalomyelitis (ADEM) secondary to transient gastroenteritis in an otherwise healthy adult (*Case Rep Neurol Med.* 2015 Jun[411]): "A 62-year-old man presented with encephalopathy and rapid neurological decline following a gastrointestinal illness. A brain MRI revealed extensive supratentorial white matter hyperintensities consistent with ADEM and thus he was started on high dose intravenous methylprednisolone. He underwent a brain biopsy showing widespread white matter inflammation secondary to demyelination. At discharge, his neurological exam had significantly improved with continued steroid treatment and four months later, he was able to perform his ADLs."

- Acute disseminated encephalomyelitis with Campylobacter gastroenteritis (*J Neurol Neurosurg Psychiatry* 2004 May[412]): "We report a case of acute disseminated encephalomyelitis (ADEM) temporally associated with Campylobacter gastroenteritis in a previously fit man. ... Two days after admission (day 16 of illness), his family reported a change in his personality and he complained of slurring of speech, intermittent diplopia, and difficulty in walking. Examination revealed mild dysarthria, left sided facial weakness, mild left pyramidal limb weakness, and decreased sensation in the left leg. Tendon reflexes were brisk but plantar responses were flexor. His gait was ataxic. ... In the majority of cases, the condition develops after systemic viral infections most commonly measles, mumps, rubella, influenza A and B, herpes simplex, Epstein-Barr virus, varicella, and vaccinia. It has also been reported following bacterial infections with Mycoplasma pneumoniae, Chlamydia, Legionella, and Streptococcus, or following immunizations for rabies, diphtheria/tetanus/pertussis, smallpox, measles and Japanese B encephalitis."

- Bickerstaff's brainstem encephalitis related to Campylobacter jejuni gastroenteritis (*J Clin Pathol.* 2007 Oct[413]): "Here we report a case of BBE following a gastrointestinal infection with Campylobacter jejuni. The patient presented with acute onset of confusion and ophthalmoplegia. The cerebrospinal fluid (CSF) showed lymphocytic pleocytosis and raised protein. This acute presentation was preceded by an episode of Campylobacter-related diarrhea as confirmed by high titers of Campylobacter-specific IgM antibodies."

- Acute encephalopathy preceding Shigella infection (*Isr Med Assoc J.* 2001 May[414]): This is a case of a 3yo girl with encephalitis which preceded mild mucus diarrhea which lead to the discovery of *Shigella sonnei.* Thus, this case is doubly unique for 1) the fact that the encephalopathy *preceded* any gastrointestinal manifestations, and 2) the gastrointestinal manifestations were impressively *mild.*

---

[409] Yamamoto et al. Bickerstaff's brainstem encephalitis associated with ulcerative colitis. *BMJ Case Rep.* 2012 Sep 21;2012
[410] The presentations to which I make reference here are specifically video presentations 1-3 wherein I describe the molecular mechanisms of dysbiosis-induced disease in our CE/CME program hosted at http://www.nutritionandfunctionalmedicine.org/lms/ and derived from the printed monograph *Human Microbiome and Dysbiosis in Clinical Disease.* International College of Human Nutrition and Functional Medicine 2015
[411] Mahdi et al. A Case of Acute Disseminated Encephalomyelitis in a Middle-Aged Adult. *Case Rep Neurol Med.* 2015;2015:601706
[412] Orr et al. Acute disseminated encephalomyelitis temporally associated with Campylobacter gastroenteritis. *J Neurol Neurosurg Psychiatry.* 2004 May;75(5):792-3
[413] Hussain et al. Bickerstaff's brainstem encephalitis related to Campylobacter jejuni gastroenteritis. *J Clin Pathol.* 2007 Oct;60(10):1161-2
[414] Somech R, Leitner Y, Spirer Z. Acute encephalopathy preceding Shigella infection. *Isr Med Assoc J.* 2001 May;3(5):384-5

Means by which inflammatory cytokines in the periphery (body) can result in inflammation in the brain
1.   Cytokines enter the brain where the blood–brain barrier (BBB) is weak or non-existent (i.e. circumventricular organs).
2.   Cytokines are transported into the brain by selective uptake systems (transporters), thus bypassing BBB.
3.   Cytokines may act directly or indirectly on peripheral nerves that can send afferent signals to the brain.
4.   Cytokines can act on peripheral tissues, inducing the secretion of molecules whose ability to penetrate the brain is not limited by the barrier. A major target appears to be endothelial cells, which bear receptors for IL-1 and endotoxin.
5.   Cytokines can be synthesized by immune cells that infiltrate the brain.
6.   Cytokines and the resultant increased ROS production can also impair mitochondrial function; impaired mitochondrial function in the periphery/body drains antioxidants (such as glutathione) and nutritive substances (such as CoQ10, tocopherols, and lipoic acid) that are important for the maintenance of cellular function and homeodynamics. Thereby, peripheral inflammation and mitochondrial impairment becomes a "sink" for draining nutrients and protectants while also becoming a "faucet" for inflammatory mediators, molecular debris and alarm signals. Increased production of glutamate, QUIN, and NO- fuel NMDAr activation and mitochondrial dysfunction. (DrV)
7.   Cytokines may be transported in a retrograde manner from the periphery, via axonal mechanisms.
8.   Cytokines may be transported in a retrograde manner from the periphery, via axonal mechanisms. (Zhang, An)
Contents 1-5 of this table are fully credited to Dunn AJ. Effects of cytokines and infections on brain neurochemistry. *Clin Neurosci Res*. 2006 Aug;6(1-2):52-68. Zhang JM, An J. Cytokines, inflammation, and pain. *Int Anesthesiol Clin*. 2007 Spring;45(2):27-37

Beyond glutamate in microbe-triggered brain inflammation: alterations in tryptophan, serotonin and additional triggering of NMDA receptors for more brain/pain activation and less inhibition

- Introduction to altered intracerebral tryptophan metabolism: Microbial, psychological, and inflammatory stressors cause elevations in IFN-g and TNF-a; "IFN-g induces the enzyme indoleamine 2,3-dioxygenase (IDO, found in immune cells such as macrophages and dendritic cells), which causes reduction in tryptophan availability, leading to a reduction in serotonin synthesis in the brain."[415] Paraphrasing the brilliantly excellent 2015 review by Jo, Zhang, Emrich, and Dietrich[416]: Following induction, IDO catabolizes/converts tryptophan into kynurenine (KYN), is converted to kynurenic acid (KA) or quinolinic acid (QUIN); "KA and QUIN have contrasting roles influencing the glutamatergic system, the first acting as antagonist and the latter as agonist of the glutamate N-methyl-D-aspartate receptor (NMDAr). Microglia are the main producers of QUIN in the brain, whereas astrocytes are the CNS-key cells involved in KA synthesis. This is explained by the fact that microglia express kynurenine 3-monooxygenase (KMO), the rate-limiting enzyme in the production of QUIN. Conversely, astrocytes exclusively express kynurenine aminotransferases, which are essential in the conversion of KYN to KA." Thus, in relevant summary, glial activation in the brain leads to cerebral tryptophan depletion, thereby depleting this important precursor of serotonin and melatonin while also leading to additional NMDAr agonism via QUIN. As such we are able to advance our understanding of this utmost-important pathophysiology that is occurring in the brain following/during inflammatory events/exposures, as illustrated and additionally detailed in the caption.

---

[415] Hurley LL, Tizabi Y. Neuroinflammation, neurodegeneration, and depression. *Neurotox Res*. 2013 Feb;23(2):131-44

[416] Jo WK, Zhang Y, Emrich HM, Dietrich DE. Glia in the cytokine-mediated onset of depression: fine tuning the immune response. *Front Cell Neurosci*. 2015 Jul 10;9:268

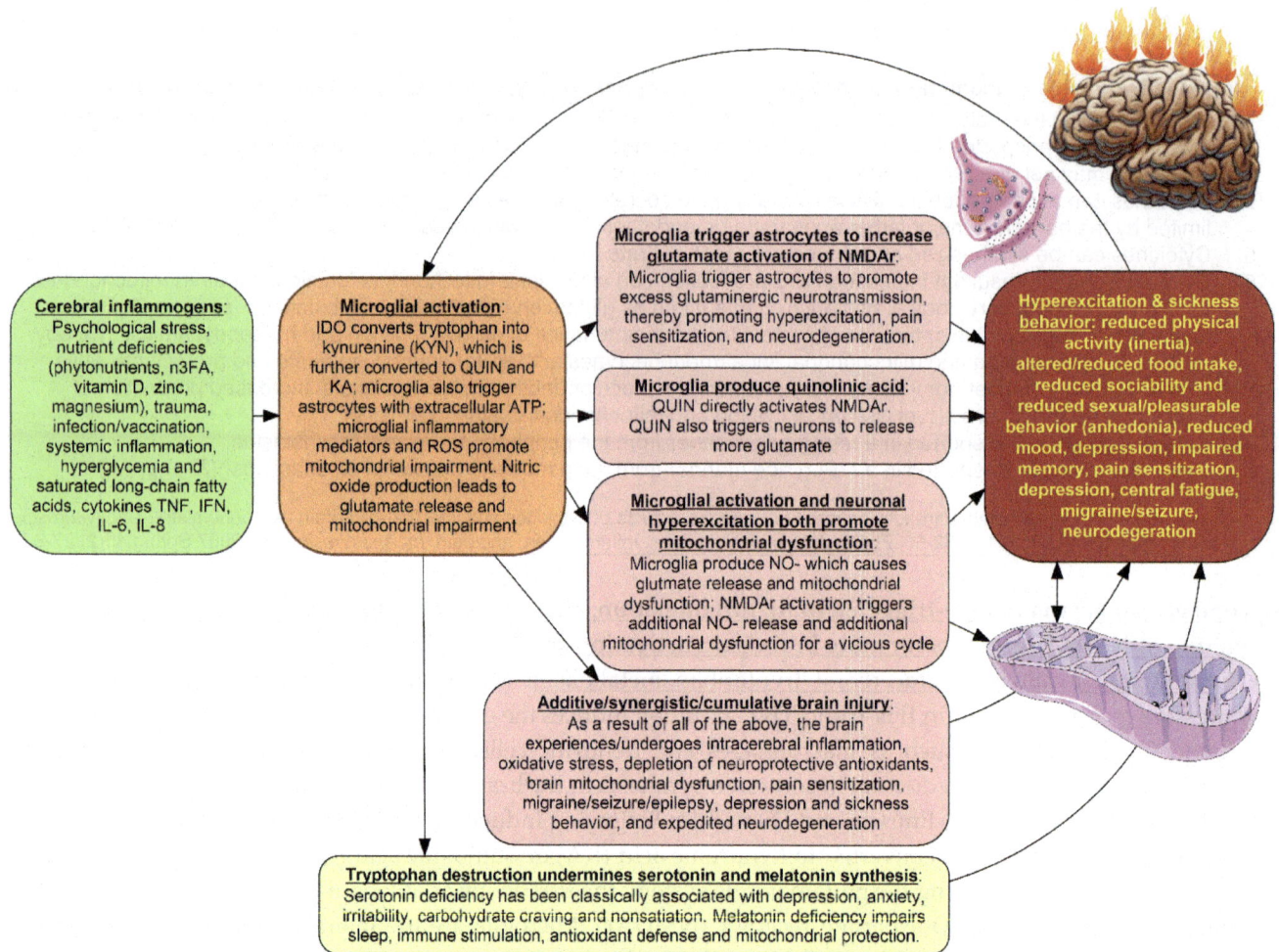

Cerebral inflammogens: Psychological stress, nutrient deficiencies (phytonutrients, n3FA, vitamin D, zinc, magnesium), trauma, infection/vaccination, systemic inflammation, hyperglycemia and saturated long-chain fatty acids, cytokines TNF, IFN, IL-6, IL-8

Microglial activation: IDO converts tryptophan into kynurenine (KYN), which is further converted to QUIN and KA; microglia also trigger astrocytes with extracellular ATP; microglial inflammatory mediators and ROS promote mitochondrial impairment. Nitric oxide production leads to glutamate release and mitochondrial impairment

Microglia trigger astrocytes to increase glutamate activation of NMDAr: Microglia trigger astrocytes to promote excess glutaminergic neurotransmission, thereby promoting hyperexcitation, pain sensitization, and neurodegeneration.

Microglia produce quinolinic acid: QUIN directly activates NMDAr. QUIN also triggers neurons to release more glutamate

Microglial activation and neuronal hyperexcitation both promote mitochondrial dysfunction: Microglia produce NO- which causes glutmate release and mitochondrial dysfunction; NMDAr activation triggers additional NO- release and additional mitochondrial dysfunction for a vicious cycle

Hyperexcitation & sickness behavior: reduced physical activity (inertia), altered/reduced food intake, reduced sociability and reduced sexual/pleasurable behavior (anhedonia), reduced mood, depression, impaired memory, pain sensitization, depression, central fatigue, migraine/seizure, neurodegeration

Additive/synergistic/cumulative brain injury: As a result of all of the above, the brain experiences/undergoes intracerebral inflammation, oxidative stress, depletion of neuroprotective antioxidants, brain mitochondrial dysfunction, pain sensitization, migraine/seizure/epilepsy, depression and sickness behavior, and expedited neurodegeneration

Tryptophan destruction undermines serotonin and melatonin synthesis: Serotonin deficiency has been classically associated with depression, anxiety, irritability, carbohydrate craving and nonsatiation. Melatonin deficiency impairs sleep, immune stimulation, antioxidant defense and mitochondrial protection.

Brain inflammation leads directly to triple enhancement of NMDAr activation (via NO-, astrocytes, and QUIN) and triple impairment of mitochondrial function (via NO-, ROS, and inflammatory barrage): Details and citations provided in the following caption. Images above by DrV. Image of brain by IsaacMao per Flickr.com via creativecommons.org/licenses/by/2.0. See educational videos and updates at www.inflammationmastery.com/pain.

- **Cerebral inflammation can be triggered by any indirect or direct insult**, including psychological stress, nutrient deficiencies (phytonutrients, n3FA, vitamin D, zinc, magnesium), trauma, infection/vaccination, systemic inflammation, hyperglycemia and saturated long-chain fatty acids, cytokines TNF, IFN, IL-6, IL-8. We need to change the way that we appreciate inflammation: we have traditionally/historically/conveniently/simplistically thought of inflammation as needing a trigger and occurring in response to that trigger; while that remains largely but not absolutely true, we need to appreciate that inflammation—especially metabolic inflammation—occurs as a manifestation of cellular dysfunction in general and mitochondrial dysfunction in particular and as such can be initiated by nutritional deficiency, including phytonutrient deficiency. For example, the fact that nutritional supplementation in physiologic subpharmacologic doses provides an antiinflammatory benefit (e.g., multivitamin/mineral[417] and vitamin D3[418]) is proof that the preexisting nutritional deficiency—even though slight and subclinical—was itself the cause of the inflammatory response. We have crystalline clarity now that peripheral inflammation leads to central/brain inflammation, whether from trauma, infection, or vaccination[419,420,421] and as such we can reasonably state—and should accept as true—that any significant inflammatory/immunologic response in the periphery is going to cause/promote central/brain inflammation and the resulting hyperexcitation, pain sensitization, and sickness behavior. Important in this conversation is that while the model of "microglial activation = astrocyte activation = neuroinflammation / central sensitization / sickness behavior" is generally accurate, this same model is actually quite nuanced and contains different variations, leading to different clinical phenotypes. Data is giving shape to the idea that different cytokines have different effects on brain cellular components, leading to different phenotypic manifestations. Taking a single example, we note the recent 2015 report showing that beta amyloid induced IL-8 mediated microglial activation, and that the resulting astrocytic activation is mediated by a different (nonIL-8) pathway; also noted is the 2015 report showing

[417] Church TS, Earnest CP, Wood KA, Kampert JB. Reduction of C-reactive protein levels through use of a multivitamin. *Am J Med.* 2003 Dec 15;115(9):702-7
[418] Timms et al. Circulating MMP9, vitamin D and variation in the TIMP-1 response with VDR genotype. *QJM.* 2002 Dec;95(12):787-96
[419] Wright CE et al. Acute inflammation and negative mood: mediation by cytokine activation. *Brain Behav Immun.* 2005 Jul;19(4):345-50
[420] Harrison NA et al. Inflammation causes mood changes through alterations in subgenual cingulate activity and mesolimbic connectivity. *Biol Psychiatry.* 2009 Sep:407-14
[421] Wilson CJ, Finch CE, Cohen HJ. Cytokines and cognition—the case for a head-to-toe inflammatory paradigm. *J Am Geriatr Soc.* 2002 Dec;50(12):2041-56

that central/brain neuroinflammation in RA is mediated by IL-1 while that in FM is mediated by IL-8. As such, we should speak of neuroinflammation<u>s</u> and glial activation<u>s</u> in the plural rather than singular forms.

- **Microglial activation drains tryptophan** by triggering IDO conversion of tryptophan into kynurenine (KYN), which is further converted to QUIN and KA.[422] Tryptophan destruction undermines serotonin and melatonin synthesis: Serotonin deficiency has been classically associated with depression, anxiety, irritability, carbohydrate craving and nonsatiation. Melatonin deficiency impairs sleep, immune stimulation, antioxidant defense and mitochondrial protection.

- **Microglia trigger astrocytes to increase glutamate activation of NMDAr**: Microglia trigger astrocytes with extracellular ATP. Microglial activation triggers astrocytes to promote excess glutaminergic neurotransmission[423], thereby promoting hyperexcitation, pain sensitization, and neurodegeneration.

- **Microglial activation and increased nitric oxide (NO-) production leads to glutamate release and mitochondrial impairment.** Microglial inflammatory mediators and ROS promote mitochondrial impairment. Readers should appreciate the implications of this vicious cycle, where in "fire in the brain" can readily burn out of control; in context with other information in this section, this understanding helps explain, for example, how immunologic triggers in the periphery such as vaccination/immunization can cause devastating brain injury, basically leading to "metabolic-inflammatory meltdown of the brain" as seen in the most horrific of vaccination responses—vaccination encephalopathy/encephalitis.[424,425] Encephalitis can also result from gastrointestinal infection. [426]

- **Microglia produce quinolinic acid (QUIN) to activate NMDAr: Microglia produce QUIN which activates NMDAr while QUIN also triggers neurons to release more glutamate, thereby leading to additional contribution to NMDAr activation.**[427] Astrocytes can produce the NMDAr agonist kynurenic acid (KA); however, in settings of glial activation, NMDAr activation clearly predominates.

- **Microglial activation and neuronal hyperexcitation both promote mitochondrial dysfunction.**[428] Microglia produce (or induce astrocytic production of*) NO- which causes glutamate release and mitochondrial dysfunction; NMDAr activation triggers additional NO- release and additional mitochondrial dysfunction for a vicious cycle. Neuronal excitation and microglial activation both promote mitochondrial dysfunction; this is physiologically disastrous because neurons need optimized mitochondrial performance generally and especially when faced with increased/dysregulated demand. Very important here is the appreciation that mitochondrial dysfunction is itself pro-inflammatory (via ROS and DAMP/PAMP receptor activation by mitochondrial fragments), thereby adding to the vicious cycle. Further, mitochondrial dysfunction triggers excess release of inflammatory cytokines from a wide range of cell types; the range of cell types showing increased pro-inflammatory cytokine release following induction of mitochondrial impairment is so wide that possibly all cells (in this conversation, including microglia and neurons) are involved/affected. *Kim and Nagai[429] noted that human microglia do not produce NO- and that NO- production in the human brain glia originates chiefly from astrocytes; still, in the context of an intact brain, we might summarize that the microglia induce NO- production by triggering astrocytes, even if human microglia—distinguished from other animal models—cannot directly produce NO-.

- **Additive/synergistic/cumulative brain injury manifesting generally and chronically as increased brain fragility**: As a result of all of the above, the brain experiences/undergoes intracerebral inflammation, oxidative stress, depletion of neuroprotective antioxidants, enhanced viral/bacterial replication/effect, brain mitochondrial dysfunction, pain sensitization, migraine/seizure/epilepsy, depression and sickness behavior, and expedited neurodegeneration. Since many of these metabolic impairments are both common and silent, these lead to the promotion of neurodegeneration and "brain fragility" (or per Morley and Seneff: "diminished brain resilience syndrome"[430]) wherein the brain is supranormally vulnerable to other insults, such as trauma, dietary insult, glyphosate/pesticide exposure, infections and vaccinations.

<u>As clinicians, pragmatists, and intellectuals, we are obligated to employ the available data</u>: We already have sufficient evidence for this model, and clinicians should move forward and implement this model in clinical practice; use of this model is considerably more attractive than ascribing the associated conditions to spontaneous generation and condemning the associated patients to eternal medicalization. For ethical and logistical reasons, we will probably never have "perfect proof" of this model, because such would require induction of disease in healthy people, and this would be clearly risky and unethical and would therefore never be approved by any competent IRB (institutional review board, tasked with approving research investigations). What we might call *perfect proof* of this would have to be established by *prospective* studies showing that ❶ administration of a sufficient total microbial load (TML)—specifically SIBO in the case of FM—causes central sensitization as assessed by some reliable

[422] Jo WK, Zhang Y, Emrich HM, Dietrich DE. Glia in the cytokine-mediated onset of depression: fine tuning the immune response. *Front Cell Neurosci.* 2015 Jul 10;9:268

[423] Béchade C, Cantaut-Belarif Y, Bessis A. Microglial control of neuronal activity. *Front Cell Neurosci.* 2013 Mar 28;7:32

[424] Alicino et al. Acute disseminated encephalomyelitis with severe neurological outcomes following virosomal seasonal influenza vaccine. *Hum Vaccin Immunother.* 2014;10(7):1969-73

[425] Lee et al. An adverse event following 2009 H1N1 influenza vaccination: a case of acute disseminated encephalomyelitis. *Korean J Pediatr.* 2011 Oct;54(10):422-4

[426] Mahdi N, Abdelmalik PA, Curtis M, Bar B. A Case of Acute Disseminated Encephalomyelitis in a Middle-Aged Adult. *Case Rep Neurol Med.* 2015;2015:601706

[427] Jo WK, Zhang Y, Emrich HM, Dietrich DE. Glia in the cytokine-mediated onset of depression: fine tuning the immune response. *Front Cell Neurosci.* 2015 Jul 10;9:268

[428] Brown GC, Bal-Price A. Inflammatory neurodegeneration mediated by nitric oxide, glutamate, and mitochondria. *Mol Neurobiol.* 2003 Jun;27(3):325-55

[429] Kim SU Nagai A. Microglia as immune effectors of the central nervous system: Expression of cytokines and chemokines. *Clin Experiment Neuroimmunol.* 2010 May; 1: 61–69

[430] Morley WA, Seneff S. Diminished brain resilience syndrome: A modern day neurological pathology of increased susceptibility to mild brain trauma, concussion, and downstream neurodegeneration. *Surg Neurol Int.* 2014 Jun ; 5: 97

technology such as functional magnetic resonance imaging (fMRI) of the brain or evidence of inflammatory changes within the cerebrospinal fluid (CSF). A prospective trial of this nature would almost certainly be considered unethical and would be almost impossible to perform, either technically (how would the microbial load be delivered safely, effectively, and *temporarily* without risk of long-term harm?) and the related near-impossibility of being passed/approved by a responsible research IRB. **Natural life provides this trial via the observation that people who naturally develop small intestine bacterial overgrowth and other forms of gastrointestinal dysbiosis frequently develop syndromes of central sensitization such as irritable bowel syndrome, fibromyalgia, and complex regional pain syndrome[431]; prospective experimental studies have shown that animals exposed to microbial inflammogens indeed develop central sensitization.** Secondarily and of lesser importance, we would also want prospective evidence that ❷ the above-mentioned microbe-induced central sensitization can be alleviated by removal of the inflammatory microbial load. Ideally, we would look for *direct* evidence of alleviation of central sensitization, again by looking at the brain and its surrounding fluid for functional/molecular evidence of normalization, but without the ideal situation, we could look for *indirect* evidence of alleviation of central sensitization by looking for alleviation of pain. **Clinical studies with humans have already shown that removing the excessive microbial load—specifically SIBO in the case of FM—alleviates the clinical manifestations of central sensitization, namely excessive pain, fatigue, and other physical and mental manifestations of the illness.** Supportively, we can appreciate data showing that ❸ mitochondrial dysfunction (mitodysfunction) and systemic inflammation in general promote central sensitization, and thereby the alleviation of either mitodysfunction or inflammation by alleviating the TML/SIBO would be expected to alleviate central sensitization. In a world of imperfect research, incomplete data, and the vast majority of doctors/researchers having had zero training in nutrition, mitochondrial optimization and treatments for dysbiosis, let us look at the support for this thesis while emphasizing the importance of incorporating the available data while recalling that absence of evidence (ie, the studies have not been performed) is neither evidence of refutation (ie, no evidence refutes the thesis) nor evidence of absence (ie, we have an abundance of supporting data, even if we are currently and perhaps always will be lacking a perfect prospective study of microbe-induced central sensitization followed by relief of same via antimicrobial/antidysbiotic interventions).

The medicomonetary reality: The goal of most research is not cure of disease, but translation of biology into drug sales: In order to further understand the nature, goals, and constraints of "biomedical research", one first needs to have some *insights into the obvious*: namely, that the general goal of *biomedical* research is to understand enough of nature and biology so that a drug can be developed to address the condition being studied. This is the *translation* of biology into the practice of medicine, and generally this culminates in the development and sales of drugs. Of note, these drugs generally do not cure

> **Basic science research and the practice of medicine are shaped by powerful financial interests**
>
> "A clinician who is unaware of the political forces that shape healthcare policy and research is analogous to a captain of an oceangoing ship not knowing how to use a compass, sextant, or coastline map. Medical science and healthcare policy are influenced by a myriad of powerful private interests motivated by their own goals, at times different from the stated goal of medicine, which purports to hold paramount the patient's welfare. Scientific objectivity and the guiding ethical principles of informed consent, beneficence, autonomy, and non-malfeasance are subject to different interpretations depending on the lens through which a dilemma is viewed. This gives rise to a disarrayed tug-of-war between factions and private interests, with paradigmatic victory often being awarded to those with the best marketing campaigns and political influence while less importance is given to safety, efficacy, and the economic burden to consumers. To be ignorant of such considerations is to be blind to the nature of research, policy, and our own biased inclinations for and against particular paradigms, assessments, and interventions. Research articles and sources of authority must be approached with an artist's delicacy and with a willingness to consider new information that may contradict deeply rooted beliefs."
>
> Vasquez A. *Musculoskeletal Pain: Expanded Clinical Strategies*. Institute for Functional Medicine, 2008

the disease nor solve the problems, but rather alleviate select and occasionally irrelevant biochemical or clinical indexes of the disease to show "improvement" and therefore justify regulatory "approval" and therefore empower drug sales. Consciously or unconsciously, this is how the system operates, and this is how people within the system generally think; in medical research centers—ie, medical research centers are almost always affiliated with hospitals or medical schools—generally everyone within these systems is a devotee of the medical paradigm, which generally holds that diseases are *idiopathic* and *need to be treated with drugs*, generally multiple drugs (polypharmacy) for

---

[431] Reichenberger et al. Establishing a relationship between bacteria in the human gut and complex regional pain syndrome. *Brain Behav Immun.* 2013 Mar;29:62-9

indefinite periods of time. The lifeblood of biomedical research centers is funding, and this is generally tied to the expectation of "advancing the practice of medicine" which by definition means using—and therefore developing for sale—more drugs. (Drugs are tangible, and drugs are profitable; drugs keep doctors employed, and they keep so-called healthcare centers [e.g., clinics and hospitals] open and profitable because patients are obligated to seek consultations and constantly renew their prescriptions—the profitability and repeat business are guaranteed when patients are told, "You have a disease that is not understood, and this disease will kill or harm you unless you take and continue to take these drugs." Drugs also maintain our power-over paradigm[432],

> **Paradigms—goals, components, needs and fears—are created to support the prevailing power structures**
>
> 248   PUBLIC OPINION
>
> consciously what facts, in what setting, in what guise he shall permit the public to know.
>
> 4
>
> That the manufacture of consent is capable of great refinements no one, I think, denies. The process by which public opinions arise is certainly no less intricate than it has appeared in these pages, and the opportunities for manipulation open to anyone who understands the process are plain enough.
>
> Lippmann W. *Public Opinion*. Harcourt & Brace, 1922

which holds that our worldview is centered on the feeling that we have *power over our problems* [rather than accepting them as they are and working with them as they are], and again we tend to seek this through concrete and obvious and simple-minded means because these are the means that have immediate appeal.) Any basic science or medical researcher who finds that a disease can be cured and the problem solved by a simple treatment will at best be the *Hero of the Day* before being forgotten (and—quite often—later fired); the doctor or researcher who finds that a drug *might* help a problem and who thereafter receives speaking opportunities at national and international medical society meetings (always directly or indirectly funded by drug companies) and who receives several hundred thousand dollars in research grants (always directly or indirectly funded by drug companies and/or the private interests tied to them) will be remembered and championed.

Limited thought—systematic addictions to searching for parts without appreciating the whole, and to disregarding the obvious as simple and therefore without merit: Within the medical paradigm is the belief that diseases are complex and serious and that therefore the treatments must be complex and serious; ironically, drug therapy is actually based on simplistic thinking evidenced by the fact that drugs almost always work on only *one single* pathway/process while complex chronic/persistent diseases are always *multifaceted*. When diseases are indeed simple or at least understandable, they must be made to appear complex and enigmatic by the confusion of research and the perpetual reenactment of ignoring previous research and starting from zero. In this manner, researchers can apply for grants using the words and phrases "new" and "innovative" and "translational" and "advancing medical science to advance patient care" and thus fall into the line of *common thought*—drug production, drug sales, medical dependency to which we are all indoctrinated and accustomed—which makes these ideas and phrases easily acceptable. A doctor or researcher who advances the idea that a disease can be treated by simple means runs the risk of appearing himself/herself as *simple* rather than *insightful*. Collectively as a society, we have created illusions of complexity on many facets of life, ranging from poverty to diabetes to perpetual war; each of these— like the majority of illnesses that bind patients and busy/occupy healthcare systems—can be understood and managed effectively, but not if we allow ourselves to be convinced that they are complex and not if we allow the profiteers to hold the reigns of conversation and intervention. I state that biomedical researchers by virtue of the society in which they live and the environments in which they work are inclined to state and perhaps believe (ie, honestly accept as their own perception) that fibromyalgia is complex, not understood, and ultimately only treatable with drugs—that is the "prescribed" line of medical thinking; we get that paradigm of thought hammered into us via reading, exams, and sleep deprivation in medical school, and medical school courses are the initial training ground for both doctors and their biomedical research colleagues (e.g., many PhD students have to take medical school courses if the PhD program is housed within a university system that contains a medical school). Thus, virtually everyone in "medicine" whether as a physician or researcher is indoctrinated with the *idiopathic-*

---

[432] Largent C, Breton D. *The Paradigm Conspiracy: Why Our Social Systems Violate Human Potential*. Hazelden, 1998

polypharmacy model. Finally, we must also appreciate the profiteering bias manifested by medical journals—who profit from sales of drug-friendly articles when drug companies pay for associated advertising and for article reprints[433]—and magazines/newspapers/websites/television that also receive more advertising money when they publish drug-friendly articles and news. In this way, research and news is inherently biased toward publishing drug-friendly articles and news.

<u>**Private control over public paradigms**</u>: Notably in the United States—the country that most strongly influences international healthcare, science, and policy—the largest media outlets for news, science, and television are owned by a small handful of multicorporation conglomerates that are interconnected—either directly, paradigmatically, or financially—with drug companies; indeed, each facet of health and healthcare in American society—including medical education itself[434] and the lack of labeling of GMO foods and the horrific failure to regulate the pesticide industry's contamination of food, air, and water[435,436]—is strongly influenced by lobbying and money from drug companies and private business interests.[437]

<u>**Denial of the obvious, especially that which is natural and immediate**</u>: Western culture has been largely built on the denial of the present moment and denial of what is natural, hence our fascination with anything new, "modern", "sophisticated", and laboratory-clean. As such, our treatment paradigms tend to avoid the *actionable* and *clear* and *natural* in favor of the passive (e.g., drugs), squeaky-clean (e.g., drugs), and the future (e.g., idiopathic now, but we are supposed to wait for future developments while postponing action and thought and in the meanwhile resign our consciousness to "the powers that be" which are supposed to make the decisions for us by their "virtue" of divine insight). Given that Western culture in its entirety is based on denial of now, natural, and actionable (except when stirred to war)—and any look at our generally passive, listless, and deferent society will confirm this—we should not be surprised that our medical paradigm is largely the same, characterized by passive drugs and passive medical care, apathy in personal thought and action (including medical professionals themselves who are taught

---

[433] Smith R. Medical Journals Are an Extension of the Marketing Arm of Pharmaceutical Companies. *PLoS Med*. 2005 May; 2(5): e138

[434] Drug-company influence on medical education in USA. *Lancet*. 2000 Sep 2;356(9232):781

[435] Bøhn T, Cuhra M, Traavik T, Sanden M, Fagan J, Primicerio R. Compositional differences in soybeans on the market: glyphosate accumulates in Roundup Ready GM soybeans. *Food Chem*. 2014 Jun 15;153:207-1 sciencedirect.com/science/article/pii/S0308814613019201

[436] Majewski MS, Coupe RH, Foreman WT, Capel PD. Pesticides in Mississippi air and rain: a comparison between 1995 and 2007. *Environ Toxicol Chem*. 2014 Jun;33:1283-93

[437] For anyone paying attention to America's political scene, especially since 1980, this statement will be self-evident and abundantly buttressed by the observance of national events that favor small numbers of rich and therefore powerful private and business interests over the interests of the American people and the overall welfare of the nation.

While some would reasonably argue that American society has always been a populist façade run amuck by a puppeteering financial elite, the population-wide data is very clear that the financial balance of the nation was essentially "inverted" in the 1980s during a time when—a fact that nobody can refute—the stated policy of the government was specifically to give more money, more power, and less responsibility to the rich at the expense of the rest of the nation; this was called "trickle-down economics" and was sold to the public via the illusion that by making the rich more rich the wealth of the nation would eventually "trickle down" to the financially lower segments of society and everyone would bathe in the wealth of the nation via the generosity and altruism of the financial elite. Obviously, this did not occur; along with the government's deregulation of industry and the demolition of public power generally and unions in particular, deceptively termed "free trade agreements" shipped American jobs overseas to nations with comparatively zero worker and environmental protections to the benefit of multinational corporations. As shown in the image from President Obama's 2015 State of the Union address, the largest section of the American population—the bottom 90%—now have access to but a small piece of the American national pie, while the top 1% own nearly 70% of the country's resources. As a result, rich individuals and companies gained even more power while the citizens saw their interests ignored; finally in 2014, the obvious was published: America no longer functioned as a democracy by and for the people but rather as an oligarchy, with the government controlled by private interests controlling policies ranging from public health to education and public transportation. Studies and press are listed below:

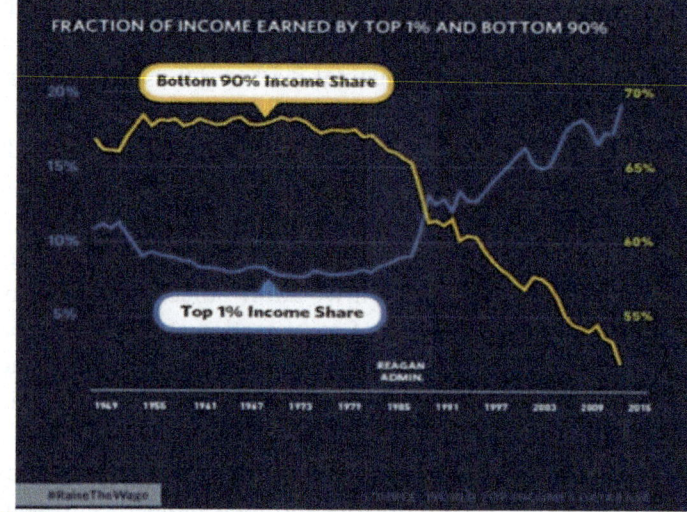

FRACTION OF INCOME EARNED BY TOP 1% AND BOTTOM 90%

Bottom 90% Income Share

Top 1% Income Share

REAGAN ADMIN.

#RaiseTheWage

1. US is an oligarchy, not a democracy. bbc.com/news/blogs-echochambers-27074746
2. America is an oligarchy, not a democracy or republic, university study finds. washingtontimes.com/news/2014/apr/21/americas-oligarchy-not-democracy-or-republic-unive/
3. The US is an oligarchy, study concludes: "Report by researchers from Princeton and Northwestern universities suggests that US political system serves special interest organisations, instead of voters." telegraph.co.uk/news/worldnews/northamerica/usa/10769041/The-US-is-an-oligarchy-study-concludes.html
4. Is the USDA Silencing Scientists? theatlantic.com/science/archive/2015/11/is-the-usda-silencing-scientists/413803/
5. One Nation, Under Monsanto. counterpunch.org/2013/02/26/one-nation-under-monsanto Of special note, this article is written by Paul Craig Roberts PhD (Economics), a former Assistant Secretary of the US Treasury and Associate Editor of the *Wall Street Journal*.

not to think but rather to defer to authority and guidelines while they focus on diagnoses and drugs[438]). In Western medicine, natural treatments whether diets or vitamins are constantly attacked and obfuscated, despite their self-evident value and importance; meanwhile, drugs in general and vaccines in particular are sacrosanct, despite their generally artificial importance, indebting/bankrupting expenses, and adverse effects that often exceed their benefit.

❹ **All other biochemical and pathophysiologic abnormalities seen in fibromyalgia can likewise be explained from the primary SIBO.**

- **Restless leg syndrome and fibromyalgia commonly co-exist, and restless leg syndrome can be alleviated by eradication of SIBO**: Restless leg syndrome (RLS) occurs in approximately 30% of FM patients and can be effectively treated by addressing SIBO with a combination of antibiotics (drugs or botanical medicines that eradicate bacteria) and probiotics (products containing beneficial bacteria, which help restore "microbial balance" in the gastrointestinal tract).[439]
- **SIBO commonly causes nutrient malabsorption and thus predisposes to subclinical selective malnutrition, specifically micronutrient deficiency**: SIBO causes nutrient malabsorption[440] and can thereby contribute to the vitamin D and magnesium deficiencies that promote pain and mitochondrial dysfunction, respectively, and which are common in fibromyalgia. Intestinal bacterial overgrowth causes nutrient malabsorption via intestinal inflammation and villus atrophy (anatomic impairment) and impairment of digestion, specifically the enzymatic degradation of mucosal peptidases and disaccharidases by bacterial proteases (biochemical impairment). As reported by McEvoy and colleagues[441], bacterial contamination [overgrowth] of the small intestine is an important cause of occult malabsorption and malnutrition, especially in the elderly.
- **SIBO can be triggered or exacerbated by emotional stress**: SIBO can be triggered in humans by reduced mucosal immunity following stressful life events, and this helps explain the link between psychoemotional stress and the SIBO-related conditions IBS and FM. Chronic mental-emotional stress causes reduced production of the antibody secretory IgA (sIgA) which is the primary line of defense against bacteria and other microorganisms in the gastrointestinal tract; thus, mental-emotional stress can reduce intestinal immunity and thereby promote SIBO. Further, stress in humans triggers enhanced microbial pathogenicity via microbial endocrinology.
- **Oxidative stress triggers exaggerated pain perception—hyperalgesia (hypersensitivity to pain) and allodynia (perception of pain from normal stimuli)**: Patients with fibromyalgia show evidence of increased free radical (oxidant) production and reduced antioxidant defenses. Increased oxidative stress can be caused by immune activation and mitochondrial dysfunction; immune activation and mitochondrial dysfunction also promote oxidative stress and depletion of antioxidants, resulting in a vicious cycle, as illustrated. In the excellent review by Cordero et al[442], the authors note that recent studies have shown that oxidative stress causes peripheral and central sensitization and alters nerve sensitivity to pain (nociception), resulting in hyperalgesia—hypersensitivity to normal stimuli. The free radical (oxidant) superoxide promotes the development of pain through direct peripheral sensitization and the release of various cytokines (such as TNF-α, IL-1β, and IL-6), the formation of peroxynitrite (ONOO-), and PARP activation. PARP—poly-ADP-ribose-polymerase—is a nuclear enzyme activated by superoxide/peroxynitrite radicals; activation of PARP promotes the development of pain syndromes, including the components of small sensory fiber neuropathy, thermal and mechanical hyperalgesia, tactile allodynia, and exaggerated pain behavior in animal models of diabetic neuropathy.[443,444]
- **Low plasma levels of L-tryptophan seen in fibromyalgia patients can be caused by degradation of dietary tryptophan by the bacterial enzyme tryptophanase**: Patients with fibromyalgia have low blood levels of the amino acid L-tryptophan[445], which is used in the body to make serotonin (important for mood maintenance,

[438] Ely et al. Analysis of questions asked by family doctors regarding patient care. *BMJ*. 1999 Aug 7;319(7206):358-61 ncbi.nlm.nih.gov/pmc/articles/PMC28191/

[439] Weinstock et al. Restless Legs Syndrome in Patients with Irritable Bowel Syndrome: Response to Small Intestinal Bacterial Overgrowth Therapy. *Dig Dis Sci* 2007 May:1252-6

[440] Elphick HL, Elphick DA, Sanders DS. Small bowel bacterial overgrowth. An underrecognized cause of malnutrition in older adults. Geriatrics. 2006 Sep;61(9):21-6

[441] McEvoy et al. Bacterial contamination of the small intestine is an important cause of occult malabsorption in the elderly. *Br Med J* 1983 Sep 17;287(6395):789-93

[442] Cordero MD, et al. Mitochondrial dysfunction and mitophagy activation in blood mononuclear cells of fibromyalgia patients. *Arthritis Res Ther*. 2010;12(1):R17

[443] Wang ZQ, Porreca F, Cuzzocrea S et al. A newly identified role for superoxide in inflammatory pain. *J Pharmacol Exp Ther*. 2004 Jun;309(3):869-78

[444] Ilnytska O, et al. Poly(ADP-ribose) polymerase inhibition alleviates experimental diabetic sensory neuropathy. *Diabetes* 2006 Jun;55:1686-94

[445] "Plasma-free tryptophan is inversely related to the severity of subjective pain in 8 patients who fulfilled criteria for a variety of non-articular rheumatism, the "fibrositis syndrome". The observation is consistent with animal and human studies suggesting a relationship between reduced brain serotonin metabolism and pain reactivity." Moldofsky H, Warsh JJ. Plasma tryptophan and musculoskeletal pain in non-articular rheumatism ("fibrositis syndrome"). *Pain*. 1978 Jun;5(1):65-71

pain alleviation, and appetite control) and melatonin (important for normal sleep, support of mitochondrial function [stimulant of ETC complexes #1 and #4], and antioxidant protection, given that melatonin is one of the most powerful antioxidants). Bacteria such as *Escherichia coli, Proteus vulgaris,* and *Bacteroides* produce the enzyme tryptophanase[446], which destroys L-tryptophan in the gut before it is absorbed from ingested foods; thus, generalized bacterial overgrowth of the small intestine could reasonably be expected to exacerbate this phenomenon. In patients with fibromyalgia, higher tryptophan levels correlate positively with serotonin levels and with less pain and better sleep, while lower tryptophan levels are associated with sleep impairment, reduced serotonin levels, and higher levels of substance P, a neurotransmitter that promotes inflammation and pain perception.[447] Fibromyalgia patients produce 31% less melatonin than do healthy controls, and "this may contribute to impaired sleep at night, fatigue during the day, and changed pain perception."[448] Thus, a likely sequence of events is that, for example, a period of stressful life events can cause impair gastrointestinal immunity leading to intestinal bacterial overgrowth, which itself causes tryptophan degradation via elaboration of bacterial tryptophanase, causing tryptophan deficiency and resultant deficiencies of serotonin (leading to pain, depression, anxiety, and food/carbohydrate craving) and melatonin (leading to sleep disturbance, impaired antioxidant defense and mitochondrial function, and impaired immune responsiveness). Enhanced degradation of tryptophan can also be effected by the liver via enhanced activation of the enzyme tryptophan pyrrolase (tryptophan 2,3-dioxygenase, TDO) in response to "stress" and increased cortisol and by immune cells such as macrophages and dendritic cells via the enzyme indoleamine 2,3-dioxygenase (IDO) which is upregulated via the Th1-type cytokine interferon-gamma (IFNg).[449] Pregnancy induces accelerated tryptophan degradation; however, for the focus of this conversation we note that most FM patients are not pregnant and thus the likely causes of tryptophan deficiency in FM patients, who show evidence of SIBO, stress, and inflammation are ❶ intraluminal bacterial tryptophanase, ❷ hepatic tryptophan pyrrolase, and ❸ immune/inflammatory 2,3-dioxygenase.

- The therapies that help fibromyalgia share mechanisms of action consistent with the model presented here: As will be reviewed below under *Therapeutic Interventions,* essentially all of the most successful therapies for fibromyalgia have effects on intestinal flora, muscle perfusion/contractility, or mitochondrial bioenergetics (biological production of cellular energy/ATP). This is true for vegetarian diets (which favorably alter gut flora and improve antioxidant defenses), supplementation with tryptophan/melatonin (which preserve mitochondrial function during bacterial LPS/endotoxin exposure), physical treatments such as acupuncture (which improves tissue perfusion), and the use of nutrients such as magnesium, acetyl-L-carnitine, D-ribose, creatine, and coenzyme Q-10—all of which support or improve mitochondrial function.

Overall and when integrated together, the research literature provides compelling evidence linking intestinal bacterial overgrowth with the genesis and perpetuation of fibromyalgia. Chronic low-dose exposure to bacterial debris such as lipopolysaccharide/endotoxin and metabolic toxins such as hydrogen sulfide and D-lactic acid from SIBO is a plausible cause of impaired cellular energy production that results in chronic, widespread muscle fatigue and soreness and which may culminate in the clinical presentation of fibromyalgia. The individual components of this model have been substantiated by mechanistic studies in animals and/or research studies in humans. CFS also shares many epidemiological and clinical similarities with FM, and a similar pathophysiology is therefore highly probable.

A consistent report from many CFS and fibromyalgia patients is that of environmental intolerance (EI) and multiple chemical sensitivity (MCS), often grouped together as EI-MCS; these are complex disorders that the medical profession has failed to appreciate and which are characterized by adverse physiological responses to ambient levels of toxic chemicals and other environmental exposures. EI-MCS can be plausibly explained by SIBO because bacterial LPS/endotoxin impairs hepatic cytochrome P450 detoxification enzymes, resulting in reduced

[446] Demoss RD, Moser K. Tryptophanase in Diverse Bacterial Species. *Journal of Bacteriology* 1969; 98: 167-171

[447] "A strong negative correlation between SP and 5-HIAA as well as between SP and TRP could be demonstrated. High serum concentrations of 5-HIAA and TRP showed a significant relation to low pain scores. Moreover, 5-HIAA was strongly related to good quality of sleep, while SP was related to sleep disturbance." Schwarz et al. Relationship of substance P, 5-hydroxyindole acetic acid and tryptophan in serum of fibromyalgia patients. *Neurosci Lett.* 1999 Jan 15;259(3):196-8

[448] "The FMS patients had a 31% lower MT secretion than healthy subjects during the hours of darkness... Patients with fibromyalgic syndrome have a lower melatonin secretion during the hours of darkness than healthy subjects. This may contribute to impaired sleep at night, fatigue during the day, and changed pain perception." Wikner J, Hirsch U, Wetterberg L, Röjdmark S. Fibromyalgia syndrome associated with decreased nocturnal melatonin secretion. *Clin Endocrinol* (Oxf). 1998 Aug;49:179-83

[449] Schröcksnadel K, Wirleitner B, Winkler C, Fuchs D. Monitoring tryptophan metabolism in chronic immune activation. *Clin Chim Acta.* 2006 Feb;364(1-2):82-90

drug metabolism and impaired clearance of xenobiotics/toxins.[450] Accumulation of xenobiotics in CFS patients[451] might therefore be explained in part by LPS-induced inhibition of xenobiotic clearance secondary to SIBO. Further, the metabolic and immunologic effects of LPS can also account for the immune activation, neurological dysfunction, and musculoskeletal complaints noted in patients with CFS, IBS, and FM. A simplified yet accurate model of fibromyalgia which accounts for the major clinical and objective abnormalities seen with this condition is presented in the diagram that follows. Following the exclusion of diagnosable and treatable conditions that can contribute to or mimic fibromyalgia, and by using an integrated model, clinicians can design treatment plans based on the previously reviewed pathogenesis and on the therapeutic considerations detailed in the following section.

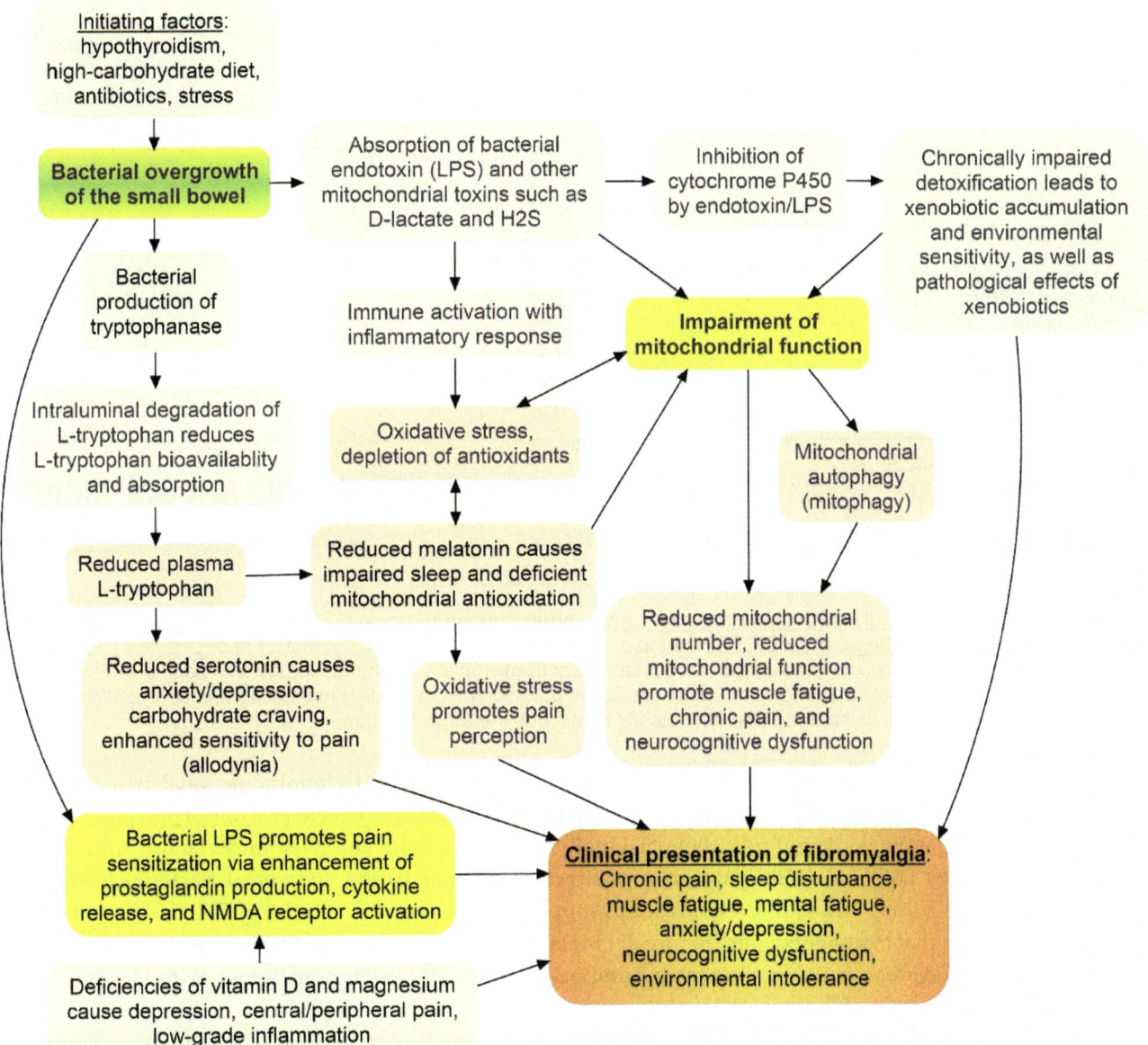

How small intestine bacterial overgrowth (SIBO) causes fibromyalgia: Bacterial overgrowth of the small bowel leads to chronic low-grade tryptophan insufficiency resulting in reduced endogenous production of serotonin (important for positive mood and relief from anxiety pain) and of melatonin (important for restful sleep and protection of mitochondria from oxidative stress). Bacterial mitochondrial toxins such as endotoxin, H2S, D-lactate cause impaired mitochondrial energy production, which leads to mitophagy, muscle fatigue, pain, and cognitive impairment. See educational videos and updates at www.inflammationmastery.com/pain

---

[450] Shedlofsky et al. Endotoxin administration to humans inhibits hepatic cytochrome P450-mediated drug metabolism. *J Clin Invest*. 1994 Dec;94(6):2209-14

[451] Dunstan et al. A preliminary investigation of chlorinated hydrocarbons and chronic fatigue syndrome. *Med J Aust*. 1995 Sep 18;163(6):294-7

Introduction to Therapeutic Approach: Rational treatment of microbe-induced pain and inflammation as seen in FM must focus on the eradication/modulation of the inflammatory microbial load as well as on the restoration of barrier defenses (e.g., the defensive lining of the skin and the gut wall) to reduce absorption of and exposure to microbial molecules (enhancing elimination of already-absorbed microbial toxins is a possibility, but is of lesser importance and is mentioned in some of my other writings). Enhancement of mitochondrial dysfunction and glial activation (brain inflammation) should also be pursued.

This section begins with a review of evidence showing important gut involvement in FM, CFS/SEID, and CRPS—all of which are variants on the same themes of microbe-induced microglial activation and mitochondrial dysfunction, as depicted in the following image, showing the relative contribution and combination of dysbiosis-induced mitochondrial impairment and brain inflammation (e.g., glial activation and central sensitization).

Microbe-induced mitochondriopathy/neurotoxicity and brain inflammation—a schematic diagram of relative contributions and combinations: In CFS/SEID, microbial induction of mitochondrial dysfunction and (D-lactate) neurotoxicity predominate, whereas fibromyalgia is a unique combination of both microbial mitochondriopathy with central sensitization. In IBS, central sensitization is potent, along with a more disruptive gut microbiome leading to bloating and constipation/diarrhea; meanwhile in CRPS, a neuroinflammatory dysbiosis clearly dominates the clinical picture.

- Patients with chronic fatigue syndrome (SEID), fibromyalgia (FM), and complex regional pain syndrome (CRPS) show evidence of increased intestinal permeability, leading to increased absorption of antigens, immunogens, inflammogens, and mitochondrial inhibitors (etc): Finally and most importantly, **antimicrobial therapy alleviates FM (and IBS) symptoms in direct proportion to the success of bacterial overgrowth eradication**, thus adding strong direct evidence in support of SIBO as a main cause of FM.[452,453] Recent clinical trials have shown that treatment of the fibromyalgia-related conditions IBS and SIBO by use of the nonabsorbed oral antibiotic rifaximin results in significant diminution of IBS-SIBO symptomatology with benefits lasting after the discontinuation of therapy.[454,455]
  - Increased intestinal permeability (IP) in patients with primary fibromyalgia (FM) and in patients with complex regional pain syndrome (CRPS) (*Rheumatology* 2008 Aug[456]): Authors of this study used well-established tests of mucosal permeability for gastroduodenal permeability (sucrose) and small intestinal permeability (lactulose and mannitol, as discussed in Chapter 1) to find that both FM and CRPS patients

[452] Wallace DJ, Hallegua DS. Fibromyalgia: the gastrointestinal link. *Curr Pain Headache Rep*.2004 Oct;8(5):364-8

[453] Pimentel et al. Improvement of symptoms by eradication of small intestinal overgrowth in FM: a double-blind study. [Abstract] *Arthritis Rheum* 1999, 42:S343

[454] Pimentel et al. The effect of a nonabsorbed oral antibiotic (rifaximin) on the symptoms of the irritable bowel syndrome. *Ann Intern Med*. 2006 Oct 17;145(8):557-63

[455] Sharara et al. A randomized double-blind placebo-controlled trial of rifaximin in patients with abdominal bloating and flatulence. *Am J Gastroenterol*. 2006 Feb;101(2):326-33

[456] Goebel et al. Altered intestinal permeability in patients with primary fibromyalgia and in patients with complex regional pain syndrome. *Rheumatology* 2008 Aug;47(8):1223-7

show increased burden of intestinal involvement; they write, "Patients with FM had a significantly higher IP than healthy volunteers. Indeed, both FM and CRPS groups had significantly higher IP values than healthy volunteers for both gastroduodenal permeability and small bowel permeability. The difference in gastroduodenal permeability between the two patient groups did not reach significance. Gastroduodenal permeability, as measured with the sucrose test, was increased in 13 patients with FM (32.5%) and in six patients with CRPS (35.3%) and in one healthy volunteer. The small bowel permeability index [using lactulose and mannitol] was increased in 15 patients with FM (37.5%), three patients with CRPS (17.6%) and in none of the volunteers." A wonderful addition to / extension of this work would have been the measurement of serum LPS levels, but this was not performed in the current study and has not been performed as of early 2015—noted and summarized immediately below is one study (Maes et al, *J Affect Disord* 2007 Apr) that measured antibodies to LPS (not LPS directly) in patients with CFS—chronic fatigue syndrome. Notably, increased IP in FM did not correlate with GI symptoms; however increased IP did correlate with serologic positivity against *Helicobacter pylori*, *Yersinia enterocolitica* and *Campylobacter jejuni*.

- Increased serum IgA and IgM against LPS of enterobacteria in chronic fatigue syndrome (CFS) shows involvement of gram-negative enterobacteria and increased gut-intestinal permeability in the etiology of CFS (*J Affect Disord* 2007 Apr[457]): These investigators measured IgA and IgM to LPS of the enterobacteria *Hafnia alvei*, *Pseudomonas aeruginosa*, *Morganella morganii*, *Proteus mirabilis*, *Pseudomonas putida*, *Citrobacter koseri*, and *Klebsiella pneumoniae* and "found that the prevalences and median values for serum IgA against the LPS of enterobacteria are significantly greater in patients with CFS than in normal volunteers and patients with partial CFS. Serum IgA levels were significantly correlated to the severity of illness, as measured by the FibroFatigue scale and to symptoms, such as irritable bowel, muscular tension, fatigue, concentration difficulties, and failing memory. The results show that enterobacteria are involved in the etiology of CFS and that an increased gut-intestinal permeability has caused an immune response to the LPS of gram-negative enterobacteria."

- Gut inflammation in chronic fatigue syndrome. (*Nutr Metab* 2010 Oct[458]): "Many CFS patients complain of gut dysfunction. In fact, patients with CFS are more likely to report a previous diagnosis of irritable bowel syndrome (IBS), a common functional disorder of the gut, and experience IBS-related symptoms. Recently, evidence for interactions between the intestinal microbiota, mucosal barrier function, and the immune system have been shown to play a role in the disorder's pathogenesis. Studies examining the microecology of the gastrointestinal (GI) tract have identified specific microorganisms whose presence appears related to disease; in CFS, a role for altered intestinal microbiota in the pathogenesis of the disease has recently been suggested. Mucosal barrier dysfunction promoting bacterial translocation has also been observed. ...For example, the administration of probiotics could alter the gut microbiota, improve mucosal barrier function, decrease pro-inflammatory cytokines, and have the potential to positively influence mood in patients where both emotional symptoms and inflammatory immune signals are elevated. Probiotics also have the potential to improve gut motility, which is dysfunctional in many CFS patients."

- Altered intestinal microbiota and organic acids may be the origin of symptoms in irritable bowel syndrome. (*Neurogastroenterol Motil.* 2010 May[459]): "Irritable bowel syndrome patients showed significantly higher counts of Veillonella and Lactobacillus than controls. They also expressed significantly higher levels of acetic acid, propionic acid, and total organic acids than controls. The quantity of bowel gas was not significantly different between controls and IBS patients. Finally, IBS patients with high acetic acid or propionic acid levels presented with significantly worse GI symptoms, QOL and negative emotions than those with low acetic acid or propionic acid levels or controls."

- Intestinal permeability and hypersensitivity in the irritable bowel syndrome. (*Pain* 2009 Nov[460]): "Here we demonstrate that diarrhea-predominant IBS (D-IBS) patients display increased intestinal permeability. We

[457] Maes et al. Increased serum IgA and IgM against LPS of enterobacteria in chronic fatigue syndrome (CFS): indication for the involvement of gram-negative enterobacteria in the etiology of CFS and for the presence of an increased gut-intestinal permeability. *J Affect Disord* 2007 Apr, 99:237–240

[458] Lakhan SE, Kirchgessner A. Gut inflammation in chronic fatigue syndrome. *Nutr Metab* (Lond). 2010 Oct 12;7:79

[459] Tana et al. Altered profiles of intestinal microbiota and organic acids may be the origin of symptoms in irritable bowel syndrome. *Neurogastroenterol Motil.* 2010 May;22(5):512-9, e114-5

[460] Zhou Q, Zhang B, Verne GN. Intestinal membrane permeability and hypersensitivity in the irritable bowel syndrome. *Pain.* 2009 Nov;146(1-2):41-6

have also found that increased intestinal membrane permeability is associated with visceral and thermal hypersensitivity in this subset of D-IBS patients. We evaluated 54 D-IBS patients and 22 controls for intestinal membrane permeability using the lactulose/mannitol method. ... We also evaluated the mean mechanical visual analogue scale (M-VAS) pain rating to nociceptive thermal and visceral stimulation in all subjects. ... Approximately 39% of diarrhea-predominant IBS patients had increased intestinal membrane permeability as measured by the lactulose/mannitol ratio. These IBS patients also demonstrated higher M-VAS pain intensity reading scale. Interestingly, the IBS patients with hypersensitivity and increased intestinal permeability had a higher Functional Bowel Disorder Severity Index (FBDSI) score (100.8 + or - 5.4) than IBS patients with normal membrane permeability and sensitivity (51.6 + or - 12.7) and controls (6.1 + or - 5.6) (p<0.001). A subset of D-IBS patients had increased intestinal membrane permeability that was associated with an increased FBDSI score and increased hypersensitivity to visceral and thermal nociceptive pain stimuli. Thus, increased intestinal membrane permeability in D-IBS patients may lead to more severe IBS symptoms and hypersensitivity to somatic and visceral stimuli."

- Antimicrobial/antibiotic treatment alleviates fibromyalgia in most FM patients, just as it also alleviates gastrointestinal symptoms in patients with irritable bowel syndrome (IBS): Finally and most importantly, **antimicrobial therapy alleviates FM (and IBS) symptoms in direct proportion to the success of bacterial overgrowth eradication**, thus adding strong direct evidence in support of SIBO as a main cause of FM.[461,462] Recent clinical trials have shown that treatment of the fibromyalgia-related conditions IBS and SIBO by use of the nonabsorbed oral antibiotic rifaximin results in significant diminution of IBS-SIBO symptomatology with benefits lasting after the discontinuation of therapy.[463,464]

  - Clinical trial: Rifaximin therapy for patients with irritable bowel syndrome without constipation (*New England Journal of Medicine* 2011 Jan[465]): Authors of this study evaluated rifaximin, a minimally absorbed antibiotic, as treatment for IBS. Subjects were given rifaximin at a dose of 550 mg or placebo, three times daily for 2 weeks and were followed for 10 weeks thereafter. "Significantly more patients in the rifaximin group than in the placebo group had adequate relief of global IBS symptoms during the first 4 weeks after treatment (40.8% vs. 31.2%). Similarly, more patients in the rifaximin group than in the placebo group had adequate relief of bloating (39.5% vs. 28.7%). In addition, significantly more patients in the rifaximin group had a response to treatment as assessed by daily ratings of IBS symptoms, bloating, abdominal pain, and stool consistency. The incidence of adverse events was similar in the two groups." Thus, among patients who had IBS without constipation, treatment with rifaximin for 2 weeks provided significant relief of IBS symptoms, bloating, abdominal pain, and loose or watery stools. *Comments by Dr Vasquez: Shortcomings of the intervention used in this IBS-rifaximin study include ❶ failure to use long-term treatment, which is often necessary in the treatment of chronic SIBO, ❷ failure to co-administer an antifungal agent to avert fungal growth in the intestines which commonly occurs as a result of antimicrobial/antibacterial drug treatment, ❸ failure to administer probiotics to re-establish beneficial flora, and ❹ failure to implement dietary modification to sustain the beneficial eradication of excess bacteria—allowing patients to continue their unhealthy diets and lifestyles is the most assured way to ensure that the condition (SIBO-IBS) will return.*

  - Review of clinical trials: Rifaximin as treatment for SIBO and IBS (*Expert Opinion on Investigational Drugs* 2009 Mar[466]): A recognized expert in the treatment of SIBO-related conditions, Dr Pimentel writes, "**Rifaximin is a broad-range, gastrointestinal-specific antibiotic that demonstrates no clinically relevant bacterial resistance**. Therefore, rifaximin may be useful in the treatment of gastrointestinal disorders associated with altered bacterial flora, including irritable bowel syndrome (IBS) and small intestinal bacterial overgrowth (SIBO)." He also notes regarding the use of rifaximin in the treatment of IBS, "Rifaximin improved global symptoms in 33 - 92% of patients and eradicated SIBO in up to 84% of patients with IBS, with results sustained up to 10 weeks post-treatment. Rifaximin caused a lower number of

[461] Wallace DJ, Hallegua DS. Fibromyalgia: the gastrointestinal link. *Curr Pain Headache Rep.* 2004 Oct;8(5):364-8

[462] Pimentel et al. Improvement of symptoms by eradication of small intestinal overgrowth in FM: a double-blind study. [Abstract] *Arthritis Rheum* 1999, 42:S343

[463] Pimentel et al. The effect of a nonabsorbed oral antibiotic (rifaximin) on the symptoms of the irritable bowel syndrome. *Ann Intern Med.* 2006 Oct 17;145(8):557-63

[464] Sharara et al. A randomized double-blind placebo-controlled trial of rifaximin in patients with abdominal bloating and flatulence. *Am J Gastroenterol.* 2006 Feb;101(2):326-33

[465] Pimentel M, Lembo A, Chey WD, et al. Rifaximin therapy for patients with irritable bowel syndrome without constipation. *N Engl J Med.* 2011 Jan 6;364(1):22-32

[466] Pimentel M. Review of rifaximin as treatment for SIBO and IBS. *Expert Opin Investig Drugs.* 2009 Mar;18(3):349-58

adverse events compared with metronidazole or levofloxacin and may have a more favorable adverse event profile than systemic antibiotics, without clinically relevant antibiotic resistance."

- <u>Results of two clinical trials of antibiotics in the treatment of fibromyalgia (*Current Pain and Headache Reports* 2004 Oct[467])</u>: This article discusses the results of two experiments using antibiotics in the treatment of FM: ❶ 96 patients with SIBO diagnosed by lactulose hydrogen breath testing (LHBT) were offered antibiotic treatment for the reduction of gastrointestinal bacteria; 25 of the 96 patients returned for a follow-up LHBT. Neomycin was the most commonly used antibiotic. Eleven of the 25 patients achieved complete transient eradication of SIBO after antibiotic treatment and experienced better improvement in more of their FM symptom scores when compared with the patients who did not achieve complete eradication. This indicates that **a direct relationship exists between the presence of SIBO and intestinal and extraintestinal symptoms in fibromyalgia, and that FM can be alleviated by effective antimicrobial/antibiotic treatment.** ❷ In this double-blind trial of eradication of SIBO in fibromyalgia, 46 patients fulfilling the established criteria for FM were tested for SIBO using LHBT. Forty-two of the 46 patients (91.3%) were positive for SIBO and were randomized to receive placebo or 500 mg of liquid neomycin (a minimally-absorbed gastrointestinal-specific antibiotic drug) twice daily for 10 days. Only six of the 20 patients (30%) in the neomycin group achieved eradication (indicating inefficacy of treatment); thus, no statistically significant difference between groups was available for analysis. Thereafter, 28 patients in the double-blind study testing positive for SIBO went on to receive open-label antibiotic treatment to eradicate SIBO, and this time 17 of the 28 patients (60.7%) achieved eradication of SIBO. When these 23 patients were compared with the 15 patients who failed to eradicate or did not undergo open-label treatment, significant improvement attributable to antibiotic treatment in the FM scores was detected. **Results show that eradication of bacterial overgrowth results in a clinically significant alleviation of FM symptoms.**

Most experienced functional medicine clinicians generally and naturopathic physicians specifically—collectively these are the clinicians with the most experience in the assessment and treatment of various forms of dysbiosis—will agree that ultimate correction of dysbiosis is no easy task. Many aspects must be addressed simultaneously, and these will be detailed in the section on *Therapeutics and Clinical Interventions*. For the here and now, I will simply outline some of the more common and important considerations, in no particular order because order implies importance, which implies effectiveness, which is dependent on the patient's response:

1. <u>Dietary optimization</u>: The diet must be diverse, varied, and plant-based in order to optimize microbial diversity and reduce intake of carbohydrates in general and simple carbohydrates in particular.

2. <u>Probiotic therapy</u>: Administering probiotics to patients who have SIBO can be effective or can cause exacerbations; patients might need to wait until other aspects are optimized before adding "good bacteria."

3. <u>Antimicrobial therapy</u>: Botanicals such as berberine, oregano oil, and others are safe and highly efficacious.

4. <u>Stimulation/normalization of peristalsis</u>: Magnesium and ascorbate can be used to promote laxation; optimization of thyroid function/status is of utmost importance. Exercise, water, relaxation, fiber are important.

5. <u>Systemic health optimization, stress reduction, sleep optimization</u>: Fatty acid intake (e.g., n3 fatty acids) and mitochondrial function need to be optimized in order to optimize gut flora. Stress promotes dysbiosis and microbial virulence; sleep deprivation impairs mitochondria, redox balance, hormones, and immunity.

In this space before diving into *Therapeutics and Clinical Interventions*, I'll briefly mention three concepts that are interrelated. ❶ Microbial identity and location are irrelevant, given that most of the adverse physiologic effects seen can be mediated by a wide range of Gram-negative bacteria; their identities and locations are irrelevant as long as they produce sufficient LPS. The only aspect that is almost entirely dependent on localization to the gut is the production of the mitochondrial neurotoxins H2S and D-lactate. ❷ Any combination of glial activation and mitochondrial dysfunction would be sufficient to induce the fibromyalgia phenotype; the agents most likely to accomplish both are pesticides and corporate toxins such as glyphosate, widely sprayed internationally and pervasive in the American food, air, and water supply. ❸ The variations in microbial combinations and total load, individual patient fragilities and vulnerabilities, nutritional status and xenobiotic permutations give rise to the nuances and variations in clinical presentations and therapeutic responses. However, the model presented

---

[467] Wallace DJ, Hallegua DS. Fibromyalgia: the gastrointestinal link. *Curr Pain Headache Rep.* 2004 Oct;8(5):364-8

throughout this section is an accurate description of the most important and common pathoetiologic considerations and clinical interventions; once these core considerations are addressed, others can be addressed with greater specific and overall efficacy.

Therapeutics and Clinical Interventions

- Overview: Treatments for FM should be ❶ science-based and should ❷ directly address the cause(s) of the disorder; treatments should be ❹ safe (generally) and ❺ effective and ❻ without potential for serious adverse effects. Drug treatment of FM does not meet these criteria; the integrative, nutritional, and functional medicine approaches outlined below can—when properly employed by a skilled clinician—address the cause(s) of FM in a way that is scientific, direct, safe, effective, and well tolerated by essentially all patients. **Treatments for FM must emphasize eradication of SIBO, prevention of SIBO recurrence, the restoration/establishment of optimal nutritional status, and specific support for optimal mitochondrial function; anything less than this will fail to be effective.** Clinical interventions for the treatment of SIBO include dietary carbohydrate restriction, normalization of slow gastrointestinal transit time (e.g., correction of hypothyroidism), selective use of probiotic supplements to normalize intestinal flora, support of mucosal immunity (with nutrients such as vitamin A, zinc, and L-glutamine), and eradication of bacterial overgrowth with drugs (such as ciprofloxacin, rifaximin, amoxicillin/Augmentin[468], metronidazole) and/or natural products (such as berberine[469], *Artemisia annua*, peppermint oil[470], and emulsified time-released oil of oregano[471])—each of these have been reviewed in greater detail elsewhere by this author.[472] Failure of any monotherapeutic approach to immediately resolve the clinical manifestations of FM can explained by the secondary metabolic, immune, and neurophysiological effects that have generally persisted over periods ranging from years to decades for most patients; in other words, the treatment program must be multifaceted in order to address the numerous major problems that cause FM, and the treatment plan must also be sustained long enough to correct the abnormal physiologic patterns that have been established by the body's response/adaptation to the disease process. The treatment program (examples provided) must be complete in order to facilitate correction of systemic oxidative damage (broad-spectrum antioxidant support), resultant nutritional deficiencies (diet optimization, vitamin and mineral supplementation), immune sensitization and induction of proinflammatory cycles (anti-inflammatory nutrition), alterations in neurotransmission and membrane receptor function (amino acid and fatty acid supplementation), and the inflammation-induced disturbances in pain reception and hypothalamic-pituitary-endocrine function (assess/correct hormonal imbalances; supplement with n-3 fatty acids and olive oil to reduce hypothalamic inflammation[473], etc.). Further, patients treated for SIBO who do not positively change their diets and lifestyles (which probably promoted the genesis and perpetuation of the disease-causing SIBO in the first place) are subject to continual recurrence until such changes are implemented and faithfully maintained.

FOOD & NUTRITION As with many rheumatologic/painful/inflammatory conditions with a strong component of gastrointestinal dysbiosis, the single best diet is a vegan or pesco-vegetarian diet free of gluten and most grains (judicious use of brown rice excepted); clearly the diet must emphasize vegetable intake and avoidance of fermentable substrate to induce quantitative reductions and qualitative improvements in microbial populations and metabolic activity. Beyond the gut, the benefits of minimized carbohydrate intake include weight loss (generally beneficial in this patient population), alleviation of physiologic and psychologic dependence on carbohydrate (over)consumption, and increased endogenous production of beta-hydroxy-butyrate which stimulates the terminal complexes of the mitochondrial electron transport chain while also promoting histone acetylation (via inhibition of histone deacetylase) for enhanced DNA transcription resulting in what has been referred to as a rejuvenative phenotype. My foundational diet-nutritional program—the 5-part "supplemented Paleo-Mediterranean Diet"—can easily be modified to pesco-vegetarian or lacto-pesco-vegetarian variants to

[468] Malik BA, Xie YY, Wine E, Huynh HQ. Diagnosis and pharmacological management of small intestinal bacterial overgrowth in children with intestinal failure. *Can J Gastroenterol*. 2011 Jan;25(1):41-5. This is a remarkable article and probably one of the most brilliant articles on the treatment of SIBO with drugs.

[469] [No authors listed] Berberine. *Altern Med Rev*. 2000 Apr;5(2):175-7

[470] "A case report of a patient with SIBO who showed marked subjective improvement in IBS-like symptoms and significant reductions in hydrogen production after treatment with ECPO is presented. While further investigation is necessary, results in this case suggest one of mechanisms by which ECPO improves IBS symptoms is antimicrobial activity in small intestine." Logan et al. Treatment of small intestinal bacterial overgrowth with enteric-coated peppermint oil: a case report. *Altern Med Rev*. 2002 Oct;7(5):410-7

[471] Force M, Sparks WS, Ronzio RA. Inhibition of enteric parasites by emulsified oil of oregano in vivo. *Phytother Res*. 2000 May;14(3):213-4

[472] Vasquez A. Nutritional and Botanical Treatments against "Silent Infections" and Gastrointestinal Dysbiosis. *Nutr Perspect* 2006; Jan: 5-21 ichnfm.academia.edu/AlexVasquez

[473] Milanski et al. Saturated fatty acids produce inflammatory response predominantly through activation of TLR4 signaling in hypothalamus. *J Neurosci*. 2009 Jan;29(2):359-70

enhance high-quality protein intake while continuing to emphasize vegetable, nut, and seed intake to maximize fiber and micronutrient intake. In particular, whey protein isolate is attractive in this patient population due to the high content of tryptophan (to correct the common tryptophan deficiency), the glutathione precursors (to alleviate oxidative stress and enhance mitochondrial function), immunoglobulins (to support mucosal defenses against bacterial overgrowth), and growth factors including whey's insulotrophic effect to promote anabolism with resultant improvements in muscle function and gut mucosal integrity. Systemic alkalinization supported by plant-based potassium citrate promotes xenobiotic excretion (reduction in total load of persistent organic pollutants and toxic metals such as lead and mercury) and endogenous production of endorphins (enhanced mood, pain relief). The increased intake of vitamins (including physiologic doses of vitamin D3), minerals, ALA, GLA, EPA, DHA, and probiotics all synergize to alleviate SIBO, oxidative stress, pain and inflammation while also promoting optimal immune and mitochondrial functions. Allergy identification and avoidance is easily achieved via the very practical and no-cost elimination-and-challenge technique. In particular for patients with fibromyalgia, magnesium intake is increased via consumption of dark green vegetables and nutritional supplements while magnesium absorption is promoted by optimized vitamin D status while renal retention of magnesium is promoted with urinary alkalinization. The consistent and pathologic secondary tryptophan deficiency is foremost corrected by eradicating the causative SIBO and the resultant intraintestinal bacterial tryptophanase-catalyzed degradation of ingested tryptophan and via dietary supplementation with L-tryptophan, 5-hydroxytryptophan, and/or whey protein isolate.

> **Dr Vasquez's summary of the medical indication for gluten-containing grains/foods**
>
> The only medical indication for the consumption of gluten-containing grains is prevention/treatment of acute starvation, assuming no other food is available.

- Diet optimization with the five-part "supplemented Paleo-Mediterranean Diet" (*Nutr Perspect* 2011 Jan[474]): The "supplemented Paleo-Mediterranean Diet" (SPMD)—the 5-part nutritional wellness protocol—as described in most of my textbooks in "chapter 2" and also in my articles available on-line at ichnfm.academia.edu/AlexVasquez should be implemented for most FM patients; exceptions to this general rule might include patients with renal insufficiency due to the risk for potassium excess (hyperkalemia [Note 475]). Because any patient might have an allergy or intolerance to any food (even a healthy food like citrus fruit, chicken or eggs), patients and doctors must be aware of the potential for food allergies and will therefore have to customize the Paleo-Mediterranean diet *for each individual patient* to exclude foods to which the patient might be allergic or sensitive/intolerant. Otherwise, this 5-part nutrition protocol is based on ❶ vegetables, nuts, seeds, (berries, fruits, and juices generally have to be avoided during treatment for SIBO due to the high content of sugars and—with juice—the rapid passage through the gastrointestinal tract) and lean sources of protein, ❷ high-potency multivitamin and multimineral supplementation, ❸ physiologic doses of vitamin D3 to optimize blood levels of vitamin D3 (measured as 25-OH-vitamin D), ❹ combination fatty acid supplementation (with flax oil [for ALA], fish oil [for EPA and DHA], and borage oil [for GLA] with oleic acid from olive oil incorporated into the diet), and ❺ probiotics—foods or supplements that contain living bacteria with beneficial qualities. The diet should emphasize strict avoidance of grains in general and gluten-containing grains *especially wheat* in particular. This diet is essential for the provision of sufficient protein, fiber, phytonutrients, and alkalinization—potassium citrate is most concentrated in vegetables and helps the body maintain proper acid-alkaline balance.[476] The diet should be low in carbohydrates to reduce fermentable substrate to intestinal bacteria. The most important books for patients to read in support of this diet are *The Paleo Diet* by Dr Loren Cordain and *Breaking the Vicious Cycle* by Elaine Gottschall.

---

[474] Vasquez A. Revisiting the Five-Part Nutritional Wellness Protocol: Supplemented Paleo-Mediterranean Diet. *Nutr Perspect* 2011 Jan ichnfm.academia.edu/AlexVasquez
[475] Because the kidneys are responsible for excreting potassium, reduced kidney function (kidney failure, renal insufficiency) implies that the kidneys may not be able to perform the function of excreting potassium; thus, consumption of a potassium-rich diet could contribute to a dangerous situation of excess potassium in the blood known as hyperkalemia (*hyper*=too much, *kal*=potassium, *emia*=blood disorder). For patients with renal insufficiency, consumption of an otherwise health-promoting diet rich in fruits and vegetables might cause a problem if potassium accumulates in the blood due to impaired excretion. Blood tests can assess renal function as well as the blood potassium level. This is one example of why a clinician/doctor should be employed by patients before implementing diet modification and nutritional supplementation.
[476] "The modern Western-type diet is deficient in fruits and vegetables and contains excessive animal products, generating the accumulation of non-metabolizable anions and a lifespan state of overlooked metabolic acidosis, whose magnitude increases progressively with aging due to the physiological decline in kidney function." Adeva MM, Souto G. Diet-induced metabolic acidosis. *Clin Nutr.* 2011 Aug;30(4):416-21

- Vegetarian diet: Fibromyalgia syndrome improved using a mostly raw vegetarian diet (*BMC Complementary and Alternative Medicine* 2001 Sep[477]): Diets high in fruits, vegetables, nuts, berries, and seeds provide ample fiber to promote laxation and can be useful as adjunctive treatment for gastrointestinal dysbiosis in general and SIBO in particular (i.e., *quantitative* reduction in GI dysbiosis). Perhaps more importantly, plant-based diets result in *qualitative* benefits by changing microbial behavior and reducing production of irritants, toxins, and bacterial metabolites, including the mitochondrial poisons D-lactate and hydrogen sulfide. Fibromyalgia patients who consume a mostly vegetarian diet have experienced significant improvements in function and reductions in FM symptomatology. Poorly designed dietary interventions that allow abundant intake of whole-grain bread, pasta, rice, and fruit juice[478] would be expected to fail because such high-carbohydrate diets feed intestinal bacteria with an abundance of substrate and would therefore be expected to sustain or exacerbate SIBO. Another advantage to a plant-based mostly-raw diet is the avoidance of dietary advanced glycation end-products (AGEs) which are inflammation-promoting chemical combinations of proteins with sugars, which can be consumed in the diet (e.g., baked deserts) or formed endogenously/internally as a result of oxidative stress and elevated blood sugar levels (e.g., diabetes mellitus). As discussed previously, FM patients show higher levels of AGEs in blood cells and muscle tissue; AGEs promote chronic pain and inflammation[479], and therefore dietary and nutritional strategies that reduce AGE intake and/or AGE formation are 1) without risk, and 2) likely to provide manifold health benefits, including but not limited to reductions in pain and inflammation.

Dr Vasquez's Nutrition Protocol: The 5-part "Supplemented Paleo-Mediterranean Diet" (5pSPMD or SMPD)

1. **Diet: Emphasize fruits, vegetables, nuts, seeds, berries, and lean sources of protein** (fish, grass-fed lamb/beef). Minimize fruit intake due to higher sugar content while treating SIBO; the goal is to deprive the bacteria and yeast in the intestines of their preferred food source (carbohydrates, sugars). Make modifications for patient-specific food allergies and sensitivities; this is especially important for patients with known allergy-related conditions such as migraine headaches. Patients with kidney disease should use caution when consuming a potassium-rich diet. Vasquez A. Revisiting the Five-Part Nutritional Wellness Protocol: The Supplemented Paleo-Mediterranean Diet. *Nutritional Perspectives* 2011 Jan

2. **Multivitamin and multimineral supplement**: Nutrient deficiencies are common and are easily treated with nutritional supplementation. Fletcher and Fairfield. Vitamins for chronic disease prevention in adults. *JAMA* 2002 Jun

3. **Vitamin D dosed at 2,000-10,000 IU per day**: The adult requirement for vitamin D3 is approximately 4,000 IU per day; some patients may achieve optimal blood levels with lower doses, but generally daily doses of 4,000-10,000 IU are necessary. Vasquez et al. Clinical Importance of Vitamin D. *Alternative Therapies in Health and Medicine* 2004 Sep

4. **Combination fatty acid supplementation**: A combination of flax oil, borage oil, and fish oil provides the health-promoting fatty acids (ALA, GLA, EPA, DHA). Patients should consume organic virgin olive oil liberally with foods. Vasquez A. New Insights into Fatty Acid Supplementation and Its Effect on Eicosanoid Production and Genetic Expression. *Nutritional Perspectives* 2005; Jan

5. **Probiotics**: Health-promoting bacteria can be consumed in the form of powders, pills, and fermented foods such as yogurt, kefir, pickles and sauerkraut.

For a video review of this foundational diet and introduction to the functional inflammology protocol, see Dr Vasquez "Functional Inflammology Protocol, part 1: Introduction and Foundational Diet" from the 2013 International Conference on Human Nutrition and Functional Medicine: https://vimeo.com/100089988 Password: "DrVprotocol_volume1"

- Vitamin B12 in the form of hydroxo-/methyl-/adenosyl-cobalamin, should be administered to all FM and CFS patients to alleviate pain, glial inflammation, accelerated neurodegeneration; reasonable doses are at least 2,000 mcg per day orally and/or 2,000 mcg per week by subcutaneous/intramuscular injection: Given that sulfur-containing molecules such as sulfite and hydrogen sulfide bind to vitamin B12[480,481], we should reasonably expect that patients with excess exposure to H2S from the gastrointestinal tract would have an increased prevalence of vitamin B12 deficiency, and indeed this has been documented; vitamin B12 deficiency in CFS and FM patients promotes fatigue and brain dysfunction via the effects of vitamin B12 deficiency directly (ie, vitamin B12 deficiency is well known to cause nerve damage and brain damage) and indirectly via impaired

[477] Donaldson et al. Fibromyalgia syndrome improved using a mostly raw vegetarian diet. *BMC Complement Altern Med*. 2001;1:7 biomedcentral.com/1472-6882/1/7
[478] Michalsen et al. Mediterranean diet or extended fasting's influence on changing the intestinal microflora, immunoglobulin A secretion and clinical outcome in patients with rheumatoid arthritis and fibromyalgia: an observational study. *BMC Complement Altern Med*. 2005 Dec 22;5:22
[479] "In the interstitial connective tissue of fibromyalgic muscles we found a more intensive staining of the AGE CML, activated NF-kappaB, and also higher CML levels in the serum of these patients compared to the controls. RAGE was only present in FM muscle." Rüster et al. Detection of elevated N epsilon-carboxymethyllysine levels in muscular tissue and in serum of patients with fibromyalgia. *Scand J Rheumatol*. 2005 Nov-Dec;34(6):460-3
[480] Añíbarro et al. Asthma with sulfite intolerance in children: a blocking study with cyanocobalamin. *J Allergy Clin Immunol*. 1992 Jul;90(1):103-9
[481] Fujita et al. A fatal case of acute hydrogen sulfide poisoning caused by hydrogen sulfide: hydroxocobalamin therapy for acute H2S poisoning. *J Anal Toxicol*. 2011 Mar:119-23

metabolism of homocysteine, which then triggers pain sensitivity and accelerated neurodegeneration via activation of NMDA receptors in the brain.

- Patients with FM and CFS have decreased vitamin B12 and increased homocysteine in the fluid surrounding the brain while blood test results are generally normal. (*Scand J Rheumatol.* 1997[482]): "Twelve outpatients, all women, who fulfilled the criteria for both fibromyalgia and chronic fatigue syndrome were rated on 15 items of the Comprehensive Psychopathological Rating Scale (CPRS-15). ... Blood laboratory levels were generally normal. The most obvious finding was that, in all the patients, the homocysteine (HCY) levels were increased in the cerebrospinal fluid (CSF). There was a significant positive correlation between CSF-HCY levels and fatigability, and the levels of CSF-B12 correlated significantly with the item of fatigability and with CPRS-15. The correlations between vitamin B12 and clinical variables of the CPRS-scale in this study indicate that low CSF-B12 values are of clinical importance. Vitamin B12 deficiency causes a deficient remethylation of HCY and is therefore probably contributing to the increased homocysteine levels found in our patient group. We conclude that increased homocysteine levels in the central nervous system characterize patients fulfilling the criteria for both fibromyalgia and chronic fatigue syndrome."

- Folic acid in the form of folinic acid or methylfolate ("5-methyltetrahydrofolate" or "5-MTHF"): Most nutrition-knowledgeable doctors do not use "folic acid" in the form of folic acid due to concerns about increased free radical generation and possible increased risk of cellular damage and malignant disease; we still use the term "folic acid" but nowadays this is—in practice—meant to imply the use of either folinic acid or methylfolate, two forms of folic acid that are considered safer, if not also more effective. Strictly speaking, "folic acid" refers to the synthetic form of the vitamin, whereas "folate" refers to derivatives of tetrahydrofolate that are found in food, especially leafy green vegetables, of which most people do not consume a sufficient amount. Some people develop antibodies against the folic acid transporter (cerebral folate receptor autoantibodies) that facilitates entry of folate into the brain, and they must receive either folinic acid or methylfolate to avoid neurologic devastation due to cerebral folate deficiency, wherein blood/serum levels of folate are normal but the brain (on the other side of the "wall" formed by the blood-brain barrier) is starved for this nutrient.[483] Folic acid from diet and/or supplementation serves many roles and thereby provides numerous benefits, largely centered on the provision of single-carbon methyl groups for metabolic processes (e.g., homocysteine metabolism) and DNA methylation, which regulates/suppresses gene transcription and thereby reduces risk of cancer and viral activation (e.g., cervical cancer following exposure to the human papilloma virus [HPV][484]). In this conversation, we are primarily concerned with optimizing folate intake to optimize "neurologic function" (i.e., generally speaking: normalization of homocysteine-mediated NMDAr activation in the brain, spinal cord and periphery) by reducing homocysteine levels because elevated homocysteine levels will cause excessive pain/fatigue/depression due to activation of the NMDA-receptor, mostly in the brain but also in the periphery. The most important nutrients for reducing homocysteine are folate (vitamin B9), pyridoxine (vitamin B6), cobalamin (vitamin B12) and the amino acid N-acetyl-cysteine (NAC); some people have a defect in their ability to convert folate into its active form via the enzyme methylenetetrahydrofolate reductase (MTHFR) and therefore need more nutritional supplementation to push this sluggish pathway to metabolic completion and reduce/normalize homocysteine levels. Increased consumption of folate from diet and/or supplements can alleviate depression, fatigue, and pain and is therefore recommended for all "pain patients", including those with migraine, fibromyalgia, and chronic fatigue syndrome. Adult doses of folate 1-5 mg (1,000-5,000 mcg) per day are reasonable and should be coadministered with a roughly equal amount of vitamin B12. Anti-seizure drugs (especially phenytoin, carbamazepine, barbiturates[485]), some of which are used in the treatment of

[482] Regland et al. Increased concentrations of homocysteine in the cerebrospinal fluid in patients with fibromyalgia and chronic fatigue syndrome. *Scand J Rheumatol.* 1997;26(4):301-7
[483] Gordon N. Cerebral folate deficiency. *Dev Med Child Neurol.* 2009 Mar;51(3):180-2
[484] Piyathilake et al. Indian women with higher serum concentrations of folate and vitamin B12 are significantly less likely to be infected with carcinogenic or high-risk (HR) types of human papillomaviruses (HPVs). *Int J Womens Health.* 2010 Aug 9;2:7-12
[485] Morrell MJ. Folic Acid and Epilepsy. *Epilepsy Curr.* 2002 Mar;2(2):31-34

migraine and chronic pain, are notorious for causing folate deficiency and homocysteine elevation[486]; obviously, the drugs would paradoxically promote pain and seizure if folate deficiency develops—coadministration of folate with anti-seizure drugs should be supervised by the prescribing physician. Diagrams illustrating these pathways tend to be repulsively complex, immemorably curvaceous, or incomplete and thereby unusable; the illustration below is perhaps the most simple for efficient understanding of the means by which nutritional supplementation lowers homocysteine levels.

- ▪ <u>Positive response to vitamin B12 and folic acid in myalgic encephalomyelitis and fibromyalgia</u> (*PLoS One.* 2015 Apr[487]): "The individual doses of B12 and folic acid, as well as the form of B12 used (i.e. hydroxocobalamin or methylcobalamin), had been due to individual decisions made by the five doctors in interplay with their patients – to a large extent following common sense in a process of trial and error – and limited by the patient's desire and the doctor's permission. It was a general experience that the patients deteriorated when returning to oral treatment, or when the injection interval was prolonged. After such a dose-finding period, they continued injective B12 therapy and learned how to self-administer the injections. In Sweden, the common form of B12 injective substrate has for more than forty years been hydroxocobalamin, provided in 1 mL ampoules with 1 mg/mL. By the end of last century, also methylcobalamin became available, in 2 mL ampoules with 5 mg/mL; i.e. an ampoule of methylcobalamin contains ten times more cobalamin than an ampoule of hydroxocobalamin. Folate in pharmacological doses is available by using tablets of folic acid (1 mg or 5 mg). ... Frequent injections of high-concentrated vitamin B12, combined with an individual daily dose of oral folic acid, may provide blood saturations high enough to be a remedy for good and safe relief in a subgroup of patients with ME/FM. Moreover, we suspect a counteracting interference between B12/folic acid and certain opioid analgesics and other drugs which have to be demethylated as part of their metabolism. Furthermore, it is important to be alert on co-existing thyroid dysfunction."

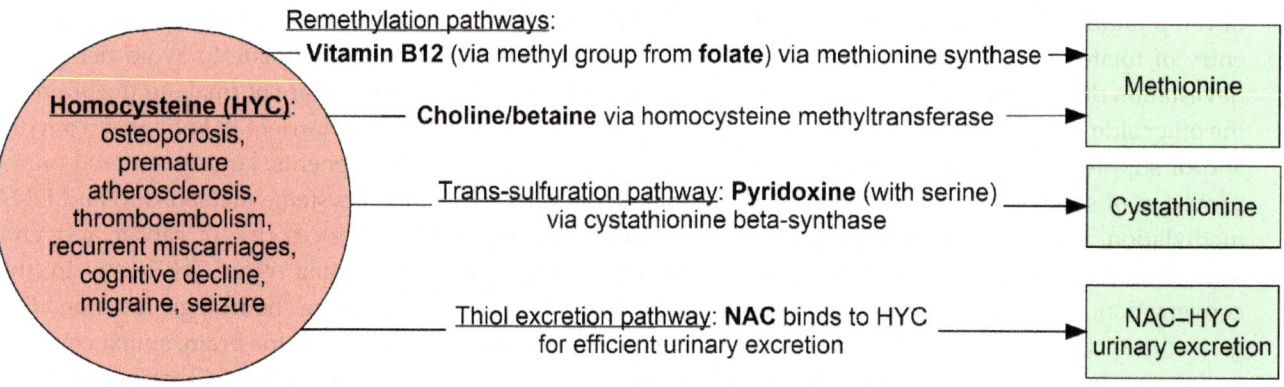

Lowering homocysteine (HYC) via nutritional supplementation: Folate gives methyl group to cobalamin (vitamin B12) to convert HYC via methionine synthase to methionine; choline/betaine can remethylate homocysteine via homocysteine methyltransferase to form methionine. Pyridoxine promotes conversion of HYC via cystathionine beta-synthase to cystathionine. The amino acid N-acetyl-cysteine (NAC) binds to HYC for efficient renal excretion of NAC-HYC.[488]

- ● **Tryptophan and 5-hydroxytryptophan (5-HTP):** Tryptophan is an amino acid found in many foods and is essential for human health and survival. Tryptophan is available as a nutritional supplement only by a doctor's prescription; it is available over-the-counter in a nonprescription supplement in the form of 5-hydroxytryptophan (5-HTP), which is commonly sourced from the seeds of *Griffonia simplicifolia*, a woody climbing shrub native to West and Central Africa. Tryptophan is the precursor to the neurotransmitter serotonin, which has antidepressant, anti-anxiety, and analgesic properties. Patients with FM are known to have low blood levels (i.e., functional nutritional insufficiency) of tryptophan, and the severity of the deficiency

---

[486] "Patients who consume antiepileptic drugs are susceptible to high levels of homocysteine and low levels of folate in the blood." Paknahad et al. Effects of Common Anti-epileptic Drugs on the Serum Levels of Homocysteine and Folic Acid. *Int J Prev Med.* 2012 Mar;3(Suppl 1):S186-90
[487] Regland et al. Response to vitamin B12 and folic acid in myalgic encephalomyelitis and fibromyalgia. *PLoS One.* 2015 Apr 22;10(4):e0124648
[488] "NAC intravenous administration induces an efficient and rapid reduction of plasma thiols, particularly of Hcy; our data support the hypothesis that NAC displaces thiols from their binding protein sites and forms, in excess of plasma NAC, mixed disulphides (NAC-Hcy) with an high renal clearance." Ventura et al. N-Acetyl-cysteine reduces homocysteine plasma levels after single intravenous administration by increasing thiols urinary excretion. *Pharmacol Res.* 1999 Oct;40(4):345-50

correlates with the severity of pain.[489,490,491] Blood levels of serotonin are often below normal in FM patients.[492] The accepted *medical-pharmacological* use of selective serotonin reuptake inhibitors (SSRI) drugs to treat the pain, depression, and anxiety associated with FM supports the use of 5-HTP to raise serotonin levels *naturally* by correcting the underlying nutritional insufficiency. As an over-the-counter nutritional supplement, the 5-hydroxylated form of tryptophan (5-HTP) has been used clinically and in numerous research studies. **Supplementation with 5-HTP has been shown to significantly alleviate symptoms of fibromyalgia.**[493] Commonly used doses range from 50 to 300 mg/d, with larger doses divided throughout the day. If tryptophan rather than 5-HTP is used, results are improved when taken on an empty stomach with carbohydrate (such as honey or fruit juice) to induce insulin secretion, which preferentially promotes uptake of tryptophan into the brain. Deficiency of either magnesium or vitamin B6 impairs conversion of 5-HTP into serotonin, and therefore the interventional program must ensure nutritional supra-sufficiency.

- Primary fibromyalgia syndrome and 5-hydroxy-L-tryptophan: a 90-day open study (*Journal of Internal Medicine Research* 1992 Apr[494]): An open 90-day study in 50 fibromyalgia patients showed significant improvement in all measured parameters (number of tender points, anxiety, pain intensity, quality of sleep, fatigue) after treatment with 5-HTP; global clinical improvement assessed by the patient and the investigator indicated a "good" or "fair" response in nearly 50% of the patients during the treatment period.

- Double-blind study of 5-hydroxytryptophan versus placebo in the treatment of primary fibromyalgia syndrome (*Journal of Internal Medicine Research* 1990 May-Jun[495]): A double-blind, placebo-controlled study using 5-HTP in 50 fibromyalgia patients showed significant improvement in all measured parameters, with only mild and transient side effects. *Note by DrV: Again, the common dose range for 5-HTP is 50 to 300 mg per day with doses greater than 100 mg generally best divided throughout the day (e.g., 50 mg thrice per day). I generally recommend starting with 50-100 mg about one hour before bedtime, then adding incremental additions of 50 mg throughout the day for a maximum daily dose of 300 mg. Effectiveness is increased with additional supplementation with magnesium, vitamin B6 (pyridoxine), and the fatty acids found in fish oil (EPA and DHA).*

- Magnesium: Magnesium deficiency is epidemic in industrialized societies due to insufficient dietary intake (e.g., from mineral water and leafy green vegetables) and concomitant metabolic-urinary acidosis, which increases urinary magnesium loss.[496,497] Additional causes of magnesium deficiency in fibromyalgia patients include vitamin D deficiency, malabsorption due to SIBO, and the stress of chronic illness. Magnesium deficiency exacerbates the symptoms of fibromyalgia by contributing to impairment of energy/ATP production in skeletal muscle, increased muscle tone and spasms (hypomagnesemic tetany), and anxiety and increased pain sensitivity—hyperalgesia via NMDA receptor overstimulation and neurocortical hyperexcitability. Magnesium deficiency also promotes constipation and intestinal stasis, which exacerbates SIBO. Magnesium supplementation (600 mg or to bowel tolerance to a limit of 1,500 mg in divided doses [bowel tolerance is defined as the dose—commonly of magnesium or vitamin C—that produces slightly loose stools due to the osmotic laxative effect]) should be used routinely in fibromyalgia patients; the primary cautions with magnesium use are renal insufficiency and the use of magnesium-sparing drugs such as the diuretic drug spironolactone. Modest benefits demonstrated in clinical trials with magnesium and malic acid[498] can easily be exceeded with concomitant interventions to address vitamin D deficiency, SIBO, and mitochondrial dysfunction.

- Vitamin C, ascorbate: Textbooks[499] and recent metaanalyses[500,501] consistently advocate use of ascorbic acid (ascorbate) 500-1,500 mg/d x50 days for the prevention of CRPS following trauma or surgery, especially to/of

[489] Moldofsky H, Warsh JJ. Plasma tryptophan and musculoskeletal pain in non-articular rheumatism ("fibrositis syndrome"). *Pain*. 1978 Jun;5(1):65-71

[490] Yunus MB, Dailey JW, Aldag JC, Masi AT, Jobe PC. Plasma tryptophan and other amino acids in primary fibromyalgia: a controlled study. *J Rheumatol*. 1992 Jan;19(1):90-4

[491] Russell IJ, Michalek JE, Vipraio GA, Fletcher EM, Wall K. Serum amino acids in fibrositis/fibromyalgia syndrome. *J Rheumatol* Suppl. 1989 Nov;19:158-63

[492] Wolfe F, Russell IJ, Vipraio G, Ross K, Anderson J. Serotonin levels, pain threshold, and fibromyalgia symptoms in the general population. *J Rheumatol*. 1997;24(3):555-9

[493] Caruso I, et al. Double-blind study of 5-hydroxytryptophan versus placebo in the treatment of primary fibromyalgia syndrome. *J Int Med Res*. 1990 May-Jun;18(3):201-9

[494] Sarzi Puttini P, Caruso I. Primary fibromyalgia syndrome and 5-hydroxy-L-tryptophan: a 90-day open study. *J Int Med Res*. 1992 Apr;20(2):182-9

[495] Caruso I et al. Double-blind study of 5-hydroxytryptophan versus placebo in the treatment of primary fibromyalgia syndrome. *J Int Med Res*. 1990 May-Jun;18(3):201-9

[496] Cordain L, et al. Origins and evolution of the Western diet: health implications for the 21st century. *Am J Clin Nutr*. 2005 Feb;81(2):341-54

[497] Rylander R, Remer T, Berkemeyer S, Vormann J. Acid-base status affects renal magnesium losses in healthy, elderly persons. *J Nutr*. 2006 Sep;136(9):2374-7

[498] Russell et al. Treatment of fibromyalgia syndrome with Super Malic: randomized, double blind, placebo controlled, crossover pilot study. *J Rheumatol*. 1995 May;22(5):953-8

[499] Papadakis, Maxine; McPhee, Stephen J.; Rabow, Michael W. *Current Medical Diagnosis and Treatment 2014*. McGraw-Hill Education.

[500] Shibuya et al. Efficacy and safety of high-dose vitamin C on complex regional pain syndrome in extremity trauma and surgery. *J Foot Ankle Surg*. 2013 Jan-Feb;52(1):62-6

[501] Meena et al. Role of vitamin C in prevention of complex regional pain syndrome after distal radius fractures. *Eur J Orthop Surg Traumatol*. 2015 May;25(4):637-41

the upper or lower limb. Mechanisms of action include the antioxidant effect[502] (thereby protecting the microvasculature following trauma) and the healing effect (promotion of bone and connective tissue repair, via hydroxyproline). Ascorbate also promotes mitochondrial function at cytochrome c, between complexes 3 and 4. My personal hypothesis is that ascorbate provides analgesic benefits via enhancement of central dopaminergic mechanisms and—via its ability to lower histamine levels (38% reduction following oral administration of ascorbate 2g/d)[503]—alleviation of neurogenic inflammation's vicious cycle, within which histamine plays a major role.[504] Appreciating its safety and efficacy in treating neuropathic, postsurgical, and migraine pain[505,506], I think all patients with pain should receive ascorbate 2-6 grams daily in divided doses. Two potential contraindications to vitamin C supplementation are iron overload and renal insufficiency.

- S-adenosylmethionine (SAMe): Studies using oral or intravenous administration of the nutritional supplement SAMe have reported conflicting results; however, the overall trend seems to indicate that SAMe (800 mg/d orally) is safe and beneficial in the treatment of fibromyalgia.[507] SAMe helps maintain mitochondrial function by preserving glutathione, and its contribution of methyl groups is important for the regulation of gene expression and neurotransmitter synthesis. *Comment: I do not regularly use this supplement, and I would only use it as a last resort if nothing else had worked or if a particular patient had a specific indication for this supplement.*

INFECTIONS & DYSBIOSIS As reviewed in a previous section, fibromyalgia patients have a remarkably high prevalence of occult SIBO, the severity of which directly correlates with the severity of FM symptomatology and the eradication of which directly correlates with alleviation of FM. SIBO is the single primary pathoetiologic mechanism that explains each and every abnormality seen in this condition; the response of fibromyalgia patients to gastrointestinal-specific nonabsorbable antimicrobial treatments such as rifaximin provides diagnostic proof of effective treatment of the causative SIBO. Jejunal aspiration is expensive, inconvenient, cumbersome, invasive, and not completely sensitive, while breath hydrogen and methane testing is also cumbersome and relatively expensive (especially when compared to making a clinical diagnosis and confirmatory treatment) and is likewise not completely reliable. Post-prandial gas and bloating is a reliable clinical indicator of SIBO, and empiric treatment of SIBO with a low-carbohydrate diet (LCD) and antimicrobial agents that results in clinical improvement (which may include alleviation of musculoskeletal pain, improved cognition, alleviation of fatigue, and—especially in elderly patients—alleviation of malabsorption and malnutrition) confirms the diagnosis. Stated more plainly, effective implementation of LCD with antimicrobial treatment is both diagnostic and therapeutic; this allows the diagnosis to be made efficiently and with high specificity, (sensitivity depends upon efficacy) and bypassing expensive/insensitive/nontherapeutic/cumbersome diagnostic methods expedites physicians' efficacy and patients' relief in a manner that is safe and cost-effective, especially when compared to perpetual nontherapeutic symptomatic polypharmacy.

- **Low-carbohydrate diet, specific-carbohydrate diet**: Patients can follow a diet that emphasizes consumption of low-carbohydrate vegetables, nuts, and seeds and excludes grains (especially wheat, which is very highly fermentable), starches from foods such as potatoes, and disaccharides such as lactose and sucrose; most of the characteristics of a competent low-carbohydrate diet can be achieved within a "Paleo diet" such as described and popularized by Cordain. Alternatively or additionally, patients can follow the specific-carbohydrate diet described and popularized by Gottschall.

- **Probiotics**: Probiotics are beneficial bacteria that can be consumed in foods or as nutritional supplements to populate the gut, particularly following antibiotic use or long-term dietary neglect. In addition to their availability in capsules and powders, probiotics are widely consumed in the form of yogurt, kefir, and other cultured foods, and they have an excellent record of safety. Probiotic supplements are available in different strengths (quantity), potencies (viability), and combinations of bacteria (diversity). Some probiotics also contain fermentable carbohydrates (prebiotics) such as fructooligosaccharides (FOS) and inulin, which are substrates to nourish the beneficial bacteria. From a practical clinical perspective, the clinician can choose probiotic foods and supplements and instruct the patient to use these on an ongoing, periodic, or rotational basis. Probiotics

502 Kapoor S. Vitamin C and its emerging role in pain management: beneficial effects in pain conditions besides post herpetic neuralgia. *Korean J Pain.* 2012 Jul;25(3):200-1
503 Johnston CS, Martin LJ, Cai X. Antihistamine effect of supplemental ascorbic acid and neutrophil chemotaxis. *J Am Coll Nutr.* 1992 Apr;11(2):172-6
504 Rosa AC, Fantozzi R. The role of histamine in neurogenic inflammation. *Br J Pharmacol.* 2013 Sep;170(1):38-45
505 Hasanzadeh Kiabi et al. Can vitamin C be used as an adjuvant for managing postoperative pain? A short literature review. *Korean J Pain.* 2013 Apr;26(2):209-10
506 Mohseni M. Use of vitamin C as placebo in anesthesiology. *Anesth Pain Med.* 2013 Winter;2(3):141
507 Leventhal LJ. Management of fibromyalgia. *Ann Intern Med.* 1999 Dec 7;131(11):850-8

(i.e., bacteria only) may have a therapeutic advantage over prebiotics or synbiotics (probiotics+prebiotics) when treating SIBO because the fermentable carbohydrate in prebiotics and synbiotics may exacerbate the preexisting bacterial overgrowth by providing already overpopulated bacteria with additional substrate. The benefits of probiotic supplementation have been demonstrated in patients with IBS, rotavirus infection, eczema and increased intestinal permeability, and SIBO associated with renal failure. To date, no studies using probiotics in the treatment of fibromyalgia have been published.

- **Antimicrobial agents**: Antimicrobial agents can be categorized as either natural or pharmaceutical, and as absorbable and systemic or nonabsorbable and gastrointestinal-specific. These can be used empirically, as such treatment for suspected SIBO is well documented in the peer-reviewed clinical medicine literature; however, clinicians must always consider risk-to-benefit ratios especially when using the pharmaceutical antimicrobials which can induce systemic adverse effects (e.g., drug allergy or Stevens-Johnson syndrome or quinolone tendonopathy) or gastrointestinal adverse effects (e.g., nonspecific diarrhea, yeast overgrowth, *Clostridium difficile* diarrhea). Clinicians must always determine the proper choice and dose of therapeutic agents per patient. Two of the best and most important articles on the subject of SIBO are "Lin HC. Small intestinal bacterial overgrowth: a framework for understanding irritable bowel syndrome. *JAMA* 2004 Aug" (concepts and system-wide pathophysiology) and "Malik et al. Diagnosis and pharmacological management of small intestinal bacterial overgrowth in children with intestinal failure. *Can J Gastroenterol* 2011 Jan" (excellent sections on clinical diagnosis and pharmacologic management emphasizing rotational implementation of gut-specific antimicrobials). I prefer to use natural antimicrobial agents continuously for an extended period of time either alone or in conjunction with pharmaceutical antibacterial drugs, which I tend to use on a rotating basis of 7-14 days. Occasionally I will use a short course of an antiparasitic drug such as metronidazole or tinidazole, and I nearly always implement an extended course of antifungal treatment—either oregano oil or nystatin as nonabsorbable agents—punctuated by fluconazole/Diflucan if I suspect treatment resistant gastrointestinal yeast or any dermatologic or sinorespiratory yeast. Clinicians should appreciate that *yeast* colonization of the intestines promotes *bacterial* colonization of the intestines via—for example—elaboration by *Candida albicans* of a sIgA-protease and gliotoxin, an appreciated immunosuppressant. The following list emphasizes the antimicrobial agents I most commonly utilize, always in conjunction with nutritional supplementation (to restore immune function and mucosal defenses) and reduction in dietary carbohydrate intake (to reduce fermentable substrate and thereby "starve the microbes"). Although some dosage and duration suggestions are provided, the clinical reality is that patients need to be treated with *"dose and duration to effect"* or *"titrate to effect"*—meaning that the milligram dose per day and the duration of treatment can and should be customized per the patient's response to treatment. Combination therapy (i.e., more than one treatment at a time), prolonged therapy (treatment of chronic [poly]dysbiosis generally requires longer duration of treatment than does treatment of acute monomicrobial infections), and periodic/punctual treatment (for exacerbations and recurrences).

  - <u>Clinical support favoring "open label" empiric antimicrobial treatment of SIBO in patients with fibromyalgia (*Current Pain and Headache Reports* 2004 Oct[508])</u>: This article discusses the results of two experiments using antibiotics in the treatment of FM: ❶ 96 patients with SIBO diagnosed by lactulose hydrogen breath testing (LHBT) were offered **antibiotic treatment** for the reduction of gastrointestinal bacteria; 25 of the 96 patients returned for a follow-up LHBT. **Neomycin** was the most commonly used antibiotic. Eleven of the 25 patients achieved complete transient eradication of SIBO after antibiotic treatment and experienced better improvement in more of their FM symptom scores when compared with the patients who did not achieve complete eradication. This indicates that a direct relationship exists between the presence of SIBO and intestinal and extraintestinal symptoms in fibromyalgia, and that FM can be alleviated by effective antimicrobial/antibiotic treatment. ❷ In this double-blind trial of eradication of SIBO in fibromyalgia, 46 patients fulfilling the established criteria for FM were tested for SIBO using LHBT. Forty-two of the 46 patients (91.3%) were positive for SIBO and were randomized to receive placebo or 500 mg of **liquid neomycin** (a minimally-absorbed gastrointestinal-specific antibiotic drug) twice daily

[508] Wallace DJ, Hallegua DS. Fibromyalgia: the gastrointestinal link. *Curr Pain Headache Rep.* 2004 Oct;8(5):364-8

for 10 days. Only six of the 20 patients (30%) in the neomycin group achieved eradication (indicating inefficacy of treatment); thus, no statistically significant difference between groups was available for analysis. Thereafter, 28 patients in the double-blind study testing positive for SIBO went on to receive **open-label antibiotic treatment** to eradicate SIBO, and this time 17 of the 28 patients (60.7%) achieved eradication of SIBO. When these 23 patients were compared with the 15 patients who failed to eradicate or did not undergo open-label treatment, significant improvement attributable to antibiotic treatment in the FM scores was detected. Results suggest that eradication of bacterial overgrowth results in a statistically and clinically significant alleviation of FM symptoms.

- Nonprescription antimicrobial agents—examples: Most of the agents listed below have their primary or exclusive area of effectiveness within the lumen of the gastrointestinal tract. These agents are generally broad-spectrum and nonspecific, which is perfectly appropriate when treating nonspecific SIBO.

- Prescription-restricted antimicrobial agents—examples: In this section specific for the SIBO of fibromyalgia, nonabsorbable agents (rifaximin, vancomycin, nystatin) are appropriate; agents with systemic absorption (Augmentin and fluconazole) are listed here due to their high efficacy and frequent clinical utilization.

  □ Rifaximin/Xifaxan: Rifaximin (gut-specific antibacterial drug) should not be confused with rifampin (systemic antibacterial drug, often used in the treatment of mycobacterium infections such as tuberculosis but also used for other bacterial infections); remember to "get your **facts/fax** right by using ri**fax**imin/Xi**fax**an" while you "use ri**famp**in **to ampl**ify the effectiveness of systemic antibiotics in the treatment of chronic infections but it also **amps up** cytochrome p450 and adverse drug effects."

  □ Vancomycin orally administered: Clinicians should consider this non/poorly-absorbed antibiotic which is effective against Gram-positive bacteria. Human studies have shown effectiveness in the treatment of IBS, constipation, and primary sclerosing cholangitis. In one particularly remarkable case of a patient with rheumatoid arthritis, I prescribed 125mg/d with great success with the intention to target Gram-positive Th17-inducing segmented filamentous bacteria.

> **A practical summary of SIBO: small intestine bacterial overgrowth**
>
> 1. Definition: Generalized nonspecific overpopulation of bacteria (commonly with other microbes such as yeast) in the small intestine (and large intestine, too).
> 2. Frequency: Very common in clinical practice and the general population.
> 3. Primary symptoms: Gas and bloating, especially after carbohydrate consumption; may also have constipation and/or diarrhea.
> 4. Secondary symptoms: Fatigue, muscle aches, difficulty with concentration and cognition ("brain fog"), nutritional deficiencies due to malabsorption, immune activation due to absorption of microbial debris and metabolites, muscle pain due to dysbiotic mitochondriopathy and LPS- and cytokine-induced central sensitization.
> 5. Diagnosis: ❶ Based on the symptoms above, ❷ jejunal aspiration is the gold standard but is expensive, cumbersome, and potentially hazardous, ❸ measurement of fermentation products (hydrogen and methane) in breath following consumption of a carbohydrate such as glucose, sucrose, or lactulose; the amount of "gas" produced is proportional to the bacterial population, ❹ may find elevated short chain fatty acids (SCFA) in stool or elevated folate in blood, but not all cases of SIBO produce high levels of SCFA or folate, ❺ clinical response to low-carbohydrate diet and/or antibiotic drugs or antimicrobial herbs. The current author (AV) uses #1 in conjunction with #5 most commonly.
> 6. Treatments: Low-carbohydrate diet with antibiotic drugs (e.g., Xifaxan/Rifaximin (200 or 550 mg each) 400-550 mg tid po [1,200-1,650 mg daily] for 10-30 days) or antimicrobial herbs (e.g., time-released emulsified oregano oil 600 mg daily for 4-6 weeks, and/or berberine 400-1,500 mg daily for 4-12 weeks). Restoration of normal flora with probiotics, plant-based dietary diversity and authentically fermented foods.

  □ Augmentin 1-2g BID: This combination of amoxicillin and clavulanate shows efficacy against more than 90% of gastrointestinal bacteria which contribute to SIBO.

  □ Nystatin 500,000 units BID-TID PO duration as needed (e.g., 1-6 months empirically or with any use of antibacterial drugs: Nystatin is a safe nonabsorbable gentle and commonly effective antifungal agent originally derived from a natural source of soil microorganisms. Its lack of significant intestinal absorption reduces the incidence of adverse effects while also prohibiting systemic antifungal effectiveness, except for reducing the total microbial load (TML) by reducing gastrointestinal fungal population. Nystatin is safe for long-term use, is inexpensive, and should generally be used anytime that antibiotic/antibacterial drugs are employed.

▫ <u>Fluconazole/Diflucan 100-150-200 mg every other day for 4-5 doses over 8-10 days</u>: The long half-life of 30 hours allows discontinuous alternate-day dosing without loss of efficacy for most routine outpatient applications. This drug is absorbed systemically with excellent tissue penetration for the delivery of multifocal antifungal effectiveness (e.g., alleviation of sinus and genitourinary fungal infections/colonization)

NUTRITIONAL IMMUNOMODULATION My use of the term and technique "nutritional immunomodulation" refers to a specific protocol designed to induce epigenetic modifications in undifferentiated Th-0 cells for their preferential promotion into the T-regulatory (Treg) FOXp3+ phenotype while shifting immune (im)balance away from the proinflammatory Th-1, Th-2, and Th-17 phenotypes. The primary components of this protocol can be safely implemented in essentially any and all patients without adverse effect; these fundamental components include low-carbohydrate plant-based diet to promote a systemic anti-inflammatory state, vitamin D3, combination fatty acid supplementation for n-3 fatty acids and GLA, probiotics (note that the first four components of the protocol are already represented in the foundational five-part nutritional protocol), vitamin A, lipoic acid, green tea, and a low-sodium diet. More assertive antidysbiotic interventions to promote healthy microbial balance in the gastrointestinal lumen may include botanical/nutritional/pharmacologic antimicrobial interventions, with some preferential utilization of orally administered vancomycin based on research supporting its effectiveness against segmented filamentous bacteria which are specific inducers of the Th-17 phenotype. Since fibromyalgia in its pure form is not directly due to an immune imbalance in the way considered here, this component of the functional inflammology protocol is not specifically relevant; however, for the many patients with concomitant diagnoses of fibromyalgia with another systemic/inflammatory/autoimmune disease (such as diabetes mellitus, rheumatoid arthritis, multiple sclerosis, or psoriasis) then of course this nutritional immunomodulation protocol should be implemented.

DYSFUNCTIONAL MITOCHONDRIA The basic view that mitochondria are the "powerhouses" of the cell responsible for the formation of cellular energy in the form of ATP is what most people learn in high school biology, and little if any additional knowledge is added to medical physicians' appreciation of the diversity of mitchondria's biologic roles in medical school. Lack of appreciation of the importance of the role of mitochondrial in general and mitochondrial dysfunction in particular in health and disease has left a huge blind spot in the therapeutic vision of most clinicians; by failing to appreciate and correct mitochondrial dysfunction, clinicians have missed a valuable component to the treatment plans of many and probably most of their patients. In addition to the well-known role that mitochondria have in the formation of energy/ATP, mitochondria also play major roles in pancreatic insulin secretion, peripheral insulin reception, microbial surveillance, and maintenance of inflammatory balance, insofar as mitochondrial dysfunction clearly contributes to a pro-diabetic and insulin-insulin resistant state, as well as enhanced pro-inflammatory responsiveness to microbial (including viral) stimuli. Fibromyalgia is clearly identified with mitochondrial dysfunction, and while the secondary mitochondrial dysfunction is one of the major causes of fibromyalgic muscle pain and fatigue, the mitochondrial dysfunction does not itself cause fibromyalgia, the primary cause of which is SIBO. Thus, SIBO's generation of LPS, D-lactate, and other mitochondrial toxins is the primary/direct cause of the mitochondrial dysfunction; effective treatment must emphasize SIBO eradication and mitochondrial resuscitation. We can compartmentalize major components of mitochondrial structure and function into these three main components: ❶ citric acid cycle, ❷ electron transport chain, ❸ and the structural integrity of the inner and outer mitochondrial membranes. The main area of clinical importance can be discussed within a conversation of the electron transport chain (ETC) since this is fed by the citric acid cycle and is structurally interwoven into the inner mitochondrial membrane and fully dependent upon the nonpermeability of the outer mitochondrial membrane for the maintenance of the electromechanical proton gradient. Primary treatment must always be directed at the primary cause of any disease—not its secondary complications; in the case of FM, the SIBO must always be treated. Among mitochondria-specific treatments for fibromyalgia, supplementation with CoQ10, melatonin, and acetyl-carnitine (preferably with lipoic acid) are the best studied and most efficacious.

- <u>Coenzyme Q10 (CoQ10)</u>: An endogenous antioxidant, vitamin-like substance, and essential component of the mitochondrial electron transport chain, oral supplementation with CoQ10 has been used therapeutically in numerous studies for the successful treatment of migraine, heart failure, hypertension, and renal failure. Additional data have shown immunomodulatory roles for CoQ10, and many clinicians employ it as adjunctive treatment for viral infections, cancer, and allergies.[509,510] The electron transport chain is the terminal step in mitochondrial energy/ATP production; as readers can see in the following diagram, each step or "complex" of the electron transport chain requires nutrients, without which energy/ATP production will be impaired, and provision of which (via supplementation) will generally enhance mitochondrial energy/ATP production. Per Cordero et al[511] in 2012, **CoQ10 levels are 40% lower in blood cells of patients with FM compared with levels in healthy persons**, and reduced levels of CoQ10 correlate with markers associated with expedited destruction of mitochondria (mitophagy).
  - <u>Clinical investigation: Mitochondrial dysfunction and mitophagy activation in blood mononuclear cells of fibromyalgia patients</u> (*Arthritis Research Therapy* 2010 Jan[512]): The authors studied 2 male and 18 female FM patients and 10 healthy controls. They evaluated mitochondrial function in blood mononuclear cells from FM patients measuring CoQ10 levels with high-performance liquid chromatography (HPLC) and measuring mitochondrial membrane potential with flow cytometry. Oxidative stress was determined by measuring mitochondrial superoxide production and lipid peroxidation in blood mononuclear cells and plasma from FM patients. Autophagy activation was evaluated in blood mononuclear cells; mitophagy was confirmed by measuring citrate synthase activity and electron microscopy examination of blood mononuclear cells. The authors **found reduced levels of CoQ10, decreased mitochondrial membrane potential, increased levels of mitochondrial superoxide in blood mononuclear cells (indicating increased oxidative stress and reduced antioxidant defense),** and increased levels of lipid peroxidation in both blood mononuclear cells and plasma from FM patients. Importantly, the authors note that "mitochondrial dysfunction was also associated with increased expression of autophagic genes and the elimination of dysfunctional mitochondria with mitophagy." *What this means in practical terms is that the biochemical aberrations that cause mitochondrial dysfunction lead to destruction of mitochondria via "mitophagy" which literally means "mitochondrial consumption", a process by which dysfunctional mitochondria are eliminated by degradative processes.*
  - <u>Case series of FM patients treated with CoQ10</u> (*Mitochondrion* 2011 Jul[513]): The authors note that CoQ10 is an essential electron carrier in the mitochondrial respiratory chain and a strong antioxidant and that **low CoQ10 levels have been detected in patients with FM.** The authors found that "**FM patients with CoQ10 deficiency showed a statistically significant reduction in symptoms after CoQ10 treatment during 9 months (300 mg/day).** Determination of deficiency and consequent supplementation in FM may result in clinical improvement." *This is a small but important study documenting 1) that CoQ10 deficiency is common in FM patients, and 2) that CoQ10 supplementation alleviates the clinical manifestations/symptoms of FM, consistent with the integrated model of FM presented in this book, which includes the components of nutrient deficiency and mitochondrial dysfunction. Although standardized blood testing for CoQ10 levels is widely available, testing for and documentation of CoQ10 deficiency is not necessary before the use of CoQ10 supplementation.*
  - <u>Clinical trial using a combination of *Ginkgo biloba* and CoQ10</u> (*Journal of Internal Medicine Research* 2002 Mar[514]): In an open trial of 23 fibromyalgia patients, the combination of 200 mg CoQ10 and 200 mg *Ginkgo biloba* (for a total dose of 48 mg flavone glycosides and 12 mg terpene lactones) daily for 84 days was shown to provide clinical benefit in 64% of patients. CoQ10 is often deficient in FM patients, and this deficiency both *causes* and *results from* mitochondrial dysfunction; stated differently, CoQ10 depletion and mitochondrial dysfunction form a vicious cycle, a relationship of reciprocal causality. *Ginkgo biloba* extract is an extensively researched botanical medicine with a long history of safe and effective clinical use for various conditions, especially those associated with reduced blood flow and impaired mitochondrial

[509] Gaby AR. The role of Coenzyme Q10 in clinical medicine: Part 1. *Altern Med Rev* 1996;1:11-17

[510] Gaby AR. The role of Coenzyme Q10 in clinical medicine: Part 2. *Altern Med Rev* 1996;1:168-175

[511] Cordero MD, De Miguel M, Moreno Fernández AM, et al. Mitochondrial dysfunction and mitophagy activation in blood mononuclear cells of fibromyalgia patients: implications in the pathogenesis of the disease. *Arthritis Res Ther.* 2010;12(1):R17

[512] Cordero et al. Mitochondrial dysfunction and mitophagy activation in blood mononuclear cells of fibromyalgia patients. *Arthritis Res Ther.* 2010;12(1):R17

[513] Cordero MD et al. Coenzyme Q(10): a novel therapeutic approach for Fibromyalgia? case series with 5 patients. *Mitochondrion.* 2011 Jul;11(4):623-5

[514] Lister. Open, pilot study to evaluate potential benefits of coenzyme Q10 combined with Ginkgo biloba extract in fibromyalgia syndrome. *J Int Med Res* 2002 Mar-Apr;30:195-9

function. *Ginkgo biloba* is a botanical/herbal medicine with a long history of human use; the three most important physiologic effects of *Ginkgo biloba* are ❶ vasodilation—improves blood circulation (which is often compromised in FM patients), ❷ improves mitochondrial function and ATP/energy production, and ❸ antioxidant benefits—quenches/absorbs free radicals, which are oxygen-containing molecules that cause damage to cell structures and body tissues. Given these therapeutic benefits, *Ginkgo* would appear to be a reasonable therapeutic agent to address the secondary pathophysiology in fibromyalgia. *Ginkgo biloba* products are generally standardized for the content of flavone glycosides (approximately 24%) and terpene lactones (approximately 6%) with adult doses ranging from 60-240 mg/d and generally 120 mg/d. *Comment by Dr Vasquez: Ginkgo biloba and CoQ10 are very safe and appropriate for use by nearly all FM patients.*

- <u>Clinical investigation and clinical trial: Oxidative stress, headache symptoms in fibromyalgia and the role of CoQ10 in clinical improvement (*PLoS One* 2012 Apr[515])</u>: The authors introduce this study by noting that FM is a chronic pain syndrome with "unknown etiology" and a wide spectrum of symptoms such as allodynia (perception of pain from stimuli that are not normally painful), debilitating fatigue, joint stiffness, and migraine headaches. The authors note a link between oxidative stress and the clinical symptoms in FM. In this study, the researchers examined oxidative stress and bioenergetic status in blood mononuclear cells (BMCs) and the association with headache symptoms in FM patients. Following this correlative analysis, the authors assessed the effects of oral CoQ10 supplementation on biochemical markers and clinical improvements. In 20 FM patients and 15 healthy controls, a variety of validated clinical and biochemical parameters was assessed; specifically for the biochemical component, measurements were performed for serum CoQ10, catalase, lipid peroxidation (LPO) levels and ATP levels in BMCs. In patients with FM, the authors found lower CoQ10 (CoQ10 deficiency), lower catalase (reduced antioxidant defenses) and lower ATP levels (reduced energy production) in BMCs while FM patients also showed elevated LPO (evidence of free-radical damage) in BMCs. Lower levels of CoQ10 and catalase levels in BMCs correlated with greater severity-frequency of headache. **In this clinical trial using CoQ10 300 mg/d for 3 months, CoQ10 supplementation caused significant reductions in pain and tender points, significant reductions in headache impact, significant elevations in cellular levels of CoQ10, a reduction in malondialdehyde (marker of lipid peroxidation) from 30nmol to 5 nmol (normal 6 nmol), an increase in catalase levels from 35 U/mg to 85 U/mg (normal 96 U/mg), and an increase in BMC production of ATP/energy from 61 nmol/mg to 191 nmol/mg (normal 202 nmol/mg).** Supplementation with CoQ10 300 mg/day divided in three doses for 3 months "restored biochemical parameters and induced a significant improvement in clinical and headache symptoms." *Note by Dr Vasquez: The dose of CoQ10 used clinically is generally approximately 100 mg per day, and occasionally a patient or doctor might decide to use a higher dose, which might be up to 300 mg per day. Higher doses generally provide better results with excellent safety, but CoQ10 tends to be one of the most expensive nutritional supplements and as such the lowest effective dose—again approximately 100 mg/d as the standard—is used. Some patients will not respond to 100 mg/d and will respond well to 300 mg/d; these more challenging patients might also need additional/different treatments, such as supplementation with synergistic nutrients, hormonal correction, xenobiotic depuration, or assertive treatment of dysbiosis/SIBO.*

---

[515] Cordero et al. Oxidative stress correlates with headache symptoms in fibromyalgia: coenzyme Q₁₀ effect on clinical improvement. *PLoS One.* 2012;7(4):e35677

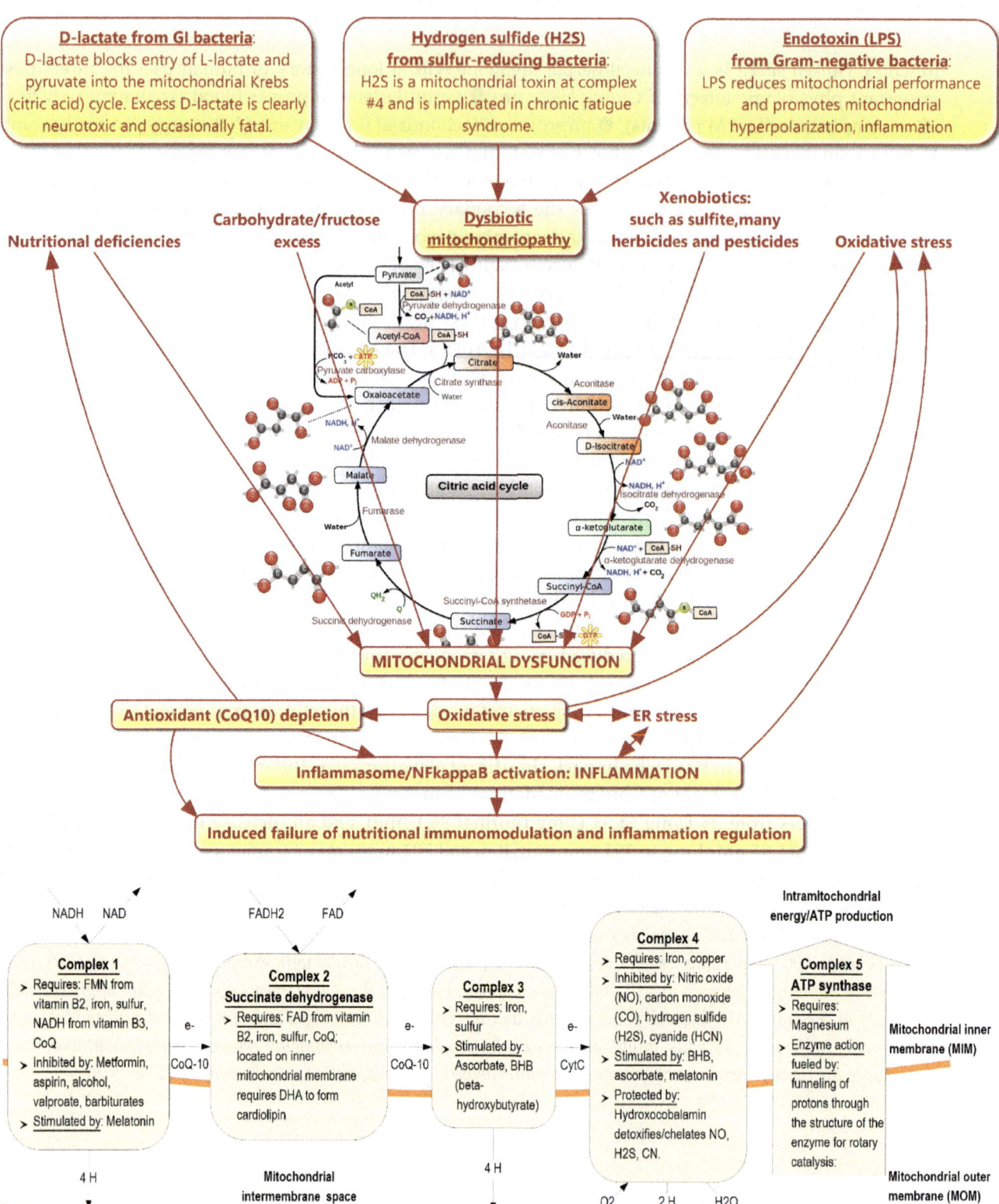

D-lactate from GI bacteria: D-lactate blocks entry of L-lactate and pyruvate into the mitochondrial Krebs (citric acid) cycle. Excess D-lactate is clearly neurotoxic and occasionally fatal.

Hydrogen sulfide (H2S) from sulfur-reducing bacteria: H2S is a mitochondrial toxin at complex #4 and is implicated in chronic fatigue syndrome.

Endotoxin (LPS) from Gram-negative bacteria: LPS reduces mitochondrial performance and promotes mitochondrial hyperpolarization, inflammation

Nutritional deficiencies

Carbohydrate/fructose excess

Dysbiotic mitochondriopathy

Xenobiotics: such as sulfite, many herbicides and pesticides

Oxidative stress

Citric acid cycle

MITOCHONDRIAL DYSFUNCTION

Antioxidant (CoQ10) depletion

Oxidative stress

ER stress

Inflammasome/NFkappaB activation: INFLAMMATION

Induced failure of nutritional immunomodulation and inflammation regulation

Intramitochondrial energy/ATP production

Complex 1
- Requires: FMN from vitamin B2, iron, sulfur, NADH from vitamin B3, CoQ
- Inhibited by: Metformin, aspirin, alcohol, valproate, barbiturates
- Stimulated by: Melatonin

Complex 2 Succinate dehydrogenase
- Requires: FAD from vitamin B2, iron, sulfur, CoQ; located on inner mitochondrial membrane requires DHA to form cardiolipin

Complex 3
- Requires: Iron, sulfur
- Stimulated by: Ascorbate, BHB (beta-hydroxybutyrate)

Complex 4
- Requires: Iron, copper
- Inhibited by: Nitric oxide (NO), carbon monoxide (CO), hydrogen sulfide (H2S), cyanide (HCN)
- Stimulated by: BHB, ascorbate, melatonin
- Protected by: Hydroxocobalamin detoxifies/chelates NO, H2S, CN.

Complex 5 ATP synthase
- Requires: Magnesium
- Enzyme action fueled by: funneling of protons through the structure of the enzyme for rotary catalysis:

Mitochondrial inner membrane (MIM)

Mitochondrial outer membrane (MOM)

Mitochondrial intermembrane space

Reduce mitochondrial protein synthesis: Tetracyclines, chloramphenicol

Cause mtDNA depletion: Adriamycin/doxorubicin, zidovudine, herpes simplex virus

Damage mitochondrial inner membrane: Roundup ® (mixture of glyphosate and solvent/inert chemicals) per *Environ Toxicol Pharmacol* 2012 Sep, *Toxicol In Vitro* 2013 Feb, *Toxicology* 2013 Nov

Microbial debris (LPS) and metabolites (D-lactate and H2S) and the subsequent inflammatory response lead to mitochondrial dysfunction: Nutritional deficiencies, genetic faults, and xenobiotic exposure/accumulation exacerbate mitochondrial impairment and also exacerbate the peripheral and central inflammatory responses. Copyright © 2015 by Dr Alex Vasquez. All rights reserved and enforced; this image may not be used, copied, or distributed without written permission. Citric acid cycle from en.wikipedia.org/wiki/Citric_acid_cycle. "Citric acid cycle with aconitate 2" by Narayanese, WikiUserPedia, YassineMrabet, TotoBaggins licensed under Creative Commons Attribution-Share Alike 3.0. See www.inflammationmastery.com/pain

- **NLRP3 inflammasome is activated in fibromyalgia and reduced by coenzyme Q10** (*Antioxid Redox Signal* 2014 Mar[516]): "Mitochondrial dysfunction was accompanied by increased protein expression of interleukin (IL)-1, NLRP3 (NOD-like receptor family, pyrin domain containing 3) and caspase-1 activation, and an increase of serum levels of proinflammatory cytokines (IL-1 and IL-18). CoQ10 deficiency induced by p-aminobenzoate treatment in blood mononuclear cells and mice showed NLRP3 inflammasome activation with marked algesia. A placebo-controlled trial of CoQ10 in FM patients has shown a reduced NLRP3 inflammasome activation and IL-1 and IL-18 serum levels. …CONCLUSION: These findings provide new insights into the pathogenesis of FM and suggest that NLRP3 inflammasome inhibition represents a new therapeutic intervention for the disease. … After CoQ10 supplementation [300 mg/day CoQ10 divided into three doses], NLRP3 and IL-1 gene were downregulated. … IL-1 and IL-18 serum levels were significantly reduced with respect to placebo." The most complete/consistent model of FMS is that it is caused by SIBO, leading to mitochondrial dysfunction, central sensitization, tryptophan/serotonin/melatonin deficiencies; these interconnections are illustrated later in this chapter and detailed elsewhere.[517]

  - **Mitochondrial dysfunction in CRPS**: Patients with CRPS show evidence of impaired oxygen diffusion and mitochondrial impairment[518], and Tan et al[519] specifically noted that mitochondrial ETC "complex II activity in the CRPS I patients was significantly lower." From a "mitochondrial micromanagement" perspective, one might consider the use of riboflavin 400 mg/d and CoQ10 100-300 mg/d to support ETC complex #2, but obviously the entire mitochondria—indeed the entire body—works together as a unit.

- Melatonin: Melatonin is a hormone produced in the pineal gland of the brain; melatonin is synthesized from the neurotransmitter serotonin, and production of both serotonin and melatonin are dependent on the nutritional availability of tryptophan and/or 5-HTP as discussed above. Patients with FM show decreased nocturnal secretion of melatonin.[520] Melatonin benefits FM patients through a wide range of mechanisms, including promotion of restful sleep and reduction in LPS-induced mitochondrial impairment. As a powerful antioxidant, melatonin scavenges oxygen and nitrogen-based reactants generated in mitochondria and thereby limits the loss of intramitochondrial glutathione, the most important component of antioxidant defense; this prevents damage to mitochondrial protein and DNA. **Melatonin increases the activity of Complexes 1 and 4 of the mitochondrial electron transport chain, improving mitochondrial respiration and increasing ATP synthesis** under various physiological and experimental conditions.[521] Successful treatment with melatonin or its precursor tryptophan/5-HTP should not deter the clinician from addressing other contributing or causative problems such as vitamin D deficiency, gastrointestinal dysbiosis including SIBO, magnesium deficiency, and chronic psychoemotional stress. The adult physiologic dose which mimics natural internal (endogenous) production is approximately 200-500 mcg [micrograms] nightly. In adults, supplementation with melatonin has a wide therapeutic index and is used safely and effectively in doses up to 20 to 40 mg [milligrams] nightly.

  - Case series (n=4): Melatonin therapy in fibromyalgia (*Journal of Pineal Research* 2006 Jan[522]): Melatonin (3–6 mg per night, administered orally 1 hour before bedtime) has been reported to normalize sleep, alleviate pain and fatigue, and resolve many other clinical manifestations of FM. The authors report, "After 15 days of treatment with melatonin, all patients developed a sleep/wake cycle that was considered normal. They also mentioned a significant reduction of pain. At this time, the patients were taken off hypnotics. Thirty days after the initiation of melatonin, other medications were withdrawn and thereafter they only took melatonin." *Comment by Dr Vasquez: These results are impressive, but—again—the other components of FM such*

---

[516] Cordero et al. NLRP3 inflammasome is activated in fibromyalgia: the effect of coenzyme Q10. *Antioxid Redox Signal.* 2014 Mar 10;20(8):1169-80

[517] Vasquez A. *Naturopathic Rheumatology and Integrative Inflammology v3.5,* 2014 and *Fibromyalgia in a Nutshell,* 2012

[518] "The mean venous oxygen saturation (S(v)O(2)) value (94.3% ± 4.0%) of the affected limb was significantly higher than S(v)O(2) values found in healthy subjects (77.5% ± 9.8%) pointing to a severely decreased oxygen diffusion or utilization within the affected limb. ... Ultrastructural investigations of soleus skeletal muscle capillaries revealed thickened endothelial cells and thickened basement membranes. Muscle capillary densities were decreased in comparison with literature data. High venous oxygen saturation levels were partially explained by impaired diffusion of oxygen due to thickened basement membrane and decreased capillary density. ...The abnormal skeletal muscle findings points to severe disuse but only partially explain the impaired diffusion of oxygen; mitochondrial dysfunction seems a likely explanation in addition." Tan et al. Impaired oxygen utilization in skeletal muscle of CRPS I patients. *J Surg Res.* 2012 Mar;173(1):145-52

[519] "We observed that mitochondria obtained from CRPS I muscle tissue displayed reduced mitochondrial ATP production and substrate oxidation rates in comparison to control muscle tissue. Moreover, we observed reactive oxygen species evoked damage to mitochondrial proteins and reduced MnSOD levels." Tan et al. Mitochondrial dysfunction in muscle tissue of complex regional pain syndrome type I patients. *Eur J Pain.* 2011 Aug;15(7):708-15

[520] Wikner J, et al. Fibromyalgia—a syndrome associated with decreased nocturnal melatonin secretion. *Clin Endocrinol* (Oxf). 1998 Aug;49(2):179-83

[521] León J, Acuña-Castroviejo D, Escames G, Tan DX, Reiter RJ. Melatonin mitigates mitochondrial malfunction. *J Pineal Res.* 2005 Jan;38(1):1-9

[522] Acuna-Castroviejo D, Escames G, Reiter RJ. Melatonin therapy in fibromyalgia. *J Pineal Res.* 2006 Jan;40(1):98-9

as SIBO and CoQ10 deficiency should also be treated assertively to reduce the risk of relapse and to treat the underlying problems; good healthcare and good self-care should extend beyond mere symptom alleviation.

- ▪ Clinical trial (n=101): Adjuvant use of melatonin for treatment of fibromyalgia (*Journal of Pineal Research.* 2011 Apr[523]): group A (24 patients) treated with 20 mg/day fluoxetine alone; group B (27 patients) treated with melatonin 5 mg alone; group C (27 patients) treated with 20 mg fluoxetine plus 3 mg melatonin; group D (23 patients) treated with 20 mg fluoxetine plus 5 mg melatonin for 8 weeks. "Using melatonin (3 mg or 5 mg/day) in combination with 20 mg/day fluoxetine resulted in significant reduction in both total and different components of Fibromyalgia Impact Questionnaire score compared to the pretreatment values. In conclusion, **administration of melatonin, alone or in a combination with fluoxetine, was effective in the treatment of patients with FMS.**"

- Acetyl-L-carnitine (ALC): Acetyl-L-carnitine is a form of the amino acid L-carnitine, most notable for its critical role in supporting mitochondrial energy/ATP production by supporting the metabolism (beta oxidation) of fatty acids in the mitochondria. A large study with 102 patients showed that ALC (administered by oral and parenteral routes, 1500 mg/d) was beneficial in patients with fibromyalgia.[524] Given the role of ALC in supporting and improving mitochondrial function, this supplement probably benefits fibromyalgia patients by compensating for LPS-induced skeletal muscle dysfunction.

- D-ribose: D-ribose is a naturally occurring pentose carbohydrate available as a dietary supplement. When administered orally (5 g thrice daily), it safely provides numerous benefits to fibromyalgia patients, according to a recent pilot study with 41 patients.[525] Improvements are seen in energy, sleep, mental clarity, pain intensity, and well-being, as well as global assessment. Among its beneficial mechanisms of action is enhancement of mitochondrial ATP production. Thus, the benefits of D-ribose supplementation may be mediated by restoration or preservation of mitochondrial impairment caused by LPS in fibromyalgia patients.

- Creatine monohydrate: Skeletal muscle levels of phosphocreatine and ATP are reduced in patients with fibromyalgia compared with normal controls; thus, oral supplementation with creatine would appear to be an obvious intervention to restore these depressed levels to normal. Artimal et al[526] reported that a patient with severe refractory fibromyalgia attained sustained alleviation of depression and pain, as well as improvements in sleep and quality of life, following oral administration of creatine monohydrate for 4 weeks (3 grams daily in the first week, then 5 grams daily). Creatine supplementation has been shown to improve ATP production and oxygen utilization in brain and skeletal muscle in humans.[527]

- Oxygen: One-hundred percent oxygen delivered by facial mask at 8 L/min for 10 minutes can help abort an attack of cluster headache. Oxygen is the required electron and proton acceptor of the mitochondrial electron transport chain (ETC) for ATP production; thus, supraphysiologic oxygen, like supraphysiologic doses of mitochondria-specific nutrients, generally improves mitochondrial energy (ATP) production. The model of pain sensitization in so-called "chronic pain syndromes"—specifically migraine, cluster headache, fibromyalgia, myofascial pain syndrome and complex regional pain syndrome (CRPS)—that I have developed includes a tripartite vicious cycle of mitochondrial dysfunction, glial activation, and neuronal hyperexcitation, all of which promote brain inflammation, central sensitization, and perpetuation and amplification of pain. Strong support for this model comes from both its biochemical and physiologic rationale as well as the efficacy of corresponding treatments that address each of the main components: mitochondrial dysfunction, glial activation, neuronal hyperexcitation, brain inflammation.

  Appreciation of the efficacy of oxygen therapy—whether as normobaric (more available and affordable) or hyperbaric (more effective and more expensive; hyperbaric oxygen therapy [HBOT])—in various pain states invites us to revisit the naturopathic profession's hierarchy of therapeutics. Symptomatic therapy clearly has a role in patient care but, in order to avoid repeated use of urgent/emergency care and the creation of unnecessary medical dependency, repeated acute care or even "maintenance therapy" should never replace treatment of the underlying cause(s). Patients need to receive treatment aimed at the underlying pathophysiology so that health is optimized and patients are moved toward better general well-being and disease-specific health. Oxygen

[523] Hussain SA, Al-Khalifa II, Jasim NA, Gorial FI. Adjuvant use of melatonin for treatment of fibromyalgia. *J Pineal Res.* 2011 Apr;50(3):267-71
[524] Rossini M, et al. Double-blind, multicenter trial comparing acetyl l-carnitine with placebo in treatment of fibromyalgia patients. *Clin Exp Rheumatol.* 2007 Mar-Apr;25:182-8
[525] Teitelbaum JE, Johnson C, St Cyr J. The use of D-ribose in chronic fatigue syndrome and fibromyalgia: a pilot study. *J Altern Complement Med.* 2006 Nov;12:857-62
[526] Amital D, Vishne T, Rubinow A, Levine J. Observed effects of creatine monohydrate in a patient with depression and fibromyalgia. *Am J Psychiatry.* 2006 Oct;163(10):1840-1
[527] Watanabe A, Kato N, Kato T. Effects of creatine on mental fatigue and cerebral hemoglobin oxygenation. *Neurosci Res.* 2002 Apr;42(4):279-85

therapy is abortive of pain and shows some contribution to breaking the vicious cycles of mitochondrial impairment (immediate treatment of headaches, current-prospective treatment of fibromyalgia and CRPS) but this therapy does not address the other aspects of mitochondrial dysfunction (e.g., CoQ10 deficiency) and does not address the cause (e.g., small intestine bacterial overgrowth [SIBO] in fibromyalgia) and therefore should remain as supplemental, abortive/acute, and adjunctive therapy not as they foundation of therapy. Obviously, hyperbaric therapy makes more money for doctors/clinics and—(except/including) when patients buy their own home hyperbaric units—will therefore receive more press and more endorsement than therapies that are curative and empowering (ie, autonomous, without medical dependence). Given that most patients with persistent inflammation and pain are antioxidant deficient and therefore at increased risk for oxygen toxicity (including subclinical damage), antioxidant repletion should occur prior to oxygen therapy; the idea of administering supraphysiologic doses of oxygen to pull more protons and electrons through an *already damaged* and *pro-inflammatory* and *ROS-generating* electron transport chain is not meritorious, although some will defend it—weakly—on the theoretic basis of hormesis.

- High-flow oxygen therapy for all types of headache (*Am J Emerg Med* 2012 Nov[528]): "We performed a prospective, randomized, double-blinded, placebo-controlled trial of patients presenting to the ED with a chief complaint of headache. The patients were randomized to receive either 100% oxygen via nonrebreather mask at 15 L/min or the placebo treatment of room air via nonrebreather mask for 15 minutes in total. ... A total of 204 patients agreed to participate in the study and were randomized to the oxygen (102 patients) and placebo (102 patients) groups. Patient headache types included tension (47%), migraine (27%), undifferentiated (25%), and cluster (1%). Patients who received oxygen therapy reported significant improvement in visual analog scale scores at all points when compared with placebo: 22 mm vs 11 mm at 15 minutes, 29 mm vs 13 mm at 30 minutes, and 55 mm vs 45 mm at 60 minutes. ... In addition to its role in the treatment of cluster headache, high-flow oxygen therapy may provide an effective treatment of all types of headaches in the ED setting.

- Hyperbaric oxygen therapy for fibromyalgia; randomized n=60, crossover n=24 (*PLoS One*. 2015 May[529]): "The HBOT protocol comprised 40 sessions, 5 days/week, 90 minutes, 100% oxygen at 2ATA. ... HBOT in both groups led to significant amelioration of all FMS symptoms, with significant improvement in life quality. Analysis of SPECT imaging revealed rectification of the abnormal brain activity: decrease of the hyperactivity mainly in the posterior region and elevation of the reduced activity mainly in frontal areas. No improvement in any of the parameters was observed following the control period. CONCLUSIONS: The study provides evidence that HBOT can improve the symptoms and life quality of FMS patients. Moreover, it shows that HBOT can induce neuroplasticity and significantly rectify abnormal brain activity in pain related areas of FMS patients." Why would (hyperbaric) oxygen provide more benefit for fibromyalgia than for migraine, given the both are largely due to mitochondrial dysfunction?—Because in migraine, the mitochondrial dysfunction is generally low, and then acute with exacerbations, and it is most notable only in the brain; in contrast, in fibromyalgia, the mitochondrial dysfunction is more moderate-severe and therefore more amenable to treatment during the course of the disease (ie, one does not have to wait for an exacerbation or attack). Also in fibromyalgia, the mitochondrial dysfunction and the pain are both central in the brain as well as peripheral in the muscles; both locations contribute partly to the pain sensations, and oxygen therapy addresses both components, therefore leading to more opportunity for symptomatic improvement.

- Hyperbaric oxygen therapy for fibromyalgia; randomized n=50 (*J Int Med Res*. 2004 May[530]): "We conducted a randomized controlled study to evaluate the effect of hyperbaric oxygen (HBO) therapy in FMS (HBO group: n = 26; control group: n = 24). Tender points and pain threshold were assessed before, and after the first and fifteenth sessions of therapy. Pain was also scored on a visual analogue scale (VAS). There was a significant reduction in tender points and VAS scores and a significant increase in pain threshold of the

[528] Ozkurt et al. Efficacy of high-flow oxygen therapy in all types of headache: a prospective, randomized, placebo-controlled trial. *Am J Emerg Med.* 2012 Nov;30(9):1760-4
[529] Efrati et al. Hyperbaric oxygen therapy can diminish fibromyalgia syndrome—prospective clinical trial. *PLoS One.* 2015 May 26;10(5):e0127012
[530] Yildiz et al. A new treatment modality for fibromyalgia syndrome: hyperbaric oxygen therapy. *J Int Med Res.* 2004 May-Jun;32(3):263-7

HBO group after the first and fifteenth therapy sessions. There was also a significant difference between the HBO and control groups for all parameters except the VAS scores after the first session. We conclude that HBO therapy has an important role in managing FMS."

- Hyperbaric oxygen therapy for complex regional pain syndrome (*J Int Med Res*. 2004 May[531]): "In this double-blind, randomized, placebo-controlled study we aimed to assess the effectiveness of hyperbaric oxygen (HBO) therapy for treating patients with complex regional pain syndrome (CRPS). Of the 71 patients, 37 were allocated to the HBO group and 34 to the control (normal air) group. Both groups received 15 therapy sessions in a hyperbaric chamber. Pain, edema and range of motion (ROM) of the wrist were evaluated before treatment, after the 15th treatment session and on day 45. In the HBO group there was a significant decrease in pain and edema and a significant increase in the ROM of the wrist. When we compared the two groups, the HBO group had significantly better results with the exception of wrist extension. In conclusion, HBO is an effective and well-tolerated method for decreasing pain and edema and increasing the ROM in patients with CRPS."

- Hyperbaric oxygen therapy for myofascial pain syndrome (*J Natl Med Assoc* 2009 Jan[532]): "Thirty patients with the diagnosis of MPS were divided into HBO (n=20) and control groups (n=10). Patients in the HBO group received a total of 10 HBO treatments in 2 weeks. Patients in the control group received placebo treatment in a hyperbaric chamber. Pain threshold and visual analogue scale (VAS) measurements were performed immediately before and after HBO therapy and 3 months thereafter. Additionally, Pain Disability Index (PDI) and Short Form 12 Health Survey (SF-12) evaluations were done before HBO and after 3 months. HBO therapy was well tolerated with no complications. In the HBO group, pain threshold significantly increased and VAS scores significantly decreased immediately after and 3 months after HBO therapy. PDI, Mental and Physical Health SF-12 scores improved significantly with HBO therapy after 3 months compared with pretreatment values. In the control group, pain thresholds, VAS score, and Mental Health SF-12 scores did not change with placebo treatment; however, significant improvement was observed in the Physical Health SF-12 test. We concluded that HBO therapy may be a valuable alternative to other methods in the management of MPS."

SOCIOLOGY, SLEEP, STRESS, SOMATIC TREATMENTS, SWEAT/EXERCISE, SPECIAL SUPPLEMENTATION Common clinical and lifestyle considerations are listed in the following sections.

- Sociology/psychology, and stress management/reduction: Everyone—patients as well as clinicians—can benefit from developing self-awareness, emotional intelligence, and other core life skill and insights; since much of our perception of stress has a psycho-epistemological basis, enhanced self-awareness in this key area can help to deconstruct the phenomenon of stress and its secondary consequences. Because this consideration is self-evident in terms of safety, efficacy, broad applicability, and life-enhancement, specific literature will not be reviewed here.

- Sleep: Sleep deprivation induces immune suppression, enhanced sensitivity to pain, and an objectively documentable proinflammatory state evidenced by increases in serum hsCRP. Patients should be encouraged to optimize sleep by avoiding late-in-the-day exercise, overstimulation, caffeine (which generally has a half-life of six hours), and overuse of bright lights following nightfall; items that are conducive to sleep are having a dark and quiet room, relaxing music or reading, and using melatonin. Enhancement of sleep quality and duration have been shown to alleviate systemic inflammation, tendency toward insulin resistance, and pain perception/sensitivity.

- Sweating and exercise: Obesity/overweight and physical inactivity are consistently associated with elevated risk for and experience of depression, low self-esteem, social isolation, systemic inflammation, cardiometabolic disease and diabetes mellitus type-2, cancers of various types, and inflammatory disorders such as asthma and psoriasis. Weight optimization and physical activity promote enhanced self-confidence, self-efficacy, skill-building, social interaction, and reductions in cause-specific and all-cause mortality. Mechanistically, exercise—defined here as physical activity of sustained duration and intensity to promote diaphoresis/sweating—promotes lipolysis (for mobilization of adipose-stored toxins, weight reduction, and enhanced BHB production

[531] Kiralp et al. Effectiveness of hyperbaric oxygen therapy in the treatment of complex regional pain syndrome. *J Int Med Res*. 2004 May-Jun;32(3):258-62
[532] Kiralp et al A novel treatment modality for myofascial pain syndrome: hyperbaric oxygen therapy. *J Natl Med Assoc*. 2009 Jan;101(1):77-80

for induction of histone acetylation and ECT stimulation), promotes glycolysis (to promote induction of enhanced mitochondrial function and insulin sensitivity), and hyperventilation which results in respiratory alkalosis and secondary urinary alkalinization (which promotes mineral retention, xenobiotic excretion, endorphin elevation, and cortisol reduction). Commonly accepted international guidelines as well as common sense advocate 30-60 minutes of daily exercise that should globally include components such as aerobic training, resistance training, skill-building, balance, and flexibility; intensity, duration, and variety are tailored to patient needs and preferences. Because this consideration is self-evident in terms of safety, efficacy, broad applicability, and life-enhancement, specific literature will not be reviewed here.

- Somatic treatments (chiropractic, acupuncture, osteopathic manipulation, qigong, balneotherapy): In a randomized, controlled clinical trial among 24 female fibromyalgia patients, balneotherapy (warm bath) in daily 20-minute sessions 5 days per week for 3 weeks (total of 15 sessions; water temperature: 96.8°F = 36°C), resulted in statistically significant reductions in measured inflammatory mediators (PGE2, interleukin-1, LTB4) and amelioration of clinical symptoms among treated FM patients.[533] The symptomatic benefits of balneotherapy for FM patients have been corroborated in other trials.[534,535,536] Chiropractic treatment (including spinal manipulation, stretching, soft tissue treatments, and therapeutic ultrasound) has shown modest symptomatic benefit in several fibromyalgia case series and clinical trials.[537,538] A short-term trial showed that osteopathic manipulative therapy with standard medical care was superior to medical care alone for FM patients.[539] Acupuncture (including traditional, nontraditional, and electrical stimulation) also has been found beneficial for fibromyalgia patients.[540,541,542] Acupuncture may relieve fibromyalgia pain by improving regional blood flow, in addition to other mechanisms.[543,544] Because specific needle placement does not appear to be important[545], the conclusion that true acupuncture is ineffective because it may not differ markedly from the results obtained by sham acupuncture[546] may not be logical. A similar conundrum is seen in other clinical trials involving physical interventions such as manual osseous manipulation, wherein authentic treatments and sham treatments may both be effective by virtue of common physiological responses.[547] Qigong was found helpful for 10 fibromyalgia patients, and benefits were still apparent at three months' follow-up.[548]

- Special treatment, somatic treatment—Intramuscular needling and anesthesia: Myofascial pain is commonly received by needing (inserting a sterile needle into the muscle), whether or not the location is specific (e.g., acupuncture) and whether or not anesthetic agents, saline, or nothing (ie, dry needling) accompany the needle; having said that, more accurate localization (e.g., available trigger points or tender points) and the use of anesthetic agents tends to yield better results.

  - Analgesic and anti-hyperalgesic effects of muscle injections with lidocaine or saline in fibromyalgia syndrome. (*Eur J Pain.* 2014 Jul[549]): "We enrolled 62 female patients with FM into a double-blind controlled study of three groups who received 100 or 200 mg of lidocaine or saline injections into both trapezius and gluteal muscles. ...[Each subject received 2 muscle injections into the center of each trapezius muscle and 2 injections into the upper medial quadrants of both gluteus maximus muscles. ...Each syringe used for muscle injections contained either 5 ml of 1% lidocaine (50 mg) or 5 ml of normal saline.] RESULTS: Primary

[533] Ardiç F, Ozgen M, Aybek H, et al. Effects of balneotherapy on serum IL-1, PGE2 and LTB4 levels in fibromyalgia patients. *Rheumatol Int.* 2007 Mar;27(5):441-6

[534] Evcik D, Kizilay B, Gökçen E. The effects of balneotherapy on fibromyalgia patients. *Rheumatol Int.* 2002 Jun;22(2):56-9

[535] Fioravanti A, Perpignano G, Tirri G, et al. Effects of mud-bath treatment on fibromyalgia patients: a randomized clinical trial. *Rheumatol Int.* 2007 Oct;27(12):1157-61

[536] Dönmez A, Karagülle MZ, Tercan N, et al. SPA therapy in fibromyalgia: a randomised controlled clinic study. *Rheumatol Int.* 2005 Dec;26(2):168-72

[537] Citak-Karakaya I, et al. Short and long-term results of connective tissue manipulation and combined ultrasound therapy in patients with fibromyalgia. *J Manipulative Physiol Ther.* 2006 Sep;29(7):524-8

[538] Blunt KL, et al. The effectiveness of chiropractic management of fibromyalgia patients: a pilot study. *J Manipulative Physiol Ther.* 1997 Jul-Aug;20(6):389-99

[539] Gamber et al. Osteopathic manipulative treatment in conjunction with medication relieves pain associated with fibromyalgia syndrome. *J Am Osteopath Assoc.* 2002 Jun:321-5

[540] Martin DP, et al. Improvement in fibromyalgia symptoms with acupuncture: results of a randomized controlled trial. *Mayo Clin Proc.* 2006 Jun;81(6):749-57

[541] Singh BB, et al. Effectiveness of acupuncture in the treatment of fibromyalgia. *Altern Ther Health Med.* 2006 Mar-Apr;12(2):34-41

[542] Deluze C, Bosia L, Zirbs A, Chantraine A, Vischer TL. Electroacupuncture in fibromyalgia: results of a controlled trial. *BMJ.* 1992 Nov 21;305(6864):1249-52

[543] Sandberg M, Larsson B, Lindberg LG, Gerdle B. Different patterns of blood flow response in the trapezius muscle following needle stimulation (acupuncture) between healthy subjects and patients with fibromyalgia and work-related trapezius myalgia. *Eur J Pain.* 2005 Oct;9(5):497-510

[544] Sandberg M, Lindberg LG, Gerdle B. Peripheral effects of needle stimulation (acupuncture) on skin and muscle blood flow in fibromyalgia. *Eur J Pain.* 2004 Apr;8(2):163-71

[545] Harris RE, Tian X, Williams DA, Tian TX, Cupps TR, Petzke F, Groner KH, Biswas P, Gracely RH, Clauw DJ. Treatment of fibromyalgia with formula acupuncture: investigation of needle placement, needle stimulation, and treatment frequency. *J Altern Complement Med.* 2005 Aug;11(4):663-71

[546] Assefi NP, et al. A randomized clinical trial of acupuncture compared with sham acupuncture in fibromyalgia. *Ann Intern Med.* 2005 Jul 5;143(1):10-9

[547] Mein EA, et al. Manual medicine diversity: research pitfalls and the emerging medical paradigm. *J Am Osteopath Assoc.* 2001 Aug;101(8):441-4

[548] Chen KW, Hassett AL, Hou F, et al. A pilot study of external qigong therapy for patients with fibromyalgia. *J Altern Complement Med.* 2006 Nov;12(9):851-6

[549] Staud et al. Analgesic and anti-hyperalgesic effects of muscle injections with lidocaine or saline in patients with fibromyalgia syndrome. *Eur J Pain.* 2014 Jul;18(6):803-12

mechanical hyperalgesia at the shoulders and buttocks decreased significantly more after lidocaine than saline injections (p = 0.004). Similar results were obtained for secondary heat hyperalgesia at the arms (p = 0.04). After muscle injections, clinical FM pain significantly declined by 38% but was not statistically different between lidocaine and saline conditions. Placebo-related analgesic factors (e.g., patients' expectations of pain relief) accounted for 19.9% of the variance of clinical pain after the injections. ... CONCLUSION: These results suggest that muscle injections can reliably reduce clinical FM pain, and that peripheral impulse input is required for the maintenance of mechanical and heat hyperalgesia of patients with FM. Whereas the effects of muscle injections on hyperalgesia were greater for lidocaine than saline, the effects on clinical pain were similar for both injectates."

- Special supplementation in the treatment of FM—targeting (micro)glia activation and glutaminergic/NMDAr-mediated neuroexcitation: In my previous publications (prior to 2015) and consistent with the bulk of the basic science and clinical research, the emphasis of my fibromyalgia protocol has been on the treatment of SIBO and mitochondrial dysfunction, and the ever-necessary fine-tuning of the treatment protocol per patient. Progressively throughout 2015 as I further developed my understanding of the nuances of glial activation and the increasingly popular "gut-brain" concept (reviewed in printed monograph[550] and CE/CME videos[551]), I have become convinced that we should be—and already have been—addressing the glial activation directly. *How can we have already been doing this if we did not know that we were doing it?*—Simply by using nutrients such as anti-inflammatory fatty acids (e.g., EPA and DHA), nutrient-dense diets with minimal/moderate carbohydrate intake, vitamin and mineral supplementation (especially pyridoxine, magnesium, zinc, and vitamin D), phytonutrients, probiotics, CoQ10 and melatonin). All of these nutrients and substances have safety and efficacy for patients generally and FM patients particularly. What we know now is that these and other nutrients lessen the severity and duration of glial activation—brain inflammation—as well, and they therefore can be used to this effect. As such, I will summarize here that central sensitization is easily understood as a combination of **microglial inflammation**, which results in a) formation of the NMDAr agonist **QUIN**, b) formation of NO- which increases glutamate release while also causing mitochondrial dysfunction, and c) astrocyte activation leading to increased glutaminergic neurotransmission. As such, addressing the microglial activation *directly* while also addressing the dysbiotic and mitochondrial components is expected to enhance efficacy of the overall protocol; further, this discussion enhances our understanding of the mechanisms of action of and the clinical rationale for these interventions.

  - Dousing glial inflammation with vitamin D, fatty acids EPA and DHA, melatonin, phytonutrients: Various specific nutritional supplements and "over the counter remedies" have evidence—per in vitro, experimental, or human studies—to reduce glial inflammation; from these can be selected interventions which safely reduce glial activation in patients. All of these have proven safety for human use; the utility in reducing clinically relevant glial activation is established by the combination of available research plus the response of individual patients. As expected given its numerous anti-inflammatory properties, **DHA** reduces (micro)glia-induced inflammation, and the effect is enhanced with aspirin; the combination of **DHA with (low-dose) aspirin** is increasingly appreciated as synergistically anti-inflammatory and proresolutory, specifically but not exclusively via enhanced production of neuroprotective and anti-inflammatory resolvins.[552] Two paradoxes are worth noting: 1) Although immunostimulatory in the periphery[553], **melatonin reduces glial activation** in experimental models of brain injury.[554] 2) **Vitamin D**

---

[550] Vasquez A. *Human Microbiome and Dysbiosis in Clinical Disease*. ICHNFM, 2015.

[551] Vasquez A. "Microbiome and Dysbiosis in Clinical Disease" available CE/CME at NutritionAndFunctionalMedicine.org and pay-per-view at vimeo.com/ichnfm/vod_pages

[552] "Docosahexaenoic Acid increased total Glutathione levels in microglia cells and enhanced their anti-oxidative capacity. It reduced production of the pro-inflammatory cytokines TNF-α and IL-6 induced through TLR-3 and TLR-4 activation. Furthermore, it reduced production of Nitric Oxide. Aspirin showed similar anti-inflammatory effects with respect to TNF-α during TLR-3 and TLR-7 stimulation. ... Combination of Aspirin and Docosahexaenoic Acid showed augmentation in total Glutathione production during TLR-7 stimulation as well as a reduction in IL-6, TNF-α and Nitric Oxide. CONCLUSIONS: Collectively, these findings highlight the combination of Docosahexaenoic Acid and Aspirin as a possible measure against inflammation of the nervous system, thus leading to protection against neurodegenerative diseases with an inflammatory etiology." Pettit LK, Varsanyi C, Tadros J, Vassiliou E. Modulating the inflammatory properties of activated microglia with Docosahexaenoic acid and Aspirin. *Lipids Health Dis*. 2013 Feb 11;12:16

[553] This is a clinical trial showing anti-infective efficacy of melatonin, while other articles have specifically documented increases in inflammatory cytokines following melatonin administration. "Administration of melatonin as an adjuvant therapy in the treatment of neonatal sepsis is associated with improvement of clinical and laboratory outcomes." Gitto et al. Effects of melatonin treatment in septic newborns. *Pediatr Res*. 2001 Dec;50(6):756-60

[554] "Melatonin administration was associated with markedly restrained microglial activation, decreased release of proinflammatory cytokines and increased the number of surviving neurons at the site of peri-contusion. Meanwhile, melatonin administration resulted in dephosphorylated mTOR pathway." Ding et al. Melatonin reduced microglial activation and alleviated neuroinflammation induced neuron degeneration in experimental traumatic brain injury. *Neurochem Int*. 2014 Oct;76:23-31

reduces glial activation[555], and this is highly consistent with the clinical benefits seen of vitamin D against depression and other neuropsychiatric conditions, clearly including chronic pain; yet, antimicrobial peptide LL-37, production of which is at least partly dependent on vitamin D adequacy, induces glial-mediated neuroinflammation[556], perhaps thereby explaining the rare and possibly transient/inconsequential exacerbation of "sickness behavior" in some patients upon commencement of vitamin D supplementation. Many **phytonutrients—especially curcumin, quercetin, green tea catechins, baicalein, and luteolin**—show anti-inflammatory and neuroprotective benefits, some of which are mediated via reducing microglial activation/inflammation; we can endlessly debate the bioavailability of agents such as curcuminoids and quercetin, or we can accept them as low-cost high-safety nutrients that merit clinical utilization based on mechanistic studies and successful multicomponent clinical trials.[557,558]

- Alleviating **NO-induced glutaminergic neurotransmission and mitochondrial dysfunction** with **vitamin B12, especially in the form of hydroxocobalamin**: Vitamin B12 in general and hydroxocobalamin in particular bind with nitric oxide (NO-); supplemental (hydroxo)cobalamin has a pharmaconutritional effect of alleviating migraine[559] and low-back pain[560,561], two conditions known to have a component of neuroinflammatory central sensitization. Likely, the clinically observed analgesic effect of (hydroxo)cobalamin is mediated partly if not largely via its "chelation" or "detoxification" of NO-, thereby reducing the mitochondrial dysfunction and NMDAr activation that would have otherwise been triggered by NO-.

- Alleviating astrocyte-induced and QUIN-triggered glutamate/NMDA receptor activation with pyridoxine, magnesium, zinc: As previously reviewed, microglial activation promotes NMDAr activation via QUIN and glutamate. Regarding glutamate's activation of the NMDAr, sufficient biochemical, experimental, and clinical data allows us to conclude that we can reduce glutamate's excitatory effect by reducing glutamate itself via supplemental pyridoxine (vitamin B6), either in its active phosphorylated form of P5P (pyridoxal 5'-phosphate) or by supporting its magnesium-dependent requirement for conversion to the active P5P form when pyridoxine itself is used. In addition to promoting conversion of pyridoxine to P5P, magnesium also partly blocks calcium passage through the NMDAr-associated calcium channel (as does zinc) and also offsets the effects of increased intracellular calcium, in addition to supporting mitochondrial function, which is easily compromised by both inflammation and increased intracellular calcium. The clinical benefit of pyridoxine supplementation in migraine headache[562], seizures/epilepsy[563], neuropsychiatric symptoms of premenstrual syndrome (depression, irritability and tiredness)[564] is likely mediated via several different mechanisms, primary among which is the enhanced conversion of glutamate to gamma-amino-butyric acid (GABA), thereby synergistically reducing neuroexcitation and enhancing neuroregulation. A generalized

[555] "According to the results of the present study, activated microglia might increase the expression of 1-α-hydroxylase and VDR. 25(OH)D3 is converted into 1,25(OH)2D3 by 1-α-hydroxylase, which then stimulates VDR signaling and inhibits the phosphorylation of p38 in activated microglia. This cascade might inhibit the inflammatory reaction of activated microglia. In conclusion, the present study suggests that vitamin D3 might have an important role in the negative regulation of microglial activation." Hur et al. Regulatory Effect of 25-hydroxyvitamin D3 on Nitric Oxide Production in Activated Microglia. *Korean J Physiol Pharmacol.* 2014 Oct;18(5):397-402

[556] "We blocked the inflammatory stimulant action of LL-37 by removing it with an anti-LL-37 antibody. The inflammatory effect was also prevented by treatment with inhibitors of PKC, PI3K and MEK-1/2 as well as with the intracellular Ca(2+)-chelator, BAPTA-AM. This indicates involvement of these intracellular pathways. Our data suggest that LL-37, in addition to its established roles, may play a role in the chronic neuroinflammation which is observed in neurodegenerative diseases such as Alzheimer's and Parkinson's disease." Lee et al. Human antimicrobial peptide LL-37 induces glial-mediated neuroinflammation. *Biochem Pharmacol.* 2015 Mar 15;94(2):130-41

[557] Blaylock RL, Maroon J. Natural plant products and extracts that reduce immunoexcitotoxicity-associated neurodegeneration and promote repair within the central nervous system. *Surg Neurol Int* 2012;3:19

[558] Bredesen DE. Reversal of cognitive decline: a novel therapeutic program. *Aging* (Albany NY). 2014 Sep;6(9):707-17

[559] "Drugs which directly counteract nitric oxide (NO), such as endothelial receptor blockers, NO-synthase inhibitors, and NO-scavengers, may be effective in the acute treatment of migraine, but are also likely to be effective in migraine prophylaxis. In the underlying pilot study the prophylactic effect of the NO scavenger hydroxocobalamin after intranasal administration in migraine was evaluated. ... 1 mg intranasal hydroxocobalamin daily. ... A reduction in migraine attack frequency of >/ or = 50% was seen in 10 of 19 patients... A reduction of > or = 30% was noted in 63% of the patients. The mean attack frequency in the total study population showed a reduction from 4.7 +/- 1.7 attacks per month to 2.7 +/- 1.6 ." van der Kuy et al. Hydroxocobalamin, a nitric oxide scavenger, in the prophylaxis of migraine: an open, pilot study. *Cephalalgia.* 2002 Sep;22(7):513-9

[560] "The efficacy and safety of parenteral Vitamin B12 in alleviating low back pain and related disability and in decreasing the consumption of paracetamol was confirmed in patients with no signs of nutritional deficiency." Mauro et al. Vitamin B12 in low back pain. *Eur Rev Med Pharmacol Sci.* 2000 May-Jun;4(3):53-8

[561] "Intramuscular methylcobalamin is both an effective and safe method of treatment for patients with nonspecific low back pain, both singly or in combination with other forms of treatment." Chiu et al. The efficacy and safety of intramuscular injections of methylcobalamin in patients with chronic nonspecific low back pain: a randomised controlled trial. *Singapore Med J.* 2011 Dec;52(12):868-73

[562] Sadeghi et al. Effects of pyridoxine supplementation on severity, frequency and duration of migraine attacks in migraine patients with aura. *Iran J Neurol.* 2015 Apr 4:74-80

[563] "An 8-year-old girl treated at our facility for superrefractory status epilepticus was found to have a low pyridoxine level at 5µg/L. After starting pyridoxine supplementation, improvement in the EEG for a 24-hour period was seen. ... A selective pyridoxine deficiency was seen in 94% of patients with status epilepticus (compared to 39.4% in the outpatients) which leads us to believe that there is a relationship between status epilepticus and pyridoxine levels." Dave et al. Pyridoxine deficiency in adult patients with status epilepticus. *Epilepsy Behav.* 2015 Nov;52(Pt A):154-8

[564] Doll H, Brown S, Thurston A, Vessey M. Pyridoxine (vitamin B6) and the premenstrual syndrome: a randomized crossover trial. *J R Coll Gen Pract.* 1989 Sep;39(326):364-8

schematic—mostly direct but very clearly clinically accurate—is provided; the illustration connects NMDAr activation with neuropsychiatric complications while providing insight into clinical remediation.

- **In the treatment of pain—including headaches and fibromyalgia—reducing the effects of glutamate-mediated neurotransmission and cellular effects is of very high importance**: Excess glutaminergic neurotransmission very clearly promotes anxiety, depression, fibromyalgia pain, myofascial pain and myofascial trigger points[565], migraine and headaches, seizures/epilepsy, and neurodegeneration. Our therapeutic goals are to 1) reduce glutamate levels with vitamin B6 and by avoiding/treating microglial activation, 2) reduce glutamate-triggered influx of calcium with zinc and magnesium, also vitamin D, alkalinization (increased consumption of base-forming foods, such as fruits and vegetables which contain citrate which is converted to bicarbonate to promote alkalinization, one effect of which is to promote magnesium retention, thereby alleviating pain[566]), omega-3 fatty acids such as from fish oil, 3) reduce the effects of glutamate/NMDA receptor activation by counterbalancing with benzodiazepine/GABA receptor activation by promoting conversion of glutamate to GABA and perhaps also by using niacinamide and the botanicals that act as ligands for the GABA receptor.

- **Reduce homocysteine levels, and recall that homocysteine may be elevated in the central nervous system (cerebrospinal fluid) of patients with chronic fatigue syndrome and fibromyalgia even when levels in blood/serum/plasma are normal[567]; safety and benefit of folate and vitamin B12 administration have been documented[568]**: Homocysteine contributes to NMDA receptor activation resulting in—identically as with glutamate—increased intracellular calcium and neurotoxicity.[569]

  - **Folinic acid or methylfolate 2-5 mg/d**: Use in combination with other vitamins, especially vitamin B12, in the form of hydroxocobalamin, adenosylcobalamin, or methylcobalamin—cyanocobalamin is obviously to be avoided because of its clinically relevant content of cyanide.

  - **Vitamin B12 >2,000 mcg per day orally, or 1-2 mg per week by injection**: Use in the form of hydroxocobalamin, adenosylcobalamin, or methylcobalamin—cyanocobalamin is obviously to be avoided because of its clinically relevant content of cyanide.

  - **Vitamin B6, pyridoxine 50-250 mg/d**: The phosphorylated form (P5P) can also be used; when the HCL form is used, additional attention must be given to magnesium status/supplementation and urinary alkalinization. As a rule, B6 supplementation should always be used with magnesium supplementation.

  - **Riboflavin 20-400 mg/d**: Small doses of 2 mg/d have been shown to significantly reduce homocysteine levels, and doses of 400 mg/d are common and well-tolerated in the treatment of migraine.

  - **Thyroid optimization**: Hypothyroidism causes elevated homocysteine and promotes insulin resistance[570] and should be treated appropriately per Chapter 1.

  - **NAC 600 mg per day and upward to 500-1,500 mg thrice daily**: Doses of NAC 4,800 mg/d have been used with success and safety in the treatment of SLE.

  - **Avoidance of homocysteine-elevating factors**: High coffee intake (>5 cups per day), ethanol, tobacco smoking, and medications/treatments (such as methotrexate, metformin, niacin and fibrate drugs); fish oil can raise homocysteine levels in some patients. Metformin is well-known to cause malabsorption of vitamin B12 and to thereby exacerbate "diabetic neuropathy" and promote depression and dementia/psychosis.

  - **Choline, phosphatidylcholine, lecithin (approximately 2.6 g choline/d)**: Each TBS (tablespoon, approximately 15 mL) of lecithin contains 275 mg of choline; thus, if the goal is to get to 2.6 g choline, one would need to use 10 TBS (150 mL) per day of granulated lecithin.

  - **Betaine, trimethylglycine 6–12 g/day**: Effects are weak/modest; likely more relevant for patients taking drugs such as metformin and fibrates that promote loss of betaine in urine.

[565] Wang et al. Spatial pain propagation over time following painful glutamate activation of latent myofascial trigger points in humans. *J Pain*. 2012 Jun;13(6):537-45

[566] Vormann et al. Supplementation with alkaline minerals reduces symptoms in patients with chronic low back pain. *J Trace Elem Med Biol*. 2001;15(2-3):179-83

[567] Regland et al. Increased concentrations of homocysteine in the cerebrospinal fluid in patients with fibromyalgia and chronic fatigue syndrome. *Scand J Rheumatol*. 1997;26(4):301-7

[568] Regland et al. Response to vitamin B12 and folic acid in myalgic encephalomyelitis and fibromyalgia. *PLoS One*. 2015 Apr 22;10(4):e0124648

[569] Abushik et al. The role of NMDA and mGluR5 receptors in calcium mobilization and neurotoxicity of homocysteine in trigeminal and cortical neurons and glial cells. *J Neurochem*. 2014 Apr;129(2):264-74

[570] Yang N et al. Novel Clinical Evidence of an Association between Homocysteine and Insulin Resistance in Patients with Hypothyroidism or Subclinical Hypothyroidism. *PLoS One*. 2015 May 4;10(5):e0125922

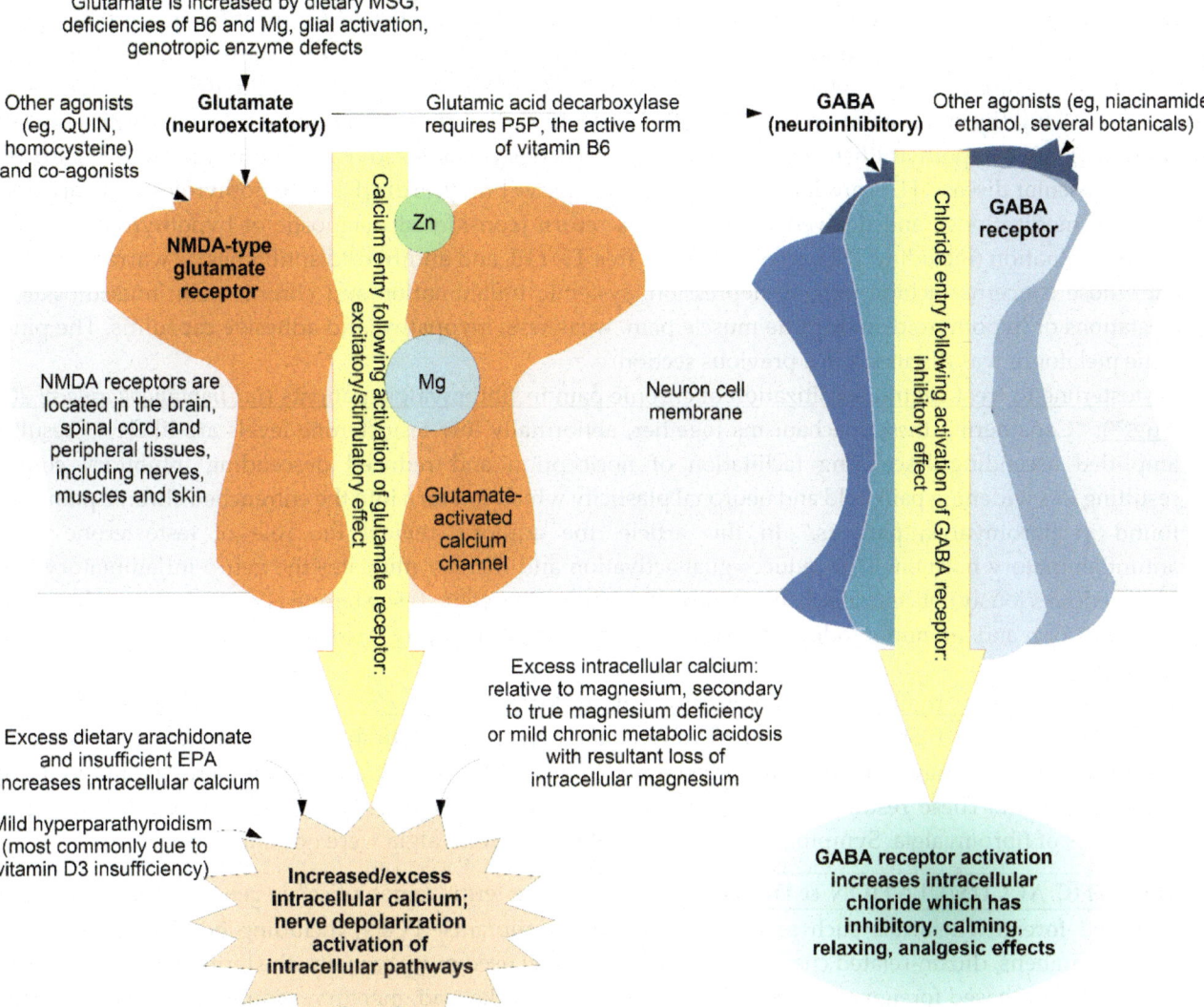

Glutamate is increased by dietary MSG, deficiencies of B6 and Mg, glial activation, genotropic enzyme defects

Other agonists (eg, QUIN, homocysteine) and co-agonists

Glutamate (neuroexcitatory)

Glutamic acid decarboxylase requires P5P, the active form of vitamin B6

GABA (neuroinhibitory)

Other agonists (eg, niacinamide, ethanol, several botanicals)

NMDA-type glutamate receptor

Zn

Mg

GABA receptor

NMDA receptors are located in the brain, spinal cord, and peripheral tissues, including nerves, muscles and skin

Neuron cell membrane

Glutamate-activated calcium channel

Calcium entry following activation of glutamate receptor: excitatory/stimulatory effect

Chloride entry following activation of GABA receptor: inhibitory effect

Excess dietary arachidonate and insufficient EPA increases intracellular calcium

Excess intracellular calcium: relative to magnesium, secondary to true magnesium deficiency or mild chronic metabolic acidosis with resultant loss of intracellular magnesium

Mild hyperparathyroidism (most commonly due to vitamin D3 insufficiency)

Increased/excess intracellular calcium; nerve depolarization activation of intracellular pathways

GABA receptor activation increases intracellular chloride which has inhibitory, calming, relaxing, analgesic effects

Glutamate receptors in the brain: Neurocortical excitation, promotion of inflammation (neuroinflammation), promotion of mitochondrial dysfunction, apoptosis/neurodegeneration

Glutamate receptors in the periphery: Glutamate receptors (including NMDAr) are located throughout the body; increased glutamate signaling promotes neurogenic inflammation, peripheral pain sensitization, muscle contraction

Central sensitization, increased pain sensitivity (hyperalgesia), depression and anxiety, migraine and seizure

Muscle contraction/hypertonicity, myofascial trigger points (MFTP), muscle cramps, hypertension due to increased peripheral resistance

Illustration of the NMDA-type glutamate receptor, its activation, effects, and nutritional modulation: The NMDA receptor is activated by glutamate, QUIN, and other substances which act as agonists (e.g., homocysteine) or co-agonists (e.g., glycine). Different forms of the NMDA receptor exist; thus, the image presented here is a generalized version that is conceptually accurate (rather than all-inclusive; for more details see reviews[571]) and clinically relevant. Neuroexcitatory glutamate is converted to neuroinhibitory GABA by the enzyme glutamic acid decarboxylase, which shows vitamin B6 dose-responsiveness in its reduction of glutamate levels. Magnesium and zinc (and perhaps copper) retard the passage of calcium through this channel, thereby mitigating some of the effects of NMDAr activation. Quenching nitric oxide (for example with hydroxocobalamin), which would otherwise trigger glutamate release, and dousing glial activation are important considerations not included in this illustration. For updates and additional information and explanations, see videos and articles at www.inflammationmastery.com/pain

---

571 Vyklicky et al. Structure, function, and pharmacology of NMDA receptor channels. *Physiol Res*. 2014;63 Suppl 1:S191-203

ENDOCRINE IMBALANCE & OPTIMIZATION Peptide-based and steroid-based hormones have wide-ranging effects beyond those with which they are classically and thus simplistically associated. The "main" hormones that we consider in most chronic inflammatory disorders are the three pro-inflammatory hormones (prolactin, estradiol, and insulin) and the three anti-inflammatory hormones (DHEA, cortisol, and testosterone); each of these hormones can be objectively assessed with serologic testing and modulated with therapeutic intervention. A full thyroid evaluation—including history, physical examination (with particular scrutiny for cold extremities [DDX: hypothyroidism, hypogonadism, vasoconstriction/vaso-obstruction, Raynaud's disorder, peripheral vascular disease, H2S-producing GI dysbiosis], relative bradycardia [DDX, hypothyroidism, heart block, beta-blocker medications], and delayed Achilles reflex return [considered diagnostic of hypothyroidism]), and laboratory evaluation (including TSH, free T4, total or free T3, rT3, and antithyroid antibodies) is warranted in any patient whose concerns include fatigue, depression, systemic inflammation and chronic pain; musculoskeletal manifestations of hypothyroidism include muscle pain, weakness, myopathy, and adhesive capsulitis. The pineal hormone melatonin was discussed in a previous section.

- Testosterone to treat central sensitization of chronic pain in fibromyalgia patients (*Int Immunopharmacol* 2015 Aug[572]): "Considering these mechanisms together, abnormally low testosterone levels are likely to result in amplified ascending/descending facilitation of nociception and reduced descending inhibitory control, resulting in a widening pain field and neuronal plasticity which can turn into the entrenched chronic pain states found in fibromyalgia patients." In this article, the author's review the role of testosterone as an antiinflammatory hormone that reduces glial activation and thereby mitigates the neuro-inflammatory basis (detailed previously) of central sensitization and the resulting pain. Testosterone is well-known to have anti-inflammatory and immunomodulatory properties with clinical utility in rheumatoid arthritis and cluster headache.

- Treatment of pain in fibromyalgia patients with testosterone gel (*Int Immunopharmacol.* 2015 Aug[573]): "Assessment of the typical symptoms of fibromyalgia by patient questionnaire and tender point exam demonstrated significant change in: decreased muscle pain, stiffness, and fatigue, and increased libido during study treatment. These results are consistent with the hypothesized ability of testosterone to relieve the symptoms of fibromyalgia. Symptoms not tightly related to fibromyalgia were not improved."

XENOBIOTIC ACCUMULATION & DETOXIFICATION The term "xenobiotics" is generally used to refer to carbon-based foreign chemicals such as persistent organic pollutants (POPs) including herbicides, pesticides, phthalates, parabens, dioxin-related chemicals, and many others; used more casually, the term may also be used to include noncarbon-based foreign substances such as toxic metals like lead, mercury, cadmium, and arsenic. Thus, "xenobiotics" has become somewhat synonymous with "toxins" in both professional-level and vernacular conversations. Laboratory assessments for chemical and metal toxins are commercially available through specialized medical laboratories and are based on analysis of blood and urine. The many biochemical and physiologic components of detoxification/depuration have been reviewed in chapter 4 of this book. Essentially everyone—all humans on the planet worldwide—have biochemical evidence of xenobiotic chemical/metal accumulation, generally with numerous xenobiotics, which have additive and synergistic adverse effects on physiology and health. Thus, scientifically, since xenobiotic accumulation is pandemic, consideration of and treatment for xenobiotic accumulation via therapeutic detoxification programs and lifestyle interventions should be routine. Easy and effective means for promoting detoxification of chemicals and metals include plant-based diet to promote bowel and renal excretion of toxins (via reduced enterohepatic recycling [better microflora, more fiber for adsorption, more frequent fecal excretion] and reduced renal resorption [urinary alkalinization], respectively), NAC for arsenic chelation and GSH production, sweating/exercise (lipolysis promotes mobilization of lipophilic toxins from adipose tissue, diaphoresis promotes direct toxin excretion), sufficient micronutrient and protein intake supports phase 1 and phase 2 of the oxidation and conjugation processes in the liver. Chemical xenobiotics can be bound in the gut during the normal process of enterohepatic recycling/recirculation with periodic or rotational use of activated charcoal, cholestyramine, and chlorella; anecdotal reports from clinical practices support the use of phytochelatin (metal-binding peptides from plants, used by plants for protection from metal toxicity) in the

---

[572] White HD, Robinson TD. A novel use for testosterone to treat central sensitization of chronic pain in fibromyalgia patients. *Int Immunopharmacol.* 2015 Aug;27(2):244-8
[573] White et al. Treatment of pain in fibromyalgia patients with testosterone gel: Pharmacokinetics and clinical response. *Int Immunopharmacol.* 2015 Aug;27(2):249-56

prevention/treatment of metal toxicity in humans but no formal clinical studies have been performed to document the effectiveness of this approach although its safety is clinically appreciated.

- Pilot study: *Chlorella pyrenoidosa* for patients with fibromyalgia syndrome (*Phytother Res* 2000 May[574]): *Chlorella pyrenoidosa* is a unicellular green alga that grows in fresh water. It is a dense source of nutrients, particularly vitamin D (500 IU vitamin D per 1.35 g *Chlorella*). *Chlorella* may have value in treating some fibromyalgia patients, but overall the efficacy is low. Thus, *Chlorella* should not be used as monotherapy for fibromyalgia, although it may be a useful adjunct either as a source of vitamin D, as a means to help modify gut flora, or as an aid in the detoxification of xenobiotics due to its ability to bind ingested and bile-excreted toxins and prevent their absorption and reabsorption in a manner similar to that of cholestyramine, a drug used to bind cholesterol in the gut, promote its excretion, and thereby lower blood cholesterol levels.[575,576,577] This "detoxifying" effect of *Chlorella* in humans is supported by 2 clinical trials showing that nursing mothers who supplement with *Chlorella* during lactation transfer less dioxin in their breast milk compared to nursing mothers who do not consume *Chlorella*.[578,579]

- Clinical investigation: Reduced exposure to xenobiotics (cosmetics) alleviates fibromyalgia (*Journal of Women's Health* 2004 Mar[580]): Women use more cosmetic products than do men, and fibromyalgia is more common in women. Cosmetic products generally contain skin-absorbable xenobiotics with potentially adverse effects; therefore this study was conducted to determine if avoidance of cosmetics would alleviate symptoms of FM. The author of this report describes a prospective, randomized, controlled trial of 48 women with FM (some of whom had a rheumatic condition) who were regular users of cosmetics was carried out to investigate if a reduced use of cosmetics would reduce the symptoms. The patients were told to avoid or completely abstain from using all ointments, creams, skin lotions, pain-relieving liniments, cleaning lotions, oil treatments, hair-coloring chemicals, and tanning lotion; they were also advised to reduce their use of soap and shampoo, both of which—like skin creams—are generally formulated with perfumes and other chemicals and applied to large regions of the body. This research showed that, after 2 years, FM patients who reduced their exposure to chemicals/xenobiotics/cosmetics experienced significant reductions in pain, sleep disturbances, and musculoskeletal stiffness (p < 0.02), together with better physical function and improved sense of well-being as measured by the Fibromyalgia Impact Questionnaire (FIQ). Thus, avoiding chemical exposure appears to provide no-cost no-risk therapeutic benefit to FM patients by alleviating pain and improving several indicators of overall health.

Conclusion: In sum, current research indicates that fibromyalgia results from impairment of cellular energy/ATP production (mitochondrial dysfunction) and induction of pain hypersensitivity (peripheral and central sensitization) due to absorbed metabolic toxins from bacterial/microbial overgrowth of the gastrointestinal tract; this is complicated by induction of tryptophan deficiency which is most likely caused by tryptophan degradation by bacterial tryptophanase activity and which leads to serotonin and melatonin insufficiencies, which lead to associated biochemical and clinical consequences, discussed previously. Available studies have shown that SIBO is ubiquitous among fibromyalgia patients and that antimicrobial interventions—whether pharmaceutical or nutritional—are efficacious. Secondary physiological effects such as mitochondrial impairment, pain sensitization, nutritional deficiencies, oxidative stress, and reduced tissue perfusion are treated with combined use of select therapeutics as reviewed previously. Patients presenting with widespread pain should be screened for causative underlying disease; if no other explanation can be found, then the diagnosis of fibromyalgia should be made, and the condition should be treated with the nondrug therapeutics discussed above. The first visit can include history, physical examination, and laboratory tests; initial laboratory assessment should include complete blood count (CBC), metabolic/chemistry panel, serum 25-hydroxyvitamin D, C-reactive protein (CRP), anti-nuclear antibodies

---

[574] Merchant RE, et al. Nutritional supplementation with Chlorella pyrenoidosa for patients with fibromyalgia syndrome: a pilot study. *Phytother Res* 2000 May;14:167-73

[575] Pore RS. Detoxification of chlordecone poisoned rats with chlorella and chlorella derived sporopollenin. *Drug Chem Toxicol.* 1984;7(1):57-71

[576] Morita K, Ogata M, Hasegawa T. Chlorophyll derived from Chlorella inhibits dioxin absorption from the gastrointestinal tract and accelerates dioxin excretion in rats. *Environ Health Perspect.* 2001 Mar;109(3):289-94

[577] Morita K, Matsueda T, Iida T, Hasegawa T. Chlorella accelerates dioxin excretion in rats. *J Nutr.* 1999 Sep;129(9):1731-6

[578] Nakano S, Noguchi T, Takekoshi H, Suzuki G, Nakano M. Maternal-fetal distribution and transfer of dioxins in pregnant women in Japan, and attempts to reduce maternal transfer with Chlorella (Chlorella pyrenoidosa) supplements. *Chemosphere.* 2005 Dec;61(9):1244-55

[579] Nakano et al. Chlorella (pyrenoidosa) supplementation decreases dioxin and increases immunoglobulin a concentrations in breast milk. *J Med Food.* 2007 Mar;134-42

[580] Sverdrup B. Use less cosmetics—suffer less from fibromyalgia? *J Womens Health* (Larchmt). 2004 Mar;13(2):187-94

(ANA), antibodies against cyclic citrullinated proteins (anti-CCP antibodies), ferritin, muscle enzymes aldolase and creatine kinase, and a complete thyroid assessment including TSH, free T4, free T3, total T3, reverse T3 (rT3), and antithyroid peroxidase and antithyroglobulin antibodies. First-day interventions can include dietary optimization, multivitamin-multimineral supplementation (including vitamin D3 and magnesium), tryptophan/5-HTP, CoQ10, mixed tocopherols, and combination fatty acids including gamma-linolenic acid (GLA), eicosapentaenoic acid (EPA) and docosahexaenoic acid (DHA). SIBO should be treated empirically; otherwise, it can be objectively assessed with breath hydrogen and methane testing, stool analysis, culture, microscopy, and parasitology. At follow-up visits, additional assessments and interventions (such as for toxic metals and chronic occult infections) can be used to fine-tune the diagnosis and further discover and define its contributors in order to maximize the patient's response to treatment and promote optimal recovery and health.

MIGRAINE HEADACHES, HYPOTHYROIDISM, AND FIBROMYALGIA:

ASSESSMENTS AND THERAPEUTIC APPROACHES USING INTEGRATIVE CHIROPRACTIC, NATUROPATHIC, OSTEOPATHIC, AND FUNCTIONAL MEDICINE

Objective *real* non-neurologic non-psychiatric abnormalities in fibromyalgia: the case against primary central sensitization.

DR. ALEX VASQUEZ
FUNCTIONALINFLAMMOLOGY.COM
INFLAMMATIONMASTERY.COM

Archive: vimeo.com/56334919

MIGRAINE HEADACHES, HYPOTHYROIDISM, AND FIBROMYALGIA:

ASSESSMENTS AND THERAPEUTIC APPROACHES USING INTEGRATIVE CHIROPRACTIC, NATUROPATHIC, OSTEOPATHIC, AND FUNCTIONAL MEDICINE

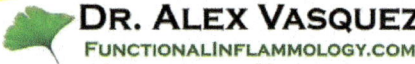

Is "central sensitization" in fibromyalgia a bunch of c.r.a.p. (Commercial Rationalization Advocating Pharmaceuticals)?

DR. ALEX VASQUEZ
FUNCTIONALINFLAMMOLOGY.COM
INFLAMMATIONMASTERY.COM

Archive: vimeo.com/56437367

Dysbiotic prototypes

Brain— dyscognition: Autointoxication, auto-brewery syndrome, hepatic encephalopathy sin hepatopathy

Brain—pain, fatigue, depression: Fibromyalgia

Inflammation— CIC, various tissues: Dysbiotic arthropathy, dermatitis, vasculitis

Inflammation— joints: Reactive arthritis

Inflammation— skin: Psoriasis

ICHNFM

Fibromyalgia

▸ One of my favorite clinical disorders because it blends 3 of my favorite topics:

1. **Dysbiosis**—these patients have a high prevalence of SIBO, which completely explains every aspect of the condition

2. **Mitochondrial dysfunction**—these patients have mitochondrial dysfunction caused by SIBO

3. **Social (in)justice**—perfectly exemplifies the extent to which the medical profession and medical practice can be easily coopted— hijacked—by the commercial interests of the pharmaceutical industry despite a mountain of research pointing directly to the cause and cure of this condition.

Archive: vimeo.com/139867947

How does small intestinal bacterial/microbial overgrowth (SIBO) cause fibromyalgia?

1. **Bacterial endotoxin/lipopolysaccharide/LPS**: causes inflammation, mitochondrial/muscle impairment, and increased sensitization to pain.

2. **Bacteria-produced D-lactic acid**: neurotoxin and metabolic poison; causes fatigue, muscle pain, dyscognition.

3. **Bacteria-produced hydrogen sulfide (H2S)**: neurotoxin and metabolic poison; causes fatigue, muscle pain, dyscognition.

4. **Bacteria-produced tryptophanase**: leads to tryptophan deficiency (documented in FM patients) and "serotonin deficiency" (pain, fatigue, carbohydrate cravings, depression) and "melatonin deficiency" (sleep disturbance, mitochondrial impairment, oxidative stress, muscle fatigue).

Archive: vimeo.com/56334918

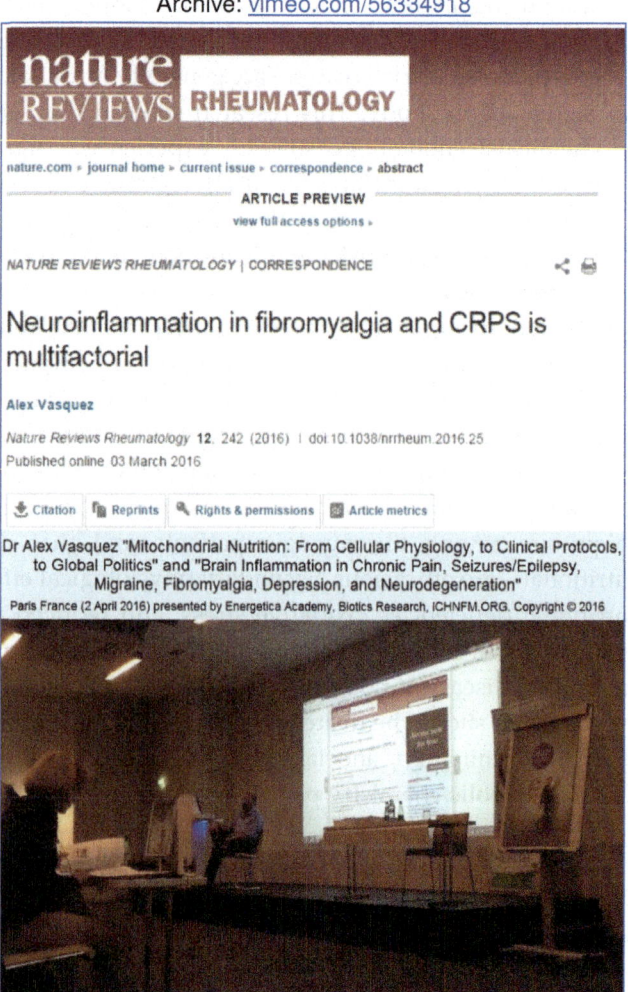

nature REVIEWS RHEUMATOLOGY

nature.com ▸ journal home ▸ current issue ▸ correspondence ▸ abstract

ARTICLE PREVIEW
view full access options ▸

NATURE REVIEWS RHEUMATOLOGY | CORRESPONDENCE

Neuroinflammation in fibromyalgia and CRPS is multifactorial

Alex Vasquez

Nature Reviews Rheumatology 12, 242 (2016) | doi:10.1038/nrrheum.2016.25
Published online 03 March 2016

Citation | Reprints | Rights & permissions | Article metrics

Dr Alex Vasquez "Mitochondrial Nutrition: From Cellular Physiology, to Clinical Protocols, to Global Politics" and "Brain Inflammation in Chronic Pain, Seizures/Epilepsy, Migraine, Fibromyalgia, Depression, and Neurodegeneration"
Paris France (2 April 2016) presented by Energetica Academy, Biotics Research, ICHNFM.ORG. Copyright © 2016

Archive: vimeo.com/161526099

Intracellular Hypercalcinosis: A Functional Nutritional Disorder with Implications Ranging from Myofascial Trigger Points to Affective Disorders, Hypertension, and Cancer

This article was originally published in *Naturopathy Digest* in 2006
naturopathydigest.com/archives/2006/sep/vasquez.php

Introduction: Let us explore the possibility that elevated levels of calcium *within the cell* (intracellular hypercalcinosis) might predispose toward a wide range of clinical problems including migraine, hypertension, myofascial trigger points, inflammation, and cancer. Further, let's review the data showing that several commonly employed nutritional interventions can be used synergistically to counteract and correct this problem. By the time readers complete this article, they will have 1) an understanding of this problem, 2) a protocol for how to correct this problem, and 3) be able to explain the biochemical rationale for using these nutritional protocols in patients who might otherwise be treated with drugs in general and calcium-channel-blocking drugs in particular.

Although prescription drugs are often used by medical doctors in a "willy-nilly manner" (according to Harvard Medical School Professor Dr. Jerry Avorn[581]), let's assume for a moment that legitimate reasons exist for the widespread use of drugs that block calcium channels in cell membranes—the "calcium-channel-blocking drugs." Although it is counterintuitive to promote health by interfering with the body's natural function, calcium-channel-blocking drugs are routinely used in pharmaceutical medicine for a broad range of problems including hypertension, heart rhythm disturbances, bipolar disorder, and anxiety/panic disorders. Widespread medical use of calcium-channel-blocking drugs appears to validate the supposition that excess intracellular calcium is an important contributor to these and perhaps other problems. Therefore, if intracellular hypercalcinosis is the problem, then any safe and cost-effective treatment that can correct this problem should be met with the same widespread acceptance given to calcium-channel-blocking drugs, which are universally accepted and utilized in the allopathic "conventional medicine" society. At the very least, we can generally state that all phenomena that contribute to calcium deficiency result in an increase in intracellular calcium levels (the "calcium paradox") due to the effect of parathyroid hormone, which specifically promotes calcium uptake in cells while mobilizing calcium from bone. Additionally, a few other nutritional influences (such as fatty acid imbalances) modulate cellular calcium balance, and these will be discussed in the section on clinical interventions.

The Problem of Excess Intracellular Calcium: Although the current author is the first to coin the phrase "intracellular hypercalcinosis", several other authors have pointed to the problem of the "calcium paradox" and the means by which *body-wide calcium deficiency* can result in *intracellular calcium overload*, which triggers a cascade of events leading to adverse health effects. Most notably, the work of Takuo Fujita[582,583] stands out in its clarity and specificity in linking intracellular hypercalcinosis with disorders such as hypertension, arteriosclerosis, diabetes mellitus, neurodegenerative diseases, malignancy, and degenerative joint disease.

Mechanisms by which intracellular hypercalcinosis contributes to disease have been defined, at least partially. However, we must remember that nutritional disorders never occur in isolation, and that the effects of intracellular hypercalcinosis observed clinically are overlaid with manifestations of the primary nutritional/metabolic disorder. Stated differently, contrary to what the pharmaceutical paradigm's monotherapeutic use of calcium-channel-blocking drugs would imply, intracellular hypercalcinosis never occurs by itself. For example, if intracellular hypercalcinosis is contributed to by vitamin D3 deficiency, then some of the observed clinical complications of that condition are due to and yet independent from the excess intracellular calcium since the primary problem (vitamin D3 deficiency) causes adverse effects and deficiency symptoms that are independent of its effect on intracellular calcium levels. To better understand the specific effects of excess intracellular calcium, a brief review of a few specific biochemical/physiologic mechanisms by which intracellular hypercalcinosis can contribute to disease is warranted. We must start by realizing that calcium is much more than

---

[581] America the Medicated. cbsnews.com/stories/2005/04/21/health/main689997.shtml
[582] Fujita T. Calcium paradox: consequences of calcium deficiency manifested by a wide variety of diseases. *J Bone Miner Metab*. 2000;18(4):234-6
[583] Fujita et al. Calcium paradox disease: calcium deficiency prompting secondary hyperparathyroidism and cellular calcium overload. *J Bone Miner Metab*. 2000;18(3):109-25

a "bone nutrient" and that it functions as an electrolyte, intracellular messenger, and regulator of cell replication and metabolism. Let's talk about five pathways by which increased intracellular calcium promotes disease:

1. <u>Adverse effects on membrane receptors and intracellular transduction</u>: The concentration of extracellular calcium exceeds the concentration of intracellular calcium by a ratio of 10,000 to one. When intracellular calcium levels rise even slightly, receptors and messaging systems in the cell membrane fail to function optimally. Thereby, increased intracellular calcium can predispose to insulin resistance (via interference with insulin receptors) and can promote neurodegeneration by amplifying the intracellular cascade of effects that follows activation of the brain's NMDA-receptors (excitoneurotoxicity). More specifically, we must note that the recently discovered "calcium-sensing receptor" (CaR, a G protein-coupled plasma membrane receptor) senses minute alterations in serum calcium levels and then ultimately translates these variations into changes in cellular function, notably alterations in cell replication (think cancer) and eicosanoid production (think inflammation).[584,585] Given that CaR are found in a wide range of cell types, including those found in bone, the kidneys, and immune system, we can see a pathway by which alterations in calcium balance could be implicated in a wide range of diseases. CaR-mediated alterations in cell function are likely to be complicated by disorders of vitamin D3 nutrition and metabolism (that commonly complicate disorders of calcium homeostasis), which affect an even wider range of cell types including those of the breast, prostate, ovary, lung, skin, lymph nodes, colon, pancreas, adrenal medulla, brain (pituitary, cerebellum, and cerebral cortex), aortic endothelium, and immune system, including monocytes, transformed B-cells, and activated T-cells. This is an example of the complexity involved in understanding nutrition in general and the effects of nutritional deficiency (always multifaceted) in particular.

2. <u>Mitochondrial failure and cell death</u>: According to the most recent edition of the classic text *Robbins Pathologic Basis of Disease* (pages 15-16), increased intracellular calcium is a major cause of cell death. When calcium levels are increased within the cell, one adverse effect is the inhibition of mitochondrial function. Since calcium is pumped out of the cell in an energy-dependent process, and because dysfunctional mitochondria pour calcium into the intracellular space, calcium-induced mitochondrial failure results in an additional increase in intracellular calcium. Further complicating this problem is the fact that the cell membrane becomes increasingly permeable to calcium as calcium levels increase. Elevated intracellular calcium levels activate enzymes such as ATPase, phospholipase, proteases, and endonucleases that promote cell death.

3. <u>Pro-inflammatory effects of intracellular calcium</u>: The recent finding that intracellular calcium activates NF-kappaB[586] has obvious implications given the pivotal role of NF-kappaB in the promotion of systemic inflammation and diseases such as rheumatoid arthritis.[587] Thus, increased intracellular calcium appears to promote inflammation. This may explain in part how vitamin D3 supplementation (which lowers intracellular calcium levels) exerts its clinically impressive anti-inflammatory and immunomodulatory benefits.[588]

4. <u>Enhanced production of lipid peroxides</u>: Fujita notes that lipid peroxides lead to an increase in cell membrane permeability to calcium, which results in increased intracellular calcium; this activates metabolic pathways that increase oxidative stress, thus leading to a vicious cycle stimulated by the production of additional lipid peroxides. Thus, intracellular hypercalcinosis promotes oxidative stress, which becomes self-perpetuating by this and other mechanisms. Of course, we all know by now that increased production of free radicals contributes to the development of many health problems, such as cancer, cardiovascular disease, arthritis, autoimmunity, diabetes, and other forms of rapid biological aging.

5. <u>Myofascial trigger points, chronic muscle spasm, and increased vascular tone (hypertension)</u>: The release of calcium from the sarcoplasmic reticulum triggers muscle contraction and plays a role in hypertension (hence the use of calcium-channel-blocking drugs in the treatment of hypertension), chronic muscle spasm

---

[584] Peterlik M, Cross HS. Vitamin D and calcium deficits predispose for multiple chronic diseases. *Eur J Clin Invest*. 2005 May;35(5):290-304

[585] Heaney RP. Long-latency deficiency disease: insights from calcium and vitamin D. *Am J Clin Nutr*. 2003 Nov;78(5):912-9

[586] "Furthermore, a calcium chelator, BAPTA-AM, attenuated the NF-kappaB activation... CONCLUSIONS: Induction of NF-kappaB within 30 min by TNF-alpha- and IL-1beta was mediated through intracellular calcium but not ROS." Chang JW, Kim CS, Kim SB, Park SK, Park JS, Lee SK. Proinflammatory cytokine-induced NF-kappaB activation in human mesangial cells is mediated through intracellular calcium but not ROS: effects of silymarin. *Nephron Exp Nephrol*. 2006;103:e156-65

[587] Tak PP, Firestein GS. NF-kappaB: a key role in inflammatory diseases. *J Clin Invest*. 2001 Jan;107(1):7-11

[588] Timms et al. Circulating MMP9, vitamin D and variation in the TIMP-1 response with VDR genotype: mechanisms for inflammatory damage in chronic disorders? *QJM*. 2002 Dec;95(12):787-96. See also: Vasquez A, Manso G, Cannell J. The clinical importance of vitamin D. *Altern Ther Health Med*. 2004 Sep-Oct;10(5):28-36

(especially when complicated by magnesium deficiency), and the perpetuation of myofascial trigger points.[589] Reducing the levels of cytosolic and sarcoplasmic calcium promotes muscle relaxation.

Nutritional Interventions to Ameliorate Intracellular Hypercalcinosis: Now that we've reviewed the data implicating intracellular hypercalcinosis as a legitimate contributor to a wide range of clinical disorders and diseases, let's explore some nutritional solutions.

1. Correction of vitamin D deficiency: Vitamin D deficiency causes calcium deficiency which increases parathyroid hormone production resulting in increased intracellular calcium levels. Vitamin D deficiency is common (40-80% of most populations) and can be established via history and more objectively by measurement of serum 25-hydroxyl-vitamin D. Replacement doses are in the range of 1,000 IU per day for infants, 2,000 IU per day for children, and 4,000 IU per day for adults.[590] Vitamin D2 (ergocalciferol) should be avoided, and vitamin D3 (cholecalciferol) should be used, preferably in emulsified form to facilitate absorption, especially in older patients and those with impaired digestion and absorption.[591]

2. Reduction in dietary arachidonic acid intake: Arachidonic acid promotes intracellular calcium uptake, as demonstrated in a recent study using human erythrocytes.[592] Rich sources of arachidonic acid include beef, liver, pork, lamb, and cow's milk.

3. Increase intake of eicosapentaenoic acid (EPA): EPA reduces intracellular calcium levels in experimental models[593] and anticancer, antihypertensive, and anti-inflammatory effects of EPA are seen clinically. One to three grams per day is reasonable for adults.

4. Urinary alkalinization: Diet-induced chronic metabolic acidosis[594] promotes loss of calcium in urine[595] and thus indirectly contributes to calcium deficiency and the resultant rise in parathyroid hormone and intracellular calcium levels. An alkalinizing plant-based Paleo-Mediterranean diet should be the foundational treatment for numerous reasons[596]; however some patients may need to supplement with vegetable culture, potassium citrate, potassium bicarbonate, and/or sodium bicarbonate either regularly or "as needed"/PRN.

5. Ensuring adequate intake of calcium: A healthy diet can supply upwards toward 1,000 mg of calcium per day, and some people may choose to supplement with an additional 500 to 1,500 mg daily. Calcium supplementation should be used with magnesium, vitamin D and other components of the supplemented Paleo-Mediterranean diet.

6. Avoiding other dietary and lifestyle factors that promote calcium loss in urine: Caffeine, sugar, alcohol/ethanol, and psychoemotional stress all increase calcium loss in urine and thus contribute to secondary hyperparathyroidism and intracellular hypercalcinosis.

Conclusions: In this brief article, I have introduced and reviewed important concepts related to diet-induced alterations in cellular calcium balance. Notice that this discussion of calcium has transcended the usual conversation of simple "deficiency" and "excess." What I've done here is review data showing that we can indirectly modulate certain aspects of intracellular nutrition to promote optimal biochemical balance within the cell in order to optimize health and prevent and correct disease and dysfunction. Next time someone tells you that there is no scientific basis for interventional nutrition, sit them down and give them a lecture on causes and treatments for intracellular hypercalcinosis. Tell them it is only the tip of the iceberg, and that they'd be wise to take interventional nutrition seriously. Just because we buy groceries and nutritional supplements without a prescription (for now), this does not mean that these choices are not powerful or lacking in scientific merit. Amazing results can be achieved with diet modification and nutritional/botanical supplementation.

[589] Simons DG. Cardiology and myofascial trigger points: Janet G. Travell's contribution. *Tex Heart Inst J*. 2003;30(1):3-7
[590] Vasquez A, Manso G, Cannell J. The clinical importance of vitamin D (cholecalciferol). *Altern Ther Health Med*. 2004 Sep-Oct;10(5):28-36
[591] Vasquez A. Subphysiologic Doses of Vitamin D are Subtherapeutic: Comment on the Study by The Record Trial Group. *The Lancet* 2005 Published on-line May 6
[592] "The Ca(2+) influx rate varied from 0.5 to 3 nM Ca(2+)/s in the presence of AA and from 0.9 to 1.7 nM Ca(2+)/s with EPA." Soldati L, Lombardi C, Adamo D, Terranegra A, Bianchin C, Bianchi G, Vezzoli G. Arachidonic acid increases intracellular calcium in erythrocytes. *Biochem Biophys Res Commun*. 2002 May 10;293(3):974-8
[593] "This is a consequence of the ability of EPA to release Ca2+ from intracellular stores while inhibiting their refilling via capacitative Ca2+ influx that results in partial emptying of intracellular Ca2+ stores and thereby activation of protein kinase R." Palakurthi SS, Fluckiger R, Aktas H, Changolkar AK, Shahsafaei A, Harneit S, Kilic E, Halperin JA. Inhibition of translation initiation mediates the anticancer effect of the n-3 polyunsaturated fatty acid eicosapentaenoic acid. *Cancer Res*. 2000 Jun 1;60(11):2919-25
[594] Maurer M, Riesen W, Muser J, Hulter HN, Krapf R. Neutralization of Western diet inhibits bone resorption independently of K intake and reduces cortisol secretion in humans. *Am J Physiol Renal Physiol*. 2003 Jan;284(1):F32-40
[595] Sellmeyer et al. Potassium citrate prevents increased urine calcium excretion and bone resorption induced by a high sodium chloride diet. *J Clin Endocrinol Metab*. 2002 May;87(5):2008-12
[596] Vasquez A. A Five-Part Nutritional Protocol that Produces Consistently Positive Results. *Nutritional Wellness* 2005 September inflammationmastery.com/reprints

Allergy—Part 1: Allergic Inflammation

Introduction:

Allergic inflammation is the second of the three major categories of inflammation: ❶ Metabolic, including neuroinflammation, ❷ Allergic, and ❸ Rheumatic/Autoimmune. While exacerbations of allergic disease might necessitate pharmacologic immunosuppression, long-term management of allergic conditions should focus on nutritional immunomodulation (detailed in Chapter 4, Section 3 of _Functional Inflammology_ / _Inflammation Mastery_. Failure to normalize the immunophenotype imbalance via nutritional immunomodulation and failure to reduce the total inflammatory load (TIL), especially the mitochondrial and dysbiotic components, are what lead to both pharmacologic dependence and pharmacologic failure in the management of allergic disease. Allergy in general and food allergy in particular are discussed in Chapter 4, Section 1 (op cit), and that information should be used in conjunction with the allergy-specific information in the following sections. Different from the other sections focusing on Clinical Applications, and appropriate for the clinical management of allergic disorders, treatments here are discussed relative to a "hierarchy of therapeutics" which—in the naturopathic medical model—prioritizes treatments which might be sequenced in first, second, third, and fourth groups. Hence the FINDSEX ® acronym and sequence has not been applied to these sections on allergy. Readers and clinicians can mentally mix and intellectually overlay the two approaches—FINSEX ® components and the sequential format here—for a skilled and flexible clinical approach.

Allergy and Food Allergy

"**Adverse food reactions**" is a broad and general category that includes food allergy, food sensitivity, and food intolerance. The term "food" here means anything that is ingested other than drugs and medications and includes food, drink, additives, preservatives, and dyes. Many studies have underestimated the true prevalence and clinical importance of food allergies because of inconsistent terminology, insensitive/inaccurate laboratory assessments[1], and the assumption that an "apparently healthy" person would only be allergic/sensitive to one or two foods—this is an erroneous assumption considering that many patients with food allergy/sensitivity/intolerance must avoid several (common range 3-10) commonly eaten foods to obtain clinical response and maximal improvement.[2,3] Clinical practice differs from basic research in that we as clinicians must often do what is effective while having neither the need nor the luxury for determining the molecular and physiologic basis for the effectiveness of each treatment in each patient. Clinical research has scientifically proven that _adverse food reactions_—regardless of the underlying mechanism(s) or classification of allergy/intolerance/sensitivity—can exacerbate a wide range of human illnesses, including thyroid disease[4], mental depression[5,6], asthma, rhinitis,[7] recurrent otitis media[8], migraine[9,10,11], attention deficit and hyperactivity disorders[12], epilepsy[13,14,15], gastrointestinal inflammation[16], hypertension[17], joint pain[18,19,20,21,22,23,24] and other health problems.

[1] Bindslev-Jensen C, Skov PS, Madsen F, Poulsen LK. Food allergy and food intolerance--what is the difference? _Ann Allergy._ 1994 Apr;72(4):317-20

[2] Grant EC. Food allergies and migraine. _Lancet._ 1979 May 5;1(8123):966-9

[3] Speer F. Multiple food allergy. _Ann Allergy._ 1975 Feb;34(2):71-6

[4] Sategna-Guidetti et al. Prevalence of thyroid disorders in untreated adult celiac disease patients and effect of gluten withdrawal. _Am J Gastroenterol._ 2001 Mar;96(3):751-7

[5] Mills N. Depression and food intolerance: a single case study. _Hum Nutr Appl Nutr._ 1986 Apr;40(2):141-5

[6] Parker G, Watkins T. Treatment-resistant depression: when antidepressant drug intolerance may indicate food intolerance. _Aust N Z J Psychiatry._ 2002;36(2):263-5

[7] Speer F. The allergic child. _Am Fam Physician._ 1975 Feb;11(2):88-94

[8] Juntti H, Tikkanen S, Kokkonen J, Alho OP, Niinimaki A. Cow's milk allergy is associated with recurrent otitis media during childhood. _Acta Otolaryngol._ 1999;119(8):867-73

[9] Monro J, Carini C, Brostoff J. Migraine is a food-allergic disease. _Lancet._ 1984 Sep 29;2(8405):719-21

[10] Egger J, Carter CM, Wilson J, Turner MW, Soothill JF.Is migraine food allergy?A double-blind controlled trial of oligoantigenic diet treatment._Lancet_1983;2:865-9

[11] Monro J, Brostoff J, Carini C, Zilkha K. Food allergy in migraine. Study of dietary exclusion and RAST. _Lancet._ 1980 Jul 5;2(8184):1-4

[12] Boris M, Mandel FS. Foods and additives are common causes of the attention deficit hyperactive disorder in children. _Ann Allergy._ 1994 May;72(5):462-8

[13] Egger J, Carter CM, Soothill JF, Wilson J. Oligoantigenic diet treatment of children with epilepsy and migraine. _J Pediatr._ 1989;114(1):51-8

[14] Pelliccia et al. Partial cryptogenetic epilepsy and food allergy/intolerance. Reflections on three clinical cases. _Minerva Pediatr._ 1999 May;51(5):153-7

[15] Frediani T, Lucarelli S, Pelliccia A, et al. Allergy and childhood epilepsy: a close relationship? _Acta Neurol Scand._ 2001 Dec;104(6):349-52

[16] Marr HY, Chen WC, Lin LH. Food protein-induced enterocolitis syndrome: report of one case. _Acta Paediatr Taiwan._ 2001;42(1):49-52

[17] Grant EC. Food allergies and migraine. _Lancet._ 1979 May 5;1(8123):966-9

[18] Golding DN. Is there an allergic synovitis? _J R Soc Med._ 1990 May;83(5):312-4

[19] Panush RS. Food induced ("allergic") arthritis: clinical and serologic studies. _J Rheumatol._ 1990 Mar;17(3):291-4

[20] Pacor ML, Lunardi C, Di Lorenzo G, Biasi D, Corrocher R. Food allergy and seronegative arthritis: report of two cases. _Clin Rheumatol._ 2001;20(4):279-81

[21] Schrander JJ, Marcelis C, de Vries MP, van Santen-Hoeufft HM. Does food intolerance play a role in juvenile chronic arthritis? _Br J Rheumatol._ 1997;36(8):905-8

[22] van de Laar MA, van der Korst JK. Food intolerance in rheumatoid arthritis. I. A double blind, controlled trial of the clinical effects of elimination of milk allergens and azo dyes. _Ann Rheum Dis._ 1992 Mar;51(3):298-302

[23] Haugen MA,Kjeldsen-Kragh J, Forre O.A pilot study of the effect of an elemental diet in the management of rheumatoid arthritis._Clin Exp Rheumatol_ 1994;12:275-9

[24] van de Laar MA, Aalbers M, Bruins FG, et al. Food intolerance in rheumatoid arthritis. II. Clinical and histological aspects. _Ann Rheum Dis._ 1992 Mar;51(3):303-6

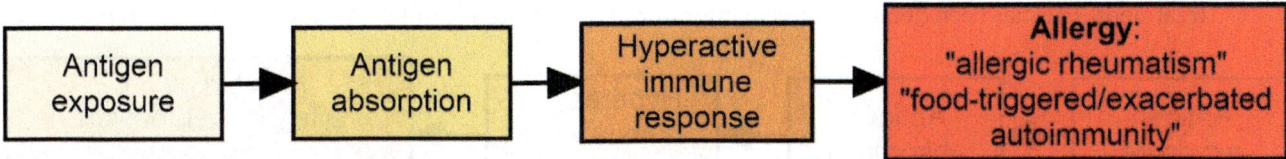

Overly simplistic ideas about allergy lead to overly simplistic drug treatments for allergic disease: This is the popular but inaccurate image that many patients and doctors have about allergy: "Allergy" and "allergic disease" do not result simply/solely from antigen exposure/absorption. The common view of allergic phenomena is incomplete and therefore inaccurate because it fails to include the prerequisite immune dysfunction and complex physiologic interconnections. Allergy should be seen as a reflection of immune dysfunction rather than a simple consequence of allergen exposure and absorption.

"**Food allergy**" generally refers to adverse food reactions that are specifically immunoglobulin-mediated. Classically, food allergy is seen with immediate-onset allergy mediated via IgE antibodies which initiate mast cell degranulation and histamine release. The classic symptoms of immediate-onset allergies are skin rash, abdominal pain, angioedema, and bronchoconstriction. However, many doctors recognize the possibility of IgG-mediated allergies and suggest that these might be responsible for the delayed-onset or "hidden" food allergies which are clinically significant but more subtle and difficult to diagnose than the classic IgE-mediated allergies.

> **Allergy is a manifestation of immune dysfunction**; except for urgent or exceptionally recalcitrant cases, simply suppressing the symptoms of this manifestation is neither rational nor adequate treatment if our goal is to provide optimal healthcare by addressing the cause of the problem
>
> "Allergic disease is a manifestation of a fundamental distortion of the mechanism through which the individual adapts itself on a cellular level to a hostile environment."
>
> Rapaport HG. What to do about the growing problem of pediatric allergy. *J Asthma Res.* 1967 Sep

The binding of antigens with immunoglobulins forms immune complexes that can deposit in parenchymal and synovial tissues where a localized immune response causes inflammation and organ dysfunction. "**Food sensitivity**" refers to immune-mediated adverse food reactions that are not antibody-mediated but are mediated by some other aspect of the immune/inflammatory system. An example of this is the increased production of specific prostaglandins in food-induced irritable bowel syndrome.[25] "**Food intolerance**" refers to adverse food reactions which are associated with poor nutritional status and/or impaired hepatic detoxification and which are *not* immune-mediated. Classic and well-known examples of this category of adverse food reaction include MSG sensitivity (associated with deficiency of vitamin B-6 and subsequent defects in hepatic transamination), tyramine intolerance that can result in hypertension and headaches, and histamine intolerance that can result in bronchoconstriction.[26] Surely, there is some overlap between allergy, sensitivity, and intolerance in some patients, and regardless of the specific mechanism(s) involved, from a practical clinical standpoint, the following facts are self-evident for any doctor working in the field of nutrition:

1. Some people have adverse food reactions from/to the foods that they eat. (This fact is obvious to anyone who has studied nutrition, but in most medical schools where nutrition is not taught, the only adverse food reaction discussed in class is the prototypic anaphylactic reaction [e.g., to peanuts] with possible mention of celiac disease while other forms of long-term and nonclassic food allergies/adversities are not discussed.)

2. Food-induced reactions may be either immediate-onset (i.e., within minutes) or delayed-onset (within days) of eating the triggering food.

3. The same patient might have immediate-onset reactions to food X with symptoms A and B and simultaneously have a delayed-onset reaction to food Y with symptom C.

4. Food X might cause symptoms D and E in one patient and symptoms F and G in another patient.

5. By avoiding allergens and/or improving or "modulating" immune function, many "diseases" resolve *without direct treatment* and the patient experiences an improved state of health.

---

[25] "Food intolerance associated with prostaglandin production is an important factor in the pathogenesis of IBS." Jones VA, McLaughlan P, Shorthouse M, Workman E, Hunter JO. Food intolerance: a major factor in the pathogenesis of irritable bowel syndrome. *Lancet.* 1982 Nov 20;2(8308):1115-7

[26] Wantke et al. Histamine in wine. Bronchoconstriction after a double-blind placebo-controlled red wine provocation test. *Int Arch Allergy Immunol.* 1996 Aug;110(4):397-400

6. Failure to identify and avoid problematic foods combined with failure to correct the underlying immune dysfunction often makes the "disease" recalcitrant to remediation even with "generally effective" treatment. This has been demonstrated in migraine, hypertension[27], and drug-resistant mental depression.[28]

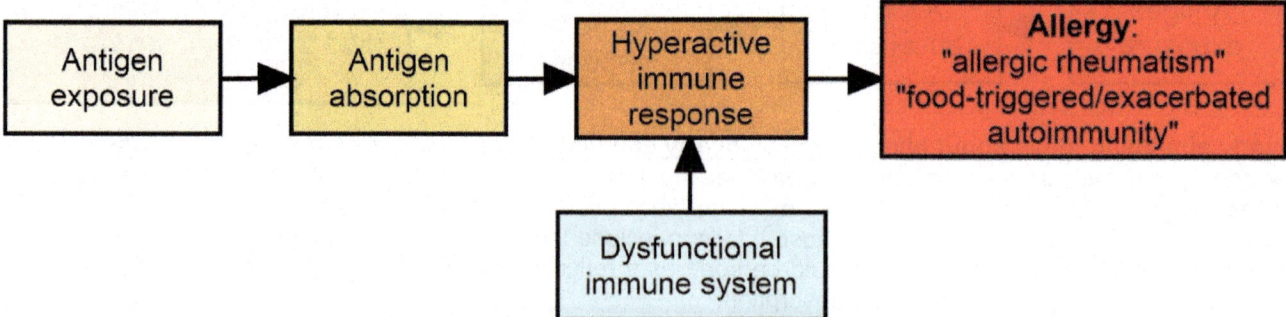

Allergy and allergic disease can only occur in the presence of preexisting immune dysfunction: Therefore, addressing the underlying immune dysfunction is the optimal treatment.

Potential roles of "food allergy" in the induction and perpetuation of autoimmunity and chronic inflammation

Food allergy both *results from* and *contributes to* immune dysfunction and a systemic proinflammatory state. Food allergy contributes to "autoimmunity" and musculoskeletal inflammation via several mechanisms, including but not limited to the following:

1. Stimulation of cytokine release: As will be discussed later, the term "superantigen" classically refers to microbial—viral, bacterial, or fungal—antigens which have the ability to induce production of excessive levels of cytokines and other inflammatory effectors[29], and superantigens appear to be involved in the pathogenesis of inflammatory musculoskeletal disorders such as rheumatoid arthritis.[30,31] In this section I propose that since food allergens appear capable of inducing cytokine production, they should in certain circumstances be considered "dietary superantigens" since they invoke cytokine release similarly as do microbial superantigens. An important distinction here, however, is that microbial superantigens generally stimulate cytokine release as an inherent property in *all* patients, whereas the production of cytokines by dietary (super)antigens is dependent on previous sensitization; thus cytokine production by allergens is patient-dependent and not an inherent property of the allergen itself. Mononuclear cells from egg-allergic patients produce much more proinflammatory cytokine (interferon) than do those from nonallergic patients.[32] Similarly, in children with autism, who commonly demonstrate immune dysfunction and neuroautoimmunity[33], exposure to food allergens greatly increases cytokine release compared to controls.[34] Food allergy, NFkB activation, cytokine release, and increased intestinal permeability form a self-perpetuating vicious cycle because consumption of dietary allergens causes damage to the intestinal mucosa and stimulates NFkB activation and cytokine release which then increases intestinal permeability, thus allowing for increased absorption of dietary and microbial immunogens for the perpetuation and

[27] "When an average of ten common foods were avoided there was a dramatic fall in the number of headaches per month, 85% of patients becoming headache-free. The 25% of patients with hypertension became normotensive." Grant EC. Food allergies and migraine. *Lancet.* 1979 May 5;1(8123):966-9

[28] "The prevalence of food intolerance as a contributing factor to depressive disorders requires clarification. Clinicians should be aware of the possible syndrome and that it may be worsened by psychotropic medication." Parker G, Watkins T. Treatment-resistant depression: when antidepressant drug intolerance may indicate food intolerance. *Aust N Z J Psychiatry.* 2002 Apr;36(2):263-5

[29] "The basis of autoimmune disorders due to superantigen is due to greater stimulation of T-lymphocytes and elaborate cytokine production." Hemalatha V, Srikanth P, Mallika M. Superantigens - Concepts, clinical disease and therapy. *Indian J Med Microbiol* 2004;22:204-211

[30] "They also suggest that the etiology of RA may involve initial activation of V beta 14+ T cells by a V beta 14-specific superantigen with subsequent recruitment of a few activated autoreactive v beta 14+ T cell clones to the joints while the majority of other V beta 14+ T cells disappear." Paliard X, West SG, Lafferty JA, Clements JR, Kappler JW, Marrack P, Kotzin BL. Evidence for the effects of a superantigen in rheumatoid arthritis. *Science.* 1991 Jul 19;253(5017):325-9

[31] "Given that binding sites for superantigens have been mapped to the CDR4s of TCR beta chains, the synovial localization of T cells bearing V beta s with significant CDR4 homology indicates that V beta-specific T-cell activation by superantigen may play a role in RA." Howell MD, Diveley JP, Lundeen KA, Esty A, Winters ST, Carlo DJ, Brostoff SW. Limited T-cell receptor beta-chain heterogeneity among interleukin 2 receptor-positive synovial T cells suggests a role for superantigen in rheumatoid arthritis. *Proc Natl Acad Sci* U S A. 1991 Dec 1;88(23):10921-5

[32] "The levels of IFN-gamma production of only IL-2-stimulated or both ovalbumin-stimulated and IL-2-stimulated peripheral blood mononuclear cells from egg-sensitive patients with atopic dermatitis was significantly higher than that of healthy children and that of egg-sensitive patients with immediate allergic symptoms." Shinbara M, Kondo N, Agata H, et al. Interferon-gamma and interleukin-4 production of ovalbumin-stimulated lymphocytes in egg-sensitive children. *Ann Allergy Asthma Immunol.* 1996;77(1):60-6

[33] "Autistic children, but not normal children, had antibodies to caudate nucleus (49% positive sera), cerebral cortex (18% positive sera) and cerebellum (9% positive sera)." Singh VK, Rivas WH. Prevalence of serum antibodies to caudate nucleus in autistic children. *Neurosci Lett.* 2004 Jan 23;355(1-2):53-6

[34] Jyonouchi H, Sun S, Itokazu N. Innate immunity associated with inflammatory responses and cytokine production against common dietary proteins in patients with autism spectrum disorder. *Neuropsychobiology.* 2002;46(2):76-84

exacerbation of allergy and immune dysfunction.[35] Generally speaking, cytokines are proinflammatory and would be expected to contribute to autoimmune disease induction via mechanisms such as bystander activation and increased autoantigen processing regardless of their original stimuli.

2. <u>Immune complex formation and deposition</u>: Dietary antigen-antibody immune complexes are formed following the consumption of allergenic foods by patients with allergy to those foods[36,37] and these anti-food and anti-IgE immune complexes contribute to allergic symptomatology by a mechanism that has been described as "chronic serum sickness."[38] These immune complexes are then deposited in the joints to localize the resultant proinflammatory response. In the study by Carini et al[39], the authors found that patients with food-induced joint pain and inflammation had anti-IgE IgG antibodies which formed large immune complexes that were detectable in synovial fluid and which probably contributed to the arthritis. Anti-IgE IgG antibodies are commonly elevated in patients with allergic/inflammatory diseases such as eczema[40], asthma[41], and Crohn's disease[42] and thus

> **Perspective & Context**
>
> This section on the protean clinical manifestations of allergy originally emphasized the relevance of allergy to systemic inflammation, including rheumatic diseases. Clinicians should keep food allergy and intolerance in mind when dealing with a wide range of conditions, including:
> - Thyroid disease
> - Mental depression
> - Fatigue
> - Asthma
> - Rhinitis
> - Recurrent otitis media
> - Migraine
> - Attention deficit and hyperactivity disorders
> - Epilepsy
> - Gastrointestinal inflammation and chronic abdominal pain
> - Hypertension
> - Joint pain and inflammation

tissue damage in these conditions appears mediated at least in part by anti-immunoglobulin immune complexes (i.e., anti-IgE IgG complexed with IgE) rather than the classic antigen-antibody immune complexes. In this way, food allergies cause joint pain and inflammation by the deposition of immune complexes into the synovium and joint cartilage.[43] Conversely, the consumption of a relatively hypoallergenic diet reduces intake of food antigens and helps reduce IgE levels. This explains, in part, the success of hypoallergenic diets in the treatment of immune-complex-mediated diseases such as mixed cryoglobulinemia[44,45], hypersensitivity vasculitis[46], and leukocytoclastic vasculitis with arthritis.[47] In patients with rheumatoid arthritis, the symptomatic and clinical improvement induced by hypoallergenic diets correlates with reductions in antibodies to food antigens.[48]

3. <u>Damage to the intestinal mucosa with resultant increased absorption of dietary and microbial antigens</u>: Consumption of food allergens increases intestinal permeability[49] and thus amplifies the absorption of intestinal contents—dietary and microbial antigens. Patients with food allergy have "leaky gut" that is

---

[35] Ma et al. TNF-alpha-induced increase in intestinal epithelial tight junction permeability requires NF-kappa B activation. Am *J Physiol Gastrointest Liver Physiol*. 2004 Mar;286(3):G367-76 ajpgi.physiology.org/cgi/content/full/286/3/G367

[36] "Antigen entry and the formation of immune complexes occur in atopic subjects after food ingestion. ...Food allergic subjects showed, after food challenge, the presence of IgE and IgG immune complexes, which correlates with the subsequent occurrence of symptoms." Carini C, Brostoff J. Evidence for circulating IgE complexes in food allergy. *Ric Clin Lab*. 1987 Oct-Dec;17(4):309-22

[37] "Following challenge, immune complexes containing IgE, IgG, and antigen are detectable in the circulation. Their appearance correlates with the production of symptoms." Carini C, Brostoff J, Wraith DG. IgE complexes in food allergy. *Ann Allergy*. 1987 Aug;59(2):110-7

[38] Marinkovich V. "Immunology and Food Allergy" in "Applying Functional Medicine in Clinical Practice" hosted by the Institute for Functional Medicine. Seattle,Wa: Mar2005

[39] "In three food-allergic patients IgG anti-IgE was detectable in a complexed form in the serum samples examined before and after food challenge. The finding of IgG anti-IgE autoantibody in a group of patients with allergic arthralgia is quite exciting." Carini et al. Immune complexes in food-induced arthralgia. *Ann Allergy*. 1987 Dec;59(6):422-8

[40] "An IgG type of antibody directed against IgE has been studied in serum from healthy and allergic individuals. ... Significantly raised levels of anti-IgE autoantibody were found in patients suffering from atopic disorders in comparison to the controls." Carini et al. IgG autoantibody to IgE in atopic patients. *Ann Allergy*. 1988 Jan;60(1):48-52

[41] "Significantly enhanced levels of IgE/anti-IgE IC were detected in children with asthma." Ritter C, Battig M, Kraemer R, Stadler BM. IgE hidden in immune complexes with anti-IgE autoantibodies in children with asthma. *J Allergy Clin Immunol*. 1991 Nov;88(5):793-801

[42] "In CD sera no food-specific IgE could be detected, but levels of immune complexes of IgE and IgG anti-IgE autoantibodies were statistically significantly increased compared to healthy controls." Huber et al. IgE/anti-IgE immune complexes in sera from patients with Crohn's disease do not contain food-specific IgE. *Int Arch Allergy Immunol*. 1998 Jan;115(1):67-72

[43] Inman RD. Antigens, the gastrointestinal tract, and arthritis. *Rheum Dis Clin North Am*. 1991 May;17(2):309-21

[44] "CONCLUSION: These data show that an LAC diet decreases the amount of circulating immune complexes in MC and can modify certain signs and symptoms of the disease." Ferri C, Pietrogrande M, Cecchetti R, et al. Low-antigen-content diet in the treatment of patients with mixed cryoglobulinemia. *Am J Med*. 1989 Nov;87(5):519-24

[45] Pietrogrande M, Cefalo A, Nicora F, Marchesini D. Dietetic treatment of essential mixed cryoglobulinemia. *Ric Clin Lab*. 1986 Apr-Jun;16(2):413-6

[46] "In three cases the vasculitis relapsed following the introduction of food additives; in one case with the addition of potatoes and green vegetables (i.e., beans and green peas) and in the last case with the addition of eggs to the diet." Lunardi et al. Elimination diet in the treatment of selected patients with hypersensitivity vasculitis. *Clin Exp Rheumatol*. 1992 Mar-Apr;10(2):131-5

[47] "Described in this report are two children with severe vasculitis caused by specific foods." Businco L, Falconieri P, Bellioni-Businco B, Bahna SL. Severe food-induced vasculitis in two children. *Pediatr Allergy Immunol*. 2002 Feb;13(1):68-71

[48] Hafstrom I, Ringertz B, Spangberg A, et al. A vegan diet free of gluten improves the signs and symptoms of rheumatoid arthritis: the effects on arthritis correlate with a reduction in antibodies to food antigens. *Rheumatology*. 2001 Oct;40(10):1175-9 rheumatology.oxfordjournals.org/cgi/content/full/40/10/1175

[49] "When compared to the control group, the 11 patients of the allergic group presented a normal mannitol urinary excretion (16.5 +/- 13.4%, p = NS, Student's t-test) and an increase in the lactulose excretion (1.36 +/- 0.92%, p < 0.001). Moreover, the allergic group showed a lactulose/mannitol ratio that was significantly different (0.105 +/- 0.071, p < 0.001)." Laudat A, Arnaud P, Napoly A, Brion F. The intestinal permeability test applied to the diagnosis of food allergy in paediatrics. *West Indian Med J*. 1994 Sep;43(3):87-8

exacerbated by consumption of allergenic foods; thus lactulose-mannitol assays can be used to assist the diagnosis of food allergy.[50,51] By increasing intestinal permeability, consumption of dietary antigens serves to exacerbate the adverse effects of gastrointestinal dysbiosis by increasing antigen and (anti)metabolite absorption. Since both dietary allergens and bacterial endotoxin stimulate production of cytokines[52], concomitant exposure to both allergens and intra-intestinal endotoxin leads to an additive increase in proinflammatory cytokine production.[53] Thus, consumption of allergenic foods in the presence of gastrointestinal dysbiosis would be expected to lead to more severe and more diverse adverse physiologic and clinical consequences than would be experienced following exposure to either allergens or dysbiosis alone.

4. <u>Dietary haptenization</u>: Dietary antigens can complex with human tissues to form *neoantigens* that are immunostimulatory. The best example of this appears to be the induction of autoimmunity by wheat-derived gliadin which haptenizes with intestinal tissue transglutaminase and other extracellular matrix proteins and results in the allergic-autoimmune disease celiac disease.[54,55] The finding that gliadin proteins haptenize with collagen and can induce the formation of anti-collagen antibodies in humans[56] makes clear the pathomechanism by which "wheat allergy" can directly precipitate systemic musculoskeletal autoimmunity. Once initiated and perpetuated by dietary gliadin from wheat, additional autoimmunity ensues (perhaps mediated directly by epitope spreading and/or indirectly by deposition of immune complexes) which is directed against various tissues, most notably the thyroid gland[57], brain[58], and musculoskeletal system.[59] Given the association between lupus and celiac disease[60,61,62], we may speculate that "allergy" becomes/triggers "autoimmunity" in certain circumstances and in susceptible patients.

5. <u>Dietary molecular mimicry</u>: Just as microbes produce structures similar to human molecules which then incite a cross-reacting immune response—molecular mimicry (discussed elsewhere in this chapter in the section on dysbiosis)—certain dietary antigens appear capable of inducing cross reactions. For example, Vojdani et al[63] recently demonstrated cross-reactivity between anti-gliadin antibodies and anti-cerebellar antibodies in an experimental model that may partly explain the anti-brain autoimmunity seen in autism. Further expanding this concept of dietary molecular mimicry is the finding that "the virulence factor of C albicans-hyphal wall protein 1 (HWP1)-contains amino acid sequences that are identical or highly homologous to known celiac disease-related alpha-gliadin and gamma-gliadin T-cell epitopes."[64] This raises three interrelated possibilities: 1) that gastrointestinal overgrowth of *Candida albicans* and the

---

[50] "After ingestion of food allergens by the patients, mean mannitol recovery fell to 11.57% and mean recovery of lactulose rose to 1.04%, both values being significantly different from those obtained in the fasting patients." Andre C, Andre F, Colin L, Cavagna S. Measurement of intestinal permeability to mannitol and lactulose as a means of diagnosing food allergy and evaluating therapeutic effectiveness of disodium cromoglycate. *Ann Allergy*. 1987 Nov;59(5 Pt 2):127-30

[51] "A provocation IPT with food induced significant L/M ratio changes only in the group in which the food was proved to be responsible for the exacerbation of skin lesions." Dupont C, Barau E, Molkhou P, Raynaud F, Barbet JP, Dehennin L. Food-induced alterations of intestinal permeability in children with cow's milk-sensitive enteropathy and atopic dermatitis. *J Pediatr Gastroenterol Nutr*. 1989 May;8(4):459-65

[52] Jyonouchi H, Sun S, Itokazu N. Innate immunity associated with inflammatory responses and cytokine production against common dietary proteins in patients with autism spectrum disorder. *Neuropsychobiology*. 2002;46(2):76-84

[53] "Thus, endotoxin and allergen acting together could play a role in up-regulating the response of the human asthmatic airway to adenosine. However, our data suggest that the interaction would be additive rather than synergistic." Karmouty Quintana H, Mazzoni L, Fozard JR. Effects of endotoxin and allergen alone and in combination on the sensitivity of the rat airways to adenosine. *Auton Autacoid Pharmacol*. 2005 Oct;25(4):167-70

[54] "Our findings firstly demonstrated that gliadin was directly bound to tTG in duodenal mucosa of coeliacs and controls, and the ability of circulating tTG-autoantibodies to recognize and immunoprecipitate the tTG-gliadin complexes." Ciccocioppo R, Di Sabatino A, Ara C, Biagi F, Perilli M, Amicosante G, Cifone MG, Corazza GR. Gliadin and tissue transglutaminase complexes in normal and coeliac duodenal mucosa. *Clin Exp Immunol*. 2003 Dec;134(3):516-24

[55] "Thus, modification of gluten peptides by tTG, especially deamidation of certain glutamine residues, can enhance their binding to HLA-DQ2 or -DQ8 and potentiate T cell stimulation. Furthermore, tTG-catalyzed cross-linking and consequent haptenization of gluten with extracellular matrix proteins allows for storage and extended availability of gluten in the mucosa." Dieterich W, Esslinger B, Schuppan D. Pathomechanisms in celiac disease. *Int Arch Allergy Immunol*. 2003 Oct;132(2):98-108

[56] "Gliadins alpha1-alpha11, gamma1- gamma6, omega1-omega3, and omega5 were substrates for tTG. tTG catalyzed the crosslinking of gliadin peptides with interstitial collagens type I, III and VI. Coeliac patients showed increased antibody titers against the collagens I, III, V and VI." Dieterich et al. Crosslinking to tissue transglutaminase and collagen favours gliadin toxicity in coeliac disease. *Gut*. 2006 Apr; 55(4): 478–484

[57] "Elevated titres of antithyroid antibodies observed in children with coeliac disease (41.1%) in comparison to control group (3.56%) indicate the need for performing the screening tests for antithyroid antibodies in children with CD." Kowalska E, Wasowska-Krolikowska K, Toporowska-Kowalska E. Estimation of antithyroid antibodies occurrence in children with coeliac disease. *Med Sci Monit*. 2000 Jul-Aug;6(4):719-2 medscimonit.com/pub/vol_6/no_4/1240.pdf

[58] Kieslich M, Errazuriz G, Posselt HG, Moeller-Hartmann W, Zanella F, Boehles H. Brain white-matter lesions in celiac disease: a prospective study of 75 diet-treated patients. *Pediatrics*. 2001 Aug;108(2):E21 pediatrics.aappublications.org/cgi/content/full/108/2/e21

[59] "JIA children have an increased prevalence of autoimmune thyroiditis, subclinical hypothyroidism and coeliac disease." Stagi S, Giani T, Simonini G, Falcini F. Thyroid function, autoimmune thyroiditis and coeliac disease in juvenile idiopathic arthritis. *Rheumatology* (Oxford). 2005 Apr;44(4):517-2

[60] Zitouni M, Daoud W, Kallel M, Makni S. Systemic lupus erythematosus with celiac disease: a report of five cases. *Joint Bone Spine*. 2004 Jul;71(4):344-6

[61] Komatireddy GR, Marshall JB, Aqel R, Spollen LE, Sharp GC. Association of systemic lupus erythematosus and gluten enteropathy. *South Med J*. 1995 Jun;88(6):673-6

[62] Rustgi AK, Peppercorn MA. Gluten-sensitive enteropathy and systemic lupus erythematosus. *Arch Intern Med*. 1988 Jul;148(7):1583-4

[63] "This cross-reaction was further confirmed by DOT-immunoblot and inhibition studies. We conclude that a subgroup of patients with autism produce antibodies against Purkinje cells and gliadin peptides, which may be responsible for some of the neurological symptoms in autism." Vojdani A, O'Bryan T, Green JA, Mccandless J, Woeller KN, Vojdani E, Nourian AA, Cooper EL. Immune response to dietary proteins, gliadin and cerebellar peptides in children with autism. *Nutr Neurosci*. 2004 Jun;7(3):151-61

[64] "Subsequently, C albicans might function as an adjuvant that stimulates antibody formation against HWP1 and gluten, and formation of autoreactive antibodies against tissue transglutaminase and endomysium." Nieuwenhuizen et al. Is Candida albicans a trigger in the onset of coeliac disease? *Lancet*. 2003;361(9375):2152-4

resultant elaboration of HWP1 and immunostimulation may result in sensitivity to gluten, particularly as HWP1 and gliadin are both substrates for transglutaminase, 2) that consumption of wheat gluten may trigger sensitivity to *Candida albicans*, and 3) that wheat gluten and *Candida albicans* must both be present for the development of celiac disease and the ensuant autoimmunity. Additional details on the ability of *C. albicans* to contribute to autoimmunity are discussed in the section on dysbiosis.

6. <u>Enhanced processing of autoantigens</u>: Food-allergic patients may produce autoimmunity-stimulating autoantigens following exposure to foods to which they are sensitized. This has been demonstrated in autistic children, exposure of lymphocytes from autistic patients to dietary antigens (gliadin and casein peptides) stimulates production of autoantigens that presumably incite and perpetuate autoimmunity.[65] Thus, at least in autistic patients, we have evidence that food allergy can segue into autoimmunity. This phenomenon is probably not restricted only to autistic patients, as suggested by the association between celiac disease and the systemic autoimmune disease lupus.[66,67,68]

7. <u>Diet-derived xenobiotic immunotoxicity</u>: Foods commonly contain trace amounts of xenobiotics such as pesticides, fungicides, fumigants, fertilizers, preservatives, military propellants such as perchlorate[69], and toxic metals such as mercury. Some of these xenobiotics have been insufficiently studied in humans, while others such as mercury are well-known immunotoxins capable of inducing immune dysfunction which may contribute to autoimmunity. Mercury poisoning/accumulation can occur in humans as a result of consumption of contaminated foods—especially seafood such as shark, swordfish, king mackerel, tilefish, and albacore ("white") tuna[70], and the immunologic effects of organic and/or inorganic mercury include immunosuppression, immunostimulation, formation of antinucleolar antibodies targeting fibrillarin, and formation and deposition of immune-complexes, resulting in a syndrome called "mercury-induced autoimmunity" which can be induced by exposure of susceptible animals to mercury.[71] Mercury/"silver" amalgam dental fillings rank highly among the most significant source of mercury exposure in humans, and implantation of mercury-silver dental amalgams in susceptible animals causes chronic stimulation of the immune system with induction of systemic autoimmunity.[72] Besides being a neurotoxin with no safe exposure limit[73], mercury is known to modify/antigenize endogenous proteins to promote autoimmunity[74], and mercury may also promote autoimmunity by contributing to a pro-inflammatory environment that awakens quiescent autoreactive immunocytes via bystander activation[75] (detailed later). For example, administration of mercury to "susceptible" mice induces autoimmunity via modification of the nucleolar protein *fibrillarin*[76]; noteworthy in this regard is the fact that antifibrillarin antibodies are characteristic of the autoimmune disease scleroderma.[77] Mercury toxicity is commonly encountered in clinical practice (diagnosis and treatment are discussed later), and a recent study published in *JAMA* showed that 8% of American women of childbearing age have sufficient levels of mercury in their bodies to produce neurologic damage in their children.[78] The mercury-based preservative thimerosol is a type-IV (delayed

[65] Vojdani A, Pangborn JB, Vojdani E, Cooper EL. Infections, toxic chemicals and dietary peptides binding to lymphocyte receptors and tissue enzymes are major instigators of autoimmunity in autism. *Int J Immunopathol Pharmacol.* 2003 Sep-Dec;16(3):189-99

[66] Zitouni M, Daoud W, Kallel M, Makni S. Systemic lupus erythematosus with celiac disease: a report of five cases. *Joint Bone Spine.* 2004 Jul;71(4):344-6

[67] Komatireddy GR, Marshall JB, Aqel R, Spollen LE, Sharp GC. Association of systemic lupus erythematosus and gluten enteropathy. *South Med J.* 1995 Jun;88(6):673-6

[68] Rustgi AK, Peppercorn MA. Gluten-sensitive enteropathy and systemic lupus erythematosus. *Arch Intern Med.* 1988 Jul;148(7):1583-4

[69] "The Bush administration has imposed a gag order on the U.S. Environmental Protection Agency from publicly discussing perchlorate pollution, even as two new studies reveal high levels of the rocket-fuel component may be contaminating the nation's lettuce supply." Peter Waldman. Rocket Fuel Residues Found in Lettuce: Bush administration issues gag order on EPA discussions of possible rocket fuel tainted lettuce. *Wall Street Journal.* See organicconsumers.org/toxic/lettuce042903.cfm rhinoed.com/epa's_gag_order.htm peer.org/press/508.html yubanet.com/artman/publish/article_13637.shtml

[70] See cfsan.fda.gov/~dms/admehg3.html for the white-washed version; see ewg.org/issues/mercury/20040319/index.php for a more complete perspective.

[71] Havarinasab S, Hultman P. Organic mercury compounds and autoimmunity. *Autoimmun Rev.* 2005;4(5):270-5 generationrescue.org/pdf/havarinasab.pdf

[72] "We hypothesize that under appropriate conditions of genetic susceptibility and adequate body burden, heavy metal exposure from dental amalgam may contribute to immunological aberrations, which could lead to overt autoimmunity." Hultman P, Johansson U, Turley SJ, Lindh U, Enestrom S, Pollard KM. Adverse immunological effects and autoimmunity induced by dental amalgam and alloy in mice. *FASEB J.* 1994 Nov;8(14):1183-90 fasebj.org/cgi/reprint/8/14/1183

[73] University of Calgary Faculty of Medicine. How Mercury Causes Brain Neuron Degeneration commons.ucalgary.ca/mercury/

[74] Havarinasab S, Hultman P. Organic mercury compounds and autoimmunity. *Autoimmun Rev.* 2005 Jun;4(5):270-5

[75] "It is therefore theoretically possible that compounds present in vaccines such as thiomersal or aluminium hydroxyde can trigger autoimmune reactions through bystander effects." Fournier et al. Induction of autoimmunity through bystander effects. Lessons from immunological disorders induced by heavy metals. *J Autoimmun.* 2001 May;16:319-26

[76] Nielsen JB, Hultman P. Mercury-induced autoimmunity in mice. *Environ Health Perspect.* 2002 Oct;110 Suppl 5:877-81

[77] "Since anti-fibrillarin antibodies are specific markers of scleroderma, the present animal model may be valuable for studies of the immunological aberrations which are likely to induce this autoimmune response." Hultman P, Enestrom S, Pollard KM, Tan EM. Anti-fibrillarin autoantibodies in mercury-treated mice. *Clin Exp Immunol.* 1989 Dec;78:470-7

[78] "However, approximately 8% of women had concentrations higher than the US Environmental Protection Agency's recommended reference dose (5.8 microg/L), below which exposures are considered to be without adverse effects. Women who are pregnant or who intend to become pregnant should follow federal and state advisories on consumption of fish." Schober et al. Blood mercury levels in US children and women of childbearing age, 1999-2000. *JAMA.* 2003 Apr 2;289(13):1667-74

hypersensitivity) sensitizing agent[79], and recent research implicates mercury as an important contributor to the clinical manifestations of autism[80,81] and eczema.[82] Preliminary clinical evidence shows that removal of mercury amalgams, particularly along with implementation of antioxidant therapy and/or mercury chelation, benefits the biochemical status and/or clinical course of autoimmune disease.[83,84] More recently, what has become very clear is that many foods are contaminated with pesticides; glyphosate for example promotes DNA damage, endocrine disruption, mitochondrial dysfunction, and—via its antibiotic effect—gastrointestinal dysbiosis.[85,86,87,88] Pesticide-contaminated foods and drinks should be avoided.

8. Diet-derived dysbiosis: Induction and exacerbation of dysbiosis following chronic consumption of allergenic foods has been reported to occur in humans; this paragraph reviews the three main types of diet induced dysbiosis: ❶ food contamination with problematic microbes, ❷ promotion of gastrointestinal bacterial overgrowth by over-consumption of carbohydrate substrate, and ❸ chronic diet-induced immunosuppression due to nutrient insufficiency or carbohydrate overconsumption. Raw vegetables and salad greens are thoroughly contaminated with bacteria and occasionally other microbes. Food can be contaminated with pathogenic microbes via improper preparation, storage, or handling by chefs with contagious diseases and poor hygiene. An inflammatory "reactive" arthritis can result from consumption of food that is contaminated by microorganisms, most commonly *Salmonella*[89,90,91] and *Campylobacter* species.[92] Long-term autoimmune/inflammatory complications of gastrointestinal infections/colonization sourced from food include Reiter's syndrome, Guillain-Barre syndrome (autoimmunity peripheral demyelinating neuropathy), uveitis, sacroiliitis, and ankylosing spondylitis. Independent and probably more common than the food contamination issues mentioned at the first half of this paragraph is the chronic gastrointestinal dysbiosis—in particular a generalized bacterial overgrowth of the small bowel—that is maintained and perpetuated by overconsumption of carbohydrates in general (starches, rice, sucrose, fructose) and difficult-to-digest carbohydrates in particular (such as those found in milk/lactose, wheat, and potatoes). High-fructose beverages are very popular, and they can promote excess colonic fermentation[93] which would be expected to result in bacterial overgrowth over time. By "feeding" intestinal bacteria with excess carbohydrate and promoting bacterial overgrowth in the intestines, the standard Western/American diet promotes dysbiosis-induced systemic inflammation and chronic musculoskeletal pain; this is particularly relevant for patients with rheumatoid arthritis or fibromyalgia.[94] Thus dietary modification taken in the interest of avoiding common allergens such as milk and wheat quite likely results

[79] "Thimerosal is an important preservative in vaccines and ophthalmologic preparations. The substance is known to be a type IV sensitizing agent. High sensitization rates were observed in contact-allergic patients and in health care workers who had been exposed to thimerosal-preserved vaccines." Westphal et al. Homozygous gene deletions of the glutathione S-transferases M1 and T1 are associated with thimerosal sensitization. *Int Arch Occup Environ Health.* 2000 Aug;73(6):384-8

[80] Vojdani A, Pangborn JB, Vojdani E, Cooper EL. Infections, toxic chemicals and dietary peptides binding to lymphocyte receptors and tissue enzymes are major instigators of autoimmunity in autism. *Int J Immunopathol Pharmacol.* 2003 Sep-Dec;16(3):189-99

[81] Geier DA, Geier MR. A comparative evaluation of the effects of MMR immunization and mercury doses from thimerosal-containing childhood vaccines on the population prevalence of autism. *Med Sci Monit.* 2004 Mar;10(3):PI33-9. Epub 2004 Mar 1. medscimonit.com/pub/vol_10/no_3/3986.pdf

[82] Weidinger et al. Body burden of mercury is associated with acute atopic eczema and total IgE in children from southern Germany. *J Allergy Clin Immunol.* 2004 Aug;114(2):457-9

[83] Prochazkova J, Sterzl I, Kucerova H, Bartova J, Stejskal VD. The beneficial effect of amalgam replacement on health in patients with autoimmunity. *Neuro Endocrinol Lett.* 2004 Jun;25(3):211-8. See also: "The MELISA Test is reproducible, sensitive, specific, and reliable for detecting metal sensitivity in metal-sensitive patients." Valentine-Thon E, Schiwara HW. Validity of MELISA for metal sensitivity testing. *Neuro Endocrinol Lett.* 2003 Feb-Apr;24(1-2):57-64. See also: "The hypothesis that metal exposure from dental amalgam can cause ill health in a susceptible part of the exposed population was supported." Lindh U, Hudecek R, Danersund A, Eriksson S, Lindvall A. Removal of dental amalgam and other metal alloys supported by antioxidant therapy alleviates symptoms and improves quality of life in patients with amalgam-associated ill health. *Neuro Endocrinol Lett.* 2002 Oct-Dec;23(5-6):459-82 nel.edu/23_56/NEL235602A12_Lindh.htm and nel.edu/pdf_w/23_56/NEL235602A12_Lindh_wr.pdf

[84] "This study documents objective biochemical changes following the removal of these fillings along with other dental materials, utilizing a new health care model of multidisciplinary planning and treatment." Huggins HA, Levy TE. Cerebrospinal fluid protein changes in multiple sclerosis after dental amalgam removal. *Altern Med Rev.* 1998 Aug;3(4):295-300

[85] Seneff S, Swanson N Li C. Aluminum and Glyphosate Can Synergistically Induce Pineal Gland Pathology: Connection to Gut Dysbiosis and Neurological Disease. *Agricultural Sciences* 2015; 6, 42-70. dx.doi.org/10.4236/as.2015.61005

[86] Krüger M, Schledorn P, Schrödl W, Hoppe HW, Lutz W, et al. Detection of Glyphosate Residues in Animals and Humans. *J Environ Anal Toxicol* 2014;4: 210

[87] Shehata AA, Schrödl W, Schledorn P, Krüger M. Distribution of glyphosate in chicken organs and its reduction by humic acid supplementation. *J Poult Sci.* 2014;51:333-7

[88] Krüger et al. Glyphosate suppresses the antagonistic effect of Enterococcus spp. on Clostridium botulinum. *Anaerobe.* 2013 Apr;20:74-8

[89] "We describe the case of a patient who became ill with Salmonella Blockley food poisoning while working in Cyprus in August 1994. As his diarrhoea resolved he began to suffer from lower limb joint pains which were diagnosed as acute salmonella reactive arthritis." Wilson IG, Whitehead E. Long-term post-Salmonella reactive arthritis due to Salmonella Blockley. *Jpn J Infect Dis.* 2004 Oct;57(5):210-1

[90] "Reactive joint symptoms after food-borne Salmonella infection may be more frequent than previously thought. The duration of diarrhea is strongly correlated with the occurrence of joint symptoms." Locht et al. High frequency of reactive joint symptoms after an outbreak of Salmonella enteritidis. *J Rheumatol.* 2002 Apr;29(4):767-71

[91] Leirisalo-Repo et al. Long-term prognosis of reactive salmonella arthritis. *Ann Rheum Dis.* 1997 Sep;56(9):516-20 ard.bmjjournals.com/cgi/content/full/56/9/516

[92] "Campylobacter jejuni is the most commonly reported bacterial cause of foodborne infection in the United States. Adding to the human and economic costs are chronic sequelae associated with C. jejuni infection--Guillian-Barre syndrome and reactive arthritis." Altekruse SF, Stern NJ, Fields PI, Swerdlow DL. Campylobacter jejuni--an emerging foodborne pathogen. *Emerg Infect Dis.* 1999 Jan-Feb;5(1):28-35

[93] "RESULTS: The incidence of colonic fermentation after ingesting sports drink, milk, and green tea was five (62.5%), six (75%), and none (0%), respectively in eight subjects." Mitsui T, Shimaoka K, Kanao Y, Kondo T. Colonic fermentation after ingestion of fructose-containing sports drink. *J Sports Med Phys Fitness.* 2001 Mar;41(1):121-3

[94] Vasquez A. *Musculoskeletal Pain: Expanded Clinical Strategies*. Gig Harbor, WA: The Institute for Functional Medicine; 2008

in benefit not only due to antigen avoidance but also due to the reduction in carbohydrate substrate that had been maintaining occult small intestine bacterial overgrowth, with its attendant systemic complications, including mitochondrial impairment and immune activation.[95] Micronutrient deficiencies, particularly of zinc and vitamins D and A, reduce immune system effectiveness and thereby promote mucosal colonization with dysbiotic bacteria; I believe this explains—at least in part—the oft experienced clinical phenomenon of significant improvement in dysbiosis-related diseases when only dietary improvement and

> **Clinical Pearl**
>
> Clinically, the most powerful "antibiotic"—antibacterial and antiviral and antifungal agent—ever discovered is the human immune system. For patients with chronic infections (including but not limited to dysbiosis), one of the first questions to ask is *"Why isn't this patient's immune system doing a better job of eliminating or controlling this infection?"* **Often, patients with chronic infections derive tremendous benefit from dietary improvement and nutritional supplementation, which allows their immune system to function more effectively and thus to clear or better control the infection/dysbiosis.**

nutritional supplementation are used: nutritional repletion empowers the immune system in general to function more effectively, thereby quantitatively and qualitatively reducing the severity of mucosal colonization. High-carbohydrate loads cause a reduction in immune surveillance that lasts for 2-3 hours after consumption.

9. <u>Diet-derived immunodysregulation</u>: Certain foods contain constituents that cause immune dysfunction and the induction or exacerbation of autoimmunity. L-canavanine sulfate is a non-protein amino acid found in alfalfa sprouts which triggers a condition similar to systemic lupus erythematosus in monkeys[96,97] and which may exacerbate SLE in humans.

10. <u>Dietary xenobiotics</u>: Artificial sweeteners, thickeners, flavor enhancers, emulsifiers, and plasticizers can be found in foods, particularly those which are manufactured and processed. Some of these chemicals have the potential to alter immune mechanisms in favor of autoimmunity. These dietary xenobiotics may be particularly relevant for initiating and promoting Crohn's disease.[98]

11. <u>Immunogenicity induced by cooking—the Maillard reaction (non-enzymatic glycosylation)</u>: Heated exposure of lysine, arginine, and tryptophan to reducing sugars such as fructose and lactose results in the non-enzymatic binding (glycosylation) of the sugar with the amino acid. If the amino acid is a component of a protein, then the structure and antigenicity of the protein is altered as it is now a glycoprotein, which may either serve as a neoantigen or may increase the allergenicity of a protein that was previously hypoallergenic, as seen with the roasting of peanuts.[99,100] Glycoproteins formed from the baking and browning of foods are also called *glycotoxins* and are capable of exacerbating inflammation in patients with diabetes.[101] Similar to the formation of glycotoxins is the formation of acrylamide, a possible carcinogen, in fried and baked foods.

Common allergy treatments advocated by the pharmaceutical industry create an overly simplistic and inaccurate view of the allergic process which obfuscates the identification and correction of the underlying processes, only two of which are antigen exposure and histamine release. Nutritionally oriented doctors, too, often emphasize the identification and elimination of allergen exposure as the sole means of addressing allergic diathesis with the presumption that allergen avoidance cures the allergy. These simplistic models and the incomplete treatments based upon them fail to address the underlying cause of the allergic phenomenon: immune dysfunction. Allergic

---

[95] "RESULTS: The incidence of colonic fermentation after ingesting sports drink, milk, and green tea was five (62.5%), six (75%), and none (0%), respectively in eight subjects." Mitsui T, Shimaoka K, Kanao Y, Kondo T. Colonic fermentation after ingestion of fructose-containing sports drink. *J Sports Med Phys Fitness*. 2001 Mar;41(1):121-3

[96] "L-Canavanine sulfate, a constituent of alfalfa sprouts, was incorporated into the diet and reactivated the syndrome in monkeys in which an SLE-like syndrome had previously been induced by the ingestion of alfalfa seeds or sprouts." Malinow MR, Bardana EJ Jr, Pirofsky B, Craig S, McLaughlin P. Systemic lupus erythematosus-like syndrome in monkeys fed alfalfa sprouts: role of a nonprotein amino acid. *Science*. 1982 Apr 23;216(4544):415-7

[97] "Occurrence of autoimmune hemolytic anemia and exacerbation of SLE have been linked to ingestion of alfalfa tablets containing L-canavanine." Alcocer-Varela J, Iglesias A, Llorente L, Alarcon-Segovia D. Effects of L-canavanine on T cells may explain the induction of systemic lupus erythematosus by alfalfa. *Arthritis Rheum*. 1985 Jan;28(1):52-7

[98] "Various food additives, especially emulsifiants, thickeners, surface-finishing agents and contaminants like plasticizers share structural domains with mycobacterial lipids. It is therefore hypothesized, that these compounds are able to stimulate by molecular mimicry the CD1 system in the gastrointestinal mucosa and to trigger the pro-inflammatory cytokine cascade." Traunmuller F. Etiology of Crohn's disease: Do certain food additives cause intestinal inflammation by molecular mimicry of mycobacterial lipids? *Med Hypotheses*. 2005;65(5):859-64

[99] "Roasted peanuts exhibited a higher level of IgE binding, which was correlated with a higher level of AGE adducts. We concluded that there is an association between AGE adducts and increased IgE binding (i.e., allergenicity) of roasted peanuts." Chung SY, Champagne ET. Association of end-product adducts with increased IgE binding of roasted peanuts. *J Agric Food Chem*. 2001 Aug;49(8):3911-6

[100] "The data presented here indicate that thermal processing may play an important role in enhancing the allergenic properties of peanuts and that the protein modifications made by the Maillard reaction contribute to this effect." Maleki et al. The effects of roasting on the allergenic properties of peanut proteins. *J Allergy Clin Immunol*. 2000 Oct;106:763-8

[101] "A study now reveals that the consumption of foods rich in browned and oxidized products (so-called glycotoxins) induces a chronic inflammatory state in diabetic individuals." Monnier VM, Obrenovich ME. Wake up and smell the maillard reaction. *Sci Aging Knowledge Environ*. 2002 Dec 18;2002(50):pe21

manifestations always require at least two factors: 1) exposure of the antigen to the immune system (antigen absorption) and 2) a dysfunctional immune system that "overreacts" to the otherwise benign antigen. Allergy treatment that fails to address the underlying immune dysfunction is incomplete. Allergy treatment that addresses the underlying immune dysfunction has the opportunity to correct the *total problem*, rather than merely reducing the manifestations of the problem. Therefore, treatment of the allergic diathesis must always address issues of antigen exposure, antigen absorption, *and the dysfunctional immune system* that results in the hyperactive immune response that we call "allergy." Elimination of either antigen exposure or antigen absorption eliminates allergic manifestations, but does not necessarily correct the underlying immune defect(s). Complete correction of the underlying immune defect obviates the need for the identification and avoidance of the allergen. In clinical practice, a combination of both approaches—allergen avoidance and immune modulation—is the most effective approach, affording relatively high effectiveness in symptom reduction even with only modest compliance.

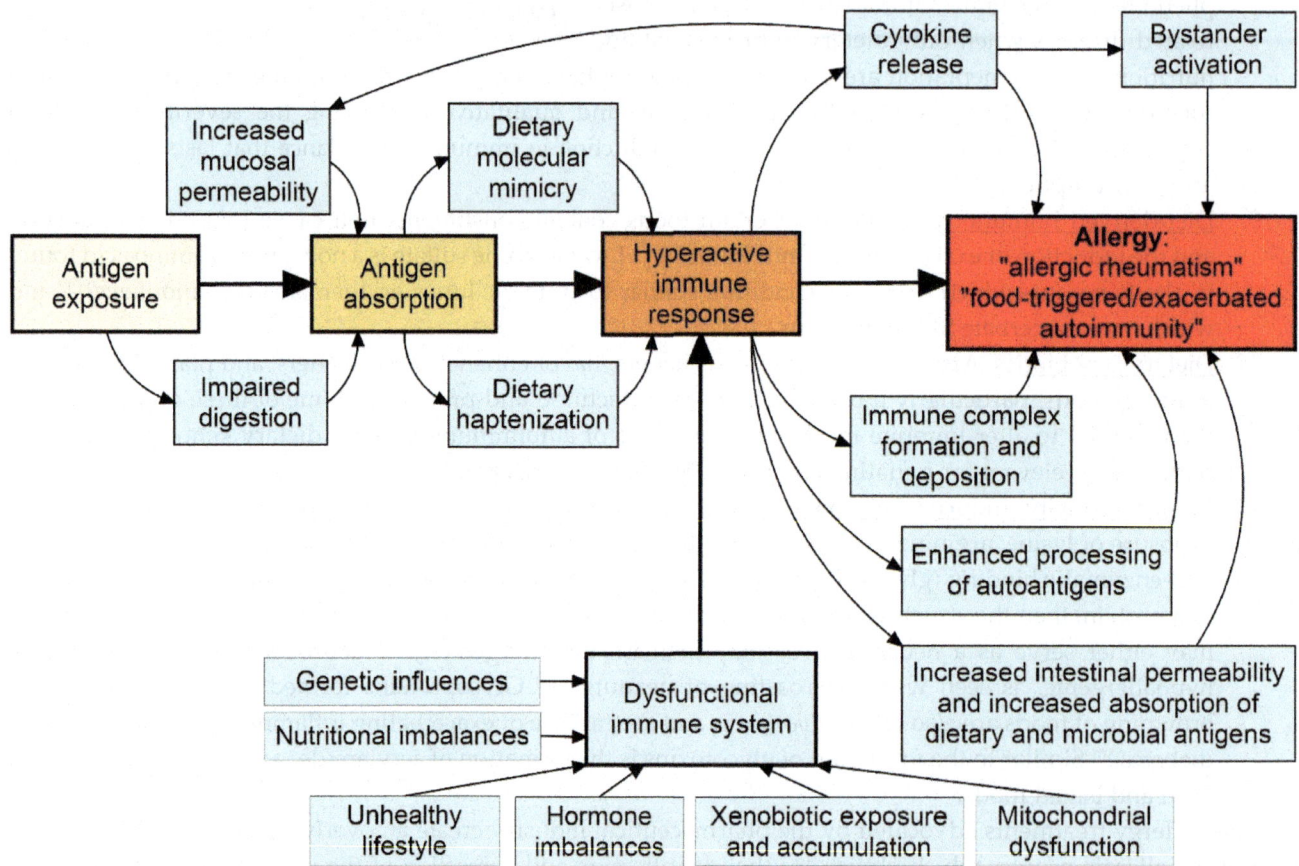

Approaching a More Comprehensive Understanding of "Allergy" and Its Contribution to Immune Dysfunction, Musculoskeletal Inflammation, Autoimmunity, and "Allergic Diseases" such as Asthma: Immune dysfunction contributes to and is perpetuated by inflammation and allergic reactions, thus forming a vicious cycle; of particular noteworthiness is the vicious cycle formed by inflammation in response to immunogen exposure that leads to increased intestinal permeability and thus to additional immunogen (e.g., dietary and microbial) exposure.

Anti-Allergy Orthomolecular Immunomodulation: The Author's Approach to Alleviating Allergy— Introduction and Perspectives Spanning more than 10 years of Protocol Development

My clinical approach to improving immune function in patients with allergy typically started/starts with supplementation of vitamin E, CoQ-10, vitamin B-12, vitamin C, bioflavonoids, honey, and fish oil; readers will appreciate that these are all anti-inflammatory nutrients/foods, all of which—like vitamin B12—have anti-allergy effects that are extensions of and/or different from their traditionally considered nutritional roles. Thereafter, I look at hormones, particularly dehydroepiandrosterone (DHEA), estrogen (quantitative and qualitative), testosterone, and cortisol. I also look at diet and bowel health with respect to putrefaction and intestinal permeability. Although rarely powerful when used in isolation, these treatments when used in combinations tailored to the individual patient often result in an impressive reduction in allergic manifestations even when allergen avoidance is either not pursued or not feasible. The process of alleviating allergic disorders is, however, arduous and time-consuming unless the doctor uses a group of protocols such as those described herein which address the most common contributing factors to allergic problems. Here I extend my previous three-step process (first published in 2005[102]) into a four-tiered approach (first published in 2009[103]), with the fourth step including selected pharmaceutical drugs. These days—starting in 2012[104] and beyond—the integration of the nutritional immunomodulation protocol (Chapter 4.3) should be used within the initial and foundational management of allergic and other inflammatory disorders; nonetheless, this previous version of the protocol serves useful purposes by providing perspectives and clinical interventions not included in the "nutritional immunomodulation protocol" described as such.

Step 1: From initial patient assessment to the first phase of treatment

In a patient with presumed "allergy" who is in otherwise good health, following a basic health assessment and exclusion of significant disease, I begin by correcting problems that are common to patients with allergy. Minor improvements in allergy symptoms as a result of a low-cost low-risk interventions can be multiplied with a specified group of interventions; we aim for a modest improvement with several treatments rather than a "silver bullet" miracle cure with a single intervention. For example, 10% improvement in symptoms may be insignificant in itself; however a 10% improvement from six interventions results in a 60% improvement and enhances patient confidence long enough for other interventions and assessments to be implemented, if necessary. The goal with the first step of treatment is to correct the most common and most likely problems, namely fatty acid imbalances, micronutrient deficiencies, phytonutrient insufficiencies, and dysbiosis.

- Avoidance of suspected food allergens: The most common allergens are wheat, cow's milk, and eggs; however any patient can be allergic to any food. It is not uncommon for patients to have to avoid up to 10 foods before attaining maximal improvement, and up to 85% of migraine patients can be cured of their headaches by the use of allergy avoidance alone.[105] Food allergy avoidance for 1 month helps achieve symptomatic relief and allows the gut to heal and the immune system to recalibrate. The diet should emphasize consumption of lean meats, fruits, vegetables, nuts, seeds, and berries to ensure a systemic anti-inflammatory effect and increased consumption of anti-inflammatory phytonutrients, especially flavonoids. High-glycemic foods are avoided as are "food additives" such as tartrazine, which is known to exacerbate allergic asthma. Some foods like tuna, certain cheeses and wines are high in histamine; frequent consumption of these foods by an allergic individual is analogous to adding fuel to a fire that the patient is simultaneously trying to extinguish. Recall that in breast-feeding infants, the mother will have to consume a hypoallergenic diet to prevent passage of allergens[106] and allergen-antibody immune complexes[107] in breast milk.

- Rotation diet: While select "offending foods" and exposures should be completely avoided, the remaining foods that are consumed should be rotated in and out of the diet with a periodicity of 3-5 days. Patients should avoid "dietary monotony"[108] by consuming a variety of foods. By rotating different foods in and out of the diet, patients are more likely to consume a nutritious diet and are less likely to develop or perpetuate food allergies.

- CoQ-10: CoQ-10 levels are low in approximately 40% of patients with allergies, according to a small study conducted by Folkers and Pfeiffer.[109] Asthmatics also have lower levels of CoQ-10 compared to healthy people.[110] In an open cross-over randomized clinical trial of patients with persistent mild-moderate asthma

---

[102] Vasquez A. Improving neuromusculoskeletal health by optimizing immune function and reducing allergic reactions: a review of 16 treatments and a 3-step clinical approach. *Nutritional Perspectives* 2005; October: 27-35, 40 https://ichnfm.academia.edu/AlexVasquez

[103] Vasquez A. *Chiropractic and Naturopathic Mastery of Common Clinical Disorders*. IBMRC, 2009

[104] Vasquez A. *Functional Immunology and Nutritional Immunomodulation: Introduction to...the new FIND SEX Acronym*. 2012

[105] Grant EC. Food allergies and migraine. *Lancet*. 1979 May 5;1(8123):966-9

[106] "In all, clinical disappearance of symptoms was observed after removal of milk from the mother's diet and/or elimination from the child's diet of any cow's-milk-based hypoallergenic formula." Barau E, Dupont C. Allergy to cow's milk proteins in mother's milk or in hydrolyzed cow's milk infant formulas as assessed by intestinal permeability measurements. *Allergy*. 1994 Apr;49(4):295-8

[107] The finding of egg-allergen immune complex in breast milk implies 1) egg protein escapes complete digestion/degradation in the gastrointestinal tract, 2) egg protein is absorbed intact through the mucosa, 3) egg protein escapes filtration by the liver, 4) egg protein stimulates formation IgA immune complexes, and 5) egg-IgA immune complexes are secreted in milk which would then expose the infant to both allergen and immune complex, possibly resulting in clinical disease. Hirose et al. Occurrence of the major food allergen, ovomucoid, in human breast milk as an immune complex. *Biosci Biotechnol Biochem*. 2001 Jun;65(6):1438-40 jstage.jst.go.jp/article/bbb/65/6/1438/_pdf

[108] Pelchat ML, Schaefer S. Dietary monotony and food cravings in young and elderly adults. *Physiol Behav*. 2000 Jan;68(3):353-9

[109] Ye CQ, Folkers K, et al. A modified determination of coenzyme Q10 in human blood and CoQ10 blood levels in diverse patients with allergies. *Biofactors*. 1988 Dec;1:303-6

[110] Gazdik et al. Decreased levels of coenzyme Q(10) in patients with bronchial asthma. *Allergy*. 2002 Sep;57(9):811-4

(n=41; ages 25-50y), daily administration of hydrosoluble CoQ10 120 mg, alpha-tocopherol 400 mg, and vitamin C 250 mg was shown to allow statistically and clinically significant reduction in the required dosage of corticosteroids; however, "Spirometric parameters did not change significantly during the study."[111] In my experience, clinical improvement is commonly seen in allergic patients after supplementation with CoQ-10, within the context of overall diet and lifestyle improvement including vitamin, mineral, and combination fatty acid supplementation. I generally prescribe at least 100 mg and preferably 200 mg per day of CoQ-10 for adults.

- Vitamin C: A clinical trial showed that 2 grams per day of ascorbic acid reduced blood histamine levels by 38%.[112] Cathcart hypothesized that high doses of vitamin C (i.e., bowel tolerance) may impair the adsorption of IgE with allergens and thus retard the allergic cascade from being initiated.[113] Either of these two mechanisms, perhaps in addition to other mechanisms such as stabilization of mast cell membranes (especially when used with bioflavonoids), may explain the anti-allergy effects of ascorbic acid.[114]

- Probiotics: Supplementation with probiotics (beneficial strains of bacteria and yeast) appears to improve intestinal barrier function, promote microecological balance in the gastrointestinal tract, modulate immune function, and thus *via several mechanisms* reduce manifestations/severity of allergic disease.[115,116,117]

- Vitamin E: Vitamin E has been shown to reduce IgE levels in humans and to reduce the manifestations of allergy-related disease.[118] I commonly prescribe 800-2,000 IU per day of mixed tocopherols with approximately 40% gamma tocopherol for patients with allergy.

- Bioflavonoids: Bioflavonoids stabilize mast cell membranes and thus reduce the liberation of histamine. Additionally, quercetin and catechin inhibit the action of histidine decarboxylase, which converts histidine into histamine. Many fruits, vegetables, herbal teas, and honey are excellent sources of flavonoids, which can also be consumed in the form of tablets, capsules, beverages, or whole foods. The efficacy of honey for reducing serum IgE is particularly noteworthy; honey consumption has been shown to significantly reduce (-34%) serum IgE levels in humans.[119] The required dose is 1.2 g of honey per kg body weight. For an individual who weighs about 220 lbs, the correct amount of honey to remain consistent with this study would be approximately 120 grams. Since one tablespoon of honey weighs 21 grams, the dose would be 5-6 tablespoons (one-third cup) of honey per day (again, this dose is for a person weighing 220 lbs). Since each tablespoon of honey contains 64 calories, six tablespoons of this powerful natural anti-inflammatory nutraceutical would add 384 calories to the daily diet; if the remainder of the patient's diet is generally low-carbohydrate (as it generally should be for most patients), then the addition of less than 400 calories is relatively insignificant, especially if the patient also exercises on a daily or near-daily basis (as most patients should). In the context of a low-carb diet and regular exercise, honey can be the before/after carbohydrate source used to fuel the workout or to provide post-exertional glycogen supercompensation. To avoid/minimize consumption of mitochondria-damaging and endocrine-disrupting pesticides, honey and other foods should be organically cultivated; commercial "mass-market" [American] honey has recently

---

[111] Gvozdjáková et al. Coenzyme Q10 supplementation reduces corticosteroids dosage in patients with bronchial asthma. *Biofactors.* 2005;25(1-4):235-40

[112] "Chemotaxis was inversely correlated to blood histamine (r = -0.32, p = 0.045), and, compared to baseline and withdrawal values, histamine levels were depressed 38% following VC supplementation. ... These data indicate that VC may indirectly enhance chemotaxis by detoxifying histamine in vivo." Johnston CS, Martin LJ, Cai X. Antihistamine effect of supplemental ascorbic acid and neutrophil chemotaxis. *J Am Coll Nutr.* 1992 Apr;11(2):172-6

[113] "Allergic and sensitivity reactions are frequently ameliorated and sometimes completely blocked by massive doses of ascorbate. I now hypothesize that one mechanism in blocking of allergic symptoms is the reducing of the disulfide bonds between the chains in antibody molecules making their bonding antigen impossible." Cathcart RF 3rd. The vitamin C treatment of allergy and the normally unprimed state of antibodies. *Med Hypotheses.* 1986 Nov;21(3):307-21

[114] Bucca C, Rolla G, Oliva A, Farina JC. Effect of vitamin C on histamine bronchial responsiveness of patients with allergic rhinitis. *Ann Allergy.* 1990 Oct;65(4):311-4

[115] Majamaa H, Isolauri E. Probiotics: a novel approach in the management of food allergy. *J Allergy Clin Immunol* 1997 Feb;99(2):179-85

[116] von der Weid T, Ibnou-Zekri N, Pfeifer A. Novel probiotics for the management of allergic inflammation. *Dig Liver Dis.* 2002 Sep;34 Suppl 2:S25-8

[117] "The administration of probiotics, strains of bacteria from the healthy human gut microbiota, have been shown to stimulate antiinflammatory, tolerogenic immune responses, the lack of which has been implied in the development of atopic disorders. Thus probiotics may prove beneficial in the prevention and alleviation of allergic disease." Rautava et al. The development of gut immune responses and gut microbiota: effects of probiotics in prevention and treatment of allergic disease. *Curr Issues Intest Microbiol* 2002 Mar;3:15-22

[118] Tsoureli-Nikita et al. Evaluation of dietary intake of vitamin E in atopic dermatitis: clinical course and evaluation of immunoglobulin E. *Int J Dermatol.* 2002 Mar;41(3):146-50

[119] "Seven men and three women received a strictly controlled regular diet during a 2-week control period, followed by the regular diet supplemented with daily consumption of 1.2 g/kg body weight honey dissolved in 250 ml of water during a 2-week test period. ... Honey reduced serum immunoglobulin E by 34%..." Al-Waili NS. Effects of daily consumption of honey solution on hematological indices and blood levels of minerals and enzymes in normal individuals. *J Med Food.* 2003 Summer;6(2):135-40

been reported as low in antioxidants and commonly contaminated with pesticides, including glyphosate.[120,121]

- <u>Vitamin B-12</u>: Vitamin B-12 has been shown to reduce physiologic manifestations of allergy in ovalbumin-sensitized mice.[122] Since vitamin B-12 is safe, non-toxic, and bioavailable when administered orally in large doses to humans, I commonly prescribe 2,500-5,000 mcg per day for allergic patients for a one-month trial. Although the benefit of vitamin B-12 in patients with sulfite-sensitive asthma is biochemically mediated rather than immunologically mediated[123], this research adds tangential support to the use of high-dose vitamin B-12 in selected patients with allergy (particularly asthma), at least for a short-term clinical trial. Hydroxocobalamin and methylcobalamin are preferred over cyanocobalamin due to the significant content of cyanide in the latter.[124]

Step 2: Additional interventions for moderate or unresponsive allergies.

For patients who do not respond sufficiently to the first phase of treatment, the following interventions can be considered.

- <u>Pancreatic and proteolytic enzymes</u>: Pancreatic enzymes have been shown to alleviate symptoms of food allergy in a controlled clinical trial.[125] Administration of enzyme preparations can alleviate intestinal and extra-intestinal manifestations of food allergy.[126] Proteolytic enzymes are safe and effective for the relief of musculoskeletal pain, as reviewed later in this text and elsewhere.[127] When taken with food, pancreatic/proteolytic enzymes facilitate hydrolysis of proteins, fats, and carbohydrates and are then absorbed into the systemic circulation for an anti-inflammatory effect. Although individual enzymes may be used in isolation, enzyme therapy is generally delivered in the form of polyenzyme preparations containing pancreatin, bromelain, papain, amylase, lipase, trypsin and alpha-chymotrypsin.

- <u>Nuclear transcription factor kappa-B (NFkB) inhibitors</u>: NFkB plays a critical role in the induction of pro-inflammatory genes and is upregulated in allergic disease; its phytonutritional modulation is detailed later in this book and elsewhere.[128] Nutrients that can be used to downregulate inflammatory responses are 1,25-dihydroxyvitamin D3[129,130], curcumin[131] (requires piperine for absorption[132]), lipoic acid[133], green tea[134],

Nutrients and foods that inhibit NFkB
- 1,25-dihydroxyvitamin D3
- Curcumin (requires piperine for absorption)
- Lipoic acid
- Green tea
- Rosemary
- Grape seed extract
- Bee propolis
- Zinc
- Selenium
- Indole-3-carbinol
- N-acetyl-L-cysteine
- Resveratrol
- Isohumulones
- CoQ-10
- Boswellia serrata
- GLA via PPAR-gamma
- Oxidized EPA via PPAR-alpha

[120] "More than 70 percent of pollen and honey samples collected from foraging bees in Massachusetts contain at least one neonicotinoid, a class of pesticide..." Feldscher K. Pesticide found in 70 percent of Massachusetts' honey samples. news.harvard.edu/gazette/story/2015/07/pesticide-found-in-70-percent-of-massachusetts-honey-samples/

[121] "Eleven of the tested honey samples were organic; five of the organic honey samples, or forty-five percent (45%), contained glyphosate concentrations above the method LOQ, with a range of 26 to 93 ppb and a mean of 50 ppb. Of the fifty-eight non-organic honey samples, thirty-six samples, or sixty-two percent (62%), contained glyphosate concentrations above the method LOQ, with a range of 17 to 163 ppb and a mean of 66 ppb." Rubio F. Survey of Glyphosate Residues in Honey, Corn and Soy Products. *Journal of Environmental & Analytical Toxicology*. 2014 Nov omicsonline.org/open-access/survey-of-glyphosate-residues-in-honey-corn-and-soy-products-2161-0525.1000249.php?aid=36354

[122] "We infer that Cbl administration significantly reduced the IL-2 concentration, and secondarily the IL-4, IgE and histamine concentrations." Funada U, Wada M, Kawata T, Tanaka N, Tadokoro T, Maekawa A. Effect of cobalamin on the allergic response in mice. *Biosci Biotechnol Biochem* 2000 Oct;64(10):2053-8

[123] Anibarro B, Caballero T, Garcia-Ara C, et al. Asthma with sulfite intolerance in children: a blocking study with cyanocobalamin. *J Allergy Clin Immunol*. 1992 Jul;90(1):103-9

[124] Freeman AG. Cyanocobalamin—a case for withdrawal: discussion paper. *J R Soc Med*. 1992 Nov;85(11):686-7

[125] Raithel M, Weidenhiller M, Schwab D, Winterkamp S, Hahn EG. Pancreatic enzymes: a new group of antiallergic drugs? *Inflamm Res*. 2002 Apr;51 Suppl 1:S13-4

[126] Gaby AR. Pancreatic enzymes block food allergy reactions. *Townsend Letter for Doctors and Patients* 2002; Nov. townsendletter.com/Nov_2002/gabyliteraturereview1102.htm

[127] Vasquez A. Improving overall health while safely and effectively treating musculoskeletal pain. *Nutr Perspect* 2005;28:34-38,40-42 ichnfm.academia.edu/AlexVasquez

[128] Vasquez A. Reducing pain and inflammation naturally - part 4: nutritional and botanical inhibition of NF-kappaB, the major intracellular amplifier of the inflammatory cascade. A practical clinical strategy exemplifying anti-inflammatory nutrigenomics. *Nutritional Perspectives*, July 2005:5-12 ichnfm.academia.edu/AlexVasquez

[129] "1Alpha,25-dihydroxyvitamin D3 (1,25-(OH)2-D3), the active metabolite of vitamin D, can inhibit NF-kappaB activity in human MRC-5 fibroblasts, targeting DNA binding of NF-kappaB but not translocation of its subunits p50 and p65." Harant H, Wolff B, Lindley IJ. 1Alpha,25-dihydroxyvitamin D3 decreases DNA binding of nuclear factor-kappaB in human fibroblasts. *FEBS Lett*. 1998 Oct 9;436(3):329-34

[130] "Thus, 1,25(OH)2D3 may negatively regulate IL-12 production by downregulation of NF-kB activation and binding to the p40-kB sequence." D'Ambrosio D, Cippitelli M, Cocciolo MG, Mazzeo D, Di Lucia P, Lang R, Sinigaglia F, Panina-Bordignon P. Inhibition of IL-12 production by 1,25-dihydroxyvitamin D3. Involvement of NF-kappaB downregulation in transcriptional repression of the p40 gene. *J Clin Invest*. 1998 Jan 1;101(1):252-62

[131] "Curcumin, EGCG and resveratrol have been shown to suppress activation of NF-kappa B." Surh et al. Molecular mechanisms underlying chemopreventive activities of anti-inflammatory phytochemicals: down-regulation of COX-2 and iNOS through suppression of NF-kappa B activation. *Mutat Res*. 2001 Sep 1;480-481:243-68

[132] Shoba et al. Influence of piperine on the pharmacokinetics of curcumin in animals and human volunteers. *Planta Med*. 1998 May;64(4):353-6

[133] "ALA reduced the TNF-alpha-stimulated ICAM-1 expression in a dose-dependent manner, to levels observed in unstimulated cells. Alpha-lipoic acid also reduced NF-kappaB activity in these cells in a dose-dependent manner." Lee HA, Hughes DA. Alpha-lipoic acid modulates NF-kappaB activity in human monocytic cells by direct interaction with DNA. *Exp Gerontol*. 2002 Jan-Mar;37(2-3):401-10

[134] "In conclusion, EGCG is an effective inhibitor of IKK activity. This may explain, at least in part, some of the reported anti-inflammatory and anticancer effects of green tea." Yang F, Oz HS, Barve S, de Villiers WJ, McClain CJ, Varilek GW. The green tea polyphenol (-)-epigallocatechin-3-gallate blocks nuclear factor-kappa B activation by inhibiting I kappa B kinase activity in the intestinal epithelial cell line IEC-6. *Mol Pharmacol*. 2001 Sep;60(3):528-33

rosemary[135], grape seed extract[136], bee propolis[137], zinc[138], high-dose selenium[139], indole-3-carbinol[140,141], N-acetyl-L-cysteine[142], resveratrol[143,144], isohumulones from *Humulus lupulus*[145], CoQ-10[146], and acetyl-11-keto-beta-boswellic acid from *Boswellia serrata*.[147] Fatty acids inhibit NF-kappaB *indirectly*; GLA activates PPAR-gamma and thereby inhibits NFkB[148], while (oxidized) EPA activates PPAR-alpha and thus inhibits NFkB.[149]

- <u>Stress reduction, psychotherapy, deconditioning</u>: Emotional and social aspects may be particularly important for some patients with allergies. "Allergic" responses to stimuli can be classically conditioned, according to replicable studies in animals[150] and humans.[151] The neurohormonal response to physical-psychological stress predisposes the immune system toward the Th-2 response with subsequent IgE antibody formation and the development of allergy.[152] Höglund et al[153] summarized by stating, "The dominance of Th2 cytokines leads to enhanced Ig class switching to IgE, recruitment of eosinophils to the airways and to down-regulation of cell-mediated immunity, features characteristic of asthmatic and allergic disease." In support of the stress-allergy link, we note published research showing, for example, increased prevalence of allergy in children exposed to the stress of international relocation.[154] Mechanisms by which physical-psychological stress can promote allergy are likely to be very complex, interactive, synergistic, self-perpetuating, and variable among individuals. Documented factors and mechanisms involved include increased mucosal permeability, alterations in flora/microbial quality (species), quantity (numerical counts) and activity (elaboration of virulence factors and changes in phenotypic expression), hypercortisolemia followed by hypocortisolemia, increased secretion of pro-inflammatory corticotrophin releasing factor, reductions in immunomodulating hormones DHEA and testosterone with an increase in pro-inflammatory estrogens and prolactin, alterations in lifestyle such as sugar and pastry binging along with dietary monotony, and the perpetuation and amplification of stress from one aspect of life to another, for example: work stress can cause financial worries which spills over into marital discord and perhaps binge eating and

---

[135] "These results suggest that carnosol suppresses the NO production and iNOS gene expression by inhibiting NF-kappaB activation, and provide possible mechanisms for its anti-inflammatory and chemopreventive action." Lo AH, Liang YC, Lin-Shiau SY, Ho CT, Lin JK. Carnosol, an antioxidant in rosemary, suppresses inducible nitric oxide synthase through down-regulating nuclear factor-kappaB in mouse macrophages. *Carcinogenesis.* 2002 Jun;23(6):983-91

[136] "Constitutive and TNFalpha-induced NF-kappaB DNA binding activity was inhibited by GSE at doses > or =50 microg/ml and treatments for > or =12 h." Dhanalakshmi et al. Inhibition of NF-kappaB pathway in grape seed extract-induced apoptotic death of human prostate carcinoma DU145 cells. *Int J Oncol.* 2003 Sep;23(3):721-7

[137] "Caffeic acid phenethyl ester (CAPE) is an anti-inflammatory component of propolis (honeybee resin). CAPE is reportedly a specific inhibitor of nuclear factor-kappaB (NF-kappaB)." Fitzpatrick LR, Wang J, Le T. Caffeic acid phenethyl ester, an inhibitor of nuclear factor-kappaB, attenuates bacterial peptidoglycan polysaccharide-induced colitis in rats. *J Pharmacol Exp Ther.* 2001 Dec;299(3):915-20

[138] "Our results suggest that zinc supplementation may lead to downregulation of the inflammatory cytokines through upregulation of the negative feedback loop A20 to inhibit induced NF-kappaB activation." Prasad AS, Bao B, Beck FW, Kucuk O, Sarkar FH. Antioxidant effect of zinc in humans. *Free Radic Biol Med.* 2004 Oct 15;37(8):1182-90

[139] Note that the patients in this study received a very high dose of selenium: 960 micrograms per day. This is at the top—and some would say over the top—of the safe and reasonable dose for long-term supplementation. In this case, th study lasted for three months. "In patients receiving selenium supplementation, selenium NF-kappaB activity was significantly reduced, reaching the same level as the nondiabetic control group. CONCLUSION: In type 2 diabetic patients, activation of NF-kappaB measured in peripheral blood monocytes can be reduced by selenium supplementation, confirming its importance in the prevention of cardiovascular diseases." Faure P, Ramon O, Favier A, Halimi S. Selenium supplementation decreases nuclear factor-kappa B activity in peripheral blood mononuclear cells from type 2 diabetic patients. *Eur J Clin Invest.* 2004 Jul;34(7):475-81

[140] Takada Y, Andreeff M, Aggarwal BB. Indole-3-carbinol suppresses NF-{kappa}B and I{kappa}B{alpha} kinase activation causing inhibition of expression of NF-{kappa}B-regulated antiapoptotic and metastatic gene products and enhancement of apoptosis in myeloid and leukemia cells. *Blood* 2005 July 15; 106(2): 641–649

[141] "Overall, our results indicated that indole-3-carbinol inhibits NF-kappaB and NF-kappaB-regulated gene expression and that this mechanism may provide the molecular basis for its ability to suppress tumorigenesis." Takada Y, Andreeff M, Aggarwal BB. Indole-3-carbinol suppresses NF-kappaB and IkappaBalpha kinase activation, causing inhibition of expression of NF-kappaB-regulated antiapoptotic and metastatic gene products and enhancement of apoptosis in myeloid and leukemia cells. *Blood.* 2005 Jul 15;106(2):641-9

[142] "CONCLUSIONS: Administration of N-acetylcysteine results in decreased nuclear factor-kappa B activation in patients with sepsis, associated with decreases in interleukin-8 but not interleukin-6 or soluble intercellular adhesion molecule-1. These pilot data suggest that antioxidant therapy with N-acetylcysteine may be useful in blunting the inflammatory response to sepsis." Paterson RL, Galley HF, Webster NR. The effect of N-acetylcysteine on nuclear factor-kappa B activation, interleukin-6, interleukin-8, and intercellular adhesion molecule-1 expression in patients with sepsis. *Crit Care Med.* 2003 Nov;31(11):2574-8

[143] "Resveratrol's anticarcinogenic, anti-inflammatory, and growth-modulatory effects may thus be partially ascribed to the inhibition of activation of NF-kappaB and AP-1 and the associated kinases." Manna SK, Mukhopadhyay A, Aggarwal BB. Resveratrol suppresses TNF-induced activation of nuclear transcription factors NF-kappa B, activator protein-1, and apoptosis: potential role of reactive oxygen intermediates and lipid peroxidation. *J Immunol.* 2000 Jun 15;164(12):6509-19

[144] "Both resveratrol and quercetin inhibited NF-kappaB-, AP-1- and CREB-dependent transcription to a greater extent than the glucocorticosteroid, dexamethasone." Donnelly et al. Anti-inflammatory Effects of Resveratrol in Lung Epithelial Cells: Molecular Mechanisms. *Am J Physiol Lung Cell Mol Physiol.* 2004 Jun 4 [Epub ahead of print]

[145] Yajima et al. Isohumulones, bitter acids derived from hops, activate both peroxisome proliferator-activated receptor alpha and gamma and reduce insulin resistance. *J Biol Chem.* 2004 Aug 6;279:33456-62 jbc.org/cgi/content/full/279/32/33456

[146] Ebadi M, Sharma SK, et al. Coenzyme Q10 inhibits mitochondrial complex-1 down-regulation and nuclear factor-kappa B activation. *J Cell Mol Med.* 2004 Apr-Jun;8:213-22

[147] "Overall, our results indicated that AKBA enhances apoptosis induced by cytokines and chemotherapeutic agents, inhibits invasion, and suppresses osteoclastogenesis through inhibition of NF-kappaB-regulated gene expression." Takada Y, Ichikawa H, Badmaev V, Aggarwal BB. Acetyl-11-keto-beta-boswellic acid potentiates apoptosis, inhibits invasion, and abolishes osteoclastogenesis by suppressing NF-kappa B and NF-kappa B-regulated gene expression. *J Immunol.* 2006 Mar 1;176(5):3127-40

[148] "Thus, PPAR gamma serves as the receptor for GLA in the regulation of gene expression in breast cancer cells." Jiang WG, Redfern A, et al. Peroxisome proliferator activated receptor-gamma (PPAR-gamma) mediates the action of gamma linolenic acid in breast cancer cells. *Prostaglandins Leukot Essent Fatty Acids.* 2000 Feb;62(2):119-27

[149] "...EPA requires PPARalpha for its inhibitory effects on NF-kappaB." Mishra A, Chaudhary A, Sethi S. Oxidized omega-3 fatty acids inhibit NF-kappaB activation via a PPARalpha-dependent pathway. *Arterioscler Thromb Vasc Biol.* 2004 Sep;24(9):1621-7. atvb.ahajournals.org/cgi/content/full/24/9/1621

[150] "In a classical conditioning procedure in which an immunologic challenge was paired with the presentation of an odor, guinea pigs showed a plasma histamine increase when presented with the odor alone. This suggests that the immune response can be enhanced through activity of the central nervous system." Russell et al. Learned histamine release. *Science.* 1984 Aug 17;225(4663):733-4

[151] "A classical Pavlovian paradigm pairing an olfactory cue with allergen challenge for a single training trial was used to produce conditioned histamine release and conditioned nasal airflow decrease in seasonal allergic rhinitis sufferers." Barrett JE, King MG, Pang G. Conditioning rhinitis in allergic humans. *Ann N Y Acad Sci.* 2000;917:853-9

[152] Montoro J, Mullol J, Jáuregui I, et al. Stress and allergy. *J Investig Allergol Clin Immunol.* 2009;19 Suppl 1:40-7 jiaci.org/issues/vol19s1/7.pdf

[153] Höglund et al. Changes in immune regulation in response to examination stress in atopic and healthy individuals. *Clin Exp Allergy.* 2006 Aug;36(8):982-92

[154] "This study suggests that unidentified factors associated with foreign relocation increase the risk of sensitization in predisposed children. Stress might be one factor." Anderzén et al. Stress and sensitization in children: a controlled prospective psychophysiological study of children. *J Psychosom Res.* 1997 Sep;43(3):259-69

drinking all of which synergize with internal neuronal and immunologic imbalances to promote the exacerbation of allergy.

- <u>Eradication of intestinal dysbiosis</u>: I have seen several patients become cured of their "allergies" once we eradicated the dysbiotic bacteria, yeast, amoebas, or other microorganisms from their gastrointestinal tract. Intestinal colonization with harmful bacteria/yeast/protozoa/amebas can cause mucosal injury and result in macromolecular absorption and thus promotes immune sensitization to dietary antigens; in these situations, correction of dysbiosis via eradication of harmful microorganisms can lead to an impressive reduction in food-associated allergic phenomena. Although many indirect mechanisms will be discussed later, the most direct means by which dysbiosis may contribute to "allergy" is via endogenous formation of histamine via bacterial histidine decarboxylase. Galland and Lee[155] reported that eradication of *Giardia lamblia* in patients with chronic digestive complaints lessened the severity of food intolerance/allergy in 54% of patients. The supremely important topic of gastrointestinal dysbiosis is detailed in Chapter 4.

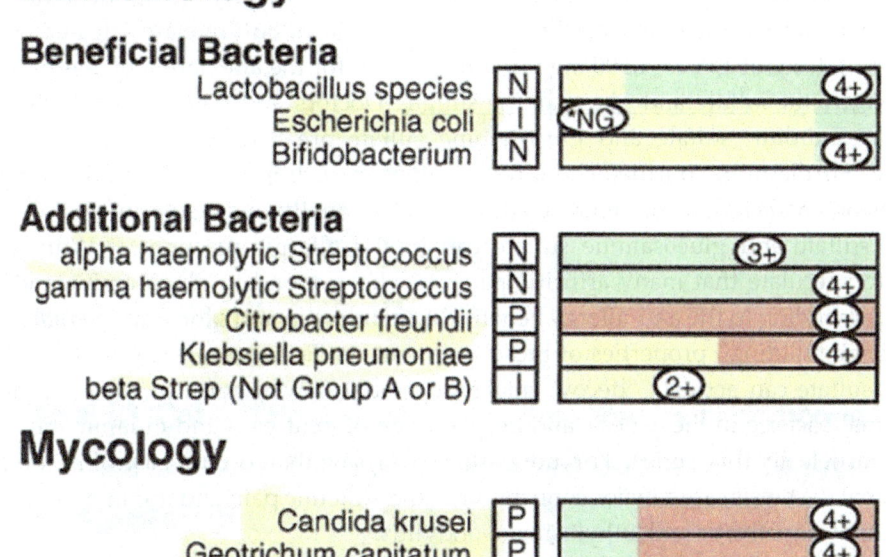

Bacteriology

Beneficial Bacteria

Lactobacillus species	N	4+
Escherichia coli	I	•NG
Bifidobacterium	N	4+

Additional Bacteria

alpha haemolytic Streptococcus	N	3+
gamma haemolytic Streptococcus	N	4+
Citrobacter freundii	P	4+
Klebsiella pneumoniae	P	4+
beta Strep (Not Group A or B)	I	2+

Mycology

Candida krusei	P	4+
Geotrichum capitatum	P	4+

<u>Intestinal dysbiosis as the causative factor in new-onset immediate hypersensitivity reactions to multiple foods, as well as physical and mental fatigue and environmental sensitivity</u>: This 25yoM patient developed numerous complaints clustering around fatigue, neurocognitive dysfunction, and multiple chemical sensitivity following a period of severe psychoemotional stress; new immediate-onset "food allergies" developed against several spices and soy/lecithin. Allergic food reactions/responses included immediate-onset (within seconds) hypersensitivity reactions in the mouth (including a blistering mucosal/labial rash) upon consumption of (previously tolerated) soy. All of the "food allergies", neurocognitive fatigue, and chemical sensitivities vanished upon successful eradication of the intestinal dysbiosis, clearly depicted per the above results on comprehensive microbiologic assessment of the stool. *Citrobacter* and *Klebsiella* are both Gram-negative bacteria implicated in pathogenic inflammatory responses, increased intestinal permeability, and impaired cytochrome p450 activity (general to endotoxin, with some additional specificity for *Klebsiella*). The *Geotrichum* is an unusual yeast associated with immunosuppression, while the *Candida* is known for producing an IgA protease that increases propensity toward dysbiosis and allergy by proteolytic degradation of the first-line IgA defense. Patient was treated with numerous antimicrobial botanicals including berberine and oregano as well as daily first-morning gastrointestinal lavage with ~30 grams ascorbic acid in one liter of water (potent osmotic laxative) with two cups of coffee (peristaltic/gastroprokinetic agent). Other testing at this time showed increased intestinal permeability via elevated lactulose-mannitol ratio, increased fecal beta-glucuronidase (leading to increased enterohepatic recycling, thereby reducing/neutralizing xenobiotic clearance), and a "pathologic" detoxification profile, characterized by (among other markers) markedly elevated caffeine clearance and brutally slow benzoate conjugation; the impaired detoxification is of course consistent with and explanatory for the patient's multiple chemical sensitivities. Among various interventions used over the seven-year course of this patient's illness, the ascorbate-coffee combination (additionally discussed in Chapter 4.2) was clearly the most effective and ultimately—and durably—curative.

---

155 Galland L, Lee M. Abstract #170 High frequency of giardiasis in patients with chronic digestive complaints. *Am J Gastroenterol* 1989;84:1181

Step 3: Treatment for severe allergies

For some patients with severe allergies, we start with selected treatments from Step 2 or Step 3 on the first visit *in addition to* the treatments included in Step 1. Implementation is customized based on history, examination, laboratory findings, and the doctor's experience and good judgment.

- Calcium and magnesium butyrate: Butyrate is a short-chain fatty acid which can be obtained from 1) a limited number of foods, namely butter, 2) intestinal fermentation of carbohydrates by probiotic bacteria, and 3) use of nutritional supplements. It is increasingly well-established that probiotic bacteria have immune-normalizing and "anti-allergy" effects, and this benefit is probably mediated at least in part by probiotic production of butyrate. The mechanisms of the anti-allergy effect of butyrate are manifold, and as a fatty acid butyrate activates peroxisome-proliferator activated receptor-alpha (PPAR-alpha) and thereby results in an immunomodulatory action and a suppressive effect on NFkB.[156,157] Butyrate is also a primary fuel for enterocytes and may improve enterocyte metabolism for the normalization of intestinal permeability. In the treatment of patients with inflammatory bowel disease, 4 grams per day of orally administered butyrate salts safely improves the action of mesalamine[158] as does topical application of butyrate (via enema) in ulcerative colitis.[159] As a normal dietary component and product of the gastrointestinal tract, supplemental calcium/magnesium salts of butyrate are safe and effective for human consumption at doses of 1,000 – 4,500 mg butyrate per day for the alleviation of allergic diseases.[160,161]

- Purified chondroitin sulfate and glucosamine sulfate: Doctors and patients everywhere should already know that chondroitin sulfate and glucosamine sulfate are safe and effective for the treatment of osteoarthritis. Furthermore, purified chondroitin sulfate is cardioprotective and that it helps to reduce the vessel occlusion characteristic of atherosclerosis.[162] Additionally, new experimental evidence shows that chondroitin sulfate and glucosamine sulfate can inhibit allergic reactions.[163] With this in mind, it is reasonable to speculate that many arthritic patients who respond to glucosamine and chondroitin may actually be responding to the anti-allergy benefits of chondroitin and glucosamine *rather than* or *in addition to* the "cartilage building" properties of these supplements. Furthermore, there is evidence that purified chondroitin sulfate can act as a "decoy" and reduce adhesion of harmful bacteria; the role of harmful gastrointestinal bacteria in the genesis and perpetuation of joint pain and inflammation will be discussed in the next article in this series. For now, suffice to say that occult gastrointestinal infections (i.e., gastrointestinal dysbiosis) are a major contributor to the systemic pain and inflammation seen in conditions such as rheumatoid arthritis and ankylosing spondylitis.

- Hormones: DHEA, progesterone, testosterone, and cortisol tend to be lower in allergic/autoimmune individuals than in healthy controls. I use either serum testing and/or 24-hour urine samples before prescribing hormones, though I will empirically use progesterone in a woman or a 3-month trial of DHEA in a man with allergies if I find sufficient indications and no contraindications. Treatment is customized per patient. I discuss the hormonal contributions to autoimmunity and chronic inflammation in Chapter 4.6 under the heading of "orthoendocrinology." Much of what applies to "allergy" also applies to "autoimmunity" and vise-versa; they are both manifestations of immune dysfunction.[164]

Step 4: Drug treatments

We must acknowledge a place for drug therapy in patients with recalcitrant or severe allergies.

- Prednisone: For patients with allergies that are inconsolable, prednisone becomes a reasonable consideration. The lowest effective dose should be used for the shortest possible period of time.

[156] Zapolska-Downar et al. Butyrate inhibits cytokine-induced VCAM-1 and ICAM-1 expression in cultured endothelial cells: the role of NF-kappaB and PPARalpha. *J Nutr Biochem.* 2004 Apr;15(4):220-8

[157] Luhrs et al. Butyrate inhibits NF-kappaB activation in lamina propria macrophages of patients with ulcerative colitis. *Scand J Gastroenterol.* 2002 Apr;37(4):458-66

[158] Vernia P, Monteleone G, Grandinetti G, Villotti G, Di Giulio E, Frieri G, Marcheggiano A, Pallone F, Caprilli R, Torsoli A. Combined oral sodium butyrate and mesalazine treatment compared to oral mesalazine alone in ulcerative colitis: randomized, double-blind, placebo-controlled pilot study. *Dig Dis Sci.* 2000 May;45(5):976-81

[159] Vernia et al. Topical butyrate improves efficacy of 5-ASA in refractory distal ulcerative colitis: results of a multicentre trial. *Eur J Clin Invest.* 2003;33(3):244-8

[160] Neesby TE. Method for desensitizing the gastrointestinal tract from food allergies. United States Patent 4,721,716. January 26, 1988

[161] Neesby TE. Method for desensitizing the gastrointestinal tract from food allergies. United States Patent 4,735,967. April 5, 1988

[162] Morrison LM, Enrick N. Coronary heart disease: reduction of death rate by chondroitin sulfate A. *Angiology.* 1973 May;24(5):269-87

[163] Theoharides TC, Bielory L. Mast cells and mast cell mediators as targets of dietary supplements. *Ann Allergy Asthma Immunol.* 2004 Aug;93(2 Suppl 1):S24-34

[164] My ideas on immunology and inflammation were first published in *Textbook of Functional Medicine* (2005, 2010) and later matured greatly in *Integrative Rheumatology* (2006), *Rheumatology v3.5* (2014) and later (2016) in the 4th Edition; the information will continue to be developed in future editions.

Discontinuation of treatment that has lasted longer than 4-7 days must be gradual in order to avoid adrenal insufficiency. Topical rather than systemic therapy should be used when appropriate.

- Sodium cromoglycate: Cromoglycate is a mast cell stabilizer which can be applied nasally for allergic rhinitis (Nasalcrom) or taken orally (Gastrocrom) by patients with food allergy to inhibit the local response to type-1 allergies.[165] The drug is poorly absorbed; therefore its anti-allergy effect is mediated at the gastrointestinal mucosa even though the benefits are systemic. Although not officially "approved" in the US for the treatment of food allergy, numerous studies support its use for this purpose.[166] Cromoglycate has been shown to reduce allergy-induced migraine[167] and eczema[168] and prevent the formation of immune complexes following the consumption of allergenic foods. In addition to preventing the allergic phenomena related directly to the consumption of allergenic foods, an additional mechanism of action of sodium cromoglycate is probably that it reduces the allergy-induced increase in intestinal permeability[169] and thereby prohibits absorption of bacterial and other microbial antigens and metabolites; stated differently, some of the manifestations attributed to "food allergy" are probably not mediated by the response to food allergens directly but result from the adverse immunologic and metabolic responses toward gut-derived microbial antigens and metabolites which are absorbed in increased amounts following the consumption of allergenic foods which increase intestinal permeability and absorption of "foreign" and "toxic" intraluminal contents which would have otherwise been excluded. Common doses for children are 100 mg 30 minutes before food (up to 400 mg per day) and 100-200 mg qid for adults 30 minutes before meals. Capsules or ampules should be mixed in plain water before consumption.

- Leukotriene antagonists: Montelukast (Singulair®, Merck) is an orally active leukotriene receptor antagonist that blocks leukotriene D4 from the cysteinyl leukotriene CysLT-1 receptor and thereby reduces vasodilation, eosinophilic inflammation, and vascular hyperpermeability. Montelukast is used in the medical treatment of asthma, rhinitis, and eczema.

Objective means for the identification of allergens: skin-prick testing, serum IgE and IgG assays, double-blind placebo-controlled food challenges, and the elimination and challenge technique

- Skin prick testing: IgE-dependent immediate-onset allergies as assessed with a **skin-prick test** are indicative of immediate-onset allergy to the particular allergen, and provide the identity of the allergen, quantification of the severity of the allergic response, *and evidence of underlying immune dysfunction*. Skin-prick testing does not assess for delayed-onset allergies thus leaving at least one class of adverse food reactions unassessed.

- Allergen-specific serum levels of IgE and IgG: Elevated serum levels of IgE and IgG, which are identified as specific for certain foods, also provide the identity of the allergen *and evidence of underlying immune dysfunction*. These "objective" tools are part of the clinician's repertoire for identifying food allergens, while keeping in mind that both skin-prick testing and serum testing are prone to both false positives and false negatives. Serum IgE testing does not assess IgG-mediated allergies, nor does it assess for sensitivity (immune but not immunoglobulin-mediated responses) or intolerance, which tends to be biochemical rather than immunologic. IgG assays and the subclasses of IgG-4 assays have not gained acceptance for their sensitivity or specificity, even though clinicians order them and patients pay for them.

- Double-blind placebo-controlled food challenge: Another commonly mentioned objective means for identifying food allergens is the "double-blind placebo-controlled food challenge" (DBPCFC) wherein food is administered a double-blind fashion with placebo control generally via either capsules or nasogastric tube. Unfortunately, DBPCFC is commonly considered the gold standard for the identification of particular allergens and the establishment of an allergic diathesis. This is unfortunate because the hospital admission

---

[165] drugs.com/MMX/Cromolyn_Sodium.html   Accessed November 24, 2005

[166] "Both the clinician's and patient's preferences and the clinician's evaluation of the specific response to challenge showed a significant benefit from SCG." Dannaeus A, Foucard T, Johansson SG. The effect of orally administered sodium cromoglycate on symptoms of food allergy. *Clin Allergy*. 1977 Mar;7(2):109-15

[167] "Immune complexes were not produced in those patients who were protected by sodium cromoglycate. These observations confirm that a food-allergic reaction is the cause of migraine in this group of patients." Monro J, Carini C, Brostoff J. Migraine is a food-allergic disease. *Lancet*. 1984 Sep 29;2(8405):719-21

[168] "The same atopic patients pretreated with oral sodium cromoglycate had less antigen entry, diminished immune-complex formation, and no atopic symptoms." Paganelli et al. Immune complexes containing food proteins in normal and atopic subjects after oral challenge and effect of sodium cromoglycate on antigen absorption. *Lancet*. 1979 Jun 16;1(8129):1270-2

[169] "It is suggested that a local IgE-mediated mechanism acts as a "trigger" for the entry of antigen and the formation of immune complexes by altering the permeability of the gut mucosa. The resulting delayed onset symptoms could be viewed as a form of serum sickness with few or many target organs affected." Carini C, Brostoff J, Wraith DG. IgE complexes in food allergy. *Ann Allergy*. 1987 Aug;59(2):110-7

and associated costs are expensive, cumbersome and therefore inaccessible for most patients. Some patients will have a false-negative response when challenged with isolated foods because of the lack of "accessory antigens", "accomplice antigens", or "bystander antigens."[170] Some patients will have adverse food reactions only when foods are eaten either with *high frequency* or in *specific combinations* or when *gastrointestinal problems* (e.g., dysbiosis or increased intestinal permeability) are present at the same time as the food challenge. For example, while the patient may tolerate eggs alone and wheat alone without the manifestation of allergic symptoms, the additive insult of the combination of both eggs and wheat may cause sufficient intestinal damage and/or immune activation that clinical manifestations become apparent. With single food challenges given with DBPCFC, "real life" situations are not reproduced, and false negative results may erroneously suggest that either the patient has no allergies or that a particular food is not offensive. Furthermore, the scientific sterility of the DBPCFC generally takes the patient out of his/her real life experience and context; the implications for this are obvious when we consider the emotional-social-psychological aspects of immune system hyper-reactivity and/or neurogenic inflammation that underlies the neuropsychological aspect of allergy, mentioned previously in the context of classical/Pavlovian conditioning of allergic responses.[171,172]

- Elimination and challenge: The "elimination and challenge" technique (more accurately described as "avoidance and challenge") requires that the patient first clear the diet of all possible offending foods, either by fasting or by consuming a simple diet of unlikely-to-be-allergenic foods, such as the classic triad of rice, lamb, and pears or a relatively hypoallergenic hydrolyzed formula such as Vivonex. After 7-14 days of elimination (i.e., avoidance) *and the clearing of symptoms thought to be allergy-mediated*, an offending food is reintroduced by intense consumption (i.e., eaten with every meal) for a period of up to two days. Every two to four days, a new food is added back into the diet, and a correlation is searched for between consumption of a given food and the exacerbation of symptoms. If the symptoms do not abate or disappear with the fasting/elimination phase, then confirming the nature of the disorder as allergic is more difficult and determining the identity of the allergen is additionally unlikely. However, in some cases, clinical signs and symptoms that are indeed allergy-mediated will fail to regress significantly during the brief washout period. This is because the underlying tissue damage is too great to be healed in such a short time. A good example is the thyroid disease induced by gluten-containing grains in people with the severe gluten allergy called celiac disease; simply avoiding gluten for 1-2 weeks does not restore endocrine function because the body needs more time to reacquire homeostasis and to heal injured tissues. A common scenario is one in which symptoms remit during fasting/elimination and then return *gradually* rather than *immediately* when the offending food is eaten. In these situations, the most likely explanations are either ❶ a threshold of time was necessary for physiologic abnormalities (e.g., immune complex deposition, increased intestinal permeability, dysbiosis, accumulative immune stimulation) to culminate in the reproduction of symptoms, or ❷ synergistic factors may have to be combined in order to produce the symptoms of allergy, such as the induction of IgE-mediated increased intestinal permeability by food R which then leads to the increased absorption of food S, to which the peripheral immune system then responds with an IgG-mediated reaction with resultant clinical manifestations. In the latter case, food R or food S *when eaten alone or on a rotation basis* may be insufficient to produce allergic manifestations, but the combination of R+S, which would not be identified with skin-prick testing, serum tests, or one-at-a-time DBPCFC, may produce allergic manifestations. Since, in real life, foods are eaten in combination when they cause allergic disease (e.g. a headache or joint pain after eating a hamburger with wheat/gluten, cheese/milk, mayonnaise/egg, and pickle/tartrazine/yeast), a reasonable conclusion is that foods will have to be avoided in specific combinations to attain maximal improvement in allergic symptoms since complex foods probably work synergistically to produce allergic manifestations in affected people. Creating chronological distance between the consumption of allergenic foods explains the success of the **rotation diets** in alleviating allergic manifestations, but it does little to address the underlying immune dysfunction other than to reduce the total allergenic load to which the immune system is exposed. **Intestinal dysbiosis** can also increase intestinal permeability and result in increased absorption of food antigens and depletion of detoxification co-factors, which can mimic or perpetuate immune-mediated food allergies. Correction of this problem can begin to normalize immune function and eliminate symptoms attributed to the consumption of specific foods.

---

[170] "The mechanisms of enhanced permeability to specific and bystander antigens have been delineated as well as the molecular events involved in the sequential phases of allergic reactions." Heyman M. Gut barrier dysfunction in food allergy. *Eur J Gastroenterol Hepatol.* 2005 Dec;17(12):1279-1285

[171] "In a classical conditioning procedure in which an immunologic challenge was paired with the presentation of an odor, guinea pigs showed a plasma histamine increase when presented with the odor alone. This suggests that the immune response can be enhanced through activity of the central nervous system." Russell M, Dark KA, Cummins RW, Ellman G, Callaway E, Peeke HV. Learned histamine release. *Science.* 1984 Aug 17;225(4663):733-4

[172] "A classical Pavlovian paradigm pairing an olfactory cue with allergen challenge for a single training trial was used to produce conditioned histamine release and conditioned nasal airflow decrease in seasonal allergic rhinitis sufferers." Barrett JE, King MG, Pang G. Conditioning rhinitis in allergic humans. *Ann N Y Acad Sci.* 2000;917:853-9

Allergy—Part 2: Asthma & Reactive Airway Disease

Introduction:

While all allergic diseases are important (particularly for the patients who suffer from them), I have chosen to detail asthma because of its increasing frequency, its debilitating nature, the many adverse effects from its medical treatment, and its life-threatening potential. Clinician readers should appreciate that many of the interventions used generally for allergy can apply to asthma, and vice-versa.

Criteria for the evaluation and classification of asthma change frequently; indeed some authorities have called for the abolition of the term "asthma" in favor of the more inclusive and "reactive airway disease" (RAD). Readers wishing to specialize in the treatment of asthma/RAD should consult more than one authoritative source (e.g., a recent clinical specialty textbook and a comprehensive peer-reviewed position paper or clinical practice guideline).

<u>Description & Pathophysiology</u>:

- "<u>Asthma</u>" (Greek: "difficult breathing") refers to a heterogeneous group of airway-pulmonary disorders characterized by the following:
  - <u>Inflammation and histologic changes</u>: Airway epithelium shows increased numbers of activated inflammatory cells including eosinophils, mast cells, macrophages, neutrophils, and T-lymphocytes which produce soluble inflammatory mediators such as cytokines, leukotrienes, and bradykinins. Airway inflammation leads to airway edema, increased vascularity, and disruption of ciliated columnar epithelium—each of these leads to perpetuation of chronic inflammation and airway obstruction. Smooth muscle hyperplasia and hypertrophy, along with increased deposition of collagen contributes to airway constriction and stiffness, both of which contribute to obstruction. Increased mucus production and goblet cell hyperplasia predispose to formation of mucus plugs, which can completely block bronchioles, thus eliminating gas exchange and promoting atelectasis in the corresponding pulmonary segment.
  - <u>Airway hyper-reactivity</u>: Airways are normally reactive to various stimuli; the distinction that characterizes asthma is the severity of the reactivity (overzealous response) and the exquisite sensitivity to triggers—asthmatic airways respond to stimuli at levels which are subthreshold for nonasthmatics. Thus, hyper-reactivity reflects overactivity of the inflammatory response and hypersensitivity to generally innocuous levels bronchoconstrictor stimuli. The speed of the inflammatory response following irritant exposure can be immediate ("immediate asthmatic response") or delayed by 4-6 hours ("late asthmatic response").
  - <u>Reversibility</u>: One of the diagnostic characteristics of asthma is its reversibility with bronchodilator challenge. However, with long-standing severe disease, airway remodeling—which includes smooth muscle hypertrophy/hyperplasia and fibrosis—becomes progressively irreversible. Irreversible airway obstruction is characteristic of COPD—chronic obstructive pulmonary disease—which includes asthma and chronic bronchitis.
  - <u>Airway obstruction</u>: Asthma primarily affects the bronchi rather than the lung parenchyma and alveoli. Thus, the clinical problem is one of *air movement* rather than *gas exchange* per se; although severely impaired air movement does necessarily impair gas exchange even when the alveoli are fully functional. Due to the dynamics of air movement during lung deflation, asthma primarily results in impaired exhalation, resulting in "air trapping" within the lungs and the resultant hyperinflation and secondarily impaired inhalation and efficient gas exchange.
  - <u>Increased prevalence during adolescence</u>: African Americans and children are most affected; the highest death rates due to asthma are seen in young African-Americans aged 15-24 years. "Asthma is the most common chronic pediatric disease."[173] Compared with adults, children show an increased prevalence of allergic/atopic disorders, which many of them will "grow out of" as they get older. Maturation of the immune system in general and the progressively increased elaboration of immunomodulating hormones cortisol, DHEA, testosterone with adrenarche (average age 6-10 years) in particular contribute to the regression of allergy/atopy as young children get older.

---

[173] Witcoff LJ. Pulmonology. In: Brown LJ, Miller LT. (Eds.) *Pediatrics Board Review Series*. Philadelphia: Lippincott Williams and Wilkins; 2005, 268-71

- Increased prevalence in industrialized societies: Asthma affects 7% of the US population (nearly 15 million people, causing more than 5,550 deaths per year), reflecting an increase of 75% from 1960 to 1994.

- Contributors to and triggers for asthma include the following:
  - Chronic sinusitis
  - Diminished β2-adrenergic receptor function: this predisposes to bronchospasm
  - Drug allergens/sensitizers, including prescription drugs with artificial colors that are known to trigger asthma
  - Dust mites and their feces
  - Food allergens
  - Fungi and mold exposure
  - Gastroesophageal reflux
  - Insects such as roaches, pet dander and saliva
  - Obesity—see Chapters 2 and 4.4 for discussion of link between obesity and inflammation
  - Pollen
  - Viral infections
  - Xenobiotic/chemical fumes including urban pollution

Clinical Presentation:

- **The classic triad of asthma includes ❶ persistent wheeze, ❷ persistent dyspnea** (shortness of breath, subjective "chest tightness"), **and ❸ persistent cough.** In the acute care setting, these same manifestations could be caused by inhalation of a foreign object, acute airway inflammation due to chemical-toxic-smoke inhalation injury, or anaphylaxis. Laboratory confirmation of asthma includes a fourth component: induction and reversibility with chemical provocation.
- **Indicators of urgency—implement immediate and aggressive treatment: difficulty talking due to dyspnea, use of accessory muscles if inspiration, pulsus paradoxus (no palpable radial pulse during inhalation), diaphoresis, mental status changes (e.g., agitation or somnolence).**
  - *Pulsus paradoxus*—the paradoxically missing peripheral pulse during inspiration—is may be seen with cardiac tamponade, pericarditis, chronic sleep apnea, croup, asthma and COPD.

Major Differential Diagnoses:

- Acute airway inflammation and angioedema due to chemical-toxic-smoke-aspiration inhalation: This can include gastroesophageal reflux, which may be otherwise asymptomatic, and which may occur unknown to the patient during sleep; relatedly, tracheoesophageal fistula should be considered in infants and post-trauma patients.
- Airway compression due to anatomic anomaly, tumor, or mediastinal lymphadenopathy:
- Allergic bronchopulmonary aspergillosis (ABPA), allergic bronchopulmonary mycosis: Skin allergy test is commonly positive to *Aspergillus fumigatus*.
- Anaphylaxis
- Antitrypsin deficiency: alpha-1-antitrypsin deficiency classically leads to emphysema and hepatic fibrosis.
- Bronchiectasis
- Bronchopulmonary dysplasia
- Cardiac disease and heart failure: "Cardiac asthma"
- Churg-Strauss vasculitis
- Cystic fibrosis
- Eosinophilic pneumonia
- Idiopathic pulmonary fibrosis: Extremely rare in children; more common (but still rare) in older adults in general and particularly those with inflammatory/autoimmune diseases
- Inhalation of a foreign object
- Pneumothorax
- Pulmonary edema: Consider congestive heart failure as a primary cause.

Clinical Assessments:
- **History/subjective:**
  - ▪ <u>HPI</u>: Episodic wheezing (reversible spontaneously or with treatment), dyspnea, subjective "chest tightness", cough, excess sputum; symptoms may be intermittent or persistent.
  - ▪ <u>Associated findings</u>: Nasal congestion, rhinorrhea, polyps; increased prevalence of eczema and otitis media.
  - ▪ <u>Common triggers</u>: URI, aspiration, gastroesophageal reflux disorder (GERD), psychoemotional and physical stress, exercise, tobacco smoke, pollution including ozone and sulfur dioxide, menses ("catamenial asthma"); assessment for the head/facial pain and post-nasal drip of chronic sinusitis is particularly important as treatment for chronic sinusitis is very effective in alleviating asthma manifestations.

> **Clinical Pearl**
> During acute exacerbations of asthma, air movement can be so severely reduced that wheezing is not present; in these situations, the more subtle physical examination findings of prolonged exhalation and a global reduction in breath sounds should be pursued.

- **Physical Examination/Objective**: Physical examination and pulmonary function may be essentially normal between exacerbations, especially in younger patients with intermittent disease.
  - ▪ <u>Lung auscultation and percussion</u>: Prolonged exhalation, tachypnea, diffuse wheezes, hyperresonance.
  - ▪ <u>Spirometry</u>: Clinical assessment of FEV1 and FVC provides the FEV1/FVC ratio, which when reduced indicates the airway obstruction typical of *but not specific for* asthma. Peak expiratory flow measurement can also be used to assess current status and response to treatment.
  - ▪ <u>BMI</u>: Overweight patients should follow a diet-exercise-lifestyle program that facilitates weight loss, with its attendant reduction in *total inflammatory load* and improved respiratory function. Weight loss in general and low-carbohydrate diets in particular help alleviate GERD, which is a well-known cause of asthma, particularly adult-onset asthma.
- **Laboratory Assessments**: Always perform a basic laboratory evaluation in essentially all patients, particularly when evaluating them for the first time or if their therapeutic progress is unsatisfactory. This basic laboratory evaluation should include CBC, chemistry/metabolic panel, urinalysis and preferably TSH, vitamin D level, CRP, and ferritin. Just because a patient has a diagnosis of "asthma" (or any other disease) and the same patient has shortness of breath (SOB) or dyspnea on exertion (DOE), this does not mean that the SOB/DOE is due to the asthma; the patient may also have iron deficiency and/or anemia as a cause of or contributor to their symptomatology.
  - ▪ <u>CBC</u>: May reveal eosinophilia. Elevated WBC, neutrophils or lymphocytes can indicate infection, whether bacterial or viral, respectively. Elevated RBC consistent with polycythemia can indicate chronic hypoxia, which may be due to chronic severe asthma or another pulmonary, renal, or myeloproliferative disorder.
  - ▪ <u>Serum total IgE levels</u>: Increased in some (not all) patients with atopy, parasitosis, ABPA
  - ▪ <u>Serum IgE levels for specific allergens</u>
  - ▪ <u>Skin testing for IgE/immediate allergy</u>
  - ▪ <u>Serum IgG4 levels for specific delayed-onset allergens</u>
  - ▪ <u>Urine sulfite</u>: A subset of asthma patients—prototypically those presenting concomitant multiple chemical sensitivity (MCS)—is sensitive to or unable to detoxify various endogenous and exogenous precursors that are ultimately reduced to sulfite. As a result, sulfite levels are increase in the urine and can be measured at abnormally high levels in affected patients. Subsequently, steps can be taken to reduce sulfite intake and/or facilitate in vivo detoxification of sulfite, such as with supraphysiologic doses of vitamin B-12, and perhaps with molybdenum supplementation.
  - ▪ <u>Sputum eosinophils</u>: Quantification of eosinophils in induced sputum can guide corticosteroid administration more effectively than clinical assessment for the prevention of exacerbations.
  - ▪ <u>Exhaled nitric oxide (eNO)</u>: Measurement of exhaled nitric oxide provides noninvasive assessment of airway inflammation, but conflicting data does not currently clarify the role of eNO in asthma management.
  - ▪ <u>Fecal antigen testing for current *Helicobacter pylori* infection</u>: A small percentage of patients with asthma—as with migraine and inflammation/autoimmunity—may have occult *H pylori* infection; eradication of this dysbiosis—especially if combined with regular implementation of the 5-part supplemented Paleo-

Mediterranean diet protocol and other anti-inflammatory health-restorative treatments may reduce their *total inflammatory load* sufficiently to provide objective and subjective improvement in their clinical status.

- **Imaging**:
  - **Chest radiograph** may show hyperinflation and can be used to assess for differential diagnoses such as foreign object, pneumonia, interstitial lung disease, pneumothorax, or lung tumor in appropriate clinical scenarios.
- **Biopsy/Procedure**: Lung biopsy is not used in the diagnosis and management of asthma *per se*; its role in this context would only be in the exclusion/confirmation of another lung disease
  - Arterial blood gases and pulse oximetry may show hypoxemia during exacerbations.
  - Spirometry can be performed in office and at home to assess response to treatment and challenge (e.g., consumption of suspected food allergen) and to monitor for exacerbations.
- **Establishing the Diagnosis**: The diagnosis of asthma is established with demonstration (clinical or historical) of reversible airway obstruction and airway hyper-reactivity. These can be provoked artificially by administration of a bronchoconstrictor (e.g., methacholine, histamine, cold air, exercise; these are considered "nonspecific" and are able to induce bronchoconstriction at levels much lower than those required to induce bronchoconstriction in nonasthmatics) and/or bronchodilator, such as albuterol or epinephrine. Iatrogenic bronchoconstriction should be undertaken only by pulmonary specialists with on-site emergency management capabilities, and such diagnostic challenge should obviously never be undertaken during an already in-process exacerbation or when FEV1 is less than 65% of predicted. **A compatible history of repeated and reversible airway obstruction based on the patient's experience is generally sufficient for diagnosis; this can be further supported with a favorable response to bronchodilator therapy.** In-office spirometry can be used to document and quantify airway obstruction. Lung volume measurements can be assessed by various methods and characteristically show hyperinflation. Arterial blood gases and pulse oximetry may show hypoxemia during exacerbations. Chest radiograph may show hyperinflation and can be used to assess for differential diagnoses such as foreign object, pneumonia, interstitial lung disease, or lung tumor in appropriate clinical scenarios.
  - *Status asthmaticus* is any severe acute exacerbation of asthma that is relatively unresponsive to expedient treatment. *Hyperacute asthma* **can be rapidly fatal**.
  - **Arterial blood gas analysis showing *progressive/absolute* hypoxemia or hypercarbia portends/indicates a medical emergency. "The combination of an increased PaCO2 and respiratory acidosis may indicate impending respiratory failure and the need for mechanical ventilation."**[174]

Disease Complications:

- Quality of life complications: Inability to participate fully in activities of daily living (ADL), impaired quality of life, social compromise, low self-esteem, lost opportunities, depression.
- Medical complications: Exhaustion, syncope, pneumothorax, respiratory failure, death

Clinical Management: Clinical management of the asthmatic patient is based on assessment of impairment and risk. In this context, impairment includes asthma severity (frequency and intensity) and the resultant functional limitations, while risk includes likelihood of acute exacerbations and chronic decline in lung function due to chronic inflammation, airway remodeling, and decompensation. Experts Chestnut, Murray, and Prendergast[175] state, "A key insight is that these two domains of control may respond differently to treatment: some patients may have minimal impairment yet remain at risk for severe exacerbations, for example, in the setting of an upper respiratory tract infection."

- Home-use peak expiratory flow (PEF) meters: Measurements can be used by patients for self-monitoring, for assessing response to challenges such as stressful events, food allergen consumption, and environmental exposure. The patient can record a daily log or "lung diary" that is given to and used by the clinician to monitor response to treatment. PEF shows diurnal variation (worst in the morning, best in the afternoon), and PEF values can be contrasted to the patient's previous values thereby serving as a true guide to patient status, whether that of improvement or exacerbation. "PEF values less than 200 L/min indicate severe airflow

[174] Chestnut et al. "Pulmonary Disorders." In: McPhee et al. (Eds.) *Current Medical Diagnosis and Treatment 2009, 48th Edition*. McGraw Hill Medical; 2009, 210-228
[175] Chestnut et al. "Pulmonary Disorders." In: McPhee et al. (Eds.) *Current Medical Diagnosis and Treatment 2009, 48th Edition*. McGraw Hill Medical; 2009, 210-228

obstruction."[176] Physicians should give patients a plan of action should pulmonary function decline significantly so that early-stage declinations can be treated before potentially developing into serious exacerbations.

- Written instructions: Patients must receive clearly written instructions for ❶ daily management including schedule of administration for their medication(s) and nutritional supplements and ❷ emergent management including additional doses of treatments and clear instructions—preferably with address, phone number, and map—to the nearest emergency care facility.
- Reserve ("back-up") medication: Patients and clinicians should ensure that treatment is available to the patient at all times and locations: at home, at school, at work, and when traveling. When traveling, patients should have reserve treatment with them, namely medications in their personal carry-on luggage as well as their checked baggage in case one of these is lost or confiscated by airport security; necessary prescriptions should be preauthorized at national pharmacies. The patient has the responsibility to inform the clinician of travel plans and to schedule any necessary office visits before traveling and with enough time for clinical evaluation and the obtainment of laboratory results.

Treatments: The two minimal goals of treatment are ❶ **expedient and efficacious control of any acute exacerbations**, and ❷ **convenient and nontoxic control of daily symptoms**. The highest goal of ❸ **optimizing endogenous inflammatory and immune balance so that the asthma resolves** is generally not a consideration in standardized allopathic medicine although is a foremost goal in naturopathic and functional medicine. Clinicians specializing in the treatment of pulmonary disorders should stay abreast with updated treatment guidelines, such as those published by the National Heart, Lung, and Blood Institute (NHLBI) nhlbi.nih.gov/guidelines/asthma and the National Asthma Education and Prevention Program (NAEPP) nhlbi.nih.gov/about/naepp. Further, treatment of status asthmaticus should be managed by emergency medicine personnel trained in and equipped for intubation, artificial ventilation, and parenteral drug administration.

- **Prescription drug treatments per asthma classification/severity**: Inhaled corticosteroids are the "default" treatment for asthma unless it is sufficiently mild and intermittent to be managed with PRN use of bronchodilators, typically inhaled beta-2 agonists (hereafter: beta2-inhaler) such as albuterol; additional drugs include leukotriene synthesis inhibitors, leukotriene receptor blockers, mast cell stabilizers, anti-IgE antibodies, and methylxanthines/theophylline. Drugs are added in a stepwise fashion depending on asthma classification, which is defined by disease frequency and severity, as shown in the following table:

Classification	Frequency & Severity	Drug Management
Intermittent	▪ Daytime symptoms: ≤ 2/wk ▪ Nighttime symptoms: ≤ 2/mo	▪ PRN short-acting beta2-inhaler
Mild persistent	▪ Daytime symptoms: 2-6/wk ▪ Nighttime symptoms: > 2/mo ▪ FEV1 ≥ 80% (normal)	▪ PRN short-acting beta2-inhaler ▪ Scheduled daily use of low-dose inhaled steroid; second-line alternatives include cromolyn, or leukotriene modulator
Moderate persistent	▪ Daytime symptoms: daily ▪ Nighttime symptoms: > 1/wk ▪ FEV1 60-80%	▪ PRN short-acting beta2-inhaler ▪ Medium-dose inhaled steroid <u>or</u> low-dose inhaled steroid and long-acting beta2-inhaler
Severe persistent	▪ Daytime symptoms: continuous ▪ Nighttime symptoms: frequent ▪ FEV1 ≤ 60%	▪ PRN short-acting beta2-inhaler -inhaler ▪ High-dose inhaled steroid ▪ Long-acting beta2-inhaler-inhaler ▪ Systemic steroids

- ▪ Cromolyn sodium: Cromolyn acts as a mast cell stabilizer, reducing the elaboration of inflammatory mediators; it is used for long-term management and is not used in the treatment of acute exacerbations.

---

[176] Chestnut et al. "Pulmonary Disorders." In: McPhee et al. (Eds.) Current Medical Diagnosis and Treatment 2009, 48th Edition. New York: McGraw Hill Medical; 2009, 210-228

- Corticosteroids: These "steroids" are either short-acting or long-acting and are delivered by oral, inhalational, and parenteral routes; although they are essential for the management of severe asthma, their chronic use can cause growth retardation in children, as well as immunosuppression, osteoporosis, and a Cushing-like syndrome and metabolic syndrome (i.e., insulin resistance, hypertension, dyslipidemia, and obesity). Importantly, corticosteroid administration increases body losses (mostly through increased urinary excretion) of calcium, magnesium, potassium, and zinc; the iatrogenic magnesium insufficiency exacerbates anxiety and bronchospasm while the zinc insufficiency impairs immune responsiveness and adversely affects hormonal immunomodulation by enhancing the effects of estrogen(s) and impairing the effects of androgens, particularly testosterone. Gvozdjáková et al[177] noted that "Long-term administration of corticosteroids has been shown to result in mitochondrial dysfunction and oxidative damage of mitochondrial and nuclear DNAs" and suggested that this iatrogenic cellular damage might be prevented or ameliorated via supplementation with coenzyme Q10, as discussed below.
- Anticholinergic drugs: Anticholinergic drugs such as atropine and ipratropium bromide block vagal/parasympathetic-mediated bronchoconstriction and thus function as bronchodilators; anticholinergic drugs can be used as second-line bronchodilators in the treatment of severe asthma.
- Anti-IgE antibody (omalizumab): Omalizumab binds to IgE and thus reduces allergic responses; the clinical safety and efficacy profiles are notably good.

- **Dietary interventions:**
  - Food allergens: Some experts would argue that the link between food allergies and asthma is so strong that failure to address the food allergy component of asthma is clinical malpractice. Among the most commonly consumed allergens that exacerbate asthma are cereal grains, "nuts" and peanuts, cow milk, eggs, chocolate (also a source of cow's milk in the case of milk chocolate), fish, tomatoes and other *Solanaceae* nightshade plants (perhaps due in part to the anti-acetylcholinesterase constituent(s)

> **Fast food (e.g., wheat, high-glycemic loads and indexes, GMO foods, AGE components, and high-dose sodium to activate Th17 inflammatory cells) increases the incidence of allergic inflammatory disease: dose-dependent response with asthma**
>
> "CONCLUSIONS: Frequent consumption of hamburgers showed a dose-dependent association with asthma symptoms, and frequent takeaway [fast food] consumption showed a similar association with bronchial hyperresponsiveness."
>
> Wickens et al. Fast foods - are they a risk factor for asthma? *Allergy*. 2005 Dec

promoting parasympathetic bronchoconstriction), food colorings (especially tartrazine [yellow dye #5] which is also found in some asthma medications, as well as some formulations of thyroxine). Early introduction of cereal grains/grasses into the childhood diet promotes development of IgE antibodies against other grasses and airborne pollens[178]; not surprisingly, the risk of atopic/allergic disease correlates directly with the number of solid foods prematurely introduced into an infant's diet.[179] Furthermore, grains are commonly contaminated with additional allergens and immunogens such as mold/fungi/yeast and insects and their feces.
  - Avoidance of proinflammatory foods: Specific food components associated with development and/or exacerbation of asthma include saturated fatty acids and high-carbohydrate calorie-dense foods. Saturated fatty acids promote systemic inflammation *in vivo* by several mechanisms not the least of which is activation of Toll-like receptor 4 which in turn activates NF-kappaB. Similarly, high glucose loads induce oxidative stress, which is well known to deplete antioxidants (some of which have immunomodulating and anti-allergy effects) and to promote systemic inflammation. Childhood food consumption patterns characterized by low intake of magnesium, vitamin E, breast milk, fruits and vegetables, and increased consumption of "fast foods", pasta, and hamburgers increase the risk of asthma.[180,181,182]

[177] Gvozdjáková et al. Coenzyme Q10 supplementation reduces corticosteroids dosage in patients with bronchial asthma. *Biofactors*. 2005;25(1-4):235-40
[178] Armentia et al. Early introduction of cereals into children's diets as a risk-factor for grass pollen asthma. *Clin Exp Allergy*. 2001 Aug;31(8):1250-5
[179] Fergusson DM, Horwood LJ, Shannon FT. Early solid feeding and recurrent childhood eczema: a 10-year longitudinal study. *Pediatrics*. 1990 Oct;86(4):541-6
[180] Hijazi N, Abalkhail B, Seaton A. Diet and childhood asthma in a society in transition: a study in urban and rural Saudi Arabia. *Thorax*. 2000 Sep;55(9):775-9
[181] Wickens K, Barry D, Friezema A, Rhodius R, Bone N, Purdie G, Crane J. Fast foods - are they a risk factor for asthma? *Allergy*. 2005 Dec;60(12):1537-41
[182] Awasthi et al. Prevalence and risk factors of asthma and wheeze in school-going children in Lucknow, North India. *Indian Pediatr*. 2004 Dec;41(12):1205-10

- <u>Health-promoting Paleo-Mediterranean Diet (previously described in this text—see Chapter 2)</u>: In 2008 Castro-Rodriguez et al[183] concluded, "The Mediterranean diet is an independent protective factor for current wheezing in preschoolers, irrespective of obesity and physical activity."

> **Paleo-Mediterranean diet (compared to standard processed food diet) protects against the development of allergy and asthma**
>
> "CONCLUSIONS: The Mediterranean diet is an independent protective factor for current wheezing in preschoolers, irrespective of obesity and physical activity."
>
> Castro-Rodriguez et al. Mediterranean diet as a protective factor for wheezing in preschool children. *J Pediatr.* 2008 Jun

- <u>Diet modification for weight loss and BMI optimization</u>: Obesity and its associated lifestyle and dietary risk factors correlates with an increased risk factor for asthma by several mechanisms, including: ❶ overconsumption of saturated fatty acids and simple carbohydrates, both of which promote systemic inflammation and oxidant stress, ❷ sedentary lifestyle, as lack of exercise causes a relative increase in systemic inflammation compared to an active lifestyle because exercising muscle releases anti-inflammatory cytokines (myokines), ❸ caloric overload is most easily accomplished by consumption of processed foods such as grain products which are inherently allergenic, ❹ physical enlargement of abdominal contents (i.e., visceral adipose) which retards diaphragmatic descent and thereby reduces respiratory efficiency, ❺ increased elaboration of inflammatory cytokines (adipokines) from adipose tissue, and ❻ enhancement of an inflammatory state via alterations in hormone levels, particularly an increase in *pro-inflammatory* estrogens and reduction in *anti-inflammatory* androgens. Delgado et al[184] wrote, "Most prospective studies show that obesity is a risk factor for asthma and have found a positive correlation between baseline body mass index and the subsequent development of asthma. Furthermore, several studies suggest that whereas weight gain increases the risk of asthma, weight loss improves the course of the illness. ... The treatment of obese asthmatics must include a weight control program."

- <u>Avoidance of sulfite-containing foods for patients with sulfite-sensitive asthma</u>: A subset of asthmatic patients are intolerant to sulfite(s) and suffer exacerbations of asthma following sulfite consumption or, possibly, increased endogenous production. Among the more commonly sulfited foods are lettuce, shrimp, dried fruits (e.g., apricots), white grape juice, dehydrated potatoes (as mashed potatoes), wine, beer, mushrooms, and candy bars (e.g., Mounds). Sodium metabisulfite is used in foods and some medications (e.g., acetaminophen) as a disinfectant, antioxidant, and preservative. Adverse food reactions following consumption of sulfited foods are not always consistent, even when the patient has confirmed sulfite sensitivity based on double-blind capsule/beverage challenge testing. Taylor et al[185] summarized, "The likelihood of a reaction is dependent on the nature of the food, the level of residual sulfite, the sensitivity of the patient, and perhaps on the form of residual sulfite and the mechanism of the sulfite-induced reaction." The clinical application of this information is to consider sulfite sensitivity in asthmatic patients, particularly those with recalcitrant disease and those with other manifestations of impaired sulfur metabolism such as multiple chemical sensitivity (MCS); in these patients, a broader therapeutic

> **Clinical Pearl: Sulfite leads to mast cell degranulation and thus "allergic inflammation" while it also impairs mitochondrial function, thereby promoting chronic/sustained inflammation and metabolic impairment**
>
> "Sulfur dioxide is 1 of 6 environmental pollutants monitored by the Environmental Protection Agency. Its ability to induce bronchoconstriction is well documented. ... Peripheral blood basophils also showed histamine release after exposure to sodium sulfite. ...
> Conclusions: **Sulfite**, the aqueous ion of sulfur dioxide, induces cellular activation, **leading to degranulation in mast cells through a non-IgE-dependent pathway**. The response also differs from IgE-mediated degranulation..."
>
> Collaco et al. Effect of sodium sulfite on mast cell degranulation and oxidant stress. *Ann Allergy Asthma Immunol.* 2006 Apr

---

[183] Castro-Rodriguez et al. Mediterranean diet as a protective factor for wheezing in preschool children. *J Pediatr.* 2008 Jun;152(6):823-8, 828.e1-2

[184] Delgado J, Barranco P, Quirce S. Obesity and asthma. *J Investig Allergol Clin Immunol.* 2008;18(6):420-5

[185] Taylor et al. Sensitivity to sulfited foods among sulfite-sensitive subjects with asthma. *J Allergy Clin Immunol.* 1988 Jun;81(6):1159-67. This is a small clinical trial of eight patients, and most of the findings were inconclusive; this study was funded in large part by the processed food industry: Supported by contributions from the Corn Refiners Association, National Fisheries Institute, National Cherry Growers and Industries Foundation, American Mushroom Institute, National Coalition of Fresh Potato Processors, Dried Fruit Association of California, Northwest Cherry Briners Association, International Food Additives Council, Villa Banfi Foundation, Inc., Frito-Lay, Inc., Del Monte Corp., Larsen Co., Pillsbury, Inc., Basic American Foods, Inc., Campbells, Inc., General Mills, Inc., Prepared Potato Co., Calreco, Inc., T. J. Lipton, Inc., Northern Star Co., Hershey Foods, Inc., R. T. French Co., Stauffer Chemical Co., Universal Foods Corp., and Mead Johnson Co.

approach might include vitamin B-12 supplementation as discussed in a following section, avoidance of sulfited foods, and perhaps more comprehensive detoxification programs.[186]

- Avoidance of excess sodium chloride: American/Westernized diets are overladen with sodium chloride. Excess sodium promotes water retention and tissue edema, especially when combined with a high-carbohydrate diet and/or insulin resistance. Sodium promotes induction of the pro-inflammatory Th17 phenotype, known to contribute to asthma.[187] The chloride ion is acidogenic and thus perturbs metabolism, disrupts homeostatic mechanisms, and promotes renal loss of calcium and magnesium—this latter effect promotes inflammation via nutrigenomic mechanisms, including but probably not limited to the development of intracellular hypercalcinosis (discussed elsewhere in this text). Avoidance of sodium chloride appears particularly relevant in the treatment of exercise-induced asthma (EIA).

  - Clinical trial: Both sodium and chloride contribute to the worsening of EIA symptoms: "The NaHCO3 diet lessened the deterioration of post-exercise pulmonary function, but not to the extent of LSD [low-salt diet]. These data suggest that both sodium and chloride contribute to the worsening of EIA symptoms seen after consuming a normal or high NaCl diet."[188] The fact that sodium bicarbonate had less impact on lung function than did sodium chloride shows that the chloride ion promotes bronchoconstriction.

  - Review: A nutritional approach to managing exercise-induced asthma: "Exercise-induced asthma (EIA) is traditionally treated with the use of pharmacotherapy. However, there is now convincing evidence that a variety of dietary factors such as elevated omega-3 polyunsaturated fatty acids and antioxidant intake, and a sodium-restricted diet can reduce this condition."[189]

  - Population-based study: Wheeze and asthma in children are associated with body mass index, sports, television viewing, and diet: "CONCLUSIONS: Our data support the hypothesis that high body weight, spending a lot of time watching television, and a salty diet each independently increase the risk of asthma symptoms in children."[190]

  - Randomized, double-blind crossover study: Dietary salt, airway inflammation, and diffusion capacity in exercise-induced asthma: "CONCLUSION: Our findings indicate that dietary salt loading enhances airway inflammation following exercise in asthmatic subjects, and that small salt-dependent changes in vascular volume and microvascular pressure might have substantial effects on airway function following exercise in the face of mediator-induced increased vascular permeability."[191]

- **Nutritional supplementation** :
  - Magnesium (oral, intravenous, inhaled/nebulized): In addition to serving as a cofactor for hundreds of biochemical enzymatic reactions including ATP production and utilization, magnesium is also necessary for muscle relaxation (implications for muscle cramps, myofascial trigger points, constipation, bronchoconstriction, hypertension, and cardiac contractility) and proper neuronal function (implications for depression, seizures, migraine, neurogenic inflammation, and NMDA receptor modulation). Given that dietary intake of magnesium is low in industrialized societies due to insufficient intake of vegetables and that urinary excretion of magnesium is increased with consumption of corticosteroids, caffeine, sugar, and alcohol, the consistent finding of laboratory-validated magnesium deficiency among a high percentage of outpatients and inpatients is to be expected. **For outpatient management and improved control of asthma and the associated anxiety and respiratory fatigue, magnesium should be a routine supplement to care given its low cost, safety, and collateral benefits.** In the acute setting, oral absorption and secondary tissue distribution would obviously be too slow to be of benefit; in the emergency setting, parenteral administration is required.

    - Clinical trial: Oral magnesium (-glycine) 300 mg/d: A double-blind randomized parallel placebo-controlled trial of children and adolescents with moderate persistent asthma (n=37; ages 7-19y) taking PRN fluticasone and salbutamol investigated the use of magnesium 300 mg/d administered

---

[186] Detoxification processes are reviewed in Chapter 4.7 of *Inflammation Mastery, 4th Edition* (2016) and later versions.
[187] Bedoya et al. Th17 Cells in Immunity and Autoimmunity. Clinical and Developmental Immunology 2013, Article 986789
[188] Mickleborough et al. Dietary chloride as a possible determinant of the severity of exercise-induced asthma. *Eur J Appl Physiol*. 2001 Sep;85(5):450-6
[189] Mickleborough TD. A nutritional approach to managing exercise-induced asthma. *Exerc Sport Sci Rev*. 2008 Jul;36(3):135-44
[190] Corbo et al. Wheeze and asthma in children: associations with body mass index, sports, television viewing, and diet. *Epidemiology*. 2008 Sep;19(5):747-55
[191] Mickleborough TD, Lindley MR, Ray S. Dietary salt, airway inflammation, and diffusion capacity in exercise-induced asthma. *Med Sci Sports Exerc*. 2005 Jun;37(6):904-14

orally in the form of Mg-glycine while the placebo group received only glycine. After 2 months of oral treatment, the Mg-group showed reduced bronchial reactivity as assessed by methacholine challenge, and skin responses to recognized antigens were also decreased. No changes were seen in forced vital capacity (FVC) or forced expiratory volume at first second (FEV1); however, the magnesium group experienced fewer asthma exacerbations and used less salbutamol compared to the placebo group.[192] Improvements in respiratory parameters seen following glycine supplementation in the "placebo" group attenuated more robust statistical differences between groups; glycine may exert therapeutic benefit in asthma ❶ by acting as an inhibitory neurotransmitter in the spinal cord and thereby modulating neurogenic inflammation, ❷ by acting as a precursor to glutathione, or ❸ or by downregulating NF-kappaB and inducible nitric oxide synthetase. In a separate study, Fogarty et al[193] researched the potential roles of amino acids in asthma and found that asthma severity was inversely related to serum glycine levels; thus glycine appears to attenuate asthma.

- <u>Clinical trial: Oral magnesium (citrate) 200-270 mg/d</u>: This randomized double-blind placebo-controlled prospective trial examined the use of magnesium (citrate) 200-290 mg/d for 12 weeks to find a statistically significant reduction in bronchodilator use, leading the authors to conclude, "Long-lasting Mg supplementation is clearly of benefit in mildly to moderately asthmatic children and is recommended as a concomitant drug in stable asthma."[194]

- <u>Clinical trial: Intravenous MgSO4</u>: In a randomized double-blind placebo-controlled study, patients with emergency acute asthma (n=135; ages 18-65y; FEV1 less than 75% predicted both before and after a single albuterol treatment) were treated with inhaled beta-agonists and intravenous (IV) steroids. Thirty minutes after entry, patients received either 2 g IV magnesium sulfate (MgSO4) or IV placebo. Overall, "Hospital admission rates were 35.3% for placebo-treated group and 25.4% for the magnesium-treated group." In patients with moderate asthma (FEV1 25-75%), hospital admission rates were 22.4% (11/49) for the placebo-treated group and 22.2% (10/25) for the magnesium-treated group; thus, no significant improvement in FEV1 was obtained in the moderate group for magnesium-treated patients. In patients with severe asthma (FEV1 < 25%), hospital admission rates were 78.6% (11/14) for the placebo-treated group and 33.3% (7/21) for the magnesium-treated group; also noted was a significant improvement in FEV1 at 120 min and 240 min among the severe asthma patients treated with magnesium. The authors concluded, "Intravenous MgSO4 decreased admission rate and improved FEV1 in patients with acute severe asthma but did not cause significant improvement in patients with moderate asthma."[195]

- <u>Systematic review: Intravenous MgSO4</u>: Review of the 7 of 27 clinical trials that met inclusion criteria lead the authors to conclude, "The use of intravenous magnesium sulfate reduces the rate of hospital admissions and improves pulmonary function in patients with severe acute asthma treated in the emergency department" while no consistent benefit was shown for patients with mild to moderate asthma.[196]

- <u>Systematic review: Intravenous MgSO4</u>: This systematic review of randomized controlled trials was limited to seven trials of acute asthma treated with intravenous magnesium sulfate versus placebo. Overall results showed that benefits of IV MgSO4 included fewer hospital admissions (especially among patients with severe asthma rather than moderate asthma) and nonsignificant improvements in peak expiratory flow rates (PEFR); FEV(1) generally improved by 10% predicted in patients with severe acute asthma. The authors concluded, "Current evidence does not clearly support routine use of intravenous magnesium sulfate in all patients with acute asthma presenting to the ED. However, **magnesium sulfate appears to be safe and beneficial for patients who present with severe acute asthma. Practice guidelines need to be changed to reflect these results.**"[197]

---

[192] Gontijo-Amaral C, et al. Oral magnesium supplementation in asthmatic children: a double-blind randomized placebo-controlled trial. *Eur J Clin Nutr* 2007;61:54–60
[193] Fogarty A, Broadfield E, Lewis S, Lawson N, Britton J. Amino acids and asthma: a case-control study. *Eur Respir J.* 2004 Apr;23(4):565-8
[194] Bede et al. Urinary magnesium excretion in asthmatic children receiving magnesium supplementation. *Magnes Res.* 2003 Dec;16(4):262-70
[195] Bloch H, Silverman R, Mancherje N, et al. Intravenous magnesium sulfate as an adjunct in the treatment of acute asthma. *Chest.* 1995 Jun;107(6):1576-81
[196] Rowe et al. Magnesium sulfate is effective for severe acute asthma treated in the emergency department. *West J Med.* 2000 Feb;172(2):96
[197] Rowe et al. Intravenous magnesium sulfate treatment for acute asthma in emergency department: a systematic review of the literature. *Ann Emerg Med.* 2000 Sep;36:181-90

- Systematic review: Inhaled/nebulized MgSO4: Six trials involving 296 patients were included in this review; four studies compared nebulized "MgSO4 + beta2-agonist" to "beta2-agonist alone", and two studies compared "MgSO4 alone" to "beta2-agonist alone." The authors concluded, "Nebulised inhaled magnesium sulfate in addition to beta2-agonist in the treatment of an acute asthma exacerbation, appears to have benefits with respect to improved pulmonary function in patients with severe asthma and there is a trend towards benefit in hospital admission."[198]

- Selenium: Selenium's (Se) prominent biological functions include ❶ antioxidant activity via its role as a cofactor for glutathione peroxidase, which regenerates reduced glutathione from glutathione disulfide, ❷ anti-inflammatory activity based on the elimination of hydroperoxide (arachidonic acid 5-hydroperoxide [5-hydroperoxyeicosatetraenoic acid, 5-HPETE] is the leukotriene-A4 precursor formed from arachidonate by 5-lipoxygenase) and downregulation of NF-kappaB, ❸ facilitating the conversion of T4 to T3, ❹ downregulation of estrogenic activity, and ❺ clinically significant antiviral effects. Routine supplemental dose is 200 mcg/d (most commonly either as selenomethionine or sodium selenite), while higher doses of approximately 800 mcg/d are also safe for long-term use but are generally reserved for acute treatment of viral infections or for the treatment of debilitating conditions such as chronic lymphedema. Given that asthmatic patients consistently show lower serum levels of selenium, reduced activity of glutathione peroxidase, and increased oxidative stress, routine supplementation with selenium is justified to reverse these negative biochemical parameters.
  - Clinical trial: Selenium 200 mcg/d for two years: A pilot study of 17 steroid-dependent asthmatics (n=17; ages 30-74y) used selenium 200 mcg/d for 24 months to effect reduced consumption of inhaled and systemic corticosteroids; clinical improvement correlated with the elevation of Se levels both in plasma and erythrocytes, and no adverse effects were noted.[199]
  - Clinical trial: Sodium selenite 100 mcg/d for 14 weeks: This double-blind clinical trial among asthmatic patients (n=24) effected significant increases in serum Se and platelet GSH-Px activity, significant reduction in the irreversible platelet aggregation induced by 5 mumol/l ADP, and significant clinical improvement in the Se-supplemented group as assessed by "assembled clinical evaluation" rather than reliance upon individual isolated parameters.[200] Sodium selenite tends to have a faster onset of action than other forms of selenium, and this—along with the use of the composite clinical evaluation rather than reliance on a single parameter—may explain the success of this clinical trial despite its low dose and short duration.
  - Clinical trial: Yeast-sourced selenium 100 mcg for 24 weeks: In a clinical trial with 197 patients, treatment with selenium 100 mcg/d for 6 months increased plasma selenium levels by 48% but provided no clinical benefit in adult asthmatic patients, the majority of whom were concomitantly treated with steroids[201]; faults with this trial include the subtherapeutic dosage (i.e., a daily dose of 800 mcg would have been more reasonable) and the fact that the selenium was sourced from yeast, to which some of the patients may have been allergic.

- Coenzyme Q10 (CoQ10): CoQ10 is an endogenous antioxidant, immunomodulator, and essential component of the mitochondrial electron transport chain; deficiency of CoQ10 may be a primary cause of or secondary effect of various disease states. Supplementation with CoQ10 has been shown in human clinical trials to ameliorate hypertension, congestive heart failure, migraine headaches, Parkinson's disease, and some cases of allergy, HIV disease, and cancer. The safety of chronic oral administration of CoQ10 in doses of 100-300 mg/d is exceedingly well established. Patients with corticosteroid-dependent asthma (n=56) were shown to have significantly lower concentrations of CoQ10 in plasma (0.34 micromol/l) and whole blood (0.33 micromol/l) compared with levels seen in healthy volunteers (0.52 and 0.50 micromol/l, respectively).[202]
  - Clinical trial: CoQ10, alpha-tocopherol, and ascorbic acid: In an open cross-over randomized clinical trial of patients with persistent mild-moderate asthma (n=41; ages 25-50y), daily administration of

[198] Blitz et al. Inhaled magnesium sulfate in the treatment of acute asthma. *Cochrane Database Syst Rev.* 2005 Oct 19;(4):CD003898

[199] Gazdik et al. Decreased consumption of corticosteroids after selenium supplementation in corticoid-dependent asthmatics. *Bratisl Lek Listy.* 2002;103(1):22-5 [Data from Medline abstract]

[200] Hasselmark L, Malmgren R, Zetterström O, Unge G. Selenium supplementation in intrinsic asthma. *Allergy.* 1993 Jan;48(1):30-6

[201] Shaheen et al. Randomised, double blind, placebo-controlled trial of selenium supplementation in adult asthma. *Thorax.* 2007 Jun;62(6):483-90

[202] Gazdík F, Gvozdjáková A, Nádvorníková R, et al. Decreased levels of coenzyme Q(10) in patients with bronchial asthma. *Allergy.* 2002 Sep;57(9):811-4

hydrosoluble CoQ10 120 mg, alpha-tocopherol 400 mg, and vitamin C 250 mg was shown to allow statistically and clinically significant reduction in the required dosage of corticosteroids; however, "Spirometric parameters did not change significantly during the study."[203]

- <u>Vitamin B6 (pyridoxine)</u>: A clear majority of young patients with asthma show endogenous defects in tryptophan metabolism, as evidenced by abnormal elevations in urinary kynurenic acid (KA) and xanthurenic acid (XA) acid following oral tryptophan administration.[204] This defect can be partially corrected by administration of high-dose pyridoxine, leading to clinical benefit.

  - <u>Clinical trial: Pyridoxine 100-200 mg/d in children</u>: The authors of this two-part study first showed that asthmatic patients had elevated urinary xanthurenic and kynurenic acid levels, which were reduced following supplementation 50-100 mg of pyridoxine; clinical benefit was seen in patients receiving pyridoxine 100 mg/d (not 50 mg/d). The second part of the study was a double-blind trial with 76 asthmatic children treated with pyridoxine 200 mg/d for five months; clinical benefits included significant improvement in asthma following pyridoxine therapy and reduction in dosage of bronchodilators and corticosteroids, leading the authors to conclude, "The data suggest that these children with severe bronchial asthma had a metabolic block in tryptophan metabolism, which was benefited by long-term treatment with large doses of pyridoxine."[205]

  - <u>Clinical trial: Pyridoxine 50 mg/d in adults</u>: Fifteen adult asthmatic patients showed lower levels of erythrocyte pyridoxal phosphate (PLP) compared to 16 control patients. Oral supplementation of seven asthmatics with pyridoxine 100 mg/d produced dramatic decreases in frequency and severity of wheezing and asthmatic attacks.[206]

- <u>Vitamin B-12 (hydroxocobalamin)</u>: Vitamin B-12 serves numerous physiologic and pharmacologic roles, and the complexities of absorption, transport, and metabolism subject this nutrient to manifold errors of metabolism as well as pervasive misunderstandings by clinicians. Relevant to the treatment of asthma, vitamin B-12 particularly its hydroxocobalamin form is a nitric oxide scavenger and sulfite chelator. A subset of asthmatic patients are intolerant to sulfite(s) and suffer exacerbations of asthma following sulfite consumption or increased endogenous production; vitamin B-12 can be used to chelate or "detoxify" sulfite and thus ameliorate asthma exacerbations. This clinical benefit to vitamin B-12 supplementation is not reliant upon the patient being vitamin B-12 deficient; thus documentation of low serum vitamin B-12 or elevated methylmalonic acid is unnecessary prior to treatment. Oral vitamin B-12 is exceptionally safe when given orally in doses of 2,000-6,000 mcg/d; fruit-tasting chewable tablets increase compliance among children and adults.

  - <u>Clinical trial: Cyanocobalamin 1,500 mcg prior to metabisulfite challenge</u>: In this small proof-of-principle study, five asthmatic children with metabisulfite intolerance confirmed by oral challenge testing were pretreated with 1.5 mg of oral cyanocobalamin prior to sulfite rechallenge. Following vitamin B-12 administration, four of the five patients were protected from metabisulfite-induced bronchospasm.[207]

- <u>Bioflavonoids</u>: As previously mentioned in the section on diet, increased intake of fruits and vegetables reduces risk and severity of asthma; certainly this occurs by many mechanisms, including ❶ increased intake of vitamin C, ❷ increased intake of magnesium, ❸ systemic alkalinization which promotes renal retention of magnesium and urinary excretion of xenobiotics, ❹ increased intake of phytonutrients and bioflavonoids, most of which have biologically relevant antioxidant and anti-inflammatory action. Given that most botanicals have an alkalinizing effect due to the virtual lack of sodium chloride and the high amounts of potassium, magnesium, and citrate (which is converted to bicarbonate in the body), and given that plants are rich sources of bioflavonoids which as a group have antioxidant and anti-inflammatory properties and respective clinical benefits, clinicians and patients can choose from a wide range of plant-based dietary patterns and plant-derived nutritional supplements. Many standardized concentrated

[203] Gvozdjáková et al. Coenzyme Q10 supplementation reduces corticosteroids dosage in patients with bronchial asthma. *Biofactors*. 2005;25(1-4):235-40

[204] Collipp PJ, Chen SY, Sharma RK, Balachandar V, Maddaiah VT. Tryptophane metabolism in bronchial asthma. *Ann Allergy*. 1975 Sep;35(3):153-8

[205] Collipp PJ, Goldzier S III, Weiss N, et al. Pyridoxine treatment of childhood bronchial asthma. *Ann Allergy* 1975;35:93–7

[206] Reynolds RD, Natta CL. Depressed plasma pyridoxal phosphate concentrations in adult asthmatics. *Am J Clin Nutr* 1985;41:684–8

[207] Añíbarro B, Caballero T, García-Ara C, et al. Asthma with sulfite intolerance in children: a blocking study with cyanocobalamin. *J Allergy Clin Immunol*. 1992 Jul;90:103-9

bioflavonoid products are commercially available as nutritional supplements, and many of the available and popular botanical medicines (e.g., *Ginkgo biloba*) and medical foods (e.g., green tea, honey) owe at least part of their clinical benefit to their flavonoid content. Among the many clinically utilized bioflavonoid products, Pycnogenol is a proprietary mixture of water-soluble bioflavonoids extracted from French maritime pine; the main constituents of

> **Clinical Pearl: Crataegus tincture for asthma**
>
> "Administration of a tincture of solid extract preparation of *Crataegus* spp to patients with asthma has proven remarkably effective in the clinical setting. ... While *Crataegus* is a powerful tool in the treatment of asthma, it should not be used alone if complete healing is expected to take place. Basic naturopathic therapies that address nutritional needs, allergies, adrenal function, and immune and liver function should always be considered."
>
> Frances D. Crataegus for asthma: case studies.
> *Journal of Naturopathic Medicine* 1998: 8; 20-24

Pycnogenol are phenolic compounds including the monomers catechin, epicatechin, and taxifolin and condensed flavonoids such as procyanidins and proanthocyanidins.

- Clinical trial: Pycnogenol 1 mg/lb/d in two divided doses: A randomized placebo-controlled double-blind trial among patients with mild-to-moderate asthma (n=60; age 6-18y) was conducted for 3 months found that patients receiving Pycnogenol 1 mg/lb/d in two divided doses had significant improvement in pulmonary functions, reductions in asthma symptoms, reduction or discontinuation of rescue inhalers, and reduction of urinary leukotrienes.[208]
- Clinical experience with *Crataegus* tincture or solid extract in the treatment of asthma: "Administration of a tincture of solid extract preparation of *Crataegus spp* to patients with asthma has proven remarkably effective in the clinical setting. ... While Crataegus is a powerful tool in the treatment of asthma, it should not be used alone if complete healing is expected to take place. Basic naturopathic therapies that address nutritional needs, allergies, adrenal function, and immune and liver function should always be considered."[209]

- "Vitamin E": "Vitamin E" intake has shown a protective inverse association with asthma in several epidemiologic studies. Food-sourced "vitamin E" would be expected to provide benefits superior to those obtained from the use of supplemental "vitamin E" when the later contains synthetic or isolated tocopherol isomers, namely DL-tocopherol or D-alpha-tocopherol, respectively, both of which may serve to promote inflammation and/or block intestinal absorption of the more potent anti-inflammatory gamma-tocopherol. Thus, the finding that "Dietary supplementation with vitamin E adds no benefit to current standard treatment in adults with mild to moderate asthma" by Pearson et al[210] in 2007 was not surprising given their use of D-alpha-tocopherol 500 mg (746 IU) per day; had the researchers used mixed tocopherols with a high concentration of gamma-tocopherol, their patients may have benefited.
- Vitamin C: Asthma patients may show a relative insufficiency of vitamin C as measured by serum vitamin C levels. Higher intakes of vitamin C protect against the development and progression of asthma.
  - Randomized, placebo controlled double-blind crossover trial: Ascorbic acid supplementation attenuates exercise-induced bronchoconstriction in patients with asthma: Eight subjects with exercise-induced bronchoconstriction (EIB) entered the study on their usual diet and were placed on either 2 weeks of ascorbic acid supplementation (1500 mg/day) or placebo, followed by a 1-week washout period, before crossing over to the non-supplemented group. "Results: The ascorbic acid diet significantly reduced (p < 0.05) the maximum fall in post-exercise FEV1 (-6.4 +/- 2.4%) compared to usual (-14.3 +/- 1.6%) and placebo diet (-12.9 +/- 2.4%). Asthma symptoms scores significantly improved (p<0.05) on the ascorbic acid diet compared to the placebo and usual diet. Post-exercise FENO, LTC4-E4 and 9alpha, 11beta-PGF2 concentration was significantly lower (p<0.05) on the ascorbic acid diet compared to the placebo and usual diet. CONCLUSION: Ascorbic acid supplementation provides a protective effect against exercise-induced airway narrowing in asthmatic subjects."[211]
  - Placebo-controlled clinical trial: Ascorbic acid lowers histamine and improves neutrophil chemotaxis: Histamine is immunosuppressive, pro-inflammatory, and capable of inducing

[208] Lau BH, Riesen SK, Truong KP, et al. Pycnogenol as an adjunct in the management of childhood asthma. *J Asthma* 2004;41:825–32
[209] Frances D. Crataegus for asthma: case studies. *Journal of Naturopathic Medicine* 1998: 8; 20-24
[210] Pearson PJ, Lewis SA, Britton J, Fogarty A. Vitamin E supplements in asthma: a parallel group randomised placebo controlled trial. *Thorax.* 2004 Aug;59(8):652-6
[211] Tecklenburg et al. Ascorbic acid supplementation attenuates exercise-induced bronchoconstriction in patients with asthma. *Respir Med.* 2007 Aug;101(8):1770-8

bronchoconstriction. Ten subjects ingested a placebo during weeks 1, 2, 5 and 6, and ==2 g/day of vitamin C== [VC] during weeks 3 and 4. "Plasma ascorbate rose significantly following VC administration compared to baseline and withdrawal values. Neutrophil chemotaxis rose 19% (NS) during VC administration, and fell 30% after VC withdrawal, but these changes were not correlated to plasma ascorbate levels. Chemotaxis was inversely correlated to blood histamine (r = -0.32, p = 0.045), and, compared to baseline and withdrawal values, ==histamine levels were depressed 38% following VC supplementation.== … These data indicate that VC may indirectly enhance chemotaxis by detoxifying histamine in vivo."[212]

- Iodine, iodide: Iodine is a nonmetal trace element (I_2) which is called iodide (I^{-1}) in the ionic form; clinicians can recall this difference in nomenclature by remembering that the elemental form of ends with "N" as in *iodine* and *natural*, whereas the ionic form in which the iodine atoms have been separated has a "D" as in *iodide* and *divided*. Both iodine and iodide can be consumed by humans, and some experts state that optimal intake of this nutrient should include both the diatomic iodine and the ionic iodide; because of this, and because of the interconversion between the diatomic and ionic forms the conjugate "iodine-iodide" will be used here while "iodide" will be used when this form is specifically cited, as it tends to be the more commonly discussed and biologically active form of this nutrient and element. Iodide has a wide range of biologic effects beyond functioning as a requisite component of thyroxine and triiodothyronine; iodide affects gene expression, hormone receptor activity, hormone metabolism, mucus viscosity, microbial survival (directly through microbicidal action and indirectly through enhanced antimicrobial effectiveness of the phagocytic respiratory burst), and oxidant-antioxidant balance. Iodide can function as an antioxidant because it is a reducing agent that can neutralize reactive oxygen species such as hydrogen peroxide via the formation of iodo-compounds. The antioxidant biochemical mechanism of iodides[213] is probably one of the most ancient mechanisms of defense from poisonous reactive oxygen species, used by blue-green algae for more than three billion years: (Iodo-Compounds* include iodo-tyrosine/histidine/lipids/carbons.)

$$2\ I^- + Peroxidase + H_2O_2 + Tyro/Hist/Lipid/Carbons \rightarrow Iodo\text{-}Compounds^* + H_2O + 2\ e^- \text{ (antioxidants)}$$

An increasing number of clinicians are using combination iodine-iodide products either in liquid or tablet form to provide approximately 12 mg/d—this is consistent with the average daily intake of iodine-iodide countries such as Japan with a high intake of seafood. Adverse effects for which to monitor include biochemical thyroid dysfunction, goiter, and acneiform skin lesions. Clinical data on the use of iodine/iodide against asthma is limited, even though it was a popular treatment among clinicians prior to onslaught of new drugs and the powerful marketing campaigns that accompanied them. Formulations of iodine/iodide are natural, nonpatentable, and of comparatively low profit for manufacturers compared to patented drugs and delivery systems.

- Letter and report of clinical experience: Iodides in bronchial asthma (*J Allergy Clin Immunol* 1981 Jun[214]): Whether administered orally or intravenously, "the iodides appeared in the saliva in about 5 to 10 minutes and in the bronchial secretions within 15 to 30 minutes. The increased salivation by these patients seemed to us to increase the probability that the iodide in adequate amounts can be effective expectorants because they are eliminated by the bronchial mucosa. Their usefulness for this purpose can be attested to by many physicians including myself who have used this drug in the treatment of asthma for many years."

- Controlled study of iodotherapy for childhood asthma (*J Allergy* 1966 Sep[215]): Patients received KI—potassium iodide—in doses of "900 and 300 mg daily." "…in the population as a whole, asthmatic symptoms were improved by KI particularly at the high dose level." The authors estimate that 64% of patients benefited from iodide supplementation.

- **Hormonal modulation**: The "Orthoendocrinology" protocol detailed in Chapter 4.6 can be reasonably employed in any patient with chronic inflammatory disease—this includes allergy and autoimmunity. In

---

[212] Johnston CS, Martin LJ, Cai X. Antihistamine effect of supplemental ascorbic acid and neutrophil chemotaxis. *J Am Coll Nutr* 1992 Apr;11(2):172-6

[213] wikipedia.org/wiki/Iodide Accessed June 29, 2009

[214] Tuft L. Iodides in bronchial asthma. *J Allergy Clin Immunol*. 1981 Jun;67(6):497

[215] Falliers CJ, McCann WP, Chai H, Ellis EF, Yazdi N. Controlled study of iodotherapy for childhood asthma. *J Allergy*. 1966 Sep;38(3):183-92

summary, serum measurement of prolactin, DHEA, cortisol, testosterone (free and total), and estradiol is performed and any abnormalities are corrected. With specific regard to allergy and asthma, DHEA has clearly received the most attention and literature support as a safe and effective intervention. Women with menstrual exacerbations of asthma may benefit from administration of progesterone either orally, by injection, or over-the-counter in transdermal preparations; progesterone has immune-modulating effects, is a precursor to cortisol, and has anti-estrogen benefits.

- ▪ Low serum dehydroepiandrosterone sulfate concentration is an indicator of adrenocortical suppression in asthmatic children treated with inhaled steroids: "In conclusion, inhaled steroid treatment suppresses dehydroepiandrosterone sulfate production in a dose-dependent manner. Monitoring of serum dehydroepiandrosterone sulfate concentrations can be used as a practical method to follow adrenocortical function and to detect its suppression during inhaled steroid treatment in children."[216] One of the important practical implications of this study is that it supports the use of serum DHEA-sulfate testing as a means for monitoring adrenal function. The ideal test for measuring adrenal reserve is the assay of serum cortisol before and after an injection of ACTH; however this test requires ACTH prescription (not available to all clinicians), ACTH injection (ACTH is often difficult to procure, and injections are poorly tolerated by many patients, especially children), and two phlebotomies for serum cortisol measurement. The simple measurement of serum DHEA-sulfate may suffice for an expedient quantification of adrenal function.
- ▪ Effects of dehydroepiandrosterone on Th2 cytokine production in peripheral blood mononuclear cells from asthmatics: "CONCLUSIONS: DHEA suppressed both Th1 and Th2 responses, with a Th1 bias, and the degree of suppression was associated with the severity of AHR [airway hyperresponsiveness] or atopy. Therefore, DHEA may be a useful therapy for asthma."[217]
- ▪ Clinical experience with low-dose DHEA in asthmatics: "I have seen two female patients with long-standing asthma who had clinical improvement after receiving 10 mg/day of DHEA. In one of these patients, chronic nasal polyps also disappeared, much to the surprise of her otolaryngologist."[218]
- ▪ Case reports: Severe premenstrual asthma alleviated with intramuscular progesterone: "Three patients with severe premenstrual exacerbations of asthma are reported. None had responded to conventional treatment, including high-dose corticosteroids. In all cases there was a striking fall premenstrually in peak flow rate. The addition of intramuscular progesterone (100 mg daily in two cases and 600 mg twice a week in one) to the regimen eliminated the premenstrual dips in peak flow, and daily doses of prednisolone were reduced in the three patients."[219]

- **Physical medicine and manipulation**: Essentially all clinical trials of manipulative therapy have shown benefit in subjective and/or objective markers of respiration. The two main problems seen in this research are ❶ the near-impossibility of having an adequate control group, and ❷ the political manipulation of the conclusions by medical journals that have a strong history of bias against natural and non-drug and non-surgical treatments. With regard to the former of these two problems, for obvious reasons clinicians should appreciate the difficulty in conducting a placebo-controlled study with manipulation, particularly if that "placebo" involves physical contact or any soft-tissue manipulation.

  - ▪ Review: Research pitfalls and manual medicine diversity versus the emerging medical paradigm (*J Am Osteopath Assoc*. 2001 Aug[220]): "Recent studies published in leading medical journals have concluded that chiropractic treatment is not particularly helpful for relieving asthma and migraine symptoms because even though study participants showed notable improvement in symptoms, those subjects who received sham manual medicine treatments also showed improvement. Yet the sham treatment received by control groups in these studies is reminiscent in many ways of traditional osteopathic manipulation. This seems to represent not only a failure to recognize the value of many manual medicine techniques but also an ignorance of the broad spectrum of manual medicine techniques used by various practitioners, from osteopathic physicians to chiropractors to physical therapists. Such blind spots compromise research

[216] Kannisto S, Korppi M, Remes K, Voutilainen R. Serum dehydroepiandrosterone sulfate concentration as an indicator of adrenocortical suppression in asthmatic children treated with inhaled steroids. *J Clin Endocrinol Metab*. 2001 Oct;86(10):4908-12

[217] Choi et al. Effects of dehydroepiandrosterone on Th2 cytokine production in peripheral blood mononuclear cells from asthmatics. *Korean J Intern Med*. 2008 Dec;23(4):176-81

[218] Gaby AR. Dehydroepiandrosterone: Biological Effects and Clinical Significance. *Alt Med Rev* 1996;1(2):60-69

[219] Beynon HL, Garbett ND, Barnes PJ. Severe premenstrual exacerbations of asthma: effect of intramuscular progesterone. *Lancet*. 1988 Aug 13;2(8607):370-2

[220] Mein EA, et al. Manual medicine diversity: research pitfalls and the emerging medical paradigm. *J Am Osteopath Assoc*. 2001 Aug;101(8):441-4

methodology with regard to manual medicine studies, which could, in turn, diminish the role of manual medicine in clinical practice."

- <u>Cochrane review: Manual therapy for asthma</u> (<u>*Cochrane Database Syst Rev* 2005 Apr</u>[221]): "AUTHORS' CONCLUSIONS: There is insufficient evidence to support the use of manual therapies for patients with asthma. There is a need to conduct adequately-sized RCTs that examine the effects of manual therapies on clinically relevant outcomes. Future trials should maintain observer blinding for outcome assessments, and report on the costs of care and adverse events. Currently, there is insufficient evidence to support or refute the use of manual therapy for patients with asthma."

- <u>Randomized controlled trial: Effects of osteopathic manipulative</u> <u>treatment (OMT) on pediatric patients with asthma</u> (<u>*J Am Osteopath Assoc* 2005 Jan</u>[222]): "The authors conducted a randomized controlled trial attempting to demonstrate the therapeutic relevance of OMT in the pediatric asthma population. With a confidence level of 95%, results for the OMT group showed a statistically significant improvement of 7 L per minute to 9 L per minute for peak expiratory flow rates. These results suggest that OMT has a therapeutic effect among this patient population."

> **An osteopathic approach to asthma**
>
> "Five areas involving asthma management are reviewed and involve a failure to do the following:
> 1. Identify disease instability and progression;
> 2. Adopt an optimal pharmacologic treatment plan;
> 3. Identify and help the patient avoid environmental triggers;
> 4. Evaluate and treat certain disruptive psychodynamic issues; and
> 5. Use essential non-pharmacologic modes of therapy such as osteopathic manipulation, nutritional considerations, physical training, and controlled breathing techniques that may help to favorably modify the asthma disease process."
>
> Rowane et al. An osteopathic approach to asthma. *J Am Osteopath Assoc.* 1999 May

- <u>Clinical trial: Quantifiable effects of osteopathic manipulative techniques on patients with chronic asthma</u> (<u>*J Am Osteopath Assoc* 2002 Jul</u>[223]): "Measurements of both upper thoracic and lower thoracic forced respiratory excursion statistically increased after osteopathic manipulative procedures compared with sham procedures. Changes in peak expiratory flow rates and asthma symptoms were not statistically significant."

- <u>Spinal manipulative therapy (SMT) is not simply a physical intervention</u> (<u>*J Manipulative Physiol Ther* 2001 Jul</u>[224]): "CONCLUSION: After 3 months of combining chiropractic SMT with optimal medical management for pediatric asthma, the children rated their quality of life substantially higher and their asthma severity substantially lower. These improvements were maintained at the 1-year follow-up assessment. There were no important changes in lung function or hyperresponsiveness at any time. The observed improvements are unlikely as a result of the specific effects of chiropractic SMT alone, but other aspects of the clinical encounter that should not be dismissed readily."

- <u>*New England Journal of Medicine* contradicts positive results with negative conclusions in study of chiropractic manipulation in the treatment of asthma</u> (<u>*N Engl J Med* 1998 Oct</u>[225]): "RESULTS: Eighty children (38 in the active-treatment group and 42 in the simulated-treatment group) had outcome data that could be evaluated. There were small increases (7 to 12 liters per minute) in peak expiratory flow in the morning and the evening in both treatment groups, with no significant differences between the groups in the degree of change from base line (morning peak expiratory flow, P=0.49 at two months and P=0.82 at four months). Symptoms of asthma and use of 3-agonists decreased and the quality of life increased in both groups, with no significant differences between the groups. There were no significant changes in spirometric measurements or airway responsiveness. CONCLUSIONS: In children with mild or moderate asthma, the addition of chiropractic spinal manipulation to usual medical care provided no benefit."

- <u>An osteopathic approach to asthma</u> (<u>*J Am Osteopath Assoc* 1999 May</u>[226]): "Five areas involving asthma management are reviewed and involve a failure to do the following: (1) identify disease instability and progression; (2) adopt an optimal pharmacologic treatment plan; (3) identify and help the patient avoid

[221] Hondras MA, Linde K, Jones AP. Manual therapy for asthma. *Cochrane Database Syst Rev.* 2005 Apr 18;(2):CD001002
[222] Guiney PA, et al. Effects of osteopathic manipulative treatment on pediatric patients with asthma: a randomized controlled trial. *J Am Osteopath Assoc.* 2005 Jan;105(1):7-12
[223] Bockenhauer et al. Quantifiable effects of osteopathic manipulative techniques on patients with chronic asthma. *J Am Osteopath Assoc.* 2002 Jul;102(7):371-5
[224] Bronfort G, et al. Chronic pediatric asthma and chiropractic spinal manipulation. *J Manipulative Physiol Ther.* 2001 Jul-Aug;24(6):369-77
[225] Balon J, et al. A comparison of active and simulated chiropractic manipulation as adjunctive treatment for childhood asthma. *N Engl J Med.* 1998 Oct 8;339(15):1013-20
[226] Rowane WA, Rowane MP. An osteopathic approach to asthma. *J Am Osteopath Assoc.* 1999 May;99(5):259-64

environmental triggers; (4) evaluate and treat certain disruptive psychodynamic issues; and (5) use essential non-pharmacologic modes of therapy such as osteopathic manipulation, nutritional considerations, physical training, and controlled breathing techniques that may help to favorably modify the asthma disease process."

- Randomized clinical trial: Chronic asthma and chiropractic spinal manipulation (*Clin Exp Allergy* 1995 Jan[227]): "Using the cross-over analysis, no clinically important or statistically significant differences were found between the active and sham chiropractic interventions on any of the main or secondary outcome measures. Objective lung function did not change during the study, but over the course of the study, non-specific bronchial hyperreactivity (n-BR) improved by 36% (P = 0.01) and patient-rated asthma severity decreased by 34% (P = 0.0002) compared with the baseline values."

- **Environmental interventions**: Beyond dietary allergen avoidance, the patient's residential, occupational, and recreational environments can be remediated to effect a reduction in immunogen exposure; effective reduction in immunogen exposure leads to pathologic and clinical improvements in asthma patients. Attention to the patient's sleeping area is particularly important and commonly overlooked; this is an area where patients spend 8-10 hours each night, and allergen exposure here can have effects throughout the day.
  - Use allergen/pollen-reducing air filters; change them on a regular basis each 1-2 months.
  - Replace old pillows and mattress with nonallergenic varieties, or have the older pillows/mattress covered with an allergen barrier, such as a vinyl enclosure.
  - Remediate or ventilate any mold-prone areas in the bathroom, kitchen, basement, attic, walls, or utility area. Use portable HEPA filtration machines in rooms where the patient spends prolonged periods of time.
  - Strongly consider removing/replacing the old carpet and pad, which might be permeated with allergens, antigens, dust mites, animal dander, etc. Hardwood, cement, laminate, or bamboo floors are much easier to keep clean of allergens/antigens than is carpet.
  - Clothes and linens can be machine washed with a detergent solution containing eucalyptus oil to eliminate dust mites. The combination of 1) hot water, 2) detergent, and 3) eucalyptus oil is an effective and method to kill dust mites and remove additional allergens. As validated by research published in *Journal of Allergy and Clinical Immunology*[228], this is an effective technique for killing and eliminating dust mites from clothing and bed sheets. Suitable detergents include "Bi-O-Klean Hand Dishwashing Liquid" or "Kit liquid dishwashing detergent concentrate" since they meet the criteria for the selection of a detergent for this purpose. 1) When mixed, the oil-detergent mixture should dissolve to form a clear homogenous solution, and 2) five mL (1 teaspoon) of the mixture stirred with 200 mL (6 oz.) of water should form a "milky, opaque solution that is stable (does not "break oil") for at least 10 minutes." Eucalyptus oil should not be applied to the skin or taken internally.
  - Use of a dehumidifier and adequate moisture ventilation can be important for homes/rooms that accumulate moisture. The steam from bathing and cooking areas should be vented outdoors so that moisture does not accumulate inside the living area. Moisture is necessary for dust mites to live and to create allergens; if the air is very moist then the allergy-producing activities of the dust mites are stimulated. Conversely, by reducing the humidity in the air, we are able to impair the dust mites and thus reduce the amount of dust mite feces—this is an important allergen for many asthmatics. In some instances, reducing the amount of moisture in the air by use of an electric dehumidifier may be necessary to help reduce the amount of both dust allergen and mold in a home.

- **Avoidance of aspirin and inhibitors of cyclooxygenase**: Inhibition of cyclooxygenase shunts free arachidonate into leukotriene formation via 5-lipoxygenase, thereby exacerbating the leukotriene-mediated inflammation of asthma.

- **Treatment of chronic sinusitis—See Chapter 4.2 subsection on sinorespiratory dysbiosis**: Chronic sinusitis exacerbates asthma by direct and indirect mechanism; the direct mechanism is the irritation of the respiratory pathway via post-nasal drip of inflammatory and antigenic secretions, while the indirect mechanism is the contribution to systemic inflammation. Treatment of chronic sinusitis effectively alleviates asthma for many patients; not surprisingly, most research studies have used pharmaceutical antibacterial drugs for this purpose.

---

[227] Nielsen et al. Chronic asthma and chiropractic spinal manipulation: a randomized clinical trial. *Clin Exp Allergy.* 1995 Jan;25(1):80-8
[228] Tovey ER, McDonald LG. A simple washing procedure with eucalyptus oil for controlling house dust mites and their allergens in clothing and bedding. *J Allergy Clin Immunol.* 1997 Oct;100(4):464-6

Clinically, the use of once-twice daily nasal lavage is very effective for the treatment of chronic sinusitis; the solution is 1 cup warm *sterile* water salinated with 0.5-1 teaspoon sodium chloride with 0.5 teaspoon baking soda administered via the nostrils by way of a bulb syringe or neti pot. Patient selection is relevant to prevent choking or aspiration; the procedure is awkward at first but becomes much more acceptable with practice. Nasal-sinus lavage is reviewed in Chapter 4 in Section 2, in the subsection on sinorespiratory dysbiosis.

- Clinical trial: Concomitant chronic sinusitis treatment in children with mild asthma: the effect on bronchial hyperresponsiveness (*Chest* 2003 Mar[229]): Among 61 children with mild asthma and allergic rhinitis, 41 were found to have chronic bacterial sinusitis, too—this finding stresses the importance of doctors' continual searching for and refining the details of their patient assessment. The treatment group received amoxicillin-clavulanate for 6 weeks and then with nasal saline solution irrigation for 6 weeks. Clinical improvement included the following: "After aggressive treatment for sinusitis, it was found that the provocative concentration of methacholine causing a 20% fall in FEV(1) of children with mild asthma and sinusitis was significantly higher after treatment. CONCLUSION: The results suggest that every asthmatic patient needs to [be] carefully evaluate[d] to determine whether the patient has concomitant sinusitis. Respiratory infections that meet criteria for sinusitis, even if they do not exacerbate asthma, should be treated. It is suggested that sinusitis should always be kept in mind as a possible inducible factor for BHR [bronchial hyperresponsiveness], and that aggressive treatment of chronic sinusitis is indicated when dealing with an asthmatic patient who shows an unpredictable response to appropriate treatment. Moreover, the findings of this study provide more evidence for an association between sinusitis and asthma with respect to BHR."

- Clinical trial: Improvement of clinical and immunopathologic parameters in asthmatic children treated for concomitant chronic rhinosinusitis (*Ann Allergy Asthma Immunol* 1997 Jul[230]): Eighteen children with moderate asthma (ages 5-12y) who were poorly controlled by high doses of inhaled corticosteroids and who also had chronic rhinosinusitis were treated with a combination of amoxicillin and clavulanate (20 mg/kg twice daily) and fluticasone propionate aqueous nasal spray (100 microg/d) for 14 days. A short course of oral corticosteroids was also prescribed (deflazacort, 1 mg/kg daily for 2 days, 0.5 mg/kg daily for 4 days, and 0.25 mg/kg daily for 4 days). "RESULTS: A negative endoscopy result was demonstrated in 15 children after treatment. Symptoms and respiratory function significantly improved after treatment and 1 month later; 8 children had intermittent asthma and 10 had mild asthma. A significant reduction of inflammatory cell numbers was detected in all asthmatic children. Interleukin 4 levels significantly decreased (P < 0.001), whereas interferon-y levels increased (P < 0.001)—[This latter finding indicates a shift from Th-2 to a Th-1 pattern of inflammation.]. CONCLUSION: Treatment of chronic rhinosinusitis is able to improve symptoms and respiratory function in asthmatic children, reducing inflammatory cells and reversing the cytokine pattern from a Th2 toward a Th1 profile."

- Clinical trial: Improvement of bronchial hyperresponsiveness in asthmatic children treated for concomitant sinusitis (*Ann Allergy Asthma Immunol* 1997 Jul[231]): This open label, randomized trial in forty-six atopic and 20 normal children used 30 days of treatment with nasal saline, sulfamethoxazole-trimethoprim, antihistamine/decongestant, and five days of prednisone. "RESULTS: The only patients with increase in methacholine PC20 were patients with rhinitis and asthma with opacified maxillary sinuses at entry and who at 30 days had normal sinus radiographs (P < .05). CONCLUSION: In this study, children with allergic rhinitis and sinusitis with asthma improved their bronchial hyperresponsiveness to methacholine and decreased their symptoms with appropriate response of their sinuses to clinical therapy." In sum, this study showed that asthmatic patients with occult sinusitis achieved clinical benefit—improved lung function—following resolution of the sinusitis with the 30-day use of nasal saline, oral antibiotics, antihistamine/decongestant, and five days of prednisone.

- **Psychosocial interventions**: Stress reduction, relationship optimization, resolution of past hurts and dysfunctional relationships should be included in any *truly* holistic healthcare plan for any condition, and of course this includes asthma.

---

[229] Tsao et al. Concomitant chronic sinusitis treatment in children with mild asthma: the effect on bronchial hyperresponsiveness. *Chest*. 2003 Mar;123(3):757-64

[230] Tosca et al. Improvement of clinical and immunopathologic parameters in asthmatic children treated for concomitant chronic rhinosinusitis. *Ann Allergy Asthma Immunol*. 2003 Jul;91(1):71-8

[231] Oliveira et al. Improvement of bronchial hyperresponsiveness in asthmatic children treated for concomitant sinusitis. *Ann Allergy Asthma Immunol*. 1997 Jul;79(1):70-4

- Clinical trial—Humorous movie (*Physiol Behav* 2004 Jun[232]): In this cross-over placebo-controlled trial of asthmatic patients (asthma n=35; control n=35) who were sensitive to either house dust mite (n=20) or epigallocatechin gallate (EGCg) (n=15), reduced bronchial responsiveness was noted among the asthmatic patients but not the control patients following watching a humorous movie. The author concluded, "Viewing a humorous film significantly reduced bronchial responsiveness to methacholine or EGCg, while viewing a nonhumorous film failed to do so in [asthma] patients…. These findings indicate that viewing a humorous film may be useful in the treatment and study of BA [bronchial asthma]." This study was published in 2004; the humorous film used was "Modern Times" featuring Charlie Chaplin released in 1936.
- Systematic review of psychological interventions for children with asthma (*Pediatr Pulmonol* 2007 Feb[233]): "Twelve studies, involving 588 children, were included in the review; however, study quality was poor and sample sizes were frequently small. A meta-analysis was performed on two studies, examining the effects of relaxation therapy on PEFR which favored the treatment group (SD 0.82, CI 0.41-1.24). … This review was unable to draw firm conclusions for the role of psychological interventions for children with asthma. … The absence of an adequate evidence base is demonstrated, highlighting the need for well-conducted RCTs in this area."

---

[232] Kimata H. Effect of viewing a humorous vs. nonhumorous film on bronchial responsiveness in patients with bronchial asthma. *Physiol Behav*. 2004;81(4):681-4
[233] Yorke et al. A systematic review of psychological interventions for children with asthma. *Pediatr Pulmonol*. 2007 Feb;42(2):114-24

Rheumatoid Arthritis, RA

Introduction:

Rheumatoid arthritis (RA) is one of the most common and "most classic" systemic autoimmune diseases. Despite its name, RA affects much more than the musculoskeletal system: rheumatoid lung, rheumatoid kidney disease, and other systemic, vasculitic, and (sub)cutaneous complications are not uncommon. Readers should begin to recognize the "patterns of inflammation" that result in distinct diagnostic labels are simply "variations on a theme" based on a finite number of identifiable and modifiable factors, which are largely amenable to nonpharmacologic interventions.

Rheumatoid arthritis and psoriasis are very similar conditions—different patterns of inflammation—and these conditions and their respective assessments and treatments should be viewed as prototypical for other conditions; as such, and especially considering that these conditions are very common in clinical practice, a reasonable assumption will be made that readers will have studied these sections so that some facts and concepts will not have to be unnecessarily repeated throughout the book for each condition that follows a similar pattern of pathogenesis and resolution.

Description/pathophysiology:

- **Description in a nutshell:** RA is a relatively common, persistent, symmetric, destructive, systemic inflammatory "autoimmune" disease chiefly characterized by peripheral arthritis but which may also affect the proximal joints (e.g., hips and shoulders), the axial skeleton (e.g., spine—notably the atlantoaxial joint—as well as the sacroiliac joints), and internal organs (e.g., "rheumatoid lung") and vascular system (e.g., rheumatoid vasculitis).

- **Basic pathology:** A pathogenic hallmark of the disease is immune complex formation and intra-articular deposition with resultant release of cytokines and other pro-inflammatory mediators. Immune complexes are important instigators of rheumatoid arthritis and vasculitis, and rheumatoid factor (RF) antibodies are important contributors to these immune complexes.[1,2] The chronic/sustained inflammation leads to synovial thickening, villous hypertrophy (pannus formation), and intraarticular colonization with activated lymphocytes and plasma cells. The localized immunocytes cause inflammation and tissue destruction via elaboration of matrix metalloproteinases (including collagenases), prostaglandins, and cytokines such as IL-1.

- **Prevalence:** Affects 0.8-1% of all populations: considered the second most common rheumatic diagnosis[3] after "osteoarthritis", many cases of which are actually genetic hemochromatosis, one of the most common hereditary conditions in humans (heterozygote frequency: 1:7; homozygote frequency 1:200-250).

  - **Musculoskeletal disorders and iron overload disease** (*Arthritis Rheum* 1996 Oct[4]—full text provided within this textbook): "Arthropathy affects up to 80% of iron-overloaded patients and is often the only manifestation of the disease. ... Thus, since iron overload affects such a large portion of the population and arthropathy is a common manifestation of this disorder, patients with musculoskeletal symptoms should be screened for iron overload."

- **Introduction to standard allopathic medical perspective and treatment:** From the allopathic perspective, RA is seen as a chronic "idiopathic" inflammatory disorder primarily affecting the peripheral joints but also affecting the axial skeleton and internal organs; it is generally treated with NSAIDs and other "anti-inflammatory" and immunosuppressive drugs, which are palliative and have no chance of providing cure. The standard sequential protocol is as follows: NAIDs and acetaminophen, prednisone, methotrexate, (perhaps sulfasalazine and hydroxychloroquine), then—ever more commonly prescribed—the "biologics", which may be followed by newer experimental and immunoparalytic drugs; this routine protocol has value in the acute suppression of inflammation, but it is notoriously expensive, wrought with adverse effects, and ineffective for the authentic treatment of rheumatoid arthritis, as noted in the landmark 2012 article cited here:

  - **Sustained rheumatoid arthritis remission is uncommon in *medical* practice** (*Arthritis Res Ther* 2012 Mar[5]): "This study shows that in clinical practice, a minority of RA patients are in sustained remission. ... Other studies have described sustained remission in daily practice as uncommon, being reached by only

---

[1] Beers MH, Berkow R (eds). *Merck Manual. 17th Edition*. Whitehouse Station; Merck Research Laboratories: 1999, page 416

[2] Jonsson T, Valdimarsson H. What about IgA rheumatoid factor in rheumatoid arthritis? *Ann Rheum Dis*. 1998 Jan;57(1):63-4 ard.bmjjournals.com/cgi/content/full/57/1/63

[3] Hardin JG, Waterman J, Labson LH. Rheumatic disease: Which diagnostic tests are useful? *Patient Care* 1999; March 15: 83-102

[4] Vasquez A. Musculoskeletal disorders and iron overload disease: comment on the American College of Rheumatology guidelines for the initial evaluation of the adult patient with acute musculoskeletal symptoms. *Arthritis Rheum*. 1996 Oct;39(10):1767-8. See full-text at ichnfm.academia.edu/AlexVasquez

[5] Prince et al. Sustained rheumatoid arthritis remission is uncommon in clinical practice. *Arthritis Res Ther*. 2012 Mar 19;14(2):R68 arthritis-research.com/content/14/2/R68

17% to 36% of RA patients for up to 6 months. These studies did not evaluate time in remission beyond 6 months. A recent study investigated the probability of remaining in remission up to 24 months, according to the ACR/EULAR, SDAI, and CDAI remission criteria in two different cohorts. They also concluded that long-term remission is rare, considering that probability of a remission lasting 2 years was 6-14%." Despite the constant barrage of new drugs, shiny brochures, polished advertisments, and self-agrandizing announcements of "progress", medical drug-based treatment of autoimmunity is impressively ineffective for long-term management and generally makes zero attempt to accomplish cure of these medically-proclaimed "incurable" conditions. Medical practice has largely been co-opted by the pharmaceutical sales model; most doctors these days do not look for authentic solutions to complex problems, and they have been convinced that "medical management" (i.e., diagnosis and testing followed by long-term medicalization and polypharmacy) is the epitome and axiom of medical practice.[6]

- Introduction to naturopathic medicine and functional medicine perspective and treatment: From the perspective of naturopathic medicine and functional medicine, the condition is considered highly amenable to treatment provided that such treatment is multifaceted and addresses the allergic, dysbiotic, nutritional, mitochondrial, endocrinologic, and immunophenotypic components of this multifaceted phenomenon.

- Etiological considerations include:
  - Genetic predisposition and HLA-DR: HLA-DR4 is positive in 70% of RA patients, compared to 28% of control patients. "Genetic risk factors do not fully account for the incidence of RA, suggesting that environmental factors also play a role in the etiology of the disease. ...[C]limate and urbanization have a major impact on the incidence and severity of RA in groups of similar genetic background."[7]
  - Urbanization / Western lifestyle: Urbanization is a risk factor for the development of rheumatic disease.[8,9] Urbanization is associated with increased risk of vitamin D deficiency and increased exposure to nutritionally-depleted multiallergenic genetically-modified AGE-laden phytonutrient-deficient prohyperglycemic "convenience foods", sleep disturbances, and exposure to particulate debris (i.e., pollution from diesel and other petrochemical combustion); each of these factors has been shown in animal models or human trials to promote systemic inflammation.
  - Female gender / estrogen: Women are affected 2-3x more often than men. Male RA patients tend to have relative reductions in DHEA and testosterone and relative excess of estrogen and prolactin. Predisposing factors for women include vitamin D deficiency, higher prolactin and estrogen/dysestrogenism (pro-inflammatory) with "relative insufficiency" of testosterone (anti-inflammatory), and the anatomically shorter urethra which predisposes the female urinary tract to recurrent microbial colonization.
  - Tobacco/cigarette smoke: Habitual tobacco/cigarette smoking increases exposure to reactive oxygen species, vasoactive/vasoconstrictive substances, carcinogens, and bacterial endotoxin. Tobacco leaves are noted for their high surface area which—unfortunately for smokers—serves as a deposition reservoir for both ambient radioactive particles[10,11] as well as Gram-negative bacteria, Gram-positive bacteria, and fungi[12]; thereby, tobacco smoking increases exposure to radioactive particles as well as microbial debris (e.g., endotoxin, exotoxin, and bacterial DNA). Thus, the finding that tobacco smoking—particularly from cigarette smoke which is inhaled deeply into the lungs in contrast with cigar smoke which is generally inhaled only into the mouth and pharynx—is a major risk factor for the development of

[6] Ely et al. Analysis of questions asked by family doctors regarding patient care. *BMJ*. 1999 Aug 7;319(7206):358-61

[7] Fauci AS, Braunwald E, Isselbacher KJ, et al., eds. *Harrison's Principles of Internal Medicine. 14th Ed*. New York, NY: McGraw-Hill; 1998, page 1881

[8] "In particular, a significantly lower prevalence of RA in rural areas compared with urban cohorts has led to the hypothesis that environmental factors associated with urbanization may be involved in disease pathogenesis." Adebajo A, Davis P. Rheumatic diseases in African blacks. *Semin Arthritis Rheum*. 1994 Oct;24(2):139-53

[9] "The general impression is that rheumatoid arthritis (RA) has a lower prevalence and a milder course in developing countries. Epidemiological studies from different regions show that varying prevalence is possibly related to urbanization." Kalla et al. Rheumatoid arthritis in the developing world. *Best Pract Res Clin Rheumatol*. 2003 Oct;17(5):863-75

[10] "Tobacco leaves are large and have sticky exudates that retain the radon decay products once they deposit on the leaves." Savidou A, Kehagia K, Eleftheriadis K. Concentration levels of 210Pb and 210Po in dry tobacco leaves in Greece. *J Environ Radioact*. 2006;85(1):94-102

[11] "Leaf tobacco contains minute amounts of lead 210 (210Pb) and polonium 210 (210Po), both of which are radioactive carcinogens and both of which can be found in smoke from burning tobacco. Tobacco smoke also contains carcinogens that are nonradioactive. People who inhale tobacco smoke are exposed to higher concentrations of radioactivity than nonsmokers. Deposits of 210Pb and alpha particle-emitting 210Po form in the lungs of smokers, generating localized radiation doses far greater than the radiation exposures humans experience from natural sources. This radiation exposure, delivered to sensitive tissues for long periods of time, may induce cancer both alone and synergistically with nonradioactive carcinogens." Kilthau GF. Cancer risk in relation to radioactivity in tobacco. *Radiol Technol*. 1996 Jan-Feb;67(3):217-22

[12] "Cured tobacco in diverse types of cigarettes is known to harbor a plethora of bacteria (Gram-positive and Gram-negative), fungi (mold, yeast), spores, and is rich in endotoxin (lipopolysaccharide). Reviewed herein are recent observations of the authors' team and other investigators that support the hypothesis that lung inflammation of long-term smokers may be attributed in part to tobacco-associated bacterial and fungal components that have been identified in tobacco and tobacco smoke." Pauly et al. Review: Is lung inflammation associated with microbes and microbial toxins in cigarette tobacco smoke? *Immunol Res*. 2010 Mar;46(1-3):127-36

rheumatoid arthritis and other systemic inflammatory/autoimmune/autoinflammatory disorders is consistent with the microbial/dysbiotic model discussed later in this section.

- Cigarette smoking and inflammation (*J Dent Res* 2012 Feb[13]): **"CS [cigarette smoking] impairs innate defenses against pathogens, modulates antigen presentation, and promotes autoimmunity.** ... Potential mechanisms by which CS promotes rheumatoid arthritis include the release of intracellular proteins from ROS-activated or injured cells, augmentation of auto-reactive B-cell function, altered presentation of antigens by CS-impaired antigen-presenting cells, altered regulatory T-cell functions, and T-cell activation by antigens found in CS." Additionally, tobacco use can alter the oral microbiome and/or promote gingivitis which promotes microbial translocation; the oxidative stress of smoked tobacco promotes nutrient deficiency via oxidative destruction/utilization of immunomodulating nutrients such as ascorbate and tocopherols.

o Occult viral, bacterial or parasitic infections/colonizations are common in autoimmune diseases:
  - Viral: **Cytomegalovirus and rubella viruses have been cultured from the synovium in patients with rheumatoid arthritis.** "...some viral diseases, such as parvovirus, chronic hepatitis B virus and hepatitis C virus infections, can produce long-lasting rheumatic symptoms. ... Some evidence suggests hepatitis C virus as a possible trigger to rheumatoid arthritis."[14] The implications of this data are not perfectly clear; however, possibilities (which may coexist) include: 1) virus *directly* provoking joint destruction, 2) virus *indirectly* provoking joint destruction, such as via immune complexes, 3) noncausal, coincidental finding, 4) inability of RA patients to clear this infection due to immunologic deficits which accompany immune dysfunction. Remember, "Unhealthy people are unhealthy" which is to say that they generally demonstrate multiple abnormalities in addition to their index disease, and an *associated* abnormality does not imply a *causal* relationship. Sick people—those who are metabolically/immunologically impaired— tend to enter vicious cycles that can amplify the original illness and lead to the genesis of new, additive health problems. Additionally, given that nutritional deficiencies—pandemic in the general population and even more common in patients with chronic illness (due to malabsorption, hypermetabolism of immune activation, and nutrient losses and malabsorption due to pharmaceutical drugs, etc)—promote viral mutagenesis and replication, the possibility exists that enhanced viral replication in patients with RA/autoimmunity is a surrogate marker for nutritional deficiency; relatedly, enhanced viral replication might be a surrogate marker for enhanced activity of the NFkB pathway, which is upregulated in inflammatory responses and which promotes viral replication. More likely from this author's perspective is the probability that increased viral replication/presence is—regardless of primary etiology—a likely contributor to the total microbial load (TML) and total inflammatory/antigenic load (TIL, TAL) that perpetuates chronic/sustained immune activation and which thus drives systemic inflammation and the clinical manifestation of autoimmunity.
  - Bacterial (specific species and generalized SIBO—small intestine bacterial overgrowth): RA is associated with gastrointestinal and genitourinary colonization with *Proteus mirabilis*.[15,16] Approximately 40% of patients with rheumatoid arthritis have bacterial overgrowth of the small bowel, and the severity of bacterial overgrowth correlates positively with the severity of the musculoskeletal inflammation, suggesting the probability of a causal relationship.[17] Relatedly, clinicians should recall that peptidoglycans, bacterial cell wall debris, endotoxins, indole, skatole and numerous other gut-derived "toxins" can promote joint inflammation.[18,19] **Animal models have demonstrated that gut-derived metabolites can cause inflammatory degenerative**

Prototypic multifocal dysbiosis in RA
• Nasopharynx: *Streptococcus pyogenes*
• Gastrointestinal: *Eubacterium aerofaciens* and (likely) segmented filamentous bacteria, in addition to generalized SIBO; some patients will have a specific "parasitic rheumatism" to a particular microbe, such as *Citrobacter* or *Endolimax*
• Genitourinary: *Proteus mirabilis*

[13] Lee et al. Cigarette smoking and inflammation: cellular and molecular mechanisms. *J Dent Res*. 2012 Feb;91(2):142-9 ncbi.nlm.nih.gov/pmc/articles/PMC3261116/

[14] Siegel LB, Gall EP. Viral infection as a cause of arthritis. *Am Fam Physician* 1996 Nov 1;54(6):2009-15

[15] Ebringer A, Rashid T, Wilson C. Rheumatoid arthritis: proposal for the use of anti-microbial therapy in early cases. *Scand J Rheumatol* 2003;32(1):2-11

[16] Rashid et al. Proteus IgG antibodies and C-reactive protein in English, Norwegian and Spanish patients with rheumatoid arthritis. *Clin Rheumatol* 1999;18(3):190-5

[17] "Eight (32%) of the patients with RA had hypochlorhydria or achlorhydria... A high frequency of small intestinal bacterial overgrowth was found in patients with RA; it was associated with a high disease activity and observed in patients with hypochlorhydria or achlorhydria and in those with normal acid secretion." Henriksson AE, Blomquist L, Nord CE, Midtvedt T, Uribe A. Small intestinal bacterial overgrowth in patients with rheumatoid arthritis. *Ann Rheum Dis*. 1993 Jul;52(7):503-10

[18] Simelyte et al. Bacterial cell wall-induced arthritis: chemical composition and tissue distribution of four Lactobacillus strains. *Infect Immun*. 2000 Jun;68(6):3535-40

[19] Toivanen P. Normal intestinal microbiota in the aetiopathogenesis of rheumatoid arthritis. *Ann Rheum Dis*. 2003 Sep;62(9):807-11 ard.bmjjournals.com/cgi/reprint/62/9/807

arthritis that resembles rheumatoid arthritis.[20,21] **The dysbiotic contribution to rheumatoid arthritis is likely to be both** *qualitative* **(related to specific inciting microbes) and** *quantitative* **(related to total, nonspecific bacterial overgrowth of the gut and multifocal mucosal colonization).** Accordingly, research published in 2007 showed that dietary modification was comparable in benefit to prednisolone, supporting the model that gastrointestinal dysfunction—namely, food allergic reactions (and probably intestinal dysbiosis)—is a major etiologic component of rheumatoid arthritis, at least in its initial stages; the authors concluded, "**This study supports the concept that rheumatoid arthritis may be a reaction to a food antigen(s) and that** the disease process starts within the intestine."[22]

- Parasitic: Gastrointestinal parasite infections, such as with *Endolimax nana*[23] and other microbes such a *Giardia lamblia*, can induce a systemic inflammatory response that mimics rheumatoid arthritis and is cured with parasite eradication.

Clinical presentations:

- Course: Variable course with exacerbations and remissions; the general trend is one of progressive joint destruction and systemic inflammation-induced damage.
- Presentation: The disease begins slowly in 2/3 of patients and can be slow to reach a diagnostic threshold—generally takes 9 months between initial onset and diagnosis; may affect only one joint initially. 10% have acute-onset polyarthritis. RA can affect any age, either gender, and clinical presentations will vary.
  - 2-3x more common in women than men.
  - Age of onset is typically 25-50 years of age.
  - "Peripheral symmetric polyarthropathy" is a classic description for RA; but this same description can be applied to many cases of hemochromatosis and SLE as well.
  - Palpable joint swelling with synovitis and effusion.
  - Morning stiffness > 1 hour.
  - Typical autoimmune systemic manifestations: fatigue, malaise, low-grade fever, anorexia, and weight loss—note that all of these clinical presentations are manifestations of immune activation in general and increased cytokine production in particular.
- Musculoskeletal:
  - The joints most commonly affected are the wrists, MCP, PIP, MTP (metatarsophalangeal) joints, and knees (Baker's cyst is common). In severe or advanced disease, essentially any joint in the body—including the TMJ and upper cervical spine—can be involved.
  - Most common at PIP, MCP joints, wrists (i.e., "knuckles and wrists").
  - Upper cervical spine involvement can lead to atlantoaxial instability—upper cervical spine manipulation is contraindicated until atlantoaxial instability has been excluded clinically or radiographically.
  - Periarticular muscle atrophy and osteoporosis—due to inflammation and disuse.
  - Generalized osteoporosis is common due to inflammation, disuse/deconditioning, hypogonadism, and drug effects.
  - Advanced complications include radial deviation of the wrists and ulnar deviation of the fingers, swan neck deformity (PIP hyperextension with DIP hyperflexion), and boutonniere deformity (PIP hyperflexion with DIP hyperextension).
- Skin: Rheumatoid nodules (subcutaneous inflammatory granulomas) are seen in up to 30% of patients. These are also rarely seen in patients with hemochromatoic arthropathy mimicking RA.[24]
- Arteries and vessels: Rheumatoid vasculitis leads to impaired circulation, causing necrosis of affected tissues/organs: fingers, skin, internal organs, and nerves (peripheral neuropathy).
- Pulmonary manifestations: Dyspnea, pulmonary nodules, fibrosis; more common in men.
- Eye: Complications are seen in 1% of patients but can lead to rapid blindness.
- Other autoimmune diseases: Up to 20% of patients with RA develop Sjogren's syndrome. SLE, MS, Hashimoto's thyroiditis, and mixed connective tissue disease can easily co-exist with RA.

---

[20] Nakoneczna I, Forbes JC, Rogers KS. The arthritogenic effect of indole, skatole and other tryptophan metabolites in rabbits. *Am J Pathol.* 1969 Dec;57(3):523-38
[21] Rogers KS, Forbes JC, Nakoneczna I. Arthritogenic properties of lipophilic, aryl molecules. *Proc Soc Exp Biol Med.* 1969 Jun;131(2):670-2
[22] Podas et al. Is rheumatoid arthritis a disease that starts in intestine? Pilot study comparing an elemental diet with oral prednisolone. *Postgrad Med J.* 2007 Feb;83(976):128-31
[23] "Endolimax nana grew on stool culture. Both the patient's diarrhea and arthritis responded effectively to therapy with metronidazole. The diagnosis of parasitic rheumatism was made in retrospect." Burnstein SL, Liakos S. Parasitic rheumatism presenting as rheumatoid arthritis. *J Rheumatol.* 1983 Jun;10(3):514-5
[24] "These manifestations which are common to rheumatoid arthritis may be seen in hemochromatotic arthropathy." Bensen WG, Laskin CA, Little HA, Fam AG. Hemochromatotic arthropathy mimicking rheumatoid arthritis. A case with subcutaneous nodules, tenosynovitis, and bursitis. *Arthritis Rheum.* 1978 Sep-Oct;21(7):844-8

Major differential diagnoses:

- Osteoarthritis (OA): OA tends to be monoarticular or oligoarticular rather than polyarticular; OA is generally only minimally inflammatory (except after the progression of joint destruction) whereas RA is clearly more inflammatory as assessed clinically and serologically (with ESR or CRP). OA is more likely to be asymmetric whereas RA is nearly always symmetric (except in cases of stroke, paralysis, or peripheral nerve lesion due to interference with neurogenic inflammation). Lab tests such as ANA, RF, and CCP antibodies are expected to be normal in OA; CRP and ESR may be moderately elevated in severe OA but inflammatory markers are generally much lower than the levels seen in RA.

- SLE: Differentiated by nonerosive arthritis, anti-DS-DNA antibodies, anti-Smith antibodies, low serum complement, the classic "butterfly rash", and an earlier and more frequent development of mucosal, serosal, vasculitic and renal complications.

- Septic arthritis: Differentiated by monoarthritis, fever, and purulent joint aspiration.
  - **Septic arthritis may complicate pre-existing rheumatoid arthritis**, and patients with RA appear to be predisposed to septic arthritis: Reasons for this septic predisposition include immune dysfunction, use of prednisone or other immunosuppressant medications, and concomitant obesity and/or diabetes. **Patients may lack the classic systemic manifestations of septic arthritis (fever, chills, leukocytosis) due to age, disease, or pharmaceutical immunosuppression.**[25,26] Patients may have concomitant respiratory or urinary tract infections, which makes the clinical presentation even more unclear. Treatment may require systemic antibiotics (oral or intravenous) and joint lavage with antibiotics.[27] **Failure to diagnose and treat septic arthritis promptly may result in deformity, disability, or death.**

- Hemochromatosis and iron overload: Given its high frequency and multifarious clinical presentations, iron overload is an essential diagnostic consideration in patients with rheumatic disease.[28,29] Doctors must test serum ferritin and transferrin saturation (along with CRP) as discussed in Chapter 1.

- Reactive arthritis: Differentiated by the recent history of infection, greatly increased prevalence of HLA-B27, and the presence of uveitis/iritis, sacroiliac and lumbar involvement, predominant acute/subacute-onset inflammation of the heels, knees, hips. *Perspective from DrV: I think rheumatoid arthritis should be considered a variant of reactive arthritis, with RA being triggered by multifocal dysbiosis (several subclinical infections) whereas the latter is triggered by a single true infection.*

- Gout and other crystal-induced arthropathy: Asymmetric arthritis, negatively birefringent crystals demonstrated with joint aspiration.

- Arthritis related to viral infection: Such as parvovirus and hepatitis C[30]; clinical correlation with appropriate serologies are warranted.

- Psoriatic arthritis: Skin lesions, nail pitting, asymmetric arthritis, negative RF and CCP. Rarely, the joint inflammation of psoriatic arthritis precedes the expected dermatologic lesions: well-demarcated erythematous patches covered with silvery scales.

- Adult Still's disease: Diagnosis relies on *all of the following*: high fevers (>102.2°F), arthralgia/arthritis, RF<80, ANA<1:100, *plus two of the following*: skin rash (generalized and confluent red papules and plaques), pleuritis/pericarditis, WBC count >15,000 cells/mm³, and hepatomegally/spenomegally/lymphadenopathy.

- Ewing's sarcoma: An aggressive bone malignancy that typically presents in children and young adults with periarticular bone pain and fever which can mimic inflammatory monoarthritis.

---

[25] "Many patients lacked distinctive features of joint sepsis (fever, chills) and only one half had leukocytosis." Blackburn WD Jr, Dunn TL, Alarcon GS. Infection versus disease activity in rheumatoid arthritis: eight years' experience. *South Med J*. 1986 Oct;79(10):1238-41

[26] "Pain and loss of motion in the affected joint were prominent, but toxic features of pyogenic infections—hectic fever, chills, sweats, local warmth, or erythema--were conspicuously absent. Two patients had moderate fever and three patients had mild leukocytosis." Kraft SM, Panush RS, Longley S. Unrecognized staphylococcal pyarthrosis with rheumatoid arthritis. *Semin Arthritis Rheum*. 1985 Feb;14(3):196-201

[27] Septic arthritis complicating rheumatoid arthritis was due to Staphylococcus aureus (12 cases) and Escherichia coli (1 case). Recommended treatment: "The authors recommend as the treatment of choice: systemic antibiotic therapy and immediate arthrotomy followed by through-and-through irrigation with fluid containing the appropriate antibiotics." Gristina AG, Rovere GD, Shoji H. Spontaneous septic arthritis complicating rheumatoid arthritis. *J Bone Joint Surg Am*. 1974 Sep;56(6):1180-4

[28] Vasquez A. Musculoskeletal disorders and iron overload disease: comment on the American College of Rheumatology guidelines for the initial evaluation of the adult patient with acute musculoskeletal symptoms. *Arthritis Rheum*. 1996 Oct;39(10):1767-8

[29] "These manifestations which are common to rheumatoid arthritis may be seen in hemochromatotic arthropathy." Bensen WG, Laskin CA, Little HA, Fam AG. Hemochromatotic arthropathy mimicking rheumatoid arthritis. A case with subcutaneous nodules, tenosynovitis, and bursitis. *Arthritis Rheum*. 1978 Sep-Oct;21(7):844-8

[30] Siegel LB, Gall EP. Viral infection as a cause of arthritis. *Am Fam Physician* 1996 Nov 1;54(6):2009-15

Clinical assessment:

- **History/subjective**:
  - Systemic manifestations (eg, fatigue, lassitude) with symmetric peripheral polyarthropathy.
  - Morning stiffness lasting more than 30-60 minutes is common.
- **Physical examination/objective**:
  - Assess joints, especially the distal/peripheral joints of the wrists/hands and ankles/feet. Remember that the initial manifestation of RA, like all inflammatory arthropathies, can affect any joint in the body, including the atlantoaxial joint. Flexion contractures and ulnar deviation of the fingers are common, classic findings of developed disease.
  - Clinically assess patient for exclusion of other diseases. Some patients with RA will develop other autoimmune diseases, especially hypothyroidism and Sjogren's syndrome.
- **Laboratory assessments**: Goals of laboratory testing are 1) exclude serious life-threatening conditions (e.g., septic arthritis), 2) quantitatively and qualitatively assess patient's health status, 3) determine nature and severity of underlying diseases and disorders for which correction can contribute to an overall improvement in immune function and reduction in total inflammatory load.
  - **CCP: Cyclic citrullinated protein antibody; Citrullinated protein antibodies (CPA); anti-CCP antibodies: anti-cyclic citrullinated peptide antibody**: Anti-CCP antibodies have 95-98% specificity for RA[31] and has become the laboratory standard for evaluating the diagnosis and prognosis of RA.[32] The best current data indicates that anti-CCP antibodies are sensitive and specific for RA[33], and clinicians should use this test in the diagnosis of RA.[34] Anti-CCP antibodies with a positive rheumatoid factor (RF) is termed "composite/conjugate seropositivity" and appears to be more specific than isolated anti-CCP or RF positivity.[35]
  - C-reactive protein: CRP can be used to support the diagnosis (as it indicates inflammation) and can be used to monitor the disease and the response to treatment.[36]
  - Erythrocyte sedimentation rate: ESR is elevated in 90% of patients and can be used to support the diagnosis (as it indicates inflammation) and can be used to monitor the disease and the response to treatment.[37]
  - Complete blood count: CBC may reveal anemia of chronic disease, anemia due to NSAID-related gastrointestinal bleeding, or suggest nutritional deficiencies (namely B12 and folic acid as discussed in Chapter 1); elevated WBC suggests infection and requires clinical correlation.
  - Ferritin: As an acute phase reactant, serum ferritin is elevated by inflammation; as a marker for iron status, serum ferritin is elevated by iron overload and lowered by iron deficiency. Transferrin saturation and serum iron should be low in RA due to inflammation, whereas they are commonly elevated in patients with iron overload. In order to determine the acute phase contribution to an elevated ferritin level, an independent marker of inflammation such as CRP or ESR should be tested simultaneously. When in doubt, iron overload can be excluded with diagnostic phlebotomy, liver MRI, liver

> **CCP antibodies: the single best laboratory test for the early detection, diagnosis, and monitoring of RA**
>
> "The anti-CCP test is more specific than the commonly used RF test (95% versus less than 90%) and has a comparable sensitivity (more than 70%). ... In conclusion, testing for anti-CCP autoantibodies is widely accepted as an indispensable tool for diagnosis and early treatment in the management of rheumatoid arthritis patients."
>
> van Venrooij et al. *Ann N Y Acad Sci* 2008 Nov

---

[31] Hill J, Cairns E, Bell DA. The joy of citrulline: new insights into the diagnosis, pathogenesis, and treatment of rheumatoid arthritis. *J Rheumatol*. 2004 Aug;31(8):1471-3

[32] "We conclude that, at present, the antibody response directed to citrullinated antigens has the most valuable diagnostic and prognostic potential for RA." van Boekel MA, et al. Autoantibody systems in rheumatoid arthritis: specificity, sensitivity and diagnostic value. *Arthritis Res*. 2002;4(2):87-93 arthritis-research.com/content/4/2/87

[33] "Serum antibodies reactive with citrullinated proteins/peptides are a very sensitive and specific marker for rheumatoid arthritis." Migliorini P, Pratesi F, Tommasi C, Anzilotti C. The immune response to citrullinated antigens in autoimmune diseases. *Autoimmun Rev*. 2005 Nov;4(8):561-4

[34] "The anti-CCP test is more specific than the commonly used RF test (95% versus less than 90%) and has a comparable sensitivity (more than 70%). ... In conclusion, testing for anti-CCP autoantibodies is widely accepted as an indispensable tool for diagnosis and early treatment in the management of rheumatoid arthritis patients." van Venrooij WJ, van Beers JJ, Pruijn GJ. Anti-CCP Antibody, a Marker for the Early Detection of Rheumatoid Arthritis. *Ann N Y Acad Sci*. 2008 Nov;1143:268-85

[35] "...our findings suggest that a positive anti-CCP antibody result does not necessarily exclude SLE in African American patients presenting with inflammatory arthritis. In such patients, the additional assessment of IgA-RF or IgM-RF isotypes may be of added value since composite seropositivity appears to be nearly exclusive to patients with RA." Mikuls et al. Anti-cyclic citrullinated peptide antibody and rheumatoid factor isotypes in African Americans with early rheumatoid arthritis. *Arthritis Rheum*. 2006 Sep;54:3057-9

[36] Gabay C, Kushner I. Acute-phase proteins and other systemic responses to inflammation. *N Engl J Med*. 1999 Feb 11;340(6):448-54

[37] Klippel JH (ed). *Primer on the Rheumatic Diseases. 11th Edition*. Atlanta: Arthritis Foundation. 1997 page 94

biopsy (especially if liver enzymes are elevated), or the response to therapeutic phlebotomy.[38]

o <u>Rheumatoid factor</u>: RF is positive in 70-80% of patients with RA but is not specific and is not necessary for the diagnosis of RA. RF provides "supportive evidence" for the diagnosis of RA only in the presence of corresponding clinical manifestations. High RF levels indicate more severe disease and worse prognosis. IgA-RF appears to have clinical superiority over other forms of RF.[39] RF is seen in 5% of apparently healthy people, and it is present in some patients with iron overload, thus making the distinction between RA and hemochromatoic arthropathy all the more difficult.[40] Diseases (other than RA) associated with RF positivity include iron overload, chronic infections, hepatitis, sarcoidosis, and bacterial endocarditis.

o <u>Thyroid assessment</u>: Hypothyroidism can mimic systemic rheumatic disease by causing an inflammatory oligoarthropathy and myopathy, complete with elevations of CRP and ESR.[41] Overt or imminent hypothyroidism is suggested by TSH greater than 2 mU/L[42] or 3 mU/L[43], low T4 or T3, and/or the presence of anti-thyroid peroxidase antibodies (anti-TPO).[44] This author's current practice is—for the laboratory evaluation of hypothyroidism—to assess the full spectrum of thyroid indexes: THS, free T4, free or total T3, reverse T3 (rT3), and the antithyroid antibodies: anti-thyroglobulin and anti-thyroid peroxidase (anti-TPO).

o <u>Complete hormone assessment</u>: Patients with RA commonly show elevations of prolactin and estradiol along with insufficiencies of testosterone, cortisol, and DHEA. These can be tested in serum, and early-morning serum cortisol is more accurate than late-day cortisol. Other options and details are provided in the following section under *Treatments* and in the section in Chapter 4 on *Orthoendocrinology*.

o <u>Lactulose-mannitol assay for "leaky gut"</u>: Increased intestinal permeability (IP) is a common contributor to and complication of many inflammatory/rheumatic/chronic diseases including psoriasis[45], Behcet's disease[46], ankylosing spondylitis[47] and seronegative spondyloarthritis[48], enteropathic spondyloarthropathy and oligoarticular juvenile idiopathic arthritis[49], lupus[50], and chronic congestive heart failure.[51] This test may be used for the evaluation of gastrointestinal mucosal integrity, which simultaneously serves as a barometer of overall health and when elevated can indicate the presence of a variety of intestinal disorders, including celiac disease, food allergies, and GI dysbiosis. Thus, an elevated lactulose:mannitol ratio is *sensitive* but not *specific* for the presence of intestinal disorders. See discussion in Chapter 1. Use of this test in RA is at the discretion of the clinician and patient, as most patients can be reasonably assumed to have increased intestinal permeability and thereafter treated empirically; the value—if any—of this test in RA is in monitoring response to treatment.

o <u>Comprehensive stool analysis and comprehensive parasitology with bacterial and fungal culture and sensitivity</u>: **All patients with rheumatoid arthritis should be considered to have gastrointestinal dysbiosis until proven otherwise** by ❶ <u>dysbiosis laboratory assessment</u> (including comprehensive stool testing with parasitology *performed by a specialty laboratory*), and ❷ <u>response to anti-dysbiosis treatment</u>

[38] "Therapeutic phlebotomy is used to remove excess iron and maintain low normal body iron stores, and it should be initiated in men with serum ferritin levels of 300 microg/L or more and in women with serum ferritin levels of 200 microg/L or more, regardless of the presence or absence of symptoms." Barton et al. Management of hemochromatosis. Hemochromatosis Management Working Group. *Ann Intern Med*. 1998 Dec 1;129(11):932-9

[39] Jonsson T, Valdimarsson H. What about IgA rheumatoid factor in rheumatoid arthritis? *Ann Rheum Dis*. 1998 Jan;57(1):63-4 ard.bmjjournals.com/cgi/content/full/57/1/63

[40] "These manifestations which are common to rheumatoid arthritis may be seen in hemochromatotic arthropathy." Bensen WG, Laskin CA, Little HA, Fam AG. Hemochromatotic arthropathy mimicking rheumatoid arthritis. A case with subcutaneous nodules, tenosynovitis, and bursitis. *Arthritis Rheum*. 1978;21(7):844-8

[41] Bowman et al. Bilateral adhesive capsulitis, oligoarthritis and proximal myopathy as presentation of hypothyroidism. *Br J Rheumatol*. 1988;27(1):62-4

[42] Weetman AP. Hypothyroidism: screening and subclinical disease. *BMJ*. 1997 Apr 19;314(7088):1175-8 bmj.bmjjournals.com/cgi/content/full/314/7088/1175

[43] "Now AACE encourages doctors to consider treatment for patients who test outside the boundaries of a narrower margin based on a target TSH level of 0.3 to 3.0. AACE believes the new range will result in proper diagnosis for millions of Americans who suffer from a mild thyroid disorder, but have gone untreated until now." American Association of Clinical Endocrinologists (AACE). 2003 Campaign Encourages Awareness of Mild Thyroid Failure, Importance of Routine Testing aace.com/pub/tam2003/press.php November 26, 2005

[44] Beers MH, Berkow R (eds). *Merck Manual. 17th Edition*. Whitehouse Station; Merck Research Laboratories 1999 Page 96

[45] Humbert P, Bidet A, Treffel P, Drobacheff C, Agache P. Intestinal permeability in patients with psoriasis. *J Dermatol Sci*. 1991 Jul;2(4):324-6

[46] Fresko I, et al. Intestinal permeability in Behcet's syndrome. *Ann Rheum Dis*. 2001 Jan;60(1):65-6

[47] Vaile et al. Bowel permeability and CD45RO expression on circulating CD20+ B cells in patients with ankylosing spondylitis and their relatives. *J Rheumatol* 1999 Jan:128-35

[48] Di Leo et al. Effect of Helicobacter pylori and eradication therapy on gastrointestinal permeability. Implications for patients with seronegative spondyloarthritis. *J Rheumatol*. 2005 Feb;32(2):295-300

[49] Picco P, et al. Increased gut permeability in juvenile chronic arthritides. A multivariate analysis of the diagnostic parameters. *Clin Exp Rheumatol*. 2000 Nov-Dec;18(6):773-8

[50] "Fourteen cases of primary lupus-associated protein-losing enteropathy have now been reported in the English-language literature." Peredina DA, Curosh NA. Lupus-associated protein-losing enteropathy. *Arch Intern Med*. 1990 Sep;150(9):1806-10

[51] "Chronic heart failure patients had a 35% increase of small intestinal permeability (lactulose/mannitol ratio: 0.023 vs. 0.017 ..., p = 0.006), a 210% increase of large intestinal permeability (sucralose excretion: 0.62 ... vs. 0.20), and a 29% decrease of D-xylose absorption, indicating bowel ischemia (26.7% vs. 37.4%, p = 0.003)." Sandek A, Bauditz J, Swidsinski A, et al. Altered intestinal function in patients with chronic heart failure. *J Am Coll Cardiol*. 2007 Oct 16;50(16):1561-9

which minimally includes the combination of anti-dysbiosis dietary modification (nutritional supplementation, plant-based diet, low-fermentation, high-fiber, superadequate protein and phytonutrients) with antimicrobial drugs or botanicals, commonly including berberine (500mg BID-TID for 3 months), emulsified time-released oil of oregano (200mg TID for 6 weeks[52]), Augmentin (2,000mg BID for variable durations of days to months to years—supportively, note successful use of long-term penicillin in the treatment of psoriasis[53]), azithromycin (500mg every other day for variable durations of days to months to years[54]), ciprofloxacin (short course only to avoid exacerbation/induction of tendonopathy), and metronidazole. Since 2013, I have become impressed by the efficacy of low-dose oral vancomycin 125-250mg PO QD; as a nonabsorbed antibiotic, the drug remains in the gut and is effective against segmented filamentous bacteria (SFB) which have been shown in several animal experiments to induce Th-17 effector cells which promote chronic arthritis/autoimmunity. A three-sample comprehensive stool analysis and parasitology examination performed by a specialty laboratory is strongly recommended as a minimal component of basic care. In lieu of *or preferably in addition to* a comprehensive parasitology test, patients can be treated for 4-8 weeks with broad-spectrum antimicrobial treatment (including an anti-dysbiosis diet) that is effective against gram-positive and gram-negative bacteria, aerobes and anaerobes, yeast, protozoa and amebas. For additional details, see Chapter 4.2 for details on dysbiosis.

- **Imaging**:
  - Radiographic changes are not seen in early disease and only have utility for clarifying diagnostic uncertainty later in the disease, screening for complications such as atlantoaxial instability, or for pre-operative assessment in patients who are candidates for joint repair or replacement.
  - Radiographic findings when clustered are relatively specific in developed disease: soft tissue swelling, periarticular osteoporosis, joint space narrowing due to loss of cartilage, **marginal erosions**, ulnar/lateral deviation of the fingers, and subluxation and dislocation may occur.

- **Establishing the diagnosis**:
  - The diagnosis is established by pattern recognition of the typical clinical manifestations and laboratory abnormalities and reasonable exclusion of protean diseases such as hepatitis C, SLE, and iron overload.

Complications:

- Disease complications are common and range from the inconveniences of pain and inflammation for patients with milder disease to the major complications of joint deformity, occupational and social disability, serious cardiovascular/renal/pulmonary/cerebral complications (due mostly to inflammation, fibrosis, and vasculitis), infections (especially septic arthritis), depression, and suicide. Adding drug side-effects atop these manifold

---

2010 American College of Rheumatology/European League against Rheumatism classification criteria

Screening: Patients with at least 1 joint and definite clinical synovitis which is not explained by another disease.

A score of ≥6 is needed for classification of definite RA:
- Score 1 large joint: 0
- 2–10 large joints: 1
- 1–3 small joints (with or without large joints): 2
- 4–10 small joints (with or without large joints): 3
- >10 joints (at least 1 small joint): 5

Serology: At least 1 test is needed:
- Negative RF (rheumatoid factor) and negative ACPA (anticitrullinated protein antibody): 0
- Low positive RF or low positive ACPA: 2
- High positive RF or high positive ACPA: 3

Acute phase reactants: At least 1 result is needed.
- Normal CRP (C-reactive protein) and normal ESR: 0
- Abnormal CRP or ESR: 1

Duration of symptoms: (self-reported)
- <6 weeks: 0
- ≥6 weeks: 1

Although patients with a score <6/10 are not classifiable as having RA, their status can be reassessed and the criteria might be fulfilled cumulatively over time.

onlinelibrary.wiley.com/doi/10.1002/art.27580/pdf
ncbi.nlm.nih.gov/pmc/articles/PMC3077961/pdf/nihms266537.pdf
unboundmedicine.com/5minute/view/5-Minute-Clinical-Consult/116053/all/Arthritis_Rheumatoid__RA

---

[52] "Oil of Mediterranean oregano *Oreganum vulgare* was orally administered to 14 adult patients whose stools tested positive for enteric parasites, *Blastocystis hominis*, *Entamoeba hartmanni* and *Endolimax nana*. After 6 weeks of supplementation with 600 mg emulsified oil of oregano daily, there was complete disappearance of *Entamoeba hartmanni* (four cases), *Endolimax nana* (one case), and *Blastocystis hominis* in eight cases. Also, *Blastocystis hominis* scores declined in three additional cases. Gastrointestinal symptoms improved in seven of the 11 patients who had tested positive for *Blastocystis hominis*." Force M, Sparks WS, Ronzio RA. Inhibition of enteric parasites by emulsified oil of oregano in vivo. *Phytother Res.* 2000 May;14(3):213-4

[53] Saxena VN, Dogra J. Long-term use of penicillin for the treatment of chronic plaque psoriasis. *Eur J Dermatol.* 2005 Sep-Oct;15(5):359-6

[54] Saxena VN, Dogra J. Long-term oral azithromycin in chronic plaque psoriasis: a controlled trial. *Eur J Dermatol.* 2010 May-Jun;20(3):329-33

disease complications makes managing the disease more difficult for doctors, and enduring the disease more difficult for patients.

- Mild disease results in mild symptoms and manageable impact on ADL (activities of daily living) and QOL (quality of life). Severe disease is painful, less responsive to treatment, disfiguring and generally devastating. Treatments that are inefficacious, unavailable, prohibitively expensive, or complicated by significant side effects contribute to despair. **RA patients are at increased risk for social isolation, depression, and suicide**[55]; these sociopsychiatric complications can be attributed to chronic pain, neuropsychiatric effects of inflammatory cytokines, therapeutic nihilism, adverse drug effects (e.g., NSAID- and steroid-induced psychosis), cerebral vasculitis, and nutritional deficiencies (e.g., EPA, DHA, vitamin D, zinc) in patients not cared for by competent integrative clinicians.
- Decreased life expectancy by 3-7 years, mostly due to infection, gastrointestinal bleeding, and cardiorenal complications.
- Patients with systemic inflammatory diseases are at increased risk for cardiovascular disorders (including hypertension, accelerated atherosclerosis, vasculitis) and renal complications (secondary to hypertension, vasculitis, immune complex deposition, NSAIDs and other drugs).

Clinical management:

- <u>Routine assessment, surveillance for complications, compliance, consultation, laboratory follow-up, access to treatments</u>: Clinical visits should include surveillance for subjective and objective indicators of disease progression/remission, treatment compliance (including overzealous compliance with its risk of adverse toxic effects or unnecessary expense, or undercompliance with attendant hazards of inefficacy and disease exacerbation), and overall health status. Questions are answered, and problems addressed. Necessary consultations are scheduled as needed; the referring provider sends a narrative letter and ensures that the patient has a scheduled appointment. Review and anticipatory scheduling of laboratory tests should be performed. Access to treatments should be verified. Appropriate documentation is mandatory.
- <u>Standard medical treatments</u>:
  - o <u>Discouraging the discouragement of "nutritional quackery"</u>: According to the <u>Merck Manual (1999)</u>, "Food and diet quackery is common and should be discouraged."[56] In contrast to this allopathic rhetoric, the biomedical literature strongly supports the use of nutritional interventions for **direct benefits** (e.g., anti-inflammatory, analgesic, immunomodulatory, and drug-sparing effects) and **indirect benefits** (e.g., cardiorenal protection, alleviation of depression).
  - o <u>NSAIDs as first-line treatment</u>: NSAIDS provide temporary pain relief while contributing to increased intestinal permeability, gastrointestinal hemorrhage, liver toxicity (dose-response relationship), renal toxicity (dose-response relationship) possible exacerbation of food allergies[57], and accelerated destruction of articular structures (especially indomethacin).[58,59,60]
  - o <u>Immunosuppression with prednisone, methotrexate, or other DMARD (disease-modifying antirheumatic drugs)</u>: **Despite the clinical drawbacks, philosophical inadequacies, and steep financial consequences, pharmacologic immunosuppression has a role in the management of patients with autoimmunity when their disease flares and threatens vital structures, particularly the heart, kidneys, and nervous system.** A common sequence of medicalization used by rheumatologists is:

---

[55] "Rheumatoid arthritis (RA) is a somatic disorder, which is known to be associated with major depression, and prevalences exceeding even 40% have been reported [5, 6]. Recently, Treharne et al. [7] showed that 11% of hospital out-patients with RA had experienced suicidal ideation." Timonen M, Viilo K, Hakko H, Särkioja T, Ylikulju M, Meyer-Rochow VB, Väisänen E, Räsänen P. Suicides in persons suffering from rheumatoid arthritis. *Rheumatology*. 2003 Feb;42(2):287-91
[56] Beers MH, Berkow R (eds). *The Merck Manual. 17th Edition*. Whitehouse Station; Merck Research Laboratories: 1999, page 419
[57] Abbreviations: cow's milk beta-lactoglobulin absorption (BLG), acetylsalicylic acid (ASA), disodium chromoglycate (DSCG). "ASA administration strongly increased BLG absorption, not prevented by DSCG pretreatment. ... Our results suggest that prolonged treatment with nonsteroidal anti-inflammatory drugs induces an increase of food antigen absorption, apparently not related to anaphylaxis mediator release, with possible clinical effects." Fagiolo U, Paganelli R, Ossi E, Quinti I, Cancian M, D'Offizi GP, Fiocco U. Intestinal permeability and antigen absorption in rheumatoid arthritis. Effects of acetylsalicylic acid and sodium chromoglycate. *Int Arch Allergy Appl Immunol*. 1989;89(1):98-102
[58] "At...concentrations comparable to those... in the synovial fluid of patients treated with the drug, several NSAIDs suppress proteoglycan synthesis... These NSAID-related effects on chondrocyte metabolism ... are much more profound in osteoarthritic cartilage than in normal cartilage, due to enhanced uptake of NSAIDs by the osteoarthritic cartilage." Brandt KD. Effects of nonsteroidal anti-inflammatory drugs on chondrocyte metabolism in vitro and in vivo. *Am J Med*. 1987 Nov 20; 83: 29-34
[59] "The case of a young healthy man, who developed avascular necrosis of head of femur after prolonged administration of indomethacin, is reported here." Prathapkumar KR, Smith I, Attara GA. Indomethacin induced avascular necrosis of head of femur. *Postgrad Med J*. 2000 Sep; 76(899): 574-5
[60] "This highly significant association between NSAID use and acetabular destruction gives cause for concern, not least because of the difficulty in achieving satisfactory hip replacements in patients with severely damaged acetabula." Newman et al. Acetabular bone destruction related to non-steroidal anti-inflammatory drugs. *Lancet*. 1985; 2: 11-4

- Begin first-visit treatment with daily/PRN low-dose prednisone (5-7.5 mg/day) and weekly methotrexate (7.5-15 mg/week, with daily folic acid to improve efficacy and reduce toxicity),
- Eventually add hydroxychloroquine and/or sulfasalazine as disease progresses,
- When the patient becomes "resistant to treatment" add either an oral immunosuppressant or one of the "biologics" such as the parenterally-administered TNF/cytokine blockers: etanercept, infliximab, adalimumab, etc.

Such a drug protocol might easily cost $50,000 per year and carry complications such as increased risk and severity of opportunistic infections (especially tuberculosis), exacerbation of heart failure, and increased risk for lymphoma and—less commonly—SLE and CNS demyelination similar to multiple sclerosis. Immunosuppression with corticosteroids/prednisone promotes bacterial overgrowth of the small bowel in humans[61], and animal studies have demonstrated increased bacterial translocation following prednisone administration[62]; recall that intestinal bacterial overgrowth/translocation are both pro-inflammatory and arthritogenic. Prednisone also causes mitochondrial dysfunction, which exacerbates fatigue and inflammation.

- Surgery: Surgery is used for deformities and other orthopedic complications, including atlantoaxial instability and protrusio acetabuli.

- **FOOD & NUTRITION: 5-part "supplemented Paleo-Mediterranean diet" (SPMD, 5pSPMD)** The 5-part "supplemented Paleo-Mediterranean diet" (SPMD—reviewed in Chapter 4) consists of ❶ foundational plant-based low-carbohydrate diet of fruits, vegetables, nuts, seeds, berries and lean sources of protein, ❷ multivitamin and multimineral supplementation, ❸ physiologic doses of vitamin D3 (range 2,000-10,000 IU/d), ❹ combination fatty acid therapy (CFAT) with n3-ALA, n6-GLA, n3-EPA, n3-DHA, and phytochemical-rich olive oil which contains n9-oleate, and ❺ probiotics.

  - Avoidance of pro-inflammatory foods: Pro-inflammatory foods act *directly* and *indirectly* to promote and exacerbate systemic inflammation. *Direct* mechanisms include the activation of Toll-like receptors and NFkB, while *indirect* mechanisms include depleting the body of anti-inflammatory nutrients and dietary displacement of more nutrient-dense anti-inflammatory foods. Arachidonic acid (found in cow's milk, beef, liver, pork, and lamb) is the direct precursor to pro-inflammatory prostaglandins and leukotrienes[63] and pain-promoting isoprostanes.[64] Saturated fats promote inflammation by activating/enabling pro-inflammatory Toll-like receptors, which are otherwise "specific" for inducing pro-inflammatory responses to microorganisms.[65] Consumption of saturated fat in the form of cream creates marked oxidative stress and lipid peroxidation that lasts for at least 3 hours postprandially.[66] Corn oil rapidly activates NFkB (in hepatic Kupffer cells) for a pro-inflammatory effect[67]; similarly, consumption of PUFA and linoleic acid promotes antioxidant depletion and may thus promote oxidation-mediated inflammation via activation of NFkB. Linoleic acid causes intracellular oxidative stress and calcium influx and results in increased NFkB-stimulated transcription of pro-inflammatory genes.[68] High glycemic foods cause oxidative stress[69,70] and inflammation via activation of NFkB and other mechanisms—e.g.,

---

[61] "A 63-year-old man with systemic lupus erythematosus and selective IgA deficiency developed intractable diarrhoea the day after treatment with prednisone, 50 mg daily, was started. The diarrhoea was considered to be caused by bacterial overgrowth and was later successfully treated with doxycycline." Denison H, Wallerstedt S. Bacterial overgrowth after high-dose corticosteroid treatment. *Scand J Gastroenterol.* 1989 Jun;24(5):561-4

[62] "These bacteria also translocated to the mesenteric lymph nodes in mice injected with cyclophosphamide or prednisone." Berg RD, Wommack E, Deitch EA. Immunosuppression and intestinal bacterial overgrowth synergistically promote bacterial translocation. *Arch Surg.* 1988 Nov;123(11):1359-64

[63] Vasquez A. New Insights into Fatty Acid Supplementation and Eicosanoid Production and Genetic Expression. *Nutr Perspect* 2005; Jan:5-16 ichnfm.academia.edu/AlexVasquez

[64] Evans et al. Isoprostanes, novel eicosanoids that produce nociception and sensitize rat sensory neurons. *J Pharmacol Exp Ther.* 2000 Jun;293(3):912-20

[65] Lee et al. Saturated fatty acids not unsaturated fatty acids induce expression of cyclooxygenase-2 mediated through Toll-like receptor 4. *J Biol Chem* 2001 May;276:16683-9

[66] "The increase in ROS generation lasted 3 h after cream intake and 1 h after protein intake." Mohanty et al. Both lipid and protein intakes stimulate increased generation of reactive oxygen species by polymorphonuclear leukocytes and mononuclear cells. *Am J Clin Nutr.* 2002 Apr;75(4):767-72

[67] Rusyn et al. Corn oil rapidly activates nuclear factor-kappaB in hepatic Kupffer cells by oxidant-dependent mechanisms. *Carcinogenesis.* 1999 Nov;20(11):2095-100

[68] "Exposing endothelial cells to 90 micromol linoleic acid/L for 6 h resulted in a significant increase in lipid hydroperoxides that coincided wiih an increase in intracellular calcium concentrations." Hennig B, et al. Linoleic acid activates nuclear transcription factor-kappa B (NF-kappa B) and induces NF-kappa B-dependent transcription in cultured endothelial cells. *Am J Clin Nutr.* 1996 Mar;63(3):322-8 ajcn.org/cgi/reprint/63/3/322

[69] Mohanty et al. Glucose challenge stimulates reactive oxygen species (ROS) generation by leucocytes. *J Clin Endocrinol Metab.* 2000 Aug;85(8):2970-3 Glucose/carbohydrate and saturated fat consumption appear to be the two biggest offenders in the food-stimulated production of oxidative stress. The effect by protein is much less. "CONCLUSIONS: Both fat and protein intakes stimulate ROS generation. The increase in ROS generation lasted 3 h after cream intake and 1 h after protein intake. Cream intake also caused a significant and prolonged increase in lipid peroxidation." Mohanty et al. Both lipid and protein intakes stimulate increased generation of reactive oxygen species by polymorphonuclear leukocytes and mononuclear cells. *Am J Clin Nutr.* 2002 Apr;75(4):767-72

[70] Koska et al. Insulin, catecholamines, glucose and antioxidant enzymes in oxidative damage during different loads in healthy humans. *Physiol Res.* 2000;49 Suppl 1:S95-100

white bread causes inflammation[71] as does *a high-fat high-carbohydrate fast-food-style breakfast.*[72] High glycemic foods suppress immune function[73,74] and thus promote the perpetuation of microbial colonization and dysbiosis. Delivery of a high carbohydrate load to the gastrointestinal lumen promotes bacterial overgrowth[75,76], which is inherently pro-inflammatory[77,78] and which appears to be myalgenic in humans[79] at least in part due to the ability of endotoxin to impair muscle function.[80] Overconsumption of high-carbohydrate low-phytonutrient grains, potatoes, and manufactured foods displaces phytonutrient-dense foods such as fruits, vegetables, nuts, seeds, and berries which contain more than 8,000 phytonutrients, many of which have antioxidant and thus anti-inflammatory actions.[81,82]

- o Avoidance of allergenic foods: **Gluten-free vegetarian diets benefit patients with rheumatoid arthritis.**[83] Any patient may be allergic to any food, even if the food is generally considered a health-promoting food. Generally speaking, the most notorious allergens are wheat, citrus (especially citrus *juice* due to the industrial use of fungal hemicellulases), cow's milk, eggs, peanuts, chocolate, and yeast-containing foods. According to a study in patients with migraine, some patients will have to avoid as many as 10 specific foods in order to become symptom-free.[84] **Celiac disease can present with inflammatory oligoarthritis that resembles rheumatoid arthritis and which remits with avoidance of wheat/gluten.** The inflammatory arthropathy of celiac disease has preceded bowel symptoms and/or an accurate diagnosis by as many as 3-15 years.[85,86] Clinicians must explain to their patients that celiac disease and wheat allergy are two different clinical entities and that exclusion of one does not exclude the other, and in neither case does mutual exclusion obviate the promotion of intestinal bacterial overgrowth (i.e., pro-inflammatory dysbiosis) by indigestible wheat oligosaccharides.

- o Gluten-free vegetarian/vegan diet: **Gluten-free vegetarian diets benefit patients with rheumatoid arthritis.**[87] Vegetarian/vegan diets show high safety and variable efficacy in the treatment of various inflammatory disorders.[88,89,90,91] The benefits of gluten-free vegetarian diets are well documented, and the mechanisms of action are well elucidated, including reduced intake of pro-inflammatory linoleic[92] and

---

[71] "The present study shows that high GI carbohydrate, but not low GI carbohydrate, mediates an acute proinflammatory process as measured by NF-kappaB activity." Dickinson et al. High glycemic index carbohydrate mediates an acute proinflammatory process as measured by NF-kappaB activation. *Asia Pac J Clin Nutr.* 2005;14 Suppl:S120

[72] Aljada et al. Increase in intranuclear nuclear factor kappaB and decrease in inhibitor kappaB in mononuclear cells after a mixed meal. *Am J Clin Nutr.* 2004 Apr;79(4):682-90

[73] Sanchez A, Reeser JL, Lau HS, et al. Role of sugars in human neutrophilic phagocytosis. *Am J Clin Nutr.* 1973 Nov;26(11):1180-4

[74] "Postoperative infusion of carbohydrate solution leads to moderate fall in the serum concentration of inorganic phosphate. ... The hypophosphatemia was associated with significant reduction of neutrophil phagocytosis, intracellular killing, consumption of oxygen and generation of superoxide during phagocytosis." Rasmussen A, Segel E, Hessov I, Borregaard N. Reduced function of neutrophils during routine postoperative glucose infusion. *Acta Chir Scand.* 1988 Jul-Aug;154(7-8):429-33

[75] Ramakrishnan T, Stokes P. Beneficial effects of fasting and low carbohydrate diet in D-lactic acidosis associated with short-bowel syndrome. *JPEN J Parenter Enteral Nutr.* 1985 May-Jun;9(3):361-3

[76] Gottschall E. *Breaking the Vicious Cycle: Intestinal Health through Diet.* Kirkton Press; Rev edition (August 1, 1994)

[77] Lin HC. Small intestinal bacterial overgrowth: a framework for understanding irritable bowel syndrome. *JAMA.* 2004 Aug 18;292(7):852-8

[78] Lichtman et al. Reactivation of arthritis induced by small bowel bacterial overgrowth in rats. *Infect Immun.* 1995 Jun;63(6):2295-301

[79] Pimentel et al. A link between irritable bowel syndrome and fibromyalgia may be related to findings on lactulose breath testing. *Ann Rheum Dis.* 2004 Apr;63:450-2

[80] Bundgaard et al. Endotoxemia stimulates skeletal muscle Na+-K+-ATPase and raises blood lactate under aerobic conditions in humans. *Am J Physiol Heart Circ Physiol.* 2003 Mar;284(3):H1028-34 ajpheart.physiology.org/cgi/reprint/284/3/H1028

[81] "We propose that the additive and synergistic effects of phytochemicals in fruit and vegetables are responsible for their potent antioxidant and anticancer activities, and that the benefit of a diet rich in fruit and vegetables is attributed to the complex mixture of phytochemicals present in whole foods." Liu RH. Health benefits of fruit and vegetables are from additive and synergistic combinations of phytochemicals. *Am J Clin Nutr.* 2003 Sep;78(3 Suppl):517S-520S

[82] Seaman DR. The diet-induced proinflammatory state: a cause of chronic pain and other degenerative diseases? *J Manipulative Physiol Ther.* 2002;25(3):168-79

[83] "The immunoglobulin G (IgG) antibody levels against gliadin and beta-lactoglobulin decreased in the responder subgroup in the vegan diet-treated patients, but not in the other analysed groups." Hafstrom et al. A vegan diet free of gluten improves the signs and symptoms of rheumatoid arthritis: the effects on arthritis correlate with a reduction in antibodies to food antigens. *Rheumatology* (Oxford). 2001 Oct;40(10):1175-9 rheumatology.oxfordjournals.org/cgi/content/abstract/40/10/1175

[84] Grant EC. Food allergies and migraine. *Lancet.* 1979 May 5;1(8123):966-9

[85] "We report six patients with coeliac disease in whom arthritis was prominent at diagnosis and who improved with dietary therapy. Joint pain preceded diagnosis by up to three years in five patients and 15 years in one patient." Bourne et al. Arthritis and coeliac disease. *Ann Rheum Dis.* 1985 Sep;44(9):592-8

[86] "A 15-year-old girl, with synovitis of the knees and ankles for 3 years before a diagnosis of gluten-sensitive enteropathy, is described." Pinals RS. Arthritis associated with gluten-sensitive enteropathy. *J Rheumatol.* 1986 Feb;13(1):201-4

[87] "The immunoglobulin G (IgG) antibody levels against gliadin and beta-lactoglobulin decreased in the responder subgroup in the vegan diet-treated patients, but not in the other analysed groups." Hafstrom et al. A vegan diet free of gluten improves the signs and symptoms of rheumatoid arthritis: the effects on arthritis correlate with a reduction in antibodies to food antigens. *Rheumatology* (Oxford). 2001 Oct;40(10):1175-9 rheumatology.oxfordjournals.org/cgi/content/abstract/40/10/1175

[88] "After four weeks at the health farm the diet group showed a significant improvement in number of tender joints, Ritchie's articular index, number of swollen joints, pain score, duration of morning stiffness, grip strength, erythrocyte sedimentation rate, C-reactive protein, white blood cell count, and a health assessment questionnaire score." Kjeldsen-Kragh et al. Controlled trial of fasting and one-year vegetarian diet in rheumatoid arthritis. *Lancet.* 1991 Oct 12;338(8772):899-902

[89] "During fasting, arthralgia was less intense in most subjects. In some types of skin diseases (pustulosis palmaris et plantaris and atopic eczema) an improvement could be demonstrated during the fast. During the vegan diet, both signs and symptoms returned in most patients, with the exception of some patients with psoriasis who experienced an improvement." Lithell et al. A fasting and vegetarian diet treatment trial on chronic inflammatory disorders. *Acta Derm Venereol.* 1983;63(5):397-403

[90] Tanaka et al. Vegetarian diet ameliorates symptoms of atopic dermatitis through reduction of the number of peripheral eosinophils and of PGE2 synthesis by monocytes. *J Physiol Anthropol Appl Human Sci.* 2001 Nov;20(6):353-61 jstage.jst.go.jp/article/jpa/20/6/20_353/_article/-char/en

[91] "For the patients who were randomised to the vegetarian diet there was a significant decrease in platelet count, leukocyte count, calprotectin, total IgG, IgM rheumatoid factor (RF), C3-activation products, and the complement components C3 and C4 after one month of treatment." Kjeldsen-Kragh J, Mellbye OJ, Haugen M, Mollnes TE, Hammer HB, Sioud M, Forre O. Changes in laboratory variables in rheumatoid arthritis patients during a trial of fasting and one-year vegetarian diet. *Scand J Rheumatol.* 1995;24(2):85-93

[92] Rusyn et al. Corn oil rapidly activates nuclear factor-kappaB in hepatic Kupffer cells by oxidant-dependent mechanisms. *Carcinogenesis.* 1999 Nov;20(11):2095-100

arachidonic acids[93], iron[94], common food antigens[95], gluten[96] and gliadin[97,98], pro-inflammatory sugars[99] and increased intake of omega-3 fatty acids, micronutrients[100], and anti-inflammatory and antioxidant phytonutrients.[101] Vegetarian diets also effect subtle yet biologically and clinically important changes—both *qualitative* and *quantitative*—in intestinal flora[102,103] that correlate with clinical improvement.[104] Patients who rely on the Paleo-Mediterranean diet (which is inherently omnivorous) can use vegetarian *meals* on a daily basis or for days at a time—for example, by having a daily vegetarian meal, or one week per month of vegetarianism. Some (not all) patients can use a purely vegetarian diet long-term provided that nutritional needs (especially protein and cobalamin) are consistently met.

o Routine carbohydrate restriction, periodic short-term fasting: Whether the foundational diet is Paleo-Mediterranean, vegetarian, vegan, or a combination of all of these, autoimmune/inflammatory patients will still benefit from periodic fasting, whether on a weekly (e.g., every Saturday), monthly (every first week or weekend of the month, or every other month), or yearly (1-2 weeks of the year) basis. The diet should generally be low in carbohydrates in order to promote ketogenesis and to retard SIBO. Since consumption of food—particularly "unhealthy" (i.e., high-fat, high-sugar, allergenic, nutritionally depleted, AGE-laden) foods—induces an inflammatory effect[105], abstinence from food provides a relative anti-inflammatory effect. Fasting indeed provides a distinct anti-inflammatory benefit and may help "re-calibrate" metabolic and homeostatic mechanisms by breaking self-perpetuating "vicious cycles"[106] that autonomously promote inflammation independent of pro-inflammatory stimuli. Water-only fasting is completely hypoallergenic (assuming that the patient is not sensitive to chlorine, fluoride, or other contaminants), and subsequent re-introduction of foods provides the ideal opportunity to identify offending foods. Fasting deprives intestinal microbes of substrate[107], stimulates intestinal B-cell immunity[108], improves the bactericidal action of neutrophils[109], reduces lysozyme release and leukotriene formation[110], and ameliorates intestinal hyperpermeability.[111] Fasting and carbohydrate avoidance also promote endogenous production of beta-hydroxybutyrate (bHB) which promotes histone acetylation for induction of a rejuvenative phenotype while bHB also stimulates complexes 3 and 4 of the mitochondrial

[93] Vasquez A. New Insights into Fatty Acid Supplementation and Its Effect on Eicosanoid Production and Genetic Expression. *Nutritional Perspectives* 2005; January: 5-16

[94] Dabbagh AJ, Trenam CW, Morris CJ, Blake DR. Iron in joint inflammation. *Ann Rheum Dis*. 1993 Jan;52(1):67-73

[95] Hafstrom et al. A vegan diet free of gluten improves the signs and symptoms of rheumatoid arthritis: the effects on arthritis correlate with a reduction in antibodies to food antigens. *Rheumatology* (Oxford). 2001 Oct;40(10):1175-9 rheumatology.oxfordjournals.org/cgi/reprint/40/10/1175

[96] "The data provide evidence that dietary modification may be of clinical benefit for certain RA patients, and that this benefit may be related to a reduction in immunoreactivity to food antigens eliminated by the change in diet." Hafstrom I, Ringertz B, et al. A vegan diet free of gluten improves the signs and symptoms of rheumatoid arthritis: the effects on arthritis correlate with a reduction in antibodies to food antigens. *Rheumatology* (Oxford). 2001 Oct;40(10):1175-9

[97] "Despite the increased AGA [antigliadin antibodies] positivity found distinctively in patients with recent-onset RA, none of the RA patients showed clear evidence of coeliac disease." Paimela L, Kurki P, Leirisalo-Repo M, Piirainen H. Gliadin immune reactivity in patients with rheumatoid arthritis. Clin Exp Rheumatol. 1995 Sep-Oct;13(5):603-7

[98] "The median IgA antigliadin ELISA index was 7.1 (range 2.1-22.4) for the RA group and 3.1 (range 0.3-34.9) for the controls (p = 0.0001)." Koot et al. Elevated level of IgA gliadin antibodies in patients with rheumatoid arthritis. *Clin Exp Rheumatol*. 1989 Nov-Dec;7(6):623-6

[99] Seaman DR. The diet-induced proinflammatory state: a cause of chronic pain and other degenerative diseases? *J Manipulative Physiol Ther*. 2002 Mar-Apr;25(3):168-79

[100] Hagfors L, Nilsson I, Skoldstam L, Johansson G. Fat intake and composition of fatty acids in serum phospholipids in a randomized, controlled, Mediterranean dietary intervention study on patients with rheumatoid arthritis. *Nutr Metab* (Lond). 2005 Oct 10;2:26 nutritionandmetabolism.com/content/2/1/26

[101] Liu. Health benefits of fruit and vegetables from additive and synergistic combinations of phytochemicals. *Am J Clin Nutr* 2003:517S-520S ajcn.org/cgi/content/full/78/3/517S

[102] "Significant alteration in the intestinal flora was observed when the patients changed from omnivorous to vegan diet. ... This finding of an association between intestinal flora and disease activity may have implications for our understanding of how diet can affect RA." Peltonen et al. Changes of faecal flora in rheumatoid arthritis during fasting and one-year vegetarian diet. *Br J Rheumatol*. 1994 Jul;33(7):638-43

[103] Toivanen P, Eerola E. A vegan diet changes the intestinal flora. *Rheumatology* (Oxford). 2002 Aug;41(8):950-1 rheumatology.oxfordjournals.org/cgi/reprint/41/8/950

[104] "We conclude that a vegan diet changes the faecal microbial flora in RA patients, and changes in the faecal flora are associated with improvement in RA activity." Peltonen et al. Faecal microbial flora and disease activity in rheumatoid arthritis during a vegan diet. *Br J Rheumatol*. 1997 Jan;36(1):64-8 rheumatology.oxfordjournals.org/cgi/reprint/36/1/64

[105] Aljada et al. Increase in intranuclear nuclear factor kappaB and decrease in inhibitor kappaB in mononuclear cells after a mixed meal. *Am J Clin Nutr*. 2004 Apr;79(4):682-90

[106] "The ability of therapeutic fasts to break metabolic vicious cycles may also contribute to the efficacy of fasting in the treatment of type 2 diabetes and autoimmune disorders." McCarty MF. A preliminary fast may potentiate response to a subsequent low-salt, low-fat vegan diet in the management of hypertension - fasting as a strategy for breaking metabolic vicious cycles. *Med Hypotheses*. 2003 May;60(5):624-33

[107] Ramakrishnan et al. Beneficial effects of fasting and low carbohydrate diet in D-lactic acidosis associated with short-bowel syndrome. *JPEN J Parenter Enteral Nutr*. 1985 May-Jun;9(3):361-3

[108] Trollmo C, Verdrengh M, Tarkowski A. Fasting enhances mucosal antigen specific B cell responses in rheumatoid arthritis. *Ann Rheum Dis*. 1997 Feb;56(2):130-4

[109] "An association was found between improvement in inflammatory activity of the joints and enhancement of neutrophil bactericidal capacity. Fasting appears to improve the clinical status of patients with RA." Uden AM, Trang L, Venizelos N, Palmblad J. Neutrophil functions and clinical performance after total fasting in patients with rheumatoid arthritis. *Ann Rheum Dis*. 1983 Feb;42(1):45-51

[110] "We thus conclude that a reduced ability to generate cytotaxins, reduced release of enzyme, and reduced leukotriene formation from RA neutrophils, together with an altered fatty acid composition of membrane phospholipids, may be mechanisms for the decrease of inflammatory symptoms that results from fasting." Hafstrom et al. Effects of fasting on disease activity, neutrophil function, fatty acid composition, and leukotriene biosynthesis in patients with rheumatoid arthritis. *Arthritis Rheum*. 1988 May;31(5):585-92

[111] "The results indicate that, unlike lactovegetarian diet, fasting may ameliorate the disease activity and reduce both the intestinal and the non-intestinal permeability in rheumatoid arthritis." Sundqvist T, et al. Influence of fasting on intestinal permeability and disease activity in patients with rheumatoid arthritis. *Scand J Rheumatol*. 1982;11(1):33-8

electron transport chain (mETC) for enhanced mitochondrial function and efficiency. **In case reports and clinical trials, short-term fasting (or protein-sparing fasting) has been documented as safe and effective treatment for SLE[112], RA[113], and non-rheumatic diseases such as chronic severe hypertension[114], moderate hypertension[115], obesity[116,117], type-2 diabetes[118], and epilepsy.[119]**

o **Broad-spectrum fatty acid therapy with ALA, EPA, DHA, GLA and oleic acid:** Fatty acid supplementation should be delivered in the form of combination therapy with ALA, GLA, DHA, and EPA. Given at doses of 3,000 – 9,000 mg per day, ALA from flaxseed oil has impressive anti-inflammatory benefits demonstrated by its ability to halve prostaglandin production in humans.[120] **Numerous studies have demonstrated the benefit of GLA in the treatment of rheumatoid arthritis when used at doses between 500 mg – 4,000 mg per day.[121,122] Fish oil provides EPA and DHA which have well-proven anti-inflammatory benefits in rheumatoid arthritis[123,124,125] and lupus.[126,127]** ALA, EPA, DHA, and GLA need to be provided in the form of supplements; when using high doses of therapeutic oils, *liquid* supplements that can be mixed in juice or a smoothie are generally more convenient and palatable than are *capsules*. For example, at the upper end of oral fatty acid administration, the patient may be consuming as much as one-quarter cup per day of fatty acid supplementation; this same dose administered in the form of pills would require at least 72 capsules to attain the equivalent doses of ALA, EPA, DHA, and GLA. Therapeutic amounts of oleic acid can be obtained from generous use of olive oil, preferably on fresh vegetables. Supplementation with polyunsaturated fatty acids warrants increased intake of antioxidants from diet, from fruit and vegetable juices, and from properly formulated supplements. Since patients with systemic inflammation are generally in a pro-oxidative state, consideration must be given to the timing and starting dose of fatty acid supplementation and the need for antioxidant protection; some patients should start with a low dose of fatty acid supplementation until inflammation and the hyperoxidative state have been reduced. Clinicians must realize that fatty acids are not clinically or biochemically interchangeable and that one fatty acid does not substitute for another; each of the health-promoting fatty acids—ALA, GLA, EPA, DHA, and oleic acid—must be supplied in order for its benefits to be obtained; imbalanced supplementation causes or exacerbates biochemical imbalances and produces suboptimal results.[128]

o **Vitamin D3 supplementation with physiologic doses and/or tailored to serum 25(OH)D levels:** Vitamin D deficiency is common in the general population and is even more common in patients with chronic illness and chronic musculoskeletal pain.[129] Correction of vitamin D deficiency supports normal immune function against infection and provides a clinically significant anti-inflammatory[130] and analgesic benefit

[112] Fuhrman et al. Brief case reports of medically supervised water-only fasting associated with remission of autoimmune disease. *Altern Ther Health Med* 2002 Jul-Aug:112,110-1

[113] "Association was found between improvement in inflammatory activity of joints and enhancement of neutrophil bactericidal capacity. Fasting appears to improve the clinical status of patients with RA." Uden et al. Neutrophil functions and clinical performance after total fasting in patients with rheumatoid arthritis. *Ann Rheum Dis* 1983 Feb:45-51

[114] "The average reduction in blood pressure was 37/13 mm Hg, with the greatest decrease being observed for subjects with the most severe hypertension. Patients with stage 3 hypertension (those with systolic blood pressure greater than 180 mg Hg, diastolic blood pressure greater than 110 mg Hg, or both) had an average reduction of 60/17 mm Hg at the conclusion of treatment." Goldhamer A, Lisle D, Parpia B, Anderson SV, Campbell TC. Medically supervised water-only fasting in the treatment of hypertension. *J Manipulative Physiol Ther.* 2001 Jun;24(5):335-9 healthpromoting.com/335-339Goldhamer115263.QXD.pdf

[115] "RESULTS: Approximately 82% of the subjects achieved BP at or below 120/80 mm Hg by the end of the treatment program. The mean BP reduction was 20/7 mm Hg, with the greatest decrease being observed for subjects with the highest baseline BP." Goldhamer et al. Medically supervised water-only fasting in the treatment of borderline hypertension. *J Altern Complement Med.* 2002 Oct;8(5):643-50

[116] Vertes V, Genuth SM, Hazelton IM. Supplemented fasting as a large-scale outpatient program. *JAMA.* 1977 Nov 14;238(20):2151-3

[117] Bauman WA, et al. Early and long-term effects of acute caloric deprivation in obese diabetic patients. *Am J Med.* 1988 Jul;85(1):38-46

[118] Goldhamer AC. Initial cost of care results in medically supervised water-only fasting for treating high blood pressure and diabetes. *J Altern Complement Med.* 2002 Dec;8(6):696-7 healthpromoting.com/Articles/pdf/Study%2032.pdf

[119] "The ketogenic diet should be considered as alternative therapy for children with difficult-to-control seizures. It is more effective than many of the new anticonvulsant medications and is well tolerated by children and families when it is effective." Freeman JM, Vining EP, Pillas DJ, Pyzik PL, Casey JC, Kelly LM. The efficacy of the ketogenic diet-1998: a prospective evaluation of intervention in 150 children. *Pediatrics.* 1998 Dec;102(6):1358-63 pediatrics.aappublications.org/cgi/reprint/102/6/1358

[120] Adam et al. Effect of alpha-linolenic acid in human diet on linoleic acid metabolism and prostaglandin biosynthesis. *J Lipid Res.* 1986 Apr;27:421-6 jlr.org/cgi/reprint/27/4/421

[121] "Other results showed a significant reduction in morning stiffness with gamma-linolenic acid at 3 months and reduction in pain and articular index at 6 months with olive oil." Brzeski et al. Evening primrose oil in patients with rheumatoid arthritis and side-effects of non-steroidal anti-inflammatory drugs. *Br J Rheumatol.* 1991 Oct;30(5):370-2

[122] Rothman D, DeLuca P, Zurier RB. Botanical lipids: effects on inflammation, immune responses, and rheumatoid arthritis. *Semin Arthritis Rheum.* 1995 Oct;25(2):87-96

[123] Adam O, et al. Anti-inflammatory effects of a low arachidonic acid diet and fish oil in patients with rheumatoid arthritis. *Rheumatol Int.* 2003 Jan;23(1):27-36

[124] Lau CS, Morley KD, Belch JJ. Effects of fish oil supplementation on non-steroidal anti-inflammatory drug requirement in patients with mild rheumatoid arthritis--a double-blind placebo controlled study. *Br J Rheumatol.* 1993 Nov;32(11):982-9

[125] Kremer et al. Fish-oil fatty acid supplementation in active rheumatoid arthritis. A double-blinded, controlled, crossover study. *Ann Intern Med.* 1987 Apr;106(4):497-503

[126] Walton AJ, et al. Dietary fish oil and the severity of symptoms in patients with systemic lupus erythematosus. *Ann Rheum Dis.* 1991 Jul;50(7):463-6

[127] Duffy et al. The clinical effect of dietary supplementation with omega-3 fish oils and/or copper in systemic lupus erythematosus. *J Rheumatol.* 2004 Aug;31(8):1551-6

[128] Vasquez A. New Insights into Fatty Acid Supplementation and Its Effect on Eicosanoid Production and Genetic Expression. *Nutritional Perspectives* 2005; January: 5-16

[129] Plotnikoff GA, Quigley JM. Prevalence of severe hypovitaminosis D in patients with persistent, nonspecific musculoskeletal pain. *Mayo Clin Proc.* 2003 Dec;78(12):1463-70

[130] Timms PM, Mannan N, Hitman GA, Noonan K, Mills PG, Syndercombe-Court D, Aganna E, Price CP, Boucher BJ. Circulating MMP9, vitamin D and variation in the TIMP-1 response with VDR genotype: mechanisms for inflammatory damage in chronic disorders? *QJM.* 2002 Dec;95(12):787-96 qjmed.oxfordjournals.org/cgi/content/full/95/12/787

in patients with back pain[131] and limb pain.[132] Reasonable daily doses for children and adults are 1,000-2,000 and 4,000 IU, respectively.[133] Deficiency and response to treatment are monitored with serum 25(OH)vitamin D while safety is monitored with serum calcium; inflammatory granulomatous diseases and certain drugs such as hydrochlorothiazide greatly increase the propensity for hypercalcemia and warrant increment dosing and frequent monitoring of serum calcium. Vitamin D2 (ergocalciferol) is not a human nutrient and should not be used in clinical practice.

- **INFECTIONS & DYSBIOSIS: ❶ antimicrobial treatments, ❷ immunorestoration, ❸ immunotolerance via Treg induction** Essentially all autoimmune/rheumatic disorders are associated with microbial colonization and intolerance to same; the presence of persistent microbial colonization is *prima facie* evidence of immunosuppression. The eight areas of multifocal dysbiosis are: ❶ sinorespiratory, ❷ orodental, ❸ gastrointestinal, ❹ genitourinary, ❺ tissue/blood, ❻ dermal, ❼ environmental, and ❽ endomicrobial.

  o Gastrointestinal dysbiosis: **All patients with rheumatoid arthritis have gastrointestinal dysbiosis until proven otherwise by the combination of 1) three-sample comprehensive parasitology examinations performed by a specialty laboratory and 2) clinical response to at least two 2-4 week courses of broad-spectrum antimicrobial treatment.** Yeast, bacteria, and parasites are treated as indicated based on identification and sensitivity results from comprehensive parasitology assessments. Patients taking immunosuppressant drugs such as corticosteroids/prednisone have increased risk of intestinal bacterial overgrowth and translocation.[134,135] Dysbiotic loci should be investigated as discussed in Chapter 4.2.

    ▪ Cell wall fragments from major residents of the human intestinal flora induce chronic arthritis in rats (*J Rheumatol* 1989 Aug[136]): "A single intraperitoneal injection of cell wall fragments from *Eubacterium aerofaciens* or *Bifidobacterium* species induced persistent chronic arthritis, in contrast to those from *Eubacterium rectale*, *Clostridium species* and *Lactobacillus leichmanii*. The results show that cell wall fragments of major residents from the human fecal flora can induce chronic arthritis in the rat and support the hypothesis that normal human intestinal flora plays a role in the induction of arthritis in man."

    ▪ Normal intestinal microbiota in the etiopathogenesis of rheumatoid arthritis (*Ann Rheum Dis* 2003 Sep[137]): The ability of bacterial cell walls to induce chronic, erosive arthritis was first described in the rat by using *Streptococcus pyogenes*. Self-perpetuating arthritis, closely resembling human rheumatoid arthritis by histological criteria, develops in susceptible rat strains after a single intraperitoneal injection of the bacterial cell wall. In addition to *Streptococcus pyogenes*, several bacterial species representing *Lactobacillus*, *Bifidobacterium*, *Eubacterium*, *Collinsella*, and *Clostridium* have been observed to have a similar ability.

  o Orodental dysbiosis: The systemic inflammatory response triggered by subclinical oral/dental "infections" is now believed to exacerbate conditions associated with inflammation, such as cardiovascular disease and diabetes mellitus.[138] Patients with RA have heightened antibody levels against common oral bacteria. IgG levels against *Porphyromonas gingivalis*, *Prevotella melaninogenica*, *Bacteroides forsythus*, and *Prevotella intermedia* were found to be significantly higher in RA patients when compared with those of controls.[139] In the first human clinical trial to test the hypothesis that treatment of orodental dysbiosis would provide subjective and objective clinical benefits for patients with RA, AlKatma et al[140] showed that **periodontal treatment consisting of scaling/root planing and oral hygiene instruction reduced symptom scores and ESR levels in patients with RA.**

---

[131] Al Faraj S, Al Mutairi K. Vitamin D deficiency and chronic low back pain in Saudi Arabia. *Spine*. 2003 Jan 15;28(2):177-9

[132] Masood et al. Persistent limb pain and raised serum alkaline phosphatase earliest markers of subclinical hypovitaminosis D. *Indian J Physiol Pharmacol*. 1989 Oct-Dec; 259-61

[133] Vasquez et al. Clinical importance of vitamin D: paradigm shift for all healthcare providers. *Altern Ther Health Med*. 2004 Sep;10(5):28-36 ichnfm.academia.edu/AlexVasquez

[134] "A 63-year-old man with systemic lupus erythematosus and selective IgA deficiency developed intractable diarrhoea the day after treatment with prednisone, 50 mg daily, was started. The diarrhoea was considered to be caused by bacterial overgrowth and was later successfully treated with doxycycline." Denison H, Wallerstedt S. Bacterial overgrowth after high-dose corticosteroid treatment. *Scand J Gastroenterol*. 1989 Jun;24(5):561-4

[135] "These bacteria also translocated to the mesenteric lymph nodes in mice injected with cyclophosphamide or prednisone." Berg RD, Wommack E, Deitch EA. Immunosuppression and intestinal bacterial overgrowth synergistically promote bacterial translocation. *Arch Surg*. 1988 Nov;123(11):1359-64

[136] Severijnen AJ, et al. Cell wall fragments from major residents of the human intestinal flora induce chronic arthritis in rats. *J Rheumatol*. 1989 Aug;16(8):1061-8

[137] Toivanen P. Normal intestinal microbiota in the aetiopathogenesis of rheumatoid arthritis. *Ann Rheum Dis*. 2003 Sep;62(9):807-11

[138] Amar S, Han X. The impact of periodontal infection on systemic diseases. *Med Sci Monit*. 2003 Dec;9(12):RA291-9 medscimonit.com/pub/vol_9/no_12/3776.pdf

[139] Ogrendik M, Kokino S, Ozdemir F, Bird PS, Hamlet S. Serum antibodies to oral anaerobic bacteria in patients with rheumatoid arthritis. *MedGenMed*. 2005 Jun 16;7(2):2

[140] "There was a statistically significant difference in DAS28 (4.3 +/- 1.6 vs. 5.1 +/- 1.2) and erythrocyte sedimentation rate (31.4 +/- 24.3 vs. 42.7 +/- 22) between the treatment and the control groups." Al-Katma MK, et al. Control of periodontal infection reduces the severity of active rheumatoid arthritis. *J Clin Rheumatol*. 2007 Jun;13(3):134-7

○ <u>Genitourinary dysbiosis</u>: Microbial contamination of the genitourinary tract can cause a systemic pro-inflammatory arthritogenic response in susceptible individuals; **in a study of 234 patients with inflammatory arthritis, 44% of patients had subclinical genitourinary colonization, mostly due to *Chlamydia, Mycoplasma*, or *Ureaplasma*.**[141]

- ┃**NUTRITIONAL IMMUNOMODULATION: Treg induction for modulation of Th-1/2/17 inflammation**┃
  Nutrients and therapeutic approaches that promote Treg or IL-10 induction and/or Th-17, IL-17 suppression include 1) mitochondrial optimization and mTOR suppression, 2) biotin, 3) vitamin E, 4) sodium avoidance, 5) transgenic/GMO food avoidance, 6) probiotics, 7) lipoic acid, 8) vitamin A, 9) inflammation reduction, 10) vitamin D, 11) fatty acid supplementation with GLA and n3, 12) infection and dysbiosis remediation, 13) green tea EGCG. Acronym: MiBESTPLAIDFIG, as detailed and substantiated in Chapter 4.

- ┃**DYSMETABOLISM & DYSFUNCTIONAL MITOCHONDRIA: MitoDys, ERS-UPR, AGE/RAGE, hyperglycemia and ceramide**┃ The major clinical considerations in this section are mitochondrial dysfunction, endoplasmic reticulum stress, unfolded protein response, TLR activation, and the dysmetabolic effects of sustained hyperglycemia and hyperinsulinemia and resultant oxidative stress, inflammation, RAGE activation, and accumulation of AGE, palmitate and ceramide. The review of this information in Chapter 4 covered approximately 30 interventions relevant to dysmetabolism, mitochondrial dysfunction, ERS-UPR, etc; these will not be reviewed here except to mention those most commonly, easily, empirically, synergistically, and effectively used: 1) low-carbohydrate diet with 2) moderate exercise, 3) CoQ-10, 4) acetyl-carnitine with 5) lipoic acid, 6) NAC, 7) resveratrol, and 8) melatonin.

- ┃**STYLE OF LIVING (LIFESTYLE) & SPECIAL CONSIDERATIONS: <u>S</u>leep optimization, <u>S</u>ocioPsychology, <u>S</u>tress management/avoidance, <u>S</u>omatic treatments, <u>S</u>pecial <u>S</u>upplementation, <u>S</u>weat/exercise, <u>S</u>auna/detoxification, <u>S</u>urgery, <u>S</u>tamp your passport and vacate current reality, <u>S</u>ensory deprivation therapy**┃
  This is a buffet of mostly lifestyle-based interventions yet also including considerations such as somatic treatments, additional supplementation, and surgery.
  - ○ <u>Self-expression and therapeutic writing</u>: Limited evidence indicates that self-expressive writing can significantly reduce symptomatology in patients with RA.[142]

- ┃**ENDOCRINE IMBALANCE & OPTIMIZATION: Prolactin, Insulin, Estrogen, DHEA, Cortisol, Testosterone, Thyroid**┃ Common hormonal imbalances seen among autoimmune/inflammatory patients are: ❶ *elevated* prolactin, ❷ *elevated* estrogen, ❸ *elevated* insulin, and ❹ *reduced* DHEA, ❺ *reduced* cortisol, and ❻ *reduced* testosterone; see Chapter 4 for discussion of these hormones and respective interventions. Thyroid evaluation (patient + labs) should be comprehensive, as discussed in Chapter 1, with a low threshold for empiric treatment.
  - ○ <u>Estradiol</u>: Men with rheumatoid arthritis show an excess of estradiol and a decrease in DHEA, and the excess estrogen is proportional to the degree of inflammation.[143]
  - ○ <u>Testosterone (insufficiency)</u>: Androgen deficiencies predispose to, are exacerbated by, and contribute to autoimmune/inflammatory disorders. **A large proportion of men with SLE or RA have low testosterone**[144,145] and suffer the effects of hypogonadism: fatigue, weakness, depression, slow healing, low libido, and difficulties with sexual performance. Testosterone levels may rise following DHEA

---

[141] "Urogenital swab cultures showed a microbial infection in 44% of the patients with oligoarthritis (15% Chlamydia, 14% Mycoplasma, 28% Ureaplasma), whereas in the control group only 26% had a positive result (4% Chlamydia, 7% Mycoplasma, 21% Ureaplasma)." Erlacher et al. Reactive arthritis: urogenital swab culture is the only useful diagnostic method for the detection of the arthritogenic infection in extra-articularly asymptomatic patients with undifferentiated oligoarthritis. *Br J Rheumatol.* 1995 Sep;34(9):838-42

[142] "Rheumatoid arthritis patients in the experimental group showed improvements in overall disease activity (a mean reduction in disease severity from 1.65 to 1.19 [28%] on a scale of 0 [asymptomatic] to 4 [very severe] at the 4-month follow-up; P=.001), whereas control group patients did not change." Smyth JM, Stone AA, Hurewitz A, Kaell A. Effects of writing about stressful experiences on symptom reduction in patients with asthma or rheumatoid arthritis: a randomized trial. *JAMA.* 1999 Apr 14;281(14):1304-9

[143] "RESULTS: DHEAS and estrone concentrations were lower and estradiol was higher in patients compared with healthy controls. DHEAS differed between RF positive and RF negative patients. Estrone did not correlate with any disease variable, whereas estradiol correlated strongly and positively with all measured indices of inflammation." Tengstrand B, Carlstrom K, Fellander-Tsai L, Hafstrom I. Abnormal levels of serum dehydroepiandrosterone, estrone, and estradiol in men with rheumatoid arthritis: high correlation between serum estradiol and current degree of inflammation. *J Rheumatol.* 2003 Nov;30(11):2338-43

[144] Karagiannis A, Harsoulis F. Gonadal dysfunction in systemic diseases. *Eur J Endocrinol.* 2005 Apr;152(4):501-13 eje-online.org/cgi/content/full/152/4/501

[145] "...patients with rheumatoid arthritis showed significantly lower serum testosterone and derived free testosterone concentrations and significantly higher serum LH and FSH concentrations compared with controls." Gordon et al. Androgenic status and sexual function in men with rheumatoid arthritis and ankylosing spondylitis. *Q J Med* 1986 Jul;671-9

supplementation (especially in women) and can be elevated in men by the use of anastrozole/Arimidex. Transdermal testosterone such as Androgel, Testim, or compounded formula can be applied as indicated.

- o **DHEA (insufficiency / supraphysiologic supplementation):** DHEA is an anti-inflammatory and immunoregulatory hormone that is commonly deficient in patients with autoimmunity and inflammatory arthritis.[146] DHEA levels are suppressed by prednisone[147], and DHEA supplementation has been shown to reverse the osteoporosis and loss of bone mass induced by corticosteroid treatment.[148] DHEA shows no acute or subacute toxicity even when used in supraphysiologic doses, even when used in sick patients. For example, in a study of 32 patients with HIV, DHEA doses of 750 mg – 2,250 mg per day were well-tolerated and produced no dose-limiting adverse effects.[149] This lack of toxicity compares favorably with any and all so-called "antirheumatic" drugs, nearly all of which show impressive comparable toxicity. **When used at doses of 200 mg per day, DHEA safely provides clinical benefit for patients with various autoimmune diseases, including ulcerative colitis, Crohn's disease[150], and SLE.[151]** In patients with SLE, DHEA supplementation allows for reduced dosing of prednisone (thus avoiding its adverse effects) while providing symptomatic improvement.[152] Optimal clinical response appears to correlate with serum levels that are supraphysiologic[153], and therefore treatment may be implemented with little regard for initial/baseline DHEA levels provided that the patient is free of contraindications, particularly high risk for sex-hormone-dependent malignancy. Other than mild adverse effects predictable with any androgen (namely voice deepening, transient acne, and increased facial hair), DHEA supplementation does not cause serious adverse effects[154], and it is appropriate for routine clinical use particularly when 1) the dose of DHEA is kept as low as possible, 2) duration is kept as short as possible, 3) other interventions are used to address the underlying cause of the disease, 4) the patient is deriving benefit, and 5) the risk-to-benefit ratio is favorable. Astute clinicians should anticipate that DHEA supplementation can increase testosterone and estradiol levels—the former with benefit and the latter with detriment in patients with autoimmunity; thus, serum levels of DHEA, testosterone, and estradiol (and potentially other estrogen metabolites) need to be reevaluated if DHEA is added to the daily regimen. Commonly, rheumatic patients will show an increase in estradiol following use of DHEA, and these over-producers of estrogen ("rapid converters") should be co-treated with an aromatase inhibitor if DHEA supplementation elevates estrogen levels, especially if testosterone levels are low.
- o **Prolactin and antiprolactin treatments:** Patients with RA and SLE have higher basal and stress-induced levels of prolactin compared with normal controls.[155,156] Men with RA have higher serum levels of prolactin, and these levels correlate with the severity and duration of the disorder.[157,158] Serum prolactin

[146] "DHEAS concentrations were significantly decreased in both women and men with inflammatory arthritis (IA) (P < 0.001)." Dessein et al. Hyposecretion of the adrenal androgen dehydroepiandrosterone sulfate and its relation to clinical variables in inflammatory arthritis. *Arthritis Res.* 2001;3(3):183-8 arthritis-research.com/content/3/3/183

[147] "Basal serum DHEA and DHEAS concentrations were suppressed to a greater degree than was cortisol during both daily and alternate day prednisone treatments. ...Thus, adrenal androgen secretion was more easily suppressed than was cortisol secretion by this low dose of glucocorticoid, but there was no advantage to alternate day therapy." Rittmaster et al. Effect of daily and alternate day low dose prednisone on serum cortisol and adrenal androgens in hirsute women. *J Clin Endocrinol Metab.* 1988 Aug;67(2):400-3

[148] "CONCLUSION: Prasterone treatment prevented BMD loss and significantly increased BMD at both the lumbar spine and total hip in female patients with SLE receiving exogenous glucocorticoids." Mease PJ, Ginzler EM, Gluck OS, Schiff M, Goldman A, Greenwald M, Cohen S, Egan R, Quarles BJ, Schwartz KE. Effects of prasterone on bone mineral density in women with systemic lupus erythematosus receiving chronic glucocorticoid therapy. *J Rheumatol.* 2005 Apr;32(4):616-21

[149] "Thirty-one subjects were evaluated and monitored for safety and tolerance. The oral drug was administered three times daily in doses ranging from 750 mg/day to 2,250 mg/day for 16 weeks. ... The drug was well tolerated and no dose-limiting side effects were noted." Dyner TS, Lang W, Geaga J, et al. An open-label dose-escalation trial of oral dehydroepiandrosterone tolerance and pharmacokinetics in patients with HIV disease. *J Acquir Immune Defic Syndr.* 1993 May;6(5):459-65

[150] "CONCLUSIONS: In a pilot study, dehydroepiandrosterone was effective and safe in patients with refractory Crohn's disease or ulcerative colitis." Andus T, et al. Patients with refractory Crohn's disease or ulcerative colitis respond to dehydroepiandrosterone: a pilot study. *Aliment Pharmacol Ther.* 2003 Feb;17(3):409-14

[151] "CONCLUSION: The overall results confirm that DHEA treatment was well-tolerated, significantly reduced the number of SLE flares, and improved patient's global assessment of disease activity." Chang DM, Lan JL, Lin HY, Luo SF. Dehydroepiandrosterone treatment of women with mild-to-moderate systemic lupus erythematosus: a multicenter randomized, double-blind, placebo-controlled trial. *Arthritis Rheum.* 2002 Nov;46(11):2924-7

[152] "CONCLUSION: Among women with lupus disease activity, reducing the dosage of prednisone to < or = 7.5 mg/day for a sustained period of time while maintaining stabilization or a reduction of disease activity was possible in a significantly greater proportion of patients treated with oral prasterone, 200 mg once daily, compared with patients treated with placebo." Petri et al. Effects of prasterone on corticosteroid requirements of women with systemic lupus erythematosus. *Arthritis Rheum.* 2002 Jul;46(7):1820-9

[153] "CONCLUSION: The clinical response to DHEA was not clearly dose dependent. Serum levels of DHEA and DHEAS correlated only weakly with lupus outcomes, but suggested an optimum serum DHEAS of 1000 microg/dl." Barry NN, McGuire JL, van Vollenhoven RF. Dehydroepiandrosterone in systemic lupus erythematosus: relationship between dosage, serum levels, and clinical response. *J Rheumatol.* 1998 Dec;25(12):2352-6

[154] Tierney ML. McPhee SJ, Papadakis MA. *Current Medical Diagnosis and Treatment 2006. 45th edition.* New York; Lange Medical Books: 2006, page 1721

[155] Dostal et al. Serum prolactin stress values in patients with systemic lupus erythematosus. *Ann Rheum Dis.* 2003 May;62(5):487-8 ard.bmjjournals.com/cgi/content/full/62/5/487

[156] "RESULTS: A significantly higher rate of elevated PRL levels was found in SLE patients (40.0%) compared with the healthy controls (14.8%). No proof was found of association with the presence of anti-ds-DNA or with specific organ involvement. Similarly, elevated PRL levels were found in RA patients (39.3%)." Moszkorzova L, Lacinova Z, Marek J, Musilova L, Dohnalova A, Dostal C. Hyperprolactinaemia in patients with systemic lupus erythematosus. *Clin Exp Rheumatol.* 2002 Nov-Dec;20(6):807-12

[157] "CONCLUSION: Men with RA have high serum PRL levels and concentrations increase with longer disease evolution and worse functional stage." Mateo L, Nolla JM, Bonnin MR, Navarro MA, Roig-Escofet D. High serum prolactin levels in men with rheumatoid arthritis. *J Rheumatol.* 1998 Nov;25(11):2077-82

[158] "Male patients affected by RA showed high serum PRL levels. The serum PRL concentration was found to be increased in relation to the duration and the activity of the disease. Serum PRL levels do not seem to have any relationship with the BMD, at least in RA." Seriolo B, Ferretti V, Sulli A, Fasciolo D, Cutolo M. Serum prolactin concentrations in male patients with rheumatoid arthritis. *Ann N Y Acad Sci.* 2002 Jun;966:258-62

is the standard assessment of prolactin status. Since elevated prolactin may be a sign of pituitary tumor, assessment for headaches, visual deficits, and other abnormalities of pituitary hormones (e.g., GH and TSH) should be performed; CT or MRI must be considered. Patients with prolactin levels less than 100 ng/mL and normal CT/MRI findings can be managed conservatively with effective prolactin-lowering treatment and annual radiologic assessment (less necessary with favorable serum response).[159, see review 160] Specific treatment options include the following:

- Thyroid hormone: Hypothyroidism frequently causes hyperprolactinemia which is reversible upon effective treatment of hypothyroidism. Obviously therefore, thyroid status should be evaluated in all patients with hyperprolactinemia. Thyroid assessment and treatment is reviewed in Chapter 4 and later in this section.
- *Vitex astus-cagnus* and other supporting botanicals and nutrients: **Vitex lowers serum prolactin in humans**[161,162] **via a dopaminergic effect.**[163] Vitex is considered safe for clinical use; mild and reversible adverse effects possibly associated with Vitex include nausea, headache, gastrointestinal disturbances, menstrual disorders, acne, pruritus and erythematous rash. No drug interactions are known, but given the herb's dopaminergic effect it should probably be used with some caution in patients treated with dopamine antagonists such as the so-called antipsychotic drugs.[164,165] Bone[166] stated that daily doses can range from 500 mg to 2,000 mg DHE (dry herb equivalent) and can be tailored to the suppression of prolactin. Due at least in part to its content of L-dopa, *Mucuna pruriens* **shows clinical dopaminergic activity** as evidenced by its effectiveness in Parkinson's disease[167]; up to 15-30 gm/d of mucuna has been used clinically but doses will be dependent on preparation and phytoconcentration. **Triptolide and other extracts from** *Tripterygium wilfordii* **Hook F exert clinically significant anti-inflammatory action in patients with rheumatoid arthritis**[168,169] **and also offer protection to dopaminergic neurons.**[170,171] Ironically, even though tyrosine is the nutritional precursor to dopamine with evidence of clinical effectiveness (e.g., narcolepsy[172], enhancement of memory[173] and cognition[174]), **supplementation with tyrosine appears to actually increase rather**

[159] Beers MH, Berkow R (eds). *Merck Manual. 17th Edition.* Whitehouse Station; Merck Research Laboratories 1999 Page 77-78
[160] Serri O, Chik CL, Ur E, Ezzat S. Diagnosis and management of hyperprolactinemia. *CMAJ.* 2003 Sep 16;169(6):575-81 cmaj.ca/cgi/content/full/169/6/575
[161] "Since AC extracts were shown to have beneficial effects on premenstrual mastodynia serum prolactin levels in such patients were also studied in one double-blind, placebo-controlled clinical study. Serum prolactin levels were indeed reduced in the patients treated with the extract." Wuttke W, Jarry H, Christoffel V, Spengler B, Seidlova-Wuttke D. Chaste tree (Vitex agnus-castus)--pharmacology and clinical indications. *Phytomedicine.* 2003 May;10(4):348-57
[162] German abstract from Medline: "The prolactin release was reduced after 3 months, shortened luteal phases were normalised and deficits in the luteal progesterone synthesis were eliminated." Milewicz A, Gejdel E, Sworen H, Sienkiewicz K, Jedrzejak J, Teucher T, Schmitz H. [Vitex agnus castus extract in the treatment of luteal phase defects due to latent hyperprolactinemia. Results of a randomized placebo-controlled double-blind study] *Arzneimittelforschung.* 1993 Jul;43(7):752-6
[163] "Our results indicate a dopaminergic effect of Vitex agnus-castus extracts and suggest additional pharmacological actions via opioid receptors." Meier B, Berger D, Hoberg E, Sticher O, Schaffner W. Pharmacological activities of Vitex agnus-castus extracts in vitro. *Phytomedicine.* 2000 Oct;7(5):373-81
[164] "The majority of patients in each group discontinued their assigned treatment owing to inefficacy or intolerable side effects or for other reasons." Lieberman JA, Stroup TS, McEvoy JP, Swartz MS, Rosenheck RA, Perkins DO, Keefe RS, Davis SM, Davis CE, Lebowitz BD, Severe J, Hsiao JK; Clinical Antipsychotic Trials of Intervention Effectiveness (CATIE) Investigators. Effectiveness of antipsychotic drugs in patients with chronic schizophrenia. *N Engl J Med.* 2005 Sep 22;353(12):1209-23
[165] Whitaker R. The case against antipsychotic drugs: a 50-year record of doing more harm than good. *Med Hypotheses.* 2004;62(1):5-13
[166] "In conditions such as endometriosis and fibroids, for which a significant estrogen antagonist effect is needed, doses of at least 2 g/day DHE may be required and typically are used by professional herbalists." Bone K. New Insights into Chaste Tree. *Nutritional Wellness* 2005 November nutritionalwellness.com/archives/2005/nov/11_bone.php
[167] "CONCLUSIONS: The rapid onset of action and longer on time without concomitant increase in dyskinesias on mucuna seed powder formulation suggest that this natural source of L-dopa might possess advantages over conventional L-dopa preparations in the long term management of PD." Katzenschlager R, et al. Mucuna pruriens in Parkinson's disease: a double blind clinical and pharmacological study. *J Neurol Neurosurg Psychiatry.* 2004 Dec;75(12):1672-7
[168] "The ethanol/ethyl acetate extract of TWHF shows therapeutic benefit in patients with treatment-refractory RA. At therapeutic dosages, the TWHF extract was well tolerated by most patients in this study." Tao X, Younger J, Fan FZ, Wang B, Lipsky PE. Benefit of an extract of Tripterygium Wilfordii Hook F in patients with rheumatoid arthritis: a double-blind, placebo-controlled study. *Arthritis Rheum.* 2002 Jul;46(7):1735-43
[169] "The EA extract of TWHF at dosages up to 570 mg/day appeared to be safe, and doses > 360 mg/day were associated with clinical benefit in patients with RA." Tao et al. A phase I study of ethyl acetate extract of the Chinese antirheumatic herb Tripterygium wilfordii hook F in rheumatoid arthritis. *J Rheumatol.* 2001 Oct;28(10):2160-7
[170] "Our data suggests that triptolide may protect dopaminergic neurons from LPS-induced injury and its efficiency in inhibiting microglia activation may underlie the mechanism." Li et al. Triptolide, a Chinese herbal extract, protects dopaminergic neurons from inflammation-mediated damage through inhibition of microglial activation. *J Neuroimmunol.* 2004 Mar;148(1-2):24-31
[171] "Moreover, tripchlorolide markedly prevented the decrease in amount of dopamine in the striatum of model rats. Taken together, our data provide the first evidence that tripchlorolide acts as a neuroprotective molecule that rescues MPP+ or axotomy-induced degeneration of dopaminergic neurons, which may imply its therapeutic potential for Parkinson's disease." Li FQ, Cheng et al. Neurotrophic and neuroprotective effects of tripchlorolide, an extract of Chinese herb Tripterygium wilfordii Hook F, on dopaminergic neurons. *Exp Neurol.* 2003 Jan;179(1):28-37
[172] "Of twenty-eight visual analogue scales rating mood and arousal, the subjects' ratings in the tyrosine treatment (9 g daily) and placebo periods differed significantly for only three (less tired, less drowsy, more alert)." Elwes et al. Treatment of narcolepsy with L-tyrosine: double-blind placebo-controlled trial. *Lancet.* 1989 Nov 4;2(8671):1067-9
[173] "Ten men and 10 women subjects underwent these batteries 1 h after ingesting 150 mg/kg of L-tyrosine or placebo. Administration of tyrosine significantly enhanced accuracy and decreased frequency of lost retrieval on the working memory task during the multiple task battery compared with placebo." Thomas JR, Lockwood PA, Singh A, Deuster PA. Tyrosine improves working memory in a multitasking environment. *Pharmacol Biochem Behav.* 1999 Nov;64(3):495-500
[174] "Ten subjects received five daily doses of a protein-rich drink containing 2 g tyrosine, and 11 subjects received a carbohydrate rich drink with the same amount of calories (255 kcal)." Deijen et al. Tyrosine improves cognitive performance and reduces blood pressure in cadets after one week of a combat training course. *Brain Res Bull.* 1999 Jan 15;48(2):203-9

than decrease prolactin levels[175]; therefore tyrosine should be used cautiously (if at all) in patients with systemic inflammation and elevated prolactin. Furthermore, the finding that **high-protein meals stimulate prolactin release**[176] may partly explain the benefits of vegetarian diets in the treatment of systemic inflammation; since vegetarian diets are comparatively low in protein compared to omnivorous diets, they may lead to a relative reduction in prolactin production due to lack of protein-induced prolactin stimulation.

- Bromocriptine: Bromocriptine has long been considered the pharmacologic treatment of choice for elevated prolactin.[177] Typical dose is 2.5 mg per day (effective against lupus[178]); gastrointestinal upset and sedation are common.[179] Clinical intervention with bromocriptine appears warranted in patients with RA, SLE, reactive arthritis, psoriatic arthritis, and probably multiple sclerosis and uveitis.[180] Data supporting bromocriptine vicariously supports cabergoline, the preferred agent.

- Cabergoline/Dostinex: Cabergoline/Dostinex is a newer dopamine agonist with few adverse effects; typical dose starts at 0.5 mg per week (0.25 mg twice per week).[181] Several studies have indicated that cabergoline is safer and more effective than bromocriptine for reducing prolactin levels[182] and the dose can often be reduced after successful prolactin reduction, allowing for reductions in cost and adverse effects.[183] Although fewer studies have been published supporting the antirheumatic benefits of cabergoline than bromocriptine, its antirheumatic benefits have been documented in a case report of a patient with unremitting RA[184] and more recently in a controlled trial.[185]

- **XENOBIOTIC ACCUMULATION & DETOXIFICATION: Chemical avoidance, nutritional support for detoxification pathways, urine alkalinization** The clinical relevance and pathogenic mechanisms of xenobiotic accumulation are irrefutably well documented and described. Clinical assessments include history, physical examination, and laboratory assessment (using serum, whole blood, urine or—rarely yet accurately—fat biopsy), and response to treatment. Treatments include nutritional support for Phases 1 and 2 of detoxification (e.g., oxidation and conjugation) and excretion via bile and urine; for the latter, urinary alkalinization is generally recommended. Chemical toxins can be bound in the gut using activated charcoal, cholestyramine, or *Chlorella*—all of these three treatments have documented safety and effectiveness for promoting removal/clearance of chemical xenobiotics. Clinically and empirically, phytochelatin (plant-derived peptides that bind toxic metals) concentrates appear safe and effective despite lack of conclusive published data supporting clinical use.

---

[175] "Tyrosine (when compared to placebo) had no effect on any sleep related measure, but it did stimulate prolactin release." Waters et al. A comparison of tyrosine against placebo, phentermine, caffeine, and D-amphetamine during sleep deprivation. *Nutr Neurosci.* 2003;6(4):221-35

[176] "Whereas carbohydrate meals had no discernible effects, high protein meals induced a large increase in both PRL and cortisol; high fat meals caused selective release of PRL." Ishizuka et al. Pituitary hormone release in response to food ingestion: evidence for neuroendocrine signals from gut to brain. *J Clin Endocrinol Metab.* 1983 Dec;57(6):1111-6

[177] Beers MH, Berkow R (eds). *Merck Manual. 17th Edition.* Whitehouse Station; Merck Research Laboratories 1999 Page 77-78

[178] "A prospective, double-blind, randomized, placebo-controlled study compared BRC at a fixed daily dosage of 2.5 mg with placebo... Long term treatment with a low dose of BRC appears to be a safe and effective means of decreasing SLE flares in SLE patients." Alvarez-Nemegyei et al. Bromocriptine in systemic lupus erythematosus: a double-blind, randomized, placebo-controlled study. *Lupus.* 1998;7(6):414-9

[179] Serri O, Chik CL, Ur E, Ezzat S. Diagnosis and management of hyperprolactinemia. *CMAJ.* 2003 Sep 16;169(6):575-81 cmaj.ca/cgi/content/full/169/6/575

[180] "...clinical observations and trials support the use of bromocriptine as a nonstandard primary or adjunctive therapy in the treatment of recalcitrant RA, SLE, Reiter's syndrome, and psoriatic arthritis and associated conditions unresponsive to traditional approaches." McMurray RW. Bromocriptine in rheumatic and autoimmune diseases. *Semin Arthritis Rheum.* 2001 Aug;31(1):21-32

[181] Serri O, Chik CL, Ur E, Ezzat S. Diagnosis and management of hyperprolactinemia. *CMAJ.* 2003 Sep 16;169(6):575-81 cmaj.ca/cgi/content/full/169/6/575

[182] "CONCLUSION: These data indicate that cabergoline is a very effective agent for lowering the prolactin levels in hyperprolactinemic patients and that it appears to offer considerable advantage over bromocriptine in terms of efficacy and tolerability." Sabuncu T, Arikan E, Tasan E, Hatemi H. Comparison of the effects of cabergoline and bromocriptine on prolactin levels in hyperprolactinemic patients. *Intern Med.* 2001 Sep;40(9):857-61

[183] "Cabergoline also normalized PRL in the majority of patients with known bromocriptine intolerance or -resistance. Once PRL secretion was adequately controlled, the dose of cabergoline could often be significantly decreased, which further reduced costs of therapy." Verhelst et al. Cabergoline in the treatment of hyperprolactinemia: a study in 455 patients. *J Clin Endocrinol Metab.* 1999 Jul;84(7):2518-22 jcem.endojournals.org/cgi/content/full/84/7/2518

[184] Erb N, Pace AV, Delamere JP, Kitas GD. Control of unremitting rheumatoid arthritis by the prolactin antagonist cabergoline. *Rheumatology* (Oxford). 2001 Feb;40(2):237-9 rheumatology.oxfordjournals.org/cgi/content/full/40/2/237

[185] Mobini et al. The effect of cabergoline on clinical and laboratory findings in active rheumatoid arthritis. *Iran Red Crescent Med J.* 2011 Oct;13(10):749-50

Clinical Case **Exemplary case of clinical and laboratory evidence of reversal of "severe, aggressive, drug-resistant" rheumatoid arthritis in a 51yoWF following implementation of the Functional Inflammology Protocol**: This summarizes the 13-month clinical outcome of the first patient treated with the updated functional inflammology protocol after its revision and expansion in March 2012.[186] After being diagnosed accurately by a rheumatologist—for this patient very clearly met diagnostic criteria—this patient presented for care following notably inefficacious treatment with the full medicopharmaceutical antirheumatic protocol comprised of NSAIDs, prednisone (she had only minimal response to prednisone >60mg/d), methotrexate, hydroxychloroquine, and "biologics" including etanercept/Enbrel; she was now being recommended to start newer "experimental" drugs. Following the failure of medical treatment, the patient was treated at the teaching clinic of a naturopathic college where her treatments included a clinician-supervised 26-day water-only fast, which resulted in the loss of 30 pounds (13.6 kilograms) but provided no clinical benefit for the rheumatoid arthritis. [Note: I/Dr Vasquez treat this patient at no charge. Dr William J Beakey of Professional Co-Op Services (Professionalco-op.com) generously donated these laboratory tests for collaborative/research purposes. Biotics Research Corporation (BioticsResearch.com) generously donated nutritional supplements for this patient.]

March 2012—severe symptoms and CCP >250: Patient reports suffering significantly with joint pain and lower extremity edema; foundational nutritional protocol[187] is implemented with antidysbiotic/antimicrobial intervention limited to emulsified oregano oil 600mg/d, mitochondrial support and the nutritional immunomodulation protocol. CCP level at this time is beyond laboratory testing limits, measured simply as "greater than" 250 units.

```
CCP Antibodies IgG/IgA          >250    High        units           0 - 19
                                                Negative               <20
                                                Weak positive      20 - 39
                                                Moderate positive  40 - 59
                                                Strong positive        >59
```

January 2013—mild symptoms and CCP 195: Few modifications are made for the first 9 months and patient feels progressively better, but wants to "move to the next level of improvement" because—despite feeling and functioning significantly better solely with dietary and nutritional interventions—patient still notes exacerbations of pain, particularly following extended manual farm labor. At this time, labs are drawn showing an impressive reduction in CCP levels from "greater than" 250 units to 195 units, correlating with a reduction of at least 22%. At this time, patient was commenced on additional treatments including cabergoline, oral vancomycin, and azithromycin.

```
CCP Antibodies IgG/IgA           195    High        units           0 - 19
                                                Negative               <20
                                                Weak positive      20 - 39
                                                Moderate positive  40 - 59
                                                Strong positive        >59
```

April 2013—virtually normal, CCP 54: Patient continues to improve clinically; her subjective and objective clinical improvements (including additional loss of 30 pounds [13.6 kilograms] and reduction in hand swelling necessitating resizing of wedding ring) correlate nicely with the reduction in CCP levels, which have reduced from >250 units to 54 units, for a reduction of more than 78%.Thus, by objective physical and laboratory criteria, this patient appears to be experiencing authentic reversal—cure—of her disease due to the functional inflammology protocol.

```
CCP Antibodies IgG/IgA            54    High        units           0 - 19
                                                Negative               <20
                                                Weak positive      20 - 39
                                                Moderate positive  40 - 59
                                                Strong positive        >59
```

---

[186] Vasquez A. *Functional Immunology and Nutritional Immunomodulation*. 2012 createspace.com/3899760 and updated as *F.I.N.D. S.E.X® The Easily Remembered Acronym for the Functional Inflammology Protocol*. 2013 createspace.com/4234627

[187] Vasquez A. Revisiting the Five-Part Nutritional Wellness Protocol: Supplemented Paleo-Mediterranean Diet. *Nutr Perspect* 2011 Jan ichnfm.academia.edu/AlexVasquez

Psoriasis & Psoriatic Arthritis

Introduction:

Psoriasis is my favorite condition to treat; successful implementation of the Functional Inflammology protocol can lead to such rapid resolution of long-term skin lesions that objective improvement is clearly and objectively demonstrable—providing irrefutable proof of efficacy while immediately improving the patient's quality of life, sense of efficacy, and self-esteem.

From this chapter onward, readers should use the information in Chapter 4—detailing the concepts and implementation of the Functional Inflammology protocol—and apply those concepts and interventions to the clinical conditions in the book and encountered in clinical practice.

Description/pathophysiology:

- Psoriatic arthritis is an inflammatory arthropathy seen in patients with psoriasis that can have both peripheral (e.g., hands and feet) and axial (i.e., spine and sacroiliac joints) manifestations. This condition has frequently been referred to as *psoriatic rheumatism* or *rheumatic psoriasis*.

- Similar to reactive arthritis and rheumatoid arthritis; strongly associated with streptococcal infections as well as staphylococcal infections.[188] Although many researchers have contributed to the literature which establishes psoriasis as a disease of multifocal dysbiosis, to the best of my knowledge the work of Patricia W. Noah PhD is exceptionally noteworthy; her 1990 review published in *Seminars in Dermatology*[189] is required reading for doctors wishing to gain independent *peer-reviewed* confirmation that **multifocal dysbiosis is the major initiator and perpetuator of this systemic autoimmune inflammatory disorder.** In this particular article, Dr Noah documents the experience of her group at the College of Medicine at the University of Tennessee, their anti-dysbiosis protocol, and its success in the treatment of psoriasis.

- **Psoriasis and psoriatic arthritis must be considered an autoimmune diseases** based on the findings of autoantibodies directed against dermal structures—stratum corneum[190] and keratinocytes[191]—and antibody-dependent and antibody-independent immune-mediated tissue destruction. Although stratum corneum antibodies are found in healthy patients without consequence, what makes them uniquely pathogenic in psoriasis is their tissue penetration in lesioned skin, their ability to bind with autoantigens, and their activation of complement.[192,193]

Clinical presentations:

- Dermal lesions are generally described as well demarcated erythematous patches with silvery scales. Lesions may be widespread or comparatively minor. Patients may have *hidden* dermal lesions on scalp or in gluteal cleft; clinical examination in patients with oligoarthritis can search for dermal psoriatic lesions while assessing for cutaneous dysbiosis. Rarely, nail pitting is the only cutaneous lesion.

- Chronologic association of *dermal psoriasis* with *psoriatic arthritis*:
  - 7-30% of patients with (dermal) psoriasis develop psoriatic arthritis
  - In 70% of patients, *dermal psoriasis* precedes *psoriatic arthritis* by several years
  - In 15% of patients, *dermal psoriasis* and *psoriatic arthritis* occur at the same time

---

[188] Klippel JH (ed). *Primer on the Rheumatic Diseases. 11th Edition*. Atlanta: Arthritis Foundation. 1997 page 176

[189] Noah PW. The role of microorganisms in psoriasis. *Semin Dermatol*. 1990 Dec;9(4):269-76

[190] "… titers of IgG anti-SC autoantibodies in psoriatic patients were not specifically higher than in normal controls but were more variable, indicating that their circulating levels are dependent on a delicate balance between consumption at inflammatory sites and a secondary increase due to SC-antigen release following inflammation." Tagami H, Iwatsuki K, Yamada M. Profile of anti-stratum corneum autoantibodies in psoriatic patients. *Arch Dermatol Res*. 1983;275(2):71-5

[191] "It seems that autoantibodies, although they do not appear to participate in the pathogenesis of psoriasis, are an important feature, and that skin antigens, which appear in lesional immature keratinocytes, cross-react with S. pyogenes and contribute to the autoimmune process in psoriasis." Perez-Lorenzo et al. Autoantibodies to autologous skin in guttate and plaque forms of psoriasis and cross-reaction of skin antigens with streptococcal antigens. *Int J Dermatol*. 1998 Jul;37(7):524-31. The authors found that all psoriasis patients had dermal autoantibodies and that these antibodies reacted specifically with endogenous dermal antigens; thus their finding that "Deposits of immunoglobulin G (IgG) were not detected in the lesions" is unexpected and inexplicable. This statement from their research is inconsistent with the findings of other research groups, and—specifically—must be placed in a context of other articles, most notably "… titers of IgG anti-SC autoantibodies in psoriatic patients were not specifically higher than in normal controls but were more variable, indicating that their circulating levels are dependent on a delicate balance between consumption at inflammatory sites and a secondary increase due to SC-antigen release following inflammation." Tagami et al. Profile of anti-stratum corneum autoantibodies in psoriatic patients. *Arch Dermatol Res*. 1983;275(2):71-5.

[192] "The stratum corneum (SC) antibodies are present in all human sera as seen by indirect immunofluorescent (IF) staining… IF tests with proper controls showed that the SC antigen in psoriatic scales is coated not only with IgG but in a majority of the lesions also with complement." Beutner EH, Jarzabek-Chorzelska M, Jablonska S, Chorzelski TP, Rzesa G. Autoimmunity in psoriasis. A complement immunofluorescence study. *Arch Dermatol Res*. 1978 Apr 7;261(2):123-34

[193] "Indirect immunofluorescent (IF) tests on sections of normal human skin reveal presence of antibodies to stratum corneum in most normal human sera. …Direct IF tests of psoriatic lesions revealed presence of in vivo bound IgG as well as other immunoglobulins and complement in stratum corneum." Beutner et al. Studies in immunodermatology. VI. IF studies of autoantibodies to stratum corneum and of in vivo fixed IgG in stratum corneum of psoriatic lesions. *Int Arch Allergy Appl Immunol*. 1975;48(3):301-23

- o In 15% of patients, *psoriatic arthritis* precedes *dermal psoriasis*—this 'reverse presentation' is particularly common in children
- Onset may be gradual (70%) or acute (30%)
- In some patients the onset and disease can be of such severity that hospitalization is required.
- Peripheral joint involvement is more common in women; spinal involvement is more common in men, particularly in association with HLA-B27
- Peak onset age 30-55 years
- Musculoskeletal manifestations: prevalence: hands > feet > sacroiliac > spine
  - o Oligoarticular peripheral arthropathy—distal interphalangeal (DIP) joints are notably affected
  - o Peripheral polyarthritis: distribution may be symmetric or asymmetric
  - o Arthritis mutilans: total destruction of the phalanges and meta-tarsals/carpals
  - o Spinal and sacroiliac involvement: may affect any portion of the spine in a random fashion—lumbar spondylitis and sacroiliitis are more common than atlantoaxial instability; spinal involvement is more common in patients positive for HLA-B27
  - o Enthesitis: inflammation at the junction of tendons to bones, classically noted at the Achilles tendon
- Systemic manifestations and complications
  - o Conjunctivitis, uveitis: seen in 30%
  - o Nail pitting may or may not be present; other findings may include transverse ridging, thickening, flaking and brittleness
  - o Aortic insufficiency
  - o Pulmonary fibrosis
  - o Swelling of the fingers and hands

Major differential diagnoses:
- <u>Ankylosing spondylitis</u>: does not occur with dermal psoriatic lesions
- <u>Rheumatoid arthritis</u>: differentiated from rheumatoid arthritis by 1) skin lesions, 2) absence of rheumatoid nodules, 3) negative rheumatoid factor
- <u>Hemochromatosis</u>: non-inflammatory peripheral arthropathy
- <u>Reactive arthritis</u>: does not classically occur with dermal psoriatic lesions
- <u>Septic arthritis</u>: e.g., infected psoriatic skin lesion predisposing to septicemia with resultant joint infection
- <u>HIV infection</u>: increased prevalence of psoriasis[194] especially associated with "an explosive onset of psoriasis and psoriatic arthritis"[195]

Clinical assessments:
- **History/subjective**:
  - o Inquire about the clinical presentations listed above
  - o Family and personal history of psoriasis is often positive
  - o Historical risk factors for psoriasis include bacterial pharyngitis and stressful life events[196]
- **Physical examination/objective**:
  - o Psoriasis—sharply demarcated erythematous plaque with silver scales
  - o Neuromusculoskeletal examination as indicated—see *Integrative Orthopedics*[197]
  - o Assess blood pressure and perform screening physical examination

---

[194] Beers MH, Berkow R (eds). *Merck Manual. 17th Edition*. Whitehouse Station; Merck Research Laboratories 1999 page 448
[195] Klippel JH (ed). *Primer on the Rheumatic Diseases. 11th Edition*. Atlanta: Arthritis Foundation. 1997 page 176
[196] "The study confirmed that recent pharyngeal infection is a risk factor for guttate psoriasis... Finally, the study added evidence to the belief that stressful life events may represent risk factors for the onset of psoriasis." Naldi et al; Psoriasis Study Group of Italian Group for Epidemiological Research in Dermatology. Family history of psoriasis, stressful life events, and recent infectious disease are risk factors for first episode of acute guttate psoriasis: results of a case-control study. *J Am Acad Dermatol*. 2001 Mar:433-8
[197] Vasquez A. *Integrative Orthopedics, 3rd Edition*, 2012

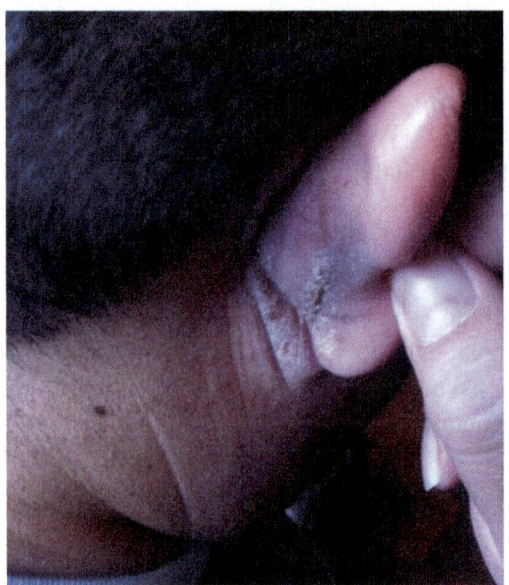 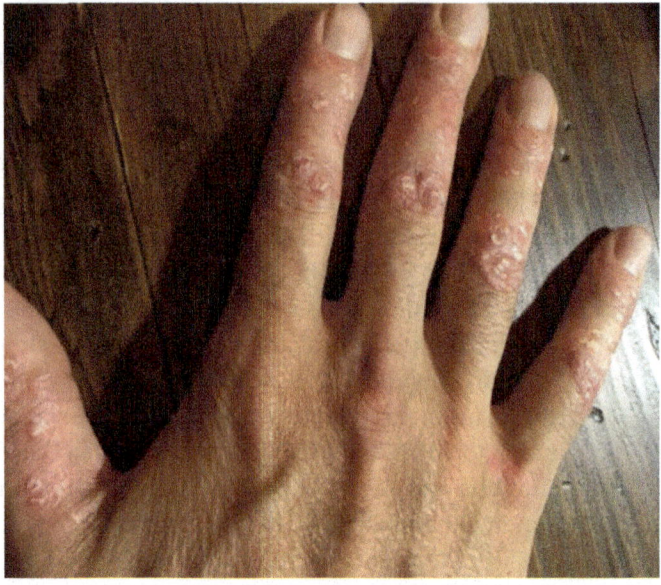

Images of Psoriasis with Two Different Types of Arthritis—Both Cases Present the Classic Dermal Manifestations of Erythematous Patches with While/Silvery Scales, Indicating Dermal Hyperproliferation: *Image left*: 34yoM with a solitary psoriasis patch virtually hidden behind his right ear, previous diagnosis was confirmed by dermatologist as a "classic psoriasis flare" after the patient was given a single dose of "penicillin" (possibly amoxicillin) for dental procedure prophylaxis; of very important note is that this patient also had confirmed rheumatoid arthritis with seropositivity for both RF and CCP, portending more aggressive disease; this patient also has thyroid autoimmunity, for a total of three different autoimmune diseases: 1) psoriasis, 2) rheumatoid arthritis, and 3) thyroiditis. *Image left*: 39yoM with psoriasis and psoriatic arthritis; nail pitting was evident in the toenails, but not the fingernails.

- **Laboratory assessments**:
  - <u>ANA</u>: Antinuclear antibodies are present in 47% of patients with psoriatic arthritis, further supporting the "autoimmune" description of this disease.[198]
  - <u>Rheumatoid factor</u>: RF is negative: positive RF suggests concomitant RA along with psoriasis.
  - <u>Chemistry/metabolic panel with uric acid</u>: Assess for overall status and elevated uric acid, the latter may be increased due to rapid skin turnover.
  - <u>Cardiovascular risk factors, especially homocysteine</u>: Patients with psoriasis have increased incidence of cardiovascular disease and as such should receive additional screening and care with regard to cardiovascular risk—including lifestyle risks such as obesity, sedentariness, smoking—and especially homocysteine.
  - <u>Ferritin</u>: Assess ferritin preferably with transferrin saturation and CRP to exclude iron overload, especially with any arthropathy.
  - <u>CRP</u>: Generally elevated; can be used to track progression/remission of the disease
  - <u>HLA-B27</u>: Present in 40% of patients with psoriatic arthritis; correlates with increased severity of disease, including increased CRP, increased propensity for sacroiliitis, and more extensive joint destruction.[199]
  - <u>HIV serologic testing</u>: Especially for patients with severe disease and/or sudden onset.
  - <u>Lactulose/mannitol assay for "leaky gut"</u>: Patients with psoriasis have increased intestinal permeability.[200]
  - <u>Dysbiosis assessments</u>
    - <u>Gastrointestinal dysbiosis</u>: Comprehensive stool and parasitology testing must include bacterial/yeast culture; antigen or antibody testing for *H. pylori* is recommended; patients with psoriasis have shown a greatly increased prevalence of *H. pylori* compared with controls[201], and the

---

[198] "RESULTS: 44/94 (47%) patients with PsA were ANA positive (>/=1/40); 13/94 (14%) had a clinically significant titre of >/=1/80. Three per cent had dsDNA antibodies, 2% had RF and anti-Ro antibodies, 1% had anti-RNP antibodies, and none had anti-La or anti-Smith antibodies." Johnson et al. Autoantibodies in biological agent naive patients with psoriatic arthritis. *Ann Rheum Dis*. 2005 May;64(5):770-2

[199] Tsai et al. Relationship between human lymphocyte antigen-B27 and clinical features of psoriatic arthritis. *J Microbiol Immunol Infect*. 2003 Jun;36(2):101-4

[200] "The 24-h urine excretion of 51Cr-EDTA from psoriatic patients was 2.46 +/- 0.81%. These results differed significantly from controls (1.95 +/- 0.36%; P less than 0.05)." Humbert et al. Intestinal permeability in patients with psoriasis. *J Dermatol Sci*. 1991 Jul;2:324-6

[201] "In the current study, 20 (40%), psoriatic patients and 5 (10%) patients of control group demonstrated H. pylori antibodies... Although our study supports a causal role of H. pylori in the pathogenesis of psoriasis..." Qayoom S, Ahmad QM. Psoriasis and helicobacter pylori. *Indian J Dermatol Venereol Leprol* 2003;69:133-134 ijdvl.com/

authors of this study suggested a causal association; likewise intestinal colonization with yeasts including *Candida albicans* and *Geotrichum candidum* are found much more commonly in psoriatics than controls.[202] Stressing the importance of this association, Waldman et al[203] wrote, "Our results reinforce the hypothesis that *C. albicans* is one of the triggers to both exacerbation and persistence of psoriasis. We propose that in psoriatics with a significant quantity of *Candida* in feces, an antifungal treatment should be considered as an adjuvant treatment of psoriasis."

> **Microbial colonization contributes to psoriasis**
>
> "We have repeatedly observed psoriatic flares associated with microbial infection, sequestered antigen, and colonization. **Removal of these microbial foci results in clearing of the disease.**"
>
> Noah P. The role of microorganisms in psoriasis. *Semin Dermatol*. 1990 Dec

- **Dermal dysbiosis**: Skin/nail culture, Giemsa staining, culture lesioned skin on blood agar, MacConkey agar, Sabouraud plates.[204]
- **Sinorespiratory dysbiosis**: Nasal swab and culture, throat culture for bacteria and yeasts.[205]
- **Genitourinary dysbiosis**: Culture and sensitivity testing for all organisms from clean catch specimens; assessment of sexual partners is advised.[206]
- **Orodental dysbiosis**: Culture of dentures and oral cavity for yeast and bacteria.
- **Environmental dysbiosis**: Examination, culture, and/or thorough cleaning of wigs, shoes, furniture, whirlpool/pool water.[207]

- **Imaging**:
  - Imaging is generally unnecessary. Radiographic findings of advanced joint disease are characteristic and can aid in differential diagnosis; findings such as the osteolytic "pencil-in-cup" and "marginal erosions" are characteristic and differentiate psoriatic arthropathy from other conditions. Radiographic changes in the spine may be severe even when the patient has mild or no symptoms—assess the spine radiographically before initiating spinal manipulative therapy. Note that inflammatory changes such as facet ankylosis and atlantoaxial instability may occur and could potentially complicate manipulative therapy.[208] Myelocompressive atlantoaxial subluxation has been reported as the presenting manifestation of psoriatic arthropathy.[209] Remarkably, Lee and Lui[210] published that, "...atlantoaxial subluxation without high cervical myelopathy has been reported in 45% of cases of psoriatic spondylitis."
- **Establishing the diagnosis**:
  - **Psoriasis**: Clinical exam reveals erythematous patches with silvery scales—this classic finding is common and may present as a singular lesion in an obscure location, such as behind the ear, at the hairline at the back of the neck, or in the gluteal cleft.
  - **Psoriatic arthritis**: Psoriasis with arthritis after the exclusion of RA, iron overload, AS, and HIV; psoriatic arthritis classicall associates with pitting of the nails.

---

[202] Candida albicans (and other yeasts) was detected in 68% of psoriatics, 70% of eczematics, 54% of the controls. Qualitative analysis revealed a predominance of Candida albicans. Geotrichum candidum occurred in 22% of psoriatics, 10% of eczematics, and 3% of controls. Buslau et al. Fungal flora of human faeces in psoriasis and atopic dermatitis. *Mycoses*. 1990 Feb;33(2):90-4

[203] "Our results reinforce the hypothesis that C. albicans is one of the triggers to both exacerbation and persistence of psoriasis. We propose that in psoriatics with a significant quantity of Candida in faeces, an antifungal treatment should be considered as an adjuvant treatment of psoriasis." Waldman et al. Incidence of Candida in psoriasis--a study on the fungal flora of psoriatic patients. *Mycoses*. 2001 May;44(3-4):77-8

[204] Noah PW. The role of microorganisms in psoriasis. *Semin Dermatol*. 1990 Dec;9(4):269-76

[205] Noah PW. The role of microorganisms in psoriasis. *Semin Dermatol*. 1990 Dec;9(4):269-76

[206] Noah PW. The role of microorganisms in psoriasis. *Semin Dermatol*. 1990 Dec;9(4):269-76

[207] Noah PW. The role of microorganisms in psoriasis. *Semin Dermatol*. 1990 Dec;9(4):269-76

[208] Laiho K, Kauppi M. The cervical spine in patients with psoriatic arthritis. *Ann Rheum Dis*. 2002 Jul;6:650-2 ard.bmjjournals.com/cgi/content/full/61/7/650

[209] "We report severe upward axial dislocation and acquired basilar impression as a presenting manifestation of psoriatic arthropathy." Kaplan et al. Atlantoaxial subluxation in psoriatic arthropathy. *Ann Neurol*. 1988 May;23(5):522-4

[210] "...atlantoaxial subluxation without high cervical myelopathy has been reported in 45% of cases of psoriatic spondylitis." Lee ST, Lui TN. Psoriatic arthritis with C-1-C-2 subluxation as a neurosurgical complication. *Surg Neurol*. 1986 Nov;26(5):428-30

Vitamin D, 1,25 + 25-Hydroxy

Test	Low	Normal	High	Reference Range	Units
Calcitriol(1,25 Di-Oh Vit D)			115.8	10.0-75.0	pg/mL
Vitamin D, 25-Hydroxy		53.1		30.0-100.0	ng/mL

Cmp14+Egfr

Test	Low	Normal	High	Reference Range	Units
Glucose, Serum		90		65-99	mg/dL
Bun		20		6-20	mg/dL
Creatinine, Serum		0.93		0.76-1.27	mg/dL
Egfr If Nonafricn Am		104		>59	mL/min/1.73
Egfr If Africn Am		120		>59	mL/min/1.73
Bun/Creatinine Ratio			22	8-19	1
Sodium, Serum		142		134-144	mmol/L
Potassium, Serum		4.8		3.5-5.2	mmol/L
Chloride, Serum		99		97-108	mmol/L
Carbon Dioxide, Total		26		18-29	mmol/L
Calcium, Serum		9.7		8.7-10.2	mg/dL

Cbc/Diff Ambiguous Default

Test	Low	Normal	High	Reference Range	Units
Wbc		5.8		3.4-10.8	x10E3/uL
Rbc		5.26		4.14-5.80	x10E6/uL

Ldh

Test	Low	Normal	High	Reference Range	Units
Ldh		123		121-224	IU/L

Homocyst(E)Ine, Plasma

Test	Low	Normal	High	Reference Range	Units
Homocyst(E)Ine, Plasma		10.7		0.0-15.0	umol/L

Laboratory results for an adult patient with psoriasis and psoriatic arthritis: Abnormally increased conversion of 25-OH-cholecalciferol to 1,25-diOH-cholecalciferol is due expression of 25-hydroxyvitamin D3-1alpha-hydroxylase (1-OHase) in inflammatory tissue/cells. Note that serum calcium is normal, so no immediate threat is present (i.e., hypercalcemia) but of course the clinician has the responsibility to ❶ monitor periodically, ❷ inform the patient of symptoms of hypercalcemia such as headache and abdominal pain, and ❸ search for any predictive risk factors such as renal insufficiency or occult leukemia/lymphoma that could precipitate hypercalcemia. Assessment for hyperparathyroidism (eg, iPTH) is reasonable but not completely necessary; likewise, cancer screening is not absolutely indicated, as it would be in the case of idiopathic hypercalcemia. Also noted is the elevated homocysteine, common in patients with psoriasis; increased cell turnover—dermal hyperproliferation—likely contributes to draining/catabolizing nutrients such as folate. Since this patient's 25-OH-D is plenty sufficient, I had the patient temporarily reduce/discontinue vitamin D supplementation to reduce risk of hypercalcemia given that he is clearly vitamin D sufficient.

<u>Complications</u>:
- Infection of skin lesions, may progress to septicemia or septic arthritis
- Atlantoaxial instability
- Cosmetic and functional deformity
- Pain
- Destructive and crippling arthritis
- Depression, social isolation, pain, reduced quality of life: **"Patients with psoriasis reported reduction in physical functioning and mental functioning comparable to that seen in cancer, arthritis, hypertension, heart disease, diabetes, and depression."**[211]

<u>Clinical management</u>:
- Referral if clinical outcome is unsatisfactory or if serious complications are evident.

<u>Treatments</u>:
- <u>Medical treatments</u>: The goal of medical treatment is to suppress inflammation and dermal proliferation; no consideration is given to searching for and addressing the underlying cause(s) of the disorder because the disease is considered idiopathic.[212] Medical textbooks describe the treatment as merely targeted toward the symptoms, e.g., "Treatment [of psoriatic arthritis] is symptomatic."[213]
  - ○ <u>For dermal psoriasis</u>:
    - ■ Prescription topical steroids
    - ■ Topical coal tars and hydrocarbons: carcinogenic
    - ■ UV-B radiation: kills active lymphocytes in skin and results in short-term superficial disappearance of psoriatic skin lesions
    - ■ PUVA: psoralen with UV-A radiation; may result in cataracts and skin cancer
    - ■ Methotrexate
    - ■ Etretinate: a severely teratogenic retinoid
  - ○ <u>For psoriatic arthritis</u>: Medical treatments for psoriatic arthritis are essentially the same as for rheumatoid arthritis[214] and are generally noncurative and "symptomatic."[215]
    - ■ <u>Etretinate</u>: a severely teratogenic retinoid
    - ■ <u>PUVA</u>: psoralen with UV-A radiation; may result in cataracts and skin cancer
    - ■ <u>Corticosteroids</u> are not highly effective
    - ■ <u>Antimalarial drugs</u> (commonly used against systemic lupus erythematosus) frequently exacerbate psoriasis
    - ■ <u>Methotrexate</u>: Used for recalcitrant psoriatic arthritis.[216]
    - ■ <u>TNF inhibitors</u>: Etanercept 25 mg subcutaneously twice weekly, or infliximab 5 mg/kg every other month. These drugs are clinically effective from the perspective of anti-inflammation, but they are associated with increased risks for lymphoma, infections, congestive heart failure, demyelinating diseases, and systemic lupus erythematosus.

- **FOOD & NUTRITION: 5-part "supplemented Paleo-Mediterranean diet" (5pSPMD)** The 5-part "supplemented Paleo-Mediterranean diet" (SPMD—reviewed in Chapter 4) consists of ❶ foundational plant-based low-carbohydrate diet of fruits, vegetables, nuts, seeds, berries and lean sources of protein, ❷ multivitamin and multimineral supplementation, ❸ physiologic doses of vitamin D3 (range 2,000-10,000 IU/d), ❹ combination fatty acid therapy (CFAT) with n3-ALA, n6-GLA, n3-EPA, n3-DHA, and phytochemical-rich olive oil which contains n9-oleate, and ❺ probiotics.

---

[211] "Patients with psoriasis reported reduction in physical functioning and mental functioning comparable to that seen in cancer, arthritis, hypertension, heart disease, diabetes, and depression." Rapp et al. Psoriasis causes as much disability as other major medical diseases. *J Am Acad Dermatol* 1999 Sep;41(3 Pt 1):401-7
[212] Lookingbill DP, Marks JG, eds. *Principles of Dermatology*. Philadelphia: W.B. Saunders, 1986: 138
[213] Tierney ML. McPhee SJ, Papadakis MA. *Current Medical Diagnosis and Treatment 2006. 45th edition*. New York; Lange Medical: 2006, pages 851-855
[214] Beers MH, Berkow R (eds). *Merck Manual. 17th Edition*. Whitehouse Station; Merck Research Laboratories 1999 page 448
[215] Tierney ML. McPhee SJ, Papadakis MA. *Current Medical Diagnosis and Treatment 2006. 45th edition*. New York; Lange Medical: 2006, pages 851-855
[216] Tierney ML. McPhee SJ, Papadakis MA. *Current Medical Diagnosis and Treatment 2006. 45th edition*. New York; Lange Medical: 2006, pages 851-855

o <u>Vitamin D3 supplementation with physiologic doses and/or tailored to serum 25(OH)D levels</u>: Vitamin D deficiency is common in the general population and is even more common in patients with chronic illness and chronic musculoskeletal pain.[217] Vitamin D3 can be applied topically and is about as effective as topical steroids in the treatment of psoriatic skin lesions.[218] Correction of vitamin D deficiency supports normal immune function against infection and provides a clinically significant anti-inflammatory[219] and analgesic benefit in patients with back pain[220] and limb pain.[221] Reasonable daily doses for children and adults are 2,000 and 4,000 IU, respectively, as defined by Vasquez, et al.[222] Deficiency and response to treatment are monitored with serum 25(OH)vitamin D while safety is monitored with serum calcium; inflammatory granulomatous diseases and certain drugs such as hydrochlorothiazide increase the propensity for hypercalcemia and warrant increment dosing and frequent monitoring of serum calcium.

o <u>Alcohol/ethanol avoidance</u>: Consumption of alcoholic beverages—even in low doses—increases intestinal permeability and exacerbates psoriasis. Psoriatics should avoid ethanol consumption[223]; wheat/grain antigens are immunogenic, ethanol exacerbates intestinal hyperpermeability, and some patients are sensitive to brewer's yeast.

o <u>Gluten-free vegetarian diet</u>: Vegetarian/vegan diets have a place in the treatment plan of all patients with autoimmune/inflammatory disorders[224], including psoriasis and psoriatic arthritis[225]; this is also true for patients for whom long-term exclusive reliance on a meat-free vegetarian diet is either not appropriate or not appealing. No legitimate scientist or literate clinician doubts the antirheumatic power and anti-inflammatory advantages of vegetarian diets, whether used short-term or long term.[226] The benefits of gluten-free vegetarian diets are well documented, and the mechanisms of action are well elucidated, including reduced intake of proinflammatory linoleic[227] and arachidonic acids[228], iron[229], common food antigens[230], gluten[231] and gliadin[232,233], proinflammatory sugars[234] and increased intake of omega-3 fatty acids and micronutrients[235], and anti-inflammatory and anti-oxidant phytonutrients[236]; vegetarian diets also effect profound changes—both *qualitative* and *quantitative*—in intestinal flora[237,238] that correlate with clinical improvement.[239] Patients who rely on the Paleo-Mediterranean Diet can use vegetarian meals, on a daily basis or for days at a time, for example, by having a daily vegetarian meal, or one week per month of vegetarianism. Of course, some (not all) patients can use a purely vegetarian diet long-term provided

[217] Plotnikoff GA, Quigley JM. Prevalence of severe hypovitaminosis D in patients with persistent, nonspecific musculoskeletal pain. *Mayo Clin Proc*. 2003 Dec;78(12):1463-70

[218] Lookingbill DP, Marks JG, eds. *Principles of dermatology*. Philadelphia: W.B. Saunders, 1986: 141

[219] Timms et al. Circulating MMP9, vitamin D and variation in TIMP-1 response with VDR genotype. *QJM*. 2002 Dec;95(12):787-96

[220] Al Faraj S, Al Mutairi K. Vitamin D deficiency and chronic low back pain in Saudi Arabia. *Spine*. 2003 Jan 15;28(2):177-9

[221] Masood et al. Persistent limb pain and raised serum alkaline phosphatase earliest markers of subclinical hypovitaminosis D. *Indian J Physiol Pharmacol* 1989 Oct:259-61

[222] Vasquez et al. The clinical importance of vitamin D (cholecalciferol): a paradigm shift for all healthcare providers. *Altern Ther Health Med*. 2004 Sep-Oct;10(5):28-36

[223] "We recommend that clinicians discourage patients with psoriasis from consuming alcohol, especially during periods of disease exacerbation." Behnam SM, Behnam SE, Koo JY. Alcohol as a risk factor for plaque-type psoriasis. *Cutis*. 2005 Sep;76(3):181-5

[224] "After four weeks at the health farm the diet group showed a significant improvement in number of tender joints, Ritchie's articular index, number of swollen joints, pain score, duration of morning stiffness, grip strength, erythrocyte sedimentation rate, C-reactive protein, white blood cell count, and a health assessment questionnaire score." Kjeldsen-Kragh et al. Controlled trial of fasting and one-year vegetarian diet in rheumatoid arthritis. *Lancet*. 1991 Oct 12;338(8772):899-902

[225] "During the vegan diet, both signs and symptoms returned in most patients, with the exception of some patients with psoriasis who experienced an improvement." Lithell et al. A fasting and vegetarian diet treatment trial on chronic inflammatory disorders. *Acta Derm Venereol*. 1983;63(5):397-403

[226] "For the patients who were randomised to the vegetarian diet there was a significant decrease in platelet count, leukocyte count, calprotectin, total IgG, IgM rheumatoid factor (RF), C3-activation products, and the complement components C3 and C4 after one month of treatment." Kjeldsen-Kragh et al. Changes in laboratory variables in rheumatoid arthritis patients during a trial of fasting and one-year vegetarian diet. *Scand J Rheumatol*. 1995;24(2):85-93

[227] Rusyn I, Bradham CA, Cohn L, Schoonhoven R, Swenberg JA, Brenner DA, Thurman RG. Corn oil rapidly activates nuclear factor-kappaB in hepatic Kupffer cells by oxidant-dependent mechanisms. *Carcinogenesis*. 1999 Nov;20(11):2095-100 carcin.oxfordjournals.org/cgi/content/full/20/11/2095

[228] Vasquez A. New Insights into Fatty Acid Supplementation and Its Effect on Eicosanoid Production and Genetic Expression. *Nutritional Perspectives* 2005; January: 5-16

[229] Dabbagh AJ, Trenam CW, Morris CJ, Blake DR. Iron in joint inflammation. *Ann Rheum Dis*. 1993 Jan;52(1):67-73

[230] Hafstrom I, et al. A vegan diet free of gluten improves the signs and symptoms of rheumatoid arthritis: the effects on arthritis correlate with a reduction in antibodies to food antigens. *Rheumatology* (Oxford). 2001 Oct;40(10):1175-9 rheumatology.oxfordjournals.org/cgi/reprint/40/10/1175

[231] "The data provide evidence that dietary modification may be of clinical benefit for certain RA patients, and that this benefit may be related to a reduction in immunoreactivity to food antigens eliminated by the change in diet." Hafstrom et al. A vegan diet free of gluten improves the signs and symptoms of rheumatoid arthritis: the effects on arthritis correlate with a reduction in antibodies to food antigens. *Rheumatology* (Oxford). 2001 Oct;40(10):1175-9

[232] "Despite the increased AGA [antigliadin antibodies] positivity found distinctively in patients with recent-onset RA, none of the RA patients showed clear evidence of coeliac disease." Paimela L, Kurki P, Leirisalo-Repo M, Piirainen H. Gliadin immune reactivity in patients with rheumatoid arthritis. Clin Exp Rheumatol. 1995 Sep-Oct;13(5):603-7

[233] "The median IgA antigliadin ELISA index was 7.1 (range 2.1-22.4) for the RA group and 3.1 (range 0.3-34.9) for the controls (p = 0.0001)." Koot et al. Elevated level of IgA gliadin antibodies in patients with rheumatoid arthritis. Clin Exp Rheumatol. 1989 Nov-Dec;7(6):623-6

[234] Seaman DR. The diet-induced proinflammatory state: a cause of chronic pain and other degenerative diseases? *J Manipulative Physiol Ther*. 2002 Mar-Apr;25(3):168-79

[235] Hagfors et al. Fat intake and composition of fatty acids in serum phospholipids in a randomized, controlled, Mediterranean dietary intervention study on patients with rheumatoid arthritis. *Nutr Metab* (Lond). 2005 Oct 10;2:26 nutritionandmetabolism.com/content/2/1/26

[236] Liu RH. Health benefits of fruit and vegetables are from additive and synergistic combinations of phytochemicals. *Am J Clin Nutr* 2003;78(3 Suppl):517S-520S

[237] "Significant alteration in the intestinal flora was observed when the patients changed from omnivorous to vegan diet. ... This finding of an association between intestinal flora and disease activity may have implications for our understanding of how diet can affect RA." Peltonen et al. Changes of faecal flora in rheumatoid arthritis during fasting and one-year vegetarian diet. *Br J Rheumatol*. 1994 Jul;33(7):638-43

[238] Toivanen P, Eerola E. A vegan diet changes the intestinal flora. *Rheumatology* (Oxford). 2002 Aug;41(8):950-1 rheumatology.oxfordjournals.org/cgi/reprint/41/8/950

[239] "We conclude that a vegan diet changes the faecal microbial flora in RA patients, and changes in the faecal flora are associated with improvement in RA activity." Peltonen et al. Faecal microbial flora and disease activity in rheumatoid arthritis during a vegan diet. *Br J Rheumatol*. 1997 Jan;36(1):64-8 rheumatology.oxfordjournals.org/cgi/reprint/36/1/64

that nutritional needs (especially protein and cobalamin) are consistently met. One particular advantage to low-protein diets in psoriasis is that the relative reduction in amino acid availability should serve to reduce polyamine formation. Formed from amino acids via ornithine decarboxylase and other enzymes, polyamines stimulate dermal hyperproliferation and are elevated in patients with psoriasis.[240] Effective psoriasis treatments are associated with a reduction in dermal/urinary polyamine levels, and, conversely, reducing polyamine formation—via either dietary manipulation or antibiologic/pharmaceutical drugs— is associated with clinical improvements in patients with psoriasis.

- **INFECTIONS & DYSBIOSIS: ❶ antimicrobial treatments, ❷ immunorestoration, ❸ immunotolerance via Treg induction** Essentially all autoimmune/rheumatic disorders are associated with microbial colonization and intolerance to same; the presence of persistent microbial colonization is *prima facie* evidence of immunosuppression. The eight areas of multifocal polydysbiosis are: ❶ sinorespiratory, ❷ orodental, ❸ gastrointestinal, ❹ genitourinary, ❺ tissue/blood, ❻ dermal, ❼ environmental, and ❽ endomicrobial.

  - <u>Psoriatogenic multifocal dysbiosis—overview of and homage to the work of Patricia Noah PhD</u>: In a very intensive investigation into the role of bacteria, yeast/fungi, and viruses in the pathogenesis of psoriasis, Noah[241] assessed microflora of 297 psoriasis patients by culture and serologic tests. Culture samples for aerobic bacteria, yeast, and dermatophytes were taken from the throat, urine, and skin surfaces from scalp, ears, chest, face, axillary, submammary, umbilical, upper back, inguinal crease, gluteal-fold, perirectal, vaginal, pubis, penis, scrotal, leg, hands, feet, finger, and toenail areas. More than 15 different microbes were causatively associated with exacerbation of psoriasis; this finding is entirely logical and is consistent with the 'idiopathic' nature of the illness and why Koch-indoctrinated researchers and clinicians have failed to understand the microbial contribution to autoimmune/inflammatory diseases. Given that each of the microbes listed (see shaded box on upcoming page) is a *common*—but not necessarily *optimal*—inhabitant of human surfaces and orifices, it is possible to see how their synergism *particularly in a genetically susceptible patient with hormonal imbalances and a proinflammatory lifestyle/diet* could tip the scales in favor of systemic inflammation and the picture/illusion of autoimmunity. Of the more than 15 categories/subspecies listed as causative microbes, what if only seven of these common "commensals" were present in a systemically-genetically-nutritionally-hormonally-emotionally predisposed patient, and each contributed only 5% to the pathophysiology of a patient's psoriasis? We would have already arrived at 35% of the psoriatic

Microorganisms causally associated with psoriasis
1. Streptococcal groups A (including Streptococcus pyogenes), B, C, D, F, G, S viridans, S pneumoniae
2. Klebsiella pneumoniae, oxytoca
3. Escherichia coli
4. Enterobacter cloacae, E aerogenes, E agglomerans
5. Proteus mirabilis, P vulgaris
6. Citrobacter freundii, C diversus
7. Morganella morganii
8. Pseudomonas aeruginosa, P maltiphilia, P putida
9. Serratia marcescens
10. Acinetobacter calbio aceticus, A luoffi
11. Flavobacterium species
12. CDC groups Ve-1, Ve-2, E-o2
13. Bacillus subtilis, B cereus
14. Staphylococcus aureus
15. Candida albicans, C parapsilosis
16. Torulopsis/Candida glabrata
17. Rhodotorula spp.
18. H. pylori*
See Noah P. The role of microorganisms in psoriasis. *Semin Dermatol.* 1990;9:269   * Qayoom S, Ahmad QM. Psoriasis and helicobacter pylori. *Indian J Dermatol Venereol Leprol* 2003;69:133-134

pathogenesis, leaving 10% each for hormones, diet, allergy, nutrition, xenobiotic accumulation (present in everyone[242,243]). While these numbers and percentages are purely speculative, I left 15% for "idiopathic" to keep researchers and clinicians alert to new possibilities and to placate the therapeutic and epidemiologic nihilists that have so far dominated the field of rheumatology with their "unknown cause" rhetoric. Each cause—each contributor to disease—may in itself be "clinically insignificant" but when additive and synergistic influences coalesce, we find ourselves confronted with an "idiopathic disease"

---

[240] "Psoriasis lesions showed increased ornithine decarboxylase activity compared with uninvolved skin." Lowe et al. Cutaneous polyamines in psoriasis. *Br J Dermatol.* 1982 Jul;107(1):21-5

[241] Noah PW. The role of microorganisms in psoriasis. *Semin Dermatol.* 1990 Dec;9(4):269-76

[242] "Although the use of HCB as a fungicide has virtually been eliminated, detectable levels of HCB are still found in nearly all people in the USA." Robinson et al. An evaluation of hexachlorobenzene body-burden levels in the general population of the USA. *IARC Sci Publ* 1986;77:183-92

[243] "Many U.S. residents carry toxic pesticides in their bodies above government assessed "acceptable" levels." Pesticide Action Network North America (PANNA). Chemical Trespass: Pesticides in Our Bodies and Corporate Accountability. panna.org/campaigns/docsTrespass/chemicalTrespass2004.dv.html

and the decision to choose between the only two available options: 1) despair in the failure of our "one cause, one disease, one drug" paradigm, or 2) appreciate that numerous influences work together to disrupt physiologic function and produce the biologic dysfunction that we experience as disease.

o Gastrointestinal dysbiosis: Patients with psoriasis have shown a greatly increased prevalence of *H. pylori*[244] and *Candida albicans*[245] and *Geotrichum candidum*.[246]

o Sinorespiratory and dermal dysbiosis: Sinorespiratory and dermal dysbiosis in patients with is *qualitatively* (increased prevalence in psoriatics compared with healthy controls) and *quantitatively* (increased prevalence of toxin-producing strains compared to those found in controls) associated with the severity of the disease.[247] Patients with psoriasis show an increased rate of nasal/dermal colonization with *Staphylococcus aureus*[248,249], a microbe known to produce several powerfully inflammatory antigens, toxins, and superantigens, and nasal colonization with which appears causally associated with the inflammatory/autoimmune disorder ANCA-associated vasculitis.[250,251] A study by Bartenjev et al[252] showed that subclinical streptococcal/staphylococcal infections were detected in 68% of psoriasis patients and in only 11 % of the control group; these authors encouraged searching for and eliminating microbial infections as an important aspect of the management of psoriasis. Supportively, other researchers[253] have found that infection with *S pyogenes* can initiate and/or exacerbate guttate psoriasis; therefore streptococcal throat infections should be treated assertively and early to avoid triggering an exacerbation of psoriasis.[254] *Streptococcus pyogenes* is a very likely trigger of psoriasis[255]; chronic penicillin treatment leads to clinical improvement of recalcitrant psoriasis.[256] Patients with guttate psoriasis have increased oropharyngeal colonization with *Streptococcus hemolyticus* compared with controls.[257] Similar to Behcet's disease[258], the dermal lesions of psoriasis are commonly colonized by

> ### Microbial antigens evoke psoriasis and autoimmunity
>
> "RESULTS: The predicted microbial product appeared heavily in lesional epidermis, but unexpectedly also as a thin deposit along the skin basement membrane zone (SBMZ) of apparently unaffected skin. Staining was negative for nonpsoriatic subjects.
> CONCLUSIONS: The findings support a direct effect of microbial antigen in psoriasis."
>
> Noah et al. Skin basement membrane zone: a depository for circulating microbial antigen evoking psoriasis and autoimmunity. *Skinmed.* 2006 Mar-Apr

---

[244] "In the current study, 20 (40%), psoriatic patients and 5 (10%) patients of control group demonstrated H. pylori antibodies... Although our study supports a causal role of H. pylori in the pathogenesis of psoriasis, a large scale study is needed to confirm the findings." Qayoom S, Ahmad QM. Psoriasis and helicobacter pylori. *Indian J Dermatol Venereol Leprol* 2003;69:133-134 ijdvl.com/

[245] "Our results reinforce the hypothesis that C. albicans is one of the triggers to both exacerbation and persistence of psoriasis. We propose that in psoriatics with a significant quantity of Candida in faeces, an antifungal treatment should be considered as an adjuvant treatment of psoriasis." Waldman et al. Incidence of Candida in psoriasis--a study on the fungal flora of psoriatic patients. *Mycoses*. 2001 May;44(3-4):77-8

[246] Candida albicans (and other yeasts) was detected in 68% of psoriatics, 70% of eczematics, 54% of the controls. Qualitative analysis revealed a predominance of Candida albicans. Geotrichum candidum occurred in 22% of psoriatics, 10% of eczematics, and 3% of controls. Buslau et al. Fungal flora of human faeces in psoriasis and atopic dermatitis. *Mycoses*. 1990 Feb;33(2):90-4

[247] "In this study, S aureus was present in more than 50% of patients with AD and PS. We found that the severity of AD and PS significantly correlated to enterotoxin production of the isolated S aureus strains." Tomi et al. Staphylococcal toxins in patients with psoriasis, atopic dermatitis, and erythroderma, and in healthy control subjects. *J Am Acad Dermatol*. 2005 Jul;53(1):67-72

[248] "In this study, S aureus was present in more than 50% of patients with AD and PS. We found that the severity of AD and PS significantly correlated to enterotoxin production of the isolated S aureus strains." Tomi et al. Staphylococcal toxins in patients with psoriasis, atopic dermatitis, and erythroderma, and in healthy control subjects. *J Am Acad Dermatol*. 2005 Jul;53(1):67-72

[249] "The nasal carriage rate of Staphylococcus aureus in psoriatics was higher than the control groups." Singh et al. Bacteriology of psoriatic plaques. *Dermatologica*. 1978:21-7

[250] Brons RH, Bakker HI, Van Wijk RT, et al. Staphylococcal acid phosphatase binds to endothelial cells via charge interaction; a pathogenic role in Wegener's granulomatosis? *Clin Exp Immunol*. 2000 Mar;119(3):566-73 blackwell-synergy.com/doi/abs/10.1046/j.1365-2249.2000.01172.x

[251] Popa et al. Staphylococcus aureus and Wegener's granulomatosis. *Arthritis Res*. 2002;4(2):77-9 arthritis-research.com/content/4/2/77

[252] "Subclinical streptococcal and/or staphylococcal infections were detected in 68 % of tested patients and in only 11 % of the control group. The results of this study indicate that subclinical bacterial infections of the upper respiratory tract may be an important factor in provoking a new relapse of chronic plaque psoriasis. Searching for, and eliminating, microbial infections could be of importance in the treatment of psoriasis." Bartenjev et al. Subclinical microbial infection in patients with chronic plaque psoriasis. *Acta Derm Venereol Suppl* (Stockh). 2000;(211):17-8

[253] "This study confirms the strong association between prior infection with S pyogenes and guttate psoriasis but suggests that the ability to trigger guttate psoriasis is not serotype specific." Telfer et al. The role of streptococcal infection in the initiation of guttate psoriasis. *Arch Dermatol*. 1992 Jan;128(1):39-42

[254] "CONCLUSIONS: This study confirms anecdotal and retrospective reports that streptococcal throat infections can cause exacerbation of chronic plaque psoriasis." Gudjonsson et al. Streptococcal throat infections and exacerbation of chronic plaque psoriasis: a prospective study. *Br J Dermatol*. 2003 Sep;149(3):530-4

[255] "These findings justify the hypothesis that S pyogenes infections are more important in the pathogenesis of chronic plaque psoriasis than has previously been recognized, and indicate the need for further controlled therapeutic trials of antibacterial measures in this common skin disease." El-Rachkidy et al. Increased Blood Levels of IgG Reactive with Secreted Streptococcus pyogenes Proteins in Chronic Plaque Psoriasis. *J Invest Dermatol*. 2007 Mar 8

[256] "Total duration of the study was two years. Initially benzathine penicillin 1.2 million units, was given I.M. AST fortnightly. After 24 weeks benzathine penicillin was reduced to 1.2 million units once a month... Significant improvement in the PASI score was noted from 12 weeks onwards. All patients showed excellent improvement at 2 years." Saxena VN, Dogra J. Long-term use of penicillin for the treatment of chronic plaque psoriasis. *Eur J Dermatol*. 2005 Sep-Oct;15(5):359-62

[257] "A high incidence of Streptococcus hemolyticus culture was observed in the guttate psoriatic group compared with the plaque psoriasis and control groups." Zhao et al. Acute guttate psoriasis patients have positive streptococcus hemolyticus throat cultures and elevated antistreptococcal M6 protein titers. *J Dermatol*. 2005;32(2):91-6

[258] "At least one type of microorganism was grown from each pustule. Staphylococcus aureus (41/70, 58.6%, p = 0.008) and Prevotella spp (17/70, 24.3%, p = 0.002) were significantly more common in pustules from BS patients, and coagulase negative staphylococci (17/37, 45.9%, p = 0.007) in pustules from acne patients. CONCLUSIONS: The pustular lesions of BS are not usually sterile." Hatemi et al. The pustular skin lesions in Behcet's syndrome are not sterile. *Ann Rheum Dis*. 2004 Nov;63(11):1450-2

proinflammatory microbes including *Staphylococcus aureus*.[259] More conclusively, Villeda-Gabriel et al[260] and Perez-Lorenzo et al[261] showed that antibodies against *Streptococcus pyogenes* cross-react (perhaps via molecular mimicry or epitope spreading) with dermal antigens; additionally, Muto et al[262] showed that antibodies against streptococcal cell wall proteins could bind with nuclei and cytoplasm of cells from skin and synovium. Thus, psoriasis is indeed a microbe-induced autoimmune disease by virtue of these cross-reacting endogenous antibodies that bind with nuclear, dermal, and articular antigens. Patients with psoriasis have elevated serum levels of antibodies against streptococcal M12 protein[263], and patients with psoriatic arthritis have a heightened inflammatory response to staphylococcal superantigens.[264]

o Antimicrobial treatments for (gastrointestinal) dysbiosis commonly include but are not limited to the following: Doses listed are for adults. Combination therapy generally allows for lower doses of each intervention to be used. Severe dysbiosis often requires weeks or months of treatment. Drugs are not necessarily more effective than natural treatments; in fact, often the botanicals work when the pharmaceuticals do not. See introductory review at the start of this chapter as well as details provided in Chapter 4 for details on anti-dysbiotic treatments.

- St. John's Wort (*Hypericum perforatum*): *Hypericum* may prove to be a useful botanical for the treatment of psoriasis due to the combination of its antidepressant and antimicrobial benefits. Hyperforin from *Hypericum perforatum* also shows impressive antibacterial action, particularly against gram-positive bacteria such as *Staphylococcus aureus*, *Streptococcus pyogenes*, *Streptococcus agalactiae*[265] and perhaps *Helicobacter pylori*.[266] Up to 600 mg three times per day of a 3% hyperforin standardized extract is customary in the treatment of depression.

- Topical antimicrobials: Treating the dermal lesions of psoriatic arthritis may help break the vicious cycles of (super)antigen absorption which perpetuates immune dysfunction. A variety of botanical and pharmaceutical creams are available. *In vitro* evidence supports the use of equal parts honey, olive oil, and beeswax against *Staph aureus* and *Candida albicans*.[267] Topical *Mahonia/Berberis* is effective for dermal psoriasis.[268] A topical gel containing artemesinin is also available for clinical use, and animal studies have demonstrated systemic absorption from topical application[269]; its use in humans with psoriasis has not been studied. Relatedly if not tangentially, topical honey is better than acyclovir against oral and genital herpes; apply *qid* for 15 minutes.[270]

---

[259] "S aureus was present in more than 50% of patients with AD and PS. We found that the severity of AD and PS significantly correlated to enterotoxin production of the isolated S aureus strains." Tomi et al. Staphylococcal toxins in patients with psoriasis, atopic dermatitis, and erythroderma. *J Am Acad Dermatol*. 2005 Jul;53(1):67-72

[260] "The recognition by immunoblot of streptococcal antigens by serum of guttate psoriasis patients, the presence of autoantibodies against their own skin, and recognition of the same skin antigens by anti-streptococcal rabbit antibodies confirm the participation of the immune system and of streptococcal infections in guttate psoriasis." Villeda-Gabriel G, et al. Recognition of Streptococcus pyogenes and skin autoantigens in guttate psoriasis. *Arch Med Res*. 1998 Summer;29(2):143-8

[261] "It seems that autoantibodies, although they do not appear to participate in the pathogenesis of psoriasis, are an important feature, and that skin antigens, which appear in lesional immature keratinocytes, cross-react with S. pyogenes and contribute to the autoimmune process in psoriasis." Perez-Lorenzo R, Zambrano-Zaragoza JF, Saul A, Jimenez-Zamudio L, Reyes-Maldonado E, Garcia-Latorre E. Autoantibodies to autologous skin in guttate and plaque forms of psoriasis and cross-reaction of skin antigens with streptococcal antigens. *Int J Dermatol*. 1998 Jul;37(7):524-31. The authors found that all psoriais paitents had dermal autoantiboes and that these antibodies reacted specifically with endogenous dermal antigens; thus their finding that "Deposits of immunoglobulin G (IgG) were not detected in the lesions" is unexpected and inexplicable. This statement from their research is inconsistent with the findings of other research groups, and—specifically—must be placed in a context of other articles, most notably "… titers of IgG anti-SC autoantibodies in psoriatic patients were not specifically higher than in normal controls but were more variable, indicating that their circulating levels are dependent on a delicate balance between consumption at inflammatory sites and a secondary increase due to SC-antigen release following inflammation." Tagami H, Iwatsuki K, Yamada M. Profile of anti-stratum corneum autoantibodies in psoriatic patients. *Arch Dermatol Res*. 1983;275(2):71-5

[262] "Monoclonal antibodies directed against type 12 Group A streptococcal cell wall antigens cross-react with nuclei and cytoplasm of cells from skin and synovium from controls, uninvolved skin of psoriatics and psoriatic plaques." Muto et al. Immune response to Streptococcus pyogenes and the susceptibility to psoriasis. *Australas J Dermatol*. 1996 May;37 Suppl 1:S54-5

[263] "Patients with psoriasis had high serum titres of antibody against the M12 (C-region) streptococcal antigen compared to controls." Muto et al. Immune response to Streptococcus pyogenes and the susceptibility to psoriasis. *Australas J Dermatol*. 1996 May;37 Suppl 1:S54-5

[264] "Our data raised the possibility that staphylococcal superantigens may also play an exacerbating role in PA." Yamamoto T, Katayama I, Nishioka K. Peripheral blood mononuclear cell proliferative response against staphylococcal superantigens in patients with psoriasis arthropathy. *Eur J Dermatol*. 1999 Jan-Feb;9(1):17-21

[265] Schempp et al. Antibacterial activity of hyperforin from St John's wort against multiresistant Staphylococcus aureus and gram-negative bacteria. *Lancet*. 1999 Jun;353:2129

[266] "A butanol fraction of St. John's Wort revealed anti-Helicobacter pylori activity with MIC values ranging between 15.6 and 31.2 microg/ml." Reichling J, Weseler A, Saller R. A current review of the antimicrobial activity of Hypericum perforatum L. *Pharmacopsychiatry*. 2001 Jul;34 Suppl 1:S116-8

[267] "Honey, beeswax and olive oil mixture (1:1:1, v/v) is useful in the treatment of diaper dermatitis, psoriasis and eczema... CONCLUSIONS: Honey and honey mixture apparently could inhibit growth of S. aureus or C. albicans." Al-Waili NS. Mixture of honey, beeswax and olive oil inhibits growth of Staphylococcus aureus and Candida albicans. *Arch Med Res*. 2005 Jan-Feb;36(1):10-3

[268] "Taken together, these clinical studies conducted by several investigators in several countries indicate that Mahonia aquifolium is a safe and effective treatment of patients with mild to moderate psoriasis." Gulliver WP, Donsky HJ. A report on three recent clinical trials using Mahonia aquifolium 10% topical cream and a review of the worldwide clinical experience with Mahonia aquifolium for the treatment of plaque psoriasis. *Am J Ther*. 2005 Sep-Oct;12:398-406

[269] "This paper reports results of pharmacokinetic studies of this preparation when applied onto a fixed area of the shaved skin of mice and rabbits. ..The drug was found to be easily absorbed from the skin." Zhao et al. [The pharmacokinetics of a transdermal preparation of artesunate in mice and rabbits] [Article in Chinese] *Yao Xue Xue Bao*. 1989;24(11):813-6

[270] Al-Waili NS. Topical honey application vs. acyclovir for the treatment of recurrent herpes simplex lesions. *Med Sci Monit*. 2004 Aug;10(8):MT94-8

- Sarsaparilla (*Smilax* spp): A clinical trial published in the *New England Journal of Medicine* in 1942 documented benefit of a sarsaparilla compound in psoriasis.[271] The proposed mechanism of action includes the binding of bacterial endotoxins, preventing their local action and systemic absorption.

  o Commonly used antibiotic/antifungal drugs: The most commonly employed drugs for intestinal bacterial overgrowth are described here.[272] Treatment duration is generally at least 2 weeks and up to 8 weeks, depending on clinical response and the severity and diversity of the intestinal overgrowth. With all anti*bacterial* treatments, use empiric anti*fungal* treatment to prevent yeast overgrowth; some patients benefit from antifungal treatment that is continued for *months* and occasionally *years*. Drugs can generally be coadministered with natural antibiotics/antifungals for improved efficacy. Treatment can be guided by identification of the dysbiotic microbes and the results of culture and sensitivity tests.

    - Penicillin: Chronic penicillin treatment leads to clinical improvement of recalcitrant psoriasis; benefits are seen when treatment is continued for at least 12 weeks, according to a clinical trial of treatment lasting for two years.[273]

    - Metronidazole: 250-500 mg BID-QID (generally limit to 1.5 g/d); metronidazole has systemic bioavailability and effectiveness against a wide range of dysbiotic microbes, including protozoans, amebas/Giardia, *H. pylori*, *Clostridium difficile* and most anaerobic gram-negative bacilli.[274] Adverse effects are generally limited to stomatitis, nausea, diarrhea, and—rarely and/or with long-term use—peripheral neuropathy, dizziness, and metallic taste; the drug must not be consumed with alcohol. Metronidazole resistance by *Blastocystis hominis* and other parasites has been noted.

    - Erythromycin: 250-500 mg TID-QID; this drug is a widely used antibiotic that also has intestinal promotility benefits (thus making it an ideal treatment for intestinal bacterial overgrowth associated with or caused by intestinal dysmotility/hypomotility such as seen in scleroderma[275,276]). Do not combine erythromycin with the promotility drug cisapride due to risk for serious cardiac arrhythmia.

Antimicrobial treatment for psoriasis

"Patients are questioned, examined, and subjected to microbiologic laboratory investigations in an attempt to identify possibly relevant microorganisms, and then are treated with antibiotics. ... Results obtained with this approach compare favorably with those achieved with more usual anti-psoriasis treatments. We recommend that a microbiologic investigation and a trial of antimicrobial treatment should precede any plan to treat psoriasis patients with anything more than the simplest topical agents."

Rosenberg EW, Noah PW, Skinner RB Jr. Microorganisms and psoriasis. *J Natl Med Assoc.* 1994 Apr

Long-term penicillin for psoriasis

"Significant improvement in the PASI score was noted from 12 weeks onwards. All patients showed excellent improvement at 2 years. Patients tolerated the therapy well. Controlled studies are needed to further confirm the benefits of long-term use of benzathine penicillin in the treatment of psoriasis."

Saxena VN, Dogra J. Long-term use of penicillin for treatment of chronic plaque psoriasis. *Eur J Dermatol.* 2005 Sep

Long-term azithromycin for psoriasis

"30 randomly selected patients with moderate to severe chronic plaque psoriasis received azithromycin for 48 weeks as a single oral 500 mg daily dose for 4 days with a gap of 10 days (total 24 such courses). ... Though the trial concluded at 48 weeks, patients in the azithromycin-arm were followed for another year to observe any relapse. A significant improvement in PASI score was noted from 12 weeks in the majority of patients in the azithromycin group. At the end of 48 weeks, 18 patients (60%) showed excellent improvement, while 6 patients (20%) showed good improvement and 4 patients (13.33%) showed mild improvement. ... An exacerbation in lesions was reported in 5 cases (16.66%) in the group receiving azithromycin. These exacerbations also responded by continuing the same treatment. ...Patients tolerated the therapy well."

Saxena VN, Dogra J. Long-term oral azithromycin in chronic plaque psoriasis. *Eur J Dermatol.* 2010 May

---

[271] Thurmon FM. The treatment of psoriasis with a sarsaparilla compound. *N Engl J Med* 1942; 227 (4): 128-33

[272] Saltzman JR, Russell RM. Nutritional consequences of intestinal bacterial overgrowth. *Compr Ther.* 1994;20(9):523-30

[273] "Total duration of the study was two years. Initially benzathine penicillin 1.2 million units, was given I.M. AST fortnightly. After 24 weeks benzathine penicillin was reduced to 1.2 million units once a month... Significant improvement in the PASI score was noted from 12 weeks onwards. All patients showed excellent improvement at 2 years." Saxena VN, Dogra J. Long-term use of penicillin for the treatment of chronic plaque psoriasis. *Eur J Dermatol.* 2005 Sep-Oct;15(5):359-62

[274] Tierney ML. McPhee SJ, Papadakis MA. *Current Medical Diagnosis and Treatment 2006. 45th edition.* New York; Lange Medical: 2006, pages 1578-1577

[275] "Prokinetic agents effective in pseudoobstruction include metoclopramide, domperidone, cisapride, octreotide, and erythromycin. ... The combination of octreotide and erythromycin may be particularly effective in systemic sclerosis." Sjogren RW. Gastrointestinal features of scleroderma. *Curr Opin Rheumatol.* 1996 Nov;8(6):569-75

[276] "Erythromycin accelerates gastric and gallbladder emptying in scleroderma patients and might be helpful in the treatment of gastrointestinal motor abnormalities in these patients." Fiorucci et al. Effect of erythromycin administration on upper gastrointestinal motility in scleroderma patients. *Scand J Gastroenterol.* 1994 Sep;29(9):807-13

- **NUTRITIONAL IMMUNOMODULATION: Treg induction for modulation of Th-1/2/17 inflammation**
Nutrients and therapeutic approaches that promote Treg or IL-10 induction and/or Th-17, IL-17 suppression include 1) mitochondrial optimization and mTOR suppression, 2) biotin, 3) vitamin E, 4) sodium avoidance, 5) transgenic/GMO food avoidance, 6) probiotics, 7) lipoic acid, 8) vitamin A, 9) inflammation reduction, 10) vitamin D, 11) fatty acid supplementation with GLA and n3, 12) infection and dysbiosis remediation, 13) green tea EGCG. Acronym: MiBESTPLAIDFIG.

- **DYSMETABOLISM & DYSFUNCTIONAL MITOCHONDRIA: MitoDys, ERS-UPR, AGE/RAGE, hyperglycemia and ceramide** The major clinical considerations in this section are mitochondrial dysfunction, endoplasmic reticulum stress, unfolded protein response, TLR activation, and the dysmetabolic effects of sustained hyperglycemia and hyperinsulinemia and resultant oxidative stress, inflammation, RAGE activation, and accumulation of AGE, palmitate and ceramide. The review of this information in Chapter 4 covered approximately 30 interventions relevant to dysmetabolism, mitochondrial dysfunction, ERS-UPR, etc; these will not be reviewed here except to mention those most commonly, easily, empirically, synergistically, and effectively used: 1) low-carbohydrate diet with 2) moderate exercise, 3) CoQ-10, 4) acetyl-carnitine with 5) lipoic acid, 6) NAC, 7) resveratrol, and 8) melatonin.
  - Carnitine / fumarate: Fumaric acid 250-500 mg 3 times a day was advocated by Wright and Gaby[277], who advised beginning with a low dose and slowly increasing the dose over a period of weeks. Flushing and hypoglycemia may occur; serial measurements of liver and kidney function tests are mandatory since fumarate has been reported to cause liver and/or renal damage. **Carnitine appears to have anti-inflammatory action via its corticosteroid receptor agonist properties[278,279] and has been reported as beneficial in a case of psoriatic arthritis.**[280]

- **STYLE OF LIVING (LIFESTYLE) & SPECIAL CONSIDERATIONS: Sleep optimization, SocioPsychology, Stress management/avoidance, Somatic treatments, Special Supplementation, Sweat/exercise, Sauna/detoxification, Surgery, Stamp your passport and vacate current reality, Sensory deprivation therapy**
This is a buffet of mostly lifestyle-based interventions yet also including considerations such as somatic treatments, additional supplementation, and surgery.
  - Folinic acid or methylfolate 5-20 mg per day: Patients with psoriasis have reduced folate status and elevated homocysteine levels.[281] Wright and Gaby recommended 50-150 mg per day of folic acid for psoriatics.[282] Folic acid has antiproliferative and anti-inflammatory effects mediated by nutrigenomic mechanisms. Folic acid, along with other vitamins and nutrients, may also help alleviate the biochemical aspect of the depression that is common in patients with psoriasis. Always supplement with vitamin B-12 in form of hydroxocobalamin or methylcobalamin (e.g., 2,000 mcg per day) when using high-dose folic acid. Most clinicians no longer use folic acid due to is causation of intracellular oxidative stress and association with malignancy; instead, folinic acid and methylated folate are preferred.
  - Topical *Berberis/Mahonia*: Topical *Berberis/Mahonia* is effective for dermal psoriasis.[283] Very obviously, topical treatments do not address the underlying problems in psoriasis and should therefore only be used for symptomatic/cosmetic improvement within the context of an overall treatment plan designed to correct the underlying/internal imbalances.
  - Topical *Capsicum annuum, Capsicum frutescens* (Cayenne pepper, hot chili pepper): Topical capsaicin has proven beneficial for alleviating the pruritus of psoriasis, presumably by depleting cutaneous neurons of

---

[277] Gaby A, Wright JV. *Nutritional Protocols*. 1998 by Nutrition Seminars
[278] "Accumulating evidence from both animal and human studies indicates that pharmacologic doses of L-carnitine (LCAR) have immunomodulatory effects resembling those of glucocorticoids (GC)." Manoli I, et al. Modulatory effects of L-carnitine on glucocorticoid receptor activity. *Ann N Y Acad Sci.* 2004 Nov;1033:147-57
[279] "Taken together, our results suggest that pharmacological doses of L-carnitine can activate GRalpha and, through this mechanism, regulate glucocorticoid-responsive genes, potentially sharing some of the biological and therapeutic properties of glucocorticoids." Alesci et al. L-carnitine: A nutritional modulator of glucocorticoid receptor functions. *FASEB J.* 2003 Aug;17(11):1553-5. Epub 2003 Jun 17 fasebj.org/cgi/reprint/02-1024fjev1
[280] Afeltra et al. Clinical improvement in psoriatic arthritis symptoms during treatment for infertility with carnitine. *Clin Exp Rheumatol.* 2004 Jan-Feb;22(1):138
[281] "The mean levels of serum tHcy, fibrinogen, fibronectin, sICAM, PAI-1 and AuAb-oxLDL were increased in patients whereas tPA, vitamin B(12) and folate levels were decreased significantly." Vanizor Kural et al. Plasma homocysteine and its relationships with atherothrombotic markers in psoriatic patients. *Clin Chim Acta.* 2003 Jun;332:23-30
[282] Gaby A, Wright JV. *Nutritional Protocols*. 1998 Nutrition Seminars
[283] "Taken together, these clinical studies conducted by several investigators in several countries indicate that Mahonia aquifolium is a safe and effective treatment of patients with mild to moderate psoriasis." Gulliver WP, Donsky HJ. A report on three recent clinical trials using Mahonia aquifolium 10% topical cream and a review of the worldwide clinical experience with Mahonia aquifolium for the treatment of plaque psoriasis. *Am J Ther.* 2005 Sep-Oct;12:398-406

substance P.[284] Very obviously, topical treatments do not address the underlying problems in psoriasis and should therefore only be used for symptomatic/cosmetic improvement within the context of an overall treatment plan designed to correct the underlying/internal imbalances.

- o Spinal manipulation: Many years ago I read a published case report of a female patient who experienced acute onset of psoriasis following trauma received during a skiing accident. Her psoriasis resolved promptly following a series of treatments of chiropractic spinal manipulative therapy.
- o Hydrotherapy, local hyperthermia: Hot bath hyperthermia (or heating pads[285]) improves skin lesions and lessens pruritus in the majority of patients with psoriasis.[286] The dermatologic improvements following hyperthermia can be objectively documented clinically and histologically/microscopically.[287]

- • **ENDOCRINE IMBALANCE & OPTIMIZATION:** **Prolactin, Insulin, Estrogen, DHEA, Cortisol, Testosterone, Thyroid** Common hormonal imbalances seen among autoimmune/inflammatory patients are: ❶ *elevated* prolactin, ❷ *elevated* estrogen, ❸ *elevated* insulin, and ❹ *reduced* DHEA, ❺ *reduced* cortisol, and ❻ *reduced* testosterone; see Chapter 4 for discussion of these hormones and respective interventions. Thyroid evaluation (patient + labs) should be comprehensive, as discussed in Chapter 1, with a low threshold for empiric treatment.

  - o Melatonin: Melatonin is a pineal hormone with well-known sleep-inducing and immunomodulatory properties, and it is commonly administered in doses of 1-40 mg in the evening, before bedtime. Its exceptional safety is well documented. Although psoriatic patients appear to have lost the physiologic nocturnal peak of melatonin[288], the role of supplemental melatonin in the treatment of patients with psoriasis has not been researched; however clinicians may reasonably decide to add this to their patients' treatment plan as appropriate. In contrast to implementing treatment with high doses of 20-40 mg, starting with a relatively low dose (e.g., 1-5 mg) and increasing as tolerated is recommended. Melatonin (20 mg hs) appears to have cured two patients with drug-resistant sarcoidosis[289] and 3 mg provided immediate short-term benefit to a patient with multiple sclerosis.[290] Immunostimulatory anti-infective action of melatonin was demonstrated in a clinical trial wherein septic newborns administered 20 mg melatonin showed significantly increased survival over nontreated controls[291]; given that psoriasis is associated with many subclinical infections, melatonin may provide therapeutic benefit by virtue of its anti-infective properties.

  - o Prolactin (excess): According to clinical trials with small numbers of patients, whether prolactin levels are high or not, treatment with prolactin-lowering treatment (such as bromocriptine[292]) appears beneficial in patients with psoriatic arthritis. Serum prolactin is the standard assessment of prolactin status. Since elevated prolactin may be a sign of pituitary tumor, assessment for headaches, visual deficits, other abnormalities of pituitary hormones (e.g., GH and TSH) should be performed and CT or MRI must be considered. Patients with prolactin levels less than 100 ng/mL and normal CT/MRI findings can be managed conservatively with effective prolactin-lowering treatment and annual radiologic assessment (less necessary with favorable serum response).[293, see review 294] Patients with RA and SLE have higher basal

[284] "CONCLUSION: Topically applied capsaicin effectively treats pruritic psoriasis, a finding that supports a role for substance P in this disorder." Ellis CN, et al. A double-blind evaluation of topical capsaicin in pruritic psoriasis. *J Am Acad Dermatol* 1993 Sep;29(3):438-42

[285] Urabe H, Nishitani K, Kohda H. Hyperthermia in the treatment of psoriasis. *Arch Dermatol.* 1981 Dec;117(12):770-4

[286] "These results indicate that simple repetitive water bath hyperthermia alone is effective in the treatment of psoriatic lesions in heatable locations." Boreham DR, Gasmann HC, Mitchel RE. Water bath hyperthermia is a simple therapy for psoriasis and also stimulates skin tanning in response to sunlight. *Int J Hyperthermia.* 1995 Nov-Dec;11(6):745-54

[287] "Electron microscopy of psoriatic skin prior to and after local hyperthermia revealed both temporary and gradual changes following treatment." Imayama S, Urabe H. Human psoriatic skin lesions improve with local hyperthermia: an ultrastructural study. *J Cutan Pathol.* 1984 Feb;11(1):45-52

[288] "Our results show that psoriatic patients had lost the nocturnal peak and usual circadian rhythm of melatonin secretion. Levels of melatonin were significantly lower than in controls at 2 a.m., and higher at 6 and 8 a.m. and at 12 noon." Mozzanica et al. Plasma melatonin levels in psoriasis. *Acta Derm Venereol.* 1988;68(4):312-6

[289] Cagnoni ML, Lombardi A, Cerinic MC, Dedola GL, Pignone A. Melatonin for treatment of chronic refractory sarcoidosis. *Lancet.* 1995 Nov 4;346(8984):1229-30

[290] "...administration of melatonin (3 mg, orally) at 2:00 p.m., when the patient experienced severe blurring of vision, resulted within 15 minutes in a dramatic improvement in visual acuity and in normalization of the visual evoked potential latency after stimulation of the left eye." Sandyk R. Diurnal variations in vision and relations to circadian melatonin secretion in multiple sclerosis. *Int J Neurosci.* 1995 Nov;83(1-2):1-6

[291] Gittoet al. Effects of melatonin treatment in septic newborns. *Pediatr Res.* 2001 Dec;50(6):756-60 pedresearch.org/cgi/content/full/50/6/756

[292] "In 2 cases of psoriatic arthritis, adding bromocriptine to gold salts and nonsteroidal anti-inflammatory drug was followed by a drastic efficacy with spectacular improvement in clinical, biological and occupational status. Because none of the cases had hyperprolactinaemia, bromocriptine acted probably had an intrinic anti-inflammatory effect independent of its antiprolactinic effect." Eulry et al. [Blood prolactin under the effect of protirelin in spondylarthropathies. Treatment trial of 4 cases of reactive arthritis and 2 cases of psoriatic arthritis with bromocriptine. French] *Ann Med Interne* (Paris). 1996;147(1):15-9

[293] Beers MH, Berkow R (eds). *Merck Manual. 17th Edition*. Whitehouse Station; Merck Research Laboratories 1999 Page 77-78

[294] Serri O, Chik CL, Ur E, Ezzat S. Diagnosis and management of hyperprolactinemia. *CMAJ.* 2003 Sep 16;169(6):575-81 cmaj.ca/cgi/content/full/169/6/575

and stress-induced levels of prolactin compared with normal controls.[295,296] A normal serum prolactin level does not necessarily exclude the use of prolactin-lowering intervention, especially since many autoimmune patients have latent hyperprolactinemia which may not be detected with random serum measurement of prolactin. Bromocriptine has long been considered the pharmacologic treatment of choice for elevated prolactin.[297] Bromocriptine appears to benefit most patients with psoriasis/psoriatic arthritis, according to a small Italian study[298] and three case reports in the French literature.[299] Typical dose is 2.5 mg per day (effective against lupus[300]); gastrointestinal upset and sedation are common.[301] Clinical intervention with bromocriptine appears warranted in patients with RA, SLE, reactive arthritis, psoriatic arthritis, and probably multiple sclerosis and uveitis.[302] A normal serum prolactin level does not necessarily exclude the use of prolactin-lowering intervention, especially since many autoimmune patients have latent hyperprolactinemia which may not be detected with random serum measurement of prolactin. Cabergoline/Dostinex is a newer dopamine agonist with few adverse effects; typical dose starts at 0.5 mg per week (0.25 mg twice per week).[303] Several

> **Estrogen promotes inflammation**
>
> "We report a patient with severe psoriatic arthritis in whom the severity of both the arthritis and psoriasis fluctuated with the menstrual cycle. These features failed to improve with standard therapy, but there was a prompt response to treatment which suppressed estrogen secretion."
>
> Stevens et al. Cyclical psoriatic arthritis responding to anti-oestrogen therapy. *Br J Dermatol.* 1993 Oct

studies have indicated that cabergoline is safer and more effective than bromocriptine for reducing prolactin levels[304] and the dose can often be reduced after successful prolactin reduction, allowing for reductions in cost and adverse effects.[305] Although fewer studies have been published supporting the antirheumatic benefits of cabergoline than those supporting bromocriptine; its antirheumatic benefits have indeed been documented.[306]

o Estrogen (excess): Although the classic pattern in patients with autoimmunity is elevated estrogen (generally considered immunodysregulatory) and reduced testosterone (generally considered anti-inflammatory and immunoregulatory), data in patients with psoriatic arthritis is inadequate to extend this otherwise consistent and successful generalization to this group. On the contrary, Stevens et al[307] published a case report of a woman with recalcitrant psoriasis and psoriatic arthritis who responded very well to anti-estrogen treatment. The small amount of data available actually suggests that estrogen may be beneficial (reduction in skin lesions with pregnancy) and that testosterone (in one woman who developed psoriasis following a testosterone-containing hormonal implant following oophorectomy) could exacerbate the disease.

o Testosterone (insufficiency): Androgen deficiencies predispose to, are exacerbated by, and contribute to autoimmune/inflammatory disorders. Female patients with psoriasis have lower levels of testosterone

[295] Dostal C, et al. Serum prolactin stress values in patients with systemic lupus erythematosus. *Ann Rheum Dis.* 2003 May;62(5):487-8

[296] "RESULTS: A significantly higher rate of elevated PRL levels was found in SLE patients (40.0%) compared with the healthy controls (14.8%). No proof was found of association with the presence of anti-ds-DNA or with specific organ involvement. Similarly, elevated PRL levels were found in RA patients (39.3%)." Moszkorzova L, Lacinova Z, Marek J, Musilova L, Dohnalova A, Dostal C. Hyperprolactinaemia in patients with systemic lupus erythematosus. *Clin Exp Rheumatol.* 2002 Nov-Dec;20(6):807-12

[297] Beers MH, Berkow R (eds). *Merck Manual. 17th Edition.* Whitehouse Station; Merck Research Laboratories 1999 Page 77-78

[298] "Bromocriptin was shown to be effective in 13 of our 18 psoriatic patients." Valentino A, Fimiani M, Bilenchi R, Castelli A, Francini G, Gonnelli S, Gennari C, Andreassi L. [Therapy with bromocriptine and behavior of various hormones in psoriasis patients] *Boll Soc Ital Biol Sper.* 1984 Oct 30;60(10):1841-4. Italian.

[299] "All three were treated with bromocriptine (5 mg/d in 2 doses) after verification of normal baseline and protirelin-stimulation prolactin levels. There was a beneficial effect in nocturnal pain relief, morning stiffness, the Lee and Ritchie scores and biological markers of inflammation." Eulry F, Mayaudon H, Lechevalier D, Bauduceau B, Ariche L, Ouakil H, Crozes P, Magnin J. [Treatment of rheumatoid psoriasis with bromocriptine] *Presse Med.* 1995 Nov 18;24(35):1642-4. French.

[300] "A prospective, double-blind, randomized, placebo-controlled study compared BRC at a fixed daily dosage of 2.5 mg with placebo... Long term treatment with a low dose of BRC appears to be a safe and effective means of decreasing SLE flares in SLE patients." Alvarez-Nemegyei J, Cobarrubias-Cobos A, Escalante-Triay F, Sosa-Munoz J, Miranda JM, Jara LJ. Bromocriptine in systemic lupus erythematosus: a double-blind, randomized, placebo-controlled study. *Lupus.* 1998;7(6):414-9

[301] Serri O, Chik CL, Ur E, Ezzat S. Diagnosis and management of hyperprolactinemia. *CMAJ.* 2003 Sep 16;169(6):575-81 cmaj.ca/cgi/content/full/169/6/575

[302] "...clinical observations and trials support the use of bromocriptine as a nonstandard primary or adjunctive therapy in the treatment of recalcitrant RA, SLE, Reiter's syndrome, and psoriatic arthritis and associated conditions unresponsive to traditional approaches." McMurray RW. Bromocriptine in rheumatic and autoimmune diseases. *Semin Arthritis Rheum.* 2001 Aug;31(1):21-32

[303] Serri O, Chik CL, Ur E, Ezzat S. Diagnosis and management of hyperprolactinemia. *CMAJ.* 2003 Sep 16;169(6):575-81

[304] "CONCLUSION: These data indicate that cabergoline is a very effective agent for lowering the prolactin levels in hyperprolactinemic patients and that it appears to offer considerable advantage over bromocriptine in terms of efficacy and tolerability." Sabuncu T, Arikan E, Tasan E, Hatemi H. Comparison of the effects of cabergoline and bromocriptine on prolactin levels in hyperprolactinemic patients. *Intern Med.* 2001 Sep;40(9):857-61

[305] "Cabergoline also normalized PRL in the majority of patients with known bromocriptine intolerance or -resistance. Once PRL secretion was adequately controlled, the dose of cabergoline could often be significantly decreased, which further reduced costs of therapy." Verhelst et al. Cabergoline in the treatment of hyperprolactinemia: a study in 455 patients. *J Clin Endocrinol Metab.* 1999 Jul;84(7):2518-22 jcem.endojournals.org/cgi/content/full/84/7/2518

[306] Erb et al. Control of unremitting rheumatoid arthritis by the prolactin antagonist cabergoline. *Rheumatology.* 2001 Feb;40(2):237-9

[307] "We report a patient with severe psoriatic arthritis in whom the severity of both the arthritis and psoriasis fluctuated with the menstrual cycle. These features failed to improve with standard therapy, but there was a prompt response to treatment which suppressed oestrogen secretion." Stevens HP, Ostlere LS, Black CM, Jacobs HS, Rustin MH. Cyclical psoriatic arthritis responding to anti-oestrogen therapy. *Br J Dermatol.* 1993 Oct;129(4):458-60

compared to those seen in healthy controls.[308] A large proportion of men with lupus or RA have low testosterone[309] and suffer the effects of hypogonadism: fatigue, weakness, depression, slow healing, low libido, and difficulties with sexual performance. Testosterone levels may rise following DHEA supplementation (especially in women) and can be elevated in men by the use of anastrozole/Arimidex. Otherwise, transdermal testosterone such as Androgel or Testim can be applied as indicated.

- o DHEA: DHEA is an anti-inflammatory and immunoregulatory hormone that is commonly deficient in patients with autoimmunity and inflammatory arthritis.[310] However, the role of DHEA in psoriatic arthritis *en masse* is unclear due to conflicting data. One study showed that patients with psoriasis did not show evidence of DHEA insufficiency[311], while other studies—especially in the German literature—have consistently documented low serum and intracellular levels of DHEA.[312] DHEA levels should be measured in these patients—especially those with severe disease, deficiencies should be treated unless contraindicated, and therapeutic trials are not unreasonable.

- • XENOBIOTIC ACCUMULATION & DETOXIFICATION: Chemical avoidance, nutritional support for detoxification pathways, urine alkalinization The clinical relevance and pathogenic mechanisms of xenobiotic accumulation are irrefutably well documented and described. Clinical assessments include history, physical examination, and laboratory assessment (using serum, whole blood, urine or—rarely yet accurately— fat biopsy), and response to treatment. Treatments include nutritional support for Phases 1 and 2 of detoxification (e.g., oxidation and conjugation) and excretion via bile and urine; for the latter, urinary alkalinization is generally recommended. Chemical toxins can be bound in the gut using activated charcoal, cholestyramine, or *Chlorella*—all of these three treatments have documented safety and effectiveness; clinically and empirically, phytochelatin (plant-derived peptides that bind toxic metals) concentrates appear safe and effective despite lack of conclusive published data supporting clinical use.

  - o Detoxification support: Cytochrome P450 (Cyp450) defects (phenotypic—not genotropic—in this research) have been noted in patients with psoriasis and correlate with the severity of the disease.[313] Assuming a causal relationship, one can speculate as to the nature and direction of that relationship:

    - ▪ Cause of disease: Perhaps the detoxification defects lead to xenobiotic accumulation which alters immune function in favor of xenobiotic immunotoxicity: resulting in immune impairment and exaggerated inflammatory response.
    - ▪ Effect of disease: Perhaps the inflammation or oxidative stress or nutritional deficiencies of psoriasis is/are the cause of the detoxification defects.
    - ▪ Shared causality: Perhaps the increased total bacterial load impairs Cyp450 via LPS and also causes the inflammatory dysfunction that precipitates psoriasis.
    - ▪ Nonexclusivity, additive/synergistic effects: All of the above.

---

[308] "The testosterone levels and LH/FSH ratio were significantly lower in the psoriatic group." Pietrzak A, Lecewicz-Torun B, Jakimiuk A. Lipid and hormone profile in psoriatic females. *Ann Univ Mariae Curie Sklodowska* [Med]. 2002;57(2):478-83

[309] Karagiannis A, Harsoulis F. Gonadal dysfunction in systemic diseases. *Eur J Endocrinol*. 2005 Apr;152(4):501-13 eje-online.org/cgi/content/full/152/4/501

[310] "DHEAS concentrations were significantly decreased in both women and men with inflammatory arthritis (IA) (P < 0.001)." Dessein PH, et al. Hyposecretion of the adrenal androgen dehydroepiandrosterone sulfate and its relation to clinical variables in inflammatory arthritis. *Arthritis Res*. 2001;3(3):183-8 arthritis-research.com/content/3/3/183

[311] "Assessing the patients by group, the mean DHEAS level was markedly lower in the pemphigoid/pemphigus than in the psoriasis and OA patients (geometric mean 600 vs. 2130 and 2100 nmol/l, respectively; p < 0.001)." de la Torre B, Fransson J, Scheynius A. Blood dehydroepiandrosterone sulphate (DHEAS) levels in pemphigoid/pemphigus and psoriasis. *Clin Exp Rheumatol*. 1995 May-Jun;13(3):345-8

[312] "The effects of this dehydroepiandrosterone deficiency are changes in the humoral regulation of events in growth and proliferation in patients with psoriasis." Holzmann H, Benes P, Morsches B. [Dehydroepiandrosterone deficiency in psoriasis. Hypothesis on the etiopathogenesis of this disease. German] *Hautarzt*. 1980 Feb;31(2):71-5

[313] "Low CYP2C activity was associated with severe psoriasis, poor metaboliser status occurring in 50% of the severe group, but in none of the mild cases, p < 0.01." Helsby NA, et al. Hepatic cytochrome P450 CYP2C activity in psoriasis: studies using proguanil as a probe compound. *Acta Derm Venereol* 1998 Mar;78(2):81-3

Systemic Lupus Erythematosus: "SLE" or "Lupus"

Introduction:
As was said to me once by a Vice President of one of the largest hospital systems in Texas, SLE is a "big league" disease with numerous and potentially fatal complications; it is not to be taken lightly. Best interests of both doctor and patient are served by having a rheumatologist and/or internist as part of the care team. SLE is the prototype of multiorgan autoimmunity, mediated by a combination of cellular and humoral factors especially including immune-complex deposition and localized inflammation in the vascular system (vasculitis), skin (dermatitis), joints (arthritis) and kidneys (nephritis).

Description/pathophysiology:

- SLE as the prototype of multisystem autoimmune disease: SLE is the prototype of multisystem autoimmune disease, characterized by a chronic progressive course with remissions and relapses; as the prototype of multiorgan "idiopathic" autoimmunity, SLE will serve to model facts and concepts that are applicable to other conditions. The skin, joints, kidneys, serosal membranes (pleura, pericardium, peritoneum), and vascular system are the most prominent targets of inflammatory attack; however, any cell and tissue may be damaged, either directly or indirectly. Autoantibodies (and resultant immune complexes) against a wide range of

Immune complex pathophysiology
Consecutive linking of antigen and antibody results in formation of immune complexes which are predisposed for deposition in joints, skin, kidneys, and vasculature. Immune complex deposition results in focal and atopic (distant from site of antigen exposure) inflammatory damage of surrounding tissue via local activation of complement pathway and local inflammation, including recruitment of neutrophils and monocytes which release free radicals and autolytic lysosomal enzymes.

endogenous/self targets are pathogenic in SLE; however, **the current pathologic paradigm places ultimate responsibility on CD4+ helper T-cells—i.e., e.g., the Th1, Th2, Th17, and Treg cells discussed in Chapter 4—** rather than the antibody-producing B-cells/plasma cells. Tissue damage in SLE is largely mediated by **autoantibodies—particularly anti-nuclear antibodies (ANA)—**and the resulting **immune complexes,** cryoglobulins, and the subsequent inflammatory cascade.[314,315,316,317] **Patients with SLE have impaired ability to clear immune complexes via hepatic and splenic routes**[318,319]; therapeutic implications are discussed below. **SLE is considered a type-3 hypersensitivity disease because it is largely mediated by immune complex deposition** and secondary activation of the complement cascade and other inflammatory pathways.

- Allopathic perspective = "idiopathic": This condition is generally considered "idiopathic" in most cases, though in some patients the disease is induced by pharmaceutical drugs (especially hydralazine, procainamide, D-penicillamine) and is then generally reversible upon discontinuation of the drug. Most people with complement deficiencies (a group of congenital immune defects) develop SLE. Other precipitating/contributing factors include ultraviolet light exposure, chemical exposure, and possibly consumption of alfalfa sprouts (based on animal data[320] and very little human data). Abnormal hormone metabolism has also been noted and may play a role in the pathogenesis as described in the section on *orthoendocrinology*—Chapter 4.6.

- Integrative/functional/naturopathic perspective = multifactorial: Numerous—not innumerable—factors contribute to SLE pathogenesis; these are well represented within the FINDSEX™ of the functional inflammology protocol.

- The role of microbes, especially viral infections: The cytokine pattern and many of the pathogenic features of SLE have pointed toward "a viral etiology" for many years; one is simultaneously challenged with the paradox

[314] Tierney ML. McPhee SJ, Papadakis MA (eds). *Current Medical Diagnosis and Treatment 2006. 45th edition*. New York; Lange Medical Books: 2006, pages 833-837

[315] Suzuki et al. Development of pathogenic anti-DNA antibodies in patients with systemic lupus erythematosus. *FASEB J.* 1997 Oct;11:1033-8 fasebj.org/cgi/reprint/11/12/1033

[316] "Pisetsky DS. Antibody responses to DNA in normal immunity and aberrant immunity. *Clin Diagn Lab Immunol.* 1998 Jan;5(1):1-6 cvi.asm.org/cgi/reprint/5/1/1

[317] Sikander FF, Salgaonkar DS, Joshi VR. Cryoglobulin studies in systemic lupus erythematosus. *J Postgrad Med* [serial online] 1989 [cited 2005 Nov 2];35:139-43

[318] "These observations support the hypothesis that IC handling is abnormal in SLE." Davies KA, Peters AM, Beynon HL, Walport MJ. Immune complex processing in patients with systemic lupus erythematosus. In vivo imaging and clearance studies. *J Clin Invest.* 1992 Nov;90(5):2075-83

[319] "These results indicate that Fc-mediated clearance of ICs is defective in patients with SLE and suggest that ligation of ICs by Fc receptors is critical for their efficient binding and retention by the fixed MPS in the liver." Davies et al. Defective Fc-dependent processing of immune complexes in patients with systemic lupus erythematosus. *Arthritis Rheum.* 2002 Apr;46(4):1028-38

[320] "L-Canavanine sulfate, a constituent of alfalfa sprouts, was incorporated into the diet and reactivated the syndrome in monkeys in which an SLE-like syndrome had previously been induced by the ingestion of alfalfa seeds or sprouts." Malinow et al. Systemic lupus erythematosus-like syndrome in monkeys fed alfalfa sprouts: role of a nonprotein amino acid. *Science.* 1982 Apr 23;216(4544):415-7

of wanting to accept this as plausible and wanting to reject it as yet another *undefined* and therefore *useless* and therefore *idiopathic* allopathic description of disease pathogenesis. With more currently available research however, I think the viral hypothesis—or more accurately the *poly*viral and polymicrobial model—is gaining credible and clinically usable merit. I will outline this territory as I see it:

- <u>Increased and/or altered total microbial load (TML)</u>: Some evidence has shown that SLE patients have evidence of increased microbial loads—both bacterial and viral. For example, patients with SLE, psoriasis, Wegener's, and eczema have all shown increased nasal carriage of *Staphylococcus aureus*. Even if no immune abnormalities were present, increased antigenic exposure would be expected to result in increased humor antibody response and the formation of more—perhaps a pathogenic "excess" of—immune complexes; if the immune system were hyperresponsive, say due to vitamin D deficiency and the resulting lack of Treg induction, then the situation would only get worse as the causes of immune hyperresponsiveness become additive or synergistic. Obviously, the TML contributes directly and powerfully to the TIL—total inflammatory load.

- <u>Impaired immune complex clearance</u>: Impaired clearance of immune complexes would—of course—complicate the aforementioned problems associated with increased TML and TIL; in fact, the result would be a positive/upward dissociation of the TIL from the TML as the inflammatory consequences become greater than normal/proportionate.

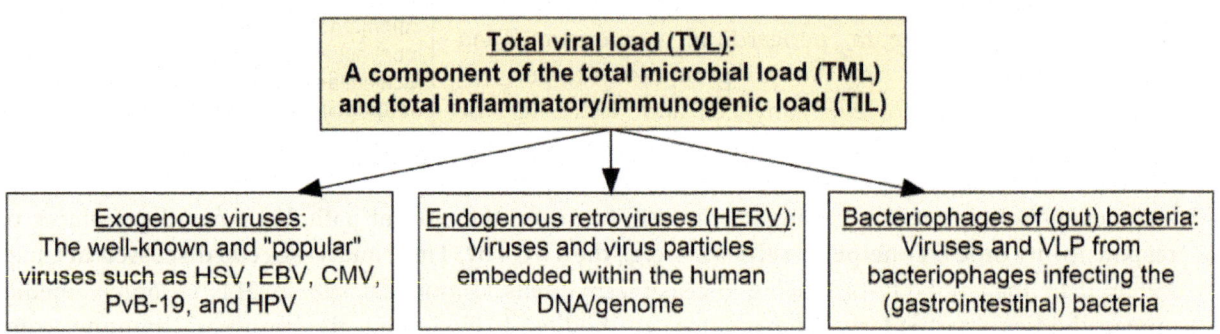

The total viral load (TVL): TVL contributes to TML (total microbial load) and thus to the TIL (total inflammatory load), to which are added the TCL (total carbohydrate load) and TXL (total xenobiotic load).

- <u>Viruses, part 1—Known/popular "epigenomic" viruses</u>: I categorize as "known" and/or "popular" those viruses that we commonly consider, such as Epstein-Bar virus (EBV), parvovirus B-19 (PvB19), cytomegalovirus (CMV), human papilloma virus (HPV) and other such viruses as we generally consider clinically and/or studied in whatever medical school we as clinicians attended. These have been described as epigenomic and/or exogenous viruses because they are close to but not part of the human genome— "epi" is a Greek-derived prefix denoting "above, on, over, nearby, upon"; these *epigenomic* viruses are contrasted with the *endogenous* viruses that are integrally "built in" to the human DNA. All four viruses mentioned in the previous sentence have been associated with autoimmunity; more recently has arrived the data supporting our new appreciation that "autoimmune patients" *may well be* and *generally are* "actively infected" with many of these viruses simultaneously—this is well-documented now in scleroderma, patients with which show active and "ectopic" (unusual locations) infections simultaneously with EBV, PvB19, and CMV. *Helicobacter pylori* may play a powerful role as a synergistic bioagent via its ability to *simultaneously* and *paradoxically* cause immunosuppression (thereby allowing other microbes to flourish) and systemic inflammation[321]; in this manner, the bacterial infection is permissive to and perhaps necessary for the autoimmune-inducing vasculopathic and fibrogenic viral infections (see section on Scleroderma for pathology details). An important concept to remember is that viral infections promote other viral infections—transactivation—via direct genomic enhancement of viral replication, by promoting a favorable cytokine environment for viral replication, and/or by stimulating

---

[321] "Infectious agents such as Helicobacter pylori (Hp) may cause chronic inflammation and autoimmune reactivity in susceptible subjects. The results of in vitro experiments performed with lymphocytes from Hp infected patients indicate that Hp can cause immunosuppression which might be eliminated by successful eradication therapy." Hybenova et al. The role of environmental factors in autoimmune thyroiditis. *Neuro Endocrinol Lett.* 2010;31(3):283-9

NFkB which is commonly "hijacked" by viruses to promote viral replication; therefore activation or suppression of any virus can be said to contribute *indirectly* to the activation or suppression, respectively, of other viral populations.[322] Relatedly and as will be discussed in the following section on endogenous viruses, replication of exogenous/epigenomic viruses—such as influenza virus and herpes simplex type-1—increases expression of endogenous viruses.

- Epstein-Barr virus in the pathogenesis of some autoimmune disorders (*Eur J Microbiol Immunol* 2011 Dec[323]): "Moreover, many observations indicate that EBV contributes also to the pathomechanism of SLE. However, this contribution differs from the relationship between EBV and MS, as shown by the lack of any increase in the risk of SLE after IM [infectious mononucleosis]. In SLE, EBV serology is quantitatively and qualitatively different from the normal response - that is, EBV viral load is higher and a strong cross-reaction can be detected between certain EBV antigens and autoantigens of pathological importance."

- Lupus and Epstein-Barr (*Curr Opin Rheumatol* 2012 Jul[324]): "SLE patients have a dysregulated immune response against EBV. EBV antigens exhibit structural molecular mimicry with common SLE antigens and functional molecular mimicry with critical immune-regulatory components. SLE patients, from a number of unique geographic regions, are shown to have higher rates of EBV seroconversion, especially against early EBV antigens, suggesting frequent viral reactivation. SLE patients also have increased EBV viral loads and impaired EBV-specific CD8 cytotoxic T cells, with impaired cytokine responses to EBV in lupus patients. ... Recent advances demonstrate SLE-specific serologic responses, gene expression, viral load, T-cell responses, humoral fine specificity, and molecular mimicry with EBV, further supporting potential roles for EBV in lupus etiology and pathogenesis."

- HTLV (human T-lymphotropic virus) in SLE (*Clin Immunol.* 2002 Feb[325]): "SLE patients produce high titer antibodies to various retroviral proteins, including Gag, Env, and Nef of HIV and HTLV (human T-lymphotropic virus), in the absence of overt retroviral infection. ... In particular, we consider the role of HTLV-1-related endogenous sequence (HRES-1) in SLE. We propose that molecular mimicry between HRES-1 and the small ribonucleoprotein complex initiates the production of autoantibodies, leading to immune complex formation, complement fixation, and pathological tissue deposition."

o Viruses, part 2—Human endogenous retroviruses (endoretroviruses, HERVs or ERVs): Human DNA is "pre-loaded" with remnants of viral infections that have coursed through and been transmitted from parents to offspring for millions of years; these endogenous viral genomes implanted into human DNA are now known to undergo reactivation with the production of immunogenic viral remnants and the anticipated inflammatory immune response. As mentioned previously related to exogenous viral transactivation, replication of exogenous/epigenomic viruses—such as influenza virus and herpes simplex type-1—increases expression of endogenous viruses[326]; as such, one method to reduce/control activation of HERVs is to suppress replication of exogenous viruses. HERV activation is inhibited by

---

Rationale for anti-viral therapy for treating autoimmunity

"Cited epidemiologic and experimental evidence suggests that increased replication of epigenomic viral pathogens such as Epstein-Barr Virus (EBV) in chronic human autoimmune diseases such as rheumatoid arthritis (RA), systemic lupus erythematosus (SLE), and multiple sclerosis (MS) may activate endogenous human retroviruses (HERV) as a pathologic mechanism."

Dreyfus DH. Autoimmune disease: A role for new anti-viral therapies? *Autoimmun Rev.* 2011 Dec

---

[322] White et al. Reciprocal transactivation between HIV-1 and other human viruses. *Virology.* 2006 Aug 15;352(1):1-13

[323] Füst G. The role of the Epstein-Barr virus in the pathogenesis of some autoimmune disorders - Similarities and differences. *Eur J Microbiol Immunol* (Bp). 2011 Dec;1:267-78

[324] James JA, Robertson JM. Lupus and Epstein-Barr. *Curr Opin Rheumatol.* 2012 Jul;24(4):383-8

[325] Adelman MK, Marchalonis JJ. Endogenous retroviruses in systemic lupus erythematosus: candidate lupus viruses. *Clin Immunol.* 2002 Feb;102(2):107-16

[326] "Since viral infections have previously been reported to transactivate retroviral long terminal repeat regions we examined the basal expression of HERV-W elements and following infections by influenza A/WSN/33 and Herpes simplex 1 viruses in human cell-lines. ... Subsets of HERV-W elements were transactivated by viral infection in the different cell-lines. Transcriptional activation of these elements, including that encoding syncytin, was dependent on viral replication and was not induced by antiviral responses." Nellaker et al. Transactivation of elements in the human endogenous retrovirus W family by viral infection. *Retrovirology.* 2006 Jul 6;3:44

DNA methylation; conversely, DNA hypomethylation is consistently associated with SLE in humans and animals.[327,328]

- ▪ Human endogenous retroviruses in the development of autoimmune diseases (*Int Rev Immunol* 2010 Aug[329]): In 2010, Balada et al provided a succinct and authoritative summary of HERVs and their relationship to the pathogenesis of autoimmunity: "Retroviruses can exist in an endogenous form, in which viral sequences are integrated into the human germ line and are vertically transmitted in a Mendelian fashion. Human endogenous retroviruses (HERVs), probably representing footprints of ancient germ-cell retroviral infections, occupy about 1% of the human genome. ... Although some of these elements show mutations and deletions, some HERVs are transcriptionally active and produce functional proteins. Some medical conditions, such as cancer and autoimmune diseases, are linked to the transcription of some of the HERVs genes, to the expression of HERVs proteins (that may act as superantigens, for example), and/or to the development of antibodies against them that might cross-react with our own proteins. Their genetic sequences may also be, totally or partially, integrated into genes that regulate the immune response. These mechanisms could give rise to autoimmune diseases, such as lupus erythematosus, insulin-dependent diabetes mellitus, multiple sclerosis, Sjögren's syndrome, and rheumatoid arthritis, among others."

> **HERV-autoimmunity associations**
> - Rheumatoid arthritis: expression of multiple ERVs detected in RA patients; HERV-K10 shows molecular mimicry
> - Juvenile RA: HERV-K10
> - Multiple sclerosis: MS-associated retroviral element (MRSV)-type HERV-W; increased expression of the env RNA and protein expression in the blood and brain cells of MS patients; also clear increase in HERV-H/F family HERV-Fc1 activity and RNA production; HERV-K18 on chromosome 1 is a risk factor for MS
> - Psoriasis: Increased expression of HERV-W, K, E, and variant ERV-9/HERV-W
> - Lupus: Hypomethylation of HERV-E and HERV-K
>
> Mechanisms for HERV-induced autoimmune diseases:
> - Molecular mimicry (HERV-K10)
> - Superantigen production (HERV-K)
> - LTR (long terminal repeat)-mediated alterations of gene expression
> - Antigenicity and immune complex formation
>
> Activation of HERVs:
> - DNA hypomethylation
> - Transactivation

Clear and complete as that is, readers might reasonably want additional sources of support, and I have provided samples of such here:

- ▪ Human endogenous retroviruses in the pathogenesis of autoimmune diseases (*Med Sci Monit* 2012 Jun[330]): "This theory takes into account the existence in the human genome, since approximately 40 million years, of so-called human endogenous retroviruses (HERVs), which are transmitted to descendants vertically by the germ cells. It was recently established that these generally silent sequences perform some physiological roles, but occasionally become active and influence the development of some chronic diseases like diabetes, some neoplasms, chronic diseases of the nervous system (e.g., sclerosis multiplex), schizophrenia and autoimmune diseases."

- ▪ Endogenous retroviral pathogenesis in lupus (*Curr Opin Rheumatol* 2010 Sep[331]: "ERV proteins may trigger lupus through structural and functional molecular mimicry, whereas the accumulation of ERV-derived nucleic acids stimulates interferon and anti-DNA antibody production in SLE."

- ▪ Autoimmune disease treatment with anti-viral therapies (*Autoimmun Rev* 2011 Dec[332]): "Cited epidemiologic and experimental evidence suggests that increased replication of epigenomic viral pathogens such as Epstein-Barr Virus (EBV) in chronic human autoimmune diseases such as rheumatoid arthritis (RA), systemic lupus Erythematosus (SLE), and multiple sclerosis (MS) may activate endogenous human retroviruses (HERV) as a pathologic mechanism. ... Other [drug] anti-viral therapies of chronic autoimmune diseases, such as retroviral integrase inhibitors, could be effective, although not without risk." This article provides support and rationale for using antiviral

---

[327] "This raises the possibility that HERV demethylation participates in the pathogenesis of SLE." Renaudineau et al. Epigenetics and autoimmunity, with special emphasis on methylation. *Keio J Med*. 2011;60(1):10-6

[328] "Hypomethylation of HERV-E and HERV-K was also observed in SLE patients." Katoh et al. Association of endogenous retroviruses and long terminal repeats with human disorders. *Front Oncol*. 2013 Sep 11;3:234

[329] Balada E et al. Implication of human endogenous retroviruses in the development of autoimmune diseases. *Int Rev Immunol*. 2010 Aug;29(4):351-70

[330] Brodziak et al. The role of human endogenous retroviruses in the pathogenesis of autoimmune diseases. *Med Sci Monit*. 2012 Jun;18(6):RA80-8

[331] Perl et al. Endogenous retroviral pathogenesis in lupus. *Curr Opin Rheumatol*. 2010 Sep;22(5):483-92

[332] Dreyfus DH. Autoimmune disease: A role for new anti-viral therapies? *Autoimmun Rev*. 2011 Dec;11(2):88-97

therapies in the treatment of autoimmunity; since anti-viral drugs nearly always have limited effectiveness and an excess of adverse effects and high cost while natural antiviral agents are safer and more broadly effective, the therapeutic choice is very clear.

- Role of endogenous retroviruses in murine SLE—an established animal model of human SLE[333] (*Autoimmun Rev* 2010 Nov[334]): "Among the principal targets of the autoantibodies produced in murine SLE are nucleic acid-protein complexes and the envelope glycoprotein gp-70 of endogenous retroviruses. Recent studies have revealed that the innate receptor TLR-7 plays a pivotal role in the development of a wide variety of autoimmune responses against DNA- and RNA-containing nuclear antigens... Moreover, the demonstration that TLR-7 is involved in the acute phase expression of serum gp70 uncovers an additional pathogenic role of TLR7 in murine lupus nephritis by promoting the expression of nephritogenic gp-70 autoantigen." Thus this animal model proves with molecular detail the cause-and-effect relationship between ERVs and SLE and further points to TLR-7 as a necessary byway for nephritogenic autoantigen expression; parallels to human SLE and according therapeutic interventions are likely. While most readers should already appreciate that TLRs recognize pathogen-associated molecular patterns (PAMPs) expressed on infectious agents (and saturated fatty acids for TLR-4, as discussed in Chapter 4) and mediate the specific PAMP-TLR expression of inflammatory cytokines for immune defense responses, what is important to note here is that TLR-7 recognizes single-stranded RNA in endosomes, a common feature of viral genomes internalized within macrophages and dendritic cells; in this manner, TLR-7 is poised to be the mediator of virus-induced HERV transactivation with resultant production of pathogenic autoantigens.

- Selective antibody reactivity with peptides from human endogenous retroviruses—HERVs—and nonviral poly(amino acids) in patients with systemic lupus erythematosus (*Arthritis Rheum* 1996 Oct[335]): "Measurement by immunoassay revealed increased frequencies of antiretroviral antibodies against 2 peptides derived from the env gene of the type C-like class, which includes ERV-9 and HERV-H, and against 2 peptides from the gag region of human T-lymphotropic virus type I-related endogenous sequence 1, in patients with SLE. Antibodies to 2 nonviral peptides, polyhistidine and polyproline, were also overrepresented in patient sera. In 1 patient, longitudinal data obtained over a period of 12 years indicated that the concentrations of certain antiretroviral antibodies varied according to disease activity. CONCLUSION: Reactivity to certain type C HERV-derived antigens was found among patients with SLE. This reactivity could be explained by increased exposure to cross-reactive epitopes from essentially complete type C HERVs."

- Endogenous retroviruses in systemic lupus erythematosus: candidate lupus viruses (*Clin Immunol.* 2002 Feb[336]): "SLE patients produce high titer antibodies to various retroviral proteins, including Gag, Env, and Nef of HIV and HTLV (human T-lymphotropic virus), in the absence of overt retroviral infection. ... In particular, we consider the role of HTLV-1-related endogenous sequence (HRES-1) in SLE. We propose that molecular mimicry between HRES-1 and the small ribonucleoprotein complex initiates the production of autoantibodies, leading to immune complex formation, complement fixation, and pathological tissue deposition."

Thus given that HERVs are 100% pervasive among humans and give rise to active transcription to HERV proteins, superantigens and the resulting antibodies—noting that microbial proteins + superantigens + antibodies = the perfect recipe for immune complex disease, made even worse among persons (e.g., lupus patients) with an inability to clear immune complexes—the most important question then becomes *what steps can be taken to suppress/repress/hamper HERV replication? Can we use the same effective antiviral treatments which already have available (in the previously listed antiviral protocol)?* Obviously, since we are not dealing with free viral particles, some of the previously mentioned antiviral treatments will

---

[333] "Murine models are useful tools for the study of the etiology of lupus. A multitude of models exist, each sharing a subset of attributes with SLE observed in humans. In addition, each model affords the study of different aspects of lupus pathogenesis." Perry et al. Murine Models of Systemic Lupus Erythematosus. *J Biomed Biotech* 2011; 271694
[334] Baudino et al. Role of endogenous retroviruses in murine SLE. *Autoimmun Rev.* 2010 Nov;10(1):27-34
[335] Bengtsson et al. Selective antibody reactivity with peptides from human endogenous retroviruses and nonviral poly(amino acids) in patients with systemic lupus erythematosus. *Arthritis Rheum.* 1996 Oct;39(10):1654-63
[336] Adelman MK, Marchalonis JJ. Endogenous retroviruses in systemic lupus erythematosus: candidate lupus viruses. *Clin Immunol.* 2002 Feb;102(2):107-16

have no effect because the mechanisms are irrelevant (such as selenium's prevention of immune-escape by reducing viral mutagenesis) or cannot reach within the nucleus to have effect (such as the virucidal activity of zinc ions, or the binding-inactivating effect of glycyrrhetinic acid to HSV particles). Given that "the virus" is already and permanently embedded/encoded within the human genome, the most immediate and obvious solutions would be those of promoting DNA methylation to silence HERV long terminal repeats (LTR, not to be confused with TLR for Toll-like receptors) and to prevent/reduce active transcription of those HERV LTR via transcription factors like NFkB and/or a pro-inflammatory cytokine milieu. This is to say, the means would most likely have to be ❶ *contra* DNA transcription, most notably via the promotion of DNA methylation, ❷ reducing any contribution of viral transactivation, ❸ reducing any contribution of inflammatory (e.g., TLR-7 pathway) and stress-induced (trans)activation.

- Blocking HERV transcription by promoting DNA methylation: "There has been a reasonable prediction that aberrant LTR activation could trigger malignant disorders and autoimmune responses if epigenetic changes including DNA hypomethylation occur in somatic cells. ... Hypomethylation of HERV-E and HERV-K was also observed in SLE patients."[337]

  - Clinical implementation of optimal DNA methylation: For optimization of DNA methylation, methyl-donating/transferring nutrients such as folate (used clinically as folinic acid and/or methylfolate), betaine, and (methyl)cobalamin are necessary but not sufficient. Other nutrients—particularly vitamin D3—play critical and complex roles, promoting methylation of some DNA regions and demethylation of others[338]; in the case of vitamin D, we note consistent epidemiologic and clinical experimental research showing that vitamin D3 protects against and treats inflammatory/autoimmune diseases. The complexity of nutrients, in this case vitamin D3, is demonstrated by the observation that vitamin D causes complex changes in gene expression at different locations and likely under different circumstances; vitamin D and activation of its receptor correlate with DNA methylation and the *conceptual opposite* DNA demethylation (occurring at different DNA sites), while also promoting histone acetylation of some regions and histone deacetylation of others.[339] Lastly and very importantly, clinicians have to think beyond nutrients and methylating nutrients to fully appreciate and optimize DNA methylation, given that this process is potently impacted by numerous environmental factors, including xenobiotic/toxin exposure, ultraviolet (UV) light exposure, and drug exposure (e.g., procainamide, hydralazine); again noted is the fact that SLE patients show global hypomethylation of DNA[340] therefore suggesting that the patients need a combination of nutritional optimization (adding methyl-active nutrients such as folinic acid, cobalamin, and cholecalciferol) and environmental optimization (subtracting injurious agents such as UV light, xenobiotics and drugs) in order to optimize DNA methylation patterns and balance.

- Blocking HERV transcription by blocking exogenous virus replication—Rationale for autoimmune disease treatment with anti-viral therapies: "Cited epidemiologic and experimental evidence suggests that increased replication of epigenomic viral pathogens such as Epstein-Barr Virus (EBV) in chronic human autoimmune diseases such as rheumatoid arthritis (RA), systemic lupus

---

[337] Katoh et al. Association of endogenous retroviruses and long terminal repeats with human disorders. *Front Oncol.* 2013 Sep 11;3:234

[338] "Alterations in DNA methylation lead to aberrant gene expression and disruptions of genomic integrity, which contribute to development and progression of diseases. Vitamin D can regulate these processes; the mechanisms behind need further investigations." Fetahu et al. Vitamin D and the epigenome. *Front Physiol.* 2014 Apr 29;5:164

[339] "These changes involve the methylation of genomic DNA and/or reversible post-translational modifications of histone proteins, such as acetylation or deacetylation at exposed lysine residues." Carlberg C. Genome-wide (over)view on the actions of vitamin D. *Front Physiol.* 2014 Apr 29;5:167

[340] "The mechanisms causing altered DNA methylation in autoimmunity, aging and carcinogenesis are incompletely characterized but include exposure to environmental agents and drugs, diet, altered signaling in pathways regulating DNA methyltransferase expression and changes in endogenous regulatory mechanisms. ... Initial studies demonstrated that T cells from patients with active lupus had globally hypomethylated DNA. ... Treating normal T cells with DNA methylation inhibitors is sufficient to cause a lupus-like disease in animal models, so exposure to exogenous DNA methylation inhibitors might similarly contribute to the development of autoimmunity. In support of this, the two drugs most frequently implicated in causing a lupus-like disease, procainamide and hydralazine, have been reported to inhibit DNA methylation...and induce autoreactivity in human and murine T lymphocytes." Richardson BC. Role of DNA methylation in the regulation of cell function: autoimmunity, aging and cancer. *J Nutr.* 2002 Aug;132(8 Sup):2401S-2405S

Erythematosus (SLE), and multiple sclerosis (MS) may activate endogenous human retroviruses (HERV) as a pathologic mechanism."[341]

- **Blocking HERV transcription by blocking exogenous virus replication**: "Herpes simplex viruses are known to transactivate retroviral regulatory LTR regions of both exogenous and endogenous human retroviruses..."[342]

- **Blocking HERV transcription by blocking nonspecific cellular stress and inflammation**: "Induction of cellular stress responses through serum deprivation did however, to some extent, mimic the effects of virus infection in terms of transcription of HERV-W elements. ... Environmental stressors can modulate the transcriptional activities of certain HERV-W elements which could thereby be markers for such insults."[343]

o **Viruses, part 3— Bacteriophages, especially of the gastrointestinal bacteria**: The fact that the lumen of the gastrointestinal tract is loaded with bacteria is well known; progressively, all healthcare providers and researchers are appreciating that bacterial imbalances (quantitative) and metabolic/behavioral disturbances (qualitative) contribute to various disease via multiple mechanisms, as reviewed in the section on dysbiosis in Chapter 4. The next step in our understanding of dysbiosis is what I have referred to previously as microbial dysbiosis—infections within microbes. Bacteriophages are viruses that infect bacteria, and the gastrointestinal bacteria, which are themselves susceptible to innumerable quantitative and qualitative imbalances, are susceptible to viral infections. Thus, any complete understanding of

Bacteriophages (also called "phages" or "virus-like particles" or VLP): mechanisms of contribution to dysbiosis, inflammation, and autoimmunity
• Bacteriophages ("viruses that infect bacteria") are the most abundant biological entities on earth; they outnumber bacteria by 10x; more than 1,200 genotypes found within the human gastrointestinal tract
• The gut virome is dominated by these prokaryotic viruses that prey on gut bacteria; since the reproductive capability of all phage particles is unknown, describing them as "viruses" is discouraged in preference for "virus-like particles" (VLP)
• Bacteriophages influence bacterial diversity and "population structure" via "destabilization of bacterial communities"; the infectious and lytic nature of bacteriophages will obviously influence survival and death of specific populations of bacteria while the effects of lysogeny result directly in more viral particles and death of bacteria with release of bacterial and viral immunogens. Conversely, human gut bacteriophage populations do not change impressively with the corresponding bacterial colonizations (exception seen with *Faecalibacterium prausnitzii* which has a proportionate phage population) within physiologic norms (longitudinal stability); the majority of phages seem to correspond (34-41%) to the *Firmicutes* phylum of bacteria.
• Bacteriophages participate in gene transfer and genome reorganization; they also carry numerous antibiotic resistance genes: multidrug efflux transporters (n = 355), vancomycin resistance genes (n = 129), tetracycline resistance genes (n = 18), and beta-lactamases (n = 16).
• VLP sequences represent 4% to 17% of the total DNA from human stool; this quantitative minority of DNA material could have profound pathological implications for conditions characterized by anti-nuclear antibodies and the resulting immune complexes. Viral particles from intestinal bacteriophages are certainly absorbed and would thereafter contribute to 1) primary inflammation, and almost certainly to 2) transactivation of HERVs, 3) cross-reactivity to DNA (e.g., ANA), and 4) immune complex deposition.
• Patients with the "autoimmune disease" Crohn's disease harbor many more bacteriophages per biopsy sample (2.1-4.1 billion) than do healthy controls (1.2 billion).
• Phage populations are modified via dietary change (*Genome Res* 2012 Oct); but the implications are not clear.

dysbiosis must also consider the role of bacteriophages; these will be reviewed via the following survey of the literature.

- **Dysbiosis in inflammatory bowel disease via bacteriophages (*Gut*. 2008 Mar[344])**: In this excellent and brief report by Lepage et al, the authors propose that bacteriophage-mediated or bacteriophage-induced inflammatory dysbiosis may play a role in inflammatory bowel disease; and they note that bacteriophages outnumber bacteria 10-fold "in many natural ecosystems." Bacteriophages are diverse, with more than 1,200 genotypes found within the human gastrointestinal tract; per biopsy

[341] Dreyfus DH. Autoimmune disease: A role for new anti-viral therapies? *Autoimmun Rev*. 2011 Dec;11(2):88-97

[342] Nellaker et al. Transactivation of elements in the human endogenous retrovirus W family by viral infection. *Retrovirology*. 2006 Jul 6;3:44

[343] Nellaker et al. Transactivation of elements in the human endogenous retrovirus W family by viral infection. *Retrovirology*. 2006 Jul 6;3:44

[344] Lepage et al. Dysbiosis in inflammatory bowel disease: a role for bacteriophages? *Gut*. 2008 Mar;57(3):424-5

sample from the human gastrointestinal tract, an average of 1.2 billion (1.2×10^9) virus-like particles (VLP) are quantifiable and dominated by the families *Siphoviridae*, *Myoviridae* and *Podoviridae*. Patients with the "autoimmune disease" Crohn's disease (CD) harbor many more VLP per biopsy sample (2.1-4.1 billion) than do healthy controls (1.2 billion).

- Human gut virome: inter-individual variation and response to diet (*Genome Res.* 2011 Oct[345]): "VLP sequences represent a minority of the total DNA from stool, in the range of from 4% to 17%"; while this may be a *numerical* minority the physiologic and immunogenic significance could be massive. This article provides technical information and demonstrates phage response to diet, but the clinical implications and the authors' presentation of data are not clear.

o <mark>Viruses, part 4—Bacterial synergism via NFkB activation and immunosuppression</mark>:

- Bacterial promotion of viral replication via inflammatory pathways: Bacterial debris such as DNA and LPS are known to trigger inflammatory responses via TLR and NFkB; activation of NFkB—the proinflammatory transcription factor often "hijacked" by viruses to promote their own replication—promotes viral replication. Thus, increased total bacterial load (TBL, such as SIBO) would be expected to promote viral replication.

- Bacterial promotion of viral replication via immunosuppression: As a specific example, *Helicobacter pylori* may play a powerful role as a synergistic bioagent for the microbial promotion of autoimmunity via its ability to *simultaneously* and *paradoxically* cause immunosuppression (thereby allowing other microbes to flourish) and systemic inflammation[346]; in this manner, the bacterial infection is permissive to and perhaps necessary for the autoimmune-inducing vasculopathic and fibrogenic viral infections (see section on Scleroderma for pathology details).

Clinical presentations:

- Subtypes and overlapping presentations: As shown in the diagram below, SLE has several subtypes which can present exclusively or in combination, ie, a patient may have classic SLE with no skin lesions, skin lesions without fulminant SLE, or classic SLE with one or more types of skin lesions.

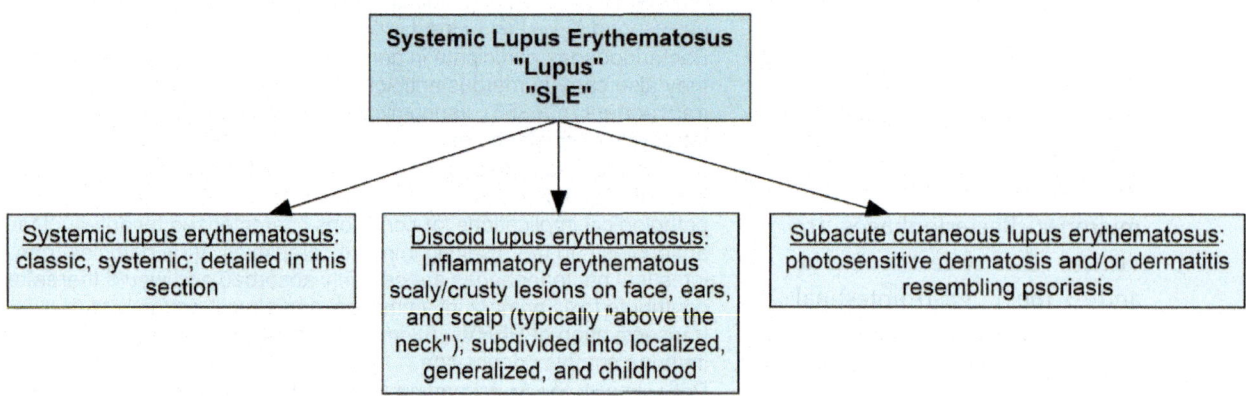

Graphic above illustrating different disease subtypes that fall under the label of SLE/lupus

- Gender: 85-90% of new patients are women in their childbearing years (frequency: 1 per 700 women); the ratio of women to men is 9:1 except among prepubertal children and older/postmenopausal men and women in which the ratio is 2:1.[347] The much higher prevalence of the disorder among women of childbearing age compared to men of the same age (11:1) implicates sex hormones and hormonal fluctuations as causative factors that predispose young women to this disorder.

- 4x more common in women of African descent (1 per 250) than Caucasian women (1 per 1000).[348] The increased prevalence of SLE in dark-skinned women may be due at least in part to their higher prevalence of vitamin D

---

[345] Minot et al. The human gut virome: inter-individual variation and dynamic response to diet. *Genome Res.* 2011 Oct;21(10):1616-25

[346] "Infectious agents such as Helicobacter pylori (Hp) may cause chronic inflammation and autoimmune reactivity in susceptible subjects. The results of in vitro experiments performed with lymphocytes from Hp infected patients indicate that Hp can cause immunosuppression which might be eliminated by successful eradication therapy." Hybenova et al. The role of environmental factors in autoimmune thyroiditis. *Neuro Endocrinol Lett.* 2010;31(3):283-9

[347] Manzi S. Epidemiology of systemic lupus erythematosus. *Am J Manag Care.* 2001 Oct;7(16 Suppl):S474-9 ajmc.com/files/articlefiles/A01_131_2001octManziS474_9.pdf

[348] Tierney ML. McPhee SJ, Papadakis MA. *Current Medical Diagnosis and Treatment 2006. 45th edition*. New York; Lange Medical Books: 2006, pages 833-837

deficiency, which unquestionably predisposes to inflammation, immune dysfunction, and the clinical manifestation of autoimmunity.[349] Although administration of vitamin D3 to cholecalciferol-deficient adults clearly has anti-inflammatory action[350,351], important windows of opportunity appear to occur *in utero* and within the first few postnatal months and years; for example, administration of vitamin D to **infants** reduces the subsequent incidence of type-1 *autoimmune-mediated* diabetes by 78%.[352] Vitamin D sufficiency appears to support immune function and thereby reduce the acquisition of infectious diseases[353]; thus, vitamin D may exert an anti-*rheumatic* benefit by exerting an anti-*infectious* benefit; i.e., by preventing the dysbiotic infections that may serve to trigger autoimmunity. Given the strength of evidence supporting the routine use of vitamin D3 supplementation in infants, children, and adults, healthcare providers should ensure adequate vitamin D status in their patients[354,355,356] for the treatment and prevention of long-latency deficiency diseases[357] and alleviation of systemic inflammation.[358]

- Positive family history of the disease is common: daughters of a mother with SLE have a 1 in 40 prevalence of SLE, whereas sons have a 1 in 250 prevalence
- Clinical course may be slow or acute, involving many organ systems or only one, and is characterized by exacerbations and remissions
- **Classic autoimmune systemic manifestations: fatigue, malaise, low-grade fever, anorexia, weight loss, peripheral polyarthritis.** Septicemia and septic arthritis should always be considered in patients with SLE, especially those taking immunosuppressive drugs and those experiencing what appears to be an exacerbation of the disease.
  - o <u>Skin</u>:
    - Malar "butterfly" rash over the cheeks and bridge of the nose: this is a classic manifestation of the disease but is seen in less than half of SLE patients
    - Photosensitivity: erythematous skin rash develops readily on sun-exposed areas
    - Hair loss
    - Nail infarcts, periungual erythema, splinter hemorrhages
    - Purpura
  - o <u>Musculoskeletal</u>:
    - 90% of patients have polyarthralgia—most commonly affecting the peripheral joints of the hands, wrists, knees, feet
    - Polymyalgia, myositis, and myopathy; avascular necrosis due to corticosteroids
  - o <u>Renal/kidney</u>:
    - <u>Immune complex-mediated glomerulonephritis</u>: 50% of patients have clinical nephritis, hematuria, and proteinuria; renal function commonly declines during exacerbation of disease and then improves with disease remission
    - **Renal failure is a leading cause of death in patients with SLE**[359]
  - o <u>CNS</u>:
    - 70% have EEG abnormalities
    - <u>**Neuropsychiatric lupus (secondary to vasculitis, neuroinflammation, and immune-mediated alterations in [dopaminergic] neurotransmission) requires specialist care and has been described as a medical emergency**</u>[360]: Characteristics include psychosis, seizures, transient ischemic attacks, severe depression, delirium, confusion. Exclude adverse drug effect (especially corticosteroid psychosis), infection, hypertension, and hyponatremia.

---

[349] Cantorna MT. Vitamin D and autoimmunity: is vitamin D status an environmental factor affecting autoimmune disease prevalence? *Proc Soc Exp Biol Med*. 2000;223:230-3
[350] Timms et al. Circulating MMP9, vitamin D and variation in TIMP-1 response with VDR genotype: mechanisms for inflammatory damage chronic disorders? *QJM* 2002:787-96
[351] Van den Berghe G, et al. Bone turnover in prolonged critical illness: effect of vitamin D. *J Clin Endocrinol Metab*. 2003;88(10):4623-32
[352] "Children who regularly took recommended dose of vitamin D (2000 IU daily) had a RR of 0.22 (0.05-0.89) compared with those who regularly received less than recommended amount." Hypponen et al. Intake of vitamin D and risk of type 1 diabetes: birth-cohort study. *Lancet* 2001;358:1500-3: very important article
[353] Wayse V, et al. Association of subclinical vitamin D deficiency with severe acute lower respiratory infection in Indian children under 5 y. *Eur J Clin Nutr*. 2004;58(4):563-7
[354] Vasquez A, Manso G, Cannell J. The clinical importance of vitamin D (cholecalciferol). *Altern Ther Health Med*. 2004 Sep;10(5):28-36 ichnfm.academia.edu/AlexVasquez
[355] Heaney RP. Vitamin D, nutritional deficiency, and the medical paradigm. *J Clin Endocrinol Metab*. 2003 Nov;88(11):5107-8
[356] Hollis BW, Wagner CL. Assessment of dietary vitamin D requirements during pregnancy and lactation. *Am J Clin Nutr*. 2004 May;79:717-26
[357] Heaney RP. Long-latency deficiency disease: insights from calcium and vitamin D. *Am J Clin Nutr*. 2003;78(5):912-9 jcem.endojournals.org/cgi/content/full/88/11/5107
[358] Timms et al. Circulating MMP9, vitamin D and variation in the TIMP-1 response with VDR genotype. *QJM*. 2002;95:787-96
[359] Suzuki et al. Development of pathogenic anti-DNA antibodies in patients with systemic lupus erythematosus. *FASEB J* 1997 Oct;11:1033-8
[360] McInnes I, Sturrock R. Rheumatological emergencies. *Practitioner*. 1994 Mar;238(1536):220-4

- Headaches, migraine, stroke
- Peripheral and cranial neuropathies, transverse myelitis
- Increased risk for meningitis when immunosuppressive therapy is used.
  o Cardiovascular and circulation:
    - Vasculitis
    - Thrombosis and **increased risk for myocardial infarction**
    - Pericarditis, myocarditis: may result in sudden death, heart failure, arrhythmias
    - Hypertension due to renal injury
    - Raynaud's phenomenon—periodic vasospasm affecting the hands and fingers
    - Antiphospholipid antibody syndrome—a major cause of complications
  o Lungs/pulmonary:
    - Pneumonitis: presents with fever, cough, dyspnea—important to **assess with radiographs and exclude infection**
    - Pleurisy, pleural effusion; **alveolar hemorrhage can be life-threatening**
  o Hematologic/CBC abnormalities:
    - Leukopenia, lymphopenia, thrombocytopenia, anemia
    - Immune complexes: Immune complexes are elevated in patients with active SLE[361]
  o Gastrointestinal:
    - Nausea
    - Diarrhea
    - **Intestinal/mesenteric vasculitis and infarct—surgical emergency**—postprandial abdominal pain, cramps, vomiting, diarrhea
    - Pancreatitis
    - Increased intestinal permeability, occasionally protein-losing enteropathy results[362]
  o Eyes:
    - **Retinal vasculitis** (look for exudates with fundoscopic examination) can cause blindness in days—**treat as an emergency**
    - Other manifestations include conjunctivitis, photophobia, blurred vision
  o Other:
    - Edema—may be seen with cardiac or renal damage
    - Lymphadenopathy
    - Mucocutaneous ulcerations
    - Increased risk of miscarriage and congenital heart block

Major differential diagnoses:

- Infection
- Cancer, lymphoma
- RA or other autoimmune disease such as scleroderma, vasculitis, sarcoidosis
- Iron overload
- Fibromyalgia
- Porphyria cutanea tarda
- Drug hypersensitivity and drug-induced lupus: SLE is differentiated from drug-induced lupus by the following characteristics of drug-induced lupus: 1) temporal association with drug/medication use; remission of disease following drug discontinuation, and 2) lack of fully characteristic pattern of clinical and laboratory manifestations: lack of renal and CNS involvement, lack of hypocomplementemia and anti-native DNA antibodies. Clinicians must exclude drug-induced lupus before making diagnosis of SLE.

---

[361] Suzuki N, Mihara S, Sakane T. Development of pathogenic anti-DNA antibodies in patients with systemic lupus erythematosus. *FASEB J.* 1997 Oct;11(12):1033-8
[362] "Fourteen cases of primary lupus-associated protein-losing enteropathy have now been reported in the English-language literature." Perednia DA, Curosh NA. Lupus-associated protein-losing enteropathy. *Arch Intern Med.* 1990 Sep;150(9):1806-10

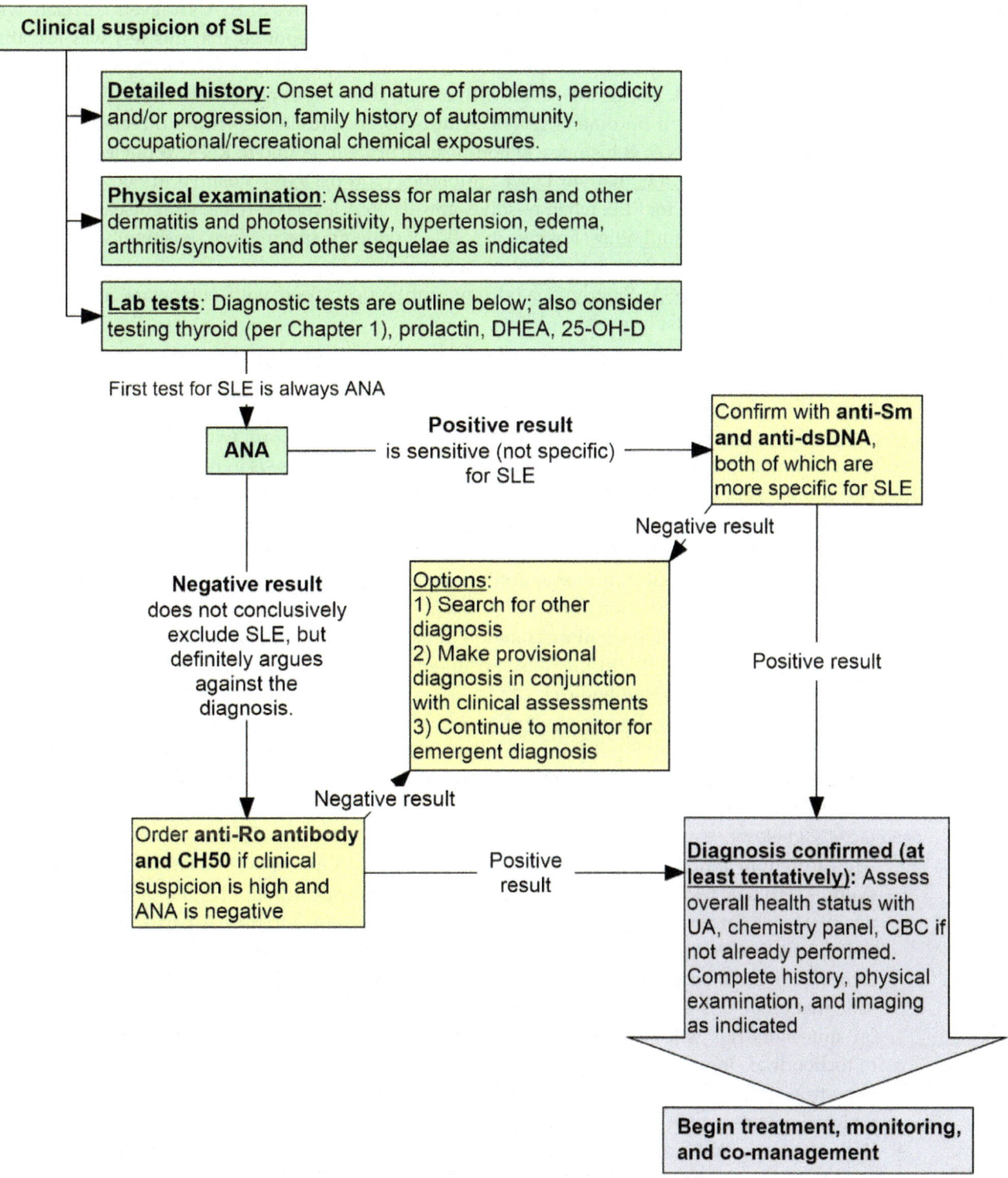

Algorithm for use of initial laboratory testing for SLE: This diagram is to be used in conjunction with other information presented in this book and any new published guidelines; however, this information will likely always remain clinically relevant and reasonably useful.

<u>Clinical assessments</u>:
- **History and physical examination**: consistent with the clinical presentations listed previously
- **Laboratory assessments**:
  - o <u>Comprehensive laboratory evaluation</u>: Use other tests (e.g. and especially, metabolic/chemistry panel, UA, CBC, etc.) to assess for complications and concomitant disease.

- ANA—anti-nuclear antibodies: ANA is the best screening test and has been described as positive in 100% of SLE patients[363] despite the acknowledged existence of ANA-negative SLE. ANA levels correlate with disease activity. Previous editions of standard medical textbooks reported that this test was less than 100% sensitive for SLE; it may be that improvements in laboratory analysis now account for the 100% sensitivity. A positive ANA test result—even with a high titer—does not necessarily indicate that the patient has SLE, especially if no other signs or symptoms are present. ANA are directed against the following four targets: ❶ DNA, ❷ histones, ❸ non-histone proteins bound to RNA, ❹ nucleolar antigens.
  - Anti-double stranded (DS, native) DNA antibodies (anti-dsDNA): Positive in ~60% of patients; specific (not sensitive) for SLE; when positive, anti-dsDNA levels correlate with disease activity.
  - Anti-Sm (anti-Smith) antibodies: Positive in ~30% of patients; specific (not sensitive) for SLE.[364]
  - Anti-histone antibodies: Seen in drug-induced lupus.
  - Anti-Ro antibodies (SSA: Sjogren's syndrome antibodies): Seen with cutaneous SLE, Sjogren's syndrome, and neonatal lupus.[365]
- CRP: Sensitive indicator of inflammation *except in SLE* where CRP levels can be normal even with severe active disease.[366,367]
- ESR: Not useful in all patients with SLE.[368]
- Complement levels (CH50): Complement levels are lowered in accord with complement pathway activation by immune complexes; levels tend to normalize when disease is in remission.
- Inherited complement deficiencies: 6% of SLE patients has an inherited/genetic deficiency in one or more complement proteins. Deficiency of C1q, C2, or **C4** appears to result in inability to clear immune complexes and thus results in exacerbation of disease manifestations due to immune complex deposition. C1q deficiency may impair clearance of apoptotic cells and thus promote antigenicity toward nuclear debris via—for example—activation of DAMP (damage-associated molecular pattern) receptors.
- HLA-DR2 and HLA-DR3: These are more common in patients with SLE than in the general population.
- Serologic testing for syphilis (VDRL): A false-positive test for syphilis is characteristic of SLE and is a reflection of antiphospholipid antibodies.
- Antiphospholipid and Anticardiolipin antibodies: Antiphospholipid antibodies (directed against plasma proteins complexed to phospholipids) are seen in 40-50% of SLE patients. Antiphospholipid antibodies are associated with significantly increased risk for venous and arterial thrombosis. In SLE patients with antiphospholipid antibodies, treatment with anticoagulants such as warfarin/coumadin are commonly used (see INR below):
  - Anticardiolipin antibodies: This is one of several types of antiphospholipid antibodies; also used in syphilis serologic testing, and therefore SLE patients with anticardiolipin antibodies may have false positive result for syphilis. Anticardiolipin antibodies interfere with the PT (partial thromboplastin) test and are thus occasionally called "lupus anticoagulant"—this factitious anticoagulation is purely an *in vitro* phenomenon and is misleading since these same patients actually have a hypercoagulable state that predisposes them to arterial and venous thromboses. Readers attentive to the information on mitochondrial will have also noted that the phospholipid cardiolipin is located on the mitochondrial inner membrane, where it serves as an anchor for the enzyme succinate dehydrogenase; this data suggests an important role for mitochondrial dysfunction in SLE: a fact which is now very well proven, although not widely known by many practicing clinicians.
  - INR: International Normalized Ratio is a standardized quantification of Prothrombin Time (PT), which is a measure of clotting/bleeding tendency. INR is used to monitor dosing of warfarin/coumadin; generally the INR should be kept between 2.0-3.0.[369]
- Comprehensive testing for celiac disease and wheat allergy: Some patients diagnosed with "systemic lupus erythematosus" actually have autoimmunity and systemic inflammation due to occult celiac

[363] Tierney ML. McPhee SJ, Papadakis MA. *Current Medical Diagnosis and Treatment 2006. 45th edition*. New York; Lange Medical Books: 2006, pages 833-837
[364] Shojania K. Rheumatology: 2. What laboratory tests are needed? *CMAJ*. 2000 Apr 18;162(8):1157-63 cmaj.ca/cgi/content/full/162/8/1157
[365] Shojania K. Rheumatology: 2. What laboratory tests are needed? *CMAJ*. 2000 Apr 18;162(8):1157-63
[366] Deodhar SD. C-reactive protein: the best laboratory indicator available for monitoring disease activity. *Cleve Clin J Med* 1989 Mar-Apr;56(2):126-30
[367] Gabay C, Kushner I. Acute-phase proteins and other systemic responses to inflammation. *N Engl J Med*. 1999 Feb 11;340(6):448-54
[368] Klippel JH (ed). *Primer on the Rheumatic Diseases. 11th Edition*. Atlanta: Arthritis Foundation. 1997 page 94
[369] Tierney ML. McPhee SJ, Papadakis MA. *Current Medical Diagnosis and Treatment 2006. 45th edition*. New York; Lange Medical Books: 2006, pages 833-837

disease. These patients achieve clinical remission after avoiding gluten/gliadin-containing grains such as wheat.[370,371] More than 23% of patients with SLE have anti-gliadin antibodies.[372] In addition to IgA and IgG anti-gliadin antibodies, serologic testing for celiac disease includes IgA and IgG antiendomysial and anti-transglutaminase antibodies which should be interpreted along with a test for total serum IgA to identify those patients with selective IgA deficiency.

- **Imaging**:
  - o Imaging is used to in the assessment of complications and exclusion of concomitant diseases.
  - o The arthritis of SLE is typically mild (compared to rheumatoid arthritis) and is nondeforming.

Establishing the diagnosis:
- Clinical presentation and lab tests; more positives = more confident diagnosis.

Qualification for a diagnosis of SLE requires quantification of <u>at least four</u> of these <u>eleven</u> criteria:
1. Malar/cheek rash
2. Discoid rash
3. Photosensitivity
4. Ulcerations of oral mucosa
5. Joint pain and inflammation not attributable to other disease or trauma
6. Serositis: Inflammation of the serous tissues, which line the lungs (pleura), heart (pericardium), and the inner lining of the abdomen (peritoneum) and associated organs
7. Renal disease (any of the following): >3+ proteinuria measured by dipstick; cellular casts; proteinuria >0.5 grams per day
8. CNS involvement: seizures or psychosis without other cause
9. Hematologic abnormalities (any of the following): hemolytic anemia, leucopenia (45%), lymphopenia, thrombocytopenia (30%), anemia of chronic disease
10. Positive ANA
11. Additional serologic tests (any of the following):
o Positive LE cell prep
o Anti-native DNA antibody (50%)
o Anti-Sm antibody (20%)
o False-positive test for syphilis (25%)

Life-threatening complications and medical urgencies/emergencies:
- **Infection**—Infections are now the leading cause of death in patients with SLE[373]
- **SLE complications: renal failure and CNS involvement**
- **Stroke, myocardial infarction**—Increased risk with male gender and antiphospholipid antibodies
- Septic arthritis
- Thromboembolism
- 10-year survival is >85%[374]

Overview of clinical management:
- **The clinical course of the disease is variable, marked by exacerbations and remissions. Life-threatening complications can develop rapidly and must be managed effectively to prevent patient morbidity and practitioner liability.**
- Treat patient safely and effectively. If you cannot get good results, refer them to someone who can. Refer if clinical outcome is unsatisfactory or if serious complications are possible. Stable patients are seen every 3-6

---

[370] "The immunological profile of IgA deficiency and/or raised double stranded DNA in the absence of antinuclear factor together with raised inflammatory markers and symptoms suggestive of an immune diathesis should alert the physician to the possibility of gluten sensitivity." Hadjivassiliou et al. Gluten sensitivity masquerading as systemic lupus erythematosus. *Ann Rheum Dis.* 2004 Nov;63(11):1501-3 ard.bmjjournals.com/cgi/content/full/63/11/1501

[371] "Villous atrophy on duodenal biopsy specimens with a favorable response to a gluten-free diet was noted in all five patients." Zitouni et al. Systemic lupus erythematosus with celiac disease: a report of five cases. *Joint Bone Spine.* 2004 Jul;71(4):344-6

[372] "Twenty-four of 103 (23.3%) systemic lupus erythematosus patients tested positive for either antigliadin antibody, whereas none of the 103 patients tested positive for antiendomysial antibody." Rensch et al. The prevalence of celiac disease autoantibodies in patients with systemic lupus erythematosus. *Am J Gastroenterol.* 2001 Apr;96(4):1113-5 For the authors to state that these patients did not have celiac disease simply because their intestinal biopsies were normal is inconsistent with the modern paradigm of celiac disease which acknowledges that the disease can be present in the absence of gastrointestinal lesions.

[373] Tierney ML. McPhee SJ, Papadakis MA. *Current Medical Diagnosis and Treatment 2006. 45th edition.* New York; Lange Medical Books: 2006, pages 833-837

[374] Tierney ML. McPhee SJ, Papadakis MA. *Current Medical Diagnosis and Treatment 2006. 45th edition.* New York; Lange Medical Books: 2006, pages 833-837

months for monitoring of disease activity, re-examination, and treatment recalibration.[375] Patients must understand that acute exacerbations and/or new symptoms—especially fever—must be evaluated promptly.

- Treatment must be customized to the patient and must be flexible to accommodate the natural exacerbations and remissions of the disease.
- To the extent possible, discourage use of NSAIDs since these drugs exacerbate joint destruction, renal impairment, and increased intestinal permeability which increases exposure to dietary and microbial antigens.

Treatments: The standard medical protocol centers on and starts with (new drugs are always being developed and added): prednisone, Plaquenil and immunoparalytic and immunosuppressive drugs.

- Drug treatments:
  - **NSAIDs:** For joint pain[376] despite adverse effects on the gut[377], joints[378,379,380] and kidneys.
  - **Antimalarial drug: hydroxychloroquine/Plaquenil**): Adverse effects include retinal damage, neuropathy, myopathy. As with anticonvulsant drugs, hydroxychloroquine/Plaquenil interferes with conversion of 25-hydroxycholecalciferol to the more active 1-25-dihydroxycholecalciferol[381]; this would be expected to exacerbate immune dysfunction, inflammation, hypertension, and depression.
  - **Danazol is an androgenic corticosteroid:** particularly used against thrombocytopenia
  - **Immunosuppression** with prednisone (promotes bacterial overgrowth and osteoporosis), cyclophosphamide (especially for renal involvement), mycophenolate mofetil, azathioprine, or other DMARD (disease-modifying antirheumatic drugs) is commonly used, particularly for the more serious complications of the disease such as those affecting the brain, heart, lungs, and kidneys. **Despite the clinical drawbacks and philosophical inadequacies, pharmacologic immunosuppression has a role in the management of patients with autoimmunity when their disease flares and threatens vital structures, particularly the heart, brain, and kidneys.**
  - **Anticoagulant drugs such as warfarin** are used for patients with antiphospholipid antibodies and resultant thrombotic complications.

- **FOOD & NUTRITION: 5-part "supplemented Paleo-Mediterranean diet" (SPMD)** The 5-part "supplemented Paleo-Mediterranean diet" (SPMD—reviewed in Chapter 4) consists of ❶ foundational plant-based low-carbohydrate diet of fruits, vegetables, nuts, seeds, berries and lean sources of protein, ❷ multivitamin and multimineral supplementation, ❸ physiologic doses of vitamin D3 (range 2,000-10,000 IU/d), ❹ combination fatty acid therapy (CFAT) with n3-ALA, n6-GLA, n3-EPA, n3-DHA, and phytochemical-rich olive oil which contains n9-oleate, and ❺ probiotics.
  - Gluten avoidance: Celiac disease can present with inflammatory oligoarthritis that resembles rheumatoid arthritis and which remits with avoidance of wheat/gluten; the inflammatory arthropathy of celiac disease has preceded bowel symptoms and/or an accurate diagnosis by as many as 3-15 years.[382,383] Some patients diagnosed with "systemic lupus erythematosus" actually have autoimmunity and systemic inflammation due to occult celiac disease, and they achieve remarkable improvement—complete remission of systemic inflammation and the ability to discontinue all anti-inflammatory drugs—after

[375] Manzi S. Epidemiology of systemic lupus erythematosus. *Am J Manag Care* 2001 Oct;7(16Sup):S474-9 ajmc.com/files/articlefiles/A01_131_2001octManziS474_9.pdf
[376] Tierney ML. McPhee SJ, Papadakis MA. *Current Medical Diagnosis and Treatment 2006. 45th edition*. New York; Lange Medical Books: 2006, pages 833-837
[377] Abbreviations: cow's milk beta-lactoglobulin absorption (BLG), acetylsalicylic acid (ASA), disodium chromoglycate (DSCG). "ASA administration strongly increased BLG absorption, not prevented by DSCG pretreatment. In normal controls treated with a single dose of ASA we obtained similar results. Our results suggest that prolonged treatment with nonsteroidal anti-inflammatory drugs induces an increase of food antigen absorption, apparently not related to anaphylaxis mediator release, with possible clinical effects." Fagiolo et al. Intestinal permeability and antigen absorption in rheumatoid arthritis. Effects of acetylsalicylic acid and sodium chromoglycate. *Int Arch Allergy Appl Immunol.* 1989;89(1):98-102
[378] "At…concentrations comparable to those… in the synovial fluid of patients treated with the drug, several NSAIDs suppress proteoglycan synthesis…." Brandt KD. Effects of nonsteroidal anti-inflammatory drugs on chondrocyte metabolism in vitro and in vivo. *Am J Med.* 1987 Nov 20; 83(5A): 29-34
[379] "This highly significant association between NSAID use and acetabular destruction gives cause for concern, not least because of the difficulty in achieving satisfactory hip replacements in patients with severely damaged acetabula." Newman NM, Ling RS. Acetabular bone destruction related to non-steroidal anti-inflammatory drugs. *Lancet.* 1985 Jul 6; 2(8445): 11-4
[380] Vidal y Plana et al. Articular cartilage pharmacology: In vitro studies on glucosamine and non steroidal anti-inflammatory drugs. *Pharmacol Res Commun.* 1978 Jun;10:557-69
[381] "Half the SLE and FM patients had 25(OH)-vitamin D levels < 50 nmol/l, a level at which PTH stimulation occurs. Our data suggest that in SLE patients HCQ might inhibit conversion of 25(OH)-vitamin D to 1,25(OH)2-vitamin D." Huisman et al. Vitamin D levels in women with systemic lupus erythematosus and fibromyalgia. *J Rheumatol.* 2001 Nov;28(11):2535-9
[382] "We report six patients with coeliac disease in whom arthritis was prominent at diagnosis and who improved with dietary therapy. Joint pain preceded diagnosis by up to three years in five patients and 15 years in one patient." Bourne JT, et al. Arthritis and coeliac disease. *Ann Rheum Dis.* 1985 Sep;44(9):592-8
[383] "A 15-year-old girl, with synovitis of the knees and ankles for 3 years before a diagnosis of gluten-sensitive enteropathy, is described." Pinals RS. Arthritis associated with gluten-sensitive enteropathy. *J Rheumatol.* 1986 Feb;13(1):201-4

avoiding gluten/gliadin-containing grains, most notoriously, wheat.[384] In a study of 103 SLE patients, more than 23% of SLE patients had anti-gliadin antibodies.[385]

o Short-term fasting: In case reports and clinical trials, short-term fasting (or protein-sparing fasting) has been documented as safe and effective treatment for SLE[386], RA[387], and non-rheumatic diseases such as chronic severe hypertension[388], moderate hypertension[389], obesity[390,391], type-2 diabetes[392], and epilepsy.[393] The combination of energy restriction and fish oil supplementation was shown highly beneficial in an animal model of SLE.[394]

o Broad-spectrum fatty acid therapy with ALA, EPA, DHA, GLA and oleic acid: Fish oil provides EPA and DHA which have well-proven anti-inflammatory benefits when used in the treatment of SLE.[395,396,397] Fatty acid supplementation should be delivered in the form of combination therapy with ALA, GLA, DHA, and EPA. Given at doses of 3,000 – 9,000 mg per day, ALA from flax oil has impressive anti-inflammatory benefits demonstrated by its ability to halve prostaglandin production in humans.[398] Numerous studies have demonstrated the benefit of GLA in the treatment of rheumatoid arthritis when used at doses between 500 mg – 4,000 mg per day.[399,400] Fish oil provides EPA and DHA which have well-proven anti-inflammatory benefits in RA[401,402,403] and SLE.[404,405]

o Vitamin D3 supplementation with physiologic doses and/or tailored to serum 25(OH)D levels: Vitamin D deficiency is common in the general population and is even more common in patients with chronic illness and chronic musculoskeletal pain.[406] **At least 50% of patients with SLE are deficient in vitamin D[407]**, and even more would be found deficient if stricter and more appropriate criteria are used.

---

[384] "The immunological profile of IgA deficiency and/or raised double stranded DNA in the absence of antinuclear factor together with raised inflammatory markers and symptoms suggestive of an immune diathesis should alert the physician to the possibility of gluten sensitivity." Hadjivassiliou M, Sanders DS, Grunewald RA, Akil M. Gluten sensitivity masquerading as systemic lupus erythematosus. *Ann Rheum Dis.* 2004 Nov;63(11):1501-3 ard.bmjjournals.com/cgi/content/full/63/11/1501

[385] "Twenty-four of 103 (23.3%) systemic lupus erythematosus patients tested positive for either antigliadin antibody, whereas none of the 103 patients tested positive for antiendomysial antibody." Rensch et al. The prevalence of celiac disease autoantibodies in patients with systemic lupus erythematosus. *Am J Gastroenterol.* 2001 Apr;96(4):1113-5. For the authors to state that these patients did not have celiac disease simply because their intestinal biopsies were normal seems to indicate that the authors were ignorant of the modern paradigm of celiac disease which acknowledges that the disease can be present in the absence of gastrointestinal lesions.

[386] Fuhrman et al. Brief case reports of medically supervised, water-only fasting associated with remission of autoimmune disease. *Altern Ther Health Med.* 2002 Jul;8:112, 110-1

[387] "An association was found between improvement in inflammatory activity of the joints and enhancement of neutrophil bactericidal capacity. Fasting appears to improve the clinical status of patients with RA." Uden AM, Trang L, Venizelos N, Palmblad J. Neutrophil functions and clinical performance after total fasting in patients with rheumatoid arthritis. *Ann Rheum Dis.* 1983 Feb;42(1):45-51

[388] "The average reduction in blood pressure was 37/13 mm Hg, with the greatest decrease being observed for subjects with the most severe hypertension. Patients with stage 3 hypertension (those with systolic blood pressure greater than 180 mg Hg, diastolic blood pressure greater than 110 mg Hg, or both) had an average reduction of 60/17 mm Hg at the conclusion of treatment." Goldhamer et al. Medically supervised water-only fasting in the treatment of hypertension. *J Manipulative Physiol Ther.* 2001 Jun;24(5):335-9

[389] "RESULTS: Approximately 82% of the subjects achieved BP at or below 120/80 mm Hg by the end of the treatment program. The mean BP reduction was 20/7 mm Hg, with the greatest decrease being observed for subjects with the highest baseline BP." Goldhamer AC, Lisle DJ, Sultana P, Anderson SV, Parpia B, Hughes B, Campbell TC. Medically supervised water-only fasting in the treatment of borderline hypertension. *J Altern Complement Med.* 2002 Oct;8(5):643-50

[390] Vertes V, Genuth SM, Hazelton IM. Supplemented fasting as a large-scale outpatient program. *JAMA.* 1977 Nov 14;238(20):2151-3

[391] Bauman WA, Schwartz E, Rose HG, et al. Early and long-term effects of acute caloric deprivation in obese diabetic patients. *Am J Med.* 1988 Jul;85(1):38-46

[392] Goldhamer AC. Initial cost of care results in medically supervised water-only fasting for treating high blood pressure and diabetes. *J Altern Complement Med.* 2002 Dec;8(6):696-7

[393] "The ketogenic diet should be considered as alternative therapy for children with difficult-to-control seizures. It is more effective than many of the new anticonvulsant medications and is well tolerated by children and families when it is effective." Freeman et al. The efficacy of the ketogenic diet-1998: a prospective evaluation of intervention in 150 children. *Pediatrics.* 1998 Dec;102(6):1358-63 pediatrics.aappublications.org/cgi/reprint/102/6/1358

[394] "In conclusion, our data strongly indicate that ER and FO maintain antioxidant status and GSH:GSSG ratio, thereby protecting against renal deterioration from oxidative insults during ageing." Kelley et al. A fish oil diet rich in eicosapentaenoic acid reduces cyclooxygenase metabolites, and suppresses lupus in MRL-lpr mice. *J Immunol.* 1985 Mar;134(3):1914-9

[395] "No major side effects were noted, and it is suggested that dietary modification with additional marine oil may be a useful way of modifying disease activity in systemic lupus erythematosus." Walton et al. Dietary fish oil and the severity of symptoms in patients with systemic lupus erythematosus. *Ann Rheum Dis.* 1991 Jul;50(7):463-6

[396] "CONCLUSION: In the management of SLE, dietary supplementation with fish oil may be beneficial in modifying symptomatic disease activity." Duffy et al. The clinical effect of dietary supplementation with omega-3 fish oils and/or copper in systemic lupus erythematosus. *J Rheumatol.* 2004 Aug;31(8):1551-6

[397] "Oral supplementation of EPA and DHA induced prolonged remission of SLE in 10 consecutive patients without any side-effects. These results suggest that n-3 fatty acids, EPA and DHA, are useful in the management of SLE and possibly, other similar collagen vascular diseases." Das UN. Beneficial effect of eicosapentaenoic and docosahexaenoic acids in the management of systemic lupus erythematosus and its relationship to the cytokine network. *Prostaglandins Leukot Essent Fatty Acids.* 1994 Sep;51(3):207-13

[398] Adam O, Wolfram G, Zollner N. Effect of alpha-linolenic acid in the human diet on linoleic acid metabolism and prostaglandin biosynthesis. *J Lipid Res.* 1986 Apr;27(4):421-6

[399] "Other results showed a significant reduction in morning stiffness with gamma-linolenic acid at 3 months and reduction in pain and articular index at 6 months with olive oil." Brzeski et al. Evening primrose oil in patients with rheumatoid arthritis and side-effects of non-steroidal anti-inflammatory drugs. *Br J Rheumatol.* 1991 Oct;30(5):370-2

[400] Rothman D, DeLuca P, Zurier RB. Botanical lipids: effects on inflammation, immune responses, and rheumatoid arthritis. *Semin Arthritis Rheum.* 1995 Oct;25(2):87-96

[401] Adam et al. Anti-inflammatory effects of a low arachidonic acid diet and fish oil in patients with rheumatoid arthritis. *Rheumatol Int.* 2003 Jan;23(1):27-36

[402] Lau et al. Effects of fish oil supplementation on non-steroidal anti-inflammatory drug requirement in patients with mild rheumatoid arthritis. *Br J Rheumatol* 1993 Nov:982-9

[403] Kremer et al. Fish-oil fatty acid supplementation in active rheumatoid arthritis. A double-blinded, controlled, crossover study. *Ann Intern Med.* 1987 Apr;106(4):497-503

[404] Walton et al. Dietary fish oil and the severity of symptoms in patients with systemic lupus erythematosus. *Ann Rheum Dis.* 1991 Jul;50(7):463-6

[405] Duffy et al. The clinical effect of dietary supplementation with omega-3 fish oils or copper in systemic lupus erythematosus. *J Rheumatol.* 2004 Aug;31(8):1551-6

[406] Plotnikoff GA, Quigley JM. Prevalence of severe hypovitaminosis D in patients with persistent, nonspecific musculoskeletal pain. *Mayo Clin Proc.* 2003 Dec;78(12):1463-70

[407] "Half the SLE and FM patients had 25(OH)-vitamin D levels < 50 nmol/l, a level at which PTH stimulation occurs. Our data suggest that in SLE patients HCQ might inhibit conversion of 25(OH)-vitamin D to 1,25(OH)2-vitamin D." Huisman et al. Vitamin D levels in women with systemic lupus erythematosus and fibromyalgia. *J Rheumatol.* 2001 Nov;28(11):2535-9

- **INFECTIONS & DYSBIOSIS: ❶ antimicrobial treatments, ❷ immunorestoration, ❸ immunotolerance via Treg induction** Essentially all autoimmune/rheumatic disorders are associated with microbial colonization and intolerance to same; the presence of persistent microbial colonization is *prima facie* evidence of immunosuppression. The eight areas of dysbiosis (multifocal) are: ❶ sinorespiratory, ❷ orodental, ❸ gastrointestinal, ❹ urogenital/genitourinary, ❺ parenchymal/tissue, ❻ microbial, ❼ dermal/cutaneous, and ❽ environmental. Dysbiotic loci should be investigated as discussed previously in Chapter 4. Recall that patients with lupus have abnormal gastrointestinal bacteria (decreased colonization resistance[408]), and some evidence suggests that gastrointestinal bacteria in these patients may translocate into the systemic circulation to induce formation of antibodies that cross-react with double-stranded DNA to produce the clinical manifestations of the disease.[409,410] Each cause—each contributor to disease—may in itself be "clinically insignificant" but when numerous "insignificant" additive and synergistic influences coalesce, we find ourselves confronted with an "idiopathic disease." We must then decide between the only two available options: 1) despair in the failure of our "one cause, one disease, one drug" paradigm, or 2) appreciate that numerous influences work together to disrupt physiologic function and produce the biologic dysfunction that we experience as disease. Experimental evidence shows that exposure to single-stranded bacterial DNA can provoke formation of antibodies to single-stranded mammalian DNA. Human patients with SLE have a reduced ability to bind bacterial DNA with antibodies, thus allowing normal/ambient levels of bacterial DNA to provoke an ongoing inflammatory response.[411] Recall from Chapter 4 that stimulation of inflammation by bacterial DNA is one of the 17 pathomechanisms of autoimmune/inflammation induction by multifocal dysbiosis
  - Sinorespiratory/nasopharyngeal and dermal dysbiosis: **Increased nasal colonization with *Staphylococcus aureus* has been noted in patients with SLE.**[412]
  - Gastrointestinal dysbiosis: Yeast, bacteria, and parasites are treated as indicated based on identification and sensitivity results from comprehensive parasitology assessments.

- **NUTRITIONAL IMMUNOMODULATION: Treg induction for modulation of Th-1/2/17 inflammation** Nutrients and therapeutic approaches that promote Treg or IL-10 induction and/or Th-17, IL-17 suppression include 1) mitochondrial optimization and mTOR suppression, 2) biotin, 3) vitamin E, 4) sodium avoidance, 5) transgenic/GMO food avoidance, 6) probiotics, 7) lipoic acid, 8) vitamin A, 9) inflammation reduction, 10) vitamin D, 11) fatty acid supplementation with GLA and n3, 12) infection and dysbiosis remediation, 13) green tea EGCG. Acronym: MiBESTPLAIDFIG as reviewed in Chapter 4.

- **DYSMETABOLISM & DYSFUNCTIONAL MITOCHONDRIA: MitoDys, ERS-UPR, AGE/RAGE, hyperglycemia and ceramide** The major clinical considerations in this section are mitochondrial dysfunction, endoplasmic reticulum stress, unfolded protein response, TLR activation, and the dysmetabolic effects of sustained hyperglycemia and hyperinsulinemia and resultant oxidative stress, inflammation, RAGE activation, and accumulation of AGE, palmitate and ceramide. The review of this information in Chapter 4 covered approximately 30 interventions relevant to dysmetabolism, mitochondrial dysfunction, ERS-UPR, etc; these will not be reviewed here except to mention those most commonly, easily, empirically, synergistically, and effectively used: 1) low-carbohydrate diet with 2) moderate exercise, 3) CoQ-10, 4) acetyl-carnitine with 5) lipoic acid, 6) NAC, 7) resveratrol, and 8) melatonin.
  - Mitochondrial hyperpolarization and ATP depletion in patients with systemic lupus erythematosus (*Arthritis Rheum* 2002 Jan[413]): "Mitochondrial hyperpolarization and the resultant ATP depletion sensitize T cells for necrosis, which may significantly contribute to inflammation in patients with SLE."

---

[408] "Colonization Resistance (CR)...tended to be lower in active SLE patients than in healthy individuals. This could indicate that in SLE more and different bacteria translocate across the gut wall due to a lower CR. Some of these may serve as polyclonal B cell activators or as antigens cross-reacting with DNA." Apperloo-Renkema et al. Host-microflora interaction in systemic lupus erythematosus (SLE): colonization resistance of the indigenous bacteria of the intestinal tract. *Epidemiol Infect.* 1994;112(2):367-73

[409] "The lower IgG antibacterial antibody titres in active SLE might possibly result from sequestration of these IgG antibodies in immune complexes, indicating a possible role for antibacterial antibodies in exacerbations of SLE." Apperloo-Renkema et al. Host-microflora interaction in systemic lupus erythematosus (SLE): circulating antibodies to the indigenous bacteria of the intestinal tract. *Epidemiol Infect.* 1995 Feb;114(1):133-41

[410] Pisetsky DS. Antibody responses to DNA in normal immunity and aberrant immunity. *Clin Diagn Lab Immunol.* 1998 Jan;5(1):1-6 cdli.asm.org/cgi/content/full/5/1/1

[411] Pisetsky DS. Antibody responses to DNA in normal immunity and aberrant immunity. *Clin Diagn Lab Immunol.* 1998 Jan;5(1):1-6 cdli.asm.org/cgi/content/full/5/1/1

[412] Medline abstract from Polish research: "In 9 from 14 patients with (64.3%) a.b. very massive growth of Staphylococcus aureus in culture from vestibulae of the nose swab was, in other cultures very massive growth of physiological flora was seen. ...clinical significance of asymptomatic bacteriuria and pathogenic bacteria colonisation of nostrils as a precedence to symptomatic infections needs further investigations." Koseda-Dragan et al. [Asymptomatic bacteriuria in women diagnosed with systemic lupus erythematosus (SLE)] *Pol Arch Med Wewn.* 1998 Oct;100(4):321-30.

[413] Gergely et al. Mitochondrial hyperpolarization and ATP depletion in patients with systemic lupus erythematosus. *Arthritis Rheum.* 2002 Jan;46(1):175-90

- **STYLE OF LIVING (LIFESTYLE) & SPECIAL CONSIDERATIONS: <u>S</u>leep optimization, <u>S</u>ocioPsychology, <u>S</u>tress management/avoidance, <u>S</u>omatic treatments, <u>S</u>pecial <u>S</u>upplementation, <u>S</u>weat/exercise, <u>S</u>auna/detoxification, <u>S</u>urgery, <u>S</u>tamp your passport and vacate current reality, <u>S</u>ensory deprivation therapy**

This is a buffet of mostly lifestyle-based interventions yet also including considerations such as somatic treatments, additional supplementation, and surgery.

- o <u>Cardiovascular disease (CVD) risk reduction</u>: Patients with SLE have an increased risk of cardiovascular disease due to the synergistic effects of inflammation, oxidative stress, antiphospholipid antibodies, and elevated homocysteine. Obviously, the risk for CVD will be exacerbated if the SLE patient has other risk factors such as tobacco use, diabetes, obesity, hypertension, or physical inactivity. Therapeutic and interventional considerations specific to the prevention of cardiovascular disease include but are not limited to the following:
    - <u>Cardioprotective diet</u>: Paleo-Mediterranean diet
    - <u>Fatty acid supplementation</u>: Combination fatty acid supplementation with ALA, GLA, EPA, DHA[414,415]
    - <u>Magnesium supplementation</u>: > 200 mg up to bowel tolerance
- o <u>Treatments to lower homocysteine</u>: Doses given here for various treatments are for adults:
    - <u>Folic acid</u>: 5-10 mg, should be used with high-dose vitamin B-12
    - <u>Hydroxocobalamin</u>: 2,000-6,000 mcg/d orally, or 1,000-4,000 mcg/wk by injection
    - <u>Pyridoxine</u>: 250 mg/day with meals, co-administered with magnesium (e.g., >200 mg/d)
    - <u>NAC</u>: 600 mg tid
    - <u>Betaine/ trimethylglycine</u>: 1-2 grams tid (>6 grams daily when used alone)
    - <u>Lecithin</u>: 2.6 g choline/d (as phosphatidylcholine) decreased mean fasting plasma homocysteine by 18%.[416] Attaining this high dose might require as many as 45 capsules of commercially available supplements; an equivalent dose in the form of powdered lecithin granules delivered in a smoothie may be better tolerated than the capsules.
- o **N-Acetyl-Cysteine (NAC) for antioxidant, antiviral, and mitochondrial-protective benefits**: NAC provides cysteine for GSH production. NAC also inhibits NFkB. NAC inhibits viral replication (e.g., HIV) more effectively than and independently from its conversion to GSH. Recently, NAC at relatively high doses of 4,800mg/d in divided doses was shown to modulate mitochondrial hyperpolarization (by dissociating the generally resultant mTOR activation) and lead to very important clinical and immunological improvements in patients with SLE; NAC was shown to be safe and well-tolerated by all SLE patients up to 2.4g/d with reversible nausea in 33% of patients receiving 4.8g/d. This study by Lai, Hanczko, Bonilla, et al[417] is truly a landmark contribution and advance in the field

> **Mechanistic and clinical proof of anti-rheumatic benefit of NAC**
>
> "Similar to the effect of rapamycin, **suppression of mTOR by NAC was accompanied by increased FoxP3 expression in CD4+/CD25+ T cells**. These results suggest that the effect of NAC on the immune system is 1) cell type-specific and 2) it occurs through disconnecting the activation of mTOR from the elevation of Δψm in lupus T cells, similar to the effect of rapamycin."
>
> Lai et al. N-acetylcysteine reduces disease activity by blocking mammalian target of rapamycin in T cells from systemic lupus erythematosus patients. *Arthritis Rheum.* 2012 Sep

of rheumatology and immunology because it proves 1) that mitochondrial dysfunction directly leads to an autoimmune phenotype, and 2) that inhibition of mTOR by NAC is safe and effective in patients with SLE; important insights from this remarkable work are as follows:

- NAC 4,800mg/d proved safe and clinically beneficial in patients with SLE, leading to reductions in disease activity and ANA levels.

---

[414] Vasquez A. New Insights into Fatty Acid Supplementation and Its Effect on Eicosanoid Production and Genetic Expression. *Nutritional Perspectives* 2005; January: 5-16

[415] Laidlaw M, Holub BJ. Effects of supplementation with fish oil-derived n-3 fatty acids and gamma-linolenic acid on circulating plasma lipids and fatty acid profiles in women. *Am J Clin Nutr.* 2003 Jan;77(1):37-42 ajcn.org/cgi/content/full/77/1/37

[416] Olthof MR, Brink EJ, Katan MB, Verhoef P. Choline supplemented as phosphatidylcholine decreases fasting and postmethionine-loading plasma homocysteine concentrations in healthy men. *Am J Clin Nutr.* 2005 Jul;82(1):111-7

[417] Lai et al. NAC reduces disease activity by blocking mammalian target of rapamycin in T cells from systemic lupus erythematosus patients. *Arthritis Rheum* 2012 Sep:2937-46

- Mitochondrial hyperpolarization (MHP) causes mTOR activation which in turn suppresses the expression of the FoxP3 transcription factor necessary for induction of T-regulatory cells. Note that the mTOR activation is the cause of the FoxP3 suppression; ironically, NAC actually increases MHP but dissociates it from mTOR by having a greater effect on and via mTOR suppression. The nutritional supplement NAC works in a similar manner as does the immunosuppressive drug rapamycin, with a mechanism of suppression of mTOR and the effect of enhancing endogenous anti-inflammatory immunomodulation via CD4+ CD25+ FoxP3+ T-regulatory cells. Stated again and differently, NAC paradoxically worsens mitochondrial hyperpolarization in patients with SLE but does so at the same time that it has a more significant impact on mTOR; NAC's rapamycin-like targeting of mTOR dissociates mitochondrial hyperpolarization from mTOR activation. The reduction in mTOR activity (which is of greater consequence than the increase in MIM polarization) allows enhanced expression of FoxP3 for increased elaboration of T-regulatory cells, thereby providing endogenous immunoregulation.

- "MHP of lupus T cells, which most prominently affects DN [double-negative, autoimmunity-promoting] T cells, was associated with resistance to activation-induced apoptosis. In 27 SLE patients receiving daily NAC doses of 1.2 g, 2.4 g, and 4.8 g considered together, both **spontaneous and CD3/CD28-induced apoptosis of DN T cells were markedly increased** and the **expansion of these cells was effectively reversed**. The **elimination of DN T cells, which are known promote anti-DNA autoantibody production by B cells**, is likely to contribute to reduced anti-DNA titers and to the efficacy of NAC.

- "The therapeutic importance of NAC for SLE is reflected by: 1) achieving clinical improvement in two validated disease activity scores within 3 months; 2) diminishing fatigue (21), which is considered the most disabling symptom in a majority of SLE patients (22); 3) absence of significant side-effects; and 4) affordability of this medication. A monthly supply of 600-mg NAC capsules (120–240 capsules) costs $15–$30 on the retail market. This sharply contrasts with average annual direct medical costs estimated to be ~$22,580 per patient in 2009.Thus, the cost of NAC at $180–$360/year would be negligible in comparison to the overall expenditures to society and the expected benefit in reducing the need for vastly more expensive medications burdened with potentially serious side-effects."

o Oral enzyme therapy with proteolytic/pancreatic enzymes: Polyenzyme supplementation is used to ameliorate the pathophysiology induced by immune complexes, such as the related condition rheumatoid arthritis.[418]

o CoQ10 (antihypertensive, renoprotective, and probably immunomodulatory): CoQ10 is a powerful antioxidant with a wide margin of safety and excellent clinical tolerability. At least four studies have documented its powerful blood-pressure-lowering ability, which often surpasses the clinical effectiveness of antihypertensive drugs.[419,420,421,422] Furthermore, at least two published papers[423,424] and one case report[425] advocate that CoQ10 has powerful renoprotective benefits. CoQ10 levels are low in patients with allergies[426], and the symptomatic relief that many allergic patients experience following supplementation with CoQ10 suggests that CoQ10 has an immunomodulatory effect. Common doses start at > 100 mg per day with food; doses of 200 mg per day are not uncommon, and doses up to 1,000 mg per day are clinically well tolerated though the high financial toll resembles that of many pharmaceutical drugs.

[418] Galebskaya et al. Human complement system state after wobenzyme intake. *Vestnik Moskovskogo Universiteta (Seriya 2: Khimiya).* 2000:41(6 Suppl): 148-149 chem.msu.ru/eng/journals/vmgu/00add/148.pdf
[419] Burke et al. Randomized, double-blind, placebo-controlled trial of coenzyme Q10 in isolated systolic hypertension. *South Med J.* 2001 Nov;94(11):1112-7
[420] Singh et al. Effect of hydrosoluble coenzyme Q10 on blood pressures and insulin resistance in hypertensive patients coronary artery disease. *J Hum Hypertens* 1999 Mar:203-8
[421] Digiesi et al. Coenzyme Q10 in essential hypertension. *Mol Aspects Med.* 1994;15 Suppl:s257-63
[422] Langsjoen P, Langsjoen P, Willis R, Folkers K. Treatment of essential hypertension with coenzyme Q10. *Mol Aspects Med.* 1994;15 Suppl:S265-72
[423] Singh et al. Randomized, double-blind placebo-controlled trial of coenzyme Q10 in chronic renal failure: discovery of a new role. *J Nutr Environ Med* 2000;10:281-8
[424] Singh et al. Randomized, Double-blind, Placebo-controlled Trial of Coenzyme Q10 in Patients with End-stage Renal Failure. *J Nutr Environ Med* 2003;13: 13–22
[425] Singh RB, Singh MM. Effects of CoQ10 in new indications with antioxidant vitamin deficiency. *J Nutr Environ Med* 1999; 9:223-228
[426] Ye CQ, Folkers K, et al. A modified determination of coenzyme Q10 in human blood and CoQ10 blood levels in diverse patients with allergies. *Biofactors.* 1988 Dec;1:303-6

o <u>Anti-autoantibody interventions</u>: Patients with SLE have impaired ability to clear immune complexes via hepatic and splenic routes.[427,428] Given that anti-DNA and related immune complexes and cryoglobulins are considered the most fundamental abnormalities in the pathogenesis of this disorder, we can explore at least three routes of clinical intervention based on this limited focus. First, therapeutic interventions might be used that inhibit the *de novo* formation of autoantibodies, particularly those that are directed against double-stranded DNA. This could be accomplished via bio-logical immunomodulation, pharmacologic/anti-biological immunosuppression, or by removing the underlying stimuli and predisposing factors ("etiologic approach"). Second, treatments might be implemented to nullify or diminish the adverse effects of these antibodies. Third, we might use interventions that remove the autoantibodies that are formed so that they are not significantly available to contribute to disease pathogenesis. As discussed previously in the section on treatments for multifocal dysbiosis, at least two primary mechanisms exist for the removal of autoantibody-containing immune complexes, namely 1) phagocytosis and proteolytic degradation by macrophages embedded in the liver and spleen, and 2) transport via hepatocytes directly into the bile for excretion. IgG double-stranded DNA antibodies are consumed and proteolytically/oxidatively/enzymatically degraded by monocytes/phagocytes[429] while IgA-containing immune complexes are preferentially consumed by hepatocytes and exported intact into the bile for excretion.

- **ENDOCRINE IMBALANCE & OPTIMIZATION: Prolactin, Insulin, Estrogen, DHEA, Cortisol, Testosterone, Thyroid** Hormonal imbalances seen among autoimmune/inflammatory patients are: ❶ *elevated prolactin*, ❷ *elevated* estrogen, ❸ *elevated* insulin, and ❹ *reduced DHEA*, ❺ *reduced* cortisol, and ❻ *reduced testosterone*; see Chapter 4 for discussion of these hormones and respective interventions. Thyroid evaluation (patient + labs) should be comprehensive, as discussed in Chapter 1, with a low threshold for empiric treatment.
  o <u>Melatonin</u>: Melatonin is a pineal hormone with well-known sleep-inducing and immunomodulatory properties, and it is commonly administered in doses of 1-40 mg in the evening, before bedtime. Starting with a relatively low dose (e.g., 1-5 mg) and increasing as tolerated is recommended. Melatonin (20 mg hs) appears to have cured two patients with drug-resistant sarcoidosis[430] and 3 mg provided immediate short-term benefit to a patient with multiple sclerosis.[431]
  o <u>Prolactin (excess)</u>: **Prolactin has proinflammatory and immunodysregulatory actions and is commonly elevated—either overtly or latently—in patients with inflammatory/autoimmune disease.** Accordingly prolactin-lowering treatment shows safety and effectiveness in the treatment of numerous inflammatory/autoimmune diseases; often these results are noted even when the patient's prolactin level was not initially elevated, suggesting the alleviation of latent hyperprolactinemia and/or an inherent anti-inflammatory action of the prolactin-lowering treatment. According to clinical trials with small numbers of patients, whether prolactin levels are high or not, prolactin-lowering treatment (such as bromocriptine) appears highly beneficial when used with other anti-rheumatic treatments ("...**drastic efficacy with spectacular improvement** in clinical, biological and occupational status..."[432]) in patients with psoriatic arthritis. Serum prolactin is the standard assessment of prolactin status. Since elevated prolactin may be a sign of pituitary tumor, assessment for headaches, visual deficits, other abnormalities of pituitary hormones (e.g., GH and TSH) should be performed and CT or MRI must be considered. Patients with

[427] "These observations support the hypothesis that IC handling is abnormal in SLE." Davies et al. Immune complex processing in patients with systemic lupus erythematosus. *J Clin Invest.* 1992 Nov;90(5):2075-83

[428] "These results indicate that Fc-mediated clearance of ICs is defective in patients with SLE and suggest that ligation of ICs by Fc receptors is critical for their efficient binding and retention by the fixed MPS in the liver." Davies et al. Defective Fc-dependent processing of immune complexes in patients with systemic lupus erythematosus. *Arthritis Rheum.* 2002 Apr;46(4):1028-38

[429] "In the presence of U937 [monocytic] cells, both the AHP-anti-dsDNA and C3b-opsonized ICs were rapidly removed from the erythrocytes; at 37 degrees C, more than half of the complexes were removed in 2 minutes." Craig et al. Clearance of anti-double-stranded DNA antibodies: the natural immune complex clearance mechanism. *Arthritis Rheum.* 2000 Oct;43(10):2265-75

[430] Cagnoni ML, Lombardi A, Cerinic MC, Dedola GL, Pignone A. Melatonin for treatment of chronic refractory sarcoidosis. *Lancet.* 1995 Nov 4;346(8984):1229-30

[431] "...administration of melatonin (3 mg, orally) at 2:00 p.m., when the patient experienced severe blurring of vision, resulted within 15 minutes in a dramatic improvement in visual acuity and in normalization of the visual evoked potential latency after stimulation of the left eye." Sandyk R. Diurnal variations in vision and relations to circadian melatonin secretion in multiple sclerosis. *Int J Neurosci.* 1995 Nov;83(1-2):1-6

[432] Abstract from article in French: "In 2 cases of psoriatic arthritis, adding bromocriptine to gold salts and nonsteroidal anti-inflammatory drug was followed by a drastic efficacy with spectacular improvement in clinical, biological and occupational status. Because none of the cases had hyperprolactinaemia, bromocriptine acted probably had an intrinic anti-inflammatory effect independent of its antiprolactinic effect." Eulry et al. [Blood prolactin under the effect of protirelin in spondylarthropathies. Treatment trial of 4 cases of reactive arthritis and 2 cases of psoriatic arthritis with bromocriptine] *Ann Med Interne* (Paris). 1996;147(1):15-9. French

prolactin levels less than 100 ng/mL and normal CT/MRI findings can be managed conservatively with effective prolactin-lowering treatment and annual radiologic assessment (less necessary with favorable serum response).[433, see review 434] **Patients with RA and SLE have higher basal and stress-induced levels of prolactin compared with normal controls.**[435,436] A normal serum prolactin level does not necessarily exclude the use of prolactin-lowering intervention, especially since many autoimmune patients have **latent hyperprolactinemia** which may not be detected with random serum measurement of prolactin. Vitex lowers serum prolactin in humans[437,438] via a dopaminergic effect.[439] Due at least in part to its content of L-dopa, *Mucuna pruriens* shows clinical dopaminergic activity as evidenced by its effectiveness in Parkinson's disease[440]; up to 15-30 gm/d of mucuna has been used clinically but doses will be dependent on preparation and phytoconcentration. Clinical intervention with bromocriptine appears warranted in patients with RA, SLE, reactive arthritis, psoriatic arthritis, and probably multiple sclerosis and uveitis.[441] A normal serum prolactin level does not necessarily exclude the use of prolactin-lowering intervention, especially since many autoimmune patients have latent hyperprolactinemia which may not be detected with random serum measurement of prolactin. Cabergoline/Dostinex is a newer dopamine agonist with few adverse effects; typical dose starts at 0.5 mg per week (0.25 mg twice per week).[442] Several studies have indicated that cabergoline is safer and more effective than bromocriptine for reducing prolactin levels[443] and the dose can often be reduced after successful prolactin reduction, allowing for reductions in cost and adverse effects.[444] Although fewer studies have been published supporting the antirheumatic benefits of cabergoline than those supporting bromocriptine; its antirheumatic benefits have indeed been documented.[445]

o <u>Cruciferous vegetables, DIM, I3C</u>: In a short-term study using I3C in patients with SLE, I3C supplementation at 375 mg per day was well tolerated and resulted in modest treatment-dependent clinical improvement as well as favorable modification of estrogen metabolism away from 16-alpha-hydroxyestrone and toward 2-hydroxyestrone.[446]

o <u>DHEA</u>: DHEA is an anti-inflammatory and immunoregulatory hormone that is commonly deficient in patients with autoimmunity, including polymyalgia rheumatica, SLE, RA, and inflammatory arthritis.[447,448] DHEA levels are suppressed by prednisone[449], and DHEA has been shown to reverse the

[433] Beers MH, Berkow R (eds). *Merck Manual. 17th Edition*. Whitehouse Station; Merck Research Laboratories 1999 Page 77-78

[434] Serri O, Chik CL, Ur E, Ezzat S. Diagnosis and management of hyperprolactinemia. *CMAJ*. 2003 Sep 16;169(6):575-81 cmaj.ca/cgi/content/full/169/6/575

[435] Dostal et al. Serum prolactin stress values in patients with systemic lupus erythematosus. *Ann Rheum Dis*. 2003 May;62(5):487-8 ard.bmjjournals.com/cgi/content/full/62/5/487

[436] "RESULTS: A significantly higher rate of elevated PRL levels was found in SLE patients (40.0%) compared with the healthy controls (14.8%). No proof was found of association with the presence of anti-ds-DNA or with specific organ involvement. Similarly, elevated PRL levels were found in RA patients (39.3%)." Moszkorzova L, Lacinova Z, Marek J, et al. Hyperprolactinaemia in patients with systemic lupus erythematosus. *Clin Exp Rheumatol*. 2002 Nov-Dec;20(6):807-12

[437] "Since AC extracts were shown to have beneficial effects on premenstrual mastodynia serum prolactin levels in such patients were also studied in one double-blind, placebo-controlled clinical study. Serum prolactin levels were indeed reduced in the patients treated with the extract." Wuttke W, Jarry H, Christoffel V, Spengler B, Seidlova-Wuttke D. Chaste tree, Vitex agnus-castus—pharmacology and clinical indications. *Phytomedicine*. 2003 May;10(4):348-57

[438] German abstract from Medline: "The prolactin release was reduced after 3 months, shortened luteal phases were normalised and deficits in the luteal progesterone synthesis were eliminated." Milewicz et al. [Vitex agnus castus extract in the treatment of luteal phase defects due to latent hyperprolactinemia. Results of a randomized placebo-controlled double-blind study] *Arzneimittelforschung*. 1993 Jul;43(7):752-6

[439] "Our results indicate a dopaminergic effect of Vitex agnus-castus extracts and suggest additional pharmacological actions via opioid receptors." Meier B, Berger D, Hoberg E, Sticher O, Schaffner W. Pharmacological activities of Vitex agnus-castus extracts in vitro. *Phytomedicine*. 2000 Oct;7(5):373-81

[440] "CONCLUSIONS: The rapid onset of action and longer on time without concomitant increase in dyskinesias on mucuna seed powder formulation suggest that this natural source of L-dopa might possess advantages over conventional L-dopa preparations in the long term management of PD." Katzenschlager et al. Mucuna pruriens in Parkinson's disease: a double blind clinical and pharmacological study. *J Neurol Neurosurg Psychiatry*. 2004 Dec;75(12):1672-7

[441] "...clinical observations and trials support the use of bromocriptine as a nonstandard primary or adjunctive therapy in the treatment of recalcitrant RA, SLE, Reiter's syndrome, and psoriatic arthritis and associated conditions unresponsive to traditional approaches." McMurray RW. Bromocriptine in rheumatic and autoimmune diseases. *Semin Arthritis Rheum*. 2001 Aug;31(1):21-32

[442] Serri O, Chik CL, Ur E, Ezzat S. Diagnosis and management of hyperprolactinemia. *CMAJ*. 2003 Sep 16;169(6):575-81 cmaj.ca/cgi/content/full/169/6/575

[443] "CONCLUSION: These data indicate that cabergoline is a very effective agent for lowering the prolactin levels in hyperprolactinemic patients and that it appears to offer considerable advantage over bromocriptine in terms of efficacy and tolerability." Sabuncu et al. Comparison of the effects of cabergoline and bromocriptine on prolactin levels in hyperprolactinemic patients. *Intern Med*. 2001 Sep;40(9):857-61

[444] "Cabergoline also normalized PRL in the majority of patients with known bromocriptine intolerance or -resistance. Once PRL secretion was adequately controlled, the dose of cabergoline could often be significantly decreased, which further reduced costs of therapy." Verhelst et al. Cabergoline in the treatment of hyperprolactinemia: a study in 455 patients. *J Clin Endocrinol Metab*. 1999 Jul;84(7):2518-22 jcem.endojournals.org/cgi/content/full/84/7/2518

[445] Erb N, Pace AV, Delamere JP, Kitas GD. Control of unremitting rheumatoid arthritis by the prolactin antagonist cabergoline. *Rheumatology* (Oxford). 2001 Feb;40(2):237-9

[446] "Women with SLE can manifest a metabolic response to I3C and might benefit from its antiestrogenic effects." McAlindon TE, Gulin J, Chen T, Klug T, Lahita R, Nuite M. Indole-3-carbinol in women with SLE: effect on estrogen metabolism and disease activity. *Lupus*. 2001;10(1):779-83

[447] "The low levels found in patients with PM:TA are in accordance with those previously reported in immune-mediated diseases such as systemic lupus erythematosus (SLE) and rheumatoid arthritis, suggesting that diminution of DHEAS is a constant endocrinologic feature in these categories of patients." Nilsson et al. Blood dehydroepiandrosterone sulphate (DHEAS) levels in polymyalgia rheumatica/giant cell arteritis and primary fibromyalgia. *Clin Exp Rheumatol*. 1994 Jul-Aug;12(4):415-7

[448] "DHEAS concentrations were significantly decreased in both women and men with inflammatory arthritis (IA) (P < 0.001)." Dessein et al. Hyposecretion of the adrenal androgen dehydroepiandrosterone sulfate and its relation to clinical variables in inflammatory arthritis. *Arthritis Res*. 2001;3(3):183-8 arthritis-research.com/content/3/3/183

[449] "Basal serum DHEA and DHEAS concentrations were suppressed to a greater degree than was cortisol during both daily and alternate day prednisone treatments. ...Thus, adrenal androgen secretion was more easily suppressed than was cortisol secretion by this low dose of glucocorticoid, but there was no advantage to alternate day therapy." Rittmaster et al. Effect of daily and alternate day low dose prednisone on serum cortisol and adrenal androgens in hirsute women. *J Clin Endocrinol Metab*. 1988 Aug;67(2):400-3

osteoporosis and loss of bone mass induced by corticosteroid treatment.[450] DHEA shows no acute or subacute toxicity even when used in supraphysiologic doses, even when used in sick patients. For example, in a study of 32 patients with HIV, DHEA doses of 750 mg – 2,250 mg per day were well-tolerated and produced no dose-limiting adverse effects.[451] This lack of toxicity compares favorably with any and all so-called "antirheumatic" drugs, nearly all of which show impressive comparable toxicity. High-dose supplemental DHEA has benefits in the treatment of SLE that are comparable to those obtained with antimalarial drugs.[452] When used at doses of 200 mg per day, DHEA safely provides clinical benefit for patients with various autoimmune diseases, including ulcerative colitis, Crohn's disease[453], and SLE.[454] In patients with SLE, DHEA supplementation allows for reduced dosing of prednisone (thus avoiding its adverse effects) while providing symptomatic improvement.[455] Optimal clinical response appears to correlate with serum levels that are supraphysiologic[456], and therefore treatment may be implemented with little regard for initial/baseline DHEA levels provided that the patient is free of contraindications, particularly high risk for sex-hormone-dependent malignancy. Other than mild adverse effects predictable with any androgen (namely voice deepening, transient acne, and increased facial hair), DHEA supplementation does not cause serious adverse effects[457], and it is appropriate for routine clinical use particularly when 1) the dose of DHEA is kept as low as possible, 2) duration is kept as short as possible, 3) other interventions are used to address the underlying cause of the disease, 4) the patient is deriving benefit, and 5) the risk-to-benefit ratio is favorable.

- **XENOBIOTIC ACCUMULATION & DETOXIFICATION: Chemical avoidance, nutritional support for detoxification pathways, urine alkalinization** | The clinical relevance and pathogenic mechanisms of xenobiotic accumulation are irrefutably well documented and described. Clinical assessments include history, physical examination, and laboratory assessment (using serum, whole blood, urine or—rarely yet accurately—fat biopsy), and response to treatment. Treatments include nutritional support for Phases 1 and 2 of detoxification (e.g., oxidation and conjugation) and excretion via bile and urine; for the latter, urinary alkalinization is generally recommended. Chemical toxins can be bound in the gut using activated charcoal, cholestyramine, or *Chlorella*—all of these three treatments have documented safety and effectiveness; clinically and empirically, phytochelatin (plant-derived peptides that bind toxic metals) concentrates appear safe and effective despite lack of conclusive published data supporting clinical use. Mercury exposure via working in a dental office is one of the greatest occupational risks ever identified for the development of SLE in humans.

[450] "CONCLUSION: Prasterone treatment prevented BMD loss and significantly increased BMD at both the lumbar spine and total hip in female patients with SLE receiving exogenous glucocorticoids." Mease et al. Effects of prasterone on bone mineral density in women with systemic lupus erythematosus receiving chronic glucocorticoid therapy. *J Rheumatol*. 2005 Apr;32(4):616-21

[451] "Thirty-one subjects were evaluated and monitored for safety and tolerance. The oral drug was administered three times daily in doses ranging from 750 mg/day to 2,250 mg/day for 16 weeks. ... The drug was well tolerated and no dose-limiting side effects were noted." Dyner et al. An open-label dose-escalation trial of oral dehydroepiandrosterone tolerance and pharmacokinetics in patients with HIV disease. *J Acquir Immune Defic Syndr*. 1993 May;6(5):459-65

[452] Tierney ML. McPhee SJ, Papadakis MA. Current Medical Diagnosis and Treatment 2006. 45th edition. New York; Lange Medical Books: 2006, pages 833-837

[453] "CONCLUSIONS: In a pilot study, dehydroepiandrosterone was effective and safe in patients with refractory Crohn's disease or ulcerative colitis." Andus et al. Patients with refractory Crohn's disease or ulcerative colitis respond to dehydroepiandrosterone: a pilot study. *Aliment Pharmacol Ther*. 2003 Feb;17(3):409-14

[454] "CONCLUSION: The overall results confirm that DHEA treatment was well-tolerated, significantly reduced the number of SLE flares, and improved patient's global assessment of disease activity." Chang DM, Lan JL, Lin HY, Luo SF. Dehydroepiandrosterone treatment of women with mild-to-moderate systemic lupus erythematosus: a multicenter randomized, double-blind, placebo-controlled trial. *Arthritis Rheum*. 2002 Nov;46(11):2924-7

[455] "CONCLUSION: Among women with lupus disease activity, reducing the dosage of prednisone to < or = 7.5 mg/day for a sustained period of time while maintaining stabilization or a reduction of disease activity was possible in a significantly greater proportion of patients treated with oral prasterone, 200 mg once daily, compared with patients treated with placebo." Petri et al; GL601 Study Group. Effects of prasterone on corticosteroid requirements of women with systemic lupus erythematosus: a double-blind, randomized, placebo-controlled trial. *Arthritis Rheum*. 2002 Jul;46(7):1820-9

[456] "CONCLUSION: The clinical response to DHEA was not clearly dose dependent. Serum levels of DHEA and DHEAS correlated only weakly with lupus outcomes, but suggested an optimum serum DHEAS of 1000 microg/dl." Barry et al. Dehydroepiandrosterone in systemic lupus erythematosus: relationship between dosage, serum levels, and clinical response. *J Rheumatol*. 1998 Dec;25(12):2352-6

[457] Tierney ML. McPhee SJ, Papadakis MA. *Current Medical Diagnosis and Treatment 2006. 45th edition*. New York; Lange Medical Books: 2006, page 1721

Scleroderma & Systemic Sclerosis

Introduction:

Scleroderma and systemic sclerosis are related conditions of either dermal or dermal+systemic fibrosis, respectively. A reasonable conceptualization is that of an inflammation/ROS-driven fibrotic response; the solution then—of course—is to address the disease-specific and patient-specific causes of excess inflammation and immune imbalance. The vicious cycles of nutritional deficiency, gastrointestinal dysbiosis, and persistent active viral infections must be addressed.

Description/pathophysiology:

- Overview: Generally considered "idiopathic" from the allopathic medical perspective; for example, a 2008 article published by the American Academy of Family Physicians introduces the topic in this manner, providing a brief description along with undermining any possible desire to treat the cause of the illness via the promulgation that the cause is officially declared to be unknown: "Systemic sclerosis (systemic scleroderma) is a chronic connective tissue disease of unknown etiology that causes widespread microvascular damage and excessive deposition of collagen in the skin and internal organs."[458] The terms *scleroderma* and *systemic sclerosis* are used somewhat interchangeably; yet, as these terms suggest, *scleroderma* is properly assigned to disease that is limited to the skin, while *systemic sclerosis* denotes visceral involvement in addition to skin changes. *Scleroderma* will be the default term in this section for linguistic expediency; because the initials "SS" can equally suggest Sjogren's syndrome as well as systemic sclerosis, the initials *SSc* will be used to denote systemic sclerosis—again interchangeably with *scleroderma*.
- **Characterized by fibrosis of the skin and internal organs, including the esophagus, intestines, lung, heart, and kidneys.** The condition can be mild and limited to the skin only, or it can be systemic and rapidly fatal due to internal organ involvement.
- Main subtypes:
  1. Limited, cutaneous scleroderma—60% of cases: Primarily affecting the skin, especially of the fingers and face; distribution often described as distal to the neck, elbows and knees; major complications are GERD, Raynaud's, and pulmonary hypertension, notably "Patients with limited cutaneous systemic sclerosis have the greatest risk of pulmonary arterial hypertension."[459]
     - CREST syndrome—variant of limited/cutaneous scleroderma: Calcinosis, Raynaud's phenomenon, esophageal dysmotility/dysfunction, sclerodactyly, telangiectasia
  2. Diffuse, systemic sclerosis—35% of cases: Characterized by systemic fibrosis of skin and internal organs, especially interstitial lung disease; may rapidly progress to death via scleroderma renal crisis.
  3. Systemic sclerosis sine scleroderma—approximately 5% of patients with systemic sclerosis: Characteristic internal organ manifestations of the disease without skin thickening.
  4. Localized/linear scleroderma and morphea: Primarily affects children, not associated with Raynaud phenomenon or significant internal organ involvement.
  5. Mixed connective tissue disease and "overlap syndromes"—less common: Combination of scleroderma with another autoimmune disease, such as dermatomyositis (sclerodermatomyositis) or RA, SLE, etc.
  6. Scleroderma secondary to xenobiotic immunotoxicity—rare: Scleroderma can result from exposure to vinyl chloride, silicone, petroleum products, toxic oil syndrome, solvents, cocaine, and pesticides.
- Patients with scleroderma have evidence of **increased oxidative stress** demonstrated by a doubling of urinary isoprostane excretion.[460] Oxidative stress *results from* and *contributes to* systemic inflammation because 1) increased immune activity results in elaboration of oxidants, and 2) oxidative stress upregulates NFkB (and other pathways) for additive immune activation; oxidative stress and inflammation both contribute to tissue fibrosis.

---

[458] Hinchcliff M, Varga J. Systemic sclerosis/scleroderma: a treatable multisystem disease. *Am Fam Physician*. 2008 Oct 15;78(8):961-8

[459] Hinchcliff M, Varga J. Systemic sclerosis/scleroderma: a treatable multisystem disease. *Am Fam Physician*. 2008 Oct 15;78(8):961-8

[460] "CONCLUSION: This study provides evidence of enhanced lipid peroxidation in both SSc and UCTD, and suggests a rationale for antioxidant treatment of SSc." Cracowski et al. Enhanced in vivo lipid peroxidation in scleroderma spectrum disorders. *Arthritis Rheum* 2001 May;44(5):1143-8

Clinical presentations:

- <u>Classic presentation</u>: "The typical patient is a young or middle-age woman with a history of Raynaud phenomenon who presents with skin induration and internal organ dysfunction."[461] 4x more common in women, general age of onset is 20-40 years. More than 95% of scleroderma/SSc patients have Raynaud's phenomenon, thereby giving this clinical manifestation a considerable degree of importance in the initial/historical assessment.
- <u>Skin changes</u>: Hyperpigmentation, tightness, tightness and thickening of the face results in "mask-like face", telangiectasia, may also have depigmentation; dermal pitting (mild) and ulceration (more severe) of fingertips; swelling and thickening of the fingers is termed sclerodactyly.
- <u>Soft tissue calcification</u>: Especially in the hands; systemic calcification is also seen.
- <u>Polyarthralgia</u>: Affects 90% of patients; flexion contractures of the joints due to fibrosis is also common.
- <u>Autonomic dysfunction: Raynaud's phenomenon</u>: Seen in 90% of patients and often precedes sclerodermatous manifestations by a period of up to 5 years; the high level of overlap among these two conditions suggests a common etiology—the factor most strongly associated with both conditions and especially Raynaud's is *H pylori* infection, discussed later in this section on SSc and also in the section on Raynaud's.
- <u>Pulmonary</u>: Dyspnea, pulmonary hypertension.
- <u>Cardiac</u>: Arrhythmias, CHF, hypertension, ECG abnormalities—may be fatal.
- <u>Renal</u>: Renal failure is a leading cause of death—see renal assessments in Chapter 1. "Scleroderma renal crisis develops in 3 to 10 percent of all patients with systemic sclerosis and in 10 to 20 percent of those with rapidly progressive diffuse cutaneous systemic sclerosis; the greatest risk occurs within the first three years of the disease. ... Patients with scleroderma renal crisis characteristically present with sudden-onset accelerated hypertension that is often associated with progressive oliguric renal failure with proteinuria, microangiopathic anemia, and microscopic hematuria. Ten to 15 percent of patients with scleroderma renal crisis are normotensive, but hypertensive when compared with their baseline blood pressure measurements."[462]
- <u>GI disturbances</u>:
  - Esophageal dysfunction and dysphagia eventually occur in most patients; histologic/biopsy examination reveals degeneration of intestinal nerves, vessels, and smooth muscle.[463]
  - Greatly increased risk for Barrett's esophagus (33% of all scleroderma patients) with a notably low risk of esophageal adenocarcinoma.
  - Slow intestinal transit—intestinal hypomotility in scleroderma promotes bacterial overgrowth of the small bowel, which probably contributes to the pathogenesis of the disease via the pro-inflammatory and immune activating effects discussed in Chapter 4. Treatment of bacterial overgrowth with antibiotics (ciprofloxacin 500 mg bid[464]) or promotility drugs (octreotide[465]) is effective treatment for scleroderma according to published case reports; **such research supports the hypothesis that intestinal dysbiosis— namely bacterial overgrowth—is an important contributor to the perpetuation of scleroderma.**

Major differential diagnoses:

- <u>Parkinson's disease</u>: Mask-like face
- <u>Other autoimmune disorders</u>: Overlap syndromes, mixed connective tissue diseases
- <u>Amyloidosis</u>: Primary or secondary forms; often leads to skin thickening due to amyloid deposition however skin generally remains soft and more edematous-like than induration-like
- <u>Nephrogenic systemic fibrosis</u>: "Nephrogenic systemic fibrosis (NSF) is a fibrosing disorder, recently described in patients with advanced chronic kidney disease, usually after exposure to gadolinium (Gd)-based contrast agents, characterized by progressive fibrotic involvement mainly of the skin. At clinical examination, the

---

[461] Hinchcliff M, Varga J. Systemic sclerosis/scleroderma: a treatable multisystem disease. *Am Fam Physician*. 2008 Oct 15;78(8):961-8

[462] Hinchcliff M, Varga J. Systemic sclerosis/scleroderma: a treatable multisystem disease. *Am Fam Physician*. 2008 Oct 15;78(8):961-8

[463] "We found ultrastructural signs of axonal degeneration and cytoskeletal abnormalities in the bundles of unmyelinated fibers. There was also focal degeneration of smooth muscle cells, often in association with the presence of partially degranulated mast cells." Malandrini et al. Autonomic nervous system and smooth muscle cell involvement in systemic sclerosis: ultrastructural study of 3 cases. *J Rheumatol*. 2000 May;27(5):1203-6

[464] Over KE, Bucknall RC. Regression of skin changes in a patient with systemic sclerosis following treatment for bacterial overgrowth with ciprofloxacin. *Br J Rheumatol*. 1998 Jun;37(6):696 rheumatology.oxfordjournals.org/cgi/reprint/37/6/696a

[465] "After 8 months of treatment, normal weight was obtained and skin induration was spectacularly reduced and pigmentation returned to a normal state." Descamps et al. Global improvement of systemic scleroderma under long-term administration of octreotide. *Eur J Dermatol* 1999 Sep;9(6):446-8

cutaneous findings of NSF may partly resemble those of systemic sclerosis. However, the different topographic distribution of the skin thickening and hardening, usually involving the limbs and trunk, whilst sparing the face, the lack of serologic abnormalities and the distinctive histopathological findings allow this new disease entity to be distinguished from systemic sclerosis and other scleroderma-like fibrosing disorders (scleromyxedema, scleredema, eosinophilic fasciitis, etc.)."[466]

- Vinyl chloride disease: exposure to vinyl chloride (VC) monomer, a volatile substance mostly used for polyvinyl chloride (PVC) synthesis produces a scleroderma-like disorder that may be complicated by vasculitic and neurologic sequelae.[467,468,469]
- Dermal infections and other diseases: Zygomycosis, sporotrichosis, cutaneous lymphoma
- Toxic oil syndrome: A syndrome of incapacitating myalgias, marked peripheral eosinophilia, pulmonary infiltrates, and increased prevalence of scleroderma and neurologic disorders following consumption of contaminated oil.[470]

Clinical assessments:

- **History/subjective**:
  - o Symptoms and complications from dermal induration/hardening and fibrosis
  - o Intestinal and digestive complaints
  - o Areas affected, ROM, ADL, QOL
  - o Xenobiotic exposure: Occupational exposure to silica is associated with scleroderma; some cases appear to be linked to silicone breast implants[471] (controversial[472]) and anti-silicate antibodies may be valuable for documenting humoral response to silicone.[473] Clinicians should ask about any history of iatrogenic, occupational, recreational or domestic xenobiotic exposure, such as to organic solvents[474], pesticides, epoxy resins[475], and other immunotoxins.[476] Use of cocaine may cause or exacerbate scleroderma.[477]
- **Physical examination/objective**: routine, including the following:
  - o Dermal exam, including nailfold capillaroscopy: Symptoms and complications from dermal induration/hardening, swelling, fibrosis, and calcium deposition: swollen fingers, tight skin on face and hands, dermal ulcerations and hypopigmentation. The "colors of Raynaud's phenomenon" are white (vasospasm), blue-purple (ischemia), and red (hyperemia).
    - ▪ Nailfold capillaroscopy—viewed clinically with magnifying lens: Reveals microvascular changes consistent with autoimmunity and autoimmune-expedited cardiovascular disease. Per Cutolo et al[478], "Raynaud's phenomenon (RP) represents the most frequent clinical aspect of cardio/microvascular involvement and is a key feature of several autoimmune rheumatic diseases. Moreover, RP is associated in a statistically significant manner with many coronary diseases. In normal conditions or in primary RP (excluding during the cold-exposure test), the normal nailfold

[466] Rota et al. Nephrogenic systemic fibrosis: an unusual scleroderma-like fibrosing disorder. *Rheumatol Int.* 2010 Aug;30(10):1389-91

[467] "Occupational exposure to vinyl chloride monomers is known to induce Raynaud's phenomenon, periportal fibrosis, liver angiosarcoma and scleroderma-like syndrome." Serratrice et al. A case of polymyositis with anti-histidyl-t-RNA synthetase (Jo-1) antibody syndrome following extensive vinyl chloride exposure. *Clin Rheumatol* 2001;20:379-82

[468] "An unusual case of systemic sclerosis occurring in a patient exposed to the vinyl chloride monomer (VCM) is presented." Ostlere et al. Atypical systemic sclerosis following exposure to vinyl chloride monomer. A case report and review of the cutaneous aspects of vinyl chloride disease. *Clin Exp Dermatol.* 1992 May;17(3):208-10

[469] "Angiosarcoma of the liver, Raynaud's phenomenon, scleroderma-like lesions, acroosteolysis and neuritis are known to be typical vinyl chloride-associated manifestations (VC disease)." Magnavita N, Bergamaschi A, Garcovich A, Giuliano G. Vasculitic purpura in vinyl chloride disease: a case report. *Angiology.* 1986 May;37(5):382-8

[470] "In 1981, in Spain, the ingestion of an oil fraudulently sold as olive oil caused an outbreak of a previously unrecorded condition, later known as toxic oil syndrome (TOS), clinically characterized by intense incapacitating myalgias, marked peripheral eosinophilia, and pulmonary infiltrates." Gelpi et al; WHO/CISAT Scientific Committee for the Toxic Oil Syndrome. The Spanish toxic oil syndrome 20 years after its onset: multidisciplinary review of scientific knowledge. *Environ Health Perspect.* 2002 May;110(5):457-64

[471] "...idiopathic form of scleroderma and related conditions. CONCLUSION. These findings suggest that ANA positivity is relatively common in individuals with silicone breast implants, and may support the existence of autoimmune mechanisms in the pathogenesis of the clinical manifestations seen in this population." Cuellar ML, Scopelitis E, Tenenbaum SA, et al. Serum antinuclear antibodies in women with silicone breast implants. *J Rheumatol.* 1995 Feb;22(2):236-40

[472] "Neither the case-control studies nor the other epidemiologic data support the hypothesis that scleroderma is associated with or causally related to breast implants." Whorton D, Wong O. Scleroderma and silicone breast implants. *West J Med* 1997 Sep;167(3):159-65

[473] Shen GQ, Ojo-Amaize EA, Agopian MS, Peter JB. Silicate antibodies in women with silicone breast implants: development of an assay for detection of humoral immunity. *Clin Diagn Lab Immunol.* 1996 Mar;3(2):162-6 cdli.asm.org/cgi/reprint/3/2/162?view=reprint&pmid=8991630

[474] "We describe a sclerodermatous syndrome in a middle-aged man who had worked with a wide variety of organic solvents over a prolonged period." Bottomley WW, et al. A sclerodermatous syndrome with unusual features following prolonged occupational exposure to organic solvents. *Br J Dermatol* 1993 Feb;128(2):203-6

[475] "A new occupational disorder characterized by skin sclerosis is described. This disease developed acutely in workmen exposed to the vapor of epoxy resins." Yamakage A, et al. Occupational scleroderma-like disorder occurring in men engaged in the polymerization of epoxy resins. *Dermatologica.* 1980;161(1):33-44

[476] "There is growing concern about the association between systemic sclerosis and certain environmental and occupational risk factors, including exposures to vinyl chloride, adulterated cooking oils, L-tryptophan, silica, silicone breast implants, organic solvents, and other agents such as epoxy resins, pesticides, and hand/arm vibration." Nietert PJ, Silver RM. Systemic sclerosis: environmental and occupational risk factors. *Curr Opin Rheumatol* 2000 Nov;12(6):520-6

[477] "It has been reported that cocaine may initiate scleroderma in an already susceptible individual or unmask it at an earlier age in subclinical disease." Attoussi S, Faulkner ML, Oso A, Umoru B. Cocaine-induced scleroderma and scleroderma renal crisis. *South Med J* 1998 Oct;91(10):961-3

[478] Cutolo M, Sulli A, Secchi ME, Paolino S, Pizzorni C. Nailfold capillaroscopy is useful for the diagnosis and follow-up of autoimmune rheumatic diseases. A future tool for the analysis of microvascular heart involvement? *Rheumatology* (Oxford). 2006 Oct;45 Suppl 4:iv43-6 rheumatology.oxfordjournals.org/content/45/suppl_4/iv43.full.pdf

capillaroscopic pattern shows a regular disposition of the capillary loops along with the nailbed. On the contrary, in subjects suffering from secondary RP, one or more alterations of the capillaroscopic findings should alert the physician of the possibility of a connective tissue disease not yet detected. Nailfold capillaroscopy (NV) represents the best method to analyze microvascular abnormalities in autoimmune rheumatic diseases. Architectural disorganization, giant capillaries, hemorrhages, loss of capillaries, angiogenesis and avascular areas characterize >95% of patients with overt scleroderma (SSc)."

- o Range of motion (ROM): Limited range of motion is characteristic secondary to a "straight jacket" effect secondary to tightened and fibrotic skin; reduced neck extension is termed "platysma sign"
- o Abdominal exam: Abdominal exam, gastrointestinal motility
- o Pulmonary exam: Pulmonary examination and auscultation; needs to be complemented by additional diagnostic testing. "Dyspnea is a late manifestation of systemic sclerosis–related lung disease; however, lung involvement is common and is the leading cause of death in patients with systemic sclerosis. ... Thus, routine screening with pulmonary function tests and Doppler echocardiography in all patients is essential for the early detection of interstitial lung disease and pulmonary arterial hypertension, respectively."[479]
- o Cardiovascular exam: Assessment for hypertension is mandatory
- **Laboratory assessments**: *lab assessments are only minimally supportive for the diagnosis, but are helpful to monitor for complications*
  - o Urinalysis: Screen for renal compromise as previously detailed
  - o Chemistry panel: Assess for renal and liver status, electrolytes, etc.
  - o CBC: May reveal anemia due to malabsorption-induced deficiencies of B12, folate, iron, hypoproliferation due to inflammation (i.e., the anemia of chronic disease).
  - o Rheumatoid factor: positive in 33%
  - o Breath hydrogen/methane for SIBO: This test is used to assess for bacterial overgrowth; it is not a perfect test and it delays treatment (dietary, antimicrobial) that should generally be implemented regardless of the results of this test.
  - o Lactulose and mannitol assay for "leaky gut" and malabsorption: Abnormal results are likely due to bacterial overgrowth and/or celiac disease with resultant malabsorption and increased intestinal permeability.[480]
  - o Fecal calprotectin—assessment for gastrointestinal involvement: "Fecal calprotectin (F-calprotectin) is increased in a majority of patients with SSc. It correlates with objective and clinically important features of GI disease, and fecal concentrations do not vary with plasma concentrations. We suggest that F-calprotectin is a promising objective non-invasive biomarker of GI involvement in SSc."[481]
  - o Leukocyte antigens: Increased prevalence of HLA-DR5 and HLA-DR1
  - o *Helicobacter pylori* detection: Given the increased prevalence of *Helicobacter pylori* infection[482,483], the addition of antigen testing onto a comprehensive stool analysis and comprehensive parasitology examination is recommended.
  - o Comprehensive stool analysis and comprehensive parasitology: essential
  - o **ANA (nucleolar): Positive in up to 96% of patients with scleroderma;** nucleolar pattern is most specific
  - o **Anticentromere antibody**: Positive in 50% with CREST; generally—relatively speaking—portends disease course more limited to dermal involvement[484]; correlates with and requires monitoring for pulmonary arterial hypertension

[479] Hinchcliff M, Varga J. Systemic sclerosis/scleroderma: a treatable multisystem disease. *Am Fam Physician*. 2008 Oct 15;78(8):961-8

[480] "Coeliac disease may account for malabsorption in scleroderma patients even when test suggest bacterial overgrowth." Marguerie C, Kaye S, Vyse T, Mackworth-Young C, Walport MJ, Black C. Malabsorption caused by coeliac disease in patients who have scleroderma. *Br J Rheumatol*. 1995 Sep;34(9):858-61

[481] Andréasson et al. Faecal calprotectin: a biomarker of gastrointestinal disease in systemic sclerosis. *J Intern Med*. 2011 Jul;270(1):50-7

[482] "Thus, risk for gastric diseases caused by HP infection is enhanced in patients with systemic sclerosis compared with white healthy, asymptomatic persons examined in other studies." Reinauer et al. Helicobacter pylori in patients with systemic sclerosis: detection with the 13C-urea breath test and eradication. *Acta Derm Venereol*. 1994 Sep;74(5):361-3

[483] "Patients with SSc have H. pylori infection at a higher prevalence than the general population." Yazawa et al. High seroprevalence of Helicobacter pylori infection in patients with systemic sclerosis: association with esophageal involvement. *J Rheumatol*. 1998 Apr;25(4):650-3

[484] Ho KT, Reveille JD. The clinical relevance of autoantibodies in scleroderma. *Arthritis Res Ther*. 2003;5(2):80-93 arthritis-research.com/content/5/2/80

- o **Anti-SCL-70 antibodies = anti-topoisomerase-1 antibodies**: Positive in 20-30% of patients; specific for scleroderma; portends disease course with internal organ involvement, particularly of the lungs; correlates with rapidly progressive skin thickening, scleroderma renal crisis, pulmonary fibrosis
  - o Antifibrillarin antibodies: seen in a small portion (~4%) of patients with scleroderma and correlates with internal organ involvement[485]
  - o Antimitochondrial antibodies, assessment for primary biliary cirrhosis: 225 Japanese SSc patients were retrospectively examined for PBC-associated autoantibodies, anti-mitochondrial M2 antibodies (AMA), anti-sp100 antibodies (anti-sp100), and anti-gp210 antibodies (anti-gp210); findings included that "37 (16.4%) had AMA, 13 (5.8%) had anti-sp100, and 3 (1.3%) had anti-gp210. Three patients were positive for both AMA and anti-sp100, and 2 were positive for both AMA and anti-gp210. PBC was found in 22 (9.8%) patients positive for AMA with or without anti-sp100 or anti-gp210, but not in those with anti-sp100 or anti-gp210 without AMA. Furthermore, 13 patients lacking these three antibodies were diagnosed with or suspected of PBC by liver biopsy and/or their clinical manifestation. Multivariable analysis revealed that AMA and anti-centromere antibodies were independently associated with PBC in SSc patients, while anti-sp100 and anti-gp210 were not. CONCLUSIONS: This study has demonstrated even higher prevalence of both PBC-associated autoantibodies and PBC in the Japanese SSc population than in the Caucasian SSc population. AMA and anti-centromere antibodies are likely to indicate increasing risk of PBC in SSc patients."[486]
- **Imaging**:
  - o ECG abnormalities are common and can include ventricular ectopy, which is correlated with sudden cardiac death
  - o Radiography, pulmonary function tests, and CT imaging may be used to detect fibrosing alveolitis and scleroderma-associated pulmonary decline
- **Establishing the diagnosis**:
  - o Clinical assessment is sufficient in patients with classic full-blown disease
  - o Combination of serologic evidence of autoimmunity and dermal induration

Complications:
- **General**: **Generalized fibrosis leads to thickening of skin (most obvious), obliteration of the lumen of small arteries (most pathologic), and reduced intestinal motility.**
- Cardiopulmonary and renal: Sudden cardiac death, pulmonary fibrosis/hypertension/failure, hypertension secondary to scleroderma-induced renal damage, renal insufficiency/failure.
- Gastrointestinal: 33% of patients will develop Barrett's esophagus and are at increased risk for cancer; periodic endoscopic surveillance is warranted; referral to gastroenterologist is recommended. To the extent possible, acid-blocking (proton pump-inhibiting) drugs should be avoided because the iatrogenic hypochlorhydria will exacerbate the small bowel bacterial overgrowth and thereby perpetuate the systemic inflammatory state. Malabsorption and resultant malnutrition are due to intestinal hypomotility and SIBO/dysbiosis; from the medical perspective—which in this case is largely correct except for failure to include dietary modification, "Antibiotics, including rifaximin (Xifaxan), and correction of nutritional deficiencies are the mainstays of therapy for intestinal overgrowth."[487] Nonpharmacologic treatments for SIBO include dietary modification especially exclusion of high-fermentation foods (such as sucrose, lactose, wheat, potatoes), berberine 1,000-1,500 mg/d, oregano oil (time-released emulsified) 300-600 mg/d, and ascorbate and magnesium to promote bowel clearance.
- Cancer: Increased incidence of breast and lung cancer

---

[485] "AFA identifies young SSc patients with frequent internal organ involvement, especially pulmonary hypertension, myositis and renal disease." Tormey VJ, Bunn CC, Denton CP, Black CM. Anti-fibrillarin antibodies in systemic sclerosis. *Rheumatology*. 2001 Oct;40(10):1157-62 rheumatology.oxfordjournals.org/cgi/content/full/40/10/1157

[486] Imura-Kumada et al. High prevalence of primary biliary cirrhosis and disease-associated autoantibodies in Japanese patients with systemic sclerosis. *Mod Rheumatol*. 2012 Nov;22(6):892-8

[487] Hinchcliff M, Varga J. Systemic sclerosis/scleroderma: a treatable multisystem disease. *Am Fam Physician*. 2008 Oct 15;78(8):961-8

Clinical management:

- Address underlying causative contributors; apply Functional Inflammology protocol.
- Monitor for complications such as systemic hypertension, pulmonary hypertension, renal failure.
  - All patients with systemic sclerosis are advised to check their blood pressure at home on a regular basis. Any persistent elevations should prompt medical evaluation and treatment with ACEi.
- Referral if clinical outcome is unsatisfactory or if serious complications are possible/evident.
- Treat complications such as HTN and GERD.

> **Diagnostic evaluation for SSc: Additional rationale for specialist comanagement**
>
> "Clinical evaluation and laboratory testing, along with pulmonary function testing, Doppler echocardiography, and high-resolution computed tomography of the chest [single-photon emission CT for detection of cardiocirculatory abnormalities], establish the diagnosis and detect visceral involvement."
>
> Hinchcliff, Varga. *Am Fam Physician*. 2008 Oct

Treatments:

- Drug treatments: "Treatment of progressive systemic sclerosis is symptomatic and supportive. ... Prednisone has little or no role in the treatment of scleroderma."[488] Per 2008 review, "No disease-modifying agent has been proven to prevent or reverse fibrosis, although retrospective studies and case series show that d-penicillamine (Cuprimine), mycophenolate mofetil (Cellcept), and cyclophosphamide (Cytoxan) may be effective in some patients"[489]; other allopathic treatments have been reviewed in articles freely available on-line.[490]
  - Prednisone or other corticosteroid is used for myositis, MCTD, and arthritis; known to exacerbate renal disease when administered in high doses, i.e., greater than 15 mg/d.
  - Penicillamine started at 250 mg/d and gradually increased to 0.5-1.0 g/d can reduce dermal and systemic involvement
  - Tetracycline: one gram per day for bacterial overgrowth[491]
  - ACE inhibitors are the drugs of choice for scleroderma renal disease and hypertension
  - Calcium channel blockers and angiotensin-II receptor blockers for Raynaud phenomenon
  - Endothelin-1 receptor blockers and phosphodiesterase-5 inhibitors for pulmonary arterial hypertension
- **FOOD & NUTRITION: 5-part "supplemented Paleo-Mediterranean diet" (SPMD)** The 5-part "supplemented Paleo-Mediterranean diet" (SPMD—reviewed in Chapter 4) consists of ❶ foundational plant-based low-carbohydrate diet of fruits, vegetables, nuts, seeds, berries and lean sources of protein, ❷ multivitamin and multimineral supplementation, ❸ physiologic doses of vitamin D3 (range 2,000-10,000 IU/d), ❹ combination fatty acid therapy (CFAT) with n3-ALA, n6-GLA, n3-EPA, n3-DHA, and phytochemical-rich olive oil which contains n9-oleate, and ❺ probiotics.
  - Supplemented Paleo-Mediterranean diet: The health-promoting diet of choice for the majority of people is a diet based on abundant consumption of fruits, vegetables, seeds, nuts, omega-3 and monounsaturated fatty acids, and lean sources of protein such as lean meats, fatty cold-water fish, soy and whey proteins. Although this diet is the most-nutrient dense diet available, rational supplementation with vitamins, minerals, and health promoting fatty acids (i.e., ALA, GLA, EPA, DHA) makes this the best practical diet that can possibly be conceived and implemented. **For scleroderma patients whose diets have habitually been low in fiber, dietary improvement which increases fiber consumption should be implemented slowly to avoid phytobezoar formation and intestinal obstruction[492]; consumption of water/fluids with meals is reasonable, as is periodic or regular use of osmotic laxative and stool-softening agents such as magnesium and ascorbate.** The specifications of the specific carbohydrate diet detailed by Gottschall[493] are met with adherence to the Paleo diet by Cordain.[494] The combination of both approaches will give patients an excellent combination of informational

[488] Tierney ML. McPhee SJ, Papadakis MA (eds). *Current Medical Diagnosis and Treatment. 35th edition*. Stamford: Appleton and Lange, 1996 page 747
[489] Hinchcliff M, Varga J. Systemic sclerosis/scleroderma: a treatable multisystem disease. Am Fam Physician. 2008 Oct 15;78(8):961-8
[490] Sapadin AN, Fleischmajer R. Treatment of scleroderma. *Arch Dermatol*. 2002 Jan;138(1):99-105. archderm.ama-assn.org/cgi/content/full/138/1/99
[491] Beers MH, Berkow R (eds). *Merck Manual. 17th Edition*. Whitehouse Station; Merck Research Laboratories 1999 Page 433
[492] Gough et al. Dietary advice in systemic sclerosis: the dangers of a high fibre diet. *Ann Rheum Dis*. 1998;57(11):641-2 ard.bmjjournals.com/cgi/content/full/57/11/641
[493] Gottschall E. *Breaking the Vicious Cycle: Intestinal health though diet*. Kirkton Press; Rev edition (August, 1994) scdiet.com
[494] Cordain L: *The Paleo Diet*. John Wiley & Sons Inc., New York 2002 thepaleodiet.com/

understanding and culinary versatility. In accord with both of these dietary programs, the diet must remain free of gluten-containing grains such as wheat, since **some patients with scleroderma have celiac disease**[495,496], and since **wheat, like most grains (except rice), promotes bacterial overgrowth of the intestine due to its high quantity of indigestible oligosaccharides.**[497] Patients with facial involvement and resulting restricted oral aperture will need to use smaller bites of food; consider using a food processor, smoothies—same applies for patients with esophageal dysmotility or restriction.

- o Overt malnutrition, micronutrient deficiencies, increased oxidative stress are common in SSc: SSc patients often show overt malnutrition, deficiencies of folate, cobalamin, lipoate, iron, copper, selenium, ascorbic acid, tocopherols, carnitine, and beta-carotene, and enhanced oxidative stress.[498] Very importantly, deficiency of antioxidants in general and selenium in particular is expected to result in enhanced viral replication and mutagenicity, an important realization considering the important role that viral infections appear to play in disease pathogenesis. From a practical clinical standpoint, iron status should be tested with ferritin while other nutritional deficiencies are—generally—treated empirically as discussed in chapters 1 and 4; individual testing of each nutrient is impractical, unnecessarily expensive, and an inappropriate use of time/effort/focus/money. Testing for vitamin B-12 status is notoriously inaccurate, and empiric treatment with 2,000 mcg/d PO is generally warranted for patients with suspected deficiency; however, given the high prevalence of malabsorption in patients with scleroderma/SSc, consideration should be given to laboratory assessments and parenteral administration.

- o Daily use of a broad-spectrum high-potency multivitamin and multimineral supplement: **Vitamin and mineral supplementation is important for patients with scleroderma.** Vitamin supplementation (particularly with pyridoxine and riboflavin) appears warranted in patients with **systemic sclerosis** based on a small (n=5) study that documented the normalization of aberrant tryptophan metabolism in most patients following the administration of pyridoxine with riboflavin; the authors concluded that this was evidence of combined vitamin deficiency in patients with scleroderma.[499] This combined deficiency is not surprising given the high incidence of bacterial overgrowth and malabsorption in scleroderma patients. Deficiencies of ascorbate and selenium have also been documented in patients with scleroderma.[500] Reduced folate and cobalamin and elevated homocysteine have also been noted in patients with scleroderma.[501]

- o Avoidance of allergenic foods: Any patient may be allergic to any food, even if the food is generally considered a health-promoting food. Generally speaking, the most notorious allergens are wheat, citrus (especially juice due to the industrial use of fungal hemicellulases), cow's milk, eggs, peanuts, chocolate, and yeast-containing foods; according to a study in patients with migraine, some patients will have to avoid as many as 10 specific foods in order to become symptom-free.[502] **Celiac disease is not uncommon in patients with scleroderma, and their scleroderma diagnosis may precede the recognition of celiac disease by many years.**[503,504] Clinicians must explain to their patients that celiac disease and wheat allergy

[495] "Coeliac disease may account for malabsorption in scleroderma patients even when test suggest bacterial overgrowth." Marguerie et al. Malabsorption caused by coeliac disease in patients who have scleroderma. *Br J Rheumatol.* 1995 Sep;34(9):858-61

[496] Gomez-Puerta et al. Coeliac disease associated with systemic sclerosis. *Ann Rheum Dis.* 2004 Jan;63(1):104-5 ard.bmjjournals.com/cgi/content/full/63/1/104

[497] "Short-chain fructooligosaccharides occur in a number of edible plants, such as chicory, onions, asparagus, wheat... Short-chain fructooligosaccharides, to a large extent, escape digestion in the human upper intestine and reach the colon where they are totally fermented mostly to lactate, short chain fatty acids (acetate, propionate and butyrate), and gas, like dietary fibres." Bornet et al. Nutritional aspects of short-chain fructooligosaccharides: natural occurrence, chemistry, physiology and health implications. *Dig Liver Dis.* 2002 Sep;34 Suppl 2:S111-20

[498] "Half of the patients had a subnormal arm muscle circumference, and two patients also had a subnormal triceps skinfold thickness, indicating severe malnutrition. The concentration of ascorbic acid, alpha-tocopherol, carotene, selenium, and also the proportion of linoleic acid (18:2) in serum phosphatidylcholine was lower in patients than in control subjects." Lundberg et al. Dietary intake and nutritional status in patients with systemic sclerosis. *Ann Rheum Dis.* 1992 Oct;51(10):1143-8 "Selenium levels were lower in patients than in controls (p=0.012). Within the patient cohort, copper correlated inversely with the total skin score (r=-0.52, p=0.03). Our findings provide further evidence that lipid peroxidation is increased and antioxidant capacity is reduced in SSc." Tikly et al. Lipid peroxidation and trace elements in systemic sclerosis. *Clin Rheumatol.* 2006 May;25(3):320-4. "In Raynaud's phenomenon (RP) and Systemic Sclerosis (SSc), a reduced concentration of ascorbic acid, alpha-tocopherol and beta-carotene as well as low values of Selenium have been reported." Simonini et al. Emerging potentials for an antioxidant therapy as a new approach to the treatment of systemic sclerosis. *Toxicology.* 2000 Nov 30;155(1-3):1-15. Famularo et al. Carnitine deficiency in scleroderma—letter. *Immunology Today* 1999 May; 246

[499] "But the simultaneous administration of pyridoxine and nicotinamide to three of these patients normalized the excretory picture after tryptophan loading." De Antoni et al. Tryptophan metabolism "via" nicotinic acid in patients with scleroderma. *Acta Vitaminol Enzymol.* 1976;30(4-6):134-9

[500] "Plasma ascorbic acid was reduced in all 3 groups of patients: median level 10.6 mg/l in controls, 4.8 mg/l in PRP (p < 0.01), 2.5 mg/l in ISSc (p < 0.01) and 6.8 mg/l in dSSc (p < 0.05). A reduction in serum selenium was especially found in dSSc (median 75 micrograms/l compared to 100 micrograms/l in controls, p < 0.05)." Herrick et al. Micronutrient antioxidant status in patients with primary Raynaud's phenomenon and systemic sclerosis. *J Rheumatol.* 1994 Aug;21(8):1477-83

[501] "Patients with SSc had higher Hcy and vWF concentrations than those with RP or controls. Folic acid and vitamin B12 were lower in SSc than in RP or controls." Marasini et al. Homocysteine concentration in primary and systemic sclerosis associated Raynaud's phenomenon. *J Rheumatol.* 2000 Nov;27(11):2621-3

[502] Grant EC. Food allergies and migraine. *Lancet.* 1979 May 5;1(8123):966-9

[503] Gomez-Puerta et al. Coeliac disease associated with systemic sclerosis. *Ann Rheum Dis.* 2004 Jan;63(1):104-5 ard.bmjjournals.com/cgi/content/full/63/1/104

[504] "Coeliac disease may account for malabsorption in scleroderma patients even when test suggest bacterial overgrowth." Marguerie et al. Malabsorption caused by coeliac disease in patients who have scleroderma. *Br J Rheumatol.* 1995 Sep;34(9):858-61

are two different clinical entities and that exclusion of one does not exclude the other, and in neither case does mutual exclusion obviate the **promotion of intestinal bacterial overgrowth (i.e., proinflammatory dysbiosis) by indigestible wheat oligosaccharides**. Rapid implementation of high fiber diets may precipitate bowel obstruction.[505]

o Vitamin D3 supplementation with physiologic doses and/or tailored to serum 25(OH)D and serum calcium levels : Vitamin D deficiency is common in the general population and is even more common in patients with chronic illness and chronic musculoskeletal pain.[506] Correction of vitamin D deficiency provides a clinically significant anti-inflammatory and immunomodulatory benefit.[507] **Oral administration of active vitamin D3 (1,25-dihydroxyvitamin D) has led to clinical improvement in patients with scleroderma**.[508] Reasonable daily doses for children and adults are 2,000 and 4,000 IU, respectively, as defined by Vasquez, et al.[509] Deficiency and response to treatment are monitored with serum 25(OH)vitamin D while safety is monitored with serum calcium; inflammatory granulomatous diseases and certain drugs such as hydrochlorothiazide greatly increase the propensity for hypercalcemia and warrant increment dosing and frequent monitoring of serum calcium.

o Broad-spectrum fatty acid therapy with ALA, EPA, DHA, GLA and oleic acid: "Sophisticated manipulation of EFA metabolism" may prove clinically beneficial for **scleroderma** patients according to a review by the late David Horrobin[510]; however, a six-month clinical trial of fatty acid supplementation showed no benefit[511], thus proving the ineffectiveness of one-dimensional intervention and of fatty acid supplementation in a condition known to have a high prevalence of untreated malabsorption. Nonetheless, as part of a *comprehensive program*, fatty acid supplementation should be delivered in the form of combination therapy with ALA, GLA, DHA, and EPA. Fish oil provides EPA and DHA which have well-proven anti-inflammatory benefits in rheumatoid arthritis[512,513,514] and lupus.[515,516] ALA, EPA, DHA, and GLA need to be provided in the form of supplements; when using high doses of therapeutic oils, liquid supplements that can be mixed in juice or a smoothie are generally more convenient and palatable than capsules. Therapeutic amounts of oleic acid can be obtained from generous use of olive oil, preferably on fresh vegetables. Supplementation with polyunsaturated fatty acids warrants increased intake of antioxidants from diet, fruit and vegetable juices, and properly formulated supplements; since patients with systemic inflammation are generally in a pro-oxidative state, consideration must be given to the timing and starting dose of fatty acid supplementation and the need for antioxidant protection.

o Probiotics for the treatment of systemic sclerosis-associated gastrointestinal bloating/ distention (*Clin Exp Rheumatol.* 2011 Mar[517]): "We compared the GIT 2.0 scores at baseline and after 2 months of use of Align (Bifidobacterium infantis; 10^9 CFU per capsule) or Culturelle (Lactobacillus GG; 10^9 CFU per capsule) using paired t-test and calculated effect size (ES). Significant improvement in total GIT 2.0 score (ES = 0.82), reflux (ES = 0.33), bloating/distention (ES = 1.76), and emotional scales (ES = 0.18) were reported after two months of daily probiotic use. This pilot study suggests probiotics significantly improve the reflux, distention/ bloating, and total GIT scales in SSc patients. As hypothesized, the largest effect was seen in distention/bloating scale. Probiotics may be useful for treatment of SSc-associated distention/ bloating."

---

505 Gough et al. Dietary advice in systemic sclerosis: the dangers of a high fibre diet. *Ann Rheum Dis.* 1998 Nov;57(11):641-2 ard.bmjjournals.com/cgi/content/full/57/11/641
506 Plotnikoff GA, Quigley JM. Prevalence of severe hypovitaminosis D in patients with persistent, nonspecific musculoskeletal pain. *Mayo Clin Proc.* 2003 Dec;78(12):1463-70
507 Timms et al. Circulating MMP9, vitamin D and variation in the TIMP-1 response with VDR genotype: mechanisms for inflammatory damage in chronic disorders? *QJM.* 2002 Dec;95(12):787-96 qjmed.oxfordjournals.org/cgi/content/full/95/12/787
508 "After the treatment period (6 months to 3 years), a significant improvement, as compared with baseline values, was observed. No serious side-effects were observed." Humbert et al. Treatment of scleroderma with oral 1,25-dihydroxyvitamin D3: evaluation of skin involvement using non-invasive techniques. *Acta Derm Venereol.* 1993 Dec;73(6):449-51
509 Vasquez et al. Clinical importance of vitamin D: a paradigm shift with implications for all healthcare providers. *Altern Ther Health Med.* 2004 Sep-Oct;10(5):28-36
510 "Controlled clinical trials of supplementation with gamma-linolenic acid (GLA) as evening primrose oil (Efamol) in both primary Sjogren's syndrome and systemic sclerosis have given positive results." Horrobin DF. Essential fatty acid and prostaglandin metabolism in Sjogren's syndrome, systemic sclerosis and rheumatoid arthritis. *Scand J Rheumatol* Suppl 1986;61:242-5
511 "Dietary essential fatty acids have no role in the treatment of vascular symptoms in established systemic sclerosis." Stainforth et al. Clinical aspects of the use of gamma linolenic acid in systemic sclerosis. *Acta Derm Venereol* 1996 Mar;76(2):144-6
512 Adam et al. Anti-inflammatory effects of a low arachidonic acid diet and fish oil in patients with rheumatoid arthritis. *Rheumatol Int.* 2003 Jan;23(1):27-36
513 Lau et al. Effects of fish oil supplementation on non-steroidal anti-inflammatory drug requirement in patients with mild rheumatoid arthritis. *Br J Rheumatol.* 1993 Nov:982-9
514 Kremer et al. Fish-oil fatty acid supplementation in active rheumatoid arthritis. A double-blinded, controlled, crossover study. *Ann Intern Med.* 1987 Apr;106(4):497-503
515 Walton et al. Dietary fish oil and the severity of symptoms in patients with systemic lupus erythematosus. *Ann Rheum Dis.* 1991 Jul;50(7):463-6
516 Duffy et al. The clinical effect of dietary supplementation with omega-3 fish oils and/or copper in systemic lupus erythematosus. *J Rheumatol.* 2004 Aug;31(8):1551-6
517 Frech et al. Probiotics for the treatment of systemic sclerosis-associated gastrointestinal bloating/ distention. *Clin Exp Rheumatol.* 2011 Mar-Apr;29(2 Suppl 65):S22-5

- <u>**INFECTIONS & DYSBIOSIS:**</u> ❶ **antimicrobial treatments,** ❷ **immunorestoration,** ❸ **immunotolerance via Treg induction** Essentially all autoimmune/rheumatic disorders are associated with microbial colonization and intolerance to same; the presence of persistent microbial colonization is *prima facie* evidence of immunosuppression. The eight areas of dysbiosis (multifocal) are: ❶ sinorespiratory, ❷ orodental, ❸ gastrointestinal, ❹ urogenital/genitourinary, ❺ parenchymal/tissue, ❻ microbial, ❼ dermal/cutaneous, and ❽ environmental. What emerges from the research on SSc and microbes is a complex model of microbial interplay where in some microbes infect vascular cells (e.g., parvovirus B19, EBV, CMV) where as other microbes promote the necessary cytokine response to promote fibrosis (e.g., EBV, *H pylori,* parvovirus B19); readers will find in the following table sufficient evidence to justify testing for viral and bacterial infections and treating, either specifically or empirically. See antiviral protocol in Chapter 4.2, second section, which is reprinted from my book *Antiviral Strategies and Immune Nutrition* (2014). Microbial contributions to scleroderma/SSC include:
  - **Gastrointestinal dysbiosis and SIBO** (small intestinal bacterial overgrowth): "The prevalence of SIBO was 43.1% in our SSc patients. ... Our study underscores that SIBO often occurs in SSc patients."[518] A growing body of literature implicates infectious agents in the etiology of **scleroderma.**[519] Regarding dermal dysbiosis, several articles by Cantwell et al[520,521] suggest epidermal and/or intradermal dysbiosis with pleomorphic bacteria, specifically acid-fast cell-wall-deficient mycobacteria. Regarding gastrointestinal dysbiosis, at the very least, we must acknowledge that 1) **bacterial overgrowth of the small bowel is common (33%) in patients with scleroderma**[522] due to impaired gastrointestinal motility, 2) **scleroderma patients show increased levels of deconjugating bacteria**[523], which inactivate bile acids and promote enterohepatic recirculation of endogenous and exogenous toxins, 3) **these patients have a high incidence of *Helicobacter pylori* infection (66% of patients with scleroderma, 78% of patients with scleroderma and Sicca syndrome**[524]), and 4) approximately **44% of scleroderma patients have esophageal overgrowth of *Candida albicans.*[525]** For these and other reasons (detailed in Chapter 4), **patients with scleroderma are presumed to have gastrointestinal dysbiosis until proven otherwise by the combination of 1) three-sample comprehensive parasitology examinations performed by a specialty laboratory and 2) clinical response to at least two 2-4 week courses of broad-spectrum antimicrobial treatment.** Yeast, bacteria, and parasites are treated as indicated based on identification and sensitivity results from comprehensive parasitology assessments. Breath hydrogen/methane testing is inferior to stool testing because it does not allow for identification and sensitivity testing of microbes. Other dysbiotic loci should be investigated as discussed in Chapter 4 in the section on multifocal dysbiosis. Attentive readers may have already surmised that treatment of gastrointestinal dysbiosis in patients with long-standing scleroderma is likely to be particularly difficult due to the neuropathic and myopathic **intestinal dysmotility**[526] **that will serve to perpetuate bacterial overgrowth and dysbiosis, thus necessitating vigilant and long-term treatment;** understanding and due persistence on the part of physician and patient are necessary to see this treatment through to completion—a combination of

---

[518] Marie et al. Small intestinal bacterial overgrowth in systemic sclerosis. *Rheumatology* (Oxford). 2009 Oct;48(10):1314-9

[519] "...increasing evidence has accumulated to implicate infectious agents in the etiology of systemic sclerosis (SSc)... ...increased antibody titers, a preponderance of specific strains in patients with SSc, and evidence of molecular mimicry inducing autoimmune responses suggest mechanisms by which infectious agents may contribute to the development and progression of SSc." Hamamdzic et al. The role of infectious agents in the pathogenesis of systemic sclerosis. *Curr Opin Rheumatol.* 2002 Nov;14(6):694-8

[520] Disabling pansclerotic morphea (DPM): "The organism could be identified as Staphylococcus epidermidis, but it also had stages of growth with morphologic forms more characteristic of a Corynebacterium-like or actinomycetelike microbe." Cantwell et al. Pleomorphic, variably acid-fast bacteria in an adult patient with disabling pansclerotic morphea. *Arch Dermatol.* 1984 May;120(5):656-61

[521] "Variably acid-fast coccoid forms, suggestive of cell wall deficient forms of mycobacteria, were observed in the dermis in microscopic sections of skin from six patients with generalized scleroderma, 10 patients with localized scleroderma (morphea), and four patients with lichen sclerosus et atrophicus (LSA)." Cantwell AR Jr. Histologic observations of pleomorphic, variably acid-fast bacteria in scleroderma, morphea, and lichen sclerosus et atrophicus. *Int J Dermatol.* 1984 Jan-Feb;23(1):45-52

[522] "Eight patients (33%) had significant bacterial counts: > 10(5) colony forming units per ml (cfu/ml) of jejunal fluid." Kaye et al. Small bowel bacterial overgrowth in systemic sclerosis: detection using direct and indirect methods and treatment outcome. *Br J Rheumatol.* 1995 Mar;34(3):265-9

[523] "Our results demonstrated that some of the bacterial species that overgrow in the upper small intestine of patients with progressive systemic sclerosis can deconjugate bile acids, and that a shift to neutral pH in gastric juice, may promote the bacterial overgrowth related to their impaired peristaltic activity." Shindo et al. Deconjugation ability of bacteria isolated from the jejunal fluid of patients with progressive systemic sclerosis and its gastric pH. *Hepatogastroenterology.* 1998 Sep-Oct;45(23):1643-50

[524] "Urease test demonstrated the presence of HP in 23 patients out of 35 (66%); 12 of them were negative to colonization. A Sicca syndrome, with abnormal Schirmers test and dry mouth was detected in 66% of the patients. 78% of the patients with Sicca syndrome had a concomitant HP infection..." Farina et al. High incidence of Helicobacter pylori infection in patients with systemic sclerosis: association with Sicca Syndrome. *Int J Immunopathol Pharmacol.* 2001 May;14(2):81-85

[525] "Esophageal mucosal brushings from 51 consecutive patients with progressive systemic sclerosis (PSS) (group I), 18 PSS patients continuously treated with high-dose ranitidine or omeprazole (group II), 34 controls referred to the outpatient clinic for endoscopy (group III), and 10 patients receiving long-term potent antireflux therapy for idiopathic gastroesophageal reflux (group IV) were cultured for Candida albicans. There were 44%, 89%, 9%, and 0% Candida albicans culture-positive patients in groups I through IV, respectively." Hendel et al. Esophageal candidosis in progressive systemic sclerosis: occurrence, significance, and treatment with fluconazole. *Scand J Gastroenterol.* 1988 Dec;23(10):1182-6

[526] "We found ultrastructural signs of axonal degeneration and cytoskeletal abnormalities in the bundles of unmyelinated fibers. There was also focal degeneration of smooth muscle cells, often in association with the presence of partially degranulated mast cells." Malandrini et al. Autonomic nervous system and smooth muscle cell involvement in systemic sclerosis: ultrastructural study of 3 cases. *J Rheumatol.* 2000 May;27(5):1203-6

pharmaceutical/botanical antimicrobials and promotility agents, including the universally safe and effective osmotic laxative magnesium, is reasonable. By this time, readers should appreciate the clinical implications of SIBO (as discussed in Chapter 4), including but not limited to malabsorption due to damage to the intestinal mucosa and mucosal enzymes, increased intestinal permeability, increased bacterial translocation, microbial mitochondriopathy, systemic inflammation, activation of DAMP, PAMP, and TLR receptors—all of these pro-inflammatory effects should be expected to promote the oxidative stress, autoimmunity, and fibrosis that characterize SSc.

- Octreotide (prescription drug): Descamps et al[527] describe the case of a 53-year-old black woman with progressive and severe systemic scleroderma, with diffuse skin sclerosis, myositis with intestinal pseudo-obstruction and bacterial overgrowth who experienced a "spectacular" normalization of clinical status and skin induration following several months of octreotide (75 mug/d). This drug is a somatostatin analog used in the treatment of acromegaly[528] and it also promotes intestinal motility and thus reduces dysbiotic intestinal bacterial overgrowth in patients with scleroderma.[529] Efficacy of octreotide in improving clinical manifestations of scleroderma is probably mediated *at least in part* by reducing the pro-inflammatory effects of dysbiotic intestinal bacterial overgrowth, which can be addressed by other means as well.

- Ciprofloxacin: Over and Bucknall[530] published a case report of a progressive scleroderma patient who experienced marked clinical improvement and biopsy-proven regression of skin changes following administration of ciprofloxacin 500 mg bid which was eventually reduced to 250 mg/d. This case report strongly supports the theory that intestinal dysbiosis is a major contributor to scleroderma. As with all antibacterial treatments, use empiric antifungal treatment with Nystatin 500,000 units bid and/or emulsified oregano 150 mg tid-qid.[531,532]

- *Artemisia annua*: Artemisinin has been safely used for centuries in Asia for the treatment of malaria, and it also has effectiveness against anaerobic bacteria due to the pro-oxidative sesquiterpene endoperoxide.[533,534] I commonly use artemisinin at 200 mg per day in divided doses for adults with dysbiosis. Evidence of past/current *H. pylori* infection is common (~40-60%) in patients with scleroderma[535], and some doctors—such as Jonathan V Wright MD—have reported anecdotally that *Artemisia annua* helps eradicate *H. pylori*. Conversely, we might reasonably look for a non-pro-oxidative treatment alternative to Artemisia, such as mastic.

- Erythromycin: 250-500 mg TID-QID; this drug is a widely used antibiotic that also has intestinal promotility benefits (thus making it an ideal treatment for intestinal bacterial overgrowth associated with or caused by intestinal dysmotility/hypomotility such as seen in scleroderma[536,537]). Do not combine erythromycin with the promotility drug cisapride due to risk for serious cardiac arrhythmia.

- Nystatin: Nystatin 500,000 units bid with food; duration of treatment begins with a minimum duration of 2-4 weeks and may continue as long as the patient is deriving benefit.

o **Cytomegalovirus—Induction of vasculopathy via direction infection and induction of pro-inflammatory cytokines, molecular mimicry**: CMV causes experimental vasculopathy resembling SSc; interestingly and consistent with my (DrV) model of dysbiosis which appreciates immunosuppression as (pre)requisite, experimental CMV-induced vasculopathy requires immunosuppression: "A viral agent known for its

---

[527] "After 8 months of treatment, normal weight was obtained and skin induration was spectacularly reduced and pigmentation returned to a normal state." Descamps et al. Global improvement of systemic scleroderma under long-term administration of octreotide. *Eur J Dermatol* 1999 Sep;9(6):446-8

[528] us.sandostatin.com/info/about/home.jsp Accessed December 16, 2005

[529] "Octreotide stimulates intestinal motility in normal subjects and in patients with scleroderma. In such patients, the short-term administration of octreotide reduces bacterial overgrowth and improves abdominal symptoms." Soudah et al. Effect of octreotide on intestinal motility and bacterial overgrowth in scleroderma. *N Engl J Med* 1991 Nov:1461-7

[530] Over et al. Regression of skin changes in a patient with systemic sclerosis following treatment for bacterial overgrowth with ciprofloxacin. *Br J Rheumatol*. 1998 Jun;37(6):696

[531] Stiles JC, Sparks W, Ronzio RA. The inhibition of Candida albicans by oregano. *J Applied Nutr* 1995;47:96–102

[532] Force M, Sparks WS, Ronzio RA. Inhibition of enteric parasites by emulsified oil of oregano in vivo. *Phytother Res*. 2000 May;14(3):213-4

[533] Dien et al. Effect of food intake on pharmacokinetics of oral artemisinin in healthy Vietnamese subjects. *Antimicrob Agents Chemother*. 1997 May;41(5):1069-72

[534] Giao et al. Artemisinin for treatment of uncomplicated falciparum malaria: is there a place for monotherapy? *Am J Trop Med Hyg*. 2001 Dec;65(6):690-5

[535] "Patients with SSc have H. pylori infection at a higher prevalence than the general population." Yazawa et al. High seroprevalence of Helicobacter pylori infection in patients with systemic sclerosis: association with esophageal involvement. *J Rheumatol*. 1998 Apr;25(4):650-3

[536] "Prokinetic agents effective in pseudoobstruction include metoclopramide, domperidone, cisapride, octreotide, and erythromycin. ... The combination of octreotide and erythromycin may be particularly effective in systemic sclerosis." Sjogren RW. Gastrointestinal features of scleroderma. *Curr Opin Rheumatol*. 1996 Nov;8(6):569-75

[537] "Erythromycin accelerates gastric and gallbladder emptying in scleroderma patients and might be helpful in the treatment of gastrointestinal motor abnormalities in these patients." Fiorucci et al. Effect of erythromycin administration on upper gastrointestinal motility in scleroderma patients. *Scand J Gastroenterol*. 1994 Sep;29(9):807-13

ability to damage vessel walls is cytomegalovirus (CMV). ... Infected immunocompetent animals exhibited only perivascular inflammation, suggesting that infection and immunosuppression were co-requisites of [vasculopathy] neointima formation. ... Induction of TGF-β1, the canonical pro-fibrotic cytokine, by human CMV (HCMV) was reported by other authors (16), implicating that a primary endothelial cell infection by HCMV may induce myofibroblast activation in the vessel wall under the effect of this cytokine."[538] "...higher prevalence of IgA antihuman cytomegalovirus antibodies in patients with SSc. ... CMV infection may play a part in SSc pathogenesis due to its ability to infect both endothelial and monocyte/macrophage cells and through the upregulation of fibrogenic cytokines and induction of immune dysregulation. ... association between increased serum levels of CMV-specific antibodies and the prevalence of SSc-related autoantibodies in patients with SSc. ... Molecular mimicry is a mechanism that may explain the pathogenicity of antibodies against viral proteins in SSc. Infection with HCMV may generate a host-antiviral response that is self-reactive toward autoantigens and endothelial cells."[539] Vulnerably to CMV-induced SSc may include genetic factors and fetomaternal/transfusional microchimerism, noted to be more common in women with SSc.

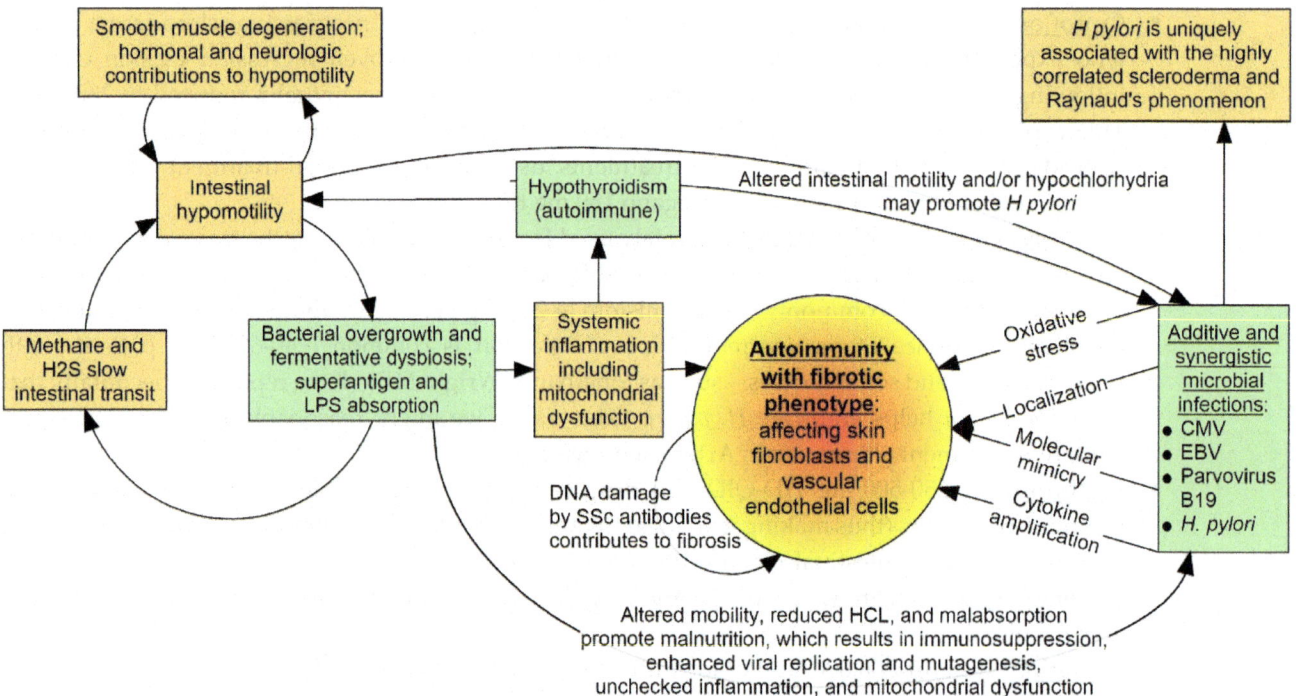

Polymicrobial and inflammatory aspects of scleroderma: diagram by Vasquez; quotes from Radić et al and Svegliati et al: "Systemic sclerosis is an autoimmune disease characterized by vascular obliteration, excessive extracellular matrix deposition and fibrosis of the connective tissues of the skin, lungs, gastrointestinal tract, heart, and kidneys. The pathogenesis of systemic sclerosis is extremely complex; at present, no single unifying hypothesis explains all aspects. Over the last 20 years increasing evidence has accumulated to implicate infectious agents in the etiology of systemic sclerosis. Increased antibody titers, a preponderance of specific strains in patients with systemic sclerosis, and evidence of molecular mimicry inducing autoimmune responses suggest mechanisms by which infectious agents may contribute to the development and progression of systemic sclerosis."[540] "Trichostatin A, an HDAC inhibitor, prevented WIF-1 loss, β-catenin induction, and collagen accumulation in an experimental fibrosis model. Our findings suggest that oxidative DNA damage induced by SSc autoreactive antibodies enables Wnt activation that contributes to fibrosis."[541]

[538] Moroncini et al. Role of viral infections in the etiopathogenesis of systemic sclerosis. *Clin Exp Rheumatol.* 2013 Mar-Apr;31(2 Suppl 76):3-7
[539] Radić et al. Infectious disease as aetiological factor in the pathogenesis of systemic sclerosis. *Neth J Med.* 2010 Nov;68(11):348-53
[540] Radić M, Martinović Kaliterna D, Radić J. Infectious disease as aetiological factor in the pathogenesis of systemic sclerosis. *Neth J Med.* 2010 Nov;68(11):348-53
[541] Svegliati et al. Oxidative DNA damage induces ATM-mediated transcriptional suppression of Wnt inhibitor WIF-1 in systemic sclerosis and fibrosis. *Sci Signal* 2014 Sept;ra84

○ **Epstein-Barr virus**—Localized infection in skin fibroblasts and endothelial cells, upregulation of cytokine production: "Here we show that EBV establishes infection in the majority of fibroblasts and endothelial cells in the skin of SSc patients, characterized by the expression of the EBV noncoding small RNAs (EBERs) and the increased expression of immediate-early lytic and latency mRNAs and proteins. We report that EBV is able to persistently infect human SSc fibroblasts in vitro, inducing an aberrant innate immune response in infected cells. EBV-Toll-like receptor (TLR) aberrant activation induces the expression of selected IFN-regulatory factors (IRFs), IFN-stimulated genes (ISGs), transforming growth factor-β1 (TGFβ1), and several markers of fibroblast activation, such as smooth muscle actin and Endothelin-1, and all of these genes play a key role in determining the profibrotic phenotype in SSc fibroblasts. These findings imply that EBV infection occurring in mesenchymal, endothelial, and immune cells of SSc patients may underlie the main pathological features of SSc including autoimmunity, vasculopathy, and fibrosis, and provide a unified disease mechanism represented by EBV reactivation."[542]

○ **Parvovirus B19**—Induction of fibrosis: "The presence of parvovirus B19 DNA was demonstrated in a significant percentage of bone marrow biopsies from SSc patients and was never detected in the control group. ... These patients showed the most severe active endothelial injury and perivascular inflammation. ...incubation with parvovirus B19-containing serum induced an invasive phenotype in normal human synovial fibroblasts."[543] Note that bone marrow-derived fibrocytes are involved in the pathogenesis of SSC; therefore, the strong positive correlation between B19 positivity and SSc and the negative correlation seen with B19 negativity and health suggests a likelihood of direct cause and effect.

○ *Helicobacter pylori*, especially the virulent CagA strain— Induction of systemic inflammation and cytokine response: "...despite the absence of a difference in *H. pylori* infection rates between SSc patients and control subjects, 90% of patients with SSc were infected with the virulent CagA strain compared with only 37% of the infected control subjects..." "Our data suggest that *H. pylori* infection correlates with severity of skin, gastrointestinal, and joint/tendon involvement in SSc patients. *H. pylori*-positive SSc patients showed higher severity score compared to *H. pylori*-negative. Therefore, *H. pylori* infection may play a role in the pathogenesis of SSc and also can provide some prognostic information."[544] "There are two general lines of evidence implicating bacterial infections in the pathogenesis of SSc. One is anecdotal evidence that treatment with antibiotics relieves SSc symptoms in some patients. The other is that graft-versus-host disease, which is recognized as having many similarities to SSc, cannot be induced in germ-free animals

---

CMV meets pathogenic criteria for SSc

- Direct infection of endothelial cells and immune cells
- Induction of pro-fibrotic cytokines
- Higher levels of CMV antibodies in SSc patients
- Exact molecular mimicry between HCMV late protein UL94 and human endothelial cell surface integrin–NAG-2 protein complex
- Cross-reacting CMV-endothelial antibodies kill endothelial cells and cause fibrosis
- Anti-UL94 antibodies bind to dermal fibroblasts and convert them to a scleroderma phenotype

Moroncini et al. *Clin Exp Rheumatol.* 2013 Mar

EBV meets pathogenic criteria for SSc

- Majority of SSc patients show active infection in vascular and dermal cells
- Virus-induced gene induction promotes the profibrotic scleroderma phenotype

Farina et al. *J Invest Dermatol.* 2014 Apr

PvB19 meets pathogenic criteria for SSc

- Direct infection of endothelial cells, immune cells, and dermal epithelial cells
- Induction of pro-fibrotic cytokines
- Bone marrow infection is seen in many SSc patients, correlates directly with disease severity, and is never noted in health patients; bone marrow fibrocytes contribute to SSc.
- PvB19 infection triggers formation of multiple autoantibodies: nuclear antigens (ANA), rheumatoid factor (RF), neutrophils cytoplasmic antigens, mitochondrial antigens (AMA), smooth muscle, gastric parietal antigens and phospholipids.

Moroncini et al. *Clin Exp Rheumatol.* 2013 Mar

---

[542] Farina et al. Epstein-Barr virus infection induces aberrant TLR activation pathway and fibroblast-myofibroblast conversion in scleroderma. *J Invest Dermatol.* 2014 Apr:954-64
[543] Radić et al. Infectious disease as aetiological factor in the pathogenesis of systemic sclerosis. *Neth J Med.* 2010 Nov;68(11):348-53
[544] Radić et al. Is Helicobacter pylori infection a risk factor for disease severity in systemic sclerosis? *Rheumatol Int.* 2013 Nov;33(11):2943-8

and is significantly reduced in children pre-treated with antibiotics to eradicate their normal bacterial flora."[545]

- o ***Toxoplasma gondii* and hepatitis B virus**: "Patients with SSc had elevated IgM and IgG against *Toxoplasma gondii* and against CMV. Higher titers were also detected against the hepatitis B virus core protein (recombinant HBc antigen) using MONOLISA anti-HBc Plus commercial kit (Bio-Rad). A significantly higher rate of IgM antibodies against the capsid antigen of the EBV was detected in SSc patients compared with healthy controls, as well."[546]
- o **<u>Clinical implications of polymicrobial dysbiosis in scleroderma</u>**: At the risk of redundancy and stating what should be obvious by now to readers who have studied the material in this book—especially chapter 4—here I will outline the implications of the information presented up to this point in this section on scleroderma/SSc. Quite obviously, the typical patient with scleroderma has multiple active microbial infections/colonizations and is therefore—by definition—demonstrating immunosuppression. Thus, two of the three components of my three-part dysbiosis model are established in SSC, and the third component—nutritional immunomodulation—is discussed in the following section. Given the solid data demonstrating polyviral activity for what I will describe as "popular viruses"—EBV, CMV, PvB19—we should reasonably assume that increased transcription of other viruses such as HSV (type-1 in 50% of the adult population; type-2 in 20% of the adult population) and the HERVs—human indigenous retroviruses—is also occurring. Serologic, newer generation PCR testing, and specialty tests—such as western blot for HSV infections—should ideally be performed to assess for the presence and severity/level of viral replication. Per previous discussions, clinicians must appreciate the total microbial load (TML) and not simply the presence/absence of these infections; bacterial quantifications—especially *H pylori*—must also be made if the initial laboratory evaluation is to be considered partly complete. Thereafter, the antimicrobial mission becomes on of search and destroy, using a combination of direct antiviral/antimicrobial agents as well as immunorestoration. My opinion and perspective is that antiviral pharmaceutic drugs—which by definition target single pathways in single viruses and are therefore easily bypassed by viral mutations and which have limited efficacy on the total viral load (TVL), respectively—are of limited clinical value but may still be used if found efficacious in individual patients; any failure of pharmacologic antiviral intervention in autoimmunity does not refute the viral etiology of autoimmunity but is rather to be expected from the failure to effectively address the larger viral load and to restore various aspects of disturbed homeodynamics. Attention should be directed toward a global or generalized antiviral approach to reduce TVL for various categories of viruses *concretely* and TVL *conceptually*, reasonably described here as ❶ common/popular viruses—these are the common viruses most commonly considered by clinicians and patients and for which we have readily available diagnostic tests, namely HIV, HBV, HCV, HSV 1 and 2, CMV, EBV, PvB19; readers should note from the above that SSC patients show viral infections that are not simply *more active* but are *active in different locations* compared to nonSSC persons, ❷ <u>human endogenous retroviruses</u>—viruses permanently embedded in the human genome, for which laboratory assessments are generally not clinically available; clinicians should consider this category to be an occult contributor to the TVL and thus TML and thus TIL—total inflammatory/immunogenic load, ❸ <u>bacteriophage load</u>—the total bacterial load (TBL) of the body and in particular the biomass in the intestines houses the bacteria-specific viruses known as bacteriophages, and these viruses-specific-for-bacteria contribute significantly to the TML of the gut in particular; thus, consideration to reducing/improving TBL in the gut would be expected to reduce the TVL as well, benignly promoting a reduction in the TIL, ❹ <u>other means of reducing TVL—reducing inflammation and bacterial load</u>: Bacterial debris such as LPS/endotoxin, other viral infections (via "transactivation"), and any other inflammatory stimuli that activate NFkB would be expected to promote viral replication via the NFkB pathway and other pathways that are "hijacked" or reappropriated[547] by viruses to promote their replication. In this manner, reducing the TBL lowers the TVL and thus the TIL. Extending the

---

[545] Radić et al. Infectious disease as aetiological factor in the pathogenesis of systemic sclerosis. *Neth J Med.* 2010 Nov;68(11):348-53

[546] Arnson et al. The role of infections in the immunopathogensis of systemic sclerosis--evidence from serological studies. *Ann N Y Acad Sci.* 2009 Sep;1173:627-32

[547] "As viruses evolve under the highly selective pressures of the immune system, they acquire the capacity to target critical steps in the host cell life, hijacking vital cellular functions to promote viral pathogenesis. Many viruses have evolved mechanisms to target the NF-kB pathway to facilitate their replication, cell survival, and evasion of immune responses." Hiscott et al. Hostile takeovers: viral appropriation of the NF-kappaB pathway. *J Clin Invest.* 2001 Jan;107(2):143-51

understanding and implications: Understanding this helps clinicians and researchers make sense of the confusion seen particularly in the research on CFS [caused by SIBO and GI dysbiosis] which is commonly complicated by evidence of increased viral replication; what I think is occurring here is that bacterial debris/LPS from SIBO is promoting viral replication via pathways including NFkB. Problematically, the LPS from SIBO also contributes to other problems such as impairment of cytochrome p450 which leads to xenobiotic accumulation and the resulting multiple chemical sensitivity [MCS], the persistent low-grade inflammatory and oxidative state which impairs the HPA axis and mitochondrial function; SIBO can cause deficiency of tryptophan and thus serotonin and perhaps melatonin via bacterial tryptophanase and deficiency of vitamin B-12 due to increased binding/chelation of B-12 with H2S.

- **NUTRITIONAL IMMUNOMODULATION: Treg induction for modulation of Th-1/2/17 inflammation** Nutrients and therapeutic approaches that promote Treg or IL-10 induction and/or Th-17, IL-17 suppression include 1) mitochondrial optimization and mTOR suppression, 2) biotin, 3) vitamin E, 4) sodium avoidance, 5) transgenic/GMO food avoidance, 6) probiotics, 7) lipoic acid, 8) vitamin A, 9) inflammation reduction, 10) vitamin D, 11) fatty acid supplementation with GLA and n3, 12) infection and dysbiosis remediation, 13) green tea EGCG. Acronym: MiBESTPLAIDFIG.
  - o <u>Vitamin E</u>: Morelli et al[548] describe a 60-year-old woman with **systemic sclerosis** complicated by hypertension, renal failure, and heart failure; although allopathic drug treatments were of no benefit, **the addition of "vitamin E (600 mg daily)" lead to rapid and significant clinical improvement.** Ayres and Mihan[549] wrote that vitamin E was effective in the clinical management of scleroderma, discoid lupus erythematosus[550], porphyria cutanea tarda, several types of vasculitis, and polymyositis.[551] Given that vitamin E is not a single compound but rather a family of closely related tocopherols, most clinicians prefer to use a source of "mixed tocopherols" inclusive of alpha, beta, delta, and—perhaps most importantly—gamma tocopherol.[552] Vitamin E has a wide margin of safety and although daily doses are kept in the range of 400-1200 IU, doses up to 3,200 IU are generally considered non-toxic. Tocopherols are now known to provide an anti-inflammatory immunomodulatory effect by elevating cAMP and thereby reducing TNF-alpha and increasing IL-10 as reviewed in Chapter 4 in the section on Nutritional Immunomodulation.

- **DYSMETABOLISM & DYSFUNCTIONAL MITOCHONDRIA: MitoDys, ERS-UPR, AGE/RAGE, hyperglycemia and ceramide** The major clinical considerations in this section are mitochondrial dysfunction, endoplasmic reticulum stress, unfolded protein response, TLR activation, and the dysmetabolic effects of sustained hyperglycemia and hyperinsulinemia and resultant oxidative stress, inflammation, RAGE activation, and accumulation of AGE, palmitate and ceramide. The review of this information in Chapter 4 covered approximately 30 interventions relevant to dysmetabolism, mitochondrial dysfunction, ERS-UPR, etc; these will not be reviewed here except to mention those most commonly, easily, empirically, synergistically, and effectively used: 1) low-carbohydrate diet with 2) moderate exercise, 3) CoQ-10, 4) acetyl-carnitine with 5) lipoic acid, 6) NAC, 7) resveratrol, and 8) melatonin.
  - o <u>Mitochondrial dysfunction in scleroderma—a cause of a fibrotic phenotype</u>: My (DrV) intuitive sense is that mitochondrial dysfunction—likely induced by bacteria, viruses and/or xenobiotic exposure—induces a fibrotic phenotype in scleroderma patients; research data supporting this concept is indirect.

---

[548] "Casually, vitamin E (600 mg daily) was added. After 6 months, clinical manifestations of heart failure were disappeared and the echocardiogram showed a normally-sized left ventricle with normal wall motion." Morelli et al. Systemic sclerosis (scleroderma). A case of recovery of cardiomyopathy after vitamin E treatment. *Minerva Cardioangiol.* 2001 Apr;49(2):127-30

[549] "Among the diseases that were successfully controlled were a number in the autoimmune category, including scleroderma, discoid lupus erythematosus, porphyria cutanea tarda, several types of vasculitis, and polymyositis." Ayres S Jr, Mihan R. Is vitamin E involved in the autoimmune mechanism? *Cutis.* 1978 Mar;21(3):321-5

[550] "Despite conflicting opinions, our personal experience and a number of reviewed clinical reports indicate that vitamin E, properly administered in adequate doses, is a safe and effective treatment for chronic discoid lupus erythematosus, and may be of value in treating other types of the disease." Ayres S Jr, Mihan R. Lupus erythematosus and vitamin E: an effective and nontoxic therapy. *Cutis.* 1979;23(1):49-52, 54

[551] "She then made a dramatic improvement when large doses of vitamin E (d, alpha-tocopheryl acetate) were administered." Killeen RN, Ayres S Jr, Mihan R. Polymyositis: response to vitamin E. *South Med J.* 1976 Oct;69(10):1372-4

[552] Jiang et al. gamma-tocopherol, the major form of vitamin E in the US diet, deserves more attention. *Am J Clin Nutr.* 2001 Dec;74(6):714-22 ajcn.org/cgi/content/full/74/6/714

However, noted is the observation that worsening systemic inflammation (measured by hsCRP) correlates with antimitochondrial antibodies in patients with scleroderma.[553]

- o Liver giant mitochondria: an almost constant lesion in systemic scleroderma (*Virchows Arch A Pathol Anat Histol 1977 Jun*[554]): "Liver electron microscopic studies were performed in 14 patients with systemic scleroderma. In 13 of these patients, giant mitochondria were demonstrated in the hepatocytes. This ultrastructural abnormality was present whatever the type and duration of the disease and was also present even when the liver was histologically normal. The mechanism of formation of giant mitochondria in systemic scleroderma is unknown."
- o Carnitine: According to the final sentence in a short report by Famularo et al[555], "Interestingly, early uncontrolled studies reported that the administration of L-carnitine had a favorable impact on the course of the disease in and this improvement was paralleled by a reduction in serum immunoglobulin levels." The use of carnitine is reviewed in Chapter 4 in the section on mitochondrial dysfunction.

- **STYLE OF LIVING (LIFESTYLE) & SPECIAL CONSIDERATIONS:** This is a buffet of mostly lifestyle-based interventions including considerations such as somatic treatments, additional supplementation, and surgery.
  - o Special supplementation—PABA (para-amino benzoic acid): **Ninety percent of patients treated with PABA experience clinical benefit, especially skin softening.[556] PABA therapy prolongs survival in patients with scleroderma.[557]** "Potaba" is a well-tolerated prescription form of PABA.[558] Wright and Gaby[559] recommend "PABA, 2-3 g, 4 times a day." A 2006 review by Gaby[560] noted that PABA administered as potassium para-aminobenzoate (KPAB) was able to preserve pulmonary function and improve survival at five years (88.5% versus 69.8%) and 10 years (76.6% versus 56.6%) among patients treated with 12-12.5 g per day for three months to 20.6 years (average, 4.2 years). Adverse effects attributable to PABA are dose-dependent and include low blood sugar, rash, fever, and liver damage; one case of fatal toxic hepatitis has been reported. Adverse effects may be seen with doses approximating or exceeding eight grams per day; thus serial serum chemistries (e.g., monthly at first, then bimonthly, then quarterly) are warranted, especially when using high doses.
  - o Special supplementation—*Centella asiatica* (Gotu cola): This botanical has been reported to favorably influence scleroderma.[561] Available forms include teas, tinctures, standardized capsules/tablets, topical ointments, and injectable preparations. The **proprietary product "Madecassol" containing madecassic acid, asiatic acid and asiaticoside has been used in several studies and has demonstrated clinical benefit in scleroderma**[562]; some preparations of this product apparently contain nitrofural, a topically and orally active antibiotic. Contact dermatitis has been reported.
  - o CoQ10: CoQ10 is a powerful antioxidant with a wide margin of safety and excellent clinical tolerability. **At least four studies have documented its powerful blood-pressure-lowering ability, which often surpasses the clinical effectiveness of antihypertensive drugs.[563,564,565,566] Furthermore, at least two published papers[567,568] and one case report[569] advocate that CoQ10 has powerful renoprotective and**

[553] "Occurrence rate of anti-mitochondria antibody in high-sensitivity CRP elevated SSc patients (8/14, 57.1%) was significantly elevated compared with that of high-sensitivity CRP low SSc patients (3/26, 11.5%) (P < 0.01). These results led us to conclusion that elevated high-sensitivity CRP shows relation to the occurrence of anti-mitochondria antibody." Ohtsuka T. Relation between elevated high-sensitivity C-reactive protein and anti-mitochondria antibody in patients with systemic sclerosis. *J Dermatol.* 2008 Feb:70-5

[554] Feldmann et al. Hepatocyte giant mitochondria: an almost constant lesion in systemic scleroderma. *Virchows Arch A Pathol Anat Histol.* 1977 Jun 23;374(3):215-27

[555] Famularo et al. Carnitine deficiency in scleroderma—letter. *Immunology Today* 1999 May; 246

[556] "Ninety percent of 224 patients treated with KPAB experienced mild, moderate, or marked skin softening." Zarafonetis CJ, Dabich L, Skovronski JJ, DeVol EB, Negri D, Yuan W, Wolfe R. Retrospective studies in scleroderma: skin response to potassium para-aminobenzoate therapy. *Clin Exp Rheumatol.* 1988 Jul-Sep;6(3):261-8

[557] "For the entire group an estimated 81.4% survived 5 years from diagnosis and 69.4% survived 10 years. …adequate treatment with potassium para-aminobenzoate (Potaba KPAB) was associated with improved survival (p less than 0.01); 88.5% 5 year survival rate and 76.6% 10 year survival rate for adequately treated patients." Zarafonetis et al. Retrospective studies in scleroderma: effect of potassium para-aminobenzoate on survival. *J Clin Epidemiol.* 1988;41(2):193-205

[558] glenwood-llc.com/potaba.html

[559] Gaby A, Wright JV. *Nutritional Protocols.* 1998 by Nutrition Seminars.

[560] Gaby AR. Natural remedies for scleroderma. *Altern Med Rev.* 2006 Sep;11(3):188-95

[561] "Titrated extract of Centella asiatica (TECA) contains three principal ingredients, asiaticoside (AS), asiatic acid (AA), and madecassic acid (MA). These components are known to be clinically effective on systemic scleroderma, abnormal scar formation, and keloids." Hong et al. Advanced formulation and pharmacological activity of hydrogel of the titrated extract of C. asiatica. *Arch Pharm Res.* 2005 Apr;28(4):502-8

[562] "Madecassol is effective and well tolerated and therefore recommended for oral and local use in combined treatment of SS adn FS." Guseva et al. [Madecassol treatment of systemic and localized scleroderma]. *Ter Arkh.* 1998;70(5):58-61. Article in Russian; information from abstract.

[563] Burke et al. Randomized, double-blind, placebo-controlled trial of coenzyme Q10 in isolated systolic hypertension. *South Med J.* 2001 Nov;94(11):1112-7

[564] Singh et al. Effect of hydrosoluble coenzyme Q10 on blood pressures and insulin resistance in hypertensive patients with CAD. *J Hum Hypertens.* 1999 Mar;13(3):203-8

[565] Digiesi et al. Coenzyme Q10 in essential hypertension. *Mol Aspects Med.* 1994;15 Suppl:s257-63

[566] Langsjoen P, Langsjoen P, Willis R, Folkers K. Treatment of essential hypertension with coenzyme Q10. *Mol Aspects Med.* 1994;15 Suppl:S265-72

[567] Singh et al. Randomized, double-blind placebo-controlled trial of coenzyme Q10 in chronic renal failure: discovery of a new role. *J Nutr Environ Med* 2000;10:281-8

[568] Singh et al. Randomized, Double-blind, Placebo-controlled Trial of Coenzyme Q10 in Patients with End-stage Renal Failure. *J Nutr Environ Med* 2003:13;13–22

[569] Singh RB, Singh MM. Effects of CoQ10 in new indications with antioxidant vitamin deficiency. *J Nutr Environ Med* 1999; 9:223-228

renorestorative benefits. CoQ10 levels are low in patients with allergies[570], and the symptomatic relief that many allergic patients experience following supplementation with CoQ10 suggests that CoQ10 has an immunomodulatory effect. Common doses start at > 100 mg per day with food; doses of 200 mg per day are not uncommon, and doses up to 1,000 mg per day are clinically well tolerated though the high financial toll approximates that of many pharmaceutical drugs.

- ▪ Coenzyme Q supplementation in pulmonary arterial hypertension (*Redox Biol* 2014 Jul[571]): In this controlled clinical trial, 300 mg daily of the reduced form of CoQ-10 were given to eight PAH patients. "Cardiac parameters improved with CoQ supplementation, although 6-minute walk distances and BNP levels did not significantly change. Consistent with improved mitochondrial synthetic function, hemoglobin increased and red cell distribution width (RDW) decreased in PAH patients with CoQ, while hemoglobin declined slightly and RDW did not change in healthy controls. In contrast, metabolic and redox parameters, including lactate, pyruvate and reduced or oxidized glutathione, did not change in PAH patients with CoQ. In summary, CoQ improved hemoglobin and red cell maturation in PAH, but longer studies and/or higher doses with a randomized placebo-controlled controlled design are necessary to evaluate the clinical benefit of this simple nutritional supplement."

- ○ N-acetyl-cysteine (NAC): **Oxidative stress promotes a fibrotic phenotype in scleroderma fibroblasts, which was normalized by administration of NAC** *in vitro*.[572] NAC is well-tolerated, inhibits NFkB, functions as an antioxidant, is a powerful and clinically important antiviral agent, and promotes detoxification via hepatoprotection and glutathione conjugation. In patients with scleroderma/SSC, studies using oral and IV NAC have been performed; benefits include improved hepatic (one-day study[573]), renal (one-day study[574]), and brachial/digital (three-year study[575]) perfusion following IV NAC.

  - ▪ Measurement of clinical change in progressive systemic sclerosis: a 1 year double-blind placebo-controlled trial of N-acetylcysteine (*Ann Rheum Dis.* 1979 Aug[576]): "Identically appearing 500 mg capsules of NAC or placebo were dispensed. ... Therapy was begun with 2-4 capsules daily and increased to a maximum of 20 capsules daily given in equally divided doses over a 2-month period. If the full dose was not tolerated, the highest tolerated dose was used. ... In the NAC-treated group, [pulmonary] residual volume increased significantly. Oral aperture increased significantly in the NAC-treated group and latex titers decreased statistically significantly."

  - ▪ Long-term N-acetylcysteine therapy in systemic sclerosis interstitial lung disease (*Int J Immunopathol Pharmacol* 2011 Jul[577]): "The primary endpoints of this study were changes between baseline and month 24 in single-breath carbon monoxide diffusing capacity (DLco). The secondary endpoints were: vital capacity (VC), forced expired volume in 1 sec (FEV1), total lung capacity (TLC), scores of high resolution computed tomography (HRCT) of the chest, number of adverse effects. In this study, we retrospectively investigated data from SSc patients who had undergone therapy with high-dose *intravenous* N-acetylcysteine (NAC) at a dosage of 15 mg/Kg/h for 5 consecutive hours every 14 days. After NAC therapy median values of DLco (69.5 vs 77.7%), VC (99 vs 101.3%) and TLC (93 vs 98.3%) significantly increased. We did not observe any significant changes from baseline in FEV1 value and HRTC score. The improvement in lung function was more evident in SSc patients

[570] Ye CQ, Folkers K, et al. A modified determination of coenzyme Q10 in human blood and CoQ10 blood levels in diverse patients with allergies. *Biofactors.* 1988 Dec;1:303-6

[571] Sharp et al. Coenzyme Q supplementation in pulmonary arterial hypertension. *Redox Biol.* 2014 Jul 31;2:884-91

[572] "Treatment of SSc fibroblasts with the membrane-permeant antioxidant N-acetyl-L-cysteine inhibited ROS production, and this was accompanied by decreased proliferation of these cells and down-regulation of alpha1(I) and alpha2(I) collagen messenger RNA." Sambo et al. Oxidative stress in scleroderma: maintenance of scleroderma fibroblast phenotype by the constitutive up-regulation of reactive oxygen species generation through the NADPH oxidase complex pathway. *Arthritis Rheum* 2001 Nov;44(11):2653-64

[573] "In an open-label study 40 patients with systemic sclerosis (SSc) were treated with 15 mg/kg/hour intravenous N-acetylcysteine for 5 consecutive hours in a single day. ... The results of our study demonstrate that NAC is able to increase HFV and total liver perfusion after a single infusion in SSc patients with low disease activity and severity scores." Rosato et al. N-acetylcysteine infusion improves hepatic perfusion in the early stages of systemic sclerosis. *Int J Immunopathol Pharmacol.* 2009 Jul-Sep;22(3):763-72

[574] "In an open-label study 40 patients with systemic sclerosis (SSc) were treated with N-acetylcysteine (NAC) iv infusion over 5 consecutive hours, at a dose of 0.015 g x kg(-1) x h(-1). ... In patients with low disease severity NAC ameliorates vascular renal function." Rosato et al. N-acetylcysteine infusion reduces the resistance index of renal artery in the early stage of systemic sclerosis. *Acta Pharmacol Sin.* 2009 Sep;30(9):1283-8

[575] "The aim of this study was to report long-term outcome (median follow-up 3 years) in a prospective study of a cohort of 50 consecutive patients with SSc who received N-acetylcysteine (NAC) infusional therapy every 2 weeks. ... In conclusion, long-term therapy with NAC, in patients with SSc, has a durable effectiveness on ischemic ulcers and Raynaud's phenomenon." Rosato et al. The treatment with N-acetylcysteine of Raynaud's phenomenon and ischemic ulcers therapy in sclerodermic patients: a prospective observational study of 50 patients. *Clin Rheumatol.* 2009 Dec;28(12):1379-84

[576] Furst et al. Measurement of clinical change in progressive systemic sclerosis. *Ann Rheum Dis.* 1979 Aug;38(4):356-61

[577] Rosato et al. Long-term N-acetylcysteine therapy in systemic sclerosis interstitial lung disease: a retrospective study. *Int J Immunopathol Pharmacol.* 2011 Jul-Sep;24:727-33

without radiological signs of pulmonary fibrosis than in patients with pulmonary fibrosis. In SSc patients with mild-moderate pulmonary fibrosis intravenous NAC administration slows the rate of deterioration of DLco, VC and TLC. In conclusion, this retrospective study demonstrates that long-term therapy with intravenous NAC ameliorates pulmonary function tests in SSc patients."

- o Comprehensive antioxidation: **As previously mentioned, patients with scleroderma have evidence of increased oxidative stress demonstrated by a doubling of urinary isoprostane excretion.**[578] Oxidative stress results from and contributes to systemic inflammation because 1) increased immune activity results in elaboration of oxidants, and 2) oxidative stress upregulates NFkB (and other pathways) for additive immune activation. *Antioxidant supplementation* alone is clinically and biochemically inferior to a *comprehensive program* that includes both antioxidant supplementation and dietary modification (i.e., the supplemented Paleo-Mediterranean diet, as described previously) that includes heavy reliance upon fruits, vegetables, low-glycemic juices, nuts, seeds, and berries for their additive and synergistic antioxidant benefits.[579]

  - ▪ In vitro modulation of collagen type I, fibronectin and dermal fibroblast function and activity, in systemic sclerosis by the antioxidant epigallocatechin-3-gallate (*Rheumatology* 2010 Nov[580]): Dermal fibroblasts from a cell line (AG), healthy individuals (CON) and SSc patients were treated with EGCG, one of the main constituents of green tea. "The results suggest that the antioxidant, EGCG, can reduce ECM production, the fibrotic marker CTGF and inhibit contraction of dermal fibroblasts from SSc patients. Furthermore, EGCG was able to suppress intracellular ROS, ERK1/2 kinase signaling and NFkB activity. Taken together, EGCG may be a possible candidate for therapeutic treatment aimed at reducing both oxidant stress and the fibrotic effects associated with SSc."

- o Oral enzyme therapy with proteolytic/pancreatic enzymes: Polyenzyme supplementation is used to ameliorate the pathophysiology induced by immune complexes.[581] Immune complexes are detected in the majority of patients with scleroderma[582] and correlate with disease severity and visceral involvement.[583] Orally administered polyenzyme preparations have an "immune stimulating" action[584] and promote degradation of microbial biofilms and increased immune and antimicrobial penetration into infectious foci.[585] Given that maldigestion, malabsorption, and pancreatic insufficiency are not uncommon in patients with scleroderma[586], enzymes may be given with food for optimal benefit.

- o Esophageal dysfunction and GERD in scleroderma—specific treatments:

  - ▪ Low carbohydrate diet, specific carbohydrate diet: The gastroesophageal dysfunction that contributes to the high incidence of Barrett's esophagus is likely the result of a confluence of different factors: neurogenic, myogenic, and dysbiotic. With regard to the latter, clinicians must be diligent in the eradication of small intestine bacterial overgrowth, since microbial products of fermentation lead to relaxation of the so-called lower esophageal sphincter.[587,588] This is why diets low in carbohydrate and fermentable fibers (such as those found in grains)—in other words: "**low fermentation diets**"—are effective in the treatment of esophageal reflux; low-carbohydrate diets deprive gut microbes of substrate for fermentation into metabolites that relax the lower esophageal

---

[578] "CONCLUSION: This study provides evidence of enhanced lipid peroxidation in both SSc and UCTD, and suggests a rationale for antioxidant treatment of SSc." Cracowski et al. Enhanced in vivo lipid peroxidation in scleroderma spectrum disorders. *Arthritis Rheum* 2001 May;44(5):1143-8

[579] Liu RH. Health benefits of fruit and vegetables are from additive and synergistic combinations of phytochemicals. *Am J Clin Nutr*. 2003 Sep;78(3 Suppl):517S-520S

[580] Dooley et al. Modulation of collagen type I, fibronectin and dermal fibroblast function and activity, in systemic sclerosis by the antioxidant epigallocatechin-3-gallate. *Rheumatology* 2010 Nov;49(11):2024-36

[581] Galebskaya et al. Human complement system state after wobenzyme intake. *Vestnik Moskovskogo Universiteta (Seriya 2: Khimiya)*. 2000:41(6 Suppl): 148-149 chem.msu.ru/eng/journals/vmgu/00add/148.pdf

[582] "Serum immune complexes were measured in 92 patients with progressive systemic sclerosis, and elevated levels were found as follows: Raji cell assay 72% (59% after pronase treatment of Raji cell), agarose gel electrophoresis 52%, and C1q binding 24%." Seibold JR, Medsger TA Jr, Winkelstein A, Kelly RH, Rodnan GP. Immune complexes in progressive systemic sclerosis (scleroderma). *Arthritis Rheum*. 1982 Oct;25(10):1167-73

[583] "Patients with SS showed an incidence of circulating immune complexes comparable to that found in SLE, with 20 patients (58.5%),...associated with both elevation of serum IgG and IgA levels and extensive visceral involvement by the disease." Hughes et al. Immune complexes in systemic sclerosis; detection by C1q binding, K-cell inhibition and Raji cell radioimmunoassays. *J Clin Lab Immunol*. 1983 Mar;10(3):133-8

[584] Zavadova et al. Stimulation of reactive oxygen species production and cytotoxicity in human neutrophils in vitro and after oral administration of a polyenzyme preparation. *Cancer Biother*. 1995 Summer;10(2):147-52

[585] "The enzymes were shown to inhibit the biofilm formation. When applilied to the formed associations, the enzymes potentiated the effect of antibiotics on the bacteria located in them." Tets VV, et al. [Impact of exogenic proteolytic enzymes on bacteria][Article in Russian] *Antibiot Khimioter*. 2004;49(12):9-13

[586] Of 20 patients: "Three patients had very low levels of tryptic activity in their intestinal juice and only nine had results which were unequivocally normal." Cobden I, Axon AT, Rowell NR. Pancreatic exocrine function in systemic sclerosis. *Br J Dermatol* 1981 Aug;105(2):189-93

[587] "Colonic fermentation of indigestible carbohydrates increases the rate of TLESRs [transient lower esophageal sphincter relaxations], the number of acid reflux episodes, and the symptoms of GERD." Piche et al. Colonic fermentation influences lower esophageal sphincter function in gastroesophageal reflux disease. *Gastroenterology*. 2003 Apr;124(4):894-902

[588] Piche et al. Modulation by colonic fermentation of LES function in humans. *Am J Physiol Gastrointest Liver Physiol*. 2000 Apr;278(4):G578-84

sphincter and thereby contribute to symptomatic improvement in patients with gastroesophageal reflux.[589] This is part of the reason why the diet for these patients must be as low as possible in the difficult-to-digest and easy-to-ferment carbohydrates that are common in the Standard American Diet (SAD) from corn, potatoes, wheat, and disaccharides such as lactose and sucrose; see *Breaking the Vicious Cycle*[590] by Elaine Gottschall for more details and recipes for the specific carbohydrate diet. Similarly, a low-carbohydrate Atkins-type diet[591] might also be considered, particularly for short-term use and particularly if modified away from proinflammatory saturated fats and arachidonic acid. As emphasized previously, high-fiber diets increase the risk for bowel obstruction in scleroderma patients, especially if implemented rapidly; slow implementation of dietary fiber increase along with an osmotic stool softener such as magnesium and/or ascorbate is advised.

- Alginate: Alginate is a processed extract from seaweed that is the active ingredient in the FDA-approved OTC anti-heartburn drug Gaviscon.[592] When mixed with stomach acid, alginate forms a foam "raft" that creates a barrier of protection for the esophagus, and it significantly reduces the number of acidic reflux events. Clinical studies have proven the effectiveness of alginate for treating GERD; however pure supplements of sodium alginate may be preferred over Gaviscon due to the latter's inclusion of aluminum (hydroxide)[593], a metal correlated with adverse effects and increased risk for neurologic disease. Alginate is also said to bind toxic metals and may therefore reduce enterohepatic recirculation of these proinflammatory immunotoxins.

- Betaine hydrochloric acid (betaine HCL): Many patients with gastroesophageal reflux are cured with the administration of supplemental HCL. Although the addition of acid rather than the suppression of acid goes against the well-funded acid-blocking drug paradigm, the truth remains that—*physiologically*—gastric emptying is promoted by acidification and—*clinically*—the treatment works for a significant number of patients with GERD. Furthermore, correction of hypochlorhydria by supplementation with betaine HCL helps to reduce bacterial/yeast counts in the stomach and upper intestine, thereby alleviating GERD by reducing the bacteria/yeast available for fermentation; recall that microbial fermentation is one of the primary driving influences for GERD/reflux.[594]

- GLA: Numerous studies have documented the anti-cancer effects of GLA, and these have specifically been documented in esophageal cancer cell lines.[595] Thus, GLA consumption may help protect against the development of esophageal cancer, in addition to its important anti-inflammatory and vasodilating actions.

- Vitamin B12: Vitamin B-12 levels are low in patients with malabsorption, and vitamin B-12 administration (4,000 mcg/d orally, or 1,000-2,000 mcg intramuscularly/ 2-3 times weekly) can promote intestinal motility.

- Raynaud's phenomenon—specific treatments: See section/minimonograph toward the end of this chapter.

- **ENDOCRINE IMBALANCE & OPTIMIZATION: Prolactin, Insulin, Estrogen, DHEA, Cortisol, Testosterone, Thyroid** Common hormonal imbalances seen among autoimmune/inflammatory patients are: ❶ *elevated* prolactin, ❷ *elevated* estrogen, ❸ *elevated* insulin, and ❹ *reduced* DHEA, ❺ *reduced* cortisol, and ❻ *reduced* testosterone; see Chapter 4 for discussion of these hormones and respective interventions. Thyroid evaluation (patient + labs) should be comprehensive, as discussed in Chapter 1, with a low threshold for empiric treatment.

---

[589] "The 5 individuals described in these case reports experienced resolution of GERD symptoms after self-initiation of a low-carbohydrate diet." Yancy et al. Improvement of gastroesophageal reflux disease after initiation of a low-carbohydrate diet: five brief case reports. *Altern Ther Health Med*. 2001 Nov-Dec;7(6):120, 116-9

[590] Gotschall E. *Breaking the Vicious Cycle: Intestinal health though diet*. Kirkton Press; Rev edition (August, 1994) scdiet.com/

[591] Atkins RC. *Dr. Atkins' New Diet Revolution (revised and updated)*. New York: Avon Books, 1999

[592] "For this population, sodium alginate was assessed as significantly superior by both investigators and patients at week two (p < 0.001 and p = 0.004, respectively) and at week four (p = 0.001 and p < 0.001, respectively)." Chatfield S. A comparison of the efficacy of the alginate preparation, Gaviscon Advance, with placebo in the treatment of gastro-oesophageal reflux disease. *Curr Med Res Opin*. 1999;15(3):152-9

[593] gaviscon.com/info.htm

[594] "Colonic fermentation of indigestible carbohydrates increases the rate of TLESRs [transient lower esophageal sphincter relaxations], the number of acid reflux episodes, and the symptoms of GERD." Piche et al. Colonic fermentation influences lower esophageal sphincter function in gastroesophageal reflux disease. *Gastroenterology*. 2003 Apr;124(4):894-902

[595] "A statistically highly significant growth-suppressive effect of the prostaglandin precursor gamma-linolenic acid (GLA) on MG63 human osteogenic sarcoma and oesophageal carcinoma cells in culture was found." Booyens et al. The effect of gamma-linolenic acid on the growth of human osteogenic sarcoma and oesophageal carcinoma cells in culture. *S Afr Med J*. 1984 Feb 18;65(7):240-2

- High incidence of thyroid disorders in systemic sclerosis (*J Clin Endocrinol Metab* 2013 Jul[596]): "Our study shows a high incidence of new cases of hypothyroidism and thyroid dysfunction in female sclerodermic patients. Female sclerodermic patients, who are at high risk (a borderline high [even if in the normal range] TSH value, anti-thyroperoxidase antibody positivity, and a hypoechoic and small thyroid) should have periodic thyroid function follow-up."
- Low DHEA sulphate serum levels in premenopausal systemic sclerosis (*Clin Exp Rheumatol* 2001 Jan[597]): "Mean serum levels of DHEAS in SSc women of childbearing age were significantly lower than in controls (0.87 +/- 0.85 microgram/ml versus 2.75 +/- 0.42 micrograms/ml; p < 0.001). On the contrary, no difference was found between postmenopausal women and controls. A reduction below the 95% confidence limits was found in 10 out of 11 patients of childbearing age and in 8 out of 29 postmenopausal women, respectively. In 5 out of 11 patients of childbearing age taking steroids for their SSc (< 10 mg/daily) DHEAS levels were significantly lower than in patients not taking steroids (p = 0.01). ... Our data show that, as in other autoimmune diseases, low serum DHEAS is a feature of premenopausal SSc patients. More extensive prospective studies are needed to define the exact role of DHEAS dysregulation in SSc."
- High prolactin and low dehydroepiandrosterone sulphate serum levels correlate with disease activity in patients with severe systemic sclerosis (*Br J Rheumatol.* 1997 Apr[598]): "Compared to SSc with <9 disease manifestations, patients with > or =9 disease manifestations had higher PRL (P = 0.044), higher soluble interleukin 2 receptor (sIL-2R, P = 0.004) and vascular cell adhesion molecule (sVCAM, P = 0.044), and lower DHEAS (P = 0.029). PRL (R(Rank) = 0.490, P = 0.003) and DHEAS (R(Rank) = -0.399, P = 0.013) were significantly correlated with the number of disease manifestations. The inverse correlation between PRL and DHEAS showed a trend (P = 0.059). PRL correlated with sIL-2R (R(Rank) = 0.553, P = 0.001) and sVCAM (R(Rank) = 0.520, P = 0.002). The number of disease manifestations and sIL-2R correlated significantly (R(Rank) = 0.463, P = 0.006)."
- Melatonin: **In an *in vitro* study with fibroblasts from normal and scleroderma patients, melatonin was shown to inhibit fibroblast proliferation**[599]; future trials may demonstrate that melatonin has an antifibrotic/antisclerodermatous benefit. Melatonin is a pineal hormone with well-known sleep-inducing and immunomodulatory properties, and it is commonly administered in doses of 1-40 mg in the evening, before bedtime. Its exceptional safety is well documented. In contrast to implementing treatment with high doses of 20-40 mg, starting with a relatively low dose (e.g., 1-5 mg) and increasing as tolerated is recommended. Melatonin (20 mg hs) appears to have cured two patients with drug-resistant sarcoidosis[600] and 3 mg provided immediate short-term benefit to a patient with multiple sclerosis.[601] Immunostimulatory anti-infective action of melatonin was demonstrated in a clinical trial wherein septic newborns administered 20 mg melatonin showed significantly increased survival over nontreated controls[602]; **given that scleroderma is associated with subclinical "infections", melatonin may provide therapeutic benefit by virtue of its anti-infective properties.**
- Estrogen (excess): **Research suggests that estrogen is immunodysregulatory and an important contributor to autoimmune disease**, perhaps explaining the greatly higher incidence of autoimmune diseases in women compared to men. So-called **"estrogen-replacement therapy" used in postmenopausal women increases the risk for lupus and scleroderma.**[603] Men with rheumatoid arthritis show an excess of estradiol and a decrease in DHEA, and the excess estrogen is proportional to the degree of inflammation.[604] Serum estradiol is commonly used to assess estrogen status; estrogens can also be

[596] Antonelli et al. Incidence of thyroid disorders in systemic sclerosis: results from a longitudinal follow-up. *J Clin Endocrinol Metab.* 2013 Jul;98(7):E1198-202

[597] La Montagna, et al. Dehydroepiandrosterone sulphate serum levels in systemic sclerosis. *Clin Exp Rheumatol.* 2001 Jan-Feb;19(1):21-6

[598] Straub et al. High prolactin and low dehydroepiandrosterone sulphate serum levels in patients with severe systemic sclerosis. *Br J Rheumatol.* 1997 Apr;36(4):426-32

[599] "These results suggest that MLT, at higher dosages, is a potent inhibitor of the proliferation of fibroblasts derived from the skin of healthy and SSc patients." Carossino AM, et al. Effect of melatonin on normal and sclerodermic skin fibroblast proliferation. *Clin Exp Rheumatol.* 1996 Sep-Oct;14(5):493-8.

[600] Cagnoni et al. Melatonin for treatment of chronic refractory sarcoidosis. *Lancet.* 1995 Nov 4;346(8984):1229-30

[601] "...administration of melatonin (3 mg, orally) at 2:00 p.m., when the patient experienced severe blurring of vision, resulted within 15 minutes in a dramatic improvement in visual acuity and in normalization of the visual evoked potential latency after stimulation of the left eye." Sandyk R. Diurnal variations in vision and relations to circadian melatonin secretion in multiple sclerosis. *Int J Neurosci.* 1995 Nov;83(1-2):1-6

[602] Gitto et al. Effects of melatonin treatment in septic newborns. *Pediatr Res.* 2001 Dec;50(6):756-60 pedresearch.org/cgi/content/full/50/6/756

[603] "These studies indicate that estrogen replacement therapy in postmenopausal women increases the risk of developing lupus, scleroderma, and Raynaud disease..." Mayes MD. Epidemiologic studies of environmental agents and systemic autoimmune diseases. *Environ Health Perspect.* 1999 Oct;107 Suppl 5:743-8

[604] "DHEAS and estrone concentrations were lower and estradiol was higher in patients compared with healthy controls. DHEAS differed between RF positive and RF negative patients. Estrone did not correlate with any disease variable, whereas estradiol correlated strongly and positively with all measured indices of inflammation." Tengstrand et al. Abnormal levels of serum dehydroepiandrosterone, estrone, and estradiol in men with rheumatoid arthritis: high correlation between serum estradiol and current degree of inflammation. *J Rheumatol.* 2003 Nov;30(11):2338-43

measured in 24-hour urine samples. Interventions to combat high estrogen levels may include any effective combination of the following:

- **Weight loss and weight optimization**: In overweight patients, weight loss is the means to attaining the goal of weight optimization; the task is not complete until the body mass index is normalized/optimized. Excess adiposity and obesity raise estrogen levels due to high levels of aromatase (the hormone that makes estrogen) in adipose tissue; weight optimization and loss of excess fat helps normalize hormone levels and reduce inflammation.
- **Avoidance of ethanol**: Estrogen production is stimulated by ethanol intake.
- **Consider surgical correction of varicocele in affected men**: Men with varicocele have higher estrogen levels due to temperature-induced alterations in enzyme function in the testes; surgical correction of the varicocele lowers estrogen levels.
- **"Anti-estrogen diet"**: Foods and supplements such as green tea, DIM, I3C, licorice, and a high-fiber "anti-estrogenic diet" can also be used; monitoring clinical status and serum estradiol will prove or disprove efficacy.
- **Anastrozole/Arimidex**: In our office, we commonly measure serum estradiol in men and administer the aromatase inhibitor anastrozole/Arimidex 1 mg (2-3 doses per week) to men whose estradiol level is greater than ~20 picogram/mL; we consider estradiol 10-24 picogram/mL to be optimal for a man.[605] Clinical studies using anastrozole/Arimidex in men have shown that aromatase blockade lowers estradiol and raises testosterone[606]; generally speaking, this is exactly the result that we want in patients with severe systemic autoimmunity. Frequency of dosing is based on serum and clinical response. Letrozole/Femara is another aromatase inhibitor, one that should generally be avoided due to its underreported and underappreciated ability to block androgen receptors.

- **XENOBIOTIC ACCUMULATION & DETOXIFICATION: Chemical avoidance, nutritional support for detoxification pathways, urine alkalinization** The clinical relevance and pathogenic mechanisms of xenobiotic accumulation are irrefutably well documented and described. Clinical assessments include history, physical examination, and laboratory assessment (using serum, whole blood, urine or—rarely yet accurately— fat biopsy), and response to treatment. Treatments include nutritional support for Phases 1 and 2 of detoxification (e.g., oxidation and conjugation) and excretion via bile and urine; for the latter, urinary alkalinization is generally recommended. Chemical toxins can be bound in the gut using activated charcoal, cholestyramine, or *Chlorella*—all of these three treatments have documented safety and effectiveness; clinically and empirically, phytochelatin (plant-derived peptides that bind toxic metals) concentrates appear safe and effective despite lack of conclusive published data supporting clinical use.
  - Xenobiotic immunotoxicity: Given that **antifibrillarin antibodies are specifically seen in patients with scleroderma**[607] and that **mercury exposure induces antifibrillarin autoimmunity in susceptible mice**[608], clinicians may be justified in searching for and treating evidence of mercury exposure in patients with autoimmunity in general and scleroderma in particular. Detailed history, dental examination for mercury-containing amalgams, and post-DMSA urine metal analysis are suggested.

---

[605] Male Hormone Modulation Therapy, Page 4 Of 7: lef.org/protocols/prtcl-130c.shtml Accessed October 30, 2005

[606] "These data demonstrate that aromatase inhibition increases serum bioavailable and total testosterone levels to the youthful normal range in older men with mild hypogonadism." Leder et al. Effects of aromatase inhibition in elderly men with low or borderline-low serum testosterone levels. *J Clin Endocrinol Metab.* 2004 Mar;89:1174-80

[607] "Since anti-fibrillarin antibodies are specific markers of scleroderma, the present animal model may be valuable for studies of the immunological aberrations which are likely to induce this autoimmune response." Hultman et al. Anti-fibrillarin autoantibodies in mercury-treated mice. *Clin Exp Immunol.* 1989 Dec;78(3):470-7

[608] Nielsen et al. Mercury-induced autoimmunity in mice. *Environ Health Perspect.* 2002 Oct;110 Sup 5:877-81 ehp.niehs.nih.gov/docs/2002/suppl-5/877-881nielsen/abstract.html

Vasculitic Diseases

Introduction:

Vasculitic diseases are largely considered to be mediated by deposition of circulating immune complexes (CIC) into/on the vascular endothelium, resulting in a localized activation of cell-mediated inflammation and activation of the complement cascade. From an allopathic perspective, these conditions are generally considered idiopathic and thus necessarily requiring long-term immunosuppression, in various forms.

From the perspective of logic and with a desire to deconstruct complex clinical phenomena, one can approach diseases that are mediated by immune complex deposition by deciphering the components into their elemental parts. For example, given that most vasculitic disease are mediated by endothelial deposition of immune complexes, and that immune complexes are chains of antigens and antibodies, one can then ask "*What are the major sources of antigens to which the immune system is exposed*?" and the correct answers are: "*Self, diet, microbes.*" One can then ponder the source of the antibodies, and ask if the presumed overproduction of antibodies is a *qualitative* problem or a *quantitative* problem, i.e., "Is the immune system 'wrong' in making antibodies to an antigen to which it is exposed [qualitative problem, error in action], *or* is the immune system 'correct' in its action but simply over-producing antibodies to perhaps otherwise benign antigens, whether these are self, diet, and/or microbes [quantitative problem, error in regulation]? From these questions, we arrive at answers other than crisis management and perpetual medicalization and pharmacologic immunosuppression; we arrive at the opportunity to reduce exposure to antigens from self (via antioxidant therapy to prevent molecular alteration of "self" structures), food (via food allergy avoidance and healing of intestinal hyperpermeability, and microbes (reducing dysbiosis and total microbial load [TML]) while also reducing the likely overzealous production of corresponding immunoglobulins via nutritional immunomodulation: induction of Treg for the reciprocal inhibition Th1, Th2, and Th17.

Description/pathophysiology, and clinical presentations:

- "Vasculitis" refers to a heterogeneous group of inflammatory disorders primarily affecting blood vessels, particularly the arteries and arterioles. Although the underlying pathomechanisms are similar among different disorders, these diseases differ in the location/size and number of affected vessels, and thus the clinical presentations and complications differ accordingly. Polymyalgia rheumatica / giant cell arteritis, ANCA vasculitis, and Behcet's disease are subtypes of vasculitis that are discussed in their respective chapters. As shown in the table at the right, several subtypes of vasculitis can be categorized based on the size/location of the vessel affected, and whether or not the cause of the vasculitis has been determined.
- Systemic manifestations are comparable to many other autoimmune disorders: insidious onset of fever, malaise, weight loss, generalized aches/pains.
- The autoimmune and immune-mediated pathogenesis of the vasculitides includes the following:
  - Antibody-antigen binding: *Example*: Goodpasture syndrome.
  - Delayed hypersensitivity reactions: Especially in lesions characterized with granulomas formation. *Example*: temporal arteritis.
  - Deposition of circulating immune complexes: The majority of the vasculitides are characterized by intra-arterial deposition of circulating immune complexes, which provoke activation of the complement cascade and leukocyte migration and activation for the resultant vascular damage, which often includes necrosis, fibrinous occlusion, and thrombosis. *Example*: acute arteritis in SLE.

Overview of common vasculopathic disorders

Primary vasculitides

Large vessel diseases
- Takayasu's arteritis
- Behcet's disease

Medium vessel diseases
- Polyarteritis nodosa
- Buerger's disease
- Giant cell arteritis

Small vessel diseases
Immune-complex mediated
- Cutaneous leukocystoclastic vasculitis
- Henoch-Schonlein purpura
- Cryoglobulinemia

ANCA-associated disorders
- ANCA vasculitis
- Microscopic polyangiitis: microscopic polyarteritis, leukocytoclastic vasculitis ; variants include allergic granulomatosis and angiitis also known as Churg-Strauss syndrome

Secondary vasculitides
- Infections, dysbiosis
- Other autoimmune disease
- Crohn's disease or ulcerative colitis
- Cancer
- Drug reactions
- Food allergies

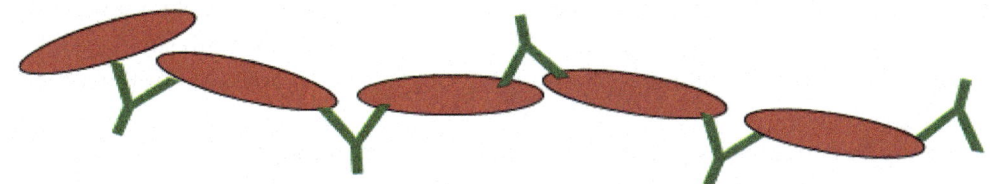

Schematized illustration of an immune complex: Immunoglobulins/antibodies—represented by the Y-shaped molecule—and antigens such as molecular fragments and peptides—represented by the ovoid molecule—form "chains" of alternating antigens-and-antibodies which in the circulation become lodged in the skin (dermatitis), vascular endothelium (vasculitis), kidney (nephritis), serosal surfaces (serositis), and synovial joints (arthritis). Readers must note that the location of the immune complex deposition is "innocent"; in immune complex disease, the location of the inflammation and complement activation (i.e., skin, vascular endothelium, kidney, synovial joints, serosa, and synovial joints) is simply a convenient molecular depot for the circulating immune complexes (CIC). Once deposited and following sufficient accumulation, immune complexes incite activation of the complement cascade and a local cell-mediated immune response, which causes local tissue inflammation and progressive destruction. Thus, for example, the joint or the skin or the kidney will be inflamed, but the actual problem of excess antigen exposure originated elsewhere, and the corresponding excess antibody production may have simply been a normal physiologic response to antigen exposure or may have been facilitated by a pro-inflammatory state and—synergistically yet distinctly—immunophenotypic imbalance.

Major differential diagnoses:

- Infection
- Cancer, especially leukemia, lymphoma, and multiple myeloma
- Autoimmunity: Concomitant or independent
- Trauma or abuse: Numerous unexplainable bruises/purpura may indicate abuse
- Adverse drug reaction
- Atherosclerosis, peripheral vascular disease, aneurysm

Clinical assessments:

- **History/subjective**:
    - See clinical presentations
- **Physical examination/objective**:
    - General physical examination with emphasis placed on symptomatic regions, circulatory examination, and dermal lesions
- **Laboratory assessments**:
    - Chemistry/metabolic panel: Assess for complications, especially renal insufficiency
    - Urinalysis: Assess for renal involvement
    - CRP/ESR: Generally elevated
    - Serum immune complexes: Most vasculopathies are due to immune complex deposition: Immune Complexes Reference Range (Raji cell technique, quantitative analysis):
        - Normal: ≤ 15.0 µg Eq/mL
        - Equivocal: 15.1-19.9 µg Eq/mL
        - Positive: ≥20.0 µg Eq/mL
    - Testing for multifocal dysbiosis: As discussed in Chapter 4
    - ANA
    - CH50: Complement levels may be low during exacerbations of immune complex mediated disease as the complement cascade is activated and complement proteins are consumed in the process, thus leading to a reduction in serum levels.
    - ANCA: Many of the vasculopathies, particularly those affecting the small vessels, are characterized by the presence of anti-neutrophilic cytoplasmic autoantibodies (ANCA), which can be segregated into two distinct subtypes: ❶ **cytoplasmic-ANCA** (C-ANCA, major antigen: proteinase 3) associated with Wegener granulomatosis, and ❷ **perinuclear-ANCA** (P-ANCA, major antigen: myeloperoxidase)

associated with microscopic polyangiitis, or Churg-Strauss syndrome. Clinicians should note that neither P-ANCA nor C-ANCA is specific for a particular diagnosis, and that 10% of patients with biopsy-proved small vessel vasculitis do not show either ANCA subtype. In patients with small vessel vasculitis, levels of ANCA correlate with disease severity, especially C-ANCA in patients with Wegener granulomatosis.

- **Imaging and biopsy**:
  - o Angiography is commonly used in the evaluation of vasculitic syndromes affecting larger vessels; Doppler ultrasound imaging can also be used.
  - o Biopsy of dermal lesions, superficial arteries, and other tissues can support the diagnosis
- **Establishing the diagnosis**:
  - o Based on clinical, laboratory, and biopsy/imaging findings

Major complications:

- Tissue necrosis: Complications depend on location of hypoxia and can include dermal necrosis, myocardial infarction, stroke, and intestinal infarction
- Infection secondary to immunosuppression
- Renal damage

Clinical management:

- Exacerbations are best managed pharmaceutically with appropriate immunosuppression. Patients may require hospital admission.
- An overview/survey of various inflammatory vascular disorders is presented on the following two pages.

> **Timely referral and comanagement**
> Generally speaking, patients with these conditions should be co-managed with a specialist (e.g., Internal Medicine, Rheumatology) because complications such as transverse myelitis and vascular occlusion leading to distal tissue ischemia—blindness, digital necrosis, mesenteric ischemia—can present quickly and require immediate immunosuppression in a hospital setting.

Overview of Vasculitic Diseases

Vasculitis subtype	Unique characteristics	Assessment and treatment considerations
Giant Cell (Temporal) Arteritis (outlined here and detailed in following subsection before the therapeutics section): Three subtypes exist along a continuum: ▪ Granulomatous vasculitis (2/3 of cases) ▪ Leukocytic infiltration of vessel wall ▪ Intimal fibrosis with lumenal narrowing	▪ GCA is the most common form of vasculitis; elevated ESR is classic ▪ Granulomatous inflammation of medium and small arteries, particularly of the head; involvement of the aorta (giant cell aortitis) is a rare variant ▪ Jaw claudication is highly suggestive ▪ Classic presentation includes headache and facial pain; 50% of patients have PMR: polymyalgia rheumatica	▪ Biopsy is the gold standard for diagnosis, although it may be normal in one-third of patients due to lesion focality/locality. ▪ **Patients can transition from asymptomatic to blind—vision loss due to occlusion of ophthalmic artery—within days; therefore, this condition is generally considered a medical emergency/urgency mandating immediate implementation of prednisone, typically starting at 60 mg/d or 1 mg/kg/d.**
Wegener granulomatosis (outlined here and detailed in following subsection before the therapeutics section): ▪ Affects small arteries all the way through to veins	▪ Granulomatous vasculitis affecting the upper respiratory tract	▪ Most patients have C-ANCA (cytoplasmic anti-proteinase 3 antibodies); small percentage of patients have P-ANCA (perinuclear anti-myeloperoxidase antibodies)

Overview of Vasculitic Diseases —*continued*

Vasculitis subtype	Unique characteristics	Assessment and treatment considerations
Takayasu arteritis: "pulseless disease" <ul><li>Leukocytic infiltration of the vasa vasorum followed by medial fibrosis and granulomatosis</li></ul>	<ul><li>Granulomatous vasculitis of large and medium arteries</li><li>Fibrous thickening of the aortic arch and occlusion of large arteries</li><li>Presentation typically includes neuro-ocular disturbances, reduced arm pulses; may include aortic valve insufficiency, and hypertension due to renal artery stenosis</li></ul>	<ul><li>Clinical assessment with aortogram</li></ul>
Polyarteritis nodosa (PAN): <ul><li>Immune-complex vasculitis</li><li>10-30% of patients have Hepatitis B—testing for hepatitis B is mandatory[609]</li><li>Generally fatal if untreated; estimated 5-year survival 13%</li><li>Without treatment, only 20% of patients survive 5 years; with treatment, survival improves to 60-90% at 5 years</li></ul>	<ul><li>Necrotizing vasculitic ischemia of numerous systems, thrombosis and ischemia at sites distal to lesion</li><li><u>Gut</u>: abdominal pain, nausea, vomiting exacerbated by eating (due to ischemia)</li><li><u>Nerves</u>: mononeuritis multiplex, vasculitic neuropathy; foot drop is most common manifestation</li><li><u>Skin</u>: dermal lesions include sharply-demarcated nodules, erythema, and ulceration; lesions are **non-palpable** and are in **different stages** of development</li><li><u>Kidneys</u>: hypertension due to renal involvement</li><li>*Pulmonary involvement is rare*</li><li>Can be categorized as *infectious and ANCA-negative* or *noninfectious and P-ANCA-positive*</li></ul>	<ul><li>Clinical presentation is varied depending on location of arterial lesion(s) and severity of systemic inflammation; typical population is young adults</li><li>Anemia, elevated ESR, leukocytosis</li><li>Autoantibodies commonly normal or low-positive</li><li>Diagnosis is established with biopsy or angiogram</li><li><u>Pharmacotherapy</u>: prednisone: 60 mg/d; pulsed methylprednisolone: 1 gram IV daily for 3 days; cyclophosphamide or other immunosuppressant drug</li><li>Plasmapheresis</li><li>Treatment of underlying hepatitis: must balance immunosuppression with anti-infective treatments</li></ul>
Mixed cryoglobulinemia: <ul><li>Many patients have underlying hepatitis C</li><li>Many patient respond to avoidance of foods to which they are allergic</li></ul>	<ul><li>Purpura</li><li>Peripheral neuropathy</li><li>Glomerulonephritis</li><li>Abdominal pain</li><li>Hepatitis</li><li>May have pulmonary involvement</li></ul>	<ul><li>Diagnosis is based on clinical picture and serology for cryoglobulins</li><li>Testing for and treatment of underlying hepatitis is essential</li><li>Immunosuppression may exacerbate viral replication</li><li>**Avoidance of food allergens is highly beneficial**[610,611]</li></ul>

[609] Tierney ML. McPhee SJ, Papadakis MA (eds). *Current Medical Diagnosis and Treatment 2006. 45th edition*. New York; Lange Medical Books: 2006, pages 844-850
[610] "CONCLUSION: These data show that an LAC diet decreases the amount of circulating immune complexes in MC and can modify certain signs and symptoms of the disease." Ferri C, Pietrogrande M, Cecchetti R, et al. Low-antigen-content diet in the treatment of patients with mixed cryoglobulinemia. *Am J Med*. 1989 Nov;87:519-24
[611] Pietrogrande M, Cefalo A, Nicora F, Marchesini D. Dietetic treatment of essential mixed cryoglobulinemia. *Ric Clin Lab*. 1986 Apr-Jun;16(2):413-6

Overview of Vasculitic Diseases—*continued*

Vasculitis subtype	Unique characteristics	Assessment and treatment considerations
Henoch-Schonlein purpura: IgA vasculitis Note: These terms are easy to intermix and confuse: ▪ **Buerger's disease:** thromboangiitis obliterans ▪ **Berger's disease:** IgA nephropathy	▪ Dermal purpura ▪ Abdominal pain ▪ Arthritis ▪ Hematuria associated with renal involvement; IgA nephropathy (Berger's disease) is generally considered a glomerular variant of Henoch-Schonlein purpura	▪ The disease is generally self-limiting to 1-6 weeks, subsiding without complications if renal involvement is mild ▪ Monitor renal function ▪ No generally effective allopathic treatment is known
Microscopic polyangiitis, microscopic polyarteritis, leukocytoclastic vasculitis: ▪ Affects small arterioles, capillaries, and venules; affected organs may include skin, lung, brain, heart, and kidneys (necrotizing glomerulonephritis) ▪ Associated with relatively acute events, such as infection (including dysbiosis), drug administration, cancer, or administration of foreign protein	▪ Necrotizing vasculitis ▪ Dermal lesions are differentiated from those of PAN because lesions of leukocytoclastic vasculitis are all at the **same stage of development** (due to acute event) and these lesions are **palpable due to acute inflammation** ▪ P-ANCA is generally positive ▪ Immune complexes are *not* characteristic of the vascular lesions	▪ P-ANCA is generally positive ▪ "In general, the disease responds well to removal of the offending agent."[612]
Churg-Strauss syndrome, allergic granulomatous angiitis: affects small arteries all the way through to veins; variant of leukocytoclastic vasculitis	▪ Eosinophilia with bronchial asthma and sinusitis; mimics allergic sinusitis and allergic asthma ▪ Pulmonary and splenic vessel involvement; granulomas ▪ Associated with Henoch-Schonlein purpura, essential mixed cryoglobulinemia, and vasculitis of malignancy	▪ ANCA, particularly P-ANCA ▪ Eosinophilia
Kawasaki disease; mucocutaneous lymph node syndrome: affects small-large arteries, classically the coronary arteries of children	▪ Arteritis of the coronary arteries in children ▪ Mucocutaneous lymph node syndrome	▪ Coronary angiography ▪ High-dose aspirin therapy

---

[612] Mitchell RN, et al. *Pocket Companion to Robbins and Cotran Pathologic Basis of Disease, 7th Edition*. Philadelphia; Saunders Elsevier: 2006, page 279

Brief Mention / Additional Emphasis

Polymyalgia Rheumatica (PMR),
Giant Cell Arteritis (GCA, previously Temporal Arteritis)

Introduction:
Giant cell arteritis (previously called temporal arteritis) and polymyalgia rheumatica are related conditions characterized histopathologically by inflammatory occlusion of small arteries and arterioles in the upper body: head, neck, shoulders. The possibility of arterial occlusion leading to blindness due to occlusion of the ophthalmic artery mandates early implementation of immunosuppressive prednisone (generally at 60mg/d or 1mg/kg/d). These patients must be co-managed with an Internal Medicine or Rheumatology specialist, while components of the Functional Inflammology protocol are appropriately applied.

Description/pathophysiology:
- This group of tightly related and largely synonymous disorders is described as "idiopathic" by medical textbooks.
- **Polymyalgia rheumatica (PMR)**: This disorder typically presents with painful inflammation of the shoulder/neck and hip muscles along with systemic manifestations of fever, malaise, and weight loss. When present in isolation (i.e., not with giant cell arteritis), it does not lead to blindness, and the condition responds to low-dose (10-20 mg) prednisone.
- **Giant Cell Arteritis (GCA)**: When treated allopathically, GCA requires higher daily doses (40-60 mg) of prednisone than PMR. GCA can result in rapid-onset blindness and therefore any evidence of ocular involvement in a patient with GCA must be treated as a medical emergency. Indeed, the diagnosis of GCA itself is considered urgent due to ability of blindness to occur rapidly and without warning. GCA was previously called temporal arteritis. Approximately 50% of patients with GCA have PMR.

Clinical presentations:
- Pain and stiffness in proximal muscle groups: shoulders, neck, and hips; weakness—if any—is secondary to pain, disuse atrophy, drug side-effect (e.g., "steroid myopathy"), or other concomitant disorder. Presentations are consistent with muscle/tissue ischemia due to the underlying panarteritis which results in vessel occlusion: head pain, jaw claudication, blindness.
- Generally presents after age 50 years. The later age of onset helps distinguish PMR from fibromyalgia, which generally affects young adult patients between the ages of 20-40 years.
- 2x more common in women than in men.
- Typical autoimmune systemic manifestations: fatigue, malaise, fever, anorexia, and weight loss.
- Patients may have high fever and chills with disease initiation and/or exacerbation.

Major differential diagnoses:
- Fibromyalgia: ESR is normal, age of onset is nearly always before 50 years.
- Dermatomyositis, polymyositis: These conditions cause muscle weakness, which is characteristically absent in patients with PMR. Muscle enzymes are elevated in patients with dermatomyositis/polymyositis but are normal in patients with PMR.
- Cancer, particularly multiple myeloma
- Hypothyroidism: Hypothyroidism can easily mimic PMR by producing an inflammatory myopathy that affects the shoulder muscles and which remits following normalization of thyroid status.
- Rheumatoid arthritis, SLE, vasculitis, or other autoimmune disorder
- Infection: WBC count is normal in GCA/PMR and is generally elevated in patients with severe infection.
- Cervical spondylosis: Normal ESR and no anemia

Clinical assessments:

- **History/subjective**:
  - See clinical presentations
- **Physical examination/objective**:
  - Palpate pulses for strength and symmetry:
    - Carotid artery in the anterior neck
    - Axillary/brachial in the axilla and inner arm, respectively
    - Radial pulse at the distal radius
    - Aorta in the abdomen
    - Femoral pulses in the groin
    - Dorsalis pedis and posterior tibial arteries at the ankle/foot
- **Laboratory assessments**:
  - <u>ESR</u>: Most patients will have a very high ESR > 50 mm/h.
  - <u>CBC</u>: Anemia is common.
  - <u>Chemistry/metabolic panel</u>: Hepatic alkaline phosphatase is elevated in 20% of patients.
  - <u>RF</u>: generally negative
  - <u>Muscle enzymes</u>: are almost always normal.
  - <u>Protein in urine, serum protein electrophoresis</u>: No evidence of proteinuria or monoclonal gammopathy, as seen in MM.
- **Imaging**:
  - Not generally indicated except when looking for complications or concomitant disease
- **Establishing the diagnosis**:
  - PMR is a clinical diagnosis based on 1) painful inflammation of the shoulder/neck and hip muscles along with 2) systemic manifestations of fever, malaise, and weight loss and 3) the absence of evidence supporting an alternate diagnosis.[613]
  - GCA is classically diagnosed following biopsy of the temporal artery.
  - Pattern recognition (proximal muscle pain with no other explanation) and evidence of inflammation in an elderly patient when other diseases have been ruled out.

Complications:

- **GCA can lead to blindness.**
- Dry cough is seen in some patients and may be the presenting complaint.
- Mononeuritis multiplex may cause (shoulder) paralysis.
- Aneurysms of the thoracic aorta are 17x more common in patients with GCA than the general population

Clinical management:

- Assess for temporal arteritis—educate patient about the significance of the onset of eye symptoms, headache, and jaw claudication.
- A few patients treated with prednisone will have permanent remission within 2 years.

<u>Treatments</u>: Use this section in association with previously mentioned assessments and interventions.

Drug treatments: This condition requires early implementation of prednisone immunosuppression; comanagement with a specialist—Internal Medicine or Rheumatology—is mandatory.

- <u>Prednisone</u>: 10-20 mg per day for PMR should result in "dramatic improvement" within 72 hours.[614] Prednisone dose for GCA is typically 60 mg per day at the start of treatment in order to prevent one of the most feared complications—blindness. Dose is tapered after clinical remission. Low-dose aspirin appears to reduce the risk of blindness and stroke in GCA patients.

---

[613] Tierney ML. McPhee SJ, Papadakis MA. *Current Medical Diagnosis and Treatment. 35th edition*. Stamford: Appleton and Lange, 1996 page 751. Tierney ML. McPhee SJ, Papadakis MA (eds). *Current Medical Diagnosis and Treatment 2006. 45th edition*. New York; Lange Medical Books: 2006, pages 486

[614] Tierney ML. McPhee SJ, Papadakis MA (eds). *Current Medical Diagnosis and Treatment 2006. 45th edition*. New York; Lange Medical Books: 2006, pages 487

Brief Mention / Additional Emphasis

ANCA-associated vasculitis, ANCA vasculitis (formerly known as Wegener's granulomatosis)

Introduction:
ANCA-associated vasculitis, formerly named Wegener's granulomatosis and here abbreviated as "ANCA vasculitis" avoid the unnecessary redundancy of the word "associated", is a granulomatous and vasculitic disease with a high mortality. Insight into the molecular basis of the condition—electrostatic haptenization of the *Staphylococcus aureus* enzyme acid phosphatase with endothelial cells—provides brilliant insight into the disease and its treatment. The possible role of other microbes, along with other factors such as immunophenotype imbalance should be intuitive by this time to readers who have read the other chapters.

Description/pathophysiology:

* This inflammatory condition generally begins with granulomatous involvement of the upper or lower respiratory tract and then progresses to systemic vasculitis and glomerulonephritis.
* Biopsy of nasopharyngeal/pulmonary/renal lesions reveals granulomatous/inflammatory tissue.
* Allopathic textbooks generally describe this condition as *idiopathic*, although the condition is increasingly associated with occult sinorespiratory dysbiosis with *Staphylococcus aureus*.[615,616] Additionally, *Klebsiella aerogenes, Haemophilus influenzae,* and *Bacillus subtilis* have been implicated.[617]
* Immune complexes contribute to pathophysiology

Clinical presentations:

* Twice as common in males as in females
* Sinorespiratory symptoms:
  * Mucosal ulcerations/friability, hemorrhagic rhinorrhea
  * Persistent sinusitis; increased incidence of otitis media
  * Cough, hemoptosis due to intraalveolar hemorrhage, pleuritis
* Renal complications are inevitable without effective/immunosuppressive treatment
* Typical autoimmune systemic manifestations: fatigue, malaise, low-grade fever, anorexia, and weight loss, polyarthritis.

> **Eponymic retractions: replacing of Reiter's syndrome with "reactive arthritis" and of Wegener's granulomatosus with "ANCA-associated vasculitis" or "granulomatosis with polyangiitis"**
>
> Reiter and Wegener were both actively involved in war crimes and support of Nazi atrocities during World War 2, and they have both been stripped of their eponymic recognition.
> * Reiter's syndrome is now "reactive arthrtitis",
> * Wegener's granulomatosus is now "ANCA-associated vasculitis" or "granulomatosis with polyangiitis"
>
> Scheinberg MA. Nazi past and changes in disease names: the Wegener's disease case. *Rev Bras Reumatol* 2012 Mar. Panush et al. Retraction of the suggestion to use the term "Reiter's syndrome" sixty-five years later. *Arthritis Rheum* 2007 Feb

Major differential diagnoses:

* Extramedullary plasmacytoma of multiple myeloma (typically occurs in the nasopharyngeal region)
* Sinus infection
* Lung cancer
* Tuberculosis
* Septicemia or septic arthritis
* Lymphoma
* Other systemic/inflammatory disorder such as lupus (ANA and low complement)
* Bacterial endocarditis

Clinical assessments:

* **History/subjective**: See clinical presentations.

---

[615] Brons RH, Bakker HI, Van Wijk RT, et al. Staphylococcal acid phosphatase binds to endothelial cells via charge interaction; a pathogenic role in Wegener's granulomatosis? *Clin Exp Immunol.* 2000 Mar;119(3):566-73 blackwell-synergy.com/doi/abs/10.1046/j.1365-2249.2000.01172.x
[616] Popa ER, et al. Staphylococcus aureus and Wegener's granulomatosis. *Arthritis Res.* 2002;4(2):77-9 arthritis-research.com/content/4/2/77
[617] George J, et al. Infections and Wegener's granulomatosis—a cause and effect relationship? *QJM.* 1997 May;90(5):367-73 qjmed.oxfordjournals.org/cgi/reprint/90/5/367

- **Physical examination/objective**:
  - Examination of oral and nasal mucosa
  - Pulmonary auscultation
  - Dermatologic screen for cutaneous vasculitis
- **Laboratory assessments**:
  - Urinalysis for assessment of renal status
  - Chemistry/metabolic panel for BUN and creatinine, etc.
  - Microbial assessments—reviewed in Chapters 1 and 4.
  - Nasal culture for *Staphylococcus aureus*[618] and other bacterial or fungal contaminants
  - Complement levels are normal or elevated
  - ESR/CRP is elevated
  - CBC may reveal leukocytosis and anemia
  - **ANA (antinuclear antibodies) are generally absent**
  - **ANCA are almost always present and strongly support the diagnosis of this condition. The finding of the more specific C-ANCA is 97% specific for the diagnosis of ANCA vasculitis.**[619] Interestingly, ANCA can also be induced by gastrointestinal parasitic infections.
- **Imaging**: Generally not required; only indicated as needed
- **Establishing the diagnosis**: Based on clinical, serologic, and biopsy findings.
  - Respiratory tract symptoms and mucosal lesions; biopsy of granulomas.
  - C-ANCA: Positive C-ANCA result can replace biopsy in a patient with a clinical picture of ANCA vasculitis.[620]

Complications:

- Severe anemia requiring blood transfusion
- Secondary bacterial infections on ulcerated mucosa
- Respiratory and renal failure
- Hypoxic complications due to vasculitis

Clinical management:

- Referral to internist/rheumatologist for additional treatment and defensive management as indicated. Unless you are a specialist, you need to have a specialist as part of the care team who can help you manage acute exacerbations which can occur with any autoimmune/inflammatory disease.

Therapeutic considerations: Medical treatment routinely includes the following:[621]

- Cyclophosphamide: 1-2 mg/kg/d PO or IV: associated with increased risk for cancer, particularly bladder cancer
- Prednisone: 1 mg/kg/d po; use the lowest dose possible
- Methotrexate: pulse treatment < 20-30 mg per week po
- **Antibiotic treatment: Bactrim / trimeth-sulfa 160/800 up to 480/2400 mg/d po**
- Blood transfusions for anemia
- **Assessment for multifocal dysbiosis: emphasis on gastrointestinal and sinorespiratory dysbiosis**
  - ***Staphylococcus aureus*: Produces an antigenic acid phosphatase which haptenizes with endothelial cells for the induction of autoimmune vasculitis in ANCA vasculitis.**[622]
    - Drugs: Antimicrobial treatment—typically with Bactrim—to eradicate *Staphylococcus aureus* results in clinical remission of the "autoimmune" disease, thus proving the microbe-rheumatic link.[623]
    - Herbs: Hyperforin from *Hypericum perforatum* shows in vitro effectiveness against *Staphylococcus aureus*.[624]

[618] Brons RH, Bakker HI, Van Wijk RT, et al. Staphylococcal acid phosphatase binds to endothelial cells via charge interaction; a pathogenic role in Wegener's granulomatosis? *Clin Exp Immunol*. 2000 Mar;119(3):566-73 blackwell-synergy.com/doi/abs/10.1046/j.1365-2249.2000.01172.x P

[619] Beers MH, Berkow R (eds). *The Merck Manual. Seventeenth Edition*. Whitehouse Station; Merck Research Laboratories 1999 Page 443

[620] Shojania K. Rheumatology: 2. What laboratory tests are needed? *CMAJ*. 2000 Apr 18;162(8):1157-63 cmaj.ca/cgi/content/full/162/8/1157

[621] Beers MH, Berkow R (eds). *Merck Manual. 17th Edition*. Whitehouse Station; Merck Research Laboratories 1999 Page 443

[622] Brons et al. Staphylococcal acid phosphatase binds to endothelial cells via charge interaction in Wegener's granulomatosis? *Clin Exp Immunol*. 2000 Mar;119(3):566-73

[623] Popa ER, et al. Staphylococcus aureus and Wegener's granulomatosis. *Arthritis Res*. 2002;4(2):77-9 arthritis-research.com/content/4/2/077

[624] Schempp et al. Antibacterial activity of hyperforin from St John's wort, against multiresistant Staphylococcus aureus and gram-positive bacteria. *Lancet*. 1999 Jun;353:2129

- Topical antiseptic: Intranasal 5% povidone iodine is highly effective against *Staphylococcus aureus*; Among 1,697 patients undergoing arthroplasty or spine fusion surgery, 5% povidone iodine proved better tolerated, safer, less expensive and more effective with greater compliance compared with intranasal mupirocin.[625]
    - *Entamoeba histolytica*: *Entamoeba histolytica* induces formation of antineutrophil cytoplasmic antibodies (ANCA).[626] Stool testing with a specialty laboratory is recommended.
    - Other microbes such as *Klebsiella aerogenes, Haemophilus influenzae* and *Bacillus subtilis*: These have also been implicated in ANCA vasculitis.[627]
- Vitamin D3 supplementation with physiologic doses and/or tailored to serum 25(OH)D levels: Since ANCA vasculitis is a *granulomatous* disease, caution and frequent monitoring must be employed when optimizing vitamin D status to avoid hypercalcemia; ANCA vasculitis can result in hypercalcemia mediated by elevated 1,25-dihydroxyvitamin D [1,25(OH)2D].[628] A reasonable clinical approach would be to start with testing of serum 25(OD)D, serum 1,25(OH)2D, and serum calcium (See Chapter 1 for review of Laboratory Association); thereafter, if necessary, start with a relatively low dose cholecalciferol 1,000-2,000 IU/d following the exclusion of hypercalcemia. Thereafter, serum calcium can be measured at 2 weeks, 4 weeks, 6 weeks, 8 weeks, and monthly/periodically thereafter.
- Assess for heavy metals, especially mercury: Exposure to mercury and lead is associated with increased risk of developing ANCA vasculitis.[629] Consider urine toxic metal assessment following 10-30 mg/kg DMSA as described in Chapter 4 and as described elsewhere for the assessment of heavy metals in patients with autism.[630]
- Proteolytic enzymes: ANCA vasculitis is mediated in large part by IgG and IgA immune complexes, which directly contribute to vasculitis and nephritis.[631] Polyenzyme supplementation has been used to ameliorate the pathophysiology induced by immune complexes in other conditions.[632]

- FOOD & NUTRITION: 5-part "supplemented Paleo-Mediterranean diet" (SPMD) The 5-part "supplemented Paleo-Mediterranean diet" (SPMD—reviewed in Chapter 4) consists of ❶ foundational plant-based low-carbohydrate diet of fruits, vegetables, nuts, seeds, berries and lean sources of protein, ❷ multivitamin and multimineral supplementation, ❸ physiologic doses of vitamin D3 (range 2,000-10,000 IU/d), ❹ combination fatty acid therapy (CFAT) with n3-ALA, n6-GLA, n3-EPA, n3-DHA, and phytochemical-rich olive oil which contains n9-oleate, and ❺ probiotics.
    - Avoidance of allergenic, inflammatory, and SIBO-promoting foods: Hypoallergenic diets can benefit patients with immune-complex-mediated diseases such as mixed cryoglobulinemia[633,634], hypersensitivity vasculitis[635], and leukocystoclastic vasculitis with arthritis.[636] Any patient may be allergic to any food, even if the food is generally considered a health-promoting food. Generally speaking, the most notorious allergens are wheat, citrus (especially juice due to the industrial use of fungal hemicellulases), cow's milk, eggs, peanuts, chocolate, and yeast-containing foods. According to a study

[625] London S. Nasal povidone-iodine cuts postop infections. *Internal Medicine News Digital Network* 2012 Nov. internalmedicinenews.com/news/conference-news/idweek-2012/single-article/nasal-povidone-iodine-cuts-postop-infections/fabb79e1a44f38b7318f060284a6018f.html

[626] George J, Levy Y, Kallenberg CG, Shoenfeld Y. Infections and Wegener's granulomatosis—a cause and effect relationship? *QJM*. 1997 May;90(5):367-73

[627] George J, Levy Y, Kallenberg CG, Shoenfeld Y. Infections and Wegener's granulomatosis—a cause and effect relationship? *QJM*. 1997 May;90(5):367-73

[628] "Furthermore, in view of this case and two other recently reported cases, we believe that Wegener's granulomatosis must be definitively added to the list of granulomatous diseases that are responsible for 1,25(OH)2D-mediated hypercalcemia." Bosch et al. Vitamin D metabolite-mediated hypercalcemia in Wegener's granulomatosis. *Mayo Clin Proc*. 1997 May;72(5):440-4

[629] "Results suggest that mercury and perhaps lead exposure were positively associated with WG as compared with either control group, although the number of patients exposed was small... CONCLUSION: We conclude that heavy metal exposure and a prior history of allergy may play a role in the etiopathogenesis of Wegener's granulomatosis." Albert D, et al. Wegener's granulomatosis: Possible role of environmental agents in its pathogenesis. *Arthritis Rheum*. 2004 Aug 15;51(4):656-64

[630] Bradstreet et al. A case-control study of mercury burden in children with autistic spectrum disorders. *J Am Physicians Surgeons* 2003; 8: 76-79 jpands.org/vol8no3/geier.pdf

[631] "RESULTS: Four of 11 biopsies taken at initial presentation and four of 21 biopsies taken at the onset of a relapse of WG showed IgG and/or IgA containing immune deposits in the subepidermal blood vessels. ...CONCLUSION: A substantial number of skin biopsies showed immune deposits during active disease. These results could support the hypothesis that immune complexes may trigger vasculitic lesions in WG." Brons et al. Detection of immune deposits in skin lesions of patients with Wegener's granulomatosis. *Ann Rheum Dis*. 2001 Dec;60(12):1097-102 ard.bmjjournals.com/cgi/content/full/60/12/1097

[632] Galebskaya et al. Human complement system state after wobenzyme intake. *Vestnik Moskovskogo Universiteta (Seriya 2: Khimiya)*. 2000:41(6 Suppl): 148-149 chem.msu.ru/eng/journals/vmgu/00add/148.pdf

[633] "CONCLUSION: These data show that an LAC diet decreases the amount of circulating immune complexes in MC and can modify certain signs and symptoms of the disease." Ferri C, Pietrogrande M, Cecchetti R, et al. Low-antigen-content diet in the treatment of patients with mixed cryoglobulinemia. *Am J Med*. 1989 Nov;87:519-24

[634] Pietrogrande M, Cefalo A, Nicora F, Marchesini D. Dietetic treatment of essential mixed cryoglobulinemia. *Ric Clin Lab*. 1986 Apr-Jun;16(2):413-6

[635] "In three cases the vasculitis relapsed following the introduction of food additives; in one case with the addition of potatoes and green vegetables (i.e., beans and green peas) and in the last case with the addition of eggs to the diet." Lunardi et al. Elimination diet in the treatment of selected patients with hypersensitivity vasculitis. *Clin Exp Rheumatol*. 1992 Mar-Apr;10(2):131-5

[636] "Described in this report are two children with severe vasculitis caused by specific foods." Businco et al. Severe food-induced vasculitis in two children. *Pediatr Allergy Immunol*. 2002 Feb;13(1):68-71

in patients with migraine, some patients will have to avoid as many as 10 specific foods in order to become symptom-free.[637] The severe wheat allergy *celiac disease* can present with inflammatory oligoarthritis[638,639], and celiac disease can also present as cryoglobulinemia and vasculitis[640], cutaneous leukocystoclastic vasculitis[641], including cerebral vasculitis[642] and pediatric stroke.[643] High glycemic foods suppress immune function[644,645] and thus promote the perpetuation of infection/dysbiosis. Delivery of a high carbohydrate load to the gastrointestinal lumen promotes bacterial overgrowth[646,647], which is inherently pro-inflammatory[648,649] and which promotes immune complex formation. Wheat consumption induces formation for immune complexes in virtually everyone (i.e., people who are "apparently healthy")[650], including as expected (but certainly not limited to) patients with dermatitis herpetiformis.[651] Vegetarian/vegan diets have a place in the treatment plan of all patients with autoimmune/inflammatory disorders[652,653]; this is also true for patients for whom long-term exclusive reliance on a meat-free vegetarian diet is either not appropriate or not appealing. No legitimate scientist or literate clinician doubts the antirheumatic power and anti-inflammatory advantages of vegetarian diets, whether used short-term or long term.[654] Patients who rely on the Paleo-Mediterranean Diet can use vegetarian meals, on a daily basis or for days at a time, for example, by having a daily vegetarian meal, or one week per month of vegetarianism. Of course, some (not all) patients can use a purely vegetarian diet long-term provided that nutritional needs (especially protein and cobalamin) are consistently met.

Wheat and circulating immune complexes in "healthy" disease-free persons: clinical findings relevant to vasculitis

- Circulating immune complexes (CICs) in blood are associated with autoimmune-diseases such as systemic lupus erythematosus, immune complex glomerulonephritis, rheumatoid arthritis and vasculitis. However, slightly increased serum concentrations of such CICs are sometimes also found in healthy individuals. The objective of the current study was to assess whether food antigens could play a role in the formation of CICs.

- MATERIAL AND METHODS: A total of **352 (265 F, 87 M), so far, healthy individuals** were tested for CICs containing C1q and immunoglobulin G (IgG) as well as for gliadin IgG antibodies using the ELISA technique.

- RESULTS: In our study, 15.3% (54/352) of the patients presented with elevated CIC concentrations (above 50 microg/ml) and 6.5% (23/352) of the study population were positive for gliadin IgG antibodies (above 20 U/ml). **CIC concentration levels were significantly higher in the group with elevated gliadin IgG antibodies** (CIC median: 49.0 microg/ml) **compared with the group with normal levels of gliadin IgG antibodies** (CIC median: 30.0 microg/ml; Mann-Whitney U-test, U=1992; p <0.001). …

- CONCLUSIONS: **The results of this study indicate that certain food antigens (e.g. gluten) could play a role in the formation of CICs.** …

Eisenmann et al. *Scand J Gastroenterol.* 2009

---

[637] Grant EC. Food allergies and migraine. *Lancet.* 1979 May 5;1(8123):966-9

[638] "We report six patients with coeliac disease in whom arthritis was prominent at diagnosis and who improved with dietary therapy. Joint pain preceded diagnosis by up to three years in five patients and 15 years in one patient." Bourne et al. Arthritis and coeliac disease. *Ann Rheum Dis.* 1985 Sep;44(9):592-8

[639] "A 15-year-old girl, with synovitis of the knees and ankles for 3 years before a diagnosis of gluten-sensitive enteropathy, is described." Pinals RS. Arthritis associated with gluten-sensitive enteropathy. *J Rheumatol.* 1986 Feb;13(1):201-4

[640] "Immunosuppressive treatment led to a normalization of transaminase levels and resolved the cryoglobulinaemic vasculitis. In addition, the patient exhibited low ferritin and iron levels, which led to the diagnosis of coeliac disease." Biecker E, Stieger M, Zimmermann A, Reichen J. Autoimmune hepatitis, cryoglobulinaemia and untreated coeliac disease: a case report. *Eur J Gastroenterol Hepatol.* 2003 Apr;15(4):423-7

[641] "A 38 year old female, with chronic uncontrolled coeliac disease, presented with the rare complication of cutaneous leucocytoclastic vasculitis." Meyers S, Dikman S, Spiera H, Schultz N, Janowitz HD. Cutaneous vasculitis complicating coeliac disease. *Gut.* 1981 Jan;22(1):61-4

[642] "A 51-year-old white man with celiac disease presented with seizures unresponsive to medical therapy." Rush PJ, Inman R, Bernstein M, Carlen P, Resch L. Isolated vasculitis of the central nervous system in a patient with celiac disease. *Am J Med.* 1986 Dec;81(6):1092-4

[643] "Because celiac disease is a potentially treatable cause of cerebral vasculopathy, serology-specifically antitissue transglutaminase antibodies-should be included in the evaluation for cryptogenic stroke in childhood, even in absence of typical gut symptoms." Goodwin et al. Celiac disease and childhood stroke. *Pediatr Neurol* 2004 Aug;31:139-42

[644] Sanchez A, Reeser JL, Lau HS, et al. Role of sugars in human neutrophilic phagocytosis. *Am J Clin Nutr.* 1973 Nov;26(11):1180-4

[645] "Postoperative infusion of carbohydrate solution leads to moderate fall in the serum concentration of inorganic phosphate. ... The hypophosphatemia was associated with significant reduction of neutrophil phagocytosis, intracellular killing, consumption of oxygen and generation of superoxide during phagocytosis." Rasmussen A, Segel E, Hessov I, Borregaard N. Reduced function of neutrophils during routine postoperative glucose infusion. *Acta Chir Scand.* 1988 Jul-Aug;154(7-8):429-33

[646] Ramakrishnan T, Stokes P. Beneficial effects of fasting and low carbohydrate diet in D-lactic acidosis associated with short-bowel syndrome. *JPEN J Parenter Enteral Nutr.* 1985 May-Jun;9(3):361-3

[647] Gottschall E. *Breaking the Vicious Cycle: Intestinal Health through Diet*. Kirkton Press; Rev edition (August 1, 1994)

[648] Lin HC. Small intestinal bacterial overgrowth: a framework for understanding irritable bowel syndrome. *JAMA.* 2004 Aug 18;292(7):852-8

[649] Lichtman et al. Reactivation of arthritis induced by small bowel bacterial overgrowth in rats: role of cytokines, bacteria, and bacterial polymers. *Infect Immun.* 1995 Jun;63(6):2295-301

[650] Eisenmann A, Murr C, Fuchs D, Ledochowski M. Gliadin IgG antibodies and circulating immune complexes. *Scand J Gastroenterol.* 2009;44(2):168-71

[651] Zone JJ, et al. Induction of IgA circulating immune complexes after wheat feeding in dermatitis herpetiformis patients. *J Invest Dermatol.* 1982 May;78(5):375-80

[652] "After four weeks at the health farm the diet group showed a significant improvement in number of tender joints, Ritchie's articular index, number of swollen joints, pain score, duration of morning stiffness, grip strength, erythrocyte sedimentation rate, C-reactive protein, white blood cell count, and a health assessment questionnaire score." Kjeldsen-Kragh J, et al. Controlled trial of fasting and one-year vegetarian diet in rheumatoid arthritis. *Lancet.* 1991 Oct 12;338(8772):899-902

[653] "During the vegan diet, both signs and symptoms returned in most patients, with the exception of some patients with psoriasis who experienced an improvement." Lithell H, et al. A fasting and vegetarian diet treatment trial on chronic inflammatory disorders. *Acta Derm Venereol.* 1983;63(5):397-403

[654] "For the patients who were randomised to the vegetarian diet there was a significant decrease in platelet count, leukocyte count, calprotectin, total IgG, IgM rheumatoid factor (RF), C3-activation products, and the complement components C3 and C4 after one month of treatment." Kjeldsen-Kragh et al. Changes in laboratory variables in rheumatoid arthritis patients during a trial of fasting and one-year vegetarian diet. *Scand J Rheumatol.* 1995;24(2):85-93

- <u>**INFECTIONS & DYSBIOSIS: ❶ antimicrobial treatments, ❷ immunorestoration, ❸ immunotolerance via Treg induction**</u> Essentially all autoimmune/rheumatic disorders are associated with microbial colonization and intolerance to same; the presence of persistent microbial colonization is *prima facie* evidence of immunosuppression. The eight areas of dysbiosis (multifocal) are: ❶ sinorespiratory, ❷ orodental, ❸ gastrointestinal, ❹ urogenital/genitourinary, ❺ parenchymal/tissue, ❻ microbial, ❼ dermal/cutaneous, and ❽ environmental. The following survey of the literature serves to remind clinicians of possible underlying infectious contributions to vasculitic diseases:

  o <u>Viral infections associated with Kawasaki disease</u> (*J Formos Med Assoc*. 2014 Mar[655]): "We enrolled 226 children with KD and 226 age- and sex-matched healthy children from February 2004 to March 2010. Throat and nasopharyngeal swabs were taken for both viral isolation and polymerase chain reaction (PCR) for various viruses. …Cases of KD had a significantly higher positive rate of viral isolation in comparison with the control group (7.5% vs. 2.2%, p = 0.02). Compared with the control group, cases of KD were more likely to have overall positive rates of viral PCR (50.4% vs. 16.4%, p < 0.001) and for various viruses including enterovirus (16.8% vs. 4.4%, p < 0.001), adenovirus (8.0% vs. 1.8%, p = 0.007), human rhinovirus (26.5% vs. 9.7%, p < 0.001), and coronavirus (7.1% vs. 0.9%, p = 0.003)."

  o <u>Ischemic retinal vasculitis in an 18-year-old man with chickenpox infection</u> (*Clin Ophthalmol*. 2014 Feb[656]): "We report a case of a healthy 18-year-old man who presented with unilateral ischemic retinal vasculitis 10 days after the onset of chickenpox. … Fundus imaging, optical coherence tomography, fundus fluorescence angiography, and electrophysiologic studies confirmed the diagnosis of retinal vasculitis, which led to generalized retinal ischemia."

  o <u>Antineutrophil cytoplasmic antibody-associated vasculitis associated with Epstein-Barr virus infection</u> (*Infection* 2014 Jun[657]): "Although a previous study indicated that there was a high positive rate of ANCA in the sera positive for IgM antibodies to EBV and EBV infection might trigger the relapse of AAV, this is the first case of incipient AAV associated with acute EBV infection. One possible explanation might be that EBV infection stimulated the production of ANCA."

  o <u>Cytomegalovirus-related necrotizing vasculitis mimicking Henoch-Schönlein syndrome</u> (*Clin Exp Rheumatol*. 2014 May[658]): "The causative role of viral infection was revealed by the presence of CMV DNA in patient's blood and positive IgG titer against the virus. … Our report suggests that CMV vasculitis is probably more frequent than previously thought, even in immunocompetent patients, with a protean clinical presentation, mimicking other types of vasculitides."

  o <u>Hepatitis C virus infection and its rheumatologic implications.</u> *Gastroenterol Hepatol* 2014 May[659]): "Symptoms of HCV infection and rheumatic diseases may be similar and include arthralgia, myalgia, arthritis, and vasculitis. …It is imperative to distinguish whether symptoms such as arthralgia, myalgia, and arthritis occur in patients with HCV infection due to primary chronic HCV infection or to a newly developed rheumatologic disease process."

  o <u>Vasculitis and anaphylactoid shock induced in mice by cell wall extract of the fungus Candida metapsilosis</u> (*Pol J Microbiol*. 2014[660]): "Our results show that intraperitoneal injection of cell wall extracts induced severe coronary arteritis, and intravenous injection induced acute anaphylactoid shock similar to extracts from Candida albicans (C. albicans)."

  o <u>Varicella zoster virus in the temporal artery of a patient with giant cell arteritis</u> (*J Neurol Sci*. 2013 Dec[661]): "We recently detected varicella zoster virus (VZV) in the temporal arteries (TA) of 5/24 patients with clinically suspect giant cell arteritis (GCA) whose TAs were GCA-negative pathologically; in those GCA-negative, VZV+TAs, virus antigen predominated in the arterial adventitia, but without medial necrosis and multinucleated giant cells. During our continuing search for VZV antigen in GCA-negative TAs, in

[655] Chang et al. Viral infections associated with Kawasaki disease. *J Formos Med Assoc*. 2014 Mar;113(3):148-54
[656] Poonyathalang et al. Ischemic retinal vasculitis in an 18-year-old man with chickenpox infection. *Clin Ophthalmol*. 2014 Feb 24;8:441-3
[657] Xu et al. Antineutrophil cytoplasmic antibody-associated vasculitis associated with Epstein-Barr virus infection: a case report and review of the literature. *Infection*. 2014 Jun;42(3):591-4
[658] D'Alessandro et al. Cytomegalovirus-related necrotising vasculitis mimicking Henoch-Schönlein syndrome. *Clin Exp Rheumatol*. 2014 May-Jun;32(3 Suppl 82):S73-5
[659] Sayiner et al. Hepatitis C virus infection and its rheumatologic implications. *Gastroenterol Hepatol* 2014 May;10(5):287-93
[660] Tada et al. Vasculitis and anaphylactoid shock induced in mice by cell wall extract of the fungus Candida metapsilosis. *Pol J Microbiol*. 2014;63(2):223-30
[661] Nagel et al. Varicella zoster virus in the temporal artery of a patient with giant cell arteritis. *J Neurol Sci*. 2013 Dec 15;335(1-2):228-30

the TA of one subject, we found abundant VZV antigen, as well as VZV DNA, in multiple regions (skip areas) of the TA spanning 350 [micrometers], as well as in skeletal muscle adjacent to the infected TA."

- o Is giant cell arteritis an infectious disease? (*Presse Med.* 2004 Nov[662]): "Simultaneous occurrence of peaks of GCA/PMR and respiratory infections have been observed in Denmark. Several viruses have been suspected as triggers and assessed by serological testing, PCR or immunostaining on temporal artery biopsies, or both techniques: the hepatitis B virus can be ruled out, as well as Herpes simplex 1 and 2, Herpes varicellae, Epstein-Barr virus and cytomegalovirus. Recent studies focused on parainfluenza virus, Parvovirus B19 and Chlamydia pneumoniae. Immunological studies suggest, at the origin of the inflammatory reaction leading to the typical pathological features of giant cell arteritis, the existence of a triggering antigen of unknown nature activating T-cells in the artery wall."

> **Endocrine imbalance in PMR/GCA**
>
> "Patients with PMR/GCA with new-onset active disease before steroid treatment have inappropriately normal cortisol levels regarding the ongoing inflammation, and significantly lower levels of DHEAS compared to the age- and sex-matched healthy control subjects. These data support the existence of a relative adrenal hypofunction in PMR and GCA."
>
> Narvaez et al. *J Rheumatol* 2006;33:1293-8

- **NUTRITIONAL IMMUNOMODULATION: Treg induction for modulation of Th-1/2/17 inflammation** Nutrients and therapeutic approaches that promote Treg or IL-10 induction and/or Th-17, IL-17 suppression include 1) mitochondrial optimization and mTOR suppression, 2) biotin, 3) vitamin E, 4) sodium avoidance, 5) transgenic/GMO food avoidance, 6) probiotics, 7) lipoic acid, 8) vitamin A, 9) inflammation reduction, 10) vitamin D, 11) fatty acid supplementation with GLA and n3, 12) infection and dysbiosis remediation, 13) green tea EGCG. Acronym: MiBESTPLAIDFIG.

- **DYSMETABOLISM & DYSFUNCTIONAL MITOCHONDRIA: MitoDys, ERS-UPR, AGE/RAGE, hyperglycemia and ceramide** The major clinical considerations in this section are mitochondrial dysfunction, endoplasmic reticulum stress, unfolded protein response, TLR activation, and the dysmetabolic effects of sustained hyperglycemia and hyperinsulinemia and resultant oxidative stress, inflammation, RAGE activation, and accumulation of AGE, palmitate and ceramide. The review of this information in Chapter 4 covered approximately 30 interventions relevant to dysmetabolism, mitochondrial dysfunction, ERS-UPR, etc; these will not be reviewed here except to mention those most commonly, easily, empirically, synergistically, and effectively used: 1) low-carbohydrate diet with 2) moderate exercise, 3) CoQ-10, 4) acetyl-carnitine with 5) lipoic acid, 6) NAC, 7) resveratrol, and 8) melatonin. See extensive review in Chapter 4.4.

- **STYLE OF LIVING (LIFESTYLE) & SPECIAL CONSIDERATIONS:** This is a buffet of mostly lifestyle-based interventions yet also including considerations such as somatic treatments, additional supplementation, and surgery. See Chapter 4, Section 5 for details.

- **ENDOCRINE IMBALANCE & OPTIMIZATION: Prolactin, Insulin, Estrogen, DHEA, Cortisol, Testosterone, Thyroid** Common hormonal imbalances seen among autoimmune/inflammatory patients are: ❶ *elevated* prolactin, ❷ *elevated* estrogen, ❸ *elevated* insulin, and ❹ *reduced* DHEA, ❺ *reduced* cortisol, and ❻ *reduced* testosterone; see Chapter 4 for discussion of these hormones and respective interventions. Thyroid evaluation (patient + labs) should be comprehensive, as discussed in Chapter 1, with a low threshold for empiric treatment.

  - o Orthoendocrinology and Dysendocrinism: Assess prolactin, cortisol, DHEA, free and total testosterone, serum estradiol, and thyroid status (e.g., TSH, T4, *and* anti-thyroid peroxidase antibodies). Correct as indicated (see Chapter 4). **Prolactin levels are typically elevated in patients with PMR and correlate with clinical symptomatology.**[663] Adrenal hypofunction in patients with PR/GCA is suggested by the relative insufficiencies of cortisol and DHEA.[664] **DHEA (insufficiency and supraphysiologic supplementation):** Patients with autoimmunity should be tested for DHEA insufficiency by

---

[662] Duhaut P, Bosshard S, Ducroix JP. Is giant cell arteritis an infectious disease? *Presse Med.* 2004 Nov 6;33(19 Pt 2):1403-8
[663] Straub RH, Georgi J, Helmke K, Vaith P, Lang B. In polymyalgia rheumatica serum prolactin is positively correlated with the number of typical symptoms but not with typical inflammatory markers. *Rheumatology* (Oxford). 2002 Apr;41(4):423-9 rheumatology.oxfordjournals.org/cgi/content/full/41/4/423
[664] "Patients with PMR/GCA with new-onset active disease before steroid treatment have inappropriately normal cortisol levels regarding the ongoing inflammation, and significantly lower levels of DHEAS compared to the age- and sex-matched healthy control subjects. These data support the existence of a relative adrenal hypofunction in PMR and GCA." Narvaez et al. Low serum levels of DHEAS in untreated polymyalgia rheumatica/giant cell arteritis. *J Rheumatol.* 2006 Jul;33(7):1293-8. Epub 2006 Jun 15

measurement of serum DHEA-sulfate; insufficiencies should generally be corrected except in cases of concomitant hormone-responsive cancer such as breast cancer or prostate cancer. The rationale for using high-dose DHEA in patients with autoimmune diseases is reviewed in Chapter 4.

- **XENOBIOTIC ACCUMULATION & DETOXIFICATION: Chemical avoidance, nutritional support for detoxification pathways, urine alkalinization** The clinical relevance and pathogenic mechanisms of xenobiotic accumulation are irrefutably well documented and described. Clinical assessments include history, physical examination, and laboratory assessment (using serum, whole blood, urine or—rarely yet accurately—fat biopsy), and response to treatment. Treatments include nutritional support for Phases 1 and 2 of detoxification (e.g., oxidation and conjugation) and excretion via bile and urine; for the latter, urinary alkalinization is generally recommended. Chemical toxins can be bound in the gut using activated charcoal, cholestyramine, or *Chlorella*—all of these three treatments have documented safety and effectiveness; clinically and empirically, phytochelatin (plant-derived peptides that bind toxic metals) concentrates appear safe and effective despite lack of conclusive published data supporting clinical use.

Spondyloarthropathies: Axial Inflammatory Conditions
Ankylosing spondylitis
Reactive arthritis (previously Reiter's syndrome)
Enteropathic spondyloarthropathy, enteropathic arthritis

Axial inflammation as yet another *pattern of inflammation*

Spinal/axial inflammatory conditions are patterns of inflammation with etiologic factors consistent with the pattern reviewed throughout this textbook and surveyed in Chapter 4; likewise therefore, similar therapeutic concepts are applicable. As always, pharmacologic immunosuppression may be urgently needed if a patient experiences exacerbation or inflammatory complication; however, routine "chronic" pharmacologic immunosuppression offers no hope of authentically curing the disease and correcting the underlying imbalances: it only suppresses manifestations of underlying physiologic imbalances.

<u>Description/pathophysiology</u>:

- Inflammatory arthropathies affecting the spine and sacroiliac joints are termed "spondyloarthropathies" and like other arthritic conditions are termed *seronegative* if not related to rheumatoid arthritis in general and RF positivity in particular. **The spondyloarthropathies differ in some aspects of their etiologies, affected populations, clinical presentations, and treatment; however—regarding etiology and treatment—the similarities far outnumber the differences.** Regarding clinical management, from both allopathic and integrative/naturopathic perspectives, the treatment and management of these different conditions is virtually identical, save for a few important nuances.

- Spondyloarthropathies and reactive arthritis differ from the classic pattern of other autoimmune conditions in that 1) most patients affected are male, 2) they are highly correlated with HLA-B27, 3) serologic evidence of autoimmunity is generally absent, 4) they are strongly associated with dysbiosis, infections, and/or occult or overt enteropathy.[665,666]

- Some variation exists in the conditions that are included under the heading of *Spondyloarthropathies*. Most medical textbooks include four disorders under the heading of spondyloarthropathies: 1) ankylosing spondylitis, 2) psoriatic arthritis, 3) reactive arthritis, and 4) enteropathic spondyloarthropathy (ES), while a few others go on to include 5) juvenile spondyloarthropathy, and 6) rheumatoid arthritis. Psoriatic arthritis (PsA) and rheumatoid arthritis (RA) are detailed in their own chapters in this book and therefore will not be discussed in great detail here.

- Although ankylosing spondylitis (AS) is the prototype of the spondyloarthropathies, reactive arthritis (ReA) is the best-known and most well accepted model for microbe-induced musculoskeletal autoimmunity. Despite nearly overwhelming research demonstrating that all of these conditions are triggered by exposure to microbes, major medical textbooks[667] still describe these conditions as *idiopathic*. Enteropathic arthritis and enteropathic spondyloarthropathy (EAES) demonstrate how gastrointestinal dysbiosis, hormonal imbalances, increased intestinal permeability ("leaky gut"), and non-musculoskeletal systemic inflammation can spill-over into peripheral and axial arthritis. As detailed in the separate chapter on psoriasis and psoriatic arthritis (PsA), PsA is clearly a microbe-triggered disease, and its similarity to AS suggests a common physiologic etiology. The common themes that weave these disorders together are 1) dysbiosis-induced musculoskeletal inflammation, 2) hormonal imbalances, and 3) increased intestinal/mucosal permeability—the latter is the most voluminous route of absorption of arthritogenic antigens, immunogens, and antimetabolites—see Chapter 4 for overview and details.

- All of these conditions are *systemic* inflammatory disorders that show clear evidence of immune-mediated tissue damage and are therefore worthy of being dubbed *autoimmune*. The systemic nature of these disorders carries important clinical implications because both doctor and patient need to be aware of *non-musculoskeletal*

---

[665] Colmegna I, Cuchacovich R, Espinoza LR. HLA-B27-associated reactive arthritis: pathogenetic and clinical considerations. *Clin Microbiol Rev.* 2004 Apr;17(2):348-69
[666] Ringrose JH. HLA-B27 associated spondyloarthropathy, an autoimmune disease based on crossreactivity between bacteria and HLA-B27? *Ann Rheum Dis.* 1999 Oct;:598-610
[667] Klippel JH (ed). *Primer on the rheumatic diseases. 11th edition.* Atlanta: Arthritis Foundation; 1997, page 181

complications. Non-musculoskeletal complications of these disorders include renal failure secondary to amyloidosis[668,669], cardiovascular and pulmonary complications, and increased risk of trauma, violent death, poisonings, and alcohol misuse.[670,671,672] Not surprisingly, the risk of pulmonary, renal, neurologic, ocular and cardiac complications is increased in patients with long-standing and severe disease.

Differentiating Characteristics of the Spondyloarthropathies

Condition	Etiopathogenesis	Unique presentation	Specific emphasis
Ankylosing spondylitis	• *Allopathic*: idiopathic • *Integrative*: dysbiosis is paramount	• Insidious onset of low-back pain in young patient • Ankylosis begins in lumbopelvis and can progress to thorax, neck, hips and knees. • 90% positive HLA-B27	• *Allopathic*: anti-inflammatory drugs • *Integrative*: Antidysbiosis and orthoendocrinology are treatment cornerstones
Reactive arthritis (previously Reiter's syndrome[673])	• *Allopathic*: infection-triggered arthritis • *Integrative*: infection-triggered arthritis in a patient with dietary and endocrinologic predispositions.	• Classically associated with a recent infection, particularly a genitourinary infection or gastrointestinal infection. • Inflammation is characteristically located at the low-back, iris, and heels. • 75% positive HLA-B27	• Antimicrobial treatment for acute and chronic infections is the mainstay of treatment although in a large percentage of patients the arthropathy continues despite apparent clearance of the primary infection.
Enteropathic spondylo-arthropathy, enteropathic arthritis	• *Allopathic*: idiopathic • *Integrative*: dysbiosis-triggered arthritis in a patient with dietary and endocrinologic predispositions	• Arthropathy of the peripheral joints and/or spine in a patient with inflammatory bowel disease—Crohn's disease or ulcerative colitis • 50% positive HLA-B27	• *Allopathic*: anti-inflammatory drugs • *Integrative*: Antidysbiosis and orthoendocrinology are treatment cornerstones • Treatment is similar to other treatments except with a greater focus on addressing the intestinal lesions

---

[668] "The mechanism of death in these patients was secondary amyloidosis in 19, cardiovascular complications in six, fracture of the spine in one, and it was not known in one patient. Excess deaths due to circulatory, gastrointestinal and renal diseases, and violence were also observed." Lehtinen K. Mortality and causes of death in 398 patients admitted to hospital with ankylosing spondylitis. *Ann Rheum Dis*. 1993 Mar;52(3):174-6

[669] "During an outbreak of Yersinia pseudotuberculosis III, one of two HLA-B27 positive brothers developed reactive arthritis (ReA), mild at first, but later severely destructive and ultimately fatal. The reactivation of ReA was possibly triggered by an oral polio vaccine. The cause of death was severe secondary amyloidosis." Yli-Kerttula T, Mottonen T, Toivanen A. Different course of reactive arthritis in two HLA-B27 positive brothers with fatal outcome in one. *J Rheumatol*. 1997 Oct;24(10):2047-50

[670] "A marked sex-associated effect was noted among deaths caused by injuries/poisoning, since 6 of the deaths occurred in men and only 1 was in a woman. CONCLUSION: Patients with PsA are at an increased risk of death compared with the general population." Gladman DD, Farewell VT, Wong K, Husted J.Mortality studies in psoriatic arthritis: results from a single outpatient center. II. Prognostic indicators for death. *Arthritis Rheum*. 1998 Jun;41(6):1103-10

[671] "The 4 leading causes of death were diseases of the circulatory (36.2%) or respiratory (21.3%) system, malignant neoplasms (17.0%), and injuries/poisoning (14.9%). The SMR for the female cohort was 1.59, and for the men, it was 1.65, indicating a 59% and 65% increase in the death rate, respectively. Deaths due to respiratory causes were particularly increased in these patients." Wong K, Gladman DD, Husted J, Long JA, Farewell VT. Mortality studies in psoriatic arthritis: results from a single outpatient clinic. I. Causes and risk of death. *Arthritis Rheum*. 1997 Oct;40(10):1868-72

[672] "Subjects with ankylosing spondylitis (AS) have an increased incidence of deaths from accidents and violence, which is due in part, but perhaps not entirely, to the vulnerability of the affected spine to fractures... Uncontrolled use of alcohol is an important determinant in the surplus of deaths from accidents and violence in Finnish patients with AS." Myllykangas-Luosujarvi et al. Increased incidence of alcohol-related deaths from accidents and violence in subjects with ankylosing spondylitis. *Br J Rheumatol*. 1998 Jun;37(6):688-90

[673] The term "Reiter's syndrome" has fallen out of favor due to the increasing acknowledgement that Dr Hans Reiter was affiliated with Nazi atrocities during World War II. See the following for additional information: "During World War II, Reiter, a physician leader of the Nazi party, authorized medical experiments on concentration camp prisoners." Lu DW, Katz KA. Declining use of the eponym "Reiter's syndrome" in the medical literature, 1998-2003. *J Am Acad Dermatol*. 2005 Oct;53(4):720-3 and "There is more than ample evidence that Hans Reiter, whose name has been eponymously linked to a rheumatologic syndrome, was a Nazi war criminal. He was responsible for heinous atrocities that violated the precepts of humanity, ethics, and professionalism." Panush et al. The tainted legacy of Hans Reiter. *Semin Arthritis Rheum*. 2003 Feb;32(4):231-6

Condition	Etiopathogenesis	Unique presentation	Specific emphasis
Juvenile spondylo-arthropathy	• *Allopathic*: idiopathic • *Integrative*: dysbiosis[674]	• Generally occurs in boys aged 8-18 years • Peripheral arthritis (90%) is more common than spondylitis (50%)	• *Allopathic*: anti-inflammatory drugs • *Integrative*: Antidysbiosis
Psoriatic arthritis	• *Allopathic*: idiopathic • *Integrative*: Food allergies and dysbiosis are paramount	• Arthropathy of the peripheral joints and/or spine in a patient with psoriasis • 50% positive HLA-B27	• *Allopathic*: anti-inflammatory drugs • *Integrative*: Antidysbiosis and orthoendocrinology are treatment cornerstones
Rheumatoid arthritis	• *Allopathic*: idiopathic • *Integrative*: dysbiosis-triggered arthritis in a patient with dietary and endocrinologic predisposition	• Inflammatory peripheral arthropathy generally precedes axial joints • Sacroiliac joints are generally spared • RF is frequently positive	• *Allopathic*: anti-inflammatory drugs • *Integrative*: Antidysbiosis and orthoendocrinology are treatment cornerstones

Clinical presentations:

- Musculoskeletal:
  - <u>Pain and limited motion in the low-back sacroiliac joints</u>: This is an aspect of all of the spondyloarthropathies, especially AS and ReA. Back pain is generally worse in the morning and alleviated by motion, including passive motion such as spinal manipulation.
  - <u>Thoracic spine pain and decreased rib expansion/excursion</u>: Although it typically begins in the lumbar spine and sacroiliac joints, AS commonly progresses to involve the thoracic spine and rib cage. Decreased mobility of the ribs limit respiration, and thus respirometry is used in the clinical assessment of patients with AS.
  - <u>Neck pain</u>: particularly common in RA and AS, two conditions associated with spontaneous atlantoaxial instability
  - <u>Atlantoaxial instability</u>: May be the presenting manifestation of AS[675] and is a common long-term complication of RA. Particularly in patients with neck pain and/or long-standing inflammation, cervical radiographs including APOM and measurement of the atlantodental interval should be performed before the clinical use of forceful cervical spine manipulation as well as esophageal/tracheal endoscopy.
  - <u>Enthesopathies</u>: Inflammation at the site of ligament insertion into bone—classically seen at the insertion of the Achilles' tendon at the calcaneus—is a characteristic finding and complaint in patients with ReA.
  - <u>Non-erosive asymmetrical peripheral arthritis</u>: 50% of patients with AS experience a temporary peripheral arthritis, while in 25% of patients the peripheral arthritis is permanent.
- Pulmonary: Pleurisy (painful inflammation of the pleural lining of the internal thoracic cavity) may be a complication of nearly all rheumatic/inflammatory disorders. Patients with AS may develop pulmonary fibrosis.
- Cardiac: "Spondylitic heart disease" is seen in patients with AS and commonly includes atrioventricular conduction defects and aortic regurgitation.[676]

---

[674] "Our findings provide clear evidence of ReA diagnosis following an acute M. pneumoniae infection that in four patients progressed to chronic jSpA. Our results suggest that detecting M. pneumoniae-specific antibodies in serological screening of jSpA patients might be useful." Harjacek et al. Juvenile spondyloarthropathies associated with Mycoplasma pneumoniae infection. *Clin Rheumatol*. 2006 Jan 4;:1-6

[675] Thompson et al. Spontaneous atlantoaxial subluxation as a presenting manifestation of juvenile ankylosing spondylitis. A case report. *Spine* 1982 Jan-Feb;7(1):78-9

[676] Tierney ML. McPhee SJ, Papadakis MA (eds). *Current Medical Diagnosis and Treatment 2006. 45th edition*. New York; Lange Medical Books: 2006, pages 851-855

- <u>GI tract</u>: Oral ulcers, intestinal inflammation, increased intestinal permeability
- <u>Skin/mucosal lesions</u>: Dermal lesions are particularly common in patients with ReA and PsA. Psoriatic lesions are typically well-demarcated erythematous patches with white/silvery scales. Dermal lesions of ReA can include pustular lesions on the feet and hands (palmoplantar pustulosis) in addition to genital lesions in patients with sexually transmitted diseases.
- <u>Renal complications</u>: These can be seen in nearly all rheumatic disorders, either as a result of the systemic inflammation (particularly immune complexes), amyloidosis, or as a result of NSAIDs or other pharmaceutical drugs.
- <u>Neurological complications</u>: Cerebral necrosis, corticosteroid psychosis, and transverse myelitis may occur. Atlantoaxial subluxation can present with myelopathic signs.
- <u>Ocular complications</u>: Anterior uveitis is seen in ~25% of patients with AS and is a characteristic finding in patients with ReA.

Major differential diagnoses:

- Initial evaluation of patients with spondyloarthropathy must include consideration of numerous differential diagnoses which may mimic or co-exist with inflammatory spondyloarthropathy. See table of *Differential Diagnoses* at the end of this chapter, as well as *algorithm for patient assessment and management*. Useful categories during the evaluation of low-back pain include the following:
  - o <u>Serious organic diseases requiring immediate attention</u>: Metastatic disease, viscerosomatic referral, osteomyelitis/discitis, aortic aneurysm.
  - o <u>Serious musculoskeletal disorders requiring immediate attention</u>: Recent fracture (pathologic fracture, osteoporosis, compression fracture, fall from a height, major motor vehicle accident), cauda equina syndrome, and severe radiculopathy (i.e., severe pain or progressive muscular deficits).
  - o <u>Rheumatologic disorders affecting the low back and pelvis</u>: Ankylosing spondylitis, reactive arthritis, enteropathic spondyloarthropathy, psoriatic arthritis, rheumatoid arthritis, and fibromyalgia.
  - o <u>Psychogenic</u>: Emotional overlay, symptom amplification, secondary gain, depression.
  - o <u>Benign musculoskeletal disorders requiring conservative treatment and monitoring</u>: Muscle spasm, facet irritation, disc injuries causing radiculitis or radiculopathy, self-limiting inflammation due to injury.
  - o <u>Functional, metabolic, allergic or nutritional causes of low-back pain</u>: Food allergies, obesity leading to a systemic inflammatory state as well as biomechanical stress on the lumbar spine, vitamin D deficiency[677], acidifying diet[678] (i.e., the Standard American Diet[679,680]).

---

[677] Al Faraj S, Al Mutairi K. Vitamin D deficiency and chronic low back pain in Saudi Arabia. *Spine*. 2003 Jan 15;28(2):177-9
[678] "The results show that a disturbed acid-base balance may contribute to the symptoms of low back pain. The simple and safe addition of an alkaline multimineral preparate was able to reduce the pain symptoms in these patients with chronic low back pain." Vormann et al. Supplementation with alkaline minerals reduces symptoms in patients with chronic low back pain. *J Trace Elem Med Biol*. 2001;15(2-3):179-83
[679] Seaman DR. The diet-induced proinflammatory state: a cause of chronic pain and other degenerative diseases? *J Manipulative Physiol Ther*. 2002 Mar-Apr;25(3):168-79
[680] Cordain L. *The Paleo Diet*. John Wiley & Sons Inc., New York 2002

Low Back Pain: Differential Diagnostic Considerations

	DDX Category	Examples:
V	Vascular	Aortic aneurysm
	Visceral referral	Pancreatic disease/cancer
I	Infectious	Ankylosing spondylitis, reactive arthritis
	Inflammatory	Rheumatoid arthritis
	Immunologic	Psoriatic arthritis
		Enteropathic spondyloarthropathy
		Lymphoma, leukemia
		Bone/ tissue infections
		Gastrointestinal disease
		Kidney infection
		Psoriatic arthritis
		Herpes zoster
N	Neurologic	Metastatic disease, primary bone tumors, multiple myeloma
	Nutritional	Herpes zoster
	New growth: neoplasia, pregnancy	Cauda equina syndrome
D	Deficiency	Degenerative joint/spine disease
	Degenerative	Congenital malformations of bones/ viscera
	Developmental	Scoliosis
		Postural syndromes
		Disc herniation
		Varicose veins in the leg mimicking sciatica
I	Iatrogenic (drug related)	Anticoagulants predispose to epidural or spinal cord bleeding[681]
	Intoxication	Prednisone use promotes osteoporosis and spinal fractures
	Idiosyncratic	Excess alcohol consumption[682]
C	Congenital	Congenital malformations of bones: hemivertebrae, leg length inequality, etc.
A	Allergy	Ankylosing spondylitis
	Autoimmune	Fractures, injuries
	Abuse	
T	Trauma	Fractures: injuries to vertebrae, ribs, muscles
E	Endocrine	Diabetes mellitus
	Exposure	
S	"Subluxation", somatic dysfunction	Segmental dysfunction of lumbar spine and pelvis
	Structural	Muscle tension
	Stress	
	Secondary gain	
M	Mental	Anxiety
	Malpractice	Depression
	Mental disorder	Endometriosis, hematocolpos[683]
	Malignancy	Ovarian tumor
	Metabolic disease	Nephrolithiasis
	Menstrual	Metastasis to spine
	Myofascial	Myofascial trigger points in quadratus lumborum, piriformis, iliacus, psoas

---

[681] Souza TA. *Differential Diagnosis for the Chiropractor: Protocols and Algorithms*. Gaithersburg: Aspen Publications. 1997 page 110
[682] "Alcohol abuse was significantly more frequent among the male low back patients." Sandstrom J, Andersson GB, Wallerstedt S. The role of alcohol abuse in working disability in patients with low back pain. *Scand J Rehabil Med*. 1984;16(4):147-9
[683] London NJ, Sefton GK. Hematocolpos. An unusual cause of sciatica in an adolescent girl. *Spine*. 1996 Jun 1;21(11):1381-2

Specific differential diagnoses

- Mechanical low back pain, traumatic low back pain, spinal strain/sprain
- Cauda equina syndrome
- Vitamin D deficiency: Vitamin D deficiency causes inflammation and low-back pain. Measure 25(OH)vitamin D in serum or supplement with 4,000-10,000 IU daily for at least three months[684] unless contraindicated by drugs (e.g., hydrochlorothiazide) or hypercalcemic condition (e.g., sarcoidosis, cancer, or hyperparathyroidism, etc.).[685]
- Spinal degeneration, degenerative arthritis of the spine
- Spinal fracture: Patients with AS may experience fracture following trivial "injury" such as rolling over in bed: **"Fracture should be suspected whenever a [AS] patient complains of new back pain."**[686]
- Osteitis condensans ilii
- Cancer, malignant disease
- Vertebral osteomyelitis, infectious discitis
- Developmental/congenital sacralization of the lumbar vertebrae
- Other autoimmune disease
- Lung disease: Asthma, COPD, bronchitis, tuberculosis
- Iron overload: Hemochromatosis may resemble ankylosing spondylitis clinically and radiographically.[687]
- Fibromyalgia: ESR, CRP, thyroid tests, ANA and most other 'basic' tests are normal; assess and treat for bacterial overgrowth of the small bowel.[688]
- Diffuse idiopathic skeletal hyperostosis (DISH): DISH generally affects the longitudinal ligaments of the spine rather than the intervertebral discs. Cervical involvement generally precedes that of the lumbar spine, and the condition is strongly associated with diabetes mellitus.

Clinical assessments:

- **History/subjective**: See clinical presentations
  - **Typical presentation is that of dull achy pain in the low-back—worse in the morning and improving as the day progresses and/or with activity.**
  - **Systemic manifestations may or may not be present in the early stages of disease.**
- **Physical examination/objective**:
  - ROM, neurologic assessments; orthopedic assessments
  - Specialty examinations may be indicated:
    - Eye exam: For retinal and anterior chamber abnormalities; external exam for scleritis
    - Genital examination and/or assessment for UTI and STDs: Indicated in patients with ReA due to high association with sexually transmitted diseases. Urethral swab for culture and DNA probes are commonly indicated.
    - Cardiopulmonary assessment: Common considerations include auscultation, measurement of thoracic excursion, and spirometry. Chest radiographs may be indicated.
    - Neurologic examination: A screening neurologic examination should be performed as part of the initial assessment of all patients and more detailed examinations are carried out when indicated.
    - Schober test: Draw a line over the spinous process of L5, then mark a line 10 cm above and 5 cm below; with lumbar flexion, the total distance should increase from 15 cm to 20 cm—less than 5 cm excursion indicates spinal rigidity, consistent with AS.
    - Occiput-to-wall distance: This assessment can be used to quantify progression/regression of cervical flexion in patients with AS.
    - Chest expansion: Use tape measure around lower thorax; measure chest circumference before and after inhalation; use along with spirometry to monitor thoracic stiffness in patients with AS.

---

[684] Al Faraj S, Al Mutairi K. Vitamin D deficiency and chronic low back pain in Saudi Arabia. *Spine*. 2003 Jan 15;28(2):177-9
[685] Vasquez et al. The clinical importance of vitamin D: a paradigm shift with implications for all healthcare providers. *Altern Ther Health Med*. 2004 Sep-Oct;10(5):28-36
[686] Harley JB, Scofield RH. The spectrum of ankylosing spondylitis. *Hosp Pract (Off Ed)* 1995 Jul 15;30(7):37-43, 46
[687] Bywaters EGL, Hamilton EBD, Williams R. The spine in idiopathic hemochromatosis. *Ann Rheum Dis* 1971; 30: 453-65
[688] Pimentel M, et al. A link between irritable bowel syndrome and fibromyalgia may be related to findings on lactulose breath testing. *Ann Rheum Dis*. 2004 Apr;63:450-2

- **Laboratory assessments:**
  - ESR or CRP: These are generally elevated, and neither test is superior to the other in the assessment of patients with AS. One study[689] used a unique approach to differentiate active disease from inactive disease in patients with AS; they added ESR value (mm/h) and CRP value (mg/L) and classified patients as having active inflammatory disease if the total was greater than thirty (30).
  - Rheumatoid factor (RF): Characteristically **negative** *by definition* in patients with sero**negative** spondyloarthropathies. Positivity suggests rheumatoid spondylitis or concomitant RA with another spondyloarthropathy.

  > **Microorganisms clinically or molecularly associated with induction of seronegative spondyloarthropathy, ankylosing spondylitis, and reactive arthritis**
  > - *Campylobacter* spp
  > - *Chlamydia trachomatis*
  > - *Citrobacter freundii*
  > - *E. coli*
  > - *Giardia lamblia*
  > - *Helicobacter pylori*
  > - *Klebsiella pneumoniae*
  > - *Mycoplasma* spp
  > - *Proteus mirabilis*
  > - *Salmonella typhimurium*
  > - *Shigella flexneri*
  > - *Shigella sonnei*
  > - *Staphylococcus aureus*
  > - *Streptococcus pyogenes*
  > - *Ureaplasma* spp
  > - *Yersinia enterocolitica*

  - CBC: Look for evidence of true *infection* (in contrast to *dysbiosis*); also assess for anemia, which may be secondary to renal failure, NSAID gastropathy, chronic inflammation, or nutritional inadequacy.
  - Comprehensive metabolic panel: Assess as indicated for complications and concomitant disease.
  - Comprehensive stool analysis with comprehensive parasitology: **All patients with AS, RA, and PsA have gastrointestinal dysbiosis until proven otherwise.** Use of comprehensive stool tests should be the standard of care for all patients with AS, RA, PsA, and of course those with enteropathic spondyloarthropathy. Patients with ReA due to gastroenteritis or those whose primary infection has not been identified/eliminated are also obvious candidates for stool testing; the most commonly implicated microbes are *Salmonella*, *Shigella*, and *Yersinia*. Regarding the etiopathogenesis of AS, the most commonly implicated microbes are *Klebsiella* and *E. coli*. However, it is more accurate to see that microbes incite autoimmunity/inflammation by numerous mechanisms and that exposure to numerous microbes—each one of which *in isolation* may be innocuous—in combination leads to additive and synergistic proinflammatory effects, as reviewed in Chapter 4 in the section on multifocal dysbiosis and elsewhere in a recent publication by the current author.[690]
  - Serologic and genital tests for sexually transmitted diseases: These tests are particularly indicated in patients with ReA due to the frequent association of this disorder with genitourinary infections, particularly those caused by *Chlamydia*. Numerous articles have shown that patients with long-term idiopathic oligoarthritis harbor "silent infections"—otherwise known as dysbiosis—in the genitourinary and gastrointestinal tracts; the most commonly identified organisms are *Chlamydia trachomatis*, *Yersinia*, *Salmonella*, *Mycoplasma*, and *Ureaplasma*.[691,692]
  - Serum vitamin D: Measure 25(OH)vitamin D in all patients and/or begin empiric treatment with physiologic doses of vitamin D3. Emulsified cholecalciferol is particularly efficacious in older patients and those with malabsorption due to enteropathy.[693] According to research by Falkenbach et al[694], **"Patients with ankylosing spondylitis may have extremely low levels of 25(OH)D."** Vitamin D deficiency appears common in patients with low-back pain[695], limb pain[696], chronic persistent

[689] Maki-Ikola O, Lehtinen K, Nissila M, Granfors K. IgM, IgA and IgG class serum antibodies against Klebsiella pneumoniae and Escherichia coli lipopolysaccharides in patients with ankylosing spondylitis. *Br J Rheumatol* 1994 Nov;33(11):1025-9

[690] Vasquez A. Nutritional Botanical Treatments against "Silent Infections" and Gastrointestinal Dysbiosis. *Nutritional Perspectives* 2006; Jan ichnfm.academia.edu/AlexVasquez

[691] "Urogenital swab cultures showed a microbial infection in 44% of the patients with oligoarthritis (15% Chlamydia, 14% Mycoplasma, 28% Ureaplasma), whereas in the control group only 26% had a positive result (4% Chlamydia, 7% Mycoplasma, 21% Ureaplasma)." Erlacher et al. Reactive arthritis: urogenital swab culture is the only useful diagnostic method for the detection of the arthritogenic infection in extra-articularly asymptomatic patients with undifferentiated oligoarthritis. *Br J Rheumatol.* 1995 Sep;34(9):838-42

[692] Fendler C, et al. Frequency of triggering bacteria in patients with reactive arthritis and undifferentiated oligoarthritis and the relative importance of the tests used for diagnosis. *Ann Rheum Dis.* 2001 Apr;60(4):337-43 ard.bmjjournals.com/cgi/content/full/60/4/337

[693] Vasquez A. Subphysiologic Doses of Vitamin D are Subtherapeutic: Comment on the Study by The Record Trial Group. *The Lancet* Published on-line May 6, 2005

[694] "Patients with ankylosing spondylitis may have extremely low levels of 25(OH)D." Falkenbach et al. Serum 25-hydroxyvitamin D and parathyroid hormone in patients with ankylosing spondylitis before and after a three-week rehabilitation treatment at high altitude during winter and spring. *Wien Klin Wochenschr.* 2001 Apr 30;113(9):328-32

[695] Al Faraj S, Al Mutairi K. Vitamin D deficiency and chronic low back pain in Saudi Arabia. *Spine.* 2003 Jan 15;28(2):177-9

[696] Masood H, Narang AP, Bhat IA, Shah GN. Persistent limb pain and raised serum alkaline phosphatase the earliest markers of subclinical hypovitaminosis D in Kashmir. *Indian J Physiol Pharmacol.* 1989 Oct-Dec;33(4):259-61

musculoskeletal pain[697], and in general medical patients.[698] [699] In our review of the literature[700], we concluded that **optimal serum 25(OH)-vitamin D levels should be defined as 40 – 65 ng/mL (100 - 160 nmol/L)** and that, "Until proven otherwise, the balance of the research clearly indicates that oral supplementation in the range of 1,000 IU per day for infants, 2,000 IU per day for children and **4,000 IU per day for adults** is safe and reasonable to meet physiologic requirements, to promote optimal health, and to reduce the risk of several serious diseases. Safety and effectiveness of supplementation are assured by periodic monitoring of serum 25(OH)D and serum calcium." Vitamin D supplementation 5,000 – 10,000 IU per day for adults was shown to alleviate low-back pain after 3 months in nearly all patients with low initial serum levels of vitamin D.[701]

- o <u>Testing for multifocal dysbiosis</u>: If the intestinal and genitourinary tracts appear clear of infection following direct testing, then empiric antimicrobial treatment should be considered. Following this, searching for other loci of infection—namely the mouth, throat, nose, sinuses, lungs, and skin—should be pursued as discussed in Chapter 4.
- o <u>HLA-B27</u>: This marker is seen with increased prevalence in patients with AS and ReA. The test can be used to support the diagnosis, particularly early in the course of the illness when radiographs are *negative.*
- o <u>Hormone assessments</u>: These should be performed as detailed in Chapter 4.6 and/or as indicated per patient.
- **Imaging**:
  - o <u>Plain radiographs</u>: In contrast to most of the other rheumatic disorders wherein radiographs are generally unnecessary in early stages of the disease, plain radiographs are of tremendous value in the assessment of spondylitis and sacroiliitis and are generally diagnostic once the diagnostic threshold has been crossed; i.e., they may be negative in early disease, but become positive after a given amount of time, which varies per patient and per disease. Characteristic initial findings in AS are lumbar syndesmophytes and sacroiliitis.
  - o <u>MRI and CT imaging</u>: Generally reserved for the evaluation of spinal stenosis and inflammatory myelopathy. **CT imaging is more sensitive than plain radiography for the initial evaluation of sacroiliitis.**[702] Also used for assessment of other complications as indicated.
- **Establishing the diagnosis**:
  - o Inflammatory spondyloarthropathy as a general term can be diagnosed with a combination of serologic, clinical, and radiographic findings. The subtype of spondyloarthropathy—AS, ReA, PsA, RA, ES, etc—is then distinguished based on the details of the clinical history (e.g., inflammatory bowel disease or recent infection), presentation, clinical findings, serologic tests, and radiographic characteristics.

<u>Complications</u>:
- Chronic pain, significant physical limitations and significant morbidity
- Renal failure, secondary to amyloidosis or medications such as sulfasalazine or NSAID's
- Spinal fracture (in patients with spinal ankylosis following minor trauma)
- Respiratory insufficiency
- Permanent disability due to rigid spinal flexion secondary to bony ankylosis resulting in loss of spinal motion
- Neurologic compromise: due to spinal stenosis, transverse myelopathy, atlantoaxial subluxation, cauda equina fibrosis, or cauda equina syndrome

<u>Clinical management</u>:
- Referral if clinical outcome is unsatisfactory or as otherwise indicated.

[697] Plotnikoff GA, Quigley JM. Prevalence of severe hypovitaminosis D in patients with persistent, nonspecific musculoskeletal pain. *Mayo Clin Proc.* 2003 Dec;78(12):1463-70
[698] Thomas et al. Hypovitaminosis D in medical inpatients. *N Engl J Med.* 1998 Mar 19;338(12):777-83
[699] Kauppinen-Makelin et al. A high prevalence of hypovitaminosis D in Finnish medical in- and outpatients. *J Intern Med.* 2001 Jun;249(6):559-63
[700] Vasquez A, Manso G, Cannell J. The Clinical Importance of Vitamin D (Cholecalciferol). *Alternative Therapies in Health and Medicine* InflammationMastery.com/reprints
[701] Al Faraj S, Al Mutairi K. Vitamin D deficiency and chronic low back pain in Saudi Arabia. *Spine.* 2003 Jan 15;28(2):177-9
[702] Tierney ML. McPhee SJ, Papadakis MA. *Current Medical Diagnosis and Treatment 2006. 45th edition.* New York; Lange Medical Books: 2006, pages 851-855

- NSAIDs, especially indomethacin 25-50 mg thrice daily—"side effects" of indomethacin include headache, giddiness, psychosis, depression, nausea, vomiting, gastric ulcer, and renal impairment. Sulfasalazine: 1,000 mg twice daily.
- Corticosteroids are notably ineffective in the treatment of spondyloarthropathy, though they are commonly used against complications such as uveitis.
- TNF inhibitors: Etanercept 25 mg subcutaneously twice weekly, or infliximab 5 mg/kg every other month. These drugs are clinically effective from the perspective of anti-inflammation, but they are associated with increased risks for lymphoma, serious infections including pulmonary tuberculosis, congestive heart failure, demyelinating diseases, and systemic lupus erythematosus.
- Methotrexate: Used for recalcitrant psoriatic arthritis.[704]

- **FOOD & NUTRITION: 5-part "supplemented Paleo-Mediterranean diet" (SPMD)** The 5-part "supplemented Paleo-Mediterranean diet" (SPMD—reviewed in Chapter 4) consists of ❶ foundational plant-based low-carbohydrate diet of fruits, vegetables, nuts, seeds, berries and lean sources of protein, ❷ multivitamin and multimineral supplementation, ❸ physiologic doses of vitamin D3 (range 2,000-10,000 IU/d), ❹ combination fatty acid therapy (CFAT) with n3-ALA, n6-GLA, n3-EPA, n3-DHA, and phytochemical-rich olive oil which contains n9-oleate, and ❺ probiotics.

  o The use of a low starch diet in the treatment of patients suffering from ankylosing spondylitis: alleviation of dysbiosis and immune complex formation via nutritional intervention (*Clin Rheumatol* 1996 Jan[705]): "The majority of ankylosing spondylitis (AS) patients not only possess HLA-B27, but during active phases of the disease have elevated levels of total serum IgA, suggesting that a microbe from the bowel flora is acting across the gut mucosa. .... Furthermore AS patients from 10 different countries have been found to have elevated levels of specific antibodies against Klebsiella bacteria. It has been suggested that these Klebsiella microbes, found in the bowel flora, might be the trigger factors in this disease and therefore reduction in the size of the bowel flora could be of benefit in the treatment of AS patients. Microbes from the bowel flora depend on dietary starch for their growth and therefore a reduction in starch intake might be beneficial in AS patients. A "low starch diet" involving a reduced intake of "bread, potatoes, cakes and pasta" has been devised and tested in healthy control subjects and AS patients. The "low starch diet" leads to a reduction of total serum IgA in both healthy controls as well as patients, and furthermore to a decrease in inflammation and symptoms in the AS patients."

- **INFECTIONS & DYSBIOSIS: ❶ antimicrobial treatments, ❷ immunorestoration, ❸ immunotolerance via Treg induction** Essentially all autoimmune/rheumatic disorders are associated with microbial colonization and intolerance to same; the presence of persistent microbial colonization is *prima facie* evidence of immunosuppression. The eight areas of dysbiosis (multifocal) are: ❶ sinorespiratory, ❷ orodental, ❸ gastrointestinal, ❹ urogenital/genitourinary, ❺ parenchymal/tissue, ❻ microbial, ❼ dermal/cutaneous, and ❽ environmental.

  o Rational assumption of polymicrobial dysbiosis: The association of spondyloarthropathies and reactive arthritis with microbial infection/colonization is so strong and consistent throughout decades of research that a review or substantiation here, notwithstanding a few relevant samples, would be superfluous; rather, the 3-part anti-dysbiosis protocols and concepts reviewed in Chapter 4 should be implemented. See also the laboratory (microbial) assessments and concepts in Chapter 1. The examples that follow should be viewed concretely for the data provided, but also as metaphorical and representative of the microbe-autoimmunity connection.

  o Helicobacter pylori eradication therapy on gastrointestinal permeability in seronegative spondyloarthritis (*J Rheumatol.* 2005 Feb[706]): "Disruption of intestinal barrier function, followed by increased antigen load, may possibly trigger joint inflammation. In seronegative spondyloarthritis (SpA)

---

[703] Tierney ML. McPhee SJ, Papadakis MA. *Current Medical Diagnosis and Treatment 2006. 45th edition*. New York; Lange Medical Books: 2006, pages 851-855

[704] Tierney ML. McPhee SJ, Papadakis MA. *Current Medical Diagnosis and Treatment 2006. 45th edition.* New York; Lange Medical Books: 2006, pages 851-855

[705] Ebringer A, Wilson C. The use of a low starch diet in the treatment of patients suffering from ankylosing spondylitis. *Clin Rheumatol*. 1996 Jan;15 Suppl 1:62-66

[706] Di Leo et al. Effect of Helicobacter pylori and eradication therapy on gastrointestinal permeability. Implications for patients with seronegative spondyloarthritis. *J Rheumatol.* 2005 Feb;32(2):295-300

both gut inflammation and altered intestinal permeability have been reported. We evaluated ...20 SpA patients, 30 patients with endoscopic gastritis (EndG), and 35 healthy controls... H. pylori affected GI permeability in both SpA and EndG patients. After eradication therapy, sucrose excretion remained increased in SpA and reverted to normal in EndG patients, whereas lactulose/mannitol test became comparable to controls in both groups. SpA patients taking chronic NSAID had increased gastroduodenal permeability only when H. pylori-positive. In SpA patients, GI permeability did not correlate with clinical activity or biochemical inflammation. CONCLUSION: In SpA, H. pylori and NSAID contribute to impaired GI permeability. Eradication therapy may help to maintain epithelial barrier function and possibly influence clinical improvement in patients with SpA."

o Reactive arthritis responding to antiretroviral therapy in an HIV-1-infected individual (*Int J STD AIDS.* 2012 May[707]): "Reactive arthritis (ReA) is an autoimmune seronegative spondyloarthropathy that occurs in response to a urogenital or enteric infection. Several studies have reported a link between ReA and HIV infection. We report a case of an HIV-1-infected patient diagnosed with a disabling ReA who failed to respond to conventional therapy but whose symptoms resolved rapidly after starting antiretroviral therapy (ART)."

o Human immunodeficiency virus associated spondyloarthropathy (*Ann Rheum Dis.* 2001 Jul[708]): "In this case report a patient is described with severe HIV associated reactive arthritis, who on magnetic resonance imaging and sonographic imaging of inflamed knees had extensive polyenthesitis and adjacent osteitis. The arthritis deteriorated despite conventional antirheumatic treatment, but improved dramatically after highly active antiretroviral treatment, which was accompanied by a significant rise in CD4 T lymphocyte counts."

o Reactive arthritis: urogenital swab culture is the only useful diagnostic method for the detection of the arthritogenic infection in extra-articularly asymptomatic patients with undifferentiated oligoarthritis (*Br J Rheumatol.* 1995 Sep[709]): "Reactive arthritis (ReA) is a seronegative oligoarthritis triggered by a preceding extra-articular infection. ... In a retrospective study, we evaluated the usefulness of urogenital swab cultures, serology and stool culture to identify infections in 234 patients with undifferentiated oligoarthritis. One hundred and forty-four patients complaining about joint pain who had no sign or history of inflammatory arthritis served as controls. Urogenital swab cultures showed a microbial infection in 44% of the patients with oligoarthritis (15% Chlamydia, 14% Mycoplasma, 28% Ureaplasma), whereas in the control group only 26% had a positive result (4% Chlamydia, 7% Mycoplasma, 21% Ureaplasma). A Chlamydia IgG-antibody titer > or = 1:256 was found in 22% of the patients in the oligoarthritis group and in 9% of the controls (P < 0.01). However, for only half of Chlamydia IgG-positive patients could a Chlamydia infection be confirmed by urogenital swab culture. Twenty-one per cent of patients with oligoarthritis vs 23% of the controls had positive antibody titers for Salmonella (not significant), 15% vs 5% for Yersinia (P < 0.05) and 17% vs 3% for Borrelia IgG (P < 0.01). In two patients, stool cultures were positive for Campylobacter. Urogenital swab culture is a sensitive diagnostic method to identify the triggering infection in ReA."

• **NUTRITIONAL IMMUNOMODULATION: Treg induction for modulation of Th-1/2/17 inflammation** Nutrients and therapeutic approaches that promote Treg or IL-10 induction and/or Th-17, IL-17 suppression include 1) mitochondrial optimization and mTOR suppression, 2) biotin, 3) vitamin E, 4) sodium avoidance, 5) transgenic/GMO food avoidance, 6) probiotics, 7) lipoic acid, 8) vitamin A, 9) inflammation reduction, 10) vitamin D, 11) fatty acid supplementation with GLA and n3, 12) infection and dysbiosis remediation, 13) green tea EGCG. Acronym: MiBESTPLAIDFIG.

• **DYSMETABOLISM & DYSFUNCTIONAL MITOCHONDRIA: MitoDys, ERS-UPR, AGE/RAGE, hyperglycemia and ceramide** The major clinical considerations in this section are mitochondrial dysfunction, endoplasmic reticulum stress, unfolded protein response, TLR activation, and the dysmetabolic effects of

---

[707] Scott et al. Reactive arthritis responding to antiretroviral therapy in an HIV-1-infected individual. *Int J STD AIDS.* 2012 May;23(5):373-4

[708] McGonagle et al. Human immunodeficiency virus associated spondyloarthropathy. *Ann Rheum Dis.* 2001 Jul;60(7):696-8

[709] Erlacher et al. Reactive arthritis: urogenital swab culture is the only useful diagnostic method for the detection of the arthritogenic infection in extra-articularly asymptomatic patients with undifferentiated oligoarthritis. *Br J Rheumatol.* 1995 Sep;34(9):838-42

sustained hyperglycemia and hyperinsulinemia and resultant oxidative stress, inflammation, RAGE activation, and accumulation of AGE, palmitate and ceramide. The review of this information in Chapter 4 covered approximately 30 interventions relevant to dysmetabolism, mitochondrial dysfunction, ERS-UPR, etc; these will not be reviewed here except to mention those most commonly, easily, empirically, synergistically, and effectively used: 1) low-carbohydrate diet with 2) moderate exercise, 3) CoQ-10, 4) acetyl-carnitine with 5) lipoic acid, 6) NAC, 7) resveratrol, and 8) melatonin.

- **STYLE OF LIVING (LIFESTYLE) & SPECIAL CONSIDERATIONS:** Sleep optimization, SocioPsychology, Stress management/avoidance, Somatic treatments, Special Supplementation, Sweat/exercise, Sauna/detoxification, Surgery, Stamp your passport and vacate current reality, Sensory deprivation therapy This is a buffet of mostly lifestyle-based interventions yet also including considerations such as somatic treatments, additional supplementation, and surgery.

- **ENDOCRINE IMBALANCE & OPTIMIZATION:** Prolactin, Insulin, Estrogen, DHEA, Cortisol, Testosterone, Thyroid Common hormonal imbalances seen among autoimmune/inflammatory patients are: ❶ *elevated* prolactin, ❷ *elevated* estrogen, ❸ *elevated* insulin, and ❹ *reduced* DHEA, ❺ *reduced* cortisol, and ❻ *reduced* testosterone; see Chapter 4 for discussion of these hormones and respective interventions. Thyroid evaluation (patient + labs) should be comprehensive, as discussed in Chapter 1, with a low threshold for empiric treatment.

- **XENOBIOTIC ACCUMULATION & DETOXIFICATION:** Chemical avoidance, nutritional support for detoxification pathways, urine alkalinization The clinical relevance and pathogenic mechanisms of xenobiotic accumulation are irrefutably well documented and described. Clinical assessments include history, physical examination, and laboratory assessment (using serum, whole blood, urine or—rarely yet accurately— fat biopsy), and response to treatment. Treatments include nutritional support for Phases 1 and 2 of detoxification (e.g., oxidation and conjugation) and excretion via bile and urine; for the latter, urinary alkalinization is generally recommended. Chemical toxins can be bound in the gut using activated charcoal, cholestyramine, or *Chlorella*—all of these three treatments have documented safety and effectiveness; clinically and empirically, phytochelatin (plant-derived peptides that bind toxic metals) concentrates appear safe and effective despite lack of conclusive published data supporting clinical use.

Sjögren Syndrome/Disease

Introduction:

Sjögren Syndrome/Disease is a sustained inflammatory disorder characterized by inflammatory and destructive lymphocytic infiltrates in exocrine organs, leading to failure of these glands and the resultant complications reviewed in the section that follows. Common to other inflammatory and autoimmune disorders, the condition is multifactorial in accord with most of the categories addressed by the Functional Inflammology protocol and recalled by the FINDSEX acronym detailed in Chapter 4 and the accompanying videos. Readers are expected to have read Chapters 1 and 4 so that this chapter can focus on the more salient points specific for Sjögren Syndrome/Disease. The condition is inaccurately named a "syndrome"—implying that it is a "group of symptoms that collectively indicate or characterize a disease or disorder"; however, this condition—like fibromyalgia—has distinct clinical and histopathological findings and is therefore more accurately described and legitimized as a "disease", which it properly is.

Description/pathophysiology:

- **Autoimmune condition affecting the exocrine glands; mucosal surfaces become dry, irritated and prone to microbial colonization.** Clinically manifested as "*sicca* syndrome" which implies a group of symptoms caused by *dryness* of mucosal surfaces.
- Like most conditions, it is generally described as "idiopathic" by medical textbooks and journal articles.[710] More common than SLE, less common than RA; Sjogren's syndrome is considered by some references to be as common as RA.
- Occurs in two general forms:
  - Primary—only Sjogren's/Sicca syndrome *without evidence of systemic autoimmunity*
  - Secondary—the occurrence of Sjogren's syndrome *along with another autoimmune disease*, especially rheumatoid arthritis, but also SLE, systemic sclerosis, primary biliary cirrhosis, polymyositis, Hashimoto's thyroiditis, polyarteritis, interstitial pulmonary fibrosis

Clinical presentations:

- Much more common in women—90% of patients with Sjögren's disease are female[711]
- Average age of onset is 50 years (typical range 40-60 years)
- **"Sicca syndrome"** denotes dryness of mucus membranes:
  - Dry eyes, keratoconjunctivitis sicca: Lymphocyte and plasma cells cause destruction of lacrimal glands; subjective complaints are more prominent than objective evidence: dry eyes, burning, itching, inability to wear contact lenses, thick mucus, photophobia, corneal ulceration—the latter can lead to infection, vision loss.
  - Dry mouth, xerostomia: this is generally more problematic than keratoconjunctivitis sicca; dental carries ("cavities") are greatly increased; 33% of patients will have parotid gland tenderness (can be treated with analgesics) and fluctuations in gland size.
  - Nose, throat, bronchi, and vagina may also be affected.
- Joint pain: Similar distribution to RA but less severe and nondestructive; minimal swelling: PIP and knees most common
- Classic presentation: Woman (90%) aged 40-60 years with dry mouth, dry eyes, and arthritis that mimics RA; other common presentations include:
  - Photosensitivity, skin rash, hair loss
  - Mouth lesions, carries
  - Chest pain (caused by pleurisy) or breathlessness
  - Raynaud's phenomenon

---

[710] "In spite of [the fact that we have no evidence-based solutions to the etiology and pathogenesis of autoimmune diseases], consensus is often taken as a truth, which may hamper the production, funding and/or publication of new and original ideas and views." Konttinen YT, Kasna-Ronkainen L. Sjogren's syndrome: viewpoint on pathogenesis. One of the reasons I was never asked to write a textbook chapter on it. *Scand J Rheumatol Suppl* 2002;(116):15-22

[711] Tierney ML. McPhee SJ, Papadakis MA. *Current Medical Diagnosis and Treatment 2006. 45th edition*. New York; Lange Medical Books: 2006, pages 842-843

Major differential diagnoses:

- Dehydration, exposure to excessively dry air (furnaces, dehumidifiers, etc.)
- Another autoimmune disease may mimic or occur concomitantly: RA, SLE, scleroderma, polymyositis, autoimmune thyroid disease, arteritis—none of these conditions by itself will cause sicca/dryness.
- Medication side effects (dry eyes and dry mouth are common side effects of many drugs)
- Systemic illness: HIV, lymphoma, sarcoidosis
- Hepatitis C—may possibly induce Sjogren's syndrome[712]
- Mumps (swollen parotid glands)
- Menopause
- Normal aging
- Salivary gland atrophy/fibrosis due to previous radiation to head and neck

Clinical assessments:

- **History/subjective**:
  - See clinical presentations
- **Physical examination/objective**:
  - <u>Schirmer test</u>: Use filter paper to assess adequacy of lacrimation for 5 minutes; less than 5 mm of wetness is abnormal
  - <u>Rose Bengal staining</u>: Used to assess the health of the cornea and to thus search for objective evidence of keratoconjunctivitis sicca
- **Laboratory assessments**:
  - <u>ANA</u>: positive in >95%
    - If ANA is negative, consider HIV, lymphoma, sarcoidosis, hepatitis C.
    - Supportive evidence with **anti-SS-A (anti-Ro)** and **anti-SS-B (anti-La)**, neither of which are specific
    - Autoimmunity directed toward glands/tissues such as stomach, adrenal, and neurons may also be noted[713]
  - <u>RF</u>: Positive in 70%
  - <u>ESR</u>: Elevated in 70%
  - <u>CBC</u>: Shows anemia (33%), leukopenia and eosinophilia (25%)
  - <u>Thyroid disorders</u>: Thyroid autoimmunity is common in patients with Sjogren's syndrome; test anti-thyroid peroxidase antibodies and anti-thyroglobulin antibodies along with TSH, T4, and perhaps T3—see Chapter 1 for discussions on thyroid assessments and interventions.
  - <u>HLA markers</u>: DR2 and DR3 are more common in patients who have Sjogren's syndrome *without rheumatoid arthritis.*
  - <u>Schirmer test</u>: Measures quantity of tears and thus objectively quantifies keratoconjunctivitis sicca.
  - <u>Salivary gland biopsy</u>: Not commonly performed except for atypical presentations such as unilateral involvement and to exclude malignancy.
  - <u>Anti-parietal cell antibodies</u>: Noted in various autoimmune conditions (e.g., approximately 33% of patients with Hashimoto thyroiditis); leads to gastric atrophy and associated hypochlorhydria, cobalamin malabsorption, and microbial overgrowth.
  - Assess patient as indicated for other conditions and complications.
- **Imaging**: Used as indicated per patient; generally not part of assessment
- **Establishing the diagnosis**: Both of the following must be present:
  1. <u>Autoantibodies—ANA or variant</u>: Preferably in combination with the gold standard in allopathic medicine: salivary gland biopsy—this is necessary for "definite diagnosis" but is not necessary for clinical purposes based on "probable diagnosis."
  2. <u>Evidence of exocrine damage</u>: keratoconjunctivitis sicca and/or xerostomia.

---

[712] Siegel LB, Gall EP. Viral infection as a cause of arthritis. *Am Fam Physician* 1996 Nov 1;54(6):2009-15
[713] Rehman HU. Sjogren's syndrome. *Yonsei Med J*. 2003 Dec 30;44(6):947-54 eymj.org/2003/pdf/12947.pdf

<u>Complications</u>:
- Vision impairment, vision loss due to corneal lesion, ulceration and secondary infection
- Dental carries
- Malnutrition, especially vitamin B-12 deficiency
- Inflammatory polyarthropathy
- Salivary stones
- Pneumonia: can be fatal
- Pancreatitis
- Raynaud's phenomenon is seen in ~20%
- Sensory neuropathy, peripheral neuropathy: immune complex neuropathy, nutrient/B12 deficiencies
- Renal tubular acidosis
- Renal insufficiency and failure: can be fatal
- Nephritis (immune complex disorder)
- Vasculitis (immune complex disorder)
- Cryoglobulinemia (immune complex disorder)
- **Lymphoma: Up to 3-10% of patients with Sjogren's syndrome develop lymphoma**; risk is increased in patients with severe dryness and systemic complications such as vasculitis, splenomegaly, and cryoglobulinemia.
- Waldenstrom's macroglobulinemia

<u>Clinical management</u>:
- <u>Medical treatment</u>: "Treatment is symptomatic and supportive."[714] "There is no specific [allopathic] treatment for the basic process. Local manifestations can be treated symptomatically."[715]
- Referral if clinical outcome is unsatisfactory or if serious complications are possible.

<u>Treatments</u>:
- Drug treatments include pilocarpine (5 mg 4 times daily) and/or cevimeline (30 mg three times daily) to promote salivation. Associated rheumatic diseases are treated as indicated; prednisone is commonly used.
- <u>Eye drops</u>: Consider vitamin-A-containing eye drops, available OTC or by a compounding pharmacist
- <u>For dry mouth</u>:
  - Sip fluids throughout the day.
  - Chew sugarless gum to promote saliva flow; xylitol chewing gum can stimulate saliva flow and inhibit the growth of cariogenic bacteria.
  - Saliva substitute with carboxymethylcellulose.
  - Fastidious oral hygiene (brushing, flossing, oral antiseptics) and regular dental care are important.
  - Liquid folic acid supplementation swished in the mouth may help alleviate mouth sores; likewise, topical vitamin E and glutamine may help (as they do with chemotherapy-induced mucositis); chewable deglycyrrhizinated licorice benefits some patients.
  - Acupuncture improves salivary flow rates in patients with Sjogren's syndrome.[716,717]

- **FOOD & NUTRITION: 5-part "supplemented Paleo-Mediterranean diet" (SPMD)** The 5-part "supplemented Paleo-Mediterranean diet" (SPMD—reviewed in Chapter 4) consists of ❶ foundational plant-based low-carbohydrate diet of fruits, vegetables, nuts, seeds, berries and lean sources of protein, ❷ multivitamin and multimineral supplementation, ❸ physiologic doses of vitamin D3 (range 2,000-10,000 IU/d), ❹ combination

---

[714] Tierney ML. McPhee SJ, Papadakis MA. *Current Medical Diagnosis and Treatment. 35th edition*. Stamford: Appleton and Lange, 1996 page 749 and Tierney ML. McPhee SJ, Papadakis MA. *Current Medical Diagnosis and Treatment 2006. 45th edition*. New York; Lange Medical Books: 2006, pages 842-843
[715] Beers MH, Berkow R (eds). *The Merck Manual. Seventeenth Edition*. Whitehouse Station; Merck Research Laboratories 1999 Page 424
[716] "CONCLUSIONS: This study shows that acupuncture treatment results in statistically significant improvements in SFR in patients with xerostomia up to 6 months. It suggests that additional acupuncture therapy can maintain this improvement in SFR for up to 3 years." Blom M, Lundeberg T. Long-term follow-up of patients treated with acupuncture for xerostomia and the influence of additional treatment. *Oral Dis* 2000 Jan;6(1):15-24
[717] "A majority of the patients subjectively reported some improvement after treatment, and a significant increase in paraffin-stimulated saliva secretion was found after treatment." List et al. The effect of acupuncture in the treatment of patients with primary Sjogren's syndrome. A controlled study. *Acta Odontol Scand* 1998 Apr;56(2):95-9

fatty acid therapy (CFAT) with n3-ALA, n6-GLA, n3-EPA, n3-DHA, and phytochemical-rich olive oil which contains n9-oleate, and ❺ probiotics.

- o <u>Avoidance of allergenic foods</u>: Any patient may be allergic to any food, even if the food is generally considered a health-promoting food. Generally speaking, the most notorious allergens are wheat, citrus (especially juice due to the industrial use of fungal hemicellulases), cow's milk, eggs, peanuts, chocolate, and yeast-containing foods. **Patients with celiac disease have an increased prevalence of Sjogren's syndrome[718], and patients with Sjogren's syndrome have an increased prevalence of celiac disease.[719] In one study, the estimated prevalence of celiac disease in Sjogren's patients was nearly 1 in 20.[720]** Celiac disease can present with inflammatory oligoarthritis that resembles rheumatoid arthritis and which remits with avoidance of wheat/gluten; the inflammatory arthropathy of celiac disease has preceded bowel symptoms and/or an accurate diagnosis by as many as 3-15 years.[721,722] Clinicians must explain to their patients that celiac disease and wheat allergy are two different clinical entities and that exclusion of one does not exclude the other, and in neither case does mutual exclusion obviate the promotion of intestinal bacterial overgrowth (i.e., proinflammatory dysbiosis) by indigestible wheat oligosaccharides.

- o <u>Broad-spectrum fatty acid therapy with ALA, EPA, DHA, GLA and oleic acid</u>: Fatty acid supplementation should be delivered in the form of combination therapy with ALA, GLA, DHA, and EPA. Given at doses of 3,000 – 9,000 mg per day, ALA from flax oil has impressive anti-inflammatory benefits demonstrated by its ability to halve prostaglandin production in humans.[723] **Patients with Sjogren's syndrome have lower levels of GLA/DGLA[724] and fatty acid supplementation—particularly with GLA (along with vitamin C)—is safe and may be beneficial (positive reports[725,726], neutral report[727], negative report[728]).**

- o <u>Vitamin D3 supplementation with physiologic doses and/or tailored to serum 25(OH)D levels</u>: **Vitamin D insufficiency has been reported in patients with Sjogren's syndrome, presumably due to reduced intake and/or malabsorption.** Vitamin D deficiency is common in the general population and is even more common in patients with chronic illness and chronic musculoskeletal pain.[729] Correction of vitamin D deficiency supports normal immune function against infection and provides a clinically significant anti-inflammatory[730] and analgesic benefit in patients with back pain[731] and limb pain.[732] **Vitamin D status is inversely associated with inflammation in patients with Sjogren's syndrome.[733,734]** Reasonable daily doses for children and adults are 2,000 and 4,000 IU, respectively, as defined by Vasquez, et al.[735] Deficiency

---

[718] "Sjogren's syndrome occurred in 3.3% of coeliac patients and in 0.3% of controls." Collin et al. Coeliac disease—associated disorders and survival. *Gut.* 1994 Sep;35:1215-8.

[719] "Further, our study shows that anti-tTG is more prevalent in SS than in other systemic rheumatic diseases." Luft et al. Autoantibodies to tissue transglutaminase in Sjogren's syndrome and related rheumatic diseases. *J Rheumatol.* 2003 Dec;30(12):2613-9

[720] "The frequency of CD in the SS population was significantly higher than in the non-SS European population (4.5:100 vs 4.5-5.5:1,000)." Szodoray et al. Coeliac disease in Sjogren's syndrome--a study of 111 Hungarian patients. *Rheumatol Int.* 2004 Sep;24(5):278-82

[721] "We report six patients with coeliac disease in whom arthritis was prominent at diagnosis and who improved with dietary therapy. Joint pain preceded diagnosis by up to three years in five patients and 15 years in one patient." Bourne et al. Arthritis and coeliac disease. *Ann Rheum Dis.* 1985 Sep;44(9):592-8

[722] "A 15-year-old girl, with synovitis of the knees and ankles for 3 years before a diagnosis of gluten-sensitive enteropathy, is described." Pinals RS. Arthritis associated with gluten-sensitive enteropathy. *J Rheumatol.* 1986 Feb;13(1):201-4

[723] Adam et al. Effect of alpha-linolenic acid in the human diet on linoleic acid metabolism and prostaglandin biosynthesis. *J Lipid Res.* 1986 Apr;27(4):421-6

[724] "We found MD levels of 20:3n6 (dihommo-gamma-linolenic acid), and basal and indomethacin-enhanced NK cell activity significantly reduced, in 10 primary Sjogren's syndrome patients as compared with 10 healthy controls." Oxholm P, Pedersen BK, Horrobin DF. Natural killer cell functions are related to the cell membrane composition of essential fatty acids: differences in healthy persons and patients with primary Sjogren's syndrome. *Clin Exp Rheumatol.* 1992 May-Jun;10(3):229-34

[725] "An attempt to treat humans with Sjogren's syndrome by raising endogenous PGE1 production by administration of essential fatty acid PGE1 precursors, of pyridoxine and of vitamin C was successful in raising the rates of tear and saliva production." Horrobin DF, Campbell A. Sjogren's syndrome and the sicca syndrome: the role of prostaglandin E1 deficiency. Treatment with essential fatty acids and vitamin C. *Med Hypotheses.* 1980 Mar;6(3):225-32

[726] "Efamol treatment improved the Schirmer-I-test..." Manthorpe R, Hagen Petersen S, Prause JU. Primary Sjogren's syndrome treated with Efamol/Efavit. A double-blind cross-over investigation. *Rheumatol Int.* 1984;4(4):165-7. The duration of this study was ridiculously short—only 3 weeks.

[727] "The objective ocular status, evaluated by a combined ocular score, including the results from Schirmer-I test, break-up time and van Bijsterveld score, improved significantly during Efamol treatment when compared with Efamol start-values (p less than 0.05), but not when compared with placebo values (p less than 0.2)." Oxholm P, Manthorpe R, Prause JU, Horrobin D. Patients with primary Sjogren's syndrome treated for two months with evening primrose oil. *Scand J Rheumatol.* 1986;15:103-8

[728] "There was no significant improvement in any of the patients during the treatment period compared to assessments done pre and post treatment." McKendry RJ. Treatment of Sjogren's syndrome with essential fatty acids, pyridoxine and vitamin C. *Prostaglandins Leukot Med.* 1982 Apr;8(4):403-8

[729] Plotnikoff GA, Quigley JM. Prevalence of severe hypovitaminosis D in patients with persistent, nonspecific musculoskeletal pain. *Mayo Clin Proc.* 2003 Dec;78(12):1463-70

[730] Timms PM, et al. Circulating MMP9, vitamin D and variation in the TIMP-1 response with VDR genotype. *QJM.* 2002 Dec;95(12):787-96

[731] Al Faraj S, Al Mutairi K. Vitamin D deficiency and chronic low back pain in Saudi Arabia. *Spine.* 2003 Jan 15;28(2):177-9

[732] Masood H, Narang AP, Bhat IA, Shah GN. Persistent limb pain and raised serum alkaline phosphatase the earliest markers of subclinical hypovitaminosis D in Kashmir. *Indian J Physiol Pharmacol.* 1989 Oct-Dec;33(4):259-61

[733] "In conclusion the inverse correlations found between levels of 25 OH D and measures of clinical and immunoinflammatory status support the notion that vitamin D metabolism may be involved in the pathogenesis of primary SS." Bang B, Asmussen K, Sorensen OH, Oxholm P. Reduced 25-hydroxyvitamin D levels in primary Sjogren's syndrome. Correlations to disease manifestations. *Scand J Rheumatol.* 1999;28(3):180-3

[734] "Among patients with increased concentrations of IgM rheumatoid factor there was a significant negative correlation between the serum titres of IgM rheumatoid factor and 25-OHD3 concentrations." Muller K, et al. Abnormal vitamin D3 metabolism in patients with primary Sjogren's syndrome. *Ann Rheum Dis.* 1990 Sep;49(9):682-4

[735] Vasquez et al. The clinical importance of vitamin D: a paradigm shift with implications for all healthcare providers. *Altern Ther Health Med.* 2004 Sep-Oct;10(5):28-36

and response to treatment are monitored with serum 25(OH)vitamin D while safety is monitored with serum calcium; inflammatory granulomatous diseases and certain drugs such as hydrochlorothiazide greatly increase the propensity for hypercalcemia and warrant increment dosing and frequent monitoring of serum calcium.

- o <u>Green tea, green tea extract (EGCG), and other phytonutritional antioxidants and anti-inflammatories</u>: Very interestingly, an *in vitro* study[736] showed that epigallocatechin gallate inhibited the expression of major autoantigens, including those which are characteristic of Sjogren's syndrome: SS-B/La, SS-A/Ro. Given its antioxidant properties and anti-inflammatory actions (specifically via inhibition of NFkB[737]), green tea and related supplements may prove beneficial for patients with Sjogren's syndrome.

- o <u>High-dose short-term oral vitamin A</u>: Szocsik et al[738] administered vitamin A 100,000 IU per day for two weeks and obtained improved immune function, such as improved natural killer cell function, in patients with Sjogren's syndrome. Vitamin A is necessary for induction of T-regulatory cells; see Chapter 4.3.

- **INFECTIONS & DYSBIOSIS: ❶ antimicrobial treatments, ❷ immunorestoration, ❸ immunotolerance via Treg induction** Essentially all autoimmune/rheumatic disorders are associated with microbial colonization and intolerance to same; the presence of persistent microbial colonization is *prima facie* evidence of immunosuppression. The eight areas of dysbiosis (multifocal) are: ❶ sinorespiratory, ❷ orodental, ❸ gastrointestinal, ❹ urogenital/genitourinary, ❺ parenchymal/tissue, ❻ microbial, ❼ dermal/cutaneous, and ❽ environmental.

  - o <u>T-cell epitope mimicry between Sjögren's syndrome Antigen A (SSA)/Ro60 and oral, gut, skin and vaginal bacteria</u> (*Clin Immunol.* 2014 May[739]): "Amongst these, a peptide from the von Willebrand factor type A domain protein (vWFA) from the oral microbe *Capnocytophaga ochracea* was the most potent activator. Further, Ro60-reactive T cells were activated by recombinant vWFA protein and whole *Escherichia coli* expressing this protein. These results demonstrate that peptides derived from normal human microbiota can activate Ro60-reactive T cells."

  - o <u>Epstein-Barr virus in Sjögren's syndrome salivary glands drives local autoimmunity</u> (*Nat Rev Rheumatol.* 2014 Jul[740]): Paraphrasing from the original article: "Ectopic lymphoid structures (ELS) within the salivary glands of patients with Sjögren's syndrome serve as niches for latency and reactivation of EBV and contribute to the activation and differentiation of plasma cells. ... EBV is aberrantly expressed in the salivary glands of patients with Sjögren's syndrome, specifically in those glands that displayed ELS, as revealed by the presence of EBV-encoded small RNA (EBER) transcripts and EBER+ cells within infiltrating cells. ... EBV reactivation occurs in a substantial proportion of perifollicular plasma cells that produce anti-Ro52 antibodies."

  - o <u>Epstein-Barr Virus Infection in Disease-Specific Autoreactive B Cell Activation in Ectopic Lymphoid Structures of Sjögren's Syndrome</u> (*Arthritis Rheumatol.* 2014 Sep[741]): "Active EBV infection is selectively associated with ELS in the salivary glands of patients with SS and appears to contribute to local growth and differentiation of disease-specific autoreactive B cells."

  - o <u>Epstein-Barr Virus Infection, Vitamin D Deficiency, and Steps to Autoimmunity: A Unifying Hypothesis</u> (*Autoimmune Dis.* 2012[742]): Per this model, "Autoimmunity is postulated to evolve in the following steps: (1) CD8+ T-cell deficiency, (2) primary EBV infection, (3) decreased CD8+ T-cell control of EBV, (4) increased EBV load and increased anti-EBV antibodies, (5) EBV infection in the target organ, (6) clonal

[736] "EGCG inhibited the transcription and translation of major autoantigens, including SS-B/La, SS-A/Ro, coilin, DNA topoisomerase I, and alpha-fodrin. These findings, taken together with green tea's anti-inflammatory and antiapoptotic effects, suggest that green tea polyphenols could serve as an important component in novel approaches to combat autoimmune disorders in humans." Hsu et al. Inhibition of autoantigen expression by (-)-epigallocatechin-3-gallate (the major constituent of green tea) in normal human cells. *J Pharmacol Exp Ther.* 2005 Nov;315(2):805-11

[737] "In conclusion, EGCG is an effective inhibitor of IKK activity. This may explain, at least in part, some of the reported anti-inflammatory and anti-cancer effects of green tea." Yang et al. The green tea polyphenol (-)-epigallocatechin-3-gallate blocks nuclear factor-kappa B activation by inhibiting I kappa B kinase activity in the intestinal epithelial cell line IEC-6. *Mol Pharmacol.* 2001 Sep;60(3):528-33

[738] "Patients with Sjogren's syndrome were treated with vitamin A (100,000 U) daily during a two-week period. The vitamin treatment significantly elevated their ADCC and NK activity." Szocsik et al. Effect of vitamin A treatment on immune reactivity and lipid peroxidation in patients with Sjogren's syndrome. *Clin Rheumatol.* 1988 Dec;7(4):514-9

[739] Szymula et al. T cell epitope mimicry between Sjögren's syndrome Antigen A (SSA)/Ro60 and oral, gut, skin and vaginal bacteria. *Clin Immunol.* 2014 May-Jun;152(1-2):1-9

[740] Onuora S. Connective tissue diseases: Epstein-Barr virus in Sjögren's syndrome salivary glands drives local autoimmunity. *Nat Rev Rheumatol.* 2014 Jul;10(7):384

[741] Croia et al. Implication of Epstein-Barr Virus Infection in Disease-Specific Autoreactive B Cell Activation in Ectopic Lymphoid Structures of Sjögren's Syndrome. *Arthritis Rheumatol.* 2014 Sep;66(9):2545-57

[742] Pender MP. CD8+ T-Cell Deficiency, Epstein-Barr Virus Infection, Vitamin D Deficiency, and Steps to Autoimmunity. *Autoimmune Dis.* 2012;2012:189096

expansion of EBV-infected autoreactive B cells in the target organ, (7) infiltration of autoreactive T cells into the target organ, and (8) development of ectopic lymphoid follicles in the target organ [which drive the tissue damage and autoantibody production as recently demonstrated per *Nat Rev Rheumatol* 2014 Jul[743] and *Arthritis Rheumatol* 2014 Sep[744]]. It is also proposed that deprivation of sunlight and vitamin D at higher latitudes facilitates the development of autoimmune diseases by aggravating the CD8+ T-cell deficiency and thereby further impairing control of EBV." Congratulations to this author—Pender—for predicting two years in advance the research that would later support this model.

- o Aryl hydrocarbon receptor-mediated induction of EBV reactivation as a risk factor for Sjögren's syndrome (*J Immunol* 2012 May[745]): This is very impressive research, connecting xenobiotic exposure with viral reactivation. "The aryl hydrocarbon receptor (AhR) is a ligand-activated transcription factor that mediates a variety of biological effects by binding to environmental pollutants, including 2,3,7,8-tetrachlorodibenzo-p-dioxin (TCDD or dioxin). ... This study evaluated the possibility that ligand-activated AhR reactivates EBV. ... TCDD enhanced BZLF1 transcription, which mediates the switch from the latent to the lytic form of EBV infection in EBV-positive B cell lines and in a salivary gland epithelial cell line. Moreover, TCDD-induced increases in BZLF1 mRNA and EBV genomic DNA levels were confirmed in the B cell lines. Saliva from SS patients activated the transcription of both CYP1A1 and BZLF1. Additionally, there was a positive correlation between CYP1A1 and BZLF1 promoter activities. AhR ligands elicited the reactivation of EBV in activated B cells and salivary epithelial cells, and these ligands are involved in SS." This is stunning research: it provides direct links between infections, xenobiotic exposure, and autoimmunity; further, by extension, this research also suggests that xenobiotic exposure could also enhance transcription of HERVs (directly, or indirectly via viral transactivation) which also contributes to autoimmunity.

- o Assess for and treat dysbiosis: Insufficient flow of saliva and other fluids promotes microbial colonization of mucosal surfaces, particularly the digestive and respiratory tracts. Gastrointestinal infection/dysbiosis can cause nutrient malabsorption, and the resultant nutritional insufficiencies can exacerbate the sicca symptoms.[746] Patients with Sjogren's syndrome may have an increased prevalence of infection/colonization with *H. pylori*[747], an organism known to incite systemic inflammation and to produce pro-inflammatory endotoxin and antigens; eradication of this microbe—or others per patient—may alleviate clinical manifestations by addressing one of the inciting causes. Of particular note is that *H. pylori* promotes gastric autoimmunity, sicca syndrome, as well as intestinal lymphoma—all of which are noted in Sjogren's syndrome.

  - ▪ *H pylori* and gastrointestinal cancer: "*H. pylori* infection is a major cause of gastric (stomach) cancer, specifically non-cardia gastric cancer (cancer in all areas of the stomach, except for the top portion near where it joins the esophagus). *H. pylori* infection also causes gastric mucosa-associated lymphoid tissue (MALT) lymphoma. *H. pylori* infection is associated with a decreased risk of some other cancers, including gastric cardia cancer (cancer in the top portion of the stomach) and esophageal adenocarcinoma."[748]

- • **NUTRITIONAL IMMUNOMODULATION: Treg induction for modulation of Th-1/2/17 inflammation**
  Nutrients and therapeutic approaches that promote Treg or IL-10 induction and/or Th-17, IL-17 suppression include 1) mitochondrial optimization and mTOR suppression, 2) biotin, 3) vitamin E, 4) sodium avoidance, 5) transgenic/GMO food avoidance, 6) probiotics, 7) lipoic acid, 8) vitamin A, 9) inflammation reduction, 10) vitamin D, 11) fatty acid supplementation with GLA and n3, 12) infection and dysbiosis remediation, 13) green tea EGCG. Acronym: MiBESTPLAIDFIG (2014) and MiBESTPLAIDFIGNaC (2016)—as reviewed in Chapter 4.3.

---

[743] Onuora S. Connective tissue diseases: Epstein-Barr virus in Sjögren's syndrome salivary glands drives local autoimmunity. *Nat Rev Rheumatol*. 2014 Jul;10(7):384

[744] Croia et al. Implication of Epstein-Barr Virus Infection in Disease-Specific Autoreactive B Cell Activation in Ectopic Lymphoid Structures of Sjögren's Syndrome. *Arthritis Rheumatol*. 2014 Sep;66(9):2545-57

[745] Inoue et al. Aryl hydrocarbon receptor-mediated induction of EBV reactivation as a risk factor for Sjögren's syndrome. *J Immunol*. 2012 May 1;188(9):4654-62

[746] Bosman et al. Sicca syndrome associated with Tropheryma whipplei intestinal infection. *J Clin Microbiol*. 2002 Aug;40(8):3104-6

[747] "Patients with SS are more prone to have H. pylori infection in comparison to other connective tissue diseases. Serum antibody titer to H. pylori correlated with index for clinical disease manifestations, age, disease duration and CRP." El Miedany et al. Sjogren's syndrome: concomitant H. pylori infection and possible correlation with clinical parameters. *Joint Bone Spine*. 2005 Mar;72(2):135-41

[748] cancer.gov/cancertopics/factsheet/Risk/h-pylori-cancer

- o <u>IL-17-producing T cells are expanded in the peripheral blood, infiltrate salivary glands and are resistant to corticosteroids in patients with primary Sjogren's syndrome</u> (*Ann Rheum Dis*. 2013 Feb[749]): "It has been recently observed that a T-cell subset, lacking of both CD4 and CD8 molecules and defined as <mark>double negative (DN), is expanded in the blood of patients with systemic lupus erythematosus, produces IL-17</mark> and accumulates in the kidney during nephritis. Since IL-17 production is enhanced in salivary gland infiltrates of primary Sjögren's syndrome (SS) patients, we investigated whether DN T cells may be involved in the pathogenesis of salivary gland damage. ... CD3(+)CD4(-)CD8(-) <mark>DN T cells were major producers of IL-17 in SS and expressed ROR-γt.</mark> They were expanded in the peripheral blood, <mark>spontaneously produced IL-17 and infiltrated salivary glands.</mark> In addition, the expansion of αβ-TCR(+) DN T cells was associated with disease activity. Notably, IL-17-producing DN T cells from SS patients, but not from healthy controls, were strongly resistant to the in vitro effect of dexamethasone." Readers should by now (following discussion in Chapter 4) appreciate that IL-17 production and tissue infiltration are synonymous with autoimmune-type tissue damage and inflammation.

- • DYSMETABOLISM: MitoDys, ERS-UPR, mTOR inhibition The major clinical considerations in this section are mitochondrial dysfunction, endoplasmic reticulum stress, unfolded protein response, TLR activation, and the dysmetabolic effects of sustained hyperglycemia and hyperinsulinemia and resultant oxidative stress, inflammation, RAGE activation, and accumulation of AGE, palmitate and ceramide. The review of this information in Chapter 4 covered approximately 30 interventions relevant to dysmetabolism, mitochondrial dysfunction, ERS-UPR, etc; these will not be reviewed here except to mention those most commonly, easily, empirically, synergistically, and effectively used: 1) low-carbohydrate diet with 2) moderate exercise, 3) CoQ-10, 4) acetyl-carnitine with 5) lipoic acid, 6) NAC, 7) resveratrol, and 8) melatonin.

- • STYLE OF LIVING (LIFESTYLE) & SPECIAL CONSIDERATIONS This is a buffet of mostly lifestyle-based interventions yet also including considerations such as additional supplementation and surgery.
  - o <u>Individualized homeopathy</u>: A small randomized placebo-controlled trial found homeopathy beneficial for xerostomia.[750]
  - o <u>Replacement of gastric HCL</u>: Tablets/capsules of betaine HCL may improve digestion, nutrient assimilation, and also alleviate intestinal microbial overgrowth; antiparietal cell antibodies may be noted.

- • ENDOCRINE IMBALANCE & OPTIMIZATION: Prolactin, Insulin, Estrogen, DHEA, Cortisol, Testosterone, Thyroid Common hormonal imbalances seen among autoimmune/inflammatory patients are: ❶ *elevated* prolactin, ❷ *elevated* estrogen, ❸ *elevated* insulin, and ❹ *reduced* DHEA, ❺ *reduced* cortisol, and ❻ *reduced* testosterone; see Chapter 4 for discussion of these hormones and respective interventions. Thyroid evaluation should be comprehensive, as discussed in Chapter 1, with a low threshold for empiric treatment.
  - o <u>Endocrine alterations in primary Sjogren's syndrome</u> (*J Autoimmun*. 2012 Dec[751]): "Heightened serum and salivary gland tissue <mark>prolactin</mark> levels in primary SS patients have been also suggested as contributors in disease pathogenesis. Finally, <mark>autoimmune thyroid disease (ATD) occurs quiet commonly in the setting of primary SS</mark> and subclinical hypothyroidism is the main functional abnormality observed in these patients."
  - o <u>DHEA in Sjogren's syndrome—a hormonal deficiency and potential treatment in search of clinical significance</u>: Generally, the finding of low DHEA and the correction/normalization of low DHEA in patients with autoimmunity/inflammation/autoinflammation correlates with clinical improvement; such has not been the situation with Sjogren's syndrome, which has been consistently resistant to improvement following DHEA administration, a fact which I have noted since the first publication of *Integrative Rheumatology* in 2006. I think what is likely here is that the DHEA deficiency is important, but that isolated DHEA supplementation is insufficient to elicit a significant clinical improvement as monotherapy.

---

[749] Alunno et al. IL-17-producing CD4-CD8- T cells are expanded in the peripheral blood, infiltrate salivary glands and are resistant to corticosteroids in patients with primary Sjogren's syndrome. *Ann Rheum Dis*. 2013 Feb;72(2):286-92

[750] "Our results suggest that individually prescribed homeopathic medicine could be a valuable adjunct to the treatment of oral discomfort and xerostomic symptoms." Haila et al. Effects of homeopathic treatment on salivary flow rate and subjective symptoms in patients with oral dryness: a randomized trial. *Homeopathy*. 2005 Jul;94(3):175-81

[751] Mavragani et al. Endocrine alterations in primary Sjogren's syndrome: an overview. *J Autoimmun*. 2012 Dec;39(4):354-8

- Low serum dehydroepiandrosterone sulfate in women with primary Sjögren's syndrome as an isolated sign of impaired HPA axis function (*J Rheumatol.* 2001 Jun[752]): "The results show that women with pSS have intact cortisol synthesis but decreased serum concentrations of DHEA-S and increased cortisol/DHEA-S ratio compared with healthy controls. The findings may reflect a constitutional or disease mediated influence on adrenal steroid synthesis. The thyroid axis and gonadotropin secretion were similar in patients and controls."
  - DHEA versus placebo for Sjögren's syndrome (*Arthritis Rheum.* 2004 Aug[753]): "A 24-week randomized, double-blinded, pilot trial of oral DHEA (200 mg/day) versus placebo was conducted. ... Apart from changes over the trial in dry mouth symptoms, no significant differences were noted between the DHEA and placebo groups for dry eye symptoms, objective measures of ocular dryness, stimulated salivary flow; IgG, or ESR. ... DHEA showed no evidence of efficacy in SS. Without evidence for efficacy, patients with SS should avoid using unregulated DHEA supplements, since long-term adverse consequences of exposure to this hormone are unknown."
  - Dehydroepiandrosterone (DHEA) treatment for severe fatigue in DHEA-deficient patients with primary Sjögren's syndrome (*Arthritis Care Res* 2010 Jan[754]): "A multicenter, investigator-based, powered, randomized controlled clinical trial (crossover, washout design) using fatigue as the primary outcome measure was performed on patients with primary SS (n = 107) who had a general fatigue score > or =14 on the 20-item Multiple Fatigue Inventory (MFI-20), combined with age- and sex-adjusted serum DHEAS values below the mean. .. Similar to earlier results using pharmacologic doses, substitution treatment with 50 mg of DHEA in DHEA-deficient and severely tired primary SS patients does not help against fatigue better than placebo."

- **XENOBIOTIC ACCUMULATION & DETOXIFICATION: Chemical avoidance, nutritional support for detoxification pathways, urine alkalinization** The clinical relevance and pathogenic mechanisms of xenobiotic accumulation are irrefutably well documented and described. Clinical assessments include history, physical examination, and laboratory assessment (using serum, whole blood, urine or—rarely yet accurately— fat biopsy), and response to treatment. Treatments include nutritional support for Phases 1 and 2 of detoxification (e.g., oxidation and conjugation) and excretion via bile and urine; for the latter, urinary alkalinization is generally recommended. Chemical toxins can be bound in the gut using activated charcoal, cholestyramine, or *Chlorella*—all of these three treatments have documented safety and effectiveness; clinically and empirically, phytochelatin (plant-derived peptides that bind toxic metals) concentrates appear safe and effective despite lack of conclusive published data supporting clinical use.
  - Aryl hydrocarbon receptor-mediated induction of EBV reactivation as a risk factor for Sjögren's syndrome (*J Immunol* 2012 May[755]): This is very impressive research, connecting xenobiotic exposure with viral reactivation. "The aryl hydrocarbon receptor (AhR) is a ligand-activated transcription factor that mediates a variety of biological effects by binding to environmental pollutants, including 2,3,7,8-tetrachlorodibenzo-p-dioxin (TCDD or dioxin). ... This study evaluated the possibility that ligand-activated AhR reactivates EBV. ... TCDD enhanced BZLF1 transcription, which mediates the switch from the latent to the lytic form of EBV infection in EBV-positive B cell lines and in a salivary gland epithelial cell line. Moreover, TCDD-induced increases in BZLF1 mRNA and EBV genomic DNA levels were confirmed in the B cell lines. Saliva from SS patients activated the transcription of both CYP1A1 and BZLF1. Additionally, there was a positive correlation between CYP1A1 and BZLF1 promoter activities. AhR ligands elicited the reactivation of EBV in activated B cells and salivary epithelial cells, and these ligands are involved in SS." This is stunning research: it provides direct links between infections, xenobiotic exposure, and autoimmunity; further, by extension, this research also suggests that xenobiotic exposure could also enhance transcription of HERVs (directly, or indirectly via viral transactivation) and thereby contribute to autoimmunity.

---

[752] Valtysdóttir et al. Low serum dehydroepiandrosterone sulfate in women with primary Sjögren's syndrome as an isolated sign of impaired HPA axis function. *J Rheumatol.* 2001 Jun;28(6):1259-65
[753] Pillemer et al. Pilot clinical trial of dehydroepiandrosterone (DHEA) versus placebo for Sjögren's syndrome. *Arthritis Rheum.* 2004 Aug 15;51(4):601-4
[754] Virkki et al. Dehydroepiandrosterone (DHEA) substitution treatment for severe fatigue in DHEA-deficient patients with primary Sjögren's syndrome. *Arthritis Care Res* (Hoboken). 2010 Jan 15;62(1):118-24
[755] Inoue et al. Aryl hydrocarbon receptor-mediated induction of EBV reactivation as a risk factor for Sjögren's syndrome. *J Immunol.* 2012 May 1;188(9):4654-62

Raynaud's Phenomenon

Introduction:

Raynaud's Phenomenon is a disorder of periodic vasoconstriction mainly affecting the hands/fingers; it is a manifestation of autonomic dysfunction associated with and often preceding autoimmune diseases, especially scleroderma. Per the 2010 criteria for fibromyalgia (FM), Raynaud's is now associated with that condition as well; this may be absurd except that both Raynaud's and FM are causatively associated with microbial dysbiosis, especially in the intestines, i.e., *Helicobacter pylori* with Raynaud's and SIBO with FM. The condition responds poorly to medical/pharmacologic treatment that focuses on vasodilation; the condition responds very well to integrative treatment, especially that which focuses on dysbiosis eradication, antioxidant supplementation, hormonal correction/supplementation, and other components of the Functional Inflammology protocol. I am increasingly interested in approaching Raynaud phenomenon from the perspective of alleviating neurogenic inflammation.

Introduction and Diagnosis

- Introduction and terminology: Raynaud's phenomenon is periodic recurrent severe vasoconstriction-induced hypoperfusion accompanied by discomfort most commonly affecting the fingers.
  - Primary Raynaud's phenomenon—formerly "Raynaud's disease": Not associated with a concomitant disease; therefore, in this case the vasospasm is considered its own problem, hence the previously used term "disease" when describing primary Raynaud's phenomenon.
  - Secondary Raynaud's phenomenon—formerly "Raynaud's syndrome": Associated with a concomitant disease, especially autoimmunity, especially scleroderma.
- Diagnosis and Evaluation: Assessment for the presence/absence of systemic disease is important; Raynaud's can precede systemic autoimmunity by several years, for example in scleroderma.
  - Digital artery blood pressure: A decrease of > 15 mmHg is consistent with vasoconstriction.
  - Doppler ultrasound: Can be used to measure blood flow.
  - Routine labs: CBC, chemistry/metabolic panel, ANA, CRP, and the full thyroid evaluation in Chapter 1..
  - Nailfold capillaroscopy: Reveals microvascular changes consistent with autoimmunity and autoimmune-expedited cardiovascular disease. Per Cutolo et al[756], "Raynaud's phenomenon (RP) represents the most frequent clinical aspect of cardio/microvascular involvement and is a key feature of several autoimmune rheumatic diseases. Moreover, RP is associated in a statistically significant manner with many coronary diseases. In normal conditions or in primary RP (excluding during the cold-exposure test), the normal nailfold capillaroscopic pattern shows a regular disposition of the capillary loops along with the nailbed. On the contrary, in subjects suffering from secondary RP, one or more alterations of the capillaroscopic findings should alert the physician of the possibility of a connective tissue disease not yet detected. Nailfold capillaroscopy (NV) represents the best method to analyze microvascular abnormalities in autoimmune rheumatic diseases. Architectural disorganization, giant capillaries, hemorrhages, loss of capillaries, angiogenesis and avascular areas characterize >95% of patients with overt scleroderma (SSc)."
- Complications: Long-term recurrent vasoconstriction can result in atrophy of the skin and subcutaneous tissues including muscle; digital ulceration and ischemic gangrene can result. Recurrent vasospasm-induced tissue hypoxia appears to increase inflammation via oxidative stress and possibly via elaboration of damage-associated molecular patterns.

Clinical Applications and Interventions

- Raynaud's phenomenon—specific treatments: Treatment of Raynaud's phenomenon should not be trivialized as merely symptomatic; the pain experienced by some patients with Raynaud's phenomenon is truly excruciating. Additionally, a wonderfully insightful comment by Simonini et al[757] in 2000 stated that the tissue

---

[756] Cutolo et al. Nailfold capillaroscopy is useful for the diagnosis and follow-up of autoimmune rheumatic diseases. A future tool for the analysis of microvascular heart involvement? *Rheumatology* (Oxford). 2006 Oct;45 Suppl 4:iv43-6 rheumatology.oxfordjournals.org/content/45/suppl_4/iv43.full.pdf

[757] "...daily episodes of hypoxia-reperfusion injury, produces several episodes of free radicals-mediated endothelial derangement. These events results in a positive feedback effect of luminal narrowing and ischemia and therefore to the birth of a vicious cycle of oxygen free radicals (OFR) generation, leading to endothelial damage, intimal thickening and fibrosis." Simonini et al. Emerging potentials for an antioxidant therapy as a new approach to the treatment of systemic sclerosis. *Toxicology*. 2000 Nov 30;155(1-3):1-15

ischemia induced by Raynaud's phenomenon is *pathogenic* because it promotes oxidative stress and the vicious cycle of inflammation; the recurrent ischemia and reperfusion of hypoxic Raynaud's phenomenon could be thought of somewhat as a "recurrent, mild heart attack [or stroke] of the hands" causing tissue damage and cell apoptosis/necrosis leading to release of damage-associated molecular patterns (DAMP) and the resultant immune activation, systemic inflammation, mitochondrial dysfunction, proinflammatory immunophenotype switch toward Th1/Th2/Th17 and resultant fibrosis and autoimmunity. Remarkably, Mahoney et al[758] proposed a similar model in 2011 when they wrote, "We propose that a recent change in the conception of the role of type 1 interferon and the identification of adventitial stem cells suggests a unifying hypothesis for scleroderma. This hypothesis begins with vasospasm. Vasospasm is fully reversible unless, as proposed here, the resulting ischemia leads to apoptosis and activation of type 1 interferon. The interferon, we propose, initiates immune amplification, including characteristic scleroderma-specific antibodies." Thus, treatments to maintain vasodilation and quench the free radicals resultant from recurrent hypoxic events are necessary. Antioxidants have been discussed previously and should be common knowledge to readers of this text. Vasodilation in Raynaud's phenomenon can be supported with any/all of the following:

- o Eradication of *Helicobacter pylori*: Eradication of *Helicobacter pylori* is one of the most effective treatments of Raynaud's disease/syndrome/phenomenon and should therefore be pursued in all affected patients.
  - Helicobacter pylori eradication ameliorates primary Raynaud's phenomenon (*Dig Dis Sci* 1998 Aug[759]): "Forty-six patients affected by primary Raynaud's phenomenon were evaluated. *H. pylori* infection was assessed by [13C]urea breath test. Eradication therapy was given to infected patients for seven days. … **Attacks of Raynaud's phenomenon completely disappeared in 17% of the patients with *H. pylori* eradication. Discomfort and the duration and frequency of attacks of Raynaud's phenomenon were significantly reduced in 72% of the remaining patients.** … The study shows that *H. pylori* eradication causes a significant decrease in clinical attacks of Raynaud's disease. The reduction of vasoactive substances determined by the eradication of the bacterium may be the pathogenetic mechanism underlying the phenomenon."
- o Inositol hexaniacinate: 3,000-4,000 mg/d *po* in divided doses[760,761,762]
- o *Ginkgo biloba*: Ginkgo reduces the number of daily Raynaud's attacks in patients with primary Raynaud's disease[763], and it is also an excellent antioxidant with potent anti-inflammatory benefits.
- o Magnesium: 300-500 mg/d or bowel tolerance; systemic alkalinization to achieve urine alkalinity of 7.5 promotes renal retention of magnesium and systemic cellular uptake.
- o Combination fatty acid therapy: must include GLA (minimum 500 mg) and EPA (minimum 2,000 mg)
- o L-arginine: L-arginine is the biochemical precursor to nitric oxide, which has vasodilating actions. L-arginine supplementation in patients with Raynaud's phenomenon showed benefit in one study[764] and no benefit in another.[765] However, arginine supplementation was tremendously beneficial in 4 case reports of scleroderma patients with Raynaud's-induced digital necrosis.[766] Excess arginine supplementation may lead to an overproduction of nitric oxide, which can be harmful in excess due to its free radical behavior and its contribution to peroxynitrite. Additionally, metabolism of arginine requires methyl groups, and therefore supplementation with methyl donors such as methylfolate/folinate, cobalamin, betaine, et al should be used anytime supplemental arginine is used for long periods of time; homocysteine levels should occasionally be measured.

---

[758] Mahoney et al. A unifying hypothesis for scleroderma: identifying a target cell for scleroderma. *Curr Rheumatol Rep*. 2011 Feb;13:28-36

[759] Gasbarrini A et al. Helicobacter pylori eradication ameliorates primary Raynaud's phenomenon. *Dig Dis Sci*. 1998 Aug;43(8):1641-5

[760] "It appears to be a safe and well tolerated drug, which, together with other symptomatic measures, merits to be used in the management of vasospastic disease of the extremities even in the presence of partial obliteration of the microcirculation." Holti G. An experimentally controlled evaluation of the effect of inositol nicotinate upon the digital blood flow in patients with Raynaud's phenomenon. *J Int Med Res*. 1979;7(6):473-83

[761] "Although the mechanism of action remains unclear Hexopal is safe and is effective in reducing the vasospasm of primary Raynaud's disease during the winter months." Sunderland et al. A double blind randomised placebo controlled trial of hexopal in primary Raynaud's disease. *Clin Rheumatol*. 1988 Mar;7(1):46-9

[762] "It is suggested that long-term treatment with nicotinate acid derivatives may produce improvement in the peripheral circulation by a different mechanism than the transient effect detected by short-term studies." Ring et al. Quantitative thermographic assessment of inositol nicotinate therapy in Raynaud's phenomena. J Int Med Res. 1977;5(4):217-22

[763] "Ginkgo biloba phytosome may be effective in reducing the number of Raynaud's attacks per week in patients suffering from Raynaud's disease." Muir et al. The use of Ginkgo biloba in Raynaud's disease: a double-blind placebo-controlled trial. *Vasc Med*. 2002;7(4):265-7

[764] "After therapy, patients with Raynaud's phenomenon secondary to systemic sclerosis showed: (1) higher digital vasodilation after local warming, (2) cold-induced digital vasodilation, and (3) increase of plasma levels of tissue-type plasminogen activator." Agostoni et al. L-arginine therapy in Raynaud's phenomenon? *Int J Clin Lab Res*. 1991;21(2):202-3

[765] "L-arginine supplementation, however, had no significant effect on vascular responses to acetylcholine and sodium nitroprusside." Khan F, Belch JJ. Skin blood flow in patients with systemic sclerosis and Raynaud's phenomenon: effects of oral L-arginine supplementation. *J Rheumatol*. 1999 Nov;26(11):2389-94

[766] "We report two cases in which oral L-arginine reversed digital necrosis in Raynaud's phenomenon and two additional cases in which the symptoms of severe Raynaud's phenomenon were improved with oral L-arginine." Rembold et al. Oral L-arginine can reverse digital necrosis in Raynaud's phenomenon. *Mol Cell Biochem*. 2003 Feb;244:139-41

o <u>NAC 500-1,500mg *po tid ic*</u>: NAC is pleiotropically beneficial, via antiviral, antioxidant, GSH-supporting, and mTOR inhibiting actions.

- <u>Intravenous N-acetylcysteine for treatment of Raynaud's phenomenon secondary to systemic sclerosis</u> (*J Rheumatol* 2001 Oct[767])—paraphrased/quoted as follows: "Twenty-two patients with RP secondary to SSc were enrolled in a multicenter, open clinical trial lasting 11 weeks and conducted in winter. Primary outcome measures were frequency and severity of RP attacks, and number of digital ulcers. Secondary outcome measure was improvement in digital cold challenge test assessed by photoelectric plethysmography. Patients received a continuous 5 day intravenous infusion of NAC starting with a 2 h loading dose of 150 mg/kg subsequently adjusted to 15 mg/kg/h. RESULTS: … Both frequency and severity of RP attacks decreased significantly compared to pretreatment values. Active ulcers were significantly less numerous at all follow-up visits (25% of baseline count on Day 33 from the beginning of infusion). In the cold challenge test, mean recovery time fell by 69%, 67%, 71%, and 71% on Days 12, 19, 33, and 61 from the beginning of treatment. Side effects were minor, easily controlled, and reversible. CONCLUSION: N-acetylcysteine appears to be safe for the treatment of RP secondary to SSc. These preliminary data warrant further controlled studies."

o <u>Acupuncture, biofeedback, counseling, stress reduction, cold avoidance, smoking cessation</u>: Since stressful events, cold exposure, and cigarette smoking are all vasoconstrictive, these should be avoided/modified to the highest extent possible. Stress reduction and modification of inter- and intra-personal socioemotional exchange would be beneficial for anyone.

- <u>Biofeedback treatment of Raynaud's disease and phenomenon</u> (*Biofeedback Self Regul.* 1981 Sep[768]): "Six Raynaud's disease [primary] and four Raynaud's phenomenon [secondary] patients were treated with 12 sessions of finger temperature biofeedback. The mean frequency of vasospastic attacks was reduced to 7.5% of that reported during the pretreatment baseline and was maintained for a 1 year follow-up period. … Raynaud's phenomenon [secondary] patients showed significantly greater temperature increases during feedback periods than Raynaud's disease [primary] patients."

o <u>Hormonal interventions</u>: Annotated below:

- <u>Treatment of Raynaud's phenomenon with large doses of triiodothyronine [T3]</u> (*Ann Rheum Dis.* 1987 Dec[769]): Triiodothyronine was prescribed at a dosage of 80 mcg/d to 9 female patients with autoimmunity (SLE, SSc, RA, overlap syndrome [OS]); they all experienced safe and significant remission of their Raynaud's symptoms. Patients who could not tolerate 80 mcg/d due to anticipated heat intolerance and palpitations were treated with lower doses of 40-60 mcg/d. "In all patients, blood pressure, pulse pressure, and pulse rate remained essentially unchanged and thyroid function tests were confirmatory of drug compliance. … In the first place, every one of them described a substantial, if not dramatic, improvement in their condition. … Large dosages of T3 were found in this study to be a highly effective treatment for Raynaud's phenomenon and one principally free from side effects."

- <u>Treatment of Raynaud's phenomenon with triiodothyronine [T3] corrects co-existent autonomic dysfunction</u> (*Postgrad Med J* 1992 Apr[770]): Nine female patients with autoimmunity and Raynaud's phenomenon showed a high prevalence of cardiovascular autonomic dysfunction as assessed by five standard non-invasive tests (3 of heart rate and 2 of blood pressure). "The subjects were given triiodothyronine, 60 to 80 micrograms per day, for vasospastic attacks. … Test results [of autonomic function] showed a considerable improvement. … Adverse side effects to triiodothyronine occurred in a single subject and were readily controlled. … Triiodothyronine may have corrected autonomic dysfunction by increasing blood flow to ischemic peripheral nerves or by acting on the autonomic system more directly."

---

[767] Sambo et al. Intravenous N-acetylcysteine for treatment of Raynaud's phenomenon secondary to systemic sclerosis: a pilot study. *J Rheumatol.* 2001 Oct;28(10):2257-62

[768] Freedman et al. Biofeedback treatment of Raynaud's disease and phenomenon. *Biofeedback Self Regul.* 1981 Sep;6(3):355-65

[769] Dessein PH, Gledhill RF. Treatment of Raynaud's phenomenon with large doses of triiodothyronine: a pilot study. *Ann Rheum Dis.* 1987 Dec;46(12):944-5

[770] Gledhill et al. Treatment of Raynaud's phenomenon with triiodothyronine corrects co-existent autonomic dysfunction. *Postgrad Med J.* 1992 Apr;68(798):263-7

- Successful treatment of Raynaud's phenomenon with L-thyroxine [T4] (*Med Hypotheses* 2003 Mar[771]):"A 50-year old patient a 15-year history of Raynaud's phenomenon developed thyroid deficiency with exacerbation of the symptoms of Raynaud's. After substitution therapy with L-thyroxine, the patient became euthyroid and the symptoms of Raynaud's phenomenon disappeared. Similarly, several patients with Raynaud's phenomenon were found to be hypothyroid and replacement therapy again eliminated the symptoms."
- 7-oxo-DHEA contra Raynaud's phenomenon (*Med Hypotheses* 2003 Mar[772]): The authors of this report basically provide a review of the literature on Raynaud's phenomenon—its assessments and treatments—and then provide a single case report of improvement; the dose and duration of treatment are not provided. "An initial result is encouraging. A 46-year old patient had increasingly frequent vasospastic attacks accompanied by pain and pallor in her left fingers except the thumb. Precipitating factors included being in an excessively air-conditioned environment, touching cold objects, and digging in cold, wet earth. The episodes were less than 10 min duration. The patient had no other complaints, denied other illnesses, and does not take any prescription medications. The patient does not smoke, and consumes minimal amounts of alcohol occasionally. On examination, her hands were without any abnormalities with normal skin and color appearance. These vasospastic attacks did not occur after taking 7-oxo-DHEA but returned within one week of discontinuing the medication, and disappeared again on resuming the medication." Obviously that is a pretty weak case report, but nonetheless, clinicians might consider using this generally considered as safe nonprescription agent in conjunction with the treatments aforementioned.

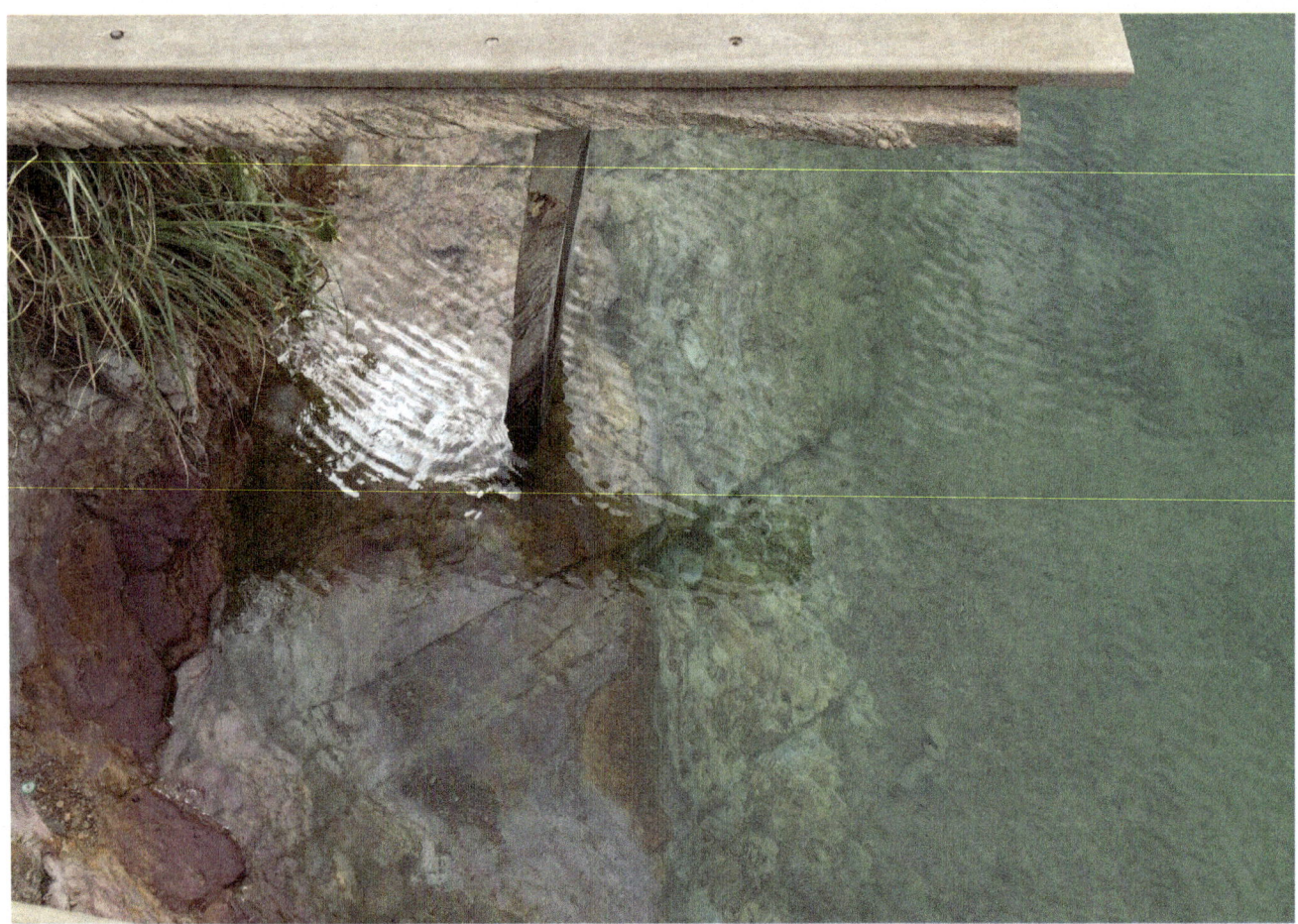

Lago Azul (Blue Lake) near Villa de Leyva, Colombia: 2014 photo by DrV

---

[771] Ihler et al. 7-oxo-DHEA and Raynaud's phenomenon. *Med Hypotheses.* 2003 Mar;60(3):391-7
[772] Ihler et al. 7-oxo-DHEA and Raynaud's phenomenon. *Med Hypotheses.* 2003 Mar;60(3):391-7

Clinical Notes on Additional Conditions:
Behçet's Disease, Sarcoidosis, Dermatomyositis and Polymyositis

---

Introduction:

The sections that follow are original to *Integrative Rheumatology* 2006/2007; later versions of my books were too large to allow inclusion of these sections per limitations of the publisher's printing capacity, and thus the sections were not updated. Here, they are presented with few modifications, mostly the removal of redundant material presented in the previous sections. The overall clinical approach is generally as outlined previously since all autoimmune/autoinflammatory diseases have the same basic components as recalled per the F.I.N.D.S.E.X.® acronym. I strongly agree with Throeau's statement that "What is once done well is done forever" (*Civil Disobedience*, page 13), and I consider the previous reviews to be at least reasonable and the research from which it was derived no less valuable simply because it has acquired a few years without updated reinforcement; the updates made to the overall protocol should generally suffice, along with the following details and nuances.

Behçet's Disease/Syndrome

<u>Description/pathophysiology</u>:
- **A relapsing systemic/multiorgan autoimmune disease associated with vasculopathy and ulcerations of the oral and genital mucosa**
- "Idiopathic"[773]; etiopathogenic associations include:
  - ○ Occult **bacterial**/viral/fungal/parasitic infections with resultant molecular mimicry and stimulation of autoreactive T-cells[774]: as summarized by Verity et al[775], "…the evidence indicates that **the underlying immune events in BD are triggered by a microbial antigen** and subsequently driven by genetic influences which control leukocyte behavior and the coagulation pathways."
  - ○ Associated with HLA-B51 in Japan and Mediterranean areas
- Considered **uncommon in the US**

<u>Clinical presentations</u>:
- Two-fold more common in men than in women
- Age of onset is generally in 20's and 30's; may occur in children
- Painful oral and genital ulcers: resembles recurrent aphthous stomatitis, most commonly the first manifestation of the disease
- Ocular complaints: pain, photophobia, blurred vision, iridocyclitis
- Skin lesions in 80% of patients: papules, pustules, vesicles, folliculitis, erythema nodosum-like lesions, "exaggerated" inflammatory reactions to minor skin trauma
- Joint pain: nondestructive arthritis in 50% of patients
- Vasculitis and thrombophlebitis: can affect any organ
- Neurocognitive disturbances and central nervous system involvement
- Abdominal pain and intestinal involvement: some patients have evidence of enteropathy

<u>Major differential diagnoses</u>:
- Aphthous stomatitis (DDX: oral herpes)
- Autoimmunity in general, vasculitis in particular
- Infection: conceivably possible to confuse oral ulcers with Koplic's spots
- Crohn's disease—multisystemic disease, oral ulcerations

---

[773] Beers MH, Berkow R (eds). *Merck Manual. 17ᵗʰ Edition*. Whitehouse Station; Merck Research Laboratories 1999 Page 424
[774] Sakane et al. Etiopathology of Behcet's disease: immunological aspects. *Yonsei Med J*. 1997 Dec;38(6):350-8 eymj.org/1997/pdf/12350.pdf
[775] Verity et al. Behcet's disease: from Hippocrates to the third millennium. *Br J Ophthalmol*. 2003 Sep;87(9):1175-83 bjo.bmjjournals.com/cgi/reprint/87/9/1175

Clinical assessments:

- **History/subjective**:
  - See clinical presentations
- **Physical examination/objective**:
  - Oral, ocular, and genital examinations
  - Other examinations as indicated
- **Laboratory assessments**:
  - ESR: elevated
  - CBC: mild leukocytosis
  - HLA-B51: may or may not be positive, but is associated with increased likelihood of the disease
  - Homocysteine: Patients with Behcet's syndrome have elevated homocysteine which exacerbates arterial and venous occlusion which underlies many of the clinical complications of the disease.[776,777]
  - Lactulose/mannitol assay: Patients with Behcet's disease have increased intestinal permeability.[778] Whether this is due in an individual patient to gastrointestinal dysbiosis or is simply a gastrointestinal reflection of systemic inflammation should be determined on a per-patient basis. Dysbiosis is so common in patients with the combination of 1) autoimmunity and 2) "leaky gut" that such patients should be presumed to have dysbiosis until proven otherwise by comprehensive parasitology assessment by a specialty laboratory.
  - Oxidant/antioxidant assessment: Numerous studies have documented increased oxidative stress and decrease antioxidant defenses in patients with Behcet's disease.[779] Vitamin C deficiency has been documented.[780] Broad-spectrum antioxidant therapy with diet and supplements is indicated.
  - Assessment for occult infections and dysbiosis: Research suggests the probability that Behcet's disease is stimulated by occult bacterial/viral/fungal/parasitic infections with resultant molecular mimicry and stimulation of autoreactive T-cells.[781] **Bacteria that have been most consistently associated with this disease are *Streptococcus sanguis*, *Escherichia coli*, *Staphylococcus aureus*[782], and *Chlamydia pneumoniae*,** as discussed in the Treatment section that follows. **The fact that antimicrobial/penicillin administration reduces the severity and frequency of the disease clearly indicates that the disease is perpetuated at least in part by an occult infection.**[783] Additional support for a microbial contribution to the pathogenesis of this disease comes from studies showing **exacerbations of the disease following exposure to streptococcal antigens**.[784] There is no consistent evidence of *B. burgdorferi*[785] (Lyme disease), varicella zoster[786], or viral hepatitis[787] in most patients with Behcet's.
  - Xenobiotic depuration: Impairment in acetylation has been demonstrated[788] and may contribute to the pathogenesis of Behcet's disease by leading to the accumulation of xenobiotics or the haptenization of

---

[776] "CONCLUSION: Homocysteine may play a role in ocular involvement of BD. Chronic inflammation can induce hyperhomocysteinemia, thereby leading to thrombosis in the retinal vascular bed in a way similar to that recently proposed for the pathogenesis of coronary artery disease." Okka et al. Plasma homocysteine level and uveitis in Behcet's disease. *Isr Med Assoc J*. 2002 Nov;4(11 Suppl):931-4

[777] "CONCLUSION: Hyperhomocysteinaemia may be assumed to be an independent risk factor for venous thrombosis in BD. Unlike the factor V Leiden mutation, hyperhomocysteinaemia is a correctable risk factor. This finding might lead to new avenues in the prophylaxis of thrombosis in BD." Aksu et al. Hyperhomocysteinaemia in Behcet's disease. *Rheumatology* (Oxford). 2001 Jun;40(6):687-90 rheumatology.oxfordjournals.org/cgi/reprint/40/6/687

[778] "The intestinal permeability in BS was significantly more than that seen among the healthy controls." Fresko et al. Intestinal permeability in Behcet's syndrome. *Ann Rheum Dis*. 2001 Jan;60(1):65-6 ard.bmjjournals.com/cgi/reprint/60/1/65

[779] Kose et al. Lipid peroxidation and erythrocyte antioxidant enzymes in patients with Behcet's disease. *Tohoku J Exp Med*. 2002 May;197(1):9-16 jstage.jst.go.jp/article/tjem/197/1/9/_pdf

[780] Noyan et al. The serum vitamin C levels in Behcet's disease. *Yonsei Med J*. 2003 Oct 30;44(5):771-8 eymj.org/2003/pdf/10771.pdf

[781] Sakane et al. Etiopathology of Behcet's disease: immunological aspects. *Yonsei Med J*. 1997 Dec;38(6):350-8 eymj.org/1997/pdf/12350.pdf

[782] Direskeneli H. Behcet's disease: infectious aetiology, new autoantigens, and HLA-B51. *Ann Rheum Dis*. 2001 Nov;60(11):996-1002 ard.bmjjournals.com/cgi/reprint/60/11/996

[783] "CONCLUSION: Penicillin treatment was demonstrated to offer adjunctive benefits in the prevention of arthritis episodes which are not obtainable with colchicine monotherapy. This finding could provide additional evidence for antigen triggering in the pathogenesis of Behcet's disease." Calguneri et al. The effect of prophylactic penicillin treatment on the course of arthritis episodes in patients with Behcet's disease. A randomized clinical trial. *Arthritis Rheum*. 1996 Dec;39(12):2062-5

[784] "Interestingly, the induction of systemic Behcet's disease symptoms was observed after the streptococcus skin test in 15 of 85 cases tested, but no case of induction by the other bacteria was observed. Our study supports the possible pathogenetic role of certain streptococcal antigens in Behcet's disease." Behcet's Disease Research Committee of Japan. Skin hypersensitivity to streptococcal antigens and the induction of systemic symptoms by the antigens in Behcet's disease. *J Rheumatol*. 1989 Apr;16(4):506-11

[785] "CONCLUSION: These results suggest no association between Behcet's disease and B. burgdorferi infection." Onen et al. Seroprevalence of Borrelia burgdorferi in patients with Behcet's disease. *Rheumatol Int*. 2003 Nov;23(6):289-9

[786] "The serological positivity for VZV IgG and IgM antibodies in BD was not statistically different from other skin diseases." Akdeniz et al. The seroprevalence of varicella zoster antibodies in Behcet's and other skin diseases. *Eur J Epidemiol*. 2003;18(1):91-3

[787] "HGV-RNA was detected in two patients with BD and in none of the healthy controls. In conclusion, BD does not seem to be associated with hepatitis viral infections including hepatitis B, C, or G." Ozkan et al. Is there any association between hepatitis G virus (HGV), other hepatitis viruses (HBV, HCV) and Behcet's disease? *J Dermatol*. 2005 May;32(5):361-4

[788] "As a result of this study we conclude the NAT2 slow acetylator status may be a determinant in susceptibility to Behcet's disease. This finding may have implications for the theories of the pathogenesis of the disease as well as for therapeutic aspects." Tamer et al. N-acetyltransferase 2 polymorphisms in patients with Behcet's disease. *Clin Exp Dermatol*. 2005 Jan;30(1):56-60

endogenous antigens by reactive intermediates. Assessment of detoxification with caffeine-benzoate-aspirin-acetaminophen challenge may provide therapeutic insight when working with individual patients, particularly those with a history of xenobiotic exposure and/or multiple chemical sensitivity.

- **Imaging**:
  - Only for monitoring complications and excluding other diseases
- **Establishing the diagnosis**: Clinical assessment based on published criteria[789]
  - Recurrent oral/genital mucosal lesions: at least 3 times in one 12-month period, *plus two of the following*:
    - Eye lesions: Anterior uveitis, posterior uveitis, or retinal vasculitis
    - Skin lesions: Erythema nodosum, pseudofolliculitis, papulopustular lesions, or acneiform nodules
    - Positive pathergy test: Exaggerated inflammatory skin response 24–48 hours following otherwise benign injury/trauma to the skin
  - Diagnosis is additionally supported by:
    - Elevated ESR
    - Systemic/multiorgan relapsing disease, and associated clinical presentations and findings
    - Exclusion of other diseases: this is "relative" rather than "absolute" due to the nonspecific nature of Behcet's disease

Complications:

- **Blindness**: Patients with ocular involvement are at risk for blindness—urgent/emergency referral/immunosuppression may be necessary
- Paralysis
- Vena cava obstruction

Clinical management:

- Referral if clinical outcome is unsatisfactory or if serious complications are evident.
- **Medical approach per *Merck Manual* up to 1999**: "The syndrome is generally chronic and manageable... Symptomatic treatment is relatively successful." [790]

Treatments:

- Medical/pharmaceutical treatments:
  - Colchicine: 0.5 mg BID or TID for the treatment of oral/genital ulcers[791]
  - Topical corticosteroids: For oral and ocular involvement; oral corticosteroid therapy does not alter the course of the disease[792]
  - High-dose oral prednisone: 60-80 mg/d is indicated for severe uveitis, CNS involvement, or other urgent complications; cyclosporine immunosuppression is indicated for patients who do not respond to prednisone[793]
- Antioxidant therapy: Such as with mixed tocopherols[794] or Chinese herbal formula called "BG-104"[795] and any combination of antioxidants such as lipoic acid and phytonutrients. Recall that the Paleo-Mediterranean diet is inherently antioxidative due to the low glycemic indexes and loads and the additive and synergistic effects of phytonutrients from fruits, vegetables, nuts, seeds, and berries.[796]
- Orthoendocrinology: On an individual basis, clinicians and patients may find it valuable to assess prolactin, cortisol, DHEA, free and total testosterone, serum estradiol, and thyroid status (e.g., TSH, T4, *and* anti-thyroid peroxidase antibodies). Some studies have shown that patients with Behcet's disease have higher levels of

[789] Verity et al. Behcet's disease: from Hippocrates to the third millennium. *Br J Ophthalmol*. 2003 Sep;87(9):1175-83 bjo.bmjjournals.com/cgi/reprint/87/9/1175
[790] Beers MH, Berkow R (eds). *Merck Manual. 17th Edition*. Whitehouse Station; Merck Research Laboratories 1999 page 425
[791] Beers MH, Berkow R (eds). *Merck Manual. 17th Edition*. Whitehouse Station; Merck Research Laboratories 1999 page 425
[792] Beers MH, Berkow R (eds). *Merck Manual. 17th Edition*. Whitehouse Station; Merck Research Laboratories 1999 page 425
[793] Beers MH, Berkow R (eds). *Merck Manual. 17th Edition*. Whitehouse Station; Merck Research Laboratories 1999 page 425
[794] Kokcam I, Naziroglu M. Effects of vitamin E supplementation on blood antioxidants levels in patients with Behcet's disease. *Clin Biochem*. 2002 Nov;35(8):633-9
[795] "The treatment with BG-104 and/or vitamin E significantly enhanced the plasma SSA in all disorders studied. Both the erythrocyte sedimentation rates, the absolute number of neutrophils, as well as C-reactive protein levels were significantly lower in patients treated with BG-104 and/or vitamin E than those without these drugs." Pronai et al. BG-104 enhances the decreased plasma superoxide scavenging activity in patients with Behcet's disease, Sjogren's syndrome or hematological malignancy. *Biotherapy*. 1991;3(4):365-71
[796] Liu RH. Health benefits of fruit and vegetables are from additive and synergistic combinations of phytochemicals. *Am J Clin Nutr*. 2003 Sep;78(3 Suppl):517S-520S

proinflammatory ==prolactin== than do normal controls[797], while other groups have contradicted these findings.[798,799]

- Antimicrobial treatments and assessment for dysbiosis: **Assess for occult infections; treat as indicated.** In patients for whom no specific microbes are detected with specialty testing such as stool testing or mucosal culture, clinicians should treat for presumptive bacterial overgrowth of the small bowel.

  - Orodental dysbiosis: Since ==oral infection with variant strains of *Streptococcus sanguis* are the most likely and most consistently identified single source of antigenic stimulation in patients with Behcet's disease==[800], all patients should use potent antimicrobial mouthwashes daily. Obviously, extracts from berberine-containing botanicals such as *Hydrastis canadensis* are first-line therapy due to their potency against oral *Streptococcus* species.[801] Since non-berberine constituents—flavonoids—from *Hydrastis* are synergistically antimicrobial and increase the effectiveness of berberine against oral pathogens[802], the ideal antimicrobial in this regard would be a broad-spectrum extract standardized for its content of berberine. Berberine/Hydrastis powder can be used in a "swish, hold, and swallow" mouth rinse—the initial taste is quite bitter but it becomes tolerable; patients may prefer a comparatively better-tasting antimicrobial mouthwash such as Listerine or its generic equivalent. Warm water nasal lavage with Berberine/Hydrastis powder, salt and baking soda (sodium chloride and sodium bicarbonate) can be used twice daily and is well-tolerated. **Patients with orodental/sinus dysbiosis should get into the habit of ❶ cleaning their sinuses (ie, nasal lavage) when ❷ brushing their teeth and ❸ using antimicrobial mouthwash, a tripartite event that should occur at least twice daily.**

  - Gastrointestinal dysbiosis: Although patients with Behcet's disease appear to have a similar prevalence of *Helicobacter pylori* as the rest of the population, ==eradication of gastrointestinal *H. pylori* infection leads to clinical improvement and resolution of genital and oral ulcers in these patients, thus showing that gastrointestinal dysbiosis is an underlying pathoetiologic factor in this condition.==[803]

  - Sinorespiratory dysbiosis: **Recent research has clearly demonstrated evidence of chronic *Chlamydia pneumoniae* infections in Behcets patients.**[804] Per Ben-Yaakov et al[805], "Because there is as yet no standardization of serological criteria for persistent infection, we considered antibody titers of > 1/20 in the IgA fraction, together with **IgG titers of 1/64 to 1/256, to be indicative of persistent infection.**"

    ```
    Chlamydia pneumoniae IgG     >1:256   High        Neg:<1:16
    Chlamydia pneumoniae IgM     <1:10                Neg:<1:10
    ```

    Elevated titers to *Chlamydia/Chlamydophila pneumoniae* suggesting chronic persistent infection—improvement with azithromycin and NAC: Following detection of the elevated antibody titer, the patient started on azithromycin and NAC, which resulted in a short-term (12-hour) exacerbation of symptoms followed by complete and sustained resolution of sinus congestion and improved energy levels and exercise endurance.

  - Cutaneous dysbiosis: Recent research implicates the skin as a loci of dysbiosis: **pustules of patients with Behcet's disease are not sterile**[806] and are contaminated with bacteria that are distinct from those seen in regular acne and which are productive of antigens and superantigens that are capable of perpetuating

---

[797] "The mean prolactin levels in all subgroups of patients with BD were higher than normal, but no statistically significant difference was shown between these subgroups. CONCLUSION: Hyperprolactinemia occurred in a small number of patients with BD and its significance remained unclear. Serum PRL level did not correlate with disease manifestations and activity." Houman et al. Prolactin levels in Behcet's disease: no correlation with disease manifestations and activity. *Ann Med Interne* (Paris). 2001 Apr;152(3):209-11

[798] "However, we found no such correlation in Behcet's disease. On the contrary, prolactin levels were lower in attacks than in remissions." Apaydin et al. Serum prolactin levels in Behcet's disease. *Jpn J Ophthalmol.* 2000 Jul-Aug;44(4):442-5

[799] "We found that mean PRL levels in patients with clinically active BS, were not significantly higher than patients with clinically inactive BS and healthy controls." Keser et al. Serum prolactin levels in Behcet's Syndrome. *Clin Rheumatol.* 1999;18(4):351-2

[800] Direskeneli H. Behcet's disease: infectious aetiology, new autoantigens, and HLA-B51. *Ann Rheum Dis.* 2001:996-1002 ard.bmjjournals.com/cgi/content/full/60/11/996#B26

[801] "Thus, berberine sulfate interferes with the adherence of group A streptococci by two distinct mechanisms: one by releasing the adhesin lipoteichoic acid from the streptococcal cell surface and another by directly preventing or dissolving lipoteichoic acid-fibronectin complexes." Sun et al. Berberine sulfate blocks adherence of Streptococcus pyogenes to epithelial cells, fibronectin, and hexadecane. *Antimicrob Agents Chemother.* 1988 Sep;32(9):1370-4

[802] "Berberine (3) exhibited an additive antimicrobial effect when tested against S. mutans in combination with 1." Hwang et al. Antimicrobial constituents from goldenseal (the Rhizomes of Hydrastis canadensis) against selected oral pathogens. *Planta Med.* 2003 Jul;69(7):623-7

[803] "In 13 patients with BD, the number and size of oral and genital ulcers diminished significantly and various clinical manifestations regressed after the eradication of HP. CONCLUSION: HP may be involved in the pathogenesis of BD." Avci et al. Helicobacter pylori and Behcet's disease. *Dermatology.* 1999;199(2):140-3

[804] "These finding provide serological evidence of chronic C. pneumoniae infection in association with Behcet's disease." Ayaslioglu et al. Evidence of chronic Chlamydia pneumoniae infection in patients with Behcet's disease. *Scand J Infect Dis.* 2004;36(6-7):428-30

[805] Ben-Yaakov et al. Prevalence of antibodies to Chlamydia pneumoniae in an Israeli population without clinical evidence of respiratory infection. *J Clin Pathol.* 2002 May:355-8

[806] "At least one type of microorganism was grown from each pustule. Staphylococcus aureus (41/70, 58.6%, p = 0.008) and Prevotella spp (17/70, 24.3%, p = 0.002) were significantly more common in pustules from BS patients, and coagulase negative staphylococci (17/37, 45.9%, p = 0.007) in pustules from acne patients. CONCLUSIONS: The pustular lesions of BS are not usually sterile." Hatemi et al. The pustular skin lesions in Behcet's syndrome are not sterile. *Ann Rheum Dis.* 2004 Nov;63(11):1450-2

the disease via proinflammatory immunodysregulation. Furthermore, there is **a direct relationship between number of pustules and the severity of arthritis**[807] which suggests that proinflammatory immunodysregulation may result from microbial antigens and superantigens from cutaneous dysbiosis.

  - o Clinical implementation: In patients with established Behcet's disease, clinicians may be faced with the task of simultaneously treating numerous dysbiotic loci—mouth and gastrointestinal tract, sinus and lungs, and skin. Indeed, treatment should be orchestrated to address different loci with as few treatments as possible and as broadly as possible—**all loci should be treated simultaneously**. This may require co-administration of botanical and pharmaceutical antimicrobials, with the latter chosen for their systemic bioavailability. Patients should generally implement the alkalinizing supplemented Paleo-Mediterranean diet (with broad-spectrum fatty acid supplementation, probiotics, vitamin D, etc.) to effect a down-regulation of inflammation for the purpose of gaining some stability before facing aggressive antimicrobial treatment, which can trigger a "die off" Herxheimer-type reaction due to increased microbial (endo)toxin production.[808] Since the treatment of large/systemic bacterial infections can lead to a dramatic increase in endotoxin release[809], prophylactic treatment with NFkB inhibitors, or other potent anti-inflammatory treatments (such as single-dose prednisone) might be considered.

- <u>Treatments to lower homocysteine</u>: Patients with Behcet's syndrome have elevated homocysteine which exacerbates arterial and venous occlusion which underlies many of the clinical complications of the disease.[810,811] See previously detailed section—most recently updated in sections on migraine and fibromyalgia.
- *Ginkgo biloba*: Ginkgo may be of therapeutic value due to its anticoagulant, vasodilating, antioxidant, and anti-inflammatory actions. *In vitro* studies demonstrate an antioxidant benefit of ginkgo in erythrocytes of Behcets patients.[812]

---

[807] Diri et al. Papulopustular skin lesions are seen more frequently in patients with Behcet's syndrome who have arthritis: a controlled and masked study. *Ann Rheum Dis.* 2001 Nov;60(11):1074-6 ard.bmjjournals.com/cgi/reprint/60/11/1074

[808] "There is clear experimental evidence that antibiotics increase the bioavailability of endotoxin from Gram-negative bacteria." Hurley JC. Antibiotic-induced release of endotoxin. A therapeutic paradox. *Drug Saf.* 1995 Mar;12(3):183-95

[809] "A three- to 20-fold increase in the total concentration of endotoxin occurs as a consequence of antibiotic action on gram-negative bacteria both in vitro and in vivo." Hurley JC. Antibiotic-induced release of endotoxin: a reappraisal. *Clin Infect Dis.* 1992 Nov;15(5):840-54

[810] "CONCLUSION: Homocysteine may play a role in ocular involvement of BD. Chronic inflammation can induce hyperhomocysteinemia, thereby leading to thrombosis in the retinal vascular bed in a way similar to that recently proposed for the pathogenesis of coronary artery disease." Okka et al. Plasma homocysteine level and uveitis in Behcet's disease. *Isr Med Assoc J.* 2002 Nov;4(11 Suppl):931-4

[811] "CONCLUSION: Hyperhomocysteinaemia may be assumed to be an independent risk factor for venous thrombosis in BD. Unlike the factor V Leiden mutation, hyperhomocysteinaemia is a correctable risk factor. This finding might lead to new avenues in the prophylaxis of thrombosis in BD." Aksu et al. Hyperhomocysteinaemia in Behcet's disease. *Rheumatology* (Oxford). 2001 Jun;40(6):687-90 rheumatology.oxfordjournals.org/cgi/reprint/40/6/687

[812] "These data indicate that an oxidative damage is present in erythrocytes obtained from Behcet's patients, and EGb 761 [Ginkgo biloba extract], which may strengthen the antioxidant defense system, may contribute to the treatment of BD." Kose et al. In vitro antioxidant effect of Ginkgo biloba extract (EGb 761) on lipoperoxidation induced by hydrogen peroxide in erythrocytes of Behcet's patients. *Jpn J Pharmacol.* 1997 Nov;75(3):253-8

Sarcoidosis

Description/pathophysiology:

- A multisystem granulomatous disease; symptoms are dependent upon the site of involvement, most common of which is the mediastinum as well as central and peripheral lymph nodes.
- Sarcoidosis is not a *classic* autoimmune disease except that 1) endogenous immune mechanisms contribute to tissue destruction and clinical manifestations, and 2) approximately 20% of patients have endocrine autoimmunity.[813]
- Spontaneous improvement and resolution may occur in as many as 50-80% of patients.
- Like many inflammatory conditions, sarcoidosis was considered "idiopathic"[814]; new research is suggesting that—as with other disorders of sustained inflammation—occult infections (i.e., dysbiosis) are the underlying trigger.[815] The proposal that the condition has an infectious etiology is somewhat supported by cure of the disease in two case reports following administration of melatonin[816], which has potent immunostimulatory and anti-infective actions.[817]

Clinical presentations:

- Typical age of onset is between 20-40 years
- More common in Northern Europeans and African Americans (two groups with pandemic vitamin D deficiency)
- Typical autoimmune systemic manifestations: fatigue, malaise, low-grade fever, anorexia, and weight loss
- Hypercalcemia—due to a combination of hyperparathyroidism and granulomatous conversion of 25-hydroxycholecalciferol (the less active form of vitamin D) to 1,25-dihydroxycholecalciferol (the much more active form of vitamin D)
- Hyperparathyroidism
- Lymphadenopathy
- Dermal plaques and nodules in chronic disease
- Erythema nodosum—a nonspecific dermatologic manifestation characterized by erythema and subcutaneous nodules—this is considered a positive/beneficial finding in sarcoidosis because it is the best predictor of benign course of disease
- Hepatic granulomas are found in 70% of patients and may be present despite normal levels of serum liver enzymes
- **Granulomatous uveitis occurs in 15% of patients and can result in bilateral blindness—this must be treated as a medically urgent condition.**
- Cardiac involvement—seen in 5-10% of patients—can result in heart failure
- Peripheral polyarthropathy or oligoarthropathy
- CNS involvement and cranial nerve palsies: **neurosarcoidosis has been associated with a 10% mortality[818] and must therefore be treated as a medically urgent condition.**

Major differential diagnoses:

- Lymphoma
- Tuberculosis

---

[813] "In conclusion, a high frequency of endocrine autoimmunity in patients with sarcoidosis, occurring in about 20% of the cases, was demonstrated. Thyroid autoimmunity and polyglandular autoimmune syndromes occurred most frequently." Papadopoulos et al. High frequency of endocrine autoimmunity in patients with sarcoidosis. *Eur J Endocrinol* 1996 Mar;134(3):331-336

[814] Beers MH, Berkow R (eds). *Merck Manual. 17th Edition.* Whitehouse Station; Merck Research Laboratories: 1999, pages 2482-85

[815] "But now the inflammation of sarcoidosis has succumbed to antibiotics in two independent studies. This review examines the cell wall deficient (antibiotic resistant) bacteria which have been found in tissue from patients with sarcoidosis." Marshall TG, Marshall FE. Sarcoidosis succumbs to antibiotics--implications for autoimmune disease. *Autoimmun Rev.* 2004 Jun;3(4):295-300

[816] Cagnoni et al. Melatonin for treatment of chronic refractory sarcoidosis. *Lancet.* 1995 Nov 4;346(8984):1229-30

[817] Gitto et al. Effects of melatonin treatment in septic newborns. *Pediatr Res.* 2001 Dec;50(6):756-60 pedresearch.org/cgi/content/full/50/6/756

[818] "Neurosarcoidosis carries a mortality of 10 per cent, over twice that of sarcoidosis overall." James DG. Life-threatening situations in sarcoidosis. *Sarcoidosis Vasc Diffuse Lung Dis* 1998 Sep;15(2):134-9

- **Fungal infection of the lungs: histoplasmosis, coccidioidomycosis, aspergillosis, cryptococcosis**— appropriate management of sarcoidosis requires exclusion of these conditions before the administration of prednisone or other immunosuppressants.
- Rheumatoid arthritis with pulmonary involvement
- Idiopathic pulmonary fibrosis

Clinical assessments:
- **History/subjective**: See clinical presentations.
- **Physical examination/objective**:
    - As indicated—see clinical presentations
    - Skin examination
    - Cardiopulmonary examination
- **Laboratory assessments**:
    - Leukopenia: common
    - Elevated serum uric acid: without gout
    - Alkaline phosphatase and GGT: elevated with liver involvement
    - Assessment for any and all types of dysbiosis and/or the implementation of empiric clinical trials of systemic antimicrobial treatments appears warranted based on emerging evidence that occult infections are a primary perpetuating factor in this disease.[819]
    - Creatine kinase: may be elevated in patients with sarcoid myopathy
    - Intestinal permeability (IP) assessment with lactulose and mannitol: Increased intestinal permeability in patients with active sarcoidosis has been documented.[820] The clinical implications of this are not perfectly clear, since the increased mucosal permeability may simply reflect systemic inflammation and does not necessarily point to an enterogenic problem. However, as discussed previously in Chapter 4, increased intestinal permeability alone is sufficient to perpetuate systemic inflammation via increased antigen absorption and bacterial translocation. Some doctors use IP testing as a barometer of overall health and thus IP testing can be used to objectively quantify overall health.
    - Endocrine autoimmunity is very common (20%) in patients with sarcoidosis[821] and is detected by appropriate serologic tests and clinical assessments:
        - Hashimoto's thyroiditis: elevated anti-thyroid peroxidase enzymes, normal or elevated TSH
        - Grave's disease: elevated thyrotropin-receptor antibodies; suppressed TSH, elevated T4
        - Addison's disease: increased ACTH, low cortisol, failure to increase cortisol production following ACTH injection, anti-adrenal antibodies[822]
        - Insulin-dependent diabetes mellitus: hyperglycemia with hypoinsulinemia
        - Premature ovarian failure: anovulation, hypoestrogenemia, infertility, elevated FSH and LH
- **Imaging and biopsy**:
    - **Chest radiographs are abnormal in 90% of patients and are an excellent and commonly employed screening test—characteristic findings include mediastinal lymphadenopathy and "ground glass" pulmonary infiltration**
    - **Biopsy results** of pulmonary nodules, liver, or lymph nodes
    - **Whole-body gallium scanning shows pathognomonic signs**—false negative results due to prednisone/immunosuppression should be avoided

---

[819] "But now the inflammation of sarcoidosis has succumbed to antibiotics in two independent studies. This review examines the cell wall deficient (antibiotic resistant) bacteria which have been found in tissue from patients with sarcoidosis." Marshall TG, Marshall FE. Sarcoidosis succumbs to antibiotics—implications for autoimmune disease. *Autoimmun Rev.* 2004 Jun;3(4):295-300

[820] "Patients with active pulmonary sarcoidosis exhibited a marked increased IP to 51Cr-EDTA (4 +/- 0.54%), which was not found in patients with inactive sarcoidosis." Wallaert et al. Increased intestinal permeability in active pulmonary sarcoidosis. *Am Rev Respir Dis.* 1992 Jun;145(6):1440-5

[821] "In conclusion, a high frequency of endocrine autoimmunity in patients with sarcoidosis, occurring in about 20% of the cases, was demonstrated. Thyroid autoimmunity and polyglandular autoimmune syndromes occurred most frequently." Papadopoulos et al. High frequency of endocrine autoimmunity in patients with sarcoidosis. *Eur J Endocrinol* 1996 Mar;134(3):331-336

[822] "Autoantibodies in patients with isolated Addison's disease are directed against the enzymes involved in steroid synthesis, P45oc21, P45oscc and P45oc17." Martin Martorell et al. Autoimmunity in Addison's disease. *Neth J Med.* 2002 Aug;60(7):269-75. Review. Erratum in: *Neth J Med.* 2002 Oct;60(9):378 zuidencomm.nl/njm/getpdf.php?id=159

- **Establishing the diagnosis**: any one of the following:
  - Characteristic radiographic findings and clinical presentation
  - Biopsy results of pulmonary nodules (50-80% positive), liver (70% positive), or palpable lymph nodes (> 85% positive)
  - Pathognomonic signs with whole-body gallium scanning
- **Complications**: 10% of patients develop serious disability, including or due to pulmonary insufficiency, cardiac insufficiency, blindness, fatigue and debility. Granulomatous uveitis occurs in 15% of patients with sarcoidosis and can result in bilateral blindness—this must be managed as a medically urgent condition.

Clinical management:
- Serial pulmonary function tests are recommended—consider referral to pulmonologist or other specialist.
- **Pulmonary fungal infections should be conclusively excluded—referral to pulmonologist or other specialist is advised**.
- **Granulomatous uveitis occurs in 15% of patients with sarcoidosis and can result in bilateral blindness**—this must be managed as a medically urgent condition.
- Referral if clinical outcome is unsatisfactory or if serious complications are evident.

Therapeutic considerations:
- Drug treatments[823]:
  - Prednisone may be initiated at 20-60 mg/d po and tapered to 5 mg/d po for relief of symptoms; this treatment does not alter long-term outcome. **Prednisone and any immunosuppressant medication must only be employed following exclusion of an infectious differential diagnosis—administration of corticosteroids to a patient with occult pulmonary infections could result in a fatal outcome.**
  - Methotrexate at 2.5 mg per week can be initiated in patients unresponsive to prednisone; CBC and liver enzymes are measured every six weeks.
- Vitamin D3 supplementation tailored to serum 25(OH)D levels and serum calcium levels: **Sarcoidosis is the classic exemplification of a granulomatous disease that can cause hypercalcemia due to "vitamin D hypersensitivity."** [824,825] **Vitamin D supplementation—if used at all in these patients—must be supervised with care to avoid hypercalcemia.** Deficiency and response to treatment are monitored with serum 25(OH)vitamin D while **safety is monitored with serum calcium; inflammatory granulomatous diseases—** *sarcoidosis being the classic example*—**and certain drugs such as hydrochlorothiazide greatly increase the propensity for hypercalcemia and warrant incremental dosing and frequent monitoring of serum calcium**.
- Orthoendocrinology: No characteristic patterns of hormonal abnormalities have been described nor researched in patients with sarcoidosis. However, on an individual basis, clinicians and patients may find it valuable to assess prolactin, cortisol, DHEA, free and total testosterone, serum estradiol, and thyroid status (e.g., TSH, T4, *and* anti-thyroid peroxidase antibodies). **Melatonin (20 mg hs)** appears to have cured two patients with drug-resistant sarcoidosis.[826] Immunostimulatory anti-infective action of melatonin was demonstrated in a clinical trial wherein septic newborns administered 20 mg melatonin showed significantly increased survival over nontreated controls[827]; given that sarcoidosis is associated with many subclinical infections, melatonin may provide therapeutic benefit by virtue of its anti-infective properties.
  - Melatonin is a safe and effective treatment for chronic pulmonary and extrapulmonary sarcoidosis. (*J Pineal Res.* 2006 Sep[828]): "Melatonin was given for 2 yr (20 mg/day in the first year, 10 mg/day in the second year) to 18 CS patients. Pulmonary function tests, chest X rays, pulmonary computed tomography, Ga(67) scintigraphy and angiotensin-converting enzyme (ACE) were assayed at baseline and in the follow-up. Normalization of ACE, improvement of pulmonary parameters and resolution of skin involvement were found in the patients given melatonin. After 24 months of melatonin therapy, hylar adenopathy completely resolved in eight patients and parenchymal lesions were markedly improved in all patients;

[823] Beers MH, Berkow R (eds). *Merck Manual. 17th Edition*. Whitehouse Station; Merck Research Laboratories: 1999, pages 2482-85
[824] Vasquez et al. The clinical importance of vitamin D: a paradigm shift with implications for all healthcare providers. *Altern Ther Health Med*. 2004 Sep-Oct;10(5):28-36
[825] Sharma OP. Vitamin D, calcium, and sarcoidosis. *Chest*. 1996 Feb;109(2):535-9 http://www.chestjournal.org/cgi/reprint/109/2/535
[826] Cagnoni et al. Melatonin for treatment of chronic refractory sarcoidosis. *Lancet*. 1995 Nov 4;346(8984):1229-30
[827] Gitto et al. Effects of melatonin treatment in septic newborns. *Pediatr Res*. 2001 Dec;50(6):756-60 http://www.pedresearch.org/cgi/content/full/50/6/756
[828] Pignone et al. Melatonin is a safe and effective treatment for chronic pulmonary and extrapulmonary sarcoidosis. *J Pineal Res*. 2006 Sep;41(2):95-100

in the five patients with reduced diffusion capacity of the lung for carbon monoxide, the values normalized after 6 months of therapy and remained stable until month 24. After 24 months, Ga(67) pulmonary and extra-pulmonary uptake was totally normalized in seven patients and, at month 12 months, ACE was normalized in six patients in which the values were high at the baseline. Skin lesions, present in three patients, completely disappeared at month 24 months. No side effects were experienced and no disease relapse was observed during melatonin treatment. Melatonin may be an effective and safe therapy for CS when other treatments fail or cause side effects."

- <u>Antibacterial therapies with systemic bioavailability</u>: The 2004 monograph by Marshall and Marshall[829] reviewed research implicating cell wall deficient (antibiotic resistant) bacteria as the major causative factor in sarcoidosis, evidenced by remission of the disease following antimicrobial treatment and the incitement of a rather **severe Jarisch-Herxheimer reaction** as the bacteria increase their production of endotoxin in response to exposure to antimicrobial agents. Also in 2004, Bachelez et al[830] published results of a small clinical trail using minocycline and/or doxycycline in 12 patients with sarcoidosis—ten of twelve patients showed a positive response.

  o <u>Minocycline</u>: **The study by Bachelez et al used 200 mg/d minocycline for 12 months for the treatment of sarcoidosis.**

  o <u>Doxycycline</u>: **Alternate treatment by Bachelez et al was 200 mg/d doxycycline for the treatment of sarcoidosis.**

  o *Artemisia annua*: Artemisinin has been safely used for centuries in Asia for the treatment of malaria, and it also has effectiveness against anaerobic bacteria due to the pro-oxidative sesquiterpene endoperoxide.[831,832] I commonly use artemisinin at 200 mg per day in divided doses for adults with dysbiosis. Whether from dried herb, teas, or standardized extracts, **artemisinin is systemically bioavailable** and has an excellent record of safety. However, its usefulness in sarcoidosis based on the treatment of occult infections has not been documented.

  o St. John's Wort (*Hypericum perforatum*): Hyperforin from *Hypericum perforatum* shows *in vitro* antibacterial action, particularly against gram-positive bacteria such as *Staphylococcus aureus*, *Streptococcus pyogenes*, *Streptococcus agalactiae*[833] and perhaps *Helicobacter pylori*.[834] Up to 600 mg three times per day of a 3% hyperforin standardized extract is customary in the treatment of depression, and such **high doses may result in serum hyperforin levels that are systemically antimicrobial.** The safety and antidepressant effectiveness of Hypericum extracts are exceedingly well documented. The usefulness of hyperforin in sarcoidosis based on the treatment of occult infections has not been documented.

- <u>Fumaric acid esters</u>: **Three patients with drug-resistant cutaneous sarcoidosis were successfully treated with fumaric acid esters** (Fumaderm®).[835] Adverse effects of oral fumarate have been reported, namely renal failure.[836]

- <u>Oral enzyme therapy with proteolytic/pancreatic enzymes</u>: Polyenzyme supplementation is used to ameliorate the pathophysiology induced by immune complexes.[837] Approximately 60% of sarcoid patients have CIC (circulating immune complexes)[838] and these are particularly relevant in patients with concomitant vasculitis.[839]

---

[829] "But now the inflammation of sarcoidosis has succumbed to antibiotics in two independent studies. This review examines the cell wall deficient (antibiotic resistant) bacteria which have been found in tissue from patients with sarcoidosis." Marshall TG, Marshall FE. Sarcoidosis succumbs to antibiotics--implications for autoimmune disease. *Autoimmun Rev.* 2004 Jun;3(4):295-300

[830] Bachelez et al. The use of tetracyclines for the treatment of sarcoidosis. *Arch Dermatol.* 2001 Jan;137(1):69-73

[831] Dien et al. Effect of food intake on pharmacokinetics of oral artemisinin in healthy Vietnamese subjects. *Antimicrob Agents Chemother.* 1997 May;41(5):1069-72

[832] Giao et al. Artemisinin for treatment of uncomplicated falciparum malaria: is there a place for monotherapy? *Am J Trop Med Hyg.* 2001 Dec;65(6):690-5

[833] Schempp et al. Antibacterial activity of hyperforin from St John's wort, against multiresistant Staphylococcus aureus and gram-positive bacteria. *Lancet.* 1999 Jun 19;353(9170):2129

[834] "A butanol fraction of St. John's Wort revealed anti-Helicobacter pylori activity with MIC values ranging between 15.6 and 31.2 microg/ml." Reichling et al. A current review of the antimicrobial activity of Hypericum perforatum L. *Pharmacopsychiatry.* 2001 Jul;34 Suppl 1:S116-8

[835] "CONCLUSIONS: On the basis of our findings FAE therapy seems to be a safe and effective regimen for patients with recalcitrant cutaneous sarcoidosis." Nowack et al. Successful treatment of recalcitrant cutaneous sarcoidosis with fumaric acid esters. *BMC Dermatol* 2002 Dec 24;2(1):15 http://www.biomedcentral.com/1471-5945/2/15

[836] "The case of a 38 year old woman who was treated with fumaric acid (420 mg bid) for 5 years before she complained of fatigue and weakness. According to clinical laboratory she had developed severe proximal tubular damage." Raschka C, Koch HJ. Longterm treatment of psoriasis using fumaric acid preparations can be associated with severe proximal tubular damage. *Hum Exp Toxicol* 1999 Dec;18(12):738-9

[837] Galebskaya et al. Human complement system state after wobenzyme intake. *Vestnik Moskovskogo Universiteta (Seriya 2: Khimiya).* 2000:41(6 Suppl): 148-149 chem.msu.ru/eng/journals/vmgu/00add/148.pdf

[838] "Complexes were detected in 29 (58%) patients." Johnson et al. Circulating immune complexes in sarcoidosis. *Thorax.* 1980 Apr;35(4):286-9

[839] "Circulating immune complexes were demonstrated and may have been important in the pathogenesis of both types of skin lesion." Johnston C, Kennedy C. Cutaneous leucocytoclastic vasculitis associated with acute sarcoidosis. *Postgrad Med J.* 1984 Aug;60(706):549-50

Polymyositis, Dermatomyositis, Dermatopolymyositis, Dermatomyositis sine myositis

Description/pathophysiology:

- **Autoimmune disease associated with immune complexes, autoantibodies, and cell-mediated muscle destruction.** Although both conditions are characterized by polymyopathy, skin involvement is a characteristic of **dermatomyositis (DM)** and not **polymyositis (PM)**. Unless articles/textbooks specifically refer to either PM or DM, the hyphenation PM-DM will be used to acknowledge that data probably applies to both conditions. The term **dermatopolymyositis** is somewhat outdated and not commonly used in contemporary literature. **Dermatomyositis sine myositis** is a rare variant of dermatomyositis characterized by inflammation of the skin *without overt myopathy*. Endogenous antigens targeted for autoimmune attack include human **Glycyl-tRNA synthetase**[840] and—not surprisingly—**myosin** from skeletal muscle.[841]

- Tissue damage is caused in large part by muscle infiltration by lymphocytes and macrophages. Lymphocytes from patients with PM-DM produce a "lymphotoxin" that causes muscle necrosis.[842]

- Despite the *idiopathic* label which is inappropriately applied to these disorders, several medical textbooks and numerous journal articles readily acknowledge that underlying viral infections[843,844], bacterial infections[845], parasitic infections[846], and malignancy[847] can contribute to the development of PM-DM. Interestingly and specifically supportive of the hypothesis that dysbiosis plays an etiologic role in the development of PM-DM, two of the endogenous autoantigens in PM share amino acid homology (molecular mimicry) with **histidyl-tRNA synthetase** and **alanyl-RNA synthetase** from *E. coli*.[848] Furthermore, myosin in human skeletal muscle shares amino acid homology with M5 protein from *Streptococcus pyogenes*.[849] Limited evidence suggests that DM may be triggered or exacerbated by bacterial infections/dysbiosis—particularly with *Staphylococcus aureus*[850,851] and *Streptococcus pyogenes*.[852,853] Patients with DM have an exaggerated response to streptococcal M5 protein[854] as well as streptococcal M12 protein.[855] Streptococcal infections may precipitate or exacerbate DM via mechanisms including molecular mimicry[856,857]; furthermore, streptococcal M protein acts as a superantigen and

Microorganisms causatively or molecularly associated with induction of polymyositis and dermatomyositis
• *Streptococcus pyogenes*
• *Staphylococcus aureus*
• *Toxoplasma gondii*
• *Mycoplasma pneumoniae*
• *Borrelia burgdorferi*
• *Coxsackie B virus*
• *Mycoplasma hominis*
• *Haemophilus influenzae*
• *Helicobacter pylori*
• *Escherichia coli*
• *Bacillus subtilis*

---

[840] Ge et al. Primary structure and functional expression of human Glycyl-tRNA synthetase, an autoantigen in myositis. *J Biol Chem*. 1994 Nov 18;269(46):28790-7 jbc.org/cgi/reprint/269/46/28790

[841] Massa et al. Self epitopes shared between human skeletal myosin and Streptococcus pyogenes M5 protein are targets of immune responses in active juvenile dermatomyositis. *Arthritis Rheum*. 2002 Nov;46(11):3015-25

[842] Ichimiya et al. Association between elevated serum antibody levels to streptococcal M12 protein and susceptibility to dermatomyositis. *Arch Dermatol Res*. 1998 Apr;290(4):229-30

[843] Beers MH, Berkow R (eds). *Merck Manual. 17th Edition*. Whitehouse Station; Merck Research Laboratories 1999 Page 434

[844] Siegel LB, Gall EP. Viral infection as a cause of arthritis. *Am Fam Physician* 1996 Nov 1;54(6):2009-15

[845] Massa et al. Self epitopes shared between human skeletal myosin and Streptococcus pyogenes M5 protein are targets of immune responses in active juvenile dermatomyositis. *Arthritis Rheum*. 2002 Nov;46(11):3015-

[846] "We report a case of polymyositis and myocarditis in a 13-year old immunocompetent girl with toxoplasmosis. The patient presented with proximal muscle weakness, dysphagia, palms and soles rash and elevated serum levels of muscle enzymes, with liver and myocardial involvement." Paspalaki et al. Polyomyositis and myocarditis associated with acquired toxoplasmosis in an immunocompetent girl. *BMC Musculoskelet Disord*. 2001;2:8. Epub 2001 Nov 20 biomedcentral.com/1471-2474/2/8

[847] Tierney ML. McPhee SJ, Papadakis MA (eds). *Current Medical Diagnosis and Treatment 2006. 45th edition*. New York; Lange Medical Books: 2006, pages 840-842

[848] "The amino acid sequences of Escherichia coli histidyl-tRNA synthetase and alanyl-tRNA synthetase, two proteins recently identified as autoantigens in polymyositis, were compared by a computer alignment procedure with those of the 3600 proteins tabulated in the National Biomedical Research Foundation protein sequence database. Both proteins contain sequences long enough to function as epitopes that match sequences on viral and muscle proteins." Walker EJ, Jeffrey PD. Polymyositis and molecular mimicry, a mechanism of autoimmunity. *Lancet*. 1986 Sep 13;2(8507):605-7

[849] Massa et al. Self epitopes shared between human skeletal myosin and Streptococcus pyogenes M5 protein are targets of immune responses in active juvenile dermatomyositis. *Arthritis Rheum*. 2002 Nov;46(11):3015-25

[850] Lane et al. Dermatomyositis following chronic staphylococcal joint sepsis. *Ann Rheum Dis*. 1990 Jun;49(6):405-6

[851] Moore et al. Staphylococcal infections in childhood dermatomyositis--association with the development of calcinosis, raised IgE concentrations and granulocyte chemotactic defect. *Ann Rheum Dis*. 1992 Mar;51(3):378-83

[852] Massa et al. Self epitopes shared between human skeletal myosin and Streptococcus pyogenes M5 protein are targets of immune responses in active juvenile dermatomyositis. *Arthritis Rheum*. 2002 Nov;46(11):3015-25

[853] Ichimiya et al. Association between elevated serum antibody levels to streptococcal M12 protein and susceptibility to dermatomyositis. *Arch Dermatol Res*. 1998 Apr;290(4):229-30

[854] Massa et al. Self epitopes shared between human skeletal myosin and Streptococcus pyogenes M5 protein are targets of immune responses in active juvenile dermatomyositis. *Arthritis Rheum*. 2002 Nov;46(11):3015-25

[855] Ichimiya et al. Association between elevated serum antibody levels to streptococcal M12 protein and dermatomyositis. *Arch Dermatol Res*. 1998 Apr;290(4):229-30

[856] Ichimiya et al. Association between elevated serum antibody levels to streptococcal M12 protein and dermatomyositis. *Arch Dermatol Res*. 1998 Apr;290(4):229-30

[857] Ichimiya et al. Association between elevated serum antibody levels to streptococcal M12 protein and dermatomyositis. *Arch Dermatol Res*. 1998 Apr;290(4):229-30

may enhance expression of endogenous autoantigens.[858] Young patients with calcific dermatomyositis have at least one immune defect (impaired granulocyte chemotaxis) that impairs their ability to fight *Staphylococcus aureus* infections/colonization/dysbiosis; this defect in chemotaxis is associated with and may be caused by elevations in serum IgE, some of which is specific for *Staphylococcus aureus*.[859] A relatively complete list of microorganisms associated with induction of PM-DM in humans includes *Staphylococcus aureus*[860,861], *Streptococcus pyogenes*[862,863], *Toxoplasma gondii*[864,865,866,867], *Mycoplasma pneumoniae*[868,869], *Borrelia burgdorferi*[870,871], and *Coxsackie B virus*.[872] Microorganisms that share amino acid homology with human skeletal muscle myosin include *Streptococcus pyogenes*, *Borrelia burgdorferi*, *Mycoplasma hominis*, *Haemophilus influenzae*, *Helicobacter pylori*, *Escherichia coli*, and *Bacillus subtilis*.[873]

- Like other disorders, PM-DM may occur with other autoimmune diseases, in which case it is described as an **overlap syndrome**. This is not surprising since the underlying characteristic of all autoimmune disorders is *immune dysfunction*; the protean consequences of immune dysfunction can morph without regard for the anthropocentric labels that we affix to different patterns of disordered expression. As with all autoimmune disorders, the course is variable and marked by exacerbations and remissions; yet the general trend is one of progressive decline. Spontaneous remission may occur.

- These conditions are commonly described as "idiopathic." The 2006 edition of <u>Current Medical Diagnosis and Treatment</u> refers to these two disorders as "idiopathic inflammatory myopathies"—a title no longer worthy of codification since 1) we have clear evidence of microbial induction/exacerbation of these disorders, 2) the hormonal aspects of these disorders (like most other autoimmune disorders) is increasingly recognized (for the most recent example, see Sereda and Werth[874]), and 3) the intentional overuse of the term *idiopathic* is leveraged by drug companies and other pharmaceutical/medical interests to justify endless medicalization in lieu of more profound assessments and effective treatments. One of the consequences of the pharmaceutically-influenced *idiopathicization* of otherwise understandable and treatable diseases is that doctors are no longer trained to *cure* disease by addressing the underlying problems; rather, they are trained to *medicate* disease indefinitely by *additive and infinite pharmacotherapy* and **symptom exchange**—trading symptoms of the disease for the side

---

[858] Ichimiya et al. Association between elevated serum antibody levels to streptococcal M12 protein and dermatomyositis. *Arch Dermatol Res*. 1998 Apr;290(4):229-30

[859] Moore et al. Staphylococcal infections in childhood dermatomyositis--association with the development of calcinosis, raised IgE concentrations and granulocyte chemotactic defect. *Ann Rheum Dis*. 1992 Mar;51(3):378-83

[860] Lane et al. Dermatomyositis following chronic staphylococcal joint sepsis. *Ann Rheum Dis*. 1990 Jun;49(6):405-6

[861] Moore et al. Staphylococcal infections in childhood dermatomyositis--association with the development of calcinosis, raised IgE concentrations and granulocyte chemotactic defect. *Ann Rheum Dis*. 1992 Mar;51(3):378-83

[862] Massa et al. Self epitopes shared between human skeletal myosin and Streptococcus pyogenes M5 protein are targets of immune responses in active juvenile dermatomyositis. *Arthritis Rheum*. 2002 Nov;46(11):3015-25

[863] Ichimiya et al. Association between elevated serum antibody levels to streptococcal M12 protein and susceptibility to dermatomyositis. *Arch Dermatol Res*. 1998 Apr;290(4):229-30

[864] "The case of a patient who developed an acute dermatomyositis-like syndrome upon infection by Toxoplasma gondii is reported." Saberin et al. Dermatomyositis-like syndrome following acute toxoplasmosis. *Bull Soc Sci Med Grand Duche Luxemb*. 2004;(2):109-19

[865] "We report a case of polymyositis and myocarditis in a 13-year old immunocompetent girl with toxoplasmosis. The patient presented with proximal muscle weakness, dysphagia, palms and soles rash and elevated serum levels of muscle enzymes, with liver and myocardial involvement." Paspalaki et al. Polyomyositis and myocarditis associated with acquired toxoplasmosis in an immunocompetent girl. *BMC Musculoskelet Disord*. 2001;2:8. Epub 2001 Nov 20 biomedcentral.com/1471-2474/2/8

[866] "The patient improved over the next six months and has been followed for approximately a five year period. During this time, antibody levels to the toxoplasma antigen have significantly decreased but the patient has developed a chronic myositis indistinguishable from polymyositis." Adams EM, Hafez GR, Carnes M, Wiesner JK, Graziano FM. The development of polymyositis in a patient with toxoplasmosis: clinical and pathologic findings and review of literature. *Clin Exp Rheumatol*. 1984 Jul-Sep;2(3):205-8

[867] "The serologic data suggested that inflammatory muscle disease was associated with recent active toxoplasma infection in certain patients." Phillips PE, Kassan SS, Kagen LJ. Increased toxoplasma antibodies in idiopathic inflammatory muscle disease. A case-controlled study. *Arthritis Rheum*. 1979 Mar;22(3):209-14

[868] "We describe the case of a 10-year-old girl who developed polymyositis associated with a Mycoplasma pneumoniae infection." Aihara Y, Mori M, Kobayashi T, Yokota S. A pediatric case of polymyositis associated with Mycoplasma pneumoniae infection. *Scand J Rheumatol*. 1997;26(6):480-1

[869] "Polymyositis, transverse myelitis, ascending polyneuritis, bilateral optic neuritis, and hearing loss developed in a patient with high complement-fixing antibody titers to Mycoplasma pneumoniae." Rothstein TL, Kenny GE. Cranial neuropathy, myeloradiculopathy, and myositis: complications of Mycoplasma pneumoniae infection. *Arch Neurol*. 1979 Aug;36(8):476-7

[870] "Lyme disease with muscle involvement can mimic or trigger dermatomyositis and should be considered in the differential diagnosis of dermatomyositis." Hoffmann et al. Lyme disease in a 74-year-old forest owner with symptoms of dermatomyositis. *Arthritis Rheum*. 1995 Aug;38(8):1157-60

[871] "We report the first case of dermatomyositis that appears to have been triggered by B. burgdorferi. This case involved an individual from Westchester County, NY, who presented with skin lesions suggestive of erythema migrans and who was seropositive for Lyme disease. He soon developed a clinical syndrome suggestive of dermatomyositis: periorbital edema, dysphagia, proximal muscle weakness, and a markedly elevated level of creatine phosphokinase." Horowitz et al. Dermatomyositis associated with Lyme disease: case report and review of Lyme myositis. *Clin Infect Dis*. 1994 Feb;18(2):166-71

[872] "These data suggest that the host response to coxsackie B virus might be related to the pathophysiology of JDM." Christensen et al. Prevalence of Coxsackie B virus antibodies in patients with juvenile dermatomyositis. *Arthritis Rheum*. 1986 Nov;29(11):1365-70

[873] Massa et al. Self epitopes shared between human skeletal myosin and Streptococcus pyogenes M5 protein are targets of immune responses in active juvenile dermatomyositis. *Arthritis Rheum*. 2002 Nov;46(11):3015-25

[874] "Using antiestrogen medication in women with DM may result in a significant improvement in their rash, possibly via the inhibition of TNF-alpha production by immune or other cells." Sereda D, Werth VP. Improvement in dermatomyositis rash associated with the use of antiestrogen medication. *Arch Dermatol*. 2006 Jan;142(1):70-2

effects of the drugs used to treat the disease.[875] Consequently, the top questions that doctors ask themselves during clinical encounters are 1) "What is the cause of symptom X?", 2) "What is the dose of the 'appropriate' drug?", and 3) "How should I manage disease or finding X?"[876] Notice that the internal dialogue of the allopathically trained physicians centers on symptoms, drugs, and management rather than any attempt to discover and address the underlying cause(s) of the symptoms or any attempt at authentic cure. Convincing doctors that *endless additive medicalization* is synonymous with *effective patient care* has been the major goal of the pharmaceutical companies[877] and is one that they accomplish by influencing medical school curricula[878,] sources of biomedical information[879], and by 'educating' doctors and patients with an incessant barrage of infomercials.[880]

Clinical presentations:

- **Bilateral symmetrical proximal muscle weakness most commonly affecting the shoulders, neck, and hips:** This weakness is reflective of the underlying autoimmune myopathy and may not be markedly present at the beginning of the disease process although it is eventually noted in all PM-DM patients. Characteristic difficulties include rising from a chair or squatting position (indicating weakness of glutei, quadriceps, and other intrinsic hip muscles), and upholding the arms (such as to comb hair) or lifting objects overhead (deltoids and rotator cuff muscles).
- **Skin/dermatologic abnormalities:**
  - **Heliotrope/purple facial/cheek rash:** "Periorbital edema with a heliotrope hue (purplish appearance) is pathognomonic."[881]
  - **Gottron's sign:** scaly patches over the metacarpophalangeal (MCP) and PIP joints of the hands—considered highly suggestive (not quite pathognomonic) of the disease.
  - Generalized skin rash and erythema, particularly over the shoulders ("shawl sign") and eyelids
  - Cuticular telangiectasias
  - Photosensitivity
- Polyarthralgia: pain and swelling, generally mild
- Muscle tenderness
- Raynaud's phenomenon: most commonly in patients with other autoimmune disease
- Fatigue
- Weight loss
- Soft tissue calcification: seen in PM-DM and scleroderma
- Cardiac involvement
- 2:1 more common in women than in men
- More common in persons of African descent, which is probably due at least in part to the higher incidence of vitamin D deficiency in this population. Vitamin D insufficiency predisposes toward inflammation, immune dysfunction, autoimmunity, and increased susceptibility to infections.
- Seen in children (5-15 years: "juvenile dermatomyositis/polymyositis") and adults (40-60 years)
- Rapid or slow onset; often preceded by infection

---

[875] "It begins on the first day of medical school… It starts slowly and insidiously, like an addiction, and can end up influencing the very nature of medical decision-making and practice… Attempts to influence the judgment of doctors by commercial interests serving the medical industrial complex are nothing if not thorough." Editorial. Drug-company influence on medical education in USA. *Lancet.* 2000 Sep 2;356(9232):781

[876] ""What is the cause of symptom X?" "What is the dose of drug X?" and "How should I manage disease or finding X?"" Ely et al. Analysis of questions asked by family doctors regarding patient care. *BMJ.* 1999 Aug 7;319(7206):358-61 http://bmj.bmjjournals.com/cgi/content/full/319/7206/358

[877] Angell M. *The Truth About the Drug Companies: How They Deceive Us and What to Do About it.* Random House; August 2004

[878] "It begins on the first day of medical school… It starts slowly and insidiously, like an addiction, and can end up influencing the very nature of medical decision-making and practice… Attempts to influence the judgment of doctors by commercial interests serving the medical industrial complex are nothing if not thorough." Editorial. Drug-company influence on medical education in USA. *Lancet.* 2000 Sep 2;356(9232):781

[879] "…despite lush advertisements from companies with obvious vested interests, and authoritative testimonials from biased investigators who presumably believe in their own work to the point of straining credulity and denying common sense… (translate: economic improvement, not biological superiority)." Stevens CW, Glatstein E. Beware the Medical-Industrial Complex. *Oncologist* 1996;1(4):IV-V theoncologist.alphamedpress.org/cgi/reprint/1/4/190-iv.pdf

[880] "…many ads may be targeted specifically at women and older viewers. Our findings suggest that Americans who watch average amounts of television may be exposed to more than 30 hours of direct-to-consumer drug advertisements each year, far surpassing their exposure to other forms of health communication." Brownfield et al. Direct-to-consumer drug advertisements on network television: an exploration of quantity, frequency, and placement. *J Health Commun.* 2004 Nov-Dec;9(6):491-7

[881] Beers MH, Berkow R (eds). *Merck Manual. 17th Edition.* Whitehouse Station; Merck Research Laboratories 1999 Page 435

<u>**Major differential diagnoses**</u>:

- <mark><u>Cancer</u>: All patients with PM-DM must be screened (in a patient-specific manner) for cancer.</mark>
- <u>Celiac disease, gluten sensitivity</u>
- <u>Corticosteroid myopathy</u>
- <u>Drug toxicity</u>: Numerous drugs can cause muscle weakness and elevated serum levels of muscle enzymes. All of the following drugs can cause proximal muscle weakness, and the drugs that are underlined can also cause elevated muscle enzymes: corticosteroids, alcohol, clofibrate, penicillamine (very commonly reported cause of polymyositis), hydroxychloroquine, <u>colchicine</u> (especially in older patients with renal failure), <u>HMG-CoA reductase inhibitors—"statins"</u>, especially when combined with gemfibrozil, cyclosporine, niacin, erythromycin, azole antifungals, and protease inhibitors, <u>Zidovudine</u>, and <u>AZT</u>.
- <u>Hepatitis and viral hepatitis</u>: Elevated AST and ALT may be seen in PM-DM and hepatitis.
- <mark><u>Hypothyroidism</u>: Hypothyroidism can almost perfectly mimic PM-DM with periorbital edema, dermatitis, and "hypothyroid myopathy" with proximal muscle weakness, and elevated CK.[882]</mark>
- <u>Inclusion body myositis (IBM)</u>: Earlier editions of some medical books discussed inclusion body myositis as a subset of polymyositis; more recent editions clearly distinguish inclusion body myositis as a distinct entity, hence its inclusion here under the category of differential diagnoses. Clinically, **IBM tends to present with *distal* muscle involvement rather than the *proximal* localization of early PM-DM**. Furthermore, muscle involvement is likely to be *asymmetrical* with IBM, differentiating IBM from PM-DM in which muscle involvement is typically symmetric.
- <u>Infection</u>: viral infection, bacterial infection, toxoplasmosis, HIV polymyositis, postviral rhabdomyolysis.
- <u>Lambert-Eaton myasthenic syndrome</u>: A disorder with pathophysiology similar to myasthenia gravis—autoantibodies directed to neuromuscular junction (voltage-gated calcium channels at terminal of alpha motor neuron); clinical presentation similar to PM-DM with proximal limb weakness. May also present with dry mouth and dry eyes (DDX: **Sjogren's syndrome**), eye ptosis and diplopia (DDX: **myasthenia gravis**), and exacerbations caused by heat (DDX: **multiple sclerosis**). Lambert-Eaton myasthenia is like PM-DM commonly associated with occult malignancy (especially small cell lung cancer) and therefore all patients with Lambert-Eaton myasthenia must be comprehensively screened for cancer. Diagnosis of Lambert-Eaton myasthenia is performed with serum tests for antibodies, supported by EMG, and followed with comprehensive cancer screening, which should include CT of lungs and biopsy of suspicious lung lesions.
- <u>Multiple sclerosis</u>: Diagnosis based on clinical presentation, findings such as internuclear ophthalmoplegia and optic neuritis, and characteristic MRI brain lesions. DDX: celiac encephalopathy.
- <u>Myasthenia gravis (MG)</u>: Presents with muscle weakness; however MG presents with facial and ocular weakness which are not characteristic of PM-DM; caused by autoantibodies directed to neuromuscular junction (acetylcholine receptor of the motor end plate).
- <u>Myocardial infarction</u>: Both MI and PM-DM have elevated CK-MB.
- <u>Neuropathy and radiculopathy</u>: Both can cause muscle weakness that can mimic PM-DM.
- <u>Polymyalgia rheumatica</u>: In these patients, muscle pain predominates over muscle weakness.
- <u>SLE</u>: Both SLE and DM can present with systemic inflammation, fatigue, butterfly heliotrope facial rash, and positive ANA. Elevated CK and aldolase are characteristic of DM but are uncommon in SLE.

<u>**Clinical assessments**</u>:

- **History/subjective**: See clinical presentations
- **Physical examination/objective**:
  - Assess muscle strength
    - Shoulders: flexion and abduction.
    - Neck: flexion, extension, and lateral bending.
    - Hips: use a combination of direct muscle testing as well as functional assessments such as "squat and rise" and rising from a chair.

---

[882] Bowman et al. Bilateral adhesive capsulitis, oligoarthritis and proximal myopathy as presentation of hypothyroidism. *Br J Rheumatol* 1988;27(1):62-4

- **Laboratory assessments**:
  - ESR/CRP: Normal in 50% of patients.
  - CBC: Assess for anemia (uncommon), infection, and possible nutritional deficiencies
  - Metabolic/chemistry panel: Elevated AST and ALT may be seen and can be confused with hepatitis.
  - Muscle enzymes: These are useful for establishing the diagnosis and monitoring the course of disease and response to treatment. Both tests should be performed together, especially at the initial evaluation.
    - Creatine kinase (CK) (previously called creatine phosphokinase (CPK): CK is generally elevated but may normalize in patients with active disease and widespread muscle atrophy[883] in a manner similar to the reduction of liver enzymes with the progression of hepatic cirrhosis.
    - Aldolase
  - ANA: Positive in many patients[884] especially those with another autoimmune disorder—overlap syndrome.[885]
  - Anti-Jo-1: Seen mostly with lung disease.
  - Serum IgE: Young DM patients affected by calcinosis have elevated serum IgE.[886]
  - Serologic testing for *Toxoplasma gondii*: Serologic testing for *Toxoplasma gondii* has been recommended because of the association between this infection and the development of PM-DM.[887]
  - Testing for celiac disease: This is especially important in PM-DM patients who have malabsorption.[888]
  - Dysbiosis testing: Assess for multifocal dysbiosis.
- **Imaging and biopsy**:
  - **Skin/muscle biopsy is necessary for definitive diagnosis**.
  - Imaging is not generally indicated except when looking for complications or concomitant disease, such as chest radiographs for associated interstitial lung disease.
  - Electromyographic assessment may be used to support the diagnosis and to exclude/evaluate concomitant disorders; this is generally unnecessary.
- **Establishing the diagnosis**:
  - The following should be present:
    - Proximal muscle weakness
    - Skin rash
    - Increased levels of muscle enzymes in serum
    - Muscle biopsy findings—specific, mandatory for definite diagnosis
    - EMG abnormalities are supportive

Complications:

- Occult malignancy—up to 25% of patients with dermatomyositis have an occult malignancy. Evaluation for underlying/occult malignancy is mandatory in all adult patients with dermatomyositis.[889] Assessment for malignancy should include complete physical examination and routine blood tests (CBC, chemistry/metabolic panel, serum protein electrophoresis, serum ferritin); additional assessments are chosen per the patient's individual profile based on age, gender, family history, and other risk factors. Measuring PSA in middle aged and older men and CA-125 in adult women would be very reasonable, as would a colonoscopy in any PM-DM patient over age 40 years. Radiographs and CT imaging are warranted for any PM-DM patient with pulmonary symptoms or history of exposure to inhaled carcinogens, including asbestos and tobacco smoke.
  - **Up to 20% of women with dermatomyositis develop ovarian cancer**
  - **Breast cancer** and **lung cancer** are also more common

883 Klippel JH (ed). *Primer on the Rheumatic Diseases. 11th Edition*. Atlanta: Arthritis Foundation. 1997, page 277
884 Tierney ML. McPhee SJ, Papadakis MA (eds). *Current Medical Diagnosis and Treatment 2006. 45th edition*. New York; Lange Medical Books: 2006, pages 840-842
885 Tierney LM. Saint S, Whooley MA (Eds). *Current Essentials of Medicine. 3rd Edition*. New York; Lange Medical Books: 2005, page 165
886 Moore et al. Staphylococcal infections in childhood dermatomyositis--association with the development of calcinosis, raised IgE concentrations and granulocyte chemotactic defect. *Ann Rheum Dis*. 1992 Mar;51(3):378-83
887 "We report a case of polymyositis and myocarditis in a 13-year old immunocompetent girl with toxoplasmosis. The patient presented with proximal muscle weakness, dysphagia, palms and soles rash and elevated serum levels of muscle enzymes, with liver and myocardial involvement." Paspalaki et al. Polyomyositis and myocarditis associated with acquired toxoplasmosis in an immunocompetent girl. *BMC Musculoskelet Disord*. 2001;2:8. Epub 2001 Nov 20 .biomedcentral.com/1471-2474/2/8
888 "Based on our findings, we further emphasize that an evaluation for celiac disease, including anti-gliadin antibodies, anti-endomysium antibody and tissue trans-glutaminase antibodies should be considered in PM/DM patients presenting with unusual and unexplained gastrointestinal features." Marie I, Lecomte F, Hachulla E, Antonietti M, Francois A, Levesque H, Courtois H. An uncommon association: celiac disease and dermatomyositis in adults. *Clin Exp Rheumatol*. 2001 Mar-Apr;19(2):201-3
889 Tierney ML. McPhee SJ, Papadakis MA. *Current Medical Diagnosis and Treatment 2006. 45th edition*. New York; Lange Medical Books: 2006, pages 840-842

- o Associated cancers have **poor prognosis**
- o **Appropriate screening includes the following**[890]:
  - **History**
  - **Physical examination**
  - **CBC**
  - **Chemistry/metabolic panel**
  - **Serum protein electrophoresis**
  - **Urinalysis**
  - **Age-, gender-, and risk-appropriate screening tests**
  - **Follow-up for cancers that become evident within the next few months**
- Vasculitis with necrosis of internal organs, especially intestines
- Dyspnea due to weakness of respiratory muscles may progress to respiratory failure
- Dysphagia due to weakness of muscles of upper pharynx
- Cardiac involvement
- Renal failure secondary to rhabdomyolysis
- Intestinal ulcerations with bleeding
- Corticosteroid myopathy
- Muscle inflammation begins with weakness and progresses to fibrosis and contractures

Clinical management:
- Referral if clinical outcome is unsatisfactory or if serious complications are possible or evident.

Treatments:
- *Medical/drug treatments*[891,892]
  - o <u>Prednisone</u>: Generally started at 40-60 mg/g, then tapered.
  - o <u>Methotrexate</u>, <u>azathioprine</u>, or <u>intravenous immune globulin</u>: Used for patients who do not respond to corticosteroids.
- <u>Vitamin E</u>: Several articles have shown benefit of vitamin E supplementation in different autoimmune conditions. Conditions that may respond to vitamin E supplementation include scleroderma, discoid lupus erythematosus[893], porphyria cutanea tarda, **polymyositis**, and vasculitis.[894,895,896] Given that vitamin E is not a single compound but rather a family of closely related tocopherols, most clinicians prefer to use a source of "mixed tocopherols" inclusive of alpha, beta, delta, and—perhaps most importantly—gamma tocopherol.[897] Vitamin E has a wide margin of safety and although daily doses are kept in the range of 400-1200 IU, doses up to 3,200 IU are generally considered non-toxic.
- <u>Avoidance of allergenic foods</u>: **Celiac disease can present with a clinical picture that closely mimics polymyositis; the "'disease" remits with gluten avoidance.**[898] Any patient may be allergic to any food, even if the food is generally considered a health-promoting food. Generally speaking, the most notorious allergens are wheat, citrus (especially juice due to the industrial use of fungal hemicellulases), cow's milk, eggs, peanuts, chocolate, and yeast-containing foods. According to a study in patients with migraine, some patients will have

[890] Tierney ML. McPhee SJ, Papadakis MA. *Current Medical Diagnosis and Treatment 2006. 45th edition*. New York; Lange Medical Books: 2006, pages 840-842
[891] Tierney ML. McPhee SJ, Papadakis MA. *Current Medical Diagnosis and Treatment 2006. 45th edition*. New York; Lange Medical Books: 2006, pages 840-842
[892] Tierney LM. Saint S, Whooley MA (Eds). *Current Essentials of Medicine. 3rd Edition*. New York; Lange Medical Books: 2005, page 165
[893] "Despite conflicting opinions, our personal experience and a number of reviewed clinical reports indicate that vitamin E, properly administered in adequate doses, is a safe and effective treatment for chronic discoid lupus erythematosus, and may be of value in treating other types of the disease." Ayres S Jr, Mihan R. Lupus erythematosus and vitamin E: an effective and nontoxic therapy. *Cutis*. 1979 Jan;23(1):49-52, 54
[894] "She then made a dramatic improvement when large doses of vitamin E (d, alpha-tocopheryl acetate) were administered." Killeen RN, Ayres S Jr, Mihan R. Polymyositis: response to vitamin E. *South Med J*. 1976 Oct;69(10):1372-4
[895] "Casually, vitamin E (600 mg daily) was added. After 6 months, clinical manifestations of heart failure were disappeared and the echocardiogram showed a normally-sized left ventricle with normal wall motion." Morelli et al. Systemic sclerosis (scleroderma). A case of recovery of cardiomyopathy after vitamin E treatment. *Minerva Cardioangiol*. 2001 Apr;49(2):127-30
[896] "Among the diseases that were successfully controlled were a number in the autoimmune category, including scleroderma, discoid lupus erythematosus, porphyria cutanea tarda, several types of vasculitis, and polymyositis." Ayres S Jr, Mihan R. Is vitamin E involved in the autoimmune mechanism? *Cutis*. 1978 Mar;21(3):321-5
[897] Jiang Q, Christen S, Shigenaga MK, Ames BN. gamma-tocopherol, the major form of vitamin E in the US diet, deserves more attention. *Am J Clin Nutr*. 2001 Dec;74:714-22
[898] "Treatment with gluten-free diet resolved all clinical and laboratory abnormalities." Evron et al. Polymyositis, arthritis, and proteinuria in a patient with adult celiac disease. *J Rheumatol*. 1996 Apr;23(4):782-3

to avoid as many as 10 specific foods in order to become symptom-free.[899] **Several cases of co-existent celiac disease with PM-DM have been reported**.[900] Regardless of the absence of allergy in a particular patient, clinicians must explain to their patients that celiac disease and wheat allergy are two different clinical entities and that exclusion of one does not exclude the other, and in neither case does mutual exclusion obviate the promotion of intestinal bacterial overgrowth (i.e., pro-inflammatory dysbiosis) by indigestible wheat oligosaccharides.

- o Dermatomyositis associated with celiac disease responsive to a gluten-free diet. (*Can J Gastroenterol.* 2006 Jun[901]): "A ... case of concomitant dermatomyositis and celiac disease in a 40-year-old woman is presented. After having been diagnosed with dermatomyositis and iron deficiency anemia, this patient was referred to the gastroenterology clinic to exclude a gastrointestinal malignancy. Blood tests revealed various vitamin deficiencies consistent with malabsorption. The results of gastroscopy with duodenal biopsy were consistent with celiac disease. After she was put on a strict gluten-free diet, both nutritional deficiencies and the dermatomyositis resolved. The patient's human leukocyte antigen haplotype study was positive for DR3 and DQ2, which have been shown to be associated with both juvenile dermatomyositis and celiac disease. It is suggested that patients with newly diagnosed dermatomyositis be investigated for concomitant celiac disease even in the absence of gastrointestinal symptoms."

- Vitamin D3 supplementation with physiologic doses and/or tailored to serum 25(OH)D levels: Vitamin D deficiency is common in the general population and is even more common in patients with chronic illness and chronic musculoskeletal pain.[902] Correction of vitamin D deficiency supports normal immune function against infection and provides a clinically significant anti-inflammatory[903] and analgesic benefit in patients with back pain[904] and limb pain.[905] Reasonable daily doses for children and adults are 1,000-2,000 and 4,000 IU, respectively.[906] Deficiency and response to treatment are monitored with serum 25(OH)vitamin D while safety is monitored with serum calcium; inflammatory granulomatous diseases and certain drugs such as hydrochlorothiazide greatly increase the propensity for hypercalcemia and warrant increment dosing and frequent monitoring of serum calcium. Vitamin D2 (ergocalciferol) is not a human nutrient and should not be used in clinical practice.

- **Assessment for dysbiosis: Given the numerous links between PM-DM and various microorganisms, testing for and treating multifocal dysbiosis (as outlined in Chapter 4) is strongly encouraged.** Yeast, bacteria, and parasites are treated as indicated based on identification and sensitivity results from comprehensive parasitology assessments. Patients taking immunosuppressant drugs such as corticosteroids/prednisone have increased risk of intestinal bacterial overgrowth and translocation.[907,908] Other dysbiotic loci should be investigated as discussed in Chapter 4 in the section on multifocal dysbiosis.

Microorganisms causatively or molecularly associated with induction of polymyositis/dermatomyositis
• *Streptococcus pyogenes*
• *Staphylococcus aureus*
• *Toxoplasma gondii*
• *Mycoplasma pneumoniae*
• *Borrelia burgdorferi*
• Coxsackie B virus
• *Mycoplasma hominis*
• *Haemophilus influenzae*
• *Helicobacter pylori*
• *Escherichia coli*
• *Bacillus subtilis*

- Orthoendocrinology: Assess prolactin, cortisol, DHEA, free and total testosterone, serum estradiol, and thyroid status (e.g., TSH, T4, *and* anti-thyroid peroxidase antibodies).

  - o Prolactin (excess): The role of prolactin in PM-DM has not been studied. However, prolactin is increasingly well-known as a proinflammatory and

[899] Grant EC. Food allergies and migraine. *Lancet.* 1979 May 5;1(8123):966-9

[900] "Based on our findings, we further emphasize that an evaluation for celiac disease, including anti-gliadin antibodies, anti-endomysium antibody and tissue trans-glutaminase antibodies should be considered in PM/DM patients presenting with unusual and unexplained gastrointestinal features." Marie et al. An uncommon association: celiac disease and dermatomyositis in adults. *Clin Exp Rheumatol.* 2001 Mar-Apr;19(2):201-3

[901] Song et al. Dermatomyositis associated with celiac disease: response to a gluten-free diet. *Can J Gastroenterol.* 2006 Jun;20(6):433-5

[902] Plotnikoff GA, Quigley JM. Prevalence of severe hypovitaminosis D in patients with persistent, nonspecific musculoskeletal pain. *Mayo Clin Proc.* 2003 Dec;78(12):1463-70

[903] Timms et al. Circulating MMP9, vitamin D and variation in the TIMP-1 response with VDR genotype: mechanisms for inflammatory damage in chronic disorders? *QJM.* 2002 Dec;95(12):787-96 qjmed.oxfordjournals.org/cgi/content/full/95/12/787

[904] Al Faraj S, Al Mutairi K. Vitamin D deficiency and chronic low back pain in Saudi Arabia. *Spine.* 2003 Jan 15;28(2):177-9

[905] Masood et al. Persistent limb pain and raised serum alkaline phosphatase the earliest markers of subclinical hypovitaminosis D in Kashmir. *Indian J Physiol Pharmacol.* 1989 Oct-Dec;33(4):259-61

[906] Vasquez et al. The clinical importance of vitamin D: a paradigm shift with implications for all healthcare providers. *Altern Ther Health Med.* 2004 Sep-Oct;10(5):28-36

[907] "A 63-year-old man with systemic lupus erythematosus and selective IgA deficiency developed intractable diarrhoea the day after treatment with prednisone, 50 mg daily, was started. The diarrhoea was considered to be caused by bacterial overgrowth and was later successfully treated with doxycycline." Denison H, Wallerstedt S. Bacterial overgrowth after high-dose corticosteroid treatment. *Scand J Gastroenterol.* 1989 Jun;24(5):561-4

[908] "These bacteria also translocated to the mesenteric lymph nodes in mice injected with cyclophosphamide or prednisone." Berg et al. Immunosuppression and intestinal bacterial overgrowth synergistically promote bacterial translocation. *Arch Surg.* 1988 Nov;123(11):1359-64

immunodysregulatory hormone. Serum levels of prolactin tend to be higher in patients with autoimmunity, and therapeutic lowering of prolactin levels results in clinically significant anti-inflammatory benefits. Among women with hyperprolactinemia, 75% of them show serologic evidence of asymptomatic autoimmunity.[909] As discussed elsewhere, patients with RA and SLE have higher basal and stress-induced levels of prolactin compared with normal controls[910,911], and men with RA have higher serum levels of prolactin that correlate with the severity and duration of the disorder.[912,913] Serum prolactin is the standard assessment of prolactin status. Since elevated prolactin may be a sign of pituitary tumor, assessment for headaches, visual deficits, and other abnormalities of pituitary hormones (e.g., GH and TSH) should be performed; CT or MRI must be considered. Patients with prolactin levels less than 100 ng/mL and normal CT/MRI findings can be managed conservatively with effective prolactin-lowering treatment and annual radiologic assessment (less necessary with favorable serum response).[914, see review 915]

> **Antiestrogen treatments are generally antiinflammatory**
>
> "Using **antiestrogen medication** in women with **dermatomyositis** may result in a significant improvement in their rash, possibly via the inhibition of TNF-alpha production by immune or other cells."
>
> Sereda D, Werth VP. *Arch Dermatol.* 2006 Jan

o Estrogen (excess): Men with rheumatoid arthritis show an excess of estradiol and a decrease in DHEA, and the excess estrogen is proportional to the degree of inflammation.[916] Estrogen status can be assessed using serum estradiol or a 24-hour urine sample. Interventions to combat high estrogen levels may include any effective combination of the following:

- Anastrozole/Arimidex: In a 2006 case report, administration of anastrozole lead to clinical improvement in a woman with dermatomyositis; per the (lack of) details in the case report, the dose was not provided but was likely 1 mg/d since this is the standard dose for the treatment of breast cancer, with which the patient was diagnosed in 2003 after developing dermatomyositis in 1998.[917] In our office, we commonly measure serum estradiol in men and administer the aromatase inhibitor anastrozole/arimidex 1 mg (2-3 doses per week) to men whose estradiol level is greater than 32 picogram/mL. The Life Extension Foundation[918] advocates that the optimal serum estradiol level for a man is 10-30 picogram/mL. Clinical studies using anastrozole/arimidex in men have shown that aromatase blockade lowers estradiol and raises testosterone[919]; generally speaking, this is exactly the result that we want in patients with severe systemic autoimmunity. Our practice has been to use the 1 (one) mg dose, with the frequency of dosing based on serum and clinical response.

o Thyroid (insufficiency or autoimmunity): Because PM-DM can be convincingly mimicked by asymptomatic hyperthyroidism, hypothyroidism, and thyroid autoimmunity (including Grave's disease and Hashimoto's thyroiditis), all patients with PM-DM should receive a comprehensive thyroid evaluation including thyroid gland palpation and serum measurements of TSH, T4, anti-thyroid peroxidase antibodies, and possibly free T3. Overt or imminent hypothyroidism is suggested by TSH

---

[909] "Twenty-five of 33 (75.7%) HPRL women were found to have at least one autoantibody, while none of the 19 women with normal PRL had any. Yet none of the HPRL women whose serum was found to contain high titers of autoantibodies presented with symptoms related to the respective autoimmune disorders." Buskila et al. Autoantibody profile in the sera of women with hyperprolactinemia. *J Autoimmun.* 1995 Jun;8(3):415-24

[910] Dostal et al. Serum prolactin stress values in patients with systemic lupus erythematosus. *Ann Rheum Dis.* 2003 May;62(5):487-8 ard.bmjjournals.com/cgi/content/full/62/5/487

[911] "RESULTS: A significantly higher rate of elevated PRL levels was found in SLE patients (40.0%) compared with the healthy controls (14.8%). No proof was found of association with the presence of anti-ds-DNA or with specific organ involvement. Similarly, elevated PRL levels were found in RA patients (39.3%)." Moszkorzova et al. Hyperprolactinaemia in patients with systemic lupus erythematosus. *Clin Exp Rheumatol.* 2002 Nov-Dec;20(6):807-12

[912] "CONCLUSION: Men with RA have high serum PRL levels and concentrations increase with longer disease evolution and worse functional stage." Mateo et al. High serum prolactin levels in men with rheumatoid arthritis. *J Rheumatol.* 1998 Nov;25(11):2077-82

[913] "Male patients affected by RA showed high serum PRL levels. The serum PRL concentration was found to be increased in relation to the duration and the activity of the disease. Serum PRL levels do not seem to have any relationship with the BMD, at least in RA." Seriolo et al. Serum prolactin concentrations in male patients with rheumatoid arthritis. *Ann N Y Acad Sci.* 2002 Jun;966:258-62

[914] Beers MH, Berkow R (eds). *Merck Manual. 17th Edition.* Whitehouse Station; Merck Research Laboratories 1999 Page 77-78

[915] Serri et al. Diagnosis and management of hyperprolactinemia. *CMAJ.* 2003 Sep 16;169(6):575-81 cmaj.ca/cgi/content/full/169/6/575

[916] "RESULTS: DHEAS and estrone concentrations were lower and estradiol was higher in patients compared with healthy controls. DHEAS differed between RF positive and RF negative patients. Estrone did not correlate with any disease variable, whereas estradiol correlated strongly and positively with all measured indices of inflammation." Tengstrand et al. Abnormal levels of serum dehydroepiandrosterone, estrone, and estradiol in men with rheumatoid arthritis: high correlation between serum estradiol and current degree of inflammation. *J Rheumatol.* 2003 Nov;30(11):2338-43

[917] "Using antiestrogen medication in women with DM may result in a significant improvement in their rash, possibly via the inhibition of TNF-alpha production by immune or other cells." Sereda D, Werth VP. Improvement in dermatomyositis rash associated with the use of antiestrogen medication. *Arch Dermatol.* 2006 Jan;142(1):70-2

[918] Male Hormone Modulation Therapy, Page 4 Of 7: lef.org/protocols/prtcl-130c.shtml Accessed October 30, 2005

[919] "These data demonstrate that aromatase inhibition increases serum bioavailable and total testosterone levels to the youthful normal range in older men with mild hypogonadism." Leder et al. Effects of aromatase inhibition in elderly men with low or borderline-low serum testosterone levels. *J Clin Endocrinol Metab.* 2004 Mar;89(3):1174-80 jcem.endojournals.org/cgi/reprint/89/3/1174

greater than 2 mU/L[920] or 3 mU/L[921], low T4 or T3, and/or the presence of anti-thyroid peroxidase antibodies.[922] Hypothyroidism can cause an inflammatory myopathy that can resemble polymyositis, and hypothyroidism is a frequent complication of any and all autoimmune diseases. Specific treatment considerations are detailed in Chapter 1:

- Comprehensive antioxidation: Patients with PM-DM may have reduced antioxidant defenses amenable to antioxidant supplementation.[923] Oxidative stress results from and contributes to systemic inflammation because 1) increased immune activity results in elaboration of oxidants, and 2) oxidative stress upregulates NFkB (and other pathways) for additive immune activation. *Antioxidant supplementation* alone is clinically and biochemically inferior to a *comprehensive program* that includes both antioxidant supplementation and dietary modification (i.e., the supplemented Paleo-Mediterranean diet, as described previously) that includes heavy reliance upon fruits, vegetables, low-glycemic juices, nuts, seeds, and berries for their additive and synergistic antioxidant benefits.[924]

- Sunscreen: To protect against photosensitivity.

---

[920] Weetman AP. Hypothyroidism: screening and subclinical disease. *BMJ*. 1997 Apr 19;314(7088):1175-8 bmj.bmjjournals.com/cgi/content/full/314/7088/1175

[921] "Now AACE encourages doctors to consider treatment for patients who test outside the boundaries of a narrower margin based on a target TSH level of 0.3 to 3.0. AACE believes the new range will result in proper diagnosis for millions of Americans who suffer from a mild thyroid disorder, but have gone untreated until now." American Association of Clinical Endocrinologists (AACE). 2003 Campaign Encourages Awareness of Mild Thyroid Failure, Importance of Routine Testing aace.com/pub/tam2003/press.php November 26, 2005

[922] Beers MH, Berkow R (eds). *Merck Manual. 17th Edition*. Whitehouse Station; Merck Research Laboratories 1999 Page 96

[923] "Fifty patients with low GSH-Px levels were treated with tablets containing 0.2 mg selenium as Na2SeO3 and 10 mg tocopheryl succinate. The GSH-Px levels increased slowly within 6-8 weeks of treatment." Juhlin et al. Blood glutathione-peroxidase levels in skin diseases: selenium and vitamin E treatment. *Acta Derm Venereol*. 1982;62(3):211-4

[924] Liu RH. Health benefits of fruit and vegetables are from additive and synergistic combinations of phytochemicals. *Am J Clin Nutr*. 2003 Sep;78(3 Suppl):517S-520S

Do the Benefits of Botanical and Physiotherapeutic Hepatobiliary Stimulation Result From Enhanced Excretion of IgA Immune Complexes?

This article was originally published in *Naturopathy Digest* 2006
InflammationMastery.com/reprints/2006IgAhepatobiliary.html

Antigen-IgA complexes are phagocytized by hepatocytes and delivered largely intact directly into the bile. This is the most efficient means of disposing of antigens resistant to hydrolytic degradation due either to their size or physiochemical configuration. IgA immune complexes are taken up by hepatocytes and then secreted into the bile for elimination. The fact that bile duct obstruction retards systemic clearance of IgA immune complexes and that restoration of bile flow reduces serum IgA levels by enhancing biliary IgA excretion in animals and humans proves the importance of ensuring optimal hepatobiliary function and supports the use of botanical and physiological therapeutics that facilitate bile flow. Evidence from journals such as the *Archives of Internal Medicine* suggests the primary physiotherapeutic intervention for the stimulation of bile flow is the enema. Enemas are differentiated from colonics in that enemas generally are delivered as a single insertion of water with a modest volume (generally 1-2 quarts [1-2 liters]), whereas colonics generally employ numerous insertions and removals of water, the total volume of which might exceed several gallons (>4-8 liters). Relatedly, the purpose of an enema is to stimulate normal function, while colonics are used to mechanically cleanse the bowel of debris in a manner analogous to the removal of dirt by hand-washing under running water. Colon irrigations were endorsed by the American Medical Association for the adjunctive treatment of numerous health problems as late as 1932, when Bastedo published a review in *Journal of the American Medical Association* endorsing and encouraging their use. In that same year, the *New England Journal of Medicine* documented the value of colon irrigation in the treatment of mental disease. In 1939, Snyder wrote a review article published in the prestigious *Medical Clinics of North America* in which he extolled the clinical benefits of colonics and enemas and lamented the decline in their use, which he attributed to doctors and nurses not having the time or inclination to administer the procedure.

Treatments to reduce the adverse effects of autoantibodies and immune complexes: a conceptual overview with interventional considerations

Goal	Strategic means	Technical means
Reduce *de novo* formation of autoantibodies	→ Biological immunomodulation	→ Orthoendocrinology, particularly supraphysiologic DHEA supplementation → Anti-inflammatory hypoallergenic diet → Anti-inflammatory nutrition: ALA, GLA, EPA, DHA, cholecalciferol, antioxidants, NFkB inhibitors, and anti-inflammatory botanicals → Xenobiotic detoxification
	→ Pharmacologic immunosuppression	→ Prednisone and other corticosteroids → Antibiologics such as hydroxychloroquine which exert their clinical benefits via interfering with normal immunologic function, not by improving overall health or addressing underlying etiologic factors
	→ Removal/correction of primary stimuli for antibody formation *per patient*	→ Orthoendocrinology → Xenobiotic detoxification → Mitochondrial resuscitation → Antidysbiotic interventions: assessment and correction of multifocal dysbiosis
Reduce effects of autoantibodies	→ Anti-inflammatory treatments	→ Anti-inflammatory nutrition: ALA, GLA, EPA, DHA, cholecalciferol, antioxidants, NFkB inhibitors, and anti-inflammatory botanicals

Goal	Strategic means	Technical means
Reduce effects of autoantibodies —*continued*	→ Proteolytic enzymes	→ Proteolytic/pancreatic enzymes appear to reduce *de novo* formation of immune complexes
Enhance clearance of autoantibodies	→ Allopathic interventions	→ Immunoadsorption[925] → Plasmapheresis[926,927]
	→ Naturopathic interventions (theoretical[928])	→ Choleretic and cholagogic botanicals: beets, ginger[929], curcumin[930], *Picrorhiza*[931], milk thistle[932], *Andrographis paniculata*[933] and *Boerhaavia diffusa*.[934] → Low-volume enemas to stimulate bile flow and liver clearance[935]

Multifocal Dysbiosis: Pathophysiology, Relevance for Inflammatory and Autoimmune Diseases, and Treatment With Nutritional and Botanical Interventions

This article was originally published in *Naturopathy Digest* 2006
The complete text is available at InflammationMastery.com/reprints/2006dysbiosis.html

At least 70 percent of patients with chronic arthritis are carriers of "silent infections," according to a 1992 article published in the peer-reviewed medical journal *Annals of the Rheumatic Diseases*. A 2001 article in that same journal which focused exclusively on five bacteria showed that 56 percent of patients with idiopathic inflammatory arthritis had gastrointestinal or genitourinary dysbiosis. Indeed, published research strongly and consistently indicates that bacteria, yeast/fungi, amoebas, protozoa, and other "parasites" (rarely including helminths/worms) are underappreciated causes of neuromusculoskeletal inflammation. In my own clinical practice, gastrointestinal dysbiosis is so common in patients with autoimmune/inflammatory disorders that I consider all of these patients to have dysbiosis until proven otherwise. We perform stool testing with a specialty laboratory, and I am rarely "disappointed" with the finding of normal stool analysis and parasitology. Overall, including patients without autoimmune/inflammatory disorders, I estimate that in my practice, approximately 80 percent of stool and parasitology examinations return with at least one clinically relevant abnormality that, when corrected, provides either subjective or objective improvement in the patient's primary complaint. My experience is consistent with that of other authors and researchers, who note a prevalence of dysbiosis in the range of 70 percent to 100 percent in patients with inflammatory disorders. Recognizing the need to appreciate and transcend the contributions by Koch and Pasture, I've defined dysbiosis as "a relationship of non-acute non-infectious host-microorganism interaction that adversely affects the human host." When used without additional specification, the term "dysbiosis" generally is meant to imply "gastrointestinal dysbiosis." However, as research has continued to progress in this arena, clinicians are now obligated to appreciate the concept of "multifocal dysbiosis" because patients might have dysbiosis in extra-intestinal sites, namely their skin, mouth, sinuses, respiratory tract, genitourinary tract, surrounding environment, and parenchymal tissues. We might reasonably describe multifocal dysbiosis as "a

[925] Braun et al. Immunoadsorption onto protein A induces remission in severe systemic lupus erythematosus. *Nephrol Dial Transplant*. 2000 Sep;15(9):1367-72

[926] Santos-Ocampo AS, Mandell BF, Fessler BJ. Alveolar hemorrhage in systemic lupus erythematosus: presentation and management. *Chest*. 2000 Oct;118(4):1083-90

[927] Choi BG, Yoo WH. Successful treatment of pure red cell aplasia with plasmapheresis in a patient with systemic lupus erythematosus. *Yonsei Med J*. 2002 Apr;4):274-8

[928] Vasquez A. Do Benefits of Botanical and Physiotherapeutic Hepatobiliary Stimulation Result From Enhanced Excretion of IgA Immune Complexes? *Naturo Digest* 2006 Jan

[929] "Further analyses for the active constituents of the acetone extracts through column chromatography indicated that [6]-gingerol and [10]-gingerol, which are the pungent principles, are mainly responsible for the cholagogic effect of ginger." Yamahara et al. Cholagogic effect of ginger and its active constituents. *J Ethnopharmacol*. 1985;13:217-25

[930] "On the basis of the present findings, it appears that curcumin induces contraction of the human gall-bladder." Rasyid A, Lelo A. The effect of curcumin and placebo on human gall-bladder function: an ultrasound study. *Aliment Pharmacol Ther*. 1999 Feb;13(2):245-9

[931] "Significant anticholestatic activity was also observed against carbon tetrachloride induced cholestasis in conscious rat, anaesthetized guinea pig and cat. Picroliv was more active than the known hepatoprotective drug silymarin." Saraswat B, Visen PK, Patnaik GK, Dhawan BN. Anticholestatic effect of picroliv, active hepatoprotective principle of Picrorhiza kurrooa, against carbon tetrachloride induced cholestasis. *Indian J Exp Biol*. 1993 Apr;31(4):316-8

[932] Crocenzi et al. Preventive effect of silymarin against taurolithocholate-induced cholestasis in the rat. *Biochem Pharmacol*. 2003 Jul 15;66(2):355-64

[933] Shukla B, Visen PK, Patnaik GK, Dhawan BN. Choleretic effect of andrographolide in rats and guinea pigs. *Planta Med*. 1992 Apr;58(2):146-9

[934] Chandan BK, Sharma AK, Anand KK. Boerhaavia diffusa: a study of its hepatoprotective activity. *J Ethnopharmacol*. 1991 Mar;31(3):299-307

[935] Garbat AL, Jacobi HG. Secretion of Bile in Response to Rectal Installations. *Arch Intern Med* 1929; 44: 455-462

clinical condition characterized by a patient's simultaneously having more than one foci/location of dysbiosis; generally the adverse physiologic and clinical consequences are additive and synergistic." Although different foci of dysbiosis generally require different types of treatment (e.g., oral versus topical versus environmental), the pathophysiologic mechanisms and clinical consequences are largely identical. Thus, sinorespiratory dysbiosis or genitourinary dysbiosis can be just as devastating as gastrointestinal dysbiosis, and therefore requires appropriate clinical consideration, particularly in patients with autoimmune/inflammatory disorders such as lupus, rheumatoid arthritis, psoriasis, polymyositis, ankylosing spondylitis, and various types of vasculitis.

Dysbiotic Emphases and Therapeutic Prioritization and Contextualization

With the concepts and data that I have presented in Chapters 1, 4, and here in 5, readers are hopefully gaining an appreciation of 1) the great importance of dysbiosis in inflammatory and autoimmune disorders, and 2) the relative importance of the various types and combinations of dysbiosis that are more compellingly implicated in various conditions. Hopefully, clinicians will also not lose sight of the fact that patient-specific variations on these themes clearly exist; yet despite the importance of patient specificity and biochemical individuality, clear patterns do exist, and I have roughly represented these emphases and relationships in the image that follows. Again, clear delineations are impossible in complex living systems affected simultaneously by all of these (and other) variables.

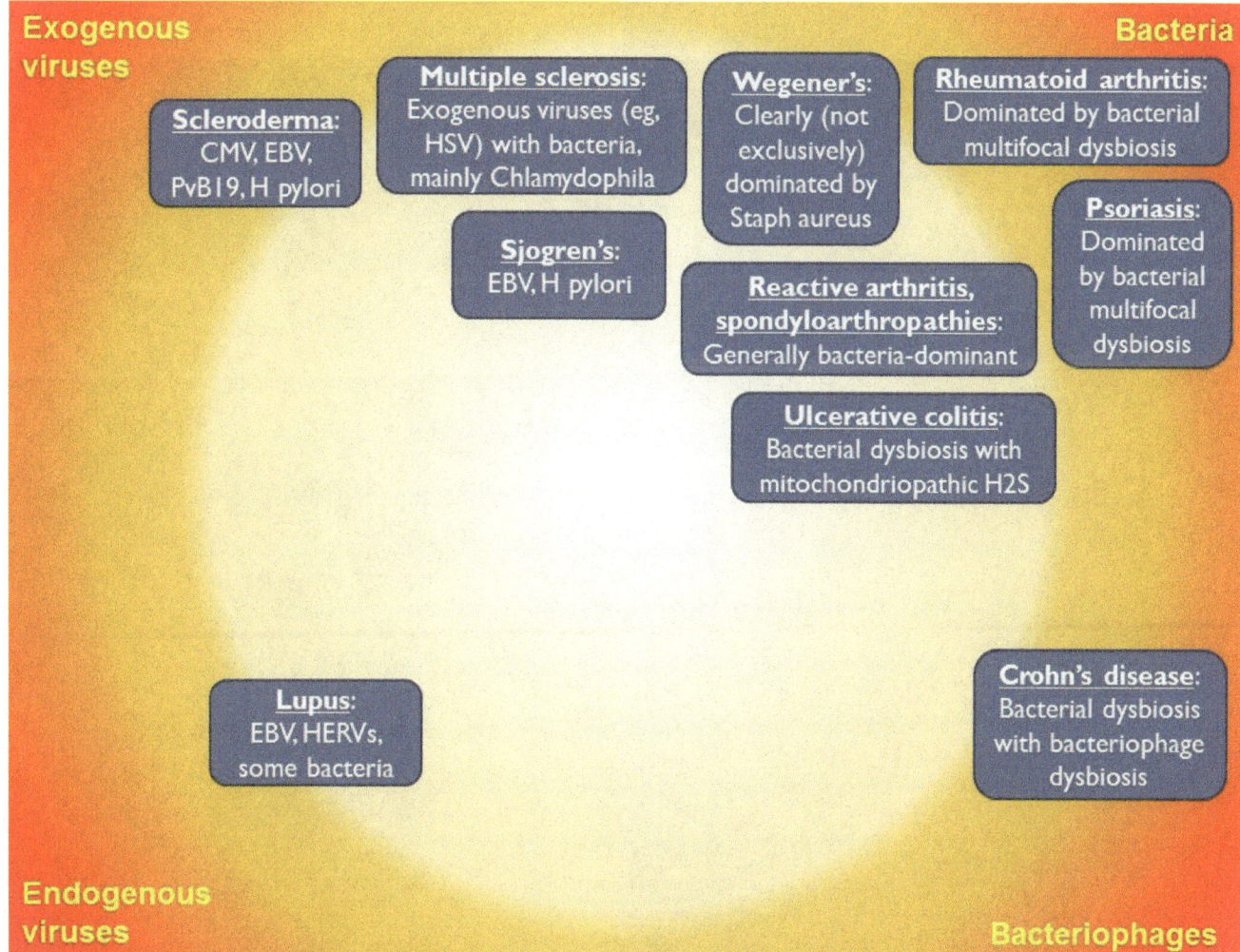

Dysbiotic emphases in various disease states: A rough estimates based on overview of research literature and clinical experience; my hope is that readers will appreciate the disease-specific information presented in this book within its disease-specific context and then break free from that context to see how the information applies to other diseases generally and individual patients specifically.

- "It was during the years of my lowest vitality that I ceased to be a pessimist. The instinct of self restoration forbade me a philosophy of poverty and discouragement. As it were, that is how those years appear to me now. I soon discovered life anew…including myself. I turned my will to health, to life, into a philosophy….into the will to power."
- "The time is now past when accidents could befall me; and what **could** now fall to my lot which has not already be my own!? It returns only, it comes home to me at last—mine own Self. And such of it as has been long abroad, and scattered among things and accidents. And one thing more do I know: I stand now before my last summit, and before that which has been longest reserved for me."
- "You have within you the power to merge everything you have lived through – attempts, false starts, errors, delusions, passions, your loves and your hopes – into your highest goal, with nothing left over."
- "At every step one has to wrestle for truth; one has to surrender for it almost everything to which the heart, to which our love, our trust in life, cling otherwise. That requires greatness of soul: the service of truth is the hardest service…"
- "With your love go into your isolation and with your creativity, my brother; and only later will justice limp after you.
- "What makes a person heroic?" Answer: "To simultaneously face one's greatest fear and one's highest hope."
- "My principle article of faith is that one can only flourish among people who share the identical ideas and the identical will."
- "Not around the inventors of new noise but around the inventors of new values does the world revolve."

Friedrich Nietzsche (German classical Scholar, Philosopher and Critic of culture, 1844-1900)

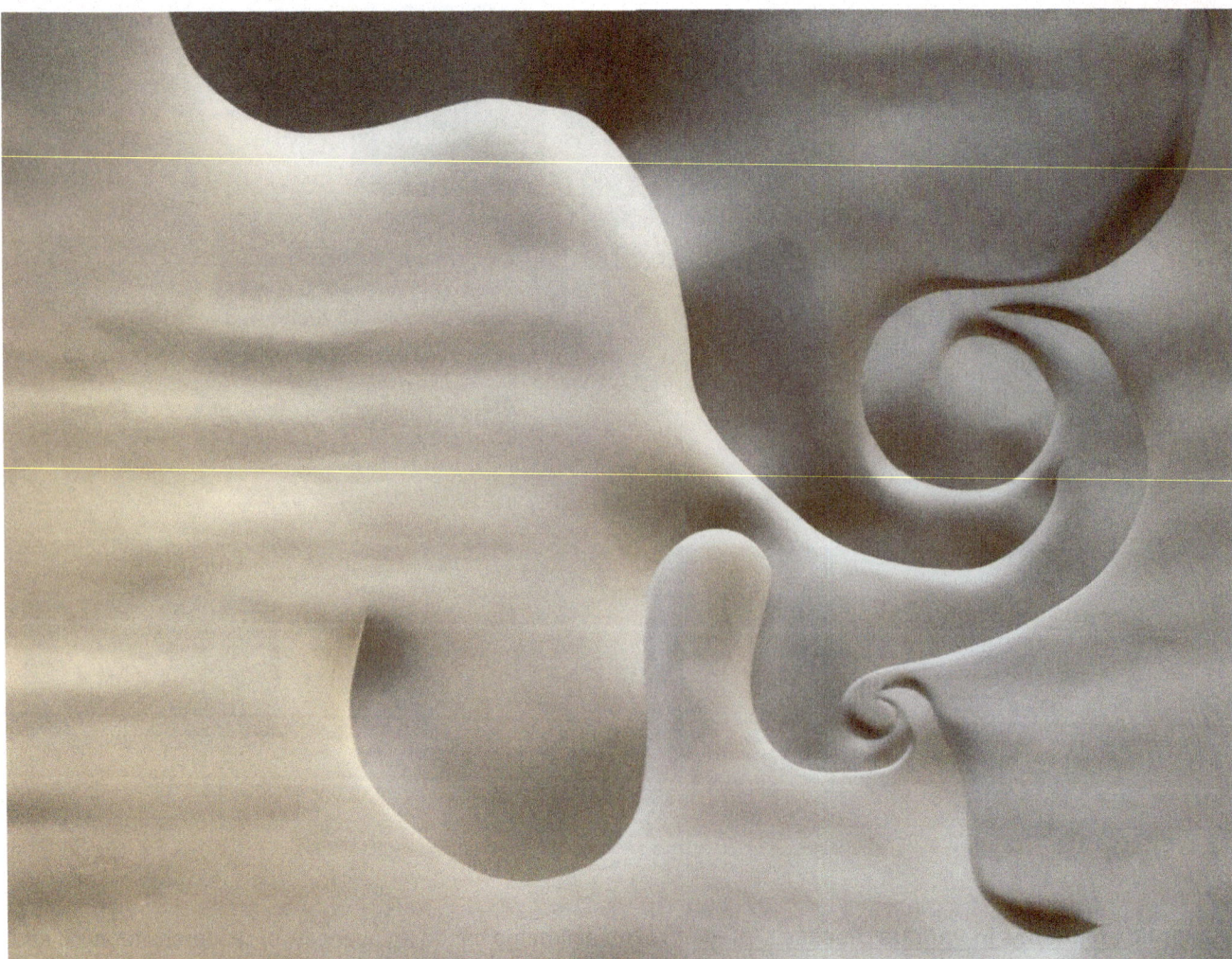

Ceiling of Café de La Pedrera in Barcelona: 2014 photo by DrV

How did Colombians overturn laws mandating the destruction of their grains, their mining, (ie, their food and ways of living)?

- Organization, protests and strikes in many cities
- 648 arrests of protesters, 262 detentions (overturned)
- 660 human rights violations
- 485 wounded
- 12 people killed during protests

That is the cost of freedom from GMO monopolization, more accurately described as GMO neocolonization. See reporting at youtube.com/watch?v=9Vz0tiRKvD0

ICHNFM.org • Colombia • Spain • United States

"Early in September, 2013, the Colombian government was forced to partially concede to the demands of a nationwide general strike instigated by farmers of the largely agrarian nation. The three week long protests and blockades that shut down much of the nation were supported by thousands of miners, truckers, students, bus drivers, and Colombian citizens, blocking roads and clashing with police. Close to 650 arrests were made, 485 injuries were reported, 12 people killed, and over 600 cases of human rights violations reported. Coverage of the nationwide protests feature rural peoples and urban demonstrators in the typical contest against body-armor clad, state riot police armed with gas, rubber bullets, flash-bang grenades and batons, beating people and dispersing women and children in clouds of smoke. ... Implementation of seed control was described by Colombian president Juan Manuel Santos as 'having Colombia tuned up to international reality.' This statement is, of course, completely true. The trending international reality is exactly this, trojan horse conquest of national food sovereignty by means of international corporate/government treaties and agreements sponsored by international governing bodies and the bottomless coiffeurs of the companies that benefit directly from such trade agreements. The shift to this international model of farming simply does not make economic or common sense for the people of most nations. Author and self-proclaimed 'economic hitman' John Perkins wrote about this type of imperial foreign occupation by corporate influence in his critical book, '*Confessions of an Economic Hitman*.' It is the newest means of international conquest. The international drive toward the monopolization of seed, the global reduction of seed diversity, and the abolishment of small scale farming is being seen all over the world."

globalresearch.ca/colombians-successfully-revolt-against-seed-control-and-agricultural-tyranny/5352534

"Tensions have been rising between the Colombian government and the agricultural sector since the regulations imposed by the **U.S.-Colombia Free Trade Agreement**, which went into effect in May 2012. ... But farmers have bristled at the **requirement that they use genetically modified seeds, engineered by international conglomerates like Monsanto and Du Pont, and pay an annual fee to do so**."

rollingstone.com/politics/news/will-colombias-farmers-get-what-they-want-20131118

The question that needs to be asked is: "Why is the US government enforcing the international adoption of genetically modified/manipulated foods, when this is clearly in the interest of private industry (unless corporate interests now rule international politics) and at the risk of destabilizing other countries (unless the goal is to destabilize those countries)?"

Prostaglandin E-3, 362
Prostaglandin F2-alpha, 369
Prostaglandin G2, 369
Prostaglandin G-3, 362
Prostaglandin H2, 369
Prostaglandin H-3, 362
Prostaglandin I2, 368
Prostaglandin I-3, 362
Prostaglandin synthase complex, 373
Protect & prevent re-injury, 254
Protein - calculation of daily intake, 206, 268, 328
Proteolytic enzymes (used in the treatment of dysbiosis), 535
Proteolytic enzymes, 273, 594
Proteus mirabilis, 471
PRRs, 417
Pseudomonas aeruginosa, 94, 471
Psoriasis, main chapter, 1038
Psoriatic rheumatism, 1038
Putrescine, 413, 929
Pyridoxine lowers serum/blood glutamate levels, 886
Pyridoxine, 288, 689, 885
Pyruvate dehydrogenase complex, 894
Qigong, 791, 973
Quorum sensing, 439
Raynaud's phenomenon in scleroderma, 1094, 1129
Raynaud's phenomenon, 94, 1129, 1133
Reactive arthritis, 93, 466, 1110
Reasons to avoid the use of nonsteroidal anti-inflammatory drugs (NSAIDs), 247, 249
Referred pain with compression, 274
REFLEXES – grading scale, 24
Relative rest - definition and application in basic holistic care, 254
Renal artery (renovascular) stenosis, 740
Renal disease survey, 743
Renal failure, cause of death in patients with SLE, 1061
Renal injury and failure caused by NSAIDs, 250
Resolvins, 363
Restless leg syndrome, 949
Retinal vasculitis, 1062
Review of systems, 12
Rheumatic psoriasis, 1038
Rheumatoid Factor - interpretation, 80
Rib manipulation, 282
Riboflavin, 290
Rifaxamin, 496
Rifaximin as treatment for SIBO and IBS, 954
Rifaximin, 954, 964
ROS: review of systems, 12
Rosacea, 482
Rose Bengal staining, 1121
Roseburia intestinalis, 427
Rosemary, 308, 377, 389, 996
Saccharomyces boulardii, 492, 719
SAD: Standard American Diet, 757

S-adenosyl-methionine, 576, 962
Safe patient + safe treatment = safe outcome, 110
Salivary gland biopsy, 1121
Salmonella, 93
SAMe, 576
Sarcoidosis, 1138
Savella, 913
Schirmer test, 1121
Schober test, 1114
Scleraderma, 741
Scleroderma secondary to xenobiotic immunotoxicity, 1074
Scleroderma, 1074
Screening laboratory tests in the evaluation of patients with musculoskeletal complaints, 25
Secondary Hemochromatosis, 160
Secretory IgA, 103, 488
SEID, 479
Selective estrogen receptor modulators inhibit Ebola virus infection, 572
Selenium, 573
Septic arthritis, 121, 125, 126
Septic arthritis, in rheumatoid arthritis, 1023
Seropositivity, 81, 1024
Serotonin synthesis, 211
Serum IgE and IgG assays, 391
Shigella, 93
Short-chain fatty acids, 104, 488
SIBO, 922
Sicca syndrome, 1120
Sick role, 265
Silibinin/silybin from Silymarin marianum, 593
Silymarin, 168
Sinorespiratory dysbiosis, 508
Sjögren Syndrome/Disease, 550, 1120
Skatole, 413, 929
Skin taping to increase afferent stimuli, 296
Skin-prick testing, 391, 999
SLE, 1053
Sleep apnea, 741
Sleep, 199
Slipped capital femoral epiphysis, 124
Small intestinal bacterial/microbial overgrowth, 473
Small intestine bacterial overgrowth in fibromyalgia, 923
Social history, 13
Sodium avoidance, 613
Sodium benzoate, 212
Sodium chloride, 763
Sodium hypochlorite, 516
Somatic dysfunction, 149
Somatostatin analog, 1083
Special considerations in the evaluation of children, 112
Spinal accessory nerve, 23
Spinal cord compression, 2, 120
Spinal manipulation, 605
Spironolatone, 812
SPMD, 717

Sporothrix schenckii, 570
St. John's Wort, 533
Standard Medical Treatment for Fibromyalgia, 912
Staphylococcus aureus, 531
Stearidonic acid, 360
Stool analysis and comprehensive parasitology, 487
Stool analysis, 103
Streptococcal infections, 94
Streptococcus pyogenes, 531
Stress is a "whole body" phenomenon, 222
Stress management and authentic living, 221
Subluxation, 742
Superantigens, 411
Supercompensation (carbohydrates), 211
Supplemented Paleo-Mediterranean Diet, 219, 256
Syndemic obesity, inflammation, cardiometabolic syndrome, and brain dysfunction, 652
Synthroid, 696
Systemic exertion intolerance disease, 479
Systemic Lupus Erythematosus, main chapter, 1053
Systemic Sclerosis, 741, 1074
Systolic hypertension, 788
Syzygium species, 534
Takayasu arteritis, 1098
Tanacetum parthenium, 897
Tartaric acid, 413, 929
Tartrazine, 212
Television, 191
Temporal arteritis, 119, 1100
Testing for Occult Infections and Dysbiosis, 86
Testosterone, 694
Tetanus toxoid, 427
Tetracycline, 497
Th17 cells, 609
Therapeutic dependency - defined, 265
Therapeutic exercise, 266
Therapeutic Interventions, 956
Therapeutic passivity - defined, 265
Thrombocytopenia, 719
Thromboxane A-2, 368
Thromboxane A-3, 362
Thromboxane B2, 368
Thrust vectors, 279
Thyme, 534
Thymus vulgaris, 534
Thyroid (insufficiency or autoimmunity), 696, 697
Thyroid disease, 742
Thyroid glandular—nonprescription T3, 697
Thyroid hormone, 689
Thyroid stimulating hormone - interpretation, 64
Thyroid testing, 745
Thyrolar, 697
Tinidazole, 495

Observance is made here—with selected highlights of common allergens and immunogens—of potential allergens to which patients may respond; by use of this information, clinicians can make better choices regarding the selection or avoidance of particular vaccines in patients with known allergies or possible hypersensitivity reactions. For example, according to the recent study by Zug et al[1], among 883 North American children approximately 60% have positive (ie, allergic) responses to substances via patch testing, and neomycin sulfate (a component of come vaccines) sensitivity is one of the more common allergies/hypersensitivities. Thus this list helps clinicians identify potential hypersensitivity reactions that might be triggered by vaccine ingredients. This document is available as of early 2016 via the CDC website at this location: http://www.cdc.gov/vaccines/pubs/pinkbook/downloads/appendices/B/excipient-table-2.pdf

Vaccine Excipient & Media Summary
Excipients Included in U.S. Vaccines, by Vaccine

This table includes not only vaccine ingredients (e.g., adjuvants and preservatives), but also substances used during the manufacturing process, including vaccine-production media, that are removed from the final product and present only in trace quantities.
In addition to the substances listed, most vaccines contain Sodium Chloride (table salt).

Last Updated February 2015
All reasonable efforts have been made to ensure the accuracy of this information, but manufacturers may change product contents before that information is reflected here. If in doubt, check the manufacturer's package insert.

Vaccine	Contains	Source: Manufacturer's P.I. Dated
Adenovirus	sucrose, D-mannose, D-fructose, dextrose, potassium phosphate, plasdone C, anhydrous lactose, micro crystalline cellulose, polacrilin potassium, magnesium stearate, cellulose acetate phthalate, alcohol, acetone, castor oil, FD&C Yellow #6 aluminum lake dye, human serum albumin, fetal bovine serum, sodium bicarbonate, human-diploid fibroblast cell cultures (WI-38), Dulbecco's Modified Eagle's Medium, monosodium glutamate	March 2011
Anthrax (Biothrax)	aluminum hydroxide, benzethonium chloride, formaldehyde, amino acids, vitamins, inorganic salts and sugars	May 2012
BCG (Tice)	glycerin, asparagine, citric acid, potassium phosphate, magnesium sulfate, Iron ammonium citrate, lactose	February 2009
DT (Sanofi)	aluminum potassium sulfate, peptone, bovine extract, formaldehyde, thimerosal (trace), modified Mueller and Miller medium, ammonium sulfate	December 2005
DTaP (Daptacel)	aluminum phosphate, formaldehyde, glutaraldehyde, 2-Phenoxyethanol, Stainer-Scholte medium, modified Mueller's growth medium, modified Mueller-Miller casamino acid medium (without beef heart infusion), dimethyl 1-beta-cyclodextrin, ammonium sulfate	October 2013
DTaP (Infanrix)	formaldehyde, glutaraldehyde, aluminum hydroxide, polysorbate 80, Fenton medium (containing bovine extract), modified Latham medium (derived from bovine casein), modified Stainer-Scholte liquid medium	November 2013
DTaP-IPV (Kinrix)	formaldehyde, glutaraldehyde, aluminum hydroxide, Vero (monkey kidney) cells, calf serum, lactalbumin hydrolysate, polysorbate 80, neomycin sulfate, polymyxin B, Fenton medium (containing bovine extract), modified Latham medium (derived from bovine casein), modified Stainer-Scholte liquid medium	November 2013
DTaP-HepB-IPV (Pediarix)	formaldehyde, gluteraldehyde, aluminum hydroxide, aluminum phosphate, lactalbumin hydrolysate, polysorbate 80, neomycin sulfate, polymyxin B, yeast protein, calf serum, Fenton medium (containing bovine extract), modified Latham medium (derived from bovine casein), modified Stainer-Scholte liquid medium, Vero (monkey kidney) cells	November 2013
DTaP-IPV/Hib (Pentacel)	aluminum phosphate, polysorbate 80, formaldehyde, sucrose, gutaraldehyde, bovine serum albumin, 2-phenoxethanol, neomycin, polymyxin B sulfate, Mueller's Growth Medium, Mueller-Miller casamino acid medium (without beef heart infusion), Stainer-Scholte medium (modified by the addition of casamino acids and dimethyl-beta-cyclodextrin), MRC-5 (human diploid) cells, CMRL 1969 medium (supplemented with calf serum), ammonium sulfate, and medium 199	October 2013
Hib (ActHIB)	ammonium sulfate, formalin, sucrose, Modified Mueller and Miller medium	January 2014
Hib (Hiberix)	formaldehyde, lactose, semi-synthetic medium	March 2012
Hib (PedvaxHIB)	aluminum hydroxphosphate sulfate, ethanol, enzymes, phenol, detergent, complex fermentation medium	December 2010

---

[1] Zug et al. Patch testing in children from 2005 to 2012: results from the North American contact dermatitis group. *Dermatitis*. 2014 Nov-Dec;25(6):345-55

Vaccine	Contains	Source: Manufacturer's P.I. Dated
Hib/Hep B (Comvax)	yeast (vaccine contains no detectable yeast DNA), nicotinamide adenine dinucleotide, hemin chloride, soy peptone, dextrose, mineral salts, amino acids, formaldehyde, potassium aluminum sulfate, amorphous aluminum hydroxyphosphate sulfate, sodium borate, phenol, ethanol, enzymes, detergent	December 2010
Hib/Mening. CY (MenHibrix)	tris (trometamol)-HCl, sucrose, formaldehyde, synthetic medium, semi-synthetic medium	2012
Hep A (Havrix)	aluminum hydroxide, amino acid supplement, polysorbate 20, formalin, neomycin sulfate, MRC-5 cellular proteins	December 2013
Hep A (Vaqta)	amorphous aluminum hydroxyphosphate sulfate, bovine albumin, formaldehyde, neomycin, sodium borate, MRC-5 (human diploid) cells	February 2014
Hep B (Engerix-B)	aluminum hydroxide, yeast protein, phosphate buffers, sodium dihydrogen phosphate dihydrate	December 2013
Hep B (Recombivax)	yeast protein, soy peptone, dextrose, amino acids, mineral salts, potassium aluminum sulfate, amorphous aluminum hydroxyphosphate sulfate, formaldehyde, phosphate buffer	May 2014
Hep A/Hep B (Twinrix)	formalin, yeast protein, aluminum phosphate, aluminum hydroxide, amino acids, phosphate buffer, polysorbate 20, neomycin sulfate, MRC-5 human diploid cells	August 2012
Human Papillomavirus (HPV) (Cerverix)	vitamins, amino acids, lipids, mineral salts, aluminum hydroxide, sodium dihydrogen phosphate dehydrate, 3-O-desacyl-4' Monophosphoryl lipid A, insect cell, bacterial, and viral protein	November 2013
Human Papillomavirus (HPV) (Gardasil)	yeast protein, vitamins, amino acids, mineral salts, carbohydrates, amorphous aluminum hydroxyphosphate sulfate, L-histidine, polysorbate 80, sodium borate	June 2014
Human Papillomavirus (HPV) (Gardasil 9)	yeast protein, vitamins, amino acids, mineral salts, carbohydrates, amorphous aluminum hydroxyphosphate sulfate, L-histidine, polysorbate 80, sodium borate	December 2014
Influenza (Afluria)	beta-propiolactone, thimerosol (multi-dose vials only), monobasic sodium phosphate, dibasic sodium phosphate, monobasic potassium phosphate, potassium chloride, calcium chloride, sodium taurodeoxycholate, neomycin sulfate, polymyxin B, egg protein, sucrose	December 2013
Influenza (Agriflu)	egg proteins, formaldehyde, polysorbate 80, cetyltrimethylammonium bromide, neomycin sulfate, kanamycin, barium	2013
Influenza (Fluarix) Trivalent and Quadrivalent	octoxynol-10 (Triton X-100), α-tocopheryl hydrogen succinate, polysorbate 80 (Tween 80), hydrocortisone, gentamicin sulfate, ovalbumin, formaldehyde, sodium deoxycholate, sucrose, phosphate buffer	June 2014
Influenza (Flublok)	monobasic sodium phosphate, dibasic sodium phosphate, polysorbate 20, baculovirus and host cell proteins, baculovirus and cellular DNA, Triton X-100, lipids, vitamins, amino acids, mineral salts	March 2014
Influenza (Flucelvax)	Madin Darby Canine Kidney (MDCK) cell protein, MDCK cell DNA, polysorbate 80, cetyltrimethylammonium bromide, β-propiolactone, phosphate buffer	March 2014
Influenza (Fluvirin)	nonylphenol ethoxylate, thimerosal (multidose vial–trace only in prefilled syringe), polymyxin, neomycin, beta-propiolactone, egg proteins, phosphate buffer	February 2014
Influenza (Flulaval) Trivalent and Quadrivalent	thimerosal, formaldehyde, sodium deoxycholate, egg proteins, phosphate buffer	February 2013
Influenza (Fluzone: Standard (Trivalent and Quadrivalent), High-Dose, & Intradermal)	formaldehyde, octylphenol ethoxylate (Triton X-100), gelatin (standard trivalent formulation only), thimerosal (multi-dose vial only) , egg protein, phosphate buffers, sucrose	2014

Centers for Disease Control and Prevention
Epidemiology and Prevention of Vaccine-Preventable Diseases, 13th Edition   April, 2015

From: http://www.cdc.gov/vaccines/pubs/pinkbook/downloads/appendices/B/excipient-table-2.pdf on 2016 January

Vaccine	Contains	Source: Manufacturer's P.I. Dated
Influenza (FluMist) Quadrivalent	ethylene diamine tetraacetic acid (EDTA), monosodium glutamate, hydrolyzed porcine gelatin, arginine, sucrose, dibasic potassium phosphate, monobasic potassium phosphate, gentamicin sulfate, egg protein	July 2013
Japanese Encephalitis (Ixiaro)	aluminum hydroxide, Vero cells, protamine sulfate, formaldehyde, bovine serum albumin, sodium metabisulphite, sucrose	May 2013
Meningococcal (MCV4-Menactra)	formaldehyde, phosphate buffers, Mueller Hinton agar, Watson Scherp media, Modified Mueller and Miller medium, detergent, alcohol, ammonium sulfate	April 2013
Meningococcal (MCV4-Menveo)	formaldehyde, amino acids, yeast extract, Franz complete medium, CY medium	August 2013
Meningococcal (MPSV4-Menomune)	thimerosal (multi-dose vial only), lactose, Mueller Hinton casein agar, Watson Scherp media, detergent, alcohol	April 2013
Meningococcal (MenB – Bexsero)	aluminum hydroxide, *E. coli*, histidine, sucrose, deoxycholate, kanomycin	2015
Meningococcal (MenB – Trumenba)	polysorbate 80, histidine, *E. coli*, fermentation growth media	October 2015
MMR (MMR-II)	Medium 199 (vitamins, amino acids, fetal bovine serum, sucrose, glutamate) , Minimum Essential Medium, phosphate, recombinant human albumin, neomycin, sorbitol, hydrolyzed gelatin, chick embryo cell culture, WI-38 human diploid lung fibroblasts	June 2014
MMRV (ProQuad)	sucrose, hydrolyzed gelatin, sorbitol, monosodium L-glutamate, sodium phosphate dibasic, human albumin, sodium bicarbonate, potassium phosphate monobasic, potassium chloride, potassium phosphate dibasic, neomycin, bovine calf serum, chick embryo cell culture, WI-38 human diploid lung fibroblasts, MRC-5 cells	March 2014
Pneumococcal (PCV13 – Prevnar 13)	casamino acids, yeast, ammonium sulfate, Polysorbate 80, succinate buffer, aluminum phosphate, soy peptone broth	January 2014
Pneumococcal (PPSV-23 – Pneumovax)	phenol	May 2014
Polio (IPV – Ipol)	2-phenoxyethanol, formaldehyde, neomycin, streptomycin, polymyxin B, monkey kidney cells, Eagle MEM modified medium, calf serum protein, Medium 199	May 2013
Rabies (Imovax)	Human albumin, neomycin sulfate, phenol red indicator, MRC-5 human diploid cells, beta-propriolactone	April 2013
Rabies (RabAvert)	β-propiolactone, potassium glutamate, chicken protein, egg protein, neomycin, chlortetracycline, amphotericin B, human serum albumin, polygeline (processed bovine gelatin), sodium EDTA, bovine serum	March 2012
Rotavirus (RotaTeq)	sucrose, sodium citrate, sodium phosphate monobasic monohydrate, sodium hydroxide, polysorbate 80, cell culture media, fetal bovine serum, vero cells *[DNA from porcine circoviruses (PCV) 1 and 2 has been detected in RotaTeq. PCV-1 and PCV-2 are not known to cause disease in humans.]*	June 2013
Rotavirus (Rotarix)	amino acids, dextran, sorbitol, sucrose, calcium carbonate, xanthan, Dulbecco's Modified Eagle Medium (potassium chloride, magnesium sulfate, ferric (III) nitrate, sodium phosphate, sodium pyruvate, D-glucose, concentrated vitamin solution, L-cystine, L-tyrosine, amino acids solution, L-glutamine, calcium chloride, sodium hydrogenocarbonate, and phenol red) *[Porcine circovirus type 1 (PCV-1) is present in Rotarix. PCV-1 is not known to cause disease in humans.]*	May 2014
Smallpox (Vaccinia – ACAM2000)	human serum albumin, mannitol, neomycin, glycerin, polymyxin B, phenol, Vero cells, HEPES	September 2009

Vaccine	Contains	Source: Manufacturer's P.I. Dated
Td (Decavac)	aluminum potassium sulfate, peptone, formaldehyde, thimerosal, bovine muscle tissue (US sourced), Mueller and Miller medium, ammonium sulfate	March 2011
Td (Tenivac)	aluminum phosphate, formaldehyde, modified Mueller-Miller casamino acid medium without beef heart infusion, ammonium sulfate	April 2013
Td (Mass Biologics)	aluminum phosphate, formaldehyde, thimerosal (trace), ammonium phosphate, modified Mueller's media (containing bovine extracts)	February 2011
Tdap (Adacel)	aluminum phosphate, formaldehyde, glutaraldehyde, 2-phenoxyethanol, ammonium sulfate, Stainer-Scholte medium, dimethyl-beta-cyclodextrin, modified Mueller's growth medium, Mueller-Miller casamino acid medium (without beef heart infusion)	March 2014
Tdap (Boostrix)	formaldehyde, glutaraldehyde, aluminum hydroxide, polysorbate 80 (Tween 80), Latham medium derived from bovine casein, Fenton medium containing a bovine extract, Stainer-Scholte liquid medium	February 2013
Typhoid (inactivated – Typhim Vi)	hexadecyltrimethylammonium bromide, formaldehyde, phenol, polydimethylsiloxane, disodium phosphate, monosodium phosphate, semi-synthetic medium	March 2014
Typhoid (oral – Ty21a)	yeast extract, casein, dextrose, galactose, sucrose, ascorbic acid, amino acids, lactose, magnesium stearate. gelatin	September 2013
Varicella (Varivax)	sucrose, phosphate, glutamate, gelatin, monosodium L-glutamate, sodium phosphate dibasic, potassium phosphate monobasic, potassium chloride, sodium phosphate monobasic, potassium chloride, EDTA, residual components of MRC-5 cells including DNA and protein, neomycin, fetal bovine serum, human diploid cell cultures (WI-38), embryonic guinea pig cell cultures, human embryonic lung cultures	March 2014
Yellow Fever (YF-Vax)	sorbitol, gelatin, egg protein	May 2013
Zoster (Shingles – Zostavax)	sucrose, hydrolyzed porcine gelatin, monosodium L-glutamate, sodium phosphate dibasic, potassium phosphate monobasic, neomycin, potassium chloride, residual components of MRC-5 cells including DNA and protein, bovine calf serum	February 2014

A table listing vaccine excipients and media *by excipient* can be found in:

Grabenstein JD. *ImmunoFacts: Vaccines and Immunologic Drugs* – 2013 (38th revision). St Louis, MO: Wolters Kluwer Health, 2012.

From: http://www.cdc.gov/vaccines/pubs/pinkbook/downloads/appendices/B/excipient-table-2.pdf on 2016 January

CPSIA information can be obtained
at www.ICGtesting.com
Printed in the USA
BVOW07s0220121217
501881BV00038B/10/P